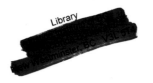
DATE DUE

BRODART, CO.   Cat. No. 23-221

29/3

SECOND EDITION

Ciottone's DISASTER MEDICINE

GREGORY R. CIOTTONE, MD, FACEP

Director, Beth Israel Deaconess Medical Center Fellowship
in Disaster Medicine
Director, Disaster Preparedness Program, Harvard
Humanitarian Initiative
Associate Professor of Emergency Medicine
Harvard Medical School
Boston, Massachusetts

ASSOCIATE EDITORS

Paul D. Biddinger, MD, FACEP, FAAEM
Robert G. Darling, MD
Saleh Fares, MD, MPH, FRCPC, FACEP, FAAEM
Mark E. Keim, MD, MBA
Michael Sean Molloy, MB, Dip SpMed (RCSI), EMDM,
MFSEM(UK), FCEM, FFSEM (RCSI)
Selim Suner, MD, MS, FACEP

ELSEVIER

ELSEVIER

1600 John F. Kennedy Blvd.
Ste 1800
Philadelphia, PA 19103–2899

CIOTTONE'S DISASTER MEDICINE, SECOND EDITION   ISBN: 978-0-323-28665-7

Notices

Knowledge and best practice in this field are constantly changing. As new research and experience broaden our understanding, changes in research methods, professional practices, or medical treatment may become necessary.

Practitioners and researchers must always rely on their own experience and knowledge in evaluating and using any information, methods, compounds, or experiments described herein. In using such information or methods they should be mindful of their own safety and the safety of others, including parties for whom they have a professional responsibility.

With respect to any drug or pharmaceutical products identified, readers are advised to check the most current information provided (i) on procedures featured or (ii) by the manufacturer of each product to be administered, to verify the recommended dose or formula, the method and duration of administration, and contraindications. It is the responsibility of practitioners, relying on their own experience and knowledge of their patients, to make diagnoses, to determine dosages and the best treatment for each individual patient, and to take all appropriate safety precautions.

To the fullest extent of the law, neither the Publisher nor the authors, contributors, or editors, assume any liability for any injury and/or damage to persons or property as a matter of products liability, negligence or otherwise, or from any use or operation of any methods, products, instructions, or ideas contained in the material herein.

Previous edition copyrighted 2006.

Library of Congress Cataloging-in-Publication Data
Disaster medicine (Ciottone)
  Disaster medicine/[edited by] Gregory R. Ciottone ; associate editors, Paul D. Biddinger, Robert G. Darling, Saleh Fares, Mark E. Keim, Michael S. Molloy, Selim Suner. – Second edition.
  p.; cm.
  Includes bibliographical references and index.
  ISBN 978-0-323-28665-7 (hardcover : alk. paper)
  I. Ciottone, Gregory R., editor. II. Title.
  [DNLM: 1. Disaster Planning–methods.   2. Bioterrorism–prevention & control.   3. Disaster Medicine–methods.   4. Disasters.   5. Emergency Medical Services–methods.   6. Radioactive Hazard Release–prevention & control. WA 295]
  RC86.7
  362.18–dc23
                                                                        2015002957

Executive Content Strategist: Kate Dimock
Senior Content Development Specialist: Ann Anderson
Publishing Services Manager: Patricia Tannian
Senior Project Manager: Sharon Corell
Manager, Art and Design: Julia Dummitt

Printed in China.

Last digit is the print number: 9   8   7   6   5   4   3   2   1

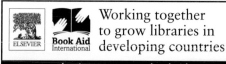

This book is dedicated to the memory of Richard V. Aghababian, MD,
and his pioneering work in the field of disaster medicine.
He was a teacher, mentor, and good friend.

ACKNOWLEDGMENTS

This book could not have been possible without the selfless devotion, unending support, and eternal encouragement of my dear wife, Amalia, and our children, Vigen and Robert. They are my keel in a churning sea and every reason for my being. I love you all very much.

–Gregory R. Ciottone

To the professionals who study how to best prepare for adversity, who strive to learn how we can all do better, and who tirelessly give of themselves to help alleviate the suffering of others in the worst of circumstances.

–Paul D. Biddinger

I wish to thank my incredible family for all their love and support—my beautiful wife, Shari, and our three incredible daughters, Natalia, Briann, and Katrina.

–Robert G. Darling

I want to express my sincere appreciation to all authors who, in their selfless and tireless efforts, were instrumental in and dedicated to the creation and publication of this landmark work. Most importantly, a special thank you goes to Dr. Gregory Ciottone for giving me the opportunity to participate.

–Saleh Fares

Dedicated to my wife, Kelly, and daughter, Cassidy.

–Mark E. Keim

Ní Neart go cur le chéile—there is no strength without unity—an old Irish proverb which resonated during our disaster response missions and in completing this work. I dedicate this manuscript to the memory of my father who encouraged me to write from a very young age. I am privileged to have an understanding family who allows me to spend time in the "writing cave." They know I like them very much—Maria my wife, Cate, Michael (the real Mick Molloy), and especially Sean who helped me order pages. Thank you for all your support. Thanks also to all the authors who gave so much time in the editing and reediting process. Without you this would not be possible.

–Michael Sean Molloy

I have been lucky to attend amazing schools like Robert College High School in Istanbul and Brown University. I enjoyed the friendly mentorship of great minds, particularly Mr. Mallinder, Gary Kleinman, John Donoghue, and Gregory Jay. Above all, nothing happens without the support and love of family and close friends. Deb and Kaya: Thank You.

For I have seen suffering at suffering's worst; the best in people have prevailed.

–Selim Suner

ASSOCIATE EDITORS

Majed Aljohani, MD
Emergency and Disaster Medicine
  Consultant
National Guard Hospital
Assistant Professor
King Saud bin Abdulaziz University for
  Health Sciences
Riyadh, Saudi Arabia

Bader Alotaibi, MD
Consultant of Emergency and Disaster
  Medicine
Chairman, Disaster Management
  Department
King Fahd Medical City
Assistant Professor
King Saud bin Abdulaziz University for
  Health Sciences
Riyadh, Saudi Arabia

Abdulrahman S. Alqahtani, MD, MS
Consultant, Emergency Medicine
Chairman, Emergency Department
King Saud Medical City
Riyadh, Saudi Arabia

Michelangelo Bortolin, MD
Emergency Physician
118 Servizio Emergenza Territoriale Torino
  (Torino EMS)
Adjunct Professor
Univeriity of Torino
Torino, Italy
Adjunct Professor
Università Vita-Salute San Raffaele
Milan, Italy

Jonathan L. Burstein, MD, FACEP
Assistant Professor of Emergency Medicine
Harvard Medical School
Massachusetts State EMS Medical Director
Boston, Massachusetts

David W. Callaway, MD, MPA
Director, Operational and Disaster Medicine
Emergency Medicine
Carolinas Medical Center
Charlotte, North Carolina

**Srihari Cattamanchi, MBBS, MD,
HAFDMEM**
Faculty, Disaster Preparedness Program
Harvard Humanitarian Initiative
Cambridge, Massachusetts
Faculty, Fellowship in Disaster Medicine
Beth Israel Deaconess Medical Center

Boston, Massachusetts
Director, Operational Medicine
"Child in Hand"
Port-au-Prince, Haiti

Edward W. Cetaruk, MD, FACMT
Assistant Professor, Medical Toxicology
University of Colorado School of Medicine
Assistant Professor, Medical Toxicology
  Fellowship
Rocky Mountain Poison Center
Physician Partner
Toxicology Associates, LLC
Denver, Colorado

Francesco Della Corte, MD
Director, Research Centre in Emergency and
  Disaster Medicine and Computer Science
  Applied to Medical Practice
Università del Piemonte Orientale
Novara, Italy

**Irving "Jake" Jacoby, MD, FAAEM,
FACEP, FACP**
Emeritus Professor of Emergency Medicine
University of California, San Diego, School
  of Medicine
La Jolla, California
Attending Physician, Emergency Medicine
USCD Medical Center
San Diego, California
Unit Commander
CA-4 Disaster Medical Assistance Team
U.S. Department of Health and Human
  Services/ASPR/OEM
National Disaster Medical System
Washington, DC

David G. Jarrett, MD, FACEP
Colonel, U.S. Army Medical Corps (Ret.)
Chemical, Biological, Radiological, Nuclear
  Incident Independent Consultant
Human Effects and Medical Response
Derwood, Maryland
Previously: Director, Armed Forces
  Radiobiology Research Institute
Medical Director, Chemical and Biological
  Defense Programs, Department of
  Defense
Bethesda, Maryland

**James M. Madsen, MD, MPH, FCAP,
FACOEM**
Adjunct Associate Professor of Preventive
  Medicine and Biometrics
Assistant Professor of Military and
  Emergency Medicine

Assistant Professor of Pathology
Uniformed Services University of the
  Health Sciences
Bethesda, Maryland
Deputy Director of Academics and
  Training Chemical Casualty Care
  Division
U.S. Army Medical Research Institute of
  Chemical Defense (USAMRICD)
APG-South, Maryland

Selwyn E. Mahon, MD, FACEP
Director of International EMS
Division of Disaster Medicine
Emergency Medicine
Beth Israel Deaconess Medical Center
Boston, Massachusetts

Jerry L. Mothershead, MD, FACEP
Senior Physician Advisor
Medical Readiness and Response
Battelle Memorial Institute
Columbus, Ohio
Assistant Professor
Operational and Emergency Medicine
Uniformed Services University of the
  Health Sciences
Bethesda, Maryland

James P. Phillips, MD, EMT-T
Instructor
Harvard Medical School
Director of Tactical Medicine
Emergency Medicine
Beth Israel Deaconess Medical Center
Boston, Massachusetts

James J. Rifino, DO
Associate Director, Emergency Medical
  Services
Emergency Medicine
Beth Israel Deaconess Medical Center
Boston, Massachusetts

Michael Rubin, MD, FAAEM
Faculty, Beth Israel Deaconess Medical
  Center Fellowship in Disaster
  Medicine
Harvard Medical School
Boston, Massachusetts
Attending Physician
Department of Emergency Medicine
The Ottawa Hospital—The University of
  Ottawa
Ottawa, Ontario

Leon D. Sanchez, MD, MPH
Vice Chair for Operations
Emergency Medicine
Beth Israel Deaconess Medical Center
Associate Professor of Emergency Medicine
Harvard Medical School
Boston, Massachusetts

Ritu R. Sarin, MD, MS
Attending Physician
Beth Israel Deaconess Medical Center

Instructor of Emergency Medicine
Harvard Medical School
Boston, Massachusetts

Charles Stewart, MD, EMDM, MPH
Emergency Physician
Visiting Professor
European Master in Disaster Medicine
   Program
Tulsa, Oklahoma

Eric S. Weinstein, MD, FACEP
Emergency Department
Carolinas Hospital System
Florence, South Carolina
Medical Director
Emergency Response Task Force
South Carolina Division of Fire and Life Safety
Columbia, South Carolina

CONTRIBUTORS

Yasser A. Alaska, MBBS
Consultant
Emergency Medicine
King Saud University
Riyadh, Saudi Arabia

Abdulaziz D. Aldawas, MBBS, SBEM
Consultant of Emergency and Disaster
Medicine
Emergency Medicine
King Abdulaziz Medical City
Riyadh, Saudi Arabia

Saleh Ali Alesa, MBBS
Saudi Board of Emergency Medicine
Consultant
Emergency Medicine
Security Forces Hospital
Head of EMS Section
Emergency Medicine
Special Security Forces Medical Services
Riyadh, Saudi Arabia
Fellow
Disaster Medicine
Brown University
Providence, Rhode Island

George A. Alexander, Major General (Ret.), MD
President and Chief Executive Officer
GA Alexander Solutions, LLC
Alexandria, Virginia

Hazem H. Alhazmi, MBBS
Disaster Medicine Fellow
Emergency Medicine
Beth Israel Deaconess Medical Center/
Harvard Medical School
Boston, Massachusetts
Pediatric Emergency Medicine Fellow
Pediatric Emergency Medicine Staff
Emergency Medicine
King Abdulaziz Medical City/King Khalid
National Guard Hospital
Jeddah, Western Region, Saudi Arabia

Nawfal Aljerian, MBBS, SBEM
Assistant Professor of Emergency
Medicine
King Saud bin Abdulaziz University for
Health Sciences
Consultant of Emergency Medicine and
Emergency Medical Services
Head Division of Emergency Medical
Services
King Abdulaziz Medical City
Riyadh, Saudi Arabia

Majed AlJohani, MD, SBEM
Emergency and Disaster Medicine Consultant
National Guard Hospital
Assistant Professor
King Saud bin Abdulaziz University for
Health Sciences
Riyadh, Saudi Arabia

Khaldoon H. AlKhaldi, MD
Emergency Physician
Emergency Medicine
Tawam Hospital
AlAin, Abu Dhabi, United Arab Emirates
Disaster Medicine Fellow
Emergency Medicine
Beth Israel Deaconess Medical Center
Boston, Massachusetts

Bryant Allen, MD
Emergency Medicine
Division of Operational and Disaster Medicine
Carolinas Medical Center
Charlotte, North Carolina

Bader S. Alotaibi, MD
Consultant of Emergency and Disaster
Medicine
Chairman
Disaster Management Department
King Fahd Medical City
Assistant Professor
King Saud bin Abdulaziz University for
Health Sciences
Riyadh, Saudi Arabia

Mohammad Alotaibi, MD
Disaster Medicine Fellow
Emergency Medicine
Rhode Island Hospital
Cranston, Rhode Island

Evan Avraham Alpert, MD
Attending Physician
Emergency Medicine
Shaare Zedek Medical Center
Jerusalem, Israel

Rakan S. Al-Rasheed, MBBS, SBEM, ArBen
Director
Clinical Skills and Simulation
Assistant Professor of Emergency Medicine
King Saud bin Abdulaziz University for
Health Sciences
Consultant
Emergency Medicine
King Abdulaziz Medical City

King Saud bin Abdulaziz University for
Health Sciences
Riyadh, Saudi Arabia

Mai Alshammari, MBChB
Disaster Medicine Fellowship
Beth Israel Deaconess Medical Center
Boston, Massachusetts

Asaad Alsufyani, MD
Emergency Physician (PGY-2 Resident)
Emergency Medicine
University of Toledo
Toledo, Ohio

Siraj Amanullah, MD, MPH
Assistant Professor
Emergency Medicine and Pediatrics
Director
PEM Fellowship Research and Research
Education
The Warren Alpert Medical School of Brown
University
Hasbro Children's Hospital
Providence, Rhode Island

Ali Ardalan, MD, PhD
Associate Professor and Chair
Disaster and Emergency Health Academy
National Institute of Health Research
School of Public Health
Tehran University of Medical Sciences
Tehran, Iran
Visiting Scientist
Department of Global Health and
Population
Fellow
Harvard Humanitarian Initiative
Harvard University
Cambridge, Massachusetts

Andrew W. Artenstein, MD
Chair
Department of Medicine
Baystate Health
Chair of Medicine
Tufts University School of Medicine at
Baystate Medical Center
Professor of Medicine
Tufts University School of Medicine
Boston, Massachusetts
Adjunct Professor of Medicine and Health
Services, Policy, and Practice
The Warren Alpert Medical School of Brown
University
Providence, Rhode Island

Miriam Aschkenasy, MD, MPH
Deputy Director
Global Disaster Response
Center for Global Health
Massachusetts General Hospital
Clinical Instructor
Harvard Medical School
Boston, Massachusetts
Associate Faculty
Harvard Humanitarian Initiative
Harvard School of Public Health
Cambridge, Massachusetts

Matthew R. Babineau, MD
Attending Physician
Emergency Department
Beth Israel Deaconess Medical Center
Clinical Instructor
Harvard Affiliated Emergency Medicine
    Residency
Harvard Medical School
Boston, Massachusetts

Kavita Babu, MD, FACEP, FACMT
Associate Professor
Emergency Medicine
University of Massachusetts Medical School
Worcester, Massachusetts

Olivia E. Bailey, MD, FACEP
Clinical Associate Professor of Emergency
    Medicine
Emergency Medicine
University of Iowa Hospitals and Clinics
Iowa City, Iowa

Gregory T. Banner, MS, MMAS
Regional Emergency Coordinator
U.S. Department of Health and Human
    Services
Boston, Massachusetts

Fermin Barrueto Jr., MD
Clinical Associate Professor
Emergency Medicine
University of Maryland School of Medicine
Baltimore, Maryland
Chairman
Emergency Medicine
Upper Chesapeake Health Systems
Bel Air, Maryland

Susan A. Bartels, MD, MPH, FRCPC
Clinical Scientist
Emergency Medicine
Queen's University
Kingston, Ontario, Canada

Bruce M. Becker, MD, MPH, FACEP
Professor
Emergency Medicine and Behavioral and
    Social Science

The Warren Alpert Medical School of
    Brown University
Providence, Rhode Island

Paul D. Biddinger, MD, FACEP, FAAEM
Vice Chairman for Emergency Preparedness
Emergency Medicine
Massachusetts General Hospital (MGH)
Medical Director for Emergency
    Preparedness
MGH and Partners Healthcare
Director
Harvard School of Public Health Emergency
    Preparedness and Response Exercise
    Program (EPREP)
Associate Professor of Emergency Medicine
Harvard Medical School
Senior Preparedness Fellow
Harvard TH Chan School of Public Health
Boston, Massachusetts

Eike Blohm, MD
Chief Resident
Emergency Medicine
University of Massachusetts Medical Center
Worcester, Massachusetts

Susan R. Blumenthal, PhD
Managing Director
Gracewood Associates
Charlotte, North Carolina

Stephen W. Borron, MD, MS
Medical Director
West Texas Regional Poison Center
Professor of Emergency Medicine and
    Medical Toxicology
Emergency Medicine
Paul L. Foster School of Medicine
Texas Tech University Health Sciences
    Center—El Paso
El Paso, Texas

Michelangelo Bortolin, MD
Emergency Physician
118 Servizio Emergenza Territoriale Torino
    (Torino EMS)
Adjunct Professor
University of Torino
Torino, Italy
Adjunct Professor
Università Vita-Salute San Raffaele
Milan, Italy

Michael Bouton, MD, MBA
Director of Pediatric Emergency Medicine
Pediatric and Emergency Deparatment
Harlem Hospital
New York, New York

Peter Brewster, BS
Program Manager
Strategic Planning and Quality

Office of Emergency Management
Veterans Health Administration
Martinsburg, West Virginia

Churton Budd, RN, EMTP
Programmer/Developer
Information Technology
Promedica
Staff Nurse
Emergency Services
University of Toledo Medical Center
Nurse/Paramedica
OH1 DMAT
National Disaster Medical System
Toledo, Ohio

James M. Burke, MD
Staff Physician
Glendale Adventist Medical Center
Glendale, California
Lieutenant Commander
U.S. Naval Reserve
Fleet Hospital
Fort Dix, New Jersey

**Frederick M. Burkle Jr., MD, MPH,
DTM**
Senior Fellow and Scientist
Harvard Humanitarian Initiative
Harvard University
Cambridge, Massachusetts
Senior International Public Policy Scholar
Woodrow Wilson International Center for
    Scholars
Washington, DC

**Lynne Barkley Burnett, MD, EdD,
LLB(c)**
Medical Advisor
Fresno County Sheriff's Department
Vice Chairman
Medical Ethics
Community Medical Centers
Adjunct Professor of Forensic Medicine and
    Forensic Pathology
National University
Adjunct Instructor
EMS Operations and Planning for WMD
Texas A&M University
Fresno, California

Nicholas V. Cagliuso Sr., PhD, MPH
Emergency Preparedness Analyst
Office of Emergency Management
The Port Authority of New York
    and New Jersey
Jersey City, New Jersey

John D. Cahill, MD, DTM&H
Assistant Professor/Senior Attending
    Physician
Infectious Diseases and Emergency
    Medicine

Icahn School of Medicine at Mount Sinai/
Mount Sinai Roosevelt Hospital Center
New York, New York

David W. Callaway, MD, MPA
Director Operational and Disaster
Medicine
Emergency Medicine
Carolinas Medical Center
Charlotte, North Carolina

Duane C. Caneva, MD, MS, FACEP
Senior Medical Advisor
Customs and Border Protection
Department of Homeland Security Office of
Health Affairs
Washington, DC

David M. Canther, MDiv
Faculty
Beth Israel Deaconess Medical Center
Fellowship in Emergency Management and
Disaster Medicine
Ooltewah, Tennessee

**Srihari Cattamanchi, MBBS, MD,
HAFDMEM**
Faculty
Disaster Preparedness Program
Harvard Humanitarian Initiative
Cambridge, Massachusetts
Faculty
Fellowship in Disaster Medicine
Beth Israel Deaconess Medical Center
Boston, Massachusetts
Director
Operational Medicine
"Child in Hand"
Port-au-Prince, Haiti

Edward W. Cetaruk, MD, FACMT
Assistant Professor
Medical Toxicology
University of Colorado School of Medicine
Assistant Professor
Medical Toxicology Fellowship
Rocky Mountain Poison Center
Physician Partner
Toxicology Associates, PLLC
Denver, Colorado

James C. Chang, BS, MS
Director of Safety and Environmental Health
Safety
University of Maryland Medical Center
Baltimore, Maryland

Zeno L. Charles-Marcel, MD
Associate Professor of Medicine (Adj)
Department of Internal Medicine
Loma Linda University School of Medicine

Loma Linda, California
Adjunct Professor
Public Health
Andrews University
Berrien Springs, Michigan
Professor of Medicine and Public Health
Faculty of Health Sciences
Montemorelos University
Montemorelos, Nuevo Leon, Mexico
Vice President for Medical Affairs and Health
Services
Medical and Health Services
Wildwood Lifestyle Center and Hospital
Wildwood, Georgia

Anna I. Cheh, MD
Attending Physician
Santa Ana Health Care Providers
Santa Ana, California
Emergency Medicine Physician
Kaiser Permanente South Bay Medical Center
Harbor City, California

David T. Chiu, MD, MPH
Instructor and Attending Physician
Emergency Medicine
Harvard Medical School
Beth Israel Deaconess Medical Center
Boston, Massachusetts

Teriggi J. Ciccone, MD
Attending Physician and Medical
Director
Urgent Care Clinic at Winchester
Hospital
Medical Director
Winchester Fire Department
Wilmington Fire Department
Winchester, Massachusetts

Gregory R. Ciottone, MD, FACEP
Director
Beth Israel Deaconess Medical Center
Fellowship in Disaster Medicine
Director
Disaster Preparedness Program
Harvard Humanitarian Initiative
Associate Professor of Emergency Medicine
Harvard Medical School
Boston, Massachusetts

Jonathan Peter Ciottone, Esq.
Partner
McGivney & Kluger, PC
Hartford, Connecticut

Robert A. Ciottone, PhD
Affiliate
Psychiatry and Pediatrics
University of Massachusetts Medical Center
Affiliate professor

Psychology
Clark University
Worcester, Massachusetts

Diana Clapp, RN, CCRN, BSN, NRP
Quality Improvement Coordinator and
EMS Liaison
R. Adams Cowley Shock Trauma Center
University of Maryland Medical System
Baltimore, Maryland

Raphael G. Cohen, PA-C, MPAS
Physician Assistant (Special Operations)
Federal Bureau of Investigation
Quantico, Virginia

Kathe M. Conlon, BSN, RN, CEM, MSHS
Burn Community Outreach and Disaster
Preparedness Director
The Burn Center at Saint Barnabas
Saint Barnabas Medical Center
Livingston, New Jersey

Joanne Cono, MD, SCM
Director of the Office of Science Quality
Office of the Associate Director for
Science
Centers for Disease Control and Prevention
Atlanta, Georgia

Hilarie Cranmer, MD, MPH
Director
Global Disaster Response
Massachusetts General Hospital
Center for Global Health
Department of Emergency Medicine
Massachusetts General Hospital
Assistant Professor
Harvard Medical School
Harvard School of Public Health
Boston, Massachusetts

**Cord W. Cunningham, Lieutenant
Colonel, U.S. Army, MD, FACEP,
FAAEM**
Fellow
EMS and Disaster Medicine
San Antonio Uniformed Services
Health Education Consortium
Fort Sam Houston
San Antonio, Texas
Assistant Professor
Department of Military and Emergency
Medicine
Uniformed Services University
Bethesda, Maryland

Steven O. Cunnion, MD, MPH, PhD
Emergency Medicine
PENN Travel Medicine
Hospital of the University of Pennsylvania
Philadelphia, Pennsylvania

Alison Sisitsky Curcio, MD
Emergency Medicine Physician
Newton Wellesley Hospital
Newton, Massachusetts

Robert G. Darling, MD
Chief Medical Officer
Patronus Medical Corporation
Chief of Telemedicine
Vitalyze.Me
Assistant Professor
Military and Emergency Medicine
Uniformed Services University of the Health
    Sciences
F. Edward Hébert School of Medicine
Bethesda, Maryland

Neil B. Davids, MD, MPH
Medical Director
Critical Care Flight Paramedic Program
Army Medical Department Center and School
Fort Sam Houston
San Antonio, Texas

Timothy E. Davis, MD, MPH
Chief Medical Officer
National Disaster Medical System
Branch Chief
Operational Medicine (HHS/ASPR/OEM/
    NDMS/OPMED)
Assistant Professor of Emergency Medicine
Emory University School of Medicine
Atlanta, Georgia

Scott Deitchman, MD, MPH, USPHS
Assistant Surgeon General
Associate Director for Environmental Health
    Emergencies
National Center for Environmental Health
    and Agency for Toxic Substances and
    Disease Registry
Centers for Disease Control and Prevention
Atlanta, Georgia

John B. Delaney Jr., MA, EMT-P
Captain
Arlington County Fire Department
Arlington, Virginia

Francesco Della Corte, MD
Director
Research Centre in Emergency and Disaster
    Medicine and Computer Science Applied
    to Medical Practice
Università degli Studi del Piemonte Orientale
Novara, Italy

Gerard DeMers, DO, DHSc, MPH
Commander
Medical Corps
United States Navy

Navy Medicine West EMS/Disaster Medical
    Director
Emergency Management Executive
    Committee Chair
Department of Emergency Medicine
Naval Medical Center San Diego
San Diego, California
Adjunct Assistant Professor
Department of Military and Emergency
    Medicine
F. Edward Hébert School of Medicine
Uniformed Services University
Bethesda, Maryland

William E. Dickerson, MD
Colonel
Medical Corps
United States Air Force
Director of Military Medical Operations
Staff Radiological Oncologist
Armed Forces Radiobiology Research Institute
Bethesda, Maryland

Sharon Dilling, BA
Director of Communications
inVentiv Health
Clinical Division
Marketing and Communication
Princeton, New Jersey

Ahmadreza Djalali, MD, EMDM, PhD
Research Associate
Università degli Studi del Piemonte Orientale
Novara, Italy

Joseph Donahue, MD
Chief Resident
Emergency Medicine
Metropolitan Hospital
Associate Professor
New York Medical College
Valhalla, New York

K. Sophia Dyer, MD
Associate Professor
Emergency Medicine
Boston University School of Medicine
Boston, Massachusetts

Benjamin Easter, MD
Denver Health Residency in Emergency
    Medicine
Denver, Colorado

Laura Ebbeling, MD
Harvard Affiliated Emergency Medicine
    Residency
Resident Physician
Emergency Medicine
Beth Israel Deaconess Medical Center
Boston, Massachusetts

Nir Eyal, DPhil
Associate Professor of Global Health and
    Populaton
Deparatment of Global Health and Populaton
Harvard T.H. Chan School of Public Health
Associate Professor of Global Health and
    Social Medicine
Harvard Medical School Center for Bioethics
Boston, Massachusetts

Andrew J. Eyre, MD
Resident
Emergency Medicine
Brigham and Women's Hospital/
    Massachusetts General Hospital
Boston, Massachusetts

**Saleh Fares, MD, MPH, FRCPC,
FACEP, FAAEM**
Head
Emergency Department
Zayed Military Hospital
Founder and President
Emirates Society of Emergency Medicine
    (ESEM)
Abu Dhabi, United Arab Emirates

Katherine Farmer, MD
The Warren Alpert Medical School of
    Brown University
Providence, Rhode Island

Denis J. FitzGerald, MD
Chief Medical Officer
Counter-Narcotics and Terrorism
    Operational Medical Support
    (CONTOMS) Program
Casualty Care Research Center
Uniformed Services University of the Health
    Sciences
U.S. Department of Defense
Washington, DC

Elizabeth Foley, MD
Harvard Affiliated Emergency Medicine
    Residency
Beth Israel Deaconess Medical Center
Clinical Fellow in Emergency Medicine
Harvard Medical School
Boston, Massachusetts

Kerry Fosher, PhD
Director of Research
Thanslational Research Group
Marine Corps University
Quantico, Virginia

David Freeman, MS, NRP
Clinical Instructor
Emergency Medicine
University of Maryland School of Medicine
Baltimore, Maryland

Robert L. Freitas, MHA
Senior Director of Business Development
Emergency Medicine
Harvard Medical Faculty Physicians
Co-Director
International Emergency Department
    Leadership Institute
Boston, Massachusetts

Franklin D. Friedman, MD, MS, FACEP
Director of Prehospital Care and Emergency
    Preparedness
Emergency Medicine
Tufts Medical Center
Assistant Professor
Emergency Medicine
Tufts University School of Medicine
Boston, Massachusetts

Frederick Fung, MD, MS, JD
Clinical Professor
Internal Medicine/Occupational Medicine
University of California, Irvine
Irvine, California
Medical Director
Occupational Medicine
Sharp Rees Stealy Medical Group
San Diego, California

Fiona E. Gallahue, MD
Associate Professor
Program Director
The University of Washington
Seattle, Washington

Lucille Gans, MD
Emergency Medicine
UMass Medical Center
Worcester, Massachusetts

Stephanie Chow Garbern, MD
Beth Israel Deaconess Medical Center
Boston, Massachusetts

Mark E. Gebhart, MD, CPM
Associate Professor of Community Health
    Concentration
Director
Emergency Preparedness
Department of Community Health
Boonshoft School of Medicine
Wright State University
Dayton, Ohio

James Geiling, MD, FACP
Associate Professor of Medicine
Dartmouth Medical School
Assistant Director
New England Center for Emergency
    Preparedness
Dartmouth-Hitchcock Medical Center

Hanover, New Hampshire
Chief
Medical Service
Veterans Affairs Medical Center
White River Junction, Vermont

Brian C. Geyer, MD, PhD, MPH
Department of Emergency Medicine
Center for Vascular Emergencies
Massachusetts General Hospital
Boston, Massachusetts

Mary Jo Giordano, BA
Homeland Security Specialist
Arlington Police Department
Arlington, Texas

William A. Gluckman, DO, MBA, FACEP
President and CEO
FastER Urgent Care
Morris Plains, New Jersey

J. Scott Goudie, MD
Attending Physician
Cambridge Health Alliance, Whidden
    Memorial Hospital
Cambridge, Massachusetts

Robert M. Gougelet, MD
Subject Matter Expert: Emergency
    Preparedness
Department of Health and Human Services
Division of Public Health
State of New Hampshire
Concord, New Hampshire

Benjamin Graboyes, MD
Division of Operational and Disaster Medicine
Emergency Medicine
Carolinas Medical Center
Charlotte, North Carolina

Michael I. Greenberg
Emergency Medical Department
King Saud University Medical City
Riyadh, Saudi Arabia

P. Gregg Greenough, MD, MPH
Assistant Professor of Emergency Medicine
Harvard Medical School
Assistant Professor of Global Health and
    Population
Harvard School of Public Health
Research Director
Division of International Emergency
    Medicine and Humanitarian Programs
Department of Emergency Medicine
Brigham and Women's Hospital
Boston, Massachusetts
Faculty
Harvard Humanitarian Initiative
Harvard University
Cambridge, Massachusetts

Ashley L. Greiner, MD, MPH
Physician
Emergency Medicine
Beth Israel Deaconess Medical Center
Instructor of Medicine
Harvard Medical School
Boston, Massachusetts

Mark Greve, MD
Clinical Assistant Professor
Emergency Medicine
Brown University
Providence, Rhode Island

Stephen Grosse, MD
Chief Resident
Emergency Medicine
Beth Israel Deaconess Medical Center
Clinical Fellow in Medicine
Harvard Medical School
Boston, Massachusetts

Shamai A. Grossman, MD, MS
Assistant Proofessor, Medicine
Harvard Medical School
Director
Cardiac Emergency Center and Clinical
    Decision Unit
Emergency Medicine
Beth Israel Deaconess Medical Center
Boston, Massachusetts

Tee L. Guidotti, MD, MPH, DABT
Vice President
HSE/Sustainability
Medical Advisory Services
Rockville, Maryland

Jason B. Hack, MD
Director
Division of Medical Toxicology
Associate Professor
Emergency Medicine
Rhode Island Hospital
The Warren Alpert Medical School of Brown
    University
Providence, Rhode Island

Matthew M. Hall, MD
Emergency Medicine Resident
Emergency Medicine
Beth Israel Deaconess Medical Center
Boston, Massachusetts

John W. Hardin, MD
Attending Physician
Emergency Medicine
St. Vincent Hospital Emergency
    Department
Beth Israel Deaconess Medical Center
    Ultrasound Fellow
Boston, Massachusetts

John L. Hick, MC, FACEP
Associate Professor of Emergency Medicine
University of Minnesota
Faculty Physician
Associate Medical Director for Hennepin
County Emergency Medical Services
Medical Director for Emergency
Preparedness
Hennepin County Medical Center
Minneapolis, Minnesota

Nishanth S. Hiremath, MD
Head of the Department and Consultant
Emergency Medicine
Bhagwan Mahaveer Jain Hospital
Vasanth Nagar, Bangalore, India

Steven Horng, MD, MMsc
Assistant Director of Informatics
Emergency Medicine
Beth Israel Deaconess Medical Center
Boston, Massachusetts

**Geoffrey D. Horning, NRP/CCMTP-P,
BA, MPH**
Head of Development and Improvement
Projects
Training Department
Al-Ghad International Colleges
Riyadh, Saudi Arabia

Kurt R. Horst, MD
Emergency Room Physician
Athens Regional Medical Center
Athens, Georgia

Ali A. Hosin, MBBS, BSc (Hons)
School of Medicine
Imperial College London
London, Great Britain

Amer Hosin, MD
Chief Executive Officer
Emergency Medicine Academy Project
Affiliate of Brigham and Women's Hospital
Boston, Massachusetts
Abu Dhabi Police GHQ
United Arab Emirates

Hans R. House, MD, MACM
Professor
Department of Emergency Medicine
University of Iowa
Iowa City, Iowa

Pier Luigi Ingrassia, MD, EMDM, PhD
Researcher and Vice-Director
Research Centre in Emergency and Disaster
Medicine and Computer Science Applied
to Medical Practice
Università degli Studi del Piemonte Orientale
Novara, Italy

Patrick M. Jackson, MD
Department of Emergency Medicine
Division of Operational and Disaster
Medicine
Carolinas Medical Center
Charlotte, North Carolina

**Irving "Jake" Jacoby, MD, FACP,
FACEP, FAAEM**
Emeritus Clinical Professor of Emergency
Medicine and Surgery
University of California
San Diego
School of Medicine
La Jolla, California
Attending Physician
Emergency Medicine and Hyperbaric
Medicine
USCD Medical Center
San Diego, California
Commander
CA-4 Disaster Medical Assistance Team
U.S. Department of Health and Human
Services/ASPR/OEM
National Disaster Medical System
Washington, DC

Rajnish Jaiswal, MS, MD
Attending Physician
Emergency Medicine
Metropolitan Hospital
Associate Professor
New York Medical College
Valhalla, New York

Adam J. Janicki, MD
Emergency Medicine
Rhode Island Hospital
The Warren Alpert Medical School of Brown
University
Providence, Rhode Island

Gregory Jay, MD, PhD
Professor
Emergency Medicine
Division of Engineering
The Warren Alpert Medical School of Brown
University
Providence, Rhode Island

Miriam John, MD
Emergency Room Physician
Newark Beth Israel Medical Center
Newark, New Jersey

Shawn E. Johnson, BS
OMS-II
Virginia College of Medicine
Blacksburg, Virginia

James R. Johnston Jr., BSHS, NREMT-P
Special Forces
U.S. Army 18 Zulu, DMT, MFFJM, SLJM
East Tennessee State University
Quillen College of Medicine
Johnson City, Tennessee

Jerrilyn Jones, MD
Fellow
Boston EMS
Emergency Medicine
Boston Medical Center
Boston, Massachusetts

Michael D. Jones, MD
Brooke Army Medical Center
SAUSHEC EM Residency Program
Fort Sam Houston
San Antonio, Texas

Josh W. Joseph, MD
Physician
Emergency Medicine
Beth Israel Deaconess Medical Center
Harvard University
Boston, Massachusetts

Patrice Joseph, MD, MSc
Clinical Trial Site Leader/Project Coordinator
Infectious Diseases
Gheskio Centers
Port-au-Prince, Haiti

Alexis Kearney, MD, MPH
Emergency Medicine
Rhode Island Hospital
Providence, Rhode Island

Donald Keen, MD
Fellow
EMS and Disaster Medicine
San Antonio Uniformed Services
Health Education Consortium
Fort Sam Houston, Texas

Mark E. Keim, MD, MBA
Chief Executive Officer
DisasterDoc, LLC
Atlanta, Georgia
Faculty
Beth Israel Deaconess Medical Center
Fellowship in Disaster Medicine
Boston, Massachusetts
Adjunct Faculty
Emory University
Rollins School of Public Health
Atlanta, Georgia
Vice President for Partnerships
World Association of Disaster and
Emergency Medicine
Madison, Wisconsin

Elizabeth Kenez, MD
Resident Physician
Emergency Medicine
University of Maryland
Baltimore, Maryland

Katharyn E. Kennedy, MD
Assistant Professor of Emergency Medicine
Department of Emergency Medicine
University of Massachusetts Medical
    School
Director of Emergency Medicine
Marlborough Hospital
Worcester, Massachusetts

Anas A. Khan, MBBS, MHA
Emergency Medical Department
King Saud University Medical City
Riyadh, Saudi Arabia

Chetan U. Kharod, MD, MPH, FACEP, FAAEM
Fellow
EMS and Disaster Medicine
San Antonio Uniformed Services
Health Education Consortium
Fort Sam Houston, Texas
Assistant Professor
Department of Military and Emergency
    Medicine
Uniformed Services University
Bethesda, Maryland

Sylvia H. Kim, MD
Attending Physician and Medical Director
Goleta Valley Cottage Hospital
Santa Barbara, California

Kevin King, MD
Chair
Emergency Medicine
Residency Program Director
Kendall Regional Medical Center
Miami, Florida

Mark A. Kirk, MD, FACMT
Director
Chemical Defense Program
Office of Health Affairs
Department of Homeland Security
Washington, DC

Leo Kobayashi, MD
Associate Professor
Emergency Medicine
The Warren Alpert Medical School of Brown
    University
Providence, Rhode Island

Lara K. Kulchycki, MD, MPH
Assistant Medical Director
Emergency Medicine

Santa Clara Valley Medical Center
San Jose, California

Rick G. Kulkarni, MD
Medical Director, eMedicine
New York, New York
Attending Physician
Adult Emergency Department
Yale-New Haven Hospital
New Haven, Connecticut

Joseph Lauro, MD, EMT-P
Assistant Professor (Clinical)
Emergency Medicine
The Warren Alpert Medical School of Brown
    University
Providence, Rhode Island

Benjamin J. Lawner, DO, MS, EMT-P, FACEP
Assistant Professor
Emergency Medicine
University of Maryland School of Medicine
Deputy Medical Director
Baltimore City Fire Department
Baltimore, Maryland

David V. Le, MD
Emergency Medicine
UT Health Science Center at San Antonio
San Antonio, Texas

Debra Lee, MD, FACEP
Emergency Medicine
University of Maryland School of Medicine
Baltimore, Maryland

Terrance T. Lee, MD
Chemical Defense Program
Office of Health Affairs
Department of Homeland Security
Washington, DC

Jay Lemery, MD, FACEP, FAWM
Associate Professor of Emergency Medicine
University of Colorado School of Medicine
Aurora, Colorado

Jeanette A. Linder, M.D.
Chief
Radiation Oncology
Sinai Hospital of Baltimore
Baltimore, Maryland

Lawrence S. Linder, MD, FACEP, FAEM
Director
Emergency Department
Senior Vice President/Chief Medical Officer
Baltimore Washington Medical Center
Glen Burnie, Maryland

Michael A. Loesch
Adjunct Faculty

Disaster Medicine Fellowship
Beth Israel Deaconess Medical Center
Boston, Massachusetts

Heather Long, MD
Attending Physician
Department of Emergency Medicine
North Shore University Hospital
Manhasset, New York

Kate Longley-Wood, MSc
Marine Biologist
Boston, Massachusetts

Michael D. Mack, DO, EMT-T, ERT, Maj, USAF, FS, MC
Staff Emergency Medicine Physician
Former Special Operations Operational
    Support Medic
Former Tactical Medic and Assistant
    Medical Director for the Warren
    County
SWAT
Eglin AFB, Florida

John M. Mackay, MD
Vice Chair and Assistant Professor
Emergency Medicine
Texas Tech University Health Science
    Center—El Paso
Paul L. Foster School of Medicine
El Paso, Texas

Laura Macnow, MD
Instructor
Emergency Medicine
Harvard Medical School
Attending Physician
Emergency Department
Beth Israel Deaconess Medical Center
Boston, Massachusetts

James M. Madsen, MD, MPH, FCAP, FACOEM
Adjunct Associate Professor of Preventive
    Medicine and Biometrics
Assistant Professor of Military and
    Emergency Medicine
Assistant Professor of Pathology
Uniformed Services University of the Health
    Sciences
Bethesda, Maryland
Deputy Director of Academics and
    Training
Chemical Casualty Care
Division
U.S. Army Medical Research Institute of
    Chemical Defense (USAMRICD)
APG-South, Maryland

Brian J. Maguire, Dr.PH, MSA, EMT-P
Professor
School of Medical and Applied Sciences
Central Queensland University
Rockhampton, Australia

Patrick J. Maher, MD
Chief Resident
Emergency Medicine
The University of Washington
Seattle, Washington

Selwyn E. Mahon, MD, FACEP
Director of International EMS
Emergency Medicine
Division of Disaster Medicine
Beth Israel Deaconess Medical Center
Boston, Massachusetts

John D. Malone, MD, FACP, FIDSA
Professor of Medicine
Uniformed Services University of the Health
    Sciences
F. Edward Hebert School of Medicine
Department of Preventive Medicine and
    Biometrics
Bethesda, Maryland

Marco Mangini, MD
Resident
Post-Graduate School in Anesthesia and
    Intensive Care
University of Florence
Florence, Italy

**Paul M. Maniscalco, MS, MPA,
PhD, LP**
President Emeritus
International Association of EMS Chiefs
Washington, DC
Deputy Chief Paramedic (Ret.)
Fire Department, City of New York
New York, New York

**Pietro D. Marghella, DHSc, MSc, MA,
CEM, FACCP**
Director
Medical and Public Health
    Preparedness
Hassett Willis and Company
Washington, DC

Jeff Matthews, AS, BS
EMT-D/Captain
Charlotte Fire Department
Charlotte, North Carolina
President
Technical Rescue Consultants, LLC
Associate
Element Rescue
Voting Member, NFPA 1006

Committee on Professional Qualifications for
    Technical Rescuers
Clover, South Carolina

Peter McCahill, MD
Operational and Disaster Medicine Fellow
Emergency Medicine
Carolinas Medical Center
Charlotte, North Carolina

Sean D. McKay, EMT-P/T
Associate and Member
Asymmetric Combat Institute, LLC
Executive Board Member
Committee for Tactical Emergency
    Casualty Care
National Tactical Officers Association TEMS
    Instructor
Associate/Editor
Element Rescue
DHS/FEMA Active Shooter and IED
    Working Group
AA, AS Emergency Medical Services
Greenville, South Carolina

C. Crawford Mecham, MD, MS, FACEP
Professor
Emergency Medicine
Perelman School of Medicine at the
    University of Pennsylvania
Philadelphia, Pennsylvania

Mandana Mehta, MBBS, DTMIH
PhD Fellow
Centre for Research on the Epidemiology of
    Disasters
Institute of Health and Society
Université Catholique de Louvain
Brussels, Belgium

Patricia L. Meinhardt, MD, MPH, MA
Adjunct Associate Professor
Department of Environmental and
    Occupational Health
Drexel University School of Public Health
Drexel University
Philadelphia, Pennsylvania

Laura Diane Melville, MD
Emergency Room Physician
New York Methodist Hospital
Brooklyn, New York

Angela M. Mills, MD
Associate Professor and Vice Chair of Clinical
    Operations
Emergency Medicine
University of Pennsylvania
Philadelphia, Pennsylvania

Andrew M. Milsten, MD, MS, FACEP
Clinical Assistant Professor

Emergency Medicine
University of Maryland
College Park, Maryland
Assistant Medical Director
Anne Arundel County Fire Department
Medical Director
Expresscare Critical Care Transport and Mass
    Gathering Events
Newsletter Editor, Disaster Medical Section
ACEP
Ann Arundel County, Maryland

Clifford S. Mitchell, MS, MD, MPH
Director
Environmental Health Bureau
Prevention and Health Promotion
    Administration
Maryland Department of Health and Mental
    Hygiene
Baltimore, Maryland

Dale M. Molé, DO, FACEP
Captain
Medical Corps
United States Navy (Ret.)
Chief Executive Officer
Scheer Memorial Hospital
Kathmandu, Nepal

**Michael Sean Molloy, MB, Dip SpMed
(RCSI), EMDM, MFSEM(UK), FCEM,
FFSEM (RCSI)**
Research Director
Beth Israel Deaconess Medical Center
    Fellowship in Disaster Medicine
Boston, Massachusetts
Consultant Emergency Physician
Bon Secours Hospital
Tralee, Ireland
Consultant Emergency Physician
Hermitage Medical Clinic
Lucan, Ireland
Chairman
Medical Advisory Committee
Pre-Hospital Emergency Care Council
Naas, Ireland

John Moloney, MBBS
Head
Trauma Anaesthesia
The Alfred Hospital
Senior Field Emergency Medical Officer
State Health Emergency Response Plan
Associate Professor
Department of Anaesthesia
Department of Community Emergency
    Health and Paramedic Practice
Monash University
Melbourne, Victoria, Australia

Ilaria Morelli, MD
Emergency Physician

San Raffaele Hospital
Adjunct Professor
Vita-Salute San Raffaele University
Milan, Italy
Adjunct Professor
University of Torino
Torino, Italy
Adjunct Faculty Member
Disaster Medicine Fellowship
Beth Israel Deaconess Medical Center
Boston, Massachusetts

Jerry L. Mothershead, MD
Senior Physician Advisor
Medical Readiness and Response
Battelle Memorial Institute
Columbus, Ohio
Assistant Professor
Operational and Emergency Medicine
Uniformed Services University of the
     Health Sciences
Bethesda, Maryland

**John Mulhern, RGN, RNP, HDip, MSc
(candidate), PGrad Critical Care**
Cardio-Respiratory and Urgent Care
     Manager
Cardiology/Urgent Care
Bon Secours Hospital
Tralee, County Kerry, Ireland

**Nicole F. Mullendore, MSN, CRNP,
CEN**
Nurse Practitioner
Adult Emergency Department
University of Maryland Medical Center
Baltimore, Maryland

Larry A. Nathanson, MD
Director
Emergency Medicine Informatics
Beth Israel Deaconess Medical Center
Assistant Professor of Emergency
     Medicine
Harvard Medical School
Boston, Massachusetts

Amelia Marie Nelson, RN, BSN
Disaster Fellow Nurse
Emergency Department
Beth Israel Deaconess Medical Center
Boston, Massachusetts

Erica L. Nelson, MD, PhM
Resident Physician
Emergency Medicine
Harvard Associated Emergency Medicine
     Residency
Brigham and Women's Hospital
Massachusetts General Hospital
Boston, Massachusetts

Lewis S. Nelson, MD
Professor and Vice Chair for Academic Affairs
Ronald O. Perelman Department of
     Emergency Medicine
New York University School of Medicine
Director
Fellowship in Medical Toxicology
New York City Poison Control Center
Professor
Emergency Medicine
New York University School of Medicine
New York, New York

Carey Nichols, MD
Division of Operational and Disaster
     Medicine
Emergency Medicine
Carolinas Medical Center
Charlotte, North Carolina

Mariann Nocera, MD
Fellow
Emergency Medicine
Rhode Island Hospital/Hasbro Childen's
     Hospital
Providence, Rhode Island

Erin E. Noste, MD
Attending Faculty
Emergency Medicine
Carolinas Medical Center–Main
Charlotte, North Carolina

Catherine Y. Ordun, MPH
Associate
Strategic Innovation Group
Booz Allen Hamilton
Washington, DC

Peter D. Panagos, MD, FAHA, FACEP
Director
Neurovascular Emergencies
Associate Professor
Emergency Medicine and Neurology
Washington University
St. Louis, Missouri

Robert Partridge, MD, MPH
Adjunct Associate Professor
Emergency Medicine
The Warren Alpert Medical School of Brown
     University
Providence, Rhode Island

Jeffrey S. Paul
Director
Morris County Office of Emergency
     Management
Tactical Operations Captain
Public Information Officer (Ret.)
Morris County Prosecutor's Office
Morristown, New Jersey

Catherine Pettit, MD
Assistant Professor
Emergency Medicine
The Warren Alpert Medical School of Brown
     University
Rhode Island Hospital
Providence, Rhode Island

James Pfaff, MD
Staff Emergency Physician
San Antonio Uniformed Services Health
     Education Consortium Emergency
     Medicine Residency
Brooke Army Medical Center
Fort Sam Houston
San Antonio, Texas

James P. Phillips, MD, EMT-T
Instructor
Harvard Medical School
Director of Tactical Medicine
Emergency Medicine
Beth Israel Deaconess Medical Center
Boston, Massachusetts

Jason Pickett, MD, EMT-P/T
Assistant Professor
Division of Tactical Emergency
     Medicine
Wright State University
Dayton, Ohio

William Porcaro, MD, MPH, FACEP
Associate EMS Medical Director and
     Co-Chair of Disaster Committee
Instructor in Medicine
Harvard Medical School
Department of Emergency Medicine
Mount Auburn Hospital
Cambridge, Massachusetts

Thérèse M. Postel, MA
United States Foreign Service Officer
Middle Village, Queens, New York

Charles N. Pozner, MD
Medical Director
Neil and Elise Wallace STRATUS Center for
     Medical Simulation
Brigham and Women's Hospital
Associate Professor
Emergency Medicine
Harvard Medical School
Boston, Massachusetts

**Vidyalakshmi PR, MBBS, DNB(Med),
FNB(ID)**
Junior Consultant
Infectious Disease Department
Apollo Specialty Hospital
Chennai, Tamilnadu, India

Lawrence Proano, MD
Clinical Associate Professor
Emergency Medicine
The Warren Alpert Medical School of
    Brown University
Providence, Rhode Island

Peter B. Pruitt, MD
Resident Physician
Emergency Medicine
Brigham and Women's Hospital
Massachusetts General Hospital
Boston, Massachusetts

Jeffrey S. Rabrich, DO, FACEP
Medical Director
Emergency Department
Mount Sinai St. Luke's Hospital
New York, New York

Jeffrey D. Race, FF/EMT, MEP
FDNY Captain HazTac (Ret.)
Charlotte, North Carolina

Luca Ragazzoni, MD, PhD
Research Associate
Research Center in Emergency and
    Disaster Medicine
Università degli Studi del Piemonte
    Orientale
Novara, Italy

Najma Rahman-Kahn, MD
Attending Physician
Lutheran Hospital
Brooklyn, New York

Kristin Allyce Reed, RN, BSN
Disaster Nurse Fellow
Emergency Departement
Beth Israel Deaconess Medical Center
Boston, Massachusetts

Wende R. Reenstra, MD, PhD
Emergency Medicine
Beth Israel Deaconess Medical Center
Boston, Massachusetts

Paul P. Rega, MD, FACEP
Assistant Professor
Public Health and Preventive Medicine
Emergency Medicine
University of Toledo College of Medicine
Toledo, Ohio

Michael J. Reilly, DrPH, MPH, CEM
Director
Center for Disaster Medicine
Associate Professor
New York Medical College
Valhalla, New York

Andrew T. Reisner, MD
Attending Physician
Assistant Professor
Emergency Medicine
Massachussetts General Hospital
Harvard Medical School
Boston, Massachusetts

Marc C. Restuccia, MD
Associate Clinical Professor
Emergency Medicine
UMass Memorial Health Care
University of Massachusetts Medical
    School
Worcester, Massachusetts

James J. Rifino, DO
Associate Director
Emergency Medical Services
Emergency Medicine
Beth Israel Deaconess Medical Center
Boston, Massachusetts

James Michael Riley, REMT-P
Senior Security Analyst
Office of Security and Investigations
U.S. Citizenship and Immigration
    Services
Washington, DC

Paul M. Robben, MD, PhD
Major
U.S. Army Medical Corps
96th Civil Affairs Battalion (Airborne)
Fort Bragg, North Carolina

Kevin M. Ryan, MD
Disaster Medicine Fellow
Beth Israel Deaconess Medical Center
Harvard Humanitarian Initiative
Affiliated Fellow
Boston, Massachusetts

Heather Rybasack-Smith, MD, MPH
Emergency Medicine Physician
Brown University
Rhode Island Hospital
Providence, Rhode Island

Leon D. Sanchez, MD, MPH
Vice Chair for Operations
Emergency Medicine
Beth Israel Deaconess Medical Center
Associate Professor
Emergency Medicine
Harvard Medical School
Boston, Massachusetts

Ritu R. Sarin, MD, MS
Attending Physician
Emergency Medicine
Beth Israel Deaconess Medical Center

Instructor of Emergency Medicine
Harvard Medical School
Boston, Massachusetts

Debra D. Schnelle, MS
Chief Operations Officer
Trifecta Solutions
Reston, Virginia

Valarie Schwind, MD
Emergency Medicine
Division of Operational and Disaster
    Medicine
Carolinas Medical Center
Charlotte, North Carolina

Malcolm Seheult, JD, PhD, FRSA
President
GR3 Inc.
Ooltewah, Tennessee

Kinjal N. Sethuraman, MD, MPH
Assistant Professor
Emergency Medicine
University of Maryland
Baltimore, Maryland

Geoffrey L. Shapiro, BSHS, EMT-P
Director
EMS and Operational Medicine Training
School of Medicine and Health Sciences
The George Washington University
Washington, DC

Marc J. Shapiro, MD
University Emergency Medicine
    Foundation
Emergency Medicine
The Warren Alpert Medical School of Brown
    University
Providence, Rhode Island

Sam Shen, MD, MBA, FACEP
Clinical Associate Professor
Emergency Medicine
Stanford University School of Medicine
Stanford, California

Suzanne M. Shepherd, MD, DTM&H
Emergency Medicine
PENN Travel Medicine
Hospital of the University of Pennsylvania
Philadelphia, Pennsylvania

William H. Shoff, MD, DTM&H
Emergency Medicine
PENN Travel Medicine
Hospital of the University of Pennsylvania
Philadelphia, Pennsylvania

Craig Sisson, MD, RDMS
University of Texas

Health Science Center at San Antonio
San Antonio, Texas

Alexander P. Skog, BA
Research Assistant
Emergency Medicine
University of Maryland School of Medicine
Baltimore, Maryland

Jonathan E. Slutzman, BSE, MD
Assistant Professor
Emergency Medicine
University of Massachusetts Medical School
Attending Physician
Emergency Medicine
University of Massachusetts Memorial
    Medical Center
Worcester, Massachusetts

Devin M. Smith, MD
Emergency Medicine Residency Program
The Warren Alpert Medical School of Brown
    University
Providence, Rhode Island

E. Reed Smith, MD, FACEP
Operational Medical Director
Arlington County Fire Department
Arlington, Virginia
Assistant Professor of Emergency
    Medicine
The George Washington University School of
    Medicine
Washington, DC

Jack E. Smith II, MA, EMT-P
Senior Program Manager
National Center for Medical Readiness
Adjunct Faculty
College of Education and Human Servces
Wright State University
Dayton, Ohio

Peter B. Smulowitz, MD
Attending Physician and Academic Faculty
    Chair
Governmental Affairs Committee for
    Massachusetts College of Emergency
    Physicians
Northside Hospital
Atlanta, Georgia

Angela M. Snyder, BA, MPH
Department of Community Health
Boonshoft School of Medicine
Wright State University
Dayton, Ohio

Joshua J. Solano, MD
Resident Physician
Emergency Medicine
Beth Israel Deaconess Medical Center
Boston, Massachusetts

John Sorenson, PhD
Distinguished Research and Development
    Staff
Oak Ridge National Laboratory
Oak Ridge, Tennessee

Kimberly A. Stanford, MD
Resident Physician
Emergency Medicine
Brigham and Women's Hospital
Massachusetts General Hospital
Boston, Masschusetts

Charles Stewart, MD, EMDM, MPH
Emergency Physician
Visiting Professor
European Master in Disaster Medicine
    Program
Tulsa, Oklahoma

M. Kathleen Stewart, MSCIS, MSLA, MPH, MS(c)DM, NRP
Paramedic
Mercy Regional EMS
Owasso, Oklahoma

Carol Sulis, MD
Associate Professor of Medicine
Boston University School of Medicine
Boston, Massachusetts

Robert J. Tashjian, AB, VMD, DSc(Hon)
President
American Veterinary Medical Frontiers
West Boylston, Massachusetts

Elizabeth S. Temin, MD, MPH
Attending Physician
Director of Prehospital Care
Emergency Medicine
Massachusetts General Hospital
Boston, Massachusetts

Andrea G. Tenner, MD, MPH, FACEP
Assistant Professor
Emergency Medicine
University of Maryland
Baltimore, Maryland

Craig D. Thorne, MD, MPH, FACP, FACOEM
Vice President/Medical Director
Erickson Living
Adjunct Assistant Professor
Department of Environmental Health
    Sciences
Johns Hopkins Bloomberg School of
    Public Health
Baltimore, Maryland

Jason A. Tracy, MD
Chief of Emergency Medicine
South Shore Hospital
South Weymouth, Massachusetts

Milana Trounce, MD, FACEP
Clinical Associate Professor of Surgery
Emergency Medicine
Stanford Medical School
Stanford, California

Jonathan Harris Valente, MD
Assistant Professor
Emergency Medicine
Brown University School of Medicine
Rhode Island Hospital and Hasbro
    Children's Hospital
Providence, Rhode Island

Alice Venier, MD
Neurosurgery
San Raffaele Hospital
Milan, Italy

Faith Vilas, PhD
Senior Scientist
Project Scientist–Atsa Suborbital Observatory
Planetary Science Institute
Tucson, Arizona

Gary M. Vilke, MD, FACEP, FAAEM
President
UCSD Academy of Clinician Scholars
Medical Director
Risk Management
UC San Diego Health System
Professor of Clinical Emergency
    Medicine
Director
Clinical Research for Emergency
    Medicine
University of California, San Diego
San Diego, California

Janna H. Villano, MD
Attending Physician
Emergency Medicine
Division of Toxicology
University of California, San Diego
San Diego, California

Barbara Vogt, PhD
Senior Research Staff
Oak Ridge National Laboratory
Oak Ridge, Tennessee

Amalia Voskanyan, RN
Co-Director
Fellowship in Disaster Medicine
Beth Israel Deaconess Medical Center
Disaster Preparedness Program

Harvard Humanitarian Initiative
Boston, Massachusetts
Chief of Staff
Abu Dhabi Emergency Medicine
   Academy
Brigham and Women's Hospital
Abu Dhabi, United Arab Emirates

Scott G. Weiner, MD, MPH
Director of Research
Emergency Medicine
Tufts Medical Center
Boston, Massachusetts

Brielle Weinstein, BA, BS, MD Candidate
College of Medicine
Medical University of South Carolina
Charleston, South Carolina

Eric S. Weinstein, MD, FACEP
Emergency Department
Carolinas Hospital System
Florence, South Carolina
Medical Director
Emergency Response Task Force
South Carolina Division of Fire and Life
   Safety
Columbia, South Carolina

Scott D. Weir, MD
Medical Director
Fairfax County Fire and Rescue
   Department
Emergency Physician
Best-Practices
Assistant Professor
Emergency Medicine
Virginia Commonwealth University School
   of Medicine
INOVA Campus
Fairfax, Virginia

Roy Karl Werner, MD, MS, FAAEM
Community First Medical Center
Presence Medical Group

Our Lady of the Resurrection Medical Center
Huntley, Illinois

Sage W. Wiener, MD
Assistant Professor of Emergency Medicine
Director of Medical Toxicology
Emergency Medicine
SUNY Downstate Medical Center
Kings County Hospital Center
Brooklyn, New York

Kenneth A. Williams, MD
Associate Professor
Emergency Medicine
The Warren Alpert Medical School of Brown
   University
Providence, Rhode Island

Robyn Wing, MD
Emergency Medicine and Pediatrics
The Warren Alpert Medical School of Brown
   University
Hasbro Children's Hospital/Rhode Island
   Hospital
Providence, Rhode Island

Wendy Hin-Wing Wong, MD, MPH
Emergency Medicine
The Warren Alpert Medical School of Brown
   University
Rhode Island Hospital
Providence, Rhode Island

Richard E. Wolfe, MD
Associate Professor of Emergency Medicine
Beth Israel Deaconess Medical Center
Associate Professor of Medicine
Harvard Medical School
Boston, Massachusetts

Stephen P. Wood, ACNP
Associate Medical Director for EMS
Winchester Emergency Medical Associates
Winchester, Massachusetts

Robert H. Woolard, MD
Professor
Emergency Medicine and Biomedical
   Sciences
Texas Tech University Health Sciences Center
El Paso, Texas

Prasit Wuthisuthimethawee, MD, FRCST
Chief
Emergency Medicine
Songklanagarind Hospital
Assistant Professor
Faculty of Medicine
Prince of Songkla University
Hat-Yai, Songkhla, Thailand

Kevin Yeskey, MD, FACEP
Senior Advisor
MDB Inc.
Garrett Park, Maryland

Sami A. Yousif, MD, SBEM
Assistant Professor of Emergency
   Medicine
King Saud bin Abdulaziz University for
   Health Sciences
Emergency Medicine and Disaster Medicine
   Consultant
King Abdulaziz Medical City-Riyadh
Riyadh, Saudi Arabia

Nadine A. Youssef, MD
Assistant Professor
Emergency Medicine
Tufts University School of Medicine
Boston, Massachusetts

Brian J. Yun, MD, MBA
Emergency Medicine
Brigham and Women's Hospital
Massachusetts General Hospital
Harvard Medical School
Boston, Massachusetts

Dorothy Parker innocently said in response to a query from Alexander Wolcott: "What could be rarer than a first edition by Alexander Wolcott?" Parker: "A second edition."

I think the events of the years since the first edition of this book have cemented in a harsh reality the need to be concerned with disasters. Not only have we had an all too steady diet of the mayhem produced by war and attempts at revolution, but we have had an unending number of natural disasters with serious problems caused by major storms, tornados, earthquakes, and volcanic eruptions. Adding in the not so natural disasters that also seem to have occurred with ever increasing frequency, such as nuclear plant spills, industrial pollutions, and industrial explosions and fires, there is such a profusion of disasters that it seems that not only a second edition, but many other editions thereafter, will be necessary.

One thing that has changed is the realization that no matter how well intentioned, without organization, there simply is no way to respond to a disaster, whether it be small enough to be handled locally or so huge that, without outside help, there is no way to help restore life toward being normal.

The logistics are formidable: how to bring in the correct supplies and personnel, without any information about what is most necessary, and how to in fact shelter and house the disaster team and maintain their supplies so that they do not further deplete the resources that have been destroyed by the disaster.

There are numerous organizations that have been developed to respond quickly to disasters. Due to the sheer numbers and characteristics of these, they have in turn sometimes produced more damage to add to that of the disaster.

The local politics can be very frustrating, because no country wishes to admit that it is unprepared or incapable of responding to any event, and yet, of course, the very definition of disaster is that the event has overwhelmed available resources.

Many humanitarian volunteers mean well but have never experienced a truly austere environment, and often they have no idea what dangers they risk by underestimating the need for security, food, water, and shelter as they attempt to give help. Ethical difficulties arise—who to help, and how familiar medical care may be a death sentence for someone in the austere disaster environment, such as amputation of a lower limb of a child whose family has been completely lost to an earthquake.

Many valuable and truly helpful nongovernmental organizations (NGOs) have evolved, but alongside the useful ones are always those with a more political mission than strictly bringing aid and resources to the disaster area. Even when the NGO is trying to be useful, it can be accused of preying on the population that has been damaged, such as trying to arrange adoptions for recently created orphans.

Another area of disaster that we had known about, but not paid much attention to, is the increase in communicable diseases due to the breakdowns of housing, sanitation, and space for shelter. Combined with sexual violence, the upsurge of sexually transmitted disease is often not considered a product of a natural disaster, but all too often 6 months to a year after the initial incident, these infections spike. Along with viral diseases, such as hepatitis, it often seems like there will never be an end to the misfortune caused by any single event.

It has become apparent that, although no one can predict the specific character of the next event, we know there will be more than one. Many of the more fortunate countries have been willing to expend some resources to put together disaster teams and units that have a maintained inventory of supplies, as well as a group of trained personnel who are willing to be called upon to serve for varying periods of time.

Moreover, there has been construction of some redundancy in the communications services and water and food supplies so that even though the exact quality of the disaster isn't known, there is advance preparation in place to respond.

What is fascinating is the willingness of one country to respond to a disaster and rebuild while others are so affected by the event that they never seem to recover. Earthquakes in Kobe and San Francisco occurred at about the same time, yet despite the greater resources of the United States compared with Japan, Kobe recovered from its earthquake in about a quarter of the time it took to rebuild in San Francisco.

We still haven't resolved how to respond to disasters that are induced by acts of terror. Although the response to 9/11 was truly magnificent, one can only shudder to contemplate how it would have been affected had there been a bioterror agent in play along with the building attacks.

Consideration of the possible magnitude of the sarin attacks in Tokyo makes one very grateful that the terroristic society that introduced the sarin didn't have a better delivery system. We will not continue to be so lucky.

Yet we still suffer from an inability to share intelligence about coming events. Interagency rivalries exist everywhere, not just in the United States, and we have yet to figure out how to overcome the jealousies of the individual agencies so as to enable preparation and efficient response. Many of the police agencies in Tokyo were on alert for an attack, but no one notified the hospitals, so they didn't know what biologic agent they were facing until physicians in a smaller community that had already suffered an attack saw what was happening on TV and called their colleagues.

I still wonder if we would have recognized the anthrax attacks in the United States so readily if they had not occurred in such close proximity to 9/11. I still believe that if a bioterror attack occurs, we won't recognize it until it has caused a large number of casualties unless the attackers give us some information by taking public credit for the attack.

Despite all these problems, and despite all the times when the situation truly seems hopeless, we have made significant advances not only locally but internationally. This book certainly can teach us much about the current state of affairs, and it provides a great resource for where to look for information to assist with one's own planning. I find it very helpful that we have seen a literature develop on disaster planning and management and that some very good minds have been working on responses to all of these problems.

It is also clear that very special kinds of training are needed, not just the medical emergency science of how to deal with multiple major problems. The diplomacy, language skills, organizations with which one must interact, and political constraints involved in every event are real issues that one must prepare for so there is no need to reinvent a response with each disaster.

There is also a growing literature on many of the ethical problems of the disaster situations, as well as the changes that are necessary to be able to respond to the situations where there are more casualties than available resources. The kind of triage logic that is necessary in these situations is indeed different from working in any trauma care institution in any country, and without thinking about how to respond to these situations, no one is emotionally or intellectually prepared to deal with the problems.

Once again, a good place to start is with the information that is found in this book. It has advanced in leaps since the first edition, and I think that anyone who found the first edition useful will be pleased to look at this edition and see how far we have come.

There is simply no substitute for preparation, and as much as we dread the next event, we will be able to respond better if we continue to train, not just for individual team responses, but to attempt to make our communities more disaster proof.

Peter Rosen, MD
Senior Lecturer
Emergency Medicine
Harvard Medical School
Emergency Medicine Attending Physician
Beth Israel Deaconess Medical Center
Visiting Clinical Professor
Emergency Medicine
University of Arizona
Professor Emeritus
Emergency Medicine
University of California San Diego

Welcome to the second edition of *Ciottone's Disaster Medicine*. This book is the culmination of an enormous amount of work by a great many intelligent and experienced people who have dedicated their efforts toward building a core curriculum around this new specialty called *Disaster Medicine*. The idea to write the first edition came to me as a responder to the 9/11 attacks. I recall walking slowly toward Ground Zero as commander of one of the first Federal Disaster Medical Assistance Teams sent into the World Trade Center disaster area and being initially struck by a sense of helplessness at the sight of the devastation. As the plumes of smoke rose from the undulating piles of destruction, we all had a sense that the disaster before us was so vast and our task so enormous that we would never be able to mount an effective response. This feeling of helplessness did not abate until we resorted to our training and took up our role in the overall disaster response. We were a cog in a very large machine, placed precisely where we would be supported by the other parts and function in such a specialized way as to keep the machine running. At that moment of realization, the concept behind this book was born.

The philosophy behind the writing of this textbook is to bring resources together necessary for the development of a comprehensive understanding of disaster medicine and its role in emergency management. Now the release of the second edition comes as Ebola continues to ravage West Africa and several years after two devastating natural disasters. The Haiti earthquake killed nearly 300,000 people and injured another 300,000, and the complex multiple-modality disaster in Japan struck a crippling blow to that country. Disaster strikes without warning, is indiscriminate in its choice of victims, and has the potential to overcome even the most prepared of systems. If there is no other justification for a book such as this, it must be said that these recent events demand that we, as health care professionals, develop an understanding of the basics of disaster medicine and stand ready to integrate into the response system if and when disaster should strike close to home.

This book is designed to serve as both a comprehensive text and a quick resource. Part I introduces the many topics of disaster medicine and management with an emphasis on the multiple disciplines that come together in the preparation for and response to such catastrophic events. It is the integration of these various response and preparedness modalities that makes disaster medicine such a unique field. This section is meant to be a comprehensive approach to the study of the discipline of disaster medicine and should be used by health care professionals to develop and expand their knowledge base. The chapters may introduce topics that are unfamiliar to the reader, as most practitioners will not be versed in some of the nonmedical subjects discussed. Although much of the information may be very new, it may also be crucial if a disaster unexpectedly strikes nearby.

Part II of the book, or the "event" chapters, introduces the reader to every conceivable disaster scenario and the management issues surrounding each. This part of the text can be used both for reference and for real-time consultation for each topic. The reader will find very detailed and specific events described in these chapters. Some disaster scenarios discussed have historical precedence whereas others are considered to be at risk for future occurrence. Many describe natural and accidental events, and some are dedicated to very specific terrorist attacks.

There is also an entirely new section in this edition dealing with topics unique to terrorist attacks and high-threat disaster response scenarios. There is no easy way to discuss these topics. In particular, terrorist events may cause a sense of unease as one reads the chapter. The chapters related to terrorism in this section and the very specific attack scenarios discussed in Part II of the book attempt to account for every possible modality terrorist operatives are thought to currently possess or may acquire in the future, as well as the unique and evolving ways they are being deployed. In some cases the scenarios may prove true, and in many they may not. It is imperative, however, that all possible modalities of attack be discussed so that, if needed, proper preparedness and response can be mounted. The term "attack" has been deliberately used in many of these chapters to emphasize the point that, if these agents and scenarios are purposefully unleashed, it will, in fact, be in the form of an attack. The need for including such terminology in an academic medical textbook underscores the climate in which this text has been written. After such events as the September 11, 2001, attacks, the London bombings of 2005, the ISIS attacks throughout the Middle East in 2014, and the Paris shootings in 2015, the need for a thorough understanding of deliberate attacks is apparent. Part II of this text discusses these scenarios in as complete a way as possible, while respecting the dignity of those afflicted by past events. In a way it is the pain and suffering of both victims and survivors of such events that have contributed most to this text, and it is in celebration of their spirit that it has been written.

Finally, I must mention the outstanding group of editors and contributors you will find within these pages. I went to great lengths to find individuals who are experts in their field, not only because they have studied it, but because they have done it. These are the doers as well as the thinkers. These are the men and women who leave their families when disaster strikes and integrate into the response systems. They are the experts called upon on a regional, national, and international level to prepare for disasters, always learning from the past and planning for the future. This edition is more than 2 years in the making, partly because during that time the editors and authors were all too often deployed for lengthy periods to disaster zones around the world. In the study of disaster medicine, perhaps like none other, knowledge born from experience makes for a very robust textbook. You will feel that experience jump from these pages, and you will be rewarded by having learned from the best.

Because of the ubiquitous nature of disaster, society is indebted to those who choose to learn and practice in this field. As a member of that society, I would like to personally thank you for doing so.

Gregory R. Ciottone, MD, FACEP

CONTENTS

SECTION FIVE Mechanical Operations in Disasters

SECTION SIX Post-Event Topics

SECTION SEVEN Topics Unique to Terrorist Events and High-Threat Disaster Response

SECTION EIGHT Operational Medicine

PART I

Overview of Disaster Management

1 CHAPTER

Introduction to Disaster Medicine

Gregory R. Ciottone

What exactly is disaster medicine? If you have decided to purchase and read this book, it is likely a question you have wrestled with. Disaster itself is not an easily defined entity, thus the new medical specialty evolving around it is continuously undergoing metamorphosis. Because a disaster is a local event, throughout history, the local medical responders have cared for the victims of disaster. The same medical personnel who provide health care on a daily basis also assume the responsibility of providing care to patients with illness or injury resulting from a disaster. Unlike other areas of medicine, however, the care of casualties from a disaster requires the health care provider to integrate into the larger, predominantly nonmedical multidisciplinary response. This demands a knowledge base far greater than medicine alone. To operate safely as part of a coordinated disaster response, either in a hospital or in the field, an understanding of the basic principles of emergency management is necessary. Now we begin to see the evolution of the specialty of disaster medicine. To respond properly and efficiently to disasters, all health care personnel should have a fundamental understanding of the principles of disaster medicine (which incorporates emergency management in its practice) and what their particular role would be in the response to the many different types of disasters.

In the mid-1980s, disaster medicine began to evolve from the union of disaster management (now called emergency management) and emergency medicine. Although disaster medicine is not yet an accredited medical subspecialty, those who practice it have been involved in some of the most catastrophic events in human history. Practitioners of present-day disaster medicine have responded to the aftermaths of the tsunami in Southeast Asia,[1] Hurricane Andrew,[2] the Haiti Earthquake,[3] the Madrid Train Bombings,[4] and the World Trade Center Attacks,[5] to name a few. During the past several decades, we have seen the first applications of basic disaster medicine principles in real-time events, and as demonstrated by the devastation caused by Hurricane Sandy in 2012 and the devastating Ebola Outbreak of 2014-2015, there is sure to be continued need for such applications.

The impetus for this text grew from a realization that as the specialty of emergency medicine grows, emergency physicians must take ownership of this new field of disaster medicine and ensure that it meets the rigorous demands put upon it by the very nature of human disaster. If we are to call ourselves disaster medicine specialists and are to be entrusted by society to respond to the most catastrophic human events, it is imperative that we pursue the highest level of scholarly knowledge and moral conduct in this very dynamic area. Until there is oversight from a certifying board, it is our responsibility to the public to maintain this high level of excellence. As in medical ethics, where patients rely on the virtue of their physicians to compel them to abide by moral standards, so must we exercise virtue in how we conduct the medical response to disaster.

THE DISASTER CYCLE

Because disasters strike without warning, in areas often unprepared for such events, it is essential for all emergency services personnel to have a foundation in the practical aspects of disaster preparedness and response. The first step is to understand that disaster can strike here at home. I can assure you the people of Haiti minutes before the earthquake of 2010 and the people of Japan minutes before the earthquake and tsunami of 2011 all were going about their normal daily routine, not expecting disaster to strike. Then it did.

As is discussed in other chapters throughout this text, emergency responders have an integrated role in disaster management. All disasters follow a cyclical pattern known as the disaster cycle (Figure 1-1), which describes four reactionary stages: preparedness, response, recovery, and mitigation or prevention. Emergency medicine specialists have a role in each part of this cycle. As active members of their community, emergency specialists should take part in mitigation and preparedness on the hospital, local, and regional levels. Once disaster strikes, their role continues in the response and recovery phases. By participating in the varied areas of disaster preparation and response, including hazard vulnerability analyses, resource allocation, and creation of disaster legislation, the emergency medicine specialist integrates into the disaster cycle as an active participant. Possessing a thorough understanding of the disaster medicine needs of the community allows one to contribute to the overall preparedness and response mission.

NATURAL AND HUMAN-MADE DISASTERS

Over the course of recorded history, natural disasters have predominated in frequency and magnitude over human-made ones. Some of the earliest disasters have caused enormous numbers of casualties, with resultant disruption of the underlying community infrastructure. *Yersinia pestis* caused the death of countless millions in several epidemics over hundreds of years. The etiologic agent of bubonic plague, *Y. pestis*, devastated Europe by killing large numbers of people and leaving societal ruin in its wake.[6] During the writing of this chapter, an Ebola outbreak raged in West Africa, along with concern that a worldwide pandemic might ensue.[7] The 2014 and 2015 Ebola and Middle East respiratory syndrome (MERS) outbreaks have proven that, despite the passage of time and the great advances in medicine, the world continues to be affected by disease outbreaks. In addition, diseases that have been eradicated have the potential of being reintroduced into society, either accidentally from the few remaining sources in existence around the world, as in the 2015 measles outbreak in the United States, or by intentional release. Such events have the potential of devastating results, as the baseline intrinsic immunity the world population developed during the natural presence of the disease has faded over time,

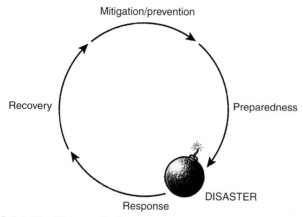

FIG 1-1 The Disaster Cycle.

putting much larger numbers of people at risk. Finally, with the advent of air travel allowing people to be on the opposite side of the world in a matter of hours, the bloom effect of an outbreak is much harder to predict and control. Disease outbreaks that were previously controlled by natural borders, such as oceans, no longer have those barriers, making the likelihood of worldwide outbreak much greater now than it was hundreds of years ago. We saw evidence of this in 2014, with Ebola-infected patients arriving in Spain and the United States from West Africa. During that outbreak, naysayers to intrusive actions such as quarantine and travel restrictions cited following the "science" learned since the disease emerged in central Africa in the 1970s. The problem with such logic was that Ebola had never before been seen in urban settings such as Nigeria, New York City, and Dallas, Texas. Transmission parameters in such settings were truly uncharted waters for the medical community.

In addition to epidemics, with each passing year, natural disasters in the form of earthquakes, floods, and deadly storms batter populations. One need only to remember the destruction in terms of both human life and community resources caused by the Indian Ocean Earthquake and Tsunami of 2004, the Haiti Earthquake in 2010, or the earthquake, tsunami, and radiation disaster in Japan in 2011 to understand the need for preparedness and response to such natural events. Considering that the earthquakes that caused these tsunamis occurred hours before the devastation, it is difficult to understand how today's advanced society, able to travel far into space among other great achievements, was unable to mitigate against some of the most deadly natural events in recent history. The realization that disaster can strike without warning and inflict casualties on the order of the 2004, 2010, and 2011 earthquakes and tsunamis, despite our many technological advances, serves as a warning that mitigation, preparedness, response, and recovery to natural disaster must continue to be studied and practiced vigorously.

Today, the possibility of terrorist attack threatens populations across the globe. Both industrialized and developing countries have witnessed some of the most callous and senseless taking of life, for reasons not easily fathomed by civilized people. It is unusual to read an Internet news article or watch a television newscast without learning of a terrorist attack in some part of the world. With the advent of more organized groups such as the Islamic State of Iraq and Syria (ISIS), Boko Haram, the Revolutionary Armed Forces of Colombia (FARC), and the Epanastatikos Agonas (EA), these attacks are more frequent and deadly, often using horrifying means of execution. The commonplace nature of a terrorist attack in modern society ensures it is unquestionably something that will continue long into the future, and will very likely escalate in scale and frequency.

The multilayered foundation on which ideological belief evolves into violent attack is beyond the scope of analysis that this book

ventures to undertake. These ongoing events do demonstrate, however, that the principles studied in the field of disaster medicine must include those that are designed to prepare for and respond to a terrorist attack. Because there are very intelligent minds at work designing systems to bring disaster on others, equally there must be as robust an effort to prepare for and respond to those disasters. Such response involves the deployment of law enforcement, evidence collection, and military personnel and equipment, which are typically not seen in the response to a natural disaster. The integration of these unique assets into the overall response is essential for the success of the mission. The disaster medicine specialist must have a thorough understanding of the role of each.

DEFINING DISASTER

A thorough discussion of disaster preparedness and response must be predicated on a clear definition of what, in fact, constitutes a disaster. Used commonly to describe many different events, the word *disaster* is not easily defined. The Indian Ocean Tsunami in 2004 and the Haiti Earthquake in 2010, each killing significantly more than 200,000 people, would certainly meet the criteria for disaster. However, the 2015 flood in Peru that killed 20 people and tropical storm in Madagascar that killed 14 have also been called disasters. Likewise, the 2003 explosion of the space shuttle *Columbia* on reentry into Earth's atmosphere that killed the crew of seven astronauts onboard has often been referred to as the *Columbia* Disaster in the lay press. How can an event resulting in the loss of seven people be placed in the same category as one that kills hundreds of thousands? Herein lies the paradox of disaster. What is it? Who defines it, and by what criteria?

It is difficult to dispute that an event causing thousands of casualties should be considered a disaster, but let us analyze why that is the case. What is it about the sheer number of dead and injured that allows the event to be called a disaster? In terms of medical needs, it is simply because there is no health care system on Earth that can handle that number of casualties. Therefore an event of such magnitude is a disaster because it has overwhelmed the infrastructure of the community in which it occurred. Following this logic, we can then also make the statement that any event that overwhelms existing societal systems is a disaster. This definition is close to the definition of *disaster* given by the United Nations International Strategy for Disaster Reduction (UNISDR)[8]:

A serious disruption of the functioning of a community or a society involving widespread human, material, economic, or environmental losses and impacts, which exceeds the ability of the affected community or society to cope using its own resources.

A similar definition is used by the World Health Organization (WHO). By applying these definitions, one can understand how an event in a rural area with 10 to 20 casualties may also be considered a disaster because the limited resources in that area may prevent an adequate response without outside assistance.

The widely accepted UNISDR and WHO definitions of *disaster* justify describing both the 2010 Haiti Earthquake and the 2015 flood in Peru as disasters. However, what about the destruction of the space shuttle *Columbia* on reentry? Clearly, this definition does not allow one to justify the use of *disaster* in describing that horrific accident, which brings to light a discrepancy in how disaster specialists and the public term events. The *Columbia* accident, as an example, does not meet any accepted criteria of disaster. It was, however, an exceedingly tragic event, seen by millions on television, as it was unfolding. It was tragic by the word's very definition in the *Cambridge Dictionary*: "A very sad event, especially one involving death or suffering." Public perception of such events may cause this misnomer, with a tragic incident being termed a disaster. Much like disaster, tragedy can also have a profound and lasting effect on society, especially a tragedy that is widely viewed through modern media outlets. This text, however, will follow the UNISDR and WHO definitions when discussing disaster.

DISASTER MEDICINE

Disaster medicine is a discipline resulting from the marriage of emergency medicine and disaster management. The role of medicine and emergency medical services in disaster response has abundant historical precedence. Responsibility for the care of the injured from a disaster has been borne by the emergency specialist or its equivalent throughout history. Therefore disaster medical response, in its many forms, has been around for thousands of years. Whenever a disaster has struck, there has been some degree of a medical response to care for the casualties. In the United States, much of the disaster medical response has followed a military model, with lessons learned through battlefield scenarios during the last two centuries.[9] The military experience has demonstrated how to orchestrate efficient care to mass casualties in austere environments. However, it does not translate directly into civilian practice. For instance, scenarios encountered on the battlefield with young, fit soldiers injured by trauma are vastly different from those encountered in a rural setting, where an earthquake may inflict casualties on a population with baseline malnutrition or advanced age. With this realization came the need to create disaster medicine as an evolution from the military practice. This recent organization of the medical role in disasters into a more formalized specialty of disaster medicine has enabled practitioners to define further their role in the overall disaster preparedness and response system.

Disaster medicine is truly a systems-oriented specialty, and disaster specialists are required to be familiar and interact with multiple responding agencies. The reality is there is no "disaster clinic." No practitioners leave home in the morning intent on seeing disaster patients. Disaster medical care is often thrust upon the practitioner and is not necessarily something that is sought out. The exception to this is the medical specialist who becomes part of an organized (usually federal) disaster team, such as a disaster medical assistance team (DMAT). In this case, one may be transported to a disaster site with the intention of treating the victims of a catastrophic event. In all other circumstances, however, the disaster falls on an unsuspecting emergency responder who is forced to abandon his or her normal duties and adopt a role in the overall disaster response.

Unlike the organized disaster team member, if an emergency provider treats casualties from a disaster, it will most likely be because of an event that has occurred in his or her immediate area. Because of the random nature of disaster, it is not possible to predict who will be put into that role next. Therefore it is imperative for all who practice in emergency health services to have a working knowledge of the basics of disaster medicine and disaster management. In addition, especially with natural disease outbreaks and the escalation in perceived and real terrorist threats of 2014-2015, there are several possible natural or attack scenarios that may involve dangerous chemical, biological, or nuclear agents and modalities. A response to these events may also require a robust public health system and knowledgeable health care practitioners spanning all specialties. Most clinicians will have a very limited knowledge of many of these agents, so it is therefore important to educate our potential disaster responders on their specifics.

The field of disaster medicine involves the study of subject matter from multiple medical disciplines. Disasters may result in varying injury and disease patterns, depending on the type of event that has occurred. Earthquakes can cause entrapment and resultant crush syndrome; tornados may cause penetrating trauma from flying debris; and infectious disease outbreak, either natural or intentional, can result from many different bacteria, viruses, and fungi. Because of the potential variability in casualty scenarios, the disaster medicine specialist must have training in the many injury and illness patterns seen in disaster victims. Even though the expanse of knowledge required is vast, the focus on areas specifically related to disaster medicine allows the science to be manageable. The study of disaster medicine should not be undertaken without prerequisite medical training. A disaster medicine specialist is always a practicing clinician from another field of medicine first and a disaster specialist second. By integrating these many disciplines, one is better prepared for the variety of injury and illness patterns that may be faced.

Finally, disaster medicine presents unique ethical situations not seen in other areas of medicine. Disaster medicine is predicated on the principle of providing care to the most victims possible, as dictated by the resources available and by patient condition and likelihood of survival. This amounts to a balance of needs versus assets, an equation that can change over time as more resources are pulled into the response. Thus the triage of patients in disasters is fluid and should be repeated regularly. Disaster triage involves assigning patients into treatment categories based on their predicted survivability. This triage process may dictate that the most severely injured patient is not given medical care but rather, it is given to a less critically injured patient. To the best of his or her ability, the triage officer must make a determination as to whether, in the environment of the specific disaster and the availability of resources, a given patient has a significant probability of survival or does not. If it is the latter, disaster triage principles mandate that care be given to the patient with a higher likelihood of survival. This basic disaster triage principle can have a profound psychological effect on the care provider. As a physician, one is trained to render care to the sick and not to leave the side of a needy patient. To deny care to a critically ill or injured patient can be one of the most emotionally stressful tasks a disaster medicine specialist performs.

The unique and ever-changing circumstances under which disaster medicine specialists operate mandate the continued evolution and vigorous pursuit of academic excellence in this new specialty. A comprehensive approach that unifies medical principles with a sound understanding of disaster management procedures will yield a well-rounded and better-prepared disaster responder. If emergency medicine providers around the world can develop a basic understanding of the fundamental principles of this specialty, great advances in the systems included in the disaster cycle will surely follow. The more widely dispersed this knowledge becomes, the better prepared we are as a society to respond to the next catastrophic event.

REFERENCES

1. Wattanawaitunechai C, Peacock SJ, Jitpratoom P. Tsunami in Thailand-disaster management in a district hospital. *N Engl J Med*. 2005;352 (10):962–964.
2. Nufer KE, Wilson-Ramirez G. A comparison of patient needs following two hurricanes. *Prehospital Disaster Med*. 2004;19(2):146–149.
3. Kirsch T, Sauer L, Guha Sapir D. Analysis of the international and US response to the Haiti Earthquake: recommendations for change. *Disaster Med Public Health Prep*. 2012;6(3):200–208.
4. Gutierrez de Ceballos JP, Turegano Fuentes F. Casualties treated at the closest hospital in the Madrid, March 11, terrorist bombings. *Crit Care Med*. 2005;33(1 Suppl):S107–S112.

5. Simon R, Teperman S. The World Trade Center attack: lessons for disaster management. *Crit Care*. 2001;5(6):318–320.

6. Lowell JL, Wagner DM, Atshaber B, et al. Identifying sources of human exposure to plague. *J Clin Microbiol*. 2005;43(2):650–656.

7. Timen A, Sprenger M, Edelstein M, Martin-Moreno J, McKee M. The Ebola crisis: perspectives from European Public Health. *Eur J Public Health*. 2015.

8. United Nations International Strategy for Disaster Reduction. Available at: http://www.unisdr.org/we/inform/terminology.org.master.com/texis/ master/search/mysite.txt?q=disaster+preparedness&order=r& id=60413a1214953850&cmd=xml.

9. Dara SI, Ashton RW, Farmer JC, Carlton Jr. PK. Worldwide disaster medical response: an historical perspective. *Crit Care Med*. 2005; 33(1 Suppl):S2–S6.

2 | CHAPTER

Public Health and Disasters

Ali Ardalan, Catherine Y. Ordun, and James Michael Riley

INTRODUCTION TO PUBLIC HEALTH

Definition, Scope, and Achievements of Public Health

According to the World Health Organization, *public health* "refers to all organized measures—whether public or private—to prevent disease, promote health, and prolong life among the population as a whole."[1] As this definition stipulates, the focus of public health activities is on the health of entire populations, not on individual patients. Dimensions of health accordingly encompass "a state of complete physical, mental, and social well-being and not merely the absence of disease or infirmity."[2] The domain of public health activities extends from local to national levels. Moreover, global public health responses involve cross-border health risks, including pandemics, climate change, famine, and displaced populations.

Public health has roots in ancient history; examples of such include initiatives by the Chinese and Romans. About 1000 BC, Chinese doctors developed the practice of variolation (inoculation of fluid from pustules as an attempt to immunize against disease), following a smallpox epidemic. Further, as early as 310 BC, the Romans exhibited a public health philosophy. They believed that cleanliness would lead to good health and thus made links between causes of disease and methods of prevention. For example, during this time, an association was made between the increased death rate of persons living near swamps and sewage. As a result, the Roman Empire began working on two major public health projects in sanitation control: the building of aqueducts to supply clean water to the city, and a sewage system to eliminate waste from the streets. Nowadays, programs promoting hand washing, breast-feeding, vaccinations, and distribution of condoms to control the spread of sexually transmitted diseases are examples of common public health measures.

Today, the benefits of public health infrastructure in the United States and abroad continue to strengthen the well-being of society. The effect of interventions has been great. In the twentieth century, the 10 greatest public health achievements have been documented, as follows[3]:

1. Vaccination programs (i.e., eradication of smallpox, elimination of poliomyelitis in the Americas, and control of measles, rubella, tetanus, diphtheria, and other diseases around the world)
2. Motor vehicle safety
3. Safer workplaces
4. Control of infectious diseases
5. Decline in deaths from coronary heart disease and stroke
6. Safer and healthier foods
7. Healthier mothers and babies
8. Family planning
9. Fluoridation of drinking water
10. Recognition of tobacco use as a health hazard

Public Health System and Infrastructure

A *public health system* is defined as "all public, private, and voluntary entities that contribute to the delivery of essential public health services within a jurisdiction."[4] Hospitals, clinics, and primary health care centers are the frontline of public health service delivery; however, the public health system goes beyond the health facilities alone. In fact, it encompasses all of the sectors that have effects on the health of populations. These include housing, agriculture, the economy, etc. The term *social determinants of health* (SDH) addresses the conditions in which people are born, grow, live, work, and age.[5] To work in such a multidisciplinary context, contemporary public health practice requires multidisciplinary education, training, and participation of scientists and professionals from other disciplines, such as sociology, community development, communications, geography, climatology, ethics, and law.[6]

Many efforts have been made to institutionalize public health policies and practices. Public health legislation began to be consolidated in the mid-eighteenth century in Europe and North America. The American Public Health Association (APHA), founded in 1872, is recognized as the oldest organization of public health professionals worldwide. However, the World Health Organization (WHO), established in 1948, is the lead agency on global public health issues.

Although the private sector, along with the charities and nongovernmental organizations (NGOs), plays a significant role in provision of health care to communities, the ultimate responsibility for the overall performance of a country's health system lies with the government.[7] Most countries have their own governmental public health agencies, sometimes known as ministries of health (MoH) or ministries of public health (MoPH). Other examples are the Ministry of Health & Family Welfare in India and the Ministry of Health and Medical Education (MoHME) in Iran that resulted from integration of the MoH and higher education system of health sciences. In Canada, the Public Health Agency (PHA) of Canada, reporting to the Minister of Health, is the national agency responsible for public health. This responsibility lies with the National Health Services (NHS) in England, under the Department of Health.

Formal public health programs in the United States have existed for well over 200 years. For example, the origins of the U.S. Public Health Service (USPHS) (initially known as the Marine Hospital Service) may be traced to the passage of an act in 1798 that provided for the care and relief of sick and injured merchant seamen. After its inception, and over the next 200 years, the Marine Hospital Service was restructured to provide a wider variety of essential services. Now the USPHS is recognized worldwide and is working alongside its other federal partners and state agencies, including the Department of Health and Human Services (DHHS) and its agencies, such as the Centers for Disease Control and Prevention (CDC), the Food and Drug Administration (FDA), and the U.S. Department of Agriculture (USDA). The USPHS encompasses a broad integration of commercial, public, government, and nongovernment entities. It is as diverse as the very population it serves. It includes government public health agencies operating on federal, regional, state, and local levels; health care delivery infrastructure, such as hospitals and clinics; public health and health science academic institutions; community entities, such as schools, organizations, and religious congregations; commercial businesses; and the media.[8] Public health is also augmented by its partnerships and increasing collaboration with expert military health institutions, such as the U.S. Army Medical Research Institute of Infectious Diseases (USAMRIID) and other defense agencies; national institutions such as the National Institute for Allergy and Infectious Diseases (NIAID) under the National Institutes of Health (NIH); law enforcement and emergency responder communities on federal (Federal Bureau of Investigation) and local levels; and the medical-legal community, which is composed of national medical examiners offices and forensic scientists.

Public Health Essential Services

The mission of public health is to fulfill society's desire to create conditions such that people can be healthy. The public health—at any level of operations—relies on the following main interdependent and cyclical pillars: (1) assessment of the population's health, (2) formulation of public policies, and (3) assurance of the population's access to appropriate and cost-effective care.[8] These pillars have been extended by the U.S. National Public Health Performance Standards (NPHPS). They are described as the 10 essential public health services, which include the following[4]:

1. Monitoring health status to identify and solve community health problems
2. Diagnosing and investigating health problems and health hazards in the community
3. Informing, educating, and empowering people about health issues
4. Mobilizing community partnerships and action to identify and solve health problems
5. Developing policies and plans that support individual and community health efforts
6. Enforcing laws and regulations that protect health and ensure safety
7. Link people to needed personal health services and assure the provision of health care when otherwise unavailable
8. Assuring a competent public and personal health care workforce
9. Evaluating the effectiveness, accessibility, and quality of personal and population-based health services
10. Researching for new insights and innovative solutions to health problems

Similar to traditional programs in public health, ranging from maternal and reproductive health to injury control and prevention, the public health relation with disaster management also fulfills the above-mentioned essential services. This introductory chapter explains why disasters are important to public health and how the public health system interacts with the disaster-management cycle. In the subsequent chapters of this textbook, the reader may find elaborative information on applications of the public health functions in disasters, including needs assessment, surveillance, public information management, safety of health workers, etc.

PUBLIC HEALTH CONSEQUENCES OF DISASTERS

Each year millions of people worldwide suffer from disasters, both in developed and less-developed countries. Disasters affect the health of populations not only directly but also indirectly, via damages to health care systems, infrastructures, and disruption of social and living conditions. The effects vary disaster by disaster and depend on the type and intensity of the hazard, population density, extent of damage, and response operations. The effects of disasters on public health can be classified in the following four categories,[9] as summarized in Table 2-1.

Direct Effect on the Health of Population

Death and physical injury are the most significant effects of disasters on health. From 2000 to 2013, natural disasters killed about 1.2 million people worldwide.[10] Different disasters result in different levels of mortality. The highest rate of mortality usually occurs following earthquakes, flash floods, and tsunamis.

Mechanisms and patterns of injury vary by disaster. Some natural disasters have predictable injury patterns, as described in more detail elsewhere in this book. Earthquakes and high-wind events can lead to severe blunt- and penetrating-trauma injuries requiring intensive care.[11] Further, crush syndrome occurs commonly following earthquakes, requiring responders to provide robust dialysis capabilities. Building collapse is the most common cause of injury and death from earthquakes. In tropical cyclones, drowning from storm surges occurs frequently. Flooding and mudflows are also expected causes of death following the storms. In high-wind events, flying debris causes blunt trauma and the structural

TABLE 2-1 Effects of Disasters on Public Health

	PPOPULATION'S HEALTH	HEALTH CARE SYSTEM
Direct effect	• Physical injury and death • Increased risk of communicable diseases • Acute illness (carbon monoxide poisoning, respiratory problems, etc.) • Heat-related illness, hypothermia, and burns • Increased morbidity and/or mortality in chronic diseases • Emotional or psychological effects	• Structural and nonstructural damages to hospitals, clinics, and health care centers • Injury, illness, death, and loss of personnel • Disruption of service delivery • Overload of trauma cases
Indirect effect	• Impaired or delayed access to health services because of service interruption or overload • Loss of normal living conditions (damage to housing, business, social life, etc.)	• Damage to external infrastructure that health system relies upon, including road and transportation, electricity, water, natural gas, and telecommunications

Adapted from Shoaf KI, Rothman SJ. Public health impact of disasters. *AJEM.* 2000;58-63.

collapse of buildings, which can kill people.[9] Blasts caused by terrorism activities or other types of human-made disasters also are capable of producing high fatality rates and severe injuries.

Disasters can also generate acute illnesses in an exposed population. Examples include coccidioidomycosis caused by exposure to soil containing spores,[12] pulmonary alveolar proteinosis caused by exposure to dust following an earthquake,[13] asthma attack following dust storms,[14] and respiratory and ocular problems caused by exposure to ash and smoke from volcanoes and wildfires.[9] Climate extremes can cause hypothermia or heat-related illness.[15] Asthma and allergic problems including rhinitis, dermatitis, and conjunctivitis have been reported as consequences of human-made disasters such as oil spills.[16]

In addition to acute illnesses, chronic problems also have been reported as consequences of disasters: a well-studied example is the thyroid cancer and leukemia in children resulting from the Chernobyl nuclear accident.[17] Moreover, long-term disabilities from severe physical injuries are also consequences of both natural and human-made disasters.

Stress caused by disasters is a risk factor for some chronic diseases. People with heart disease, hypertension, and diabetes are at risk of higher morbidity and/or mortality after natural disasters.[18–21] Increased risk of hospitalization for heart disease was also observed following the World Trade Center disaster.[22]

Disasters can potentially increase the risk of communicable diseases, particularly in developing countries. This happens because of damage to sanitation services, poor hygiene, overcrowding in shelters, exposure to extreme weather conditions, damage to the health sector, and difficult access to the health facilities. However, the occurrence of outbreaks after natural disasters has been relatively rare.[11] The association of dead bodies and outbreaks is also a myth.[23] In fact, occurrences of outbreaks after disasters depend on the existence of the disease in the community before the event.[11] Nevertheless, complex emergencies accompanied by large population displacement in chaotic situations and a lack of public health infrastructure have the potential for outbreaks to occur.

Disasters can provoke specific emotional reactions that take on a variety of different psychological responses, affecting both the primary victims (those directly involved in the disaster) and the secondary victims (such as relatives, coworkers, and schoolmates). In addition, relief workers can also experience mental health issues.[24] The mental health ramifications are possibly greater for those who witness or are involved with certain experiences from a disaster. Some examples include loss of loved ones, life-threatening danger or physical harm, exposure to gruesome death, extreme environmental or human violence, and the loss of a home.[24]

Direct Effect on the Health Care System

Health facilities and their personnel may become victims of disasters when their services are in highest demand.[25,26] It is important to preserve the ability of the health care system to continue its essential functions after disasters.

Disasters are capable of damaging the physical components and functions of hospitals, clinics, and primary health care centers.[25,27] Although structural damage significantly affects the health system, many health facilities fail to continue their operations because of damage to nonstructural components, such as electricity, water, heating and ventilation systems, and medical equipment.[25,28,29] Overload of hospitals with trauma cases can also hinder appropriate service delivery.

Similar to the general population, health personnel can be killed or injured during disasters. In addition, acute illnesses, such as respiratory problems following dust storms, may lead to absence from work.[27] Moreover, health personnel might not be able to report to work because of the severe weather conditions, destruction of roads, transportation stoppage,

or security concerns around a disaster. Disruption of the medical staff hinders the functions of a health care system during disasters.

Indirect Effect on the Health of the Population

Indirect effects of disasters on a population's health are associated with disruption of normal societal functions, living conditions, and routine health care.[9] Disasters cause damage to neighborhoods, homes, and property and thus often expose the affected population to stressors related to living in temporary settlements. The death of family members and friends causes additional stress. Further, disasters may change or destroy the social network and support systems that existed before the event. Damage to the economy and livelihoods has adverse effects on society, families, and individuals, as well as the quality of life of the survivors. The recovery of those affected depends on the community resilience and the assistance they may receive.[30] Vulnerable people, such as the elderly, disabled, and those with low socioeconomic status, are at higher risk of late or incomplete recovery.

Destruction or overload of the health facilities beyond their surge capacities adversely affects the health of populations.[31] In addition, inadequate preparedness by providers and patients for disastrous situations increases the adverse effects of disasters. These conditions hinder delivery of primary health services, such as vaccination, maternal and childcare, and management of chronic diseases: for instance, increased hospitalization rates were observed among dialysis patients following Hurricane Katrina because of disruption of planned care.[32]

Other examples of indirect disaster effects on a population's overall health include problems with contaminated water from damage to water pipelines, malnutrition and famine because of damage to agriculture, and food insecurity following droughts or complex emergencies. Further, carbon monoxide poisoning caused by fuel-burning equipment and toxicity from gasoline exposure were reported following Hurricane Sandy.[33,34]

Indirect Effect on the Health Care System

Even when a health facility is not directly affected by a disaster, damage to other infrastructure systems hampers its functionality. The systems that are essential to the operations of health facilities include roads and transportation, water supply, electrical power, telecommunications, natural gas, and steam energy.[35] Further, interdependencies among the infrastructure systems should be considered because systems do not operate in isolation of one another.[36] For instance, telecommunications depends on electricity. Health facilities are among the most dependent systems on other infrastructures, so their functions are affected by damage to other systems.[37]

PUBLIC HEALTH AND THE DISASTER-MANAGEMENT CYCLE

To minimize the public health consequences of disasters, understanding the interconnectivity of public health and disaster management helps people to choose the appropriate interventions. Timely and effective disaster response and recovery is necessary. Public health professionals must take a proactive approach to reduce the risk of disasters. This approach centers on disaster-mitigation and preparedness activities for the health facilities and the community exposed to natural and human-made hazards. This approach also best fits with the core principles of primary and secondary preventions.

This section explains how public health functions can be applied in each of the four phases of disaster management, which include prevention/mitigation, preparedness, response, and recovery. Box 2-1 summarizes these functions.

BOX 2-1   Public Health Functions in the Disaster-Management Cycle

Prevention and Mitigation
- Conduct the risk assessment of health facilities
- Contribute in the community-disaster-risk-assessment process
- Monitor the risks and vulnerability of health facilities and the population over time
- Manage structural and nonstructural mitigations in health facilities
- Support public awareness on disaster risks and mitigation measures
- Ensure that the disaster risk reduction is considered in environmental policies and is operationalized by the relevant sectors
- Ensure that land-use regulations are in place to prevent population settlement and construction of health facilities in high-risk zones
- Ensure that all health facilities, other infrastructures, and houses are insured

Preparedness
- Conduct the risk assessment of health facilities
- Contribute in the community disaster risk assessment process
- Establish early-warning systems
- Develop the emergency response operations plan and conduct the associated activities
- Provide education and training of health authorities and personnel
- Conduct drills and exercises
- Monitor community preparedness for disasters
- Provide public awareness programs

Response
- Conduct the rapid health-needs assessment of the affected population
- Conduct damage assessment of health facilities and ensure the continuity of their services
- Ensure the mental health and physical safety of health personnel
- Provide emergency medical and trauma care
- Establish disease surveillance and emergency information systems
- Monitor the environmental health and conduct environmental decontamination
- Monitor the food safety
- Provide other primary health care, including communicable diseases management, sexual and reproductive health care, management of noncommunicable and chronic diseases, and mental health services
- Provide risk communications and issue health advisories

Recovery
- Repair and reconstruction of damaged health facilities
- Replace damaged equipment and supplies
- Recover the damaged health care services and functions
- Provide physical rehabilitation services to trauma cases
- Provide psychological rehabilitation services to survivors

Prevention and Mitigation

Prevention is the avoidance of adverse effects of disasters and the associated hazards.[38] Prevention is not feasible in many circumstances; therefore, mitigation measures (i.e., strategies and activities that would lessen or limit the adverse effects of hazards must be taken). Examples of preventive measures are dams or embankments that eliminate flood risks and land-use regulations that prohibit settlement in high-risk zones.[38] These measures save both health infrastructures and the population.

The main strategies of disaster mitigation include risk assessment, risk reduction, and insuring against risk[39]:

- *Risk assessment* is essential to prioritize the response in hazards and high-risk zones. The risk assessment process not only evaluates the magnitude and likelihood of potential losses but also provides understanding of the vulnerability conditions, causes, and effects of the losses.[40] Public health agencies are required to contribute actively in the process of community risk assessment by providing health-related indicators and information. Further, the public health system should monitor the vulnerability status of the community over time. In addition to participation in the community risk assessment process, those within the public health system must assess the disaster risks at their health facilities. Disaster risk assessment requires multihazard engineering science and advanced technology. In addition, however, less-sophisticated and easy-to-use methods and tools are available. Examples include the Kaiser Permanente Hazard Vulnerability Assessment (HVA) tool that allows staff in medical centers to prioritize potential events based on risk as calculated using probability and severity; and the Hospital Safety Index (HSI), developed by the WHO. It assesses the safety level of the hospital in three main components (i.e., functional capacity, structural safety, and nonstructural safety).[41]

- Examples of risk-reduction measures are hazard-resistant construction and using nonstructural safety techniques. To be sustainable, risk-reduction regulations should be embedded in environmental policies and enforced by law. In the context of climate change policies, mitigation can be achieved by the reduction of greenhouse gas emissions. Public awareness, as a key public health strategy, is also essential to enhance the culture of safety and mobilize community participation in risk-reduction activities.

- To minimize the consequences of financial loss caused by disasters, it is important that private and public structures be provided with affordable insurance.[39] However, this is not easy to achieve. For instance, in China, only 3% to 5% of properties are insured against natural disasters. Insuring against disasters will help the affected community to prevent further damages that might be caused by the initial loss of property and livelihood. Further, insured health facilities will be able to repair the physical destruction and replace the damaged equipment and supplies; in turn, their functions will recover faster than if they lacked secure financial resources.

Preparedness

As defined by the United Nations International Strategy for Disaster Reduction (UNISDR), *preparedness* is the knowledge and capacities that would enable an organization, community, household, or individual to anticipate, respond to, and recover effectively from the effects of disasters.[38] Preparedness activities begin with the assessment of risks and capacities, and continue with the development of an emergency-response plan (ERP) and associated training and exercises. Activities related to the ERP include the development of command, control, and coordination mechanisms; surge capacity protocols; information management; and plans for communications, evacuation, public information, safety, and security, as well as the stockpiling of equipment and supplies. Formal institutional, legal, and budgetary capacities are needed to support the implementation of an ERP.

The establishment of early-warning systems for natural hazards, such as tsunami, storms, floods, and drought, is also a key component of the preparedness phase. Early warning is used to predict the likely conflicts and complex emergencies; early detection of infectious diseases in a hospital setting or reporting parameters and a system for the detection of bioterrorism events are other examples. End-to-end, early warning offers the benefit of a rapid response and reduction in morbidity and mortality. Effectively linking the health facilities to the warning process might give facilities enough time to get ready before a disaster strikes.

An "all-hazard/whole-health" approach is recommended when planning for disasters.[42] The term *all-hazard* concerns arrangements for managing the large range of possible effects of risks and emergencies. Although many risks require specific sets of actions, they can cause similar problems and, in turn, require similar interventions. A "whole-health approach" entails the following components: (1) establishment of a unified preparedness and response platform for all categories of health risks; (2) inclusion of all health-related capabilities available by governmental and nongovernmental organizations, the private sector, and the military; and (3) assure that all aspects of public health, including emergency medical care, pharmaceuticals, environmental health, communicable disease control, management of chronic diseases, mental health, reproductive health, and nutrition, are well addressed.

Public health personnel must be integrated and participate with other response agencies during drills and exercises to better familiarize each stakeholder with their respective roles and abilities. In addition, this is the phase in which public health agencies would develop interagency agreements, memoranda of understanding (MOUs), and external support contracts.

The public health system is also required to ensure that communities, households, and individuals are prepared for disasters. The system not only acts as a preventive strategy to reduce the number of deaths and injuries but also reduces the number of people who need emergency health and trauma care during a disaster. This requires monitoring of the community disaster preparedness and conducting public awareness programs. There are examples of the public health programs that have effectively enhanced the household disaster preparedness and community-based early-warning systems.[43,44]

Response

In the response phase, each agency and section with responsibility to respond activates its ERP to the specific threat or situation. Responses can incorporate those at the local, regional, and national levels. Public health emergency-response functions must be coordinated with the other sectors involved in the response operations. To achieve this, public health functions should be consistent with principles, organizational processes, and guidance defined by the overall community response framework and the incident management system. This consistency can improve operations and service delivery to the affected population.

According to the whole-health approach, as presented above, the public health system must ensure that all aspects of the populations' health are considered during response operations. However, priority should be given to the most vulnerable people, including the elderly, the disabled, dialysis patients, the homebound, minorities, and the nonnative-speaking and transient populations, such as tourists and migrant workers.[45]

As soon as a disaster occurs, conducting a rapid needs and damage assessment is the first step that should be taken. The assessment addresses the population's health needs and damage to infrastructure and health care facilities. The subsequent public health activities include providing emergency medical and trauma care; ensuring the mental health and physical safety of health personnel; establishing disease surveillance and emergency information systems; conducting communicable disease control programs, including vaccination, medical treatment of infected cases, and outbreak investigation; providing sexual and reproductive health care, including maternal, newborn, and child health care plus the care related to violence and sexual abuse; managing noncommunicable and chronic diseases; providing mental health services; monitoring environmental health (water, sanitation, and hygiene); conducting environmental decontamination measures; monitoring food safety, including food items provided by relief organizations; and issuing health advisories as needed.[42,45]

The CDC has enlisted the ongoing public health emergency functions and associated tasks relevant to the acute phase of an emergency (i.e., the first 24 hours).[46] The acute phase is divided into the following timeframes: immediate (hours 0 to 2), intermediate (hours 2 to 6 and 6 to 12), and extended (hours 12 to 24). The ongoing functions and tasks may need to be implemented during a disaster beyond the acute phase of the response and can be applied during both natural and human-made disasters. However, the order of performance may vary according to the specific incident.[46]

Recovery

The recovery tasks of rehabilitation and reconstruction begin soon after the emergency phase has ended. However, the division between some response actions and the subsequent recovery stage is not clear-cut[38] Examples include the supply of temporary housing and psychosocial supports that may extend into the recovery phase.

Public health agencies must identify what resources might be available to assist in restoring the operation and address other physically and emotionally affected populations. Public health recovery operations are multidisciplinary and involve multiple sectors of society (law enforcement, military, public policy, public works, etc.), and they vary depending on the extent of the disaster's effect on the society. Further, recovery efforts comprise several components, some of which are reinstitution of medical services if clinics and hospitals are destroyed; and establishment of corrupted lifelines, such as sanitation, electricity, and water. The international public health operation during the 2010 Haiti Earthquake was an example of multilateral and global relief. The recovery from this disaster and other large disasters is ongoing and likely will last several years.

PUBLIC HEALTH IN NATIONAL DISASTER FRAMEWORKS: THE CASE OF THE UNITED STATES

The Federal Emergency Management Agency (FEMA), established in 1978, is responsible for determining the U.S. federal government's role in all phases of disaster management, including prevention/mitigation, preparedness, response, and recovery. These responsibilities apply for all types of disasters, whether natural or human-made, including acts of terror. Following the September 11, 2001, attacks, Congress passed the Homeland Security Act of 2002, which created the Department of Homeland Security (DHS) for better coordination among the different federal agencies. In 2003, FEMA became part of the DHS.[47]

In line with FEMA's mission, five national frameworks (NFs) have been developed, one for each preparedness mission area addressed in Presidential Policy Directive-8.[48] These national frameworks address the mission areas of prevention, protection, mitigation, response, and recovery. This part of the chapter provides an overview on how the U.S. public health system, under the leadership of DHHS, interacts with other partners within the NFs.

National Prevention Framework

This framework was developed to ensure that the nation is prepared to prevent imminent acts of terrorism. Under the president's lead, the following departments and agencies have specific roles regarding terrorism prevention: the Department of Defense, DHS, Department of Justice, Federal Bureau of Investigation, Office of the Director of National Intelligence, and Department of State. However, to be successful, any approach to the delivery of prevention capabilities will require a national approach including all levels of government, the private and nonprofit sectors, and individuals.[49]

Public health and health system leaders are among the intended audiences of this framework, and their role in bio-surveillance tasks, including medical, public health, animal health, and environmental tasks, is critical to identify, discover, or locate imminent terrorist threats. It is placed under the core capability of the national prevention framework (NPF) of "screening, search, and detection."[49]

National Mitigation Framework

The national mitigation framework (NMF) covers the capabilities necessary to reduce the loss of life and property by lessening the effects of disasters. DHHS has been assigned as a member of the Mitigation Framework Leadership Group of the NMF, where it collaborates with other members, including local, state, tribal, and territorial representatives and the Department of Agriculture, Department of Commerce, Department of Defense, Department of Energy, Environmental Protection Agency, General Services Administration, DHS, Department of Housing and Urban Development, Department of the Interior, Department of Justice, Small Business Administration, and Department of Transportation.[50] NMF considers an intact health and medical system as a requirement for an effective recovery process in a disaster-affected community. The health system requires taking disaster-mitigation measures in environmental health departments, hospitals and hospital associations, and behavioral health services.[50]

National Response Framework

The national response framework (NRF) provides a context for how the whole community works together during a disaster response and how the response efforts relate to other parts of national preparedness.[51] The framework comprises 15 emergency support functions (ESFs), including Public Health and Medical Services (i.e., ESF-8), where DHHS serves as the coordinating and primary agency. The following departments and agencies contribute in the ESF-8 as the supporting organizations: the Department of Agriculture, Department of Commerce, Department of Defense, Department of Energy, DHS, Department of the Interior, Department of Justice, Department of Labor, Department of State, Department of Transportation, Department of Veterans Affairs, Environmental Protection Agency, General Services Administration, U.S. Agency for International Development, U.S. Postal Service, and American Red Cross.[51]

ESF-8 provides supplemental assistance to local, state, tribal, territorial, and insular area resources in response to emergencies and disasters in the following core functional areas[51]:

- Assessment of public health and medical needs
- Health surveillance
- Medical surge
- Health, medical, and veterinary equipment and supplies
- Patient movement
- Patient care
- Safety and security of drugs, biologics, and medical devices
- Blood and tissues
- Food safety and defense
- Agriculture safety and security
- All-hazards public health and medical consultation, technical assistance, and support
- Behavioral health care
- Public health and medical information
- Vector control
- Guidance on potable water, wastewater, and solid-waste disposal
- Mass fatality management, victim identification, and decontaminating remains
- Veterinary medical support

NATIONAL DISASTER RECOVERY FRAMEWORK

The national disaster recovery framework (NDRF) addresses guidance that enables effective recovery support to disaster-impacted communities. To build a more resilient nation, it focuses on how best to restore, redevelop, and revitalize the health, social, economic, natural, and environmental fabric of the community. This framework includes six recovery support functions (RSFs). DHHS has responsibilities in all of the other RSFs, except for the natural and cultural resources, as described below[52]:

- Coordinating (along with DHS) the RSF of community planning and capacity building, a common public health strategy for community empowerment, which here is applied in the context of disaster recovery
- Coordinating the RSF of health and social services and addressing the recovery efforts at public health departments, health care facilities, medical services, and also essential social services
- Supporting the RSFs of economic, housing, and infrastructure systems

CONCLUSION

Historically, promoting and managing the health of a society has been shown to increase the welfare of the society. This discipline, called public health, is a broad one, encompassing multiple sectors of the community and professional fields, government and nongovernment agencies, and local, regional, federal, and sometimes international institutions. Collectively, these groups respond to disasters to study, reduce, and develop ways to mitigate future adverse health effects.

This chapter began with a definition of *public health* and its essential services that can be applied to all types of health threats including disasters, and continued with a summary of direct and indirect impact of disasters on populations' health and health care system. It also discussed the "all-hazard-whole-health" approach and explained what the specific public health functions are in each of the four phases of disaster management. Further, this chapter emphasized that public health systems require taking a proactive approach toward disaster mitigation and preparedness of both health facilities and the community in general. Finally, the role of the U.S. health system in disaster management was explained, as an example that is well recognized worldwide.

It is recommended that the newcomer to disaster medicine and public health review the many references in this chapter and refer to resources on the Internet. It is also recommended that they read the following chapters to gain a better understanding on how public health functions can be operationalized in the context of disaster management. These are the beginning steps to achieving a more-efficient, life-saving public health role in disaster risk management.

REFERENCES

1. World Health Organization. Public health. Available at: http://www.who.int/trade/glossary/story076/en/.
2. World Health Organization. WHO definition of health. Available at: http://www.who.int/about/definition/en/print.html.
3. Centers for Disease Control and Prevention. Ten great public health achievements—United States, 1900-1999. *MMWR.* 1999;48(12):241–243.
4. Centers for Disease Control and Prevention. The public health system and the 10 essential public health services. Available at: www.cdc.gov/nphpsp/essentialservices.html.
5. World Health Organization. Social determinants of health. Available at: http://www.who.int/social_determinants/en/.

6. Joint Task Group on Public Health Human Resources. *Building the public health workforce for the 21st century.* Ottawa: Public Health Agency of Canada; 2005. Available at: www.ciphi.ca/files/documents/cpc/ccworkforce.pdf.

7. World Health Organization. What is health system? Available at: http://www.who.int/features/qa/28/en/.

8. Institute of Medicine, Committee on the Future of Public Health. *The future of public health.* Washington, DC: National Academy Press; 1988.

9. Shoaf KI, Rothman SJ. Public health impact of disasters. *AJEM.* 2000;58–63.

10. EM-DAT. The OFDA/CRED International Disaster Database. Brussels: Université Catholique de Louvain. Available at: www.emdat.be.

11. Noji EK. *Public health consequences of disaster.* NewYork, NY: Oxford University Press; 1997.

12. Schneider E, Hajjeh RA, Spiegel RA, et al. A coccidioidomycosis outbreak following the Northridge. California earthquake. *JAMA.* 1997;277(11):904–908.

13. Hisata S, Moriyama H, Tazawa R, et al. Development of pulmonary alveolar proteinosis following exposure to dust after the Great East Japan Earthquake. *Respir Investig.* 2013;51(4):212–216.

14. Merrifield A, Schindeler S, Jalaludin B, et al. Health effects of the September 2009 dust storm in Sydney, Australia: did emergency department visits and hospital admissions increase? *Environ Health.* 2013;12:32. http://dx.doi.org/10.1186/1476-069X-12-32.

15. Centers for Disease Control and Prevention. Heat-related deaths after an extreme heat event—four states, 2012, and United States, 1999-2009. *MMWR.* 2013;62(22):433–436.

16. Kim YM, Park JH, Choi K, et al. Burden of disease attributable to the Hebei Spirit oil spill in Taean. *Korea BMJ Open.* 2013;3(9):e003334. http://dx.doi.org/10.1136/bmjopen-2013-003334.

17. Moysich KB, Menezes RJ, Michalek AM. Chernobyl-related ionizing radiation exposure and cancer risk: an epidemiological review. *Lancet Oncol.* 2002;3(5):269–279.

18. Inui A, Kitaoka H, Majima M, et al. Effect of the Kobe earthquake on stress and glycemic control in patients with diabetes mellitus. *Arch Intern Med.* 1998;58(3):274–278.

19. Hung KK, Lam EC, Chan EY, et al. Disease pattern and chronic illness in rural China: the Hong Kong Red Cross basic health clinic after 2008 Sichuan earthquake. *Emerg Med Australas.* 2013;25(3):252–259.

20. Nozaki E, Nakamura A, Abe A, et al. Occurrence of cardiovascular events after the 2011 Great East Japan earthquake and tsunami disaster. *Int Heart J.* 2013;54(5):247–253.

21. Nishizawa M, Hoshide S, Shimpo M, et al. Disaster hypertension: experience from the great East Japan earthquake of 2011. *Curr Hypertens Rep.* 2012;14(5):375–381.

22. Jordan HT, Stellman SD, Morabia A, et al. Cardiovascular disease hospitalizations in relation to exposure to the September 11, 2001 World Trade Center disaster and posttraumatic stress disorder. *J Am Heart Assoc.* 2013;2(5):e000431. http://dx.doi.org/10.1161/JAHA.113.000431.

23. de Ville de Goyet C. Epidemics caused by dead bodies: a disaster myth that does not want to die. *Rev Panam Salud Publica.* 2004;15(5):297–299.

24. Dubouloz M. Mental health. In: de Boer J, Dubouloz M, eds. *Handbook of disaster medicine.* Utrecht: Van der Wees; 2000.

25. Pan-American Health Organization. Protecting new health facilities from natural hazards: guidelines for the promotion of disaster mitigation. *Prehosp Disaster Med.* 2004;19(4):326–351.

26. Milsten A. Hospital responses to acute-onset disasters: a review. *Prehosp Disaster Med.* 2000;15(1):40–53.

27. Ardalan A, Mowafi H, Khoshsabeghe HY. Impacts of natural hazards on primary health care facilities of Iran: a 10-year retrospective survey. *PLoS Curr.* 2013;5. http://dx.doi.org/10.1371/currents.dis.ccdbd870f5d1697e4edee5eda12c5ae6.

28. Whitney DJ, Dickerson A, Lindell MK. Nonstructural seismic preparedness of Southern California hospitals. *Earthq Spectra.* 2001;17(1):153–171.

29. Myrtle RC, Masri SF, Nigbor RL, et al. Classification and prioritization of essential systems in hospitals under extreme events. *Earthq Spectra.* 2005;21(3):779–802.

30. Ardalan A, Mazaheri M, VanRooyen M, et al. Post-disaster quality of life among older survivors five years after the Bam earthquake: implications for recovery policy. *Ageing Soc.* 2011;31(2):179–196.

31. Sareen H, Shoaf KI. Impact of the 1994 Northridge earthquake on the utilization and difficulties associated with prescription medications and health aids. *Prehosp Disaster Med.* 2000;15(4):173–180.

32. Howard D, Zhang R, Huang Y, et al. Hospitalization rates among dialysis patients during Hurricane Katrina. *Prehosp Disaster Med.* 2012;27(4):325–329.

33. Chen BC, Shawn LK, Connors NJ, et al. Carbon monoxide exposures in New York City following Hurricane Sandy in 2012. *Clin Toxicol.* 2013;51(9):879–885.

34. Kim HK, Takematsu M, Biary R, et al. Epidemic gasoline exposures following Hurricane Sandy. *Prehosp Disaster Med.* 2013;28(6):586–591.

35. Arboleda C, Abraham D, Richard J, et al. Vulnerability assessment of health care facilities during disaster events. *J Infrastruct Syst.* 2009;15(3):149–161.

36. Chang SE. Infrastructure resilience to disasters. 2009 frontiers of engineering symposium: session on resilient and sustainable infrastructures. Available at: http://www.nae.edu/File.aspx?id=15629.

37. Oh EH, Deshmukh A, Hastak M. Disaster impact analysis based on inter-relationship of critical infrastructure and associated industries: a winter flood disaster event. *IJDRBE.* 2010;1(1):25–49.

38. United Nations International Strategy for Disaster Reduction. *Terminology on disaster risk reduction.* Geneva: UN; 2009.

39. Federal Emergency Management Agency. What is mitigation? Available at: http://www.fema.gov/what-mitigation.

40. United Nations Development Program. Disaster risk assessment. Available at: http://www.undp.org/content/dam/undp/library/crisis%20prevention/disaster/2Disaster%20Risk%20Reduction%20-%20Risk%20Assessment.pdf.

41. World Health Organization. *Hospital safety index: Guide for evaluators.* Geneva: WHO; 2008.

42. World Health Organization. Risk reduction and emergency preparedness: WHO six-year strategy for the health sector and community capacity development. Available at: http://www.who.int/hac/techguidance/preparedness/emergency_preparedness_eng.pdf.

43. Ardalan A, Mowafi H, Malekafzali H, et al. Effectiveness of a primary health care program on urban and rural community disaster preparedness, I.R. Iran: a community intervention trial. *DMPHP.* 2013;7(5):481–490.

44. Ardalan A, Holakouie Naieni K, Mahmoodi M, et al. Flash flood preparedness in Golestan province of Iran: a community intervention trial. *Am J Disaster Med.* 2010;5(4):197–214.

45. Landesman LY. *Public health management of disasters: The pocket guide.* Washington, DC: American Public Health Association; 2006.

46. Centers for Disease Control and Prevention. *Public health emergency response guide for state, local, and tribal public health directors. Version 2.0.* 2011, Available at: www.bt.cdc.gov/.../pdf/cdcresponseguide.pdf.

47. Federal Emergency Management Agency. About the agency. Available at: http://www.fema.gov/about-agency.

48. Federal Emergency Management Agency. National planning frameworks. Available at: https://www.fema.gov/national-planning-frameworks.

49. Federal Emergency Management Agency. National prevention framework. Available at: http://www.fema.gov/national-prevention-framework.

50. Federal Emergency Management Agency. National mitigation framework. Available at: http://www.fema.gov/national-mitigation-framework.

51. Federal Emergency Management Agency. National response framework. Available at: https://www.fema.gov/national-response-framework.

52. Federal Emergency Management Agency. National disaster recovery framework. Available at: http://www.fema.gov/national-disaster-recovery-framework-0.

Role of Emergency Medical Services in Disaster Management and Preparedness

James J. Rifino and Selwyn E. Mahon

Disaster response comes in many forms. It occurs in stages and involves many different agencies over an extended period. With current technology, meteorologists track the weather patterns leading to tornados and other severe storms, thus allowing for warnings, sometimes days in advance. Certain seasons are well known for the occurrence of natural disasters in specific areas, such as hurricanes in the Caribbean Basin, thus mandating appropriate preparedness during these times. Other disasters, such as those that are human-made, rarely allow for preparation and can result in a significant increase in morbidity and mortality. Regardless of the situation or its origin, one particular responding group can significantly affect the outcome of any disaster event: emergency medical services (EMS) personnel. Having a well-prepared EMS system that has been tested in disaster response decreases the morbidity and mortality associated with the event. From the moment an event unfolds, an emergency call is made, and multiple agencies respond, including police, fire, and ambulance personnel. The medical personnel on scene determine the gravity of the situation and often have to make life-and-death decisions, because resources may be quickly depleted in large-scale events.

HISTORICAL PERSPECTIVE

EMS today are largely the product of past civilian and military experiences, with current EMS principles and practices (particularly in the United States) evolving from wartime casualty care. The first-known organized use of ambulances was on the battlefields of Crimea, and the Vietnam War brought us the concept of the modern "field medic." EMS history is undeniably rich in militaristic tradition, with practices documented as far back as 1500 BC, in Egypt. An ancient medical text known as the Edwin Smith Papyrus was used for military purposes. It describes injuries (wounds, dislocations, and fractures), presents a rational and scientific approach to the treatment of these injuries, and differentiates itself from other texts of the time, which were more based on magic than science. Each case detailed the type of injury, examination of the patient, diagnosis and prognosis, and treatment for the particular ailment. Treatments outlined included suturing wounds, controlling hemorrhage, and bandaging and splinting fractures. The document even described immobilization of the head and spinal cord in cases of injuries.[1]

Baron Dominique Jean Larrey, Napoleon's surgeon-in-chief, has been described as the father of modern military surgery. He mastered wound management, including early limb amputation (to prevent gangrene), and treated the wounded according to the severity of their wounds and not according to their rank within the military. He is also largely credited with placing the first ambulances in service (horse-drawn carts called *ambulances volantes*), more than 150 years ago,

during the Crimean War, rapidly evacuating wounded soldiers from the combat zone to aid stations and then to hospitals if needed.

During the U.S. Civil War (largely felt to be the starting point for EMS systems in the United States), a nurse named Clara Barton recognized that wounded soldiers of the Union Army were brought to facilities giving suboptimal care. She coordinated and rendered emergency care to wounded infantry, crusading tirelessly for the medical relief of sick and wounded soldiers, and quickly becoming known as the "Angel of the Battlefield."[2] After the war, Barton was introduced to the "Red Cross" in Geneva, Switzerland, and she established a branch within the United States. As the organization's first president, she directed relief work for disasters, such as famines, floods, pestilence, forest fires, hurricanes, and earthquakes, in the United States and throughout the world.

Moreover, during the Civil War, it was also recognized that ambulances could be used on a daily basis to assist those in medical need. Some of the first cities in the world to adopt the use of the "ambulance" included New York City (NYC), London, Paris, and Cincinnati. During the late 1800s, ambulances in NYC were staffed with a medical intern and equipped with medicines, splints, bandages, and an array of other medical equipment.

With the improvement of military technology during the last century, casualties increased, necessitating training soldiers themselves to deliver EMS on the battlefield. During World War I, soldiers were taught basic medical management, as well as techniques in transport. In addition, the "Thomas Traction Splint" was introduced and used to stabilize leg fractures. This procedure alone was found to decrease morbidity and mortality in the field. Aeromedical transport systems were established during World War II and further refined during the Korean conflict, to expedite transfer of the wounded.[3]

World War II resulted in a physician shortage in the United States because the doctors were pulled from ambulances and the medical community to serve their country, which abruptly resulted in untrained staff in ambulances throughout the United States. Although this shortage was problematic for urban areas, rural areas were especially hard hit, and ambulance services were commonly run by mortuary attendants. Throughout the 1950s and 1960s, it was obvious to many that there was a need to restructure the EMS model throughout the country. The Vietnam War is widely considered a time when trauma protocols and interventions helped to shape the current approach to prehospital care. The corpsman of Vietnam most closely resembled the "paramedic" of today, with personnel being well trained in a variety of advanced medical interventions. It was clearly documented that battlefield mortality rates decreased significantly with the evolution of trauma care, early advanced interventions, and expeditious transport from the front lines to definitive care via helicopter. Casualty rates for U.S. soldiers were clearly reduced as follows: 8% during World

War I, 4.5% during World War II, 2.5% during the Korean War, and less than 2% during the Vietnam conflict.[4] The shift from empiricism to the practice of evidence-based medicine and the provision of acute care in the field clearly made armed conflict much more survivable. The immense benefits of rapid, advanced field stabilization and swift transport to definitive care facilities would soon become the expectation of politicians and civilians alike in the United States.

Throughout the 1960s, numerous studies throughout the world showed that prehospital CPR with defibrillation and medication administration was found to make a difference (20% resuscitation success was reported by a group in Ireland).[5,6] Such data helped politicians, physicians, and interested parties make the case for a more integrated and sophisticated EMS system. Researchers in the United States during the early 1960s further found that an infantry soldier in Vietnam had a statistically greater chance of survival than the average citizen involved in a motor vehicle collision on any of the nation's highways had. This single disparity prompted two significant legislative acts in 1966 in the United States. First, the National Academy of Sciences-National Research Council (NAS-NRC) published *Accidental Death and Disability: The Neglected Disease of Modern Society*. This white paper put forth 24 recommendations to improve care for injured persons, and it served as a blueprint for the development of EMS. Recommendations included disaster planning, regulation of EMS by the states, development of trauma registries, the creation of various standards within EMS for training, public safety infrastructure improvements, emergency department overhauls, and the creation of "...a single nationwide number to summon an ambulance." It also went on to recommend that emergency departments be staffed with more-experienced personnel and be categorized and that they should collect data on select injuries. The second bill prepared by Congress was the Highway Safety Act of 1966. It mandated the creation of the U.S. Department of Transportation (USDOT) and the National Highway Traffic Safety Administration (NHTSA). Both entities provided legislative authority and financial assistance to EMS systems in the United States. Since the 1960s, EMS have been evolving throughout the United States, with current governance being through local, regional, and state protocols. Prehospital care is largely delivered through a variety of options, with emergency medical technicians (EMTs) and fire personnel predominantly providing this service.

Over the past 50 years, EMS systems worldwide have evolved, and they continue to evolve today. Many countries do not have a robust system such as those found in the United States, Europe, and Australia. Internationally, disasters continue to happen, resulting in an international response, because local resources are quickly outstripped. The bombings in Europe (e.g., Spain, England), the coordinated acts of 9/11, and the violence throughout Africa and some Arab countries bring to light the need for emergency preparedness and a proper disaster response to human-made disasters. Natural disasters continue to occur at an alarming rate (Haiti, 2010; Cyclone Nargis in Myanmar, 2008; the Pakistan Earthquake, 2005; Hurricane Katrina, 2005; the Tohoku Earthquake and Tsunami, 2011; the Philippines Super Typhoon, Haiyan, 2013; the New Zealand Earthquake, 2011; the East Africa Drought, 2011; the European Heat Wave, 2003), with many of the worst recorded natural disasters in the history of the world occurring in the past 20 years. Worldwide, it has been recognized that the EMS response must be coordinated and efficient, necessitating the need for training and preparedness of EMS personnel. In the United States, federal guidelines and regulations have become more integrated after 9/11 because disaster response and mitigation are both extensively discussed and drilled. In addition to having highly skilled and trained personnel, it has been well recognized that a highly organized structure for disaster response is necessary to respond in the most effective manner to any disaster situation. There is no better example of how a disaster

situation can be further negatively affected, than the historic 9/11 attack on the World Trade Center in 2001. New York City's Office of Emergency Management (OEM) was headquartered at Seven World Trade Center, with communications from the city's OEM based on the rooftop of One World Trade Center.[7,8] Less than 9 hours after the first strike, Seven World Trade Center collapsed, resulting in a lack of radio frequency interoperability among EMS, the New York Police Department, and the Fire Department of New York. Triage and transport of patients were adversely affected by the lack of coordinated communications with local and regional hospitals in the NYC metropolitan area.[9,10]

Although EMS in the United States developed largely from the frontline medical practices of the Vietnam War, the Incident Command System (ICS) was developed in the early 1970s, by fire administrators in California, to manage better the rapidly moving wildfires and operational deficits previously encountered. Specific complications cited before the creation of the ICS included too many people reporting to one supervisor, different emergency response organizational structures, lack of reliable incident information, inadequate and incompatible communications, lack of structure for coordinated planning among agencies, unclear lines of authority, terminology differences among agencies, and unclear or unspecified incident objectives. In 1980, U.S. federal officials recognized the importance of the ICS and realized that it could easily be incorporated on a national level to help with disaster response. In the United States, the National Interagency Incident Management System (NIIMS) was created. Since then, it has been adapted further for use in disaster response in the United States. The inherent flexibility of the ICS to accommodate issues of incident size and utilization of available resources has allowed the system to be used to mitigate both minor crises and major disasters exacted by nature and humans alike. As public safety personnel developed familiarity with the ICS, the federal government identified the need for the development of a body of government to establish standards of practice within increasingly complex applications of disaster management. In response to the increasing threat of terror attacks and the need to ensure a more cohesive response to large-scale incidents, federal guidelines were created to establish the role of EMS.[11,12]

In 1998, Congress issued a report underscoring concern regarding "...the real and potentially catastrophic effects of a chemical or biological act of terrorism." Legislators indicated that, although the federal government is integral in the prevention and secondary response to such incidents, state and local public safety personnel who respond initially require additional assistance. The Appropriations Act (Public Law 105-119) authorized the U.S. attorney general to aid state and local responders in acquiring specialized training and equipment to "...safely respond to and manage terrorist incidents involving weapons of mass destruction (WMD)."

Shortly after the attacks on September 11, 2001, the largest and most expensive reorganization of the U.S. federal government in history occurred, resulting in the formation of the Department of Homeland Security (DHS). While less than 4% of the total funding was allocated toward EMS, the functions of the newly created offices included incident management and oversight of preparation, response, and recovery after terrorist incidents. The Homeland Security Act of 2002 placed DHS in command of 22 government agencies, including the Federal Emergency Management Agency (FEMA).[13]

EMS INTERNATIONALLY

The terms *EMS* and *prehospital care* are often used to describe services systems at the provider, ambulance service, community, region, state, or even national levels. Comparisons of EMS systems are difficult because EMS systems have traditionally been developed based on the unique local needs of their community, which has led to the many different classifications of EMS systems in use globally. Regardless of the place on this planet, EMS systems often have common principles and practices, although the structure may be very different. Generally, EMS involve trained personnel responding to care for another person in medical need, as well as the use of a vehicle and common equipment and the need for expertise in managing emergency medical issues. Whereas new EMS systems are created both locally and internationally, and existing systems improve, implementing best practices that work globally is essential. Classifications of EMS systems are therefore necessary so that similar systems can be compared, and concepts such as quality improvement and best practices can be established.

As outlined in "EMS: A Practical Global Guidebook," EMS systems can be classified based on how the service is regulated[14]:

1. *National system:* EMS systems administered by national governments or ministries
2. *Local or regional system:* EMS systems administered by local or regional governments, often as a part of local or regional police or fire departments
3. *Private system:* Systems in which private EMS companies contract with local, regional, or national governments to provide prehospital care
4. *Hospital-based system:* EMS system based at and/or run by central or referral hospitals
5. *Volunteer system:* Common in smaller, rural areas, where the systems rely on community volunteers, who donate their time to provide local prehospital care
6. *Hybrid system:* EMS systems that combine some or all of the features of the above-mentioned systems

EMS systems can also be classified based on the level of care provided by the many types of providers in the ambulance. The service can be:

1. *Unorganized:* Common in developing countries, in these systems, the sick and injured are transported to the hospital in a nonorganized manner, by an unstructured system, and often by bystanders who have no knowledge of medicine and who transport the person via a personal vehicle. Providers may or may not have official training or certification, and the vehicles are not regulated.
2. *Basic life support (BLS):* These systems consist of essential noninvasive life-saving procedures (CPR, artificial ventilation/oxygenation, basic airway management, hemorrhage control, extremity splinting, spinal immobilization, and vital signs).
3. *Advanced life support (ALS):* BLS skills as well as more-advanced invasive life-saving procedures (advanced airway adjuncts, intravenous infusions, medication administration, defibrillation, electrocardiogram interpretation, community paramedicine, etc.) are included.
4. *Physician service:* In these systems, a physician staffs the ambulance or a car and responds as part of the ambulance crew to evaluate and provide care on scene. The physician may opt to treat on scene and not take the patient to the hospital or to take the patient into the hospital for treatment.

Even within these classifications, it is difficult to compare the quality of medical care because the providers at each level have a variety of training, and the "EMS system" differs from country to country, depending on the financial resources available. The doctors in physician-led services may not actually be emergency-trained physicians and may not even have experience as physicians before being allowed in the ambulances (they may still be interns or recent medical school graduates with no residency training). In ALS systems, EMS provider certifications vary, not only from state to state but also country to country. This can make credentialing difficult. In some local systems, physicians can mandate their own individual standards and expectations, making it difficult for EMS personnel to have a standard when treating patients in the prehospital environment. More importantly, the lack of a standardized system can result in increased morbidity and mortality for patients for a number of reasons. These include lack of skill maintenance, difficulty with maintaining quality assurance, varied authorizations to perform advanced procedures, varied medications to administer and learn, and varied "whims" by different medical directors.

EMS systems around the world can generally be divided into two main models: the Franco-German model or the Anglo-American model. The Franco-German model of EMS delivery is based on the "stay and stabilize" philosophy. The motive of this model is to bring the hospital to the patient(s). It is usually run by physicians, and they have extensive scope of practice with very advanced technology. The model utilizes many methods of transportation alongside land ambulances, such as helicopters and coastal ambulances. This model is usually a subset of the wider health care system. This philosophy is widely implemented in Europe, where emergency medicine is a relatively young field. Throughout Europe, prehospital emergency care is usually provided by "emergency physicians," although this specialty is not officially recognized in many countries as it is in the United States. The physicians in the field have the authority to make complex clinical judgment and treat patients in their homes or at the scene. Under this system, many EMS users are treated on-site and not transported to a hospital. In some systems, patients who are transported to a hospital can be directly admitted to hospital wards (including ICUs) by the attending field physician, thereby bypassing the emergency department. Countries such as Germany, France, Greece, Malta, and Austria have well-developed Franco-German EMS systems. Italy has a system made up of predominantly volunteer BLS ambulances, with physician ALS ambulances to augment with advanced interventions when it is determined that these services are needed on scene.

In contrast to the Franco-German model, the Anglo-American model is based on a "scoop and run" philosophy. This model aims to bring patients to the hospital rapidly, with fewer prehospital interventions. It is usually allied with public safety services (police or fire departments) rather than public health services and hospitals. Trained paramedics and EMTs run the system with medical oversight. The model relies heavily on land ambulances and less so on aeromedical evacuation or coastal ambulances. In countries following this model, emergency medicine is well developed and generally recognized as a separate medical specialty. Almost all patients in the Anglo-American model are transported by EMS personnel to developed emergency departments rather than hospital wards. Countries that use this model of EMS delivery include the United States, Canada, New Zealand, the Sultanate of Oman, and Australia.

Many studies have attempted to compare the two systems in terms of outcome or cost-effectiveness. This is essentially futile because each model tends to operate very differently, as the demands and expectations of the community are ultimately what must be met. In addition, the lack of unified standards between the two models makes comparison an unjustifiable exercise. There is currently no evidence that one model is "better" than the other is, and studies continue to show conflicting conclusions, despite the personal beliefs and experiences of physicians, nurses, and EMS personnel worldwide.[15,16]

Currently, most countries have no developed EMS system. International EMS systems have varied features and practices, but they all resemble the main models of EMS systems in one way or another. Countries that are recognizing emergency medicine and prehospital

TABLE 3-1   Comparison between Franco-German Model and Anglo-American Model[15]

MODEL	FRANCO-GERMAN MODEL	ANGLO-AMERICAN MODEL
No. of patients	More treated on the scene Few transported to hospitals	Few treated on the scene More transported to hospitals
Provider of care	Medical doctors supported by paramedics	Paramedics with medical oversight
Main motive	Brings the hospital to the patient	Brings the patient to the hospital
Destination for transported patients	Direct transport to hospital wards, i.e., bypassing EDs	Direct transport to EDs
Overarching organization	EMS is a part of the public health organization	EMS is a part of the public safety organization

care as new specialties and building EMS systems often find themselves having to choose between the two models. Others are more creative and use concepts of both, thus creating hybrid systems that incorporate features of both models.

The World Health Organization regards EMS systems as an integral part of any effective and functional health care system.[15,18] EMS (no matter the form) is the first point of contact globally for the majority of people to health care services during emergencies and life-threatening injuries. In many countries, EMS is the "gate-keeper" for access to specialty hospitals, according to the injury or illness identified. Emergency medical providers around the world continue to learn and utilize advanced clinical technology while they care for medical and trauma emergencies. The goal of any international EMS system must be to adapt a model and create a system that meets the local needs, works with regional health care resources, and is sensitive to the local and national customs, while working within the political and financial structure in each individual community. In addition, the EMS community must keep in mind that a well-practiced and trained EMS system is what makes all the difference in the morbidity and mortality associated with any disaster scenario (Table 3-1).

CURRENT PRACTICE

Throughout the world, many countries recognize that EMS is expected to be a first-line organized response able to bring order to an extremely chaotic situation. Disaster management may be examined in the following four phases[19]:

1. Prevention and planning
2. Preparedness
3. Response
4. Recovery/analysis

The prevention and planning phase includes the identification of specific hazards, threat assessments to life and property, and preemptive steps to minimize potential losses. The process of prevention and planning uses an effective application of the "hazard vulnerability analysis (HVA)." The HVA is a process for identifying natural and human-made hazards and the direct and indirect effect these hazards may have on an institution and/or community. Potential events are scrutinized using three categories: probability, risk, and preparedness. Probability is determined by analyzing the known direct risk, relevant historical data, and any additional pertinent statistics. The risk assessment defines potential totals among lives, property, and financial and legal stature. Finally, preparedness integrates the overall value of probability

and risk into a cohesive plan that dictates training requirements, contingency plans, and resource allocation. On completion, the HVA allows managers to consider common elements within preparedness procedures and to properly plan for an appropriate response to an overwhelming situation. Each community is tasked with the responsibility of preidentifying hazards and potential issues in the wake of a natural disaster. In general, communities are well aware of the potential natural disasters for which they are at risk, and they plan accordingly, although they often lack a "back-up plan" in case the first plan is thwarted (e.g., a tornado takes out the high school gym that was going to be used for a shelter). Most communities do not plan for the unusual disasters, and they do not plan well for the unforeseen disasters (e.g., mass shootings and other human-made disasters). The key to any disaster response is to plan and be prepared for anything. Community leaders (usually EMS leaders and elected officials) must start this very difficult conversation and engage experts in the field of disaster preparedness to assist with this planning and preparation. This preparedness ultimately reduces potential loss of life and property by lessening the impact of disasters, thus known as *disaster mitigation*. Mitigation measures also include public awareness campaigns, a keen eye by EMS and other health care personnel entering people's homes, and reporting of unusual circumstances, identification of flood zones, hurricane planning, and legislative action.

Preparedness encompasses the training and education of both public safety personnel and members of the community. In the United States, on a federal level, the Department of Health and Human Services (HHS) has specified the Office of Emergency Preparedness (OEP) as the lead agency for directing domestic preparedness efforts and creating standards for health and medical services with the Federal Response Plan. OEP also directs and manages a federally coordinated system known as the National Disaster Medical System (NDMS). The NDMS assists local and state authorities in dealing with the medical and health effects of a major disaster in the United States, by deploying teams to a disaster. Disaster Medical Assistance Teams (DMAT) and International Medical and Surgical Response Teams (IMSuRT) are deployable volunteer teams designed to respond to a major disaster, usually for 1 to 2 weeks at a time, supplementing local resources with high-quality medical care, despite the challenging environment found within disaster scenes. They are also used, at times, in advance of a disaster (hurricane), in assisting with patient evacuation. When a disaster occurs suddenly (more often the case), local EMS and resources must be self-sufficient for 72 hours because it often takes 48 to 72 hours to organize these large teams and arrange travel for them to a disaster area. Local DMAT personnel may be used to supplement health care personnel locally, until the federal response is complete, but this is not guaranteed. EMS personnel may be tasked with providing care outside their scope in more of a primary care role rather than their typical emergency-response capacity. This expansion of medical capabilities should be legislated ahead of time. Moreover, it requires the development of a strong relationship between EMS physicians, health care facilities, elected officials, and the EMS agencies themselves during the planning phase. The NDMS does ensure that teams are equipped to sustain operations for 72 hours without additional resources. EMS systems and personnel must also be equipped for and prepared to function for 24 to 48 hours, as major disaster scenes are rarely mitigated completely without a more significant time commitment.[20-22]

There are a number of federal resources available to educate individuals and communities on various disaster scenarios. One particular resource, *Emergency Responder Guidelines*, assists agencies in establishing a baseline understanding of the training necessary to respond safely and effectively to incidents involving the use of WMD. The guidelines provide an integrated compilation of baseline knowledge, skills, and responder capabilities for use as a reference by providers as well as course developers and trainers, to underscore the importance of interoperable response strategies. The *Emergency Responder Guidelines* specify training objectives and establish the baseline level of operational knowledge of three distinct levels of responsibility—awareness, performance, and management—required within specific response disciplines. Training is based on a provider's level of experience and operational accountability within the three levels of responsibility. Commonalities among specific response disciplines (e.g., law enforcement, fire, and EMS) illustrate areas in which common training and understanding can be established to ensure a more cohesive operational response.[23,24]

Awareness-level guidelines pertain to law enforcement officers, firefighters, and basic level EMTs. At a minimum, response personnel within this category are expected to be among the first to encounter an incident. Once management operations are under way, awareness-level personnel assume a supportive role. These providers are responsible for recognition and referral after encountering a hazardous environment. The training objectives establish a basic understanding of operational actions, including notification of need for additional specialized resources, maintenance of scene control, and demonstrated competence of self-protection measures.

Performance-level guidelines apply primarily to advanced-level providers on scene, including paramedics and firefighters involved in rescue or fire-suppression operations or a hazardous-materials event. Depending on the various ICS assignments in use during a given incident, the performance-level providers must efficiently multitask their primary responsibilities with additional assignments from their commander. Therefore, performance-level personnel require a strong working knowledge of the ICS and the ability to follow the Unified Command System (UCS). The provider must be able to follow procedures for the integration and implementation of each system and know how the two structures can be used to manage the incident. Procedures include establishing adequate communication capabilities to manage the incident, coordinating multiple responding agencies, and securing triage, treatment, and transport areas. The performance-level responder must also demonstrate competence in self-protection measures, rescue and decontamination operations, and evacuation procedures for managing victims.

Planning-level and management-level providers are typically service administrators, supervisors, and emergency management officials. Those who operate within these guidelines must first complete both awareness-level and performance-level objectives. Individuals responsible for training at this level will be a part of the leadership and management of subordinate emergency medical personnel during the response operation. Objectives include planning before the incident and managing resources used to conduct the event. Leadership personnel must also be capable of overseeing medical surveillance of subordinates.

The priority among EMS responders must be to render responsible prehospital care, while understanding that priorities in a disaster response are different from the everyday response. To enable this goal, responders must first drill using an ICS structure and be very familiar with this structure ahead of time. During any Mass Casualty Incident (MCI), ICS should be utilized and discussed afterward, so that larger incidents are seamless. During an actual disaster, an ICS (or equivalent system for international agencies) must be part of the response plan, to allow for effective management of any large-scale incident. During the response phase, multiple responders and agencies must be coordinated to operate effectively. A single commander must oversee the scene and coordinate all responding agencies (fire/rescue, EMS, and law enforcement). As the scale of an incident grows, the command structure must

be able to expand to meet the increasingly diverse needs, thus providing effective management. With large-scale incidents, the underlying organizational construct becomes even more critical while coordination extends to incorporate local, state, and federal resource allocation.

During the response phase in the United States, personnel must implement the ICS early and effectively. Regardless of location around the world, all responders on scene must be familiar with the structure and function of whatever plan is utilized locally. The ICS (or equivalent UCS) enables integrated communication by establishing a manageable span of control. Beneath a single incident commander (IC), subordinate commanders exercise their own span of control among context-specific divisions. In the United States, the overall structure of the system describes four divisions beneath the IC: operations, planning, logistics, and finance. With each application of the ICS, commanders may elect how to delegate these various designations among responders. The benefits of operating within the ICS structure include clearly defined roles for each responder; delegation of leadership responsibilities, which thus optimizes the ability of each officer to complete very specific tasks; and the ability to ensure that the fulfillment of every critical intervention is simplified. Triage, treatment, and transport are the highest priorities for most paramedics and emergency medical personnel, and specialized medical units with the necessary training and equipment may assume additional duties as directed by the IC.

Upon the arrival of additional local, state, federal, and private-party personnel, it is imperative that the ICS structure can be modified to accommodate the expanding operation. The concept of UC is to allow for expansion of the initial ICS structure while multiple ICs become involved with a large-scale incident. Members of the UC work together to develop a common set of incident objectives, produce strategies, share information, maximize the use of available resources, and enhance the efficiency of the individual response organizations.

The final phase of disaster management is the process of recovery/analysis. Initial and long-term recovery efforts are directed toward the reconstruction and rehabilitation of infrastructure and the community. EMS systems usually do not serve a primary role in recovery, but this final phase of management is critical for system reassessment and improvement. Analysis of specific methodologies used during incident management, including the efficacy of triage and predictive outcome assessments, is useful to the global community.[25] Initial recovery is the method by which an affected community is assisted in regaining a proper level of functioning after an incident. Long-term recovery addresses community-specific deficits of reconstruction and rehabilitation. EMS systems need to address their own logistical and psychological recovery so that they can return to a proper level of functioning after an incident. Specifically, equipment must be accounted for and repaired and, if necessary, any disposable supplies must be replaced and organized. A critical function of recovery within an EMS system must also account for responder well-being. "Critical Incident Stress Debriefing" (CISD) is an extremely important part of recovery because the mental anguish of family loss, personal loss, financial loss, and rescuer fatigue weighs on the individuals who have responded to the situation and may be victims themselves. It is not possible to resume normal operations if the infrastructure is not intact and ready to work toward full recovery. Additionally, this phase affords the EMS system the opportunity to engage in critical analysis of its own performance during the incident. The opportunity to engage in self-assessment is critical in identifying system weaknesses that may be targeted in future improvements, as well as to create the forum for commending personal actions that had a positive influence on the outcome of an incident. On completion, this analysis offers evidence supporting the use of specific methodologies.[26–29]

Analysis of significant incidents worldwide may offer some compelling data for analysis and educational opportunities concerning disaster management. There are many triage methods available and an obvious need for a uniform system, especially because international response is becoming more frequent, often adding to the chaos at times. Modeling triage methods based on the predictive value of anatomical scoring systems has revealed evidence-based, outcome-driven improvements in field triage and resource allocation. Significant analysis of the outcome among blunt and penetrating trauma patients provided the framework for the Sacco Triage Method, which has been well studied, with data from more than 100,000 trauma patients. Support for improvements in the management of disaster result comes only from effective analysis and evidence-based practice. Because of the globalization of health care and mitigation, the resulting data from events worldwide must be delivered in a useful format. Application of the Utstein template may be useful to ensure international value of data by standardizing terminology and significance. Originally created to classify data used to determine cardiac arrest survival rates and allow for international comparison of statistically similar events, the Utstein method has been applied to disaster outcomes recently. Applying sound epidemiological methods to patients after the incident management is critical to the reduction of empiricism within disaster medicine methodology.[30]

These key phases have defined the mitigation of crises of all sizes since their inception in the early 1970s. After the establishment of the DHS and ODP, both agencies issued guidelines for municipal, state, and federal responders within public safety. These guidelines, in conjunction with the serial reassessment of current practice methodologies, allow responders to ensure that the most appropriate management strategies have been selected for a given situation. Adhering to the use of this construct allows EMS systems to optimize their ability to react to disaster.[31,32]

⚠ PITFALLS

The role of EMS in a disaster is to provide responsible prehospital care to the unfortunate victims of the disaster, maximizing care to the most viable, and giving comfort to those who are doomed not to survive. In addition, EMS helps to bring a sense of order to a very chaotic situation. To facilitate this objective effectively, EMS personnel must be extremely familiar with ICS (or their own equivalent), regularly conduct drills using the system, and understand the concepts of triage in a disaster situation.

Responders who have familiarity with such massive, disruptive events understand the importance of preparing for any MCI, as well as the importance of drills. The emotional component is truly unimaginable unless the provider has had the unfortunate experience of responding to an incident and witnessing firsthand the mayhem that ensues while a scene unfolds. There is no way to recreate the panic and disruption that erupt in the wake of an actual disaster. The raw emotion is unmistakable. Despite this fact, drills are the most effective way of preparing for any MCI. It is unfortunate that widespread funding for states and communities in the United States for disaster preparation goes unused, and EMS agencies and communities continue to be inadequately prepared for mass casualty situations, failing to recognize preventable hazards and assuming a "not-in-my-backyard" attitude. Although it is assumed that the term *hazard vulnerability analysis* ought to be well understood by every leader in every community, it is still an anomaly to many. Inexperienced and unprepared EMS responders are unfortunately the majority, particularly concerning knowledge of what the "ICS" is and how it is applied. This failure in preparing leads to inadequate responses, poor treatment, increased chaos, increased mortality, and potentially further destruction of property. Finally, a well-prepared community

may find itself in a unique position of deterring someone from acting on a destructive thought in their community, if there is a perception that the response would be swift and overwhelming, with less destruction as a result.

The four phases of disaster preparedness and emergency management are often inadequately addressed. EMS systems need to prepare for major incidents, and so do hospitals and other health care facilities. Too often, health care facilities inadequately prepare for a disaster or put inexperienced people "in charge" of the committee. Many EMS systems and health care facilities operate at or near capacity on a daily basis, and they do not practice for a surge. In addition, many fail to participate in the planning process and/or to drill when asked. This leads to an entire jurisdiction that is ill prepared. Partnerships for patient transfers and supply requisition must be in place before any event. The different agencies (police, fire, DPH, EMS, hospital, etc.) must work in coordination with each other, and this can only be understood while they are made to work through scenarios by participating in drills and tabletop exercises.

EMS personnel could practice using the ICS system but often fail to do so. As a matter of practical familiarity, services should mandate the use of the ICS at every opportunity (small MCIs, specifically). The benefit to personnel at the awareness and performance levels becomes clear. With repeated use, the responders use the techniques with more certainty, regardless of incident size.

Worldwide, different systems have been implemented to fit the needs of each community, region, state, and nation. This lack of common practice and language leads to confusion and further chaos with respect to an international response, and it can lead to further morbidity and mortality for the unfortunate victims. Financially, many nations cannot afford to put a robust EMS system in place and often neglect this particular area of human services because they have issues that are more pressing, such as basic human needs, to worry about and attempt to fund. Discussions about funding for EMS are common, but follow-through continues to be an issue for many countries.

REFERENCES

1. Edwin Smith Papyrus, National Institute of Medicine Library, http://archive.nlm.nih.gov/proj/ttp/books.htm.
2. Clara B. *The Story of My Childhood*. World Digital Library. 1907. Retrieved 2013-10-09.
3. Sanders MJ. *Mosby's Paramedic Textbook*. Revised 2nd ed. St. Louis: Mosby; 2001, 2-13.
4. Committee on Trauma and Committee on Shock, Division of Medical Sciences, National Academy of Sciences, National Research Council. *Accidental Death and Disability: The Neglected Disease of Modern Society*. Washington DC: National Academy of Sciences; 1966.
5. Kouwenhoven WB, Jude JR, Knickerbocker GB. Closed chest cardiac massage. *JAMA*. 1960;173:1064.
6. Pantridge JF, Geddes JS. A mobile intensive care unit in the management of myocardial infarction. *Lancet*. 1966;1:807–808.
7. New York City Office of Emergency Management. Available at: http://www.ci.nyc.ny.us/html/oem/.
8. New York State Emergency Management Office. Available at: http://www.nysemo.state.ny.us/.
9. Simon R, Teperman S. The World Trade Center attack: lessons for disaster management. *Crit Care*. 2001;5:318–320.
10. US Department of Labor, Occupational Safety and Health Administration. Incident Command System eTool. Available at: http://www.osha.gov/SLTC/etools/ics/nrs.html.
11. National Interagency Management System. Available at: http://www.niims.net/.
12. US Department of Homeland Security. Available at: http://www.dhs.gov/dhspublic/.

13. Cuny FC. Principles of disaster management lesson 1: introduction. *Prehospital Disaster Med.* 1998;13(1):88–92.

14. Tintinalli JE, Cameron P, Holliman J. International Federation for Emergency Medicine; *EMS: A Practical Global Guidebook* 2010.

15. Al-Shaqsi S. Models of International Emergency Medical Service (EMS) Systems. *Oman Med J.* 2010;25(4):320–323.

16. Dick WF. Anglo-American vs. Franco-German emergency medical services system. *Prehosp Disaster Med.* 2003;18(1):29–35, discussion 35–37.

17. Pan American Health Organization. *Emergency Medical Services Systems. Lessons learned from the United States of America for Developing Countries* [Holtermann K-e, ed.]. Washington DC: PAHO HQ Library Cataloguing-in-publication; 2003.

18. Sasser S, Varghese M, Kellermann A, et al. *Prehospital Trauma Care Systems.* WHO; 2005.

19. de Boer J. Order in chaos: modeling medical management in disasters. *Eur J Emerg Med.* 1999;6(2):141–148.

20. Roth PB, Gaffney JK. The Federal Response Plan and Disaster Medical Assistance Teams in domestic disasters. *Emerg Med Clin North Am.* 1996;14:371–382.

21. US Department of Homeland Security, National Disaster Medical System. Available at: http://www.ndms.dhhs.gov/.

22. US Department of Homeland Security. Initial National Response Plan. Available at: http://www.dhs.gov/interweb/assetlibrary/Initial_NRP_100903.pdf .

23. Office of Domestic Preparedness. *Emergency Responder Guidelines;* 2002, 2002, Washington DC.

24. US Department of Homeland Security, Federal Emergency Management Agency. Available at: http://www.fema.gov/.

25. Abrahams J. Disaster management in Australia: the national emergency management system. *Emerg Med (Fremantle).* 2001;13(2):165–173.

26. Weddle M, Prado-Monje H. Utilization of military support in the response to hurricane Marilyn: implications for future military-civilian cooperation. *Prehospital Disaster Med.* 1999;14(2):81–86.

27. Holsenbeck LS. Joint Task Force Andrew: the 44th Medical Brigade mental health staff officer's after action review. *Mil Med.* 1994;159 (3):186–191.

28. Johnson WP, Lanza CV. After hurricane Andrew. An EMS perspective. *Prehospital Disaster Med.* 1993;8(2):169–171.

29. Branas CC, Sing RD, Perron AD. A case series analysis of mass casualty incidents. *Prehosp Emerg Care.* 2000;4(4):299–304.

30. Task Force on Quality Control of Disaster Management. Health disaster management: guidelines for evaluation and research in the Utstein style. Volume 17. *Prehospital Disaster Med.* 2003;17(suppl 3):1–177.

31. Becker B. Disaster management: problems and solutions. *RI Med J.* 1991;74 (8):383–389.

32. Alson RA, Alexander D, Leonard RD, Stringer LW. Analysis of medical treatment at a field hospital following hurricane Andrew. *Ann Emerg Med.* 1994;22(11):726–730.

Role of Emergency Medicine in Disaster Management

Richard E. Wolfe

Emergency medicine (EM) is optimally suited to lead the health care response in the hours following a disaster. By routinely providing the front line of hospital care for acutely ill and injured patients, regardless of the underlying characteristics of the pathology or the patient, emergency providers can adapt quickly to the changing conditions brought on by a mass casualty incident. In addition to having broad expertise in response to various types of emergencies, EM providers manage patient-volume surges routinely. Thus, when confronted with mass casualty incidents, they have less of a transition to make in their practice compared with any other specialist.[1]

Following a disaster, physician leaders and frontline care providers will need a wide variety of skills and knowledge to deliver care and manage resources. These may differ from one disaster to another, involving an understanding of triage of mass casualties, decontamination, resuscitation, trauma, infectious disease, hypothermia, toxicology, and management of radiation poisoning. In addition, the physician leader in a disaster must know how to interface with incident-command systems, community resources, and regional assets. Most of these skills are already integral to the practice of EM. Emergency physicians thus commonly assume a leadership role in the immediate aftermath of a disaster.

Emergency departments (EDs) serve as the key interface between the community and the hospital system. The role of the ED is to triage patients on arrival to the health care facility, and then stabilize and disposition patients to their next stage of care, which may be to an inpatient setting, an outpatient setting, or another health care facility. The basic role remains unchanged in a disaster, but the methods by which it is executed change, based on the nature and extent of the disaster and the resources available to the ED.

The definition of the word *disaster* is highly subjective. A number of papers have tried to develop a standard nomenclature that would cover events ranging from a contained mass casualty incident to a catastrophe that knocks out most of the health care system.[2,3] For the purpose of this chapter, a *disaster* will be viewed as a mass casualty incident in which the health care resources are overwhelmed and outside help is required. When properly managed in this situation, the ED expands its capacity to the limit, using hospital resources for added staffing and space, thus modifying triage prioritization to ensure the highest survival rate. Once saturated, outside resources are needed to allow the ED to be bypassed, but this role is then delegated to other emergency facilities, in the field or at remote hospitals.

By processing patients with acute illness and injuries from stabilization to disposition, the performance of the ED will be a major determinant of survival; however, this is dependent on the skills of the health care providers who staff the emergency department and the design of the ED itself. To define the role of EM in disasters fully, the role of emergency providers and that of the facility must be considered. EM providers not only deliver emergency care but also oversee prehospital care, as well as engage in leadership roles in disaster preparedness and study ways to improve outcomes following a disaster. As an example, ED data can be used in disease detection and surveillance as an early warning system to an impending pandemic.[4] Because of their unique knowledge of the prehospital world, hospital leadership, and the other medical specialties, EM providers play an integral part in communications during a disaster and in the delivery of the initial care.

Finally, in disasters, care and resources must be rationed. Under normal conditions, EM providers prioritize access to inpatient beds and diagnostic studies. This gatekeeper role is expanded in a disaster when rationing rather than prioritization is necessary.[5]

HISTORICAL PERSPECTIVE

To understand how the role of EM adapts to disaster management, it is helpful to review the development and evolution of the entire public health infrastructure, and, in particular, the specialty of EM (Box 4-1).

EDs grew rapidly along with hospital-based medicine after World War II.[6] Available staffing was driven by financial incentives because of fee-for-service reimbursement. Complaints about the quality of care and threat of liability because of inadequate staffing motivated hospitals to recruit physicians with some EM experience. With improved care and financial success, these early EDs evolved rapidly from part-time coverage by physicians without specialized training to 24-hour coverage by residency-trained, board-certified emergency physicians. The highly specialized knowledge and skills these doctors came to possess allowed EDs to dramatically expand their scope of practice, to diagnose and manage a wide range of problems, and to serve as gatekeepers for inpatient care.[7] With the growth in scope and competency, EDs became increasingly complex and versatile. A victim of this success, hospitals began allowing crowding of EDs by inpatient borders, patients who were admitted but for whom there was not an available hospital bed. This practice allowed for maximum occupancy of the inpatient services and strong operational performance without overstraining the inpatient staff. However, it resulted in growing dysfunction in the ED. The Institute of Medicine report described emergency care in 2007 as an "overburdened, underfunded and highly fragmented" system of emergency care.[8] The strain seen routinely in many tertiary centers could pose a significant liability in preparing the ED to receive victims from a disaster.[9]

By 1976, the American College of Emergency Physicians (ACEP) published a position paper on the role of the emergency physician in mass casualty and disaster management.[10] This policy was later approved (1985), reaffirmed (1997), and revised and expanded (2000). (See Box 4-2 for the full policy statement.) In this policy, "ACEP believes that emergency physicians should assume a primary role in the medical aspects of disaster planning, management, and patient care."

BOX 4-1   Timeline of Developmental and Sentinel Events

YEAR	EVENT
6 AD	The Corps of Vigiles: first professional fire service established
13th century	England: fire protection insurance becomes available
1666	Great Fire of 1666 in London; changes that took place after this disaster resulted in the model of today's fire service
1798	Marine Hospital Service created (later to become the Public Health Service)
1917	Influenza pandemic
1931	Flood in China
1932	Famine in Soviet Union
1953	U.S. Department of Health, Education, and Welfare (cabinet level)
1954	Volcanic eruption in Colombia
1961	Alexandria Plan: first full-time emergency physicians
1966	*Accidental Death and Disability* report by the National Academy of Sciences/National Research Council
1968	Foundation of ACEP established
1973	Emergency medical services created
1976	ABEM created
1979	Emergency medicine recognized as a medical specialty; Federal Emergency Management Agency formed; FIRESCOPE and Incident Command started; Public Health Service is moved to Department of Health and Human Services
1983	Critical incident stress debriefing begins
1988	ACEP forms Section of Disaster Medicine
1991	National Fire Protection Association begins standard development
1992	Hurricane Andrew
1993	World Trade Center attack
1995	Oklahoma City Bombing
1999	Federal Response Plan
2000	Disaster Mitigation Act of 2000
2001	Joint Commission on Accreditation of Health Care Organizations, standards for preparedness change; Sept. 11 attacks at the World Trade Center, Pentagon, and in Pennsylvania; Anthrax attacks
2002	Passage of the Homeland Security Act
2003	Homeland Security Presidential Directive/HSPD-5 calls for a National Incident Management System (NIMS) and a National Response Plan (NRP); Department of Homeland Security established
2004 (November)	States must file to qualify for predisaster hazard-mitigation funds; threat assessments completed
2010	Earthquake in Haiti
2012	Aurora Shooting
2013	Boston Marathon Bombing

From Bern AI. Role of emergency medicine in disaster management. In Ciottone GR, ed. *Disaster Medicine*. Philadelphia: Elsevier Mosby; 2006:26-33.

BOX 4-2   ACEP Policy Statement: Disaster Medical Services

The American College of Emergency Physicians (ACEP) believes that emergency physicians should assume a primary role in the medical aspects of disaster planning, management, and patient care. Because the provision of effective disaster medical services requires prior training or experience, emergency physicians should pursue training that will enable them to fulfill this responsibility.

A medical disaster occurs when the destructive effects of natural or human-made forces overwhelm the ability of a given area or community to meet the demand for health care.

Disaster planning, testing, and response are multidisciplinary activities that require cooperative interaction. Each agency or individual contributes unique capabilities, perspectives, and experiences. Within this context, emergency physicians share the responsibility for ensuring an effective and well-integrated disaster response.

Emergency medical services and disaster medical services share the goal of optimal acute health care; however, in achieving that goal, the two systems use different approaches. Emergency medical services routinely direct maximal resources to a small number of individuals, while disaster medical services are designed to direct limited resources to the greatest number of individuals. Disasters involving the intentional or accidental release of biological, chemical,

radiological, or nuclear agents present an extremely difficult community planning and response challenge. In addition, they may produce a far greater number of secondary casualties and deaths than conventional disasters. Because the medical control of emergency medical services is within the domain of emergency medicine, it remains the responsibility of emergency physicians to provide both direct patient care and medical control of out-of-hospital emergency medical services during disasters.

Improvement of established disaster management methods requires the integration of data from research and experience. Emergency physicians must use their skills in organization, education, and research to incorporate these improvements as new concepts and technologies emerge.

Where local, regional, and national disaster networks exist, emergency physicians should participate in strengthening them. Where they are not yet functional, emergency physicians should assist in planning and implementing them.

This policy statement was prepared by the Emergency Medical Services Committee. It was approved by the ACEP Board of Directors June 2000. It replaces one with the same title originally approved by the ACEP Board of Directors June 1985 and reaffirmed by the ACEP Board of Directors March 1997.

Reproduced with permission from American College of Emergency Physicians. Disaster medical services. *Ann Emerg Med.* 2001;38:198-199.

It also called for emergency physicians to participate in "local, regional, and national disaster networks." The University Association of Emergency Medicine echoed the call for training in disaster medicine and further called for the development of fellowship training in disaster medicine.[11] ACEP also was an advocate for emergency physician participation in the "development of comprehensive plans developed by communities" to cope with disasters, and of the National Disaster Medical System, through disaster medical assistance team (DMAT) participation (1985, revised 1999).[12] The ACEP Section of Disaster Medicine was formed in 1988. Through continued involvement and advocacy of disaster medicine, section members are participating on many levels: joining DMATs, researching and writing, and participating in educational conferences and hospital and community emergency management.

CURRENT PRACTICE

Role of Emergency Medicine Specialists

During a disaster, at the very least, emergency physicians will be expected to play a role in providing triage, emergency stabilization, and disposition of disaster victims. These basic responsibilities have led many academic emergency physicians to adopt disaster medicine as an area of expertise. They study these events to predict outcomes and improve future responses. They teach disaster preparedness, from the level of the medical school to international professional meetings. With this expertise, they often become leaders in preparing for regional and national disasters. At the time of a disaster, they often assume roles as incident commander or chief medical officer. Routine work in the ED puts EM providers into professional contact with the key specialties needed in disasters, as well as administration and nursing leadership. Emergency physicians are thus ideally suited to act as system integrators, allowing easy communication within the hospital and the prehospital sector.

The various roles of the emergency position are shown in Figure 4-1. The figure identifies nine potential interactions within the system. When a disaster strikes, emergency physicians will need to assume the roles identified as two through five, even if they possess only the basic knowledge of disaster management.

The on-duty emergency physician must provide leadership to his or her department, hospital, EM services, and community. The emergency physician's duties will depend on specific "job actions," defined through the hospital's Incident Command System (a standard required by The Joint Commission in the United States)[13] and the disaster plan implemented by the hospital. One model is the hospital emergency incident command system (HEICS).[14] The HEICS provides a flexible and expandable command structure that does not rely on specific individuals. It is ubiquitous in the fire service, EM services, military, and police agencies, thus allowing for ease of communication during event management.

Emergency physicians play a key role in disaster preparedness training and research. Disaster medicine has evolved as a subspecialty of EM, and emergency physicians with specialized training now provide much of the leadership in public health planning for disaster. Emergency physicians are also key participants in developing training modules for health care providers and in publishing studies about disasters to expand knowledge and develop new approaches to improve survival.

Role of the ED in a Disaster

The surge capacity and scope of practice of EDs vary immensely from one ED to another. Differences in rural and urban EDs and between the role and the scope of practice of EDs between countries can be striking. The location of a disaster as much as the type of disaster will have a huge influence on the ability of the EDs to improve the overall outcome of victims.

Beyond its primary role as a site for providing care, EDs routinely deliver a wide variety of additional services to other "clients," including patients' families, referring physicians, specialty consultants, hospitals, public health agencies, and society at large. EDs provide a source of reliable information for the media and state legislature about emergent health care issues. This role in public health communication continues during a disaster. EDs also serve as a safety net for the health care of patients with limited access to routine primary care, and as observation and holding units to protect inpatient beds.[6]

As the only effective connectors between the prehospital sector and hospitals, almost all of the victims of a mass casualty incident who are not pronounced dead at the scene will pass through the ED. EM providers are used to making creative use of space and resources and dealing with the unexpected. Many EDs have the ability to flex up capacity of care rapidly and to be ready to receive multiple casualties in less than an hour after being notified of the incident. The staff of the departments of EM also provides a reserve of specialized human resources ideally suited for the initial management of victims. The daily experience of

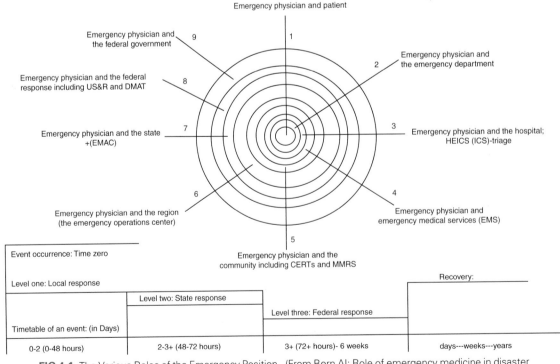

FIG 4-1 The Various Roles of the Emergency Position. (From Bern AI: Role of emergency medicine in disaster management. In: Ciottone GR, ed. *Disaster Medicine*. Philadelphia: Elsevier Mosby, 2006, pp 26-33.)

managing unstable patients with little or no prior information or warning makes the EM physicians ideally suited to act as the front line for stabilization and triage of disaster victims.

The ability of an ED to perform appropriately following a mass casualty incident is based on many factors. These include the total possible patient-care space available, the preparation and training of the EM providers, the support of the hospital, the skills of the leadership following the disaster, the resources available, and the strength and training of the security. Because of economic difficulties, hospitals routinely have insufficient inpatient beds to deal with routine workloads, which results in low prioritization of access to inpatient beds of emergency patients, leading to overcrowding and prolonged boarding of patients in the ED. Overcrowded EDs have much greater problems in flexing up capacity rapidly in the event of a mass casualty incident. Because of this, one key element in preparation for disaster is the creation of processes that can be triggered following a mass casualty incident to rapidly clear ED care spaces and free up providers for the incoming patients of the mass casualty incident. Models of this process have been developed to deal with overcrowded EDs when diversion is not an option.[15]

When building a new ED, consideration about surge capacity in a disaster should be a factor in the design.[12]

Decontamination sites, rooms with negative airflow, single patient bays that can be easily converted into multipatient-care areas, and non-patient-care areas that can be transformed into "field" patient-care areas at very short notice are all examples of ways a well-designed ED will facilitate the response to a disaster.

ORGANIZATION OF THE EMERGENCY DEPARTMENT DURING A DISASTER

In the setting of disasters and mass casualty incidents, the ability of EDs to perform depends on the severity of the disaster, resources and surge capacity of the physical plants, training and organization of the medical staff at each site, and coordination of the health care network to transport the most critical patients to the EDs rapidly and distribute these to optimize the resources.

Although disasters are a global phenomenon, the organization of emergency care is highly variable from one country to the next. There are differences in the approach to disaster management in the United States when compared with those in the rest of the world. The United States arguably has the most developed and robust network of EDs per capita. Besides the national differences in staffing and resources, the differences in disaster management might be due to the nature of historical disasters in the United States. Loss of life from disasters was substantially less in the United States before 1987. The death toll of disasters between 1865 and 1928 did not exceed 1000 victims in any disaster.[11] The one notable exception is the pandemic of 1918, in which more than 600,000 lives were lost and health care resources were completely overwhelmed. This low number of disasters is contrasted by events that have occurred in the rest of the world. The Soviet Union famine in 1932 left 5 million dead. A 1931 flood in the Republic of China resulted in the death of 3.7 million. A November 13, 1985, volcanic eruption in Colombia resulted in the death of 21,800.[16] More than 200,000 were killed in the tsunami of Southeast Asia, in December 2004. Estimates of the number of deaths during the earthquake in Haiti in 2010 exceed 100,000, and the Haitian government claims that the number is greater than 300,000.[17] Although the mortality was on a completely different scale, the 2996 deaths from the bombings in New York and Washington, DC, on September 11, 2001, were a catalyst for the United States to work aggressively on disaster management, leading to far more sophisticated preparedness in the country's EDs.

As one of the first countries to recognize EM nationally, the majority of EDs are staffed with board-certified emergency physicians who train, participate in planning, and often have experience in mass casualty incidents. Further, EM residency curriculums incorporate comprehensive disaster management as a basic part of training a specialist.[18] At present, more than 200 residencies graduate in excess of 2000 specialists a year. U.S. EDs have developed substantial capacity and resources to deal with surges in patients. The surge capacity available in the United States may only be exceeded by Israel where entire facilities are mothballed, to be ready for use in case of an overwhelming disaster. This combination of highly trained providers and extensive resources at close proximity places urban American and to a certain extent urban European EDs on the far end of the spectrum when compared with facilities in third world countries or in rural areas.

When planning for disasters, existing resources, training of the local EM staff, and the possible effects of different types of disaster events must be factored in. When preparing to receive multiple victims from a mass casualty incident, initially, lack of information and rumors make it difficult to anticipate the number and types of victims that will soon be arriving. One must therefore assume the worst-case scenario and prepare the ED to receive the largest number of patients possible, anticipating for all levels of acuity.

Unless the prehospital systems are extremely well organized and the casualties limited, the ED is often inundated with low-acuity patients before the more critical patients arrive. An additional problem following a terrorist mass casualty incident is the risk of the secondary attack on the health care facilities. A natural response for all of the hospital's health providers on hearing the news of an event is to come to the hospital to help. The natural point of gathering for these providers is often the ED, and, if not controlled, this can create confusion and delay by having the patient-care area impaired by providers and administrators without a designated role. It is critically important to mitigate for this risk by setting up robust security to control access to the ED.

Scene safety is the first rule in the prehospital setting, and it applies to the ED during mass casualty events. Security, assisted by triage officers, needs to ensure scene safety by preventing secondary assaults on the ED. Based on the type of disaster, checkpoints may be needed to screen for radioactivity, contain the spread of biological agents, and manage family members and the press.

The on-duty emergency physician, assisted by the resource nurse, will need to provide the initial leadership in organizing the department and the needed interface with the rest of the hospital, EMS, and the community. The hospital's disaster plan should clearly define specific roles for all providers, the organization of leadership structure during a disaster, and the steps to ensure adequate supplies, food, and communication. The Joint Commission requires that the hospital have an incident-command system (ICS) to be implemented in the event of a disaster. The ICS will help define the specific role of the emergency providers in the ED. The ICS should include the following steps:

- Identify the physician and nursing leadership in the department and the basic reporting structure for the disaster
- Appoint a liaison with the hospital Emergency Operations Center
- Implement the security plan for the ED rapidly

Because of the risks to the facility during terrorist events or with breakdown of the social order, security must change the usual procedures to protect the facility aggressively.[5] It may be helpful if sufficient numbers of health care providers are available, to assign some of the staff to assist security with initial screening of patients, families, and volunteers. Directing these different groups to reception and staging areas is a critical role to protect the organization of emergency care and to manage human resources.

Initiate Procedures for Clearing Emergency Department Care Space for Incoming Patients

The care space of the ED might become critically important, and freeing up space and personnel for the incoming disaster victims is essential. Patients awaiting admission to a patient bed should be moved to the inpatient hallways, even if the bed is not ready. Elective admissions and surgeries should be canceled to create inpatient space. Low-acuity admissions should be discharged rapidly once life threats have been ruled out. It may be helpful to identify specific providers, such as case managers, to create space by finding solutions for the disposition of existing ED patients. Psychiatrists may be recruited to work to move psychiatric emergencies to a mental health facility.

Set Up a Decontamination Area

Set up of the decontamination area is based on the type of disaster. It is critical when there is a threat of radiation, biological, or nerve agent attack. Moreover, it is critical to protect the ED from becoming a secondary disaster site. Plans of where and how to execute this function should be part of any hospital disaster plan.

Establishing Zones and Health Care Teams

The providers designated to be among the frontline caregivers in the ED should be organized into small health care teams, similar to trauma resuscitation teams. These teams should be zoned geographically to receive patients in a focused area of the department after triage. By having providers focus on a limited number of patients, there is less risk that anyone will be overwhelmed by the chaos and horror of a disaster. Overall performance can be enhanced, and patient and provider time optimized. The providers can generally preserve the normal patient-physician relationship. Therefore they are less likely to run into ethical problems created by rationing because their patients have already undergone triage to determine if they should receive the available resources. This team approach might also help mitigate the psychological problems that providers might experience following disasters.

Assess Functionality of Emergency Department Tracking Systems for the Impending Disaster

To prevent added confusion and distraction, shutting off electronic systems and moving to a paper-based system may be necessary. Most Emergency Department Information Systems (EDIS) today are not designed to handle mass casualties.[19] However, newer EDIS may have disaster modules that would be able to handle the surge and facilitate patient identification and tracking. New developments in ways to use the Internet and advanced "smart devices" have the potential to improve vastly the EM response to such mass casualty incident disasters through the use of specially designed EDIS.[20] Awareness of the limits and potential of the existing EDIS is essential before victims arrive, to ensure the best approach to tracking.

Alert and Organize Registration for the Incoming Victims

Patient identification and tracking are critical in avoiding errors of misidentification. Methods to accomplish this might be as high tech as EDIS systems designed to perform during disasters or as simple as medical tags or felt-tipped pen notes written directly on the patient's forehead or limbs. Registration staff should both be trained as part of the ED disaster team and positioned to collect the needed patient identifiers at the time of triage of victims.

Organize Specialty Services in the Emergency Department

Certain types of specialists may be needed in the ED to support stabilization of disaster victims. In disasters resulting in massive numbers of trauma victims, Acute Care Surgery (ACS) and Orthopedics should be alerted and called in to provide support. The ACS service should take the lead in creating a Disaster Care Service that will oversee all inpatient care of the disaster victims. The ACS service should also be charged with coordinating the ED and the OR to optimize flow and access for surgical patients. Specialty surgical services such as neurosurgery, ENT, and ophthalmology will also be critical in disasters that result in massive numbers of trauma victims. Psychiatry may play a critical role in the second phase of the disaster with not only the patients but also families and providers, in preventing posttraumatic stress disorder (PTSD). Assistance from other specialties and physicians can also be critically helpful in the early phase in helping to clear the ED to create the needed space to receive the casualties.

Management of Volunteer Providers

A common problem that occurs in the ED in the immediate aftermath of a disaster is the confusion created by the arrival of great numbers of health care volunteers. Many providers will arrive at the ED seeking to help. These volunteers may have useful skills. In particular, those credentialed at the institution and that have participated in drills may be easily incorporated into the health care teams. These providers can also serve as workforce reserves. However, a number of volunteers lack the skill and knowledge to be effective participants.[21]

The ED tends to be a natural gathering point of volunteers. The sheer number can quickly overcrowd the department, creating added confusion and dysfunction at the most inopportune time. The phenomenon of convergent volunteerism, defined as the arrival of unexpected or uninvited personnel wishing to render aid at the scene of a large-scale emergency incident, occurs in the ED, as well as at the scene of a disaster. Volunteers without a prior relationship with the ED or the institution represent a particularly difficult problem because a disaster, by definition, requires outside help. These providers may have useful skills and could potentially serve as a source of labor. However, it may be difficult to verify their credentials with the timeframe and resources available. Further, after a terrorist attack, there is a risk of infiltration of health care facilities by dangerous individuals masquerading as health care providers, with the facility serving as a secondary target.

The inverse problem occurs if the medical staff does not respond following a disaster, often because they themselves have been injured.[22-24] Unlike convergent volunteerism, failure of the medical staff to report in the hours following a disaster creates critical shortage of qualified personnel. When planning the ED response to a disaster, previsions must be taken to determine how to recruit providers if the workload exceeds the available staffing.[25] Hospital disaster plans may need to plan a call-out list to reach providers rapidly, while factoring in that cell phone networks may be shut down both because of the disaster or to prevent further detonation of bombs.

WHEN THE NUMBER OF VICTIMS BEGINS TO WIND DOWN

Emergency providers are at risk of acute stress disorders, depression, or PTSD after caring for disaster victims.[26] After the patients have all been processed or when a provider needs to be taken off duty, have someone debrief the retiring physician or nurse. This step may identify resource shortages and specific problems linked to the disaster. It may also help prevent PTSD or identify providers who are at risk and should be referred for counseling. This support is also appreciated by most providers, and it helps reinforce the team mentality and the value of the care provided. All providers should be reminded of the rules around patient confidentiality. Moreover, the rules should be emphasized to prevent breaches in social media or when being interviewed by the media.

Emergency Medicine Preparedness and Training for Disasters

Good, simple response plans can be developed for complex clinical scenarios. Local experts are best suited to design these and to evaluate ED readiness. Clinicians can be trained to follow these plans, if they are trained by *realistic* drills. These drills, which are required by regulatory and certifying bodies, take time and money and thus require government funding.[27,28]

The available evidence is insufficient to determine whether training health care providers in disaster preparedness is effective in improving knowledge and skills. Nonetheless, both disaster preparedness and appropriate disaster training for health care providers remain important national and professional priorities.[29]

Emergency physicians often serve as educators for the prehospital personnel. When training for disasters, reinforcing concepts during training such as the use of field tourniquets can profoundly affect survival rates following disasters with limb injuries, such as earthquakes and blast injuries. Team training with EMS providers can help enhance the interface between the prehospital sector and the ED.

The majority of the EM staff of most urban hospitals in the United States is residency trained or board certified in EM. At baseline, these providers will have had some training in disaster management during residency or as part of continuous medical education. They will also have good grounding in how to prepare rapidly for mass casualties, how to triage a wide variety of disaster-related presentations, and how to stabilize patients following various disasters. In 2001 the Model of the Clinical Practice of Emergency Medicine was created through the collaboration of the six largest U.S. EM organizations. This EM model provided an integrated and representative presentation of the Core Content of Emergency Medicine, and it has been updated annually. In terms of disaster management, EM specialists are expected to "understand and apply the principles of disaster and mass casualty management, including preparedness, triage, mitigation, response, and recovery."[30] This requirement is incorporated into the curriculum of training programs and in the questions asked during board examinations.

Additional training is also needed to ensure that providers have comprehensive knowledge of the types of injuries based on mechanisms seen during different disasters that are not part of routine practice. Examples include the clinical signs and treatment of cholinergic agents, pulmonary injuries secondary to blasts, the risk of penetrating trauma from shrapnel, and the types of radiation poisoning specifically seen with dirty bombs.

The ethics of patient care and the principles of triage may also be modified during a disaster, because care must be rationed to those who might benefit most, to provide for the best outcome for the largest number. This requires breaking free from the logic used at triage when there is a surplus of resources. During normal times, choices are made for prioritization rather than rationing.[2] During a disaster, however, decision making must be shifted to determine who will have access to limited resources. This determination requires that the providers are aware of the resources available and are able to ration resources to optimize the highest survival rate; such decision making can run counter to the physicians' ethical code, which focuses on striving for maximum benefit for each individual patient. Without guidelines, education, and drills, critical errors can be made during a disaster through waste of time and resources.

CONCLUSION

EM has a critical role in the early management of victims in a disaster. EM providers must be prepared to meet the challenge through education and drills. The ED, too, must be well prepared, from its design to the response the minutes before the arrival of victims, and at every level, to ensure the "greatest good for the greatest number."

❗ PITFALLS

- Delay in implementing security measures to protect the facility and organize flow of patients, families, and volunteers
- Failure to set up a decontamination site in disasters with risk of radiation, biological contagion, or nerve agents
- Lack of drills and training of the medical staff for various types of disasters
- Failure to plan for the failure or needed shutdown of EDIS tracking
- Failure to establish a reliable communication with the hospital EOC
- Poor organization and planning of how to manage volunteers
- Failure to address mental health needs of providers following a disaster
- Failure to educate and remind providers about Health Insurance Portability and Accountability Act (HIPAA) rules following a mass casualty event

REFERENCES

1. Dennis AJ, Brandt MM, Steinberg J, et al. Are general surgeons behind the curve when it comes to disaster preparedness training? A survey of general surgery and emergency medicine trainees in the United States by the Eastern Association for the Surgery for Trauma Committee on Disaster Preparedness. *J Trauma Acute Care Surg.* 2012;73(3):612–617.
2. de Boer J. Definition and classification of disasters: introduction of a disaster severity scale. *J Emerg Med.* 1990;8:591–595.
3. Koenig KL, Dinerman N, Kuehl AE. Disaster nomenclature—a functional impact approach: the PICE system. *Acad Emerg Med.* 1996;3(7):723–727.
4. American College of Emergency Physicians. Positioning America's emergency health care system to respond to acts of terrorism: report of the Terrorism Response Task Force. Available at: http://www.acep.org/webportal/PracticeResources/issues/disasters/masscas.
5. Hick JL, Hanfling D, Cantrill SV. Allocating scarce resources in disasters: emergency department principles. *Ann Emerg Med.* 2012;59(3):177–187.
6. Kellermann AL, Martinez R. The ER, 50 years on. *N Engl J Med.* 2011;364 (24):2278–2279.
7. Morganti KG, Bauhoff S, Blanchard JC, et al. *The Evolving Role of Emergency Departments in the United States.* Research Report, The Rand Corporation; 2013. Available at, http://www.rand.org/pubs/research_reports/RR280.html.
8. Institute of Medicine. Hospital-based emergency care: at the breaking point. *Consensus Report.* 2007.
9. Reeder TJ, Garrison HG. When the safety net is unsafe: real-time assessment of the overcrowded emergency department. *Acad Emerg Med.* 2001;8 (11):1070–1074.
10. The role of the emergency physician in mass casualty/disaster management. ACEP position paper. *JACEP.* 1976;5(11):901–902.
11. Auf der Heide E. *Disaster Response: The Principles of Preparation and Coordination.* St Louis: Mosby; 1989.
12. Wagner SK. Disaster preparedness. D.C. medical center unveils mass casualty design concepts. *Hosp Health Netw.* 2008;82(5):22.
13. Joint Commission Accreditation. *Comprehensive Accreditation Manual 2014: Standards of Elements of Performance Scoring Accreditation Policies (Comprehensive Accreditation Manual for Hospitals).* Publications and Education, Lslf ed. Oakbrook Terrace, Illinois: Joint Commission Resources; December 2013.
14. Zane RD, Prestipino AL. Implementing the hospital emergency incident command system: an integrated delivery system's experience. *Prehosp Disaster Med.* 2004;19(4):311–317.
15. Burke LG, Joyce N, Baker WE, et al. The effect of an ambulance diversion ban on emergency department length of stay and ambulance turnaround time. *Ann Emerg Med.* 2013;61(1):303–311.

16. The Disaster Center. The most deadly 100 natural disasters of the 20th century. Available at: http://www.disastercenter.com/disaster/TOP100K.html.

17. Weiner T. Floods bring more suffering to a battered Haitian town. *N Y Times.* May 29, 2004.

18. Allison EJ, Aghababian RV, Barsan WG, et al. Core content for emergency medicine. *Ann Emerg Med.* 1997;29(6):791–811.

19. Genes N, Chary M, Chason KW. An academic medical center's response to widespread computer failure. *J Disast Med.* 2013;8(2):145–150.

20. Chan TC, Killeen J, Griswold W, et al. Information technology and emergency medical care during disasters. *Acad Emerg Med.* 2004;11 (11):1229–1236.

21. Hodge JG, Gable LA, Calvews SH. Volunteer health professionals and emergencies: assessing and transforming the legal environment. *Biosecur Bioterr.* 2005;3(3):216–223.

22. Ukai T. The great Hanshin-Awaji earthquake and the problems with emergency medical care. *Ren Fail.* 1997;19:633–645.

23. Waeckerle JF. Disaster planning and response. *N Engl J Med.* 1991;324:815–821.

24. Uemoto M, Inui A, Kasuga M, Shindo S, Taniguchi H. Medical staff suffered severe stress after earthquake in Kobe, Japan. *BMJ.* 1996;313:1144.

25. Chen WK, Cheng YC, Ng KC, et al. Were there enough physicians in an emergency department in the affected area after a major earthquake? An analysis of the Taiwan Chi-Chi earthquake in 1999. *Ann Emerg Med.* 2001;38(5):556–561.

26. Fullerton CS, Ursano RJ, Wang L. Acute stress disorder, posttraumatic stress disorder, and depression in disaster or rescue workers. *Am J Psychiatry.* 2004;161:1370–1376.

27. Burstein JL. Smoke and shadows: measuring hospital disaster preparedness. *Ann Emerg Med.* 2008;52(3):230–231.

28. Goldberg LA, Hourvitz A, Amsalem A, et al. Lessons learned from clinical anthrax drills: evaluation of knowledge and preparedness for a bioterrorist threat in Israeli emergency departments. *Ann Emerg Med.* 2006;48 (2):194–199.

29. Williams J, Nocera M, Casteel C. The effectiveness of disaster training for health care workers: a systematic review. *Ann Emerg Med.* 2008;52 (3):211–222.

30. Chapman DM, Hayden S, Sanders AB, et al. Integrating the accreditation council for graduate medical education core competencies into the model of the clinical practice of emergency medicine. *Ann Emerg Med.* 2004;43 (6):756–769.

CHAPTER 5

Disaster Nursing

Kristin Allyce Reed and Amelia Marie Nelson

Nurses, as an integral part and the largest component of the health care team, must be prepared for disaster situations. Disasters occur all over the world, sometimes with warning and sometimes without, making it even more essential to have effective planning and preparedness training programs for nurses. As stated by Powers in *International Disaster Nursing*, "the goal of disaster nursing is ensuring that the highest achievable level of care is delivered through identifying, advocating and caring for all impacted populations throughout all phases of a disaster event, including active participation in all levels of disaster planning and preparedness."[1] Many of these duties have fallen on public health nurses and emergency department nurses; however, all nurses will be called upon when a catastrophic event occurs.

Historically, nurses have responded to the call for help when needed. Starting with times of war, this desire and sense of duty to provide care for patients in need have placed the profession on the front lines of disasters. Many of these events occurred in nurses' own backyards; however, countless others have taken it upon themselves to volunteer and travel away from home to respond. Because nursing professionals often desire to help those in need in an unconventional setting, it is our duty to prepare those who respond to disasters.

HISTORICAL PERSPECTIVE

Florence Nightingale, the pioneer of modern nursing, functioned as a disaster nurse during the Crimean War. Taking 38 other women with her to Turkey, she assumed the management responsibilities of the barracks hospital.[2] Wartime health care is similar to disaster health care in that the needs far outweigh the resources. Nightingale worked tirelessly to develop a rudimentary standard of care for the soldiers. This required adaptation of previous knowledge and skills in order to provide care to these soldiers. This ability to adapt is one of the building blocks required for disaster nurses.[3]

Clara Barton, another pioneering nurse, worked diligently during the Civil War providing care to soldiers and then founded the American Red Cross in 1881. Barton had a keen understanding of the needs of the soldiers and what she could do to help. She came to be known as "the angel of the battlefield."[4] By her example, and the establishment of the American Red Cross, a new precedent for volunteerism was set.

In modern day medicine, nurses tend to focus on the refined medical skills learned in school and practiced in normal settings. During a time of need, these innovators in disaster nursing focused on providing food, water, and shelter. Although in the twenty-first century there have been great advances in health care in disaster settings, nurses must not forget the holistic approach and importance of basic human needs. During a disaster situation, a nurse must be flexible and adaptable in order to fill whatever role is necessary at the time, ensuring the best care for all patients.

The flu pandemic of 1918-1919 affected millions of people worldwide; in all, 20 million people perished during this time. This incredible number of people affected by flu required a large number of nurses and doctors to care for them. The health care system was entirely overwhelmed, requiring the establishment of alternate care sites. In one treatment facility in Camp Dodge, Iowa, nurses were able to adapt to an exponentially rising patient population. In a twelve-day period, the number of patients quickly rose from 1254 to 7863; however, the initial nursing staff of 245 nurses only marginally increased to 442.[5] The supply of nurses could not keep up with the exceptional demands of the growing patient population, yet the nurses' adaptability and flexibility allowed them to provide the best care possible with the resources available. The ability to work outside of their normal duties and adapt to the disaster at their feet was crucial.

Over the last century the specialty of emergency nursing has developed because the rapid evaluation and treatment of patients during wartime was noted to save lives.[6] Prior to this time it would have been the responsibility of a nurse in the community to respond to a disaster. The development of the specialty of emergency medicine, emergency departments, and emergency medical systems has redirected small disasters to be cared for directly in emergency departments.

These few examples chronicle the development of disaster medicine and disaster nursing, both created out of necessity. Although these subspecialties are needed sporadically, when an event occurs they become essential. It is important to explore the relatively new subspecialties and develop the fundamental knowledge and the skill sets necessary for the nursing personnel to function at the time of disaster.

CURRENT PRACTICE

Education and Principles of Disaster Nursing

Many of the key skills that nurses perform in their day-to-day roles make for exceptional providers in disaster settings. Some of the key skills that nurses embody are the ability to prioritize and delegate tasks, think critically, be adaptable and flexible, and advocate for themselves and the patients that they care for. With these skills and further training nurses are well equipped to handle disaster situations. Each nurse maintains his or her own specialty and scope of practice, but without the combined efforts of all members of the health care team the patients suffer. This becomes even more important during disasters. Responding to disasters requires a cohesive team of individuals with comprehensive understanding of their skill sets and how to function within the team. As noted by the International Council of Nurses, "Nurses, as team members, can play a strategic role cooperating with health and social disciplines, government bodies, community groups, and non-governmental agencies, including humanitarian organizations."[7] Nurses, as an integral part of this team, require training and education in order to function successfully in these roles.

Disaster preparedness is not just being prepared and knowing what to expect when responding to a disaster but also assisting in the formulation and execution of a response plan for one's own community and workplace. Nurses should have at least a basic understanding of the following principles:

- *The Incident Command System (ICS):* In the United States the ICS is used as a standardized framework for chain of command. To function during a disaster, nurses should be well versed in the principles of ICS.
- *The local and regional disaster response plan:* Nurses must have an understanding of preexisting disaster plans in their communities and facilities. This would include knowing where and when to report during times of disaster and what role they are expected to fill within the response system.
- *Self-preparedness:* It is necessary to discuss and develop an individual and family preparedness plan. The nurse, as a responder, will be away from his or her family for an uncertain period of time, so it is essential that a well-developed family plan is devised ahead of time. One should also be mentally prepared for this separation.
- *Community resources:* Understanding of available resources allows for more effective care of those in need (i.e., available alternate care sites, blood bank capabilities, pharmacy stockpiles, and shelters).
- *Personal abilities and shortcomings:* While working in an unfamiliar setting with unfamiliar people, it is necessary to stand firm in one's knowledge base and skill sets. Being able to communicate this to the team will allow for proper delegation of tasks, therefore providing safe and effective care to patients. Prior to the occurrence of a disaster, nurses should consider and understand their emergency skill set.
- *Participation in disaster drills:* Often hospitals will run disaster drills simulating a variety of scenarios, from biological, mass casualty, and internal disasters. Nurses must be involved during these drills because they will be integral parts of a real-world disaster response.

Nursing Within the Disaster Cycle

When one thinks of disaster nursing or disaster medicine as a whole, it is often the response phase that gets most of the attention. Without mitigation and preparation, however, the response to a disaster would be disorganized at best. As defined by the World Health Organization (WHO), a disaster is "A serious disruption of the functioning of a community or a society causing widespread human, material, economic, or environmental losses which exceed the ability of the affected community or society to cope using its own resources."[8] Although many nurses have neither the desire nor the ability to travel domestically or internationally to all disasters, this does not exclude them from potentially needing to respond to a nearby event. Disasters happen every day and often in our own backyards; therefore nurses of all skills and specialties should have a basic knowledge of the four phases of the disaster cycle.

Mitigation

During mitigation it is imperative to complete accurate vulnerability assessments. It is this phase in which providers can assess a situation and make changes in order to decrease the likelihood that events, human-made or natural, will become disasters. Nurses, with a firm grasp on the abilities and resources within their communities and facilities, should be involved in the assessment and then planning of this stage. This requires close evaluation and analysis of the risks that exist

and the resources required. It is during this time that a disaster plan should be developed after a thorough hazard vulnerability analysis (HVA). Nurses should assist with the HVA in this phase.

Throughout history, and in modern day disaster settings, there are often secondary disease processes that infiltrate a disaster zone, particularly in events that occur in developing countries. As nurses, one of the interventions that should be implemented is that of vaccination. When a disaster causes gross displacement of a population and results in large-scale sheltering, there is greater risk of disease. Vaccinations not only play important roles in disease management in such settings but also help prevent pandemic events, such as influenza. Vaccinations are not the only nursing practice that can mitigate disease in a disaster. Basic knowledge of good hygiene practices, such as hand washing and use of antiseptic solutions, are important in postdisaster settings because they help to prevent the outbreak of communicable diseases. During this phase nurses are highly involved in teaching the community and fellow health care practitioners.

Preparedness

During the preparedness phase, nurses should help develop the disaster plan for their hospitals or working facilities. It is of utmost importance that nurses during this phase are involved in the discussion of surge capacity and patient care aspects of the developing disaster plan. In this phase nurses should also develop plans for their own families and encourage other medical personnel to do the same. Knowing that when a disaster strikes, health care workers will be needed to provide medical care, it is exceptionally important that all have a plan for their own families during this time.

The plans developed during the preparedness phase should be exercised regularly and include all parties that would be involved in a real disaster. It is important that the first time response plans are enacted not be during an actual disaster. Nurses should have a chance to practice their roles during drills in order to be competent in the tasks that may be outside of their normal responsibilities.

Response

Nurses are vital during the response phase. Due to the number of nurses in the health care field, they will carry out the majority of the care delivered to the injured or ill. To be successful in this phase, nurses must have a basic understanding of the disaster plan, as well as the pathophysiology of the unique diseases and injuries they may encounter. Nurses will be responsible not only for direct patient care, but also for patient flow, surge capacity operations, and the utilization of resources. The available supplies may be limited and require careful distribution and rationing. With potentially limited resources, nurses will need to be flexible and adaptable in order to optimize the quality of care delivered to the affected masses. Having a firm understanding of expected disaster operations and the ICS system within the facility or community will allow nurses to be more efficient and effective in their individual roles.

Another important role nurses may be asked to perform during this time is that of disaster triage. Triage is a skill set that nurses routinely exercise and therefore they are well suited to take on this role in a disaster. Disaster triage using the simple triage and rapid treatment (START) technique and the traditional nursing emergency severity index (ESI) triage used in the United States looks to prioritize patients based on acuity. However, in disaster triage there is the addition of the deceased/expectant category, where an individual has either expired or will likely die despite medical interventions. During a disaster it is necessary to sort the overwhelming patient population by acuity and prioritize their medical care. The WHO defines disaster triage as "a process designed to prioritize casualty care to ensure care is available to those who need it most urgently and that the greatest number of casualties survive."[9] During disaster triage, nurses must prioritize care to optimize resource utilization and ensure that the greatest number of patients survive.

Recovery

After a disaster occurs communities must return to their normal state. This process may overlap with the response phase. During this phase communities start to heal and rebuild. The length of this phase can vary considerably based on the type of disaster. The recovery process will include significantly more than the rebuilding of structures and reestablishment of the physical appearance of the community. Nurses should be aware and in tune with the needs of their patients during this phase. "The immediate drama and high profile of the relief responses can absorb and exhaust compassion and support, leaving the ongoing recovery phase without the required critical attention and funding. Thus long-term health and socioeconomic consequences are not reduced and may even result in a secondary disaster."[10] While the community rebuilds physically it is essential for nurses to closely observe how their communities heal mentally, emotionally, and physically and assist in this process. Although usually not the primary victims of disaster, health care workers must be vigilant about stress debriefing and their own personal recovery.

The disaster cycle is a continuum. Part of the recovery phase is personal reflection in order to function successfully at home, at work, and in future disasters. We must not forget, but we must also look back and learn. Shortcomings in prior disaster preparation and response should be looked at as the framework for developing an ever-growing skill set and improvement in future responses.

NURSING ROLES WITHIN DISASTER RESPONSE

Nurses who wish to participate in disaster response have a number of different organizations where they would be welcomed and their work would be beneficial. Local programs such as the Medical Reserve Corps and the American Red Cross take volunteers to assist in domestic responses. These organizations are exceptionally important when disasters occur locally. Nurses are more effective when responding as part of an organization, due to the clear direction and support provided.[11] By having nurses and other medical professionals precredentialed, there is an additional workforce that can be called upon to assist in disaster responses.

Another opportunity for nurses who wish to be involved in disaster response is through the National Disaster Medical System (NDMS). NDMS is a federally run program that responds during peacetime to disasters that occur nationally and occasionally internationally.[12] Within NDMS there are two agencies that utilize nurses in their disaster response: the Disaster Medical Assistance Team (DMAT) and the International Medical Surgical Response Team (IMSURT). These teams are regionally or state based, with most states having at least one DMAT. These teams will deploy within the United States when called up by federal orders.

For nurses with the desire to expand their skills beyond the border of the United States there are many organizations that provide disaster and humanitarian aid internationally. These organizations provide medical care, relief, and recovery during times of need in foreign countries. Most of these organizations provide information, training, and education prior to deployment. They deploy to areas with long-term needs as well as areas in crisis. Volunteering on an international level takes nurses further outside their comfort zones and stresses their ability to adapt to unfamiliar and often austere conditions. The sharp learning curve required to be successful in such an environment allows nurses to return strengthened in their routine roles. Such experiences provide nurses the opportunity to grow further as practitioners and exercise their critical thinking skills, even more so than perhaps they do in their day-to-day jobs.

As described above, for those with an interest there are a multitude of organizations and opportunities for nurses to volunteer their time in the arena of disaster medicine. Nurses play an important role in all aspects of the disaster cycle and therefore play an integral role in the responding agencies.

! PITFALLS

At present, the major pitfalls for nurses in disaster are the lack of overall disaster-related education and the absence of nurse involvement in the planning and drilling stages. The increased number of terrorist attacks combined with the ongoing occurrences of natural disasters brings to light the need for more training and education of nurses, so that they might assist in all phases of the disaster cycle. Incidents such as the Oklahoma City Bombing, 9/11, Hurricane Katrina, the Haiti earthquake, the Boston Marathon Bombing, and Typhoon Haiyan in the Philippines required nurses with emergency and critical training to step out of their normal roles. Nurses were on the front line of the 2014 Ebola outbreak and will continue to be on the front line in similar disasters long into the future. It is therefore important that nurses who respond and deploy to areas affected by disaster have the required training to be successful in caring for their patients. This training should include how to respond medically to injuries or disease processes that may be encountered, as well as having an understanding of how the ICS operates. Having nurses involved in the mitigation and planning phases allows them to have an understanding of the roles they may be asked to fill and the resources required to face disaster.

The ever-rising number of disasters makes it even more apparent that the education routinely provided to nurses is grossly inadequate. As identified in a study conducted in the 2000-2001 academic year, which looked at 348 nursing programs in the United States, 32.7% of the programs included a disaster nursing curriculum. In the post-9/11 world of nursing and disaster education, this number rose only marginally to 53%.[13] As shown in this study, the basic education surrounding disaster nursing is lacking. Although some would argue that the topic of disaster nursing is very specific and does not have a place in the fundamentals of nursing, experts in disaster nursing would disagree. It is necessary for all nurses to have a basic awareness of disaster mitigation, preparedness, response, and recovery. While this information will provide a rudimentary understanding of disasters, one must have a more in-depth competence surrounding the practices of disaster nursing.

CONCLUSION

All levels of medical providers practice disaster medicine, including physicians, nurse practitioners, physician assistants, nurses, paramedics, and emergency medical technicians (EMTs); therefore an integrated, multidisciplinary response is imperative. This can only be accomplished by education at all levels, including nursing, and the inclusion of nurse education and participation in all phases of the disaster cycle. Because nurses make up the majority of the health care workforce worldwide, they will most assuredly play a pivotal role in future disasters. Whether due to volunteer deployment to a region recently affected or a mass casualty incident in their hometown, nurses will need a fundamental knowledge of disaster preparedness and response.

REFERENCES

1. Powers R, Daily E. *International Disaster Nursing.* Cambridge University Press; 2010, 3.
2. Selanders L, Crane P. The voice of Florence Nightingale on advocacy. *OJIN Online J Issues Nurs.* 2012;17(1):1.
3. Booker C, Waugh A. *Foundations of Nursing Practice: Fundamentals of Holistic Care.* Elsevier; 2013, 34.
4. *American Red Cross History.* Available at: http://www.redcross.org/about-us/history/clara-barton.
5. Keeling A. "Alert to the necessities of the emergency": U.S. nursing during the 1918 influenza pandemic. *Public Health Rep.* 2010;125 (suppl 3):105–112.
6. Gebbie K, Qureshi K. A historical challenge: nurses and emergencies. *OJIN Online J Issues Nurs.* 2006;11(3):2.
7. ICN. *Nurses and Disaster Preparedness.* Geneva: International Council of Nurses; 2006.
8. Weiner E, Irwin M, Trangenstein P, Gordon J. Emergency preparedness curriculum in nursing schools in the United States. *Nurs Educ Perspect.* 2005;26(9):334–339.
9. WHO. Definitions: emergencies. http://www.who.int/hac/about/definitions/en/. Web access 5/14.
10. Arbon P, Zeitz K, Ranse J, et al. Putting triage theory into practice at the scene of multiple casualty vehicular accidents: the reality of multiple casualty triage. *Emerg Med J.* 2008;25(4):230–234.
11. Powers R, Daily E. *International Disaster Nursing.* Cambridge University Press; 2010, 496.
12. Powers R, Daily E. *International Disaster Nursing.* Cambridge University Press; 2010, 19.
13. Public Health Emergency. National Disaster Medical System (NDMS) Response Teams. Available at: http://www.phe.gov/Preparedness/responders/ndms/teams/Pages/default.aspx. Web access date 5/14.

CHAPTER 6

Role of Hospitals in a Disaster

Ahmadreza Djalali, Pier Luigi Ingrassia, and Luca Ragazzoni

By definition, the hospital is an institution providing medical and surgical treatment and nursing care for sick or injured people.[1] The word *hospital* comes from the Latin *hospes*, signifying a stranger or foreigner, and hence a guest.[2] The earliest documented institutions aiming to provide cures were ancient Egyptian temples. Around 100 BC, the Romans constructed buildings called *valetudinaria*, for the care of sick slaves, gladiators, and soldiers, and, around 300 AD, a hospital and medical training center existed at Gundeshapur, one of the major cities in the Khuzestan province of the Persian empire in what is current-day Iran.[2] By the late nineteenth century, the modern hospital was beginning to take shape, with a variety of public and private hospital systems.

It is unclear when hospital disaster preparedness was first taken under consideration; however, the Second World War is a major milestone. During World War II, some hospitals in England and the United States were systematically prepared to provide efficient medical services to casualties. In 1956 principles of disaster planning for hospitals were developed by the American Hospital Association, and in 1957 the Joint Committee on Accreditation of Hospitals in the United States recognized the importance of hospital disaster planning, making it a point in the scoring for accreditation, ensuring that every hospital had to have a disaster plan.[3]

An important point of progress in hospital organization for managing possible disasters was the adoption of the Incident Command System (ICS), to be used in the hospital-based response to disasters. It was later renamed the Hospital Emergency Incident Command System (HEICS) and then the Hospital Incident Command System (HICS).[4–7]

The terrorist attacks of September 11, 2001, in the United States, heightened preparedness efforts worldwide, including hospital disaster preparedness. In addition, the development of a worldwide strategy by the United Nations regarding disaster-risk reduction, the Hyogo Framework for Action 2005-2015: Building the Resilience of Nations and Communities to Disasters, was a remarkable improvement in the field of hospital disaster preparedness and safety.[8] As a result of the strategy, 2008 was nominated as the year of the "safe hospital" by the World Health Organization (WHO), and a standardized guideline was introduced by the WHO, regarding hospital safety and functional capacity.[9] In the United States, the American Society for Testing and Materials (ASTM) suggested a consensus-based product such as the "Standard Guide for Hospital Preparedness and Response, E2413-04 (Reapproved 2009)."[10] However, despite the progress in research, planning, and practice, no internationally accepted standards for hospital disaster preparedness and response exist.

HISTORICAL PERSPECTIVE

Hospitals are usually vulnerable during disasters. Past events have illuminated the destructive effects of disasters on hospital structures and/or functionality, which are not limited to developing countries.[11–14]

- From 1985 to 2001, natural events affected more than 1000 hospitals in various countries of the Americas (e.g., earthquakes affected 276 hospitals in El Salvador, Chile, and Mexico; El Niño affected 437 hospitals in Peru; 302 hospitals in Nicaragua, Dominican Republic, Honduras, Jamaica, and Costa Rica were affected by hurricanes.[15]
- According to a WHO report, from 1979 to 2009, 69 hospitals were evacuated because of either natural or human-made disasters, worldwide.[13]
- An earthquake struck Northridge, California, on January 17, 1994, and damaged a number of hospitals. Six hospitals either were partially or complete evacuated.[11]
- The Chi-Chi Earthquake in Taiwan in 1999 resulted in four hospitals being evacuated because of significant nonstructural damage.[16]
- In Iran, the Bam Earthquake in 2003 destroyed three hospitals, and approximately 130 other health facilities.[17]
- The flooding in the wake of Hurricane Katrina in 2005 left hospitals in greater New Orleans, Louisiana, and in Mississippi in crisis. Patients and staff were trapped in facilities without essential services, resulting in the largest mass hospital evacuation in U.S. history.[12]
- In June 2001, 3 feet of rain from Tropical Storm Allison fell in the Houston area in Texas, causing the flooding and complete disruption of the hospitals. One of the hospitals experienced failure of hospital systems. The water supply failed, and the sewer system stopped functioning. The vertical evacuation of 570 patients was conducted, and the hospital was closed for 38 days.[18]
- A sudden and extensive power failure occurred at Huddinge Hospital in Stockholm, Sweden, on Easter Saturday, April 7, 2007. The power failure lasted 1 hour and 22 minutes, but it took longer for activities to return to normal. It put many critically ill patients at great risk, particularly those in intensive care.[19]
- In the course of responding to the Great East Japan Tsunami, 2011, a 30-km evacuation radius was decided by the government in response to the Fukushima nuclear accidents. Therefore patients of the hospitals in this radius were transferred to other hospitals.[20]
- During the 2001 World Trade Center attack, 194 casualties were triaged and treated within the first 24 hours in Bellevue Hospital, New York City. Despite huge efforts, the hospital lost track of patients, ran out of supplies, and struggled with coordination of health care providers to ensure patient rest and safety.[21] In addition, the University Downtown Hospital received 350 patients within the first 2 hours of the World Trade Center attacks.[22] St. Vincent's Hospital treated nearly 800 victims. Because St. Vincent's shared water lines with the World Trade Center and telecommunications lines were routed through it, the functioning of these systems was affected.[23]

The examples herein are only a few of the possible effects that disasters could have on hospitals. Hospitals have collapsed or been damaged during many other events.

CURRENT PRACTICE

Public Expectation of Hospital Function

Hospitals are an integral part of the health care system and a symbol of social progress and political values in society, which contribute to the sense of security and well-being in a community. Moreover, hospitals have a significant economic effect on a society, and are a prerequisite for stability and economic development.[13,24]

Hospitals are expected to be ready to provide medical care in all circumstances. The actual purpose of a hospital, being the initial source of medical care, demands that it remain fully operational in the aftermath of any major disaster.[11] *Hospital readiness* may be defined as the ability to maintain hospital operations effectively, to sustain a medically safe environment reliably, and to address adequately the increased and potentially unexpected medical needs of the affected population.[25] To be highly prepared and able to respond effectively, hospitals must consider substantial investment in equipment, training, facilities improvements, and supplies to assure that the facility is safe and functional and that adequately trained staffing is available to provide high-quality treatment for disaster victims.[26]

However, ethical challenges with patients and relatives of casualties during disasters can be expected. The community belief is to provide medical care and to put all efforts and resources into caring for the sickest patients, but the key principle of disaster medical care is to do the greatest good for the greatest number of patients.[27]

ELEMENTS OF COMPREHENSIVE HOSPITAL PREPAREDNESS FOR DISASTERS

Preparedness is defined as the knowledge and capacities developed by the community and response and recovery organizations, such as a hospital, to anticipate, respond to, and recover effectively from the effects of disasters.[28] The preparedness process starts with planning based on risk assessment, and it requires a comprehensive approach to reach a reliable level of preparedness.[10,17]

A comprehensive hospital disaster plan follows an all-hazard approach. However, this does not mean that the hospital is prepared for every type of hazard that could occur in a particular community, including the hospital. An all-hazards approach considers things that commonly occur in many kinds of disasters, such as the need for treatment and triage of victims. These things can be addressed in a general plan, to provide the basis for responding to unexpected events.[10,17,29] The kinds of disasters that might occur must be addressed in a hospital disaster plan; however, the plan and the command and control system need to be adaptable to all events.[10,17,29]

Another aspect of a comprehensive disaster plan is considering all phases of the disaster-management cycle: (1) mitigation and prevention, (2) preparedness, (3) response, and (4) recovery and rehabilitation.[10,30]

The third aspect of a comprehensive hospital disaster plan is being part of a community disaster plan.[17,31] Hospitals will not work in isolation during disasters, and it is impossible for a hospital to respond effectively to a disaster without assimilating into the overall response system, and contribute to the disaster-management process.

Integration into the community disaster plan will also support a hospital during disasters: for example, with respect to surge capacity. Moreover, the hospitals might receive financial, informational, and business benefits from active participation in the community-focused emergency planning process. This condition might also help hospitals to contain costs by sharing expertise, training resources, and equipment. Among all external organizations, emergency medical service (EMS) is the most important one with which a hospital can have an integrated disaster-management plan; in fact, the EMS performance significantly affects the hospital workload during disasters.[32] As well as being comprehensive, a hospital disaster plan should consider some other principles, such as being predictable, simple, flexible, and concise.[33]

Hospital Vulnerability

The complexity, occupancy level, specialized services, and specific equipment of hospitals make them vulnerable to the effects of disasters. The potential effect of disasters on hospitals is of major importance for the following reasons[34-36]:

1. Hospitals must maintain their normal functions in case of a sudden surge in patients requiring varying levels of treatment following a disaster.
2. Hospitals accommodate a large number of patients who are unable to evacuate the building easily in the event of a disaster.
3. Hospitals have a network of electrical, mechanical, and sanitary facilities and expensive equipment that is essential for the routine operation of the hospital.

Generally, disasters may affect health system operations both directly and indirectly.[34] Direct effects include damaged health care facilities and damaged infrastructure across the locality, leading to the breakdown of public services that are indispensable to health facility operations. Indirect effects can include an unexpected number of deaths, injuries, or disease in the affected community, exceeding the capacity of the local health care network to provide treatment. Indirect effects also include spontaneous or organized migrations away from the affected area toward other areas where health system capacity may be overwhelmed by the new arrivals. Increases in the potential risk of a critical outbreak of communicable diseases and an increase in the risk for psychological diseases among the affected population are also indirect effects on health system operations. Additionally, food shortages leading to malnutrition and weakened resistance to various diseases can cause indirect effects on the health system.

There are three elements of vulnerability for a hospital: structural, nonstructural, and administrative and organizational.

Structural Elements

The structural elements include foundations, columns, bearing walls, beams, staircases, elevators, and floors. Evaluation of the structural vulnerability and relevant issues are specific to the type of hazard. Generally, the effect of disasters on structural elements differs from slight damage to complete destruction.[17,36]

Nonstructural Elements

The nonstructural vulnerability evaluation considers architectural elements (e.g., false ceilings, covering elements, and cornices), equipment and furnishings (e.g., medical equipment, office equipment, and furnishings), and basic installations and services (e.g., drinking water, medical gasses, and air conditioning).[35]

The consequence of damage to nonstructural elements, with regard to injury to the occupants and interfering with the performance of the facility, is categorized as low, moderate, or high.[17,36]

Administrative and Organizational Elements

The administrative and organizational elements include all physical and administrative measures required for organizing the hospital personnel to respond to disasters and to optimize the hospital capacity to function during and after a disaster.[17,35,36]

Some important issues in the context of administrative vulnerability are contracting, acquisitions, and routine maintenance, as well as the physical and functional interdependence of the different areas of the facility. Organizational aspects include an optimized organization of personnel, equipment, material, resources, and spatial organization. Regarding administrative and organizational vulnerability, the hospital functionality, during and after disasters, can be classified as good, average, or poor.[17,35,36]

It is the duty of health authorities to assess a hospital's vulnerability to disaster effects and to have an estimation of existing risk levels to ensure the safety and proper response of the hospital to the needs in a disaster response.

Hospital Safety Index

Addressing the priorities of "Hyogo Framework for Actions 2005-2015: Disaster Risk Reduction," the global campaign "Hospitals Safe from Disasters: Reduce Risk, Protect Health Facilities, Save Lives" was developed by the Secretariat of the United Nations International Strategy for Disaster Reduction (UNISDR) in partnership with the WHO in 2008 to 2009.[24] The aim of the strategy is to ensure that hospitals will not only remain standing in case of a disaster but also function effectively and without interruption.

Making all health facilities safe in the event of disasters poses a major challenge for some countries because of not only the high number of facilities and their high cost but also because there is limited information about current safety levels in hospitals.[9]

A remarkable product of this campaign was the evaluation forms for the safe hospital, the Hospital Safety Index (HSI), which was initially developed by the Pan American Health Organization.[9] The HSI is a rapid and low-cost tool to assess the probability of a hospital or health facility remaining operational in emergency situations.[9,17] The tool has been used to evaluate hospitals in various locations, such as Moldova, Iran, Sweden, and Latin America.[9,37-40]

The HSI consists of two main forms:

- Form 1, "General Information about the Health Facility," includes the name of the facility, number of beds by services or medical specialty, hospital occupancy rate, number of personnel, expansion capacity in case of disaster, etc.[9]
- Form 2, "Safe Hospitals Checklist," is used for preliminary diagnosis of the hospital safety in the event of disasters. It contains 145 variables, and each has three safety levels: low, medium, and high. It is divided into four modules: (1) geographic location of the health facility, (2) structural safety, (3) nonstructural safety, and (4) functional capacity.[9]

The sum of three modules (structural, nonstructural, and functional capacity) gives the HSI. The index is expressed as the probability that a facility will be able to continue its safety and function in a disaster situation, as detailed below.[9]

A (0.66-1): it is likely that the hospital will function in case of a disaster. It is recommended that the hospital improve response capacity and carry out preventive measures in the medium and long term to improve the safety level in case of disaster.

B (0.36-0.65): intervention measures are needed in the short term. The hospital's ability to function during and after a disaster is potentially at risk.

C (0-0.35): urgent intervention measures are needed. The hospital safety level is inadequate to protect the lives of patients and hospital staff during and after a disaster.

Hazard Vulnerability Analysis

Disaster planning begins with a risk-assessment and hazard-vulnerability analysis to identify the most likely threats to a particular hospital and to prevent or mitigate the effects of hazards on the hospital building and/or function.[10,41] The hazard vulnerability analysis (HVA) method, a useful tool to evaluate risk of hazards to a hospital was invented by the Kaiser Permanente Foundation, in the United States. Hospitals were asked to complete an annual HVA as a basis for emergency planning.[42] The method evaluates potential for incident and response among the natural, human-related, technological, and hazardous material events using the hazard-specific scale. The assumption is that each event (e.g., hurricane, earthquake, explosion, electrical failure, hazardous materials [HazMat] accident, etc.) occurs at the worst possible time (e.g., during peak patient loads). The risk of each event is defined as "probability × severity." The severity also comes from the magnitude (the effects of the event on humans, property, and businesses) and the mitigation (preparedness, internal response, and external response capabilities).

To calculate the risk, issues should be considered for each of the following components[43]:

- Probability: known risk, historical data, and manufacturer and vendor statistics
- Risk to human life: potential for staff and patient's death or injury
- Impact on property: cost to replace, repair, and recover
- Effects on business: employees unable to report to work, interruption of critical supplies, customers unable to reach facility, etc.
- Preparedness: plans, training and exercise, alternate systems, insurance, etc.
- Internal resources: types and volume of supplies on hand, staff availability, etc.
- External resources: agreements with community agencies, coordination with proximal health care facilities, etc.

Hospital Incidence Command System

A hospital disaster plan should address the role of the hospital during disasters in relation to other response organizations in the community. In addition, the overall incident organization of the hospital, based on a strategy of efficient and effective utilization of resources, should be defined, and the chain of command should be addressed as the HICS.[6,10,44] The HICS (a modification of ICS) was developed by the Orange County, California, EMS.[4-7] It is currently the most commonly used model for hospital disaster response in the United States. This model is also used in Iran, Taiwan, and Turkey.[44-48] The HICS is critical to assure the organizational and logistical support to meet incident-generated demands by getting the right personnel and supplies to the right place at the right time, to provide timely and effective patient care.[49] It uses a common organizational terminology and facilitates communication between the hospital, first responders, and other health care facilities.[50] This system is composed of a command group and four sections, including operations, planning, logistics, and finance and administration (Figure 6-1).[6]

The incident command group has the overall responsibility for the incident management activities of the hospital. It consists of the incident commander, the public information officer, the safety officer, the liaison officer, and a group of medical and technical specialists.[6]

The operations section is responsible for managing the tactical objectives outlined by the incident commander. This section consists of one department-level management part and five branches: staging management, medical care operations, infrastructure operations, security operations, business continuity operations, and hazardous material branch.[6]

The planning section is responsible for collecting, evaluating, and disseminating status reports, to display various types of information and to develop the Incident Action Plan (IAP). This section consists of four units: resource, situation, documentation, and demobilization.[6]

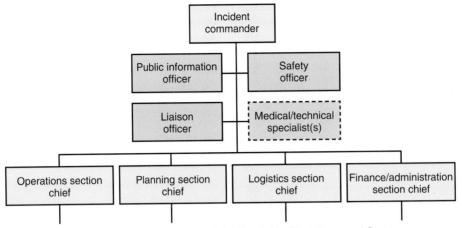

FIG 6-1 First-Level Organization of the Hospital Incident Command System.

The logistics section coordinates all activities to provide necessary resources, from internal and external sources, for hospital functions during disasters. The section has two branches: service and support.[6]

The finance and administrative section is intended to develop financial and administrative procedures to support the program before, during, and after an emergency or a disaster. The section consists of time, procurement, compensation and claims, and cost units.[6]

Each group and section consists of various positions. For each position, a job-action sheet explains the main mission and expected tasks, within immediate (0 to 2 hours), intermediate (2 to 12 hours), and extended (beyond 12 hours) operational periods. It also explains the demobilization and system recovery.[6]

Surge Capacity

In a disaster situation, no single health care facility standing alone can provide optimal care to all the victims affected. However, a hospital usually receives an influx of casualties within a few hours of an emergency, and it is not possible to receive all requirements from other hospitals. Therefore the medical facility must be able to surge its medical capacity to minimize mortality and morbidity. *Hospital surge capacity* is defined as the ability of a hospital to expand rapidly and augment services in response to one or multiple incidents,[10] and to manage patients who require unusual or very specialized evaluation or interventions (e.g., contaminated or burn patients).[51] These terms refer not only to the physical space but also the organizational structure, medical and ancillary staff, support, supply, information systems, pharmaceuticals, and other resources required to support patient care efforts, which could be summarized as S4 ("staff, stuff, space, and system").[52]

To consider the priorities for hospital activities and surge capacity during disasters, the medical services can be rated as (1) dispensable, (2) preferable, (3) necessary, (4) very necessary, and (5) indispensable (e.g., ICU as indispensable; laboratory as very necessary; and dermatology as dispensable) (Table 6-1).[35]

Disasters usually affect directly or indirectly hospitals located in the affected zone. Therefore decline of hospital capacity is expected. Moreover, it is not realistic to assume a full functional capacity for a hospital. To address surge capacity, usually, the first step is to stop all elective operations and visits to free up personnel and space for emergency management activities. The second step is to empty the current space through earlier discharge or disposition of patients to other health and medical facilities. Consequently, more space, staff, and stuff will be

TABLE 6-1 **Importance of Some Hospital Services During a Disaster**	
HOSPITAL SERVICES	**IMPORTANCE**
Emergency care (ED and OR)	Indispensable
Intensive care unit	
Trauma and orthopedic	
Urology	
Sterilization	
Diagnostic imaging	
Pharmacy	
Blood bank	
Pediatrics	Very necessary
Laboratory	
Hemodialysis	
Internal medicine	Necessary
Gynecology and obstetrics	
Administration	
Respiratory medicine	Preferable
Ophthalmology	
Dermatology	Dispensable
Oncology	
Otorhinolaryngology	
Therapy and rehabilitation	

available. Another step could be adding extra staff, stuff, and space to the hospital.

It is not possible to calculate an exact number or proportion to estimate hospital surge capacity. However, assuming the intact elements of a hospital, some methods have been suggested by researchers for surge capacity planning.[51–54] For instance, "the maximal number of victims that any hospital is reasonably capable of absorbing during a mass casualty incident is 20% of the total number of registered beds."[53] Hospital treatment capacity (HTC), the number of casualties that can be treated in the hospital in an hour, is considered 3% of the total number of beds. Whereas, hospital surgical capacity (HSC), the number of seriously injured patients that can be operated upon within a 12-hour period, is calculated as "number of operation rooms × 7 × 0.25 operations/ 12 hours."[33] A trauma center that is geographically isolated may enhance its capacity (emergency department, operation rooms, intensive care unit) up to 11%.[55]

Hospital Evacuation

Evacuation of hospitals because of imminent or impacting disasters is not a rare event. A review article revealed there were 275 hospital evacuations in the United States within 1971 to 1997.[56] It has also been reported from other areas, such as Italy, Pakistan, China, Indonesia, South American countries, and the United Kingdom, where some hospitals have been evacuated because of earthquake, flood, fire, and other disasters.[13,57]

Evacuation of a hospital is a complex process, with the goal being to safeguard the health and lives of its occupants.[13] In this situation, not only the patient but also relevant equipment and documents must be evacuated, which can results in the functional collapse of a hospital, including critical departments such as the ICU and operating rooms, which are typically in greater demand during a disaster. Hospital evacuations also produce psychological, financial, and social problems for the whole community.[13,58]

Hospital evacuation might be immediate or delayed, vertical or lateral, partial or complete, pre-event (e.g., because of impending tsunami, hurricane, or other disasters) or post-event. The determination to evacuate the hospital must be based on precise criteria and a rapid decision-making process.[58,59] Evacuation of an entire hospital is an enormous logistical undertaking, which usually requires outside capabilities. It often requires the cooperation and involvement of other organizations, such as police, fire, and EMS. Supporting organizations may provide transportation, facilities, supplies, equipment, and personnel. All of these services must be precisely orchestrated to accomplish the evacuation efficiently and safely.[11,13,58–61]

Creating a staging location is a crucial phase of the evacuation operation. Patients will be transported to alternate care facilities from the staging area. Hospitals, clinics, hotels, nursing facilities, and others could all be alternate care sites for evacuated patients.[58,59]

Patients can be categorized into three groups: (1) ambulatory and self-sufficient patients, (2) nonambulatory patients who require medical care and support but are not in critical or unstable condition, and (3) patients who need critical and continuous medical services or are fully dependent on technology (e.g., patients in the ICU or isolation rooms).[58–61]

Maintaining continuous medical services to nonambulatory patients is essential during the evacuation process. However, it may be unrealistic to keep all equipment and procedures with the patients while they are being evacuated, particularly if elevators are not working and patients must be transported by staff on stairs in a high-rise hospital. Moreover, for ethical reasons, triage in evacuation is necessary if it is not possible to evacuate some patients.[58,59]

Areas and floors in highest danger should be evacuated first; however, a top-to-bottom evacuation should be considered if there is no immediate threat to the hospital. Special equipment, stairs, and elevators are used for evacuation, depending on safety issues.[58–61]

To prepare for a successful evacuation in the event of severe damage to the hospital, the first step is to perform a pre-event assessment of the hospital infrastructure, layout, and demographic situation.[61] The second step is to estimate time needed to evacuate the hospital, both to the staging area and to transport to alternate care sites. The output will vary based on different scenarios. Number of patients, available exit routes, available resources and staff, traffic conditions, and distance to the evacuation sites are factors for determining the required time.[58–61] The third step is to estimate resources needed to evacuate the hospital, both to the staging area and to transport to alternate care sites. Resources (staff, equipment, and vehicles) are needed for both transportation and continuing the medical services in the appropriate environment, considering temperature, air condition, security, and safety.[58,59] It is important to send enough information along with the patients (e.g., name and background information, medical file, time of discharge, equipment sent with the patient, and special considerations and precautions, such as police hold, mental health, and suicide watch).[58,60]

Hospital Readiness for Hazardous Materials Emergencies

HazMat and their accidental or intentional spill are the sources of many human-made disasters. During the past decades, the number of disasters caused by industrial chemical spills, gas leaks, or industrial explosions and fires, has increased across the world.[62] The impact of HazMat incidents on hospitals is significant, and the treatment of contaminated patients is not a rare event. Hospital staffs have been injured while treating these patients, and hospital facilities have been shut down or evacuated because of secondary contamination.[63]

Since the terrorist attacks of September 11, 2001, the need to be prepared to respond to events involving HazMat contaminants in mass casualty scenarios or in situations involving smaller numbers of victims has been increasingly taken under consideration by health facilities, especially in the United States.[64,65] However, some studies report that the health system, including hospitals, is not well prepared to handle patients from such emergencies.[66–68] The necessary level of readiness for HazMat emergencies should be determined by the HVA, which takes into account geographic, demographic, historical, and industrial factors. In addition, different managerial tactics and actions might be considered if the risk comes from either terrorist attacks or industrial events. However, in terms of medical treatment, the approach to dealing with terrorist and industrial CBRN incidents will not differ in most situations. Triage, decontamination, medical treatment, and safety will be the main functions during all HazMat emergencies.[66–68]

As well as performing the risk assessment, training hospital managers and staff in HazMat emergencies is a priority for the preparedness process. In fact, the lack of awareness and knowledge by hospital managers and staff about the characteristics of HazMat events is a main bottleneck of emergency preparedness and response to such events. A basic training course for hospital managers and staff should cover some core topics (e.g., the threats of a HazMat to the staff, safety issues, and essential equipment and resources, along with medical treatment and decontamination principles).[65–71]

To list and provide essential equipment and medical resources, such as antidotes, personal protective equipment (PPE), and detection and monitoring instruments, is another important preparedness step to take.[67–70] PPE is designed to provide protection from serious injuries resulting from contact with HazMat. No single combination of protective equipment and clothing is capable of protecting against all hazards. There are four categories of PPE, and for hospital staff selection of PPE is based on the degree of protection afforded against type and severity of contamination on the casualties.[69–71]

- Level A protection should be worn when the highest level of respiratory, skin, eye, and mucous membrane protection is needed. Usually, it is not used at a hospital if it is placed in a safe zone.
- Level B protection should be selected when the highest level of respiratory protection is needed but a lesser level of skin and eye protection is needed. This level of protection is suggested for use by a hospital staff working on the decontamination of victims.
- Level C protection should be selected when the type of airborne substance is known, concentration measured, criteria for using air-purifying respirators met, and skin and eye exposure is unlikely. This level of protection is suitable for hospital staff in case of receiving HazMat incident victims. A typical Level C set includes a full-face or half mask, air-purifying respirator; chemical-resistant clothing; chemical-resistant gloves, both inner and outer; and steel toe and shank, chemical-resistant boots.

- Level D protection is primarily a work uniform used for nuisance contamination only. It requires only coveralls and safety shoes or boots. Other PPE is designated for use based on the situation, and it should not be worn where respiratory or skin hazards exist.

A safe place to treat contaminated patients is also a key element of hospital preparedness for HazMat emergencies. Two zones are needed: a warm zone and a cold zone.[71,72] The warm zone is an isolated place where contaminated victims, equipment, and waste might be present. Triage, medical stabilization, and decontamination are performed in this zone. The cold zone is an area where equipment and personnel are not expected to become contaminated.[71,72]

Development of standardized procedures and guidelines on how to manage the casualties coming from a HazMat incident (both contaminated and not) has a critical role in hospital performance during Haz-Mat events.

EDUCATION AND TRAINING

Education and training are key elements of disaster readiness of the health system, including hospitals. All staff should be familiar with standardized concepts and terms and understand the nature and consequences of possible hazards and how they might contribute to disaster-management activities.[73–76] The basic theory that supports the development of education and training programs is called instructional system design (ISD). ISD is composed of the analysis of training needs and the identification of requirements for the target audience; the design of the education and training program, schedule, and delivery methods; the development of content and instructional resources; the implementation of the educational and training program; and the evaluation and improvement activities (Figure 6-2).[17,77]

The frequency and scope of training should be sufficient to maintain educational objectives, such as knowledge and performance levels of hospital personnel.[74–76,78,79] The use of Bloom's Taxonomy is common to determine learning objectives in educational and training courses.[80] In summary, it can be classified in three levels of education for hospital staff: awareness (remembering and understanding), practice (applying), and expertise (analyzing, evaluating, and creating) in disaster management. All hospital staff must be considered for the awareness level training. Almost all medical staff and some of the nonmedical staff should be included in practice-level training; however, a few experts are needed for a hospital to be properly trained in disaster management.

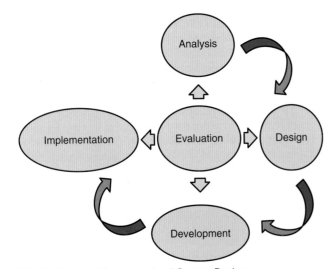

FIG 6-2 Phases of the Instructional System Design.

All training programs on hospital disaster management should be based on multidisciplinary, scenario-based, modular, and competency-based approaches.[17,79,81] The hospital staff is grouped as managers, responders, and supporters, considering their roles in response to disasters. The competencies and training needs of each group will be different but overlapping. However, the core competencies of all groups must be addressed in the disaster-training program (e.g., safety, command system, surge capacity, evacuation, etc.).[75,76,78,79,81]

Assessment of Hospital Preparedness for Disasters

The assessment of hospital disaster preparedness is critical to understand the strengths, weaknesses, gaps, and capacities of a hospital, in respect to disaster management, before the occurrence of an incident. It will help the authorities to promote the preparedness status of the hospital, mainly through diminishing vulnerabilities and enhancing capabilities.

Although it is difficult to recognize and evaluate all elements of disaster preparedness for a hospital, the items that should certainly be included in the assessment are: (1) command and control, (2) communications, (3) safety and security, (4) triage, (5) surge capacity, (6) essential services, (7) human resources, (8) resource management, and (9) recovery.[82]

Different methods, such as surveying, visiting department, implementing structured checklists, analyzing video recorded during drills and exercises, and interviewing key authorities might be used for evaluation of hospital preparedness. However, there is no consensus on both a valid and reliable tool with which to measure hospital preparedness.[30,37,41,83]

Evaluating an exercise provides more reliable and realistic results concerning readiness and performance of a hospital during a disaster. Depending on the objective, an exercise method (tabletop, computerized, functional, full-scale, and drill) can be used for simulating a disaster and then evaluating different aspects of preparedness (e.g., personal performance, managerial performance, problem solving capability, etc.).[47,83–86]

The easiest and most common method of evaluating the level of hospital preparedness for disasters is the survey. Using an international and validated tool may be useful and low cost, especially for poor communities, and it allows for standardized comparisons to national and international benchmarks. Therefore the WHO recommends a standardized checklist for assessment of the capacity of health facilities in response to emergencies and disasters.[82] The checklist consists of 92 items, classified in nine categories. For each item, there are three levels of preparedness actions: (1) due for review, (2) in progress, and (3) completed.

The main weakness of all evaluation methods regarding hospital disaster preparedness is the lack of an "outcome base." Determining whether preparedness elements decrease mortality and morbidity of disaster victims, and if so, how effective the influence is on outcomes is difficult to determine.

⚠ PITFALLS

There are possible shortcomings in disaster-preparedness planning for hospitals.[25] The following factors can have a remarkable influence on hospital preparedness.

- Funding and economic factors can be a major impediment to hospital motivation for disaster preparedness. The financial resources for hospital disaster preparedness should be provided by the hospital, community, or state and federal grants, which help to plan, organize, and provide action plans for disasters and mass casualty incidents.[25,47,87]

- Lack of a comprehensive risk perception might be a negative factor in hospital preparedness. The risk-assessment methods that only rank the hazards in their order of priority, rather than developing an understanding of vulnerability elements, do not achieve risk reduction objectives. They also may confuse inexperienced personnel creating higher risk for their hospitals.[25,53]
- Improper-planning assumptions, which come from traditional planning based on conventional wisdom rather than evidence- and experience-based research, are another obstacle to preparedness motivation at hospitals: for instance, expecting only ambulances transporting casualties, expecting that only decontaminated casualties will arrive, expecting prompt and full community assistance, etc.[25]
- Lack of legal issues might hinder hospitals' disaster preparedness in different ways: for example, if hospitals are not legally requested to be safe from disasters, are not guaranteed reimbursement for the medical care they provide during a disaster, do not receive legal memoranda of understanding to provide assistance in the event of an emergency to maintain continuity of services or to create surge capacity, etc.[88]
- The financial and personnel time cost associated with disaster preparedness can be a major challenge. Expending funds without an immediate return or economic benefit may appear as a threat to a hospital business plan. In addition, costs of maintaining an adequate state of readiness in the hospital and investing in equipment and supplies that may never be used must be considered. Further, it is often difficult for a hospital to release key employees from their daily duties to participate in disaster training and exercises, but this must be done to ensure readiness.[25,87]
- Lack of standardized measures and metrics for hospital disaster preparedness might be an important obstacle to disaster planning and preparedness. Standard measures on hospital emergency management can require a scientific, legal, and practical framework to conduct an effective hospital disaster plan.[25,37,89]
- Lack of knowledge and awareness of and the attitude among hospital personnel about concepts of disaster management, as well as an absence of those willing to be involved in disaster-management activities are barriers to planning hospital preparedness.[90]

Despite the obstacles to planning for hospital disaster preparedness, a few actions are recommended to enhance the potentiality of hospital preparedness.

- Well-designed and objectives-based research can reveal potential ways to overcome the barriers to hospital disaster preparedness. Research subjects may focus on managerial elements, operational processes, resiliency of the response system, outcome measures, etc.
- Education is a basic action on capacity building for risk reduction and a key tier of the disaster-preparedness cycle. Trained managers and staff understand the necessity of hospital preparedness and work wisely on the issue.
- Motivational interventions and strategies could improve readiness for possible disasters. However, attention directed on maintaining a safe and secure environment for patients, visitors, and staff might be more valuable.
- Preparedness guidance may help a hospital system to define and plan to capture necessary response capabilities. The guidance should be validated as effective in establishing operational level, rather than according to the usual "awareness" level competency.
- Rewarding good and effective practices in disaster-preparedness actions will motivate the managers and staff to improve plans relevant to disaster-management issues.
- Lessons learned from previous disasters could serve as a basis for hospital staff to design realistic disaster scenarios and revise key elements to enhance the preparedness condition.

- Availability of standard guidelines and measures may remove most of the uncertainties in disaster management and demonstrate the optimal performance metrics required of hospitals to operate ideally during disasters.
- Developing national policies and strategies on disaster management will help all organizations, including hospitals, to recognize their responsibilities and commitments in the community during a disaster.
- Financial support and reimbursement by the national or local government will remove an important barrier to disaster-preparedness activities for hospitals.

SUMMARY

Hospitals are usually vulnerable to disasters. Past events demonstrate the destructive effects of disasters on hospitals, and these effects are not limited to developing countries. The role of the hospital in a disaster as the place where casualties are cared for medically demands that the hospital remain operational in the aftermath of any major disaster, which requires comprehensive preparedness by the hospital. The preparedness process starts with a hazard vulnerability analysis (HVA) and risk assessment, followed by preparedness steps in response to that analysis. The HICS is a standardized organizational plan, enabling hospitals to respond efficiently to possible disasters that might require increasing their surge capacity. Regular evaluation of hospital preparedness, using standardized tools such as the WHO checklists, helps authorities to recognize possible gaps in and barriers to hospital readiness for upcoming disasters. Lack of funds and established standards, as well as legal deficiencies, could be large barriers to hospital safety and preparedness. Training programs, research on outcome-based preparedness methods, and fulfilling financial requirements are recommended to make hospitals safe and prepared for efficient disaster response.

REFERENCES

1. Oxford dictionaries. Availabe at: http://www.oxforddictionaries.com/definition/english/hospital, Accessed April 2014.
2. Wikipedia. http://en.wikipedia.org/wiki/Hospital, Accessed April 2014.
3. Chesbro WP. Disaster medical care: the basic hospital disaster plan. *Calif Med*. 1961;95(6):371–373.
4. Zane RD, Prestipino AL. Implementing the hospital emergency incident command system: an integrated delivery system's experience. *Prehosp Disast Med*. 2004;19(4):311–317.
5. *Hospital Emergency Incident Command System, Version 3*. San Mateo County Health Services Agency Emergency Medical Services; 1998. Available at: http://www.heics.com/HEICS98a.pdf, Accessed April 2014.
6. *Hospital Incident Command System Guidebook*. The California Emergency Medical Services Authority (EMSA); 2006. Available at: http://www.emsa.ca.gov/hics/, Accessed April 2014.
7. *Hospital Incident Command System (HICS)*. The California Emergency Medical Services Authority (EMSA); 2014. Available at: http://www.emsa.ca.gov/disaster_medical_services_division_hospital_incident_command_system, Accessed June 2014.
8. *Hyogo Framework for Action 2005–2015: Building the Resilience of Nations and Communities to Disasters*. United Nations/International Strategy for Disaster Reduction. Available at: http://www.unisdr.org/2005/wcdr/intergover/official-doc/L-docs/Hyogo-framework-for-action-english.pdf, Accessed April 2014.
9. *Hospital Safety Index: Guide for Evaluators*. Geneva, Switzerland: World Health Organization; 2008. Available at: http://www.paho.org/english/dd/ped/SafeHosEvaluatorGuideEng.pdf, Accessed April 2014.
10. *Historical Standard: ASTM E2413-04 Standard Guide for Hospital Preparedness and Response*. The American Society for Testing and Materials (ASTM); 2009.

11. Schultz CH, Koenig KL, Lewis RJ. Implications of hospital evacuation after the Northridge, California, earthquake. *N Engl J Med.* 2003;348 (14):1349–1355.

12. Gray BH, Hebert K. Hospitals in Hurricane Katrina: challenges facing custodial institutions in a disaster. *J Health Care Poor Underserved.* 2007;18 (2):283–298.

13. Bagaria J, Heggie C, Abrahams J, et al. Evacuation and sheltering of hospitals in emergencies: a review of international experience. *Prehosp Disaster Med.* 2009;24(5):461–467.

14. Miyamoto K, Yanev P, Salvaterra I. L'Aquila earthquake, Italy: earthquake field investigation report. *Global Risk Miyamoto.* Available at: http://www.grmcat.com/images/Italy-EQ-Report.pdf, Accessed April 2014.

15. Pan-American Health Organization, World Health Organization. Protecting new health facilities from natural hazards: guidelines for the promotion of disaster mitigation. *Prehosp Disaster Med.* 2004;19 (4):326–351.

16. Yao GC, Lin CC. Identification of earthquake damaged operational and functional components in hospital buildings. *J Chinese Inst Engrs.* 2000;23 (4):409–416.

17. Djalali AR. *Preparedness and safe hospital: medical response to disasters.* (thesis), 2012. Stockholm, Sweden: Karolinska Institutet; 2012. Available at: http://openarchive.ki.se/xmlui/handle/10616/40986, Accessed April 2014.

18. Nates JL. Combined external and internal hospital disaster: impact and response in a Houston trauma center intensive care unit. *Crit Care Med.* 2004;32:686–690.

19. Angantyr LG, Häggström E, Kulling P. KAMEDO report No. 93—the power failure at Karolinska University Hospital, Huddinge, 07 April 2007. *Prehosp Disaster Med.* 2009;24(5):468–470.

20. Yanagawa Y, Miyawaki H, Shimada J, et al. Medical evacuation of patients to other hospitals due to the Fukushima I nuclear accidents. *Prehosp Disaster Med.* 2011;26(5):391–393.

21. Wolinsky PR, Tejwani NC, Testa NN, et al. Lessons learned from the activation of a disaster plan: 9/11. *J Bone Joint Surg Am.* 2003;85:1844–1846.

22. Cushman JG, Pachter NL, Beaton HL. Two New York City hospitals' surgical response to the September 11, 2001 terrorist attack in New York City. *J Trauma.* 2003;54:147–155.

23. Feeney J, Parekh N, Blumenthal J, et al. September 11, 2001: a test of preparedness and spirit. *Bull Am Coll Surg.* 2002;87:12–17.

24. *Hospitals Safe from Disasters.* United Nations/International Strategy for Disaster Reduction (UN/ISDR). Available at: http://www.unisdr.org/2009/campaign/pdf/wdrc-2008-2009-information-kit.pdf, Accessed April 2014.

25. Barbera JA, Yeatts DJ, Macintyre AG. Challenge of hospital emergency preparedness: analysis and recommendations. *Disaster Med Public Health Prep.* 2009;3(2 suppl):S74–S82.

26. Healthcare Association of New York State. *Meeting New Challenges and Fulfilling the Public Trust: Resources Needed for Hospital Emergency Preparedness.* New York: Healthcare Association of New York State; 2001, 1–4.

27. Jenkins JL, McCarthy ML, Sauer LM, et al. Mass-casualty triage: time for an evidence-based approach. *Prehosp Disaster Med.* 2008;23(1):3–8.

28. *Terminology on Disaster Risk Reduction.* Nations/International Strategy for Disaster Reduction (UN/ISDR); 2009. http://www.unisdr.org/files/7817_UNISDRTerminologyEnglish.pdf, Accessed April 2014.

29. Waugh WL. Terrorism and the all-hazards model. In: *Emergency Management On-Line Conference, June 28–July 16, 2004.* Available at: http://www.idsemergencymanagement.com/Common/Paper/Paper_63/waugh.pdf, Accessed April 2014.

30. Adini B, Goldberg A, Laor D, et al. Assessing levels of hospital emergency preparedness. *Prehosp Disast Med.* 2006;21(6):451–457.

31. Braun BI, Wineman NV, Finn NL, et al. Integrating hospitals into community emergency preparedness planning. *Ann Intern Med.* 2006;144 (11):799–811.

32. Djalali A, Khankeh H, Ohlen G, Castrén M, Kurland L. Facilitators and obstacles in pre-hospital medical response to earthquakes: a qualitative study. *Scand J Trauma Resusc Emerg Med.* 2011;19:30.

33. *Guidelines for Hospital Emergency Preparedness Planning.* United Nations Development Programme, India. Available at: http://sdmassam.nic.in/pdf/publication/undp/guidelines_hospital_emergency.pdf, Accessed April 2014.

34. *Guidelines for Vulnerability Reduction in the Design of New Health Facilities.* Pan American Health Organization/ World Health Organization; 2004. Available at: http://www.preventionweb.net/files/628_7760.pdf, Accessed April 2014.

35. *Principles of Disaster Mitigation in Health Facilities.* Pan-American Health Organization/World Health Organization; 2000. http://www1.paho.org/english/PED/fundaeng.htm, Accessed April 2014.

36. *Health Facility Seismic Vulnerability Evaluation.* World Health Organization, Regional Office for Europe (WHO/EURO). Available at: http://www.euro.who.int/__data/assets/pdf_file/0007/141784/e88525.pdf, Accessed April 2014.

37. Djalali A, Castren M, Khankeh H, et al. Hospital disaster preparedness as measured by functional capacity: a comparison between Iran and Sweden. *Prehosp Disaster Med.* 2013;28(5):454–461.

38. Pisla M, Domente S, Chetraru L, et al. *Evaluation of Hospital Safety in the Republic of Moldova.* World Health Organization; 2010. Available at: http://www.euro.who.int/en/what-we-do/health-topics/emergencies/disaster-preparedness-and-response/news/news/2011/04/official-launch-of-the-evaluation-of-hospital-safety-inthe-republic-of-moldova-report, Accessed April 2014.

39. Ardalan A, Kandi M, Talebian MT, et al. Hospitals safety from disasters in I. R.iran: the results from assessment of 224 hospitals. *PLoS Curr.* 2014 Feb 28;6.

40. Djalali A, Ardalan A, Ohlen G, et al. Nonstructural safety of hospitals for disasters: a comparison between two capital cities. *Disaster Med Public Health Prep.* 2014;8:179–184.

41. Kaji AH, Koenig KL, Lewis RJ. Current hospital disaster preparedness. *JAMA.* 2007;298(18):2188–2190.

42. Campbell P, Trockman SJ, Walker AR. Strengthening hazard vulnerability analysis: results of recent research in Maine. *Public Health Rep.* 2011;126 (2):290–293.

43. *Kaiser Permanente Hazards and Vulnerability Analysis.* California hospital association. Available at: http://www.calhospitalprepare.org/hazard-vulnerability-analysis, Accessed April 2014.

44. Arnold JL, Dembry L, Tsai MC, et al. Recommended modifications and applications of the Hospital Emergency Incident Command System for hospital emergency management. *Prehosp Disast Med.* 2005;20(5):290–300.

45. Autrey P, Moss J. High-reliability teams and situation awareness: implementing a hospital emergency incident command system. *J Nurs Adm.* 2006;36(2):67–72.

46. Arnold J, O'Brien D, Walsh D, et al. The perceived usefulness of the Hospital Emergency Incident Command System and an assessment tool for hospital disaster response capabilities and needs in hospital disaster planning in Turkey. *Prehosp Disast Med.* 2001;16(2):s12.

47. Djalali A, Castren M, Hosseinijenab V, et al. Hospital Incident Command System (HICS) performance in Iran: decision making during disasters. *Scand J Trauma Resusc Emerg Med.* 2012;20(1):14.

48. Tsai MC, Arnold JL, Chuang CC, et al. Implementation of the Hospital Emergency Incident Command System during an outbreak of severe acute respiratory syndrome (SARS) at a hospital in Taiwan, ROC. *J Emerg Med.* 2005;28(2):185–196.

49. *Best Practices for Hospital Preparedness.* American college of emergency physicians. Available at: www.acep.org/content.aspx?id=45409, Accessed April 2014.

50. Born CT, Briggs SM, Ciraulo DL, et al. Disasters and mass casualties: I. General principles of response and management. *J Am Acad Orthop Surg.* 2007;15(7):388–396.

51. *Medical Surge Capacity and Capability: A Management System for Integrating Medical and Health Resources during Large-Scale Emergencies.* U.S. Department of Health and Human Services; 2007. Available at: https://www.phe.gov/preparedness/planning/mscc/handbook/documents/mscc080626.pdf, Accessed April 2014.

52. Hick JL, Hanfling D, Burstein JL, et al. Health care facility and community strategies for patient care surge capacity. *Ann Emerg Med.* 2004;44 (3):253–261.

53. Lynn M, Gurr D, Memon A, et al. Management of conventional mass casualty incidents: ten commandments for hospital planning. *J Burn Care Res.* 2006;27(5):649–658.

54. Abir M, Davis MM, Sankar P, et al. Design of a model to predict surge capacity bottlenecks for burn mass casualties at a large academic medical center. *Prehosp Disaster Med.* 2013;28(1):23–32.

55. Spiteri M, Calleja N, Djalali A. *Modelling of Hospital Surge Capacity for a Mass Casualty Event Response in a Small Island State Hospital* (thesis). Novara, Italy: European Master in Disaster Medicine. Available at: http://www.dismedmaster.com/, Accessed May 2014.

56. Sternberg E, Lee GC, Huard D. Counting crises: US hospital evacuations, 1971–1999. *Prehosp Disaster Med.* 2004;19(2):150–157.

57. Achour N, Miyajima M, Kitaura M, et al. Earthquake induced structural and nonstructural damage in hospitals. *Earthq Spectra.* 2011;27(3):617–634.

58. *Hospital Evacuation Decision Guide.* Agency for healthcare research and quality, U.S. department of health and human services; 2010. Available at: http://archive.ahrq.gov/prep/hospevacguide/hospevac.pdf, Accessed April 2014.

59. Iserson KV. Vertical hospital evacuations: a new method. *South Med J.* 2013;106(1):37–42.

60. Petinaux B, Yadav K. Patient-driven resource planning of a health care facility evacuation. *Prehosp Disaster Med.* 2013;28(2):120–126.

61. Hultz CH, Koenig KL, Auf der Heide E. Benchmarking for hospital evacuation: a critical data collection tool. *Prehosp Disaster Med.* 2005;20(5):331–342.

62. Arnold J. Disaster medicine in the 21st century: future hazards, vulnerabilities, and risk. *Prehosp Disaster Med.* 2002;17(1):3–11.

63. Ghilarducci DP, Pirrallo RG, Hegmann KT. Hazardous materials readiness of United States level 1 trauma centers. *J Occup Environ Med.* 2000;42(7):683–692.

64. Kollek D, Cwinn AA. Hospital emergency readiness overview study. *Prehosp Disaster Med.* 2011;26(3):159–165.

65. Niska RW, Shimizu IM. Hospital preparedness for emergency response: United States, 2008. *Natl Health Stat Report.* 2011;24(37):1–14.

66. Bennett RL. Chemical or biological terrorist attacks: an analysis of the preparedness of hospitals for managing victims affected by chemical or biological weapons of mass destruction. *Int J Environ Res Public Health.* 2006;3(1):67–75.

67. Burda P, Sein Anand J, Chodorowski Z, et al. Strategic preparedness of selected hospitals to act during massive chemical disasters. *Przegl Lek.* 2007;64(4–5):212–214.

68. Barelli A, Biondi I, Soave M, et al. The comprehensive medical preparedness in chemical emergencies: the chain of chemical survival. *Eur J Emerg Med.* 2008;15(2):110–118.

69. Koenig KL, Boatright CJ, Hancock JA, et al. Health care facilities' "war on terrorism": a deliberate process for recommending personal protective equipment. *Am J Emerg Med.* 2007;25(2):185–195.

70. *Chemical Hazards Emergency Medical Management: Information for Hospital Providers.* U.S. department of health and human services. Available at: http://chemm.nlm.nih.gov/hospitalproviders.htm. Accessed April 2014.

71. Hick JL, Penn P, Hanfling D, et al. Establishing and training health care facility decontamination teams. *Ann Emerg Med.* 2003;42(3):381–390.

72. *Hospital-Based First Receivers of Victims from Mass Casualty Incidents Involving the Release of Hazardous Substances.* Occupational Safety and Health Administration; 2005. Available at: https://www.osha.gov/dts/osta/bestpractices/firstreceivers_hospital.pdf, Accessed April 2014.

73. Ingrassia PL, Foletti M, Djalali A, et al. Education and training initiatives for crisis management in the European Union: a web-based analysis of available programs. *Prehosp Disaster Med.* 2014;29(2):115–126.

74. Burkle FM Jr. The development of multidisciplinary core competencies: the first step in the professionalization of disaster medicine and public health preparedness on a global scale. *Disaster Med Public Health Prep.* 2012;6(1):10–12.

75. Walsh L, Subbarao I, Gebbie K, et al. Core competencies for disaster medicine and public health. *Disaster Med Public Health Prep.* 2012;6(1):44–52.

76. Archer F, Seynaeve G. International guidelines and standards for education and training to reduce the consequences of events that may threaten the health status of a community. A report of an Open International WADEM Meeting, Brussels, Belgium, 29–31 October, 2004. *Prehosp Disaster Med.* 2007;22(2):120–130.

77. Banathy BH. Instructional systems design. In: Gagne RM, ed. *Instructional Technology: Foundations.* Hillsdale, NJ: Lawrence Erlbaum Associates; 1987:85–112.

78. Djalali A, Hosseinijenab V, Hasani A, et al. A fundamental, national, disaster management plan: an education based model. *Prehosp Disaster Med.* 2009;24(6):565–569.

79. Schultz CH, Koenig KL, Whiteside M, et al. Development of national standardized all-hazard disaster core competencies for acute care physicians, nurses, and EMS professionals. *Ann Emerg Med.* 2012;59(3):196–208.

80. *Revised Bloom's Taxonomy.* Available at: http://www.utar.edu.my/fegt/file/Revised_Blooms_Info.pdf, Accessed April 2014.

81. Seynaeve G, Archer F, Fisher J, et al. International standards and guidelines on education and training for the multi-disciplinary health response to major events that threaten the health status of a community. *Prehosp Disaster Med.* 2004;19(2):S17–S30.

82. *Hospital Emergency Response Checklist: An All-Hazards Tool for Hospital Administrators and Emergency Managers.* World Health Organization: Regional Office for Europe. Available at: http://www.euro.who.int/__data/assets/pdf_file/0020/148214/e95978.pdf, Accessed April 2014.

83. Kaji AH, Langford V, Lewis RJ. Assessing hospital disaster preparedness: a comparison of an on-site survey, directly observed drill performance, and video analysis of teamwork. *Ann Emerg Med.* 2008;52(3):195–201.

84. Ingrassia PL, Colombo D, Barra FL, et al. Impacto de la formación en gestión médica de desastres: resultados de un estudio piloto utilizando una nueva herramienta para la simulación in vivo. *Emergencias.* 2013;25(6):459–466.

85. Frank-Law JM, Ingrassia PL, Ragazzoni L, et al. The effectiveness of simulation based training on the Disastermed.Ca emergency department simulator for medical student training in disaster medicine. *Can J Emerg Med.* 2010;12(1):27–32.

86. Ingrassia PL, Ragazzoni L, Carenzo L, et al. Virtual reality and live simulation: a comparison between two simulation tools for assessing mass casualty triage skills. *Eur J Emerg Med.* 2014 May 23 [Epub ahead of print].

87. Liong AS, Liong SU. Financial and economic considerations for emergency response providers. *Crit Care Nurs Clin North Am.* 2010;22(4):437–444.

88. Sauer LM, McCarthy ML, Knebel A, et al. Major influences on hospital emergency management and disaster preparedness. *Disaster Med Public Health Prep.* 2009;3(2 suppl):S68–S73.

89. Lurie N, Wasserman J, Nelson CD. Public health emergency preparedness: evolution or revolution? *Health Aff.* 2006;25:935–945.

90. Chaffee M. Willingness of health care personnel to work in a disaster: an integrative review of the literature. *Disaster Med Public Health Prep.* 2009;3(1):42–56.

7 | CHAPTER

Complex Emergencies

Susan A. Bartels, Matthew M. Hall, Frederick M. Burkle Jr., and P. Gregg Greenough

CHARACTERIZATION OF COMPLEX EMERGENCIES

The characterization of complex emergencies has evolved over time, with different individuals and different organizations favoring particular definitions to highlight specific characteristics. However, there are important key features of complex emergencies that have been well documented across a wide range of crisis settings, and these are more universally accepted than any one particular definition.

Common characteristics of complex emergencies:

- Conflict and warfare are at the core of complex emergencies with most originating from widespread violence or loss of life and involving massive population displacements, as well as pervasive and extensive damage to societies, their infrastructures, and their economies.
- The underlying causes of complex emergencies are usually multifaceted and dynamic throughout the course of the crises and include political, environmental, economic, and demographic instability.[1]
- Complex emergencies are often prolonged, with the average civil war now lasting at least 10 years.[2]
- Delivery of humanitarian assistance is often hindered by political and military constraints, leading to security risks for relief workers.
- The majority of victims are civilian with morbidity and mortality highest among vulnerable and unprotected children, women, the elderly, and the disabled. In fact, civilians account for 90% of war-related deaths[3] from civil strife, genocide, and other violations of the Geneva Conventions.

As of early 2014, there were 60 countries in the world at war, involving an estimated 531 militias and separatist movements.[4] The majority of these were internal nation-state wars. State and nonstate perpetrators in these conflicts wantonly violate the Fourth Geneva Convention, which mandates the protection of civilians from attack and inhumane treatment and prohibits attacks directed at civilian hospitals and medical teams.[5] Within these contemporary wars, civilian lives are often strategically targeted through the destruction of livelihoods, forced displacement, and direct physical violence, and there is now a wealth of evidence substantiating the massive effect that war has both on individual and public health.[6,7] Direct health effects include injuries, deaths and disabilities, human rights and international humanitarian law abuses, and psychological stress. Indirect health effects actually contribute to the majority of mortality and morbidity and arise from population displacement, disruption of food supplies, and the destruction of health facilities and public health infrastructure.

A comprehensive understanding of complex emergencies requires consideration of the politics surrounding the underlying conflicts. In present-day intrastate war, there are frequently multiple warring factions with unique ideologies often inscrutable to the outside world. The combination of many armed actors, with individual identities driven by enigmatic beliefs, has prompted the international community, its policy makers, and its media to designate these conflicts generically as *chaos*.[8] The Second Congo War in the Democratic Republic of Congo (DRC) was a prime example, with at least 20 armed factions actively engaged at the height of the conflict. But contemporary conflicts are sometimes intended to be confusing, and it is important to recognize the underlying motivations for war. Chaos, for instance, can serve as a strategic cover for political and economic manipulation and for carrying out self-aligned agendas.[8] Wars are almost always functional: they serve a purpose for one or more involved parties, and those parties may have little interest in ending a conflict from which they are directly benefitting.

All manner of players within a complex emergency can manipulate humanitarian services for political purposes and self-gain. For instance, relief is sometimes withheld for economic purposes or in a malicious attempt to deprive the opponent, or perceived supporters of the opponent, of life-sustaining aid.[8] This has been a common occurrence in Syria where the government's denial of humanitarian access has greatly exacerbated and perpetuated civilian suffering. Such manipulation of humanitarian aid places relief workers at significant personal risk; undertaking humanitarian response thus requires a politically informed approach. Geoff Leone of the International Committee of the Red Cross (ICRC) advises, "Know the politics, so you can negotiate the minefield."[8] By pushing aid through to those in need, the delivery of relief services also becomes a political act that has the potential to challenge power structures. In this politically complex environment, aid organizations must balance humanitarian access with bearing witness to war crimes and crimes against humanity, understanding the stark reality that publically denouncing witnessed atrocities risks being denied future access to those in critical need.[8] Additionally, aid organizations responding to complex emergencies must always bear in mind that relief work is intended to relieve suffering and to save lives among affected populations, and that it will never be a substitute for a political solution to the underlying crisis.

Mass Population Displacement

Mass population displacement and its effects on health have been increasingly recognized since the end of the Cold War. According to a 2013 midyear report, the total "population of concern" to the United Nations (UN) High Commissioner for Refugees (UNHCR) was 38.7 million, representing the highest number on record for the agency.[9] Of these, approximately 10.5 million are refugees, defined by international conventions as "persons who cross international borders due to fear of persecution on the basis of race, religion, nationality or membership in a particular social or political group."[10] The Refugee Convention entitles those who meet this legal definition to access services that sustain health and well-being—food, water, shelter, sanitation, and health care—and assigns them certain rights within their host countries. While repatriation is usually the long-term goal for refugees, it must be on a voluntary basis when deemed safe to return to the country of origin. In international law, the principle of *non-refoulement* dictates that no refugee should be forced to return to any country where he or she is likely to face persecution or torture.

Internally displaced persons (IDPs) are individuals who leave their homes out of fear of being persecuted for reasons similar to those of refugees, but they do not cross an international border. The world's IDP population is estimated to be in excess of 20 million, far outpacing the number of refugees over the last 10 years.[9] Because they have not crossed an international border, IDPs legally remain under the protection of their own governments, even though those same governments may be responsible for their forced displacement. Therefore, IDPs are among some of the world's most vulnerable individuals. Although they do not technically fall under the mandate of the UNHCR and are therefore not guaranteed the same protections and rights as refugees, the UNHCR has been variably lending assistance to IDPs for many years.

The acute phase of mass displacement and forced migration typically results in mortality rates significantly increased above the baseline mortality rates of the population prior to displacement. Mortality surveillance systems implemented by aid agencies attempt to capture numbers of deaths, but inevitably under-report given the degree of insecurity on the ground. This is especially true for IDP mortality figures in which national authorities may prohibit access to the displaced population. The high mortality associated with this acute phase derives both directly from injuries incurred from the violence preceding or during flight, and indirectly from food scarcity, siege, and communicable disease outbreaks. One of the highest refugee mortality rates ever documented was among the almost 1 million Rwandans who fled into eastern Zaire in 1994. A cholera outbreak in the refugee camps near Goma largely contributed to this catastrophe, with a crude mortality rate of 54.5 deaths/10,000 daily[11] (prewar crude mortality rate in Rwanda was 0.6 deaths/10,000 daily).

Food Insecurity

Political instability and insecurity can have a significant adverse impact on national and local economies, including the agricultural industry. Fighting can damage irrigation systems, warring parties may intentionally destroy crops or loot harvests, and distribution systems that connect rural production zones and urban populations may completely collapse.[12] Cumulatively, these factors can lead to food scarcity and/or compromise a population's reliable access to food, and during complex emergencies the prevalence of acute malnutrition and micronutrient deficiencies can be extremely high,[13] particularly in developing countries. Such conditions may contribute to other coincident factors of food scarcity—drought, ill-fated government policy, crop failure—that result in famine, a state of widespread food scarcity accompanied by acute malnutrition, micronutrient deficiencies, and elevated mortality rates. Such has been the case in recent conflicts in Somalia, Ethiopia, and Sudan.

Sexual Violence

Documentation of wartime sexual violence has improved in recent years, leading to a focused appreciation for the magnitude of the problem. Recent conflicts in the former Yugoslavia, DRC, Darfur, Liberia, and Sierra Leone were all characterized by extensive sexual violence that was both strategic and systematic in nature. Sexual violence is used to terrorize civilian populations, forcing them to rapidly flee from their homes, leaving their belongings and livelihoods behind.[14] In conflicts motivated by ethnic cleansing, sexual violence is sometimes used as a means of "polluting" bloodlines and forcibly impregnating women to produce "ethnically cleansed" children.[14,15] In modern, intrastate warfare, sexual violence has established itself as a cheap, low-technology, and yet highly effective weapon.

Not all conflict-related sexual violence is systematic, however. Sexual abuse and exploitation by relief workers have also been reported,[16–19] and, in recent years, there have been multiple interventions to address these concerning issues. Furthermore, preexisting sexual violence is often heightened during times of war. Intimate partner violence (IPV) is one of the most common forms of gender-based violence (GBV) in displaced camp settings and in complex emergencies. Overall rates of IPV tend to be much higher than rates of sexual assault outside the home.[20] It is important to note that men and boys are also targets of sexual violence.[21,22]

HISTORICAL PERSPECTIVE

In the early post-Cold War period, humanitarian assistance was believed to be the key to effectively intervening in complex emergencies. Relief organizations, drawing on international treaties and covenants such as the Geneva Conventions, based their work on neutrality, impartiality, and the right to assistance based purely on need and without political discrimination. The global community soon realized, however, that sustained peace and development would never occur without a political solution, and that the "humanitarian imperative" driving humanitarian responses was simply not enough to adequately protect the health and well-being of civilian populations during conflict. At about the same time, variable quality of relief delivery, lack of professional standards, and lack of evidence-based practices challenged the ability of humanitarian organizations to work effectively in field operations, creating further frustration for donors, governments, and humanitarian organizations alike.[23]

In early UN emergency responses, peacekeeping forces were deployed under Chapter VI of the UN Charter to help quell the conflict and provide some semblance of security for intervening UN agencies and relief organizations. Under Chapter VI, peacekeepers lacked the resources and legal mandate to use military force in achieving their objectives and ensuring "humanitarian space." As this protected working zone became more tenuous and health care workers assumed more extraneous roles (contributing to a perception of less neutrality and less impartiality), there was an alarming increase in intentional violence and banditry against humanitarian relief agencies and peacekeeping forces.[24] This violence contributed to a decision to replace UN peacekeeping forces with peace enforcement troops under UN Charter Chapter VII. Peace enforcement troops have the resources to stop violence in order to protect civilians and are permitted to use military action to restore international peace and security. The transition from peacekeeping to peace enforcement was slow, but all UN military interventions have since been authorized under Chapter VII.[25]

After a slow and inadequate humanitarian response in Darfur in 2004, the UN Emergency Relief Coordinator and Under-Secretary General for Humanitarian Affairs commissioned the *Humanitarian Response Review*, which was aimed at closing operational gaps and augmenting the timeliness, effectiveness, and predictability of aid delivery. In the 2005 *Review*, three networks were identified to which most relief organizations belonged: UN network, Red Cross/Red Crescent Movement, and nongovernmental organizations (NGOs).[26] Additionally, to close the identified gaps and improve the delivery of humanitarian assistance, four pillars of humanitarian reform were introduced: (1) the Cluster Approach, (2) Strengthening the Humanitarian Coordination System, (3) Adequate, Flexible, and Predictable Humanitarian Financing, and (4) Building Partnerships.[27] Within the Cluster Approach, "clusters" are groups of organizations, both UN and non-UN,

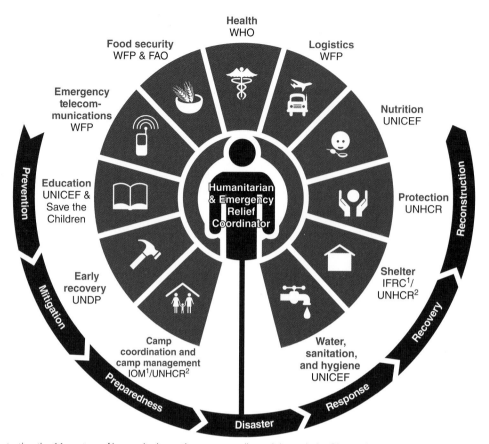

FIG 7-1 Diagram illustrating the 11 sectors of humanitarian action now coordinated through the Cluster Approach, which was introduced in 2005. (From UN Office for the Coordination of Humanitarian Affairs. Humanitarian Response 2013. Available from: http://www.humanitarianresponse.info/clusters/space/page/what-cluster-approach [accessed April 6, 2014])

designated by the Inter-Agency Standing Committee (IASC) to lead response coordination within each of the main sectors of humanitarian action (Fig. 7-1).

CURRENT PRACTICE

Humanitarian Response

It is not uncommon for NGOs and other relief organizations to be established in an unstable country long before violence garners the attention of the international community. The broader, multinational humanitarian response begins with a decision to intervene, a decision that is usually prompted by increasing violence and by mass displacement of refugees and IDPs. It is also usually preceded by weeks or months of debate within the UN Security Council before a resolution is passed directing the scope of the humanitarian assistance and defining the participating actors.

Humanitarian assistance usually comes from assets contributed by the UN Office for the Coordination of Humanitarian Affairs (OCHA) and other field operational UN agencies such as the World Food Program (WFP), the World Health Organization (WHO), and the UN Children's Fund (UNICEF). The response typically also includes the Red Cross Movement, relief organizations, and donor agencies that primarily represent the governments of industrialized nations, such as the United States Agency for International Development (USAID), the Canadian International Development Agency (CIDA), and the United Kingdom's Department for International Development (DFID). Without good coordination between the relief organizations delivering assistance, there can be many gaps and overlaps in the response.

Concern about the lack of standards and accountability among humanitarian relief personnel peaked in the mid-1990s following the Rwandan genocide. To address these growing concerns, the Humanitarian Charter and Minimum Standards (Sphere Project) was initiated in 1997 under the joint management of InterAction and the Steering Committee for Humanitarian Response (SCHR).[28] The objective of the Sphere Project is to "improve the quality of assistance delivered to people affected by disaster or conflict" and to improve "the accountability of humanitarian agencies and states towards their constituents, donors and affected populations."[28] The *Sphere Handbook* provides standardized guidelines, continually revised according to empiric evidence and consensus, for addressing the core areas of water and sanitation, nutrition, food aid, shelter, and site planning as well as health services.

Evolution of Civilian Medical Needs in Complex Emergencies

In the early phases of complex emergencies, the most urgent health concerns are often injuries resulting from direct violence. Although there will continue to be traumatic injuries, with time other health priorities will emerge. For instance, if displaced populations are sheltered in overcrowded and unsanitary conditions, it is common for air-, water-, and vector-borne communicable diseases, particularly those endemic to the region, to break out and propagate easily. The threat of preventable communicable diseases, such as measles and polio, is further exacerbated by interruptions in routine vaccination as a result of the crisis. With time, mental health and psychological distress become a priority for the population in general and medical responders in particular. With more time, food insecurity will lead to acute malnutrition, particularly among children, the disabled, and the chronically ill. In less developed countries where food insecurity and chronic undernutrition is the norm, cases of malnourishment emerge sooner. And finally, with the passage of more time, an increasing number of individuals will seek care for chronic, preexisting medical problems such as hypertension, cardiac disease, and diabetes, especially in more developed countries with advanced health systems and a high prevalence of these conditions precrisis.

Public Health Priorities

Complex emergencies have a severe impact on the health of entire communities. Malnutrition coupled with infectious disease, lack of access to emergency care, and the targeting of health care facilities/providers are all known to shorten life expectancy within crisis-affected populations.[7,12] A series of four mortality surveys in the DRC between 2000 and 2004 showed a crude mortality rate (CMR) of 2.2 deaths per 1000 persons per month, up 70% from preconflict values, indicative of excess mortality generated from the breakdown of public health infrastructure. The CMR was found to be higher still, at 2.6 deaths per 1000 persons per month, in the most affected areas of the country.[29]

Both endemic diseases and illnesses once nearly exterminated must be monitored when planning treatment programs. Malaria is such a common disease in areas affected by complex emergencies that WHO includes both rapid testing supplies and basic antimalarial treatment in their Interagency Emergency Health Kit, a prepackaged kit designed to provide basic health care for up to 10,000 people for 3 months. However, other rarer conditions can also be encountered and require monitoring. For instance, although Syria declared polio eradicated within its borders in 1999, in 2013 and 2014 it had at least 27 confirmed cases of polio in the midst of its ongoing conflict.[30] Large outbreaks of meningococcal meningitis have been documented in DRC, Sudan, and Rwanda,[31] highlighting the need to screen for previously sporadic diseases, to rapidly treat individual cases, and to implement effective monitoring and control strategies.

Public Health Indicators

Although often challenging to implement, public health and communicable disease monitoring must be integrated into initial rapid assessments in complex emergencies. Rapid assessments provide initial estimates of death rates using simple measures such as the CMR and under-5 mortality rate, which are derived from household surveys, remaining vital registration systems, grave counts, and other creative measures like distribution of burial shrouds.[11,12,29,32] These "quick and dirty" evaluations have improved since the 1990s and, despite being done quickly under difficult conditions, have gained a reputation for quality.[33] With advancements in indicator identification, epidemiological analysis, data retrieval technologies, and training of relief personnel, these critical rapid assessments continue to improve as an art and a science.

As resources and time permit, more sophisticated public health measures should be implemented. The WHO Interagency Emergency Health Kit contains materials for recording distribution of medicines and other medical supplies as they are used; the *Sphere Handbook* outlines benchmarks for health care delivery with emphases on required medical staff and facilities, essential medications, mortality rates, standardized case management for common infections, newborn/childhood health, vaccine-preventable illnesses, and mental health access.[34] Furthermore, the concept of excess deaths in a complex emergency is a critical epidemiological tool, especially in the setting of conflict and mass population movement.

It is imperative to measure the prevalence of specific diseases to allow for early intervention and targeted treatment. When diagnostic resources are limited and/or qualified health personnel are lacking, it may not be possible to specifically diagnose each case of a particular disease. For example, in Goma in 1994, cases of *Vibrio cholerae* and *Shigella dysenteriae* were differentiated simply by descriptions of "watery diarrhea" and "bloody diarrhea."[32] Similarly, if rapid malaria testing is not available, then recording the incidence of "fever and chills" is often used as a proxy for diagnosing malaria. As more resources become available, greater diagnostic accuracy can be expected. Rates of acute malnutrition should also be recorded; frequently used nutrition indicators include weight/height index and middle upper arm circumstance (MUAC) for young children and body mass index (BMI) for adults. Clinical signs of severe acute malnutrition such as edema are also used as markers of malnutrition among children.[12]

Communicable Diseases
Diarrhea

In some complex emergencies diarrheal outbreaks have caused up to 40% of deaths.[31] Many factors play into the spread of diarrheal illnesses including contaminated water sources and water transport vessels, lack of latrines, overcrowded living conditions, lack of soap, and poor hygiene. Diarrheal outbreaks can be prevented or addressed by providing acceptable latrines and encouraging their primary use for defecation, maintaining a clean water supply, providing safe water vessels, and issuing adequate soap supplies. Each case of diarrhea should be classified and reported as watery or bloody as well as by patient age and gender.[12] Patients with diarrhea should be treated with oral rehydration therapy (ORT). Critical to ORT success are the implementation of rehydration centers and the availability of skilled staff to instruct caretakers on the quantity and rate of rehydration.[12]

Measles

During the 1980s, measles was a major cause of morbidity and mortality in complex emergencies with case fatality rates as high as 33%.[31] However, since the institution of widespread vaccination programs, the virus has been much better controlled. Overcrowded conditions result in higher infectious inoculation of the virus and thus transmission, and coincident malnutrition correlates with greater disease morbidity.[31] It is imperative to institute mass immunization campaigns, regardless of prior immunization history, for all individuals aged 6 months to 15 years.[12] This will require an intact cold chain and proper needle disposal to prevent transmission of blood-borne pathogens. Measles further depletes vitamin A stores in already malnourished individuals; vitamin A supplementation, shown to reduce mortality in low-income nations, should be considered at the time of measles vaccination.[35]

Malaria

Malaria prevalence increases and malaria epidemics occur either when a population moves from an area of low endemicity to higher endemicity areas or when a population migrates from a hyper-endemic region to a less endemic area.[31] Overcrowding and poor shelter provide further hazards. Sites for refugee camps should be selected with local vector-borne risk in mind. Bed nets and other impregnated materials will help prevent the spread of disease, as does washing livestock with permethrin and eliminating standing bodies of water. Further study is required to understand if pregnant women should be empirically treated with antimalarials or if there is utility in mass malaria prophylaxis at the time of measles immunization.[12] Treatment, which is included in the WHO Emergency Kit, should consider national treatment guidelines of the host country. Diagnosis should be confirmed when possible, but empiric treatment is often the norm in emergency settings.[34]

Respiratory Illnesses

Acute respiratory infections cause a great deal of morbidity and mortality in complex emergencies. Overcrowding, inadequate shelter, inadequate blankets in cold environments, and exposure to indoor cooking fires and smoke promote the spread of respiratory infections. Diphtheria and pertussis vaccination programs can be initiated as indicated by surveillance measures. Tuberculosis (TB) is becoming increasingly common in complex emergencies particularly in areas with high HIV/AIDS prevalence.[31] Given the complexity of TB control programs, they are typically only instituted once emergencies have stabilized.[12] Vitamin A supplementation will promote innate immune defenses and protect against respiratory infections independent of measles infection.[31]

Meningitis

Although it is rarer, a high degree of suspicion must be maintained for bacterial meningitis. Outbreaks have been documented in complex emergencies, especially in the sub-Saharan Africa "meningitis belt" where *Neisseria meningitides* A and C (and increasingly serogroup W135) are the main causes.[31] Epidemic control measures are typically instituted when the incidence rate is in excess of 15 per 100,000 people per week for 2 weeks or with a doubling of cases weekly for 3 weeks.[12] Once an epidemic is confirmed, mass immunization should be conducted; if the outbreak is among a displaced population, the host community should be vaccinated as well. Prophylactic treatment has not proven effective and should not be done. In Africa, treatment of meningitis has been successful with single-dose chloramphenicol in oil.[12]

Noncommunicable Diseases
Mental Health

Conflict can lead to mental health consequences for individuals and for entire communities, with depression, anxiety, and post-traumatic stress disorder (PTSD) being most commonly noted. There is, however, disagreement surrounding the diagnosis of PTSD. Some argue that significant proportions of a population will suffer from PTSD, while others maintain that the response to warfare and displacement is a social phenomenon that should not be "medicalized."[12] Nevertheless, most agree that there is almost always a small percentage of the population who may have been exposed to more extreme violence or torture and who will require more intensive mental health treatment than the remainder of the population.[12] The WHO Interagency Emergency Health Kit anticipates the need for treatment of both newly diagnosed as well as preexisting psychiatric disease and provides antipsychotics, antidepressants, and anxiolytics.[34]

Reproductive Health

All individuals have the right to reproductive health, even in conflict settings. Women and girls are highly vulnerable in emergency settings, not only because they are at high risk for sexual violence but also because they may not be able to advocate for their rights and may not be able to access desired reproductive health services. This is particularly true in contexts where preexisting gender norms undervalue women's role in society. In some complex emergencies, dire economic need leads women and adolescent girls to engage in commercial sex work, placing them at risk of unplanned pregnancies, sexually transmitted infections, and HIV/AIDS. The Inter-Agency Working Group on Reproductive Health in Crisis has published a minimum standard of reproductive health services that should be made available to all females affected by complex emergencies and has prepackaged kits available containing the drugs and supplies required to implement priority reproductive health care.[36]

Sector-Specific Responses
Nutrition

Nutritional assessments are typically performed with population convenience samples in which newly arriving refugees or displaced persons are screened, or through cluster sample surveys in lieu of population lists. The malnutrition rate for children under age 5 ranks just below the CMR as the most specific indicator of a population's health.[37,38] The malnutrition rate helps determine the urgency for food ration delivery and requirements for supplementary feeding and therapeutic feeding centers. Except in the case of severely malnourished children with acute complications, community-based therapeutic care (CTC) is now the standard of care, and commercially prepared ready-to-use therapeutic foods (RTUF) have become the preferred feeding products. The most common RTUF in acute emergencies today is Plumpy'Nut, which requires no preparation and no water or refrigeration, contains 500 kcal per pouch, and has a 2-year shelf life.[39] Micronutrient deficiencies are also important in acute emergencies, particularly in developing countries, where they have profound effects including infection, blindness, adverse birth outcomes, growth stunting, mental retardation, and increased risk of death.[40] The most important micronutrients requiring supplementation are thiamine, riboflavin, niacin, folic acid, iron, iodine, and vitamins A, C, and D. As mentioned, vitamin A supplementation is particularly critical for children; its benefits are now so well established that it is a routine intervention.

The quantity and quality of food rations are also important determinants of health outcomes in emergency-affected populations.[12] A minimum of 2100 kcal/person is generally adopted as a reference for the daily energy requirement, although ration size needs to consider the demographics of the population, climate, and access by the population to alternative sources of food and income. Food rations in developing countries generally consist of a staple cereal such as wheat, maize, or rice, in additional to a source of dense fat such as vegetable oil and a protein source such as beans, lentils, groundnuts, or dried fish.[12] In more developed countries, food rations typically include cheese, meat, powdered orange juice, and fruit. In high-income countries, food vouchers are sometimes distributed rather than actual food items. Specific needs of at-risk groups must also be considered (for instance, pregnant and lactating women, young children, those with chronic diseases, and the disabled),[40] and breast-feeding should be strongly encouraged for children younger than 2 years of age. The Sphere Project is internationally recognized as providing benchmark levels of performance with regards to food security and nutrition.[28]

Shelter

Shelter is a primary consideration in complex emergencies because mass population displacements are common. If families are to be housed in formal settlements, smaller camps are preferred as they tend to be more secure, less crowded, and easier to manage.[12] In some instances, local politics can contribute to inappropriate decisions about camp locations. Considerations for camp sites must prioritize safety of the residents and access to clean water and cooking fuel.[12] In some conflicts, it is important to be mindful of where landmines have been laid. Because food and non-food items will have to be delivered, it is critical to have road access to the area in all climatic conditions.[12] At times, it is favorable to have displaced individuals integrated into the host community, although if there are a large number of refugees scattered in many different locations, the task of identifying and providing relief services on a regular basis can be quite challenging.

Ideally, houses should be constructed from local materials using traditional designs for the given context. Plastic sheeting or tarpaulins may be required for waterproofing. In warmer, humid climates, shelters should have optimal ventilation and should offer protection from direct sunlight.[12] In colder climates, houses need to provide insulation and sufficient bedding with auxiliary heating. Death from hypothermia, particularly in young children and the elderly, has been documented in some emergencies when weather-appropriate shelter was lacking. It is preferable, for privacy reasons, for individual families to be housed separately, and camps are often divided into sections of 5000 persons to ease service administration. The *Sphere Handbook* provides standards as to the recommended size of shelters (3.5 to 4.5 m^2 of covered area per person).[28]

Water and Sanitation

The Sphere Project also provides minimum standards for water and sanitation, with the recommended minimum quantity of water being 15 L per person per day for all domestic needs.[28] Sphere standards also recommend the provision of at least one water collection point for every 250 people, that people should not have to walk further than 500 m to the nearest collection point, and that the maximum queue time to collect water should not exceed 30 minutes.

Options for supplying water in collective settlements include surface water such as lakes, rivers, and streams in addition to springs and wells.[12] Water can be trucked in from external sites, although this introduces additional costs and can be logistically challenging. Surface water is often the most abundant (and readily available) source, but it needs to be treated before use. Shallow wells and springs need to be protected in order to ensure that the water is clean, and pumps or other mechanisms for drawing water need to be installed and maintained.[12] Deep bore wells offer the advantage of providing clean water with the convenience of having it onsite, but require drilling expertise, time to build, and specialized equipment. Recently introduced programs for the disinfection and safe storage of water at the household level in combination with behavioral change in sanitation and hygiene practices show promise in conflict-affected populations.[41,42]

Because diarrhea is the second leading cause of death among children under the age of 5 years and because 88% of these deaths can be attributed to inadequate sanitation and poor hygiene,[43] sanitation is a primary concern in emergencies, particularly in large, overcrowded camps. To address these risks, the *Sphere Handbook* recommends a minimum of 20 people per latrine, that latrines be segregated by sex, and that for security reasons latrines be located within 50 m of other dwellings.[28] Hand washing with soap, distribution of at least 250 g of soap per person per month, and community hygiene awareness programs are also of key importance.

⚠ PITFALLS

In the initial phases of an emergency, organizations commonly send teams to the affected area to assess the situation and to help plan the type of response needed. Until the mid-1990s, standardized tools for these assessments were lacking and the evaluations that were done sometimes led to contradictory information, which in turn created the potential for the implementation of unhelpful, redundant, or even harmful responses. To address this gap, in 1999 WHO published a series of standardized protocols to be employed in the rapid assessments of disasters and emergencies.[44]

The shift from interstate conflict to intrastate war has been associated with broad and frequent violations of the humanitarian space. Non-state armed combatants are sometimes unfamiliar with the Geneva Conventions; in other instances, the protections outlined for humanitarian workers are completely defied. Violence against humanitarian responders is motivated by various and often overlapping economic, criminal, and political factors.[45] Other evidence suggests that a blurring of the distinction between humanitarian assistance, counter-

insurgency, and counter-terrorism may be at least partially responsible for violence against relief workers.[46]

Complex emergencies often severely disrupt health care infrastructure. The demand for health services is typically inversely proportional to the rate at which the health care infrastructure is destroyed, but it is also dependent on the moral integrity of governance. In the early phases of a complex emergency, the need for health care may outweigh the rate at which resources can be made available.[47] The health response, similar to that of other sectors, may be ineffective if its design is based on poor quality information. It is thus critical that experienced and interdisciplinary teams conduct initial assessments of the situation as soon as it is clear that an emergency exits. Key data points include baseline data on endemic disease, mortality rates, morbidity incidence rates, nutritional status, mapped health care facilities, and the impact of the emergency on health service delivery.[28,37,44,48]

SUMMARY

Complex emergencies generally arise from conflict or insecurity, have complicated political root causes, and serve a purpose for one or more involved parties. The humanitarian response is critical in saving lives and in preventing morbidity but is not a substitute for a political solution to any crisis. The mass displacement of large populations and the protection of refugees and IDPs are critical factors when fashioning the humanitarian response, as is the provision of shelter, nutrition, medical care, and water/sanitation. Complex emergencies are often characterized by high mortality rates, generally due to collapse of the local medical and public health systems, with communicable diseases such as diarrheal illnesses, measles, malaria, and respiratory infections responsible for much of the loss of life. The humanitarian responses of today are generally coordinated among a large number of international and national organizations as well as by local actors at the country level. The response to a complex emergency must be a professional one, guided by credible data collected using the most rigorous methods feasible at the time, and with benchmarks intended to improve and standardize the assessment and delivery of assistance across the sectors that most impact the health of a crisis-affected population: water, sanitation, nutrition, food aide, shelter, site planning, and health services.

REFERENCES

1. Macias L. *Research Brief: Complex Emergencies.* The Robert S. Strauss Center for International Security and Law, University of Texas at Austin; 2013 [cited 2014 March 29]. Available from, *https://strausscenter.org/complex-emergencies-publications.html.*
2. Fearon J. *Why Do Some Civil Wars Last So Much Longer Than Others?* Department of Political Science, Stanford University; 2002 [cited 2014 March 30]. Available from, *http://www.stanford.edu/group/ethnic/workingpapers/dur3.pdf.*
3. Solana J. *A Secure Europe in a Better World: European Security Strategy.* Paris: European Union Institute for Security Studies; 2003 [cited 2014 March 30]. Available from, *http://www.iss.europa.eu/uploads/media/solanae.pdf.*
4. Wars in the World. *List of Ongoing Conflicts;* 2014 [updated March 24, 2014; cited 2014 April 1]. Available from, http://www.warsintheworld.com/?page=static1258254223.
5. International Committee of the Red Cross. *Convention (IV) Relative to the Protection of Civilian Persons in Time of War.* Geneva: International Committee of the Red Cross; 1949 [cited 2014 April 1]. Available from, *http://www.icrc.org/ihl/INTRO/380.*
6. Burkholder B, Toole MJ. Evolution of complex disasters. *Lancet.* 1995;346:1012–1015.
7. Rohini HJ, Rubenstein L. Health in fragile and post-conflict states: a review of current understanding and challenges ahead. *Med Confl Surviv.* 2012;28(5):289–316.

8. Keen D. *Complex Emergencies.* Cambridge, UK: Polity Press; 2008.

9. United Nations High Commission for Refugees. *UNHCR Mid-Year Trends;* 2013. Available from, http://unhcr.org/52af08d26.html.

10. United Nations General Assembl. *Draft Convention Relating to the Status of Refugees.* Geneva: UN General Assembly; 1950 [cited 2014 April 2]. Available from, *http://www.refworld.org/docid/3b00f08a27.html.*

11. Paquet C, Soest MV. Mortality and malnutrition among Rwandan refugees in Zaire. *Lancet.* 1994;344:823–824.

12. Toole MJ, Waldman R. Complex emergencies. In: Merson MH, Black RE, Mills AJ, eds. *Global Health: Diseases, Programs, Systems, and Policies.* 3rd ed. Burlington, MA: Jones & Bartlett Learning; 2012:539–607.

13. Young H, Borrel A, Holland D, Salama P. Public nutrition in complex emergencies. *Lancet.* 2004;364:1899–1909.

14. Gingerich T, Leaning J. *The Use of Rape as a Weapon of War in the Conflict in Darfur, Sudan;* 2004 [cited 2014 April 10]. Available from, http://physiciansforhumanrights.org/library/reports/darfur-use-of-rape-as-weapon-2004.html.

15. Reseau des Femmes pour un Developpement Associatif, Reseau des Femmes pour la Defense des Droit et la Paix, International Alert. *Women's Bodies as a Battleground: Sexual Violence against Women and Girls during the War in the Democratic Republic of Congo;* 2005 [cited 2014 April 10]. Available from, http://repositories.lib.utexas.edu/bitstream/handle/2152/4949/4053.pdf?sequence=1.

16. Naik A. Protecting children from the protectors: lessons from West Africa. *Forced Migration Review.* 2002;15:16–19.

17. Levine I, Bowden M. Protection from sexual exploitation and abuse in humanitarian crisis: the humanitarian community's response. *Forced Migration Review.* 2002;15:20–21.

18. Save the Children. *No One to Turn To: The Under-Reporting of Child Sexual Exploitation and Abuse by Aid Workers and Peacekeepers;* 2008, London [cited 2014 April 10]. Available from, http://www.un.org/en/pseataskforce/docs/no_one_to_turn_under_reporting_of_child_sea_by_aid_workers.pdf.

19. United Nations High Commission for Refugees, Save the Children—UK. *Sexual Violence and Exploitation: The Experience of Refugee Children in Guinea, Liberia and Sierra Leone;* 2002 [updated February 2002]. Available from, http://www.savethechildren.org.uk/sites/default/files/docs/sexual_violence_and_exploitation_1.pdf.

20. Holmes R, Bhuvanendra D. Preventing and responding to gender-based violence in humanitarian crisis. *Humanitarian Practice Network.* 2014;77.

21. Sivakumaran S. Lost in translation: UN responses to sexual violence against men and boys in situations of armed conflict. *Int Rev Red Cross.* 2010;92(877).

22. United Nations. *Sexual Violence Against Men and Boys in Conflict Situations;* 2013 [cited 2014 April 9]. Available from, http://ifls.osgoode.yorku.ca/wp-content/uploads/2014/01/Report-of-Workshop-on-Sexual-Violence-against-Men-and-Boys-Final.pdf.

23. Pugh M. Military intervention and humanitarian action: trends and issues. *Disasters.* 1998;22(4):339–351.

24. Sheik M, Gutierrez MI, Bolton P, Spiegel P, Thieren M, Burnham G. Deaths among humanitarian workers. *BMJ.* 2000;321.

25. Burkle FM. Complex emergencies and military capabilities. In: Maley CSW, Thakur C, eds. *From Civil Strife to Civil Society: Civil and Military Responsibilities in Disrupted States.* Tokyo and New York: United Nations University Press; 2002:68–80.

26. United Nations Emergency Relief Coordinator, Office for the Coordination of Humanitarian Affairs. *Humanitarian Response Review;* 2005, New York and Geneva [cited 2014 April 6]. Available from, http://www.unicef.org/emerg/files/ocha_hrr.pdf.

27. United Nations Office for the Coordination of Humanitarian Affairs. *The Four Pillars of Humanitarian Reform;* 2005 [cited 2014 April 6]. Available from, http://www.terzomondo.org/library/essentials/The_humanitarian_reform-Four_Pillars.pdf.

28. Sphere Project. *Humanitarian Charter and Minimum Standards in Humanitarian Response: Sphere Project;* 2014 [cited 2014 April 6]. Available from, http://www.sphereproject.org/about/.

29. Coghlan B, Ngoy P, Mulumba F, et al. Update on mortality in the democratic republic of Congo: results from a third nationwide study. *Disaster Med Public Health Preparedness.* 2009;3:88–96.

30. Centers for Disease Control and Prevention. *Polio in Syria: CDC;* 2014 [cited 2014 June 10]. Available from, http://wwwnc.cdc.gov/travel/notices/alert/polio-syria.

31. Connolly MA, Gayer M, Ryan MJ, Salama P, Speigel P, Heymann D. Communicable diseases in complex emergencies: impact and challanges. *Lancet.* 2004;364:1974–1983.

32. Goma Epidemiology Group. Public health impact of Rwandan refugee crisis: what happened in Goma, Zaire, in July, 1994? *Lancet.* 1995;345:339–344.

33. Gregg MB. *Field Epidemiology.* Oxford, U.K.: Oxford University Press; 2008.

34. World Health Organization. *The Interagency Emergency Health Kit 2011.* Geneva: World Health Organization; 2011 [cited 2014 April 7]. Available from, *http://whqlibdoc.who.int/publications/2011/9789241502115_eng.pdf?ua=1.*

35. Mayo-Wilson E, Imdad A, Kurt H, Yakoob M, Bhutta Z. Vitamin A supplements for preventing mortality, illness and blindness in children aged under 5: systematic review and meta-analysis. *BMJ.* 2011;343.

36. Inter-Agency Working Group on Reproductive Health in Crisis. *Inter-Agency Field Manual on Reproductive Health in Humanitarian Settings: 2010 Revision for Field-Testing;* 2010 [cited 2014 June 10]. Available from, http://iawg.net/resources2013/tools-and-guidelines/field-manual/-download.

37. Hakewill P, Moren A. Monitoring and evaluations of relief programs. *Trop Doct.* 1991;21(suppl 1):24–28.

38. Davis A. Targeting the vulnerable in emergency situations: who is vulnerable? *Lancet.* 1996;348:868–871.

39. Nutriset. *Plumpy'Nut;* 2014 [cited 2014 April 7]. Available from, http://www.nutriset.fr/index.php?id=92.

40. United Nations High Commission for Refugees, United Nations Children's Fund, World Food Program, World Health Organization. *Nutritional Needs in Emergencies.* World Health Organization [cited 2014 April 7]. Available from: http://www.who.int/nutrition/publications/en/nut_needs_emergencies_text.pdf.

41. Centers for Disease Control and Prevention. *The Safe Water System;* 2012 [cited 2014 April 8]. Available from, http://www.cdc.gov/safewater/.

42. Lantagne D, Clasen T. Use of household water treatment and safe storage methods in acute emergency response: case study results from Nepal, Indonesia, Kenya, and Haiti. *Environ Sci Technol.* 2012;46(20):11352–11360.

43. UNICEF, World Health Organization. *Diarrhea: Why Children Are Still Dying and What Can Be Done?;* 2009, Available through, http://www.who.int/maternal_child_adolescent/documents/9789241598415/en/ [cited 2014 April 8].

44. World Health Organization. *Rapid Health Assessment Protocols for Emergencies.* Geneva: WHO; 1999.

45. Metcalfe V, Giffen A, Elhawary S. *UN Integration and Humanitarian Space: An Independent Study Commissioned by the UN Integration Steering Group;* 2011 [cited 2014 April 6]. Available from, http://www.stimson.org/images/uploads/research-pdfs/Integration_final.pdf.

46. Sistenich V. *Briefing Note: UN Integration and Humanitarian Coordination: Policy Considerations towards Protection of the Humanitarian Space;* 2012 [cited 2014 April 6]. Available from, http://www.hpcrresearch.org/blog/vera-sistenich/2012-07-06/briefing-note-un-integration-humanitarian-coordination-policy-conside.

47. Desenclos J-C, Michel D, Tholly F, Magdi I, Pecoul B, Desve G. Mortality trends among refugees in Honduras, 1984–1987. *Int J Epidemiol.* 1990;19(2):367–373.

48. Toole MJ, Waldman R. Refugees and displaced persons: war, hunger and public health. *JAMA.* 1993;270:600–605.

CHAPTER 8

Disaster and Climate Change

Prasit Wuthisuthimethawee

INTRODUCTION

Climate change, consequent to the phenomenon of global warming resulting from the anthropogenic emission of greenhouse gases, is expected to lead to increasing temperatures and changing rainfall patterns over the next century.[1] Climate change can be both a complex and protracted hazard,[2] potentially affecting both the environment and human population by changing the distribution of various risk factors.[3] Climate change is a multifaceted (from drought to flood) and multidimensional (from local to global) hazard that has short-, medium-, and long-term effects and unknown outcomes.[2]

Global climate change is increasing the risk of extreme weather and climate events, such as droughts, floods, heat waves, and stronger storms.[2] In the 21st century, increases in frequency and severity of heat waves, cold waves, drought, and flooding are expected globally, even in temperate regions.[1] Projections of global climate change for 2100 are striking: The Intergovernmental Panel on Climate Change (IPCC) predicts an average global temperature increase in the range of 1.0-6.4 °C, a rise in sea levels by as much as one meter, and an intensification of the hydrologic cycle in a warmer atmosphere, likely making droughts and floods more frequent and intense.[4]

Climate change is intensifying the hazards that affect human livelihoods,[3] settlements, and infrastructure.[2] It is also weakening the resilience of community systems by increasing the uncertainty and frequency of disasters. Population movements in response to climate change may also result in new exposures to hazards. Furthermore, climate change can increase the vulnerability to unrelated, nonclimatic hazards, such as an urban earthquake hitting when the elderly population is already suffering from the sort of heat wave that occurred in Europe during 2003.[2]

HISTORICAL PERSPECTIVE

Disasters triggered by natural hazards are killing more people and costing more money every year.[2] A heat wave can have a large impact on human health.[5] Health care personnel are increasingly confronted with severe heat-related illnesses (such as heat exhaustion and life-threatening heatstroke), which they are often neither familiar with nor trained to treat.[1] The mortality rate from a heat wave is greater than from hurricanes, lightning, tornados, floods, and earthquakes combined[6] and is an environmental hazard that can have serious public health consequences.[7]

In the summer of 2003 a heat wave killed more than 14,800 people globally with heavy casualties and massive heat wave-related deaths recorded in Europe, the United States, and China.[1] The risk of heat-related mortality increases 2.49% for every increase of 1 °F in heat wave intensity and 0.38% for every increase of 1 day in heat wave duration.

Climate change may increase the frequency, duration, or intensity of heat waves.[5] Heat waves are discussed in more detail in Chapter 99.

Drought has an adverse effect on economies, food security, community nutritional status, and health-related issues. Malnutrition is often seen in chronic drought-affected areas.[8] The cocoliztli outbreak of hemorrhagic fever occurred in Mexico during a severe and sustained megadrought.[9] The simultaneous effect of the heat and the drought also raised the frequency of fires and caused energy blackouts.[10] Chronic drought can lead to famine, which is discussed in more detail in Chapter 102.

Projected changes in climate are expected to increase flood risk.[11] During 2000 to 2010, many countries of the world experienced natural disasters resulting from floods. Flooding is the most common natural disaster that affects developed and developing countries.[12] Standing water and sediments remaining in flooded areas are breeding grounds for various microorganisms, including fungi and bacteria, that can become airborne and be inhaled. These exposures may increase the incidence of lung disease, allergic respiratory disease, asthma, and mycotic infections in immunocompromised subjects. Bacterial growth in flooded homes can be a significant source of endotoxins, which can induce airway inflammation and dysfunction.[13] Floods are discussed in more detail in Chapter 97.

Tropical cyclones (typhoons and hurricanes) and tornados are devastating and recurring natural disasters that cause significant damage to life and property in many countries worldwide.[14] As the ocean water cycle is projected to change under global warming, tropical ocean barrier layers may change accordingly.[15] The relationship between temperature and the frequency of typhoon hazards is supported by the fact that typhoons form over tropical oceans where water temperatures reach or exceed 27 °C. Typhoon activities may also be related to ocean-atmosphere fluctuations, such as the El Niño activity and Southern Oscillation.[14] It is expected that typhoon hazards will become ever more frequent in the next century as global temperatures continue to rise.[14] Strong winds pile up the water along the shore and generate storm surges, causing coastal flooding,[16] which results in damage and fatalities in the affected areas.[17] The unprecedented disasters caused by Hurricanes Katrina and Rita in 2005 disrupted the public health and medical infrastructures in New Orleans and created many difficult environmental health challenges.[13] While the infrastructure of an affected community usually remains at least partially intact, these storms can result in mass-casualty situations for emergency and local medical facilities.[18] Tropical cyclones, hurricanes, and typhoons are discussed in more detail in Chapter 94.

The intersection between climate change, disasters, health, and development is an area of concern for community development.[19] Understanding how climate changes affect health through historical precedent is the key to preparing communities for disasters.[5] Excess mortality rates during the devastating 2003 heat wave in Europe and during the recent 2006 heat waves in the United States and Europe have shown that extreme temperatures remain a major challenge to public health preparedness.[20]

CURRENT PRACTICE

Preparedness and Prevention

Most hazards that lead to disasters cannot be prevented, but their effects can be mitigated.[2] Changes in the climate influence changes in the frequency and magnitude of those hazards. Vulnerability to these hazards is also increasing due to rising poverty, a growing global population, armed conflict, and other underlying development issues. Whereas climate change is contributing to raising disaster risk, measures to mitigate the risk need to focus on reducing vulnerability in the context of development efforts.[3] Disaster preparedness must change from a conventional response and relief to a more comprehensive risk reduction concept (Fig. 8-1).[17] To be successful in disaster reduction planning and preparedness, it is important to have an in-depth understanding of the underlying vulnerabilities to natural hazards and the basic perceptions, goals, and behaviors of the local people.[17] The local population's relationship with the environment is essential. Planners, policymakers, and development practitioners should endeavor to understand local knowledge and practices.[17] The underlying causes of vulnerability to disasters locally are often economic and societal, such as poverty, fragmentation of community cohesion, and lack of access to political representation.[3] Climate-related vulnerability is derived from a set of social, economic, political, and physical factors. The risk to a population arises from the interaction of these hazards and vulnerabilities.[2] It is important to set up a plan based on durable solutions for the protection of the population, particularly the more vulnerable, from future natural disasters.[1] The "Hyogo Framework for Action 2005-2015," which came out of the World

Conference for Disaster Reduction in 2005 and was endorsed by the United Nations General Assembly, outlines steps required for disaster risk reduction to natural disasters and promotes a strategic and systematic approach to reducing vulnerabilities and risks to hazards. It identifies ways of building the resilience of nations and communities to disaster. The efforts to reduce disaster risk must be systematically integrated into policies, plans, and programs for sustainable development and poverty reduction, and be supported through regional and international cooperation.[17]

Steps taken by human society, either as individuals or governing authorities, toward risk reduction for natural hazards may be characterized as flexible or inflexible depending on the perception of the hazard, choices available, economic efficiency, and power structure of the government. The degree of destruction is a function of the human context as much as the hazard itself because hazards of similar severity can produce dramatically different outcomes in different social and economic contexts. All of this information is vital to strategic planning and decision making.[14] Planning to reduce the impact of disasters requires many techniques to prepare for, to reduce potential losses from, and to respond and adapt to hazards. Unfortunately, poorly planned development interventions may become a source of hazards. Disaster planning is a necessary step and is needed to realize the goals of sustainable development. Because climate change is a source of multiple hazards that threaten long-term developmental actions by the international community, planning approaches that link development and disaster should extend to climate change.[2] An appropriately trained, qualified, and agile health workforce is required to improve the response to disasters.[19] Furthermore, crisis simulation exercises can be excellent opportunities to practice and modify risk reduction guidelines.[10] Successful management of disasters will also maximize the resources available to adapt to future climate change.[3]

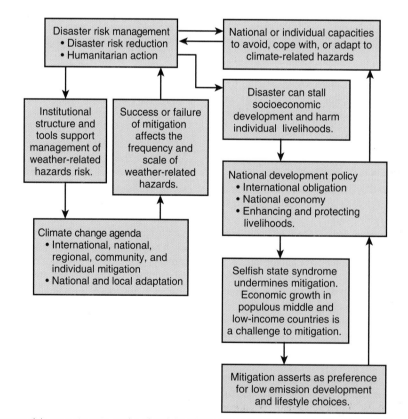

FIG 8-1 Climate change, disaster risk management, and national development policy linkage. Modified from Schipper L, Pelling M. Disaster risk, climate change and international development: scope for, and challenges to, integration. *Disasters.* 2006;30:19-38.

Information technologies can facilitate coordination in all disasters, particularly those related to climate change, environment, and weather. The intrinsic chaos caused by a disaster challenges the coordination between organizations to prevent misunderstanding and to slow collective actions. New technologies (such as the geographic information system, command and control and decision support systems, varieties of social media, and sms messaging) are used extensively in a crisis response. E-mail can be used for vertical, horizontal, and interorganizational and intraorganizational coordination by a formal or emergent response network. This method is a potentially reliable and profitable tool to support coordination in a crisis response. An ad hoc crisis management system was used effectively in the SARS outbreak in Singapore in 2003, in response to the tsunami of 2004 in Sri Lanka, and in the San Diego fires in 2007.[10] The role of informatics, mobile disaster applications, and social media in disasters is further discussed in Chapters 25, 43, and 44.

Heat waves have had debilitating effects on human mortality. Global climate models predict an increase in the frequency and severity of heat waves. Annual mortality attributable to heat waves for Chicago (using several global climate models and climate change scenarios) found that mortality will increase in the future and that a mitigation of this projected increase may be expected through a lower pathway of future carbon dioxide emissions.[21] Protective measures against heat are to withdraw from hot weather, implement widespread installation of air-conditioning in hospitals, nursing and retirement homes, and public buildings, and to facilitate their accessibility for vulnerable populations. Air-conditioning should be made affordable for low socioeconomic groups by reducing energy costs during extreme heat waves. Other steps include installing an early warning system, providing advance reports in the news media, broadcasting simple advice, and seeking out the most vulnerable and ensuring their well-being within the community.[1] These measures have already been shown to reduce morbidity and mortality during heat waves.[1] During the summer in Chicago, there are a graded series of warnings (via television, radio, and newspapers). Private and public resources (such as air-conditioned cooling centers) are mobilized, transportation is provided, the public and police are encouraged to check on their neighbors (especially the elderly and infirmed), public health officials and hospitals are alerted to look for early patterns of emergency department admissions and deaths, and a heat awareness week is set up to reduce the incidence of heat-related mortality.[6] Toronto public health uses a protocol that calls for activation of a heat warning (alert) using a threshold of a 1-day forecast of the humidex (a Canadian summer temperature and humidity index) over 40 °C. A heat alert activates the city's hot weather response plan that coordinates the efforts of the city and community agencies to provide services to socially isolated individuals (including homeless people), seniors, and medically at-risk people. This, combined with well-designed, planned community responses, can reduce the amount of heat-related morbidity and mortality.[7]

Flood management includes different water resource activities. Sustainable flood management requires an integrated consideration of economic, ecological, and social consequences of disastrous floods. There are three main stages in flood management: (a) planning, (b) flood emergency management, and (c) postflood recovery. Different alternative measures (both structural and nonstructural) are analyzed and compared for possible implementation to minimize future flood damage during the flood planning stage. In the response stage of emergency management, regular evaluation of the current flood situation and daily operations is performed. Postflood recovery involves numerous decisions regarding return to normal life. The main issues during this stage include assessment and rehabilitation of flood damage and provision of flood assistance to flood victims. In all three stages, the decision-making process takes place in a multidisciplinary and multiparticipatory environment.[22]

Several flood defense mechanisms can be used to protect a city and its population. The waterfront in New York City plays a crucial role as the first line in managing flood risk and protecting the city from future climate change and the rise in sea levels. This "greener waterfront" is also attractive for business and residents. Restrictions and enforcement of infrastructure construction (e.g., flood-proof telephones, electricity switchboards, and heating and gas installations above the base flood elevation level) can be implemented to reduce flood risk and damage.[23] Building an infrastructure like a fail-proof, low-maintenance levee has proven to protect the Japanese cities of Tokyo and Osaka. This type of flood protection offers advantages beyond the structural and flood protection aspects. The stabilized and strengthened sides can be developed to extend the urban development area to the top of the levee and allow easier visual and physical access to the water.[23]

Climate-adaptive programs should include the following: (a) modifying policies to anticipate the impacts of climate change, (b) improving resilience to climate change and the rise in sea levels, (c) changing future land use (e.g., flood zoning policies, flood insurance, and building codes) and hence the potential vulnerability of land use to flood risk, and (d) developing flood risk maps (e.g., delineating hazard areas, mapping floodways, and flood elevation and velocity).[23] The major sources of uncertainty in the hydrologic impacts of climate change should use a multimodel approach, combining the output of multiple emission scenarios, global climate models, and conceptual rainfall runoff models within the framework of the generalized likelihood uncertainty estimation to quantify uncertainty in future impacts at the catchment scale.[11]

An insurance program is important to achieve risk reduction by limiting the vulnerability of new construction to flood hazards. Insurance has been referred to as an effective tool for reducing, sharing, and spreading climate change-induced disaster risks in both developed and developing countries.[14] Government funding in flood prevention also plays a crucial role in mitigating potential flood damage. Long-term planning and sustainability with its established relationships with multiple stakeholders are well positioned to coordinate, explore, and foster the implementation of a plan.[23] Four key criteria regarding the long-term sustainability of effective insurance in natural disaster risk are contribution to risk reduction, commercial viability, affordability, and governance.[24]

In 2008 the International Federation of Red Cross and Red Crescent Societies used a seasonal forecast to implement an early warning system in West Africa. This was one of the early action strategies for enhanced flood preparedness and response. This approach improved their capacity and response; potential benefits were realized from the use of medium-to-long–range forecasts in disaster management, especially in the context of extreme weather and climate-related events due to temperature variability and change. The full potential of these forecasts will require continued effort and collaboration among the disaster managers, climate service providers, and major humanitarian donors.[4] Early warning, early action (EWEA) is one strategy that was developed to help disaster managers benefit from the various types of information, making full use of scientific information on all timescales. The EWEA concept aligns with increasing emphasis within the disaster risk management community on preparedness, awareness, and risk reduction.[4] Disaster managers will need to invest more in preparedness, early warning, and vulnerability reduction rather than focusing primarily on response.[4]

Cyclone preparedness in Bangladesh, exemplified by the existing comprehensive disaster management policies of the government and localized vulnerability factors in cyclone hazards, are also mandatory.[17] An analysis of the relationship between cyclone hazards and human behavior in coastal areas (using local-level and personalized accounts) appears to be imperative for developing improved disaster reduction strategies.[17] The locations and patterns of settlements are the most important factors when determining a coastal population's vulnerability to a tropical cyclone, followed by inappropriate land management systems, the means of livelihood, and a lack of infrastructure.[17]

Three underlying vulnerabilities to cyclone disasters are hazard risk perceptions, precyclone decisions about whether to go to shelters, and inadequate land management policies in the coastal areas of a country.[17] Typhoon hazards can be prevented and mitigated by adopting a number of measures, including stricter observance of construction guidelines, new flood barrier proposals (as well as enhanced associated flood defense), and upgraded existing pumping systems along with better management of the collection of household litter and construction refuse. Insurance can also help the vulnerable population mitigate the effects from a typhoon.[14]

Blizzards are predictable disasters with preventable health outcomes. Specific demographic, health, and cause-related information can assist health care providers and public health officials in providing more effective warnings to reduce blizzard-related morbidity and mortality in the general population.[25]

The best way to reduce vulnerability is to improve the socioeconomic standing of the most vulnerable; for this to happen, these people must have an assured income based on assets that will enable them to acquire social and economic credit worthiness within the local economy. People with resources can protect themselves economically and physically from disasters; the speed of their recovery is related to the size of their asset base. The case can be made that poverty alleviation should be the central aim of all disaster reconstruction and development programs.[26]

Response and Recovery

Capacity, including health care capacity, was one of the objective determinants identified as the most significant in influencing the adaptive capability of disaster response systems. There are several elements that can support the adaptive capacity of the health care sector, such as inclusive involvement in disaster coordination, policies in place for health workforce coordination, belief in their abilities, and strong donor support. Factors constraining adaptive capacity include weak coordination of international health personnel, lack of policies to address health worker welfare, limited human and material resources, shortages of personnel to deal with psychosocial needs, inadequate skills in field triage and counseling, and limited capacity for training.[19]

The response to a heat wave involves various types of organizations. The response network is composed of groups with specific missions and objectives, which include civil protection and public security and order in routine situations by police organizations that are charged with the additional responsibility of providing emergency services (e.g., caring for injured people and organizing rescue operations). The group of health care organizations needs to be in charge of taking care of the injured and sick. Other outsider organizations need to have significant influence on the development of a crisis response.[10] Unequal distribution of community-based resources has important implications for geographic differences in survival rates during a heat wave; this may be relevant for other disasters.[27] The risk factors in heat wave mortality are being elderly, male, sick, grossly obese, disproportionately poor, residing in an economically and socially disadvantaged neighborhood, and living in a socially isolated population.[6] A heat wave for consecutive days leads to widespread heat-related injuries and hospitalization and a rapidly increasing mortality rate. The pattern of a temperature greater than 37 °C being maintained for several consecutive days and an elevation of the minimum temperature above 25.5 °C does not allow recovery

from a severe heat-stressed experience.[1] The higher the temperature or the longer the heat wave, the more work is required for the cardiovascular system to maintain normal body temperature; therefore, a more intense or longer heat wave is likely to have greater health effects.[5]

The greatest mortalities seen in heat emergencies resulted from sudden death and cardiovascular causes.[20] Many of those who survived heatstroke were anticipated to sustain severe neurologic damage, which may culminate in death even up to 1 year or more after the illness.[1] Extreme heat also poses a salient risk to the health and well-being of the mentally ill. Elevated and fluctuating temperature may exacerbate psychiatric conditions and increase the incidence of depression and suicide.[28] Risk factors known to increase susceptibility to heat illness are social isolation of elderly people with comorbid conditions (such as psychiatric, pulmonary, or cardiovascular illnesses), the use of medications that interfere with thermoregulation, and the absence of air-conditioning.[1] Local health care providers, such as emergency medical services and hospitals, need to prepare to handle the patient surge, diagnoses, and care.[10]

Severe drought has an adverse impact on food reserves. There is a higher incidence of inadequate vitamin A status of rural preschool children, particularly those with illiterate mothers and belonging to an older age group. Communities need to provide medical care, including nutritional support and education.[8]

Data from the National Oceanographic and Atmospheric Administration (NOAA) in the United States reported more death and destruction from flood than any other hydrometeorlogic phenomenon from 1990 to 2005.[12] Flooding usually makes responses to a disaster more complex due to the damage of local infrastructure. The accessibility to the affected areas is quite difficult for all external organizations. Flash flooding is defined as flooding that occurs within 6 hours of the inciting event, such as heavy rainfall or levee or dam failure.[12] The moving water is very powerful. The lateral force of one foot of water moving 10 miles per hour is about 500 pounds, and 2 feet of water at 10 miles per hour will float virtually every car.[12]

Because flash flooding occurs so quickly, it can have lethal effects on anyone caught in its path.[12] The vulnerable groups (e.g., disabled, elderly, and children) are the first priority in a flood response. Injuries are likely to occur during the aftermath and cleanup stage, but most of them are mild, predominantly consisting of cuts, lacerations, puncture wounds, and strains/sprains to the extremities. Most medical care for flood victims is routine, such as providing refilled medicines and treating exacerbations of preexisting diseases.[12] However, in the later stage, infectious disease, arthropod bites, and violence can be overwhelming.[12] The typical infectious diseases listed in association with excess flood exposure are leptospirosis, dengue fever, malaria, measles, typhoid, viral diarrheal illnesses, pink-eye disease, and hepatitis A virus infection. Melioidosis (discussed in Chapter 137) can be included in the differential diagnosis of patients with severe community-acquired pneumonia and skin and soft-tissue infections during and after flood exposure.[12,29] Unprecedented flooding and disasters provide ample ideal niches for the growth of fungi and bacteria that result in an increased risk of exposure to some biocontaminants derived from these microorganisms.[30] The level of endotoxins was elevated in the dust collected from flood-affected homes 2 years after the floods.[30] Leptospirosis is known to be an important cause of weather disaster-related infectious disease epidemics after seasonal rains and flooding in endemic wet zones.[31] Field epidemiology is very important to identify the needs in every stage of the response and to provide information to the incident commander for decision making.

In tornado situations factors associated with seeking shelter were hearing warning sirens, having a basement in one's home, having a plan of action, and having at least a high-school education.

A tornado-warning system decreased tornado-related deaths, and it had to be coordinated with accessibility to a shelter. Storm shelters in tornado-prone areas should have quick accessibility by the residents. Seeking appropriate shelters after hearing tornado warnings is associated with reduced mortality and injury. It is recommended that people who live in tornado-prone areas without underground shelters should prepare a plan of action to immediately respond to tornado warnings in an effective manner. The engagement of tornado drills will allow the community to be familiar with safety procedures, sources of shelters in houses and outdoors, and weather updates. Public education about how to respond to tornado watches and warnings in areas with high tornado activity is mandatory.[18]

Blizzard conditions were associated with increased visits for myocardial infarction and angina even in people without preexisting heart disease. Those myocardial infarction and angina visits were primarily related to shoveling and decreased visits to a physician for asthma. The decrease in physician visits for asthma most likely resulted from asthmatic people avoiding exposure to blizzard conditions. There is an association between heavy snowfall and ischemic heart disease morbidity and mortality. Other diseases are carbon monoxide poisoning (associated with blocked vehicle exhaust pipes), drug or medication overdose, alcohol abuse, and attempted suicide.[25]

Disasters usually create a huge number of casualties, but the majority are minor casualties.[12] Most of the deaths were attributed to heat, although those affected were essentially the elderly (70% and 120% excess deaths in the age groups 75 to 94 and older than 95 years, respectively). Other deaths were related to mental illness or living in group homes for people with mental illnesses.[1] Preexisting psychologic illness can more than triple the risk of death.[28] A concept in management during a disaster, especially in the response phase, is "the greatest good for the greater number of casualties." The triage system must be implemented during the immediate response phase to prioritize the patients. Later, after resources have increased, care can be given to most of the victims, and endemic diseases can be further prevented.

Disaster research is crucial for providing valuable information for future disaster planning and prevention. A vulnerability factor is needed for the development of disaster research.[17]

⚠ PITFALLS

A lesson to be learned is to think "globalization" when considering climate change and disaster-related patient care. Climate change is a root-cause effect for many natural disasters. As such, specific risk reduction steps should not be ignored. Also, there are no longer frontiers and barriers for diseases exacerbated by temperature and weather change to travel. Simply stated, climate change is a global problem that must be adequately mitigated against.[1]

Disasters can also trigger organizational crises that aggravate coordination issues. Crisis responders can face difficulties meeting the urgent needs of those affected when they have to handle coordination problems within and between organizations.[10] Organizations should invest in information technology tools, promote "good practices" related to the use of e-mail (e.g., using codes to specify the type of action related to the message), and forward e-mails to experts rather than hierarchic superiors.[10] The electronic communications that take place in a disaster can be analyzed to determine the responsibilities and effectiveness or failures in crisis management.[10]

The lesson from Japan is to consider flood protection not as the isolated endeavor of a single agency, but as part of a larger body of work that is intertwined with urban redevelopment, open space planning, land rehabilitation, and habitat generation.[23]

There are remaining challenges in managing flood forecasting and responses. Communication and decision-making chains are not prepared to process forecast information, and difficulties remain in mobilizing donor support prior to a disaster. Early actions can be taken even earlier, and limited capacity inhibits action in the areas of finance, equipment, technology, and political and bureaucratic processes.[4]

SUMMARY

Climate change will continue to result in multiple effects on our planet, especially in terms of natural disasters. An approach is needed to underpin the incorporation of risk management into the work on climate change and the introduction of climate change into natural hazards and development planning. The key concepts in that approach should be capacity-building, resilience, and the involvement of all stakeholders.

ACKNOWLEDGMENTS

The author thanks Kingkarn Waiyanak for the literature search and retrieval and Glenn K. Shingledecker for his help in editing the manuscript.

REFERENCES

1. Abderrezak B. The 2003 European heat wave. *Intensive Care Med.* 2004;30:1–3.
2. O'Brien G, O'Keefe P, Rose J, et al. Climate change and disaster management. *Disasters.* 2006;30:64–80.
3. Schipper L, Pelling M. Disaster risk, climate change and international development: scope for, and challenges to, integration. *Disasters.* 2006;30:19–38.
4. Braman LM, van Aalst MK, Mason SJ, et al. Climate forecasts in disaster management: Red Cross flood operations in West Africa, 2008. *Disasters.* 2013;37:144–164.
5. Anderson GB, Bell ML. Heat waves in the Unites States: mortality risk during heat waves and effect modification by heat wave characteristics in 43 U.S. communities. *Environ Health Perspect.* 2011;119:210–218.
6. Franklin CM. Lessons from a heat wave. *Intensive Care Med.* 2004;30:167.
7. Pengelly LD, Campbell ME, Cheng CS, et al. Anatomy of heat waves and mortality in Toronto: lessons for public health protection. *Can J Public Health.* 2007;98:364–368.
8. Arlappa N, Venkaiah K, Brahmam GN. Severe drought and the vitamin A status of rural pre-school children in India. *Disasters.* 2011;35:577–586.
9. Acuna-Soto R, Stahle DW, Therrell MD, et al. Drought, epidemic disease, and the fall of classic period cultures in Mesoamerica (AD 750-950). Hemorrhagic fevers as a cause of massive population loss. *Med Hypotheses.* 2005;65:405–409.
10. Adrot A, Figueiredo MB. Handling coordination in an extreme situation: tensions in electronic communication and organizational emptiness during the 2003 French heat wave crisis response. *Systèmes d'Information et Management.* 2013;18:11–56.
11. Bastola S, Murphy C, Sweeney J. The sensitivity of fluvial flood risk in Irish catchments to the range of IPCC AR4 climate change scenarios. *Sci Total Environ.* 2011;409:5403–5415.
12. Llewellyn M. Floods and tsunamis. *Surg Clin North Am.* 2006;86:557–578.
13. Adhikari A, Jung J, Reponen T, et al. Aerosolization of fungi, (1→3)-beta-D glucan, and endotoxin from flood-affected materials collected in New Orleans homes. *Environ Res.* 2009;109:215–224.
14. Zong Y, Chen X. Typhoon hazards in the Shanghai area. *Disasters.* 1999;23:66–80.
15. Balaguru K, Chang P, Saravanan R, et al. Ocean barrier layers' effect on tropical cyclone intensification. *Proc Natl Acad Sci U S A.* 2012;109:14343–14347.
16. Aerts JC, Lin N, Botzen W, et al. Low-probability flood risk modeling for New York City. *Risk Anal.* 2013;33:772–788.

17. Alam E, Collins AE. Cyclone disaster vulnerability and response experiences in coastal Bangladesh. *Disasters*. 2010;34:931–954.

18. Balluz L, Schieve L, Holmes T, et al. Predictors for people's response to a tornado warning: Arkansas, 1 March 1997. *Disasters*. 2000;24:71–77.

19. Rumsey M, Fletcher SM, Thiessen J, et al. A qualitative examination of the health workforce needs during climate change disaster response in Pacific Island Countries. *Hum Resour Health*. 2014;12:9.

20. Kaiser R, Le Tertre A, Schwartz J, et al. The effect of the 1995 heat wave in Chicago on all-cause ans cause-specific mortality. *Am J Public Health*. 2007;97(S1):S158–S162.

21. Peng RD, Bobb JF, Tebaldi C, et al. Toward a quantitative estimate of future heat wave mortality under global climate change. *Environ Health Perspect*. 2011;119:701–706.

22. Akter T, Simonovic SP. Aggregation of fuzzy views of a large number of stakeholders for multi-objective flood management decision-making. *J Environ Manage*. 2005;77:133–143.

23. Aerts JC, Botzen WJ. Flood-resilient waterfront development in New York City: bridging flood insurance, building codes, and flood zoning. *Ann N Y Acad Sci*. 2011;1227:1–82.

24. Akter S, Brouwer R, van Beukering PJ, et al. Exploring the feasibility of private micro flood insurance provision in Bangladesh. *Disasters*. 2011;35:287–307.

25. Blindauer KM, Rubin C, Morse DL, et al. The 1996 New York blizzard: impact on noninjury emergency visits. *Am J Emerg Med*. 1999;17:23–27.

26. Winchester P. Cyclone mitigation, resource allocation and post-disaster reconstruction in south India: lessons from two decades of research. *Disasters*. 2000;24:18–37.

27. Browning CR, Feinberg SL, Wallace D, et al. Neighborhood social processes, physical conditions, and disaster-related mortality: the case of the 1995 Chicago heat wave. *Am Socio Rev*. 2006;71:661–678.

28. Hansen A, Bi P, Nitschke M, et al. The effect of heat waves on mental health in a temperate Australian city. *Environ Health Perspect*. 2008;116:1369–1375.

29. Apisarnthanarak A, Khawcharoenporn T, Mundy LM. Flood-associated melioidosis in a non-endemic region of Thailand. *Int J Infect Dis*. 2012;16:409–410.

30. Adhikari A, Lewis JS, Reponen T, et al. Exposure matrices of endotoxin, $(1 \rightarrow 3)$-beta-D-glucan, fungi, and dust mite allergens in flood-affected homes of New Orleans. *Sci Total Environ*. 2010;408:5489–5498.

31. Agampodi SB, Dahanayaka NJ, Bandaranayaka AK, et al. Regional differences of leptospirosis in Sri Lanka: observations from a flood-associated outbreak in 2011. *PLoS Negl Trop Dis*. 2014;8:e2626.

CHAPTER 9

Children and Disaster

Michael Bouton and Bruce M. Becker

Children, along with the elderly and pregnant women, are the most vulnerable populations in disasters. In developing countries, children also make up a disproportionate percentage of the population, as exemplified by Haiti, where over 40% of the population is under 18.[1] Physiologically and psychologically, children are less fit to survive the acute, subacute, and chronic stresses imposed by a disaster than adults are. For example, children under the age of 5 in the Ethiopian famine of 2000 had a mortality rate double that of the general population during the crisis.[2] Children depend on their parents or guardians for food, clothing, shelter, hygiene, sanitation, water, medical care, and general personal safety. Regardless of the type of disaster, inevitably, a certain percentage of surviving children will be separated from one or both of their parents or guardians. Without the appropriate stewardship of adults, the hazards imposed on children by the disaster situation are multiplied. Children are more likely than others are to suffer from malnutrition in the predisaster period and therefore are more sensitive to decreased food availability after the disaster. Children are also more likely to suffer multisystem organ injury during a disaster than adults are, as they are less likely to protect themselves, and their bodies have less protection of vital organs. In addition, they are more vulnerable to the risks of both dehydration and respiratory insufficiency from acute infection in the wake of the vast structural destruction. Disruption of the social fabric of their lives can lead to long-term depression, posttraumatic stress disorder (PTSD), interruption of normal growth and development, and lifelong disability. Sadly, orphaned children are also potential victims of unscrupulous adults who may seek to exploit them as slave workers, sex workers, or combatants in civil war and rebellion. Clearly, an entire text could be written about the proper medical and psychological care of children in disasters. This chapter will serve as an introduction and overview. References and additional readings are included at the end of the chapter for the interested reader.

Disaster response planners must consider the unique characteristics and needs of children, when designing, preparing, implementing, and assessing any disaster relief intervention. This chapter provides a historical perspective and focuses on current practices and pitfalls. It is important to be aware that many natural or human-made disasters will destroy the homes and social structures of the families of children. The children and their parents then become displaced persons or refugees, which presents them with a set of significant risks and challenges. This chapter considers a continuum of medical and psychological challenges for such children. Acute medical care must be provided in the immediate wake of the disaster, and then subacute and chronic care must be provided, locally or distantly, for displaced or refugee populations of children forced out of their domestic environment because of the disaster.

HISTORICAL PERSPECTIVE

In the past, the international community's response to disaster was disorganized, poorly monitored, and inefficient, with a focus on capital investment, structural replacement, and trans-shipment of large amounts of materials, such as medical supplies and equipment, clothing, canned food, and tents. Much of this material was outdated, culturally unacceptable, untranslated, misunderstood, and not specific to the pediatric population. Moreover, there were unintended negative outcomes resulting from improper use of pharmaceutical agents and equipment by untrained personnel. These historical problems associated with disaster relief were magnified when children were considered.

It was not until the 1980s that the emergency medical service(s) (EMS) systems in the United States began to treat children differently than adults in the prehospital setting.[3] This change came about because most of the equipment, medications, and training were not pediatric specific and therefore children were not receiving treatment based on an adequate, medically appropriate, evidence-based approach to prehospital medical care. In the same vein, the disorganized and rarely assessed response to disaster relief that existed before the mid-1980s did not fully consider the separate and important medical and psychological needs of children affected by disasters. This is especially tragic because in many developing countries, about 40% of the population is younger than 15 years,[4] and the most medically devastating natural and human-made disasters typically occur in the developing world. The level of human devastation is a direct result of inadequate intrinsic infrastructure, populations that are severely compromised and vulnerable before the disaster, and inadequate local and nationwide resources for acute and long-term responses to the disaster.

Even though many health care practitioners were eager to "do something" before there was a change in focus on children affected by disaster, few had experience, and even fewer were trained specifically in pediatric disaster medicine. Preliminary need assessments were not performed, planning was haphazard, and outcomes research was nonexistent. In the 1980s, primary health care, which was just beginning to be applied to health care development projects in developing countries, began to be applied to refugee and disaster medicine. Concepts of immunization, nutrition, oral rehydration therapy (ORT), cooperation and collaboration with the affected populations and between local and international nongovernment organizations, involvement of the local ministry of health, outcome evaluations, and appropriate information gathering, including needs assessment, were becoming more commonplace. This structured approach to disaster and refugee medical relief has been more effective.

Children routinely make up the highest mortality rates in disaster situations, and those rates are highest for children younger than 5 years.[5] Unfortunately, there are many examples of the disproportionate mortality rates among children in the disaster literature. Among Ethiopians displaced to Sudan in the mid-1980s, children younger than 5 years old were twice as likely to die as the rest of the population were.[6] In the mid-1990s, among Nicaraguan and Honduran children displaced to refugee camps because of the Contra war, infants represented 42% of all deaths, and children younger than 5 years represented 54% of all deaths.[7] During the famine of 1992 in Somalia, a horrifying 74% of children died in the town of Baidoa.[8] During the civil unrest in Rwanda in 1996, displaced Tutsi children represented 54% of all deaths among refugees in camps in Goma, Zaire,[9] with the accrued mortality 15 to 18 times greater than their baseline. More recently, in Sudanese refugee camps in 2012, pediatric deaths were 58% of the total. It is clear from the examples that children are an especially vulnerable population. These mortality rates reflect tremendous suffering and waste of human capital.

Why are children dying? The common reported causes of death of children caught up in natural and human-made disasters involving civil unrest or war and transmigration to refugee camps include acute respiratory infection, measles, malaria, severe malnutrition, diarrheal disease, injury (e.g., gunshots, mines, shrapnel, and contusions), and burns.[10] Countries experiencing armed conflict account for over 36% of the total child deaths, stillbirths, and maternal death worldwide,[11] and even in this violent setting most of these deaths are due to indirect causes such as diarrheal diseases and malnutrition.[12]

CURRENT PRACTICE

Appropriate disaster intervention aimed at decreasing the morbidity and mortality of children requires proper predisaster preparation, training, and equipment; prompt and appropriate assessment of the disaster situation; rapid intervention appropriate to the specific disaster and tailored to children's specific needs; and long-term interventions that address chronic, predictable problems associated with different forms of complex emergencies.

During the last few decades, there have been significant advances in disaster medical relief activities, and groups such as the Sphere Project have sought to rigorously analyze and standardize guidelines. This has allowed planners to prepare more appropriately for and respond to complex emergencies that arise around the world. In this process, a growing emphasis has been placed on pediatric care, reflecting its central role in disaster response. This chapter will focus on the four elements of disaster response outlined by Sphere, as each relates to the care of children: water supply; sanitation and hygiene promotion; food security and nutrition; shelter, settlement, and nonfood items; and finally health action. We also provide a separate section dealing with psychological support.

Water, Sanitation, and Hygiene

Many human-made or natural disasters interrupt the clean water supply to a population. Earthquakes may destroy wells, urban water lines, and water treatment systems. Hurricanes and tsunamis introduce fecal material, toxic chemicals, and salt water to standing water sources and wells. Combatants in war and civil unrest often destroy water sources as strategic acts of war. Despite these threats to the water supply, the minimum personal water requirement is 15 L per day,[13] and there is no evidence that children require less. Table 9-1 gives an outline of how water should be distributed across usages according to Sphere.

Even more clean water is recommended in certain situations such as collective feeding centers for children, where 30 L is recommended;

TABLE 9-1   Water Distribution across Usages

Survival needs: water intake (drinking and food)	2.5-3 liters per day	Depends on the climate and individual physiology
Basic hygiene practices	2-6 liters per day	Depends on social and cultural norms
Basic cooking needs	3-6 liters per day	Depends on food type and social and cultural norms
Total basic water needs	7.5-15 liters per day	

Adapted from Sphere Project. Humanitarian Charter and Minimum Standards in Disaster Response. Available at: http://www.sphereproject.org/.

hospitals, in which the recommended amount is 40 to 60 L; and cholera treatment, where 60 L per person per day is recommended. It is also important to pay attention to details such as the need for families to have containers for transport and storage of water. In most cultures, mothers or older female children are responsible for collecting and managing water. These same individuals are usually responsible for child care, and a remote water source is a significant drain on limited resources, which is why individuals should have access to a water source within 500 m.[14]

Sanitation is very important during and after disasters and complex emergencies. Sewage lines and sewage treatment may be disrupted by natural and human-made disasters. Many countries do not have adequate toilets, underground sewage, or sewage treatment in rural districts. Children are particularly vulnerable to fecal-oral pathogens. The so-called dirty-hands diseases, which include dysentery, cholera, typhoid, hepatitis A, polio, and helminthiasis, are transmitted because of poor hygiene and a lack of adequate clean water and soap. Providing soap and educating the population about appropriate hand washing as part of hygiene education can have a profound effect. This was demonstrated by Chinese schoolchildren, where rates of helminthic infection were decreased by 50%, after a brief education program with the provision of soap.[15] Soap distributed to refugees from Mozambique similarly decreased the incidence of diarrhea in children by almost 30%.[16]

The disaster response team should have training and experience in the assessment of the water supply and water treatment, as well as simple interventions directed at keeping the water supply safe. Short-term, rapid interventions may involve chlorination, filtration, boiling, or the provision of a mobile water supply. Long-term interventions include the drilling of deep or artesian wells that are protected from contamination by fenced wellheads. Basic hygiene items, including water containers, bathing and laundry soaps, and menstrual hygiene products, should be part of every intervention.

Responders should have an ability to assess the sanitation needs of the disaster-struck population and the cultural and sociological parameters of defecation in the affected population. In many developing countries, it is uncommon for toddlers to wear diapers or other coverings, and, even among adults, use of proper facilities may be unavailable or not used. When defecation takes place randomly throughout populated areas, it facilitates the spread of fecal pathogens. Fenced-off defecation fields, trenches, and pit latrines should be established at least 30 m from the nearest groundwater source and 1.5 m above the water table.[17] Responders must consider traditional methods and habits of defecation, as well as religious, cultural, and social mores concerning defecation and the joint use of facilities across gender and age. Decisions must be made in conjunction with appropriate local authorities and solutions implemented rapidly because large populations separated from free access to toilets will find other means and sites of relief that are fraught with the potential for spreading epidemics.

Diarrheal disease is the single most common immediately precipitating cause of death in children under the age of 5 in disaster situations,[18] and it is intimately related to the water supply. Epidemics, specifically in refugee camps, can accelerate rapidly, as was unfortunately exemplified in a Rwandan refugee camp in 1994. In a population of about 650,000 refugees in North Kivu, Democratic Republic of the Congo, an outbreak of *Shigella* and cholera caused 85% of the 50,000 deaths that were recorded in the first month.[19] Children are disproportionally affected, and it has been shown that mortality as a result of cholera is greatest in children younger than 4 years, with a 4.5-fold relative risk of death when compared with older children and adults.[20]

The mainstay of treatment for diarrheal disease in children is ORT. The UNICEF guidelines state that, per stool, children younger than 2 years should be provided ¼ to ½ of a large cup (250 mL) of ORT solution, and children 2 years or older, between ½ to 1 large cup.[21] In 2006, the World Health Organization (WHO) released a new formula for ready-to-use ORT that is available in easy-to-use packets. If these ORT packets are unavailable, a solution of 1 L of clean water with ½ tablespoon (2.5 g) of salt with 6 level teaspoons (30 g) of sugar, stirred until completely dissolved, can be used instead.[22] Vomiting is frequent, even with moderate dehydration, and oral therapy should be attempted, because vomiting will improve as the dehydration resolves. Intravenous therapy should be reserved for cases of severe dehydration ($\geq$10%) or when children have failed oral therapy. Isotonic solutions, such as normal saline or Ringer's lactate, should be used, whereas hypotonic solutions, such as D5, should be avoided. In children with severe malnutrition, ORT and intravenous hydration should be carried out carefully to avoid congestive heart failure (CHF).

Zinc supplementation is important adjunct therapy for diarrheal illness. It has been shown to reduce the duration of a diarrheal episode by about 25% and the stool volume by 30%.[23,24] All children under 5 with dysentery should receive daily treatment with elemental zinc (under 6 months, 10 mg; between 6 months and 5 years, 20 mg daily) for 2 weeks of treatment.[25]

The treatment of diarrheal illness in disasters differs from standard treatment in the United States, where antibiotics are usually avoided, partially out of concern for precipitating hemolytic uremic syndrome. WHO guidelines state that all cases of dysentery should be treated with antibiotics, and cholera patients have been shown to benefit from the treatment.[26] If possible, laboratory testing for *Vibrio cholerae* and *Shigella* should be carried out, with antibiotics tailored to the pathogen; however, presumptive treatment should begin before or even without laboratory confirmation. For treating bloody diarrhea in children, ciprofloxacin (totaling 15 mg/kg dosage [daily total] given for 3 days) is the current treatment of choice, despite the known risk of arthropathy.[27] In addition, ciprofloxacin is also effective in cholera treatment; however, a single dose of azithromycin[28] has also demonstrated effectiveness, and it is easier to implement. Surveillance is very important in managing an outbreak of diarrhea in a population of children after a disaster or a complex emergency. Surveillance should include case definitions, number and severity of cases, type of diarrhea by pathogen, age-specific and diarrhea-specific mortality, and demographics of the affected population.

Food Security and Nutrition

A disaster assessment team arriving on-site should be prepared to evaluate the pediatric population's nutritional status, using simple anthropometric measurements. Measuring the child's weight in relation to his or her height (weight-for-height [WFH]) and mid–upper-arm circumference (MUAC), and evaluating for edema are the most useful tools. A child with a WFH greater than 2 standard deviations (SDs) below the

median for age by month is said to be wasted. Weight is more sensitive than height to sudden changes in food availability, which is why WFH is used instead of height-for-age (HFA) when evaluating acute malnutrition. HFA measurements reflect chronic nutritional deficiency and HFA greater than 2 SDs below the median is referred to as stunting. When performing these measurements, children less than 86 cm should be measured in the recumbent position, and fully extended by the provider. For weights, it is helpful to have a hanging scale that can be zeroed. Both WFH and HFA measurements are compared with WHO standardized growth charts, by sex and age, by month. The results are reported as Z scores, which are the number of SDs the patient falls above or below the median when compared with a breast-fed and well-nourished population. Frequently, the child's exact age is not known, and this information can be estimated by using a local events calendar, where the family member is asked about surrounding dates, such as harvests, large storms, elections, or other memorable local events. A further advantage of WFH over HFA is that it does not suffer because of this estimation.

There are about 7 million annual deaths in children under the age of 5, and undernutrition is a primary cause in 45% of cases.[29] Severe acute malnutrition (SAM) is the most serious form of undernutrition, and it is defined by a WFH 3 SDs less than the median or by the presence of bilateral edema. SAM is one of the most serious challenges children face during disasters, and children with this condition have an 11.6-fold (hazard ratio) increase in all causes of death compared with nonmalnourished children.[30] This group requires refeeding and close medical attention because of their increased susceptibility to infectious diseases. One common and proven strategy is to provide 175 kcal per day per kg of ready-to-use therapeutic food (RUTF), such as Plumpy Nut, and to provide empiric antibiotic therapy.[31] In the past, these children were often hospitalized or kept at a refeeding center, but more recently nontoxic appearing children with SAM are being discharged home with RUTF (see Table 9-2). This helps to keep the family unit together and to relieve the burden on an already stressed medical system. An important addition to this is that if a family has multiple children, supplementary food should be provided for all children in the household, even those without SAM, to assure that the RUTF is not split among the siblings.

Children with SAM are susceptible to a multitude of conditions and environmental insults. Thermoregulation is impaired in children with SAM, and therefore extra blankets should be provided and special attention paid to keep the child warm. SAM also results in limited glucose stores and impaired gluconeogenesis, which in the setting of infection may rapidly cause clinically significant hypoglycemia. CHF can be seen secondary to fluid overload that may occur in the process of rehydrating children with gastroenteritis and dehydration. CHF may also result from severe anemia with high output failure, electrolyte disturbances, wet beriberi from thiamine deficiency, or cardiac muscle atrophy associated with prolonged protein deprivation.

Even moderate acute malnutrition (MAM) can be a significant contributor to the death of children in complex emergencies or disasters,[32,33] and children who are 0 to 5 years old are at greatest risk.[34] There is no consensus on the treatment of wasted children between −2 and −3 SDs, but, given the significant risks faced by this group, it is reasonable to supply RUTF. Malnutrition in children after a disaster is often a result of an exacerbation of preexisting chronic malnutrition. Unfortunately, this is a common condition in many developing countries in the world today. In well-nourished populations, less than 2.5% of children younger than 5 years have WFH Z scores of less than −2, and 0.15% are less than 3 SDs below the median. Rates of wasting can be much higher after a disaster, as was recently shown in Darfur, where 21.8% of children had WFH Z scores more than 2

TABLE 9-2 WHO Decision Chart for Implementation of Selective Feeding Programs	
FINDING	**ACTION REQUIRED**
Food availability at household level below 2100 kcal per person per day	Unsatisfactory situation: • Improve general rations until local food availability and access can be made adequate
Malnutrition rate 15% or more or 10%-14% with aggravating factors	Serious situation: • General rations (unless situation is limited to vulnerable groups); and • Supplementary feeding generalized for all members of vulnerable groups especially children and pregnant and lactating women • Therapeutic feeding program for severely malnourished individuals
Malnutrition rate 10-14% or 5%-9% with aggravating factors	Risky situation: • No general rations; but • Supplementary feeding targeted at individuals identified as malnourished in vulnerable groups • Therapeutic feeding program for severely malnourished individuals
Malnutrition rate under 10% with no aggravating factors	Acceptable situation: • No need for population interventions • Attention for malnourished individuals through regular community services

Source: World Health Organization, *The Management of Nutrition in Major Emergencies*, WHO, Geneva, 2000. Adapted with permission of the WHO.
Note: This chart should be adapted to local circumstances.
The malnutrition rate is defined as the percentage of the child population (6 months to 5 years) who are below either the reference median weight-for-height −2 SDs or 80% of the reference weight-for-height.
Aggravating factors:
• General food ration below the mean energy requirement
• Crude mortality rate more than 1 per 10,000 per day
• Epidemic of measles or whooping cough (pertussis)
• High incidence of respiratory or diarrheal diseases

SDs below the median (MAM), and 3.9% of children suffered from SAM.[35] It is important to note that while anthropometric data are often collected on children 6 months to 5 years, for reference purposes, all children deemed at risk should be included as part of the intervention. Testing in this younger age group is done because this group is at increased risk compared with the whole population, and therefore data from this group are a helpful early warning sign of a problem.

Micronutrient deficiencies, including iron, vitamin A, vitamin C, niacin, and thiamine, can be seen clinically in displaced children as anemia, night blindness, scurvy, pellagra, and beriberi, respectively.[36] For instance, in 2004, internally displaced children 6 months to 5 years old in Darfur had a rate of anemia of 55.2%.[37] Proper nutrition, including the promotion of protein, fruits, and vegetables, is undoubtedly central; however, targeted supplementation also has a role. For example, vitamin A supplementation has been shown to reduce mortality when administered to the community as part of a campaign, and it was particularly effective when given to measles patients.[38] One helpful

resource in the evaluation of malnutrition is the Standardized Monitoring and Assessment of Relief and Transitions (SMART) methodology. It provides a comprehensive template and free software that can be used to carry out emergency nutrition assessments.[39]

Shelter, Settlement, and Nonfood Items

Natural and human-made disasters often destroy homes and displace families. Most affected people will attempt to return home as soon as possible after a disaster, and efforts should be made to facilitate this process, if safety can be assured. Another option is to have people live with neighbors and thus keep communities intact. Providing supplementary income or food to those who are willing to shelter their neighbors may be significantly cheaper and better for the displaced than housing them in a camp setting would be. Of course, there will be instances in which it is impossible to keep families within their communities and in which emergency shelter will need to be provided.

Lack of shelter is particularly dangerous to children, whose thermoregulation is impaired, compared with that of adults, who have larger surface-to-body ratios. The disaster medical response team must consider emergency shelter as part of the intervention. Local environmental factors and cultural norms will dictate largely what types of shelters are acceptable, and the population affected and the existing authorities should be closely involved in both materials and construction design. The disaster team should bear in mind the following basic principles. In cold climates, low ceiling heights allow for a smaller space that can be kept warm more easily, whereas, in warm climates, higher ceilings allow for increased air circulation. Appropriate ventilation of cooking areas and stoves is paramount, as indoor pollution will have immediate and long-term effects on the health of children. Cooking fires are also potentially hazardous to children because fires can lead to burns or inhalational injuries, which can be avoided with appropriate design. Finally, when implementing emergency shelters, it is recommended that 3.5 m by 3.5 m of floor space be made available per person.[40]

Poorly planned and designed shelters or groups of shelters create pathogenic environments for children and families. Overcrowding and poor hygiene inevitably lead to epidemics of infectious disease. It is very difficult to predict the longevity of displacement among the affected population, and, often, initial housing will need to be repaired and upgraded. Considerations for preplanning individual and group shelters with an eye toward sustainability are important. Easy access to a reasonable supply of clean water is essential to preserve health in children, as discussed above. Environmental health risks must be considered, including stagnant open water and swamps, which should be drained or treated. One should also consider that complex emergencies and civil unrest often cause combatants from both sides to be displaced and share living spaces. Clearly, this has implications for children; they need to be protected from any incipient violence.

Health Action

Upon reaching the disaster site, the disaster response team should initiate a rapid health assessment of the children present, to determine an appropriate strategic plan for intervention. Team members should determine the major health needs of the affected children and the local response capacity. They also should determine the total number of affected children and their age and gender breakdown. The SMART methodology discussed previously regarding nutrition is useful here as well. It is important to obtain background health information and an understanding of what the main health problems of children in the region were before the disaster, including previous sources of health care; important health beliefs; the traditions of parents; the social structure of families, including decision-making pathways within the family; and the strength and coverage of public health programs at the disaster site, including immunization rates for various childhood illnesses.

The response team should use existing facilities first, whenever possible. Temporary health facilities created by the response team should have a water supply; refrigeration; heat (in a cold climate); windows with screens (in a hot climate); a generator; vaccine and vaccination equipment, including materials to maintain a cold change; and supplies of essential drugs, medical disposables (i.e., exam gloves), and nondisposables (i.e., scales). The medication and equipment should be appropriate for children, including, if possible, items such as Broselow tapes with accompanying medical packs containing sized airway and intravenous equipment, as well as standard drugs for resuscitation. Local medical personnel should be included in the relief efforts at the earliest possible stage because of their experience and familiarity with the language, culture, and sociological background of the children, as well as their familiarity with the country and intrinsic health resources. The disaster medical response team should have the ability to create a health record. It is likely that health records and vaccination forms will have been destroyed by the disaster and, therefore, will need to be recreated, either electronically or on durable materials that can be maintained after the team has left the area.

Basic medications such as antibiotics should be available in liquid form or in easily divisible, chewable tablets for weight-based pediatric dosing. Standardized case management protocols for the diagnosis and treatment of common diseases should be adopted. One such protocol that has been demonstrated to improve pediatric care[41] is the WHO's Integrated Management of Childhood Illnesses, and a few examples for common childhood illness are presented here.[42] Children with a cough and suspected pneumonia should be assessed for fast or difficult breathing and retractions. Those with fast or difficult breathing should receive an oral antibiotic, such as amoxicillin, and those with retractions should be referred to a hospital. Children with a cough and wheezing who are afebrile should not receive empiric treatment if not in respiratory distress but should receive inhaled salbutamol, using a metered dose inhaler (MDI) with spacer devices to relieve bronchoconstriction. For the evaluation of fever in malaria endemic regions, the goal is to both diagnose and treat with an appropriate antimalarial therapy, such as artemisinin-based combination therapies (ACTs) within 24 hours. Patterns of resistance geographically should govern the ultimate treatment choices. Laboratory testing is the ideal; however, children should be treated empirically, if testing facilities are not immediately available.

Malaria is especially concerning when displaced populations travel from an area of low endemicity to an area of high endemicity because the population may lack any resistance. Prevention is very important and long-lasting insecticide-treated netting should be distributed. Disaster medical relief teams should identify and attempt to decrease the opportunities for mosquito reproduction, particularly in standing water. Further, special care to cover water storage containers with lids will be especially important where dengue is also a consideration.

Reproductive health and sexually transmitted diseases cannot be ignored in disaster response activities. Sexual and gender-based violence is common in displaced populations, and this violence is often directed at children. In cases of sexual assault, postexposure prophylaxis against HIV, empiric sexually transmitted infection treatment, tetanus, and hepatitis B prevention should be provided. Emergency contraception should be offered discretely, where these practices are culturally acceptable and will not jeopardize the disaster team's ability to continue serving the community.

Finally, immunizations are of paramount importance to prevent widespread disease transmission. One of the most concerning infectious diseases in the refugee camp setting is measles, which has been identified as a leading contributor to mortality in children who are displaced after disaster. Outbreaks can have a case-fatality rate as high as 10% to 20% among malnourished children.[43] Measles is highly contagious and spread through the air by infectious droplets, causing high fever, rhinorrhea, cough, and red, watery eyes about 10 days after exposure. Small white spots inside the cheeks (Koplik spots) can occur in the initial stage, and, after a few days, a facial rash develops and spreads downward. Measles vaccination campaigns should be assigned the highest priority by response teams when predisaster vaccination coverage is less than 90% or is unknown.[44] A measles immunization program along with vitamin A supplementation are recommended in emergency settings for all children from the ages of 6 months to 5 years, and children up to 15 should also be immunized. A complete vaccination program, including catch up schedules for those not previously immunized, should be implemented in conjunction with national authorities as soon as is feasible.

Disaster relief workers should practice universal precautions and should bring HIV postexposure prophylaxis for themselves in case of needlestick or other exposure. Medical, dental, and surgical material should be disinfected and sterilized. Single use injectable doses should be used where available. The team must dispose of medical waste and sharp instruments appropriately. Many developing countries reuse sharps after sterilization procedures, and, if this is to be done, then great attention must be paid to sterilization, to prevent the spread of bloodborne pathogens. It is important that relief members not be overcome by scale of need and thus forget to implement standard safety and hygienic protocols.

Psychological Support

Disasters and complex emergencies impose a tremendous amount of psychological stress on children, who are often overwhelmed by anxiety, fear, injury, and the stress of separation from their families. About half of the Thai children affected by the devastating tsunami in 2004 exhibited PTSD, diagnosed by DSM-IV criteria, 6 weeks after the tsunami.[45] There is a direct relationship between the parents' response to disaster and the subsequent effects on their children. After an earthquake in Bolu, Turkey, researchers found that the severity of PTSD in children was mainly affected by the presence of PTSD and depression in their fathers. Fathers who had experienced the disaster and who became more irritable and detached because of these symptoms affected their children more significantly.[46]

Several researchers have reported an increase in the incidence of child abuse after natural disasters. Researchers in the United States studying the effects of the Loma Prieta Earthquake in California and Hurricane Andrew in Florida concluded that most of the evidence presented indicated that child abuse escalates after major disasters.[47] Researchers in North Carolina found that the incidence of inflicted traumatic brain injury in children increased most in counties affected by Hurricane Floyd. This increase in incidence returned to baseline levels 6 months after the disaster.[48]

It is clear that both children and parents are affected psychologically by disasters; moreover, the effect on parents can have a domino-like effect on their children. The earlier that disaster medical response teams initiate psychological counseling for the child victims of disaster, the more likely they are to circumvent the long-term development of disabling morbidity, including PTSD, anxiety, depression, and suicidal behavior. Restoring "normalizing" social structures, such as schools, playgrounds, and community centers, as well as basic human services—shelter, water, sanitation, food, and clothing—can be as effective as formal counseling in ameliorating the psychologically devastating effects of disaster.

In addition, several psychosocial concomitances of disaster and complex emergencies must be considered when focusing on children in disaster response. Disasters in which there are many adult deaths result in widespread orphaning of children. Identification and database services need to be set up soon after the medical response team arrives to try to pair children who are separated from their parents back with their parents or relatives.

! PITFALLS

- Paying attention to all the basic needs, including water supply, sanitation, and hygiene promotion; food security and nutrition; shelter, settlement, and nonfood items; and health action
- Not providing clean water and appropriate sanitation, the two most important interventions in the prevention of epidemics of potentially fatal gastrointestinal infectious diseases in children
- Not providing ORT and zinc supplementation to all dysentery cases and using antibiotics as an adjunct to therapy
- Not recognizing the impact of SAM and malnutrition, in general, after disasters and not treating children appropriately with proper nutrition and empiric antibiotics
- Not implementing effective and rapid immunization programs, especially those focusing on measles with vitamin A supplementation, which can have a widespread effects on children in the aftermath of disaster
- Ignoring psychosocial issues early in a disaster medical response and failing to mitigate long-term debilitating PTSD and depression in children

REFERENCES

1. At a glance: Haiti, Statistics section. UNICEF website, 3 Jan 2013. Available at: http://www.unicef.org/infobycountry/haiti_statistics.html.
2. Salama P, Assefa F, Talley L, Spiegel P, van Der Veen A, Gotway CA. Malnutrition, measles, mortality, and the humanitarian response during a famine in Ethiopia. *JAMA.* 2001;286(5):563–571.
3. Edgerton EA. *Institute of medicine, emergency medical services for children.* U.S Department of Health and Human Services Health Resources and Services Administration; 2006.
4. The UN Population Division's World Population Prospects. Available at: http://data.worldbank.org/indicator/SP.POP.0014.TO.ZS.
5. Toole MJ, Waldman RJ. Prevention of excess mortality in refugee and displaced populations in developing countries. *JAMA.* 1990;263:3296–3302.
6. Shears P, Berry AM, Murphy R, Nabil MA. Epidemiological assessment of the health and nutrition of Ethiopian refugees in emergency care in Sudan, 1985. *BMJ.* 1987;295:314–318.
7. Desenclos JC, Michel D, Tholly F, Magdi I, Pecoul B, Desve G. Mortality trends among refugees in Honduras, 1984–1987. *Int J Epidemiol.* 1990;19:367–373.
8. Moore PS, Marfin AA, Quenemoen LE, et al. Mortality rate in displaced and resident population of central Somalia during 1992 famine. *Lancet.* 1993;341:935–938.
9. Nabeth P, Vasset B, Derin P, Doppler B, Tectonidis M. Health situations of refugees in eastern Zaire. *Lancet.* 1997;349:1031–1032.
10. Toole MJ, Waldman RJ. The public health aspects of complex emergencies and refugee situations. *Annu Rev Public Health.* 1997;18:283–312.
11. Southhall D. Armed conflict women and girls who are pregnant, infants and children; a neglected public health challenge. What can health professionals do? *Early Hum Dev.* 2011;87:735–742.
12. Muggah R. Armed Violence in Africa: reflections on the costs of crime and conflict. *Small Arms Survey.* October 2007. UNDP. Available at: http://www.genevadeclaration.org/fileadmin/docs/regional-publications/Costs-of-Crime-and-Conflict-in-Africa.pdf.
13. Sphere Project. Water Supply Standard 1: Access and Water Quantity. Humanitarian Charter and Minimum Standards in Disaster Response. Available at: http://www.spherehandbook.org/en/water-supply-standard-1-access-and-water-quantity/.
14. Ibid. Viii.
15. Bieri FA, Gray DJ, et al. Health-education package to prevent worm infections in Chinese schoolchildren. *N Engl J Med.* 2013;368 (17):1603–1612.
16. Peterson EA, Roberts L, Toole MJ, Peterson DE. The effect of soap distribution on diarrhea: Nyamithuthu Refugee Camp. *Int J Epidemiol.* 1998;27:520–524.
17. Sphere Project. Excreta Disposal Standard 1: Environment Free from Human Feces. Humanitarian Charter and Minimum Standards in Disaster Response. Available at: http://www.spherehandbook.org/en/excreta-disposal-standard-1-environment-free-from-human-faeces/.
18. Connolly MA, Gayer M, Ryan MJ, Spiegel P, Salama P, Heymann DL. Communicable diseases in complex emergencies: impact and challenges. *Lancet.* 2004;364(9449):1974–1983.
19. Goma Epidemiology Group. Public health impact of Rwandan refugee crisis: what happened in Goma, Zaire, in July, 1994? *Lancet.* 1995;345: 339–344.
20. Swerdlow DL, Malenga G, Begkoyian G, et al. Epidemic power among refugees in Malawi, Africa: treatment and transmission. *Epidemiol Infect.* 1997;118:207–214.
21. UNICEF. *Facts for Life.* 4th ed. Available at: http://factsforlifeglobal.org/07/1.html.
22. *Guidelines for the Control of Shigellosis, Including Epidemics Due to Shigella Dysenteriae Type 1.* World Heatlh Organization; 2005.
23. Bhandari N, Bahl R, Taneja S, et al. Substantial reduction in severe diarrheal morbidity by daily zinc supplementation in young north Indian children. *Pediatrics.* 2002;109(6):e86.
24. Fonatine O. Effect of zinc supplementation on clinical course of acute diarrhoea. *J Health Popul Nutr.* 2001;19(4):339–346.
25. *Guidelines for the Control of Shigellosis, Including Epidemics Due to Shigella Dysenteriae Type 1.* World Heatlh Organization; 2005. http://www.who.int/cholera/publications/shigellosis/en/.
26. *Guidelines for the Control of Shigellosis, Including Epidemics Due to Shigella Dysenteriae Type 1.* World Heatlh Organization; 2005. http://www.who.int/cholera/publications/shigellosis/en/.
27. *Guidelines for the Control of Shigellosis, Including Epidemics Due to Shigella Dysenteriae Type 1.* World Heatlh Organization; 2005. http://www.who.int/cholera/publications/shigellosis/en/.
28. Khan WA, Saha D, Rahman A, Salam MA, Bogaers J, Bennish ML. Comparison of single-dose azithromycin and 12-dose, 3-day erythromycin for childhood cholera: a randomsed, double-blind trial. *Lancet.* 2002;360 (9347):1722–1727.
29. Black RE, Vcitora CG, Walker SP, et al. Maternal and Child Nutrition Study Group. *Lancet.* 2013;382:427–451.
30. The Lancet Series on Maternal and Child Nutrition. Launch Symposium. 2013 June 6. http://download.thelancet.com/flatcontentassets/pdfs/nutrition_2.pdf.
31. Trehan I, Golbach HS, LaGrone LN, et al. Antibiotics as part of the management of severe acute malnutrion. *NEJM.* 2013;368:425–435.
32. Rice AL, Sacco L, Hyder A, Black RE. Malnutrition as an underlying cause of childhood death associated with infectious disease in developing countries. *Bull World Health Organ.* 2000;78:1207–1221.
33. Pelletier DL, Frongillo EA Jr, Shroeder DT, Habicht JP. The effects of malnutrition on child mortality in developing countries. *Bull World Health Organ.* 1995;73:443–448.
34. Mason KB. Lessons on nutrition of displaced people. *J Nutr.* July 1, 2002;132 (7):2096S–2103S.
35. Emergency Food Security and Nutrition assessment in Darfur, Sudan, WFP, October 2004.
36. Weise Prinzo Z, de Benoist B. Meeting the challenges of micronutrient deficiencies in emergency-affected populations. *Proceedings of the Nutrition Society.* May 2002;61:251–257.
37. Emergency Food Security and Nutrition assessment in Darfur, Sudan, WFP, October 2004.
38. Fawzi WW, Chalmers TC, Herrera MG, et al. Vitamin A supplementation and child mortality. *JAMA.* 1993;269:898–903.
39. SMART. Measuring Mortality, Nutritional Status, and Food Security in Crisis Situations: SMART Mehtodology. Version 1 April 2006.

40. Sphere Project. Shelter and settlement standard 3: Covered living space. Humanitarian Charter and Minimum Standards in Disaster Response. http://www.spherehandbook.org/en/shelter-and-settlement-standard-3-covered-living-space/.

41. Arifeen SE, Blum LS, Hoque DME, et al. Integrated Management of Childhood Illness (IMCI) in Bangladesh: early findings from a cluster-randomised study. *Lancet*. 2004;364:1595–1602.

42. WHO. *Evidence For Techinical Update of Pocket Book Recommendations. Recommendations for management of common childhood conditions: Newborn conditions, dysentery, pneumonia, oxygen use and delivery, common causes of fever, severe acute malnutrition and supportive care*; 2012. http://whqlibdoc.who.int/publications/2012/9789241502825_eng.pdf.

43. Guha-Sapir D, D'Aoust O. *Demographic and health consequences of civil conflict*. Background Paper, *World Development Report 2011*. World Bank; 2011. *http://web.worldbank.org/archive/website01306/web/pdf/wdr_background_paper_sapir_d'aoust4dbd.pdf?keepThis=true&TB_iframe=true&height=600&width=800*.

44. Sphere Project. Essential health servics child health standard 1: Prevention of vaccine preventable diseases. Humanitarian Charter and Mimimum Standards in Disaster Response. http://www.spherehandbook.org/en/essential-health-services-child-health-standard-1-prevention-of-vaccine-preventable-diseases/.

45. Piyasil V, Ketumarn P, Prubrukarn R, et al. Post-traumatic stress disorder in children after the tsunami disaster in Thailand: a 5-year follow-up. *J Med Assoc Thai*. 2011;94(Suppl 3):S138–S144.

46. Kilic EZ, Ozguven HD, Sayil I. The psychological effects of parental mental health on children experiencing disaster: the experience of Bolu earthquake in Turkey. *Fam Process*. 2003;42(4):485–495.

47. Curtis T, Miller BC, Berry EH. Changes in forced incidents of child abuse following natural disasters. *Child Abuse Negl*. 2000;24(9):1151–1162.

48. Keenan HT, Marshall SW, Nocera MA, Runyan DK. Increased incidence of inflicted traumatic brain injury in children after a natural disaster. *Am J Prev Med*. April 2004;26(3):189–193.

Psychological Impact of Disaster on Displaced Populations and Refugees of Multiple Traumas

Amer Hosin

This chapter is designed to examine the impacts of disaster on displaced populations and refugees of multiple trauma events. The aims therefore are to highlight the processes of psychological triage, identify at-risk groups, and suggest treatment approaches that enhance the adjustment processes and well-being of victims and survivors. The focus is particularly on those victims who have witnessed traumatic events and experienced considerable loss.

It is hoped that this work will also answer a few important questions on how displaced populations, including children, women, and other adult family members, may react to the traumatic refugee experience, how they adjust and cope in the host culture, and what their mental health problems are. The answers provided to these questions are important to a number of professionals and emergency field workers, including emergency staff and rapid response team members, doctors, nurses, policy makers, researchers, psychiatrists, psychologists, social workers, and other mental health professionals.

The scale of refugee population movements in the world today is becoming alarming, with approximately 51.2 million people across the globe considered to be "of concern" to the United Nations High Commissioner of Refugees (UNHCR).[1] In 2013 the UNHCR suggested the reasons for large-scale refugee movements are numerous, including persecution, conflict and wars, generalized violence, and human rights abuse and violation. The same report of the UNHCR noted that 16.7 million of these displaced people were refugees in foreign host nations, whereas 33.3 million individuals became internally displaced persons (IDPs) within their own countries, and 1.2 million of the reported figures became asylum seekers. This particular report also noted that the year 2013 alone witnessed the displacement of 10.7 million individuals, of which 8.2 million were internally displaced and 2.5 million later became refugees. That is with an estimate of 32,200 individuals who leave their home daily and seek protection elsewhere.[1] It is worth noting that the majority of these displaced populations are children and women. Children below 18 years old represented 50% of the displaced population. Meanwhile the group between 18 and 50 years old represented 46% of displaced figures; individuals more than 60 years old were only 4% of the population. The majority of these displaced individuals seem to be currently living in developing countries. Major sources of countries of refugees include Afghanistan, Syria Arab Republic, Somalia, Sudan, Democratic Republic of Congo, Myanmar, Iraq, Colombia, Vietnam, and Eritrea.[1]

The 2011 civil war in Syria has contributed to one third of its population fleeing and becoming displaced in what could be described as the worst humanitarian disaster in modern times. It has also created the worst refugee crisis in the Middle East. It is estimated that 2.5 million Syrians have fled abroad and another 6.5 million have been internally displaced. Most Syrian refugees are currently living in poor conditions in tents and in neighboring countries, such as Turkey, Iraq, Jordan, and Lebanon.

As will be seen throughout this chapter, victims of war and oppression usually flee in large numbers, arriving in poor, underdeveloped countries without appropriate care or education for the young individuals. Most of these host developing countries lack the appropriate infrastructure needed to facilitate massive humanitarian needs. Similarly Iraq continues to face a long-standing, large-scale population displacement and pressing humanitarian needs for its own population, particularly in the north and west of the country. Terrorist organization attacks (Islamic State of Iraq and the Levant [ISIL]) on Mosul have forced hundreds of thousands of people of various Iraqi ethnic backgrounds to seek shelter elsewhere in Iraq. However, the services remain inadequate, overcrowded, and unsustainable.

Focusing on the literature[2-6] in this area, apart from some very limited publications, it has been suggested[7-9] there is very little attention paid to the links between reactions, losses, and adjustment of displaced populations and refugees living in a host nation.[10] Published research that links both adjustment and preflight problems, particularly among those refugees who have escaped civil strife and wars and suffered multiple traumas or displacement, is very limited.[11] An interesting study,[12] which was funded by the King's Fund (United Kingdom), on the health needs assessment of the Iraqi community in London, suggested that 53% of the adult population studied had a wide range of mental health problems, 49% had heart diseases, and 24% suffered from various types of cancers. These findings confirm results reported by similar studies.[13,14] The former examined the importance of social factors in exile among 84 Iraqi refugees and found depression in 44% of the sample. This particular study suggests that many of the most important factors in continuing morbidity can be modified in the country of exile. It has also highlighted the importance of the preflight experience and family reunion in which the survivor is separated from close relatives, including spouses and children. Meanwhile another study[14] found that 46.6% of patients included in their study had a posttraumatic stress disorder (PTSD) according to the criteria of the *Diagnostic and Statistical Manual*—Fourth Edition (DSM-IV). Age, gender, unemployment, and torture emerged as important predictors of emotional withdrawal in this study. Both of the above-mentioned studies seem to place emphasis on the multifactorial nature of risk factors in the psychological health of refugees and the need for integrated rehabilitation efforts as well as professional help to improve the social environment and the need to provide appropriate activities and support to the refugee population.

POSTMIGRATION AND ADJUSTMENT OF TRAUMATIZED REFUGEES IN HOST NATIONS

Certain research[11] has reported that reactions to direct exposure and living through war conditions may contribute to promoting negative outcomes among newly arrived refugees, including high levels of PTSD symptoms in children and adults who have survived war. This particular study further added that traumatic stressors in war are commonly multiple, diverse, chronic, and repeated. Other research in this area[15,16] has focused on parental adjustment and children's reactions to traumatic events. In fact some of these studies,[11–13,15] which were conducted in former conflict regions, such as Bosnia, Lebanon, Iraq, and South Africa, have found that adults and parental mental health, particularly that of mothers in times of conflict, was a significant predictor of children's adjustment and morbidity. Baker and those of similar work[17,18] support the above-mentioned findings and add "tortured individuals are less likely to function as parents, spouses or employees. Tortured survivors can have difficulty in establishing relationship and trust with their spouse and children and are therefore more likely to transmit their problem to their offspring."

Sourander[19] looked at the extent of damage on separated refugee minors waiting for placement in an asylum center in Finland and reported that approximately half of the minors were functioning within clinical or borderline range when evaluated with the Child Behavior Checklist. This study also claimed that very young and unaccompanied refugee minors are more vulnerable to emotional distress than older children. Hauff and Vaglium[20] suggested that the availability of a close confidante, such as a spouse, children, or close relatives, in periods of psychosocial transition has been shown to have a protective effect against psychiatric disorders. This research also noted that married refugees separated from their spouses by the flight were more emotionally distressed than other refugees on arrival. Allodi[21] indicated that emotional distress in children was related to previous traumatization of the parents and the current coping styles. Weile and colleagues stated that children of traumatized refugee families were fragile, vulnerable, and had more psychosomatic problems than age-matched native school children.[22]

LEVEL OF EXPOSURE TO VIOLENCE AND HUMAN DISASTER VERSUS VULNERABILITIES OF DISPLACEMENT

It is worth noting here that the extent of vulnerability depends on the impact of premigration exposure to violence and postmigration experience on individuals and community.[4] This may include, before migration, witnessing the death and injury of a parent or sibling and perhaps persistent exposure to death, destruction, and ultimately children separated from parents. Researchers[23,24] regard separation from family support, siblings, and friends as more stressful than exposure to bombing and injury. Hence the most vulnerable time appears to be the preschool years and early adolescence.[25,26] Other risk factors may include sudden and unanticipated death of parents or siblings during disaster, consequent radical change in family circumstances, and poor access to family support, followed by an unstable, inconsistent host environment in the dissimilar host culture. It would be fair to suggest here that rapidly changing environments with little stability as well as parental psychopathology and lack of security or protection have implications on the physical health and mental well-being of the refugee population.

Further research in this area[27–29] has looked at the factors that help children to cope with severe and stressful life events. This work indicates that a lack of immediate support, disintegration of family, and the more risk factors a child is exposed to are more likely to make children vulnerable to psychiatric or mental health problems. Williamson, Ahearn, and Athey have summarized the plight of refugees and the extent of their vulnerability and suggested "at any point in time, half of the refugees in the world are children. Most large-scale flights involve children, young adults, and women. These children often experience

malnutrition, lack of a balanced diet for normal growth, infectious diseases during the flights, exposure to crowded conditions, and poor sanitation. Many children also may lose siblings because of infectious diseases, experience separation, experience death of parents, become victims of violence, be beaten and suffer injuries, and are more likely to assume an adult role when the family structure changes through the death of parents and during illness."[30,31]

While writing on the legacies of war, atrocities, and refugees, Summerfield noted that there had been at the time an estimated 160 wars and armed conflicts in the developing world since 1945, with 22 million deaths and 3 times as many injured.[32] He quoted United Nations Children's Fund (UNICEF) figures for 1986 and suggested "in the First World War, 5% of all casualties were civilians, 50% in the Second World War, over 80% in the U.S. war in Vietnam and in present conflicts over 90%." He went further to add that 80% of all war refugees are in developing countries, many among the poorest on earth. In parts of Central America, he claimed 50% of households are headed by a woman and these are much more likely to be poor. Mortality rates during the acute phase of displacement by war are up to 60 times those of expected rates. Those at extra risk are households headed by an unprotected woman (often widowed), those without a community or marginalized in an alien culture, those at serious socioeconomic disadvantage or in severe poverty, and those with poor physical health or a disability. The emotional well-being of children remains reasonably intact for as long as their parents (or other significant figures) can absorb the continuing pressure of the situation. Once parents can no longer cope with day-to-day living, children's well-being deteriorates rapidly and infant mortality rates rise.

DISASTER AND MENTAL HEALTH TRIAGE OF REFUGEES AND SUGGESTED THERAPEUTIC APPROACHES

In a comprehensive review Westermeyer suggested that assessment and treatment should take into consideration a wider range of past experience and current life situations as well as medical history, family illnesses, and social background.[33] This should include physical examination, developmental data, prenatal and postnatal problems, social and emotional development, preflight stressors, losses, length of stay in refugee camps, and early resettlement experience. That is to say premigration, transmigration, and postmigration experiences are frequently traumatic and must be assessed.

Treatment, however, should resemble that offered to indigenous populations and should include counseling, cognitive and behavioral therapy, and pharmacotherapy, if necessary. Compliance problems and complaints regarding side effects may occur more often among refugees who are not familiar with long-term medications. These can be reduced through education and reeducation of the parents and children. Refugee problems are too complex to rely on medication to solve mental health and psychiatric problems. Doctors and therapists therefore should direct patients to counseling, social activities, play, group work, stress management, education, and recommendation of other psychotherapies available to deal with stressful and long-term problems.

Jones worked with adolescent refugees in Bosnia who experienced uprooting and various losses (i.e., losses of family, home, school, town, friends, and relatives) and suggested that greater flexibility over boundaries is required, particularly regarding time and setting.[34] In addition, therapists working in a human rights or refugee camp context should be prepared to acknowledge their own impartiality and subjectivity and allow the discussion of political and social issues within the group. It is also suggested that such support can be of use through providing a space for expressing feelings, problem-solving, and rebuilding of social ties. Eisenbruch uses the term *cultural bereavement* to describe the losses and sees this as a condition that can affect both physical and mental health.[35] Jones and Eisenbruch both agreed on the fundamental task of first rebuilding the social networks, engaging in community support, facilitating the development of problem-solving skills, and addressing the collective experience of loss rather than focusing entirely on the psychopathological impact of trauma on the individual.[34,35] It has been claimed that the most important task to accomplish during debriefing is to educate the victims and survivors about the psychological sequela frequently experienced by most refugees. This normalization of stress through debriefing can reduce people's responses to the inevitable symptoms of stress, depression, guilt, sleep disturbance, etc. The sociocultural background of the survivor may be an important consideration in the screening process. Some survivors may be from certain cultures or from certain parts of a particular country where psychotherapy is not recognized as a form of treatment. In such cases an offer of psychotherapy may be rejected by the client or, even when accepted, premature termination of treatment is always a possibility.

In refugee camps and on arrival, physical needs, such as food, water, clothes, shelter, sanitation, immunization, and care for infectious diseases should be a priority. Psychological and social needs should follow and must include reduction in uncertainty, improved education, and links with religious groups, expatriate groups, and other social agencies. Moreover, screening for problems of mental health and social adjustment should occur in school, through the social services, and perhaps through primary care clinics and hospitals. Staff in these locations should be sensitive to the special needs and problems of refugees. Woodhead summarized the needs of refugees as follows, "refugees arrive from different countries—with different historical, age, gender and cultural backgrounds—seeking safety, accommodation and security. Some arrive in considerable distress, are victims of war and torture and may have complex physical and mental health needs. However, food and a safe environment (home) is likely to be their first priority. Those who arrive from war-torn regions tend to show signs of PTSD alongside other psychiatric and health problems such as anxiety, depression, insomnia, malnutrition, intestinal problems, skin complaints, stigma, poor self esteem."[5]

Overall, refugee assessments demand special sensitivity to anxiety, fear, shyness, reassurance, clarity, and understanding. Refugees are individuals with a well-founded fear arising from one of a number of causes, including witnessing malicious violence and losses to being subject to interrogation, imprisonment, and oppression. Turner stated "despite the resilience of many refugees coming to the United Kingdom, there was a substantial proportion who have evidence of serious psychological difficulties. Newly arrived refugees not only need community support but also many will have significant mental health problems and will need access to effective mental health treatment."

Prevalence studies of refugee reactions to disaster and PTSD have revealed that approximately 25% to 30% of individuals who witness a traumatic event may develop chronic PTSD symptoms and/or other forms of mental disorders, such as depression.[36–42] Preexisting psychopathology, degree of horror, duration, frequency and level of exposure, gender, age, suddenness, controllability, inflicted damage and intensity of the disaster, perceived threat at the time, early separation from family, and availability of support would all be risk factors that determine PTSD development in both children and adults. In summary the prevalence of symptoms is related to a variety of factors, including the nature of trauma and the child's own experience, age, sex, past psychiatric illnesses, and the degree of social support received from parents at home. It should be noted, however, that a high prevalence of some forms of mental health problems is a characteristic of studies of refugee communities. For example, Brent and Harrow's survey indicated that self-reported mental health problems were more than 5 times higher in a refugee sample than in the general population sample.[43] Furthermore, other research also reported that approximately 30% of refugee children are in a severe state of mental discomfort and are in urgent need of child psychiatric or psychosocial rehabilitation.[34]

Finally Stimpson and co-workers confirmed the above findings and indicated that psychiatric disorder is common, disabling, and a burdensome source of disability after war.[44] Treatment approaches and rehabilitation of trauma must include the whole family (spouses, children) and the whole social network of the victims. However, working with refugee families and their children who may have witnessed displacement, exile, torture, atrocity, or separation is at best difficult. The stress levels suffered by such traumatized patients are chronic and sometimes severe. It is advisable to use a combination of approaches (e.g., debriefing, counseling, cognitive therapy, drugs, and other psychotherapeutic approaches) to treat the problems of decrease of social interest, isolation, chronic depression, nightmares, poor concentration, and irrational and avoidance behaviors. Dedicated professionals with the necessary energy and expertise may be able to provide specialized treatments that recognize the role of current stresses, relieving some symptoms by medication and also helping traumatized individuals to get the social, emotional, and financial support that they require. Jumaian, Hosin, and Rahmatallh touched on this issue by suggesting that the treatment approach for survivors of traumatic events often begins with debriefing.[45] Other studies suggested that there is a wide range of effective strategies, including group therapy, behavior and cognitive approaches, desensitization, flooding techniques, as well as relaxation training used for tension, anxiety, and intrusive thoughts.[46–48] Most of these techniques can help sufferers to enhance their coping skills. Sleep problems and nightmares are other aspects of PTSD symptoms among children who have witnessed disasters. Halliday found that relaxation and music before bedtime could be useful techniques for alleviating the recurrence of nightmares.[49] Other reactions that need careful intervention and therapy include depression, guilt feelings, pessimism, irritability, and anger.

Furthermore, whatever approach is used, establishing a supportive, trusted relationship and being in a safe environment are essential elements in therapy. Finally Levin indicated that professionals should consider the following aspects while assessing or offering rehabilitation programs to traumatized refugees: the type of trauma, difficult life events before the flight, experience in refugee camps, cultural and ethnic background, gender perspectives, language difficulties, and life in exile.[50]

UNACCOMPANIED CHILDREN, WOMEN, AND DISPLACED REFUGEE FAMILIES

It is understood that most of the industrial world in the past has received and still receives asylum applications from unaccompanied children. Some of these children arrive completely alone, whereas others are with relatives or nongovernmental organizations.[4] Their parents could be dead, ill, imprisoned, or simply did not have the money to flee as well. It has been suggested that most unaccompanied children and refugees come from war-torn regions, such as Syria, Iraq, Afghanistan, Somalia, Eritrea, and Ethiopia. However, more than half (53%) of all refugees worldwide come now from just three main countries: Afghanistan, the Syrian Arab Republic, and Somalia.[1]

These studies add that refugee women and their children are extremely vulnerable, as are the elderly. Rape is a common element in the pattern of persecution, terror, and ethnic cleansing that uproots refugee families from their homes and communities. The UNHCR also reports that from Somalia to Bosnia refugee families frequently cite rape or the fear of rape as a key factor in their decision to leave.[4]

It has been estimated that 20% to 30% of refugees up to 1990 have been tortured.[3,4,51,52] In a study of 104 torture survivors Domovitch observed the following mental symptoms in descending order of frequency: anxiety, insomnia, nightmares, depression, withdrawal, irritability, loss of concentration, sexual dysfunction, memory disturbance, fatigue, aggressiveness, impulsiveness, and hypersensitivity to noise.[51] Similarly Somnier and Genefke reported that the most common symptoms were sleep disturbances, nightmares, headaches, impaired memory, poor concentration, fatigue, fear and anxiety, and social withdrawal.[52] It should be emphasized here that refugee populations cannot be regarded as a homogeneous group. Although they share the experience of forced uprooting, their reactions to trauma are not necessarily similar or totally predictable. Some refugees have highly developed occupational skills, whereas others are educated and have various abilities which enable them to resettle and perhaps make a useful contribution to the new host country. Some become depressed or lack the skills to adapt quickly to a new culture. Because of their near-death experiences and exposure to violence either before or during the flight, many adults are unable to function adequately as parents, spouses, employees, or citizens and they are likely to experience a series of strained relationships as a result. In addition, their mental health problems are significantly higher when compared with the general nonrefugee population.

Good psychological adjustment among refugee families and children is more likely to manifest itself when parents are psychologically healthy and less distressed. As well as parental health, variables, such as the duration and number of years spent in the host country, the group's background, current level of social contact and support, numbers of family members sharing the household, and the nature of the traumatic experience before their flight, have been investigated. The prior-mentioned outcomes were expected and discussed within the frameworks of acculturation, culture-learning theory, U-curve theory, and the multidimensional model on acculturation discussed below.[53,54] It was claimed that such problems can be attributed to problems before displacement, the new demands of the host culture, daily stresses, unmet expectations, isolation, and perhaps lack of skills and social support in the new and unfamiliar culture.[54,55] On the other hand, the manifestation of social, emotional, and behavioral problems among children was related to their home surroundings, isolation, and lack of care provided by the suffering and traumatized parents. This research has also suggested that emotional and adjustment problems manifested among children will not disappear without proper intervention programs, and proper consideration of all risk factors, including family circumstances and previous parental psychopathology.

Indeed the challenge of learning a new language, internalizing different social norms, and finding new employment are great challenges for even the most able and creative refugees. Westermeyer, Hauff, and Vaglum confirm the above and pointed out that upon assessment it is important to take into account the conditions during exile and premigration experience, the traumatization in the host country (i.e., the acculturation stress and the pressure of assimilation during the first years of resettlement), and other predisposing factors that are not related to their experience.[4,56,57] In other words, research on the mental health of refugees should take into account the complexity of their holistic situation. That is to say the quality of life and the health situation of the refugee population demand considerable attention, including the delivery of services, which should be available, effective, and aimed at reducing stress. However, lack of social support and isolation appears to be a much stronger predictor of poor mental health and depression in the long term than severity of trauma. Indeed an early period of adjustment to a new environment and coming to terms with posttraumatic experiences need a much more sensitive approach, particularly for the most vulnerable refugees, such as victims of torture and rape, and for unaccompanied children.[58] It should also be remembered that while refugee experiences can generate a number of mental health problems, some refugees are reluctant to seek help, and their tendency to somaticize emotional problems is particularly common because they come from societies that stigmatize mental illnesses.

Almqvist and Hwang addressed the importance of parental coping and parental functioning and stated that young children will continue to cope with difficult environments as long as their parents are not pushed beyond the stress threshold level capacity.[59] This research also added that parents who are hopeful and optimistic are more likely to influence children's adjustment in the host culture. Freud and Burlingham identified the importance of the family as a buffer for stress and separation from the family as a major stress crisis period.[60]

Various writers claim that successful adjustment in an unfamiliar culture is greatly dependent on not only the individual but also on other situational factors and reasons for the exposure to the host culture (i.e., reasons for the contact), length of the stay, and culture norms and policies.[61] Furthermore, other researchers maintain that both assimilation policies and integration are facilitative strategies for adjusting into the new culture as compared with separation.[62,63] Some researchers argue that the least stress occurs during the early stage of contact with the host culture, whereas the most stress occurs during the intermediate phase of acculturation processes.[64,65] The latter relates adjustment to the duration and stages of time spent in a host culture. It involves an initial stage of optimism, which Lysgaard describes as the honeymoon period, followed by a culture shock and the process of improvement of adjustment in the host society.[65] In fact others associate an individual's reactions to the nature of the displacement to complex factors, such as personality, temperament, the extent of social support, cultural similarity, prior knowledge of the language, reasons for contact, and perceived cognitive control over the experience.[66] Using the stress model, researchers suggest that any new move to a new place creates stressful demands, and a major task confronting individuals in stressful situations is a cognitive one.[67,68] This implies the interpretation of the situation and the activation of the coping response could maximize a sense of control over the situation. Similarly others claim that an individual who possesses positive cognitive control and views the changes resulting from the acculturating experience as being constructive adapts better to the host culture.[61,63] As can be seen now, there is a somewhat complex interplay among a variety of factors that influences the extent to which successful adjustment can be made in the host culture. Having discussed all of the possible factors which may contribute to the poor psychological well-being of the refugee population, a good understanding of this complexity and the relationship between migration and mental health is essential for any assessment or rehabilitation program.

NATIONAL AND INTERNATIONAL POLICIES ON ASYLUM SEEKERS, DISPLACED POPULATIONS, AND REFUGEES OF MULTIPLE TRAUMA

Refugees arrive with a wide range of experiences, including massacres and threats of massacres, detention, beatings, torture, rape, sexual assault, witnessing death and torture of others, destruction of homes and property, and forcible eviction. Unfortunately, and despite the guidelines of the 1951 Geneva Convention, which tends to protect and care for refugees, most Western countries now are seeking to implement new deterrent policies characterized by indefinite detention of all refugees, including children, women, and young adult men who arrive at their shores and ports of entry. This is very much the case in Australia, the Netherlands, Germany, and Britain.

Many of the above-mentioned countries are aware that the 1951 Geneva Convention specifically bars countries from punishing people who have arrived directly from a country of persecution provided that they present themselves speedily to the authorities and show good cause for their illegal entry. With regard to detention and repatriation policies of failed asylum, Germany, Denmark, the Netherlands, Austria, Switzerland, and the United Kingdom have already sent refugees home. Previously in the Netherlands, five Kurds from Northern Iraq went for more than 80 days on a hunger strike protesting at the Dutch decision to deport them. The protestors were between the ages 25 and 36. According to *The Guardian* in 2001 this measure is already deployed by the Home Office and has led to a dramatic increase in the refusal rate. Further the U.K. government regulations on asylum indicate that asylum seekers can get residency in Britain only if they meet the 1951 U.N. Convention's definition of a refugee. This means they must have a "well-founded fear of persecution" on the grounds of race, religion, nationality, membership of a particular social group, or political opinion. Asylum seekers can make a verbal application for residency at a British port and then have 5 days to collect evidence to substantiate their claim. The application is then sent to the Home Office's Immigration and Nationality Directorate for a decision. If it is turned down, the asylum seeker can appeal; if that appeal is turned down by the Immigration Appeals Tribunal the asylum seeker will be deported. Britain has already called for changes, amendment, and modernization of the 1951 U.N. Convention on Refugees.

It is worth noting, people who seek refugee and asylum status are not a homogeneous population. However, previous studies have found that one in six refugees has a physical health problem severe enough to affect their life, and two thirds have experienced anxiety or depression, sleep problems, and poor memory.[7,8] Social isolation and poverty have a compounding negative impact on mental health, as can hostility and racism. Reducing isolation and dependence, having suitable accommodation, and spending time more creatively through education or work can often do much to help adjustment. Moreover, positive changes can be seen if immigrants are reunited with families and take up educational and employment opportunities. Refugee community organizations are invaluable in supporting refugees. They can provide information and orientation and reduce the isolation experienced by so many refugees. In a study of Iraqi asylum seekers, it was reported that depression was more closely linked with poor social support than with a history of torture.[13] Hence it is important for refugees to develop ongoing links and friendships and with people in the host community. Further details on the health and well-being of asylum seekers, refugees' adjustment, as well as the impact of deterrent refugee policy, detention, and impact on refugees mental health can be found in Burnett and Peel, O'Nions, Keyes, and Grant-Peterkin, Schleicher, Fazel, and co-workers.[6–8,69–71] The latter study has discussed the status of mental health and well-being of asylum seekers and refugees in immigration removal centers and suggested that evidence exists that immigration detention can be harmful to mental health, especially for people with preexisting mental health problems, such as PTSD.[71] This particular work additionally reported that time spent in a detention center was shown to be positively associated with severity of mental health. Furthermore, it was also indicated that detention precipitates mental health disorders and can cause severe relapses and substantially increase the risk of self-harm and suicide. Recommendations from this research further suggested that detainee asylum seekers are often highly vulnerable, particularly if they have mental health disorders. Thus

professionals have the duty of care to ensure that their needs are appropriately met. That is to say, medical professionals must ensure that they do not become complicit in a system that prioritizes deterrence over protection of refugees and asylum seekers. Other recommendations of this study indicate that alternatives to immigration detention exist and these should be explored by professionals before vulnerable people are placed in detention centers.

CONCLUDING REMARKS ON A REFUGEE BEING IN AN UNFAMILIAR, UNKNOWN HOST SURROUNDING

At the individual level, Berry and Hsiao-Ying consider adjustment to new and unfamiliar host culture as a psychosocial process by which the individual should achieve harmony with the new surrounding through interaction and changes in knowledge and attitudes and in cognitions.[72,73] Meanwhile Bochner relates successful adjustment to cultural learning that embraces the acquisition of appropriate social skills and behaviors necessary to conduct successful daily activities and negotiate the cultural milieu.[74,75] This of course includes general knowledge about the specific culture, length of residence in the host culture, language and communication competence, and quantity and quality of contact with the host nationals. Other factors that are relatively important for adjustment include premigration stress, cognitive reappraisal of change, personality, loneliness, and quality of social relationships. Adjustment here is discussed in terms of skills deficit and acculturative stress and a range of mediating variables that can either increase or decrease the deficit and the psychosocial stress that refugees may face. In general these influential variables can be related to the individual, cultural knowledge, self-efficacy, the available resources, social support, and host cultural relations.

Early theoretical perspective in this area was the U-curve model developed by Lysgaard.[55] The U-curve theory describes the three stages of emotional adjustment one often experiences in a host culture. The initial stage is the honeymoon period, which may be characterized by high levels of positive adjustment due to enthusiasm, excitement, and a positive expectation of being in the host culture. This is followed by decreased adjustment, frustration, and distress due to lack of interaction, culture shock, lack of understanding of the native language, and the sharp disparities between the dominant and the original culture.[76,77] However, the third stage is characterized by a gradual learning, acquisition of necessary skills, social interaction, and possible integration with the new culture. And above all else, familiarity with the customs and values system of the host culture which may promote positive and successful adjustment. Critics of the U-curve theory claimed that that because there are many variations within the process of adjustment it is difficult to see a universal pattern emerging across various situations and individuals.[75] On the other hand, cultural maintenance theory links the individual's adjustment and coping to the process of assimilation and/or integration within the host culture and to the efforts that may be made by individuals to maintain their own cultural identity alongside the host culture.[55] Attitudes that are adopted toward the host culture are fundamental factors that determine the path of adjustment among refugees.

REFERENCES

1. United Nation High Commissioner of Refugees. *War's Human Cost: UNHCR Global Trends.* Geneva, Switzerland: UNHCR Publication; 2013.
2. Aldous J, Bardsley M, Daniell R. *Refugee Health in London: Key Issues in Public Health.* East London and City Health Authority: The Health of Londoners Project; 1999.

3. Hosin AA. Children of traumatised and exiled refugee families: resilience and vulnerability. A case study report. *Med Confl Surviv.* 2001;17(2):137–145.

4. Hosin AA, ed. *Reponses to Traumatised Children.* England: Palgrave Macmillan; 2007.

5. Woodhead D. *The Health and Wellbeing of Asylum Seekers and Refugees.* London: King's Fund Report; 2000.

6. Burnett A, Peel M. What brings asylum seekers to the United Kingdom? *Br Med J.* 2001;322(7284):485–488.

7. Burnett A, Peel M. Asylum seekers and refugees in Britain, health needs of asylum seekers and refugees. *Br Med J.* 2001;322:544–547.

8. Burnett A, Peel P. Asylum seekers and refugees in Britain. The health of survivors of torture and organized violence. *Br Med J.* 2001;322:606–609.

9. Westermeyer J, Vang T, Neider J. Refugees who do and do not seek psychiatric care: an analysis of premigration and postmigration characteristics. *J Nerv Ment Dis.* 1983;171:86–91.

10. Almqvist K, Broberg AG. Mental health and social adjustment in young refugee children 3 1/2 years after their arrival in Sweden. *J Am Acad Child Adolesc Psychiatry.* 1999;38(6):723–730.

11. Smith P, Perrin S, Yule W, Rabe-Hesketh S. War exposure and maternal reactions in the psychological adjustment of children from Bosnia-Hercegovina. *J Child Psychol Psychiatry.* 2001;42(3):395–404.

12. Jafar S. *Health Needs Assessment Study of Iraqi Community in London.* London: Iraqi Community Association in cooperation with King's Fund; 2000.

13. Gorst-Unsworth C, Goldenberg E. Psychological sequelae of torture and organised violence suffered by refugees from Iraq: trauma-related factors compared with social factors in exile. *Br J Psychiatry.* 1998;172:90–94.

14. Lavik NJ, Hauff E, Skrondal A, Solberg O. Mental disorder among refugees and the impact of persecution and exile: some findings from an out-patient population. *Br J Psychiatry.* 1996;169:726–732.

15. Bryce J, Walker N, Ghorayeb F, Kanj M. Life experiences, response styles and mental health among mothers and children in Beirut, Lebanon. *Soc Sci Med.* 1989;28:685–695.

16. Dawes A, Tredoux C, Feinstein A. Political violence in South Africa: some effects on children of the violent destruction of their community. *Int J Ment Health Nurs.* 1989;18:16–43.

17. Baker R. Psychological consequences for tortured refugees seeking asylum and refugee status in Europe. In: Basoglu M, ed. *Torture and Its Consequences: Current Treatment Approaches.* Cambridge: Cambridge University Press; 1992.

18. Basoglu M, ed. *Torture and Its Consequences: Current Treatment Approaches.* New York, NY: Cambridge University Press; 1992.

19. Sourander A. Behaviour problems and traumatic events of unaccompanied refugee minors. *Child Abuse Negl.* 1998;22(7):719–727.

20. Hauff E, Vaglum P. Organised violence and the stress of exile: predictors of mental health in a community cohort of Vietnamese refugees three years after resettlement. *Br J Psychiatry.* 1995;166:360–367.

21. Allodi E. The children of victims of political persecution and torture: a psychological study of a Latin American refugee community. *Int J Ment Health.* 1998;18:3–15.

22. Weile B, Wingender LB, Bach-Mortensen N, Busch P, Lukman B, Holzer KI. Behavioural problems in children of torture victims: a sequel to cultural maladpatation or to parent torture? *J Dev Behav Pediatr.* 1990;11:79–80.

23. Black D. What happens to bereaved children? *Proc R Soc Med.* 1976;69:842–844.

24. Black D, Newman M, Harris-Hendriks J, Mezey G, eds. *Psychological Trauma: A Developmental Approach.* London: Gaskell and Royal College of Psychiatrists; 1997.

25. Bowlby J. *Attachment and Loss*; Vol 3. New York: Basic Books; 1980.

26. Rutter M. *Children of Sick Parents.* London: Oxford University Press; 1966.

27. Rutter M. Resilience in the face of adversity: protective factors and resistance to psychiatric disorder. *Br J Psychiatry.* 1985;147:598–611.

28. Garmezy N. Stress, competence and development: continuities in the study of schizophrenic adults, children vulnerable to psychopathology, and the research for stress-resistant children. *Am J Orthopsychiatry.* 1987;57(2):159–174.

29. Werner EE. High risk children in young adulthood: A longitudinal study from birth to 32 years. *Am J Orthopsychiatry.* 1989;59:72–81.

30. Williamson J. Half the world's refugees. *Refugees.* 1988;54:16–18.

31. Ahearn FL, Athey JL, eds. *Refugee Children: Theory, Research and Services.* Baltimore: Johns Hopkins University Press; 1991.

32. Summerfield D. The impact of war and atrocity on civilian populations. In three years after resettlement. *Br J Psychiatry.* 1997;166:360–367.

33. Westermeyer J. DSM-III psychiatric disorders among Hmong refugees in the United States: a point of prevalence study. *Am J Psychiatry.* 1988;145:197–202.

34. Jones L. Adolescent groups for encamped Bosnian refugees: some problems and solutions. *Clin Child Psychol Psychiatry.* 1998;3(4):541–551.

35. Eisenbruch M. Cultural bereavement and homesickness. In: Fisher S, Cooper CL, eds. *On the Move: The Psychology of Change and Transition.* London: Wiley; 1990.

36. Meichenbaum D. *A Clinical Handbook: Practical Therapist Manual for Assessing and Treating Adults with Post Traumatic Stresses Disorder.* Canada, Ontario: Institute Press; 1994.

37. Yule W, ed. *Post Traumatic Stress Disorders: Concepts and Therapy.* New York, NY: Wiley; 1999.

38. Fairbank JA, Schlenge WE, Saigh PA, et al. An epidemiological profile of post-traumatic stress disorder: prevalence, comorbidity, and risk factors. In: Friedman MJ, Charney DS, Deutch AY, eds. *Neurobiological and Clinical Consequences of Stress: From Normal Adaptation to PTSD.* Philadelphia, PA: Lippincott Williams & Wilkins; 1995.

39. Koopman C. Political psychology as a lens for viewing traumatic events. *J Polit Psychol.* 1997;18(4):831–847.

40. Resick P. *Stress and trauma.* Philadelphia, PA: Taylor & Francis; 2001.

41. Deivedi KN, ed. *Post-Traumatic Stress Disorder in Children and Adolescents.* London: Whurr; 2000.

42. Thomas TN. Acculturative stress in the adjustment of immigrant families. *J Soc Distress Homel.* 1995;4(2):131–142.

43. Brent and Harrow Refugee Survey. *London Brent and Harrow Health Agency*; 1995.

44. Stimpson N, Thomas H, Weightman AL, Dunstan F, Lewis G. Psychiatric disorder in veteran of the Persian Gulf. *Br J Psychiatry.* 2003;182:391–403.

45. Jumaian A, Hosin A, Rahmatallh A. Post-traumatic stress disorder in children: symptoms, assessment and treatment. *Arab J Psychiatry.* 1997;8(2):127–139.

46. Yule W, Udwin O. Screening child survivors for posttraumatic stress disorder. Experience from Jupiter sinking. *Br J Clin Psychol.* 1991;30:131–138.

47. Saigh PA. The development of posttraumatic stress disorder. *Behav Ther.* 1991;2:213–216.

48. Joseph SA, Brewin CR, Yule W, Williams R. Casual attributions and psychiatric symptoms in survivors of the Herald of Free Enterprise Disaster. *Br J Psychiatry.* 1991;159:245–246.

49. Halliday G. Direct psychological therapies for nightmares: a review. *Clin Psychol Rev.* 1987;7:501–523.

50. Levin L. Traumatised refugee children: a challenge for mental rehabilitation. *Med Confl Surviv.* 1999;15(4):342–351.

51. Domovitch E, Berge PB, Wawe MJ, et al. Human torture: Description and squeal of 104 cases. *Can Fam Physician.* 1984;30:827–830.

52. Somnier FE, Genefke IK. Psychotherapy for victims of torture. *Br J Psychiatry.* 1986;149:323–329.

53. Berry JW, Kim U, Power S, Young M. Bujaki M Acculturation attitudes in plural societies. *J Appl Psychol.* 1989;38:185–206.

54. Berry JW, Kim L. Acculturation and mental health. In: Dasen PR, Berry JW, Sartorius N, eds. *Health and Cross-Cultural Psychology: TouBards Applications.* Newbury Park, CA: Sage; 1988:207–238.

55. Aronowitz M. Adjustment of immigrant children as a function of parental attitudes to change. *Int Migrat Rev.* 1992;26:86–110.

56. Westermeye J. *Psychiatric Care of Migrants.* Washington, DC: American Psychiatric Press; 1989.

57. Westermeyer J. Psychiatric service for refugee children: an overview. In: Ahearn F, Athey JL, eds. *Refugee Children: Theory, Research and Services.* Baltimore: The John Hopkins University Press; 1991.

58. Clinton-Davis L, Fassil Y. Health and social problems of refugees. *Soc Sci Med*. 1992;35(4):507–513.

59. Almqvist K, Hwang P. Iranian refugees in Sweden: coping processes in children and their families. *Childhood*. 1999;6(2):167–187.

60. Freud A, Burlingham D. *Young Children in War Time*. London: George Allen & Unwin; 1943.

61. Ward C, Bochne S, Furnham A. *The Psychology of Culture Shock*. 2nd ed. Philadelphia and Hove, East Sussex: Routledge; 2001.

62. Ward C, Kennedy A. Acculturation strategies, psychological adjustment and sociocultural competence during cross-cultural transitions. *Int J Intercult Relat*. 1994;18:329–343.

63. Berry JW, Poortinga YH, Segall MH, Dasen PR. *Cross-cultural Psychology: Research and Application*. Cambridge, NY: Cambridge University Press; 1992.

64. Furnham A, Bochner S. *Culture shock: Psychological Reactions to Unfamiliar Environment*. London: Methuen; 1986.

65. Lysgaard S. Adjustment in a foreign society: Norwegian Fulbright grantees visiting the United States. *Int Soc Sci Bull*. 1955;7:45–51.

66. Noels KA, Pon G, Clement R. Language, identity and adjustment. The role of linguistic self confidence in the acculturation process. *J Lang Soc Psychology*. 1996;15(3):246–264.

67. Williams CL, Berry JW. Primary prevention of acculturation stress among refugees: Application of psychological theory and practice. *Am Psychol*. 1991;46(6):632–641.

68. Lazarus RS, Folkman S. *Stress, Appraisal and Coping*. New York, NY: Springer; 1994.

69. O'Nions H. The effects of deterrence-based policies on vulnerable, traumatized asylum seekers and refugees. In: Hosin A, ed. *Responses to Traumatised Children*. Basingstoke: Palgrave; 2007.

70. Keyes E. Mental health status in refugees: an integrative review of current research. *Issues Ment Health Nurs*. 2000;21:397–410.

71. Grant-Peterkin H, Schleicher T, Fazel M, et al. Inadequate mental health care in immigration removal centres. *Br Med J*. 2014;349:g6627.

72. Berry JW. Immigration, acculturation and adaptation. *Appl Psychol Inte Rev*. 1997;46:5–34.

73. Hsiao-Ying T. Sojourner adjustment: the case of foreigners in Japan. *J Cross Cult Psychol*. 1995;26:523–536.

74. Bochner S. The social psychology of cross-cultural relations. In: Bochne S, ed. *Cultures in Contact: Studies in Cross-Cultural Interaction*. Oxford: Pergamon; 1982.

75. Bochner S. Coping with unfamiliar cultures: adjustment or culture learning? *Aust J Psychol*. 1986;38:347–358.

76. Oberg K. Culture shock: adjusting to new cultural environments. *Pract Anthropol*. 1960;7:177–182.

77. Vaughan GM. The social distance attitudes of New Zealand students towards Maoris and fifteen other national groups. *J Soc Psychol*. 1962;57:85–92.

CHAPTER 11

Ethical Issues in Disaster Medicine

Nir Eyal

Medical practitioners and health officials train for decades to provide run-of-the-mill health services. How should their choices change in times of disaster, that is, during "a serious disruption of the functioning of a community or a society involving widespread human, material, economic, or environmental losses and impacts, which exceeds the ability of the affected community or society to cope using its own resources"?[1]

This definitional inability to cope without outside help creates a strong moral imperative for health workers, officials, and ordinary citizens from societies near and far to pitch in and help. This obligation is a matter of humanity, and sometimes justice, as well as prudence.[2] For some health workers and officials, including many local ones, helping in a disaster is part of their job.

Fortunately, people often accept the duty to assist those in a disaster, even across international borders. Donations pour in. Our "rescue mentality" inclines us to strive to save identified endangered life,[3] especially during a discrete event,[4] even at great cost. The question is how to use that aid wisely and ethically—and how to prevent and prepare for disasters in the first place.

HISTORICAL PERSPECTIVE

Toward the end of the twentieth century, two cultural processes affecting disaster response ethics have taken shape. Until that time, bioethics writing had relatively little to say on disasters.[5,6] Nowadays, a number of professional societies and international organizations have specific (sections of) documents on disaster management,[7–10] as do a number of U.S. states.[11–13] Second, the HIV/AIDS epidemic ushered in a paradigm change to public health culture in America and elsewhere. An earlier emphasis on collective health interests was replaced by emphasis on personal liberty, nonstigmatization, and checks on public health authorities' powers.[14] For example, quarantine, which used to be a staple intervention for containment of infections, is now used only esoterically, often during disasters.[14,15] Legal culture now substantially constrains the ability of public health officials to surveil disease and to mandate reporting and disclosure of disease status,[14] again making disasters the exception.

We have relatively new documents to address events that have newly become rarer in the culture of public health surrounding them. How do these documents conceive of disaster ethics? How should we conceive of it?

CURRENT PRACTICE

Disaster ethics affects conduct during the prevention, mitigation, and planning stages (Section 1). It also affects many dilemmas that arise during disaster response, especially about altered standards of care, informed consent, triage, disparities, quarantine, surveillance, research, transparency and communication, rescuers' rights, and political involvement (Section 2 to Section 11). Finally, it affects choice in the recovery process (Section 12).

Section 1. Prevention, Mitigation, and Planning

A less fortunate side of our rescue mentality is that our inclination to act before disaster events is weaker.[3,4] But it is wiser and more ethical to try to *prevent* disasters by stemming the vulnerabilities that lead to them (e.g., through safely built nuclear reactors), *mitigate* them (e.g., through building codes and zoning laws that mitigate the effects of future earthquakes and flooding, as well as insurance to minimize their economic effects), and *plan* the response, once a disaster becomes inevitable (reducing the adverse effects of disaster, e.g., through public announcements; stocking up on medications, equipment, food, etc.; and training first responders and other health personnel for effective, coordinated disaster response).[16] Some advance processes can take decades, for example, creating command chains, comprehensive guidelines, and legal frameworks for effective response, and fully training health personnel, which is a shared responsibility of medical educators and the personnel.[8,17]

Advance preparation is as important for optimizing ethical decision making during a response as it is for optimizing medical and logistical components: "Ethical rules defined and taught beforehand should complement the individual ethics of physicians."[7] Moreover, rapid ethical consulting and support can preempt health worker stress, which might otherwise later occasion unethical choices, as allegedly happened in Memorial Hospital during Hurricane Katrina in 2005.[18] It can also prevent accidental active harm by health workers: inadequate training may have contributed to the many unnecessary amputations (example courtesy of Michael Southworth) that aid workers performed following the 2010 Haiti earthquake.[19] Advance preparation permits international organizations to tailor their general plans respectfully toward local circumstances and cultures.[9] It also permits coordination across centers, organizations, and jurisdictions, increasing both efficiency and equality.

Section 2. Altered Standards of Care

Sections 2–11 focus on ethical questions that arise in disaster response. These are some of the most dramatic questions in medical ethics: Are clinicians allowed to help each patient below the standard of care or without informed consent, just to save resources and time for others? How should one ration life-saving ventilators during an avian flu pandemic? How should one decide equitably which area to protect next from spreading fire? When is it permissible, or mandatory, to force people into quarantine, to shut schools, or to evacuate an area? What are the limits of permissible surveillance, mandatory testing, and other potential transgressions of privacy? What kinds of medical trials are legitimate on vulnerable disaster victims? How should one communicate risk to a frightened public responsibly yet with ample transparency and opportunity for feedback? Do health workers deserve added protections or instead have duties to take on major personal risks? How should aid organizations balance their avowed neutrality with the urge to act for patients in political and legal battlegrounds?

The present subsection addresses the common expectation that responders, seeking to be free to help more patients, will provide less intense care per patient than is standard in normal times.[7] One way to put this is by calling for "crisis standards of care," defined as "a substantial change in usual health care operations and the level of care it is possible to deliver, which is made necessary by a pervasive (e.g., pandemic influenza) or catastrophic (e.g., earthquake, hurricane) disaster."[20] Altered practices don't just include allegiance to special algorithms and to a command hierarchy, with less plurality and more coordination than in ordinary practice. They also require greater resource stewardship, and hence reduced resource investment per patient. This can and should be avoided up to a certain point by, for example, using stockpiles and added volunteers, by repurposing patient care areas, by extending the efficacy of existing personnel (say, by cutting required administrative and clinical procedures per patient and by assigning each more patients), and by conserving, adapting, substituting, and occasionally reusing supplies.[20,21] But there can come a point when the combined medical need of services is so high that a choice must be made: standard care for some, or seriously altered care for many more. At that point, the ethical choice is usually the latter.[20]

Some disagreement exists about expressing an altered standard through legal statutes.[22] However, with rare exceptions,[23] experts agree on the legitimacy of some radical alterations to expectations from caretakers in a disaster. Even opponents of altered standards of care agree that "creating algorithms to equitably and rationally allocate scarce resources is necessary and appropriate."[22]

Such radically altered care practices are often defended as part of the transition in disasters from focus on one's own patient's care to maximizing the number of patients serviced and lives saved overall: "the guiding principles for health care delivery during catastrophes may shift from autonomy and beneficence to utility, fairness, and stewardship."[24] They could also be defended as a matter of equality: providing something to everyone is more equal than privileging only some.

The legitimacy of radically altered care raises the question whether there is any minimum to the quality of care that can be provided. Alternatively, does the acceptable level always depend on the opportunity cost in terms of other patients' needs? Some authors[25] and the SPHERE project[16] insist that even in the worst disasters, there is always a minimum standard that must be kept, defined in terms of, for example, a certain number of gallons of water per person or a certain health service, such as trauma care. On the other hand, the very definition of disaster is that not all services can be dispatched. In battlefield triage and certain disaster triage systems, some wounded patients are tagged as "black" (or, in some systems, "blue"), that is, too terminally wounded for scarce medical support, trauma care included.

What remains constant even in disasters is human dignity; in fact the need to acknowledge patients' dignity may only increase. When patients are "black" or "blue," some dignity and respect remain important, which could be expressed in different ways: palliation and sedatives, separation from other patients, or some consent and privacy rights. This is part of the reason why certain ordinary patient rights should always be safeguarded.[7,20]

Section 3. Informed Consent

It is generally recognized that "a public health disaster such as a pandemic, by virtue of severe resource scarcity, will impose harsh limits on decision-making autonomy for patients and providers."[11] The value of

provider allegiance to special algorithms and to a chain of command has already been mentioned. But part of the altered standard affects patient autonomy. According to the World Medical Association, "the most appropriate treatment available should be administered with the patient's consent. However, it should be recognized that in a disaster response there may not be enough time for informed consent to be a realistic possibility."[7] Some decisions that affect the patient's health and welfare, such as triage and, for some, mandatory quarantine (see the following discussion), do not require consent at all—although if time permits, they are best explained to the patient and performed with his or her informed consent.

The point can be summed up as follows: In a disaster, when a certain care decision must take place with great expediency (either for the patient's sake or in order to move quickly to treat others), ethics requires less by way of patient consent than in normal times (legality will change with jurisdictions). In decisions affecting only the patient's own health (e.g., amputation of an infected foot, evacuation from a dangerous area), some consent or assent remain necessary unless the patient is decisionally incapacitated and proxies are not available. Given the time constraints, fully informed consent generally remains unnecessary. Decisions about a patient's care that substantially affect the health of others (e.g., vaccination, isolation) do not require the patient's fully informed consent, yet some form of consent or assent may remain necessary if the intervention is intrusive. Even when informed consent is unnecessary, it usually remains important to be transparent and to disclose pertinent information such as treatment follow-up steps and any underlying triage principle, if only in hindsight.

Section 4. Triage

"Triage is a medical action of prioritizing treatment and management based on a rapid diagnosis and prognosis for each patient."[7] At various points in the disaster response process, not all patients who could benefit from medical assistance can receive it. Even if all could receive one type of assistance (say, full medical attention for postexposure psychological stress after having watched many hours of television coverage), that would take too many resources away from other services. Planned, sensible, and coordinated triage can keep these decisions expedient, rational, and fair.

Triage decisions are often difficult for health personnel, who usually define themselves as their patient's staunch advocates yet find themselves making hard choices between patients. Perhaps as a result, "many recent disaster responses have been characterized by a general lack of meaningful triage" (see Chapter 54). Following blast events there is a documented tendency to categorize patients with major soft-tissue injuries as highest priority, even when they lack internal bleeding and critical injuries, which can come at the expense of patients with critical injuries who could have otherwise been saved.[26] To keep triage as expedient, rational, and fair as possible, it helps to plan standard triage practices and train in them and/or delegate them to professionalized triage teams.

Triage Methods

But how to triage? Many methods are in current use. Some triage methods categorize patients into several levels of urgency—most commonly (1) immediate priority (color-coded red), (2) must wait (yellow), (3) least severe injuries, or the "walking wounded" (green), and (4) prognosis so poor that there is no justification for spending limited resources on them (black; or black or blue) (see Chapter 54).[7] Other methods consist of instructions, such as the following:

- Provide assistance first to patients with the highest improved incremental survival,[27] or (more widely) to those who stand to benefit most from assistance, medically or overall.

- Provide assistance first to the most vulnerable people,[9] or to those with the greatest or most "urgent" need, or to the worse off, medically or overall, currently or usually.
- Provide assistance first to patients who are first in line (first-come-first-served).[12]
- Provide assistance first to response personnel, such as some health workers and police.
- Provide assistance as ordained by a fair lottery.

How to decide between all these methods? One way to do so is according to the fundamental goals that triage purports to serve.

Fundamental Goals Behind Triage

What is the point of triage efforts? What are the methods described methods *for*? If you will, what would count as success in a triaging method?

1. *Utilitarianism:* One fundamental approach to judging triage is utilitarian. *Utilitarianism* is the ethical theory that we should maximize collective welfare.[28] For some, utilitarianism ought to govern disaster triage, and triage has sometimes been defined as necessarily utilitarian: "Triage is the utilitarian sorting of patients into categories of priority to rationally allocate limited resources; it is, proverbially, to do 'the greatest good for the greatest number.' " (see Chapter 54).

   In disaster triage, utilitarianism could be understood to demand maximizing the number of *lives* saved, or that of the *life years* saved, or that of the *quality-adjusted life years* (QALYs) saved, or simply the *welfare* saved. It is especially common to understand utilitarianism to support saving the most lives.[20] However, "disaster impacts may include loss of life, injury, disease, and other negative effects on human physical, mental, and social well-being, together with damage to property, destruction of assets, loss of services, social and economic disruption, and environmental degradation."[1] Saving lives is not the only relevant (health) metric from the utilitarian viewpoint of maximizing collective welfare. Clearly some of the attention of utilitarian emergency personnel should go to other matters: to helping radiation victims not only accomplish short-term survival but also live as long as possible; to minimizing amputation-related disabilities[19] or, indeed, mental morbidities; and to helping "psychologically traumatized individuals who do not require treatment for bodily harm but might need reassurance or sedation if acutely disturbed."[7] Some utilitarians would add that when the quality of life for a sufficient number of patients or enough life years are at stake, these considerations can trump a slightly greater chance of saving a single patient's life for a short period. Even when the relevant disaster triaging is for life support, some have proposed "explicitly adding considerations of 'maximizing life-years saved' to 'saving the most lives,' " which, they hold, "yields a more complete specification of accomplishing the greatest good for the greatest number."[29]

   Whether in terms of life saving or longevity, health, and welfare more broadly, questions remain as to which triaging method utilitarianism would support. Color-coding seems suitable (more so for a utilitarian approach that restricts itself to maximizing lives saved, and less for ones focused on other metrics). On the face of it, so is providing care to patients with the highest prospect of treatment benefit. But on the rare occasions in which admission or diagnosis is very long and resource intensive, utilitarianism may support even first-come first-served or a fair lottery, arbitrariness notwithstanding, due to their extreme expediency. Utilitarianism may also be thought to lend support to prioritizing response personnel, because a response worker is instrumental to the effort to assist many patients. Helping a single one of these other patients would help patients less, even if that single patient stands to benefit more from

immediate help than the worker does (see the Response Worker Prioritization section).

2. *Egalitarianism:* Another fundamental approach to judging triage methodology is egalitarian. *Egalitarianism* (from the French *égal*, meaning "equal") is an ethical theory that values equality and therefore places at least some weight on increasing or expressing equality.[30] Egalitarians, when deciding triage levels, do not always decide in favor or the patient who stands to benefit the most from the treatment. When a patient stands to benefit only a little more than others would, but they are much worse off than he or she is, egalitarians may decide in their favor.

   Egalitarianism comes in many variants. As a fundamental approach behind disaster triage, it may demand greater equality in survival or, depending on its variant, in longevity, lifetime health (expressed in, e.g., QALYs), or welfare, or greater equality in the prospects or capabilities for them. Alternatively, it can demand equalizing service availability and quality (or prospects or capabilities for *them*), or it can demand that the system express equal concern and respect for all in other ways.

   In our context, egalitarianism may support giving some priority to patients and populations who are (momentarily or usually) relatively worse off, medically or overall. Depending on the exact variant of egalitarianism, the resulting limited priority may go to patients whose contemporaneous prognosis is dire (because their medical prospects are now poor), to patients who have lived with serious disabilities for years (because their lifetime health is worse), to young patients (because dying now would make them short-lived), to socioeconomically disadvantaged patients (because their welfare prospects and resources are lower), or to those who queued up first (because first-come first-served may be thought to express equal concern).[31]

3. *Proceduralism:* A final fundamental approach to judging triage emphasizes the process of decision making. *Proceduralism* emphasizes certain preferred *procedures*: impartial and nondiscriminatory decisions; transparency about triage criteria and deliberation with stakeholders, including socially marginalized groups, about those criteria; and use of fair lotteries. Proceduralism is not directly concerned with *outcomes*, such as the number of lives saved or the equality of benefit distribution across populations.

   A worry about focusing on procedures for triage decision and not on what these decisions should be is that preferred procedures can still lead to misguided triage. A fair lottery can recommend very wasteful and inegalitarian triage, as can deliberation with stakeholders. However, some proceduralists believe that using the right procedures also tends to select the best procedures, at least in the long run. This seems plausible with regard to some procedural considerations, such as the prohibition on any personal relations between triage officers and the patients being triaged.[7] Emergency physicians should not make triage decisions about people to whom they are partial, including even their own patients (so decisions about continued ventilator support or continued surgery after initial laparotomy should usually be handled by other doctors).[26] One reason that partiality would be wrong is that it is a recipe for making biased triage decisions. However, it is less clear how other preferred procedures necessarily enhance the quality of triage decisions in the long run, and whether disaster is the time to act in the light of speculative long-term benefits.

Disability Weights, Age Weights, and Discrimination

A startling implication of one potential fundamental goal mentioned, that of maximizing health or QALYs, is that people living with a chronic condition are deprioritized for life-saving treatment, say, for ventilators during influenza pandemics. The reason is that saving each such person is expected to produce fewer QALYs and less health *per annum* than saving a similar person who is expected to remain healthy. Another implication is that older and/or terminal patients, whose remaining life expectancy tends to be lower than that of healthier, younger patients, should usually be deprioritized. The emergency preparedness documents of some U.S. states embrace similar triage practices. One states, "There are reasons to deprioritize to use resources well: e.g., age at the extremes, terminally ill, chronically ill with a life-threatening disease."[12,13]

Advocates for people living with disabilities and the elderly have protested these suggestions for deprioritization as prejudiced or unfair.[31,32] Some of their responses rest on questionable denials that even serious disabilities really tend to reduce health or quality of life. A more straightforward response is egalitarian: there is something unequal and unfair when a person who has lived with worse health is deprioritized as such for important future health benefits.

Whether or not this egalitarian response works for "reprioritizing" disabilities, egalitarianism only bolsters the case for deprioritizing the elderly as such. They have already gotten their "fair innings" and lived for many years—they are "rich" in life years. By contrast, should the young die now, they will die without having had many life years and without the key life experiences those life years enable.[33] In fact, while the elderly do not always have lower life expectancy than all young people (some young people are terminally ill), and while the elderly's potential contemporaneous vulnerability can lend them priority from some egalitarian viewpoints,[16,34] the "fair innings" argument uniformly supports giving priority to the young.[20]

Because complex philosophical considerations may deprioritize the *youngest* patients (neonates, and perhaps infants and children),[35] some have proposed that fairness gives people who are in the prime of their lives, with life plans and persons who are fully developed yet seldom fulfilled, somewhat higher priority than it does to either the very old or the very young.[35]

It may seem as although the procedural prohibition on partiality and discrimination that we mentioned renders these complexities moot. Disaster responders are often warned against any discrimination on the basis of personal relations, race, religion, economic status, geographic location, sex, and some other attributes, any of which would count as partial.[9] Does this prohibition rule out any consideration of disability status or age? A lot depends on precisely what it makes sense to deem irrelevant for disaster triage. First, the World Medical Association regards only nonmedical characteristics as irrelevant,[7] and one could argue that age or at least disability status are medical characteristics. On the other hand, for the International Federation of Red Cross and Red Crescent Societies, only "medical need" (or elsewhere: "need") should make a difference,[9] and one could argue that those living with disabilities or the elderly have an equal need to live. That having been said, it is philosophically complex whether, when the medical benefits following survival are unequal, medical needs in survival remain equal.

A second response emphasizes that "an ethical policy does not require that all persons be treated in an identical fashion, but does require that differences in treatment be based on appropriate differences among individuals." The response adds that the person's own medical need is not the only legitimate ground for favorable treatment. What matters for avoiding partiality is that "this priority should stem from … relevant factors," and these factors can transcend personal medical need. For example, they include also "important community goals, such as helping first responders or other key personnel stay at work."[20] To accept this logic would render the question whether medical need is similarly less crucial.

Response Worker Prioritization

Should disaster triage give first responders and other key personnel priority for treatment and prophylaxis? Many documents suggest as much,[12] on a number of grounds:

- Only healthy, able relief staff can help minimize morbidity and mortality for all—so all benefit from this potential inequality.
- Only well-protected relief staff are likely to want to stay in dangerous environments. For example, whether or not morally their obligation is to show up to work even during pandemic flu, health workers who know that they (and their families) are inoculated are likelier to do so.
- Response teams often face higher risk than the general population, for instance, of infection, burns (for firefighters), a building collapsing further, or a second bomb exploding. It is only fair to pool this elevated risk by providing response teams with added protection and priority for treatment, thereby reestablishing more equal chances at life.
- Response teams deserve societal gratitude for their often taxing or brave services. Priority for health services is one way to thank them.

However, some disagree that response personnel should be prioritized in every disaster situation. They warn that such automatic priority may look partial and undermine societal trust in that personnel.[36]

Nondisaster Needs

In the aftermath of the 2010 Haiti earthquake, a foreign volunteer response team faced the following dilemma: Seven-year-old Haitian twins reached the hospital, both with broken left legs. One had been trapped under rubble and debris during the earthquake and the other was not affected by the earthquake but fell off of a tree while playing (example courtesy of MGH Disaster Relief Ethics Group). Was it ethical to attend to both twins and not just to the former, although the mission had been defined, and explained to donors, as one about disaster relief?

This question arises on a larger scale as well. Many humanitarian organizations use leftover funds from one disaster response mission for others. Money earmarked for tsunami response in South Asia was sometimes used for famine relief in Africa. Would it have been preferable to use the extra funds to build improved health systems in South Asia—not exactly a matter of disaster response either?[36a]

Given that systems are overburdened during disaster, the job of disaster responders can certainly extend beyond disaster response in the strictest sense. It can include preventing escalation, for example, in terms of later food insecurity[16] and securing continuous routine immunizations, protection from mosquito exposure, and so forth.[16] While a full theory remains necessary on the exact scope of rescue work, part of the expectation is that this work will go beyond disaster response in the narrowest sense.

Repeat Triage

"Since cases may evolve and thus change category, it is essential that the situation be regularly reassessed by the official in charge of the triage."[7] One interesting implication is that patients previously triaged not to receive immediate care can later be repeat-triaged to receive care immediately. A more striking implication is that patients previously allotted care may lose that entitlement. That implication can be very hard for caretakers and families to accept. However, in a disaster, at least, "policies permitting the withdrawal of critical care treatment to reallocate to someone else based on higher likelihood of benefit may be ethically permissible."[27] The main question concerns the exact circumstances that make such reallocation permissible. Are disaster triage criteria for withdrawal of treatment strictly equivalent to the ones for its withholding[27] or moderately more complicated?[37] Either way, treatment withdrawal aimed at saving other patients will often remain appropriate in a disaster, such as during a pandemic flu in which the number of patients in need of ventilators is twice the number of available ventilators,[37a] and training should prepare health workers and triage teams for it.

Section 5. Disparities

Disasters tend to affect minorities, the poor, women, and other vulnerable or marginalized groups more than they do social elites.[38] The former are more vulnerable to disastrous events (flooding washes away hillside slums more than it does hilltop villas, and women take care of children more than their husbands do). They face greater difficulties obtaining good services—the poor may lack funds for paying private physicians or purchasing vehicles for reaching public hospitals first.

Response planners should remain "mindful of existing health disparities that may affect populations or regions"[24] and make advance plans to mitigate or redress them. They may, for example, organize added public transportation in poor neighborhoods, boost translation services, and set up regular briefings with minority representatives to glean information on barriers to equitable response efforts.[20,38] Addressing disparities at the level of individual triage is inappropriate and sometimes too late.

Section 6. Quarantine

Public health interests can be in tension with the interests, needs, liberties, or rights of individuals, and disasters can bring these tensions into sharp relief. When a disaster consists of infectious disease outbreaks, containment sometimes benefits from geographic isolation of infected individuals, social distancing measures (e.g., bans on public gatherings), border controls and travel bans, and, most controversially in modern times, quarantine, the geographic isolation of individuals considered to be at a sufficiently high likelihood of being infected.[38a]

The "health and human rights" approach tends to play down clashes between public health and individual rights. It points out the complications for public health when the individuals whose collaboration is needed for reporting, self-transport, containment, and grassroots-level mutual assistance are antagonized or fearful that collaboration might cost them direly—for example, that seeing a doctor is likely to land them in quarantine. In the 2014-2015 Ebola outbreak in West Africa, attempts to place areas under quarantine floundered: against a background of distrust as well as insufficient supplies in many quarantined areas, individuals kept breaking the quarantine. Health and human rights lawyers emphasize that quarantine has greater chances of success when individuals receive food and other supplies, there is constant attention to their evolving needs,[39] and quarantine is voluntary not mandatory.

It is true that in some ways protection of personal rights provides good collective outcomes. But it is also true that that is not always the case. Arguably, in the same West African Ebola crisis, early quarantine could have contained Ebola, as it regularly does in East Africa, where it has been used successfully against Ebola for decades.

There is no reason, of course, to make measures transgressing individual liberty or interests worse than they need be: "Any measures that limit individual rights and civil liberties must be necessary, reasonable, proportional, equitable, nondiscriminatory, and not in violation of national and international laws."[2,40] Such measures should respect due process and "least restrictive alternative" requirements.[15] They should be regularly reassessed in light of evolving evidence.[2,15] The interests of affected individuals should be promoted as much as possible, to maintain equality or reciprocity[2]—and not just by securing enough food and safety. Luxury hotels were said to work just as well for quarantine.[41] Post hoc compensation or apology can make sense.[42]

Yet there is no logical reason why there could not be clashes between collective disaster response interests and individual interests.[14]

On those rare occasions that clashes are inevitable, the approach that is common in contemporary ethics is that there are no absolute rules—including rules forbidding intrusive quarantine, etc. Utilitarians and other consequentialists recognize no rules constraining the pursuit of maximal utility and other good consequences.[28] But even nonconsequentialist thinkers, who believe that some rules should be respected, nearly always agree that these rules are not absolute.[43] Disaster situations in which scores of lives are at stake clearly are the paradigm cases in which there is a sufficient case for transgression of moral rules.

But clashes between public health interests and those of individuals are not just rare. The history of quarantine and other travel restrictions disproportionally affecting minorities and marginalized migrants has another potential lesson to tell.[15] Many seeming clashes between public health and personal rights are not genuine clashes. They could have been reconciled otherwise. One way forward is therefore to use quarantine and other measures that limit personal rights and welfare, but to do so as sparsely and as minimally as possible, while making their (continuing)[44] use subject to multiple *external* approvals, thereby guarding against partiality and prejudice. A standing international body or respected public health experts from remote regions could be appointed during disaster planning for approval positions.

Section 7. Surveillence

Postdisaster surveillance is crucial for assessing what works to overcome an infection—which is crucial so long as very regular meetings to reassess and change practice in light of new evidence actually take place. Here again, a tension arises between a public health need and a personal need—in this case, a personal need of privacy and confidentiality. How does one ensure that identifiable patient information is not accidentally divulged?[17] Should reporting be mandatory?[17] Just as we observed in relation to quarantine, here too the tension is attenuated by some overlap in public and individual needs. For example, there is also a public health interest in maintaining confidentiality, which encourages people to come forth and provide information. To some degree therefore the tension is between different factors affecting one ethical desideratum—effective disaster response that protects the public's health—and empirical studies may help settle which effect is stronger, under which circumstances.

Section 8. Research

Just as surveillance is crucial in a disaster, more rigorous studies are also crucial. Medical, implementation, and public health studies can help develop countermeasures and evaluate them safely and reliably—for the ongoing disaster and for better response in similar later situations (see Chapter 60).

In the 2014 Ebola outbreak, some scholars supported rigorous research, even if it involved individually randomized control trials.[36,44a,44b] Others proposed ways to temper scientific rigor with what they saw as compassion, and they emphasized logistical complications in individual randomization.[45,46] Further scholarship on this complex question remains necessary.[2]

Section 9. Rescuers' Rights

The American Medical Association medical code states, "Individual physicians have an obligation to provide urgent medical care during disasters. This ethical obligation holds even in the face of greater than usual risks to their own safety, health or life."[8] Different authors penned much stronger[47,47a] or much weaker[48,48a,48b] statements of physicians' and other response workers' right to prioritize personal interests and health over effective disaster response. What seems to be generally agreed is that moral "demandingness" is far higher for health workers than for the general public. Health workers will have often taken the Hippocratic oath, accepted societal esteem and benefits, and invited social trust that they will be available if needed. We all now rely on them.

Section 10. Transparency and Communication

To remain accountable, to preserve public trust, to facilitate public feedback, to allow coordination between different organizations, and to show respect to stakeholders (including voters, affected populations, and disaster personnel),[49] it is usually best to maintain transparency about disaster planning and operations,[6,49] including the rationing principles being used.[40,50] However, media relations and public health risk communication are intricate matters,[51] and it is by no means self-evident that maximal transparency will always be the most effective way to maintain public trust, cooperation, and calm. Those matter, too. During a disaster, they can translate into many lives saved. Unbridled transparency also risks violating patients' privacy,[17] presenting affected populations as helpless victims without substantial agency, and even exacerbating stereotypes against stigmatized social groups.[2,6]

What is more straightforwardly a net gain is communication flow from the public to disaster managers. Collection of public input on ethical and other aspects on disaster planning and response (e.g., a process for public comments on a website)[12] can help planners gather ideas and responders receive real-time alerts about response breakdowns.[51a]

Some have proposed a more ambitious process of public deliberation and participation in expert decision making.[2,50,52] Disaster response is the wrong time for elaborate deliberative polls, which are very time consuming. Even during the planning period, it is not clear how valuable the process as currently envisaged would be. Intense discussions over days are resource intensive and can only happen with small samples, making the findings statistically less interpretable. Even then, a couple of days' education does not create expertise on these intricate matters, yet many lives hang on these decisions. It has been said that "people will be more likely to cooperate, and accept difficult decisions made by their leaders for the common good" if community representatives are at the negotiating table.[52] But experts appointed democratically already do that, and many people will not have even heard that disaster plans rest on joint decision. Where deliberation clearly would help is in collecting diverse perspectives as input to inform expert planning. But perspectives input can be collected in the simpler ways noted earlier.

Section 11. Political Involvement

Engagement in political debates raises other complexities. On the one hand, it risks losing disaster response workers their crucial reputation for neutrality, which buys them broad support from patients, donors, and sometimes literally warring political factions. Such involvement clearly goes beyond workers' tacit mandate of disaster response in a strict sense. In fact, response workers can feel cheated and instrumentalized when their missions turn out to serve long-term organizational or political goals.[49] Although there is no absolute rule against this brand of long-term organizational or political thinking, it should remain rare. Certainly one should not compromise patient care for political gain, for example, by rejecting enemy combatants or terrorists in order to advance organizational popularity and donations.

That said, disaster responders are in a good position to advise the public on certain political decisions. They may lobby to provide generous international aid during disasters abroad, to release vaccine stockpiles for international use, and to avoid scientifically unfounded, automatic quarantining of all returning health workers.[2]

This tension, between political engagement and an image of neutrality, is genuine and hard to avoid. The IFRC embraces, among other things, a mission of changing minds and promoting a safer culture of social inclusion, and it calls for national legal preparedness and international legal cooperation through the development and promotion of disaster laws, principles, and rules. These are important agendas. They are also ones with political ramifications. In some future situations, they may turn out to threaten the organization's principle of neutrality.[9]

Section 12. Recovery

During disaster recovery, evacuees return home, regular civil services and normality are restored, and ethical tasks can be completed.

Disasters put a strain on many things we value: on societal trust in health workers, who must provide care below normal standards; on local and national sovereignty, which can be threatened by the aid coming from metropolitan national and international centers[53]; and on the dignity, standing, and perceived agency of affected populations, which will have often been presented in the media as victims, and of marginalized social groups, which will have often been blamed as the causes of the disaster. In particular, recovery provides an occasion for international organizations to return any doctors they will have hired to the local public service and to allow that service to assume responsibility for all roles—the most sustainable solution in the long run.

Disaster recovery can also be used for system improvement. Although systems will often be compromised or destroyed by the disaster, the rescue mentality, mentioned earlier, will still be there, along with some donations and psychological momentum. This is when the circumstances of disaster can be mobilized to achieve lasting, substantial increases in health and welfare—prophylactically rather than only in hindsight—so that vulnerabilities that gave rise to a disaster are removed and cost-effective interventions to improve the public's health are firmly in place.[9]

CONCLUSION

Disasters tend to appeal to our shared humanity and touch all of us, leading to an outpouring of donations and willingness to help, even across international borders. This humanitarian momentum should be leveraged both into efficient and fair interventions in the lead-up to and during disaster, as well as into creating an efficient and fair health system in normal times—part and parcel of prevention and preparedness toward future disasters.

⚠ PITFALLS

Here are some ethical pitfalls to avoid in disaster policy and response:
- Letting partiality, xenophobia, intergroup animosities, stigma, and other prejudices affect decisions
- Rushing to ration medical resources when they are not truly scarce (e.g., when existing supplies can be effectively conserved, adapted, substituted, or reused)
- Resisting rationing, or triage, when it is inevitable or only fair
- Doggedly insisting on regular standards of care in those disaster circumstances of great scarcity that make altered standards advisable for public health and fairness
- Creating, understanding the need for, and yet failing to use crisis decision procedures and chains of command
- Using the special prerogatives of executives in disasters to implement nondisaster political or personal agendas, or without ample consideration for the scientific need to breach personal rights
- Refusing to use these prerogatives against overwhelming evidence of their necessity to prevent widespread morbidity and mortality.

- Failing to monitor, collect feedback about, and surveil the crisis and the response; to invite rigorous studies that may improve current and future disaster response; or to translate the evidence coming from these investigations into better policy

Acknowledgment

For helpful comments on previous drafts, the author thanks Hanna Amanuel, Christine Baugh, Stephanie Kayden, Leah Price, and Heikki Saxen.

REFERENCES

1. Terminology: Disaster. 2007. Available at: http://www.unisdr.org/we/inform/terminology#letter-d
2. Presidential Commission for the Study of Bioethical Issues. *Ethics and Ebola: Public Health Planning and Response.* February 2015, Washington, DC.
3. Cohen IG, Daniels N, Eyal N, eds. *Identified vs. Statistical Persons.* New York, NY: Oxford University Press; 2015.
4. Rubenstein J. Distribution and emergency. *J Polit Philos.* 2007;15:296–320.
5. Halpern P, Larkin GL. Ethical issues in the provision of emergency medical care in multiple casualty incidents and disasters. In: Ciottone GR, Anderson PD, eds. *Disaster Medicine.* 1st ed. New York, NY: Elsevier; 2006.
6. Ozge Karadag C, Kerim Hakan A. Ethical dilemmas in disaster medicine. *Iran Red Crescent Med J.* 2012;14:602–612.
7. *World Medical Association. WMA Statement on Medical Ethics in the Event of Disasters.* 2006, Geneva.
8. AMA's Code of Medical Ethics 2014-15. AMA; 2014. Available at: http://www.ama-assn.org/ama/pub/physician-resources/medical-ethics/code-medical-ethics.page?.
9. *International Federation of Red Cross and Red Crescent Societies. Strategy 2020.* Geneva: International Federation of Red Cross and Red Crescent Societies (IFRC); 2015.
10. *International Federation of Red Cross and Red Crescent Societies, ICRC. The Code of Conduct for the International Red Cross and Red Crescent Movement and Non-Governmental Organisations (NGOs) in Disaster Relief.* 1992. Available at: www.ifrc.org/global/publications/disasters/ccode-of-conduct/code-english.pdf.
11. New York State Department of Health, New York State Task Force on Life & the Law. Allocation of ventilators in an influenza pandemic; 2007. Available at: www/health.state.ny.us/diseases/communicable/influenza/pandemic.ventilators/.
12. *State of Michigan Department of Community Health. Guidelines for Ethical Allocation of Scarce Medical Resources and Services During Public Health Emergencies in Michigan.* 2012, Version 2.0. Lansing, MI.
13. Vawter DE, Garrett JE, Gervais KG, et al. *For the Good of Us All: Ethically Rationing Health Resources in Minnesota in a Severe Influenza Pandemic.* 2010.
14. Bayer R. The continuing tensions between individual rights and public health. *EMBO Rep.* 2007;8:1099–1103.
15. Gostin LO, ed. *Public Health Law and Ethics: A Reader.* Rev. and updated 2nd ed. Berkeley: University of California Press; 2010.
16. Partridge RA, Proano L, Marcozzi D, eds. *Oxford American Handbook of Disaster Medicine.* New York: Oxford University Press; 2012.
17. Holt GR. Making difficult ethical decisions in patient care during natural disasters and other mass casualty events. *Otolaryngol Head Neck Surg.* 2008;139:181–186.
18. Fink S. The deadly choices at Memorial. *New York Times.* August, 25, 2009.
19. Knowlton LM, Gosney JE, Chackungal S, et al. Consensus statements regarding the multidisciplinary care of limb amputation patients in disasters or humanitarian emergencies: report of the 2011 Humanitarian Action Summit Surgical Working Group on amputations following disasters or conflict. *Prehosp Disaster Med.* 2011;26:438–448.
20. Hanfling D, Altevogt BM, Viswanathan K, et al. *Crisis Standards of Care: A Systems Framework for Catastrophic Disaster Response.* Washington, DC: Institute of Medicine; 2012.
21. Sztajnkrycer MD, Madsen BE, Alejandro Baez A. Unstable ethical plateaus and disaster triage. *Emerg Med Clin North Am.* 2006;24:749–768.
22. Schultz CH, Annas GJ. Altering the standard of care in disasters—unnecessary and dangerous. *Ann Emerg Med.* 2012;59:191–195.
23. Caro JJ, DeRenzo EG, Coleman CN, et al. Resource allocation after a nuclear detonation incident: unaltered standards of ethical decision making. *Disaster Med Public Health Prep.* 2011;5(Suppl 1):S46–S53.
24. Snyder L. American College of Physicians Ethics Manual: sixth edition. *Ann Intern Med.* 2012;156:73–104.
25. Noji EK. Public health issues in disasters. *Crit Care Med.* 2005;33:S29–S33.
26. Hick JL, Hanfling D, Cantrill SV. Allocating scarce resources in disasters: emergency department principles. *Ann Emerg Med.* 2012;59:177–187.
27. Christian MD, Devereaux AV, Dichter JR, et al. Introduction and executive summary: care of the critically ill and injured during pandemics and disasters: CHEST consensus statement. *Chest.* 2014;146(4 Suppl):8S–34S.
28. Sinnott-Armstrong W. Consequentialism. In: Zalta EN, ed. *Stanford Encyclopedia of Philosophy.* Revised ed. Available at: http://plato.stanford.edu/archives/spr2014/entries/consequentialism/. Palo Alto, CA.
29. White DB, Katz MH, Luce JM, et al. Who should receive life support during a public health emergency? Using ethical principles to improve allocation decisions. *Ann Intern Med.* 2009;150:132–138.
30. Lippert-Rasmussen K, Eyal N. Equality and Egalitarianism. In: Chadwick Ruth, ed. *Encyclopedia of Applied Ethics.* 2nd ed. San Diego, CA: Elsevier Academic Press; 2012:141–148.
31. Bognar G, Hirose I. *The Ethics of Health Care Rationing: An Introduction.* London: Routledge; 2014.
32. Kamm FM. Rationing and the disabled: several proposals. In: Eyal N, Hurst SA, Norheim OF, et al. *Inequalities in Health: Concepts, Measures, and Ethics.* New York, NY: Oxford University Press; 2013.
33. Williams A. Intergenerational equity: an exploration of the "fair innings" argument *Health Econ.* 1997;6:117–132.
34. Nord E. Concerns for the worse off: fair innings versus severity. *Soc Sci Med.* 2005;60:257–263.
35. Emanuel EJ, Wertheimer A. Public health. Who should get influenza vaccine when not all can? *Science.* 2006;312:854–855.
36. Rid A, Emanuel EJ. Ethical considerations of experimental interventions in the Ebola outbreak. *Lancet.* 2014;384(9957):1896–1899.
36a. Walker P, Maxwell DO. *Shaping the humanitarian world.* London: Routledge; 2014.
37. Eyal N, Firth P. MGH Disaster Relief Ethics Group. Repeat triage in disaster relief: questions from Haiti. *PLoS Curr Disasters.* 2012;1–8.
37a. Bartlett J, Borio L. The current status of planning for pandemic influenza and implications for the health care planning in the United States. *Clin Infec Dis.* 2008;46(6):919–925.
38. DeBruin D, Liaschenko J, Marshall MF. Social justice in pandemic preparedness. *Am J Public Health.* 2012;102:586–591.
38a. Centers for Disease Control and Prevention. About Quarantine and Isolation. Available at: cdc.gov/quarantine/quarantineandisolation.html August 28, 2014. Accessed April 25, 2015.
39. Powell A. Fewer clinics, less care. *Harvard Gazette.* August 15, 2014.
40. World Health Organization. *Pandemic Influenza Preparedness and Response.* Geneva: WHO; 2009.
41. Caplan A. Bioethicist: hotels, not quarantines, for Ebola heroes. *NBC News;* 2014.
42. Wigley S. Disappearing without a moral trace? Rights and compensation during times of emergency. *Law Philos.* 2009;28:617–649.
43. Nagel T. War and massacre. *Philos Public Aff.* 1972;1:123–144.
44. Ignatieff M. The ethics of emergency. In: Viens AM, Selgelid MJ, eds. *Emergency Ethics.* Farnham, UK: Ashgate; 2012:310–336. (2005).
44a. Joffe S. Evaluating novel therapies during the Ebola epidemic. *JAMA.* 2015;312(13):1299–300.
44b. Cox E, Borio L, Temple R. Evaluating Ebola therapies—the case for RCTs. *N Eng Jrnl of Med.* 2014; 371(25).
45. Adebamowo C, Bah-Sow O, Binka F, et al. Randomised controlled trials for Ebola: practical and ethical issues. *Lancet.* 2014;384:1423–1424.
46. Kass N, Goodman S. Trials tempered by compassion and humility. *New York Times.* December 1, 2014.
47. Emanuel EJ. The lessons of SARS. *Ann Intern Med.* 2003;139:589–591.
47a. The societies of US emergency physicians. https://www.acep.org/Clinical—Practice-Management/Code-of-Ethics-for-Emergency-Physicians/.

48. Akabayashi A, Takimoto Y, Hayashi Y. Physician obligation to provide care during disasters: should physicians have been required to go to Fukushima? *J Med Ethics.* 2012;38:697–698.

48a. Specialists (otolaryngologists) https://www.entnet.org/sites/default/files/Code%20of%20Ethics_0.pdf.

48b. Jackson BA, et al. Protecting emergency responders, vol. 3: safety management in disaster and terrorism response (Cincinnati RAND NIOSH). 2004. Available at: www.rand.org/publications/MG/MG170.

49. Clarinval C, Biller-Andorno N. Challenging operations: an ethical framework to assist humanitarian aid workers in their decision-making processes. *PLoS Curr.* 2014;6.

50. Advisory Committee to the Director of the Centers for Disease Control and Prevention. *Ethical Considerations for Decision Making Regarding Allocation of Mechanical Ventilators during a Severe Influenza Pandemic or Other Public Health Emergency.* Atlanta: Centers for Disease Control and Prevention; July 1, 2011.

51. Covello VT. Risk communication. In: Frumkin H, ed. *Environmental Health: From Global to Local.* 2nd ed. San Francisco, CA: Jossey-Bass; 2010:1099–1140.

51a. Sphere Project 2011 edition.

52. University of Toronto Joint Centre for Bioethics Pandemic Influenza Working Group. *Stand on Guard for Thee: Ethical Considerations in Preparedness Planning for Pandemic Influenza.* Toronto: University of Toronto; 2005.

53. Hussein GMA. When ethics survive where people do not. *Public Health Ethics.* 2010;3:72–77.

CHAPTER 12

Issues of Liability in Emergency Response

Jonathan Peter Ciottone

Whenever a doctor cannot do good, he must be kept from doing harm.

—*Hippocrates*

Organized and professional emergency response has become a frequent and expected reaction to the present-day disaster, be it natural, human-made, or an act of terror. Over the course of the last century, the proliferation of media technology, including television, the Internet, and handheld multimedia devices, has spawned a progressively hyperaware and instantly informed society that has come to expect that every catastrophe be met with an instant, competent, and efficiently executed response by the emergency responder. This evolving expectation has naturally led to the necessity of organized state- and federally sanctioned response teams, as well as legislation to both oversee and protect the responder regarding issues of liability, which may arise from the administration of care. Catastrophic disasters and emergencies invariably demand medical assistance from professionals and laypersons alike. Although, generally, the law does not impose an affirmative duty to assist those in peril,[1] public policy suggests that any emergency responders should be shielded from subsequent liability stemming from the aid they deliver. Accordingly, laws have been crafted to establish immunity, to encourage individuals to render aid without fear of future litigation. These laws are colloquially known as "Good Samaritan" laws. By 1980, all 50 U.S. states had enacted variations of Good Samaritan laws.[2] Although these laws were originally drafted to protect physicians, nurses, and other medical professionals,[3] most Good Samaritan laws now protect the general citizenry from liability as well.[4] Good Samaritan laws were drafted to incentivize volunteerism in emergency situations; however, the disparate application of these laws by courts to varying situations across the country has resulted in criticism from the legal community.[5] Moreover, many of these laws do not address volunteer organizations and agencies, whose sole purpose is to assist in delivering aid during and in the aftermath of disaster-like situations. Prompted by the attacks on 9/11 the World Trade Center in New York and the subsequent barrage of litigation, federal, state, and local governments have attempted to provide additional safeguards for emergency responders.[6] For instance, the Centers for Law and the Public's Health drafted the Model State Emergency Health Powers Act (MSEHPA), which proposes a series of statutes designed to assess and declare public emergencies.[7] The MSEHPA provides for more comprehensive and broader immunity for both private individuals and volunteer entities.[8] Since the MSEHPA's "Good Samaritan's" publication, several states have adopted their own legislation based upon the provisions of the MSEHPA.

Even though emergency responder law and general response infrastructure has drastically changed over the course of the last 50 years, the threat of litigation for responders remains viable. For instance, in the aftermath of Hurricane Katrina, several health professionals were forced to render aid in less-than-ideal circumstances.[9] Hospitals, dealing with the stress of the storm, including loss of power, overcrowding, and flooding, put medical personnel in difficult positions in terms of their ability to deliver proper aid. One treating physician became the target of several wrongful-death law suits, which allege that she expedited the deaths of several critically ill patients to make space for others.[10] Further evidence of the continuous threat of legal liability in emergency response can be seen in the wake of the school shooting at Sandy Hook Elementary School in Newtown, Connecticut. Although subsequently withdrawn following the public outcry of discontent, at least one civil lawsuit was filed in connection with the shootings' immediate aftermath. The lawsuit sought $100 million in damages on behalf of a 6-year-old survivor, related to the State of Connecticut's inability to render aid properly.[11] Even though emergency responder law has been a part of American jurisprudence for quite some time, the laws governing response and those who respond are constantly evolving in reaction to societal change. A proper understanding of this law and all attendant immunities is necessary before delivering emergency care. The first step in doing so requires an overview of the legal system and the various sources that comprise emergency responder law.

HISTORICAL PERSPECTIVE

History of Emergency Response Management

Governmental emergency response management is not a new concept. It was first introduced in the United States in 1803. In response to a series of fires that swept through Portsmouth, New Hampshire, and recognizing the need for an organized and coordinated response, a Congressional act was passed that contained within it the first national disaster legislation in U.S. history. Over the course of the next century, building upon the lessons of Portsmouth, Congress implemented an ad hoc approach to dealing with national disasters, enacting over 100 separate acts to deal with catastrophic events such as the Chicago Fire of 1871, the Texas Hurricane of 1900, and the San Francisco Earthquakes of 1906. Each act was enacted to respond to and deal with the unique needs of the individual events.

In the early 1930s, organized federal response to natural disasters gained a foothold with the establishment of the Reconstruction Corporation, the Flood Control Act, and the Bureau of Public Roads. Federal intervention and response became a popular and apparently necessary idea that resonated throughout the national psyche. By the 1940s, the popularity of these programs led to the creation of civil defense programs, including air raid warnings and emergency shelter systems to protect the public in the event of a military attack on American soil. In 1950, the landmark Disaster Relief Act was passed. The act for the first time granted the president the authority to issue disaster declarations, allowing for the mobilization of federal agencies to assist in both state and federal governments in the event of an emergency, catastrophe, or major disaster. The Disaster Relief Act was not designed to supersede but rather supplement and orchestrate state and local government response. Throughout the 1950s, emergency management concentrated on civil defense and wartime preparations. It was not until a series of natural disasters, occurring from the early 1960s through the early 1970s, that the federal government recognized the necessity of a specialized organized and federal response to natural disasters, and thus enacted the Disaster Relief Act of 1974, which provided the president with the authority to declare a national disaster. Though clear federal response mechanisms were then in place to deal with a broad scope of major disasters, the overall efforts of the agencies remained disjointed; with over 100 different agencies in place and in operation at any given time. Recognizing the necessity of a centralized and coordinated response system in 1979, by executive authority, President Carter enacted Executive Order 12148, creating the Federal Emergency Management Agency (FEMA), thereby centralizing disaster response under one coordinated federal effort. In its infancy, FEMA struggled with its efficiency and response, failing to come together as a cohesive organization. In 1992, following Hurricane Hugo, the Federal Response Plan (FRP) was developed in the wake of growing frustration with the lack of organization. The FRP defines the structure for coordinating, organizing, and mobilizing federal resources. Today FEMA has over 7000 employees and an annual budget of almost $11 billion.

Undoubtedly, one of the most prevalent landmark events in the evolution of organized emergency response management was the 9/11 attacks on the World Trade Center in New York City. Less than 2 weeks following the attacks, Pennsylvania Governor Tom Ridge was appointed as the country's first director of Homeland Security, despite the fact a Department of Homeland Security did not yet exist, demonstrating the political response to the public's need for a visible and dedicated federal terrorist prevention and response agency. On November 25, 2002, the Homeland Security Act was passed, establishing the Department of Homeland Security (DHS). The DHS was created with a prime directive of not only protecting the United States and its citizens from acts of terror but also responding to both human-made and natural disasters. The establishment of the DHS unified and consolidated 22 separate federal agencies under one centralized cabinet agency. On February 28, 2003, Homeland Security Presidential Directive 5 (HSPD-5) was issued, directing the secretary of Homeland Security to develop and administer a National Incident Management System (NIMS) to provide a consistent nationwide plan for government, nongovernmental organizations, and the private sector, to coordinate disaster response. HSPD-5 requires all federal departments and agencies to adopt NIMS and to use it in their individual incident management programs and activities, as well as in support of all actions taken to assist state, tribal, and local governments. In New York, an appellate court determined that failure to comply with a mandatory, nondiscretionary NIMS directive could result in civil liability in the event of injury or death. Now, response to a major disaster, terrorist attack, or natural catastrophe involves the coordination of a multitude of governmental, quasi-governmental, and private agencies, including local, state, and federal responders. A byproduct of the evolution of federal and state organized response is the expectation that a responder be held to a legally reasonable standard of care, by which that responder may be held liable under the U.S. civil legal system. Though responders are protected by rights and immunities to act within their discretion in the administration of emergency care, there has been a marked decline of the application of responder immunity and protection over the last several decades, in a further effort to emphasize a patient's rights to be

afforded proper and reasonable care under the standard. Much like a general practitioner, surgeon, or other licensed medical provider, an emergency responder is expected to deliver specialized medical care in a manner that is generally acceptable in the field that demonstrates, at a minimum, a baseline level of competency in implementation of care. The philosophy behind the application of a standard of care to emergency response is to ensure that medical care is administered in a professional, acceptable, and standard method; to heighten a responder's awareness of a patient's rights in the administration of care; and to deliver effective and competent medical treatment. Ironically, disaster response, by nature, is anything but standard. Thus the obvious paradoxical question to be posed is how can a reasonable standard of care be measured during the administration of medical care in an otherwise chaotic or catastrophic situation?

Basic Concepts of Law

As discussed previously, and more thoroughly discussed in the immunities section below, emergency responders have several legal shields that will safeguard them from the imposition of liability. However, it is important to understand the concepts of law that are evaluated by a court of law when determining an emergency responder liability. For a responder to be held liable for acts rendered in an emergency, the plaintiff will have to demonstrate that the responder acted negligently. The tenets of negligence require that the plaintiff prove the following elements as a prerequisite to a finding of liability: duty, breach, causation, and damages. With regard to duty, although it is true that most states do not require persons to deliver aid to a person in an emergency, once a responder chooses to act, she is required to do so with reasonable care. Reasonable care requires that the responder act with the degree of caution that a similarly situated ordinary person would act with under identical or similar circumstances.[12] "Similarly situated" takes into account the responder's knowledge at the time aid is delivered. Accordingly, if the responder has a heightened degree of medical knowledge, the responder's actions will be judged with that knowledge in mind. Consequently, breach is established if a court determines that the responder did not act reasonably under the circumstances. Breach of a duty of reasonable care does not necessarily mean that liability attaches. Instead, the plaintiff must prove that the emergency responder's breach caused the injury. If the plaintiff was harmed by something other than the responder's breach, then policy, fairness, and justice demand that the responder not be held liable for any injuries suffered by the plaintiff. The last element in a negligence inquiry is the harm a plaintiff suffers because of the responder's breach. The harm element requires the plaintiff have damages that can be redressed in a court of law.

Although the above discussion represents a small overview of the principles of negligence, as illustrated below, several states have created their Good Samaritan laws to circumvent a negligence analysis to incentivize responder action without fear of liability.

CURRENT PRACTICE

Basis of Law

Medical malpractice and emergency responder liability claims are rooted in tort law. A tort is a violation of a duty owed by one to another that is set in law and is other than an agreement, which would constitute a contract. When the duty is breached, the grieved party may seek compensation for damages. Medical malpractice and negligent emergency response is considered a tort under the law; the legal issue at the center of these claims is the breach of a duty owed to the patient by a medical provider. The body of law known as torts is not a product of malpractice actions, specifically but rather an evolving body of law that over time has adapted and conformed to the legal needs of an ever-changing society. The history of American tort law can be traced back to actions of trespass to both property and person, with the roots of American tort law found in English common law, from which our civil justice system was born. A medical malpractice or medical tort claim is a civil action in which a patient or party seeks compensation for the acts or omissions of a medical provider who failed to practice to the accepted standard of care.

The Judicial System

In the United States, individual rights are grounded in the U.S. Constitution, as well as individual state constitutions. The U.S. Constitution sets forth the bedrock of individual rights, whereas state constitutions may broaden or limit its citizenry's individual rights, as long as any such variation is not in direct conflict with the U.S. Constitution. Both the U.S. Constitution and state constitutions establish the framework for the implementation of executive function, governing laws, legislatures, and judicial authority on both the federal and state levels. Legal authority within this framework is derived from statutory law, treaties, administrative regulations, and common law. Overwhelmingly, state jurisprudence has governed issues arising in the medical profession, specifically in the individual state court systems, when dealing with issues of malpractice or negligence. An increased number of legal actions against medical providers have lent themselves to a continued battle over tort reform and limitation of liability in attempt to control the costs of jury awards, which has in turn, increased the costs of medical malpractice insurance and the overall costs of medical care. In the context of disaster response, however, both U.S. and state constitutional rights have been challenged on the most basic of levels when the need for government infringement of such rights is necessary for the common good (i.e., quarantine, martial law, and forced decontamination). The proliferation of disaster response over the past several decades has influenced and effected a broadening of administrative and legal authority over individual rights.

Courts

In both the federal and state systems, a tiered court system functions to interpret and apply the law of a given case. Individuals have a constitutionally protected right to have disputes and questions of law decided within the appropriate judicial system. When a dispute arises, a party may file a lawsuit with a court, invoking that court's authority over the opposing party, as well as the question of law in dispute.

All jurisdictions, both federal and state, are based upon a tiered, hierarchical court system, in which the highest court of the system may control and reverse the decisions of the lower courts. The U.S. Supreme Court is the highest court in the U.S. judicial system; it issues decisions that control and effect all rulings and decisions of the federal appellate and trial courts. The U.S. Supreme Court may also influence and control some decisions and ruling of a state court, as well, when issuing a decision regarding the U.S. Constitution or a federal law that is preemptive over state law. In contrast, however, a state's Supreme Court decisions, though controlling over its own state's appellate and trial court system, would not be controlling in a sister state or over any federal court addressing a question of federal law.

Venue

The venue is the geographic locality in which a legal question is to be adjudicated. The majority of medical malpractice cases are based upon state law, and thus are venued in state court. However, a case may be brought in federal court either if there is a diversity of citizenship, a question of federal law, or the case involves a federal employee. Diversity of citizenship exists when an individual or legal entity's residence is

of a different state than that of the individual or entity bringing the action. Individual venues also exist within individual states. State courts are often organized according to district or county on a statewide or citywide basis. Cases typically may be brought in the district or county in which a party resides or the incident at issue occurred. Juries are selected according to the district or county in which the case is venued and are commonly referred to as "jury pools." A jury pool is the geographic location from which a court may summon potential jurors for voir dire: the process of juror selection. The geographic location of a venue is often one of the deciding factors in the outcome of a given case. Both plaintiff and defense attorneys review and study the jury verdicts of differing districts or counties to determine the probability of a successful outcome in a given location. This practice has lent itself to what is commonly referred to as "forum shopping," whereby a party will labor to venue a case in the geographic location that would be most advantageous to a successful outcome of a case. In instances where a case involves parties from multiple geographic locations, the opportunity to forum shop increases. In the case of emergency-response liability, the probability of such a scenario increases, given the likelihood of multiple victims and/or responders residing in different cities and states. In addition, a party may also move to change the venue of a trial, based upon a potential prejudice of a jury, which may deny a party their constitutional right to a fair and impartial jury. More often than not, such a request is made on behalf of a defendant. By way of example, on April 19, 1995, Timothy McVeigh and Terry Lynn Nichols, using an ammonium nitrate-based explosive hidden in a moving truck, destroyed the Murrach Federal Building in Oklahoma City, Oklahoma: in the explosion, 168 people were killed. In preparation for trial, the defense made a Motion for Change of Venue, requesting the trial be moved from Oklahoma to Colorado. The defense argued to the court successfully that, given the horrific nature of the event, including the destruction of a daycare center and the killing of 15 children, McVeigh would be denied due process of law under the Fifth Amendment and his right to a trial by an impartial jury under the Sixth Amendment because the jury pool had been tainted with negative publicity and personal sentiment.

Case Law

In deciding issues of law, courts are expected to follow "common law" or precedent, case law that has been previously decided on similar or identical issues of law within the court's jurisdiction. A court will decide a case pursuant to prior rulings or decisions of the Court's jurisdiction, referred to as *stare decisis*. If there is no precedent case law directly on point within the jurisdiction in which the issue is at bar, a court may look to other jurisdictions for guidance. Reference to an alternate jurisdiction's case law is referred to as *dicta*, and, though not controlling, it can be influential in deciding a case of first impression.

Standard of Care

In an action involving an emergency responder, prior to deliberations, a jury would be instructed by the trial judge regarding the law governing the responder's actions in question and the basis upon which a jury may weigh the evidence presented at trial. This is called the "jury charge." The jury is instructed to decide, based upon the evidence presented, if the defendant's actions conformed to the standard of care commonly accepted, in the jurisdiction in which the case is venued. The standard of care may be established by way of state or federal law, regulatory law, case law of a jurisdiction, or testimony of an expert witness and is the standard by which a responder's actions are measured to be reasonable or not under the given circumstances. A responder would be negligent if the measures taken to assist a patient did not rise to the degree of care that a reasonably prudent responder would have exercised under the same circumstances.

In the absence of regulations, statutes, or common law, expert witnesses may offer testimony as to the accepted standard of care. Experts are disclosed prior to trial regarding the particular field about which they will testify. Attorneys may depose an expert witness prior to trial and, if deemed appropriate, move to preclude the expert from trial based upon the expert's lack of competency or experience regarding the expertise in which he or she was disclosed. Expert witness testimony, in the absence of controlling law, is powerful and often pivotal as to the outcome of a case. In many situations, a jury will hear evidence from several experts, often with differing opinions. It is the duty of the jury to weigh the testimony, credentials, and credibility of each expert to decide what standard is applicable to a case.

Although on its face, the concept of emergency response appears to be universal, the standard of care may differ from state to state, depending on the jurisdiction in which the action is pending. In general, the standard of care is considered the acceptable or minimal level of competency exercised by an emergency responder in response to a specific situation or applied treatment in the jurisdiction in which the case is tried. However, the legal concept of negligence, which is then applied to the standard of care, is generally consistent throughout all jurisdictions. The concept of negligence was originally developed under English common law, and it is commonly defined as failing to act as a reasonable or prudent person would do in a similar situation. Negligence does not rise to the level of wanton or reckless action, but rather to the omission of reasonableness, and it is broken down and analyzed by way of the following four elements:

1. *Duty:* Did the responder establish a relationship with the patient that created a legal obligation of the responder to the patient?
2. *Breach:* Did the responder's actions fail to meet the established standard of care, thus breaching his or her duty to the patient?
3. *Injury:* Did the responder's breach of duty to the patient result in an injury that naturally flowed from the responder's actions? Injuries may include physical or psychological injuries, damage to property, or violation of a patient's legal rights. In some circumstances, *injury* may also be defined as a third party's observations of a responder's actions, which resulted in emotional or psychological distress to the third party. The question of injury often leads to further analysis of the patient's claimed injuries—did the claimed injury predate the alleged negligent act? Could the claimed injury have naturally flowed from the responder's breach of his duty?
4. *Damages:* Assuming the responder breached his duty of care to a patient and the claimed injuries naturally flowed from the breach, what if any award should be given to compensate and "make whole" the plaintiff. The question of damages often includes a multidimensional analysis of economic and noneconomic injury (i.e., medical bills, future cost of treatment, lost wages, impaired earning capacity, and pain and suffering).

The Role of the Jury

The majority of states and all federal courts allow a party to an action to request a trial by jury, as opposed to a bench trial, in which a case is decided solely by the trial judge. Jury section, or voir dire, is the process by which jurors are selected by the lawyers involved in a particular case to serve as a member of a jury. Potential jurors are summoned from the court's geographic district for the selection process. The process of jury selection differs throughout the various jurisdictions. Either potential jurors are accepted as jurors or excused for cause, or an attorney may exercise a preemptive challenge and dismiss a juror without cause. The numbers of preemptive challenges an attorney may exercise are often limited per the rules of the jurisdiction. The federal system and the most common state court method utilizes the "in the box" method of selection, whereby a panel of potential jurors collectively

is questioned regarding any prejudices or conflicts they may have that would impede their ability to decide a case impartially. Some states' jury selection process is completed individually. In Connecticut State Court, for instance, jurors are instructed as to the general facts of a case as a group but are questioned individually as to potential conflicts. Individual voir dire is often much more time consuming than "in the box" voir dire, and it may cause the jury selection process to last for weeks rather than days. Conflicts or prejudices that may arise, which can result in the dismissal of a potential juror for cause, may include personal knowledge or relationship with a party to the action, an expert involved in the case, a fact witness, or a treating physician. Other reasons for dismissal as a juror for cause may be personal prejudice or political activism at odds with the legal issues of the case. By way of example, in the case of a medical malpractice action, a potential juror may be dismissed for cause if that juror had been treated by the defendant physician in the past. Such a relationship may cause a juror to decide the outcome of the case on their previous experience as a patient rather than the evidence presented in court.

The Role of the Trial Judge

Judges play many roles within the judicial system. In the context of a liability action, a judge is charged with the duty of recognizing, applying, and interpreting the relevant law for each specific case and has the responsibility of safeguarding the rights of both the plaintiff and the defendant throughout the litigation process. Several judges may be involved throughout the litigation process. At trial, however, a case is heard by one judge. The trial judge must at all times function as an impartial arbiter of the law and avoid any impropriety or the appearance of impropriety in all his actions throughout a case. If necessary, a trial judge must recuse himself in any situation in which he may doubt his ability to preside over a case impartially or whenever he believes his impartiality can reasonably be questioned. A trial judge is present to decide issues of law within a case; it is the role of the jury to decide the case.

The Attachment of Liability

In terms of assessing liability, the inquiry must be done on a state-by-state basis.[13] As indicated above, almost all states' legislatures have a codified Good Samaritan law. Although it is important to consult with your state law, an examination of the standards of care of various states is nonetheless instructive. Under Maryland, Alabama, Massachusetts, New Jersey, Oklahoma, Virginia, Wisconsin, West Virginia, Wyoming, Michigan, and North Dakota law, for example, liability will only attach if the emergency responder is found to be acting with gross negligence or willful misconduct.[14] This is a much higher threshold than that of reasonable care described in the foregoing section. The standard will only be satisfied upon a showing of "wanton or reckless disregard for human life or the rights of others."[15] For instance, when a paramedic was delivering aid to a plaintiff experiencing an asthma attack, yet failed to administer oxygen, which ultimately led to plaintiff's death, a Maryland court nonetheless found this conduct below the "gross negligence" standard required to impose liability.[16] Under reasonable care, however, the paramedic would have likely been subject to liability.

As illustrated above, gross negligence is the highest standard that needs to be demonstrated to support a showing of liability. Accordingly, the following standards of care require a lower burden to substantiate liability. Iowa, for example, will provide civil immunity to emergency responders if the responder acted in good faith. However, good faith can be overcome if the acts in question are found to be reckless.[17] Even though the Iowa statute does not define *reckless*, nor has case law clarified this term, it appears that any standard of negligence would qualify in order to impose liability, including a breach of reasonable care. Although Iowa is one of a number of states to provide the affirmative defense of good faith, several states, including Delaware, Montana, Nebraska, and Washington, do not provide a good faith defense. Instead, the plaintiff need only prove negligence in order to support a finding of liability; the responder's state of mind is not considered by the court.[18] Although understanding the common principles of negligence is exceedingly important to comprehending responder liability, it is essential to consult your state's law, as Good Samaritan statutes vary greatly.

Immunities

Several legal immunities serve as affirmative defenses against the threat of litigation relating to the actions of an emergency responder. Immunities do not prohibit a potential plaintiff from filing a lawsuit against a responder, but they do afford an absolute defense to the claim. Accordingly, the party asserting an affirmative defense of immunity would bear the burden of proving that the immunity is applicable.

Good Samaritan Laws

At the foundation of the immunities associated with emergency responder law are the varying Good Samaritan laws found in every state. As indicated above, these laws protect individuals who gratuitously attempt to render aid in emergencies. A Good Samaritan is an individual who assists a victim at the scene of an injury or sudden emergency, when he or she has no obligation to do so. Good Samaritan laws reduce the barrier of liability by providing immunity from liability for ordinary negligence. Originally, these laws were designed to protect physicians, but some states have extended protection to laypersons as well.[19] The Good Samaritan laws do not always exclusively apply in disaster-like situations; 24 states provide immunity for individuals who render emergency care in hospitals on a case-by-case basis.[20] It should be noted that the immunity offered via Good Samaritan laws is not absolute. For instance, should the individual rendering aid fail to exercise reasonable care, thus exacerbating the injuries, the responder could face liability.[21] There is no federal Good Samaritan law. Accordingly, it is important to understand the extent of immunity available in your state.

Federal Tort Claims Act

Emergency response measures are generally governed by federal agencies, most often the FEMA and The National Disaster Medical System (NDMS) teams. FEMA and NDMS teams are deployed to disaster-like situations to provide aid. Any potential liability stemming from the aid rendered by a federal agency is subject to the provisions of the Federal Torts Claims Act (FTCA). Under the act, federal responders are considered federal employees and are immune from lawsuits, with the federal government acting as the primary insurer. The FTCA allows for patients who have suffered injury by the negligent or wrongful actions of a federal responder to have access to compensation, without bringing a legal action against the responder directly. The FTCA so provides that "a person suffering legal wrong because of agency action or adversely affected or aggrieved by agency action is entitled to judicial review."[22] Even though the FTCA seemingly provides legal redress by those aggrieved by federal emergency responders, there are several provisions that serve to limit potential liability. For instance, the FTCA immunizes the federal government from liability for "any claim based upon the exercise or performance or the failure to exercise or perform a discretionary function or duty on the part of a federal agency."[23] Subsequent case law has cited this discretionary function provision of the FTCA to excuse federal agencies from liability in emergencies.[24]

Volunteer Protection Act

The Volunteer Protection Act (VPA) was an early act of federal legislation in the emergency responder body of law, signed into law by President Bill Clinton in 1997. The VPA attempts to provide immunity to the nonprofit organizations and governmental entities that deliver care in emergencies, and it preempts any state laws that are inconsistent with the act; a state that wishes to have more protection under the VPA may, but any state law that limits the VPA is preempted. Essentially, the VPA establishes immunity for volunteers who are providing services for a not-for-profit organization. The VPA only applies to uncompensated volunteers who provide services to 501(c)(3) and 501(c)(4) organizations. However, the VPA enumerates several prerequisites that must be fulfilled to qualify for immunity under the VPA; a volunteer must obtain relevant licenses and certifications in the state where the harm occurred.[25] Immunity is not available where the court deems that the harm was caused by "criminal misconduct, gross negligence, reckless misconduct, or a conscious, flagrant indifference to the rights or safety of the individual harmed."[26] In addition to adopting the provisions of the VPA, all 50 states have also enacted variations of their own VPAs.

The Emergency Management Assistance Compact

The Emergency Management Assistance Compact (EMAC) is a federal initiative that was drafted to assist in the coordination of disaster relief efforts between federal, state, and local governments.[27] Several provisions of this act address state and federal personnel offering and receiving assistance. The act enables states to share resources during a disaster or catastrophic event. The EMAC is administered and coordinated through the National Emergency Management Association. Employees or officials of a party state administering aid in another state are considered agents of the state requesting aid for tort liability and immunity purposes. Per the act, no party state or its employees or officials rendering aid in another state shall be liable because of any act or omission in good faith. Article VI of the EMAC specifically shields a properly licensed state official from liability associated with rendered aid.[28] Even though the EMAC provides a degree of uniformity and consistency in the assessment of liability of an emergency responder, it only applies to state officers. Accordingly, its provisions would not apply to a private citizen. The EMAC acts to complement the federal disaster response system. Moreover, the EMAC is utilized both in concert with or in lieu of federal assistance, depending on the needs of the assisted state, which theoretically ensures the continuous and uninterrupted flow of necessary aid.

The Uniform Emergency Volunteer Health Practitioners Act

Although, as noted, there is no federal Good Samaritan law that operates to immunize emergency responders uniformly, the Uniform Law Commission has drafted a model initiative entitled the Uniform Emergency Volunteer Health Practitioners Act (UEVHPA). The UEVHPA, drafted in the aftermath of Hurricane Katrina, was created in response to the overwhelming need for licensed volunteer medical providers. The act attempts to expedite the deployment of aid to emergency situations and to protect licensed responders from future liability by recognizing during a declared emergency the license of a health care provider from a sister state.[29] However, these volunteers must be registered with a federally or state-managed volunteer registry to be eligible for any legal immunity.[30] Therefore ordinary licensed medical practitioners who are not part of the registry, and laypersons, cannot find protection under the UEVHPA. The model legislation offers two alternatives for dealing with issues of liability: a state may offer clear immunity for volunteers from civil liability for acts that occur while providing health or veterinary services or, essentially, may replicate and utilize the existing liability protections found within the VPA.

A handful of states have adopted the UEVHPA in full, whereas others have adopted certain sections.[31]

The Model State Emergency Health Powers Act

As aforementioned, in response to the attacks on the World Trade Center in New York and ongoing threats of biological warfare, the MSEHPA was drafted to serve as a model for states to coordinate a timely response in the event of a disaster. Unlike the EMAC and the UEVHPA, the MSEHPA does indeed provide immunity for private individuals who deliver emergency medical care.[32] However, the MSEHPA *imposes* liability upon individuals if the aid rendered is deemed to be grossly negligent or willful.[33] Even though the MSEHPA would certainly solve the inconsistencies spawned by the Good Samaritan laws and other disparate federal laws attempting to shield volunteers, it is a piece of model legislation, not actual law. However, 33 states have introduced 133 bills, all based on the MSEHPA. Several of these bills provide immunity for emergency responders.[34] Many civil liberties organizations have opposed the model bill as written, as the bill's broad-sweeping powers allow health care providers to take such actions as forced vaccines, without voluntary or informed consent. In addition, the model bill includes provisions to allow for state militia to seize homes, cars, telephones, food, fuel, clothing, firearms, and the like, as well as to arrest, imprison, and forcibly examine, vaccinate, and medicate citizens without consent, without being held liable for any harm that may come about from the use of these powers. In an extreme example, under the MSEHPA as written, a person could be forced to accept a vaccine to which they have an allergy. In the event, if the individual died because of a reaction to the vaccine, the medical provider who administered or forced the vaccination could not be held liable.

PATIENT RIGHTS

When considering issues of medical malpractice or emergency responder liability, the most fundamental issue to address is the basic right of patient choice. In a disaster scenario, the right of choice may become problematic because a patient is unconscious, in an impaired mental state, or unable to communicate or respond. Commonly referred to as "informed" consent, an unimpaired, competent adult, of the age of majority, has the right to choose or deny medical treatment, even if such a decision would result in the denial of life saving treatments or other necessary care for the improvement or sustaining of life. The informed consent doctrine derives from the principle that every human being of adult years and sound mind has a right to determine what shall be done with his own body. However, if a person is unable to consent to or deny treatment because of incapacity, legal incompetence, or unconsciousness, the person's choice may be determined to be "implied." Implied consent can be inferred through the actions or conduct of a patient rather than direct communications. In the context of a disaster or catastrophe, obtaining express or implied consent is often an impossibility, and thus the "emergency exception" would apply. The emergency exception is based upon the implied consent exception, and it assumes that an unconscious patient would consent to emergency care if the patient were conscious and able to consent. Additionally, sometimes referred to as the "reasonable man" standard, the emergency exception assumes a patient in need would choose to accept medical treatment. The emergency exception also assumes, and only applies, if the patient has not previously put health care professionals on notice of an intent to refuse treatment (i.e., the prior execution of a health care proxy). The emergency responder may only rely upon implied consent in the absence of consent and can never reverse prior explicit rejection of care. What constitutes an emergency to trigger the emergency exception varies from state to state; however, in the context of a disaster response, invariably, the

emergency exception may apply. In a disaster scenario, the administration of direct individual medical care is only one of several measures that may be taken that brings into question patient rights. In many disaster scenarios, a patient's individual rights may be "infringed" upon for the benefit of the greater good. Consider a chemical, biological, or dirty bomb attack. In all three scenarios, disaster response would, in all likelihood, result in mass quarantine; in some instances, quarantine or isolation may result in detaining people who may not show signs of illness or disease. Though individuals may be competent to decline quarantine, isolation, or large-scale preventive care, individuals may be compelled to such measures based on federal and state laws and regulations. Confinement or quarantine of a competent individual who has expressly declined such medical intervention, in any other context, could be considered liable (i.e., false imprisonment, assault, reckless endangerment). In such circumstances, however, wherein the safety of the public is at issue, the rights and safety of the public would supersede and outweigh any assertion of individual rights contrary to greater good (i.e., denial of quarantine). Such legal power is derived from the U.S. Constitution and regulatory and statutory law, on both the state and federal levels. The federal government's power to exercise quarantine is rooted in the Commerce Clause of the Constitution and in legislation such as Section 361 of the Public Health Service Act, which authorizes the U.S. secretary of Health and Human Services to take action to prevent entry or spread of communicable disease, including the use of quarantine. Individual state quarantine laws differ from state to state, but, in general, a state's laws will offer police power to control the spread of disease within its borders. The breaking of a quarantine in most states is a criminal act; thus not only can a patient not bring a liability action for false imprisonment or assault, that patient could be found guilty of a crime for disobeying a state-issued quarantine.

NONDISCRIMINATORY RESPONSE

Human rights laws, on a domestic and global level, are present to protect against discrimination of any kind based upon race, color, creed, sex, religion, age, sexual orientation, or disability. The administration of relief aid or the medical response to a disaster must be administered in an equitable nondiscriminatory manner, based on no criteria other than the ability to provide and need. Members of ethnic or religious minority groups, the elderly, women, or indigenous people are among the classes historically at particular risk of discrimination on a global level for inequity in disaster relief.[35] The principles of human rights, as well as international and domestic laws function, to assist and guide the emergency responder in providing equality of care. The introduction of discrimination-based decisions, unintended or otherwise, in an emergency-response scenario can have dire consequences. During a disaster response, providers may be under pressure to make rapid decisions with incomplete information. The introduction of any form of discrimination into the decisions of administration of care could have serious consequences on a potentially large scale, and possibly result in loss of life.[35] Decisions regarding administration of aid and treatment must be made solely based on medical necessity and logistical ability to protect against potential discrimination and possible issues of liability regarding the same.

REGULATORY VIOLATIONS

The rules that apply to regulatory violations differ, sometimes dramatically, from state to state. For instance, depending on the jurisdiction, negligence may be established per se, if a responder's actions in and of themselves violate a regulation. A per se violation is deemed an automatically negligent act, in and of itself. For negligence per se to apply to a case, it must be found that a responder violated a regulation or statute; the regulation or statute the responder violated was designed to protect a certain group of people from harm; the patient was part of the group the regulation or statute aims to protect; and the responder's actions caused the kind of injury the statute was designed to protect. Other states adhere to the prima facie rule, which shifts the burden of proof from the patient to the responder, to demonstrate the violation of a regulation was not negligent. Regardless of the standard applied, if a regulation does not clearly define a standard, that is the legislative intent is not clear as to the creation of a safety standard, it is the burden of the injured party to prove that the violation of the regulation creates liability.

SUMMARY

Medical emergency responders now face increasingly the seemingly overwhelming and ever-evolving threat of both local and large-scale disaster, while under the ever-scrutinizing and focused eye of the law. Response, be it local, domestic, or global, should be carried out in the most professional, organized, and coordinated manner available, with a vigilant focus on providing quality of care under the mandates of the law while balancing individual patient rights with the greater good of the general public. Preparedness and training, as well as awareness of the federal, state, and local laws and regulations governing the jurisdiction in which a responder practices or will be deployed, are essential tools for providing quality and compliant care in emergency response.

⚠ PITFALLS

- Assuming that there are no legal standards of care to observe in a disaster
- Not implementing a rapid response management plan in preparation for a disaster
- Assuming a responder cannot be found civilly liable based upon the classification of an event as a disaster
- Acting outside the scope of one's field of expertise when responding to a disaster
- Failing to properly acknowledge and coordinate with chains of command and jurisdictional authority
- Failing to act within the framework of the federally and state-mandated management plan
- Not being aware of the federal, state, or local laws and regulations under which a responder is providing care
- Failing to train for and prepare in advance for deployment into a disaster area

ACKNOWLEDGMENTS

Thanks to Alysa B. Koloms and Pooja Patel for their contributions to this chapter.

REFERENCES

1. MINN. STAT. § 604A.01 (2010) (requiring an individual to provide assistance without penalty stemming therefrom); VT. STAT. ANN. tit. 12, § 519 (2010) (levying a fine upon an individual who fails to assist a person in need).
2. 745 ILL. COMP. STAT. 49/2 (2010).
3. W. PAGE KEETON ET AL., PROSSER & KEETON ON THE LAW OF TORTS § 56, at 378 (5th ed. 1984).
4. See generally Victoria Sutton, Is There a Doctor (and a Lawyer) in the House? Why our Good Samaritans Laws Are Doing More Harm Than Good for a National Public Health Security Strategy: A Fifty State Survey, 6 J. HEALTH & BIOMED. L. 261 (2010) (discussing the several nuances of Good Samaritan laws in all fifty states).
5. See generally Victoria Sutton, Is There a Doctor (and a Lawyer) in the House? Why our Good Samaritans Laws Are Doing More Harm Than Good for a National Public Health Security Strategy: A Fifty State Survey, 6 J. HEALTH & BIOMED. L. 261 (2010).
6. UTAH CODE ANN. § 78B-4-501[2] (West 2010) (providing immunity to those responders in a bioterrorism event).
7. CENTER FOR L. & PUB.'S HEALTH, MODEL STATE EMERGENCY HEALTH POWERS ACT pmbl. (2001).
8. Id. CENTER FOR L. & PUB.'S HEALTH, MODEL STATE EMERGENCY HEALTH POWERS ACT pmbl. at § 804.
9. Sheri Fink, The Deadly Choices at Memorial, N.Y. TIMES MAG., Aug. 25, 2009, available at http://www.nytimes.com/2009/08/30/magazine/30doctors.html?_r=2&ref=magazine (detailing the inabilities of New Orleans' regional hospitals to properly provide medical care in the aftermath of Hurricane Katrina).
10. Id. Sheri Fink, The Deadly Choices at Memorial, N.Y. TIMES MAG., Aug. 25, 2009.
11. Bridget Murphy, Newtown Lawsuit: Lawyer for School Shooting Survivor Says $100 Million Claim Is About Security, HUFFINGTON POST, Dec. 29, 2012, available at http://www.huffingtonpost.com/2012/12/29/newtown-lawsuit-100-million-irving-pinsky_n_2381733.html.
12. Regan v. Eight Twenty Fifth Corp., 287 N.Y. 179, 182.1941.
13. See generally Sutton, supra note 4. Sutton's article thoroughly dissects the different standards of care at play in most states throughout the country.
14. McCoy v. Hatmaker, 763 A.2d 1233, 1240 (Md. Ct. Spec. App. 2010). Maryland's Good Samaritan statutes only apply to fire, resuce, law enforcement, as well as medical personnel. See id. The law does not apply to laypersons; see also MICH. COMP. LAWS § 691.1407; (2012) N.D. CENT. CODE §32-03.1-01.(2010).
15. Id. McCoy v. Hatmaker, 763 A.2d 1233, 1240 (Md. Ct. Spec. App. 2010).
16. Tatum v. Gigliotti, 80 Md. App. 559, 568-74 (Md. Ct. Spec. App. 1989).
17. IOWA CODE § 613.17.1(1998).
18. DEL. CODE ANN. TIT. 16 § 6801(a) (2010).
19. Sutton, supra note 6, at 272 (listing those states which will not extend immunity to individuals with no medical qualifications).
20. Id. Sutton, supra at 273.
21. RESTATEMENT (SECOND) OF TORTS § 323. (1965).
22. 5 U.S.C. § 702 (2006).
23. 28 U.S.C. § 2680(a) (2006).
24. United States v. Gaubert, 499 U.S. 315, 322–24, (1991).
25. 42 U.S.C. § 14503(a). (2000) Other qualifiers demand that the volunteer was acting within the scope of his/her responsibilities, the harm was not caused by willful conduct, and the harm was not caused by the volunteer operating a vehicle for which the operator or owner of the vehicle is required to possess insurance or maintain insurance. Id.
26. 42 U.S.C. at § 14503(a).[3]
27. NAT'L EMERGENCY MGMT. ASS'N. EMERGENCY MANAGEMENT ASSISTANCE COMPACT: OVERVIEW FOR NATIONAL RESPONSE FRAMEWORK, available at http://www.fema.gov/pdf/emergency/nrf/EMACoverview-ForNRF.pdf.
28. Id. NAT'L EMERGENCY MGMT. ASS'N. EMERGENCY MANAGEMENT ASSISTANCE COMPACT: OVERVIEW FOR NATIONAL RESPONSE FRAMEWORK.
29. UNIF L. COMM'N, UNIFORM EMERGENCY VOLUNTEER HEALTH PRACTITIONERS ACT, Prefatory Note (2007).
30. Id. UNIF L. COMM'N, UNIFORM EMERGENCY VOLUNTEER HEALTH PRACTITIONERS ACT, at § 6.
31. Boatemaa Ntiri-Reid, Licensing, Credentialing, and Liability Protects for Healthcare Volunteers During Disaster, 5 J. HEALTH & LIFE SCI L. 125 (2012).
32. CENTER FOR L. & PUB'.S HEALTH, MODEL STATE EMERGENCY HEALTH POWERS ACT § 804 (2001).
33. Id. at § 804(b)2(3). However, if the emergency responder is simply providing shelter, no liability can stem therefrom. Id. at § 804(b). (1).
34. THE TURNING POINT MODEL STATE PUBLIC HEALTH ACT: STATE LEGISLATIVE, UPDATE TABLE (2007) (listing the substance of passed legislation based on the MSEHPA by several states).
35. Human Rights and Natural Disasters Operations Guidelines and Field Manual of Human Rights Protection in Situations of Natural Disaster, Brookings-Bern Project on Internal Displacement (2008) available at http://www.refworld.org/pdfid/49a2b8f72.pdf.

13 | CHAPTER

Disaster Response in the United States

Jerry L. Mothershead

Response to emergencies and disasters for the protection of life, health, safety, and the preservation of property is a government responsibility. In the United States, governors, not the president, are primarily responsible for the health and welfare of their respective citizens, and they possess broad "police powers" that include the various legal authorities to order evacuations, commandeer private property, require quarantine, and take other actions to protect public safety.[1] Emergency response is carried out by local government entities within their defined jurisdictions (e.g., towns, cities, and counties). State governments coordinate needs identified by local governments with resources available at either the state or federal level.

In this chapter, the evolution of emergency and disaster management in the United States is discussed, and an overview of disaster response as currently practiced in this country is provided.

HISTORICAL PERSPECTIVE

The Early Years: 1776 to 1945

The first recorded involvement of the federal government in disaster response dates to 1803, when the state of New Hampshire requested funding assistance after a series of devastating fires.

During the ensuing 150 years, response to major emergencies and disasters by government entities above the local level can only be characterized as reactive. Typically, a significant event would occur, outside resources would arrive from neighboring communities, and the event would be contained. Recovery operations were often slow, prompting requests to state governments for economic assistance. Only when the state was unable or unwilling to assist these local communities would the federal government become involved. At that point, federal legislation was often required to authorize the expenditure of supplemental funds to assist the state and community involved.

Certain disasters occurred with greater frequency than others did, and when the frequency and severity of these events became significant enough to draw national attention, Congress would establish an office or agency to address them. Thus during the first half of the twentieth century, the Reconstruction Finance Corporation was established to make disaster loans after certain types of disasters. The Bureau of Public Roads provided funding for transportation infrastructure damage. The Flood Control Act, which gave the U.S. Army Corps of Engineers greater authority to implement flood control projects, was also passed. This uncontrolled and disorganized approach remained in effect until after World War II.[2]

Civil Defense Era: 1945 to 1974

Although during World War II, sporadic coastal watch groups and other organizations were established in various locales for protection against possible invasion or attack, the development of modern emergency management began in the 1950s, with the passage of two pieces of federal legislation[1]: the Civil Defense Act, aimed at funding initiatives that prepared for civil defense against enemy attack (shelter programs and packaged disaster hospitals),[2] and the Disaster Relief Act, which provided funds to state and local governments for rebuilding damage to public infrastructure.[3]

During the 1950s and much of the 1960s, civil defense from enemy attack was a federal government priority, as exemplified by the threat from nuclear attack during the 1961 Cuban Missile Crisis. Moreover, state and local governments were contending with significant natural disasters, such as the Alaskan Earthquake in 1964 and Hurricanes Betsy in 1965 and Camille in 1969. Federal funding for civil defense greatly outweighed that provided for natural disasters, and federal requirements prohibited the use of civil defense funds for either preparedness or response to natural disasters.

In addition, research and guidelines for disaster response started to appear. Severe wildfires in Southern California in the early 1970s gave rise to the congressional-funded project, Firefighting Resources Organized for Potential Emergencies (FIRESCOPE), which developed the Incident Management System (IMS) concept. The first standards for disaster management were authored by the National Fire Protection Association (NFPA) and were aimed at health care facility preparedness (J. Kerr, personal communication, 2000). The "first assessment" of disaster research occurred in 1975, and it summarized the findings of the disaster research community.[4]

Coordinating State and Federal Response: 1974 to 2001

In the early 1970s, the National Governor's Association (NGA) called for streamlining the fragmentation of federal civil defense and disaster assistance programs. In 1974, Congress passed the Robert T. Stafford Disaster Relief and Emergency Assistance Act, which unified federal funding of civil defense and disaster assistance programs.[5] In 1979, President Carter established the Federal Emergency Management Agency (FEMA) to serve as the overall executive branch coordination agency for disaster response.[6] Parallel efforts at the state level resulted in the establishment of either a state emergency management agency or the assignment of similar coordination functions to other offices, such as the Adjutant General of the State National Guard.

The creation of FEMA and promulgation of various executive orders during the 1970s and 1980s improved overall federal response, but in general, authorities and responsibilities remained confusing and, on occasion, contentious. In an attempt to resolve many of these conflicts and promote a coordinated approach to disaster response, the Federal Response Plan (FRP) was developed to serve as the principal organizational guide for defining the roles and responsibilities of 26 federal member agencies and the American Red Cross, which are charged with the delivery of national-level emergency assistance during major crises.[7] Although revised several times, the FRP did not solve all response and coordination problems and, in reaction to various disasters, additional federal plans were developed, including the Federal Radiological Emergency Response Plan (FRERP) and the National Oil and Hazardous Substances Pollution Contingency Plan, more commonly referred to as the National Contingency Plan (NCP). These various plans were often at odds with other plans, resulting in confusion as to which plan should be used if criteria were met for more than one.

Problems other than coordination continued. One example was the often-significant delay in the arrival of state and federal response resources. To obviate this, a number of states entered into compacts with other specific states to provide limited services across state lines during disasters. These agreements were most often used for wildland firefighting resources in the Midwestern and Western United States. The National Governors' Association (NGA) successfully lobbied Congress to enact the Emergency Management Assistance Compact (EMAC) legislation, the first significant alteration to the model state civil defense legislation passed in the 1950s.[8] This legislation established a template for state-to-state resource sharing during disaster response.

Thus, by the turn of the century, the framework existed at the state and federal levels for coordinated response and recovery operations to disasters caused by nature or as the result of technological mishaps. Unfortunately, a new threat loomed that would again result in a major revision of the approach to disaster management.

New Millennium, New Threats: Post-2001

Terrorism arrived in the United States in the 1990s, with the first attack on the World Trade Center in 1993, followed by the bombing of the Murrah Federal Building in Oklahoma City in 1995. Internationally, terrorist organizations were growing in numbers, and terrorist acts were becoming more lethal. In addition to conventional weapons, these organizations were using chemical, biological, and radiological agents to cause greater harm, and they were turning these threats against civilians as well as the political or industrial figures attacked in the past. The Aum Shinrikyo religious sect used the nerve agent sarin unsuccessfully against several magistrates in Japan in 1994, and, in the following year, successfully attacked passengers in a Tokyo subway station. Aum Shinrikyo also attempted, unsuccessfully, to weaponize botulinum toxin. In 1995, Chechen rebels directed a reporter to a park in central Moscow, where she found a package containing 15 kg of explosives and cesium-137. U.S. interests were increasingly under attack overseas, evidenced by dual embassy bombings in Africa in 1998, which were followed by the maritime attack on the destroyer USS *Cole*.

These events drew the attention of both the executive and legislative branches of the federal government. Under the Clinton administration (1992-2000), a series of executive orders, referred to as Presidential Decision Directives (PDDs), were promulgated, and a number of federal statutes were enacted, to improve the defensive posture of and to protect the United States and its citizens against terrorist attacks. Several new offices and programs were established in federal agencies, including in the Departments of Justice, Health and Human Services, and Defense. The most significant legislation was the Defense against Weapons of Mass Destruction Act,[9] commonly referred to as the

Nunn-Lugar-Domenici legislation. One of the act's many purposes was to provide resources for equipment and the training of local response personnel for mitigating a weapons-of-mass-destruction (WMD) incident.

These initiatives, while significant, proved insufficient to prevent the terrorist attacks that totally destroyed three World Trade Center buildings in New York, significantly damaged the Pentagon, and resulted in nearly 3000 deaths on September 11, 2001. One month later, weaponized *Bacillus anthracis* (anthrax) spores were distributed through the U.S. mail system, resulting in 11 deaths and another 11 infected persons. In combination, these events resulted in some of the greatest restructuring of the federal government since its inception.

CURRENT CONCEPTS OF DISASTER RESPONSE

The terrorist events of 2001 sent shock waves throughout the U.S. government. New legislation was introduced in the first three months after the attacks that surpassed all antiterrorism legislation of the previous decade. President Bush, who had been recently elected, issued new and revised executive orders, now termed Homeland Security Presidential Directives, which called for changes in executive branch agencies to meet the current threat of terrorism. Funding to fight the "global war on terrorism" at home and abroad, beyond massive expenditures needed to fight the wars in Afghanistan and Iraq, increased by a full order of magnitude.

To understand the current emergency management system in the United States, first it is important to realize that all levels of government have certain roles and responsibilities in mitigation, preparedness, response, and recovery, and that various government entities have different functions in preparedness and response. Regardless of the government level, however, the designated emergency management agency is responsible for day-to-day coordination of mitigation and preparedness activities involving agencies and organizations at that level and for synchronization of these agencies during response and recovery phases. The designated emergency management agency also serves as the focal point for hierarchical coordination between local, state, and federal response agencies.

Local Level Emergency Management

Because there are subordinate jurisdictions within each state that are usually established by geographic boundaries, local emergency management may occur at the city, township, borough, county, or (in some states) parish level. Largely, the attention given to emergency and disaster preparedness and response will be dictated by the overall population within the jurisdiction, actual or perceived threats to the area, and population concentration. Ultimately, however, emergency management comes down to funding.

Regardless of the type of jurisdiction, an executive/managerial official will be in charge of emergency management operations. This official may be the community safety official, the fire chief, or the police chief. It is this individual's responsibility to form a multicratic organizational model within the community that brings together the disparate response and recovery organizations, including entities such as hazardous materials teams, fire services, law enforcement agencies, public works departments, and city, county, or district health departments.

State-Level Emergency Management

All 50 states and the 6 territories have emergency management agencies that fall under the executive branch of the state government. In most cases, these agencies either are independent entities or increasingly are incorporated into the agency responsible for the state's National Guard. State Emergency Management Agencies (SEMAs) are responsible for standards and the training, oversight, and guidance of emergency management organizations at lower jurisdictional levels; coordination with other state-level agencies and organizations in their preparedness and planning activities; and the administration and distribution of state or federal funds earmarked for emergency management. In some states, disaster-related organizations, such as the state emergency medical service(s) (EMS) office, are part of the SEMA, but this subordinate organization is by no means uniform across the states.

During response and recovery operations, SEMAs usually provide overall operations and support at state-level emergency operations centers, provide liaison personnel to federal coordinating officers (the on-scene federal emergency manager), receive requests for assistance from local Emergency Management Agencies (EMAs), and provide state-level resources (both personnel and material) and expertise to local emergency managers.

In addition to its own resources, a state could request outside assistance from other states that are EMAC signatories. Initially, few states signed on to this agreement, but in the wake of the terrorist attacks of 2001, many states rushed in, enabling statutes through their legislatures. As of 2014, all states and four territories have approved these compacts. Under an EMAC, an affected state may request material resources and personnel from a signatory state. If available, the assisting state will provide those resources, with the understanding that the requesting state will provide appropriate legal coverage from assisting personnel and will reimburse the assisting state for resources used. Depending on the actual wording and annexes of individual EMACs, such resources could include the National Guard or medical personnel who are not state employees. A number of states, particularly in the Northeast, have also signed international EMACs with provinces in Canada, to allow resource sharing.

Federal-Level Emergency Management

With the rare exception of a disaster that meets the criteria of a national security event, coordinated federal response to disasters usually does not occur unless the governor of the affected state requests a presidential declaration of a national disaster, which then must be approved. However, each federal agency that could be involved in disaster response is still able to exercise its autonomy and respond directly to a request for assistance outside this coordinated federal response. For example, the Environmental Protection Agency could provide expert assistance during clean-up operations from an oil spill that did not meet national emergency thresholds. Similarly, the Centers for Disease Control and Prevention could mobilize one of its Epidemiological Investigative Service teams to assist in the evaluation and containment of a contagious disease outbreak. Under these circumstances, however, the funding stream to reimburse the agencies would fall outside that which is established for presidential declarations and may have to come through either state or agency resources. The Department of Defense (DoD) is a notable exception to this. A number of specific statutes preclude autonomous response of DoD forces to disasters, beyond local events that would affect military establishments in the jurisdictional area.

Department of Homeland Security

Because of its pivotal role in overall federal-level emergency management, the current organization and functions of the Department of Homeland Security (DHS) are important to understand. Initially, DHS was authorized to serve an advisory role to the president; however, a shift toward the concept of "Homeland Security" evolved, and, through congressional efforts, DHS became the federal entity focused exclusively on this issue. In November 2002, the president signed into law H.R. 5005,[10] the Homeland Security Act of 2002, which established the DHS[11] as a cabinet-level executive agency. DHS consolidated 22 agencies and 180,000 employees (now almost 250,000) and unified many federal functions into a single agency dedicated to protecting the United States.

Agencies under the DHS include the Transportation Security Administration, the U.S. Coast Guard, and FEMA. FEMA's traditional role as the lead coordinating agency for all disaster response in the United States continues, but under the oversight of DHS. The secretary of DHS was given extraordinary powers, including the authorization to initiate a federal response under the Stafford Act, without prior consultation with the president under certain exigencies.

DHS has expanded from its original 4 primary directorates, and it is now organized at the headquarters level, into 14 different subordinate directorates, offices, and components, plus a supporting, management directorate. Additionally, it exercises operational control over seven independent federal organizations, the most important of which from a disaster management perspective are the U.S. Coast Guard and FEMA, the latter of which has absorbed many of the functions of the original Emergency Preparedness and Response Directorate.

All responses to disasters and emergencies that reach the threshold for a presidential declaration of a national disaster fall under the coordination purview of DHS. Under these circumstances, FEMA is the primary operational arm of DHS in executing response and recovery initiatives, and it does so within the framework of two documents, the National Response Framework and the National Incident Management System (NIMS).

On February 28, 2003, the president issued Homeland Security Presidential Directive #5[12] to enhance the ability of the United States to manage domestic incidents. To implement this directive, the secretary of DHS directed that a single, integrated federal Emergency Operations Plan (EOP) be developed. The resultant National Response Plan (NRP)[13] paralleled the earlier FRP in format and linked the following hazard-specific EOPs:

- FRP[14]
- U.S. Government Interagency Domestic Terrorism Concept of Operations Plan[15]
- FRERP[16]
- Mass migration response plans
- National Contingency Plan[17]

As further evolution of the shared responsibilities between local, state, and federal response agencies ensued, and as shortcomings in the NRP were highlighted by such catastrophic events as Hurricane Katrina, a shift in the focus of the overall response plan was deemed necessary by DHS leadership. With this shift of focus, the NRP was reissued as the National Response Framework (NRF), and as with its predecessor documents, under the NRF, FEMA serves as the overall coordinator for federal support. However, under the NRF construct, support is considered to fall within 15 different Emergency Support Functions (ESFs), which are listed in Table 13-1. Because resources and expertise in these various functions may exist within multiple federal agencies, each ESF response is coordinated by an ESF coordinating agency: a primary agency, which is usually the same as the coordinating agency, and a number of secondary (supporting) agencies. The NRF also identifies a number of support annexes, covering a range of topics from critical infrastructure protection to public affairs, and seven incident-specific annexes focused on events that present unique national challenges. These incident annexes include nuclear/radiological and biological incidents, mass evacuation situations, and others.[18] The DHS continues to develop additional publications and tools to assist emergency management entities, both in preparedness and response. For example, one challenge identified during response activities was ensuring that all response organizations had a common understanding of the capabilities of response resources, and that the right capability resource was requested and provided. These issues were addressed by the development of the Target Capabilities List, which identifies 36 discrete response capabilities and embedded "Universal Task Lists" that identify discrete tasks to be accomplished to specific standards.[19]

TABLE 13-1   Emergency Support Functions

ESF NO.	FUNCTIONAL AREA
1	Transportation
2	Communications
3	Public works/engineering
4	Firefighting
5	Emergency management
6	Mass care, housing
7	Resource support
8	Public health and medical services
9	Urban search and rescue
10	Oil and hazardous materials
11	Agriculture and natural resources
12	Energy
13	Public safety and security
14	Recovery and mitigation
15	External communications

In the event of a national disaster, various emergency operations centers and oversight and policy entities will be activated at the headquarters level, not only of the DHS but also of other federal agencies. The principal headquarters office responsible for interacting with state/local operations managers is the Regional Response Coordination Center (RRCC). At the local/regional level, the principal coordinating office is now termed the Joint Field Office (JFO). The JFO provides a local coordination of federal, state, local, tribal, nongovernmental, and private-sector response organizations, and, in addition to federal, defense, and state field officers, it is staffed by representatives from appropriate ESF coordinating agencies and other state representatives.

National Incident Management System

Homeland Security Presidential Directive #5 (an executive order) called for the creation of a standardized IMS to facilitate interoperability and integration among the many federal, state, and local response organizations. The NIMS[20] provides a standardized system for implementing the NRF. The NIMS provides a consistent yet flexible nationwide framework within which local, state, and federal levels of governments and the private sector can work effectively and efficiently to be aware of, prepare for, prevent, respond to, and recover from domestic incidents, regardless of their cause, size, or complexity. The NIMS is mandated for use by all agencies in the executive branch of the federal government. Although not mandatory for use by the states and local jurisdictions, federal funding for disaster and Homeland Security initiatives is directly tied with these jurisdictions' use of the NIMS in preparation, planning, and response

SUMMARY

Emergency management has evolved over the past 200 years, and it continues to evolve. With the creation of DHS as an authoritative central executive agency for oversight of all federal emergency management activities, a level of cooperation and collaboration at the federal level never before achieved is a possibility. Moreover, continued refinements of and support for emergency management initiatives at the state and local levels have improved hierarchical integration during response and recovery. *Standardization* is the watchword. Emergency management has evolved from an exercise in on-the-job training to a degreed, scientific profession at all levels.

The challenge now is to maintain the momentum. Over a decade has passed since the World Trade Centers collapsed, and, although there

have been many attempts, no major terrorist incidents have occurred in the United States since. There have been, however, major natural disasters, and these catastrophic events continue to highlight the challenges of preparedness and response. Nonetheless, budgetary constraints, especially after the "Great Recession" of 2008, have forced curtailment of funding for many programs, and disaster preparedness programs were not exempted. If the local, state, and national agencies responsible for national protection and response are to be best prepared for the next "big one," diligence within those respective organizations, as well as sufficient resourcing, remains paramount.

REFERENCES

1. Pine J. *A Review of State Emergency Management Statutes.* Washington, DC: Federal Emergency Management Agency; 1989: 8.
2. Federal Emergency Management Agency. FEMA history. Available at: http://www.fema.gov/about/history.shtm.
3. LaValla P, Stoffel R. *Blueprint for Community Emergency Management: A Text for Managing Emergency Operations.* Olympia, WA: Emergency Response Institute; 1983.
4. White GF, Haas JE. *Assessment of Research on Natural Hazards.* Cambridge: MIT Press; 1975.
5. Robert T. *Stafford Disaster Relief and Emergency Assistance Act, as amended by Pub L No. 106-390;* October 30, 2000. Available at: http://www.fema.gov/library/stafact.shtm.
6. Drabek T. The evolution of emergency management. In: Drabek T, Hoetmer G, eds. *Principles and Practices for Local Government.* Washington, DC: International City Management Association; 1991:17.
7. Federal Emergency Management Agency. *Federal Response Plan.* Washington, DC: Government Printing Office; April 1992. Document 9230.1-PL: Supersedes FEMA 229.
8. National Emergency Management Association. Emergency Management Assistance Compact. Available at: http://www.emacweb.org/.
9. Pub L No. 104-201 (Defense Against Weapons of Mass Destruction Act of 1996).
10. U.S. Citizenship and Immigration Services. HR 5005 Homeland Security Act of 2002. Available at: http://uscis.gov/graphics/hr5005.pdf.
11. U.S. Department of Homeland Security. The Department of Homeland Security. Available at: http://www.dhs.gov/interweb/assetlibrary/book.pdf.
12. The White House. Homeland Security Presidential Directive/ HSPD-5. Available at: http://www.dhs.gov/dhspublic/display?theme=42&content=496.
13. U.S. Department of Homeland Security. Initial National Response Plan fact sheet. Available at: http://www.dhs.gov/dhspublic/display?theme=43&content=1936.
14. U.S. Department of Homeland Security. Emergencies and disasters: planning and prevention: National Response Plan. Available at: http://www.fema.gov/rrr/frp/.
15. Federal Emergency Management Agency. U.S. Government Interagency Domestic Terrorism Concept of Operations Plan. Available at: http://fema.gov/pdf/rrr/conplan/conplan.pdf.
16. U.S. Department of Homeland Security. Federal Radiological Emergency Response Plan (FRERP)-Operational Plan. Available at: http://www.fas.org/nuke/guide/usa/doctrine/national/frerp.htm.
17. Environmental Protection Agency. National Contingency Plan overview. Available at: http://www.epa.gov/oilspill/ncpover.htm.
18. U.S. Federal Emergency Management Agency. National Response Framework. Available at: http://www.fema.gov/national-response-framework.
19. U.S. Department of Homeland Security. Target Capabilities List V1.1. Available at http://www.ncrhomelandsecurity.org/ncr/downloads/Target%20Capabilities%20List.pdf.
20. U.S. Department of Homeland Security. National Incident Management System. Available at: http://www.dhs.gov/dhspublic/display?theme=51&content=3423.

14 CHAPTER

Disaster Response in Europe

Michelangelo Bortolin

The important goals of disaster and mass casualty incident (MCI) response are to protect and to save life. When a disaster strikes a population, people expect that leaders, local authorities, and the national government will take actions to respond immediately and in an appropriate manner, restoring order as quickly as possible.[1]

Starting with the establishment of the European Union (EU), and in particular over the last 20 years, state members and European institutions have committed to mutual support in response to disasters. As a consequence of this commitment, the EU founded a specific institution, recognized by all state members, exclusively dedicated to humanitarian aid, supporting or supplementing national policies in the field of mutual civil protection assistance, and facilitating coordination of assistance interventions.[2,3] This institution is called the European Community Humanitarian Office (ECHO).

HISTORICAL PERSPECTIVE

From Ancient Times to the Middle Ages

Since ancient times, Europe has been stricken by multiple disasters. Examples include tsunami and earthquakes (Helike tsunami and earthquake 373 BC), fires (Great Fire of Rome 64 BC), volcanic eruptions (Minoan eruption 1628 BC), and bubonic plague (Justinian's Plague 541 AD), to mention a few.

Ancient civilizations believed that disasters are events due to the intervention of the gods or fate, and this belief was perpetuated even into modern times. Indeed, the word disaster appears to have been derived from the ancient Greek word "dus-aster" or the Latin "dis-aster" that means "bad-star" in English. Despite this belief, primitive responses, often ineffective and in some cases bizarre, were provided at the local level. The first fire brigade service was established in Ancient Rome during the second century BC. Its name notwithstanding, this service did not protect against all the fires that frequently occurred in the city, but was a profit-making business protecting private interests. Marcus Licinius Crassus became one of the wealthiest men in Ancient Rome because he imagined and organized a private fire brigade service with several hundred slaves. When notified, they rushed to the location of a fire. Once on site, they negotiated a fee with the property owner to extinguish the fire. In the event no agreement was reached, the fire brigade did not intervene. If the fire resulted in the complete destruction of the property, Crassus made an offer to buy the land at a favorable price.

Another example of ancient European disaster response is reported in the Latin literature, when Pliny the Younger described the operation of search and rescue provided by his uncle, Pliny the Elder, to save his friends and his family in Pompeii during the Vesuvius eruption of 79 AD.

With the spread of Christianity in the Mediterranean basin and throughout Europe, religious congregations provided the bulk of disaster response, particularly during epidemics. Groups organized themselves to help the infirm, usually with minimal success due to lack of medical knowledge. Medical practice at that time was largely based on the use of herbs, astrology, and local superstition, often with the consequence of spreading the outbreak among healthy people.

The plague known as the "Black Death" that spread from Central Asia to Europe in the middle of the fourteenth century AD was one of the largest pandemics in history, with an estimated 75 to 200 million deaths. Monks and priests provided care for the ill, and victims of the plague were often abandoned by their families and expelled from the community. Saint Roch from Montpellier (canonized as the special patron against contagious diseases) is still venerated for the great aid and support given during the plague.[4] The religious orders also provided strong support during the famine that struck Europe during the Middle Ages. Another frequent type of disaster in Europe during these times was war (e.g., the Hundred Years' War 1337 to 1453 AD). Early European responses to nearly all large-scale disasters were ineffective, and it was not until the modern era that the first transformations and innovations in the disaster response system were to be seen.

Modern Era

Disaster management in the modern era witnessed many important improvements. Concepts of mitigation and preparedness were combined into disaster management; the epidemiology of disaster was investigated, and a number of improvements were instituted in triage, treatment, and transport of casualties. Although disaster management was often viewed as a local issue, the nineteenth century witnessed the founding of numerous nongovernmental organizations (NGOs) created to provide assistance throughout Europe. The twentieth century marked the development of agreements between nations, national policies and laws regarding disaster response, and civil protection.

The start of the modern era in disaster preparedness and response can be considered to be the year 1755 during the Lisbon earthquake. Immediately after the first earthquake hit Lisbon and caused more than 30,000 victims, King Jose Manuel I of Portugal named the Prime Minister Marquis of Pombal as the Incident Commander to manage the disaster response and recovery. The Marquis's first innovation was to collect information from the population, and in particular from priests, regarding the tremors and the collapsed buildings, certain that these phenomena could be studied as natural events and therefore mitigated. He also established a program of disaster relief for the population with shelter and food centers, fire brigades, and mass burials to avoid disease outbreaks. He started an urban plan to rebuild the city that was based on the information collected regarding the buildings, proposing and actuating the construction of more solid structures—thus developing the first mitigation plan for a city.[4,5]

Another important milestone in disaster response occurred shortly thereafter. At the end of the eighteenth century, a French surgeon of the Napoleonic Army, Dominique Jean Larrey, after years as chief surgeon on the battlefield, took inspiration from military medicine. He established the first ambulance service to evacuate and provide aid to the wounded on the battlefield and invented the first method of triage (the word is derived from the French "trier," "sorting"). Before this ambulance service, staffed by a team of surgeons and nurses who provided some care on-scene and transported patients in a light two-wheeled carriage, casualties not able to walk often stayed on the battlefield for days before being moved to a field hospital. Many died in agony, waiting for care.[6] Larrey also introduced several changes in the medical practice of that period, including performance of immediate rather than delayed amputations as life-saving measures and the field use of positive pressure ventilation and hypothermia.[7] A few decades later, a cholera outbreak spread across London in 1854, causing more than 600 deaths. A physician, John Snow, determined that the outbreak was due to contaminated water supplied by a pump in a specific neighborhood of the city. His approach to solving this medical mystery was revolutionary. Snow analyzed data from the population and information about the water supply network and demonstrated the cause of the outbreak, how the disease was spread, and how to control spread. He applied methodologies now referred to as epidemiology.[8] In the same year, Florence Nightingale, an English woman born in Italy, instituted some of the first organized disaster relief efforts.[9] Despite coming from a rich British family, she wished to commit her efforts to the care of the sick. During the Crimean War she led a group of 38 women who treated the injured. During this war the medical facilities were very poor, and mortality rates were 10 times higher than on the battlefield.[10,11] Florence Nightingale reorganized British hospital practices by cleaning the rooms, promoting good hygiene, creating nutritional and water sanitation programs, improving health standards, and reducing mortality by two thirds. She introduced a new model of care, shaping the future of modern nursing. After her experience in the field, she established a school of nursing at Saint Thomas Hospital in London. Her efforts and work resulted in major changes regarding medical care, public health, sanitations, and military health.

In the same year, Jean Henry Dunant, a Swiss businessman, impressed with the violence of the Battle of Solverino of 1859 and the resulting number of deaths and casualties (more than 20,000), organized a medical support system for the casualties utilizing the local population, in particular young women. A few years later in 1863 he founded the International Committee of the Red Cross (ICRC).[12,13] The ICRC was the first organization that provided support to victims of war and other disasters. It was also the first internationally recognized organization that provided humanitarian relief in agreement with the principles of neutrality, independence, and impartiality.[14] Through the efforts of the ICRC, in 1864 12 European states signed the "Convention for the amelioration of the condition of the wounded in armies in the field." Signatory states committed to provide aid to the injured from war of any nationality, the field identification of health care personnel involved in medical support by displaying a red cross, and the inviolability and neutrality of persons involved in the performance of humanitarian relief and assistance.[15] Despite initial challenges, including bankruptcy in 1867, the ICRC's commitment to humanitarian relief was enormous and remains active today, ensuring decent conditions and humane treatment of prisoners, aiding populations affected by all forms of conflict and disaster, providing assistance for family reunification, supporting the poor, promoting the improvement of living conditions and a sustainable environment, and providing basic health care assistance. The ICRC played an important role as a provider of medical support, humanitarian activities, and service on the battlefield and in prisoner of war camps during the First and Second World Wars. These important efforts were internationally recognized, with the ICRC being awarded the Nobel Peace Prize in 1917, 1944, and 1963.

In 1927 several European and outside nations signed the convention establishing the International Relief Union (IRU), which became operational in 1932. The objectives of the IRU were to give first aid and support to populations stricken by disasters and to coordinate the disaster response. The IRU was active in response to several disasters until 1982, when several nations invoked the withdrawal clause of the convention and ceased their support.[16]

During and between World Wars I and II, the international response to war, and ensuing complex humanitarian disasters such as famine or displaced populations, was provided by international or local humanitarian agencies such as ICRC and Oxfam.

CONTEMPORARY ERA AND CURRENT PRACTICE

Shortly after the end of World War II, a number of European nations developed enabling legislation to support the organization of civil protection and development of programs in disaster risk reduction, preparedness, and response at local, regional, and national levels. These acts collectively resulted in improvements in disaster management and culminated in the creation of national civil protection legislation in every member state of the EU). In 1948 the British parliament passed the Civil Defense Act,[17] followed in 1950 by the French with their Ordinance (for civil protection) and the Decree Relating to Civil Defense in 1965.[18] In Slovenia during the cold war of the 1960s, a civil protection system was established, while in 1985 the Italian Ministry of the Interior established the Department of Civil Protection.

A great movement toward the development and implementation of civil protection occurred during the 1980s, especially in France and Italy because of the disasters that struck these countries.[19] In 1985 EU leaders formally agreed on the Community Cooperation in Civil Protection. After that, numerous other suggestions, resolutions, and acts were proposed to develop and improve cooperation. During the following decade, roles and responsibilities of national civil protection were clearly defined and became operational in all member states of the EU.[20,21] In 1992 the member states of the EU founded ECHO, which has the responsibility to provide coordinated humanitarian response to disasters around the world and to alleviate suffering in affected populations, in agreement with the principles of humanity, neutrality, impartiality, and independence. Today, the EU is the world's largest donor of humanitarian aid. In December 1999 the EU promulgated the concept of "community action program in the field of civil protection" to develop cooperation and to support and supplement national policies in the field of civil protection in order to increase preparedness and the ability to undertake immediate response actions.[22] In 2004 ECHO became the Directorate-General for humanitarian response, and in 2010 it was integrated into the civil protection programs of 28 EU member states, plus the former Yugoslav Republic of Macedonia, Iceland, Liechtenstein, and Norway.[23] The EU Civil Protection Mechanism was established, fostering cooperation among national civil protection authorities across Europe, and is organized at local, regional, and national levels with different authorities, organizations, and operational centers at each level. These organizations also collaborate across international borders.

Local Level Emergency Management

Disaster management at the local level is usually directed by the mayor or other municipality leader. At this level each local administration has a division of Civil Protection. Disaster response is provided by emergency service organizations: emergency medical services, fire brigades, police, public health services, local Civil Protection offices, volunteers, NGOs, and specialized teams, as delineated in the local emergency operations plan (EOP). The role of local authorities is very important in the prevention and mitigation of disasters. Another important role is in training and public awareness campaigns. The Major Incident Medical Management and Support (MIMMS) course is used in Europe for disaster health care operations.

Regional Level Emergency Management

If a disaster cannot be managed at the local level, assistance can be requested from other municipalities, and it will be managed at the regional level.[24] The regional level response (Lander Level in Germany,[25] Province Level in Belgium[26]) varies among the 32 EU member states. However, most organizations and functions are similar. Response is coordinated through a regional operating center directed by a governor or prefect who manages overall disaster response, while at the local level, the municipal authority remains in charge within his or her jurisdiction.

National Level Emergency Management

At the national level, the Minister of Interior or Internal Affairs (or the Minister of Defense in Sweden or the Prime Minister in the United Kingdom) is the head of a strategic committee, and he or she is charged with overall command, coordination, and control of the event. The committee manages the crisis in accordance with a National Disaster Plan. According to the policies in effect and decisions made by the committee, the regional and local authorities will manage the event at the site. In several states, such as Italy, the central government has the responsibility over all phases of disaster management. These include establishing criteria concerning mitigation, forecasting, prevention, preparedness, response, and recovery. The central government also contributes to the administration of material resources for disaster prevention, response management, and recovery from all types of events; coordinates and promotes training and public information campaigns; and assists in the development and preparation of operational units at local and regional levels.[27,28]

International Level Emergency Management (European Union)

When a disaster exceeds national level management capabilities, a country may request assistance from the EU. The EU Civil Protection Unit within ECHO has a key instrument for supporting a nation when a disaster strikes, referred to as the Civil Protection Mechanism (CPM). The CPM enables coordinated assistance from member states. Assistance is coordinated through the European Emergency Response Centre (ERC), which is operational at all times. The ERC is a communication hub among the member states. It receives and provides disaster-related information and supports, coordinates, and facilitates the response using resources from the 32 member states.[29,30] The member states pool and deploy staff, material resources, and experts for assessment and coordination of the response.

The EU member states may also respond to disasters outside Europe. Any nation can call on the EU CPM for assistance. Civil protection assistance often consists of highly specialized equipment and teams that are organized as "modules." Modules are emergency response units that operate within the parameters of the CPM and have a rapid activation time (maximum 12 hours). Modules are able to work independently, but also are experienced in working together. These operational units can be dispatched in Europe or worldwide by one or several countries. Using modules ensures that the response is rapid, effective, and coordinated.[31] Any European team sent from the EU to a disaster area remains under the direction of the national authorities of the affected country, which has the right to ask European teams to stand down at any time. European teams are subject to local law and should operate in conformity with national rules and procedures governing their work. In the past ECHO has provided relief and assistance to millions of people in more than 140 countries around the world. Recent major deployments include responses to the tsunami in South Asia (2004/2005), Hurricane Katrina in the United States (2005), the earthquake in Haiti (2010), and Typhoon Haiyan in the Philippines (2013).

REFERENCES

1. Federal Emergency Management Agency. *Guide for All-Hazard Emergency Operation Planning*; 1996. Available at: http://www.fema.gov/pdf/plan/slg101.pdf.
2. European Community. Official Journal of the European Communities: Council Regulation No 1257/96 of 20 June 1996. Available at: http://eur-lex.europa.eu/LexUriServ/LexUriServ.do?uri=OJ:L:1996:163:0001:0006:EN:PDF.
3. European Community. Official Journal of the European Communities: Council Decision 2001/792/EC, Euratom. Available at: http://eur-lex.europa.eu/legal-content/EN/TXT/PDF/?uri=CELEX:32001D0792&from=EN.
4. Penuel KB, Statler M. *Encyclopedia of Disaster Relief*. Thousand Oaks, CA: SAGE Publications; 2011.
5. Mendes-Victor L, Sousa Oliveira C, Azevedo J, Ribeiro A. *The 1755 Lisbon Earthquake: Revisited.* Springer eBook; 2009.
6. Nestor P. Baron Dominique Jean Larrey 1766–1842. *J Em Prim Health Care.* 2003;1(3–4).
7. Remba SJ, Varon J, Rivera A, Sternbach GL. Dominique-Jean Larrey: the effects of therapeutic hypothermia and the first ambulance. *Resuscitation.* 2010;81(3):268–271. http://dx.doi.org/10.1016/j.resuscitation.2009.11.010, Epub 2009 Dec 29.
8. Science Museum. *John Snow (1813–1858)*. Available at: http://www.sciencemuseum.org.uk/broughttolife/people/johnsnow. Accessed 21.06.14.
9. The Critical Thinking Consortium. *Globalizing Factors in the History of Disaster Relief*; 2014. Available at: http://tc2.ca/pdf/Disaster_relief.pdf, Accessed 21.06.14.
10. BBC History. *Florence Nightingale: the Lady with the Lamp*; 2011. Available at: http://www.bbc.co.uk/history/british/victorians/nightingale_01.shtml, Accessed 21.06.14.
11. BBC History. *Florence Nightingale*; 2014. Available at: http://www.bbc.co.uk/history/historic_figures/nightingale_florence.shtml, Accessed 21.06.14.
12. International Committee of the Red Cross (ICRC). *Henry Dunant.* Available at: http://www.icrc.org/eng/resources/documents/misc/57jnvq.htm, Accessed 21.06.14.
13. Nobel Prize. *Henry Dunant—biographical*; 2014. Available at: http://www.nobelprize.org/nobel_prizes/peace/laureates/1901/dunant-bio.html, Accessed 21.06.14.
14. International Committee of the Red Cross (ICRC). *The ICRC's Mandate and Mission*; 2014. Available at: http://www.icrc.org/eng/who-we-are/mandate/overview-icrc-mandate-mission.htm, Accessed 21.06.14.
15. International Committee of the Red Cross (ICRC). *Convention for the Amelioration of the Condition of the Wounded in Armies in the Field. Geneva, 22 August 1864*; 2014. Available at: http://www.icrc.org/applic/ihl/ihl.nsf/Treaty.xsp?documentId=477CEA122D7B7B3DC12563CD002D6603&action=openDocument, Accessed 21.06.14.
16. German Permanent Mission in Geneva. *The International Relief Union/PIUS*; 2014. Available at: http://www.genf.diplo.de/Vertretung/genf/en/01/union-internat-secours__en.html, Accessed 21.06.14.
17. Coppola DP. *Introduction to International Disaster Management.* Oxford: Butterworth-Heinemann; 2010.
18. European Community Humanitarian Office (ECHO). *France—Disaster Management Structure. European Commission—Humanitarian Aid and Civil Protection*; 2014. Available at: http://ec.europa.eu/echo/civil_protection/civil/vademecum/fr/2-fr-1.html, Accessed 21.06.14.

19. UNISDR. *The Structure, Role and Mandate of Civil Protection in Disaster Risk Reduction for South Eastern Europe—South Eastern Europe Disaster Risk Mitigation and Adaptation Programme*; 2009. Available at: http://www.unisdr.org/files/9346_Europe.pdf.

20. European Community Humanitarian Office (ECHO). *EU Focus on Civil Protection*. European Communities; 2012. Available at: http://ec.europa.eu/echo/civil_protection/civil/pdfdocs/focus_en.pdf, Accessed 21.06.14.

21. Ekengren M, Matzén N, Rhinard M, Svantesson M. Solidarity or sovereignty? EU cooperation in civil protection. *J Eur Integration*. 2006;28 (5):457–476.

22. European Community Humanitarian Office (ECHO). European Community (EC) (1999) Official Journal of the European Communities: Council Decision 1999/847/EC. Available at: http://ec.europa.eu/echo/civil_protection/civil/pdfdocs/1299pc0847_en.pdf; 1999.

23. European Community Humanitarian Office (ECHO). *"Presentation" European Commission—Humanitarian Aid and Civil Protection*; 2014. Available at: http://ec.europa.eu/echo/about/presentation_en.htm, Accessed 21.06.14.

24. European Community Humanitarian Office (ECHO). *Norway Emergency Planning. European Commission—Humanitarian Aid and Civil Protection*; 2014. Available at: http://ec.europa.eu/echo/civil_protection/civil/vademecum/no/2-no-2.html#cipro, Accessed 21.06.14.

25. European Community Humanitarian Office (ECHO). *Country Profile— Germany. European Commission—Humanitarian Aid and Civil Protection*;

2014. Available at: http://ec.europa.eu/echo/civil_protection/civil/vademecum/de/2-de.html, Accessed 21.06.14.

26. European Community Humanitarian Office (ECHO). *Country Profile— Belgium. European Commission—Humanitarian Aid and Civil Protection*; 2014. Available at: http://ec.europa.eu/echo/civil_protection/civil/vademecum/be/2-be.html, Accessed 21.06.14.

27. European Community Humanitarian Office (ECHO). *Country Profile— Italy. European Commission—Humanitarian Aid and Civil Protection*; 2014. Available at: http://ec.europa.eu/echo/civil_protection/civil/vademecum/it/2-it.html, Accessed 21.06.14.

28. Protezione Civile. *Strutture Operative*; 2014. Available at: http://www.protezionecivile.gov.it/jcms/it/strutture_operative.wp, Accessed 21.06.14.

29. European Community Humanitarian Office (ECHO). *EU Civil Protection— ECHO Factsheet Thematic. European Commission—Humanitarian Aid and Civil Protection*; May 2014. Available at: http://ec.europa.eu/echo/files/aid/countries/factsheets/thematic/civil_protection_en.pdf, Accessed 21.06.14.

30. European Community Humanitarian Office (ECHO). *The Community Mechanism for Civil Protection. European Commission—Humanitarian Aid and Civil Protection*; 2014. Available at: http://ec.europa.eu/echo/policies/disaster_response/mechanism_en.htm, Accessed 21.06.14.

31. European Community Humanitarian Office (ECHO). *Modules. European Commission—Humanitarian Aid and Civil Protection*; 2014. Available at: http://ec.europa.eu/echo/policies/disaster_response/modules_en.htm, Accessed 21.06.14.

Local Disaster Response

Jerry L. Mothershead

All disasters are local. Regardless of type, magnitude, or progression, disasters affect communities. Community responders will be the first on the scene and will remain for recovery operations well after supporting resources and organizations have departed.

Depending on the type of disaster, various government, public, and private organizations responsible for public safety, public security, and infrastructure maintenance will be tasked to save lives, preserve property, and identify and rebuild essential services for the population served. Prioritizing and coordinating these missions will require collaboration, cooperation, and understanding on the part of the leadership and membership of these response and recovery organizations.

In general, these services are organized in the United States within a jurisdictional framework, and overall coordination falls to the governing entity of the affected jurisdiction. Unfortunately, these government systems are not identically established throughout the United States. The general framework usually involves metropolitan areas (e.g., cities, towns) within a county, which is within a state. However, many "states" are in fact commonwealths, counties may be supplanted by parishes, and some states recognize townships or independent cities not subordinate to surrounding counties.

Thus no single description of local response can be provided that is applicable to all localities. Rather, this chapter will address functional entities and notional organizational structures, processes, and responsibilities; concepts, rather than specifics, will be emphasized.

LOCAL GOVERNANCE

Protection, prevention, and response to emergencies and disasters are well-recognized government responsibilities. Depending on a number of factors, local jurisdictions either have systems in place for emergency response or band together with neighboring communities to provide overall emergency management to a larger constituency. Certainly, jurisdictions with substantial populations tend to establish discrete offices, referred to herein as emergency management offices, to provide coordination for prevention, mitigation, planning, and response functions.

However, even in those discrete jurisdictional areas, there might be multiple government entities involved that provide similar services. Law enforcement is but one example. Cities usually have a discrete police department, with the chief of police reporting to the city governing entity (e.g., mayor, city council). However, if that city is within a recognized county, certain law enforcement responsibilities, even within city limits, may fall to the county sheriff's office, and state police might be tasked with other or overlapping duties. The city might also harbor a local Federal Bureau of Investigation (FBI) office with federal law enforcement and investigatory responsibilities, and should that community include ports of ingress, or abut an international border,

other federal law enforcement entities, such as U.S. Customs and Border Protection or U.S. Citizenship and Immigration Services, may have certain authorities within the jurisdiction.

Responsibilities become even more confusing when applied to public health and medical services. All states have a division or department of public health that usually falls within the executive branch of the state government. A public health infrastructure, which may contain regional, county, district, and city public health offices, usually exists. Members of the public health organization are usually state employees. Medical care, on the other hand, may fall within the responsibilities of a variety of organizations. There are very few public health hospitals left in the United States, and most inpatient care is provided through private, for-profit and not-for-profit, hospitals that do not limit their services to discrete jurisdictional boundaries. There are, however, many veterans and military hospitals in communities throughout the country, and these facilities could be either affected by local disasters, or have resources that could, under the right circumstances, be available to assist in response. Physician offices and independent clinics outside of any one hospital's organization are common in all communities. Increasingly, freestanding laboratories, diagnostic centers, and other health care services also exist that are not part of larger health care systems, but they do form part of the health care network. Emergency medical services (EMS) and emergency ambulance services may be provided by fire services, discrete government entities, hospitals, or contracted providers, and multiple EMS providers may support individual or multiple jurisdictions. EMS (and fire services) may be agencies with paid career staff, volunteer groups, or composites. Statewide, EMS may fall within the public health department, emergency management agency, or another state organizational construct. In addition to EMS, many jurisdictions also have private ambulance transport services with licensed or credentialed emergency medical technicians (EMTs).

Under the paradigm of the National Response Framework (NRF), there are 15 essential functions that potentially are required in the event of a disaster.[1] In the case of federal support, a discrete federal agency or organization has been identified as the primary coordinating entity for providing each functional area support to state and local governments. (Note that several states have additional, state-level essential functions beyond these 15.) These 15 essential functions, with the usual local entity responsible for their provision, are outlined in Table 15-1. What is most important is not the specific organization, because this may vary with the jurisdiction, but that, at the local level, some organization or entity has been (or should be) assigned the principal coordinating responsibility and has the necessary resources (material, manpower, and economic) to provide for the reestablishment and maintenance of these services under emergency conditions or has the processes and framework to request, acquire, and incorporate outside resources into this functional organization.

TABLE 15-1	**Community Essential Functions**
FUNCTION	**RESPONSIBLE ORGANIZATION**
Transportation	Public works department
Communications	*
Public works	Public works department
Firefighting	Fire and emergency services department
Emergency management	Local emergency management agency
Mass care	*
Public health and medical	Jurisdictional public health department
Resource support	Various
Urban search and rescue	Fire and emergency services department
Oil spills and HazMat	Fire and emergency services department
Agriculture and natural resources	*
Energy	*
Public safety and security	Jurisdictional law enforcement organizations
Recovery and mitigation	Various
External communications	Area emergency warning agency

*This function is not typically a responsibility of a local jurisdictional office or entity or is not provided by government.
Adapted from National Response Framework, 2nd Edition. Department of Homeladn Security. May 2013. Available at: http://www.fema.gov/media-library-data/20130726-1914-25045-1246/final_national_response_framework_20130501.pdf. Last checked 1/18/2014.

Perusal of Table 15-1 will make it clear that not only are multiple, disparate local government agencies and organizations crucial to emergency management, but that participation may be necessary with non-government and industry organizations if the response is to be fully effective. Power, light, and natural gas resources and services are provided almost exclusively by private corporations. Crucial communications with the public will entail cooperation by local news media organizations and telecommunications corporations.

SUPPORTING ORGANIZATIONS AND CAPABILITIES

It is clear from the discussion above that a full accounting of all local resources is imperative during preparation and planning for emergency response. The most common forum in which this occurs is through local emergency preparedness committees (LEPCs). LEPCs and state emergency response commissions (SERCs) are mandated by the Emergency Planning and Community Right-to-Know Act.[2] The act requires each state to set up an SERC.[3] All 50 states and the U.S. territories and possessions have established these commissions. Indian tribes have the option to function as an independent SERC or as part of the state SERC in the state in which the tribe is located. This can at times present complications, in that certain tribal lands fall within more than one state.

In some states, the SERCs have been formed from existing organizations, such as state environmental, emergency management, transportation, or public health agencies. In others, they are new organizations with representatives from public agencies and departments and various private groups and associations.

Duties of SERCs include the following:
- Establishing local emergency planning districts
- Coordinating activities of the LEPCs
- Reviewing local emergency response plans
- Monitoring legislation and information management concerning hazardous materials
- Maintaining situational awareness of locations of all major quantities of defined toxic industrial materials

- Establishing procedures for receiving and processing public requests for information collected under the Emergency Planning and Community Right-to-Know Act
- Taking civil action against facility owners or operators who fail to comply with reporting requirements

LEPCs normally include elected officials and representatives of law enforcement, civil defense, fire services, EMS, public health, local transportation agencies, communications and media organizations, facilities involved with the handling of toxic industrial materials, and the medical community.[4] Others from the public at large may also be included. The primary responsibility of an LEPC is to plan, prepare for, and respond to chemical emergencies. LEPCs must identify and locate all hazardous materials, develop procedures for immediate response to a chemical accident, establish ways to notify the public about actions they must take, coordinate with corporations and plants that harbor toxic industrial materials, and schedule and test response plans. An LEPC also receives emergency releases and hazardous chemical inventory information submitted by local facilities and must make this information available to the public. An LEPC serves as a focal point in the community for information and discussions about hazardous substances, emergency planning, and health and environmental risks.

LOCAL RESOURCES

The Metropolitan Medical Response System (MMRS) Program was established under federal auspices in the late 1990s. One of the many goals of the MMRS Program is to coalesce all potential public health and medical response capabilities into collaborative functional areas.[5] In the case of health and medical support, this extends far beyond the traditional boundaries of EMS, hospital-based care, and local-jurisdiction public health. Under the MMRS paradigm, one or multiple jurisdictions could join together to optimize the use of resources along a more regional approach, to the benefit of all. The ability of all functional elements of response to surge capabilities and capacity in reaction to an emergency cannot be overemphasized. Failure of complementary surge in even one sector can result in bottlenecks and lack of optimal response across the spectrum.[6]

In addition to traditional entities and organizations, there is a wealth of additional resources that could be brought to bear in the event of a public health emergency or other disaster with significant health effects. These range from private organizations, corporations, and other business ventures to the recruitment of appropriate volunteers, either from volunteer organizations or the public at large. A partial listing of these other medical or paramedical resources is included in Box 15-1. Important in local planning are the recruiting, training, and cataloging of all potential participatory organizations, entities, and individuals; cooperative planning on best use of these resources; and the training of these individuals and organizations to produce a cohesive response organization. Convergent volunteerism is an important adjunct to area emergency managers, but planning for utilization of these resources is a necessity for their optimal use.[7] Indeed, uncoordinated and uncontrolled convergent volunteerism can lead to casualties among the volunteers themselves.

One organization of particular note is the National Voluntary Organizations Active in Disaster (NVOAD).[8] NVOAD coordinates efforts by many organizations responding to disaster. These organizations provide more effective service with less duplication by getting together before disasters strike. This cooperative effort has proven to be the most effective way for a wide variety of volunteers and organizations to work together in a disaster.

An initiative recently sponsored by the U.S. Department of Health and Human Services (DHHS), through the Office of the Surgeon General, is the Medical Reserve Corps (MRC).[9] The mission of the MRC program is to establish teams of local volunteer medical and public health professionals who can contribute their skills and expertise throughout the year as well as during times of crisis. The MRC program office functions as a clearinghouse for community information and "best practices."

MRC units are made of locally based medical and public health volunteers who can assist their communities during emergencies, such as an influenza epidemic, a chemical spill, or an act of terrorism. MRC units are community based and function as a specialized component of Citizen Corps, a national network of volunteers dedicated to making sure their families, homes, and communities are safe from terrorism, crime, and disasters of all kinds. Citizen Corps, AmeriCorps, Senior Corps, and the Peace Corps are all part of the U.S.A. Freedom Corps, which promotes volunteerism and service throughout the United States.

LOCAL RESPONSE CONCEPTS OF OPERATIONS

Because no two disasters are identical, the actual concepts of operations during response will vary depending on the circumstances. There are,

however, some basic concepts that will affect operations; these basics should be well appreciated by emergency managers and planners.

Community Warning

The ability of the community to be prepared for the disaster is predicated on adequate forewarning of the impending event. Unfortunately, many disasters do not lend themselves to early detection by any form of sensor, or analysis has not reached the point that actions may be appropriately taken. It is well documented in the literature that false warnings actually impede future community actions, a classic example of "the boy crying wolf" once too often.

Most warnings are issued by government agencies. Most dissemination and distribution systems are owned and operated by private companies, and effective public-private partnerships are required. Great strides are taking place in threat detection and warning communications technology. Warnings are becoming much more useful to society as lead time and reliability are improved.

To be effective, warnings should reach, in a timely fashion, every person at risk and only those persons at risk, no matter what they are doing or where they are located. There is a window of opportunity to capture peoples' attention and encourage appropriate action. Appropriate response to warning is most likely to occur when people have been educated about the hazard and have developed a plan of action well before the warning. Warnings must be issued in ways that are understood by the many different people within our diverse society. A single, consistent, easily understood terminology should be used, which may need to be conveyed in several languages in certain communities. If warnings are not followed by the anticipated event, people are likely to disable the warning device.

Examples of failed or ineffective warnings include the following:
- *Alabama, March 27, 1994:* A tornado killed 20 worshipers at a church service. A warning had been issued 12 minutes before the tornado struck the church. Although it was broadcast over electronic media, the warning was not received by anyone in or near the church.
- *Florida, February 22-23, 1998:* Tornadoes killed 42. The National Weather Service issued 14 tornado warnings. The warnings were not widely received because people were asleep.
- *South Dakota, May 31, 1998:* A tornado killed six. Sirens failed because the storm had knocked out power.

A variety of warning devices should be used to reach people according to the activity in which they are engaged. Effective warning systems should also have redundancy.

Response Scene Operations

The immediate concern of response organizations is the preservation of life. This not only includes actions directed at victims of the disaster—search and rescue, extrication, triage, scene treatment, transportation, and definitive treatment and rehabilitation—but also at preventing further risks to the community through containment of the disaster.

The disaster must be contained. This is relatively easy to envision in the case of a spreading hazardous materials incident, but the concept applies to any disaster. Containment can be both geographic (erecting levees for flood protection) or can be internal to the disaster area. These types of actions actually represent secondary or compound disasters. In the case of a progressive communicable disease outbreak (e.g., measles, influenza, or smallpox), containment of disease spread is the principal goal of public health. Failure to contain the disaster early on will result in significantly greater losses of life and economic resources.

All the actions one would think of to rescue and treat individuals directly affected by the disaster must take priority over salvage and property protection operations. Sequentially, these actions include the following:

- *Search and rescue:* In a hazardous materials (HazMat) environment, up to an hour may pass before HazMat teams even arrive and enter the "hot zone." Thus those minimally injured may self-extract and seek treatment well before those most severely injured, resulting in a bimodal presentation to area hospitals.
- *Triage of victims:* This must be done at multiple stages of the operations. Classic triage is based on trauma, and this form of triage may not be the best for victims of chemical or biological incidents. Although most communities continue to use the simple triage and rapid treatment (START) methodology, a recent study indicates that other triage systems may be more accurate in predicting morbidity and mortality.[10]
- *Decontamination, especially in known HazMat incidents:* A study conducted several years ago revealed that only 18% of victims of HazMat incidents who were treated at hospitals underwent decontamination before arrival.[11] In the 1995 sarin attack in Tokyo, nearly 600 patients arrived at St. Luke's Hospital within the first 45 minutes of the incident. None had been decontaminated (fortunately most did not require this). Still, a number of hospital personnel developed nerve agent exposure symptoms from treating and evaluating the victims.
- *On-scene treatment of victims:* The majority of minimally injured victims do not stay at the scene long enough to receive prehospital triage and treatment. Those who remain on the scene are usually the most severely injured and are unable to escape the scene before the arrival of rescue assets. Also of interest, however, is that several studies have recently called into question the efficacy of victims waiting for responders.[12] In one study, the morbidity and mortality of those who waited for EMS agencies were significantly higher than for those who were transported to community hospitals by the most expeditious method available.
- *Transportation of victims:* This is also more complicated in a disaster situation. Although the nearest hospital might be the best equipped, if it has already been overwhelmed by the arrival of other critically ill victims, EMS will need to invoke "first-wave" protocols.[13] This occurs when the most critically ill patients are distributed among potential receiving hospitals with little regard of proximity.
- *Retriage of victims and receiving fixed-site medical treatment facilities:* Procedures and policies must be in place to handle this sudden surge of victims while still tending to already anticipated patients not involved in the mass casualty incident.

First responders will be overwhelmed in a true mass casualty incident. As mentioned, most first responders and EMS personnel have been trained in the START algorithm.[14] This algorithm, which assesses mental status, respiratory effort, and peripheral perfusion, can be performed in as little as 30 seconds and allows only minimal treatment: repositioning of the head to decrease airway resistance and bandaging of gross hemorrhage.

Ambulance and vehicle control at the scene are important considerations. In the 1979 Avianca plane crash on Long Island, so many rescue vehicles arrived unsolicited that departing vehicles could not get on the one-lane road that provided the sole ground access to the scene. All arriving vehicles should be sent to staging areas out of the way, with at least one staff member remaining with the vehicle at all times.

Contaminated vehicles pose a risk to both patients and staff as a result of residual contamination or off-gassing from patients in the confined treatment compartment. In general, patients whose conditions are stable should undergo full decontamination at the scene before transportation. Patients whose conditions are unstable may undergo gross decontamination, which may entail removal of clothing only, and be placed in nonporous patient wraps for transport. Once a vehicle

is used for a potentially contaminated patient, it should be considered contaminated until fully cleaned inside and out.

Receiving Facility Considerations

Receiving facilities must have capabilities to decontaminate potential patients and should have sufficient space to maintain these patients for a period, even if the patients are to be transferred elsewhere eventually.

First-wave protocols should be developed in communities with multiple hospitals. A first-wave protocol matches hospital resources with total victim requirements. It does a victim little good to be taken to a facility already overrun with critical patients merely because it is the nearest hospital, while other facilities that are slightly farther away remain empty. Distribution of victims throughout the entire hospital system will do the most good for the most number of patients, and this may be considered a form of transportation triage.

During planning, treatment facilities must determine how to rapidly expand their services for a surge of patients. This entails increasing staff through recall, expedient credentialing of volunteers, canceling elective procedures, and premature discharge of patients whose conditions are stable. It also means that additional bed space should be made available by using, for example, cots, litters, cafeterias, other open spaces, and same-day surgery clinics. Although, historically, few hospitals have suffered supply shortages in disasters in the United States, some caches should be available to handle the disaster until outside resources arrive.

Above all, facilities must be protected. If a facility becomes contaminated, it threatens its entire function. Facilities should have methods for expedient collective protection and must have security personnel available for access control.

Public Welfare Issues

In a disaster that involves large geographic areas, people will be displaced. Depending on the location, the socioeconomic status of the community, the type of disaster, and adequacy of the warning (that was heeded by the population), this may or may not be a problem.

- *Shelter:* Evacuees responding to hurricane warnings on the East Coast generally travel inland and stay with friends or relatives over a larger geographic area, where the impact of the surge population is not felt as greatly. Still, those who have not evacuated, or those without family support, may be forced into shelters.
- *Health care:* It must be remembered that a displaced population has additional needs due to the recent stressors, but individuals within this cohort may also have special needs in and of themselves, especially if residents of nursing homes or rehabilitation centers or significant numbers of chronically ill patients are part of the displaced population. As a group, those evacuees who arrive at shelters may have significant health conditions, many exacerbated by the evacuation.[15]
- *Family assistance programs:* These programs become important very early in a disaster. People from outside the region want to know that their loved ones are safe. Families get separated during the disaster, and relocation is an important issue. Bereavement programs for survivors must be ready for implementation during this period.

ISSUES IN LOCAL RESPONSE

There are a number of crosscut issues and functions that affect all phases of emergency response, including the following:

- The establishment and manning of emergency operations centers and command posts
- Effective unified or incident command systems operations

- Intraagency and interagency communications
- Effective resource management, both material resources and manpower
- The ability of different sectors of the response to rapidly and seamlessly integrate with outside agencies, whether locally through memoranda of understanding or through activation of state or federal emergency response plans
- The media, who will arrive almost immediately and demand information (effective media relations will pay off during after-action reviews; at the same time, the public will want information and may need both information and direction)
- Forensic issues in disasters caused by criminal or terrorist acts, as crime scene investigators and consequence management agencies work together
- Legal issues, ranging from the application of Occupational Safety and Health Administration standards to liability issues
- Law enforcement issues, depending on the particular disaster and the community's response to it, such as crowd control, vandalism protection, and other law enforcement agency functions beyond crime scene investigation

SUMMARY

Local response to disasters is where the rubber meets the road. Effective planning, preparation, and response entails identification and cataloging of all available resources, education and training of personnel from disparate organizations, and a response structure that allows seamless integration of these assets.

REFERENCES

1. U.S. Department of Homeland Security. *National Response Plan.* Available at: http://www.fema.gov/media-library-data/20130726-1914-25045-1246/final_national_response_framework_20130501.pdf. Last Accessed 18.01.15.
2. U.S. Environmental Protection Agency. *Emergency Planning and Community Right to Know Act, 42 USC 11001 et seq;* 1986. http://www2.epa.gov/laws-regulations/summary-emergency-planning-community-right-know-act. Last Accessed 18.01.15.
3. State Emergency Response Commission. Available at: http://www2.epa.gov/epcra/state-emergency-response-commissions. Last Accessed 18.01.15.
4. U.S. Environmental Protection Agency. *Local Emergency Planning Committee (LEPC) Database.* Available at: http://www2.epa.gov/epcra/epcra-sections-311-312. Last Accessed 18.01.15.
5. Metropolitan Medical Response System. Available at: https://www.fema.gov/fy-2011-homeland-security-grant-program. Last Accessed 18.01.15.
6. Hick JL, Hanfling D, Burstein JL, et al. Health care facility and community strategies for patient care surge capacity. *Ann Emerg Med.* 2004;44(3):253–261.
7. Cone DC, Weir SD, Bogucki S. Convergent volunteerism. *Ann Emerg Med.* 2003;42(6):847.
8. National Voluntary Organizations Active in Disaster. Available at: http://www.nvoad.org/. Last Accessed 18.01.15.
9. Medical Reserve Corps. Available at: https://www.medicalreservecorps.gov/HomePage. Last Accessed 18.01.15.
10. Cross KP, Cicero MX. Head-to-head comparison of disaster triage methods in pediatric, adult, and geriatric patients. *Ann Emerg Med.* 2013;61(6):668–676.
11. Okumura T, Ninomiya N, Ohta M. The chemical disaster response system in Japan. *Prehospital Disaster Med.* 2003;18(3):189–192.
12. Demetriades D, Chan L, Cornwell E, et al. Paramedic vs private transportation of trauma patients. Effect on outcome. *Arch Surg.* 1996;131(2):133–138.
13. Auf der Heide E. *Disaster Response: Principles of Preparation and Coordination.* St. Louis: Mosby; 1989.
14. Bozeman WP. Mass casualty incident triage. *Ann Emerg Med.* 2003;41(4):582–583.
15. Greenough PG, et al. Burden of disease and health status among Hurricane Katrina-displaced persons in shelters: a population-based cluster sample. *Ann Emerg Med.* 2008;51(4):426–432.

CHAPTER 16

State Disaster Response: Systems and Programs

Gregory T. Banner

This chapter outlines key points in understanding state-level emergency response functions within the United States, focusing on medical and public health operations. Emergency response systems vary from country to country. As compared to other countries, the United States, because of its federalist system, has more power delegated to lower levels of government and has less of a formally structured system directed from the national level. This form of government has certain advantages in that it empowers state and local governments, but it also has disadvantages because of the challenges in creating integrated systems across and among the states. In practice and law, many responsibilities and authorities for emergency management reside with the states. Nonetheless, a number of federal statutes, regulations, and systems provide a common framework on which states build their emergency management programs; there are more similarities than differences in state and local governmental structures, and federal funding and training have driven common practices that translate well between the states.

STATE AND LOCAL EMERGENCY MANAGEMENT ORGANIZATION

State and local emergency management, as with other governmental functions, usually falls within the authorities of the executive branch of government, and elected leaders (mayors or governors) are statutorily responsible for effective emergency preparedness and response.[1] There is usually a designated office or agency, within state or substate jurisdictional areas, responsible for specific emergency management duties. At lower jurisdictional levels, these duties may often be collateral and performed by volunteer or part-time staff; at higher levels, these become full-time responsibilities. A great part of local emergency management responsibilities involves coordination among first-response organizations, such as police departments, fire and emergency services, and emergency medical service(s) (EMS) organizations, all of which routinely practice "emergency management" while they respond to the scenes of local incidents. At the state level, this coordination occurs among such organizations as the State Department of Health, Highway Patrol, and Transportation and Safety. Throughout the country, there is a robust capability for local scene management, which can be augmented if needed by additional support from higher levels of government. Because coordination and management become more complex, the higher the level of government, there is likewise more variability at higher levels.

At the state level, there are commonly separate Homeland Security and emergency management agencies. The State National Guard also has a significant role in emergency response. These three organizations provide overlapping leadership for emergency management activities. Homeland Security offices generally address the broader political, law enforcement, and security issues involved in the prevention and investigation of human-made events. Emergency management offices may be subordinate, but, usually, they are separate and they focus on all-hazard planning, consequence management during and after a disaster, and recovery and mitigation operations. The National Guard usually has the most robust state-level resources (material and personnel) for emergency response operations. National Guard units can be mobilized by the governor, and they possess a wide variety of useful equipment and skills. These key state offices may be organized differently, or they may have different relationships, but even if structurally not aligned, they often work very closely with one another. In some states, all three organizations are subordinate to one secretary or assistant secretary who in turn reports directly to the governor. Other state-directed but related functions might also interact and have significant effects on emergency management activities. These include the state police, prison system, statewide 911 systems, and sheriff departments. Regardless of the organizations and structures involved, the State Emergency Management Agency (SEMA) is the focal point for planning and organizing emergency management within the state. An Internet search of state governments will often show the organizational structures involved with emergency management, most of which provide preparedness and planning links, tools, and products. The largest cities in the United States (e.g., New York City, Chicago, and San Antonio) often have large emergency management agency (EMA) staffs, programs, and capabilities equal to those of some states.

One of the key challenges facing every state or local EMA is the plethora of offices and partners that it must try to organize, for both planning and operations, organizations over which, for the most part, the EMA has no authority. The lack of a day-to-day system that provides a clear management structure results in challenges in planning for, or responding to, emergencies. At the state level, these stakeholder organizations include other state agencies, nongovernmental organizations (NGOs), and critical private industry (such as the entire private health care system). Below the state level, the complexity is in the different organizational structures, which account for all the important collaborates—hospitals, utility companies, local chapter of the American Red Cross, etc. In most cases, there will be different fire districts, police districts, school districts, and health districts, and each may have different jurisdictional or catchment boundaries. In some states, there are sometimes no intermediate jurisdictional levels between the state and communities, meaning that the only local EMA partners the state may have are the hundreds of community EMAs—an obvious span of control problem.

The solution to all these organizational issues is to build partnerships and response structures to coordinate across the various stakeholder offices. In many cases, the states have deliberately created regional command and control offices to subdivide their territory.

For example, New York is divided into five Emergency Management Regions.[2] A state often uses these subordinate structures to deliver grant funding, which incentivizes local consensus building and cooperation. To understand the local structure, it is usually a matter of understanding the partnerships in the area more so than the individual agencies or offices.

State EMAs operate with a day-to-day staff working on key issues, such as grants, mitigation programs, plans development, communications, and training. There are a variety of programs and funding streams, from federal sources and those internal to the states, which coalesce at the EMA from where they are then distributed to partners and local agencies. The primary focus of the state EMA is to prepare state and local response organizations to be rapidly notified, activated, and mobilized to respond to all emergencies. For actual contingencies and response, emergency operations plans (EOPs) have been put into writing, detailing the most critical information and procedures for the jurisdiction. All states have EOPs, and these are usually aligned to the National Response Framework.[3]

All of the EMAs are heavily involved in emergency response training, using both local and national programs. These range from individual courses to large training events for organizations and response units. The Minnesota Homeland Security and Emergency Management website shows an example of their training opportunities.[4]

Once an emergency or disaster has occurred, and often even prior to the event (as in the case of hurricanes, tornados, or other extreme weather) the State EMA, operating out of an emergency operations center (EOC), takes the lead in managing state response. The state EOC serves as the conduit for coordinating outside assets from the federal government, other states, or mutual aid within the state. One of the key tools used by the states is their participation in the Emergency Management Assistance Compact (EMAC). EMAC is the system of mutual aid between the states for any assets that they would lend during emergencies, including their National Guard. This important program is activated every year across the country.[5]

The states generally parallel federal organization in that they assign state agencies as the lead for specific functions, which are typically called Emergency Support Functions (ESFs). Sometimes at the state level, these are renamed State Support Functions (SSFs). ESF/SSF8, for example, usually performs the function concerned with public health and medical issues. Some states have additional SSFs addressing unique or frequent challenges within the state.[6]

STATE DEPARTMENTS OF HEALTH AND HEALTH FUNCTIONS

State health department programs are similar to those of state EMAs in terms of complexity and organizational challenges. Subordinate structures include a variety of public health programs, private partnerships, and nongovernmental organizations. Almost every state health department has created a specific office to plan for and manage emergency operations. This office must coordinate internally (e.g., epidemiology, labs, public information, community health, water and food programs, and radiation control), with other state agencies (e.g., offices of the medical examiner, mental health services, and veterinary services) and with the private medical system. In general, all of the states have developed ways to create state-level cooperative functions and regional partnerships to manage both planning and operational issues across the entire jurisdiction.[7] This would include having in place effective management structures and operational plans for dealing with emergencies of all types, either public health emergencies, specifically, or in support of broader emergencies with significant health and medical components. As with other emergency management partners, the health departments

analyze issues within their functional area and then develop plans, conduct training, and run exercises to address these issues.

There are two major funding mechanisms in the United States that support the majority of the state's health emergency programs: both under the U.S. Department of Health and Human Services (US DHHS). Under the structure of the National Response Framework, the US DHHS is the federal agency responsible for public health and medical planning and response,[8] and it manages or implements most of the applicable programs at that level. The two important programs are the Public Health Emergency Preparedness (PHEP) grant program, managed by the Centers for Disease Control and Prevention (CDC) (one of the many subordinate agencies of the US DHHS)[9]; and the Hospital Preparedness Program (HPP) grant program, through the Office of the Assistant Secretary for Preparedness and Response, US DHHS.[10] The CDC PHEP program generally focuses on public health programs, health staff, and emergency management operations, as well as some specific operational programs such as the Strategic National Stockpile. The HPP grant program focuses on facility activities, mainly but not limited to hospitals. At the state level, both of these programs typically are managed within the state Health Department Emergency Planning Office. These offices work with local partners to determine how to redistribute funds and manage regional/local activities within the state.

SPECIFIC PUBLIC HEALTH AND MEDICAL PROGRAMS

Within the states, because of common practice and available federal funding, there are certain key programs, typically using the same names across the country, which help provide the core of many activities and plans.

The Health Alert Network (HAN) provides health information to partners on emergency management health issues at both national and state level.[11] The national system transmits information to state partners; internally the states have created a variety of systems to communicate this information to stakeholders at the state or substate levels. Very often these systems are web/E-mail based, with links to text messaging, etc., and individual clinicians/offices can (should) sign up to receive the information provided.

The Strategic National Stockpile (SNS) is the major national medical emergency supply system in the country. It was created initially with the realization that it was cost-prohibitive and logistically very difficult for any locality to maintain its own stockpiles of critical medications (mainly antibiotics) to deal with large bioterrorism events. For that reason, the federal government took on the responsibility to maintain appropriate stockpiles of key medications, along with a rapid delivery system to get these anywhere in the country. The federal government will deliver the needed items, but it is up to the state to distribute them within their geographic area. Within the health departments, every state has an office dedicated to this emergency distribution function, and this includes a variety of mechanisms and partners to accomplish the mission rapidly. It is a huge logistical challenge and very complex work, with detailed and continuous planning required. Although initially focused on antibiotics, the SNS has expanded to include almost anything in the realm of medical logistics. In addition to strategically located "push packages," contracts with vendors have been established for "managed inventories." Many states also have "chempacks," which are caches of antidotes and other supplies used to treat victims of chemical events.[12]

The Laboratory Response Network (LRN) is managed by the CDC, and it links together the laboratory system in the country, in particular those that have received federal funding to be able to identify agents/diseases of interest rapidly.[13] These laboratories routinely work with law enforcement to support not only clinical but also investigative needs of any analysis.

The Medical Reserve Corps (MRC) is a national system that has supported the development, training, and use of local teams of volunteers to support medical emergency response. There are MRC units throughout the country, and they fill a number of needs through coordination with state and local health authorities.[14]

As part of normal operations, the state health departments create a number of local coalitions, such as with hospitals, the ambulance system, clinicians, pharmacies, or other specialized groups. These are planning groups that are also usually tied into the health departments' emergency response and management systems.

EMERGENCY FUNCTIONS

Once an emergency is recognized, state and local emergency management offices first respond by activating their EOCs. This is also done for planned activities, which may require coordination among public safety agencies (large parades, athletic events, political events, etc.). The Incident Command System (ICS) has emerged as the predominant management system for organizing at all levels, from the scene up to national command centers. As ICS is flexible, every location might use different pieces of the structure and different tools/forms/reports, but, in general, many common terms and concepts will be used. A network of activated EOCs will serve to divide responsibilities geographically and to manage information (up and down) and resources/requests. Any activated EOC will have a command element and a staff structure that organizes functions such as operations, plans, logistics, and administration/finance, as well as bringing in key partners. A Joint Information Center (JIC) may be organized to centralize public information and media relations. The elected officials at each level have the statutory responsibility for their jurisdictions and, therefore, take leadership roles, often becoming the public face of the response. These officials will often work out of their EOCs, monitoring events and making key decisions as necessary. State EOCs are typically purpose-built facilities with workspace, communications, and support assets, most often colocated with the state EMA offices.

Information management is a key part of any response, as well as one of the great challenges facing emergency managers. The states and national government have invested heavily in better ways to communicate with each other during activations. The tools available include satellite phones, radios, conventional telephone systems, computers, and other devices, all linked by redundant systems. Many offices have network-based systems for organizing requests and information. The goal of these systems is to have a single "common operating picture" at all levels that pulls in all available information and in turn makes it available in a useful form to all who need it.

The public health and medical functions are often critical to any response. The health department will activate its own emergency functions and those of subordinate levels as needed. There will often be a dedicated health EOC separate from the state EOC, usually at the state health department offices. Many agencies will have liaison personnel at the state EOC, but there is not enough space for all of the people needed for every emergency function. Throughout the state, key offices will have their own EOCs, or workers will perform emergency functions from their regular workspace, attending meetings as necessary or reporting as requested. The health department will have staff monitor key sectors, such as facilities, medical logistics, epidemiology, health information operations, fatality management, or medical shelters. The state health departments will most likely also communicate with clinicians and interact with the private medical system providing direct patient care. Common reasons for this communication include managing patient movement, management of supply shortage issues, or addressing facility functions such as power needs. Regulatory issues may need to be addressed to facilitate emergency response.

SUMMARY

Within the states, elected leadership is ultimately responsible for emergency response within their jurisdictions. Even though there are some similarities across all states and jurisdictions, all are different and over time have developed different structures and programs. During routine daily operations, state governments have a number of offices and officials who plan for emergencies and are in the best position to provide the needed leadership when emergencies happen. Taking any organization from day-to-day operations into emergency response is a complex business; the transition is sometimes difficult and can require a few days to accomplish. The logistical challenges can be staggering. States and state health departments, as just one component, have spent considerable time, energy, and money, and their emergency management programs continue to evolve.

REFERENCES

1. "A Governor's Guide to Homeland Security." The National Governor's Association; November 2010. Available at: http://www.nga.org/files/live/sites/NGA/files/pdf/1011GOVGUIDEHS.PDF.
2. New York State Emergency Management Regions. Available at: http://www.dhses.ny.gov/oem/about/index.cfm#OEM-regional-map.
3. Texas State Emergency Management Plan and Annexes. Available at: http://www.txdps.state.tx.us/dem/downloadableforms.htm.
4. Minnesota Homeland Security and Emergency Management training opportunities. Available at: https://dps.mn.gov/divisions/hsem/training/Pages/default.aspx.
5. The Emergency Management Assistance Compact. Available at: http://www.emacweb.org/.
6. National Response Framework. *Emergency Support Function Annexes: Introduction.* 2nd ed. U.S. Department of Homeland Security; May 2013. Available at: http://www.fema.gov/pdf/emergency/nrf/nrf-esf-intro.pdf.
7. U.S. Department of Health and Human Services, Office of the Assistant Secretary for Preparedness and Response. PHE.gov web site listing of state health department emergency offices. Available at: http://www.phe.gov/emergency/connect/Pages/default.aspx#state.
8. National Response Framework. *Emergency Support Function #8 - Public Health and Medical Services Annex.* 2nd ed. U.S. Department of Homeland Security; May 2013. Available at: http://www.fema.gov/pdf/emergency/nrf/nrf-esf-08.pdf.
9. Public Health Emergency Planning Grant. Centers for Disease Control and Prevention, U.S. Department of Health and Human Services. Available at: http://www.cdc.gov/phpr/coopagreement.htm.
10. Hospital Preparedness Program. U.S. Department of Health and Human Services, Office of the Assistant Secretary for Preparedness and Response. Available at: http://www.phe.gov/preparedness/planning/hpp/pages/default.aspx.
11. Health Alert Network Program. Centers for Disease Control and Prevention. Available at: http://emergency.cdc.gov/HAN/.
12. Strategic National Stockpile Program. Centers for Disease Control and Prevention. Available at: http://www.cdc.gov/phpr/stockpile/stockpile.htm.
13. Laboratory Response Network Program. Centers for Disease Control and Prevention. Available at: http://emergency.cdc.gov/lrn/.
14. Medical Reserve Corps Program. U.S. Department of Health and Human Services, Office of the Assistant Secretary for Preparedness and Response. Available at: http://www.phe.gov/Preparedness/planning/abc/Pages/mrc.aspx.

Selected Federal Disaster Response Agencies and Capabilities

Kevin M. Ryan, Jerry L. Mothershead, Kevin Yeskey, and Peter Brewster

Chapter 13 provides a historical account of the evolution of emergency management in America and the basic framework for current concepts of operations. This chapter discusses selected federal response organizations and agencies, supporting programs for state and local emergency managers, and response capabilities. With the near-exponential growth in disaster management capabilities and initiatives that have occurred since the terrorist attacks of 2001, it would be impossible to discuss all of the many federal capabilities to any significant degree. Thus this chapter focuses on the agencies of principal interest to public health, medical emergency managers, and health care professionals.

A more-detailed presentation of current concepts of federal operations is provided, as well as a discussion of some of the more significant issues and challenges facing the federal sector in responding to disasters or catastrophic emergencies of any type.

PRINCIPAL FEDERAL AGENCIES

Although virtually all of the federal executive branch agencies have capabilities and expertise that could be brought to bear in a disaster to save lives, reduce pain and suffering, and otherwise mitigate the effects of these events on the human condition, five stand out as supporting programs that provide the most-direct support in this endeavor:

- U.S. Department of Homeland Security (DHS)
- U.S. Department of Health and Human Services (DHHS)
- U.S. Department of Defense (DoD)
- Department of Veterans Affairs (DVA)
- American Red Cross (ARC)

Department of Homeland Security

The organizational structure and overarching functions of the DHS are described in Chapter 13. Among the many provisions of the Homeland Security Act of 2002, three important programs were initially transferred from DHHS to DHS: the National Disaster Medical System (NDMS), the Strategic National Stockpile (SNS) program, and the Metropolitan Medical Response System (MMRS).[1] Despite restructuring the organizations, after 2004, only the MMRS remains under DHS oversight, although now as part of the Homeland Security Grants Program (HSGP). In addition, even though it maintains many of its autonomous functions, the Federal Emergency Management Agency (FEMA) was transferred into the Emergency Preparedness and Response Directorate of the DHS in 2003 and was subsequently reorganized after Hurricane Katrina in 2006.[2]

Homeland Security Grants Program

As part of Homeland Security's mission of building and sustaining a secure nation, FEMA and DHS oversee the HSGP. The HSGP, reorganized in 2012, incorporates three grant programs, including the State Homeland Security Program (SHSP), Urban Areas Security Initiative (UASI), and Operation Stonegarden to support the five missions of prevention, protection, mitigation, response, and recovery. The Metropolitan Medial Response System, although previously funded as its own entity before 2012, is now incorporated into these three programs. The SHSP has made over $401,000,000 available to all 50 states, the District of Columbia, and territories of the United States, whereas the UASI made over $587,000,000 available to both high-threat and high-density urban areas. Combined, these three programs have provided over $1 billion of funding to implement the National Preparedness System.[3]

Department of Health and Human Services

The DHHS is the federal agency that has the responsibility of protecting the health of the nation and providing essential services to all U.S. citizens. The DHHS has an annual budget of $940.9 billion (2015 fiscal year) and employs more than 76,000 personnel.[4] It administers more than 300 programs in 11 operating divisions and is the parent organization for the Commissioned Corps (CC) of the U.S. Public Health Service (USPHS).

The DHHS has a long history of providing disaster response and preparedness activities both domestically and internationally.[5] The DHHS is the lead federal agency for coordinating the federal health and medical response services (Emergency Support Function #8), as described in the National Response Framework (NRF) (Box 17-1).[6] The Public Health Threats and Emergencies Act of 2002 authorizes the DHHS secretary to take appropriate actions if a public health emergency is determined to exist and to establish a Public Health Emergency Fund.[7] Other statutes authorize the U.S. Surgeon General to make and enforce regulations to "prevent the introduction, transmission, or spread of communicable diseases from foreign countries into States or possessions, or from one State or possession into any other State of possession."[8]

DHHS disaster response and preparedness activities are conducted in the Operating Divisions and the USPHS CC. Coordination is performed at the Office of the Assistant Secretary for Preparedness and Response (ASPR) within DHHS. The DHHS, along with the National Institutes of Health (NIH), also convenes the National Science Advisory Board for Biosecurity, which guides the development of systems for biosecurity-research peer review, guidelines for identification and conduct of research that might require security surveillance, professional code of conduct for scientists and laboratory workers, and materials to educate the research community about biosecurity.

National Disaster Medical System

The NDMS is a public-private partnership between the DHS, FEMA, the DHHS, DoD, DVA, and civilian hospitals and health professionals.

BOX 17-1   Emergency Support Function #8: Public Health and Medical Services

- Assessment of health and medical needs
- Surveillance of health care issues
- Acquisition and distribution of medical care personnel
- Acquisition and distribution of health and medical equipment and supplies
- Patient evacuation
- In-hospital care
- Food, drug, and medical device safety
- Worker health and safety

- Radiological monitoring
- Chemical monitoring
- Biological monitoring
- Mental health assessment
- Development and dissemination of public health information
- Vector control
- Water safety, including wastewater and solid waste disposal
- Victim identification and mortuary services

The NDMS serves two primary functions: it is a backup to military health care operations in the event of overwhelming combat casualties, referred to as the Integrated CONUS (Continental United States) Medical Operations Plan (ICMOP), and it coordinates the provision of national health care resources to casualties resulting from disasters in the United States and its territories.[9] Originally established by Memorandum of Understanding in 1984, the NDMS was codified into law in 2002. There are three components to the NDMS: (1) on-site health care operations, (2) medical evacuation, and (3) definitive care at participating hospitals in unaffected areas. The NDMS may be activated by a presidential declaration of a national emergency. It may also be activated at the direction of the secretaries of the DHS, DHHS, or DoD.

On-site augmentation to local or state health care operations are provided principally through the mobilization of any of the approximately 85 Disaster Medical Assistance Teams (DMATs). The number and capability of DMATs are evolving continually as new teams are being formed and established teams are augmenting their capabilities. Most medical teams are composed of more than 100 physicians, nurses, and allied health care personnel who are sworn in as temporary federal employees and who volunteer their time to prepare and train for emergency operations. In the event of activation, they become federal assets, with attendant liability protection. The majority of DMATs provide general clinical operations either in disaster areas or on scene or as augmentation staff to local hospitals. A number of specialty teams exist, including burn, pediatrics, crush injury, and mental health teams. Four disaster veterinary assistance teams (DVATs) and 10 Disaster Mortuary Operational Response Teams (DMORTs) are also components of the NDMS. One DMORT is specially trained in the handling of contaminated or contagious remains, with three Disaster Portable Morgue Units (DPMUs) staged in the United States to augment DMORT operations. These DPMUs contain a morgue and workstations, as well as prepackaged equipment. There are also three larger National Medical Response Teams–Weapons of Mass Destruction (NMRT-WMD) located in North Carolina, Colorado, and California. These teams are specially equipped and trained to assist local emergency response organizations in the event of terrorist events involving chemical, biological, or radiological substances. When deployed, DMATs are self-sustaining for 3 days and are supported by management support units (MSUs) for resupply.

Medical evacuation operations are coordinated by the DoD.[10] Medical regulation is managed by the Global Patient Movement Requirements Center (GPMRC) at Scott Air Force Base in Illinois. This is the same system used to evacuate military casualties in peacetime or during combat operations worldwide. Actual medical evacuation occurs primarily through the use of fixed-wing U.S. Air Force assets, such as the C-141 Starlifter and the C-17 Globemaster III (each of which can accommodate in excess of 50 litter patients), under the auspices of the Commander, the U.S. Transportation Command (USTRANSCOM). Nontraditional or Commercial Air Carrier (CAC) air evacuation platforms or ground conveyances can also be used, as required. Most DMAT members have training in basic fixed-wing and helicopter operations as they pertain to the evacuation of patients.

Definitive care is provided by the 1600 hospitals that have voluntarily agreed to support NDMS operations. In all, approximately 100,000 beds (including the staff to support them) could be made available throughout the United States. Cooperating hospitals are coordinated through regional federal coordinating centers (FCCs), which are managed by the Veterans Health Administration (VHA) or the military services hospitals.[11]

Strategic National Stockpile

The SNS, originally authorized as the National Pharmaceutical Stockpile Program by Congress in 1998, has as its goal the rapid mobilization and provision of pharmaceuticals and other medical supplies to areas affected by public health emergencies or disasters of any cause. The SNS program has a number of elements, including scientific review, education, training, and technical and logistical support. The primary material components of the SNS are the 12-hour push packages and managed inventory (MI) supplies.[12]

Twelve push packages, preconfigured and under environmental and security safeguards, are strategically placed throughout the United States. They can be deployed to arrive at a suitable airfield nearest to a disaster within 12 hours of release by the secretary of DHS or DHHS. Push packages are large caches that require more than 5000 square feet of storage space that may be transported by air or ground conveyance. Supplies include antibiotics, antiviral agents, and airway and intravenous supplies. Ventilators, stored separately, may be shipped as needed. Vaccines, also stored separately, may be shipped with or without the entire cache. In 2003 regionally placed chemical agent antidotes were established under the CHEMPACK program to provide for more timely arrival. These CHEMPACKs are provided through the SNS program, but are managed by the jurisdictions in which they are placed.

If specific supplies are known to be needed in advance of push package shipment, these may be obtained through MI stocks, which are maintained by pharmaceutical or medical supply corporations that have contracts with the federal government. The MI program was used in the wake of the Anthrax mailings shortly after 9/11. MIs were designed, however, to be follow-on packages of specifically needed supplies to arrive 24 to 36 hours after the push packages.

All states are required to develop and exercise plans for the request, acquisition, storage, staging, distribution, and dispensing of SNS caches to prophylaxis or vaccination centers or area hospitals. Caches will be accompanied by a small team of medical logisticians referred to as technical assistance response units (TARUs).

The Office of the Assistant Secretary for Preparedness and Response

Created under the Pandemic and All-Hazards Preparedness Act of 2006 and reaffirmed in 2013, this office assumed the functions of the

ASPR for Public Health Emergency Preparedness. It provides (1) interface between agencies within the DHHS and other federal departments, agencies, and offices and (2) interface between the DHHS and state and local entities responsible for public health and emergency preparedness. The ASPR ensures that health and medical vulnerabilities are identified and prioritized within the DHHS; that DHHS preparedness programs are coordinated and integrated with other federal programs; and that response activities are coordinated within the DHHS and integrated with other federal, state, and local response.[13] The ASPR also oversees the development of the National Health Security Strategy; released first in 2009, it serves to guide the nation on building community resilience and strengthening and sustaining health and emergency response systems. The office also maintains a scientific group that oversees the development and procurement of all SNS medical countermeasures.

The ASPR works with state and local officials to enhance health and medical preparedness, and it coordinates various federally funded preparedness activities. The DHHS has established guidelines, benchmarks, and competencies to serve as markers of preparedness.

The ASPR also oversees the Biomedical Advanced Research and Development Authority (BARDA) and Project BioShield. These divisions provide an integrated approach to developing medical countermeasures against chemical, biological, radiological, and nuclear threats. As part of the Pandemic and All-Hazards Preparedness Reauthorization Act of 2013, the secretary is permitted to use unapproved products during emergencies and to appropriate funds for security countermeasures of the SNS.

Agency for Healthcare Research and Quality

The Agency for Healthcare Research and Quality's (AHRQ's) mission is to improve the quality, safety, efficiency, and effectiveness of health care by sponsoring, conducting, and disseminating research that relates to the aforementioned mission.[14] The AHRQ has a number of disaster-related functions within the DHHS, with an emphasis on bioterrorism (BT)-related issues. The organization has funded BT-related research, conducted a variety of audio conferences for clinical providers, issued evidence-based practice reports, and distributed issue briefs based on the audio conferences. The AHRQ also provides technical support to the ASPR during responses.

Centers for Disease Control and Prevention

The Centers for Disease Control and Prevention (CDC) is the world's foremost public health organization. It has had significant experience in responding to disasters and public health emergencies globally.[15] It also has a major role in disaster-response mitigation through its leadership in disease-prevention activities. The CDC is the national leader in the areas of epidemic outbreak response, disease surveillance, environmental health, public health laboratory readiness, and public communications. In conjunction with the Agency for Toxic Substances and Disease Registry (ATSDR), the CDC serves as the DHHS lead for infectious disease response, chemical and hazardous materials exposure, vector control, radiological monitoring, and public (risk) communications. Moreover, the CDC has the lead scientific responsibility for the SNS.

CDC epidemiologists and other response-team personnel (usually as part of the Epidemiology Investigative Service, or EIS) deploy in support of public health incidents. These personnel perform case investigations and contact tracing, assist with surveillance, and serve as technical advisors for issues such as vector control. CDC laboratories can perform specialized assays to identify biological and chemical agents from clinical and, in some cases, environmental specimens. The CDC also manages the Laboratory Response Network (LRN), a national network of public health laboratories, each capable of performing sophisticated testing of infectious agents. Participants in the LRN program receive training, protocols, supplies, and a secure reporting system.

Public communications can occur through a variety of CDC venues. The Morbidity and Mortality Monthly Report (MMWR) has long been recognized as a periodical that serves to notify and update professionals about public health investigations and incidents. The CDC also developed two other lines of communication. The Health Alert Network (HAN) and the Epidemiologic Exchange (Epi-X) were developed as web-based communications networks. The HAN is used to distribute information through a widespread open network. The Epi-X is more secure and is directed to epidemiologists and other public health professionals at the federal, state, and local levels. The CDC also conducts provider training through on-site courses and teleconferences.

The CDC maintains a state-of-the-art emergency operations center that serves as the information-gathering center for the agency. It provides 24-hour, daily access for local, state, and federal agencies.

Food and Drug Administration

The Food and Drug Administration's (FDA's) stated public health mission is "assuring the safety, efficacy, and security of human and veterinary drugs, biological products, medical devices, our nation's food supply, cosmetics, and products that emit radiation."[16] The FDA regulates the safety of biological (including the blood supply), cosmetics, drugs (prescription and over-the-counter), foods (except meat and dairy products), medical devices, radiation-emitting electronic products, and veterinary products. The FDA also has the responsibility for animal health as it relates to food safety and security.

The FDA has investigated foodborne outbreaks and medication tampering and has supported DHHS response to domestic disasters. In recent years, the FDA has played a major role in the preparedness activities against terrorism and has organized several new offices to facilitate its activities. The Office of Crisis Management (OCM) coordinates FDA emergency response activities. The Office of Emergency Operations within the OCM coordinates FDA field and headquarters activities and maintains the FDA emergency operations center.

The FDA maintains expertise to assist in areas of food safety, including the production, processing, storage, and holding of domestic and imported foods. It has worked with other federal agencies to implement a national laboratory network capable of responding to a food security incident. The FDA uses field personnel to perform food import examinations at approximately 90 U.S. ports. It collaborates with U.S. blood banks to ensure the continuous supply of safe blood. It also works with other DHHS agencies and the pharmaceutical industry to help guide the development of new medical countermeasures for BT. New regulations have facilitated the FDA approval process for new products and medical countermeasures. The FDA works with other federal agencies in developing guidance for using the countermeasures in special populations or when there is no FDA-approved product or no approved indication for a marketed product. Devices under investigational new drug (IND) status or investigational device exemption (IDE) applications can be used during an emergency.

Health Resources and Services Administration

The Health Resources and Services Administration's (HRSA's) involvement in disaster response has largely been the issuance of grants to improve hospital BT preparedness. HRSA grants have provided funding through state health departments to address surge capacity, communications, decontamination, and exercises related to hospital operations.[17]

The Federal Occupational Health office is a component of the HRSA that provides clinical services, environmental health services, and employee assistance programs for federal workers. Personnel from this organization have provided postdisaster clinical and counseling services to federal employees at disaster field offices, regional offices, and headquarters.

Indian Health Service

The Indian Health Service (IHS) has provided leadership in addressing disasters affecting the health and medical systems directly associated with tribal nations and reservations.[18] In the Hantavirus outbreak on the Navajo Reservation, IHS medical personnel were active participants in the response. (Hantavirus disease was virtually unknown in the Americas until 1993 when a physician at the IHS in New Mexico reported that two previously healthy young people had died from acute respiratory failure.)[19] In 2007, a syphilis outbreak was first noted by the IHS and reported to the Arizona Department of Health Services, ultimately leading to the identification of 35 cases.[20] Tribal leaders and medical personnel have been actively engaged with their state counterparts in preparing for BT and emergency preparedness. The IHS Office of Urban Indian Health Programs and Office of Public Health Support address public health needs associated with disease outbreaks, as well as emergency preparedness. IHS personnel have also been deployed to domestic events.

National Institutes of Health

The NIH's role in the nation's health response system has been parsed out to a variety of its 27 institutes and centers. The NIH mission relates to the stewardship of medical and behavioral research.[21] Its National Institute of Mental Health supports research in the area of response to trauma and violence.[22] The National Institute of Environmental Health Sciences supports research directed at the health consequences of environmental toxins.[23] The NIH also supports and performs research that enhances the understanding of the basic biology and mechanisms of immunological response to particular biological agents. The National Institute of Allergy and Infectious Diseases (NIAID) has the NIH lead on many of these activities and receives substantial funding within the DHHS to accelerate development of new and improved vaccines, diagnostic tools, and therapies against potential agents of BT.[24] The NIH has also been dedicated to the expansion of the medical countermeasures for biological agents of terrorism. The NIAID has created the Integrated Research Facility at Fort Detrick in Maryland to carry out biodefense research especially directed at high-consequence infections. In addition to the research activities, the NIH sponsors regional centers for biodefense research and biocontainment laboratories.

Substance Abuse and Mental Health Services Administration

The Substance Abuse and Mental Health Services Administration (SAMHSA) provides the coordination of federal mental health services for the government. It assists in the assessment of mental health needs and the identification of mental health services that can be provided to those affected by disasters. Moreover, it provides grants to states that assist in training mental health counselors and enhancing mental health response capacity.[25] It also produces publications related to planning, preparedness, and the mental health effects of disasters, as well as training manuals for mental health responders. SAMHSA also maintains a technical assistance center that can be accessed by responders.

Commissioned Corps of the U.S. Public Health Service

Headed by the U.S. Surgeon General, the CC consists of more than 6500 commissioned officers who have degrees in health- and medical-related professions.[26] CC officers are distributed among all of the DHHS

Operating Divisions and can be assigned to other federal agencies. The CC serves as the health care corps for the U.S. Coast Guard. CC personnel have responded internationally to a full spectrum of disasters. Two specific units merit discussion: the USPHS DMAT and the CC Readiness Force (CCRF). The USPHS DMAT has been the prototype for all subsequent DMATs and has been one of the most-deployed federal medical response units to domestic disasters. However, in 2006, a tier level of CC response teams were formed and PHS-1 and PHS-2 were renamed RDF (Rapid Deployment Force) 1 and 2. Currently, five RDF teams rotate through a monthly call for incidents.[27] CCRF personnel receive training similar to that of the NDMS response teams and must meet additional requirements beyond those of other USPHS officers.

Department of Veterans Affairs

The DVA is a cabinet-level agency with three primary divisions: the Veterans Benefits Administration, National Cemetery System, and the VHA. The VHA is the largest health care system in the United States. Within its 23 Veterans Integrated Service Networks (VISNs) are more than 150 hospitals, 800 clinics, and 400 additional facilities, such as counseling centers. The VHA employs more than 14,000 physicians and nearly 200,000 other health care professionals. It principally exists to provide medical care to military veterans. VHA also has important roles in medical research and the education of the health care workforce.

The fourth mission of the VHA is that of emergency management.[28] In that capacity it supports medical operations as a backup for DoD (through the Integrated CONUS Medical Operations Plan), as a supporting agency under the NRF, as a partner to the NDMS, and for continuity of governmental operations functions. It also has a unique role in fielding emergency medical response teams for radiological emergencies.

Interagency coordination and policy matters related to emergency management and response reside at the secretary level, but day-to-day management and oversight comes from the VHA Office of Emergency Management (OEM). The OEM is headquartered in Martinsburg, West Virginia. It has a staff of 25 individuals at its headquarters in Martinsburg and Washington, DC, as well as 75 field program staff. These peripheral staff members coordinate all emergency management activities within the VISNs and subordinate facilities.

VHA personnel have deployed to the vast majority of national disasters in the last decade, including the response to the New York City terrorist attack of 2001. These personnel have also provided support to National Security Special Events (NSSE), such as presidential inaugurations and the Olympic Games.[29]

Executive order 12657 places an additional responsibility on the VHA to provide medical response to incidents involving radiological emergencies.[30] The VHA has the 30-member Medical Emergency Radiological Response Team (MERRT), which can arrive at the site of a radiological emergency and is self-sustaining. As such, it is not a first-response organization, but rather, it provides supplemental medical care at hospitals and technical assistance and guidance in decontamination and monitoring. When MERRT is deployed, it is considered a federal resource.

Another initiative within the VHA is the population of the Disaster Emergency Medical Personnel System (DEMPS) database. The DEMPS is a voluntary enrollment of both full-time and retired personnel within the Veterans Affairs (VA). Individuals register in advance of disasters and serve as a pool of personnel to be activated should an event within the VA or elsewhere occur. Current employees must be released by their local facility and VISN before being used to support other requests.

The VHA also has a role in federal disaster cache management. In addition to its role as logistical manager of SNS caches, it maintains caches for its facilities' use, and, by extension, these could be used in community-wide disasters. It also maintains caches for NSSE events, as well as a stockpile for response involving disasters that would affect the U.S. Congress.

The VHA has its greatest role in local emergency management. The VHA operates the majority of the NDMS FCCs. VHA hospitals are also charged with assisting local community health care resources in their preparedness and planning. Finally, as part of the community health care network, VHA resources would be automatically drawn into the response to a local disaster, as in Houston, Texas, in 2000, when VHA facilities accepted transferred patients from area civilian hospitals incapacitated as the result of flooding caused by Tropical Storm Allison.

Department of Defense

The DoD is identified as a support agency for nearly all of the 15 Emergency Support Functions identified in the NRF. Its component services have large amounts of material and personnel resources that could be brought to bear in response to a disaster, anywhere in the world. The Army Civil Affairs branch (primarily found in the Reserves component) even has expertise in governmental function reestablishment. In addition to the active duty component, the DoD can call on Reserve forces of all of the services, and, under certain circumstances, can federalize Army and Air Force National Guard personnel as part of its military response. To chronicle all of the many assets would far exceed the scope of this chapter.

DoD support to federal, state, or local emergency managers is governed by a number of statutes and executive orders, collectively referred to as "Military Support to Civil Authorities" (MSCA).[31] General guidance for the use of MSCA includes the following:

- Civil resources are applied first.
- DoD resources are provided only when requirements are beyond the capabilities of civil authorities.
- Specialized DoD capabilities requested for MSCA are used efficiently.
- Military operations other than MSCA will have priority over MSCA.
- National Guard forces that are not in federal service have primary responsibility for providing military assistance to state and local government agencies in civil emergencies.
- DoD and the military services will not procure or maintain any supplies, material, or equipment exclusively for providing MSCA.
- In general, DoD resources will not be used for law enforcement or intelligence-gathering functions.

Imminently serious conditions resulting from any civil emergency or attack may require immediate action by military commanders to save lives, prevent human suffering, or mitigate great property damage. When such conditions exist and time does not permit prior approval from higher headquarters, local military commanders are authorized to take necessary action to respond to requests of civil authorities. This is commonly referred to as "Immediate Response."

Under the MSCA doctrine, and in line with the NRF, requests for military support are submitted by lead federal agencies (LFAs) through FEMA to the Joint Director of Military Support (JDOMS) on the Joint Chiefs of Staff. The JDOMS has the authority to task Unified Combatant Commanders, services, and defense agencies to provide MSCA support for presidentially declared disasters and emergencies. The JDOMS validates requests for military assistance from LFAs and plans, coordinates, and executes DoD civil support activities. The JDOMS controls a joint staff to conduct operations during declared disasters.

Operationally, MSCA is directed through the U.S. Northern Command (USNORTHCOM) in Colorado Springs, Colorado, through a standing Joint Task Force-Civil Support (JTF-CS).[32] The JTF-CS was established specifically for homeland defense missions. The two continental armies of the United States (First Army and Fifth Army) have response task forces that can deploy to the vicinity of the disaster and assume operational control over all military forces assigned to the response. In addition, USNORTHCOM has CBRNE Consequence Management Response Forces (CCMRF), which can deploy as initial response forces for a CBRNE incident.

DoD resources fall into two broad categories: (1) mass resources that can augment similar capabilities in the other federal agencies and (2) unique resources that can provide expertise and technical assistance. Its mass resources of interest to civilian medical planners include the following:

- More than 75 military hospitals and more than 100,000 public health and medical professionals
- Deployable medical platforms, ranging in size from the U.S. Air Force's air transportable Expeditionary Medical Support (which can be expanded up to 25 beds each) to the two U.S. Navy 1000-bed hospital ships
- Significant air assets that can be used to evacuate casualties, as described in the section on the NDMS
- Caches of pharmaceuticals and medical supplies, referred to as wartime stocks, which would only be mobilized for MSCA missions in the most unusual circumstances
- Specialized resources[33] that may be brought to bear in the event of an overwhelming disaster:
- Deployable public health laboratories
- Specially trained response teams, such as the U.S. Army Chemical and Biological Special Medical Augmentation Response Teams (C/B-SMART), the U.S. Navy Special Psychiatric Intervention Teams (SPRINTs), or the U.S. Air Force Radiation Assessment Teams (AFRATs)
- Reach-back expertise capabilities through the U.S. Army Medical Research Institute of Infectious Disease (USAMRIID) and the Medical Research Institute for Chemical Defense (USAMRICD), the Armed Forces Radiobiological Research Institute (AFRRI), or the Armed Forces Institute of Pathology (AFIP)

The DoD is in the process of restructuring the CCMRF model, while further enhancing National Guard capabilities by integrating an in-state response capacity based on the Civil Support Teams, CBRN Emergency Response Force Packages (CERFPs) and the standup of 10 NG Regional Homeland Response Forces (HRFs), one per FEMA region. These geographically distributed HRFs will improve the ability of DoD to respond quickly in case of a major or catastrophic CBRNE CM event by providing the necessary lifesaving capabilities to the incident area within hours versus days. The CERFP teams consist of approximately 186 Soldiers and Airmen. Each team has a command and control section, decontamination element, medical element, casualty search and extraction element, and fatalities search and recovery element.[34]

Other specialized capabilities exist within the DoD because of its combat mission: for example, the Technical Escort Unit (TEU), which is trained and equipped to handle extremely hazardous materials and radiation sources, forms the nidus of the much larger Guardian Brigade, which has specific homeland defense functions. The U.S. Marine Corps includes the Chemical and Biological Incident Response Force (CBIRF), a rapid response unit trained to work in hazardous environment operations, including patient extrication, decontamination, and emergency stabilization and treatment.

American Red Cross

Chartered by Congress in 1905, the Red Cross[35] has as its mission to "carry on a system of national and international relief in time of peace and apply the same in mitigating the sufferings caused by pestilence, famine, fire, floods, and other great national calamities, and to devise and carry on measures for preventing the same." Each year, the ARC responds to more than 70,000 disasters of various sizes and complexities. The ARC is the LFA for the Mass Care Emergency Support Function of the National Response Plan (NRP), and it has supporting roles in the Public Health and Medical Services Emergency Support Function.

The ARC provides shelter, food, and health services, including mental health, to address basic human needs. Family and individual assistance is also given to those affected by disaster to enable them to resume their normal daily activities independently. It also feeds emergency workers, handles inquiries from concerned family members outside of the disaster area, provides blood and blood products to disaster victims, and helps those affected by disaster to access other available resources.

ISSUES IN FEDERAL RESPONSE TO DISASTERS

With its many resources and vast expertise, the U.S. government has the capabilities and capacities to respond effectively to virtually all but the most cataclysmic disasters imaginable. However, a number of issues remain unresolved. Some of these follow:

- Response time—identifying, activating, and mobilizing these resources may take considerable time, and local response agencies should not anticipate significant federal support to be on-site and fully operational for 24 to 48 hours, especially at remote locations or those whose transportation infrastructures (airfields, railways, or highways) have been compromised because of the disaster.
- Identification of appropriate resources—in general, federal resources have been designed for primary functions other than disaster response and relief. Therefore, no two response teams are identical in capabilities. Requests for federal resources must be in the form of a capabilities request, as opposed to a platform, and identifying specific agency resources to meet those requested needs may slow response. Resource typing, through the National Incident Management System (NIMS) seeks to alleviate these issues.
- Command and control—with the exception of forensic and other law enforcement functions in the case of a terrorist event, federal resources are to augment state and local authorities. With numerous response organizations from all levels of government, each operating by its own protocols and procedures, collaboration and integration during high-tempo operations may at times be problematic. Again, the NIMS was designed to alleviate some of the previous problems with command and control.

SUMMARY

The U.S. government, through its many federal agencies, has a wealth of capabilities and the capacity to respond to natural, technological, or terrorist-induced disasters. These resources may be accessed through a process, at the request of local or state civil authorities. Challenges continue in command and control, coordination, and attaining access to these resources in a timely manner.

REFERENCES

1. U.S. Department of Homeland Security. Homeland Security Act of 2002. Available at: https://www.dhs.gov/xlibrary/assets/hr_5005_enr.pdf. Last accessed 6 March 2015
2. Federal Emergency Management Agency. Available at: http://www.fema.gov/about-agency. Last accessed 6 March 2015.
3. Federal Emergency Management Agency. Homeland Security Grant Program. Available at: https://www.fema.gov/fy-2014-homeland-security-grant-program-hsgp. Last accessed 6 March 2015.
4. U.S. Department of Health and Human Services. Available at: http://www.hhs.gov/about/. Last accessed 6 March 2015.
5. Roth P, Gaffney J. The federal response plan and disaster medical assistance teams in domestic disasters. *Emerg Med Clin North Am*. 1996;14(2):371–382.
6. Federal Emergency Management Agency. *Department of Homeland Security National Response Plan*; 2013. Available at: http://www.fema.gov/national-response-framework Last accessed 6 March 2015.
7. Pub L No. 106-505 (The Public Health Threats and Emergencies Act of 2002).
8. USC 42 (The Public Health and Welfare Act, January 2003).
9. U.S. Department of Health and Human Services. National Disaster Medical System. Available at: http://www.phe.gov/Preparedness/responders/ndms/Pages/default.aspx. Last accessed 6 March 2015.
10. Department of Defense Directive 6010.22. National Disaster Medical Systems. Available at: http://www.dtic.mil/whs/directives/corres/pdf/601022p.pdf. Last accessed 6 March 2015.
11. U.S. Department of Homeland Security. National Disaster Medical System. Federal coordinating centers. Available at: http://www.phe.gov/Preparedness/responders/ndms/teams/Pages/recruitment-old.aspx. Last accessed 6 March 2015.
12. Centers for Disease Control and Prevention. Strategic National Stockpile. Available at: http://www.cdc.gov/phpr/stockpile/stockpile.htm. Last accessed 6 March 2015.
13. U.S. Department of Health and Human Services. Office of the Assistant Secretary for Preparedness and Response. Available at: http://www.phe.gov/about/aspr/Pages/default.aspx. Last accessed 6 March 2015.
14. Agency for Healthcare Research and Quality. Available at: http://www.ahrq.gov. Last accessed 6 March 2015.
15. Centers for Disease Control and Prevention. Available at: http://www.cdc.gov/. Last accessed 6 March 2015.
16. U.S. Food and Drug Administration. Available at: http://www.fda.gov/.
17. Health Resources and Services Administration. Available at: http://www.hrsa.gov/. Last accessed 6 March 2015.
18. U.S. Department of Health and Human Services. Indian Health Service. Available at: http://www.ihs.gov/. Last accessed 6 March 2015.
19. Health and Human Resources. Available at: http://www.hhs.gov/asl/testify/t990629c.html. Accessed 6 March 2015.
20. Centers for Disease Control. Morbidity and Mortality Weekly Report. Available at: http://www.cdc.gov/mmwr/preview/mmwrhtml/mm5906a2.htm. Last accessed 6 March 2015.
21. U.S. Department of Health and Human Services. National Institutes of Health. Available at: http://www.nih.gov/. Last accessed 6 March 2015.
22. National Institute of Mental Health. Available at: http://www.nimh.nih.gov/. Last accessed 6 March 2015.
23. National Institutes of Health. National Institute of Environmental Health Sciences. Available at: http://www.niehs.nih.gov/. Last accessed 6 March 2015.
24. National Institutes of Health. National Institute of Allergy and Infectious Diseases. Available at: http://www.niaid.gov/. Last accessed 6 March 2015.
25. U.S. Department of Health and Human Services Administration. Substance Abuse and Mental Health Services Administration. Available at: http://www.samhsa.gov/index.aspx. Last accessed 6 March 2015.
26. Mullan F. *Plagues and Politics: The Story of the United States Public Health Service*. New York: Basic Books; 1989.
27. U.S. Department of Health and Human Services. Office of Force Readiness and Deployment. Available at: http://dcp.psc.gov/ccmis/ReDDOG/REDDOG_essentials_m.aspx. Last accessed 6 March 2015.
28. Koenig KL. Homeland security and public health: role of the Department of Veterans Affairs, the U.S. Department of Homeland Security, and implications for the public health community. *Prehosp Disaster Med*. 2003;18(4):327–333.
29. Hodgson MJ, Bierenbaum A, Mather S, et al. Emergency management program operational responses to weapons of mass destruction: Veterans Health Administration, 2001-2004. *Am J Ind Med*. 2004;46(5):446–452.
30. Federal Emergency Management Agency. Executive Order 12657: Federal Emergency Management Agency Assistance in Emergency Preparedness Planning at Commercial Nuclear Power Plants. Available at:

http://www.archives.gov/federal-register/codification/executive-order/12657.html. Last accessed 6 March 2015.

31. Department of Defense Directive 3025.15. Military Assistance to Civil Authorities. Available at: http://biotech.law.lsu.edu/blaw/DOD/manual/full%20text%20documents/Agencies%20Documents/DODD-3025.15.pdf. Last accessed 6 March 2015.

32. U.S. Northern Command. Available at: http://www.northcom.mil/. Last accessed 6 March 2015.

33. Joint Publication 3-41 "Joint Doctrine for Chemical, Biological, Radiological, and Nuclear Consequence Management" June 2012. Available at: http://www.dtic.mil/doctrine/new_pubs/jp3_41.pdf. Last accessed 6 March 2015.

34. National Guard CERFP Fact Sheet, available at http://states.ng.mil/sites/MA/about/pubs/Fact_Sheets/CERFP_Fact_Sheet.pdf. Last accessed 6 March 2015.

35. American Red Cross. Available at: http://www.redcross.org/. Last accessed 6 March 2015.

CHAPTER 18

Global Disaster Response

Miriam Aschkenasy and Hilarie Cranmer

We cannot predict when or where disasters will happen, but we know they will, and they are on the rise. In 2012 there were 357 reported natural disasters affecting 120 different countries.[1] According to the United Nations Office for the Coordination of Humanitarian Affairs (UN OCHA), in that same year, 1.4 million people were affected by disasters or displaced by conflict,[2] with billions (in U.S. dollars) spent on disaster response and recovery.[1] This upward trend in numbers affected and economic burden will continue to affect populations increasingly in the future. Increased urbanization, globalization, climate change, and migration of populations because of the scarcity of and resulting competition for resources all contribute to these large-scale disasters.[3,4] Disasters can range from sudden or gradual onset "natural" occurrences, such as tsunamis, earthquakes, or droughts to "human-made" or complex emergencies that involve political upheaval and violence or technological disasters, such as chemical spills and radiation exposure. The "humanitarian space" describes the increasingly complex milieu between those needing assistance and those wishing to deliver it. This chapter focuses on the response phase of the disaster management cycle. It is important to understand the unique functions of the various response sectors, the actors, and the necessary skills, attitudes, and behaviors, or competencies, of the workforce in order to function effectively in this space. This workforce has grown at a rate of 6% per annum, and thus we are even more compelled to ensure that those responders are trained as professionals, no matter what their background or specialty.[5]

The key sectors of global disaster response are also known as clusters, essential components necessary to prioritize in order to mitigate disaster effects. In acute settings, humanitarian responders strive to provide for the immediate needs of those affected in terms of shelter, food, medical care, clean water, and sanitation. Additional sectors of logistics, protection, coordination, education, telecommunications, and food security, are just as important. Table 18-1 provides definitions of these sectors. Finally, early transition to recovery is a crucial component of early response that must also be considered.[6] During this transition, those delivering aid need to focus on sustainable interventions, mitigation, and disaster risk reduction to prepare for the future.[7]

There are a multitude of actors working in the diverse but interconnected sectors involved in humanitarian assistance. Most familiar is the United Nations (UN), created in 1945, and its member states. Article 71 of Chapter 10 of the UN charter designates a consultative role for organizations that are neither governments nor member states, referred to as nongovernmental organizations (NGOs).[8] When the UN was formed there were just 45 of these consultative organizations. Now there are well over 33,000, and many more form during crises. NGOs involved in disaster response have an ill-defined classification system. For example, the World Bank divides NGOs into operation and advocacy (or campaigning) groups. In general, NGOs deliver services and play coordination and funding roles in their area of expertise. Other actors in the response process include the military, police, donors, the diaspora, academic institutions, hospitals, and community-based organizations. With so many varied participants it is imperative that they speak a common language, share at least minimum standards, and have a common framework.

This has led to professionalization and standardization in the field of emergency response.[9,10] The ability of governments and response organizations to prepare for, mitigate, and respond to humanitarian disasters has increased, while concurrent international standards, frameworks, and guidelines have been developed and implemented.[11] Even though there are still many obstacles to overcome, there has been much progress made, especially during the past decade. The following are but a few of the examples of the transformation now occurring in disaster management:

- The formation of the Sphere standards in humanitarian response[12]
- The humanitarian accountability partnership (HAP), a multiagency initiative working to improve accountability in humanitarian actions to people affected by disasters and other crises[13]
- The progress of the transformation agenda described by the Interagency Standing Committee (IASC), a branch of the UN that is a unique interagency forum for coordination, policy development, and decision making involving the key UN and non-UN humanitarian partners[14]
- The classification and implementation of guidelines for foreign medical teams as defined by the Global Health Cluster[15]

This chapter will explore global disaster response involving humanitarian assistance as it moves toward a more professional framework. Reviewing the history of global disaster response will provide context for the current practices. The actors, sectors, and major organizations will be discussed, as will the current practice and existing standards (through frameworks) for operations. Finally, a review of the challenges in future responses will provide a way forward for our next generation of providers.

HISTORICAL PERSPECTIVE

Global disaster response has undergone a transformation since Henry Dunant, a Swiss businessman and social activist, first formulated the concept in 1863. In reaction to the horror of war he witnessed at the 1859 Battle of Solferino, Italy, Dunant became instrumental in the creation of the International Committee of the Red Cross (ICRC), incorporated by the Geneva Society for Public Welfare in 1876. The mission of the ICRC was to be the first politically neutral organization to provide humanitarian relief. In the ensuing years, continued war and conflict, natural disasters and epidemics, and the advent of modern military combat resulted in more populations being affected,

TABLE 18-1 **United Nations Office for the Coordination of Humanitarian Affairs: Cluster Coordination Sectors and Their UN-Lead Organizations and Sector Definitions***

CLUSTER	MISSION	UN-LEAD ORGANIZATION
Protection	Provide protection to internally displaced persons and other populations affected by nonrefugee emergencies	Office of the United Nations High Commissioner for Refugees (UNHCR)
Food security	Ensure physical and economic access to sufficient safe and nutritious food that meets the dietary needs of those affected by humanitarian disasters	Food and Agriculture Organization (FAO) and World Food Program (WFP)
Emergency telecommunications	Provide vital IT and telecommunications services to help humanitarian workers carry out operations efficiently and effectively	WFP
Early recovery	The restoration of basic services, livelihoods, shelter, governance, security, the rule of law, and environment and social dimensions, including the reintegration of displaced populations	United Nations Development Program (UNDP)
Education	A formal forum for coordination and collaboration on education in humanitarian crisis	United Nations Children's Fund (UNICEF) and the International Non-governmental Organization (INGO) Save the Children
Sanitation, water, and hygiene (WASH)	Improve the predictability, timeliness, and effectiveness of a comprehensive WASH response to humanitarian crisis	UNICEF
Logistics	To ensure lifesaving relief cargo reaches affected populations in time	WFP
Nutrition	Safeguard and improve the nutritional status of emergency affected populations by ensuring a coordinated, appropriate response that is predictable, timely, effective, and at scale	UNICEF
Emergency shelter	Supports country-level shelter clusters and other nonrefugee coordination mechanisms by providing predictable, effective, and timely shelter coordination services to improve humanitarian response	UNHCR and the International Federation of the Red Cross (IFCR)
Camp management and coordination	Ensure equitable access to services and protection for displaced persons living in communal settings, to improve their quality of life and dignity during displacement, and advocate for solutions while preparing them for life after displacement	UNHCR and International Organization for Migration (IOM)
Health	Strengthen system-wide humanitarian preparedness by ensuring sufficient capacity in information management; surge; normative guidance and tools; development of the capacities of national stakeholders; as well as advocacy and resource mobilization	World Health Organization (WHO)
Information management	Collecting, analyzing, and sharing information that is important for the cluster stakeholders to make informed strategic decisions	Humanitarian and Emergency Relief Coordinator

*http://www.unocha.org/what-we-do/coordination-tools/cluster-coordination.
(From the UN Office for the Coordination of Humanitarian Affairs, New York, NY, © [2014] United Nations. Reprinted with the permission of the United Nations.)

and thus to an expansion of the humanitarian aid community. This in turn brought further development and innovation to the field of disaster-response medicine, legal frameworks, and institutional organizations.[16]

The ICRC was formed based upon the humanitarian ideals of neutrality, independence, and impartiality.[17] It was the basis for the adoption of the first Geneva Convention in 1864, a treaty requiring care for wounded soldiers and establishing the use of the Red Cross emblem to protect and provide aid to those removed from combat. Natural disasters and epidemics also played an important role in the growth of aid organizations, and, consequently, regulations for assistance began to emerge.[16] This period in history saw the first international conferences and committees on issues related to disaster and epidemic response, such as the first International Sanitary Conference (1850s) and the International Health, Maritime, and Quarantine Board (1881).

World War I and the Influenza Pandemic of 1918 played a considerable role in the further development of global disaster response. A new disaster taxonomy materialized as food insecurity, pandemic spread, mass displacement, and statelessness, emerged as newer, more complex catastrophes. World War II, however, was the major turning point for the humanitarian sector. More than twice as many civilians as combatants were killed during that conflict.[18] With so many affected civilians and millions of internally displaced populations and refugees, several new humanitarian NGOs were formed, such as the International Rescue Committee (1933), Oxfam (1942), and Catholic Relief Services (1943).

It was during this time that the UN charter was formed (1945), which subsequently led to four Geneva Conventions, adopted in 1949. The Geneva Conventions and Additional Protocols are the backbone of international humanitarian law.[19] These set forth protections for civilians and aid workers, as well as the wounded, ill, and prisoners of war.[20] Another direct result of World War II was the formation of the United Nations High Commissioner for Refugees (UNCHR) in 1950. This organization was initially formed to help those displaced by the war, and it now works with over 33.9 million individuals worldwide who are internally displaced, refugees, returnees, stateless people, or asylum seekers.[21]

After World War II, the United States also addressed the need for global disaster response. Recognizing that the country needed a single agency to coordinate development and international assistance, the Foreign Assistance Act of 1961 was passed, authorizing the development of the U.S. Agency for International Development (USAID) as the single U.S. agency responsible for foreign economic development, including humanitarian assistance. The USAID Office of Foreign Disaster Assistance (OFDA) is tasked to lead the U.S. government's global disaster response.

In 1971, UN Resolution 2816 established the Office of the UN Disaster Relief Coordinator. The same year, Médecins San Frontières (MSF), translated as Doctors Without Borders, was formed. MSF was a new kind of humanitarian organization, one devoted to the principles of providing medical aid, but also committed to speaking out against the actions of the offending governments and related actors,[22] including the humanitarian sector as a whole. MSF was founded by a group of physicians and has grown to be a lead organization in the medical sector of humanitarian response, creating guidelines for refugee health, books on rapid health assessments, and clinical guidelines for working in remote settings and field hospitals.[23] Unlike the ICRC and the UN, MSF does not wait for diplomatic efforts with state governments to occur before accessing the populations in need.

During the 1980s, conflict and natural disasters continued to influence the further development of the global response field. There were ongoing challenges that included coordination, duplication of efforts, funding, communications, and civil-military interactions. As a direct result, in 1991, the UN General Assembly passed Resolution 46/182, establishing the position of Emergency Relief Coordinator (ERC) and the IASC, the Central Emergency Revolving Fund (CERF), which is now the Central Emergency Response Fund), and the Consolidated Appeal Process (CAP).[24] Resolution 46/182 "... was designed to strengthen the UN response to complex emergencies and natural disasters, while improving the overall effectiveness of humanitarian operations in the field."[25] One way to accomplish this objective was to make funds immediately available to those who were responding in the field through the CERF and the CAP.

The United Nations Office for the Coordination of Humanitarian Affairs (UN OCHA) was created in 1998. The UN OCHA is responsible for communications, coordination, needs assessments, coordinated funding appeals, and creating humanitarian policies. During this time, the NGO community was working to create common principles and frameworks for providing disaster response. The Sphere Project was launched in 1997 to develop a set of minimum standards in core areas of humanitarian assistance. In 1998 the first edition of the *Humanitarian Charter and Minimum Standards in Humanitarian Response*[26] (also known as the Sphere standards) was published. This is a handbook for humanitarian organizations created by a consensus of global response agencies striving to improve their work and have more accountability. The handbook sets forth minimum standards, guidelines, and indicators for each of the large sectors, including water, sanitation, and hygiene (WASH), and health. The most recent edition, available for free on the Internet, was revised in 2011. Most workers in the field are familiar with these guidelines, which have become an essential tool for all providers.

In 2005 the UN IASC undertook major humanitarian reforms in which they introduced the coordinated cluster, or sector, approach to humanitarian response. Using the cluster system, groups of UN and non-UN humanitarian actors in the same sector could work together more easily with a designated UN office to oversee the sectoral response at the country level, rather than in the field. At the field level, one NGO usually takes this responsibility.

CURRENT PRACTICE

As part of reforms of 2005, the Fifty-Eighth World Health Assembly revised and enacted new International Health Regulations.[27] An important new disaster-classification scheme emerged, and it was mandated that the UN members and leads act according to the defined level of the disaster.[28] These, along with the 2005 and 2011 Humanitarian Reforms of the IASC, afforded the World Health Organization (WHO) new roles and responsibility for providing leadership on issues of global health in general and disaster response in particular. These new roles included: acting as the health cluster lead during a humanitarian response; supporting member states in disaster preparedness and relief; developing performance standards; and providing technical expertise.[27] The IASC also introduced the UN Transformative Agenda in 2011 to further increase accountability and enhance strong

leadership in the field. Reform processes effected change in all humanitarian response sectors.[29] In its role as the health cluster lead agency, the WHO developed the "Emergency Response Framework" (ERF)[30] and subsequently the "... classification and minimum standards for foreign medical teams in sudden onset disasters."[15] These are the most current medical disaster-response guidelines in use today.

According to the ERF, the role of the WHO during emergencies is "... to support Member States and local health authorities to lead a coordinated and effective health sector response together with the national and international community, in order to save lives, minimize adverse health effects and preserve dignity, with specific attention to vulnerable and marginalized populations."[31]

In response to the crises of 2010, which included floods in Pakistan and India and the Haiti earthquake, the WHO, working with many other regional partners, established the Foreign Medical Teams Working Group. This group developed a classification system, minimum standards, and a registration process for foreign medical teams (FMTs) responding to sudden onset crises.[32] Notionally, an affected country can review the registered FMTs, usually with the aid of a UN partner, and choose those that are needed for the particular response. Accordingly, "The process of registration and declared commitment of registered FMTs to adhere to the principles, and comply with both core and technical standards, will assist countries affected by sudden onset disasters to select professional FMTs from their region and globally."[15] FMTs are divided into three categories based on capabilities (Table 18-2).

FMT's are groups of health professionals equipped and trained to provide health care in resource-poor arenas with additional training to deal specifically with disaster-affected communities. Having a degree in a clinical specialty does not automatically qualify an individual or group to be prepared for humanitarian medical response. This has been well articulated by Dr. Frederick Burkle, an expert in the field, when he wrote in 2010, "Those who define themselves as humanitarian professionals have doubled from a decade ago to almost 200,000 today. They are eager and well-traveled. But like us all, they do not know what they don't know."[33] Well-intentioned, ad hoc, spontaneous volunteers often converge at a disaster site ill equipped to handle the working environment and stress, resulting in the diversion of scarce resources to care for the volunteers themselves. Formal training of humanitarian responders in a set of core competencies that include knowledge of how to practice in resource constrained settings, self-sufficiency, humanitarian principles, and minimum standards, is required.[10,34,35] Responders need to master the skills of multitasking, negotiating and mediating, and team building, while understanding how to conduct a needs assessment, address security and safety issues, and comply with the tenets of international humanitarian law.[36] Finally, they need the appropriate tools for personal stress management and self-care.

There are now several options for those interested in humanitarian health to obtain the competencies, skill sets, and credentials to operate as a member of an FMT.[35] The UN, as well as nongovernmental and academic institutions, provides courses on the Sphere standards, the cluster approach, and humanitarian response. Organizations like the Enhanced Learning and Research for Humanitarian Assistance (ELRHA) and the HAP are helping to further professionalize the sector. Even though there are still responders and agencies that have yet to conform to these new standards, the momentum to move toward degree courses, core competencies, and professional credentials is building, and the role of the ad hoc volunteer who wishes to help but instead needs to be helped is diminishing.

As global disaster response has evolved so has the relationship of all of the actors. As we see the UN clearly defining its role in relation to member states and NGOs, so has it moved to define its relationships with military organizations. In 2008 UN OCHA published a document

TABLE 18-2   Classification and Minimum Standards for Foreign Medical Teams in Sudden Onset Disasters; Classification, Definition, and Minimum Standards*

TEAM CLASSIFICATION	DEFINITION	MINIMUM BENCHMARK INDICATOR
I. Outpatient emergency care	Initial outpatient emergency care of injuries or other significant health care needs	100 patients per day
II. Inpatient surgical emergency care	Inpatient acute care with general and obstetric surgery for trauma and other major conditions	1 operating theater with 1 operating room 20 inpatient beds 7 major or 15 minor operations a day
III. Inpatient referral care	Complex inpatient referral surgical care including intensive care capacity	1 operating theater with at least 2 operating rooms 40 inpatient beds 15 major or 30 minor operations per day 4-6 intensive care beds
Additional specialized care	Additional specialized care cells within type II or III or a hospital	Depending on capacity

*http://www.who.int/hac/global_health_cluster/fmt_guidelines_september2013.pdf.

that specifically addresses civil-military interactions during response to humanitarian emergencies.[37] This document, which includes operational guidelines, outlines when and how the military commanders should coordinate with humanitarian actors. This is especially relevant to the health sector as the transport of supplies, communications, logistics, and safety and security are often provided by the military if involved in a complex humanitarian response.

The U.S. government's role in humanitarian response has also evolved over the past several decades. If a sovereign government requests aid from the U.S. government, the disaster exceeds the affected countries own ability to respond, and the response is in the best interest of the U.S. government, then an OFDA assessment team may be deployed.[38] If the event is of a large scale or an extended response is anticipated, a disaster assistance response team (DART) may be deployed to assess the situation, aid in coordination, make recommendations, establish an operational base, provide funding, and conduct monitoring and evaluation.[38] The U.S. Department of State may also deploy International Medical Surgical Response Teams (IMSuRT), portable, fully equipped field hospitals, to aid in international response.

Over the past several decades, global disaster response has moved toward stronger leadership, more clearly defined roles and guidelines, and professionalization. The implementation and continued improvement of the clusters approach, Sphere standards, role of IASC, ERF,

guidelines for FMTs in humanitarian response, and civil-military engagement are all hallmarks of the current field of disaster response.

In turn, as the global disaster response health sector has grown and matured, so has the need for professionalization of the field. This is exemplified by the development of the ERF and FMT guidelines. Even though there is still much work to be done, the current practice of humanitarian health fosters increased accountability, core competencies, and coordination.

! PITFALLS

Despite significant improvement in global disaster response, some of the prior challenges continue to persist. This is seen most acutely in coordination, adherence to guidelines, working within local health structures, ethical constraints, and planning and preparedness. New challenges will arise, some predictable and some unforeseen, as climate change and rapid urbanization alter the environment.

Effective coordination is still difficult to accomplish and fraught with political and functional impediments. The cluster system and development of the standardized Multi-Cluster Initial Rapid Assessment (MIRA), which is meant to be applied within the first 2 weeks of a crisis, have helped address some of these issues, but not all actors involved in humanitarian assistance are familiar with or choose to participate in the cluster system. Although the goal of the clusters is to "… create partnerships between international humanitarian actors, national and local authorities, and civil society," it is a voluntary commitment for NGOs, civil society, and governments.[39] There are no enforceable repercussions if a country or organization determines it does not want to participate in the cluster response, as a recipient or as a participant.

This same challenge is encountered when asking organizations or individuals to adhere to a set of guidelines or principles. For example, during the Haiti earthquake response, there were over 400 medical NGOs, providing medical and surgical care through rehabilitation. Many were not registered with the government and had no prior knowledge of the UN cluster system, international humanitarian law, or the Sphere standards, and therefore frequently did not work within those parameters. This led to poor medical care, no care transition plans, and responder PTSD.[40,41]

The Haiti response also resulted in congruent but separate health structures with little integration into the existing local system. According to Dr. Jennifer Leaning and Dr. Debarati Guha-Sapir, "Sudden infusion of outside aid and expertise can compromise existing community public health operations by setting up parallel systems with different norms and resources."[42] Even with improved coordination, it has been challenging for the humanitarian aid community to properly integrate into local health systems and to adjust to norms and standards of the community. Many humanitarian practitioners must grapple with the ethical constraints of providing care in a resource-limited setting. They are challenged in adjusting their expectations and recalibrating noncrisis standards of care to move toward more sustainable interventions necessary to prevent undermining existing health care structures. The FMT guidelines, which grew out of this catastrophe, are unfortunately limited in scope and only set standards for sudden onset natural disaster scenarios. It does not encompass complex crises or technological or urbanization disasters.

In addition, an ethical dilemma facing humanitarian responders occurs when clinicians are forced to choose between providing care and speaking out against an atrocity or human rights violation. By voicing their concerns, they can put themselves or other team members in danger, may be removed from the country, or can be denied access to those in need. This is a personal and organizational decision that must be contemplated prior to deployment and be in compliance of the existing international humanitarian law. How an organization chooses to work with the government has other implications as well.

The role the government plays in planning and preparing for potential catastrophes can have a direct effect on the international community response. In many countries, there are few regulations addressing international relief efforts, which can hinder response activities, contribute to delays in mobilization, and increase costs. In 2007 the International Federation of Red Cross and Red Crescent Societies produced guidelines to help governments prepare for a global response on their soil, through development of needed systems and regulations.[11] This is a long and complicated process. Many governments are already stretched thin with limited resources and conflicting priorities and have not undertaken this planning and preparation to date.

The strain on existing governments for proper planning can also be seen in the trend toward urbanization. Urban growth is often unplanned and disorganized, and this leads to large numbers of people living without essential infrastructures in high risk areas.[4] Coupled with the increased likelihood of natural disasters, food or water shortages, and disease outbreaks related to climate change and resource scarcity,[3] there are new and extremely complicated sets of challenges for humanitarian response. Even though the humanitarian health sector is robust and dynamic, this new milieu is fraught with obstacles that further confound an already complicated field.

Global disaster medical response has evolved significantly in the past two centuries. The initial guiding principle to help those in need has not changed. When Henry Dunant established the first humanitarian space in 1846, he set into motion the development of a new field of medicine: global disaster medical response provided by professionals. In 1859 Dunant asked, "Would there not be some means of forming relief societies whose object would be to have the wounded cared for in times of war by enthusiastic, devoted volunteers, fully qualified for the task?"[43] There are such societies, and they are populated with qualified individuals who dedicate their lives to helping others.

REFERENCES

1. WHO Collaborating Center for Research on the Epidemiology of Disasters—CRED. *Annual Disaster Statistical Review 2012;* 2012. Available at, http://www.cred.be/sites/default/files/ADSR_2012.pdf.
2. United Nations Office for the Coordination of Humanitarian Affairs Policy Development and Studies Branch—UN OCHA PDSB. World Humanitarian Data and Trends 2013. Available at, https://docs.unocha.org/sites/dms/Documents/WHDT_2013%20WEB.pdf.
3. Diaz JH. The influence of global warming on natural disasters and their public health outcomes. *Am J Disaster Med.* 2007;2(1):33–42.
4. Patel RB, Burkle FM. Rapid urbanization and the growing threat of violence and conflict: a 21st century crisis. *Prehosp Disaster Med.* 2012;27(2):194–197.
5. Walker P, Russ C. *Professionalizing the Humanitarian Sector: A Scoping Study.* London, UK: Enhancing Learning and Research for Humanitarian Assistance; April 2010.
6. United Nations Inter-Agency Standing Committee. *Reference Module for Cluster Coordination at the Country Level;* 2012. Available at, https://clusters.humanitarianresponse.info/system/files/documents/files/iasc-coordination-reference%20module-en_0.pdf.
7. Board of Natural Disasters. Mitigation emerges as major strategy for reducing losses caused by natural disasters. *Science.* 1999;284:1943–1947.
8. The United Nations. Available at www.un.org/aboutun/charter. Accessed May 25, 2014.
9. Hein D. The competency of competencies. *Prehosp Disaster Med.* 2010;25(5):396–397.
10. Johnson K, Idzerda I, Baras R, et al. Competency based standardized training for humanitarian providers: making humanitarian assistance a professional discipline. *Disaster Med Public Health Prep.* 2013;7:369–372.
11. International Federation of Red Cross and Red Crescent Societies. *Introduction to the Guidelines for the Domestic Facilitation and Regulation of International Disaster Relief and Initial Recovery Assistance;* 2011. Available at, http://www.ifrc.org/PageFiles/125652/1205600-IDRL%20Guidelines-EN-LR%20(2).pdf. Accessed May 30, 2015.
12. The Sphere Project. *Humanitarian Charter and Minimum Standards.* Available at www.sphereproject.org. Accessed May 25, 2014.
13. Humanitarian Accountability Partnership (HAP). Available at www.hapinternational.org. Accessed May 25, 2014.
14. Inter-Agency Standing Committee (IASC). Available at www.humanitarianinfo.org/iasc. Accessed May 25, 2014.
15. World Health Organization Foreign Medical Team Working Group under the Global Health Cluster. *Classification and Minimum Standards for Foreign Medical Teams in Sudden Onset Disasters;* 2013. Available at, http://www.who.int/hac/global_health_cluster/fmt_guidelines_september2013.pdf. Accessed May 25, 2015.
16. Davey E, Borton J, Foley M. *A History of the Humanitarian System Western Origins and Foundations;* Humanitarian Policy Group Working Paper, 2013. Available at, http://www.academia.edu/5622470/A_History_of_the_Humanitarian_System_Western_Origins_and_Foundations. Accessed May 25, 2014.
17. International Committee for the Red Cross website. Available at http://www.icrc.org/eng/who-we-are/mandate/index.jsp. Accessed May 25, 2014.
18. The National WWII museum website. Available at http://www.nationalww2museum.org/learn/education/for-students/ww2-history/ww2-by-the-numbers/world-wide-deaths.html. Accessed May 25, 2014.
19. International Committee for the Red Cross web site. Available at http://www.icrc.org/eng/war-and-law/treaties-customary-law/geneva-conventions/index.jsp. Accessed May 25, 2014.
20. International Committee for the Red Cross. *The Geneva Conventions of 1949 and their Additional Protocols.* Available at http://www.icrc.org/eng/assets/files/publications/icrc-002–0173.pdf.
21. The United Nations High Commission for Refugees website. *A Global Humanitarian Organization of Humble Origins.* Available at http://www.unhcr.org/pages/49c3646cbc.html. Accessed May 25, 2014.
22. Medecines Sans Frontieres/Doctors Without Borders website. Available at www.msf.org.uk/founding-msf. Accessed May 25, 2014.
23. Medecines Sans Frontieres/Doctors Without Borders website. Available at http://www.refbooks.msf.org/msf_docs/en/MSFdocMenu_en.htm.
24. United Nations Office for the Coordination of Humanitarian Affairs. *OCHA on Message: General Assembly Resolution 46/182;* 2012. Available at, https://docs.unocha.org/sites/dms/Documents/120402_OOM-46182_eng.pdf.
25. United Nations Office for the Coordination of Humanitarian Affairs. *History of OCHA.* Available at www.unocha.org/about-us/who-we-are/history. Accessed May 25, 2014.
26. *2011 Sphere Handbook.* Available at http://www.sphereproject.org/resources/download-publications/?search=1&keywords=&language=English&category=22. Accessed May 25, 2014.
27. World Health Organization. *International Health Regulations.* 2005. Available at, http://whqlibdoc.who.int/publications/2008/9789241580410_eng.pdf. Accessed May 25, 2014.
28. *Humanitarian System-Wide Emergency Activation: Definition and Procedures.* IASC Working Group; 2012. Available at, file:///C:/Users/ma65/Downloads/2.%20System-Wide%20(Level%203)%20Activation%20(20Apr12)%20(4).pdf. Accessed May 30, 201.
29. IASC Transformative Agenda 2012. Available at http://www.humanitarianinfo.org/iasc/pageloader.aspx?page=content-template-default&bd=87. Accessed May 25, 2014.
30. World Health Organization. *Emergency Response Framework (ERF).* 2012, Available at, http://www.who.int/hac/about/erf_.pdf.
31. World Health Organization. *Emergency Response Framework (ERF).* 2012. Page 14. Available at, http://www.who.int/hac/about/erf_.pdf. Accessed May 25, 2015.
32. World Health Organization Foreign Medical Team Working Group under the Global Health Cluster. *Classification and Minimum Standards for Foreign Medical Teams in Sudden Onset Disasters;* 2013. Page 12. Available at, http://www.who.int/hac/global_health_cluster/fmt_guidelines_september2013.pdf. Accessed May 25, 2015.

33. Burkle F. Future humanitarian crisis: challenges for practice, policy, and public health. *Prehosp Disaster Med.* 2010;25:191–199.

34. Cranmer H, Biddinger P. Typhoon Haiyan and the professionalization of disaster response. *N Engl J Med.* 2014;370:1183–1184.

35. Burkle F, Walls A, Jeck J, et al. Academic affiliated training centers in humanitarian health, Part I: program characteristics and professionalization preferences of centers in North America. *Prehosp Disaster Med.* 2013;28(2):155–162.

36. Walker P, Hein K, Russ C, et al. A blueprint for professionalizing humanitarian assistance. *Health Aff.* 2010;28(12):2223–2230.

37. United Nations Office for the Coordination of Humanitarian Affairs. *Civil Military Guidelines and Reference for Complex Emergencies;* 2008. Available at, http://ochaonline.un.org/cmcs/guidelines. Accessed May 30, 2015.

38. United States Agency for International Development, Bureau for Humanitarian Response, Office of Foreign Disaster Assistance. *Field Operations Guide for Disaster Assessment and Response;* 2005. Available at, https://scms.usaid.gov/sites/default/files/documents/1866/fog_v4.pdf. Accessed May 30, 2015.

39. United Nations Office for the Coordination of Humanitarian Affairs website. Available at http://www.unocha.org/what-we-do/coordination-tools/cluster-coordination. Accessed May 30, 2015.

40. Redmond D, Mardel S, Taithe B, et al. A qualitative and quantitative study of the surgical and rehabilitation response to the earthquake in Haiti, January 2010. *Prehosp Disaster Med.* 2011;26(6):449–456.

41. *Disasters: Preparedness and Mitigation in the Americas.* Website for the Pan American Health Organization. Editorial: Filed Hospitals and Medical Teams in the Aftermath of Earthquakes. Oct. 2010;(issues 114). Available at http://www.paho.org/disasters/newsletter/index.php?option=com_content&view=article&id=429%3Afield-hospitals-and-medical-teams-in-the-aftermath-of-earthquakes&catid=200%3Aissue-114-october-2010-editorial&Itemid=256&lang=en. Accessed May 30, 2015.

42. Leaning J, Guha-Sapir D. Natural disasters, armed conflict, and public health. *N Engl J Med.* 2013;369:1836–1842.

43. Dunant H. *A Memory of Solferino.* American National Red Cross; 1959.

Nongovernmental Organizations in Disaster Medicine

Zeno L. Charles-Marcel, David M. Canther, Malcolm Seheult, and Patrice Joseph

NGOs serve a vital role at the local, State, and national levels by performing essential service missions in times of need.
National Response Framework (2008)

Disaster medicine specialists are expected to respond to the most catastrophic human events and attend to the medical and health care needs of those affected. Yet they are only part of the response team and cannot perform optimally without the collaboration and engagement of other essential elements. It is incumbent upon medical care providers to know who constitutes the team; their respective roles, strengths, and weaknesses; and how best to work with them for successful disaster management.

The ultimate responsibility for management of a disaster rests with the local or national government in the jurisdiction where the disaster occurs. Because disasters, by definition, overwhelm the emergency response capability of the affected community, assistance from "outside" is the rule rather than the exception. Whether we examine the historic 1889 Johnstown, Pennsylvania, disaster that took 2200 human lives or the recent 2014 Ebola outbreak in West Africa, humanitarian volunteers from "outside" collaborate with local and other government personnel on both the front lines and behind the scenes (Fig. 19-1).[1] In all disasters, multiple stakeholders are involved in all aspects of disaster response—treating victims, caring for families, communicating vital lifesaving information to communities, and consoling the bereaved. Whether in the case of an earthquake, tsunami, typhoon, terrorist attack, or volcanic eruption, the work of humanitarian aid agencies and charities—that is, nongovernmental organizations (NGOs)—is vital to the success of the deployment. In the case of the Ebola outbreak, the United Nations (UN) Office for the Coordination of Humanitarian Affairs (OCHA) reported that "NGOs had provided many essential services in this relief effort."[1] But what are these NGOs? Which essential services do they provide? How are their activities coordinated in disaster management? What are their major challenges? These are the questions that will be addressed in this chapter.

HISTORICAL PERSPECTIVE

Historically, there is evidence of both Eastern and Western humanitarian gestures, that is, the will and action to alleviate the suffering of others in response to natural and human-made disasters. Conceptually humanitarian work roughly parallels human history itself as it seems reasonable to postulate that family members, friends, relatives, and tribal brothers of the victims must have mounted some kind of relief effort based on the situation. Tribal customs and religious traditions probably dictated the response of the community to the survivors and to the disposal of the dead bodies in the aftermath of natural tragedies and war. When the first groups organized themselves to deal with such events, the involvement of NGOs in disaster management was born. Asian history points to the Han Dynasty as having one of the earliest recorded humanitarian systems with specific disaster and famine relief functions dating back to the Southern Song Dynasty (1127-1279 AD).[2]

In western history, Christians established hospitals in Jerusalem to serve traveling pilgrims centuries ago.[3] Peter, the Patriarch of Jerusalem, requested funds from Emperor Justinian to establish a hospital in the holy city in the sixth century, and Pope Gregory I founded a hospice near the Church of the Holy Sepulcher in 603 CE.[4] Other records show that specific humanitarian systems were later designed to deal with the effects of natural disasters and wars in Europe.[5] In 1767, a Society for the Recovery of the Drowned was established in Amsterdam, and by the early 1800s, humane societies specializing in the rescue and resuscitation of victims of drowning and shipwrecks had been founded on every continent.[6] The goal of these "Humane Societies" was the dissemination of new resuscitation techniques, whereas the Royal Jennerian Society (another humane society founded in 1803) had as its objective the speedy extermination of smallpox through the newly discovered methods of vaccination.[7]

Organized international humanitarian aid shows itself in the late nineteenth century in response to the Northern Chinese Famine of 1876-1879 and simultaneously the Great Famine of 1876-1878 in India, both brought about by a severe drought that claimed the lives of as many as 10 million people in China alone.[8] The Shandong Famine Relief Committee was established with the participation of diplomats, businessmen, and Protestant and Roman Catholic missionaries[9] in response to a plea from British missionary Timothy Richard, and led to collected donations of between $7 million and $10 million for the relief work in China.[10]

The terms *nongovernmental organization* (NGO) and *civil society organization* (CSO) were created in the UN charter to describe certain nonstate entities to be awarded observer status at UN assemblies and other meetings.[11] The UN further established the Committee on Non-Governmental Organizations as a standing committee of the Economic and Social Council (ECOSOC) by Council resolution 3(II) on June 21, 1946, with original terms of reference in 1950 and subsequent revisions in 1968 by resolution 1296 (XLIV) and 1996 by resolution 1996/31.[12] NGOs have been actively engaged with the UN since its inception. "They work with the United Nations Secretariat, programs, funds and agencies in various ways, including in consultation with Member States. NGOs contribute to a number of activities including information dissemination, awareness raising, development education, policy advocacy, joint operational projects, participation in intergovernmental processes and in the contribution of services and technical expertise"[13] (Box 19-1).

In general terms, an NGO is civilian-based, independent of government, and staffed by volunteers who share a common background or

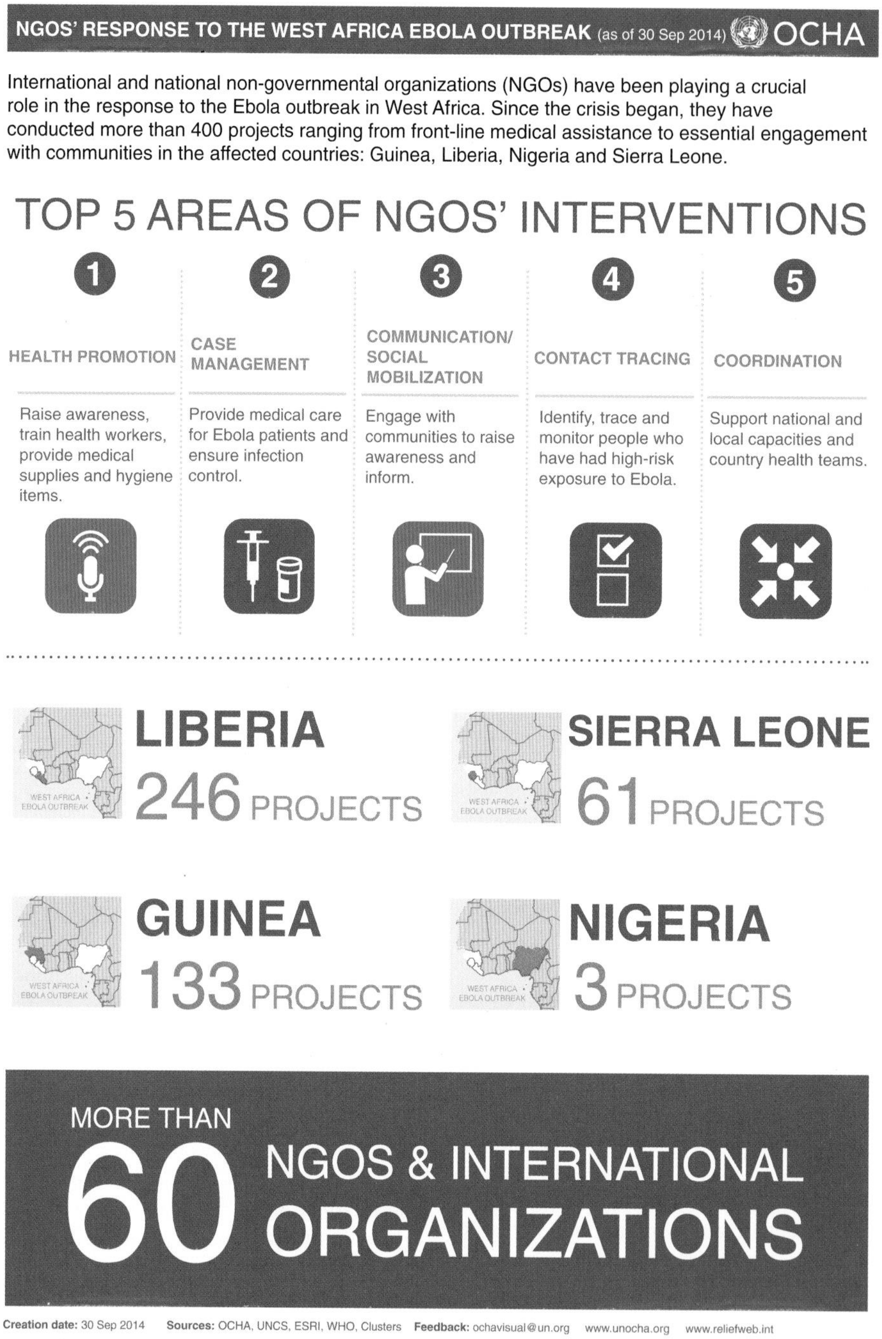

NGOS' RESPONSE TO THE WEST AFRICA EBOLA OUTBREAK (as of 30 Sep 2014) OCHA

International and national non-governmental organizations (NGOs) have been playing a crucial role in the response to the Ebola outbreak in West Africa. Since the crisis began, they have conducted more than 400 projects ranging from front-line medical assistance to essential engagement with communities in the affected countries: Guinea, Liberia, Nigeria and Sierra Leone.

TOP 5 AREAS OF NGOS' INTERVENTIONS

1 HEALTH PROMOTION Raise awareness, train health workers, provide medical supplies and hygiene items.

2 CASE MANAGEMENT Provide medical care for Ebola patients and ensure infection control.

3 COMMUNICATION/ SOCIAL MOBILIZATION Engage with communities to raise awareness and inform.

4 CONTACT TRACING Identify, trace and monitor people who have had high-risk exposure to Ebola.

5 COORDINATION Support national and local capacities and country health teams.

LIBERIA 246 PROJECTS

SIERRA LEONE 61 PROJECTS

GUINEA 133 PROJECTS

NIGERIA 3 PROJECTS

MORE THAN 60 NGOS & INTERNATIONAL ORGANIZATIONS

Creation date: 30 Sep 2014   Sources: OCHA, UNCS, ESRI, WHO, Clusters   Feedback: ochavisual@un.org   www.unocha.org   www.reliefweb.int

FIG 19-1 NGOs Response to the West African Ebola Outbreak. (From the UN Office for the Coordination of Humanitarian Affairs, New York, New York, © [2014] United Nations. Reprinted with the permission of the United Nations.)

motivations; has a primary mission that is not commercial; and depends on funding and materials from external sources. Ball and Dunn[15] outlined some of the common traits of NGOs as follows: (1) formed voluntarily; (2) they are independent of government; (3) they do not exist for private profit or gain; and (4) their principal objective is to improve the circumstances and prospects of disadvantaged people. NGOs also tend to be highly practice-oriented, prize neutrality (i.e., giving nonpartisan assistance), and are decentralized and somewhat resistant to centralization as they value their independence and have strong commitments to "their" cause.

Classifying NGOs is difficult. One useful system was described in 1989 by Brown and Korten,[16] who divide all NGOs into one of four types: (1) voluntary organizations (VOs); (2) people's organizations (POs); (3) hybrid governmental and nongovernmental organizations (co-opted NGOs, or CONGOs); and (4) public service contractors (PSCs). Yet there is a virtual alphabet soup of differing combinations and flavors of ideologies, activities, and main and subsidiary foci that defies simple characterization of NGOs (Box 19-2).

Common NGO ideologies include the golden rule, that all possible steps should be taken to alleviate human suffering arising out of calamity and conflict, an emphasis on human rights and dignity, health care as a right not a privilege, that people affected by disaster have a right to life with dignity and therefore a right to assistance, democracy for all, those who can must help those who can't help themselves, no life is less

BOX 19-1   Examples of NGOs' Primary Purposes, Scope of Action, Philosophical or Practical Orientation and Representative Objectives

Primary Purpose
- Development
- Advocacy
- Disaster relief
- Advisory
- Operations
- Education and training
- Business development
- Watchdog
- Humanitarian aid
- Medical services
- Technology sharing
- Cultural enrichment
- Human rights
- Law and justice

Scope of Action
- International
- Local
- Regional
- National

Orientation
- Faith-based
- Secular humanitarian
- Political
- Professional: technology, health, legal

Areas of Activity[14]
- International relief and development
- Democracy promotion and electoral support, human rights, and good governance
- Conflict mitigation, management, and resolution
- Civil society support and community-based services
- Education, medical, and state service replacement (traditionally formed locally to substitute or enhance lacking or nonexistent government services

BOX 19-2   NGO Alphabet Soup: A Symptom of Classification Confusion

- BINGOs: big international nongovernmental organizations
- CBOs: community-based organizations
- CB-NGOs: community-based nongovernmental organizations
- CSOs: civil society organizations
- DOs: development organizations
- DONGOs: donor nongovernmental organizations
- GONGOs: government-sponsored nongovernmental organizations
- GROs: grassroots organizations
- GRSOs: grassroots support organizations
- IDCIs: international development cooperation institutions
- INGOs: international nongovernmental organizations
- NGDOs: nongovernmental development organizations
- NNGOs: northern nongovernmental organizations
- NPOs: nonprofit organizations
- PANGO: party nongovernmental organization
- POs: people's organizations
- PSCs: public service contractors
- PVOs: private volunteer organizations
- QUANGOs: quasi-nongovernmental organizations
- SCOs: social change organizations
- SNGOs: support nongovernmental organizations
- TSOs: third sector organizations
- TNGO: transnational nongovernmental organization
- VOLAGs: voluntary organizations
- VOs: volunteer organizations
- WCOs: welfare church organizations

Adapted from Vakil AC. Confronting the classification problem: toward a taxonomy of NGOs. *World Develop.* 1997;25(12):2057-2070.

response and recovery workers) for relocation or evacuation; providing or facilitating food and water procurement and distribution; assisting in and garnering help for postdisaster sanitation and mortuary services; caring for lost children; attending to animals and pets; vector control; and linking donors with disaster relief activities.

CURRENT PRACTICE

Despite sovereign governments having the ultimate disaster management responsibility, NGOs often fill response gaps when conventional local or national emergency response personnel are negatively impacted by the disaster itself. The link between disaster medicine and NGOs is special as most expatriate medical and other health care personnel who respond to a disaster do so through or in conjunction with an NGO, be it an international NGO, a church group, or an academic or community medical facility. However, use of NGOs to provide a quick fix for short-term relief is a thing of the past. Instead, through coordination and collaboration with all stakeholders, NGOs are often involved with facilitating sustainable recovery and development which, in turn, empowers local communities to manage their own environments.[17]

Whether national or international, NGOs improve relief efforts and capacity to address a wide range of victims' needs, especially in dealing with complex emergencies. NGOs may be deployed to provide direct assistance (e.g., distribution of goods and services directly to the people), indirect assistance (e.g., services one step removed from the people, like transporting relief supplies and personnel), and even infrastructure and logistical support that may be entirely invisible to the people. Sometimes one large NGO has a diverse skill set and a great capacity, but often multiple smaller NGOs, each focused primarily on their individual mission,

valuable than any other, technical knowledge is a means to escape poverty, and geography is no fault of anyone.

Their diversity of focus spans a wide spectrum of issues: social, cultural, environmental, educational, developmental, technological, peace-building, human rights and dignity, health (public health, health services, and access), humanitarian assistance, shelter, children and youth, law and justice, disaster relief and management, and resiliency. Regarding the NGOs that have disaster relief and management as their primary focus, their scope may be local, regional, national, or international, and their competencies may be specifically well developed in one or more areas: for example, procurement and distribution of clothes, blankets, and appropriate supplies; disaster awareness and preparation; building community resiliency; assisting in search and rescue exercises; providing first aid and medical assistance to the wounded; providing shelter to disaster victims; providing psychosocial and psychospiritual care to victims, survivors, bystanders, and response personnel; assisting with or providing disaster response and recovery logistics; facilitating or providing transportation (to victims and/or complement each other, are more flexible, and collaborate better with an integrated approach. In 2002, a Regional Workshop on Networking and Collaboration among NGOs of Asian Countries in Disaster Reduction and Response was held, in which the participants agreed on a number of steps aimed at promoting and strengthening networking and collaboration among NGOs in Asia for disaster reduction and response "in recognition of the important role played by NGOs especially in Asia (the most natural disaster prone region on the planet)."[18]

As of 2008, worldwide humanitarian work was being accomplished by an estimated 210,800 humanitarian aid workers as calculated by the Active Learning Network for Accountability and Performance (ALNAP), a research and analysis agency serving organizations working in the humanitarian system. This total workforce comprises roughly 50% workers from NGOs, 25% Red Cross/Red Crescent personnel, and 25% workers from the UN system.[19] In 2014 there were more than 4 million NGOs worldwide and about 1.5 million in the United States alone. Their cumulative size, scope, and diversity make their impact almost inestimable. From the small two- or three-person local organization acceptable by U.S. law,[20] to the gigantic international and multinational behemoths such as BRAC International, which has 120,000 staff touching the lives of more than 135 million people,[21] and the International Co-operative Alliance with approximately one billion individuals in its member organizations[22]; NGOs encompass a wide array of endeavors and represent an enormous amount of resources.

The International Federation of Red Cross/Red Crescent Societies (IFRC), perhaps the most recognizable disaster-related NGO worldwide (with 189 recognized national societies, one in almost every country in the world and supported by 17 million volunteers, 80 million members, and 430,000 staff globally),[23] and other large disaster-related NGOs typically establish alliances and develop an international presence almost on par with the UN itself. The IFRC even has special status in transgovernmental international relief and disaster management circles. Large NGOs like the IFRC develop strong, long-lasting local institutional collaboration and networks that increase their influence and capacity to provide or procure immediate and highly effective response services. Smaller NGOs tend to address single needs or sets of related needs around which they have focused and refined their abilities and/or niche. This allows major humanitarian aid organizations to fund response and recovery by financially supporting "niche NGOs" that respond to the given disaster, rather than trying to do the same work using their own staff and resources. Over time, the work of the NGOs has improved the efficiency and efficacy of emergency management operations at the local, national, and, most significantly, international levels.

Nongovernmental Organizations and Volunteers

Volunteers remain essential to the functioning of many NGOs, but may or may not be of assistance in a specific circumstance depending on their background, training, and familiarity with disaster management schema. NGOs are involved in recruiting volunteers, donors, and experts from the private sector; they help orient volunteers to the field of disaster management, assist in outfitting them for the field, and provide or arrange for transportation, lodging, and sustenance in the hot zone, allowing medical and health care volunteers to "work without worry." Volunteers with unique skills who have specialized training (e.g., Community Emergency Response Team [CERT], Federal Emergency Management Agency [FEMA], Incident Command System [ICS], National Incident Management System [NIMS], OCHA, and/or International Search and Rescue Advisory Group [INSARAG] standardized procedures) are invaluable assets in disaster response. NGOs may incur liability when the spontaneous attraction of well-meaning untrained and/or unlicensed health care volunteers to disaster response efforts (convergent volunteerism)[24] also includes people who are actually imposters; this can be avoided if

licenses and background checks are required and volunteers documented. When "appropriate" and vetted volunteers are not available, NGOs (and governments) may turn to paid contractors or business partners, or develop contractual arrangements with freelance experts, academic institutions, and even "niche NGOs."

As a group, NGOs address almost every aspect of response and recovery. At the time of this writing, the websites Relief Web (www.reliefweb.int), National Volunteer Organizations Active in Disasters (www.NVOAD.org), and InterAction (http://www.interaction.org/crisis-list/) track NGOs that respond to disasters, describe specific functions carried out by each, and provide public relations and other information about the NGOs. Fig. 19-1 shows the activity of NGOs responding to the Ebola epidemic in the West African countries of Liberia, Sierra Leone, Guinea, and Nigeria and their key interventions: health promotion, case management, communication and social mobilization, contact tracing and monitoring, and coordination and support of local health teams.

When Disasters Occur

NGOs usually shine in the response and recovery phases of disaster management. In the United States, all emergencies, regardless of size or type, are local events. However, when a community's resources are insufficient to respond to an incident, local government may call upon county, state, and federal governmental agencies and also NGOs for assistance.[25] "As required under Homeland Security Presidential Directive (HSPD)-5, the NIMS enables responders from different communities with a variety of job responsibilities to better work together. Everyone has a role to play in NIMS implementation—fire and rescue, law enforcement, hospitals and health care systems, transportation systems, public works, voluntary agencies, private industry, nongovernmental organizations, and many others—not only in responding to an event, but in ongoing preparedness activities as well."[25]

According to the National Response Framework (NRF),[26] "NGOs collaborate with responders, governments at all levels, and other agencies and organizations" and contribute to the following:

- Training and managing volunteer resources
- Identifying shelter locations and needed supplies
- Providing critical emergency services to those in need, such as cleaning supplies, clothing, food and shelter, or assistance with post-emergency cleanup
- Identifying those whose needs have not been met and helping coordinate the provision of assistance

The NRF builds upon NIMS and describes how communities, the federal government, NGOs, and other voluntary agencies (VOLAGs) collaborate to coordinate the national response. "Some NGOs are officially designated as support elements to national response capabilities. E.g. American Red Cross and National Voluntary Organizations Active in Disasters (NVOAD)."[26] Some U.S. federal agencies fund disaster relief outside of the NRF, which falls exclusively under the Stafford Act. Notable recent events falling outside of the direct provisions of the NRF include the 2010 Gulf of Mexico oil spill; the responses to this event were coordinated under the provisions of the National Contingency Plan (NCP).[27] This directly impacts the funding and availability of resources for response efforts.

In an international disaster, the government of the affected nations will invoke its national disaster response program either formally or informally. The government agency responsible for disaster management may also request international assistance from allied governments and the UN Disaster Assessment and Coordination (UNDAC) unit.[28] UNDAC was created in 1993 and designed to:

- Help the UN and governments of disaster-affected countries during the first phase of a sudden-onset emergency as part of the international emergency response system for sudden-onset emergencies

- Assist in the coordination of incoming international relief at national level and/or at the site of the emergency.
- Provide teams that are able to deploy at short notice (12 to 48 hours) anywhere in the world
- Respond upon request of the UN Resident or Humanitarian Coordinator and/or the affected government
- Provide services without cost to the disaster-affected country

International NGOs may assist in information gathering and assessment in coordination with UNDAC teams in the field and assist in the overall response effort with permission or by invitation of the government of the affected country. Local NGOs assist as capacity and ability warrant and permit.

After and in Between Disasters

Because of the cyclic nature of disasters, vulnerable communities are always predisaster or postdisaster when not involved in an active event. Nonetheless, research shows that there is a low level of priority placed on disaster mitigation and preparedness.[29] Recently, Houghton stated, "... disaster preparedness/mitigation is cited as the most important issue to emerge from recent (humanitarian assistance) evaluations."[30] Interestingly, NGOs have not been as visible in the phases of preparation and mitigation or prevention as they are in response and recovery. Reasons for this were described in a Tearfund study in 2003 on donor practice and policy in natural hazard reduction. The study echoes other literature which suggests that donors still see these phases as low priority, which is reflected in relief and development planning and processes as well. The study offers three possible explanations: (1) poor understanding of what risk reduction really is; (2) lack of obvious ownership of preparedness and risk reduction; and (3) competition for mind share within the phases (response, health care, and education are much more visible and pressing).[31] Progress in this arena has been made with the formation of NGOs specifically addressing preparedness and mitigation, for example, the Los Angeles Emergency Preparedness Foundation (www.laemergencypreparednessfoundation.org), which accomplishes its mission by fostering collaborative preparedness efforts with business, government, academic institutions, other NGOs, and the communities it serves.

In the United States, all responding organizations including NGOs are expected to apply the concepts of hazard vulnerability analysis (HVA) to identify risk, estimate risk probability, and establish key components of an operative response plan. Combined efforts and pooled resources are then employed as measures to reduce potential loss of life and property. NGOs fill gaps in the local planning and in the resource pooling. The organized activities of VOLAGs, including NGOs, permit more robust planning and preparation for disaster (Table 19-1). VOLAGs participate in all aspects of the disaster cycle: some create disaster plans and train responders; others make disaster areas habitable again; still others help displaced families regain some semblance of normalcy post-event. Interweaving NGOs' activities with governmental responses as complementary or supplementary actions helps to stretch limited federal or state resources.

Regarding international disaster management in the interdisaster phases, the governments of 168 countries adopted a 10-year plan to make the world safer from natural hazards at the 2005 World Conference on Disaster Reduction, held in Kobe and Hyogo, Japan. The Hyogo Framework, as the plan is called, is a global blueprint for disaster risk reduction efforts during the decade ending in 2015. Its goal is to substantially reduce disaster losses in lives as well as the social, economic, and environmental assets of communities and countries.[32] Recognizing the prime role of local elements in moving the disaster risk reduction agenda forward, a Global Network of CSOs for Disaster Risk Reduction was initiated in 2007 with close support from the United

TABLE 19-1	Roles of NGOs in the Four Phases of the Disaster Cycle
DISASTER CYCLE PHASE	**ROLE/ACTIVITY**
Preparedness	Interinstitutional networking, contingency planning, public awareness, advocacy, needs analyses, capacity building, training and simulations, community mobilization, community-level research, fundraising, etc.
Response	Recruitment of medical and other skilled volunteers, donation procurement and execution of wills of donors, search and rescue, first aid, debris removal, disposal of dead bodies and animal carcasses, vector control, damage and needs assessment, relief mobilization and distribution, temporary shelter, inventory control, registration, comfort care, reuniting of families, information management, food and water procurement, food and water distribution, child care and diversion therapy, health care, psychological first aid, spiritual care, "employment" of survivors, education, training, responder care, disaster "myth-busting," etc.
Recovery	Housing, orphan care and placement, livelihood, skill-building, institution and organization rebuilding, ongoing public information, assisting with evacuation and sheltering, search and rescue, damage assessments, debris clearance, removal and disposal, utilities and communications restoration, temporary housing, financial management, economic impact analyses, environmental assessments, etc.
Mitigation/ Prevention	Community education, resource mobilization and pooling, outreach, training, and coordination with the public and private sectors; advising and advocating policy development or policy change; etc.

Nations International Strategy for Disaster Reduction (UNISDR) and the Special Unit for South-South Cooperation of the UN Development Program. The Hyoga Framework highlights the essential participation of the private sector, including NGOs.[33]

CHALLENGES

There are various challenges that face NGOs as a sector in relation to every phase of disaster management.

The roles of NGOs vary depending upon the location of the disaster and the predisaster conditions, policies, and infrastructure. As a group, their diversity provides strength and capability to attend to a wide spectrum of needs (Box 19-1). An important feature of NGOs is their independence and self-reliance. This allows for flexibility, innovation, and successful operations conducted by nonconventional means. Their philanthropic work is less scrutinized than that of governmental and international organizations and is perceived as disinterested benevolence rather than as serving some legal mandate or statutory requirement. Their perceived neutrality has been a factor in reducing security risks to the volunteer staff, but NGOs face a growing security threat in disasters involving armed conflict and terrorist acts. Nonetheless, their independence influences NGOs' humanitarian response operations in both positive and negative ways. In the past there was often inter-NGO competition, but better coordination and the adoption of standards of conduct have diminished this considerably. Much of the competition arose from the "pride of mission" fueled by the reality of these often resource-poor groups working hard to attract funding and to serve the perceptions of their donor base. As malignant as the aforementioned are the corruption, misappropriation and misuse of funds, and poor management with little accountability that have plagued some groups and are, unfortunately, situations not uncommon among NGOs.[34] Identifiable factors favoring corruption in humanitarian operations include lack of planning (or even the impossibility of planning), the number of humanitarian actors present, and the financial resources at stake.[35]

Nongovernmental agencies usually do not have the same authority as government agencies, but NGOs are usually under no obligation to participate in any emergency management coordination framework or mechanism; also, they often have no statutory requirements or preset societal mandated expectations from the served population. Just as governments often need NGOs, NGOs may also need government assistance, and when planning the allocation of local community emergency management resources and structures, some government organizations provide direct assistance to NGOs.[26] Whereas NGOs may have access to people that governmental agencies have difficulty reaching because of political realities, governments have the final say in permitting NGOs access to the people in their jurisdiction. In addition, governments may strategically favor one needy segment of the population over another, while a given NGO may have an agenda based on its mission that is just the opposite. Nonetheless, as demonstrated in a recent case study of a public–nonprofit partnership established during the response to the 2010 earthquake in Haiti, "... communication and trust between partnering organizations, as well as experience working together, are the most important inputs ..." for success.[36]

COORDINATION

As trust and communication are fundamental components of team-building and collaboration, so are teamwork and coordination of all stakeholders vital to the effective management of a disaster, regardless of the organization type. Coordination permits optimization of efforts in both the reach and the coverage of responding organizations. Solid coordination increases the quality and quantity of valuable information and data as well as their communication and meaningful interpretation. Coordination reduces duplication, wastage, unnecessary activity while increasing transparency, trust and accountability, collaborative exercises, and sharing of equipment, resources and valuable contacts in the field. Thoughtful coordination minimizes overlooked areas of need and coverage blackouts and serves to reduce security risks to rescue and relief personnel.

As the benefits of coordinated action outweigh the liabilities, coordination mechanisms have become more formalized and effective, but as there are differences in circumstances (e.g., affected country or region, collaborating partners like the military or some private business), there are corresponding differences in forms and mechanisms of coordination, including command and control mechanisms, to accommodate these differences. Even so, there are factors unique to each disaster which challenge the NGOs' ability to coordinate with each other and with governmental agencies operating in the hot zone. This is especially relevant when there is military involvement in benevolent work since the perceived missions of the NGO and the military are often in conflict,[37] and joint operations are often needlessly chaotic.[38]

NGOs may coordinate by location and situation under a variety of mechanisms. The physical extent of the disaster, its speed of onset, its

> ### BOX 19-3 Challenges Posed by NGO Presence in Disaster Management Efforts
>
> - Lack of organization, management, and leadership in the field
> - Lack of teamwork and collaboration
> - Duplication of efforts
> - Myth promotion
> - Self-serving rather than community serving
> - Lack of consideration for security and volunteer safety
> - Interference with other critical operations
> - Burdening the fragile support infrastructure
> - Fraud
> - Propaganda
> - Misrepresentation of capacity and capability
> - Cultural and religious insensitivity
> - Operational inefficiency
> - Social and economic disruption of the affected society
> - Proselytizing and sectarian dogmatism

scope, and the range of agencies involved in response, as well as local emergency management capacity all affect each NGO's own scope of action. The various coordination mechanisms include, but are not limited to: a local, regional, or national government emergency operations center (EOC); formal NGO-specific coordination mechanisms; UN-established coordination mechanisms; civil–military operations centers; field coordination meetings, and even designated coordination websites. Nonetheless, however difficult to accomplish, coordination of efforts is essential for both efficiency and effectiveness in disaster management, and because NGOs have no statutory obligation to participate they may sometimes prove to be more a hindrance than a help. There are some distinct challenges posed by the NGOs presence in disaster management efforts in this regard (Box 19-3).

Despite the advances in coordination among the responding NGOs and the other responding agencies, there is sometimes still a lack of cooperation and collaboration between local and international NGOs because of coexisting, yet differing multiple NGO coordination mechanisms that operate independently of each other. Different coordination mechanisms may be at the same level (local-local) or address different levels of humanitarian action (local vs. national, national vs. regional, or international). The presence of multiple coordination mechanisms generally has a negative effect on response and recovery operations because their simultaneous application favors redundant actions and service gaps, noncollaboration and hoarding, competitiveness and rivalry or "turf battles," missed opportunities for co-learning, and inconsistencies in planning and execution in the field.

Collaboration in the United States

According to Hogan and Burstein,[39] NGOs are a key part of the overall national disaster response in the United States, collaborating with first responders, with other agencies, and with government at all levels, and play a critical role when the services they provide are not otherwise available.[30] Certain NGOs are ubiquitous in the disaster management arena. For example, the American Red Cross (ARC) provides local relief and also coordinates with Emergency Support Function (ESF) #6 in mass care situations.[39] NVOAD, founded in 1970, is a consortium of about 200 faith-based, community-based, and other nonprofit groups representing thousands of professional staff and volunteers with unique skills. This organizing entity of NGOs provides a wide range of expertise and specialized services to the incident command system during disasters. During major incidents, NVOAD typically sends representatives to the FEMA's National Response Coordination Center to represent the voluntary organizations, assist in response coordination and facilitate the provision of specialized services by member NGOs.[40] Examples of NVOAD specialized training partners include ACTS World Relief's advanced disaster simulation; Global Rapid Rescue and Relief (GR3Inc.), which provides technical and psychological first aid simulations; and those of the American Radio Relay League (ARRL) of the National Association for Amateur Radio, which establishes two-way communication links with devastated communities.[41] NVOAD also contributes in the area of disaster spiritual and psychological care training, programming, and operations with partnering organizations such as "Headwaters" Relief Organization. All members are guided by the core principles of the Four Cs—cooperation, communication, coordination, and collaboration. NVOAD was included as a valuable asset in the development of the National Response Plan (NRP)[42] and advocates among its members for an in-depth understanding and the adoption of the principles of the NIMS, as outlined in a 2008 FEMA Fact Sheet of 14 key points specifically prepared for NGOs operating in U.S. territories.[25]

In international disasters, a written national disaster management plan is not always in place, or the affected areas may span several nations that have diverse plans and goals, thus making a coordinated disaster response more challenging to achieve. The UN OCHA was created to be responsible for bringing together humanitarian actors to ensure a coherent response to emergencies. Although the ultimate goal is to assist people when they most need relief or protection, a key pillar of the OCHA mandate[43] is to "coordinate effective and principled humanitarian action in partnership with national and international actors." To accomplish this, OCHA's activities include assessing situations and needs; agreeing on common priorities; developing common strategies to address issues such as negotiating access; mobilizing funding and other resources; clarifying consistent public messaging; and monitoring progress.[44]

One special "family" of NGOs is probably the most recognizable around the world, the Red Cross. The International Committee of the Red Cross (ICRC) is the oldest and largest of the NGOs. It has a mandate under The Geneva Convention to function as a religiously, politically, and ideologically neutral intermediary to protect victims of conflict and support those affected by natural disaster. It is separate from all other international humanitarian organizations and NGOs and has special status in the UN. In contrast to this Swiss-based NGO, the U.S.-based ARC, a federally chartered instrumentality of the U.S. government[26] yet not a federal agency under the NRF, is not neutral but similarly is not a member of the IFRC, the umbrella organization for all other Red Cross and Red Crescent Societies throughout the world.

Coordinating bodies like OCHA and collaboration superstructures like IFRC and NVOAD help NGOs fulfill their respective missions together. In the past NGOs have not always sought collaboration and did not have an agreed-upon humanitarian ethics conduct or maintained predetermined standards of conduct.[45] Recognizing the need for such standards, one group embarked on the Sphere Project, which produced a well-known standard of conduct (http://www.spherehandbook.org/). The Sphere Project Handbook provides detailed guiding principles for managing response and recovery requirements like sanitation, water, and shelter. Another frequently referenced code of conduct was created in 1994 by a small group of well-known, large NGOs. The Code of Conduct for NGOs in Disaster Relief,[46] as it is called, attempts to formalize the actions of the actors in humanitarian work, serves as general guidelines for all organizations involved in international disaster management, and provides a framework for organization and self-discipline among the adopters of its philosophy.

Even with these challenges, all is not dismal. Patrick Kilby's 2008 case study, "The Strength of Networks: The Local NGO Response to the Tsunami in India"[47] discusses NGO collaboration after the Asian Tsunami in 2004 and concludes that it was the trust and capacity built up through previous network activities communities that enabled the launch of an effective response to the tsunami. The lesson was that similar existing network collaborators could be effectively employed in other disaster responses around the world. Coordination and collaboration is also the key point to successful disaster management in the United States.[48]

FUTURE PERSPECTIVE

As of January 2015, another level of scrutiny was implemented for NGOs that desire to be recognized in the global arena by the Internet domain suffix ".ngo" or ".ong." The project[49] includes a transparent, systematic process for vetting organizations that wish to have this designation. The designers' aim is to create an online community that helps to garner wider visibility for nonprofits and NGOs worldwide, and whose validation process reassures Internet users worldwide that website addresses owned by organizations with domain names ending in .ngo and .ong represent bona-fide NGOs. This should clear up some of the transparency, credibility, management, and accountability issues challenging NGOs.

Before World War II, government programs to reduce environmental hazards were very limited,[50] but this has changed. So too, the future roles of NGOs in disaster medicine are great but will be different. Building on the numbers, diversity, and increasing competencies of NGO staff and volunteers, some niche NGOs are already developing expertise in training and disaster simulation, telehealth and GPS mapping, psycho-spiritual care, and posttraumatic stress disorder (PTSD) prevention. Understanding that there is no better way to deal with disasters than being well prepared in the first place, and using an all-hazards approach to disaster anticipation and prevention, NGOs stand poised to collaborate with other team members and bring resources in research and development to the table. Along with being prepared for common natural disasters like earthquakes and typhoons, communities will need to be prepared to deal with terrorist attacks only imaginable today, as well as the effects of emerging hazards like toxic fumes from dumps and red tides. Responses will need to be well coordinated but permit flexibility for innovation and creativity in the relief effort (i.e., planned innovation).[51] As essential participants in the disaster management field, NGOs can build better alliances with the communities they serve as well as with governments and the military. Better attention to assessment of disaster response needs before deployment, collection of goods and shipping of equipment and materials, and using probability-based decision making will ensure that NGOs and governments can better anticipate what and where to warehouse supplies for more rapid and appropriate deployments.

As Vye points out, ". . . reviews of major natural disaster crises show that, in by far the most cases, inadequate and inefficient relief and rescue efforts can be traced back to a lack of preparedness, at all levels, and lack of commitment on behalf of the government to establish clear and rigid policy for building in high risk areas. NGOs stand to make a difference in bridging this gap and facilitating a better understanding of what needs to be mandated in policy and how to pass this information on to the grassroots level. Essentially, those affected by the disaster directly need to be included in the planning of mitigation efforts. Although an NGO may have established a high acceptance level in a particular community, increased and improved coordination among NGOs is necessary to be taken more seriously from top-down disaster management actors . . . . Building better partnerships and professionalization of the sector is therefore of paramount importance to be taken in earnest."[17] Cronin and colleagues[52] also suggest that links with academia, in particular the scientific community, should be formed by NGOs and show the benefits of such collaborations in their study of volcanology.

Finally, as the community itself becomes recognized as a fundamental stakeholder in the process of preventative measures, community-based NGOs will have as major a stake in the mitigation and prevention phases as they currently have in the other phases of disaster management.[53]

CONCLUSION

Natural disasters occur throughout the world, but their economic and social impacts have been increasing, with greater negative effects in developing countries than in developed ones. Disasters can wipe out development gains and eclipse years of progress development.

Sovereign governments are ultimately responsible for the disaster management and prevention within their own territories; however, they often depend upon nongovernmental groups, such as academic centers, businesses, private organizations, and volunteer associations, to fill the gaps that are not or inadequately attended to by their own disaster management infrastructure. The NGO has played an important role historically and currently and has a definite niche in the future of disaster medicine.

The greatest strengths of NGOs are their numbers, diversity, and autonomy to engage in planned innovation. Their greatest weaknesses are independence, the episodic nature of many of their organizations, interagency competition, and the perpetuation of some fundamental disaster myths shared by donors.

Although their roles in disaster management in times past may have varied between "solo responders" to interference with prime objectives, there is little doubt today that their current and emerging roles are now central to any reasonable response to disasters and the essential prevention, planning, and preparation necessary in all communities BEFORE disasters occur. The IFCR, ARC, and other NGOs are respected players in most high-level international disaster forums now and will be in the foreseeable future. With the increase in global catastrophic events, the contribution of the NGO sector to international disaster management and disaster medicine is even more promising as improvements in collaboration and engagement of all stakeholders become critical to successful disaster preparedness, response, recovery, and mitigation.

REFERENCES

1. OCHA. NGOs' response to the West Africa Ebola outbreak. Available at: http://reliefweb.int/report/liberia/ngos-response-west-africa-ebola-outbreak-30-sep-2014.
2. Krebs HB. *Responsibility, Legitimacy, Morality: Chinese Humanitarianism in Historical Perspective.* HPG Working Paper, London: Overseas Development Institute; September 2014. Available at: http://www.odi.org/sites/odi.org.uk/files/odi-assets/publications-opinion-files/9139.pdf.
3. Chen-Wing R. The Knights of St. John of Jerusalem as a prototypical NGO. *Tiresias.* 2012;1:51–55. Available at: https://artsonline.uwaterloo.ca/hydra/ojs/index.php/tiresias/article/view/20/8.
4. Risse GB. *Mending Bodies, Saving Souls: A History of Hospitals.* New York, NY: Oxford University Press; 1999.
5. Davey E, Borton J, Foley M. *A History of the Humanitarian System: Western Origins and Foundations.* HPG Working PaperLondon: Overseas Development Institute; June 2013. Available at: http://www.odi.org/sites/odi.org.uk/files/odi-assets/publications-opinion-files/8439.pdf.
6. Davies T. NGOs: a long and turbulent history. *Global J.* January 24, 2013. Available at: http://theglobaljournal.net/group/global-governance/article/981/.
7. Address of the Royal Jennerian Society for the Extermination of the Small-pox: with the plan, regulations and instructions for vaccine inoculation: to which is added a list of the subscribers (1803). Available at: https://archive.org/details/cihm_47523.
8. Edgerton-Tarpley K. Pictures to draw tears from iron. Available at: http://ocw.mit.edu/ans7870/21f/21f.027/tears_from_iron/tfi_essay_03.pdf.
9. Janku A. The North-China Famine of 1876-1879: performance and impact of a non-event. In: *Measuring Historical Heat: Event, Performance, and Impact in China and the West. Symposium in Honour of Rudolf G. Wagner on His 60th Birthday, Heidelberg, November 3-4;* 2001:127–134. Available at: http://www.sino.uni-heidelberg.de/conf/symposium2.pdf.
10. China Famine Relief Fund Shanghai Committee. *The Great Famine.* Shanghai: American Presbyterian Mission Press; 1879; pp. 1, 88, 128, 157. Available at: https://archive.org/details/cu31924023248796.
11. UN Charter Chapter X Article 71. Available at: http://www.un.org/en/documents/charter/chapter10.shtml.
12. Economic and Social Council (ECOSOC) of the United Nations. Available at: http://www.un.org/esa/coordination/ngo/committee.htm.
13. United Nations. *Working with ECOSOC: An NGO Guide to Consultative Status.* 2011. Available at: http://www.un-ngls.org/IMG/pdf/ATTCPCS7.pdf.
14. Lawry L. *Guide to Nongovernmental Organizations for the Military. Originally produced as Frandsen, G. A Guide to NGOs. 2002.* Washington, DC: Center for Disaster and Humanitarian Assistance Medicine, Department of Defense; 2009. Available at: www.dtic.mil/cgi-bin/GetTRDoc?AD=ADA519436.
15. Ball C, Dunn L. *Non-Governmental Organisations in the Commonwealth: Guidelines for Good Policy and Practice.* London: The Commonwealth Foundation; 1994.
16. Brown D, Korten D. *Understanding Voluntary Organizations: Guidelines for Donors.* vol. 1. Working Paper 258. Washington, DC: World Bank, Country Economics Department. Available at: http://www-wds.worldbank.org/external/default/WDSContentServer/IW3P/IB/1989/09/01/000009265_3960928075717/Rendered/PDF/multi_page.pdf.
17. Vye E. The Role of Non Governmental Organisations in Disaster Mitigation and Response—A Case Study in Uttarakhand, Northern India. In: *Masters Thesis in partial fulfilment of the Masters in Humanitarian Action degree,* Michigan Technological University, School of Biology and Environmental Science; 2007. Available at: http://www.geo.mtu.edu/~raman/papers2/VyeRoleofNGOs.pdf.
18. Regional Workshop on Networking and Collaboration among NGOs of Asian Countries in Disaster Reduction and Response, February 20-22, 2002. Available at: http://www.adrc.asia/publications/ngo_workshop/statement.pdf.
19. Harvey P, Stoddard A, Harmer A, Taylor G. *The State of the Humanitarian System: Assessing Performance and Progress—A Pilot Study.* Available at: http://www.alnap.org/pool/files/alnap-sohs-final.pdf.
20. U.S. Department of State. Fact Sheet: Non-Governmental Organizations (NGOs) in the United States. January 12, 2012. Available at: http://www.humanrights.gov/2012/01/12/fact-sheet-non-governmental-organizations-ngos-in-the-united-states/.
21. BRAC Global Report 2013. The Story of BRAC. Available at: http://www.brac.net/sites/default/files/annual-report-2013/GlobalReportforweb011014.pdf.
22. International Co-operative Alliance. Co-operative facts and figures. Available at: http://ica.coop/en/whats-co-op/co-operative-facts-figures.
23. International Federation of Red Cross/Red Crescent Societies. Available at: http://www.ifrc.org/en/what-we-do/volunteers/global-review-on-volunteering/.
24. Cone DC, Weir SD, Bogucki S. Convergent volunteerism. *Ann Emerg Med.* 2003;41:457–462.
25. FEMA. *Fact Sheet NIMS Implementation for Nongovernmental Organizations.* Washington, DC: NIMS Integration Center; 2006. Available at: www.fema.gov/emergency/nims.
26. National Response Framework 2008. pp. 18–20. Available at: http://www.fema.gov/media-library-data/20130726-1914-25045-1246/final_national_response_framework_20130501.pdf and NRF Resource Center http://emilms.fema.gov/IS800B/lesson6/NRF0106060.htm.
27. Environmental Protection Agency. The National Oil and Hazardous Substances Pollution Contingency Plan (40 CFR 300). Available at: http://www.epa.gov/radiation/rert/ncp.html.
28. United Nations Office for the Coordination of Humanitarian Affairs (OCHA). *United Nations Disaster Assessment and Coordination (UNDAC)*

Handbook. 2006. Available at: https://ochanet.unocha.org/p/Documents/UNDAC Handbook-dec2006.pdf.

29. Benson C, Twigg J, Myers M. NGO initiatives in risk reduction: An overview. *Disasters.* 2001;25(3):199–215.

30. Houghton R. Tsunami Emergency Lessons Learned from Previous Natural Disasters. In: *Active Learning Network for Accountability and Performance in Humanitarian Action Review Series. Lessons Learned Studies,* London: ALNAP; 2005.

31. La Trobe S, Venton P. Natural Disaster Risk Reduction: The Policy and Practice of Selected Institutional Donors. In: *A Tearfund Research Project*; 2003. Available at: http://www.tearfund.org/webdocs/Website/Campaigning/Policy and research/Natural Disaster Risk Reduction research.pdf.

32. ISDR. *NGOs & Disaster Risk Reduction: A Preliminary Review of Initiatives and Progress Made (Background Paper for a Consultative Meeting on a "Global Network of NGOs for Community Resilience to Disasters,"* Geneva, 25–26; October, 2006. Available at: http://www.unisdr.org/2008/partner-netw/ngos/meeting1-october-2006/NGOs_and_DRR_Background_Paper.pdf.

33. UN/ISDR & UN/OCHA. *Disaster Preparedness for Effective Response Guidance and Indicator Package for Implementing Priority Five of the Hyogo Framework.* Geneva, Switzerland: United Nations Secretariat of the International Strategy for Disaster Reduction (UN/ISDR) and the United Nations Office for Coordination of Humanitarian Affairs (UN/OCHA).

34. Larché J. Corruption in the NGO world: what it is and how to tackle it. *Humanit Exch.* 2011;52, Available at: http://www.odihpn.org/humanitarian-exchange-magazine/issue-52/corruption-in-the-ngo-world-what-it-is-and-how-to-tackle-it.

35. Maxwell D, et al. *Preventing Corruption in Humanitarian Assistance: Final Research Report.* Humanitarian Policy Group and TI: Feinstein International Center; 2008.

36. Nolte IM, Boenigk S. Public–nonprofit partnership performance in a disaster context: the case of Haiti. *Public Admin.* 2011;89(4):1385–1402.

37. United States Institute of Peace. Guide for Participants in Peace, Stability, and Relief Operations. Available at: http://www.usip.org/node/5607.

38. Byman D. Uncertain partners: NGOs and the military. *Survival: Glob Poli Strategy.* 2001;43(2):97–114.

39. Hogan DE, Burstein JL. The United States National Response Plan. In: Hogan DE, Burstein JL, eds. *Disaster Medicine.* 2nd ed. Philadelphia, PA: Lippincott Williams & Wilkins; 2007:153.

40. US Department of Homeland Security. National Response Framework. January 2008. Available at: http://emilms.fema.gov/IS821/assets/nrf-core.pdf.

41. Amateur Radio Emergency Service. *Katrina: The Untold Story.* 2008. Available at: http://www.arrl.org/ares-el?issue=2014-08-20.

42. US Homeland Security. NRP Brochure. Available at: http://www.dhs.gov/xlibrary/assets/NRP_Brochure.pdf.

43. UN Office for the Coordination of Humanitarian Action. Who We Are. Available at: http://www.unocha.org/about-us/who-we-are.

44. UN Office for the Coordination of Humanitarian Action. Coordination. Available at: http://www.unocha.org/what-we-do/coordination/overview.

45. Global Development Research Center. *The NGO Management Toolbox.* Available at: http://www.gdrc.org/ngo/codes-conduct.html.

46. IFRC. The Code of Conduct of NGOs in Disaster Relief. Available at: http://www.ifrc.org/Docs/idrl/I259EN.pdf.

47. Kilb P. The strength of networks: the local NGO response to the tsunami in India. *Disasters.* 2008;32(1):120–130.

48. Sylves R. *Disaster Policy and Politics: Emergency Management and Homeland Security.* 2nd ed. Thousand Oaks, CA: CQ Press; 2014.

49. PIR. The Public Interest Registry. Available at: http://pir.org/about-us/.

50. Waugh W. *Living with Hazards, Dealing with Disasters: An Introduction to Emergency Management.* Sharpe: New York, NY; 2000.

51. Gabriel EJ. Making room for outside the box thinking in emergency management and preparedness. *Jt Comm J Qual Saf.* 2003;29:319–320.

52. Cronin SJ, Gaylord DR, Charley D, Alloway BV, Wallez S, Esau JW. Participatory methods of incorporating scientific with traditional knowledge for volcanic hazard management on Ambae Island, Vanuatu. *Bull Volcanol.* 2004;66:652–668.

53. Sharma VK. Disaster management strategies in India. In: *Coping with Natural Hazards: Indian Context.* Andhra Pradesh, India: Orient Longman; 2004:250–256.

SUGGESTED READINGS

1. National Disaster Management Guidelines. *Role of NGOs in Disaster Management.* New Delhi, India: National Disaster Management Authority, Government of India; September 2010.

2. FEMA Comparative Emergency Management Session 26: Nongovernmental Organizations. Available at: https://training.fema.gov/emiweb/edu/compEmMgmt/.

3. Burkle FM, Greenough PG. Impact of public health emergencies on disaster taxonomy, planning and response. *Disaster Med Public Health Prep.* 2008;2(3):192–199.

4. Pinkowski J, ed. *Disaster Management Handbook.* Boca Raton, FL: CRC Press; 2008.

5. Kapucu N, Van Wart M. The evolving role of the public sector in managing catastrophic disasters—lessons learned. *Admin Soc.* 2006;38:279.

6. Van Wart M, Berman E. Contemporary public sector productivity values: narrower scope, tougher standards, and new rules of the game. *Publ Prod Manag Rev.* 1999;22:326–347.

Disaster and Emergency Management Programs

Angela M. Snyder and Mark E. Gebhart

WHAT IS DISASTER AND EMERGENCY MANAGEMENT?

Offices of disaster and emergency management focus on providing aid to communities and other entities with prevention, preparation, and recovery from disastrous events. In order to accomplish these tasks, those involved with emergency management work with other agencies before, during, and after disasters to coordinate services through programs developed primarily to deal with the disaster itself and its consequences. Prior to disasters, emergency management offices develop or revise emergency plans and programs and also provide training, drills, and exercises to help responding agencies prepare and be ready for disasters. During disasters, emergency management offices focus on preservation of life and property. After disasters, these offices focus on recovery through the coordination of available services and resources to return communities back to the way they were, or better than they were, before the disaster. Overall, the purpose of disaster and emergency management is to work with all parties involved to ensure safety in time of disasters. Disaster and emergency management programs have four main goals: (1) saving lives, (2) preventing injury, (3) protecting property, and (4) protecting the environment.

The Emergency Management Cycle

Effective emergency management is a continuous process, frequently discussed in terms of phases of the emergency management cycle. Although this is a convenient way to categorize the many processes and actions involved with emergency management, it must be stressed that actions in each of the phases can and often are conducted simultaneously with actions in a different phase. The five phases, with examples of actions involved, are:

- *Prevention:* Create safety protocols and barriers to aid in the prevention of disasters.
  - *Examples:* Build dams, conduct security checks at airports and other high-profile public places.
- *Mitigation:* Develop ways to minimize the negative effects of disasters.
  - *Examples:* Hurricane warning systems, tornado sirens, earthquake-resistant buildings, land use management, education programs.
- *Preparedness:* Organize and prepare for disasters in coordination with response agencies.
  - *Examples:* Conduct exercises and drills, create response plans, develop memoranda of understanding between responding agencies, and establish integrated material logistical support.
- *Response:* Respond to disasters to ensure safety and the protection of victims and property.
  - *Examples:* Search and rescue, firefighting, first aid, open shelters, law enforcement, public health.
- *Recovery:* Assist communities and individuals to get things back to "normal."
  - *Examples:* Clear debris, stabilize critical infrastructure, and rebuild homes.

Why Do We Need Disaster and Emergency Management Programs?

In times of disaster, important tasks are carried out by multiple agencies to assist those in need. Most agencies and first responders are able to respond and handle small-scale emergencies on their own, such as house fires and motor vehicle crashes; however, larger disasters may require coordination across multiple agencies in a jurisdiction or integration of and collaboration with multiple jurisdictions and agencies, and a coordinating body can oversee activities of all these entities.

HISTORICAL PERSPECTIVE

History of Disaster and Emergency Management Programs

The federal government has been assisting with disaster relief since the Congressional Act of 1803 was passed in response to a large fire in New Hampshire. From the 1800s until about the 1960s and 1970s, U.S. government response can be best characterized as reactive and primarily financial. Numerous agencies had primary responsibilities, depending on the specific type of disaster. This caused relief efforts to be more complex, complicated, and, at times, not very effective.[1,2]

In the 1970s, following four major hurricanes (Hurricanes Carla 1962, Betsy 1965, Camille 1969, and Agnes 1972), the National Governors Association approached President Jimmy Carter and requested the development of a more centralized federal disaster relief program. In response, Executive Order 12127, establishing the Federal Emergency Management Agency (FEMA), was issued. FEMA assumed the bulk of disaster management responsibilities. An all-hazards approach to emergency management was developed, and an Integrated Emergency Management System (IEMS) was created to address disaster and emergency management and organize federal emergency management during natural and human-made disasters.[1,2]

From the 1970s to the 1990s, FEMA continued to provide federal disaster relief under the direction of the president. To ensure that the federal government had the constitutional authority to provide disaster response, the Robert T. Stafford Disaster Relief and Emergency Assistance Act was signed in 1988, creating the legal framework needed for FEMA to operate.[1]

Although there have been a number of outstanding directors of FEMA, James L. Witt, appointed in 1993 by President Clinton, was the first with prior experience in emergency management. Under his leadership, FEMA addressed other aspects of emergency management, specifically recovery and mitigation efforts. This was the first step toward federal involvement in all five phases of the emergency management cycle.[1]

The terrorist attacks on the World Trade Center and the Pentagon of September 11, 2001, resulted in a major turning point for FEMA. Heretofore, disaster planning had focused primarily on natural, technological, or transportation disasters. The new threat—terrorism with weapons of mass destruction—was added to the list of potential disasters. In order to be more effective in national security, the Department of Homeland Security (DHS) was established in March of 2003. DHS absorbed FEMA as well as 21 other major disaster and emergency management and national security agencies.[1] Some of these agencies included the following:[3]

- U.S. Coast Guard
- Immigration and Naturalization Service
- Transportation and Security Administration
- Federal Law Enforcement Training Center
- National Disaster Medical Center (returned to Health and Human Services 2004)
- U.S. Secret Service

The two most current pieces of legislation pertaining to FEMA were developed in 2006 and 2013. Following Hurricane Katrina, the Post-Katrina Emergency Management Reform Act was created to identify and close the major gaps that FEMA identified during the response and recovery phase of this major disaster. The Act created new leadership positions in FEMA, developed new missions, and gave FEMA administration the ability to participate in a broader range of disaster and emergency management efforts.[4] The Sandy Recovery Improvement Act of 2013 significantly modified public assistance procedures, debris removal, public transportation coordination, community disaster loans, and other disaster-related functions.[5]

CURRENT PRACTICE

Federal Programs

Community Emergency Response Team

Community Emergency Response Teams (CERTs) were developed by the Los Angeles City Fire Department in 1985 to educate, prepare, and engage civilians in disaster response and preparedness. CERT members are trained in basic response and preparedness including fire safety, light search and rescue, hazard identification, and disaster medical operations. This training gives them the ability to respond to disasters in their communities and even their workplace, if the need arises. In some disaster situations, emergency responders are not always able to access all disaster areas immediately. CERTs provide valuable services until professional emergency responders can arrive. CERT members are also encouraged to take active roles in preparedness projects and plans and communicate the importance of preparedness to family, friends, and neighbors to help grow resilience.[6]

Voluntary Organizations Active in Disaster

Voluntary Organizations Active in Disaster (VOAD) is a coalition of nonprofit organizations that form teams of volunteers to assist their communities with disaster recovery and to build disaster-resilient communities. VOAD uses the four Cs—cooperation, communication, coordination, and collaboration—to ensure that resources and knowledge are shared, planned, and deployed properly in times of disaster.[7]

National Preparedness System

The National Preparedness System provides an outlined process that communities can use when developing their preparedness plans. Inclusion of the "whole community" is highlighted throughout this process

to help achieve National Preparedness Goals while keeping all involved entities informed. This process consists of six suggested steps:

- Conduct a risk assessment: Where and what are the areas of risk for the community?
- Determine resources required: What is needed to be prepared for community risks?
- Develop required resources: What is the best way to use available resources and identify resources still needed?
- Deliver required resources: How can we coordinate with the entire community to deliver the necessary resources?
- Validate resources: What exercises can we conduct to practice using the plans and resources developed?
- Regularly review and update plans: How often and what should we do to update plans and ensure that resources still exist?

Along with this six-step process, other tools and resources are provided to assist communities in developing their preparedness plans and goals.[8]

Medical Reserve Corps

Through the Office of the Surgeon General, the Division of Civilian Medical Reserve Corps gives support to medical reserve corps (MRC) throughout the United States. An MRC consists of volunteers in the medical profession, including physicians, nurses, pharmacists, dentists, veterinarians, and epidemiologists. Along with medical and public health personnel, interpreters, religious officials, and legal advisors are also necessary.

An MRC's main priority is to make public health, emergency response, and community resilience stronger in their communities. During times of disaster or emergencies, MRCs work with FEMA and American Red Cross (ARC) representatives to provide medical assistance in emergency shelters, hospitals, and health clinics. They provide medical services that are not otherwise available or help alleviate the extra pressure on regular medical staff in a disaster area.[9]

National Disaster Medical System

The National Disaster Medical System (NDMS) is a partnership among FEMA, the Departments of Defense and Veteran Affairs, the U.S. Public Health Service, and civilian providers, ancillary personnel, and hospitals. NDMS provides supplemental assistance to all levels of government that have been overwhelmed by a federally declared disaster through the allocation of funds, equipment, and medical personnel that are trained to assist in any way possible, including on-site care and stabilization, patient transportation, and definitive care at remote facilities. During nondisaster times, the NDMS is authorized to assist in the treatment of service personnel returning from combat environments if the Military Healthcare System (MHS) is overwhelmed, through the Integrated CONUS (continental United States) Medical Operations Plan, or ICMOP. Under the National Response Framework, the Department of Health and Human Services has the lead for NDMS activities, which are deployed under Emergency Support Function #8 (ESF#8).[10]

Federal Education Programs

Federal disaster and emergency management programs offer a variety of educational opportunities for students, public officials, emergency managers, and first responders. Two major educational outlets are the Emergency Management Institute (EMI) and the Center for Domestic Preparedness (CDP), both operated by FEMA.

EMI is physically part of the National Emergency Training Center (NETC) in Emmitsburg, Maryland, and develops emergency management education and training curricula. The goal is to better the response capabilities of government officials, volunteers, and organizations in the public and private sector in order to mitigate the consequences of disasters. Course topics include natural and technological hazards, leadership, public information, and integrated emergency management. Students may attend classes, take courses online through the Independent Study Program, or participate in specialized training and drills like the Chemical Stockpile Emergency Preparedness Program.[11]

CDP, located in Anniston, Alabama, provides hands-on training for emergency service providers at the state, local, and tribal level. They offer courses in areas ranging from Emergency Management to Emergency Medical Services to Public Health and Public Works. The CDP comprises three main training facilities. The Chemical, Ordnance, Biological and Radiological Training Facility (COBRATF) provides exercises using actual toxic chemical agents to give civilians the experience of responding to real-life chemical, biological, radiological, and explosive disasters. The Noble Training Facility (NTF) is a converted army hospital now used to train health and medical professionals in the skills necessary to respond to disasters. The Advanced Responder Training Complex (ARTC) operates a mock municipality to provide responders with a realistic training environment.[12]

State Emergency Management

Each state has an Office of Emergency Management (usually called the State Emergency Management Agency, or SEMA) that develops disaster and emergency management programs similar to those of the federal government. Just as the federal government supplements the relief efforts of the state government, the state government supplements the relief efforts of local emergency management within the state. Typically this is done when local emergency management and responders have become overwhelmed by a disaster. SEMAs provide a link between the resources from the federal government or other in-state jurisdictions or facilitate interstate mutual aid through Emergency Management Assistance Compacts. Overall, state emergency management plays a crucial role in the assistance of local emergency management and liaison between federal and local relief.[13]

The governor of a state has specific responsibilities for emergency management. He or she is the sole person able to request federal aid, declare disaster areas within the state, and sign mutual aid agreements.

Local Emergency Management

Depending on the structure of the local and state government, disaster and emergency management responsibilities can fall to the county or parish, city, or other predefined region. Each section of disaster and emergency management works together with emergency responders to ensure that the necessary resources are available when needed. Other roles of local emergency management offices are to conduct hazard vulnerability assessments of their communities and to coordinate all of the disaster-related resources within the community. If additional resources are required, the local emergency manager can communicate with elected leaders to request assistance from the state disaster and emergency management office.

Nongovernment Organizations

The ARC is a worldwide volunteer organization committed to helping people in need. ARC volunteers range from medical professionals to ham radio operators to mass care and feeding personnel. The ARC provides emergency shelter, food, health and mental health services, and other disaster resources and referrals to aid victims after disasters. The ARC also supports responders during recovery operations. The ARC plays a large role in disaster planning and response with all levels of the government and is part of the National Response Framework under Emergency Support Function #6 (ESF #6).[14]

Community and Faith-Based Organizations

Organizations that work with and provide services to the community on a daily basis have gained the trust of most members of the community and therefore play a crucial role in assisting emergency management with disaster relief. Examples of community and faith-based organizations include the following:

- Functional needs support agencies
- Local church volunteer groups
- Local business volunteer groups

These organizations attempt to remain operational during and after disasters to provide information to the community. Some of these organizations can also be used as safe havens during and after a disaster for those who may not have been able to evacuate or do not trust outside organizations with their care. Another way that community and faith-based organizations assist is by providing space for mass shelters, information centers, and medical care distribution centers.[15]

University Programs

Colleges and universities have developed degree and certificate programs that focus on disaster and emergency management. Undergraduate and graduate degrees can be as general as public health or public administration with concentrations in emergency management, or as specific as counterterrorism. These programs are typically designed for students wanting to pursue a career in disaster and emergency management.[16] (Examples can be viewed at http://training.fema.gov/EMIWeb/edu/collegelist/.) Certificate programs focus on professionals wanting continuing education credits or refresher training for their current work position and duties. Most certificate programs do not require enrollment at the college or university and can typically be done online or through short courses.

Some of the skills taught in disaster and emergency management programs are the following:

- Identifying hazards and hazard vulnerability
- Creating emergency response plans
- Coordinating mutual aid
- Role of public health in emergency management
- International emergency management

Private Sector Programs

Hospitals. Hospitals use Hospital Preparedness Program (HPP) resources to assist with the development of surge capacity after disasters and to create preparedness plans to enhance response and community awareness.[17] Participating hospitals are required to develop an emergency operations plan (EOP) that includes communications, safety and security, resources and assets, staff responsibilities and support activities, response procedures, and capabilities.[18] Through skills attained as participants and the utilization of an incident management system aligned with other response organizations, hospitals are able to continue to provide the services needed for patients during and after disasters. Health care facilities also conduct certain activities in preparation for disasters, a requirement for accreditation by The Joint Commission.

Businesses. Most private-sector companies, especially those that provide essential infrastructure services, have developed highly functional emergency management programs to assist with keeping their businesses operational. When a disaster happens, businesses begin their response and recovery prior to any request from emergency management. This is beneficial because services and supplies are available at a moment's notice. In order to accomplish this, businesses create their own incident command, develop their own continuity of operations plans, and stage multiple disaster scenarios and drills.

An example of private-sector businesses participating in emergency management is the creation of emergency response teams for utility companies. Local unions are pairing with utility companies to bring in members and train them to become part of these teams. Training takes place in the classroom and the field to prepare members for the types of environments and problems they will encounter during and after disasters. For example, in Detroit, Michigan, a "storm lab" has been established to train electricians on how to properly respond to emergencies, assess damage, and use disaster-related terminology to report problems.[19]

! PITFALLS

Communication

Communication has been a problem for emergency managers and responders for quite some time. When a large-scale disaster occurs, multiple agencies from multiple jurisdictions are involved in the response. It is crucial that these agencies are able to communicate with each other throughout and following the disaster. Unfortunately, not all agencies share a common radio frequency that can be used for disasters and therefore essential communication is lost. This can result in agencies and departments not adhering to the plans of the incident commander, not knowing what the next step is to take and not knowing where and how to respond. For victims and property at stake, this lack of communication can be very harmful.

Resilience

The Household Preparedness section of the *Behavioral Risk Factor Surveillance System from 2006 to 2010* (BRFSS) states that the majority of United States citizens are under-prepared and do not have a plan in place for when a disaster strikes.[20] Improved resilience in communities would increase the effectiveness of emergency management by having a prepared community that is able to become part of the response and recovery efforts. When communities are not resilient and are not included in the emergency response plans for the community, the response and recovery will not be as effective due to lack of valuable resources and preparedness.[2,21]

Accountability

Disaster drills and training are some of the most effective ways to increase preparedness and response for emergency management and response agencies. Unfortunately, disaster drills do not always go as planned, either because the resources are not available or some agencies or responders do not take accountability for the roles they are assigned to play. Even though a disaster is not really happening, it is imperative that drills be conducted in the most professional and educational manner possible. Lack of accountability is a waste of money, resources, and human-power and needs to be addressed. The only possible way to fix this problem would be to conduct outside evaluation of each agency or response team to score how well they performed in drills. Based on these evaluations, future funding may or may not be effected. Taking disaster drills and training more seriously could improve the level of response from emergency management and responders.

Funding

The determination of whether or not a program is created or effective is often based on the amount of funding available at any given time. Since September 2001, funding for emergency management programs was initially shifted to preparing for and responding to terrorist events instead of natural hazards. This has proved illogical, as evidenced by the issues in response and recovery during hurricanes Katrina and Sandy and other major natural disasters. Another major issue with funding is time. Typically after a disastrous event, the need for preparedness, prevention, and recovery programs is brought into the spotlight, and funding becomes available from public and private sectors. Unfortunately, during the down times of need, emergency management and preparedness programs are forgotten about until the need resurfaces.[21]

Lack of Private Sector Ties

The private sector has the ability to provide resources, personnel, ideas, and models that government agencies could use for more effective emergency management. Supplies and personnel are the most important resources needed to respond to and recover from disasters. Private sectors typically have an excess of supplies ranging from demolition equipment for cleanup to stockpiles of food from local grocers to emergency medical supplies. Creating ties with organizations and businesses that are able to supply these things will help build capacity and response for emergency management.[2,21] Another way the private sector could provide beneficial assistance to emergency management programs is through surveillance measures pertaining to the products that certain businesses sell. One surveillance example that is currently in use is the tracking of thermometer sales, which can assist in predicting the projected flu cases during flu season. This same concept can be used to track the need for recovery efforts in certain areas based on the amount of building supplies purchased or the amount of food staples purchased to predict where survivors are located. Collaboration with the private sector can only increase the effectiveness of disaster response and recovery programs.

REFERENCES

1. Federal Emergency Management Agency. About the agency. Available at: http://www.fema.gov/about-agency. Accessed 16.02.14.
2. Waugh WL Jr, Streib G. Collaboration and leadership for effective emergency management. *Public Adm Rev.* 2006;(special issue):131–140. Available at: http://faculty.maxwell.syr.edu/rdenever/NatlSecurity2008_docs/Waugh_CollaborationLeadership.pdf. Accessed 28.02.14.
3. Department of Homeland Security. Who joined DHS. Available at: http://www.dhs.gov/who-joined-dhs. Accessed 16.02.14.
4. Bea K, Halchin E, Hogue H, et al. *Federal Emergency Management Policy Changes After Hurricane Katrina: A Summary of Statutory Provisions;* 2006. Available at http://www.training.fema.gov/emiweb/edu/docs/FederalEMPolicyChangesAfterKatrina.pdf. Accessed 16.02.14.
5. Federal Emergency Management Agency. Sandy Recovery Improvement Act of 2013. Available at: https://www.fema.gov/about-agency/sandy-recovery-improvement-act-2013. Accessed 16.02.14.
6. Federal Emergency Management Agency. About community emergency response teams. Available at: http://www.fema.gov/community-emergency-response-teams/about-community-emergency-response-team. Accessed 06.02.14.
7. Ready.gov. Voluntary organizations active in disaster. Available at: http://www.ready.gov/voluntary-organizations-active-disaster. Accessed 06.02.14.
8. Federal Emergency Management Agency. National preparedness system. Available at: http://www.fema.gov/national-preparedness-system. Accessed 06.02.14.
9. Medical Reserve Corps. About the Medical Reserve Corps. Available at: https://www.medicalreservecorps.gov/pageViewFldr/About. Accessed 06.02.14.
10. United States Department of Health and Human Services. National disaster medical system—PHE. Available at: http://www.phe.gov/preparedness/responders/ndms/pages/default.aspx. Accessed 16.02.14.
11. Federal Emergency Management Agency. Emergency management institute. Available at: http://training.fema.gov/aboutemi.asp. Accessed 16.02.14.
12. Department of Homeland Security. About the Center for Domestic Preparedness. Available at: https://cdp.dhs.gov/about/. Accessed 16.02.14.

13. Federal Emergency Management Agency. State organization and role in emergency management, 2006. Available at: http://training.fema.gov/EMIWeb/edu/docs/hazdem/Session17-StateRole.doc. Accessed 16.02.14.

14. American Red Cross. American Red Cross guide to services. Available at: http://www.redcross.org/images/MEDIA_CustomProductCatalog/m3140117_GuideToServices.pdf. Accessed 16.02.14.

15. City of Philadelphia Pennsylvania. Emergency management planning toolkit for community-based organizations. Available at: http://chpsw.temple.edu/cprep/sites/default/files/imce_uploads/OrganizationalToolkit.pdf. Accessed 16.02.14.

16. Federal Emergency Management Agency. Emergency Management Institute—course college list. Available at: http://training.fema.gov/EMIWeb/edu/collegelist/. Accessed 16.02.14.

17. United States Department of Health and Human Services. Hospital preparedness program (HPP)—PHE. Available at: http://www.phe.gov/preparedness/planning/hpp/Pages/default.aspx. Accessed 16.02.14.

18. California Hospital Association. Emergency operations plan—emergency preparedness. Available at: http://www.calhospitalprepare.org/emergency-operations-plan. Accessed 16.02.14.

19. International Brotherhood of Electrical Workers. Utility companies recruit wiremen for emergency response teams. *Electr Work Online*. 2013; http://www.ibew.org/articles/13ElectricalWorker/EW1310/Storm.1013.html. Accessed 01.03.14.

20. Centers for Disease and Control Prevention. Household preparedness for public health emergencies—14 states, 2006–2010. Available at: http://www.cdc.gov/mmwr/preview/mmwrhtml/mm6136a1.htm. Accessed 16.02.14.

21. Haddow G, Bullock J. The future of emergency management. Available at: http://training.fema.gov/EMIWeb/edu/docs/emfuture/FutureofEM-TheFutureofEM-HaddowandBullock.doc.

CHAPTER 21

Emergency Department Design

Robert H. Woolard, Stephen W. Borron, and John M. Mackay

In the United States, hospitals build new emergency departments (EDs) every 15 to 20 years. Renovations of existing EDs occur every 5 to 10 years. The main concerns of ED designers are providing efficient spaces for routine care, handling peak volumes, and anticipating future needs. Well-designed EDs accommodate daily, weekly, and seasonal tidal peaks and valleys in patient flow. The variety of high- and low-acuity illnesses and injuries requires EDs to prioritize care into critical, emergent, and urgent treatment. EDs meet community needs for specialized care by providing areas for unique care needs with pediatric, cardiac, trauma, geriatric, or stroke centers. Often only as a last thought do EDs include some design features for disaster and mass-casualty response.[1,2] In the wake of terror-related events, such as the Boston Marathon Bombing and the New York City World Trade Center disaster on September 11, 2001, and natural disasters, such as hurricanes Sandy and Katrina, more EDs are being designed or renovated to meet anticipated disaster needs. These designs and renovations include enhanced security, decontamination, and isolation, and addition of other specialized treatment areas, as well as expanding capacity to treat multiple victims within, or in proximity to, EDs.

When planning a new ED or a renovation, the following question should be added to the usual list of design questions: "How can the new ED better respond to disaster events?" ED designs should be planned for normal operations, as well as potential disaster events that could create increased demand and unique needs. One approach to better ED design for disaster is to organize a workshop early in the design process to address emergency preparedness, bringing together hospital administration, ED staff, other key employees, and security and community agencies to complete a risk assessment analysis. Better design can emerge from identifying potential disaster scenarios (e.g., hurricane, pandemic epidemic, or direct attack on the ED), rating their probability of occurrence (e.g., very likely, high, low, or very unlikely), and then listing the potential facility implications of each scenario.[3]

HISTORICAL PERSPECTIVE

In the aftermath of terror events and natural disasters with subsequent disaster response planning, hospital architects have begun to design EDs to better meet the needs anticipated from a terror attack, flood, or epidemic. Some ED design lessons have been learned from disaster events. From the Tokyo Sarin event, recent natural disasters and epidemic illnesses, and other routine "disasters," such as influenza

outbreaks, hospitals know they need to plan for surge capacity. Methods of alerting and preparing ED staff early and protecting emergency care providers from contamination and infection are needed, a lesson integrated into current ED staff vaccination requirements and made painfully clear by the Tokyo Sarin event, in which many emergency providers were contaminated. The Boston Marathon Bombing event illustrated the need to provide emergency and surgical care to mass casualties, requiring coordination of response between hospitals and enhanced field rescue efforts to meet high volume demands over a short time period. In New York after 9/11, the cleanup phase after the event led to prolonged increased prehospital and ED volume. Most care was provided by emergency personnel working close to ground zero. From the anthrax mailings in the wake of the World Trade Center event, planners learned to anticipate the need for accurate public information and increased ED patient volume. From the flooding and evacuation of hospitals and EDs, with the needs for medical capacity met at new sites on high ground during Katrina, planners relearned the importance of providing care throughout a larger health care system, with each hospital and ED participating uniquely, some evacuating and relocating, and others providing care to surges of relocated and new patients.

The ED remains the most available point of access to immediate health care in the United States. ED designers are now anticipating increased volumes of patients that might be generated by a disaster, epidemic, or a terror event. Although a stressed public needs information and health screenings that perhaps can be met by providers outside the ED, the ED will be accessed for counseling and screening when other services are overwhelmed, critical information is misunderstood, or delay to access is anticipated or encountered. In most disaster scenarios, shelter needs are provided outside the ED. However, loss of facilities or needs for quarantine of exposed and ill patients during bioterror events and epidemics may create shelter needs proximate to EDs.

ED design and response capability after 9/11 became a larger concern for public disaster planners, the federal government, and hospital architects. Two federally funded projects coordinated by emergency physicians, one at Washington Hospital Center (ER One) and another at the Rhode Island Disaster Initiative (RIDI), have developed and released recommendations. ER One suggests designs for a new ED that meets any and all anticipated needs of a disaster event.[4] RIDI has developed new disaster response paradigms, training scenarios, and response simulations that also can be used in ED design.[5]

Recommendations of Project ER One

Scalability

- Universal patient care rooms that are configurable for any purpose
- Single patient rooms reconfigurable to accommodate up to three patients
- Rapid conversion of nonpatient care space such as waiting rooms into clinical space for 4 to 5 times scalability

Alternate Care Sites

- Modular and mobile solutions rather than dedicated built-in equipment
- Convex multilane vehicular access
- Emphasis on portability and modularity at every scale
- Instant access to all data for any patient at any moment
- Person-to-person communications net independent of other communications systems

Capability

- All rooms with negative pressure capability and 100% nonrecirculated air
- Every room an isolation room with separate ventilation and separate toilet facilities
- Ability to isolate single rooms or entire zones and sectors
- Multimode decontamination capability in every area of the facility
- Portals for access control and threat detection
- Universal docking capability for portable external modular treatment units
- Robust real-time data sharing with local, state, and federal health authorities

Threat Mitigation

- Self-decontamination surfaces
- Offset parking away from building footprint
- Single-room and single-zone modular compartmentalized ventilation systems
- 100% air filtration
- Assured water supply with internal purification capabilities
- Blast-protection walls and blast-deflection strategies
- Elimination or encapsulation of building materials that can shatter during an event
- Built-in radiation protection
- Advanced security and intrusion detection technologies

CURRENT PRACTICE

An ED design using ER One concepts has been constructed at Tampa General Hospital in Florida. After considering highly likely disaster scenarios, specific recommendations were developed and integrated into the Tampa ED design. To address surge capacity, the State of Florida, the project architects, and hospital administration agreed on an ED that could expand from 77 treatment spaces to 210 within the ED. A parking area beneath the ED was designed to convert to a mass decontamination zone, feeding directly into the ED. The ED observation area was designed to convert into a quarantine unit, with direct access from outside the ED during epidemics. Adding these elements to create an ED that is more disaster ready increased the cost of the project by less than 5%.[6] ED design would be tremendously enhanced if a prototype "disaster-ready" ED demonstrating all the elements of ER One could be built. To date no full prototype has been constructed, and it has yet to be shown that ED designers are able to create an "all-hazards-ready" ED, given financial constraints. However, incorporating some disaster-ready suggestions when EDs are built or renovated will improve our

readiness and may be more financially feasible. New building materials, technologies, and concepts will continue to inform the effort to prepare EDs for terror attack. Urban ED trauma centers are attempting to develop the capacity to serve as regional disaster resource centers and the capability for site response to disaster events. These EDs are designed to incorporate larger waiting and entrance areas, adjacent units, or nearby parking spaces in their plans to ramp-up treatment capacity. More decontamination and isolation capacity is being built to help control the spread of toxic or infectious agents.

Information systems are being made available to provide real-time point-of-service information and any needed "just-in-time" training for potential terror threats. An example of better organized disaster information is the CO-S-TR model, a tool for hospital incident command that prioritizes action to address key components of surge capacity. There are three major elements in the tool, each with four subelements. "CO" stands for command, control, communications, and coordination and ensures that an incident management structure is implemented. "S" considers the logistical requirements for staff, stuff, space, and special (event-specific) considerations. "TR" comprises tracking, triage, treatment, and transportation.[7] Having an information system with robust capability to gather and display the detailed information needed in a preformatted and rehearsed mode such as CO-S-TR, with easy access by multiple electronic means, including wireless and handheld devices, is an important facility design feature.

The technology needed to respond to a terrorist event, such as personal protective equipment (PPE), is becoming more widely available and is stored where it is easily available in EDs. Although mass decontamination can and in general should occur close to the disaster scene, EDs are gearing up to better decontaminate, isolate, and treat individuals or groups contaminated with biologic or chemical materials upon arrival. The Tokyo Sarin episode demonstrated clearly that contaminated patients will make their way to the ED without waiting for first responders.[8] Four elements of ED design are being addressed to prepare EDs for terror events: scalability, security, information systems, and decontamination.

Scalability, Surge, and Treatment Capacity

EDs are generally designed with sufficient, but not excess, space. The number of treatment spaces needed in an ED is usually matched to the anticipated ED patient volume; roughly 1 treatment space per 1100 annual ED visits or 1 treatment space per 400 annual ED hospital admissions is recommended.[1] According to disaster planners, a major urban trauma center ED built for 50,000 to 100,000 visits per year should have surge capacity up to 100 patients per hour for 4 hours and 1000 patients per day for 4 days. One disaster-ready design challenge is to provide surge capacity to meet anticipated patient needs. Hospitals are woefully overcrowded, and EDs are routinely housing admitted patients.[9–11] To maintain surge capacity, efforts to address hospital overcrowding and eliminate the boarding of admissions in the ED must be successful.

EDs are now being designed to allow growth into adjacent space: a ground level or upper level, a garage, or a parking lot. Garage and parking lot space has been used in many disaster drills and mass exposures. Garages and parking lots can be designed with separate access to streets, allowing separation of disaster traffic and routine ED traffic. More often, needed terror-response supplies (e.g., antidotes, respirators, personal protective gear) are stored near or within the ED. The cost of ventilation, heat, air conditioning, communication, and security features often prohibits renovation of garages. More often, tents are erected over parking lots or loading areas. Modular "second EDs," tents or structures with collapsible walls (fold and stack), have been deployed by disaster responders. These can be used near the main ED, preserving the ED for critical cases during a disaster surge. Some hospitals are building capacity for beds in halls and double capacity patient rooms, and converting other nontreatment spaces to wards to increase their ability to meet patient surges during disaster. Hallways can provide usable space if constructed wider and equipped with medical gases and adequate power and lighting. Often only minimal modifications are necessary to make existing halls and lobbies dual-use spaces. Some hospitals have increased space by installing retractable awnings on the exterior over ambulance bays or loading docks. Tents are often used outside EDs as decontamination and treatment areas in disaster drills. Tents with inflatable air walls have the added benefit of being insulated for all-weather use.

In the military, the need to provide treatment in limited space has resulted in the practice of stacking patients vertically to save space and to reduce the distances that personnel walk. U.S. Air Force air evacuation flights have stacked critical patients three high, and some naval vessels may bunk patients vertically in mass-casualty scenarios. Similar bed units could be deployed for a mass event. Portable modular units are also available to help EDs meet additional space needs. Unfortunately, many EDs plan to rely on other facilities in the regional system and do not build in surge capacity. During a terror event occurring on a hospital campus, the ED function may need to be moved to a remote area within the hospital in response to a flood, fire, building collapse, bomb or bomb threat, active shooter, or other event. Many disaster plans designate a preexisting structure on campus as the "backup" ED. The area is stockpiled with equipment and has a viable plan for access. Patient and staff movement are planned and developed during drills.

In addition to increasing ED surge capacity, significant off-loading of ED volume can be accomplished by "reverse triage" of inpatients. Through such measures as delaying elective admissions and surgeries, early discharge, or interhospital transfer of stable patients, significant improvements in bed capacity can be accomplished within hours.[12,13]

Although the capacity to handle patient surges is being addressed regionally and nationally, large events with high critical care volumes will overtax the system regionally, as was the case during Hurricane Katrina. The National Disaster Medical System (NDMS) can be mobilized to move excess victims and establish field hospitals during events involving hundreds or thousands of victims. However, there are barriers to a prompt response time in the deployment of NDMS resources.[14]

The ED plan to provide treatment during disaster must include evacuation, since the event may produce an environmental hazard that contaminates, floods, or renders the ED inaccessible. Evacuation of ED patients has been addressed by ED designers. Some EDs have the capacity to more easily evacuate. In well-planned EDs, stairwells have floor lights to assist in darkness. Stairways are sufficient in size to allow backboarded and chair-bound patients to be evacuated. Ground level EDs should have access to surface streets, interior pathways, and exterior sidewalks. The communication and tracking system includes sensors in corridors and stairways. Patient records are regularly backed up and stored for web access and hence available during and after evacuation. Specially designed ambulance buses allow for the safe transfer of multiple patients of variable acuity to other facilities.

Security

Securing the function of an ED includes securing essential resources: water, gases, power, ventilation, communication, and information. ED security involves surveillance, control of access and egress, threat mitigation, and "lockdown" capacity. Surveillance exists in almost all EDs. Many ED parking and decontamination areas are monitored by cameras. The wireless tracking system can also be part of the surveillance system. A tracking system can create a virtual geospatial and temporal map of staff and patient movement. Tracking systems have been used in disaster drills to identify threat patterns. Most EDs have identification/access cards and

readers. Chemical and biologic sensors for explosives, organic solvents, and biologic agents are becoming available, but have not been used in EDs. Many EDs have metal detectors and security checkpoints prior to access by ambulatory patients and visitors. When selecting a sensor, designers consider sensitivity, selectivity, speed of response, and robustness.[15–19] Sensor technology is an area of active research that continues to yield new solutions that could be incorporated into ED security. In concept, all entrances could be designed to identify persons using scanning to detect unwanted chemicals, biologic agents, or explosives, allowing detention and decontamination when needed. Given the wide array of physicochemical properties of hazardous materials in commerce, developing sensors with sufficient sensitivity to detect threats while avoiding an excess of false positives will remain a challenge.

Most EDs have multiple entry portals for ingress of patients, visitors, staff, vendors, law enforcement personnel, and others. EDs are using screening and identification technologies at all entrances in combination with closed-circuit video monitoring. Personnel must be dedicated for prompt response when needed. Automation of identification can efficiently allow safe flow of patients, staff, and supplies. Vehicle access has been managed by bar-coding staff and visitor vehicles. At some road access points, automated scanners could monitor and control vehicle access. Modern EDs limit the number of entrances and channel pedestrian and vehicular traffic through identification control points. For the most part, points of entrance into the ED can be managed with locking doors, identification badge control points, and surveillance to allow desired access for staff and supplies. Thoughtful planning should facilitate rapid access between the functional areas, such as the ED, operating rooms, catheterization suites, and critical care units. Movement within and between buildings needs to be controlled and must allow a total lockdown when necessary.

Direct threats to the ED include blasts; chemical, biologic, and environmental contamination; and active shooting. There are several strategies to mitigate blasts. Twelve-inch-thick conventional concrete walls, using commercially available aggregates (147 lb per cubic foot), afford reasonable blast protection.[20,21] On some campuses, the space between the ED and the entrance is designed largely to prevent direct attack.[22] However, atriums are terror targets. Although atriums are useful as overflow areas, their windows and glass can create hazardous flying debris. In general, use of unreinforced glass windows, which help create a more pleasant ED environment, must be balanced against threat of injury from broken glass shards. Given the threat of blast attack, communication, gas, electric, water, and other critical services should be remote from vulnerable areas and shielded when they traverse roads and walkways. Protection against release of chemical and biologic agents inside or outside the ED requires a protective envelope, controlled air filtration in and out, an air distribution system providing clean pressurized air, a water purification system providing potable water, and a detection system. Better HVAC systems can pressurize their envelope, keeping contaminants out, and also purge contaminated areas.

Information

Anticipated computing needs for ED operations during disaster events are immense. In most EDs, large amounts of complex and diverse information are routinely available electronically. Overflow patients in hallways and adjacent spaces can be managed with mobile computing, which is available in many EDs. Wireless handheld devices can facilitate preparation for disasters and allow immediate access to information by providers in hallways and decontamination spaces. Multiple desktop and mobile workstations are available throughout most EDs. During disaster, displays of information that will aid decision making include bed status, the types of rooms available, the number of persons waiting, and ambulances coming in. Monitors now display patient vital signs, telemetry, and test results. Significant improvements in efficiency and decision making can be achieved when more real-time information is available to decision makers. Having available multiple computer screens with preformatted disaster information screens that are regularly used should enhance ED readiness.

Clinical decision tools and references, such as UpToDate,[23] make information readily available to providers. These and other just-in-time resources will be needed when practitioners treat unusual or rare diseases not encountered in routine practice. The wide variety of potential disaster scenarios argues for the availability of just-in-time information. Information specific to a disaster event should be broadcast widely on multiple screens in many areas. Cellular links and wireless portable devices should also be designed to receive and display disaster information. Access to information has been enhanced in most EDs through cell phone, texting, and other social media use. Developing apps to make local disaster information available through as many media as possible and to guide each staff member should be part of the information system disaster plan.

Diagnostic decision support systems have been demonstrated to help practitioners recognize symptom complexes that are uncommon or unfamiliar. Information systems should be capable of communicating potential terror event information regularly. Many EDs have log-on systems that require staff to read new information. In a disaster-ready ED, a list of potential threats could be posted daily. However, the utility of computer references or on-call experts is limited by the practitioner's ability to recognize a situation that requires the resource.

Computer-based patient tracking systems are available for routinely tracking patients in most EDs. Some computer-based tracking systems have a disaster mode that quickly adapts to a large influx of patients allowing for collation of symptoms, laboratory values, and other pertinent syndromic data. In many regions, EDs provide real-time data that serve as a disaster alert surveillance network. Routine data obtained on entry are passively collected and transferred to a central point for analysis (usually a health department). In the event of a significant spike in targeted patient symptom complexes, these data can trigger an appropriate disaster response. The capacity for this entry point surveillance should be anticipated and built in to any disaster-ready ED information system.[24-26] For example, data terminals allowing patients to input data at registration similar to electronic ticketing at airports could passively provide information during a surge, rather than requiring chief complaint and registration data input by staff. This self-service system could add to ED surge capacity. Similarly, real-time bed identification, availability, and reservation systems used to assist patient management in some EDs could aid ED function during disaster. Movement to an inpatient bed is a well-documented choke point recognized nationally during normal hospital operations, and implementing a plan to open access to admissions becomes an issue during disaster.

Lobby screens can facilitate family access to information during a disaster, displaying information about the event and patient status using coded names to preserve confidentiality. During disasters, family members can be given their family member's coded name and access to screens to query for medical information. Computers with Internet access that could display public event information are available in patient rooms in some EDs.

During anthrax mailings, public hysteria taxed the health care system. Posttraumatic stress, anxiety, and public concern over possible exposure to a biologic or chemical agent may generate a surge of minor patients at EDs. Within some EDs, lecture halls or media centers are available; they are generally used for teaching conferences but could provide venues for health information and media briefings during disaster. The media are an important source of public information and must be considered when planning disaster response. An adjacent conference area can serve as a media center, where information could be released to the Internet and closed-circuit screens could provide more accurate information to allay public concerns and direct the public to appropriate resources and access points for evaluation of potential exposures. Poison control centers provide an immediate source of valuable information for hazard communication and risk assessment.

Notwithstanding the tremendous potential value of computer systems in disaster management, it is important to anticipate and plan for information systems and communications failure. Failure of hospital generators, such as occurred in Hurricane Sandy, will rapidly render computers and landline telephones inoperable. Cellular telephone services are often overwhelmed during disasters. The Internet appears to be less likely to crash during disasters, due to its redundancy, but hospitals should plan for alternative methods of communication and documentation.

Isolation and Decontamination

Many EDs have patient decontamination (DECON) areas. Adequate environmental protection for patients undergoing DECON is necessary and includes visual barriers from onlookers, segregation of the sexes, and attention to personal belongings.[27,28] In many EDs, DECON areas are being added to accommodate mass exposures. EDs have added or augmented DECON facilities. DECON areas should have a separate, self-contained drainage system, controlled water temperature, and shielding from environmental hazards. Exhaust fans are used to prevent the buildup of toxic off-gassing in these decontamination areas. Most importantly, DECON facilities should be deployable within minutes of an incident, to avoid secondary contamination of the ED. For most EDs, mass DECON has been accomplished by using an uncovered parking lot and deploying heated and vented modular tent units. Uncovered parking areas adjacent and accessible to the ED have been enabled for disaster response. Other EDs use high-volume, low-pressure showers mounted on the side of a building. Serial showers allow multiple patients to enter at the same entrance and time. However, serial showers do not provide privacy, can be difficult for an ill patient to access, and can lead to contaminated water runoff. Also, persons requiring more time may impede flow and reduce the number of patients decontaminated. Parallel showers built in advance or set up temporarily in tenting offer greater privacy but require wider space and depth. Combined serial and parallel design allows the advantages of each, separating ill patients and increasing the number of simultaneous decontaminations.[29]

Often built into the ED is another DECON room for one or two patients with the following features: outside access; negative pressure exhaust air exchange; water drainage; water recess; seamless floor; impervious, slip-resistant, washable floor, walls, and ceiling; gas appliances; supplied air wall outlets for PPE use; high-input air; intercom; overhead paging; and an anteroom for DECON of isolated cases. PPE is routinely used by military and fire departments during events involving hazardous materials. Hospitals likewise must be trained for and plan to use these devices and store a reasonable number of protective ensembles (i.e., gloves, suits, and respiratory equipment), usually near the ED DECON area. DECON areas are built with multiple supplied air outlets for PPE use to optimize safety and maximize work flexibility.

Powered air purifying respirators (PAPRs) are used by many hospitals in lieu of air supplied respirators. While providing increased mobility and convenience, their utility is somewhat limited by the requirement for battery power and the need to select an appropriate filtration cartridge. Voice-controlled two-way radios facilitate communication among DECON staff with receivers in the ED. A nearby changing area is available in some EDs. The changing area is laid out to optimize medical monitoring and to ease access to the DECON area.[30-34] The need for easily accessible PPE and adequate training and practice in the use of PPE cannot be overemphasized.

Some capability to isolate and prevent propagation of a potential biologic agent has been designed into most EDs. Patients who present with undetermined respiratory illnesses are routinely sent to an isolation area. A direct entrance from the exterior to an isolation room is not usually available but has been a recent renovation in some EDs. Creation of isolation areas poses special design requirements for HVAC, cleaning, and security to ensure that infections and infected persons are contained. An isolation area should have compartmentalized air handling with high-efficiency filters providing clean air.[35-38] Biohazard contamination is particularly difficult to mitigate. Keeping the facility "clean" and safe for other patients is an extreme challenge. Biologic agents of terrorism or epidemics may resist decontamination attempts. Infected patients present a risk to staff. During the severe acute respiratory syndrome (SARS) epidemic, Singapore built outdoor tent hospitals to supplement their existing decontamination facility. Patients were evaluated outside the ED and those with fever were isolated and not allowed to enter the main hospital. This, among other measures, allowed Singapore to achieve relatively rapid control over the epidemic.[39] Few triage areas and ED rooms have been designed for decontamination. Surfaces must be able to withstand repeated decontamination. Sealed inlets for gases and plumbing have also been considered.[40] Patients who are isolated can be observed with monitoring cameras. Some isolation areas include a restroom within their space, which helps restrict patient egress.

All ED areas could have more infection control capabilities built in. Floor drains have been included in some ED rooms for easier decontamination. Infection control is improved using polymer surface coatings that are smooth, nonporous, and tolerant to repeated cleaning, creating a virtually seamless surface that is easy to clean. These coatings can be impregnated with antimicrobial properties, enhancing their biosafe capability. Silver-impregnated metal surfaces in sinks, drains, door handles, and other locations can reduce high bacterial content. Silver-impregnated metal has demonstrated antimicrobial effects.[41]

Conventional ventilation systems use 15% to 25% outside air during normal operation, thus purging indoor contaminants. Air cleaning depends on filtration, ultraviolet irradiation, and purging. HVAC design should model demand for adequately clean air and also for isolation of potential contaminants.[42] The disaster-ready ED requires protection from external contaminations as well as contagious patients. A compartmentalized central venting system without recirculation has the ability to remove or contain toxic agents in and around the ED. Compartmentalized HVAC systems allow for the sealing of zones from each other. More desirable HVAC systems electronically shut down sections, use effective filtration, and can clean contaminated air. A compartmentalized system can fail, but it only fails in the zone it is servicing; smaller zones mean smaller areas lost to contamination. These systems are less vulnerable to global failure or spread of contamination. Modular mobile HVAC units developed for field military applications have been added to existing ED isolation areas for use when needed to create safe air compartments.

⚠ PITFALLS

Cost may prohibit addressing issues like building more space or better ventilation, decontamination, and isolation facilities. If added space and facilities are not made more available, many lives may be lost during a disaster event. When funds are scarce, less money is spent for disaster readiness, since all available money is spent to support EDs' continuous function day to day. EDs in the United States are challenged to provide efficient routine care and board excess admitted patients.

However, they must also be designed to handle the consequences of a terror event, epidemic, or natural disaster. These competing functions could result in EDs with less financial support to handle routine care.

These design efforts could also lead to unnecessary increases in expenditures in anticipation of terror events that never materialize. To the extent that efforts to provide disaster care can be translated into solutions that address other more immediate hospital and ED problems, they will gain support. More access to information systems providing just-in-time training could inform staff not only of terror events but of mundane policy changes and unique patient needs such as bloodless therapy for Jehovah's Witnesses, etc. Better information access could also improve routine ED efficiency and communication with patients and families. Hopefully, these rationales will prevail when funds are made available for disaster readiness. Decontamination equipment and areas may be used for commercial hazardous materials spills. Isolation areas could be more routinely used in an effort to contain suspected contagions, such as influenza.

Lack of bed capacity in hospitals leads to ED overcrowding. Scalable EDs may offer temporary solutions in times of overburdened hospital inpatient services. However, when reserve spaces are used to solve other overcapacity problems, those spaces are no longer available for disaster operations. Thus, a new facility could "build" the capability of handling large surges of patients into adjacent spaces, only to lose it by filling these spaces with excess patients whenever the hospital is over census, which is a recurrent problem at many medical centers.

Finally, the next disaster event may be different from those for which responders prepare. The rarity of terror events creates a need for testing and practicing disaster plans, skills, and capacities in drills to maintain current competence. Drills may uncover design problems that can then be addressed, but such drills can only prepare emergency personnel for anticipated threats.

CONCLUSION

Why pour such resources into building capacity that may never be used or undertake other costly initiatives in anticipation of disaster events? Among the lessons learned from past disaster events is the need to develop disaster skills and build a disaster response system from components that are in daily use. Systems that are used routinely are more familiar and more likely to be used successfully during disaster events. Certainly the surge capacity of a disaster-ready ED could be used for natural disaster response and in disaster drills. The surge space could also be used for over-census times, public health events, immunizations, and health screenings. Newly built or renovated EDs should have excess capacity by design to serve as a community disaster resource. These capacities could be utilized routinely in response to hospital overcrowding or public service events (such as mass immunization campaigns) and should be deployed and tested regularly in disaster drills to maintain readiness in a post-9/11 world.

REFERENCES

1. Australian College for Emergency Medicine. Emergency Department Design Guidelines. Available at: http://www.acem.org.au/open/documents/ed_design.htm.
2. Emergency department design. Riggs LM, ed. *Functional and Space Programming*. Dallas, Tex: American College of Emergency Physicians:111.
3. Zilm F. Designing for emergencies. Architecture+Design: 11.01.10.
4. ER One/All-Risks-Ready Emergency Department. Available at: http://www.whcnurses.org/workfiles/EROneRelease.pdf.
5. Rhode Island Disaster Initiative. Improving disaster medicine through research. Available at: http://www.ridiproject.org/page_manager.asp.

6. Zilm F, Berry R, Pietrzak MP, Paratore A. Integrating disaster preparedness and surge capacity in emergency facility planning. *J Ambul Care Manage.* 2008 Oct-Dec;31(4):377–385.

7. Hick JL, Koenig KL, Barbisch D. Bey TA Surge capacity concepts for health care facilities: the CO-S-TR model for initial incident assessment. *Disaster Med Public Health Prep.* 2008 Sep;2(Suppl 1):S51–S57.

8. Okumura T, Hisaoka T, Yamada A, et al. The Tokyo subway Sarin attack—lessons learned. *Toxicol Appl Pharmacol.* 2005 Sep 1;207(2 Suppl):471–476.

9. Andrulis DP, Kellermann A, Hintz EA, et al. Emergency departments and crowding in US teaching hospitals. *Ann Emerg Med.* 1991;20(9):980–986.

10. Meggs WJ, Czaplijski T, Benson N. Trends in emergency department utilization, 1988-1997. *Acad Emerg Med.* 1999;6(10):1030–1035.

11. Bazarian JJ, Schneider SM, Newman VJ, Chodosh J. Do admitted patients held in the emergency department impact the throughput of treat-and-release patients? *Acad Emerg Med.* 1996;3(12):1113–1118.

12. Satterthwaite PS, Atkinson CJ. Using 'reverse triage' to create hospital surge capacity: Royal Darwin Hospital's response to the Ashmore Reef disaster. *Emerg Med J.* 2012 Feb;29(2):160–162.

13. Kelen GD, McCarthy ML, Kraus CK, et al. Creation of surge capacity by early discharge of hospitalized patients at low risk for untoward events. *Disaster Med Public Health Prep.* 2009 Jun;3(2 Suppl):S10–S16.

14. Franco C, Toner E, Waldhorn R, Maldin B, O'Toole T, Thomas V. Inglesby Systemic collapse: medical care in the aftermath of Hurricane Katrina. *Biosecur Bioterror.* 2006;4(2):135–146.

15. Physical Security Equipment Action Group (PSEAG). Department of Defense. Available at: http://www.dtic.mil/ndia/2002security/toscano.pdf.

16. Ellis AB, Nickel AL, Shaw GA, Heirseele KV. Interior/Exterior Intrusion and Chemical/Biological Detection Systems/Sensors. In: *Proceedings of the Same National Symposium on Comprehensive Force Protection, Charleston, SC. OPNAVINST 5510.1G, 45B.* November 2001.

17. Jurs PC, Bakken GA, McClelland HE. Computational methods for the analysis of chemical sensor array data from volatile analytes. *Chem Rev.* 2000;100(7):2649–2678.

18. Kissinger PT. Electrochemical detection in bioanalysis. *J Pharm Biomed Anal.* 1996;14(8–10):871–880.

19. Lonergan MC, Severin EJ, Doleman BJ, et al. Array-based vapor sensing using chemically sensitive, carbon black-polymer resistors. *Chem Mater.* 1996;8(9):2298–2312.

20. Heavy Concrete Web site. Available at: http://www.HeavyConcrete.com.

21. Nadel BA. Designing for security. *Archit Rec.* March 2002.

22. Putting Clinical Information into Practice. UpToDate Web site. Available at: http://www.uptodate.com.

23. Bennett NM, Konecki J. Emergency department and walk-in center surveillance for bioterrorism: utility for influenza surveillance [abstract]. ICEID 2002. *Emerg Infect Dis.* 2005;11(8). Available at: http://www.cdc.gov/ncidod/eid/index.htm.

24. Karpati A, Mostashari F, Heffernan R, et al. Syndromic surveillance for bioterrorism New York City, Oct-Dec 2001[abstract]. ICEID 2002. *Emerg Infect Dis.* 2005;11(8). Available at: http://www.cdc.gov/ncidod/eid/index.htm.

25. Gong E, Dauber W. *Policewomen win settlement.* Seattle Times; July 11, 1996, B1.

26. Stern J. *Fire Department Response to Biological Threat at B'nai B'rith Headquarters, Washington DC: Report 114 of the Major Fire Investigative Project.* Emmitsburg, Md: US Fire Administration; October 2001.

27. Barbera JA, Macintyre AG, DeAtley CA. *Chemically Contaminated Patient Annex (CCPA): Hospital Emergency Operations Planning Guide.* Washington, DC: United States Public Health Service; March 2001.

28. Burgess JL, Kirk M, Borron SW, Cisek J. Emergency department hazardous materials protocol for contaminated patients. *Ann Emerg Med.* 1999;34(2):205–212.

29. Centers for Disease Control and Prevention. CDC recommendations for civilian communities near chemical weapons depots. 60. *Fed Regist.* 1995;33307–33318.

30. US Department of Labor, Occupational Safety and Health Administration. *Hospitals and Community Emergency Response: What You Need to Know. Emergency Response Safety Series.* Washington DC: OSHA; 1997, 3152.

31. Macintyre AG, Christopher GW, Eitzen E Jr., et al. Weapons of mass destruction events with contaminated casualties: effective planning for health care facilities. *JAMA.* 2000;283(2):242–249.

32. Shapira Y, Bar Y, Berkenstadt H, et al. Outline of hospital organization for a chemical warfare attack. *Isr J Med Sci.* 1991;27(11–12):616–622.

33. *Guidelines for Design and Construction of Hospitals and Healthcare Facilities.* Philadelphia: The American Institute of Architects Academy of Architecture for Health; 2001.

34. Transport Canada. *Emergency Response Guidebook: A Guidebook for First Responders During the Initial Phase of a Dangerous Goods-Hazardous Materials Incident (ERG 2000).* Washington, DC: U.S. Department of Transportation, and Secretary of Transport and Communications of Mexico; 2000.

35. Department of Health and Human Services. *Metropolitan Medical Response System's Field Operation Guide.* Washington, DC: Department of Health and Human Services; November 1998.

36. *Volume I—Emergency Medical Services: A Planning Guide for the Management of Contaminated Patients.* Agency for Toxic Substances and Disease Registry; March 2001.

37. Victorian Government Health information. *Infectious Diseases Epidemiology and Surveillance.* Australia: Victoria. Available at: http://www.dhs.vic.gov.au/phb/9906058a/9906058.pdf.

38. American Institute of Architects. *Guidelines for Design and Construction of Hospital and Health Care Facilities, 1996-7.* Washington, DC: American Institute of Architects Press; 1996.

39. Seow E. SARS: experience from the emergency department, Tan Tock Seng Hospital, Singapore. *Emerg Med J.* 2003 Nov;20(6):501–504.

40. Barbera JA, Macintyre AG, DeAtley CA. *Chemically Contaminated Patient Annex: Hospital Emergency Operations Planning Guide [August 23, 2001, draft].* Washington, DC: George Washington University; 2001.

41. Deitch EA, Marino AA, Gillespie TE, Albright JA. Silver-nylon: a new antimicrobial agent. *Antimicrob Agents Chemother.* 1983;23(3):356–359.

42. Kowalski WJ, Bahnfleth WP, Whittam TS. Filtration of airborne microorganisms: modeling and prediction. Available at: *ASHRAE Transactions.* 1999;105(2):4–17.http://www.engr.psu.edu/ae/iec/abe/publications/filtration_airborne_microorganism.pdf.

CHAPTER 22

Community Hazard Vulnerability Assessment

James C. Chang

On August 23, 2011, residents in the tristate area (Maryland, Virginia, and District of Columbia) experienced an uncharacteristic event, but one relatively commonplace in the western United States and other regions of the world: an earthquake. The tristate area reported mostly minor damage from the Mineral, Virginia earthquake, with a few notable exceptions (e.g., the Washington Monument and the National Cathedral; Fig. 22-1). The National Cathedral sustained over 20 million dollars in damage when masonry structures were shaken apart.[1] In the frequently asked questions (FAQ) section of their webpage dedicated to the earthquake, the question was asked, "Why is the earthquake damage not covered by an insurance policy?" The response is illustrative:

> While we try to consider every eventuality in our stewardship of the Cathedral, it is necessary to make decisions based on the best information available at the time. Until August, the area had not seen an earthquake of this size since 1897. The combination of the improbability of an earthquake coupled with high deductibles and annual premiums made the purchase of earthquake insurance a poor financial decision. We are currently reviewing our coverage to ensure that the Cathedral is prepared in similar circumstances going forward.[1]

Similar mitigation considerations were contemplated by the Metropolitan Washington Council of Governments (MWCOG). After acknowledging that the Mineral, Virginia, earthquake was only the second event since the 1700s to register greater than a magnitude 5.0, the council recommended that local government should further standardize their response to earthquakes.[2] Both the MWCOG recommendation and the National Cathedral's FAQ insurance response seem to suggest the expenditure of effort and resources to prepare for the next earthquake event despite acknowledging the very low likelihood of an(other) earthquake event.

An even more obscure hazard example is a solar event. Solar events occur approximately every 11 years and are evidenced by waxing and waning sun spot activity. Periods of intense sun spot activity are known as solar maximum events. The most common manifestation of solar maximum events are the Northern Lights (aurora borealis) shifting southward, visible over the continental United States. Other effects are less innocuous, and these include loss of global positioning satellite (GPS) services, radio system interference, and damage to critical infrastructure (e.g., communications systems and power grids). Similar solar events in 1972 damaged phone lines, and those in 1989 blacked out a large portion of the northeast United States and Canada.[3] Despite the known vulnerability and potential severity of consequences, preparation for solar events remains relatively unheard of among most emergency planners.

The community hazard vulnerability assessment (cHVA) is a process used by many communities to identify high-probability risks. The cHVA involves the systematic examination of a multitude of hazards, as well as their individual probabilities and the consequences that may be encountered in the community. This assessment requires an in-depth knowledge of the community and is typically performed by a multidisciplinary team. The cHVA is often used as the basis for the community's emergency management program and selection of target hazards. Earthquakes and solar events are just two possible scenarios that challenge community and hospital emergency managers and elicit the question what should you plan for?

Like the health care facility hazard vulnerability assessment (HVA) presented in Chapter 23, the cHVA helps emergency planners identify potential community threats. Emergency managers and community leaders conducting cHVAs are met with similar budgeting challenges when trying to determine how best to allocate limited resources to high-risk hazards. Unlike the hospital-based HVA, the scope and performance of cHVAs are often beyond the direct control (and sometimes influence) of hospital-based planners and are conducted by local emergency management officials. Nonetheless, hospitals must engage with community planners and response agencies to develop a successful, comprehensive emergency preparedness program.

HISTORICAL PERSPECTIVE

To understand where the practice of conducting an HVA arose, one must understand the short, fragmented history of emergency management in the United States.

The Federal Civil Defense Administration (FCDA) was established by President Truman in 1949 in response to increasing Cold War concerns. The Federal Civil Defense Act of 1950 was quickly passed to give the FCDA the authority and resources to begin planning and coordinating activities. One of the most noteworthy successes of the FCDA and its director, Val Peterson, was the idea that civil defense activities such as disaster planning had peacetime value. Meanwhile, Congress continued to reinforce the role of the federal government in responding to (but not preparing for) disasters with the Federal Disaster Act of 1950. This act, intended for "getting assistance to rebuild the streets and farm-to-market highways and roads," was viewed by many as Congress establishing the legal basis for a continuing federal role in disaster relief. Subsequent acts, including the Disaster Relief Acts of 1970 and 1974, reinforced the federal government's role in disaster relief.[4]

In 1972, the Office of Civil Defense, which had been reestablished in 1961, was renamed the Defense Civil Preparedness Agency. Moreover, increasing international tensions and growing stockpiles of nuclear weapons gave rise to the concept of crisis relocation planning (CRP). The premise behind CRP was the dispersal of the populace from high-risk areas in times of heightened international tensions; in essence,

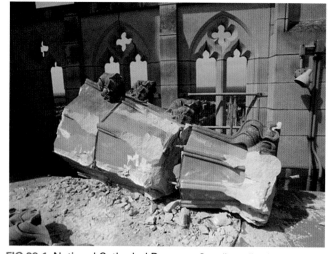

FIG 22-1 National Cathedral Damage. Standing taller than a human, this fallen pinnacle weighs thousands of pounds. (Source: John Stuhldreher, photographer, courtesy of Washington National Cathedral.)

this was an extension of existing hurricane evacuation programs that many coastal areas had successfully developed. Two years later, Congress passed the Disaster Relief Act of 1974, which specifically authorized the federal government to assist in disaster preparedness activities.

Difficulties in implementing CRP and the resulting frustrations experienced by federal, state, and local emergency planners led to a study and report by the National Governors Association (NGA) in 1978. This report called for a coordinated federal policy and approach to emergency planning. The NGA report introduced the concept of comprehensive emergency management (CEM), which is the cornerstone for emergency management today. In response to the NGA report and pressure from the constituency, President Jimmy Carter established the Federal Emergency Management Agency (FEMA) in 1979, to pull together many fragmented federal programs and implement a CEM program. Under CEM, instead of focusing on specific scenarios and their consequences (e.g., nuclear attack, earthquake, or flood), local and state agencies were encouraged to ask the following:

- What hazards confront our community?
- What resources are available? What needed resources are not available? Over what period of time could local government reasonably acquire these resources?
- What actions could be taken to mitigate future vulnerabilities?

These questions are essential to an Integrated Emergency Management System (IEMS) approach; IEMS is the tool under which FEMA implements CEM. Under IEMS, emergency managers perform systematic assessments of both hazards and response capabilities. Gaps are identified, and then multiyear remediation plans, along with hazard mitigation and recovery plans, are created to address these gaps. Implicit in the use of IEMS is the change from a reactionary to a proactive approach to emergency management. This planning approach facilitates the transition from a hazard-specific to an all-hazards approach to emergency management.[4]

Significant events in the 1980s (e.g., Three Mile Island and the Loma Prieta Earthquake) and 1990s (e.g., Hurricane Andrew) helped focus attention on the agency and its disaster planning, response, and recovery efforts. Following the terror attacks of 2001, FEMA adopted a new mission: homeland security. Working with the newly created Office of Homeland Security, the agency, using its all-hazards approach to disasters, directed billions of dollars to communities to help prepare

for the terrorism threat. In 2003, FEMA was integrated into the new Department of Homeland Security (DHS), the new agency tasked to bring a coordinated all-hazards approach to planning for and responding to both human-made and natural disasters.[5]

CURRENT PRACTICE

To properly plan for emergencies in the community, focus is applied to identifying the list of potential hazards, their probability or relative risk, and their consequences. This process helps the planning team decide which hazards merit special attention, what actions must be planned for, and what resources are likely needed.

The cHVA is composed of four critical elements:
- cHVA team membership
- Community profile
- Hazard identification
- Hazard profiling (probability and consequences)

To gain better insight into the cHVA process, we will review each of these elements in greater detail.

cHVA Team Membership[6]

A multidisciplinary team approach should be considered for both the cHVA and the development of the final Emergency Operations Plan (EOP) for many reasons, including:
- To share (synergistic) expertise
- To develop and foster teamwork and working relationships
- To ensure that a holistic view of hazards is taken
- To create a sense of ownership and commitment from all parties

The constituency of the teams will differ depending on their stated purpose (e.g., cHVA vs. plans development). Prospective members of the cHVA team may include representatives from various agencies and organizations. Examples are listed below:
- Emergency Management Agency
- Community leadership (e.g., city manager and county executive)
- Each community public safety agency (law enforcement—police department and sheriff's office, fire department, emergency medical services [EMS])
- Hospitals and other community health care facilities
- Public health agencies (local health department)
- Planning departments or agencies
- Public works
- Utilities
- Local emergency planning committee (LEPC)
- Professional groups (e.g., Certified Hazardous Materials Managers and American Society of Safety Engineers)
- National Weather Service (NWS)
- Special hazards occupancies or operations (e.g., military bases, industrial complexes, dams, and nuclear power plants)
- Major business entities
- Other emergency management planners (e.g., from local, county, regional, or state agencies or private industry)
- Volunteer agencies
- Animal welfare agencies and caretakers (i.e., shelters, farmers, Humane Society)

Development of Community Profile

A profile of the community to be assessed is the first step in the cHVA process. This profile should include information relative to the location of hazards, affected populations, community operations, and public safety. Geospatial information systems (GIS) tools are often a valuable means to accomplish this task. Examples of relevant information for a community profile are listed below.

- Demographic information
- Land use and development patterns (including master plans)
- Geographic features
- Climate
- Transportation networks
- Key industries and organizations
- Critical infrastructure
- Location of public safety agencies
- Emergency warning system coverage

Hazard Identification

Hazard identification is the exercise of identifying what kinds of emergencies have occurred or could occur within the jurisdiction. For assessment purposes, it may be helpful to divide emergencies into the following categories:

- *Naturally derived emergencies:* for example, floods, hurricanes, tornados, and winter storms
- *Technologically derived emergencies:* for example, power or utility failures, hazardous materials releases, and computing systems failures
- *Human-made emergencies:* for example, attacks involving weapons of mass destruction

A partial listing of potential emergencies is provided in Box 22-1. This listing is not all inclusive, and care must be taken to ensure that hazards are not inappropriately excluded or omitted when assembling the community's overall list of potential hazards.[6] More importantly, hazards may arise from differing sources (e.g., epidemics may be naturally occurring or the result of bioterrorism). Finally, hazards and emergencies may be linked together. For example, a hurricane may generate flooding, mudslides, and loss of utilities.

There are many potential sources of information to support the hazard identification effort; examples are listed below[7]:

- Experiences of planning team members
- Experiences of utilities or other major business entities in the community
- Local and/or state emergency management agency records
- Local emergency response agency(ies) records
- Newspaper or other historical archives (see note below)
- Experiences of similar or adjacent communities
- Hazard information maps compiled by FEMA and state emergency management agencies, the U.S. Geological Survey (USGS) and state geological surveys, the NWS, and the Federal Insurance Administration (National Flood Insurance Program)
- Maps of 10- and 50-mile emergency planning zones (EPZs) around nuclear power plants
- Maps of hazardous materials sites prepared by the LEPC
- Risk management plan submittals by users of extremely hazardous substances
- Local American Red Cross or other disaster relief agency records
- Results of any federal, state, or private hazard analyses
- Local or state historical society
- Area universities (e.g., departments of history, sociology, geography, and engineering)
- Insurance industry groups (especially highly protected risk [HPR] insurers)
- Professional or business associations (e.g., local engineers and builders)
- Engineering assessments (e.g., reliability studies and mean time between failure studies)
- Longtime community residents

BOX 22-1 Examples of Community Hazards

Naturally Derived
- Avalanche
- Drought
- Earthquake
- Epidemic
- Flood
- Hurricane (cyclone, typhoon)
- Landslide
- Mudslide
- Severe thunderstorm
- Solar storm
- Subsidence
- Temperature extremes
- Tornado
- Tsunami
- Volcanic eruption
- Wildfire
- Windstorm
- Winter storm (blizzard or ice storm)

Technologically Derived
- Airplane crash
- Dam failure
- Hazardous materials release
- Hog or other animal farm waste containment failure
- Information technology system failure
- Power failure
- Radiological release
- Train derailment
- Urban conflagration
- Utility interruption (natural gas, water, sewer, telephone, or data)
- Water supply contamination

Human-made
- Civil disturbance
- Mass casualty events
- Terrorism (chemical, biological, radiological, nuclear, or high-yield explosive [CBRNE])

Hazard Profiling (Probability, Vulnerability, and Consequences)

Once the list of possible hazards has been assembled, the next action is to profile or characterize each hazard for probability, vulnerability, and effect or consequence.

Probability Assessment

A probability assessment examines the likelihood of the hazard or emergency occurring, which is often categorized as improbable, low, medium, or high. Other related factors listed below may be helpful in assessing or describing probability.[8]

- *Frequency of occurrence:* The more frequent the occurrence, the higher the likelihood.
- *Location of the hazardous event and the region affected:* Events that occur within or proximal to the community are more likely to affect the community, whereas events that occur at some distance may be less likely to affect the community.
- *Seasonal (or other cyclical) variations:* Events that occur with some regularity may be presumed to be more probable. Commonplace examples include the occurrence of "influenza season" each fall through winter, and drought and/or floods (location-dependent) associated with El Niño.

Some hazards, such as civil disorder and terrorism, by their nature are highly unpredictable and may be difficult to properly assign to a probability level. Emergency managers may elect to use other means to assess the probabilities of these events, such as intelligence reports, increased insurgent activity, or contributing phenomena, such as economic instability that may increase chances for civil disorder.

Consequences

The consequences are the effect of the hazard on the community, and they may be categorized into human, property, and business consequences. Examples of each category are listed below (the reader should note that these are not all encompassing):

- Human impact
  - Injuries
  - Illnesses
  - Fatalities
  - Psychological impact
- Property damage
  - Damage to or loss of use of buildings, structures, or domiciles
  - Damage to or loss of use of infrastructure (e.g., roadways and utility distribution systems)
- Business loss
  - Business interruption (including recordkeeping issues arising from loss of records, inability to access, and compromise of integrity)
  - Unanticipated costs
  - Loss of revenue (from all causes, such as loss of tourism, sales tax revenue, and fees for services)
  - Decline in property values
  - Adverse publicity
  - Fines, penalties, and legal costs

The degree of the effects may be expressed qualitatively as nonexistent, low, medium, high, or catastrophic, or they may be expressed quantitatively as a numerical score. As a consideration, the cHVA team may wish to add greater weight to hazards that occur without warning (e.g., tornado strike).

Vulnerability Assessment

A vulnerability assessment asks the questions how vulnerable is the community (or portions of the community) to the hazards identified in the earlier probability and consequences assessments? Are there portions of the community that may be more vulnerable to an identified event (e.g., flood prone areas)? By overlaying the information contained within the community profile (e.g., locations of population centers and important facilities) with the details from the hazard assessment, planners can look for areas where the hazards overlap with population centers and important facilities to assess the community's vulnerabilities.[9]

Summary

The end goal of a cHVA should be a listing of hazards facing the community. Depending on the needs of the reviewer or end-user (e.g., emergency management or lead planning agency), this listing may or may not be prioritized. An example of Durham County's (NC) 2001 cHVA, excerpted from the county's EOP is presented in Box 22-2.

As mentioned earlier in this chapter, the cHVA is the foundation for the community's integrated emergency management activities, such as creation of plans, preparedness activities, hazard mitigation programs, and recovery plan development. An estimate of potential harm (usually expressed in human casualties or dollar values) will be made, and priorities can be established as to which hazards are most threatening. The highest-priority hazards are typically ones that the community

---

BOX 22-2 Example of Durham County's HVA Plan[11]

Durham County is exposed to many hazards, all of which have the potential to disrupt the community, cause damage, and create casualties. Potential hazards (natural, technological, and national security) are:

1. Major fires
2. Floods/dam failure
3. Tornados/severe thunderstorms
4. Severe winter storms
5. Hurricanes
6. Power failure
7. Drought
8. Earthquake
9. Mass casualty/fatality
10. Hazardous material
11. Fixed nuclear facility (ingestion pathway)
12. National security emergency
13. Civil disorder
14. Sabotage/terrorism
15. Aircraft crash (civilian/military)
16. Severe bridge damage
17. Public utility damage (e.g., phone, electricity, water, and sewer)

---

places more emphasis, effort, and resources (people, supplies, equipment, and funds) toward addressing.

⚠ PITFALLS

Management of Low-Probability, High-Consequence Events

In the prior edition of *Disaster Medicine* by Ciottone et al., 2006, the concept of threat assessments (terrorism-specific vulnerability assessment) was introduced. Even though a threat assessment appears similar to a cHVA in format and process, the threat assessment differs in several ways. For example, the threat assessment focuses only on the effects of malicious activities or persons in the community (vs. all hazards). More sophisticated threat assessments actually review the consequences of these malicious acts on specific targets, such as infrastructure, critical function areas, symbolic targets, or even special events (e.g., concerts). Threat assessments are typically performed by law enforcement officials (vs. a multidisciplinary team) because of their specialized knowledge and access to sensitive information.

A common question facing the cHVA team is "what should be included in our assessment?" Prior to the terrorist attacks of September 11, 2001 (commonly referred to as 9/11), the concept of terrorism-specific threat assessments was fairly limited in audience. In a post-9/11 environment, increased attention is being applied to active shooter scenarios. Shooting events such as those at the West Nickel Mines Amish School in Pennsylvania (2006), Virginia Tech, Virginia (2007), the Aurora, Colorado, Movie Theater (2012), and recently at the Sandy Hook Elementary School in Newtown, Connecticut (2012), have increased demand for inclusion of active shooter scenarios into community assessments.

Placing emphasis on a demarcation between events likely to occur versus ones unlikely to occur is an important tool. In their Knowledge Note 6-5, the World Bank suggests that events likely to occur are those that happen every 100 years or less. Events occurring less than once every 1000 years are considered unlikely to occur.[10] Based on this concept, the planning team should address hazards most likely to occur in their community, such as hazardous materials events, fires, or, for some, floods (events occurring less than once per 1000 years are considered outliers). Hazards likely to occur (within 100 years) should be identified and prioritized and resources should be allocated to manage risks at a level that community leaders find comfortable. Common risk management examples may include flood control measures, establishment of hazardous materials response teams, and evacuation planning around high-hazard chemical processing facilities.

In their review of the East Japan Earthquake (2011), the World Bank suggests that managing risks of unlikely events (events occurring less than every 1000 years) should rely on a systems strategy versus management of specific hazards. A systems approach emphasizes saving lives through the use of integrated disaster risk management strategies (vs. specific structural fixes or hardening). These strategies may include[10]:

- Emphasis on resilience
- Early warning and forecasting systems
- Evacuation planning
- Consideration if events exceed expectations
- Consideration to the "chain of events" effect
- Use of technology tools where appropriate (e.g., GIS)
This approach is in many ways consistent with the IEMS approach.

CONCLUSION

The cHVA is a critical step for any community's emergency management activities because the cHVA methodically defines the scope and breadth of hazards that may be encountered in the community. Under CEM, hazards identified (and prioritized) by the cHVA team will be addressed through a variety of means, including the development of emergency operations and response plans, hazard mitigation programs, and preparedness efforts such as training and drills. Although it is not possible to plan or prepare for every conceivable emergency, the cHVA can ensure that plans are developed to deal with higher-probability hazards or those with more significant consequences.

Management of low-probability, high-impact or high-consequence events is an area that requires special attention. No community emergency manager wants to be unprepared when a catastrophe strikes. However, emergency managers also need a response to political leaders and the public when they ask why have we not prepared for the horrific scenario depicted on the evening news? Left uncontested, emergency management planners may be asked to divert attention to hazards that although important, may not be the most appropriate for their communities; for example, the jurisdictions in the National Capital Region that rushed to implement earthquake response plans after 2011. Use of a systems-based approach with an overall goal of improving the ability to react and respond may be more beneficial than specific scenario-based preparations.

Health care facilities can both contribute to and benefit from the cHVA effort. Hospital administrators and physicians may provide expertise to community emergency managers on issues such as mass casualty management, infectious disease consequences, and surge management. At the same time, the cHVA may be utilized as a basis for external hazards in the health care facility's own HVA. For example, if the cHVA identifies mass casualties arising from a hazardous materials event as a probability, this should be reflected in the health care facility's HVA. Ultimately, it should be the goal of both community and health care facility emergency planners to have a coordinated response to maximize efficiencies and avoid duplication of efforts.

REFERENCES

1. Washington National Cathedral website. FAQs. Available at: http://www.nationalcathedral.org/dcquake/earthquakeFAQ.shtml.
2. Quake gets attention of D.C. area officials. In: Washington Post; September 14, 2011. Available at: http://www.washingtonpost.com/local/dc-politics/quake-gets-attention-of-dc-area-officials/2011/09/14/gIQAeoJqSK_story.html.
3. Solar Maximum. In: National Oceanic and Atmospheric Administration, National Weather Service, Space Weather Prediction Center. Available at: http://www.swpc.noaa.gov/info/SolarMax.pdf.
4. Federal Emergency Management Agency. State and Local Guide (SLG) 101: Guide for All-Hazards Emergency Operations Planning. Chapter 2: The Planning Process. Available at: http://www.fema.gov/pdf/rrr/2-ch.pdf.
5. Federal Emergency Management Agency. About the Agency. Available from: http://www.fema.gov/about-agency.
6. Drabek T. The evolution of emergency management. In: Drabek TE, Hoetmer GJ, eds. *Emergency Management: Principles and Practice for Local Government*. Washington, DC: International City Management Association; 1991:6–8, 10–13, 17–18.
7. The National Lessons Learned & Best Practices Information Network. Emergency Management Programs for Healthcare Facilities: Hazard Vulnerability Analysis: Comparing and Prioritizing Risks. Available at: https://www.llis.dhs.gov/frontpage.cfm.
8. Drabek TE, Hoetmer GJ, eds. Mitigation and hazard management. In: *Emergency Management: Principles and Practice for Local Government*. Washington, DC: International City Management Association; 1991:140–142.
9. Step 1 Identify Hazards and Risks. In: *Local Hazard Mitigation Planning Workbook*. Michigan Department of State Police, Emergency Management Division (EMD PUB 207): 2003. Available at: http://www.michigan.gov/documents/4-pub207_60737_7.pdf?
10. Strategies for Managing Low-probability, High-impact Events. In: *KNOWLEDGE NOTE 6-5: CLUSTER 6: The Economics of Disaster Risk, Risk Management, and Risk Financing*. The World Bank Institute. Available at: *http://wbi.worldbank.org/wbi/document/strategies-managing-low-probability-high-impact-events*
11. Basic plan. In: *Durham/Durham County Emergency Operations Plan*. Durham, NC: Durham County Emergency Management Agency; 2001:BP-2.

23 CHAPTER

Health Care Facility Hazard and Vulnerability Analysis

William A. Gluckman, Eric S. Weinstein, Kathe M. Conlon, and James C. Chang

In 1988 Jan deBoer and colleagues[1] published the first attempt to mathematically score and classify a disaster, with the intent to create data to be used prospectively during the management of a calamity. They defined a disaster as "a destructive event that caused so many casualties that extraordinary mobilization of medical services was necessary."[1] In the proposed Medical Severity Index of Disasters, the parameters needed to quantify a disaster were the casualty load (number of casualties), the severity of incident (severity of injuries sustained), and the capacity of medical services.[1] Twenty-six years later, the importance of determining the effects of a disaster on a health care facility (HCF) has heightened because HCFs have become industrial leaders in the community and, therefore, must be able to swiftly return to normal business functioning. Individual health care providers are acutely aware of the business side of their practice while at the bedside, but they are not cognizant of the ramifications that a disruption of normal HCF operations would have on the community. Business and industry emergency management principles by which HCFs can accommodate the clinical effects of a disaster are discussed in this chapter.

Disasters are events that cause significant enough damage to disrupt the normal activities or function of a community and overwhelm the local resources. What may be an easily handled event in a large urban city may be a disaster for a rural town. Although disasters are not predictable with any great accuracy, many consequences of disasters can be anticipated as part of a comprehensive emergency management plan that includes a hazard and vulnerability analysis (HVA). The HVA will help HCFs plan for these events and allow them to continue operating while assessing structural and operational damage, acquiring needed essentials, and protecting staff and patients. Much can be learned from business and industry with respect to preparedness.

Although not a new concept in business and industry, an HVA is a component in the development of a hospital disaster plan, as recognized since 2001 by The Joint Commission. The emergency management standard (EC.4.1) requires hospitals to identify specific procedures in response to a variety of disasters based on an HVA performed by the organization.[2] The HVA will assist in the mitigation and preparedness of the HCF to respond to and then recover from a disaster. A hazard can be any threat that could cause injury, fatality, property, infrastructure, or environmental damage or impair operations. An HVA is a tool used by emergency management to screen for risk and plan for strategic use of potentially limited resources.

HISTORICAL PERSPECTIVE

Many events have affected HCFs in the past. The future is certain to exhibit challenges as we move into a more technologically advanced society challenged by geopolitical terrorist threats. Hospitals inherently have to be prepared for emergencies. Preparation traditionally was based on informal HVAs and was largely dependent on perceived issues. For example, hospitals in northern climates typically planned for adverse winter weather–related issues; hospitals in the South planned for hurricanes; and hospitals in Southern California planned for forest and wildland fires and earthquakes. Failure to consider all hazards when developing the facility emergency response plan was a flaw in the informal approach.

Hazard identification relies on the collection of potential emergencies that the HCF or operation could anticipate encountering. This list may be assembled by cause, by location, or by a combination of both criteria. Causes may be divided into the following categories for assessment purposes: naturally derived emergencies, technologically derived emergencies, and humanmade emergencies (Box 23-1). HCFs experience two types of disasters: (1) those internal to the HCF, isolated to the confines of the HCF physical plant, and (2) those occurring external to the HCF that produce direct effects (casualties) and indirect effects (e.g., loss of electricity and supply due to damaged roads) to the HCF. In the past few years, several major disasters, natural external events, have affected HCFs: in 2005, Hurricane Katrina caused complete devastation of the primary hospital in New Orleans; in 2011, an F5 tornado devastated St. John's Regional Medical Center in Joplin, Missouri; and in 2012, Hurricane Sandy forced the evacuation of three large New York City medical centers. Internal disasters are similar to those encountered by business and industry, which until recently were not formally considered in an HVA. Milsten's[3] exhaustive review of direct and indirect disasters that hospitals faced from 1977 to 1997 showed that external and internal disasters are not mutually exclusive. This chapter focuses on the HVA and events specific to internal disasters, those that directly occur within the confines of the HCF, and those that indirectly affect the HCF because of consequences of a disaster.

CURRENT PRACTICE

Successful mitigation efforts and effective response plans are based on the best possible knowledge of the HCF's vulnerability in terms of deficiencies in its capacity to provide services, physical weaknesses, and organizational shortcomings in responding to emergencies. The HVA should also highlight and identify strengths within personnel, processes, plans, and other attributes. Past successes during disasters should be revisited to learn best practices.

All HVAs have some degree of subjectivity in their findings because many assumptions are made with regard to the perceived risk and even the level of preparedness if hard data are not available. Use of a multidisciplinary team should be encouraged to ensure a holistic characterization of each hazard and to help minimize the inherent subjectivity of the analysis and skewed or erroneous results. The team should be led by

BOX 23-1 Hazard Identification

Natural Events
- Drought
- Earthquake
- Flood
- Hurricane (cyclone, typhoon)
- Landslide
- Severe thunderstorm
- Temperature extremes
- Tidal wave
- Tornado
- Wildland fires
- Windstorm
- Snow/ice storms/blizzard
- Volcanic ash
- Meteor crashes
- Infestation

Technology Event
- Aircraft crash
- Medical evacuation helicopter crash
- Other aviation crash
- Loss of medical gases
- Air
- Oxygen
- Nitrogen
- Nitrous oxide
- Electrical/power shortage or failure
- Loss of backup generator(s)
- Fire: chemical, paper, wood, and other
- Computer network disruption or loss
- Loss of fire alarm/smoke detection
- Loss of steam
- Food contamination
- Pneumatic tube disruption or loss
- Food supply interruption
- Loss or leak of potable water
- Fixed facilities incidents
- Loss of suction/vacuum
- Loss of fuel oil supply or delivery
- Elevator service disruption or loss

- Hazardous material release
- Structural failure
- Natural gas/pipeline disruption
- Noxious fumes
- Sewer failure
- HVAC failure
- Loss of equipment requiring cooling
- Patient/staff at risk
- Loss of instrumentation (thermostat control/regulation)
- Supply chain interruption
- Labor dispute
- Shortage of labor
- Communication failure
- Paging: internal and external
- Emergency medical services or other radio
- Internal HCF telephone
- External telephone
- Cellular phone
- Satellite
- Transportation disruption
- Labor dispute
- Roadway/highway incident/blockage

Human Events: With or Without Political, Terrorist, or Criminal Intent
- Mass casualty incidents
- Trauma
- Civil disturbance
- CBRNE*
- Infectious disease
- Foodborne illness
- Abduction (infant, child, or adult)
- Armed or threatening intruder
- Bomb threat
- Civil disorder
- Forensic admissions
- Hostage situation
- Violent labor action
- VIP visitor
- Workplace violence

*Chemical, biological, radiological, nuclear, or high-yield explosive.

someone familiar with the HVA process and consist of representatives from at least the following areas within the HCF:
- Emergency management
- Security/safety
- Facilities (e.g., engineering, maintenance, information technology, and telecommunications)
- Operations (e.g., nursing, medical staff, laboratory, and radiology)
- Ancillary services (e.g., materials, food, housekeeping, and environmental services)
- Administration
- Finance/business

Community representatives, such as the local emergency manager, fire official, police official, and city manager, can also provide valuable input. Additional members, including the hospital administrator-at-large may be beneficial, as long as the group size remains manageable and consensus is achievable within a reasonable amount of time. Regularly scheduled meetings with a defined agenda and other

business-related models will assist the completion and maintenance of the assignment of the HVA team.

Most HVA tools come preloaded with a listing of likely hazards that the developer believes the average HCF could face. It is important that the HVA team begin by reviewing the listing of hazards in the HVA tool to ensure that it is comprehensive and applicable to the facility(s). The HVA tool should address all possible events regardless of their likelihood. The first step is to "brainstorm" and determine all possible hazards. This can be accomplished with assistance from the county local emergency preparedness committee (LEPC) in conjunction with the Office of Emergency Management for both the county and state. The hazards are then classified into categories, as described in Box 23-1.

Risk, or effect, relates to the threat a particular hazard has with respect to the effects on humans: safety of people (patients and staff); effects on property: structure(s) and property; and effects on business: the ability to continue operations. Each risk can be assigned a numerical value to allow for a comparison or relative risk. The three types of effects are averaged, and a score is assigned for each category. This will be important in the overall assessment.

Examples of each category include but are not limited to[4]:

- Effects on humans
  - Potential for injury or death to staff members
  - Potential for injury or death to visitors
  - Potential for injury, death, or adverse outcomes to patients
- Effects on property
  - Damage to the facility (up to and including loss of the facility)
  - Loss of use of the facility
  - Loss of or damage to equipment and/or supplies
  - Costs associated with replacement/repair of the facility, equipment, or services
- Effects on business
  - Business interruption
  - Unanticipated costs
  - Loss of revenue (from all causes)
  - Record keeping issues (e.g., loss of records, inability to access, and compromise of integrity)
  - Employees unable or unwilling to report for work
  - Patients unable to reach the facility
  - Damage to reputation
  - Fines, penalties, and legal costs
  - Future insurance premium increases

The degree of risk may be expressed as a numerical score or verbally with use of terms such as *nonexistent, low, medium, high,* and *catastrophic.* As a consideration, the HVA team may wish to add greater weight to hazards that occur without warning (e.g., tornado strike).

Probability relates to how likely an event is to occur at the facility or to affect the facility, based on proximity. This, too, can be assigned a numerical value and is best determined from historical data (e.g., a scale from 1 to 5, with 1 representing a low probability of occurrence and 5 a very high probability of occurrence). Looking back at historical data is critical in making an "educated guess" about the future. This is an assessment of the likelihood of a hazard or emergency occurring that is often described as improbable, low, medium, or high. Other related factors that may be helpful in assessing or describing probability include the following[5]:

- *Frequency of occurrence:* Obviously, the more frequent the occurrence, the higher the likelihood.
- *Location of the hazardous event and the region affected:* Events that occur proximal to the HCF are more likely to directly (or indirectly) affect the facility, whereas events that occur at some distance may be less likely to affect the HCF.
- *Seasonal (or other cyclic) variations:* Events that occur with some regularity may be presumed to be more probable. Commonplace examples include the occurrence of "influenza season" each fall through the winter, and drought and/or floods (location-dependent) associated with El Niño.

Where possible, probability should be based on objective data, such as historical archives, to learn of local disasters. Equipment failure rates or mean time between failure data should be available to the HVA team. Even maintenance records and expected length of service of equipment may lead to objective data that influence an HVA. Often, however, probability assessments are colored by the prior experiences of HVA team members and recent organizational memory.

Facility preparedness may be expressed explicitly in a separate category or integrated with another element (probability or risk). Intuitively, if the facility is well prepared to deal with an emergency, the effects of the emergency should be lessened. The presence of a preparedness component aids in tracking the organization's preparedness efforts and is a means to decrement HVA scores as preparedness levels increase. Preparedness also should be reported to help determine the need for improvement in areas

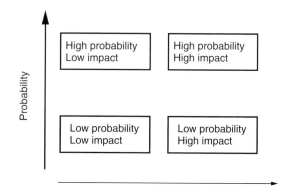

FIG 23-1 Probability versus Effect.

that have high risk and/or probability. Preparedness may be assigned a numerical value, or it simply may be a listing of what, if any, plans currently exist to address that particular event. It may also represent resources and the amount of them available (e.g., a lot, little, or none); resources can be subdivided into internal and external resources. The average of these two is the numerical value for preparedness.

Adding the numerical values of these three components (risk, probability, and preparedness) provides a value. Looking at probability versus effects graphically (Figure 23-1), one would expect higher sums for those events that fall in the high-probability–highly effected areas and lower values for those events in the low-probability–lowly effected areas.

For maximum benefit, the HVA should generate a prioritized listing of hazards with sufficient detail to characterize each one. To do this, a means to grade or rank each hazard, vulnerability, risk (consequence), and level of preparedness. This characterization may be qualitative or quantitative; each approach has pros and cons.

Qualitative assessments may be simpler and faster to perform; however, these are often more difficult to implement fully in the end. A qualitative analysis may be as simple as having HVA team members rank a listing of potential hazards in order, based on their subjective judgment. A slightly more-involved approach to qualitative assessment is found in the HVA model provided by the Emergency Management Strategic Healthcare Group (EMSHG) of the Veterans Health Administration. This model uses a scoring system from 0 (not applicable) to 3 (high) for probability and risk (consequence). Any hazard with a score of 2 or greater in either category requires action.[6] Qualitative HVA models often generate little differentiation between hazards and tend to group all hazards into one category (such as "high") or another. These models have little flexibility in implementation and do not help the organization when it is time to determine organizational priorities for emergency planning and/or allocation of resources.

Quantitative assessments can be used to provide additional flexibility in implementation by enhancing the differences between each hazard. Depending on the HVA tool chosen, the scores for each hazard may be the sum or product of probability, risk, and preparedness scores or may be derived from more complex weighting schemes. For example, the HVA model used by Duke University Hospital (Durham, North Carolina) takes the sum of the products of the probability of a hazard multiplied by the risk to people, property, and business, and then multiplies the resulting product by a facility preparedness score:

$$\sum \text{(Probability of Each Event} \times \text{Risk of Each Event)}$$
$$\times \text{Facility Preparedness Score}$$
$$= \text{Weighted Score of Event}$$

See Table 23-1 for an example of the Duke University Hospital HVA.

TABLE 23-1 Sample HVA

TYPE OF EMERGENCY	PROBABILITY RATING	HUMAN EFFECT	PROPERTY EFFECT	BUSINESS EFFECT	EFFECT RATING	INTERNAL RESOURCES	EXTERNAL RESOURCES	RESOURCES RATING	TOTAL*	EMERGENCY PLANS IN PLACE?
Score	High to Low 5↔1	High to Low 5↔1	High to Low	5↔1		Few Resources 5	Many Resources 1			
Technological Events										
Electrical failure	3	1	3	1	1.7	2	2	2.0	6.7	
Transportation failure	2	1	1	2	1.3	3	2	2.5	5.8	
Fuel shortage	2	1	1	1	1.0	1	1	1.0	4.0	
Natural gas failure	2	1	1	1	1.0	2	1	1.5	4.5	
Water failure contamination	3	1	1	1	1.0	3	3	3.0	7.0	
Sewer failure	2	1	1	1	1.0	3	3	3.0	6.0	
Steam failure	2	1	1	1	1.0	3	3	3.0	6.0	
Fire alarm failure	3	1	1	1	1.0	3	1	2.0	6.0	
Communications failure	5	3	3	3	3.0	2	2	2.0	10.0	
Medical gas failure	2	2	1	1	1.3	2	2	2.0	5.3	
Medical vacuum failure	2	3	1	1	1.7	2	2	2.0	5.7	
HVAC failure	3	2	1	2	1.7	2	2	2.0	6.7	
Information systems failure	3	3	3	3	3.0	2	2	2.0	8.0	
Fire, internal	4	4	4	4	4.0	2	1	1.5	9.5	
Hazardous materials exposure, internal	4	2	1	2	1.7	3	1	2.0	7.7	
Unavailability of supplies	3	1	1	2	1.3	2	2	2.0	6.3	
Structural damage	2	2	2	2	2.0	4	2	3.0	7.0	
Natural Events										
Hurricane	3	3	3	4	3.3	2	2	2.0	8.3	
Tornado	2	1	3	2	2.0	2	2	2.0	6.0	
Severe thunderstorms	4	2	2	2	2.0	2	2	2.0	8.0	
Snowfall	5	2	1	3	2.0	2	2	2.0	9.0	
Ice storm	4	3	2	3	2.7	2	2	2.0	8.7	
Earthquake	2	1	3	1	1.7	2	2	2.0	5.7	

Continued

TABLE 23-1 Sample HVA—cont'd

TYPE OF EMERGENCY	PROBABILITY RATING	HUMAN EFFECT	PROPERTY EFFECT	BUSINESS EFFECT	EFFECT RATING	INTERNAL RESOURCES	EXTERNAL RESOURCES	RESOURCES RATING	TOTAL*	EMERGENCY PLANS IN PLACE?
Tidal wave	1	1	2	1	1.3	2	2	2.0	4.3	
Temperature extremes	4	2	1	1	1.3	1	1	1.0	6.3	
Drought	3	2	2	2	2.0	2	2	2.0	7.0	
Flood, external	2	3	2	3	2.7	2	2	2.0	6.7	
Wildfire	2	1	1	1	1.0	1	1	1.0	4.0	
Landslide	1	1	1	1	1.0	1	1	1.0	3.0	
Volcano	1	1	1	1	1.0	1	1	1.0	3.0	
Epidemic	3	2	1	4	2.3	2	2	2.0	7.3	
Human Events										
Mass casualty incident (trauma)	5	4	1	4	3.0	3	3	3.0	11.0	
Mass casualty incident (medical)	5	4	1	4	3.0	3	3	3.0	11.0	
Mass casualty incident (hazardous materials)	4	3	1	4	2.7	3	3	3.0	9.7	
Terrorism, chemical	5	5	1	5	3.7	3	3	3.0	11.7	
Terrorism, biological	5	5	1	5	3.7	3	3	3.0	11.7	
Terrorism, nuclear	5	5	3	5	4.3	3	3	3.0	12.3	
Accidental, chemical	4	5	1	5	3.7	3	3	3.0	10.7	
Accidental, biological	1	5	1	5	3.7	3	3	3.0	7.7	
Accidental, nuclear	1	5	3	5	4.3	3	3	3.0	8.3	
VIP situation	3	1	1	1	1.0	2	2	2.0	6.0	
Infant abduction	2	4	1	3	2.7	2	2	2.0	6.7	
Hostage situation	3	3	1	3	2.3	3	2	2.5	7.8	
Civil disturbance	5	2	2	3	2.3	2	2	2.0	9.3	
Labor action	3	1	1	3	1.7	2	2	2.0	6.7	
Forensic admission	4	1	1	1	1.0	2	2	2.0	7.0	
Bomb threat	5	2	1	2	1.7	2	2	2.0	8.7	

*Total is the sum of the probability, impact rating, and resource rating.

The end result of the Duke University Hospital and similar quantitative HVA models is weighted scores that address the probability, consequences, and preparedness level of each hazard. The weighted score of the event is then used to order its priority for emergency planning purposes. An institution may choose to address potential emergencies beginning with the highest-scoring event and progress down the list until all potential events are addressed. A variation of this theme may be to address the top five (or other number) high-scoring events in year one, and presuming completion of planning, preparedness, and/or mitigation activities, address the next five highest-scoring events in year two and so on. A third alternative may be to establish a predefined threshold level; any hazard scenario exceeding this threshold value would require some type of action (i.e., planning, preparedness, and mitigation).

More sophisticated HVA tools, such as the one developed by the Kaiser Permanente health care system, take the quantitative approach one step further by generating scores (percentages) and a graphical/visual output product.[7]

The HVA is the foundation for an organization's emergency management program. It is, therefore, advantageous to expend the effort and resources to ensure that the job is done properly. The assessors should begin by developing a list of potential emergencies that the organization may face and then characterize each hazard as to its probability and consequence. An automated HVA tool is a significant time saver, both as a means to test different scenarios for each hazard and as a documentation aid. Often a quick review of actual disasters, internal and external, that the HCF faced over the past 5 to 10 years is sufficient to commence action by the HVA team. A systematic and consistent approach is needed. The team leader should ensure that all team members have equal input into the process.

The end product of the HVA should be a prioritized, all-encompassing, objective (to the extent possible) assessment of the possible, potential, or historical internal and external indirect events that may affect the HCF. The HVA produced is the foundation of the HCF's emergency management program. It is used as the basis for planning and budgeting for hazard mitigation, preparedness, and response efforts within the institution. It should be intuitive that emergencies with the highest scores or ranks should be addressed first, and lesser items handled as time and funding permit.

An annual review and revalidation of the HVA should be performed to ensure that changes to the operating environment of the facility are assessed for their effect on the facility's emergency management program. Another reason for periodically reassessing the HVA is to reflect the benefit of hazard mitigation and preparedness activities. For example, as hospital preparedness activities reduce the risk (and consequences) of an emergency, such as a power failure, the item may be moved down on the list of priorities, and other more pressing items may be moved up. Review should also be conducted after real-world events, to reexamine if the true value of a hazard has been identified. In the original HVA a hazard may receive a low or mid-level ranking; however, actual experience may demonstrate that a higher value needs to be reassigned. Conversely the opposite may also hold true. Although an HVA may have identified patient surge as a hazard, the events of 9/11 demonstrated that hospitals need to prepare to receive patient admissions in the hundreds; well beyond most estimates. Two New York City hospitals located close to the Twin Towers reported treating over nine hundred admissions resulting from that particular incident.[8]

As a final consideration, the HVA work product (including drafts and working papers) should be considered a sensitive document and be protected to the same degree as a patient record or a peer review, quality-assurance/improvement, or sensitive business document is protected. Remember that the HVA details the organization's vulnerabilities, and depending on the format used and level of supporting documentation

maintained, may describe how the facility will respond to an emergency. In the wrong hands, this information may actually increase a facility's vulnerability to attack, and, for this reason, it should not be freely disseminated (e.g., placed on the Internet). Contact the Interagency Operational Security (OPSEC) Support Staff (IOSS) (www.ioss.gov) for operational security program development guidance, training courses, and consultative support.[9]

! PITFALLS

A typical pitfall is underestimating the time required to develop an HVA and not allowing sufficient time to adequately complete the evaluation. In a large facility in a complex urban environment, an HVA may be a multiday process. A related pitfall is the gradual decline in interest as the evaluation progresses; the amount of time spent on each topic is typically directly related to how long the team has been working. Most assessments begin with an extremely thorough discussion of hazards and decline rapidly to more cursory examinations as the day progresses.

It is sometimes necessary to reiterate the sole purpose of the HVA; that is, the development of a prioritized listing of hazards to be addressed in the hospital's emergency planning process. It is not uncommon for representatives of a particular service or group to consider any mention of a hazard in their area as a personal affront. Care should be taken to ensure that this bias does not cause hazards to be arbitrarily dismissed with an "it'll never happen here" attitude.

HVAs are important in a well-designed disaster plan and thus need to be updated on a regular basis. Geographic and industrial changes will affect a hospital and need to be considered. The establishment of a new chemical company in town, for instance, may make a significant change in an institution's assessment of hazardous materials threat.

Another problem, sometimes referred to as the "paper plan syndrome," gives the illusion of true preparedness simply because a written document exists. "Disaster planning is an illusion unless: It is based on valid assumptions about human behavior, incorporates an interorganizational perspective, is tied to resources, and is known and accepted by the participants."[10] To address this concern, institutions should consider taking plans beyond the paper stage and conduct tabletop and functional exercises. It is only through actual experience that planners and participants alike begin to understand the true nature of the process and, if in fact, the plan is operational. At the conclusion of the exercise an After Action Report (AAR) should also be generated. The purpose of an AAR is to identify plan strengths and weaknesses in order to improve upon overall effectiveness. However, exercising is not without its obstacles, especially for hospitals, where daily functions such as patient care cannot be interrupted simply for training purposes. Nor is there always sufficient staff to both conduct an exercise and still carry on with daily operations

CONCLUSION

In today's resource-constrained health care environment, it is not realistic to plan for every conceivable hazard or eventuality that may befall the institution. Health care administrators need to allocate their limited resources to ensure that likely scenarios are addressed promptly, whereas the "one-in-a-million" occurrences may be held in abeyance until some later date. The HVA is a tool for HCF administrators to assess and characterize systematically the plethora of hazards that their facility may face. Failure to exercise due diligence when conducting the HVA may have adverse consequences, ranging from professional embarrassment on the part of the emergency management coordinator to loss of life, business interruption, damage to reputation, and litigation from inadequate emergency planning. Proper use of the HVA helps minimize these risks.

REFERENCES

1. deBoer J, Brismar B, Eldar R, et al. The medical severity index of disasters. *J Emerg Med*. 1989;7:269–273.
2. Joint Commission on Accreditation of Healthcare Organizations. Available at: http://www.jcaho.org/.
3. Milsten A. Hospital responses to acute-onset disasters: a review. *Prehospital Disaster Med*. 2000;15(1):32–45.
4. The National Lessons Learned & Best Practices Information Network. Emergency Management Programs for Healthcare Facilities: Hazard Vulnerability Analysis: Comparing and Prioritizing Risks. Available at: https://www.llis.dhs.gov/frontpage.cfm.
5. The National Lessons Learned & Best Practices Information Network. Emergency Management Programs for Healthcare Facilities: Hazard Vulnerability Analysis: Identifying Potential Disasters and Probability. Available at: https://www.llis.dhs.gov/frontpage.cfm.
6. Emergency Management Strategic Healthcare Group, Veterans Health Administration. Section 3.10.3—Hazard Vulnerability Analysis (HVA) Instructions. Available at: http://www1.va.gov/emshg/apps/emp/emp/hva_instructions.htm.
7. California Hospital Association. Kaiser Permanente Medical Center Hazard and Vulnerability Analysis. Available at: http://www.calhospitalprepare.org/hazard-vulnerability-analysis.
8. James GC, Pachter HL, Beaton HL. Two New York City hospitals' surgical response to the September 11, 2001, terrorist attack in New York City. *Journal of Trauma—Injury Infection & Critical Care*. January 2003;54(1):147–155.
9. Interagency OPSEC Support Staff. Available at: http://www.ioss.gov/.
10. Auf der Heide E. Disaster Response: Principles of Preparation and Coordination. Chapter 3. Available at: http://orgmail2.coe-dmha.org/dr/DisasterResponse.nsf/section/03?opendocument.

CHAPTER 24

Public Information Management

William A. Gluckman, Eric S. Weinstein, Sharon Dilling, and Jeffrey S. Paul

In the chaos and craziness that ensues during or immediately after a disaster, whether it is a suspected contagious disease, an earthquake, or the explosion of a dirty bomb, there will be two constants: (1) the public will demand information about what is happening, and (2) the media will be at the scene trying to tell them. Ever since images from Vietnam broadcast live into the living rooms of millions of Americans, the public has come to see breaking news coverage not only as a given, but as their right. The thirst for information grows with every passing minute, fueled by the ever-increasing competition within the media for advertising, sponsorship, and viewers. All of this factors heavily into disaster response. Balancing emergency care for the sick or injured with the need to disseminate accurate public information is always a challenge. Emergency responders would never think of treating a patient without having the proper medical training. Training for disaster communication is also highly important; preparation is the key. Understanding what types of information the public and the media will want and need will help mitigate the effects of the disaster, win the confidence of the media, and reassure the public. Information presented in a clear and truthful manner within a reasonable amount of time will further its effectiveness.

MEDIA HISTORY

The development of the printing press in the fifteenth century allowed inexpensively produced newspapers and books to spread information to large numbers of people.[1] When Marconi sent a wireless message in 1896, radio came alive, allowing electronic communication during World War I.[2] The newsreel brought edited pictures of World War II to moviegoers, albeit somewhat delayed. In the 1950s the "American dream" turned out to be a television as the centerpiece of every living room. By the 1960s, nearly all of America tuned in to watch the son of President John Fitzgerald Kennedy salute the flag-draped coffin of his father. Walter Cronkite became "the most trusted man in America." And, of course, there was the Vietnam War. Television coverage has arguably changed the course of history by providing a window into the harsh realities of war that had never been seen before by most of America.

By the late twentieth century, new media outlets developed, offering 24-hour-a-day news coverage, as cable television proliferated America. A few years later, as a new millennium approached, the Internet and e-mail revolutionized communication, allowing information to travel rapidly right to the desktop. This, coupled with the competitive news business, created even more demand by both the public and the media for up-to-the-minute communication. This urgency for information has surpassed accuracy and even, in some cases, reason. In 1994, millions tuned in to watch a white Ford Bronco with O.J. Simpson inside drive down a freeway. And then there was September 11,

2001. The television images could not be edited to shelter viewers. They unfolded in real time, with real heartache. The world watched again and again with the hope of somehow hitting the pause button to allow the victims an additional moment or two of peaceful existence. Viewers tuned in for days, hoping to see people emerge alive from the burning rubble. News coverage was 24 hours a day for almost two weeks. Regular programming was preempted, and viewers struggled to come to terms with what had happened. As sad as it was, this horrific tragedy is a good example of what is expected of emergency response and public information.

In the past few years the era of "Social Media" have erupted as a popular means of communication. The public's thirst for real-time data has never been stronger. Facebook, Twitter, Instagram, VK, Google, and YouTube are just a few of the popular sites used by millions of people globally. These sites were developed for communication among friends and families but have now morphed and have both pros and cons in the setting of disaster communications. The common operating picture for all of these sites is data sharing. We now live in an environment where crime scene photos and other emergency response scenes are being posted, blogged, shared, and transmitted before the first responders and other media personnel are on scene.

There are both pros and cons to social media (Table 24-1). A big advantage includes being able to reach large numbers of people in a short time with a consistent message. However, for this to be effective, that message must come from a credible source. Many local municipalities and state governments have official accounts and release generally credible information. This is not to say that local citizens do not have good information to provide. During disasters citizens become the eyes and ears to real events before first responders. During Hurricane Sandy in New Jersey, there were Good Samaritans texting pictures of emergency situations to the Morris County Office of Emergency Management (OEM); for example, police officers and firefighters could not respond to people trapped in a car because of arcing wires on the vehicle. Local power authorities present in the emergency operation center at the time were able to identify the pole and shut off the power, while OEM personnel responded back with safety directions to the civilian. During the 2007 Virginia Tech massacre, the school was delayed in getting messages out, but social media was flooded with pictures and information from students. During the 2010 Deepwater Horizon oil spill in the Gulf of Mexico, community residents texted photos and locations of oil-soaked birds to the Louisiana Bucket Brigade, whose maps helped volunteers identify areas needing cleanup.[3]

Messages that are sent should relay the important facts and provide reassurance to the community at large, while not providing detail that may be harmful to emergency personnel operating at the scene. For example, if a terrorist group has several children held hostage at a school, it would be appropriate to communicate that 20 children have

TABLE 24-1	**Pros and Cons of Social Media**
PROS	**CONS**
Able to disseminate messages to large number of people quickly	Inaccurate data may be released by noncredible sources
Allows for the public to serve as "citizen soldiers"	Not all people have smartphones or social media accounts
Reassuring to the public	Lengthy periods of power outages may preclude charging of cell phones and access
Documents hazards and important information in near real time	Cell data towers and/or cable lines may be inoperable
Helpful in rumor control	Potential for unintentional release of sensitive data
Internet access may be available even in areas of power failure	Not all information provided is accurate or helpful
Effective tool to raise relief funding	Need dedicated personnel to update constantly
Another information gathering tool for TV, print, and radio media reporters	Message size may be limited

been rescued while 8 are still being held captive. It would not be advisable, however, to communicate that 20 children are being held safely with emergency and fire crews at the Kiddie Gym at 123 Main Street. This would give the opportunity for other members of the terrorist group who may be monitoring the media to potentially attack the gym.

MEDIA AND DISASTERS

The medical management of disasters, both small and large, requires a multifaceted response to ensure timely evacuation, assessment, treatment, and recovery. This response, usually based on the Incident Command System (ICS), requires the appointment of an incident commander, a logistics chief, and others. One important and often overlooked component of the ICS and disaster management in general is an area defined as public information management. The ability to provide appropriate, timely information can significantly affect the disaster response.

The components of public information management include not only the release of information to prepare rescue workers and volunteers, but the dynamic ongoing release of information to the media and the incorporation of the media within the response mission. Effective interaction with the media can improve the accurate distribution of information that ultimately aids the response, while at the same time satisfying the needs of the media to "get the story." This applies not only to hospitals or other institutions providing support in a disaster, but also to the rapid response elements (e.g., police, fire, and emergency medical services [EMS]) and to intermediate response organizations, such as the National Disaster Medical System's disaster medical assistance teams, the U.S. Department of Health and Human Services' Medical Reserve Corps, and the Federal Emergency Management Agency, to name a few.

During a disaster, potentially significant amounts of information should be communicated to the region affected to achieve a good response. This information provides the basis for management of the disaster as well as development of the public trust in the responsible agencies. For example, if a government frequently notifies the population of potential storms and their need to evacuate immediately, and subsequently, each storm causes insignificant damage, the population will learn to not trust the local government. If a category 5 hurricane

then heads to this same region, the population may not heed requests to evacuate because they have been misled many times before and may not believe the local government or disaster coordinators. However, if the local government warns residents of only potentially dangerous storms and only requests evacuation for events that most likely will cause significant damage and injuries, while providing the details behind its decisions, the population will more likely respond to an evacuation request and, therefore, injuries and loss of life will be reduced. Obviously, the decision to warn or request evacuations is not just dependent on actual risks, but also on potential legal action or bad publicity should the disaster be worse than expected.

Further, immediately after an event, those who evacuated or had interests in the area will want to access the affected area to find family members, recover personal items, and assess the damage so that they may start to rebuild or repair. They will depend on information provided by functioning public communications systems. If this recovery action by those affected is not coordinated in a timely manner, people returning to the affected area can hamper appropriate response efforts and hinder response communications. For example, cellular phone towers may become overloaded with users and, therefore, important phone calls are not able to be placed. Providing reentry instructions contained in the evacuation order and subsequent evacuation instructions is the best strategy. Phone numbers, radio stations, websites, and other means to provide timely and accurate information to those returning to an evacuated area will reduce anxiety, potential traffic jams, and the overuse of the limited resources of response agencies that will have to divert their focus to communication with an uninformed population searching for information. Finally, information about sources of food, potable water, medical care, cash, shelters and housing, fuel, and available government assistance needs to be communicated to the residents returning to the affected area.

Effective management of information can help minimize property loss and reduce the chance of injuries, and even deaths, but also can improve the effectiveness of response teams. To do this, methods need to be developed to communicate information to the population from one reliable, consistent source. Disasters do not just include the typical natural occurrence (e.g., flooding, hurricane, tornado) or human-made acts (e.g., industrial accident or terrorism), but also include loss of infrastructure (e.g., computer information systems, power grids, potable water, sewers, job action). Even though a disaster may not result in any injuries or fatalities, the fact that "something went wrong" brings the problem into the public eye. In such cases, the news media become interested and so do the government and public. The handling of the incident by the "offending" corporation or entity (1) can provide for a good public relations (PR) review and minimize the PR effect of the disaster, or (2) if poor PR ensues, can make the disaster more significant and potentially harm the corporation.

CURRENT PRACTICES

When a disaster strikes, media flood into the area. Be prepared to share your space. As word of the planes crashing into the two World Trade Center towers and the Pentagon spread, firefighters, police, and rescuers rushed to the scene. Not far behind were reporters, photographers, and camera crews. Tune into the local television station near where a hurricane is headed and undoubtedly reporters donning bright yellow rain slickers will be broadcasting from an evacuated beachfront while waves crash around them and lightning bolts light up the seas. Turn on the radio to hear broadcasters coughing out their report as the smoke of a nearby wildfire burns brush just steps away. Pick up a newspaper to learn how a reporter interviewed a family as they crouched in a storm cellar with a tornado blowing overhead. In a competitive media market, the emphasis is not always on providing the most accurate data but rather any data. In today's social media market this is happening quicker than a press release can be developed and often leads to confusion among the public, and in some instances panic as a result of inaccurate or otherwise bad data. Castillo et al. observed that immediately after the 2010 earthquake in Chile, when information from official sources was scarce, several rumors posted and reposted on Twitter contributed to increase the sense of chaos and insecurity in the local population.[4] Accepting media presence at events is important. Reporters will not go away, so it is best to help them find their way to a place that is close enough to the action to satisfy their needs, yet far enough away to prevent them from broadening the crisis by becoming a victim, or worse, placing emergency personnel at risk. When the media shift into crisis mode, they will broadcast whatever information they have in the order in which they receive it.[5] Providing factual information to the media will allow one to effectively control the information instead of the information being in control. Reporters may or may not have time to verify the information, but they would rather report something than have nothing to report. If they have nothing to report, they probably will speculate. When the *New York Post* went to press with its July 6, 2004, headline, "Kerry's Choice," they declared Dick Gephardt as running mate to presidential candidate John Kerry. Kerry announced his choice of John Edwards for vice president that same morning. The debacle mirrored the infamous 1948 Chicago Daily Tribune headline, "Dewey Defeats Truman." In the Gephardt case, the already tarnished reputation of the *Post* took a hit, and the Kerry campaign benefited from the exposure.[6] Although a mistake by the media can hardly be deemed a crisis, it clearly illustrates the pressure that time and competition weigh on the media. In most instances, it is best to offer some information, even a small amount, to the media, as long as it is correct.

Provide the media with factual information as soon as possible; even small or minor details or known truths can be helpful. The first source often becomes the most credible. Also, remember to demonstrate empathy when providing information.[7] In the immediate aftermath of the destruction of the World Trade Center towers, New York City Mayor Rudy Giuliani spoke to the people of New York and the nation. He provided very little new information, but he told what he knew and demonstrated empathy—that he was grieving, too. "The number of casualties," he said, "will be more than any of us can bear."[8] This was not an unknown fact, and it most certainly was not a new piece of information. Giuliani had never been known for his compassion, and his behavior after the World Trade Center disaster was a turning point in his career, making him arguably the most popular mayor in the city's history.

Be honest. The truth almost always comes out anyway. There are numerous instances throughout history in which an initially dishonest action was forgiven by the public after the truth was told. If one shares inaccurate information and later the information is determined to be false, all credibility will be lost.

Time and space in the media are money. When a newspaper is put together, the first pieces to go in are the advertisements. Articles fill in the spaces around them. Space is at a premium. Select words wisely. Studies have shown that the average level of reading comprehension is at grade 6. If the message is targeted to a sixth-grader, the majority of the population will understand it; however, keep the audience in mind and adjust accordingly. For television, the rule of 27/9/3 is extremely helpful. Developed by Dr. Vincent Covello of the Center for Risk Communication, this rule suggests keeping messages to 27 words, 9 seconds, and 3 ideas or concepts for maximum comprehension.[9]

Media may not always be a friend, but they do not have to be an enemy.[5] The media have a job to do, just like those who respond to a disaster. The media may play an essential role in communicating to the public during a disaster situation by offering evacuation routes, safety tips, or other important advice. Keeping the media up-to-date in an emergency is essential and should not be overlooked. Failure to provide frequent updates may result in the media using any means to get closer to the scene to get the information firsthand or going to possibly less reliable sources. Make the media a friend, and let them relay the information you provide, as opposed to what someone else provides.

"Hope for the best but prepare for the worst" is a very applicable cliché concerning the need to have prepared public information systems in place before a disaster. Current practice for emergency preparation is to plan and drill response. This should always include testing the public information component.[10]

Medical/Emergency Medical Services/Fire Models

Disasters occur frequently, ranging from bus accidents with 10 to 20 injured persons, to hazardous material events requiring local evacuation, to regional incidents such as hurricanes. In all of these cases, the local community or larger region enters a disaster mode when the resources needed are greater than one segment can provide. EMS must redirect ambulances and rescue vehicles, hospital emergency departments must prepare for casualties, and government provides resources for scene control and forensic investigation, with preservation of evidence balanced with response and recovery. All of this must occur while the daily standard delivery of health care and maintenance of law and order are maintained and the community infrastructure is preserved. The totality of the response is dependent on the size of the disaster and the numbers affected with the dynamic match of available resources, supplies, and the specific demands.

Many events happen simultaneously during the early stages of a disaster response: EMS, fire, and police personnel are dispatched to the event and use an incident management system. Bystanders render aid, or as the word spreads, people arrive who may be able to help, but more than likely, they are not suitable responders. Plans should be made for this convergent volunteerism because it cannot be avoided (this is explored in other chapters of this text).[11] Local emergency management representatives should work with local media to prevent a situation in which the media take it upon themselves to call emergency responders for help before the responders get direction from their office. If the media are asked to communicate a call for help, specific emergency personnel, upon arrival to the disaster scene, can then be directed to a gathering place and then to their duty station. Management of volunteers can consume precious resources away from critical aspects of a timely response. By reporting certain types of information, the media can fulfill an important role in assisting health care providers travel to their workplace, ensuring that any response teams are directed to their prearranged muster stations, and helping in prevention of injuries to unnecessary volunteers. The media responding to an event must also be directed to a location that enables them to accurately report while being kept safe.

In addition, it must be recognized that each response unit from various government and nongovernment agencies will have differing perspectives, based on their interpretation of the dynamics of the event, guiding their management or role. Unfortunately, all these views can diverge and provide a confusing and inconsistent picture of events, simply because of each unit's perspective and underlying knowledge base. Caution must follow because each unit or members of each unit may be approached separately by members of the media and innocently provide inconsistent information. This can lead to misperception and loss of public trust. Further, if such misperception is acted upon by members of the command and control system, this may lead to disruption of the disaster response. Such misinformation may be a direct consequence of the real-time reporting that often occurs around disaster scenes. With media at the scene reporting in real time but missing vital elements or reporting unsubstantiated information, decisions can be rendered that can interfere with the dynamic response and recovery or divert resources, triggered by political expediency or a microphone held in someone's face under bright lights.

Effect of Media Reports

A new area of media interaction related to disaster medicine is how the public responds to news reports and images that have the potential to induce posttraumatic stress disorder (PTSD).[12] It has been reported that there is increased incidence of PTSD with intense coverage of an event, especially one associated with many images. This was reported to be especially true with the pediatric population.[13] The authors believe that intense exposure to significant events, such as the World Trade Center disaster, is associated with psychopathology.[14]

Media Communication

Several studies have looked at the public's response to uncertainty. These results can have implications for how the public will respond to media communications. One study found that a majority of respondents prefer ranges of risk estimates because they believe that these ranges make the government look more honest. However, about half just want to know whether an area is safe or unsafe. Finally, disagreement among scientists about risk, even if a majority has one opinion, tends to result in the public assuming the worst. The implications of this reinforce the need for one spokesperson for a disaster response.[15] Other studies looking at risk communication have provided goals for risk communication that could also apply to disaster communication, especially before the event. These are building trust, raising awareness, education, agreement, and motivating action. Before a hurricane or another major disaster, the development of these goals will help foster action by the community. The media become the vehicle for the communication of these goals and need to work with the public information officer (PIO) and responsible organization to develop them.[16]

Detroit Free Press Example

The media are also concerned with safety and minimizing interference with the relief effort. The *Detroit Free Press* requests that their reporters and photographers work as teams. These teams are allowed to do whatever is needed to get a story as long as they feel comfortable or safe, obviously a very large leeway for the reporter. The teams are expected to be as inconspicuous as possible and to identify themselves to responsible agencies, including the police, to reduce potential problems. Reporters and their editors want to publish information that they believe is accurate, is timely, and has been verified with multiple sources, if possible. They prefer to verify information with at least two, but preferably three, sources. In addition, they have deadlines that must be met. Finally, these teams are willing to help responsible agencies to disseminate information as long as they have access (T. Fladung, managing editor, *Detroit Free Press*, personal communication, 2004).

Lessons from Recent Disasters

Multiple disasters have occurred within the last 20 years that provide a glimpse into the do's and don'ts of public information management. These events have stemmed from airplane and train disasters, earthquakes, and terrorist actions. In each case, lessons learned have improved disaster response and have shown the importance of public information management.

Tokyo Sarin Attack, 1995

On March 20, 1995, Tokyo experienced a nerve gas poisoning attack with sarin. The first patient from this attack arrived at the hospital before ambulances began delivering patients. Approximately 2.5 hours after the event, the first press conference was held at one hospital, and the first televised news announcement was made 3 hours after the attack. At this point, most patients had reported to a local medical facility. In addition, there was no initial report to the population from an official source until all patients had left the scene. In this case, the media notification and distribution of information from an official were late, but the information after the initial conference was consistent.[17]

Oklahoma City Bombing, 1995

On April 19, 1995, a terrorist action caused an explosion that destroyed the Murrah Federal Building in Oklahoma City. The blast was felt by many in the local area and was reported by news networks very quickly. The local emergency departments (EDs) immediately became fully staffed; many medical personnel immediately offered their services to local EDs, and as the departments became staffed, personnel decided to go directly to the explosion site and provide freelance medical care and rescue efforts. In addition to the local response, the local media, without notification or request, directed those with medical training to go to the federal building to provide care. This resulted in more than 300 volunteers at the site. Even though volunteers provided evacuation assistance, the site was unsafe and the responders did not have protective gear; as a result, one volunteer died from falling debris.[18]

Some of the lessons learned from this disaster included how to request that additional health care providers go to their respective facilities and how to prevent untrained and superfluous volunteers from converging on the scene. If the need for additional support arises at the incident location, the incident management commander can request this through emergency management channels. The media can then receive a specific request for specific volunteers to be directed to a gathering, muster, or staging area for credentialing, briefing, equipping, and transportation assignments. The receiving medical facilities can then, either by direct communication or preexisting disaster protocols, have their requests met through proper channels and be prepared for the additional health care professionals, limiting resources dedicated to incorporate them into the existing staff. The media should be informed early in a disaster of set expectations of their role, any boundaries placed on them, and how they could potentially hinder the response and recovery. This partnership should be communicated to the public to build public trust. In addition, if the incident management team does not want bystanders because of safety concerns, this should also be conveyed to the media so that they might communicate this information to the public.

Haiti Earthquake, 2010

The Haiti earthquake showed how media coverage can focus a world's attention on a disaster, but when the "excitement" of the event dissipates and the media leave, the ongoing disaster can fall off the world's radar screen. The earthquake in Haiti killed an estimated 300,000 people in 2010. The consequences of this devastating event continue to cause death and suffering today. Yet, it is rare to find any news coverage of the situation today at all. The media have moved on to newer and more dramatic events, leaving Haiti to find a way to remain relevant and continue to garner the world support it so desperately needs.

⚠ PITFALLS OF MANAGING PUBLIC INFORMATION

Managing the flow of information in a crisis or disaster is no small task. There are, however, 10 common pitfalls to be avoided.

Failing to Bring in Experts

Emergency responders are supposed to respond to emergencies: physicians are supposed to take care of sick or injured patients, search and rescue teams are called in to look for trapped individuals, and firefighters battle fires. When a disaster occurs, be it large or small, an expert who can speak about it effectively should be summoned.

This is not to say that a firefighter is not the best spokesperson at the scene; it means that anyone speaking to the media, or formally to the public, should have some basic PIO training.[5] In a large-scale disaster, it is strongly recommended to have a designated key spokesperson. There are training programs available through the Centers for Disease Control and Prevention, the Federal Emergency Management Agency, and a number of private companies that specialize in crisis and risk communication.

Using Complex Language or Jargon

In a crisis situation, the listening skills of people involved are highly challenged. They often do not hear correctly, are overcome with emotion, and are experiencing high anxiety. Additionally, audiences in a crisis may vary in their level of education and comprehension. A best practice guideline is to target communications to the reading level of a sixth-grader.[19] Try to keep information clear, succinct, and to the point. Do not use acronyms or abbreviations because they may confuse the public.

Arguing, Fighting, or Losing Your Temper

Disasters by nature are stressful. It is difficult to remain calm when dealing with situations that involve extensive loss of life or property. Often, disaster workers go without proper rest for long periods, and it is easy for tempers to flare. When speaking to the public or a reporter, remaining calm is the key. Do not be afraid to politely end a conversation if it becomes heated or uncomfortable. Reporters almost always win an argument; they have the editor on their side. Offer a succinct and truthful response for best results, and stay on your message.[10] Repeat your main idea as many times as necessary. Do not deviate from your main message or key points.

Predicting

Often, questions about what will happen next will be asked after a crisis. Unless emergency responders arrive on scene with a working crystal ball, these kinds of questions should not be answered. No one can predict the future. Reassure the public that every effort is being made to mitigate the crisis or that the best possible care is being offered.[20]

Answering a Question That You Are Not Qualified to Answer

It is OK to say, "I don't know." Do not answer a question that you are not qualified to answer. In fact, when offering information to the public, be prepared to repeat the information you do know several times in several different ways. Admitting you are not qualified to answer a specific question and suggesting someone who can may even add to your credibility.[9]

Failing to Show Empathy

Empathy or sensitivity is essential in disaster communication. Whereas many first responders or health care providers often emotionally detach themselves from a crisis situation, PIOs cannot. The most effective communicator is one who cares.[9]

Lying, Clouding the Truth, or Covering Up

History has shown us, from Watergate to the Monica Lewinsky scandal to the legal woes of Martha Stewart, that it is often not the initial incident that is the problem, but rather the cover-up. Never cover or hide information. In this age of e-mail, cellular phones, and up-to-the-minute communication, the information is almost always going to get out. Of course, discretion and good judgment are factors, but avoid lying or blatant cover-ups.

Not Responding Quickly

Slow and steady do not win the race in a disaster response, be it rescuing the injured or communicating the issues.[20] Respond quickly and thoughtfully. Also, be sure to be accurate and truthful. When holding a press briefing, schedule it in a reasonable period of time and be on time. If you cancel or delay your briefings, reporters will go elsewhere for the information. If you don't feed the "beast" (the media), the beast will go somewhere else to eat.

Not Responding at All

The infamous words "no comment" bring chills to experienced PIOs everywhere. There is almost always something better to say than "no comment." Some suggestions include, "I don't know," or "I'll get back to you with an answer to that question." The main thing to remember when tempted to respond with "no comment" is that this refrain instantly makes the speaker sound as if something is being hidden or there is something dishonest about what is happening. Always remember what can be commented on and offer that instead, even if it does not answer what the reporter asked.

Failing to Practice Emergency Communications

Schools practice fire drills. Communities practice evacuations. Hospitals drill for emergency response. Communications should be an essential part of any drill. Practice is the key to success when a real disaster hits. Allow the information officer to participate in scheduled exercises, and ask local media to attend. Work with them in advance so that they may provide a more realistic scenario with the stresses that come along with the reporting of a major event.[10]

The key to managing public information is to be prepared, respond quickly with accurate information, and show empathy.

CONCLUSION

Good disaster management provides for a mass communication system with appropriate information. The goal of this system is to establish relationships between the response agencies, the media, and the public. A major underpinning for success is accurate and timely information to the public.[21] The media can be friends or foes. Mutual respect for each other will generally result in better cooperation and a smoother interaction. The provision of timely and accurate information will help keep reporters from searching for unreliable facts. The media most likely will not be the cause of any panic. Any panic by the population will be based on the incident, not the reporting of it.[22] It is recommended for organizations that may have to deal with the media to have a media policy in place before an event. In addition, a representative or PIO is needed on-site. The media also do not just want facts, but human interest stories. Establish procedures to allow responders to tell their story: highlight outstanding efforts or acts of heroism and then notify the media.[23] PIOs should consider predeveloped news release forms and develop a contact list for the area and a list of "experts" to call on to explain the situation to the public and reporters.[24] Incorporate social media into your communication plan. Even though the media can be intrusive, they also can disseminate accurate information, as well as advice or warnings.[25] Recommend that the media assist in providing accurate information to the public. Before events, have the media participate in disaster drills and network with organization leaders for disaster events.[26]

REFERENCES

1. McLuhan M. *The Gutenberg Galaxy.* Toronto: University of Toronto Press; 1962.
2. Weightman G. *Signor Marconi's Magic Box: The Most Remarkable Invention of the 19th Century and the Amateur Inventor Whose Genius Sparked a Revolution.* New York: DeCapo Press; 2003.

3. Merchant R, Elmer S, Lurie N. Integrating social media into emergency-preparedness efforts. *N Engl J Med.* 2011;365(4):289–291.

4. Castillo C, Mendoza M, Poblete B. Information credibility on Twitter. In: *Proceedings of the 20th International Conference on Worldwide Web March 28–April 1, 2011, Hyderabad, India International World Wide Web Conference Committee*; 2011:675–684.

5. Society for Healthcare Strategy and Market Development. *Crisis Communications in Healthcare: Managing Difficult Times Effectively*; 2002, Chicago.

6. Colford P. Another post exclusive. *New York Daily News.* July 7, 2004.

7. Emergency Management Laboratory of the Oak Ridge Institute for Science and Education. *Emergency Public Information Pocket Guide*; May, 2001, Oak Ridge, TN.

8. Pooley E. Time magazine person of the year 2001:mayor of the world. *Time Magazine.* Dec. 31, 2001.

9. Covello VT. *Risk Communication.* New York: Center for Risk Communication/Consortium for Risk and Crisis Communication Slides; 2004.

10. Reynolds B, Hunter-Galdo J, Sokler L. *Crisis and Emergency Risk Communication.* Atlanta: Centers for Disease Control and Prevention; 2002.

11. Cone DC, Weir SD, Bogucki S. Convergent volunteerism. *Ann Emerg Med.* 2003;41:457–462.

12. Njenga FD, Nyamai C, Kigamwa P. Terrorist bombing at the USA embassy in Nairobi: the media response. *East Afr Med.* 2003;80(3):159–164.

13. Pfefferbaum B, Seale TW, Brandt EN Jr, et al. Media exposure in children one hundred miles from a terrorist bombing. *Ann Clin Psychiatry.* 2003;15(1):1–8.

14. Ahern J, Galea S, Resnick H, et al. Television images and psychological symptoms after the September 11 terrorist attacks. *Psychiatry.* 2002;65(4):289–300.

15. Johnson BB. Further notes on public response to uncertainty in risks and science. *Risk Anal.* 2003;23(4):781–789.

16. Bier VM. On the state of the art: risk communication to the public. *Reliab Eng Syst Saf.* 2001;71:139–150.

17. Okumura T, Suzuki K, Fukuda A, et al. The Tokyo subway sarin attack: disaster management, part 2: hospital response. *Acad Emerg Med.* 1998;5:618–624.

18. Maningas PA, Robison M, Mallonee S. The EMS response to the Oklahoma City bombing. *Prehospital Disaster Med.* 1997;12(2):9–14.

19. Covello VT. Best practices in public health risk and crisis communication. *J Health Comm.* 2003;8:5–8.

20. Sandman PM. *Anthrax, Bioterrorism, and Risk Communication: Guidelines for Action.* Presented at, Atlanta: Centers for Disease Control and Prevention; November 20, 2001.

21. Quarantelli EL. Ten criteria for evaluating the management of community disasters. *Disasters.* 1997;21(1):39–56.

22. Garrett L. Understanding media's response to epidemics. *Public Health Rep.* 2001;116(suppl 2):87–91.

23. Anzur T. How to talk to the media: televised coverage of public health issues in a disaster. *Prehospital Disaster Med.* 2000;15(4):196–198.

24. Allison EJ. Media relations at major response situations. *JEMS.* December 1984;39–42.

25. Auf der Heide E, Lafond R, et al. Theme 1. Disaster coordination and management: summary and action plans. *Prehospital Disaster Med.* 2001;16(1):22–25.

26. Schultz CH, Mothershead JL, Field M. Bioterrorism preparedness I: the emergency department and hospital. *Emerg Med Clin North Am.* 2002;20:437–455.

SUGGESTED READING

1. Covello VT. *Message Mapping, Risk Communication, and Bio-terrorism.* Presented at, Geneva, Switzerland: World Health Organization Workshop on Bio-terrorism and Risk Communication; October 1, 2002.

CHAPTER 25

Informatics and Telecommunications in Disaster

Churton Budd

The United States and many other countries are threatened by a number of new crises because of terrorist activities. Behind these new threats looms the ever-present danger of a natural disaster, such as an earthquake, fire, or hurricane, and human-made or technological disasters, such as a transportation accident or loss of an electrical grid. All of these incidents generate strong demands on the collection, analysis, coordination, distribution, and interpretation of many types of health and preparedness information. Along with the increasing risk of bioterrorism, there is a greater requirement and stronger emphasis on the use of sophisticated information-gathering tools and information technologies. These tools are necessary to manage the complex surveillance and data analysis necessary to spot trends and make early identification of outbreaks, as well as allow for rapid communication of health information, mitigation strategies, and treatment modalities to health care workers in the field.

Fortunately, many of those involved in emergency management have begun to embrace technology, and, consequently, many vendors have recognized the need to produce hardware and software to meet the needs of disaster responders. Various tools have been used to help mitigate, prepare for, and respond to disasters. One of the more difficult issues during a response to a disaster is the inability to communicate. The breakdown of communications has been a recognized effect of almost every major response to a disaster. Communications issues occur at some level in almost every disaster response, no matter how large or small. As the disaster community has experienced these failing communications systems, it has found strategies to improve the systems or replace them with methods that work. Over time, the ability to accumulate, analyze, and disseminate disaster preparedness and response information has improved. Largely, this is due to advances in information technology that have taken place during the past half century.

HISTORICAL PERSPECTIVE[1]

The disaster response community got off to a slow start with embracing information technology; however, this technology is rapidly gaining momentum. Before the 1980s, computer systems were primarily used in the business, banking, and scientific communities. For the most part, anything close to emergency or disaster planning use of these systems was limited to the Department of Defense and large commercial research firms who did operation planning and simulation, or occasionally, epidemiological or sociological studies.

During the 1980s, the desktop computer, or personal computer (PC), was introduced. Data could be stored on a disk that was easily carried in a briefcase. By the mid-1980s, disaster responders could enter data into a computer so that documents could be produced, spreadsheets updated, and commodities and resources tracked, sometimes

even in the field. During the late 1980s, the Internet began to gain popularity and became more in the reach of the average person. The precursors to the Internet—BITNET and ARPANET—transformed into the World Wide Web, and at that time the average citizen began getting a dial-up Internet connection via CompuServe or America Online. Online resources at major centers of learning began to accumulate databases related to disaster management and planning. People could exchange files and documents via e-mail or by way of a number of sites that acted as file repositories, called file transfer protocol (FTP) sites (FTP is the methodology of transferring binary and text files from one computer to another). Special software programs called "gophers" (short for "go for this and that") cataloged these file repositories and allowed a person to search for them by keyword. These programs were the precursor to the big search engines such as Yahoo! and Google.

Applications such as computer-aided management of emergency operations (CAMEO) were developed in 1988 by the National Oceanic and Atmospheric Administration. CAMEO is used to assist first responders with easy access to response information. It provides a tool to enter local information and develop incident scenarios. It contains mapping, an air dispersal model, chemical databases, and other tools to help display to the emergency responder critical information in a timely fashion. Hazardous materials information and material safety data sheets (MSDS) became available on CD-ROM. Other databases also became available on CD-ROM to allow the responder access to a library of information while at the disaster site. About this time, the Centers for Disease Control and Prevention (CDC) released Epi Info (www.cdc.gov/epiinfo). Using this software, an epidemiologist or public health professional could develop a questionnaire or form, customize the data entry process, and enter and analyze data. Epi Info can be used to produce epidemiological statistics, tables, graphs, and maps.

Specialized computer mapping software called geospatial information systems (GIS) integrates data with map information. Because disasters are usually spatial events, GIS can assist in all phases of disaster management. It is often useful for disaster planners to see a map of the disaster to assist in plan development. A map will show the scope of the disaster, where damage is greatest or has the greatest impact, what property or lives are at risk, and what resources are available and where are they needed. Disaster managers, using GIS to graphically display critical information that is location based, can quickly map the disaster scene, establish priorities, and develop action plans.

In the 1990s, information exchange improved exponentially. List servers on the Internet allowed emergency managers, disaster responders, and medical providers the ability to discuss disaster response in an informal setting. It was not uncommon to see a post to a list server from a responder actually at the site of the disaster. Lessons learned could be immediately disseminated throughout the disaster response community. Agencies such as the Federal Emergency Management Agency, the Natural Hazards Center at the University of Colorado, and the CDC all began to publish large amounts of public information about disasters on their websites. The use of satellite telephone systems and cellular phone–based data networks allowed those with a laptop to stay connected in the field and collect and transmit a large amount of information to other responders and to their response agencies.

Today, it is hard to find someone in the disaster response field that has not used e-mail or some type of computer resource to do his or her job. It appears that the use of information technology is reducing operational costs and increasing productivity, although this is difficult to quantify because information technology is still growing so rapidly. Portable computers have now decreased in size. The cellular phone and personal data assistant (PDA) have merged into a smartphone. Tablet PCs and the iPad have allowed desktop computing power to become highly portable. Although still falling behind that of the corporate sector, information technology training for disaster response and management personnel is beginning to be a job requirement. Electronic commerce is allowing disaster responders to achieve real-time procurement and payment for relief supplies. Broadband and wireless networks can be set up rapidly and cheaply to allow for access to vast informational resources. The public has become far better educated, and they seek information on their own health care; manage their finances online; and now are able to research, mitigate, and prepare for disasters using the many publicly available resources on the Internet.

What does the future hold for informatics in disaster management? It is hard to tell because information technology in general continues to develop so quickly. It is likely that the disaster responder will one day use a wearable computer with a small flexible screen. It is also probable that voice and data technologies will continue to merge so that interaction with digital devices can be accomplished by voice command. Storage devices will continue to become smaller so that victims of a disaster may have their entire financial records, health records, and other personal information archived on a chip they carry in their pocket, which will allow them to save this important personal information from being destroyed by a disaster. Real-time monitoring and surveillance will assist the disaster responder to become aware of an impending disaster sooner. The ability to monitor patient flow, track resources, and perform real-time mapping and visualization of the disaster scene will allow planners and managers to "roll with the punches" during a disaster and modify the response effectively. It is likely that information technology will continue to be a stronger and stronger tool for disaster response personnel.

CURRENT PRACTICE

Various tools and elements of informatics and telecommunications are being used currently by disaster managers and responders. Some of these tools are used in the preparation and mitigation stage, and some are used during the response phase. Some tools can be used in all phases of the disaster cycle.

Computer Devices

The computer has revolutionized many aspects of modern life. Some people are so dependent on e-mail for doing their daily work that when the corporate e-mail system goes down, they find it hard to conduct business. The same is true for researchers using the Internet to access the vast amount of knowledge on the Web to do their research: when it is inaccessible, they almost feel withdrawal symptoms. There are many types of computing devices available to a disaster manager or responder, everything from corporate mainframes to wearable PCs.

The Laptop

Probably the most commonly used device other than the smartphone is the laptop. As technology improves, the speed and power of laptops have become equivalent to a desktop computer. Because memory and storage are cheap, the average laptop has a larger hard drive than it did just a few years ago. Most of the applications written for the desktop are also used on the laptop, so many laptops have memory equivalent to that of the desktop. New chipsets and microprocessors use lower power and run cooler, allowing for longer running time on batteries. Some laptops are even fanless with solid state hard drives, greatly improving battery life. Laptops are getting thinner, and many of them are bundled with all the accoutrements, such as wide theater-like screens, DVD players, CD burners, and high-speed connections, such as a High Definition Multimedia Interface (HDMI) and Universal Serial Bus (USB) connectors, for peripheral devices. Most new laptops also include wireless access technologies, such as Bluetooth and Wi-Fi. With a docking station and external keyboard, mouse, and monitor, many people are finding that they can use their laptop docked at their desk and then pop it out and take it when they travel. This takes the place of a desktop computer and provides the user all the amenities of the office or home while out in the field. See Box 25-1 for tips on traveling with a laptop.

The Tablet PC

Similar to a laptop is a specialized portable computer called a tablet PC. These are finding rapid popularity. These devices use primarily a stylus

---

BOX 25-1   Checklist for Traveling with a Laptop

- Update the antivirus and spyware protection software to the latest virus definitions, because one cannot be sure that a network used on the road is fully protected.
- Use a program that creates an image of the laptop's hard drive, so that if the hard drive crashes, it can be recovered from the image.
- Check the batteries and, if time permits, cycle them all the way down and back to full charge again. If possible, take an extra battery that is charged to extend your PC time if you are isolated without power. Consider alternative power sources, such as solar panel chargers, disposable battery replacements and power cells, and a 12-volt adapter for converting power from a car battery to use your laptop.
- Place the computer in a hard-shell padded case. It also helps to have an assortment of plugs and adapters and an extra network cable, just in case. Do not forget a power/recharge cable.

- Put everything in plastic baggies, even when the equipment is in its case. If you can find a large enough baggie for your laptop, you can protect it from moisture should your case be exposed to the elements and leak. Temperature changes can cause condensation, so if you do pack your equipment in baggies, throw a couple of silica gel desiccator packs into the baggie, too.
- Take a surge protector to prevent power spikes from damaging your devices, particularly if you know you will be in an area operating on generator power.
- Avoid, at all costs, having your laptop or computer device go through a baggage check. Make sure it can be stowed as a carry-on. Try to keep it away from metal detectors because they might erase magnetic media.
- Take a cable lock so that you can secure your laptop somewhat. Although it will not prevent a thief who really wants it, it may deter someone walking by from snatching it while you have your back turned.

or finger for the input and for data entry. Tablet PCs are finding a niche in vertical markets such as health care and on the warehouse floor. They can be extremely useful for filling out forms such as a medical record or a field survey at a disaster site that can be plugged into a GIS for mapping. Tablet PCs usually have equivalent performance to that of a laptop, with the added convenience of usually a longer battery life, a slightly smaller form, and the stylus- or finger-based input.

When selecting a laptop or tablet PC to take to the field, one will be deluged with thousands of choices. In selecting a device, it is important to consider the conditions under which the device will be used. There are many "hardened" devices, specifically designed to military standards for shock and vibration resistance, water resistance, and dust impingement. These hardened devices can be twice the price of the regular off-the-shelf laptop or tablet. If a hardened device is affordable, one can rest assured that it will more than likely survive being taken into the field and be able to keep data safe. An alternative, however, is to purchase an off-the-shelf laptop from a local computer or electronics store and an insurance policy for it. Oftentimes, a $50-per-year policy with a deductible of only a few hundred dollars is available. This would easily cover a catastrophic loss of the device (e.g., major drop, crush, or immersion), but it probably would not cover minor damage such as the disk drive door breaking off. When buying a hardened device, ask the vendor specific questions about drop and immersion tests and whether the device meets military standards (Box 25-2).

If at all possible, test a device in various types of weather, from direct sun to nighttime. Make sure the screen is readable in direct sunlight, can be dimmed for use during night operations, and is ergonomic when held and does not cause undue strain due to weight or bulkiness. Try the doors, accessory ports, and plugs to make sure that, by simply plugging a peripheral into the device, it is not rendered immobile or unwieldy or that its water resistance or another hardened standard is not rendered ineffective.

The Smartphone

Another handheld device that is usually smaller than the tablet PC is the smartphone. The smartphone has become the peripheral brain for many in the health care setting. Rather than wear or carry a laboratory coat full of plastic cards with scores and scales, quick guide books, and other reference texts, a health care provider can store all of this information in a smartphone. The information can be indexed and

referenced quickly. Smartphones utilize a number of operating systems, such as iOS for Apple devices, Android, and Microsoft Windows Mobile. Most of the major vendors are authoring software for all three platforms. Software is often downloaded from a marketplace, and most titles are very affordable, with many being free and public domain. A smartphone can be an invaluable resource for the disaster responder. Often in the field, the disaster responder does not have the luxury of ducking into the emergency department library to look up something in the *Physicians' Desk Reference* or other medical text. With a smartphone, however, one can "take" those texts to the field (Box 25-3). In many cases, searches can be done with a keyword to rapidly find the needed information. You can even do a quick consultation with another provider outside the disaster scene via e-mail, text message, or video chat.

The address book, calendar, contacts, tasks, camera, and notes are probably the more commonly used built-in applications on a smartphone. Other uses of the smartphone for disaster response include keeping track of contact information for other disaster responders and agencies. There are also a number of programs that allow for rapid form filling and database applications for recording data and creating quick ad-hoc reports. Most smartphones have built-in cameras, allowing one to rapidly document a disaster scene for later use. With accessories such as an external keyboard, one can even type full documents on the smartphone and print the documents with a wireless-capable printer.

Although smartphones may seem to be stand-alone devices, they require periodic visits to the various online sites for synchronization. During this synchronization process, vendors provide updates to software over the Internet; calendars, address books, tasks, and notes are synchronized with corporate e-mail systems; and new software can be installed from the various online application markets. If you are recording data on forms on the smartphone, this synchronization may also be required to pass the data from the forms tool on the device to an application running on a server and to the back end database.

As with the laptop, there are a number of accessories that are useful to have when traveling. An attachable or Bluetooth keyboard is helpful to type reports on the smartphone for printing later. The smartphone should have a hard-shell case, and it is advisable to pack the device in a plastic baggie for protection against the elements. The application markets have hundreds of free medical texts and references available, and sites on the Internet can be accessed and would be quite useful if a disaster responder becomes isolated from paper-based reference resources. These can be found by searching the Internet for texts and software related to health care and disaster and response; some will be free, some will be for sale. A solar battery charger is ideal for a smartphone or tablet because their batteries do not require much energy to charge. Lastly, make sure that data on the device are uploaded to a desktop or laptop computer or to a repository such as iCloud, OneDrive (formerly

---

BOX 25-2 MIL-STD 810

MIL-STD is a series of specifications set by the U.S. Department of Defense. When purchasing a hardened device for field use, look for vendor affirmation that their device meets military standards to ensure that it will survive use in a postdisaster field environment.

BOX 25-3 Useful Smartphone Programs for Disaster Responders

- *Epocrates (www.epocrates.com):* Epocrates is an enhanced drug and formulary reference with integrated ID treatment guides and tools.
- *WISER (http://wiser.nlm.nih.gov/):* WISER provides a wide range of information on hazardous substances, including substance identification support, physical characteristics, human health information, and containment and suppression advice.
- *Skyscape Books (http://www.skyscape.com):* This is a portfolio of medical references for use on handheld devices.
- *PEPID (http://www.pepid.com/):* PEPID is a physician, critical care, and nursing reference suite.

- Sites that have tablet or smartphone disaster or medical software:
  - http://www.fema.gov/smartphone-app
  - http://sis.nlm.nih.gov/dimrc/disasterapps.html
  - http://www.grabpak.com/the-ultimate-smartphone-disaster-preparedness-app-list/
  - http://lifehacker.com/how-to-use-your-smartphone-as-an-essential-part-of-your-1442683676
  - http://www.redcross.org/prepare/mobile-apps

SkyDrive) or Dropbox, and try to store critical files and information on removable memory media. In the event that power is unavailable and the device loses its charge, all the data may be lost without that backup.[2]

Like the laptop or tablet, a smartphone comes with many features and options. Pay attention to whether the device can fit into your pocket or whether you will have to carry it around in a case that you might put down and forget or not have on hand when you need it. The ideal device is small and unobtrusive; however, the device should have enough computing power, storage, and functionality to meet the user's needs. One should also consider purchasing a hardened device. Although not expensive in comparison with a hardened laptop, a smartphone or tablet that has been designed to take into the elements will still be higher priced than an off-the-shelf model. The small size and highly portable nature of the smartphone and tablet may make it a better investment because the user may be more likely to take it into the field than a laptop.

Local Area Network/Wide Area Network/Wireless Network

As emergency managers are getting more sophisticated in their use of information technology, it is not uncommon to see disaster responders establish a local area network (LAN) where their incident command is set up (e.g., in the Emergency Operations Center or in the disaster field office). This network links a group of computers and devices together and allows instant messaging, video conferencing, and the sharing of files and documents between computers; better yet, it allows the centralization of file storage to one large networked hard drive that each workstation has rights to access. Thus, a backup can be taken of just that centralized hard drive periodically, rather than each individual workstation. In many cases, a wide area network can be established, which is the linking of more than one LAN. For example, the disaster field office may be linked over a public network through a virtual private network (VPN) to the main office or headquarters. This VPN connection provides a secure tunnel through the Internet from point to point so that sites in between cannot access passing traffic. This creates a wide area network that is not limited by geography or distance, just connectivity.

Wireless networks take advantage of a network access point, which is a transceiver that communicates with a wireless transceiver card on the workstation or portable device. Essentially, this topography creates a wireless network similar to a wired one, but with the convenience of rapid setup, without the need to string network cable all over the site. Wireless networks could even be deployed in a tent city, linking treatment areas in the tents to a command tent. Unfortunately, wireless networks, like voice radio frequencies, can be fairly easily received and decrypted by an eavesdropper, thus making them fairly insecure. Sophisticated encryption methods must be put into place to protect sensitive operational security and patient information that may be transferred across a wireless network.

Communications Devices
Geographical Positioning System

The Geographical Positioning System (GPS) began as a military system in 1985 and is based on a 24-satellite configuration of transmitters. By measuring the distance to four satellites from the user location, it is possible to establish three coordinates of the user location (latitude, longitude, and altitude). Although originally developed for the U.S. Department of Defense, the not-quite-complete system was offered to the civilian community in 1983 by President Reagan after Korean Airlines flight 007 was shot down when it accidentally strayed into Soviet Union airspace. The satellite configuration was complete in the early 1990s, and the Gulf War prompted the sale of thousands of commercial GPS receivers; at that time the military had not manufactured many GPS receivers. Since then, GPS has found its way into the travel, surveying, mapping, and delivery industries. In addition, many casual users take a GPS when they are recreating in remote areas or to locate their favorite fishing spot. For the disaster responder, a GPS unit can be helpful in giving an exact location of a shelter or the location of a landing zone for helicopter evacuation and can assist in the location and mapping of resources to be used to respond to the disaster. Most modern tablets and smartphones have built-in and sophisticated GPS mapping capabilities.[3]

Cellular Devices

A smartphone or basic cell phone is probably the most common tool that people use to communicate. Many disaster response agencies consider the cellular phone to be their primary communications tool and issue them to their disaster responders. Consequently, cellular sites after a disaster may experience a high demand as the civilian population makes calls to friends and family to check on their welfare, as responders arrive and begin to arrange resources, as the media arrive and make arrangements to cover the story, and as people shift to cellular as their primary phone if their landline phone is inoperable because of a power outage or other disruption. It is reasonable to assume that a cellular phone may have difficulty in making a connection during a postdisaster response, due to the cellular site being overwhelmed. Normally, cellular providers scale their cellular sites to handle only 20% to 30% of their customer base at a time. This is fine for normal traffic, but when a disaster strikes and customers all need to make a contact in a compressed time frame, or when outside people come into the area with their cellular phones, the cellular sites may be congested into uselessness. Fortunately, a few initiatives are in place that might reduce this congestion on the cellular systems, especially for disaster responders. Cellular phone providers can deploy a trailer with a cellular antenna, repeater, and generator power, as well as a cell site on wheels (COW) that can be strategically placed in the disaster area and connected to the public telephone network to increase the availability of cellular connections. Also, a few cellular providers have enabled a capability in their systems in which an emergency worker can receive priority on the cellular phone system and get a connection sooner. Unfortunately, there is no legal requirement for them to do so, and as a result of the expense of purchasing additional hardware to make this happen, only a few providers have adopted this technology. Most have not; therefore, this is not a reliable option. After the 2003 summer blackout, only one cellular phone provider in New York City provided priority access.[4]

Satellite Phone Systems

There are a number of satellite phone system providers that use a number of different technologies. IMARSAT is probably the oldest vendor of satellite phone service; it started its service in the early 1990s. The early phone systems consisted of a fold-out, umbrella-like antenna and a briefcase-sized box with a handset. They were portable, although bulky, and the transmission of data over the phone system, if possible, was done at very slow speeds of 300 to 4800 bits per second (compared with 700 to 1500 Kbits per second on a broadband cable modem). Satellite phone costs originally were as high as $3 a minute, but most of the current vendors charge about $1 per minute. Phone size also has shrunk. The flip-up lid of the phone, similar to opening the screen of a laptop, acts as the antenna and should be pointed at an angle toward one of the satellites.

Because many of these phone systems use a geostationary orbiting satellite constellation, one must be geographically aware and point the antenna in the correct direction and at the correct inclination to get a good signal on the satellite. There are automatic antenna systems on a number of vendors' satellite phones, which can be mounted to a vehicle so that the phone can maintain a line of sight link to the satellite and be used during travel to the disaster site. Dense leaves or vegetation as well as very dense rain can reduce the signal strength. Some newer phone systems, such as Iridium and Globalstar, have a handset that is not much bigger than a cordless phone for home use. These systems use a constellation of low earth-orbiting satellites and incorporate the group special mobile (GSM) protocol for cellular phone technology, allowing the handset to connect to terrestrial GSM cellular networks while in signal range to a cellular site and then automatically switch to an orbiting satellite when out of the terrestrial GSM range. Unfortunately, satellite phone systems are very expensive to bring into service and maintain. A number of vendors have been close to bankruptcy and been saved by investors.[5]

Mobile Communications Vehicles

Many response agencies have built and deployed vehicles that are outfitted with communications and computer equipment that is capable of performing a variety of functions. These vehicles usually are equipped with their own generators for power and contain a number of different radio systems that can be programmed to communicate on many different radio frequencies. A radio operator in the vehicle can pass information between disparate radio systems and agencies and may be able to help with some of the lack of interoperability issues. These vehicles also have the ability to patch into a telephone network and the Internet. Depending on their sophistication, they may have satellite phone systems, high-frequency radio, and facsimile capability computers with scanners and printers. Specially trained teams of radio operators, both amateur and public safety dispatchers, and information technology personnel usually staff one of these vehicles. Oftentimes, the incident command staff makes use of these vehicles as part of their command post, or the vehicle can support a disaster response team or disaster field office until more permanent communications can be set up. In events such as mass gatherings or disasters of limited duration, a communication vehicle such as this can be used to provide rapidly deployed communications support in a small footprint and then be completely disassembled at the end of the event.

Radio Systems

Whole books have been written on radio communications, even specifically on disaster communications. Professional communications specialists and many amateur radio operators have spent hundreds of hours training themselves on these systems, so this chapter only gives a mile-high view of the communications systems and frequencies that may be used during a disaster response. It is a good idea for the disaster responder to be aware of what systems are in use, when they should and should not be used, and how to best take advantage of these tools.

Radio frequency (RF) is the part of the electromagnetic spectrum in which electromagnetic waves can be generated and fed through an antenna. There are a number of different modes of the RF spectrum that are most often used for voice and data transmission during a disaster response (Table 25-1). High frequency (HF) is the frequency range from 3 to 30 MHz and is classically termed "shortwave." HF radio waves are often reflected off the ionosphere, thus frequencies in this range are often used for medium- to long-range terrestrial communications. Sunspot and other solar activity, polar aurora, sunlight/darkness at the transmitting and receiving station, and even the choice of frequency within the spectrum can diminish the relative difference between the signal strength over the background noise (signal-to-noise ratio) and make communication on HF radio unusable at times. In other words, if interference increases the static (noise), a transmitter must be more and more powerful to have the transmitted signal hearable above that noise. HF radio is used in some widely dispersed populations for domestic broadcasting. HF radio is often used for HF networks of radio operators who can, in short term, pass information from one radio station to another, essentially allowing, by a number of "hops," worldwide communications. Amateur radio operators oftentimes provide the first information to the outside world when a disaster site is cut off after a hurricane or a major geological event.

For more local communications, very high frequency (VHF) may be used and ranges from 30 to 300 MHz. FM radio (88 to 108 MHz) and various television signals are included in this range. VHF is not usually reflected off the ionosphere, so it is limited to local communications. VHF is not as affected as lower frequencies by atmospheric noise and interference from electromagnetic sources; it does, however, penetrate buildings and other substantial objects more than higher frequencies. Ultra high frequency (UHF) includes frequencies from 300 to 3000 MHz. UHF also includes some frequencies dedicated for television signals (in the United States, above channel 13). UHF frequencies penetrate some densely built buildings a little better than VHF frequencies do. UHF wavelengths are very small, allowing for more compact antennas, which some people feel are more convenient and more attractive than the longer VHF antennas. In more sophisticated communications systems, there may occasionally be a super high frequency (SHF) signal, which includes microwaves transmitted from one antenna in line of sight to another. These SHF microwave signals can carry voice and data. Satellite radio bands are contained within this range of frequencies.

With a two-way radio, there are two types of uses of the frequencies. Simplex use of a frequency means that the same frequency is being used to transmit and receive; while one person is talking, nobody else can talk. Duplex use of the frequencies allows duplex conversations, like on a telephone. Additionally, duplex frequency use can allow for a repeater to be placed centrally in the disaster area. The repeater receives on one frequency and rebroadcasts out at higher power on the other frequency. The repeater is usually put in a high location or has a high antenna. Repeater antennas have a high gain, meaning they can pull in weak signals and have strong transmitters that can transmit signals

TABLE 25-1	Typical Radio Frequencies Used in Disaster Response		
BAND	**FREQUENCY**	**DESCRIPTION**	**USES/LIMITATIONS**
HF	3-30 MHz	High frequency	Good for long distance because the radio waves bounce off the ionosphere back to earth. Subject to environmental noise and interference.
VHF	30-300 MHz	Very high frequency	Line of sight, less affected by environmental noise. More easily blocked by land features than HF.
UHF	300-3000 MHz	Ultra high frequency	Line of sight, better MHz penetration of land and human-made features. Smaller wave size allows for smaller antennas.
SHF	3-30 GHz	Super high frequency	Microwaves pass more easily through the atmosphere and terrestrial features than VHF and UHF. More radio spectrum available in this band.

farther. A repeater allows the transmission of handheld radios to be extended from just a few miles to tens of miles. Frequencies that do not penetrate buildings well, such as UHF, have better transmission.[6]

Specialized Informatics Systems and Decision Support Tools

In recent years, the need for specialized information systems composed of databases, surveillance tools, personnel and patient tracking, and evidence-based medicine to support disaster response and management has been recognized. Health departments, which in many cases did not operate 24 hours a day, seven days a week and in some situations did not even have fax capability 10 years ago, now are developing and putting into place sophisticated systems to monitor for bioterrorism, emerging diseases, and ecological impact on a population.

The television news networks are often at the disaster scene, rapidly passing on information. This was the case on September 11, 2001, when millions of people witnessed the second plane hitting the World Trade Center as broadcasters were on the air covering the event in minutes. In large-scale international disasters, such as the Haiti earthquake in 2010 and Typhoon Haiyan striking the Philippines in 2013, television-based news coverage is often the only information to come from the disaster scene for days following the event. Field personnel can send hundreds of e-mails a day from the disaster site back to their agency. Resources come into play faster as response plans gear up and agencies and their personnel begin reporting their status. There are many ways to communicate, and the amount of information available to decision makers has increased and is dispersed more rapidly. Information can come into the local response center and at agency headquarters, oftentimes directly from the source. Each piece of information must be interpreted and requires a familiarity with the source. Assessments, requirements, and needs from the field may come in from many different sources, each with possibly contradictory information. Oftentimes, this can be correctly interpreted only by the local incident commander. In a wide-area disaster, this may be very difficult to consolidate and evaluate at a higher level.

The analysis of the information coming in from field responders is as important as the information flow itself. Consolidation in a meaningful manner and then appropriate communication to the headquarters should be done by someone knowledgeable enough at the local level to pass only that consolidated information gathered by their support personnel. Many examples exist of these types of decision support systems. The CDC makes its decisions based on information consolidated from state health departments. State health departments make their reports to the CDC based on information passed on by local health departments, who, in turn, received their information from the emergency department physician who, for example, may have noticed six patients with the same abnormal symptoms in the last hour. If that emergency physician were to call the CDC directly, the information would be documented but may not be further considered until the physician had passed the information through the correct channel for consolidation and communication to a higher level.[7]

Humanitarian Information Systems

Humanitarian information systems (HIS) are specialized systems linking many sources of information and consolidating and reporting them. HIS consist of an early warning and reporting system, which includes the monitoring of specific trends of values, such as rainfall amounts, vegetation mapping, crop production, and market prices, and measures of human factors, such as nutritional status, unemployment, and poverty level. In a smaller-scale disaster, this could include a severity score tabulated from a door-by-door outreach effort to rate the

occupants of a dwelling on a number of health, psychosocial, and life safety scores, and then map those using a GPS location and a GIS to plot the overall postdisaster health and safety of the community. Thus, a needs assessment is conducted to estimate the needs of the affected population. An HIS should track the resources on hand and the delivery of those resources and then gauge whether the resources are meeting their goals and being delivered to the victims in an efficient manner.[8]

Surveillance and Bioterrorism Detection Systems

Whereas an HIS is a mix of various pieces of software integrated into a single system, bioterrorism detection systems are being developed with federal funds and by private corporations that include continuous surveillance of hospital data from a number of sources. This allows for normalizing and analyzing that data for statistically significant patterns and less specific indicators and rapidly alerting health officials of a developing trend. In the recent past, public health surveillance did not occur in real time, but that has changed and data must begin to be collected often before cases are confirmed and cultures are reported positive. Often there is a narrow window of opportunity after an exposure in which treatment is most effective, such as for anthrax, and rapid identification of similar symptoms from multiple sources can be facilitated if a surveillance system is in place, where real-time reporting can take place. As technology improves, environmental biosensors can be linked to the system to provide even earlier detection before widespread infection and symptoms occur. Because most hospital information systems register every patient, deidentification can be done on patient data and the reason for visits can be easily transferred to a local database and even to a national database, such as the National Electronic Disease Surveillance System advocated by the CDC. It is more likely that the initial detection of a covert biological or chemical attack will occur at a local level. More and more local and state health agencies are developing ways to detect unusual patterns of disease and injury. Early response to such patterns is essential for ensuring a prompt response to a biological or chemical attack. Unfortunately, many of these projects are at a regional or state level. Local and even some state health agency budgets are still meager, and the cost of research and development of these systems is still out of reach for many smaller municipalities. If a system is developed, it usually lacks integration with other information systems and often relies on a person to do the daily initial data load or complex schemes of transmitting the data between systems. The Department of Defense system, ESSENCE, which downloads outpatient data from almost 300 Army, Navy, Air Force, and Coast Guard installations around the world each day, currently receives the data in one to three days of patient visits, longer than ideal for an optimal reaction to a potential outbreak. Systems that rely on a person interpreting patient visits for key indicators and inputting them into a central database are prone to variations and interpretation of how the data should be tabulated and entered, creating room for error and inconsistency. Furthermore, it has been demonstrated that early detection of just hours can make an enormous difference in a covert attack. Unfortunately, prototype automated surveillance systems have never been able to prove that they can detect a pathogen that quickly and may render a false sense of security. There are very few vendors of bioterrorism surveillance software. Currently the most promising endeavors are those funded by grants from the Department of Defense, CDC, and other federal agencies.[3]

SUMMARY

Disaster informatics and telecommunications have become indispensable tools for disaster managers and responders. As pervasive as these tools are in our daily lives, they are increasingly finding their way into the field. E-mail, instant messaging, LANs and intranets, cellular phones, two-way radios, teleconferencing, and many other sophisticated tools are becoming common in handheld devices and in the pockets of disaster responders. Information is a commodity, and the ability to analyze and distribute it to aid in the reduction of human suffering is probably the best money spent.

Device selection will probably be the disaster responder's most difficult task, because there are thousands of brands on the market for desktops, laptops, tablet PCs, and smartphones. Vendors may be of help in selecting a product that meets the user's needs, but many vendors are not familiar with the disaster responder's role and may not understand what punishment the device may endure. Generally, vendors who sell hardware that is being used in the public safety and field service fields will have a better idea of the harsh environments in which the equipment will have to operate. These vendors are a good first choice to talk with about the different devices.

Protecting the device and data is the next important task for the technologically armed disaster responder. Making sure that the device is stored in a padded, hard-shell case for shipping and travel and ensuring that there are redundant backups of the data at multiple points in the preparation, deployment, and demobilization phases are important. This includes taking backup copies of software on a CD in the event that the hardware is damaged in the field.

GPS receivers, cellular phones, radio systems, and the Internet are all tools that a disaster responder may use during a response to help establish and maintain communications with the home agency and other responders. These tools will be a lifeline for ongoing support and the reporting of events. Again, the user will be faced with trying to determine the best radio frequencies to use for any given circumstance. The disaster responder will need to locate the best vendor for cellular service near the disaster area, one that is large enough or has a large enough customer base that it is in the vendor's best financial interest to supplement local or damaged cellular stations to ensure better usability of the system after the event. Having multiple options for Internet access, such as dial-up, wireless, and fixed LAN ability, will ensure the user flexibility in plugging into whatever is available after a disaster.

As the disaster responder becomes more reliant on electronic equipment for postdisaster duties, he or she will need to consider alternative power sources and methods of recharging batteries, such as solar chargers, hand generators, and disposable power packs. He or she will need to consider taking any number of wall chargers, cords, dongles, adapters, and plugs to the disaster site. The electronic and communications demands for rapid information and assessment in the response and recovery efforts of a disaster mission will prompt the disaster responder to become more computer savvy, more electronically aware, and more technically knowledgeable, and, as a result, the disaster responder will be more productive. Reports and assessments must be rapidly tabulated and disseminated through the chain of command. Assessment efforts may rely on computerized surveillance techniques, information gathering and database development for resource tracking, and statistical analysis, all with the ability to rapidly communicate this information to various players and agencies at the disaster site in an organized and succinct manner. As pervasive as each of these technologies is getting in daily life, it is obvious that they are becoming equally so in disaster response.

REFERENCES

1. Gantz J. *40 years of IT-An Executive White Paper from IDC.* International Data Corp; 2004. Availlable at: http://edn.idc.com/prodserv/downloads/40_years_of_IT.pdf.
2. Bucklen KR. Earthquake in Iran: using the pocket PC for disaster medical relief. *Pocket PC.* June/July 2004;69–72.
3. Zubieta JC, Skinner R, Dean AG. Initiating informatics and GIS support for a field investigation of bioterrorism: the New Jersey anthrax experience. *Int J Health Geogr.* 2003;2(1):8.
4. Schumer C. Schumer reveals: when cell phones failed during blackout, only one NY cell phone company had emergency plan in place [press release]. Available at: http://schumer.senate.gov/SchumerWebsite/pressroom/press_releases/PR01953.html.
5. Requirements on Telecommunications for Disaster Relief from the International Federation of the Red Cross and Red Crescent Societies. Presented at: ITU-T Workshop on Telecommunications for Disaster Relief; 2003; Geneva.
6. Coile RC. The role of amateur radio in providing electronic communications for disaster management. *Disast Prev Manag.* 1997;6(3):176–185.
7. Henry W, Fisher I. The role of information technologies in emergency mitigation, planning, response and recovery. *Disast Prev Manag.* 1998;7(1):28–37.
8. Maxwell D, Watkins B. Humanitarian information systems and emergencies in the Greater Horn of Africa: logical components and logical linkages. *Disasters.* 2003;27(1):72–90.

SUGGESTED READINGS

1. Farrel B. *The National Communications System.* Available at: http://www.naseo.org/committees/energysecurity/energy assurance/farrell.pdf.
2. Fazio S. The need for bandwith management and QoS control when using public or shared networks for disaster relief work. Presented at: ITU-T Workshop on Telecommunications for Disaster Relief; 2003; Geneva.
3. Garshneck V. Telemedicine applied to disaster medicine and humanitarian response: history and future. Presented at: 32nd Hawaii International Conference on System Science; 1999; Hawaii. Available at: http://esd12.computer.org/comp/proceedings/hicss/1999/0001/04/00014029.PDF.
4. Teich JM, Wagner MM, Mackenzie CF, Schafer KO. The informatics response in disaster, terrorism and war. *J Am Med Inform Assoc.* 2002;9(2):97–104.
5. Brennan PF, Yasnoff WA. Medical informatics and preparedness. *J Am Med Inform Assoc.* 2002;9(2):202–203.
6. Sessa AB. Humanitarian Telecommunications. Presented at: ITU-T Workshop on Telecommunications for Disaster Relief; 2003; Geneva.
7. Garshnek V, Burkle FM, Jr. Applications of telemedicine and telecommunications to disaster medicine: historical and future perspectives. *J Am Med Inform Assoc.* 1999;6(1):26–37.
8. Zimmerman H. Communications for Decision-making in Disaster Management. Presented at: ITU-T Workshop on Telecommunications for Disaster Relief; 2003; Geneva.

Medical Simulation in Disaster Preparedness

Charles N. Pozner and Yasser A. Alaska

With increased awareness and attention to disaster and emergency preparedness, significant efforts have been directed toward enhancing pre-event training using educational exercises. This has resulted in the need to train large numbers of health care providers in a skill set that they are rarely asked to employ in their day-to-day practice.

"See one, do one, then teach one" has been one of the most common approaches to clinical education in the United States. Although its origin is unknown, it is a product of an apprenticeship model in which skill acquisition relies on the performance of clinical procedures on real patients. For obvious reasons this is not the safest educational model for patients. However, it is also flawed for learners who must gain competence in the unpredictable and often hectic clinical environment that places more and more limitations on learning. In addition to being unsafe, it has resulted in a lack of practice standardization, as well as the propagation of improper techniques when the mentor has been taught incorrectly.[1] Moreover, the unique nature of the disaster makes teaching and learning less practical using this traditional method.

In this chapter, we will introduce the concept of medical simulation as a means to educate clinician learners in a controlled and safe environment. We will describe the theory underlying its use and the different types of simulators and simulations, as well as introduce the reader to applications in the field of disaster management.

HISTORICAL PERSPECTIVE

Medical simulation is the use of a device or series of devices that emulate a real patient care situation for the purposes of training, assessment, or research. It exposes learners to both rare and common clinical situations in a predictable manner. It can enable novice learners to have mentored practice of technical skills at a pace that facilitates skill acquisition, and more-advanced learners the repetitive exposure to attain mastery.[2]

Simulators can be employed for the acquisition and assessment of cognitive, technical, and behavioral skills, and as a tool for research, product development, and process improvement. Medical simulation has likely been around for millennia, as simulation has long been recognized as a valuable educational strategy. The first modern simulators were developed in the early 1960s as a tool to teach both clinicians and the lay public the technique of cardiopulmonary resuscitation.[3] These task trainers provided learners the opportunity to practice the necessary resuscitation skills individually or while being overseen and corrected by instructors. Over the years more complex tasks have been simulated, and there are now sophisticated physiologically based whole-body simulators that enable novices and practicing clinicians to hone their skills.

Riding on the coattails of other high-reliability industries, modern medical simulation began to transcend its role in resuscitation training in the late 1980s and early 1990s. In response to the recognition that flight mishaps were typically caused by or made worse by communication failures, the aviation industry developed a set of principles, "cockpit resource management."[4] These principles were developed, learned, and assessed in flight simulators. These principles were adapted to the operative environment in a program called Anesthesia Crisis Resource Management.[5] Anesthesiologists started to teach these principles more broadly, and other disciplines rapidly began to adapt them to their specialties. In 2003 new human-patient simulators were released that changed the face of simulation forever. Prior to this, medical simulators were extraordinarily expensive. Few institutions could afford them, resulting in limited familiarity with the technology and, as a result, an impediment to further innovation. These new, more-affordable simulators brought about a dramatic increase in their availability and use, which resulted in both increased use and a corresponding increase in exploration and innovation. As team training continued to advance, increased use led to a broadening of applications. New simulation modalities were introduced, and there was also a proliferation of research in simulation. Simulation became established in a variety of health care professions, including nursing, emergency medical service(s) (EMS), other allied health fields, and increasingly in disaster preparedness.

EDUCATIONAL THEORY IN SIMULATION

Medical simulation takes advantage of adult learning theory. First described by Malcolm Knowles, the adult learner differs from the child learner.[6] The adult brings a vast experience database to each learning event. They are also very much goal and relevancy oriented; if they do not see the need for the knowledge, they are less likely to learn it. Although the "see one, do one, teach one" model also takes advantage of adult learning theory by making the training relevant and the learner goal oriented, its patient safety limitations among other limitations, has contributed to the emergence of simulation for clinical education.

Russell and Feldberg in 1999 put forth a theory that implicates human emotion as an important element in adult learning.[7] Their "Circumplex Model of Emotion" provides an excellent representation of how emotionality plays into adult learning. Although many learning opportunities, such as lectures, provide a pleasant milieu for both the learner and instructor, the learner is most often in a deactivated state. Adults learn best when they are both activated and under some degree of stress.[8] This is one of the underpinnings of the adult learning model. However, too much stress can actually be counterproductive, creating an environment that can be cognitively challenging.[9] The making of a clinical error is a frequent motivator of learning. If an error is recognized, the now motivated clinician typically seeks out the cause of the error by reading an article, looking it up on the Internet, or consulting a colleague in an attempt to avoid a similar error in the future. Another example of the importance of emotionality in learning is the enhanced motivation to learn after the debriefing of a disaster response. Not only is the identification of the error important, its effect on the emotions of the responders will influence the degree to which people are motivated to address change.[10] Simulation attempts to activate learners; commonly introducing a modicum of stress, and thus enhancing the learning experience by increasing the motivation to learn. Another illustration of how simulation can enhance learning is through its effect on the learner's perception of competence in a subject. The adult learner typically comes to the learning encounter with two levels of competence. The first is their perceived competence (how well they think they know something); the other is their actual competence (how well in reality they know it). Although in some cases the learner may actually have greater knowledge than he or she thinks, in the majority of cases, the learner's actual competence is eclipsed by his or her perceived competence. The "competence gap" is the difference between actual and perceived competence. At the conclusion of a simulated (or actual encounter for that matter), the learner is provided with a real sense of their competence. Narrowing of the "competence gap" is motivational to the adult learner. This now motivated learner has an enhanced hunger for knowledge. If the same material were being presented in a lecture format, the learner would likely remain at their initial level of perceived competence, making the learning interaction less relevant and providing less motivation to pay attention.

Ericsson, in his landmark work, theorizes that people are not naturally born with the skills necessary to become experts; they achieve expertise only after thousands of hours of practice and repetition; enhanced under the watchful eyes of a coach.[11] This is as true for clinicians as it is for athletes. In athletics, it is common for training to occur away from the competitive arena. For instance, the expert golfer has spent thousands of hours practicing and perfecting his skills under the tutelage of a coach before playing in a professional tournament. It is not unusual for surgeons to hone their skills in the operating room, let alone to do the procedure there for the first time. In fact, clinicians learn while "playing in the tournament."

Simulation offers clinicians an opportunity to learn new skills and develop a minimal level of competence prior to performing the skill on a real patient. Certainly, the honing of skills into expertise should involve practice on simulators, as well as on real people. Simulation also enables clinicians to practice rare or infrequently performed skills so that they are more prepared to perform them successfully when needed. This advantage is clearly leveraged in disaster preparedness; simulations being an often-used modality for the training and preparation for disaster response.

Debriefing, a term originating in the military, involves the review of operations at the conclusion of a mission to learn from the experience and improve future performance.[12] A critical element of scenario-based simulation, debriefing enables learners to reflect on their performance in the scenario. Integrating experiences into this process, the facilitator(s) leverages the activated and somewhat stressed state that the scenario has generated into an effective learning experience. It is postulated that this activated, interactive, and self-reflective experience creates an advantageous milieu for durable learning to occur.[12] Even though a degree of nervous tension is intended, the development of frank anxiety is thought to impede the process, making the development and framing of the experience a critical element.

TYPES OF SIMULATORS

Prior to the use of one of the first cardiopulmonary resuscitation training simulators called Resusci-Anne, patient care had been simulated using both cadaver and animal models. Although to some extent diminishing, the use of both of these continues to this day. Another well-accepted mode of simulation incorporates the use of standardized patients. Actual actors (or more commonly untrained volunteers) have been used extensively to simulate large-scale disaster responses. Although the fidelity of the clinician-patient interaction may be excellent, the introduction of accurate pathophysiological patient responses to changes in disease states or interventions is difficult to produce. Medical simulators have evolved considerably since the development of Resusci-Anne. We now have the capacity to create a pathophysiological presentation that is much more realistic, by altering the simulators anatomy and/or physiology. However, what has been gained in physiological fidelity is offset by loss of the interactive fidelity that a standardized patient can provide. Besides full-body mannequins, simulators include part-task trainers, screen-based simulators, virtual reality simulators, low-resource simulators, and hybrid simulation.

Full-body simulators come in two varieties: high-fidelity and medium fidelity. Although Resusci-Anne was developed as a full-body simulator, she was actually a part-task trainer used exclusively for the practice of CPR. These simulators enable learners to interact with, assess, and perform a variety of procedures on a simulated patient that through a variety of anatomical and physiological modifications controlled by the instructor behaves as would an actual patient. Depending on the level of fidelity, these simulators breathe, speak, and have pulses and heart and lung sounds, and they can display a wide variety of physiological parameters on their monitors. Some high-fidelity simulators employ a physiologically based platform that can mimic sophisticated physiology parameters; those that a human may exhibit under similar clinical circumstances. Depending on the fidelity of the simulator, clinicians may perform a number of procedures in response to anatomical and/or physiological presentations. These include airway management, IV fluid and medication administration, thoracostomy, and urinary catheterization, among others. Most of these mannequins may be preprogrammed to ensure that subsequent participants are exposed to the same patient, or they can be "run on the fly," during which the physiology is manipulated during the scenario. Full-body simulators may be employed in disaster-response preparation; requiring responders to not only identify a victim but provide needed care as part of a training exercise.

Part-task trainers are designed to enable the learner to perform one or several procedures on the device for both procedural introduction and ongoing practice. These may be as simple as an IV arm to practice IV insertion, or as sophisticated as an ultrasound phantom with pulsatile arteries and collapsible veins that enables a learner to perform ultrasound-guided central venous catheter insertion. The technology has become so sophisticated that simulators exist that enable the learner to perform endoscopy and laparoscopy, as well as a variety of other procedures. These simulators enable the learner to gain a certain level of competence prior to performing a procedure on an actual patient. They can also be useful in the assessment of procedural competence, and they provide an opportunity to practice low-frequency procedures such as those that may be required during a disaster response.

Screen-based simulators employ computer software that enables the user to interface with preprogrammed clinical scenarios. These programs typically enable the learner to obtain a history and perform a physical examination leading to interventions that the program responds to physiologically. There have been numerous programs designed; however, the first professional, large-scale product is being used to provide online cardiopulmonary resuscitation education.[13] Screen-based simulations often enable the learner to interface with a teaching module as a means of providing feedback on the progression of the scenario. There are several limitations of this technology. Although these programs afford learners the ability to employ their cognitive skills, because they are screen-based, the learner cannot perform the actual procedure. Screen-based simulations do not offer learners the opportunity to interact with co-providers; eliminating the possibility to practice the important nontechnical skills that underpin and influence our cognitive and technical performance. Some programs are now web-based, and they enable learners in a different (or same) location to provide care as a virtual team, offering an opportunity to practice nontechnical skills in this learning environment. Table-top simulations, a tried-and-true modality for disaster-response preparation, have slowly begun to incorporate screen-based simulations as a means of enhancing fidelity, ease of implementation, and interactivity.

Virtual reality simulators are another form of screen-based simulation. Many procedures now employ digital or fiber optic technology to enable the performance of less-invasive procedures. Laparoscopic surgery enables surgeons to perform operative procedures without the need for large incisions. Endoscopy is another procedure that utilizes real-time imaging to visualize and perform a variety of procedures on deep anatomic structures. In virtual reality simulation, using a functional replica of the actual user interface, the operator performs the procedure using sophisticated computer graphics that mimic the process that one would perform in the actual clinical environment. To enhance fidelity, some of these graphical interfaces employ haptics, a technology that recreates the sense of touch. If video imaging is used in an actual procedure, simulating it is now possible using these technologies.

Other modalities of simulation include low-fidelity and hybrid simulators. Low-fidelity simulators may be proprietary products or products that are created locally to meet the specific needs of the user. Examples of this include the "tried-and-true" use of an orange or grapefruit to enable learners to practice administering intramuscular injections. The authors have used papayas to simulate cervical dilation and endometrial curettage. However, there is an as yet unsettled debate regarding the level of fidelity necessary to meet the educational needs of the learner or participant.[14] Hybrid simulation employs different modes of simulation to enhance learning. For instance, one may develop a scenario with both a human-patient simulator and a standardized patient. Another example of hybrid simulation is the integration of an IV simulator with a standardized patient. In this case, the fidelity of the simulated patient-clinician interaction is maximized, and the participant may initiate intravenous access and administer medications as part of the scenario. Disaster training may use hybrid simulation, employing standardized patients, as well as a part-task simulator.

USE OF SIMULATION IN DISASTER PREPAREDNESS

As stated earlier, the use of simulation in disaster preparedness is not a new concept. Table-top and full-scale drills of varying scope and fidelity have been employed for decades. The use of simulation for the training of low-frequency, high-acuity events in health care translates effectively to the disaster realm. As with any educational endeavor, one must determine the goals and objectives of the experience prior to developing curriculum and selecting the appropriate modality(s) that will enable the organizers to meet these predetermined goals and objectives. Other issues to consider include the level of fidelity possible and needed, resources available, and cost. It is only after this deliberate planning process that the simulation-based disaster drill can be successfully developed and implemented. Possible aims of the exercise may include the training or assessment of individuals and/or teams, the assessment of new or modified processes, the testing of new technologies, and, in some cases, the reenactment of a prior disaster or drill in order to determine the root cause of problems encountered. The value of the exercise will depend on the assessment of actions taken, effective debriefing of participants, and thoughtful implementation of strategies learned from it. In the end, time spent planning the exercise is time well spent.

Table-top exercises, a traditional model of disaster simulation, are typically informal gatherings of individuals representing entities that may be involved in a response to a potential disaster. These can be limited to specific segments of the response or be of broad scope; bringing together all potential stakeholders. They are designed to assist in the testing of the response to a hypothetical situation, such as a natural or human-made disaster, to evaluate the group's ability to cooperate and work together and test their readiness to respond.[15] They familiarize participants with current plans, policies, and procedures, or they may be used to develop new plans, policies, agreements, and procedures. These may include paper-based scenarios or increasingly may be digitized, enabling more-robust presentations and interactions. Because they are static, they do not assess individual skills or delve deeply into processes. They provide an overview of the response, and the conclusions reached may dictate the need for change or enhancement of a disaster plan.

Operations-based simulated exercises can also assess plans, policies, and procedures, but because these exercises require active participation, they can also enable assessment of individuals and the systems in which they operate. This requires the actual deployment of people and resources; therefore the planning required for and the cost of these exercises can be substantial. Thus many of these are of limited scope. Operations-based exercises may test a single specific function or operation within a single group or they may be large in scale and much broader in scope, bringing together multiple agencies from different disciplines.

The level of fidelity of simulation in operations-based exercises may vary significantly. In some cases merely placing a piece of paper with a description of an injury for responders to find is used to simulate injuries, which is sufficient to test various elements of the response. In other cases volunteers play the role of the patients injured during the event. To enhance realism, volunteers may be "moulaged" (the application of simulated injuries), so that simulated injuries must be detected and then assessed, and patients are triaged and subsequently transported to the hospital. Depending on the scope of the exercise, triage at the hospital may take place with patients being admitted to the emergency department. These exercises may involve other areas of the hospital, enabling identification of hospital strengths and vulnerabilities. In all of these cases, because healthy people are used as patient surrogates, the level of fidelity and the ability to clinically intervene are limited. There is now growing experience in which high-fidelity human-patient simulators are employed during these exercises, enabling clinicians to not only assess the "patient" but implement clinical interventions.[16] This level of fidelity enables the assessment of systems, processes, and individual care providers. Controlling responses to treatment can enable systems deeper within the hospital to be challenged in a more-authentic manner, enabling assessment of hospital systems, transitions of care, and individual practitioners.

THE FUTURE SIMULATION IN DISASTER PLANNING

As the use of simulation as a learning modality grows in popularity and the availability of simulators and staff to operate them becomes more prevalent, it is clear that medical simulation for disaster preparedness will also grow. These simulators have become more portable, making their use in austere environments easier. Although the cost of simulation has moderated to some extent, it is still an expensive technology that needs to be used thoughtfully and with specific aims in mind. The fidelity of simulation will also continue to be enhanced over time. The improvement in realism will enable more genuine replication of clinical care, including critical transitions in care. Team training, a staple of many simulation programs at all levels of education, should also result in an expansion in the number of clinicians who have more-highly developed nontechnical skills, resulting in even more-efficient, collaborative care during these low-frequency, high-acuity events.

Additional futuristic modalities in simulation are sure to be developed that will likely enhance disaster preparation. One such technology is the development of virtual environments. Through the use of high-speed photography, space can now be recreated. One can imagine the value of this technology in recreating environments digitally that can be manipulated, in which people could simulate events. Simulation's historical place in disaster preparedness will continue to grow and be used as a means to train, assess, and assist in process improvement.

REFERENCES

1. Vozenilek J, Huff JS, Reznek M, Gordon JA. See one, do one, teach one: advanced technology in medical education. *Academic Emergency Medicine.* 2004;11:1149–1154.
2. Nishisaki A, Keren R, Nadkarni V. Does simulation improve patient safety? Self-efficacy, competence, operational performance, and patient safety. *Anesthesiol Clin.* 2007;25:225–236.
3. Cooper JB, Taqueti VR. A brief history of the development of mannequin simulators for clinical education and training. *Postgrad Med J.* 2008;84:563–570.
4. Gaba DM, DeAnda A. A comprehensive anesthesia simulation environment: re-creating the operating room for research and training. *Anesthesiology.* 1988;69:387–394.
5. Gaba DM, Fish KJ, Howard SK. *Crisis Management in Anesthesiology.* New York: Churchill Livingstone; 1994.
6. Knowles MS. Andragogy, not pedagogy. *Adult Leadersh.* 1968;16 (10):350–352, 386.
7. Russell JA, Barrett LF. Core affect, prototypical emotional episodes, and other things called emotion: dissecting the elephant. *J Pers Soc Psychol.* 1999;76:805–819.
8. Nater UM, Moor C, Okere U, et al. Performance on a declarative memory task is better in high than low cortisol responders to psychosocial stress. *Psychoneuroendocrinology.* 2007;32:758–763.
9. Elzinga BM, Bakker A, Bremner JD. Stress-induced cortisol elevations are associated with impaired delayed, but not immediate recall. *Psychiatry Res.* 2005;134:211–223.
10. Engel KG, Rosenthal M, Sutcliffe KM. Residents' responses to medical error: coping, learning, and change. *Acad Med.* 2006;81:86–93.
11. Ericsson KA. Deliberate practice and the acquisition and maintenance of expert performance in medicine and related domains. *Acad Med.* 2004;79 (10 suppl):S70–S81.
12. Fanning RM, Gaba DM. The role of debriefing in simulation-based learning. *Simul Healthc.* 2007;2:115–125.
13. The HeartRescue Project. Available at: http://www.heartrescuenow.com/; Accessed 01.08.14.
14. Rodgers DL, Securro S Jr., Pauley RD. The effect of high-fidelity simulation on educational outcomes in an advanced cardiovascular life support course. *Simul Healthc.* 2009 Winter;4(4):200–206.
15. Federal Emergency Management Agency website, Emergency Planning Exercises. Available at: http://www.fema.gov/emergency-planning-exercises; Accessed 01.08.14.
16. Gillett B, Peckler B, Sinert R, et al. Simulation in a disaster drill: comparison of high-fidelity simulators versus trained actors. *Acad Emerg Med.* 2008;15:1144–1151.

27 | CHAPTER

Disaster Mitigation

Robert M. Gougelet

The definition of mitigation includes a wide variety of measures taken before an event occurs that will prevent illness, injury, and death and limit the loss of property. Taking steps to mitigate potential hazards has taken on increasing favor in disaster preparedness circles, particularly in the international arena, where the pursuit of disaster risk reduction (DRR) and disaster risk management (DRM) is emphasized above efforts focused simply on disaster event response. The absolutely stunning loss of life, illnesses, injury, psychological impact, displacement from home and community, and social and financial consequences of a disaster, coupled with its disproportionate impact on the already disadvantaged, makes it imperative to fully implement the best principles and practices of disaster mitigation.[1] These principles and practices fall into two types:

1. *Disaster Risk Reduction (DRR)* aims to reduce the damage caused by natural hazards like earthquakes, floods, droughts, and cyclones, through the ethic of prevention.[2]
2. *Disaster Risk Management (DRM)* includes management activities that address and seek to correct or reduce disaster risks that are already present.[3]

HYOGO FRAMEWORK FOR ACTION

The Hyogo Framework for Action[4] offers guiding principles, priorities for action, and practical means to achieve disaster resilience for vulnerable communities. Priorities for action include the following:

1. Ensure that DRR is a national and local priority with a strong institutional basis for implementation
2. Identify, assess, and monitor disaster risks and enhance early warning
3. Use knowledge, innovation, and education to build a culture of safety and resilience at all levels
4. Reduce the underlying risk factors
5. Strengthen disaster preparedness for effective response at all levels

Although the primary emphasis on the Hyogo Framework is natural disasters, the processes discussed and framework for community resiliency and partnerships have application to all types of hazard responses.

ENGAGING THE WHOLE COMMUNITY

The Federal Emergency Management Agency (FEMA) reinforces the importance of engaging "not only FEMA and its federal partners, but also local, tribal, state and territorial partners; non-governmental faith-based and nonprofit organizations, and private sector industry; to individuals, families and communities, who continue to be the nation's most important assets as first responders during a disaster." Engaging local communities and a diverse set of partners ensures that the "unique and diverse needs of a population" are met and helps communities become more resilient after a disaster.[5]

Some specific medical response mitigation activities commonly include the following:

- Conduct health care facility and community hazard vulnerability analysis
- Conduct general efforts to support community resistance and resiliency
- Recruit and support staff (local citizens are more likely to support response and recovery efforts closer to home)
- Establish Memorandums of Understanding, which outline legal protections and authorities with local and regional nongovernmental organizations (NGOs), public agencies, faith-based groups, and private partnerships
- Develop training and educational activities to maintain skills and motivate staff
- Conduct organized Homeland Security Exercise and Evaluation Program (HSEEP) exercises
- Structure social media and other nontraditional methods of community outreach to communicate with individuals before, during, and after a disaster
- Implement technologies to support patient tracking, communications, data collection, and command and control.

INTRODUCTION OF MITIGATION IN THE UNITED STATES

It is of critical importance that emergency planners incorporate the basic elements of mitigation and have the authority and resources to incorporate these changes into their agency, organization, facility, or community. Emergency planners should have a working knowledge of the concepts of mitigation through their experience in natural disasters over the years. The federally mandated transition to the all-hazards approach for disaster event planning has also given a new perspective on mitigation.[6] Although it is not necessary to redefine mitigation, it is essential to understand how the scope and complexity of mitigation, risk reduction, and risk management strategies have evolved as the United States adapts to new threats.

For example, what measures can be taken in advance to protect the population and infrastructure from an earthquake, flood, ice storm, pandemic, or improvised nuclear device? As with each mass casualty event, the answers to this question are location-specific and heavily dependent on the circumstances surrounding the event. However, a common understanding of the goals and concepts of mitigation along with knowledge of its policy history and current practices will help a community develop mitigation strategies that are both locally effective and economically sustainable.

This chapter illustrates how mitigation strategies have evolved, outlines key historical elements of U.S. mitigation policy, highlights critical current mitigation practices, and describes common pitfalls that can hamper mitigation efforts. The realm of mitigation planning is far-reaching and complex. Therefore the emphasis of this chapter is on the continuity of medical care during a mass casualty event within a community.

GOALS AND CONCEPTS OF MITIGATION

In the simplest of terms, mitigation means to lessen the possibility that a mass casualty event can cause harm to people or property. However, this definition covers a broad range of possible activities. For example, an effort to ensure that essential utilities, such as electricity and phone service, continue to be available throughout a natural disaster is very different from efforts to minimize the economic damage of postdisaster recovery from a major flood or attempts to educate the public on how to reduce their risk of exposure during a pandemic.

Mitigation strategies can range from focusing exclusively on "hardening" to focusing more on resiliency. Hardening of targets is best described as measures that are taken to physically protect a facility, such as bolting down equipment, securing power and communications lines, installing backup generators, placing blast walls, or physically locking down and securing a facility. Mitigation through hardening has only limited use in systems or facilities such as hospitals where open access to the surrounding community is the hallmark of their operations. In these circumstances, a resilient system capable of flexing to accommodate damage and the ability to maintain or even expand current operations will make that system ultimately more secure. These efforts are solidly based within the community and their importance is emphasized by policy and supporting documentation from Presidential Policy Directive (PPD)-8: National Preparedness, FEMA, the Assistant Secretary of Preparedness and Response (ASPR) in the Department of Health and Human Services, the U.S. Centers for Disease Control and Prevention (CDC), the National Association of County and City Health Officials (NACCHO), and The Joint Commission (formerly the Joint Commission on Accreditation of Health Care Organizations, or JCAHO).

Mitigation through resiliency also has limitations. In many cases, hardening structures is most appropriate, particularly when many citizens may be quickly affected without prior notice or warning. This may include hardening structures in earthquake zones, protecting and monitoring the food chain and drinking water systems, and physically securing and protecting nuclear power plants. In these cases, resiliency may come too late to prevent illness and death in large numbers of patients, and planners should target hardening to whatever degree is practically and financially feasible.[7] The threats of nuclear, radiological, chemical, and biological attacks present new challenges for emergency planners. The potentially covert nature of the attacks, the wide variety of possible agents (including contagious agents), and soft civilian targets make planning efforts exponentially more difficult than in the past. This complexity has also eroded the distinction between mitigation and response activities.

Although it is never possible to mitigate or plan responses for all contingencies, we do know that there is a basic common response framework. This framework includes coordination, communication to enable interagency information sharing, and flexibility to rapidly adapt emergency plans to different situations.[8,9]

RECENT HISTORICAL PERSPECTIVE

Traditionally, mitigation in the United States has focused on natural disasters; however, early mitigation planning against human-made disasters included civilian fallout shelters and the evacuation of target cities if a nuclear attack was imminent. FEMA states:

Mitigation is the effort to reduce loss of life and property by lessening the impact of disasters. Mitigation is taking action *now*—before the next disaster—to reduce human and financial consequences later (analyzing risk, reducing risk, insuring against risk).[10] Risk Reduction works to reduce risk to life and property through land use planning, floodplain management, [and] the adoption of sound building practices . . . Mitigation projects that reduce risk include elevating, relocating, or acquiring properties located in floodplains and returning them to open space, and the reinforcing of buildings in earthquake-prone areas.[10a]

Mitigation begins with local communities assessing their risks from recurring problems and making a plan for creating solutions to these problems and reducing the vulnerability of their citizens and their property to risk.[11] However, since the mid-1990s, mitigation planning has become increasingly more complex. Terrorist attacks, industrial accidents, and new or reemerging infectious diseases are just a few of the threats that have started to consume more planning time and resources. The growing scope of threats that must be addressed in mitigation strategies challenges all aspects of planning and response at all levels of government.[12-14]

The importance of sharing intelligence information, for example, at the earliest possible stage of a terrorist attack, is recognized in national policy as a critical mitigation asset. Fusion centers have been implemented in jurisdictions across the United States.[15,16] It is imperative that first responders and hospitals receive notification at the earliest indication of a contagious biological attack. Early notification allows state, regional, and local communities to implement appropriate responses that provide isolation, treatment, prophylaxis, and stockpiling and staging of federal resources, which, when rapidly implemented, could contain a potentially widespread event. This intelligence sharing must become a larger part of mitigation efforts aimed at also limiting the impact of natural and human-made disasters. The elevated status of intelligence within the National Incident Management System (NIMS) establishes the importance of early and effective intelligence sharing. The challenge is to establish these sharing relationships before a disaster by incorporating them into an ongoing hazard monitoring process, drills, exercises, and day-to-day activities to ensure that this critical resource is operational when needed to mitigate the consequences of a disaster.[17] A similar analogy can be made with the early warning given to the medical community when a surveillance system detects an unusual cluster of illnesses, which triggers an investigation leading to increased awareness, training, laboratory recognition, and possible identification of a sentinel case long before the initial diagnosis may be confirmed at a physician's office or health care facility.

The Disaster Mitigation Act of 2000 (DMA-2000)[18] emphasized the importance of mitigation planning within communities by authorizing the funding of certain mitigation programs and by involving the Office of the President. Under DMA-2000, the President may authorize funds to communities or states that have identified natural disasters within their borders and have demonstrated public–private natural disaster mitigation partnerships. DMA-2000 promotes awareness and education by providing economic incentives for states, local communities, and tribes.

DMA-2000 Federal assistance priorities include the following:
- Forming effective community-based partnerships for hazard mitigation purposes
- Implementing effective hazard mitigation measures that reduce the potential damage from natural disasters
- Ensuring continued functionality of critical services
- Leveraging additional nonfederal resources in meeting natural disaster resistance goals
- Making commitments to long-term hazard mitigation efforts to be applied to new and existing structures

This important legislation sought to identify and assess the risks to states and local governments (including Indian tribes) from natural disasters. The funding would be used to implement adequate measures to reduce losses from natural disasters and to ensure that the critical services and facilities of communities would continue to function after a natural disaster.

Further evidence of the expanding complexity of mitigation efforts can be found in the Terrorism Insurance Risk Act of 2002. This act fills a gap within the insurance industry, which typically does not provide insurance coverage for large-scale terrorist events. The federal government promptly passed this act in the wake of the September 11, 2001, attacks to address concerns about the potential widespread effect of insured losses due to terrorism on the economy. The act provides a transparent shared public–private program that compensates insured losses as a result of acts of terrorism. The purpose is to "protect consumers by addressing market disruptions and ensure the continued widespread availability and affordability of property and casualty insurance for terrorism risk; and to allow for a transitional period for the private markets to stabilize, resume pricing of such insurance, and build capacity to absorb any future losses, while preserving State insurance regulation and consumer protections."[19,20] Now, effective mitigation planning is expected to include many different aspects of private industry.

Private industry is a critical partner; its involvement may range from being a potential risk to the community, such as a chemical plant, to providing assistance in responding to an event. This is especially true in the area of health care; most health care in the United States is provided by the private sector. It is important to note that the National Fire Protection Association (NFPA) recently released NFPA 1600, Standard on Disaster/Emergency Management and Business Continuity Programs, 2013 edition. This standard establishes a common set of criteria and best practices to help local, regional, and national governments, agencies, and organizations plan for disaster management, emergency management, and business continuity. Planners may use these criteria to assess or develop programs or to respond to and recover from a disaster.[21]

Although mitigation planning has become an essential feature of nearly every industry and institution in the wake of 9/11, health care settings are disproportionately affected by new challenges and complexities in mitigation. The severe acute respiratory syndrome (SARS) outbreak shook the foundation of mitigation and prevention in health care when health care workers and first responders in China and Canada died in 2003 after caring for patients infected with the SARS virus. Access to several Toronto area hospitals was significantly limited for several months because of illness, quarantined staff, and concerns about contamination. The economic costs to the city of Toronto were in the billions of dollars. Hospitals and their communities were thrown into a complex mitigation and prevention crisis. Like SARS, the steady spread of Middle East respiratory syndrome coronavirus (MERS-CoV) in Saudi Arabia since 2012 poses similar threats and has disproportionately affected health care workers, who remain most vulnerable to contagious emerging and reemerging infectious diseases.

The Association of State and Territorial Health Officials (ASTHO) released specific guidelines and checklists to help prepare states and communities for a possible outbreak.[22] Pan-influenza planning closely parallels SARS planning, with considerable effort toward preventive vaccination of the population and emphasis on protecting health care workers.[23] Effective strategies were learned during the Toronto SARS outbreak, although it was definitely a "learn-as-you-go-along" situation. The most effective mitigation strategies to prepare for the consequences of an outbreak would be to plan for the home quarantine of patients, establish public information strategies to reduce public concern, close affected facilities until conditions permit their safe reopening, plan for a coordinated information and command and control center, and have preestablished protocols and procedures in place to protect the health of health care workers and first responders.[24]

Vaccination is an essential component of hospital and community mitigation planning. During the fall of 2002, the U.S. government requested that all states prepare for a smallpox attack. The preparations called for each state to present plans to vaccinate all persons within the state, within a 10-day period, starting with health care workers.[25] Each facility and community needs to look at the risk of a disease, the effect of vaccination on health care workers, and the ability to maintain continuity of care. One outcome of the 2009 H1N1 pandemic was that several organizations, including the Society for Healthcare Epidemiology of America (SHEA), the Association for Professionals in Infection Control and Epidemiology (APIC), and the Infectious Disease Society of America (IDSA) recommended that health care workers be mandated to receive yearly influenza vaccinations, which helps to minimize the risk that they will transmit influenza to high- and low-risk patients and bring influenza home to their families. If properly informed and vaccinated, health care workers could respond and treat patients without risk to themselves or their families. The availability of a vaccine and the ability to mass-vaccinate the majority of the population should be considered in all community response plans. The plans for both SARS and pan-influenza now need to address the availability and possible stockpiling of antiviral agents as well as procedures for mass vaccination of the population, if a vaccine were to become available.

Nonpharmaceutical interventions (NPIs) are also of critical importance in preventing the spread of pandemic illnesses such as the H1N1 pandemic of 2009. Communities can enact policies promoting NPIs that reduce the risk of spreading disease, such as encouraging flexible sick leave and offering telework for employees, closing schools temporarily, and encouraging those who are ill to stay home until they are well.[26] Social media, such as a local health department's Twitter or Facebook account and the CDC's Flu Activity & Surveillance webpage,[27] help individuals stay informed on the status of an outbreak and provide recommendations tailored to community members or populations at higher risk for complications.

We have learned from the many earthquakes, tornadoes, hurricanes, fires, and floods that the United States has experienced, but it is extremely difficult to plan for massive terrorist and natural events that happen without notice and can quickly overwhelm communities, states, and even the nation. These historical events, policy developments, and shifts in public attention have created a very complex planning and operating environment. The next section of this chapter addresses some of the key current practices that mitigation strategists should consider.

CURRENT PRACTICE

Current mitigation strategies are as varied as the circumstances in which they are formed. This section illustrates the impact of mitigation through a comparison of responses to two earthquakes that were broadly separated both in geography and degree of community preparedness. These examples are followed by a discussion of critical elements of mitigation and risk reduction practice in three broad categories: coordination with other organizations and jurisdictions, hospital concerns, and mitigation strategies based in community health promotion and surveillance.

The first step for protecting communities and their critical facilities against earthquakes is a comprehensive risk assessment based on current seismic hazard mapping. This determination of location should also include the assessment of underlying soil conditions, the potential for landslides, and other potential hazards.[28] Communities located on seismic fault lines must also develop and enforce strict building codes.

After the Bam, Iran, earthquake in 2003, a large section of the city looked at first glance like a burned forest with only the bare trees left standing. It soon became clear that these "trees" were steel vertical beams standing upright in mounds of concrete rubble. In comparison, after the Northridge, California, earthquake in 1994, many of the buildings were structurally compromised but did not collapse upon their occupants. Undoubtedly, this was the result of the strict building codes and enforcement throughout the state of California. For the victims of the Bam earthquake, the most important lifesaving measures might have been the development and enforcement of strict building codes.[29] Building codes are minimum standards that protect people from injury and loss of life from structural collapse; they do not ensure that normal community functioning might continue after a significant event.[30]

The structural issues, generator failures, flooding, and sewage problems experienced by hospitals during hurricanes Sandy and Katrina were widely and dramatically displayed by the press across the world. With over half of the 16,000 hospitals in Latin America and the Caribbean in high-risk disaster zones, the Pan American Health Organization (PAHO) has developed extensive guidance for hospital preparedness.[31]

Structural protection of facilities requires the active role of qualified and experienced structural engineers during planning, construction, remodeling, and retrofitting. The immediate response of a structural engineer after a disaster is to assess building damage and to assist in determining the need for evacuation and the measures needed to ensure continuity of function. Extensive analysis of seismic data taken during an earthquake and compared with subsequent building damage has given structural engineers valuable information on structural failures of buildings. This information allows communities to rebuild with better and stronger facilities.[32]

The following measures to protect the structural integrity of a facility should be in place before an incident[33]:

- A contract with a structural engineering firm to participate in planning, construction, retrofitting, and remodeling
- A contractual agreement guaranteeing the response, after an event, of a structural engineer (with appropriate redundancy) to ensure structural stability, assess the need for evacuation, and take additional measures to ensure the continuity of essential functions
- An inventory and classification of all buildings
- A vulnerability assessment
- Strict code compliance
- Determination of public safety risks
- Determination and prioritization of structural reinforcement needs
- Lists of vulnerable structures for use in evacuation and damage assessment.

Extensive resources and technical assistance for structural earthquake protection are available on the Internet. FEMA's website itemizes these resources into three major categories: earthquake engineering research centers and National Earthquake Hazards Reduction Program-funded centers, earthquake engineering and architectural organizations, and codes and standards organizations.[34] FEMA has also released the Risk Management Series publications, which provide very specific guidance to architects and engineers about protecting buildings against terrorist attacks.[35] The Institute for Business and Home Safety is also an excellent source of incident-specific information for both businesses and homes.[36]

The protection of facilities from earthquake damage also involves protecting the facility's nonstructural elements so that the fundamental structure of the building and operations are not compromised (Box 27-1). Primary damage to nonstructural elements may be the result

BOX 27-1 Nonstructural Elements

- Cabinets
- Compressed gas tanks
- Fuel tanks
- Generators
- Equipment and supplies
- Signs and pictures
- Electrical lines
- Communication and information technology lines
- Bookshelves
- Windows
- Electrical fixtures
- Storage containers
- Hazardous materials
- Lockers
- Building parapets and facings
- Computer and IT networks

of overturning, swaying, sliding, falling, deforming, or internal vibration on sensitive instruments. Relatively simple measures that do not require a structural engineer may be taken to prevent damage to or from nonstructural elements. These measures may include fastening loose items and structures, anchoring top-heavy items, tethering large equipment, or using spring mounts. Other elements, such as stabilizing a generator from vibration damage by placing it on spring mounts or from sliding damage by having slack in attached fuel and power lines, may require the assistance of an engineer.

Hospitals and other medical care facilities are especially vulnerable to damage from nonstructural elements. Consider the placement of routine medical care items such as intravenous poles, monitors and defibrillators, and pharmaceutical agents and medical supplies on shelves. Loss of emergency power to key services, such as computed tomography scanners, laboratory equipment, electronic medical records, and dialysis units, may also significantly affect the continuity of medical care.[37,38] Loss of generator power may be due to failure of crossover switches, loss of cooling, or loss of connection of power and fuel lines. A process for the continual review of the power needs of new and critical equipment should be a part of a hospital's emergency planning process.

Cooperating with the federal government and understanding the resources, structure, and timeframe within which federal resources are available are critical to appropriate mitigation planning.[39] NIMS and the National Response Plan are described elsewhere in this book. Each document describes in detail the organizational structure and response authority of the federal government in the time of a disaster.[40] Health care organizations, communities, and states are mandated to ensure that their strategies for mitigation, response, and recovery are developed in coordination with these national models. Homeland Security Presidential Directive (HSPD) 5 mandated that by fiscal year 2005, "the Secretary shall develop standards and guidelines for determining whether a State or Local entity has adopted the NIMS,"[41] and all mitigation and risk reduction strategies should be designed accordingly.

In addition to efforts to coordinate with federal plans, mitigation strategists must also build functional partnerships within communities and across jurisdictional lines. This point has been emphasized in several recently published planning guides.[42-44] These guides help hospitals and their communities plan for mass casualty events by incorporating key features of planning, risk assessment, exercises, communications, and command and control issues into functional and operational programs.

Hospitals also present special challenges. HSPD 8 specifies that hospitals qualify as first responders.[45] As such, they have important mitigation activities to consider. What does mitigation mean for a hospital? In the current threat environment, it means minimizing the impact of an event on the institution and ensuring continuity of care.

Accessibility to the public 24 hours a day, 7 days a week has been a hallmark of hospital emergency care. However, one of the most important mitigation strategies a hospital can adopt is the ability to limit and control access to patients and families during the time of a mass casualty or a hazardous materials event. Additionally, facilities must have plans and the ability to decontaminate patients, protect essential staff and their families, handle a surge of patients with complementary plans for the forward movement of patients to surrounding areas, set up alternative treatment facilities within the community, train staff in early recognition and treatment of illness or injury related to weapons of mass destruction, and ensure continuity of care and financial stability during and after an event.

Although hospitals will always form the cornerstone for medical treatment of patients during mass casualty events, best practices for hospitals must now also incorporate health care resources within the community.[46] Hospitals will have to work with other first responders within the community to conduct drills and exercises that realistically test the whole hospital's ability to respond to a mass casualty event.[47] Hospitals also will have to ensure that staff members have the proper training to complete hazard vulnerability assessments[48] and to set up and staff outpatient treatment facilities to ensure continuity of care.[49] Even with very careful planning, most communities will be overwhelmed for the first minutes to hours or possibly days after a massive event, until an effective and prolonged response can occur. Communities must also look at the continuity of medical care as a community-wide issue and not just emphasize the hospital or emergency medical services aspects of medical care. The loss of community-based clinics, private medical offices, nursing homes, dialysis units, pharmacies, and visiting nurse services can significantly increase the number of patients seeking care at hospitals during a mass casualty event. Risk communication and education specifically aimed at protecting the affected population can help prevent surges of medical patients.[50]

Hospitals now have enormous community responsibilities in terms of preparing for and mitigating mass casualty events. Hospitals in hurricane, flood, earthquake, and tornado zones have prepared for many years against these threats. However, a pattern of repeated systems failures within hospitals continues and includes communications and power loss, with additional physical damage to the facility.[51] To prevent such failures, hospitals need to recognize that mitigation and risk reduction planning must approach a level of detail and logistical support that parallels military planning.

Surveillance is another key mitigation strategy for hospitals and public health emergencies. Early recognition of sentinel cases in biological events can significantly affect the outcome, particularly in contagious events. States are funded and required to participate in the surveillance programs mandated in CDC and Health Resources and Services Administration (HRSA) guidelines.[52,53] The earlier an event is recognized, especially if it involves a contagious disease, the earlier treatment can begin and preventive measures can be taken to prevent the spread of illness to health care workers and responders, as well as the rest of the community. Local and state public health departments are critical to establishing relationships between local providers and their communities. Local, state, and federal public health agencies must ensure that effective surveillance at the community level occurs. These agencies can also assist in awareness-level and personal protection training for hospital staff, emergency medical service employees, and law enforcement first responders.

NEW HAMPSHIRE CRITICAL CARE AND SUPPLEMENTAL OXYGEN PROGRAM (NHCCSOP)

The State of New Hampshire was faced with the task of increasing the state's capacity and capability to provide for critical care and supplemental oxygen during widespread pandemic events or overwhelming local or sub-state regional events. The first phase involved the placement of high-performance, transport-capable ventilators within hospitals and emergency medical services across the state. The decision to place the ventilators with end users accomplished the goals of having the ventilators in the field where they would be readily available and maintained and could be utilized in day-to-day emergent interfacility and intrafacility transports. The supplemental oxygen component of the program provides low-flow oxygen within the community-based alternate care facilities that are supported by state legislation during mass casualty events and public health emergencies. Critical to this effort was state support and legislation as well as the effective use of sub-state public health regions to support planning and command and control response activities. Within the regions, coalitions supporting this effort included a core group of critical partners providing medical control and subject matter expertise and multiple supportive agencies and NGOs. Space included public schools, college facilities, community centers, and NGO facilities. Staff comprised community volunteer groups, the state Metropolitan Medical Response System (MMRS) team, hospitals, private practices, and other practitioners. Supplies included a combination of state-purchased equipment and supplies, with an emphasis on high-priority coordination with state and local vendors for oxygen equipment and supplies. Sustainability, the effective utilization of regionally based and local resources, appears to be an effective strategy for this important capability after a series of HSEEP-certified workshops and exercises across the thirteen regions of the state.[54]

COMMON PITFALLS

Motivating health care facilities to take part in mitigation is one of the largest challenges in disaster medicine. It is always best to take measures beforehand to minimize property damage and prevent injury and death. In the case of hospitals, some preliminary research indicates that four factors affect an institution's motivation to mitigate: influence of legislation and regulation, economic considerations, the role of "champions" within the institution, and the impact of disasters and imminent threats on agenda-setting and policy making. It was discovered during this research that "mitigation measures were found to be most common when proactive mitigation measures were mandated by regulatory agencies and legislation."[55] Tax incentives, government assistance grants, and building code and insurance requirements may also serve to motivate administrators and decision makers to put the necessary time and effort into mitigation planning.[30]

The Hospital Preparedness Program (HPP), designed to provide leadership and funding through grants to and cooperative agreements with states, territories, and eligible municipalities to improve surge capacity and enhance community and hospital preparedness for public health emergencies,[52] has undergone significant cuts over the past few years that threaten to undo progress made in the last decade. HPP appropriations have decreased from $426 million in FY2010 to $255 million in FY2014, including a one-third cut in the FY2014 omnibus.[56] HPP provides financial incentives to ensure that hospitals are able to coordinate, cooperate, and reduce loss of life during an emergency. The program allowed the coalition in Boston to practice two 24-hour disaster simulations involving several area hospitals before the 2013 Boston Marathon Bombing. The planning and efficiency of the hospitals after the attack were major factors in saving the lives of the 264 individuals injured in the bombings, and there were no additional deaths after the three on-site fatalities.[57] The loss of an estimated 46,000 state and local public health jobs since 2008[58] also has the potential to damage the progress made in all-hazards preparedness since 9/11. With little prospect of increased national funding in the immediate future, it is necessary for local communities to develop sustainability strategies to ensure every dollar is well spent in helping their communities prepare for disasters.[59] The CDC Capability 10: Medical Surge publication encourages the widespread collaboration and allocation of resources in community-wide surge capacity efforts and has been helpful in focusing these efforts in a realistic and operational manner.[60]

CONCLUSION

Extensive mitigation activities are a necessary prerequisite for the response and recovery activities that must follow a large-scale mass casualty event. It is very difficult, as well as disturbing, to plan for the potential number of casualties in the United States that we are preparing for today. We do have the threat of an enemy who will strike within the United States with the purpose of inflicting mass numbers of casualties on the civilian population. We must maintain the perspective that even the smallest chance of such an incredibly devastating event, whether human-made or natural, warrants our full attention. If there is no other motivating factor, the possibly of such an event must suffice. 9/11, SARS, H1N1, the 2013 Boston Marathon Bombing, the anthrax attacks, hurricanes Katrina and Irene, and Superstorm Sandy are all recent events that have impacted a wide range of areas from dense urban to very rural with a wide range of injury, illness, death, and destruction.

REFERENCES

1. World Bank. *Natural Hazards and UnNatural Disasters; the economics of effective prevention.* The International Bank for Reconstruction and Development/The World Bank; 2010. Overview available at: http://www.gfdrr.org/sites/gfdrr.org/files/nhud/files/NHUD-Overview.pdf. Accessed 04.26.15.
2. The United Nations Office of Disaster Risk Reduction. *What Is Disaster Risk Reduction?* Available at: http://www.unisdr.org/who-we-are/what-is-drr. Accessed 04.26.15.
3. UNISDR. The United Nations Office for Disaster Risk Reduction. *Terminology.* Available at: http://www.unisdr.org/we/inform/terminology. Accessed 04.26.15.
4. UNISDR. Hyogo framework for action 2005-2015: building the resilience of nations and communities to disasters 2005-2015. Available at: http://www.unisdr.org/we/inform/publications/1037. Accessed 04.26.15.
5. Federal Emergency Management Agency. *Whole Community.* Available at: http://www.fema.gov/whole-community. Accessed 04.26.15.
6. New England Center for Emergency Preparedness. *Modular Emergency Medical System: A Regional Response for All-Hazards Catastrophic Emergencies.* Available at: http://www.dmsnecep.org/files/mems.pdf. Accessed 04.26.15.
7. Aur der Heide E. Principles of hospital disaster planning. In: Hogan DE, Burstein JL, eds. *Disaster Medicine.* Philadelphia: Lippincott Williams & Wilkins; 2002.
8. Department of Homeland Security. *National Response Framework.* Available at: http://www.fema.gov/pdf/emergency/nrf/nrf-core.pdf. Accessed 04.26.15.
9. Federal Emergency Management Agency. *National Incident Management System.* Available at: http://www.fema.gov/national-incident-management-system. Accessed 04.26.15.
10. FEMA. What is Mitigation? Available at: http://www.fema.gov/what-mitigation. Accessed 04.26.15.
10a. FEMA Fact Sheet. http://www.fema.gov/media-library-data/20130726-1621-20490-7885/fima_2012.txt. Accessed 04.26.15.
11. State of Vermont Emergency Management Agency/Vermont Department of Public Safety. *State of Vermont Hazard Mitigation Plan.* Available at: http://vem.vermont.gov/sites/vem/files/VT_SHMP2013%20FINAL%20APPROVED%20ADOPTED%202013%20VT%20SHMP_scrubbed_cleanedMCB.pdf. Accessed 04.26.15.
12. Centers for Disease Control and Prevention. *Smallpox Response Plan And Guidelines* (Version 3.0). Available at: http://www.bt.cdc.gov/agent/smallpox/response-Plan/index.asp. Accessed 04.26.15.
13. Centers for Disease Control and Prevention. *Severe Acute Respiratory Syndrome (SARS).* Available at: http://www.cdc.gov/sars/index.html/. Accessed 04.26.15.
14. Centers for Disease Control and Prevention. Biological and chemical terrorism: strategic plan for preparedness and response. Recommendations of the CDC Strategic Planning Workgroup. *Morb Mortal Wkly Rep.* April 2000;49(RR-4). Available at: http://www.cdc.gov/mmwr/preview/mmwrhtml/rr4904a1.htm. Accessed 04.26.15.
15. White House. *National Security Strategy.* Available at: http://www.whitehouse.gov/sites/default/files/rss_viewer/national_security_strategy.pdf. Accessed 04.26.15.
16. Department of Homeland Security. *State and Major Urban Area Fusion Centers: National Network of Fusion Centers.* Available at: http://www.dhs.gov/state-and-major-urban-area-fusion-centers. Accessed 04.26.15.
17. Federal Emergency Management Agency. *NIMS Intelligence/Investigations Function: Guidance and Field Operations Guide.* October 2013. Available at: http://www.fema.gov/media-library-data/1382093786350-411d33add2602da9c867a4fbcc7ff20e/NIMS_Intel_Invest_Function_Guidance_FINAL.pdf. Accessed 04.26.15.
18. Federal Emergency Management Agency. *Disaster Mitigation act of 2000.* Available at: http://www.fema.gov/media-library/assets/documents/4596. Accessed 04.26.15.
19. U.S. Department of the Treasury. H.R. 3210. Terrorism risk insurance act of 2002. Available at: http://www.treasury.gov/resource-center/fin-mkts/Documents/hr3210.pdf. Accessed 04.26.15.
20. Manns J. Insuring against terror? *Yale Law J.* 2003;112(8):2509–2551. Available at: http://www.yalelawjournal.org/note/insuring-against-terror. Accessed 04.26.15.
21. *National Fire Protection Association.* 2013. *NFPA 1600®: Standard on Disaster/Emergency Management and Business Continuity Programs.* Available at: http://www.catalog.nfpa.org/2013-NFPA-1600-Standard-on-Disaster-Emergency-Management-and-Business-Continuity-Programs-P1438.aspx?link_type=buy_box&pid=160013&icid=B484&cookie_test=1.
22. Hopkins RS, Misegades L, Ransom J, Lipson L, Brink EW. SARS Preparedness Checklist for State and Local Health Officials. *Emerg Infect Dis.* 2004;10(2):369–372. Available at: http://wwwnc.cdc.gov/eid/article/10/2/pdfs/03-0729.pdf. Accessed 04.26.15.
23. Gensheimer KF, Meltzer MI, Postema AS, Strikas RA. Influenza Pandemic Preparedness. *Emerg Infect Dis.* 2003;9(12):1645–1648. Available at: http://wwwnc.cdc.gov/eid/article/9/12/pdfs/03-0289.pdf. Accessed 04.26.15.
24. Gopalakrishna G, Choo P, Leo YS, et al. SARS Transmission and Hospital Containment. *Emerg Infect Dis.* 2004;10(3):395–400. Available at: http://www.ncbi.nlm.nih.gov/pmc/articles/PMC3322797/. Accessed 04.26.15.
25. Centers for Disease Control and Prevention. *CDC Guidance for Post-Event Smallpox Planning.* Available at: http://www.bt.cdc.gov/agent/smallpox/prep/post-event-guidance.asp. Accessed 04.26.15.
26. Centers for Disease Control and Prevention. *Nonpharmaceutical Interventions (NPIs).* Available at: http://www.cdc.gov/nonpharmaceutical-interventions/. Accessed 04.26.15.
27. Centers for Disease Control and Prevention. *Flu Activity & Surveillance.* Available at: http://www.cdc.gov/flu/weekly/fluactivitysurv.htm. Accessed 04.26.15.
28. *Local Mitigation Planning Handbook.* FEMA. 2013. Available at: http://www.dhses.ny.gov/oem/mitigation/documents/fema-local-mitigation-handbook.pdf. Accessed 04.26.15.
29. Personal observations during deployment: DMAT NM#-1 Northridge Earthquake 1994, IMSURT-East Bam, Iran 2004.
30. Auf der Heide E. Community medical disaster planning and evaluation guide: an interrogatory format. Dallas, TX: *Am Coll Emerg Phys.* 1995. Available at:

http://books.google.com/books/about/Community_Medical_Disaster_Planning_and.html?id=5UkOywAACAAJ. Accessed 04.26.15.

31. Pan American Health Organization. *The Hospital Safety Index*. Available at: http://www.paho.org/disasters/index.php?option=com_content&task=view&id=964&Itemid=911. Accessed 04.26.15.

32. Hays W. *Presented at: International Workshop on Earthquake Injury Epidemiology for Mitigation and Response. Data acquisition for earthquake hazard mitigation—abstract*. Baltimore: Johns Hopkins University; 1989, July 10-12 Accessed 04.26.15.

33. State of California, Governor's Office of Emergency Services. Hospital earthquake preparedness guide. Available at: http://preventionweb.net/go/6939. Accessed 04.26.15.

34. Federal Emergency Management Agency. National Earthquake Hazards Reduction Program. Available at: http://www.fema.gov/national-earthquake-hazards-reduction-program. Accessed 04.26.15.

35. Federal Emergency Management Agency. Security Risk Management Series Publications. Available at: https://www.fema.gov/what-mitigation/security-risk-management-series-publications. Accessed 04.26.15.

36. Insurance Institute for Business and Home Safety. Available at: http://www.ibhs.org/. Accessed 04.26.15.

37. AHA solutions: Disaster Recovery Solutions (Agility). Available at: http://www.aha-solutions.org/partners/agility.shtml. Accessed 04.26.15.

38. FEMA. Non-Structural Earthquake Mitigation Guidance Manual. Available at: http://www.fema.gov/media-library/assets/documents/19087. Accessed 04.26.15.

39. Federal Emergency Management Agency. Response and recovery. A Guide to the Disaster Declaration Process and Federal Disaster Assistance. Available at: https://www.fema.gov/media-library/assets/documents/6094. Accessed 04.26.15.

40. Federal Emergency Management Agency. National Response Plan. Available at: https://www.dhs.gov/xlibrary/assets/NRP_Brochure.pdf. Accessed 04.26.15.

41. U.S. Department of Homeland Security. Homeland Security Presidential Directive/HSPD-5: Management of Domestic Incidents. Available at: http://www.dhs.gov/sites/default/files/publications/Homeland%20Security%20Presidential%20Directive%205.pdf. Accessed 04.26.15.

42. New England Center for Emergency Preparedness. Modular emergency medical system: a regional response for all-hazards catastrophic emergencies. Available at: http://www.dmsnecep.org/files/mems.pdf. Accessed 04.26.15.

43. FEMA. Public-Private Partnerships. Available at: http://www.fema.gov/public-private-partnerships. Accessed 04.26.15.

44. State of California. Medical Care and Public Health Surge Plan, All-Hazard Response to Disasters. California Emergency Medical Services Authority. Available at: http://bepreparedcalifornia.ca.gov/CDPHPrograms/PublicHealthPrograms/EmergencyPreparednessOffice/EPOProgramsandServices/Surge/SurgeProjectBackground/Documents/DRAFTSURGEPLANRevised121506.pdf. Accessed 04.26.15.

45. Homeland Security. Presidential Policy Directive/PPD-8: National Preparedness. Available at: http://www.dhs.gov/presidential-policy-directive-8-national-preparedness. Accessed 04.26.15.

46. Joint Commission on Accreditation of Healthcare Organizations. Health Care at the Crossroads: Strategies for Creating and Sustaining Community-wide Emergency Preparedness Systems. Available at: http://www.jointcommission.org/assets/1/18/emergency_preparedness.pdf. Accessed 04.26.15.

47. The Joint Commission. Clarifications and Expectations: Environment of Care Management Plans. Available at: http://www.jointcommission.org/assets/1/6/EOCManagementPlans.pdf. Accessed 04.26.15.

48. The Joint Commission. Case Study: Multiple-site Ambulatory Organization Performs Hazard Vulnerability Analysis. Available at: http://www.jointcommission.org/assets/1/18/ECN-2003-March_Case_Study.pdf. Accessed 04.26.15.

49. New England Center for Emergency Preparedness. Modular Emergency Medical System: (p.6: MEMS Structure and Operational Overview). Available at: http://www.dmsnecep.org/files/mems.pdf. Accessed 04.26.15.

50. Aur der Heide E. Principles of hospital disaster planning. In: Hogan DE, Burstein JL, eds. *Disaster Medicine*. Philadelphia, PA: Lippincott Williams & Wilkins; 2002.

51. Milsten A. Hospital responses to acute-onset disasters: a review. *Prehospital Disaster Med*. 2000;15(1):32–45.

52. U.S. Department of Health and Human Services, Public Health Emergency. Health Resources and Services Administration. Hospital Preparedness Program. Overview Available at: http://www.phe.gov/Preparedness/planning/hpp/Pages/overview.aspx. Accessed 04.26.15.

53. Centers for Disease Control and Prevention. Continuation Guidance Budget Year Five. Available at: http://www.cdc.gov/phpr/documents/coopagreement-archive/FY2004/readiness-attacha.pdf; see Section II; page 3. Accessed 04.26.15.

54. Budde K, Gougelet R. Developing low-flow oxygen capacity in alternate care sites: a collaborative approach to strengthening medical surge capability. Poster Presentation, Preparedness Summit, Atlanta, Georgia, April 2014.

55. Connell, RP. Disaster Mitigation in Hospitals: Factors Influencing Organizational Decision-Making on Hazard Loss Reduction. Thesis. Available at: http://ns.bvs.hn/docum/crid/HospitalesSeguros/MULTIMEDIA/PDF/doc16_connell_thesis.pdf. Accessed 04.26.15.

56. Trust for America's Health. Public Health Emergency Preparedness Cooperative Agreement (CDC). Hospital Preparedness Program (ASPR) Fiscal Year 2015 Appropriations Request. Available at: http://healthyamericans.org/health-issues/wp-content/uploads/2014/03/FY2015-PHEP-HPP.pdf. Accessed 04.26.15.

57. ABC News. Drills That Readied Boston Hospitals, EMS for Bombings Face Funding Cuts. April 26, 2013. Available at: http://abcnews.go.com/Health/emergency-drills-readied-boston-bombings-face-funding-cuts/story?id=19044714. Accessed 04.26.15.

58. Association of State and Territorial Health Officials and National Association of County and City Health Officials. Letter to Majority Leader Reid and Minority Leader McConnell. May 7, 2012. Available at: http://www.astho.org/WorkArea/DownloadAsset.aspx?id=6977. Accessed 04.26.15.

59. Health Affairs Blog. Health Care Preparedness Funding: Are We Inviting Disaster? Available at: http://healthaffairs.org/blog/2013/12/31/health-care-preparedness-funding-are-we-inviting-disaster/. Accessed 04.26.15.

60. CDC. *Capability 10: Medical Surge*. Available at: http://www.cdc.gov/phpr/capabilities/capability10.pdf. Accessed 04.26.15.

SUGGESTED READINGS

1. Pan American Health Organization and World Health Organization. Guidelines for Vulnerability Reduction in the Design of New Health Facilities. Available at: www.paho.org/english/dd/ped/vulnerabilidad.htm. Accessed 04.26.15.

2. Pan American Health Organization and World Health Organization. Principles of Disaster Mitigation in Health Facilities. Available at: http://www.paho.org/English/PED/fundaeng.htm. Accessed 04.26.15.

3. U.S. Department of Health and Human Services. Medical Surge Capacity and Capability: Available at: http://www.phe.gov/Preparedness/planning/mscc/handbook/Documents/mscc080626.pdf. Accessed 04.26.15.

4. Pan American Health Organization and World Health Organization. Protecting New Health Care Facilities from Disasters. Available at: http://www.paho.org/english/dd/ped/proteccion.htm. Accessed 04.26.15.

CHAPTER 28

Disaster Risk Management

Rajnish Jaiswal, Joseph Donahue, and Michael J. Reilly

OVERVIEW OF DISASTER RISK MANAGEMENT

Risk, as it relates to the health care system during and following a disaster, has several meanings that health care emergency managers, hospital administrators, and physician leaders should consider when performing comprehensive risk management as part of disaster planning at a health care facility. The different definitions of risk that are appropriate for hospital emergency planners to consider include the following:

- Risk of damage to the physical structure or infrastructure of the health care facility
- Risk to patients, visitors, and staff from the hazard of concern
- Risk of loss of revenue from cancellation of elective procedures or patients choosing other facilities for services in the future because the facility was not well protected and was damaged or contaminated
- Risk of liability and monetary damage from insurance claims or litigation related to the actions or inactions of the hospital or its staff during or following an event

Physicians and health care administrators have an ethical, moral, and professional obligation to provide clinical care consistent with the appropriate standards of care and to provide safe facilities where ill and injured victims of disasters, terrorism, or public health emergencies can receive care. Although clinical competence and facility readiness are paramount in the health system's response to a disaster event, whenever care is provided, it is often subject to scrutiny and sometimes litigation following a disaster, as evidenced by the civil and criminal proceedings concerning the care provided in New Orleans-based health care facilities following hurricanes Katrina and Rita in 2005. Although physician leaders and health care administrators might find it counterintuitive, there underlies a complex web of liability and malpractice concerns unique to the delivery of patient care during and following disasters.

Although some federal and state laws exist that waive certain requirements and make it easier for the health care system to operate during a major disaster, including certain liability protections for health professionals who may choose to volunteer, gaps remain that rarely indemnify health care providers or facilities from all risk and liability during a disaster response. Considering these situations during disaster planning activities and involving physician leaders, hospital administration, and legal counsel in planning activities will promote a discussion of risk management that may allow for the better preparation for risk reduction activities by medical staff when responding to the community's health care needs during a disaster. There are three main areas of consideration related to risk management and minimization related to health care emergency preparedness: ethical, legal, and operational. Each of these areas is discussed in more detail in the sequel.

Ethical Considerations

Most ethical challenges related to the provision of patient care during or following a disaster, act of terrorism, or public health emergency are related to two primary concepts: (1) our duty to act, and (2) our obligation as health care professionals to above all, do no harm. As patients present to health care facilities, emergency departments (EDs), urgent care centers, or physicians' offices seeking care for disaster-related illness or injury, providers can typically handle a specific number or volume of patients at a certain level of acuity before they become overwhelmed by the numbers or severity of cases that present. This fundamental concept of supply and demand is pertinent to the study of disaster science. Disasters, by nature, are emergencies where the resources needed to respond to or manage an event exceed what is readily available to meet that need. If four moderately injured victims from a car accident present in a hospital ED, most facilities would be able to handle these injuries with the number of physicians, nurses, diagnostic services, operating suites, and inpatient resources that an acute care hospital would routinely possess.

However, if we modified this scenario to the collapse of a section of bleachers at a college football game where 400 patients were injured, it is unlikely that this same hospital would be as effective at attending to all of the victims from this event without needing to alter some standards of care. The concept of altered standards of care is discussed further in this chapter; however, the ethical principle of the allocation of scarce resources is a significant issue that should be considered by hospital emergency planners and ethics committees during mass casualty incidents (MCI). When the needs of multiple patients exceed the clinical or physical resources of the health care facility, and transfer is not an option, how should the hospital address the needs of patients in a manner that allows for the largest number of individuals to survive? This question leads to a discussion of the differences between day-to-day ED triage, where the measurement of priority of care is acuity, compared to disaster triage, where those with injuries or illnesses that are most likely to recover or survive would be treated in lieu of patients whose conditions place them in a high likelihood of mortality.

There are a few specific ethical considerations for health care emergency planners that typically come up during disaster planning. All are associated, in some way, with the allocation of scarce resources.

Ventilator Allocation

Acute care hospitals typically have a fixed number of ventilators available for patients. Some of these are located on critical care units, others in the operating suites, and others in the ED. If patients come to a hospital with syndromes of illness that progress to respiratory failure or other conditions that require intubation and ventilator therapy, what would be the triage procedure for determining which patients would receive a ventilator versus which patients would not? This question is particularly salient in the setting of pandemics, severe acute respiratory syndrome (SARS), and other emerging infectious disease threats, including those from bioterrorism.

What guidance could the medical leadership, the general counsel of the hospital, and the ethics committee give to attending physicians to assist in making this determination when there is a finite number of ventilators and many patients require ventilator therapy? Conceivably the astute clinician would be able to prevent the need for some patients to be intubated by using aggressive medication therapy, and the use of noninvasive continuous positive airway pressure (CPAP)- or bi-level positive airway pressure (BiPAP)-type devices. However, as with all scarce resource events, there is inevitably a tipping point where demand exceeds availability and physicians will need to provide supportive therapy only to a certain subpopulation of patients, while placing others on ventilators. This decision is one that should be supported by clear guidance that is medically sound, ethically appropriate, and legal defensible.

Critical Care Admission Thresholds

Acute care hospitals may have one or more critical care inpatient units. This may vary in sophistication from a single intensive care unit (ICU) within a small community hospital to a number of ICUs and intermediate care units in larger tertiary medical centers. Typically, due to the severity and clinical acuity of the patients admitted to these units, the patient-to-staff ratios are kept low, so that changes in status are rapidly identified and patients who require more intensive treatments or procedures are attended to by an appropriate number of nurses, mid-level practitioners, and physicians. During a disaster, act of terrorism, or public health emergency, there may be a larger number of patients who require critical care admission than there are available beds. Medical leadership along with hospital administration and the hospital ethics committee should develop a rapid discharge tool for attending physicians to use in situations where it is prudent to move certain patients to subacute care floors, or discharge them to other facilities in order to create more critical care surge capacity within the facility. A second aspect of critical care surge management is the adjustment of the staff-to-patient ratio. If critical care units possess beds that are unfilled because of staffing levels, these beds should be used or, as space permits, beds could be added and the ratio of nurses and house staff to patients increased. This would require more staff; however, it may allow for a temporary ability to handle more admissions to critical care units during or following disasters.

Triage of Pharmaceuticals and Medical Countermeasures

As with the discussion above of ventilator allocation, hospitals may not have an endless supply of pharmaceuticals or medical countermeasures to an agent of concern during a calamity, especially in an austere setting. Many hospitals write preparedness plans which specify that they would contact other hospitals to obtain necessary medications, or use caches of medical equipment and supplies such as the Strategic National Stockpile (SNS), or even enter into preferred vendor agreements where vendors would maintain an inventory of supplies that are earmarked for a specific hospital. This strategy is helpful for a local or geographically limited event; however, in a regionwide event where all health care facilities need the same types of supplies, a shortage is likely to develop, and hospitals may not be able to keep sufficient stock of medical countermeasures specific to the illness or agent of concern. In this case, if alternative countermeasures are not appropriate or clinically effective, it may be necessary for the physician leadership, pharmacist-in-charge, and the ethics committee to develop an appropriate formulary tool that goes beyond the indications for use promulgated by the health department or the Centers for Disease Control (CDC). This is one reason that The Joint Commission has required

facilities to adopt the 96-hour rule of self-sufficiency before relying upon external resources during a disaster.[1]

Elective Procedures and Outpatient Units

Elective procedures are often rescheduled or delayed during a disaster or public health emergency that requires the hospital to activate its emergency plan. Outpatient units provide useful space for housing patients, and the additional medical staff is useful in supplementing the needs on inpatient floors or at alternate care sites (ACSs) within the facility. Access to imaging, additional ventilators, operating suites, and ancillary services can contribute positively to a hospital's ability to handle a surge during or following a disaster. Trigger points on when to make these decisions are ones that should be discussed by hospital administration, emergency planners, and medical leadership in advance of a disaster, and clear guidance on when and how this will be done should be present in emergency plans and understood by decision makers. Staff should be instructed on their alternate functional roles within the hospital should this plan be activated.

Legal Considerations
Altered Standards of Care

In the spectrum of medical malpractice and negligence, the concept of standard of care has caused much confusion, yet ironically often serves as the basis of a legal action. An acceptable definition might be

> *The law exacts of physicians and surgeons in the practice of their profession only that they possess and exercise that reasonable degree of skill, knowledge, and care ordinarily possessed and exercised by members of their profession under similar circumstances, and does not exact from them the utmost degree of care and skill attainable or known to the profession.*[2]

Most physicians are held to the standard of care of what a reasonable physician would do under like circumstances.[3] The anatomy of a successful lawsuit requires that the four basic tenets of negligence—duty, breach of duty, harm, and causation—be satisfied. Treatment or therapy that deviates from the principal of standard of care is tantamount to breach of duty. Though seemingly straightforward in its description, the standard of care concept leaves much room for varied interpretation. These pitfalls are only exaggerated during a disaster and MCI. There exists no universally accepted definition of standard of care.

In large-scale catastrophes, resources are scarce. The demand-and-supply ratio to equipment, medications, supplies, and human resources is unfavorably skewed. Even the very setting of care provided may be outside a hospital or clinic. Within such a drastically altered climate, it would be impossible to provide the same care as in nondisaster situations. Table 28-1 highlights the changing standards as a disaster situation evolves.

In the aftermath of September 11, 2001, an expert panel recommended the formulation and implementation of alterations to the concept of standard of care.[4] The panel suggested having a robust action plan that ensures that the health care system stays functional, involves local community and regional agencies, ensures patient safety and privacy, and provides adequate legal shielding for the volunteers involved. Furthermore, having prior knowledge of and training that applies these altered standards would inevitably lead to better care as opposed to letting volunteers navigate these matters on their own with no planning, prior guidance, or assistance.[5]

The proposed alteration or revision of these standards raises questions of its own. Why should these standards be altered or changed during a disaster? This question remains a legal and ethical hotbed for debate. The counterargument asserts that such an alteration would

TABLE 28-1	**The Changing Standards as a Disaster Situation Evolves**			
	LEVEL OF STANDARDS			
STAGE OF DISEASE IN POPULATION	**NORMAL MEDICAL CARE STANDARDS**	**NEAR NORMAL MEDICAL CARE STANDARDS (ALTERNATE SITES OF CARE, USE OF ATYPICAL DEVICES, EXPANDED SCOPE OF PRACTICE)**	**FOCUS ON KEY LIFESAVING CARE (CANNOT OFFER EVERYONE HIGHEST LEVEL BUT CAN OFFER LIFESAVING CARE)**	**TOTAL SYSTEM/ STANDARDS ALTERATION (QUESTIONS ASKED ABOUT WHO GETS ACCESS TO WHAT RESOURCES)**
Prerelease of agent	✓			
Release of responses	✓	✓		
Symptomatic		✓	✓	
Illness			✓	✓
Death			✓	✓

Data from Dr Michael Allswede, University of Pittsburgh, UPMC Health System.

promote deviation from necessary care, and that alteration of standards essentially means a deterioration of standards. Furthermore, the very definition of standards of care permits extenuating circumstances and hence requires no further changes.[6] An extrapolation of this argument in legal parlance predicts that any alteration would be detrimental to patient care and that physicians should be awarded no special considerations or immunity even during catastrophic circumstances[7] Altered standards of care can be defined as a substantial change in usual health care operations and the level of care it is possible to deliver, made necessary by a pervasive (e.g., pandemic influenza) or catastrophic (e.g., earthquake, hurricane) disaster.[8]

In 2009 The Institute of Medicine proposed guidelines for "Crisis Standards of Care" that allow for some deviation from the norm yet encourage evidence-based, legally sound, and ethically commensurate practices.[9] These propositions were formed after extensive analysis of previous disaster responses, assessing their shortcomings and pitfalls and incorporating new research and development in the field. These guidelines also take into account the ever-changing circumstances of a disaster and allow a transition from conventional standards to contingency and crisis care. Thus they provide an operational framework for responders. These guidelines, however sound, have not been universally accepted.

In a further attempt to demystify this concept, some states like Massachusetts have proposed formal, concise guidelines as to how and when the standard of care may be altered during public emergencies and disasters.[10] These guidelines allow such alterations only in areas that have been designated as disaster zones by the Governor, implemented only when deemed necessary and for a finite period of time. Such conditions would be reevaluated continually. The guidelines also accommodate physician discretion.

Critics of altered standards of care postulate that these alterations are counterproductive and would have unfavorable consequences, most notably for the patients and victims involved. Such alterations are viewed as deteriorations in standards of care, and compliance with them as providing inferior care, though no evidence of such outcomes exists. Furthermore it is hypothesized that such practices would cause more confusion and place greater burden on implementation while removing any accountability of providers in disaster care, making the situation "a race to the bottom."[11] Another counterpoint argues that the fear of litigation and liability is overstated and is not substantiated by real cases. These criticisms, however, fail to acknowledge the gaps that exist in the legal framework of disaster care and understate the liability on providers. Litigation continues to be a justifiable concern for emergency technicians, volunteers, and physicians; these altered standards provide some protection.

Quality health care is a byproduct of competent physicians, nurses, auxiliary supporting staff, and appropriate resources that are administered in a secure and safe environment. Some or most of these components are critically deficient in large-scale catastrophic events. The goals and objectives of disaster care are also different. The focus is not on heroic resuscitations to save an individual but on saving the maximum number of lives with limited resources. This changed focus alters the medical management and disposition of critical patients. Disaster preparedness and response efforts must reflect these alterations and so should the standards of care.

Disaster planning starts well before any impending catastrophe. The greatest tool for management is planning and preparation. Having a well-executed, cogent, pragmatic, and realistic plan forms the basis of disaster care. Designation and allocation of responsibility are critical as all actors involved need to know their roles. Furthermore, collaboration is an integral part of the disaster response. Communicating and cooperating with state, federal, regional, and local agencies itself can be a challenge, and mechanisms must be in place to facilitate such efforts.

Triage Protocols

The word triage comes from French word *trier* (to sort or separate), a military concept born on the battlefields of the Napoleonic wars. Today it is an integral part of most EDs around the country. Though military medicine has its own defined triage protocols, civilian triage of MCIs is somewhat different. In his memoirs, Dominique Jean Larrey, Chief Surgeon of Napoleon's Imperial guard and the father of military and triage medicine, stated that "those who are dangerously wounded should receive the first attention, without regard to rank or distinction."[12] The basic purpose of triage still remains the same as Larrey envisioned, to risk-stratify patients and prioritize resource allocation, medical and nonmedical, to those who are likely to receive the most benefit. To paraphrase a famous quote, it is the "the greatest good for the greatest number."[13] An ideal triage system would be easy to understand, identify and deliver resources in a timely manner, be adaptive and evolve with the rapid change in surroundings, optimize resource allocation, neither underestimate the injuries of a critical patient (undertriage), nor divert unnecessary resources by overstating the patient's condition (overtriage). Overtriage has been shown to actually worsen patient outcomes.[14]

No system is perfect, and triage protocols continue to advance. Many triage systems exist, some borrowed from the military like the North America Treaty Organization triage protocol,[15] while others like the simple triage and rapid treatment (START) protocol were designed for use by untrained or minimally trained individuals for civilian use in an MCI.[16] START and its pediatric version, JumpSTART, continue to be popular systems whereby patients are essentially distributed under a color coded scheme, red being the most urgent and black being those who are beyond saving ("expectant") or already deceased.

Triage systems continue be region specific and operator dependent. These discrepancies are magnified during a large-scale catastrophe, and hence MCI triage guidelines are critical to future response scenarios. These criteria would include general considerations, global sorting, life-saving interventions, and assignment of triage categories.[17] In an effort to standardize and universalize mass casualty triage, an expert committee performed a detailed analysis and review of existing triage systems and proposed the SALT (sort, assess, lifesaving intervention, transport) system.[18] This is one of the most exhaustive and detailed analyses of all existing triage systems in place. After much deliberation, the committee proposed the Model Uniform Core Criteria (MUCC) protocol for mass casualty triage. MUCC include 24 specific criteria that are detailed yet easy to implement, allow greater interoperator consistency, and permit further modifications. Most triage systems, including SALT, currently use 15 of these criteria. Though MUCC was well received in the disaster preparedness community, its formal acceptance and implementation nationwide remains a challenge. As of 2010, only 18 states in the United States had implemented statewide MUCC-compliant mass casualty triage protocols.[19] SALT was conceived so as to make triage easy to understand across jurisdictions, avoid confusion, and improve outcomes. Although it appears effective in principle, further research needs to be undertaken to establish the efficacy of such a system in large-scale disasters. The National Disaster Life Support Foundation (NDLSF) offers training in SALT along with other methodologies for disaster preparedness.

In most hospital emergency departments, triage tends to be administered by an experienced nurse. During an MCI, triage ideally should be under the supervision of a trained physician; however, resources may not always permit this. Along with medical decision making, disaster triage also presents many ethical dilemmas, sometimes counterintuitive to the essence of being a physician. The sickest patients may not always get priority if they are deemed unlikely to benefit from the finite resources available. These people may be considered "beyond emergency care." Such patients should be treated with empathy, dignity, and compassion and may benefit from sedation and analgesia.[20]

The concepts of "expectant" patients and "reverse triage" led to one of the most well-known cases of litigation in the aftermath of Hurricane Katrina. Dr. Anna Pou, a practicing surgeon, and her nursing team were assisting in the evacuation of critical patients from Memorial Medical Center. With no imminent help, resources, or guidance, her team decided to reverse-triage evacuees. Those who were unlikely to survive the process were given palliative care with sedation and analgesia. Although there were no specific guidelines to do so, Dr. Pou exercised her clinical judgment in these cases. Volunteer physicians are routinely asked to make such tough choices and expected to formulate, design, and implement such criteria or algorithms, placing an extra burden on them and their ability to care for patients.[21] In one of its most controversial decisions yet, the Louisiana Attorney General's office decided to pursue criminal charges against Dr. Pou and her team for administering palliative doses of sedatives and analgesics to expectant patients. Dr. Pou was a salaried employee, as were her nurses, and thus not considered a volunteer worker, which disqualified her from the legal shield of the Uniform Emergency Volunteer Health Practitioners Act (UEVHPA). (We discuss UEVHPA and other regulations in more detail below.) As stated previously, no laws exist to shield care providers from willful or negligible acts of malpractice. The case against Dr. Pou was subsequently dropped, although civil cases lingered until they were dismissed later. In response, Dr. Pou championed the cause of better protection for health care volunteers and physicians in the State of Louisiana,[22] including salaried and paid workers participating in disaster care. Though such laws were later implemented and have brought better clarity and improved protection in Louisiana, the rest of the nation still lags behind.

Triage is the first step in disaster response and the most crucial. Having a well-executed plan that involves all agencies is the first step in effective triage. These plans must be implemented under controlled settings to identify deficiencies and pitfalls and must learn and evolve from mistakes. Having a dedicated Triage Committee is beneficial. Such a committee can routinely assess the effectiveness of current triage protocols, design and implement routine exercises for all responders and volunteers, liaise with local and state emergency planning committees, and maintain a vigilant review of MCI triage success and failures. Committee members themselves should attend workshops and seminars to keep abreast of the latest developments in this field. Such practices would not only ensure the best possible delivery of care but also mitigate risk management.

Modified Scopes of Practice

Physician Assistants. During the physician shortage in the United States in the 1960s, a movement to create and promote the use of nonphysician health care providers was established. Physician assistant (PA) and nurse practitioner (NP) programs have flourished and today form an integral tool for delivering quality health care, with disaster situations being no exception. The American Academy of Physician Assistants (AAPA) has a detailed position paper that delineates the role of PAs in disasters and large-scale emergencies and addresses issues of scope of practice, reciprocity, licensure, and legal protection.[23]

The AAPA position paper states that disaster care begins with effective and competent training and discourages untrained volunteers to participate in response efforts. It also recommends that PAs register in advance with accredited relief agencies such as the Red Cross or Disaster Medical Assistance Teams (DMATs) created as part of the National Disaster Medical System (NDMS). This allows verified and credentialed personnel to be readily deployed in a disaster scenario. Communication with physicians and nurses in the response team is essential as PAs bring their own set of skills and expertise that must be maximally used. Defining their role and expectations is critical, as sometimes PAs may be the most skilled and capable personnel in a response team that includes physicians and nurses. The AAPA also advises its members to familiarize themselves with local, state, and federal laws regarding disaster care and take the initiative to understand the existing legal framework. Such knowledge serves as an important tool in negotiating the risk management landscape.

Advanced Practice Nurses. Born in the battlegrounds of the Crimean War and pioneered by Florence Nightingale, the profession of nursing has been an intricate part of health care delivery and continues to enjoy great prominence and advancing scope of practice. Wartime experiences with nursing demonstrated the critical services nurses provide when dealing with the sick and injured. The First and Second World Wars actively mobilized and deployed volunteer nurses, predominantly with the Red Cross, mostly women.[24] Nursing became an independent service of its own for the Red Cross in 1909.[25] Their experience and learning have shaped the course of modern day emergency nursing. Today nurses form the largest group of the health care workforce.[26] Although training and education of nurses have improved and evolved, disaster preparedness continues to be a critical deficiency.[27] Columbia University developed emergency preparedness core competencies for hospital workers in 2003 that have been widely cited throughout the literature. These deserve review when considering emergency preparedness content for nursing education.[28]

NPs were trained as physician extenders primarily to shoulder the burden of primary and preventative care. Their scope of practice continues to broaden as the nation struggles to meet its demands for qualified health care personnel. NPs are likely to also be crucial in disaster preparing and planning. As the physician extender's responsibilities grow in the United States, the NPs' positions in the community allow them to serve as a great medium to transmit awareness and model preparedness. NPs are trained to be exceptional planners, and this role should be maximized within the interdisciplinary emergency preparedness team in all communities.[29]

Allied health and mid-level provider volunteers are subject to the same laws and regulations as physician volunteers and are also afforded the similar legal protections. NPs have proven to be highly reliable and efficient workers in such measures.[30] Qualified and competent mid-level providers have been shown to decrease medical liability,[31] although whether this trend extends to disaster situations remains unclear.

Advanced Prehospital Providers (Paramedics).

Advanced practice prehospital providers, specifically paramedics, possess a skill set similar or superior to that of an ED's registered nurse and can perform similar procedures with little supervision and under direct or standing orders from a physician. Not all disasters or public health emergencies require a robust prehospital response; for example, in the case of a pandemic or an emerging infectious disease, emergency medical services providers can be a useful surge workforce augmenting traditional health care professionals. Studies have shown that the clinical competencies of paramedics are quite congruent with those of ED and critical care registered nurses. This could be a useful consideration for the inclusion of paramedics as part of health care facility surge staffing plans, particularly in facilities that employ paramedics as part of a hospital-based emergency medical services system.[32,33]

Health Profession Students.

There is limited experience with health profession students acting beyond the expectations of lay volunteers in disaster care, particularly medical students. Undergraduate medical school curriculums usually are insufficient in addressing disaster medicine and preparedness.[34] Nursing students, however, have been used by health departments and hospitals as both "victims" during disaster drills and exercises and as vaccinators and clerical staff during point of dispensing (POD) exercises. The use of undergraduate health profession students, particularly nursing students, in drills and exercises, as well as by departments of health in medical countermeasure plans has been well documented in the medical and allied health literature. Important considerations for risk management in any situation where health profession students are used include supervision, malpractice liability, and scope of practice.

Students who are not specifically trained to deal with the professional and personal challenges that accompany such work are unlikely to provide quality care and in some cases may engender unfortunate consequences for themselves or their patients.[35] A recent example from events in Kashmir highlighted these issues. Volunteer medical students were unprepared for the complex medical, surgical, and psychosocial issues that arose; they would have benefited from prior training and preparation. Third- and fourth-year medical students may be particularly suited to participate in such measures[36] and are usually eager to learn.[37] However, as mentioned previously, students should always work under qualified supervisors, not just for legal precautions but as an ethical and professional obligation toward patients.

Credentialing of Volunteer Health Care Providers.

Catastrophic events routinely overwhelm the resources of a health care system for mounting an effective disaster response[38] A substantial portion of the disaster response team, including physicians, nurses, and mid-level providers, may come from adjacent or nearby regions as well as other states and occasionally from other countries. The aftermath of the 9/11 attacks saw an unprecedented volunteer response, as physicians, mid-level providers, nurses, and students from all backgrounds arrived offering their help.

Additionally, untrained individuals walked into secure areas wearing scrubs and rendered "medical" aid without verification of credentials or even the identity of the individual.[39] Conventional methods to scrutinize training and offer privileges was not feasible in such a situation and would have taken too much time, a luxury most disasters do not permit. The government was required to make sure that all survivors and victims would be put in the care of people who had the right background, experience and training to help them. In 2006, as part of the Pandemic and All-Hazards Preparedness Act, the federal government introduced the Emergency System for Advance Registration of Volunteer Health Professionals (ESAR-VHP).[40] This act was introduced to eliminate obstacles in mobilizing health care forces across state lines. It functions under a four-level system of credentialing and is administered by Assistant Secretary for Preparedness and Response (ASPR). Another attempt at precredentialing of health and medical volunteers prior to a disaster was the formation of the Medical Reserve Corps.

In 1996 Congress confirmed the Emergency Management Assistance Compact (EMAC) in an effort to provide a legal framework for the transfer of aid, resources, and personnel to a governor-declared disaster zone from another state or territory. Not since the Civil Defense Compact of 1950 had there been a nationwide disaster compact ratified by Congress. In 2005 EMAC allowed over 2000 health care professionals from 28 states to treat over 160,000 patients.[41] Although it stands as the nation's premier mutual aid delivery platform, EMAC has its own limitations. It only allows preregistered state or federal employees to contribute toward aid efforts, thus excluding private or unregistered volunteers from participation. Furthermore, only health care volunteers registered with EMAC are afforded protection under the Federal Torts Claims Act (FTCA), which provides legal immunity for such workers. These limitations were tragically obvious during the Gulf Coast hurricanes of the late 90s and early 2000s. FTCA was preceded by the Federal Volunteer Protection Act (FVPA) of 1997, which provided legal immunity to volunteer workers from nonprofit organizations, provided they did not receive any remuneration over $500 per year.[42] A consideration in using out-of-state workers under EMAC agreements is the need to secure malpractice coverage and verify credentialing to minimize risk and liability exposure.

In 2005 the National Conference of Commissioners on Uniform State Laws (NCCUSL) proposed UEVHPA. This act was envisioned with idea of providing a legal platform for interstate cooperation between government and private sectors by allowing qualified volunteers to provide much-needed assistance to disaster-stricken regions. UEVHPA maintains a database of preregistered volunteers who can be effectively deployed to provide care without excessive delays for state credentialing, background checks, etc. It also allows expedited registration during an emergency for volunteers who are not already in the system. Most states receiving these volunteers (host states) reserve the right to determine the role and capacity of these volunteers and usually do not permit any activity outside their scope of practice. In 2007 NCCUSL approved further amendments to the UEVHPA regarding civil liability protection for volunteer workers, providing more specific language regarding the application of this law.[43] As is the case with all these laws, acts of willful, wanton misconduct or criminal activity are exempt from these scenarios.

As these efforts continue, the legal community argues over immunity for volunteer physicians. One school of thought proposes that there is no evidence that shows that lack of, or unclear, immunity for physicians hampers volunteer participation in disasters, although some studies find otherwise.[44] An extrapolation of this point of view is that altruistic physicians are rarely deterred in such cases, and shielding volunteer physicians creates a division of those who can be held accountable versus those who cannot. Not all physicians who deliver care during crises are volunteers. Non-volunteer physicians are compensated and remunerated for their services and are held liable for malpractice. Non-volunteers tend to treat patients who are financially sounder, whereas volunteers are likely to treat the indigent and destitute. Giving volunteers immunity would take away any legal recourse for the most indigent and destitute should they receive substandard care. Protecting volunteer physicians has been called "unwise, unnecessary and unjust."[8]

These arguments, however, are an overt simplification and idealization of existing laws and procedures. They ignore the fact that volunteer health professionals risk their lives, livelihoods and their own well-being in disasters; to ignore the legal ramifications that these volunteers may be faced with or to deny them any protection will ultimately be detrimental to the future of disaster response.[45]

Waiver of State and Federal Health Care Laws and Regulations

Health Insurance Portability and Accountability Act. In 1996 Congress passed the Health Insurance Portability and Accountability Act (HIPAA) to legislate the transmission and release of protected health information held by the so-called covered entities, along with health care access, portability, and renewability. These entities include health care providers, health insurers, and health care clearing houses. Under this law, the exchange or disclosure of personal health information without the patient's consent would be considered a civil or criminal offense.[46] In a disaster or declared emergency, however, observing privacy rules can be challenging. According to the Department of Health and Human Services (DHHS), HIPAA is not suspended during declared emergencies, although certain provisions such as obtaining consent prior to sharing information with family members may be waived.[47] Provisions are also allowed for "covered entities" to share private information with other disaster relief organizations including those from the private sector.[48] These waivers are not generalized or indefinite and apply to specific areas of declared emergencies and to explicit hospitals where disaster protocols have been activated for an explicit time period, usually 72 hours. The Office of Civil Rights (OCR) oversees HIPAA compliance and offers a "Decision Tool" for advanced planning for relief organizations to further guide and clarify what HIPAA waivers and provisions can be allowed in disasters. At the time of publication there has not been verification by the Office of Civil Rights of any reported HIPAA violations related to release of PHI during a disaster response.

Emergency Medical Treatment and Active Labor Act. Enacted in 1986, the Emergency Medical Treatment and Active Labor Act (EMTALA) was conceived to prevent hospitals and emergency rooms from withholding or refusing care to the uninsured or transferring such patients to other facilities. EMTALA is a federal law that is regulated under the Center for Medicaid Services (CMS). In brief, it requires all Medicare-participating hospitals with dedicated emergency departments to provide a medical screening exam (MSE) to all those who seek care at their emergency room and determine if an emergency medical condition (EMC) exists. Should an EMC be identified, the hospital is obligated to stabilize the patient and, if deemed necessary, transfer him or her to another hospital that has the means and capacity to provider further care to that patient.[49]

In its original format, EMTALA made no provisions for MCIs or disasters, placing the burden of compliance on emergency departments even if overwhelmed with patients. In the wake of 9/11 and multiple flu pandemics, CMS introduced an amendment that would provide waivers for patient transfers during declared disasters in emergency areas; such transfers would not be considered EMTALA violations even if they do not meet the guidelines.[50] No provisions were made for the MSE component of the law.

As a direct consequence of the terrorist attacks of 9/11, a year later Congress enacted the Public Health Security and Bioterrorism Response Act, which added Section 1135 to the Social Security Act. Under Section 1135, the Secretary of DHHS is allowed to waive certain Medicare and Medicaid requirements, including EMTALA, during emergencies. These waivers apply to transfer and redirection of patients from the emergency department.[51] These waivers, however, only apply to certain regions that have been declared a disaster region by the U.S. President or the Secretary of DHHS for a finite period of time. Local and state emergencies do not qualify for Section 1135.[52] Such a declaration was made on September 4, 2005, in response to Hurricane Katrina. The waiver addressed specific issues such as HIPAA, EMTALA, state licensure, and credentialing, among other things.[53]

CMS has introduced additional guidelines for hospitals responding beyond surge capacity in a pandemic that do not qualify for federal waivers. It delineates administration of MSEs at alternative health facilities that are hospital controlled and reiterates when and where EMTALA waivers apply.[54] It is customary for CMS to announce additional disaster-specific guidelines for EMTALA through its regional offices during active crises. In the spring of 2009, CMS advised New York City hospitals—particularly those experiencing significant increases in emergency department visits—that they could permissibly send patients seeking a flu screening to a specific area of the hospital without violating EMTALA.[55]

Medical Licensing. Licensing and regulation of health care workers are usually the purview of state medical boards or licensing agencies, with no federal involvement. Each medical board has its own unique requirements commensurate with state and local laws that must be satisfied before privileges to practice in health care are granted. In disasters and large-scale emergencies, these processes are too slow and cumbersome to license out-of-state health care professionals. After the 9/11 attacks, North General Hospital received a significant number of patients that overwhelmed the existing providers. A number of volunteer physicians who were not credentialed at the hospital were allowed to provide care under New York State's education law that permits for licensed physicians to provide emergency care.[56] In response to multiple disasters, The Joint Commission formulated guidelines for hospitals regarding credentialing and privileges for a volunteer licensed independent practitioner (LIP) that allows temporary privileges to external practitioners when the hospital's emergency management plan has been activated.[57] These standards have now been adopted by most states, including New York.[58]

In contrast to these waivers to state licensing regulations, New York State has also prohibited the use of paramedics in ACSs within the state that are set up during public health emergencies. The rationale is that paramedics are certified, not licensed, and limitations on their certification prohibit them from operating within a fixed health care facility.

This has placed a significant burden on local and county health departments, which need staff who can establish intravenous lines and administer intravenous medications during a public health emergency and do not have the numbers of registered nurses to staff these sites appropriately.[59] A potential solution to this is a formal request to the State Commissioner of Health for a waiver during the duration of a declared public health emergency. Although, many state agencies will not issue waivers prospectively, it is likely they would consider them during an actual event.

As discussed earlier, the EMAC and UEVHPA are legislative platforms that can be used in large-scale operations and provide liability protection to volunteer workers. EMAC has been criticized for not including private sector resources, and UEVHPA is only applicable in a few states in the country, leaving much room for discrepancy and inconsistency. Efforts are being made to centralize or federalize a nationwide uniform system that would allow for the expedited licensing of volunteers. The American College of Emergency Physicians (ACEP) recommends that all hospitals have an emergency credentialing protocol in place should a need to arise to credential nonfacility physicians in a disaster situation.[60]

Operational Considerations

Disasters create a wide range of challenges on an operational level for hospitals. In order to mitigate an event, ranging from the most straightforward component of finding staff and space to see to the surge of patients associated with a natural disaster, pandemic condition, or terrorist event, to the more complex considerations of supply chains and providing adequate food for patients and staff, extensive planning should take place prior to the event. Surveys of staff, tabletop exercises, and simulated disasters all play a role in the development of disaster plans and stockpiles. Advance warning of an event such as Hurricane Sandy in New York City or the 2009 H1N1 influenza pandemic allows for specific measures to be taken just prior to the event. Alternatively, sudden events such as the terrorist attacks on 9/11 or the theater shooting in Aurora, Colorado, rely on systems already in place to run efficiently. Reflecting on prior events provides a framework to prepare for the future.

Reducing Nonessential Hospital Operations. In the setting of an emergency, providing and planning for patient care become the absolute priority. It has become standard for hospitals to designate essential versus nonessential personnel. Essential personnel include all employees with patient care responsibilities, food services, and maintenance and facility management, among others. Reducing nonessential personnel assures that the limited resources available can be dedicated to enhancing surge capacity or caring for current patients. In certain settings, nonessential personnel may be reassigned to essential roles. For example, a greeter or volunteer may be assigned to assist with patient flow. A physician who acts primarily as a researcher or in the clinic may be reassigned to assist with ED overflow areas.[61] Employees should be clearly assigned as essential or nonessential and reporting guidelines should be established before an event to assure proper staffing.

Closing Outpatient Services. Outpatient services serve an important role in hospital operations and support the practices of physicians affiliated with the hospital. However, they also use a large number of nursing, physician, laboratory, and other resources that may be strained in an event that limits access or increases utilization of these resources. Hurricane Sandy, which struck New York City in October of 2012, is an example where hospitals proactively closed outpatient services to focus efforts on an anticipated need for increased surge capacity. Many of these clinics remained closed because of damage or to allow staff to assist in evacuation efforts after the event.[62] The resources of an outpatient services center, including physicians and nurses, can be reassigned to assist in other areas in such a setting.

Alternatively, outpatient clinics may also serve as a useful buffer for emergency services if used appropriately. Children's Hospital of Philadelphia was faced with a large surge volume of influenza-like illnesses during the H1N1 outbreak in 2009. As the first cases of H1N1 were reported in Philadelphia, an integrated plan involving their outpatient after-hours call program, outpatient clinics, inpatient teams, and EDs was put into place. Routine and preventative visits were cancelled, but many clinics remained open with increased availability for sick visits. Pediatric specialty clinics were at times cancelled, with the space used for ED overflow patients, or saw influenza patients in addition to their normal schedule. These interventions were estimated to decrease ED visits by 11 to 44 per day.[63]

Cancellation of Elective Procedures. Just as outpatient services may be suspended or adapted in preparation or response to an event, establishing a protocol to cancel or delay outpatient surgeries is another way to provide staff to enhance surge capacity or to deal with a large number of casualties caused by an event. Clearly in the setting of an MCI like the 2013 Boston Marathon Bombing or the shootings in Aurora, the large number of casualties requiring surgical intervention would take precedence over an elective procedure. For the expected event of Hurricane Sandy, hospitals suspended elective surgeries for 2 days to increase available staff for emergent cases and to assist with surge capacities.[62]

In the correct setting, surgeries do not have to be cancelled in anticipation of an event, but plans can be made should the surge capacity hit a critical level. Disaster plans for Children's Hospital of Philadelphia during the H1N1 pandemic called for cancellation of elective procedures only when surge capacity hit a critical level, with reassignment of the staff in that event. While the surge capacity was significant, the threshold to cancel outpatient and elective procedures was never surpassed, thereby avoiding the need to delay and reschedule these procedures.[61]

Surge Capacity and Capability

The influx of patients following a disaster can overwhelm the most prepared hospitals. Clearly established plans to identify and treat additional patients require finding space and providers in the ED as well as inpatient and intensive care units. Established protocols through tabletop exercises and simulated events help to identify ways to expand the hospital's capacity.

Emergency Department Surge Capacity. The ED serves as the frontline for the patient surge during and immediately following a disaster. Studies on referral patterns of patients from disasters report that over two thirds of patients from disasters that refer to hospital EDs will not arrive via ambulance.[64] Following Hurricane Sandy, ED volumes increased by 20%; other events such as the H1N1 pandemic have demonstrated similar levels of stress on the department.[62,63,65] Various approaches can be used to mitigate these stresses, depending on the resources of a given hospital and the nature of the event.

ED staffing may be augmented in several ways to increase the capacity and capability of the department to see patients. Additional shifts or volunteer shifts may be added. It may be possible to bring physicians from other departments such as internal medicine, family medicine, or pediatrics to staff extra shifts. In the setting of a closed hospital or other health care facility, credentialing displaced physicians may offset the patient load. Rapid or emergency credentialing is another way to increase staffing. Any of these methods in various combinations may be appropriate for a particular setting, but having established plans in place will allow for a more rapid response.[62,63]

Volumes may also be managed by adapting typical ED workups in the emergency setting to facilitate more rapid discharge. Avoiding nonemergent laboratory tests, will decrease the burden on the laboratory and facilitate rapid return of other, more critical laboratory tests. In other cases, such as a low-acuity influenza, it may be appropriate to forego sending labs or giving intravenous (IV) hydration that would be considered if more resources were available. It may also be possible to facilitate a rapid discharge by condensing workups, such as using a single troponin test or a second troponin test 2 hours later to rule out a cardiac event in an apparent low-risk chest pain patient. These rapid discharges free up nursing, ancillary staff, and physicians to focus on evaluating and treating the sickest patients in the surge. Rapid discharge does not come without risk, and it is important to remember to provide patients with appropriate discharge instructions and return precautions.[66]

Medical/Surgical Beds and Step-Down. Beyond the ED, inpatient wards will also have to deal with the influx of additional patients. Anticipating the surge associated with Hurricane Sandy, New York hospitals proactively managed their inpatient census, discharging 10% to 25% of patients who were safe to send home at that time. When two large hospitals were forced to close because of flooding, this decreased both the number of transfers necessary and allowed other hospitals to accept more patients. Notably, hospitals had significant difficulties arranging for skilled nursing facilities to accept patients on short notice.[62] Similar steps may be taken if there is no advance warning of a disaster, but it would present additional challenges to rapidly discharge inpatients while accepting surge patients.

The physical space of the medical and surgical floors may present challenges or delays in care of the patients. Doubling up patients in rooms or transforming common areas into makeshift care areas or holding areas for newly admitted patients may increase the available space. Hallway spaces, especially as temporary holding areas for newly admitted patients, may be of use as well. These methods can also be used to decrease boarding time for admitted patients in the ED, freeing space for the evaluation of new patients.

Step-down or intermediate care units may also play a valuable role in increasing surge capability. Depending on the particular needs of the event, they can serve lower-acuity admissions overflowing from the inpatient wards. Alternatively, they can accommodate lower-acuity ICU patients and mechanically ventilated patients to increase critical care beds.

Critical Care Surge Capability

Critical care beds are a very limited resource that may be stretched by the surge capability of a disaster. In simulations of MCIs, the first bottleneck that occurred was lack of availability of beds in intensive care units (ICUs).[67] In addition to appropriately identifying the patients who would be best served by these beds, findings ways to safely expand the capacity for critical patients may be necessary.

Similarly to discharging appropriate patients from medical or surgical beds, downgrading the most appropriate patients to a floor bed or step-down unit will free up some of the space in the ICU. Boarding of critical patients in an alternate ICU, such as a patient with acute respiratory distress syndrome (ARDS) in the surgical or cardiac ICU, is the easiest way to increase bed availability. The pediatric ICU may be used to care for younger adult patients, while older pediatric patients may need to be cared for in the medical or other ICU.

If additional critical care beds are needed, then additional space must be found. Transfer of patients to another hospital may be appropriate in some settings. The postanesthesia care unit (PACU) may have critical care capacity in most hospitals. During planning for the H1N1 pandemic surge, plans were made to transfer surgical patients to the PACU in order to free up additional beds on the floor or ICU.[61] Each hospital must carefully consider its available resources to determine the safest way to accommodate an increased flux of critical patients.

Transforming Nonpatient Care Areas into Subacute Holding Areas. When faced with a surge of patients, physical space may become a barrier to department throughput. In this case, urgent care areas have been used to increase acute care areas. Hospital lobbies have been converted to ED patient care areas or waiting rooms. It may also be helpful to create holding areas for admitted patients or to minimize boarding times by expediting transfer to the medical and surgical floors.[62] Challenges associated with these methods include a lack of basic supplies such as oxygen (typically immediately available in the ED setting) so it is necessary to select appropriate acuity patients for these areas.

Mobile Solutions, Tents, etc. In some instances, the physical space available in the hospital may not be enough to accommodate the entire surge. Physical damage to a part of the facility may not be enough to shut down the entire hospital, but could severely reduce the capacity and capability of the hospital. In these settings, various mobile solutions or ACSs may be deployed. Some hospitals have added overflow space designed to increase outpatient or ED volume by building clinics that do not meet all of the building requirements to operate on a daily basis, but that may be used as a place to evaluate patients during an emerging infectious disease outbreak. Tents were deployed to care for lower-acuity injuries and illnesses in the 2013 Boston Marathon Bombing and in Pennsylvania during the influenza epidemic of 2013. In a large-scale event, a federal medical station may be set up to assist a hospital. Federal medical stations are part of the SNS and are designed to assist damaged or overwhelmed existing medical facilities. They include supplies and pharmaceuticals to treat 250 patients for up to 3 days for both emergency and lower-acuity inpatients. They also provide some support for critical care and specialized units.[68]

Supply Chain Issues. Supply chains are vital to the successful delivery of medical care in a hospital. Both small-scale surge events and major incidents that disrupt basic services compromise the ability of the facility to continue to provide care in a safe and efficient manner. Through a combination of stockpiling within a hospital, interfacility and supplier agreements, and the use of national stockpiles, it is possible to mitigate some of the difficulties caused by these disruptions.

Medical Equipment and Supplies. Basic medical supplies are critical to the effective delivery of medical care. There are many supplies that are commonly needed in disasters, such as intravenous fluids, airway management equipment, medications, cardiac monitors, and syringes and needles. Whether dealing with pandemic flu, explosives, radiation, or another event, these common supplies will be necessary, and a local stockpile within the hospital should be considered.[69] Beyond the first 12 to 24 hours, additional supplies should become available through the SNS.

In addition to basic medical supplies, other medical equipment must be available in an emergency. Items such as batteries must be available and charged. Personal protective equipment and masks, wheelchairs, beds, oxygen tanks, flashlights, etc., should be considered while making disaster plans. Another critical resource, ventilators, may be in short supply in a disaster. The SNS includes 4000 ventilators in the managed inventory that can arrive at a given location within 24 to 36 hours following a federal disaster declaration and request from the State Department of Health for the assets.[70] As space may become an issue in an overcrowded unit, smaller models or units that can be placed on a bed may be of increased value in this setting.

Linen. Basic necessities that are given in normal situations can become a precious resource in a disaster setting. Extra sheets, pillows, blankets, and towels are a given resource in normal operating conditions that may become scarce in the setting of a surge or disrupted supply chains. External laundering services may not be available to provide clean linen to a hospital. Disrupted water supplies may prevent laundering in-house. Limited supplies may not be adequate in the setting of a surge. For these reasons it is important to include linen in a hospital's disaster plans.

Dirty or improperly cleaned linen may be a source of infection or contamination in a disaster. In a Louisiana hospital, an outbreak of mucormycosis over an 11-month period led to five pediatric deaths. The source of the infection was determined to be linen that was not handled appropriately; 26 of 62 environmental samples of clean linen were found to be contaminated.[71] In the setting of a biological or chemical attack or contamination, strict adherence to protocols for proper laundering becomes even more important.

A comprehensive plan for management of hospital linens in the setting of a disaster should include several components. A reasonable stockpile of clean linen to support the surge capacity of the hospital should be available at all times.[72] Clear guidelines for increasing turnaround times for in-house laundering should be in place. If available, preexisting plans for mutual aid from local area hospitals or with local laundry businesses may be of use.[73] An extremely conservative use of linens should be considered, with changes of linens only when absolutely necessary and a strict limit of linen use for patient care. Hospital staff and permitted patient family members should provide their own linen when possible for their sleeping quarters so as to reserve hospital linen for patient care. Clean linen should not be used to clean spills or mitigate flooding or leaks. If circumstances demand, it is acceptable to consider using soiled linen for these purposes, but contaminated linen should not be used for this at any time.[72]

Pharmaceuticals and Medical Countermeasures. Disasters, whether naturally occurring or terrorist in nature, result in a rapid need for medications that could rapidly overwhelm a hospital's normal usage. Additionally, biological, radiological, and chemical incidents require medications and vaccinations rarely used in routine clinical practice. As a consequence, the stockpiling of pharmaceuticals and medical countermeasures has become a critical component of disaster preparedness.

In 1979 the first federally mandated stockpiles were created. The focus at this time was on naturally occurring diseases such as smallpox. Following the Sarin attacks in Japan in 1995, along with the threat of biological weapon production by multiple foreign governments, the federal government created the national pharmaceutical stockpile program, now the SNS program. These resources are intended to augment local stockpiles within a medical facility.[68,74]

The most readily available component of the SNS is the 12-hour push package. This premade package contains 50 tons of medical supplies, pharmaceutical agents, and equipment designed to begin 10-day regimens for up to 300,000 patients. The contents of this package include oral and IV antibiotics, airway management equipment, resuscitation equipment, analgesics, and other emergency supplies. These packages are stored at secret locations around the country and are designed to arrive at the site of a disaster within 12 hours of request by state government or federal agency. A 5- to 7-person Technical Advisory Response Unit is also deployed to assist local authorities in the implementation of the push pack.[68,75]

In addition to the 12-hour push pack, the government has managed inventory supplies. Instead of a preassembled unit, these supplies are specific to the event and are designed to arrive within 24 to 36 hours of request. The managed inventory may be used to augment push pack supplies. It also contains vaccines, antitoxins, chelating agents, ventilators, and additional antibiotics. In smaller scale disasters that do not warrant a full push pack, managed inventory supplies can be requested alone.[68]

Extensive financial investments by the government have been made to generate vaccines and treatments; $4.7 billion has been contributed to the production of cell-based vaccine technology and stockpiling with another $1.4 billion for oseltamivir.[76] Stockpiles of smallpox vaccine are now adequate to vaccinate the entire population of the United States.[77] Additional specific antidotes include the Chempack, which is stored locally in all of the states and contains atropine, pralidoxime, and diazepam. These units are designed to be at the site of an emergency within 1 hour.[78]

Obtaining and maintaining stockpiles of pharmaceuticals and medical countermeasures is an expensive and complicated undertaking. A detailed plan to effectively deploy the countermeasures must be established. The H1N1 influenza pandemic of 2009 serves as an important reminder. While the public health measures undertaken to decrease the spread of disease are suspected to have been largely successful, the deployment of oseltamivir—an antiviral to treat influenza—met with unexpected challenges. Because of cost-saving and shelf life concerns, the Mexican government invested in a dried oral powder requiring reconstitution, with a plan to ship locally for reconstitution. When the pandemic was identified, officials sent the medication, only to learn that local laboratories did not have the necessary components to reconstitute the medication and the medication would have to be shipped back and reconstituted centrally. This with other factors led to a delay of 11 days before the first doses of oseltamivir could be administered.[79]

Food Services. Another critical area of disaster preparation is ensuring an adequate food supply for patients in the setting of limited resources or availability. Loss of water and electricity is the most common problem concerning food services, according to a survey of food service directors, yet the majority of the directors polled were unable to identify alternative water sources or procedures to sanitize the lines if they become contaminated.[80] Hospitals should consider a stockpile of food and water for a minimum of 96 hours, planning for one quart of water per person per day, taking surge capacity into account. In the setting of advance notice of a potential event, consider expanding reserves to a 5- to 7-day supply. Whenever possible, a normal meal schedule should be maintained, though it may be necessary to adapt menus to supplies. Donations may be accepted if necessary. Drinking water should be preserved, and toilets should be flushed only with nonpotable water. Hospital food supplies should be reserved for patients, and physicians or families should plan to bring their own food supplies. Food stockpiles may be rotated for items with limited shelf life to minimize waste. Interfacility transfer agreements should consider transfer of food and water with the patient. Agreements between suppliers can be made in advance to supply hospitals with additional food in these settings. Food and nutritional services employees are critical employees in a disaster, and planning should directly involve the director of food services.[72]

Alternative Care Sites

Developing alternative systems to deliver emergency health services during a pandemic or public health emergency is essential to preserving the operation of acute care hospitals and the overall health care infrastructure. ACSs can serve as areas for primary screening and triage or short-term medical treatment, assist in diverting nonacute patients from hospital EDs, and manage non–life-threatening illnesses in a systematic and efficient manner. In addition to diverting patients to an alternative location where limited medical care can be provided, such as influenza-type care (hydration, bronchodilator therapy, antibiotics and antivirals, etc.) patients could be discharged from acute hospitals to this location prior to returning home. This would allow the health system to handle a surge beyond its original capacity, and in a far-reaching public health emergency allow for the recovery of the health system. Maintaining consistent standards of care in these settings is essential to a uniform approach to the medical management of a public health emergency.

The ACS/community based care center operations use the ACS facility to treat patients with specific clinical needs that can be cared for in a nonacute care hospital setting. This strategy may relieve hospitals of new admissions and allow them to focus on patients in need of either emergency care or more sophisticated (critical) care than could be provided in an ACS. In order to use the limited resources at the ACS to treat the most appropriate patients, it is necessary to adopt a model where patients from the community can receive a medical evaluation at another location, where a determination can be made as to the patient's clinical acuity and where the patient can be most appropriately treated (i.e., home, hospital, or ACS/community-based care center). Public health agencies across the country are working on this model, and states such as New York have adopted statewide models for ACSs to augment the traditional health system during a public health emergency.

SUMMARY

Disaster risk management is an integral and necessary component of disaster care. Meticulous planning and preparation are the backbone of this concept. Disaster plans must be field tested frequently, updated and scrutinized regularly, subject to expert review and incorporate lessons from other sources and events. Ideally, these tasks should be undertaken by a disaster committee within a health care facility. Engaging the health care volunteer workforce and local community members and educating them about disaster care and legal protections is highly recommended. Committee members should be well informed about the federal, state, and local laws regarding disasters and be versed in the ethical, legal, and operational challenges associated with health care emergency management.

REFERENCES

1. Storbakken S, Lackey C, Kendall S. Strategies for 96-hour critical infrastructure compliance. Available at: http://www.hfmadv.org/documents/Strategiesfor96hourcriticaloperation.pdf. Accessed August 4, 2014.
2. Drechsler CT. Duty of care: liability for malpractice. Vol. 61, Section 206. In: *American Jurisprudence: Physicians, Surgeons, and Other Healers.* 2nd ed. St Paul, MN: West Press; 1999.
3. Restatement of Torts, Second. Section 283, as reported by William L Prosser, University of California, Hastings College of Law, John W. Wade, Vanderbilt University School of Law American Law Institute.
4. AHRQ. *Altered Standards of Care in Mass Casualty Events.* Prepared by Health Systems Research Inc. under Contract No. 290-04-0010. AHRQ Publication No. 05-0043. Rockville, MD: Agency for Healthcare Research and Quality. April 2005.290-04-0010. AHRQ Publication No. 05-0043. Rockville, MD: Agency for Healthcare Research and Quality; April 2005.
5. Merin O, Ash N, Levy G, Schwaber MJ, Kreiss Y. The Israeli field hospital in Haiti—ethical dilemmas in early disaster response. *N Engl J Med.* 2010;362:e38–e38.
6. Rothstein M. Malpractice immunity for volunteer physicians in public health emergencies: adding insult to injury. *J Law Med Ethics.* 2010;38(1):149–153.
7. Pezzino G, Simpson SQ Guidelines for the use of Modified Healthcare Protocols in Acute Care Hospitals During Public Health Emergencies, Kansas Dept. of Health and Environment. Available at: http://www.kdheks.gov/cphp/download/Crisis_Protocols.pdf.
8. Louisiana Department of Health & Hospitals. *ESF-8 Health & Medical Section, State Hospital Crisis Standard of Care, Guidelines in Disasters, Version 2.0.* August, 2013.
9. Institute of Medicine. *Establishing Crisis Standards of Care for Use in Disaster Situations.* Committee on Disaster Care Standards, 2009.
10. Levin D, Cadigan RO, Biddinger PD, Condon S, Koh HK. Altered standards of care during an influenza pandemic: identifying ethical, legal, and practical principles to guide decision making. *Disaster Med Public Health Prep.* 2009;3(Suppl 2):S132–S140.
11. Schultz CH, Annas GJ. Altering the standard of care in disasters—unnecessary and dangerous. *Ann Emerg Med.* 2012;59(3):191–195.
12. Hall RW. *Memoirs of Military Surgery and Campaigns of the French Armies, on the Rhine, in Corsica, Catalonia, Egypt, and Syria; at Boulogne, Ulm, and Austerlitz, in Saxony, Prussia, Poland, Spain, and Austria. From the French of D.J. Larrey.* Baltimore: Joseph Cushing; 1814.
13. Bentham's Commonplace Book. In: *Collected Works,* x, p 142.
14. Frykberg ER. Medical management of disasters and mass casualties from terrorist bombings: how can we cope? *J Trauma.* 2002;53:201–212.
15. Burkle FM Jr, Orebaugh S, Barendse BR. Emergency Medicine in the Persian Gulf War—Part 1: Preparations for Triage and Combat Casualty Care. *Ann Emerg Med.* 1994;23(4):742–747.
16. Super G. *START: A Triage Training Module.* Newport Beach, CA: Hoag Memorial Hospital.
17. American Academy of Pediatrics, American College of Emergency Physicians, American College of Surgeons—Committee on Trauma, et al. Model uniform core criteria for mass casualty triage. *Disaster Med Public Health Prep.* 2011;5(2):125-128. doi:10.1001/dmp.2011.41.
18. Lerner EB, Schwartz RB, Coule PL, et al. Mass casualty triage: an evaluation of the data and development of a proposed national guideline. *Disaster Med Public Health Prep.* 2008;2(Suppl 1):S25–S34.
19. MIEMSS. *Maryland Survey: Mass Casualty Triage System as of July 24, 2008.* Unpublished results provided to FICEMS Preparedness Committee, 2010.
20. Policy Announcement, WMA Statement on Medical Ethics in the Event of Disasters, *57th WMA General Assembly, Pilanesberg, South Africa.* October 2006. http://www.wma.net/en/30publications/10policies/d7.
21. Merin O, Ash N, Levy G, Schwaber MJ, Kreiss Y. The Israeli field hospital in Haiti—ethical dilemmas in early disaster response. *N Engl J Med.* 2010;362:e38–e38.
22. Okie S. Dr. Pou and the hurricane—implications for patient care during disasters. *N Engl J Med.* 2008;358:1–5.
23. AAPA. The Physician Assistant in Disaster Response: Core Guidelines (adopted 2006 and amended 2010). American Academy of Physician Assistants. http://www2.wpro.who.int/internet/files/eha/toolkit/web/Technical%20References/Human%20Resources/The%20Physician%20Assistant%20in%20Disaster%20Response%20Guidelines.pdf. Accessed 28/05/14.
24. MacDonald L. *The Roses of No Man's Land, Micheal Joseph London;* 1980: 3–10 [chapter 3].
25. Evans GD. Clara Barton: teacher, nurse, Civil War heroine, founder of the American Red Cross. *Int Hist Nurs J.* 2003;7(3):75–82.
26. Department of Labor. Bureau of Labor Statistics Chartbook Occupational employment and wages, May 2009. Available at: http://www.bls.gov/oes/2009/may/chartbook_occupation_focus.htm#figure1. Updated November 10, 2010. Accessed May 2014.
27. Weiner E, Irwin M, Trangenstein P, Gordon J. Emergency preparedness curriculum in US nursing schools, Survey Results. *Nurs Educ Perspect.* 2005;26(6):334–339.
28. Center for Public Health Preparedness Columbia University Mailman School of Public Health, Center for Health Policy Columbia University School of Nursing. *Emergency Preparedness and Response Competencies for Hospital Workers.* July 2003. Available at: http://www.gnyha.org/eprc/general/guidelines/EmergencyPrepHospComps.pdf. Accessed 28/05/14.
29. Spain KM, Clements PT, DeRanieri JT, Holt K. Emergency preparedness for nurse practitioners. *J Nurse Pract.* 2012;8(1):38–44.
30. Spain KM, Clements PT, DeRanieri JT, Holt K. When disaster happens: emergency preparedness for nurse practitioners. *J Nurse Pract.* 2012;8(1): 38–44.

31. Hooker RS, Nicholson JG, Le T. Does the employment of physician assistants and nurse practitioners increase liability? *J Med Lic Discipl.* 2009;95(2):6–16.

32. Reilly M, Markenson D. Utilizing paramedics for in-patient critical care surge capacity. *Am J Disaster Med.* 2010;5(2):163–168.

33. Markenson D, Reilly MJ, Dimaggio C. Public health department training of emergency medical technicians for bioterrorism and public health emergencies: results of a national assessment. *J Public Health Manag Pract.* 2005;11(6 Suppl):S68–S74.

34. Kaiser HE, Barnett DJ, Hsu EB, Kirsch TD, James JJ, Subbarao I. Perspectives of future physicians on disaster medicine and public health preparedness: challenges of building a capable and sustainable auxiliary medical workforce. *Disaster Med Public Health Prep.* 2009;3(4):210–216. http://dx.doi.org/10.1097/DMP.0b013e3181aa242a.

35. Sabri A, Qayyum M. Why medical students should be trained in disaster management: our experience of the Kashmir earthquake. *PLoS Med.* 2006;3(9):e382.

36. Sauser K, Burke RV, Ferrer RR, Goodhue CJ, Chokshi NC, Upperman JS. Disaster preparedness among medical students: a survey assessment. *Am J Disaster Med.* 2010;5(5):275–284.

37. Ragazzoni L, Ingrassia PL, Gugliotta G, Tengattini M, Franc JM, Corte FD. Italian medical students and disaster medicine: awareness and formative needs. *Am J Disaster Med.* 2013;8(2):127–136. http://dx.doi.org/10.5055/ajdm.2013.0119.

38. Kovács G, Spens KM. Humanitarian logistics in disaster relief operations. *Intl J PhysDistrib Logistics Mgmt.* 2007;37(2):99–114.

39. Cone D, Weir SD, Bogucki S. Convergent volunteerism. *Ann Emerg Med.* 2003;41:457–462.

40. Pandemic and All-Hazards Preparedness Reauthorization Act of 2013, Section 203, 113th Congress by Rep Mike Rogers (R-MI) (2013-2014).

41. *2005 Hurricane Season Response After-Action Report* for the Emergency Management Assistance Compact (EMAC), by the National Emergency Management Association.

42. United States Code, Title 42, Chapter 139, p. 14501, 2006.

43. UNIFORM EMERGENCY VOLUNTEER HEALTH PRACTITIONERS ACT, Amendment 2007- drafted by National Conference of Commissioners of Uniform State Laws.

44. United States Government Accountability Office, Congressional Report, June 2008. http://www.gao.gov/new.items/d08668.pdf. Accessed 03/06/15.

45. Gostin LO, Hanfling D, Hodge JG Jr, Courtney B, Hick JL, Peterson CA. Standard of care—in sickness and in health and in emergencies. *N Engl J Med.* 2010;363:1378–1380.

46. United States Code, Title 42, Chapter 7, Subchapter XI, Part C § 1320d–5.

47. Health Information Privacy: US Dept of Health and Human Services. Available at: http://www.hhs.gov/ocr/privacy/hipaa/faq/disclosures_in_emergency_situations/1068.html. Accessed April 4, 2014.

48. See 45 CFR 164.510(b)(4).

49. Department of Health and Human Services: Centers for Medicare & Medicaid Services 42 CFR Parts 413, 482, and 489.

50. CFR § 489.24(a)(2).

51. 116 Stat. 594, Public Law 107-188.

52. The EMTALA Technical Advisory Group ("TAG"). *Report Number Five to the Secretary of U.S. Department of Health and Human Services from the Emergency Medical Treatment and Labor Act Technical Advisory Group,* November 2-3, 2006 (issued February 6, 2007).

53. Michael O. *Leavitt, Secretary, Dep't of Health and Human Servs., Waiver Under Section 1135 of the Social Security Act;* September 4, 2005. http://www.hhs.gov/katrina/ssawaiver.html. Accessed 03/06/15.

54. Emergency Medical Treatment and Labor Act (EMTALA) & Surges in Demand for Emergency Department (ED) Services During a Pandemic, Department of Health & Human Services Centers for Medicare & Medicaid Service.

55. GNYHA. http://www.gnyha.org/ResourceCenter/NewDownload/?id=252&type=1. Accessed March 2014.

56. Public Health Law Article 30, Section 3000-a. Emergency medical treatment.

57. Joint Commission on Accreditation of Healthcare Organizations, Medical Staff Standards, Emergency Management EM 02.02.13.

58. ML-139, NYSDOH Position paper on JCHAO Standard regarding disaster privileges.

59. New York State Department of Health. Community-Based Care Center Toolkit. New York State Department of Health, 2011.

60. Hospital disaster physician privileging: revised and approved by the ACEP Board of Directors titled, "Hospital Disaster Physician Privileging," January 2010. Available at: http://www.acep.org/Clinical---Practice-Management/Hospital-Disaster-Physician-Privileging/. Accessed January 14, 2015.

61. Fieldston E, Scarfone R, Briggs L, Zorc J, Coffin S. Pediatric integrated delivery system's experience with pandemic influenza A (H1N1). *Am J Manag Care.* 2012;18(10):635–644.

62. Adalja A, Watson M, Bouri N, Minton K, Morhard R, Toner E. Absorbing citywide patient surge during Hurricane Sandy: a case study in accommodating multiple hospital evacuations. *Ann Emerg Med.* 2014;64(1):66–73.

63. Scarfone RJ, Coffin S, Fieldston ES, Falkowski G, Cooney MG, Grenfell S. Hospital-based pandemic influenza preparedness and response: strategies to increase surge capacity. *Pediatr Emerg Care.* 2011;27(6):565–572.

64. Reilly MJ, Markenson D. Referral patterns of patients during a disaster: who is coming through your hospital doors? *Disaster Med Public Health Prep.* 2010;4(3):226–231.

65. Redlener I, Reilly MJ. Lessons from Sandy—preparing health systems for future disasters. *N Engl J Med.* 2012;367(24):2269–2271.

66. Shah V, Pierce L, Roblin P, Walker S, Sergio M, Arguilla B. Waterworks, a full-scale chemical exposure exercise: interrogating pediatric critical care surge capacity in an inner-city tertiary care medical center. *Prehosp Disaster Med.* 2014;29(1):100–106.

67. Abir M, Davis M, Sankar P, Wong A, Wang S. Design of a model to predict surge capacity bottlenecks for burn mass casualties at a large academic medical center. *Prehosp Disaster Med.* 2013;28(1):23–32.

68. Stewart A, Cordell G. Pharmaceuticals and the strategic national stockpile program. *Dent Clin N Am.* 2007;857–869.

69. Bayram JD, Sauer LM, Catlett C, et al. Critical resources for hospital surge capacity: an expert consensus panel. *PLoS Curr.* 2013;5.

70. Malatino E. Strategic national stockpile: overview and ventilator assets. *Respir Care.* 2008;53(1):91–95.

71. Duffy J, Harris J, Gade L. Mucormycosis outbreak associated with hospital linens. *Pediatr Infect Dis J.* 2014;33:472–476.

72. Disaster Prep Plan Template. *Novation;* 2014. Available at: https://www.novationco.com/media/safety/. Accessed April 11, 2014.

73. Mincer M, Quinlisk P. *Iowa Department of Public Health Attachment 11: Guidelines for Hospital Surge Capacity Management;* May 2006. Available at: http://www.cidrap.umn.edu/sites/default/files/public/php/190/190_guidelines_hospitals.doc. Accessed April 11, 2014.

74. Noah D, Huebner K, Darling RG, Waeckerle JF. The history and threat of biological warfare and terrorism. *Emerg Med Clin North Am.* 2002;20:255–271.

75. USDHHS. *Strategic National Stockpile.* 2013. Available at: http://www.remm.nlm.gov/sns.htm. Accessed April 2, 2014.

76. Gostin L. Medical countermeasures for pandemic influenza: ethics and the law. *JAMA.* 2006;295(5):554–556.

77. Russell P, Gronvall G. US Medical countermeasure development since 2001: a long way yet to go. *Biosecur Bioterror.* 2012;10(1):66–76.

78. CDC. *Public Health Preparedness and Response for Bioterrorism— Chempack Program Description.* June 14, 2004. Available at: http://www.cdc.gov/phpr/documents/coopagreement-archive/FY2004/chempack-attachj.pdf. Accessed April 2, 2014.

79. Gutierrez-Mendoza L, Schwartz B, de Jesus Mendez de Lira J, Wirtz V. Oseltamivir storage, distribution and dispensing following the 2009 H1N1 influenza outbreak in Mexico. *Bull World Health Organ.* 2012;90:782–787.

80. Gerald B. Water safety and disaster management procedures reported by Louisiana health care food service directors. *J Environ Health.* 2005;67(10):30–34.

29 | CHAPTER

Vaccines

Michael Bouton

HISTORICAL BACKGROUND

Immunization is the method of artificially inducing immunity to prevent the development of disease. The artificial induction of immunity was first demonstrated by Edward Jenner in 1796[1] after he observed that milkmaids who had contracted cowpox were immune to smallpox. He developed the practice of vaccination, inoculating fluid from cowpox lesions into the skin of susceptible individuals. Inoculated individuals typically developed only mild illness. Vaccination in the United States started shortly thereafter, and the first law to require smallpox vaccination was passed in 1809 in Massachusetts.[2] In a ruling that would become the basis for public health laws to this day, the Supreme Court in 1905 upheld the rights of states to enforce compulsory vaccination laws, with Justice Harlan writing in the majority opinion that "the possession and enjoyment of all rights are subject to such reasonable conditions as may be deemed by the governing authority of the country essential to the safety, health, peace, good order and morals of the community."[3]

Vaccines have proven extremely effective at reducing the global burden of naturally occurring disease. Measles, for example, has been virtually eliminated among those vaccinated in the United States, but continues to devastate displaced populations in developing countries where immunization is less prevalent.[4] In disaster situations vaccination programs are of the utmost importance to prevent outbreaks of infectious diseases.

More concerning, particularly in recent years, has been the use of viruses and bacteria as weapons of terrorism and war. The Biological and Toxin Weapons Convention was established in 1972 and produced a treaty that prohibits the development, production, stockpiling, and acquisition of biologic weapons. This was the first comprehensive, international effort to ban biologic and chemical weapons since the Geneva Protocol in 1925, and it was the first international treaty to ban an entire class of weapons. The treaty was signed by 144 nations, including the United States and the Soviet Union, which had the largest stockpiles of such weapons at the time. To this day, however, there is no mandatory monitoring program in place.

On October 4, 2001, a case of inhalational anthrax was reported in Florida.[5] Epidemiologists at the Centers for Disease Control and Prevention (CDC) later identified and confirmed 22 cases: 11 cases of inhalational anthrax and 11 cases of cutaneous anthrax.[6] The dissemination of these anthrax spores via letters through the U.S. mail appeared to be an intentional act of bioterrorism. In the aftermath of the Al-Qaida attacks on the World Trade Center and Pentagon buildings, this act illustrated a vulnerability to terrorist attacks involving biologic weapons. In response to the terrorist attacks, the U.S. government passed the USA Patriot Act in October 2001 and the Public Health Security and Bioterrorism Preparedness and Response Act in June 2002. These acts created the Department of Homeland Security and empowered the Department of Health and Human Services (DHHS) to begin efforts to protect the civilian population against future attacks with biologic weapons by enhancing surveillance and promoting preparedness.

DHHS, in conjunction with the CDC and National Institutes of Health, convened members of the research community to discuss the development of a research agenda and strategic plan for biodefense research. These efforts to counter bioterrorism focused on a group of microbes that included *Yersinia pestis* (plague), *Francisella tularensis* (tularemia), *Bacillus anthracis* (anthrax), *Variola major* virus (smallpox), *Clostridium botulinum* (botulism), and the hemorrhagic fever viruses.[7] Smallpox, eradicated in 1977 from natural transmission, was particularly feared because of its high mortality rate, the absence of specific therapy, and the highly susceptible general population.[8] Current CDC plans focus on targeted vaccination, contact tracking, and isolation and quarantine.[9] There was initial debate on whether the entire population should be vaccinated to eliminate the threat of a future attack, or whether to institute a targeted vaccination program only after an attack occurs or if the likelihood of an attack is deemed high by government officials. CDC officials decided to support a "ring vaccination" approach after a case of smallpox was identified.[10] This vaccination approach focuses on a surveillance and containment strategy. It involves the identification of smallpox cases, isolating those individuals, and vaccinating contacts and household contacts of those contacts.[9] The plan does not recommend mass vaccination in response to a documented case.

A well-developed, country-level vaccination program is probably the best protection against an intentional or spontaneous outbreak, because the infrastructure of the vaccine program can be rapidly adapted to meet the new challenge. For example, if there were an outbreak of a new strain of influenza in the United States, the yearly flu vaccine may provide some immunity, and the well-developed cold chain and delivery mechanism in place could be scaled to meet the needs.

IMMUNITY

Immunization can be induced via active or passive methods. Active immunization typically involves the administration of a vaccine, such as the rabies vaccine, to induce the host to produce an immune response against a particular microorganism. Passive immunization refers to the practice of providing temporary protection by passively transferring an exogenously produced antibody, such as rabies immune globulin, to a susceptible host. Immunizing agents include vaccines, toxoids, antitoxins, and antibody-containing solutions.

The initial response of the immune system to the introduction of an antigen occurs after the primary exposure. Circulating antibodies do not typically develop for 7 to 10 days. If an antigen is presented for a second time, an exaggerated humoral- or cell-mediated response occurs, called an "amnestic response." These amnestic responses usually result in antibody formation within 4 to 5 days.

There are multiple determinants of immunogenicity including the physiological state (e.g., nutrition, immune status, age) and the genetic characteristics (e.g., major histocompatibility complex polymorphism) of the host, the manner in which the immunizing agent is presented (e.g., route, timing of doses, use of adjuvants), and the composition and degree of purity of the antigen.

VACCINES

The ideal vaccine should possess the following characteristics[11]:
- It should be easy to produce in well-standardized preparations that are readily quantifiable and stable in immunobiological potency.
- It should be easy to administer.
- It should not produce disease in the recipient or susceptible contacts.
- It should induce long-lasting (ideally permanent) immunity that is measurable by available and inexpensive techniques.
- It should be free of contaminating and potentially toxic substances.
- It should cause minimal adverse reactions that are minor in consequences.

Current vaccines do not typically meet all of these criteria. Most possess limited efficacy or have unwanted side effects.

Vaccines typically consist of live-attenuated or killed-inactivated microbiological agents. Many viral vaccines contain live-attenuated virus (e.g., measles, mumps, rubella, oral polio). The vaccines for some viruses and most bacteria are killed-inactivated, subunit preparations or are conjugated to immunobiologically active proteins (e.g., tetanus toxoids). Live-attenuated vaccines tend to elicit a broader and more durable immunological response on behalf of the recipient. Killed-inactivated vaccines, which typically have a lesser antigenic effect, require booster vaccinations.

Currently licensed vaccines are generally both effective and safe; however, adverse events are associated with vaccine administration. Adverse events can be both trivial and life threatening. Examples include injection site reactions, fever, irritability, and hypersensitivity reactions. Administration of live viruses can sometimes lead to disseminated infection and therefore is contraindicated in immunocompromised populations and when the risk of disease is low.

Oral polio vaccine is one such live-attenuated vaccine that, while creating more immunity than the dead virus injected form, is no longer used in developed countries because in the setting of low disease prevalence, the risk of the vaccine inducing clinical polio was greater than the benefit. The development of the oral polio vaccine had a profound initial impact on childhood morbidity and mortality.[12] In the early 1950s there were approximately 16,000 cases of polio each year in the United States,[13] but after vaccination the last naturally occurring case was in 1993.[14] From 1980 through 1999 in the United States when oral polio vaccine was still in use, there were 162 confirmed cases of paralytic polio and 154 of these cases were vaccine-associated.[15] The United States has now transitioned to the dead virus injectable form that is not able to transform. The oral live-attenuated polio vaccine, although able to transform, is still used internationally because of its increased immunogenicity. On the whole it is thought to prevent disease, despite outbreaks such as occurred in 2006 when 70 children in Nigeria were found to have vaccine-associated paralytic polio.[16]

The National Childhood Vaccine Injury Act was passed by Congress in 1986. This act required the reporting of certain vaccine adverse events to the secretary of the DHHS. It also led to the creation of the Vaccine Adverse Events Reporting System.[17] The system's primary function is to investigate and study new vaccine adverse events or changes in the frequency of known vaccine adverse events. The reporting system has helped identify rare adverse events, including intussusceptions associated with the initial rotavirus vaccine,[18] ischemic cardiac events among smallpox vaccine recipients,[19] and viscerotropic and neurotropic disease after yellow fever virus administration.[20]

Vaccine Storage

Maintaining a cold chain from manufacture to delivery of a vaccine is usually the most difficult part of a vaccination program. Whereas each vaccine should be evaluated for specific requirements, as a general rule the cold chain should be able to maintain temperatures between 2 and 8 °C without allowing freezing (Table 29-1). The live-attenuated influenza vaccine and varicella are two exceptions to this rule and are stored frozen at −15 °C. Stand-alone refrigerators are preferred to combination freezer/refrigerator units because the former has a more uniform temperature throughout the area where vaccines will be stored. Certain vaccines contain an aluminum adjuvant that precipitates when exposed to freezing temperature, and if this precipitate is noted then the vaccine should be discarded. Not all vaccines have this property, however, and a normal appearance does not assure reliability. According to the CDC, temperatures should be documented twice daily and a thermometer with an accuracy of ± 0.5 °C used. It is important that the thermometer have a certificate of traceability and calibration testing.

In many instances refrigeration may not be available on transport to the end user. If nonfrozen vaccines are to be brought into the field the following protocol is recommended[21]:
1. Use a hard-sided insulated cooler with walls at least 5 cm (2 inches) thick.
2. First place at least a 5-cm (2-inch) layer of coolant packs that have been left at room temperature for 1 to 2 hours in the base of the container. Completely frozen coolant can freeze vaccine.
3. Place an insulating barrier such as bubble wrap on top of the coolant packs.
4. Then place a thermometer as well as vaccines on insulating barrier.
5. Place another layer of insulation on top of the vaccines and then a second 5-cm (2-inch) layer of coolant packs.
6. Finally, place a layer of insulating material on top of coolant packs and firmly secure cooler lid.

CURRENT PRACTICE

Potential Bioterrorism Agents

The CDC has designated three categories of biologic agents according to their potential as weapons of terrorism.[22] Category A agents were given the highest priority because they are easily disseminated or transmitted, associated with high mortality rates, can cause panic and social disruption, and require special action for public preparedness. Category B agents are moderately easy to disseminate, cause moderate morbidity and low mortality, and require enhanced diagnostic capacity and disease surveillance. Category C agents include emerging pathogens that have the potential for becoming biologic weapons in the future.

Category A

Anthrax (Bacillus anthracis). Anthrax is a potentially devastating bioterrorism weapon and is discussed in detail in Chapter 124. During the 2001 anthrax events, a total of 11 cases of inhalation anthrax were identified with a case fatality rate of 45%, despite intensive care

TABLE 29-1   Vaccine Storage Temperature Requirements

35-46 °F (2-8 °C)		≤5 °F (−15 °C)	
INSTRUCTIONS	VACCINE	INSTRUCTIONS	VACCINE
Do not freeze or expose to freezing temperatures. Contact state or local health department or manufacturer for guidance on vaccines exposed to temperatures above or below the recommended range.	Diphtheria-, tetanus-, or pertussis-containing vaccines (DT, DTap, Td) *Haemophilus* conjugate vaccine (Hib)* Hepatitis A (HepA) and hepatitis B (HepB) vaccines Inactivated polio vaccine (IPV) Measles, mumps, and rubella (MMR) vaccine in the lyophilized (freeze-dried) state† Meningococcal polysaccharide vaccine Pneumococcal conjugate vaccine (PCV) Pneumococcal polysaccharide vaccine (PPV) Trivalent inactivated influenza vaccine (TIV)	Maintain in continuously frozen state with no freeze-thaw cycles. Contact state or local health department or manufacturer for guidance on vaccines exposed to temperatures above the recommended range.	Live attenuated influenza vaccine (LAIV) Varicella vaccine

*ActHIB (Aventis Pasteur, Lyon, France) in the lyophilized state is not expected to be affected detrimentally by freezing temperatures, although no data are available.
†MMR in the lyophilized state is not affected detrimentally by freezing temperatures.
From Vaccination in acute humanitarian emergencies: a framework for decision making. http://www.who.int/immunization/sage/meetings/2012/november/FinalFraft_FrmwrkDocument_SWGVHE_23OctFullWEBVERSION.pdf.

management.[23] BioThrax is the only human vaccine for the prevention of anthrax in the United States. Licensed in 1970, the vaccine was formerly known as Anthrax Vaccine Adsorbed (AVA). The vaccine is prepared from a cell-free culture filtrate of a nonencapsulated, attenuated strain of *B. anthracis*.[24] The most recent immunization schedule from 2008 involves five immunizations. The vaccine is administered intramuscularly in a 0.5-mL dose at 0 then 4 weeks and 6, 12, and 18 months, with an annual booster recommended thereafter.[25] The available vaccine is recommended for select laboratory workers and military personnel.[26]

In 1998, the U.S. Department of Defense recommended vaccinating military recruits against anthrax; since then about 8 million military personnel have been vaccinated. Opposition by some recruits was voiced because of a fear of unwanted side effects, and currently only personnel operating in high risk areas are mandated to receive the vaccine. Adverse events from vaccination include injection site reactions, fever, chills, myalgia, and hypersensitivity reactions.

The vaccine has proven effective for the prevention of cutaneous disease in adults, but no conclusive evidence exists that it is protective against the more dangerous inhalation form.[27] There are studies in nonhuman primates, however, that suggest it confers protection from inhalational disease as well.[28] In the event of an inhalation anthrax event the CDC recommends 60 days of appropriate antimicrobial prophylaxis, such as ciprofloxacin, combined with three doses of vaccine administered at 0, 2, and 4 weeks postexposure.[29] In high risk exposures, it is recommended that both pregnant women and children adhere to the same schedule.

Botulism (Clostridium botulinum). There are four major types of botulism: foodborne, wound, adult colonization, and infantile (*Clostridium botulinum* is discussed more thoroughly in Chapter 154). There is also

theoretical concern that botulism could be aerosolized and cause an inhalational form of disease. In each case the bacteria forms a toxin that is carried in heat-resistant spores and causes a neuroparalytic illness. There is no person-to-person transmission. Therapy for each includes passive immunization with antitoxin and supportive care. From the standpoint of a bioterrorism threat, contamination of the food supply causing the foodborne form of illness is the most concerning. Unusually large numbers of patients presenting with acute, descending flaccid paralysis and prominent cranial nerve involvement should be considered a sign of a potential bioterrorism event. Symptom onset is usually within 36 hours of exposure, however, a latency period of up to 10 days is possible. This delay in onset may make it more difficult to identify botulism as the causative agent event early on, when the antitoxin is most useful. A retrospective study demonstrated that the administration of antitoxin within 24 hours of onset of symptoms was associated with an overall mortality rate of 10%, compared with 15% in patients in whom antitoxin was administered after 24 hours of symptoms and 46% in patients who did not receive antitoxin at all.[30]

Heptavalent botulinum antitoxin (HBAT) is the only available antitoxin in the United States for foodborne and wound botulism and is available through the CDC. Human-derived botulinum (BIG-IV) is indicated for use in cases of infant botulism.[31] Treatment only prevents progression of paralysis because the antitoxin neutralizes toxin molecules that have not yet bound to nerve endings. While many patients will recover when the neuromuscular connections regenerate, this process may take up to two months of ventilator support and stress our health care resources. There is no licensed botulism vaccine.

Smallpox (Variola major). The last case of endemic smallpox in the United States occurred in 1949 and worldwide in 1977 in Somalia. With no natural reservoir or host other than humans, the only known stocks of variola virus are in research laboratories in the United States and Russia. Concern for its use as an agent of bioterrorism remains especially high because of fear that not all isolates were properly guarded during the chaotic fall of the USSR. Furthermore, the United States and world population lacks immunity to smallpox, because routine vaccination against the virus ceased in the United States in 1972 and worldwide in 1982.[32]

Unfortunately, the onset of symptoms begin vaguely, with fever and myalgias after an incubation period of 7 to 17 days. After a few days of illness, macular/papular lesions that are most prominent on the face and extremities develop into characteristic vesicular and then pustular lesions. Groups of lesions at different stages of development across the body are classic and help differentiate smallpox from chickenpox. Patients remain contagious until all lesions are crusted and separated from the skin.

Smallpox can be spread from person to person by droplet,[33] but can also be spread by contact, as demonstrated by its use as an agent of bioterrorism during the 1700s, when infected blankets were distributed to Native American populations with devastating effect.[34] Among nonimmunized populations the case fatality rate in the 1960s was about 30%,[35] and it is unclear if this would be substantially different with modern intensive care.

When administered early in the incubation period the vaccine is believed to be highly efficacious,[36,37] and the CDC now stocks enough for every American.[38] The vaccine is administered with the use of a bifurcated needle. A droplet of vaccine is held by capillary action between the two tines. The needle is introduced into the epidermis and 15 perpendicular strokes are rapidly made in a 5-mm area. A skin lesion known as a Jennerian pustule forms with an area of crusting and edema at the site of inoculation about 5 days after inoculation and represents successful vaccination.[39] The lesions scab and leave a scar.

The smallpox vaccine is a live virus vaccine made from the related vaccinia virus. It is considered safe, but adverse events have been described. Vaccination programs for smallpox among military personnel and health care providers have been limited because the public has come to see the vaccine itself as potentially more harmful than the possibility of disease.[40] Injection site pain and myalgia and other minor side effects are common. Complications include postvaccinial encephalitis (12.3/1 million primary vaccinations), progressive vaccinia (1.5/1 million primary vaccinations), eczema vaccinatum (38.5/1 million primary vaccinations), generalized vaccinia (241.5/1 million primary vaccinations), inadvertent inoculation (529.2/1 million primary vaccinations), rashes (1/3700 vaccinated), Stevens-Johnson syndrome (rare), and myopericarditis (<1/12,000 vaccinated persons).[41,42] Death occurs as a result of life-threatening reaction to the vaccine in about 1 per 1 million primary vaccinations.[42] Vaccinia immune globulin (VIG) and cidofovir may be used to treat patients with serious adverse reactions. In the event of a bioterrorism event any exposed person, including pregnant women and children, should be vaccinated. Smallpox is discussed in more detail in Chapter 147.

Plague (Yersinia pestis). Rodents are the primary natural reservoir for plague, and it is typically spread to humans by the bite of a flea. In the 1300s a plague pandemic caused the death of about one third of all Europeans. During that same period were the first reports of its use as a biological weapon when catapults were used to launch corpses of those killed by plague into cities under siege. In World War II the Japanese dropped infected fleas from airplanes, causing outbreaks in Chinese villages.[43] It is suspected that both the United States and Russia have aerosolized versions that no longer require fleas for transmission. There are three main categories of plague: bubonic, bloodstream septicemic, and pneumonic. The vector of exposure is primarily responsible for determining which clinical manifestations will predominate. For example, inhalational exposure will cause pneumonic plague. Clinically, the disease resembles a rapidly progressing pneumonia that can develop into acute respiratory distress syndrome (ARDS).

Antibiotics such as streptomycin and gentamicin, when administered early in the course of disease, are effective in conjunction with aggressive supportive care to reduce the case fatality rate to 5% to 14%.[44] There is no current vaccine available. However, until 1999 there was a formaldehyde-killed whole-cell bacilli vaccine available. It was not effective against pneumonic plague, but it did have some protective effect against bubonic disease.[45,46] Research is ongoing regarding a new vaccine.[47] See Chapter 125 for a more thorough discussion of *Yersinia pestis.*

Tularemia (Francisella tularensis). In the 1950s the U.S. military aerosolized *F. tularensis* for use as a biological weapon, and it is speculated that Russia has similar stores.[48] Inhalation tularemia causes a nonspecific febrile illness without prominent respiratory symptoms or findings in the early phase.[49] Antibiotics are generally effective therapy, along with supportive care. There is an experimental vaccine carried by the U.S. Department of Defense and under review by the Food and Drug Administration. Vaccination is not currently recommended for postexposure prophylaxis because of its limited efficacy and available alternative treatment. More information on *Francisella tularensis* can be found in Chapter 126.

Hemorrhagic fever viruses. Hemorrhagic fever viruses are discussed in more detail in Chapters 142 to 145. They are divided into four distinct families of viruses that each cause fever and a bleeding diathesis. The four families (including examples) are Filoviridae (Ebola), Arenaviridae (Lassa virus), Bunyaviridae (hantavirus), and Flaviviridae (dengue and yellow fever). These viruses are typically spread by arthropod vectors, aerosols, or direct contact. Human to human transmission is possible for most, with the notable exception of Flavivirida viruses. Research on the weaponization of these viruses was performed by both the USSR and the United States.[50] There are no licensed vaccines for any of the hemorrhagic fever viruses, except for yellow fever. The yellow fever vaccine was initially licensed in 1953.[51] It is a live-attenuated vaccine that is highly effective in travelers to endemic areas.[52] It is not recommended for postexposure prophylaxis because of the virus's short incubation period.

Category B

Food safety threats (e.g., Salmonella species, Chapter 134; Escherichia coli O157:H7, Chapter 139; Shigella, Chapter 133). Typhoid is predominantly a concern in developing countries. There are three typhoid (*Salmonella typhi*) vaccines that are currently licensed for use in the United States. The first is an oral live-attenuated vaccine that was licensed for use in 1990.[52] It is indicated for children age 6 and older, as well as for adults.[53] Individuals ingest one enteric-coated capsule every other day for a total of four doses. The manufacturer recommends a new complete series every 5 years.[53] The oral vaccine is associated with minimal unwanted side effects. Reported side effects include abdominal discomfort, nausea, vomiting, fever, headache, and rash.[53] The second available option is parenteral heat-phenol-inactivated vaccine that was first licensed for use in 1917.[53] This vaccine is very effective, but has higher rates of adverse reactions and requires two injections 4 weeks apart. The third option is a Vi capsular polysaccharide vaccine, which is indicated for individuals age 2 and older.[53] The main advantage of this vaccine is that it is administered as a single intramuscular injection. Booster doses are recommended by the manufacturer every 2 years.[53] Adverse effects associated with the parenteral vaccine include fever (0% to 1%), headache (1.5% to 3%), and injection site reactions (7%).[53] The demonstrated efficacy of these vaccines ranges from 50% to 80% after a primary series.[52] Immunization is currently recommended for travelers to endemic areas, people with an exposure to a documented *Salmonella typhi* carrier, and laboratory workers with frequent contact with *S.*

typhi.[52] General contraindications include children younger than 2, pregnant women, and people with a history of a hypersensitivity reaction to the vaccine. The oral Ty21a vaccine should not be administered to individuals actively taking antibiotics, especially sulfonamides or mefloquine.[52] One should allow the individual to stop taking these medications for at least 24 hours before administering the vaccine. The oral vaccine, which is a live-attenuated virus, should not be administered to immunocompromised individuals.[52] No human vaccine is currently available for the prevention of illness caused by *Escherichia coli* O157:H7, *Shigella dysenteriae*, or salmonellosis.

Water safety threats (e.g., Vibrio cholerae, Chapter 132). There are now multiple oral cholera vaccines available,[53] including next generation vaccines such as the rBS-WC vaccine. In a mass immunization campaign from 2003 to 2004 in a region of Mozambique where cholera is endemic, the rBS-WC vaccine was shown to decrease rates of cholera by 78%.[54] While the World Health Organization and CDC do not generally advise immunization for individuals traveling to or from cholera-infected regions, vaccination may play a role in preventing and containing outbreaks among vulnerable populations.

For the other Category B diseases, no human vaccine is currently available: Q fever (*Coxiella burnetii*, Chapter 128), brucellosis (*Brucella* species, Chapter 127), glanders (*Burkholderia mallei*, Chapter 136), melioidosis (*Burkholderia pseudomallei*, Chapter 137), viral encephalitis (alphaviruses, e.g., Venezuelan equine encephalitis, eastern equine encephalitis, western equine encephalitis, Chapter 140), typhus fever (*Rickettsia prowazekii*, Chapter 129), toxins (e.g., ricin, Chapter 158; epsilon of *Clostridium perfringens*, Chapter 155; staphylococcal enterotoxin B, Chapter 153), and psittacosis (*Chlamydia psittaci*, Chapter 138). Similarly, no human vaccine is available for Category C emerging threats: Nipah virus (Chapter 151) and hantavirus (Chapter 150).

Vaccinations for displaced persons. Of foremost concern in a refugee camp setting is control of communicable diseases. Vaccinations, along with proper water sanitation settlement design, are necessary to achieve this goal. Outbreaks of measles can have a case fatality rate as high as 10% to 20%[55] and spread rapidly by droplet transmission. Measles vaccination campaigns should be undertaken by response teams when predisaster vaccination coverage is less than 90% or is unknown.[56] A measles immunization program along with vitamin A supplementation is recommended in emergency settings, with first priority given for children from the ages of 6 months to 5 years, and then if supplies are available, children up to 15 years old should also be immunized.

Cholera epidemics from the Democratic Republic of the Congo to Haiti have demonstrated the devastation that it can cause among displaced persons.[57] While the prime treatment for cholera remains oral rehydration therapy (ORT), zinc supplementation, and antibiotics, vaccination is becoming a viable adjunct in combating this disease.

The decision on what vaccines to provide to displaced populations is complex and depends on both general risk factors of the population and disease-specific risk factors. General risk factors for a population to consider are nutritional status, burden of chronic diseases, age distribution, access to health services, and finally sanitation, water supply, and degree of overcrowding. Disease-specific factors that must also be considered include the environmental conditions allowing for transmission, population immunity (innate or vaccine induced) against the disease, and burden of the specific disease prior to emergence. Each of the above parameters are graded as low, medium, or high risk based on criteria developed by the World Health Organization (WHO) and then entered into a classification table shown in Table 29-2.[58] This can help inform the decisions on whether a particular vaccine should be implemented.

Influenza. The flu causes about 1 billion clinical cases and an estimated 300,000 to 500,000 deaths worldwide.[59] The commonly used

TABLE 29-2 Epidemiological Risk Assessment Classification for Any VPD*

		LEVEL OF RISK DUE TO GENERAL FACTORS		
		HIGH	**MEDIUM**	**LOW**
RISK DUE TO FACTORS SPECIFIC TO VPD	HIGH	Definitely consider	Definitely consider	Possibly consider
	MEDIUM	Definitely consider	Possibly consider	Do not consider
	LOW	Definitely consider	Do not consider	Do not consider

*VPD, Vaccine preventable disease.
From http://www.cdc.gov/mmwr/preview/mmwrhtml/figures/m242a6t1.gif.

inactivated, injectable vaccine is grown in embryonated chicken eggs. The cycle from identification of strain, growth in the egg medium, inactivation, packaging, and distribution usually takes months and makes response to new strains or an emerging pandemic slow. Typically, the vaccine has been trivalent, containing the strains of influenza A H3N2, influenza A H1N1, and influenza B strains deemed most likely to circulate in the upcoming influenza season.[60] Work is now under way for a quadrivalent vaccine that will likely include an additional influenza B strain.[61] Vaccination is now recommended for all persons over 6 months who do not have contraindications. Inactivated, live-attenuated, and recombinant hemagglutinin (HA) vaccines are all available and each vaccine has its own set of contraindications. The most commonly used inactivated, injectable vaccine, IIV, is contraindicated for individuals with a history of severe allergic reaction to any component of the vaccine, including egg protein, or after a previous dose of any influenza vaccine, and caution is advised in those with moderate to severe illness with or without fever and those with a history of Guillain-Barré syndrome within 6 weeks of receipt of influenza vaccine. IIV is the vaccination of choice for pregnant women. The recombinant HA vaccine RIV3 can be administered to those allergic to egg and is licensed for use in patients 18 through 49 years.[61]

The opportune time to vaccinate people in the United States is by October, because the peak influenza season is typically December through March. The vaccine typically offers protection for 4 to 6 months with an estimated efficacy of 30% to 80%, depending on how well the vaccine is matched to the circulating strains.[62] Local reactions occur in 10% of individuals 13 years or older.[62] A slight increase in Guillain-Barré syndrome was seen in vaccine recipients.[62] This resulted in an excess rate of approximately 1 per 1 million people immunized.[62]

⚠ PITFALLS

- Failure to consider the immunization needs of a community after a disaster
- Use of vaccination as monotherapy when supportive care is an essential part of treatment
- Failure to maintain a cold chain in the effort to deliver immunization rapidly to a community in need

ACKNOWLEDGMENT

I would like to thank Kent J. Stock who wrote this chapter for the previous edition and whose work contributed greatly to this text.

REFERENCES

1. Hopkins DR. *Princes and Peasants*. Chicago: University of Chicago Press; 1983.

2. Orenstein WA, Hinman AR. The immunization system in the United States—the role of school immunization laws. *Vaccine*. 1999;17(suppl 3): S19–S24.

3. Jacobson v Massachusetts, 197 U.S. 11(1905).

4. Kouadio IK, Kamigaki T, Oshitani H. Measles outbreaks in displaced populations: a review of transmission, morbidity and mortality associated factors. *BMC Int Health Hum Right*. 2010 Mar 19;10:5. http://dx.doi.org/10.1186/1472-698X-10-5.

5. Centers for Disease Control and Prevention. Ongoing investigation of anthrax—Florida. October 2001. *Morb Mortal Wkly Rep*. 2001;50:877.

6. Centers for Disease Control and Prevention. Update: investigation of bioterrorism-related anthrax—Connecticut, 2001. *Morb Mortal Wkly Rep*. 2001;50(48):1077–1079.

7. Lane HC, La Montagne J, Fauci AS. Bioterrorism: a clear and present danger. [erratum in: Nat Med. 2002;8:87]. *Nat Med*. 2001;7:1271–1273.

8. Henderson DA, Inglesby TV, Bartlett JG, et al. Smallpox as a biologic weapon: medical and public health management. *JAMA*. 1999; 281:2127–2137.

9. Centers for Disease Control and Prevention. *Interim Smallpox Response Plan and Guidelines: Version 3.0*. Atlanta: Centers for Disease Control and Prevention; November 26, 2002. Available at, http://www.bt.cdc.gov/agent/smallpox/response-plan/index.asp.

10. Centers for Disease Control and Prevention. *Interim Smallpox Response Plan and Guidelines: Draft 2.0*. Atlanta: Centers for Disease Control and Prevention; November 21, 2001.

11. Dennehy PH, Peter G. Active immunizing agents. In: Feigin RD, Cherry JD, Demmler GJ, et al. eds; 2004. Textbook of Pediatric Infectious Diseases; vol. 2. Atlanta, Georgia: Elsevier Health Sciences; 2004.

12. Centers for Disease Control, Prevention. Impact of vaccines universally recommended for children—United States, 1990–1998. *Morb Mortal Wkly Rep*. 1999;48:243–248.

13. Pickering LK, Baker CJ, Overturf GD, et al. Active and passive immunization. In: *Red Book: 2003 Report of the Committee on Infectious Diseases*. 26th ed. Elk Grove Village, IL: American Academy of Pediatrics; 2003:2.

14. Centers for Disease Control and Prevention. *Vaccines and Immunizations: Polio Disease-Questions and Answers*. Available at: http://www.cdc.gov/vaccines/vpd-vac/polio/dis-faqs.htm.

15. Centers for Disease Control and Prevention. *Vaccines and Immunizations: Polio Disease-Questions and Answers*. Available at: http://www.cdc.gov/vaccines/vpd-vac/polio/dis-faqs.htm.

16. Willyard C. Polio eradication campaign copes with unusual outbreak. *Nat Med*. 2007;13:1394.

17. National Childhood Vaccine Injury Act of 1986, at Section 2125 of the Public Health Service Act as codified at 42 USC Section 300aa-26.

18. Centers for Disease Control and Prevention. Intussusception among recipients of rotavirus vaccine: United States, 1998–1999. *Morb Mortal Wkly Rep*. 1999;48:577–581.

19. Centers for Disease Control and Prevention. Cardiac adverse events following smallpox vaccination: United States, 2003. *Morb Mortal Wkly Rep*. 2003;52:248–250.

20. Centers for Disease Control and Prevention. Adverse events associated with 17D-derived yellow fever vaccination: United States, 2001–2002. *Morb Mortal Wkly Rep*. 2002;51:989–993.

21. CDC, National Center for Immunization and Respiratory Diseases. Vaccine Storage and Handling Toolkit. United States: 96–97. Available at, http://www.cdc.gov/vaccines/recs/storage/toolkit/storage-handling-toolkit.pdf. Accessed 21.01.14.

22. Centers for Disease Control and Prevention. Biologic and chemical terrorism: strategic plan for preparedness and response. Recommendations of the CDC Strategic Planning Workgroup. *MMWR Recomm Rep*. 2000;49 (RR-4):1–14.

23. Jernigan DB, Raghunathan PL, Bell BP, et al. Investigation of bioterrorism-related anthrax, United States, 2001: epidemiologic findings. *Emerg Infect Dis*. 2002;8:1019–1028.

24. Michigan Department of Public Health. *Anthrax Vaccine Adsorbed*. Lansing: Michigan Department of Public Health; 1978.

25. Wright JG, Quinn CP, Shadomy S, Messonnier N. CDC. Use of anthrax vaccine in the United States, Recommendations of the Advisory Committee (ACIP), 2009. *MMWR Recomm Rep*. July 2010;59:1–30. Available at, http://www.cdc.gov/mmwr/preview/mmwrhtml/rr5906a1.htm, Accessed 20.01.14.

26. Centers for Disease Control and Prevention. Notice to readers: use of anthrax vaccine in response to terrorism: supplemental recommendations of the Advisory Committee on Immunization Practices. *Morb Mortal Wkly Rep*. 2002;51:1024–1026.

27. Donegan S, Bellamy R, Gamble CL. Vaccines for preventing anthrax. *Cochrane Database Syst Rev*. 2009;(2). http://dx.doi.org/10.1002/14651858.CD006403.pub2, CD006403.

28. Ivins BE, Fellows P, Mitt ML, et al. Efficacy of standard human anthrax vaccine against *Bacillus anthracis* aerosol spore challenge in rhesus monkeys. *Salisbury Med Bull*. 1996;87:125–126.

29. Wright JG, Quinn CP, Shadomy S, Messonnier N. CDC. Use of anthrax vaccine in the United States, Recommendations of the Advisory Committee (ACIP), 2009. *MMWR Recomm Rep*. July 2010;59:1–30. Available at, http://www.cdc.gov/mmwr/preview/mmwrhtml/rr5906a1.htm, Accessed 20.01.14.

30. Tacket CO, Shandera WX, Mann JM, et al. Equine antitoxin use and other factors that predict outcome in type A foodborne botulism. *Am J Med*. 1984;76:794–798.

31. Arnon SS, Schechter R, Maslanka SE, Jewell NP, Hatheway CL. Human botulism immune globulin for the treatment of infant botulism. *N Engl J Med*. 2006;354:462–471.

32. Fenner F, Henderson DA, Arita I, Jezek Z, Ladnyi ID. *Smallpox and Its Eradication*. Geneva: World Health Organization; 1988. Accessed April 5, 2002, at, http://www.who.int/emc/diseases/smallpox/Smallpoxeradication.html.

33. Wehrle PF, Posch J, Richter KH, Henderson DA. An airborne outbreak of smallpox in a German hospital and its significance with respect to other recent outbreaks in Europe. *Bull World Health Organ*. 1970;43:669–679.

34. Stearn EW, Stearn AE. *The Effect of Smallpox on the Destiny of the Amerindian*. Boston, Mass: Bruce Humphries; 1945.

35. Fenner F, Henderson DA, Arita I, Jezek Z, Ladnyi ID. *Smallpox and Its Eradication*. Geneva, Switzerland: World Health Organization; 1988, 1460.

36. Dixon CW. Tripolitania, 1946: an epidemiological and clinical study of 500 cases, including trials of penicillin treatment. *J Hyg*. 1948;46:351–377.

37. Earl PL, Americo JL, Wyatt ES, et al. Immunogenicity of a highly attenuated MVA smallpox vaccine and protection against monkeypox. *Nature*. 2004;428:182–185.

38. Centers for Disease Control, Small Pox Executive Summary. http://www.bt.cdc.gov/agent/smallpox/response-plan/files/exec-sections-i-vi.pdf.

39. Reman J, Enderson D. Diagnosis and managmetn of smallpox. *N Engl J Med*. 2002;346(17).

40. Chen RT, Rastogi SC, Mullen JR, et al. The Vaccine Adverse Event Reporting System (VAERS). *Vaccine*. 1994;12:542–550.

41. Centers for Disease Control and Prevention. *Executive Summary: Smallpox Response Plan*. Available at: http://www.bt.cdc.gov/agent/smallpox/response-plan/files/exec-sections-i-vi.pdf.

42. Centers for Disease Control and Prevention. *Adverse Reactions Following Smallpox Vaccination*. Available at: http://www.bt.cdc.gov/agent/smallpox/vaccination/reactions-vacc-clinic.asp.

43. Harris SH. *Factories of Death*. New York, NY: Routledge; 1994: 78, 96.

44. Inglesby TV, Dennnis DT, et al. Plague as a biological weapon; medical and public health management. *JAMA*. May 2000;283:17.

45. Speck RS, Wolochow H. Studies on the experimental epidemiology of respiratory infections: experimental pneumonic plague in Macacus rhesus. *J Infect Dis*. 1957;100:58–69.

46. Centers for Disease Control and Prevention. Prevention of plague: recommendations of the Advisory Committee on Immunization Practice (ACIP). *Morb Mortal Wkly Rep*. 1996;45(RR-14):1–15.

47. Titball RW, Eley S, Williamson ED, et al. Plague. In: Plotkin S, Mortimer EA, eds. *Vaccines*. Philadelphia: WB Saunders; 1999:734–742.

48. Christopher GW, Cieslak TJ, et al. Biological warefare: a historical perspective. *JAMA.* 1997;278.

49. Dennis DT, Inglesby TV, et al. Tularemia as a biological weapon; medical and public health management. *JAMA.* 2001;285(21).

50. Center for Nonproliferative Studies. *Chemical and biological weaspons; possession and programs past and present.* March 2008, Available at, http://cns.miis.edu/cbw/possess.htm, Accessed 13.02.14.

51. Orenstein WA, Wharton M, Bart KJ, et al. Immunization. In: Mandell GL, Bennett JE, Dolin R, eds. *Principles and Practice of Infectious Diseases.* 5th ed: 2000:3211.

52. Monath TP. Yellow fever: an update. *Lancet Infect Dis.* 2001;1:11–20.

53. Pickering LK, Baker CJ, Overturf GD, et al. Summaries of infectious diseases. In: *Red Book Report of the Committee on Infectious Diseases.* 26th ed. Elk Grove Village, IL: American Academy of Pediatrics; 2003:245, 386–391, 557, 688.

54. Lucas M, Deen JL. Effectiveness of mass oral cholera vaccination in Beira, Mosambique. *N Engl J Med.* 2005;352:757–777.

55. Guha-Sapir D, D'Aoust O, World Bank. Demographic and Health Consequences of Civil Conflict October 2010. World Bank Development Report 2011. Available at: http://web.worldbank.org/archive/website01306/web/pdf/wdr_background_paper_sapir_d'aoust4dbd.pdf?keepThis=true&TB_iframe=true&height=600&width=800.

56. The Sphere Project. *Essential Health Services—Child Health Standard 1: Prevention of Vaccine—Preventable Diseases. Humanitarian Charter and Minimum Standards in Humanitarian Response.* Available at http://www.spherehandbook.org/en/essential-health-services-child-health-standard-1-prevention-of-vaccine-preventable-diseases/.

57. Goma Epidemiology Group. Public health impact of Rwandan refugee crisis: what happened in Goma, Zaire, in July, 1994? *Lancet.* 1995;345:339–344.

58. *Vaccination in Acute Humanitarian Emergencies: A Framework for Decision Making.* World Health Organization; 2013.

59. Girard MP, Cherian T, Pervikov Y, Kieny MP. A review of vaccine research and development: human acute respiratory infections. *Vaccine.* 2005;23:5708–5724.

60. Lambert L, Fauci AS. Influenza vaccines for the future. *N Engl J Med.* 2010;363:2036–2044.

61. Grohskopf LA, Shay DK, et al. Prevention and control of seasonal influenza with vaccines: recommendations of the Advisory Committee on Immunization Practices—United States, 2013–2014. *MMWR Recomm Rep.* 2013;62(7).

62. Cifu A, Levinson W. Influenza. *JAMA.* 2000;284:2847–2849.

Occupational Medicine: An Asset in Time of Crisis

Tee L. Guidotti

Disasters, by definition, are more than just "large-scale" incidents or events with multiple casualties. They differ qualitatively from routine medical emergencies and public health threats.[1]

This qualitative difference arises from the disruption of normal support systems and saturation of available residual capacity and capability, which is much degraded from normal operations: supply of resources exceeds demands of the disaster. It manifests itself in inaccessibility of routine system dependent resources and impediments to operations such as communication failures. Reliance on routine standard operating procedures becomes counterproductive, yielding highly individualistic on-the-spot innovation and improvisation risks causing confusion, thus making matters worse. Accompanying the disaster is the emergency management equivalent of "the fog of war," a condition of knowledge privation resulting not only from shortages of information but also from miscommunication, unfamiliar vocabulary (especially in industrial or chemical disasters), distortions, preconceived notions that have not yet been corrected in the event, and the seductive but often misleading tendency to rely on the experience from the most recent similar event.

In a disaster, the strategy of protecting the individual necessarily gives way to that of protecting the population. In other words, medical care gives way in priority to public health, and the system needs the versatility to manage this transition smoothly. To achieve this, occupational medicine (OM), and the occupational health service (OHS) that provides both primary and preventive care, wellness programs, and management services in health, is the pivot point within employer organizations.[2] (See Box 30-1 for a list of acronyms used in this chapter.) Corporations and other large institutions became deeply concerned with continuity of operations and the security of their personnel after 9/11 and have maintained this concern since, reinforced by natural disasters, such as Hurricane Katrina. For effective response to a disaster, responders need to have the appropriate tools and training for the mission. For effective response to the unpredictable and especially the unexpected, responders must be prepared for multiple events, have flexible approaches, be cross-trained, and have the capacity and capability to deal with "all threats" rather than one type of emergency at a time.

Among the responses to these threats has been the idea to strengthen and repurpose the OHS and to increase participation of occupational health professionals, particularly physicians, in the employer's disaster planning and emergency management response. A management model developed by Jean-Pierre Robin, at Noranda, an aluminum producer, suggests that any organization that creates wealth and adds value cannot rely on routine operations and public services for protection against catastrophic disruption and that sustainability must rest on a foundation that includes special functions designed to assure its security and continuity of operations. The OHS is key to continuity and therefore sustainability, and, to be effective, its functions are integrated with other protective services within the company, in a hierarchical manner. (See Fig. 30-1 for a graphic representation of the model.[2])

The imperatives of continuity of operations and disaster response have invigorated and reemphasized the role of OM, one of the oldest recognized medical specialties, in emergency management.[2–4] In the past and especially during wartime mobilization, physicians were regularly more involved by employers in disaster planning. That ebbed until the present era, stimulated by the threat of terrorism, and this role has now returned as a central function of corporate physicians.[5,6] The OHS cannot rescue the entire company in the event of catastrophe but that is not its mission. It adds its value in preparedness and planning, and advance networking with community-based public services. Historically, OHSs have always been most active in disaster planning but not the first-line resource in disaster response.

Box 30-2 presents the usual functions of a corporate medical department, provided or supervised by occupational physicians.[3,5,7,8] These functions have traditionally been clustered in a few broad missions: to protect health, to support productivity, to reduce loss and liability, to manage health affairs, and to ensure compliance with regulations and best practice for the industry. These functions have traditionally been viewed as support functions, not part of the business operations of the organization. Indeed, this is why these functions were subject to outsourcing throughout the private and government sectors during the 1980s and 1990s. Disaster management, by its nature, does not lend itself well to outsourcing and so virtually every major employer has some form of emergency management and disaster response plan, contingency, or capacity built into its global operations plan.[7]

OHSs are perhaps most familiar in the manufacturing sector, public safety services, and in the setting of a plant medical clinic. Typically, such services include at least one occupational health nurse (also a professional specialization), an occupational physician (typically on contract), and support staff, all of whom report on a regular basis to a plant manager and are responsible professionally to a corporate medical director, who serves as a traveling troubleshooter, an in-house resource on health issues, and an auditor for health affairs. This physician-led, health-centered team typically is engaged in regular interaction and problem solving in collaboration with an industrial hygienist and safety officer, who are usually oriented more toward process and plant operations, documenting regulatory compliance, and identifying and measuring health hazards. These hazard-oriented professionals usually report through a different manager or directly to the plant manager. This basic pattern was once the norm in industry, but

BOX 30-1 **Glossary of Acronyms**

ACOEM	American College of Occupational and Environmental Medicine	OSHA	Occupational Safety and Health Administration, Department of Labor
DHS	Department of Homeland Security	PPE	Personal protective equipment (includes respirators, eye protection, etc.)
EPCRA	Emergency and Community Right-to-Know Act, enabling legislation for LEPCs		
ISAC	Information Sharing and Analysis Center	SARS	"Severe acute respiratory syndrome," a novel viral disease originating in China and disseminated from Hong Kong that caused an intercontinental outbreak in 2002 and 2003; travel restrictions were imposed by many multinational employers at the time to protect their workers and prevent spread of the disease
LEPC	Local Emergency Planning Committees		
OH-CG	Occupational Health Coordinating Group, a steering committee for worker protection across critical industries that was housed within the ISAC for the health care and public health ISAC; OH-CG is regarded in OM as a missed opportunity for worker protection in critical industries		
		SDS	"Safety data sheet," which is a summary of the hazard of chemicals that must be provided by the manufacturer and distributor for all chemicals sold in the United States and many other countries; the SDS replaced the "material safety data sheet" and indicates that the document conforms to the Globally Harmonized System of Classification and Labeling of Chemicals
OHDEN	Occupational Health Disaster and Emergency Network, the platform for worker protection in disaster and emergency response developed by the OH-CG and initially funded by ACOEM; after some initial success in "proof of concept" it stopped operations around 2007, due to lack of support and interest on the part of industry partners		

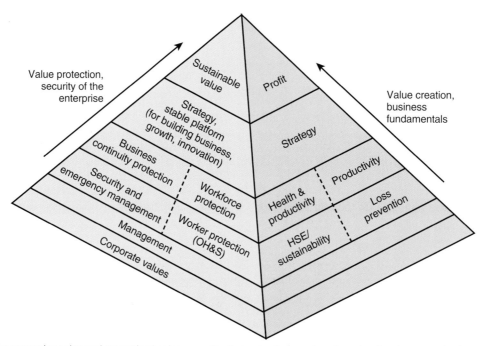

FIG 30-1 Schema for preserving value and protecting business continuity in a business enterprise, showing the strategic placement of business continuity protection and occupational health, after Jean-Pierre Robin. (Reprinted with permission from Guidotti TL. Emergency management at the enterprise level. In: Guidotti TL, ed. *Occupational Health Services: A Practical Approach*, 2nd ed. London, UK: Routledge; 2013, 389–403.)

the dramatic reorganization in industry, the management focus on core business, and the rise of the service sector have forged a new pattern, in which services are outsourced to contractors and consultants.[8]

The full-time, physician-led, fully staffed on-site medical facility has been mostly replaced in sectors by a leaner model, in which physicians contract with multiple employers to provide services at various facilities on a part-time basis or send workers out to see designated physicians in the local community. Large employers, with bigger operations and more at risk, are much more likely to have fully staffed OHSs, as well as the capacity and capability to respond during a disaster.[3] However, whichever pattern is followed in a particular enterprise, the essentials are in place in most large operations for a response to protect health in a disaster: a means of monitoring the health of workers, a system

for documenting their health, a system for documenting and evaluating hazards, a mechanism for responding to emergencies, and access to a panel of health consultants.[3]

An in-house, corporate, or on-site plant-level OHS usually is already involved within the organization in planning the medical response to emergencies, networking with local hospitals and health agencies, and providing services for casualties who can be helped with available resources, and diverting them away from local hospitals with limited capacity. They also deploy resources for dealing in the first instance (especially triage) with serious injuries and mass casualties, and provide health protection for key personnel (such as diabetic personnel) as required. This existing resource provides the platform that large organizations need to respond to disasters and to protect the security and

BOX 30-2 The Core Functions of an Occupational Health Service

1. Acute care for injured employees
   - Providing care on site
   - Monitoring care given off site
2. Preplacement evaluations that assess fitness to work
   - Assessing functional capacity to do the job
   - Assessing need for accommodation under the Americans with Disabilities Act
3. Functional evaluation of employees after hire
   - Fitness-to-work evaluations that assess the recovery and functional capacity of injured employees to return to work, as well as the accommodations they may need
   - Impairment evaluation for injured workers who are the subject of workers' compensation claims
   - Certification of time off work for workers with a nonoccupational illness or injury. (This is often performed by other physicians.)
4. Review of workers' compensation claims for causation
5. Periodic health surveillance of employees exposed to a particular hazard such as noise, chemicals, dusts, or radiation. (This often takes the form of a medical examination, often conducted annually.)
6. Investigation of exceptional hazards, disease outbreaks, unusual injuries, fatalities, or other emerging issues
7. Prevention, health promotion, and educational programs designed to enhance the health of employees and increase productivity
8. Management of the health problems of employees on site, to reduce absence and disability
9. Advice and consultation to management on issues of health, health and workers' compensation insurance, and regulatory issues in occupational health
10. Disaster planning and emergency management on site
11. External communications on health issues, as with local public health agencies and local physicians
12. Managing relations between the organization and local hospitals and the medical community
13. Employee assistance programs, for employees with problems involving alcohol and drug abuse or other addictive behaviors, such as gambling, that interfere with work
14. Executive wellness programs, such as special medical evaluations or monitoring health problems among senior executives

Larger and more complex organizations may also involve the occupational physician in managing environmental risks, product safety, contracting for health services, representing the organization in industry-wide health activities, and proactive programs for preparedness, risk management, and other senior management functions.

continuity of operations.[9] Involvement of the OHS in emergency management is a natural extension of the existing mission of the OHS. Disaster medicine involves only an increment of further training and preparation for consequence management and mitigation activities (as described in this textbook), preparedness for a response within the physical plant, and planning for the management of risks inherent to the operation of the specific industrial site and processes.[3,10]

The most obvious role for the OHS in a disaster mode is as a "poste médicale avancé," a forward medical position.[1] In an emergency, casualties may be brought for triage; minor wounds treated; the injured stabilized for transport; and the worried may be examined, counseled, and, importantly, kept away from the nearest hospital, which should be reserved for seriously injured casualties. This clinical role is often assumed by managers to be the obvious role for the OHS. In practice, this is usually impractical because of insufficient staffing, although some large companies, especially in manufacturing and industries in which there is a high potential risk of injury, do have this advanced OHS. However, the true value lies elsewhere, and this is where the pivot from medical care to the public health model comes into play.

The value of the OHS is much greater in public health protection, before the response phase (especially periodic health surveillance for the protection of first responders) and in the health management functions of planning and mitigation. These functions apply directly to continuity of operations.[3,7,9,11] The usefulness of a trained, well-informed, prequalified medical resource for dealing with incidents on site is obvious. These may include, but are certainly not limited to, sending infectious material through the mail to company personnel, using company equipment (such as airplanes or, potentially, chemical plants or storage facilities) as instruments of assault, and managing the psychological consequences of an assault. As well, the occupational physician, who is trained in hazard assessment, may assume the responsibility of determining when a site is safe to reenter or a facility to be reopened. This physician may also be responsible, independently or with the employee health service, for managing the psychological consequences of an assault.

Less obvious, but equally valuable, is the role that such occupational physicians may play in both managing the consequences of widespread disruption of business operations due to major threats and protecting the business, the product, and the brand against catastrophe. In time of crisis, the occupational physician may help get the community back on its feet by helping to keep an employer open or critical infrastructure functioning.[12] For example, a little known and almost completely undocumented story of the 9/11 tragedy was how occupational physicians were able to care for vulnerable employees, many older and in ill-health, during the stress and logistical strain of the temporary relocation of the nation's financial services industry to sites outside Manhattan.

Similarly, the occupational physician is now regularly called upon to manage the corporate response to serious health-related issues, such as travel to areas in which SARS and other emerging infections were a risk, rapid investigation of suspicious outbreaks of disease, following exposure to potential hazards, and determining when reentry and reoccupancy is possible in contaminated facilities, such as post office facilities contaminated with anthrax.[9] Several companies, including Cathay Pacific, participated in an informal monitoring network during the SARS epidemic, to share observed trends and experience when the information they needed was not forthcoming from conventional sources. Procter and Gamble, alerted to the emerging problem by its own corporate medical leader for China, instituted SARS precautions a month before any official warnings were advised.

The occupational physician also has an important place at the table as an active member of the management team, interacting with local prehospital care providers and hospitals on the Local Emergency Preparedness Committee (LEPC). LEPCs are charged, under the 1986 Emergency Planning and Community Right-to-Know Act (EPCRA), with developing emergency response plans, reviewing them annually, and providing information about chemicals in the community at the request of citizens (which obviously needs balance against the threat of terrorism). They bring together first responders (police, fire, and emergency medical technicians), civil defense and emergency management, facility and agency heads and key managers, public health authorities, media, and community representatives. The community emergency response plans have several required elements, each of which has obvious implications for employers, the workforce, and occupational health protection (adapted from the Environmental Protection Agency)[13]:

- Identification of facilities holding and transportation routes for the movement of extremely hazardous substances
- Descriptions of emergency response procedures, on and off a given site
- Designation of a community coordinator and facility emergency coordinator(s) to implement the plan
- Outline of emergency notification procedures
- Description of the method by which the probable area and population affected by releases will be determined (e.g., air modeling)
- Inventory and description of local emergency equipment and facilities and the persons responsible for them
- Evacuation plans
- Training plan for emergency responders (including schedules)
- Simulation and drill schedules for exercising emergency response plans

These functions build on the traditional involvement of occupational physicians in disaster planning, as well as health protection for employees.[3,6,8,10] The occupational physician has usually assumed responsibility within the organization for planning the medical response to emergencies, identifying facilities and resources for dealing with serious injuries and mass casualties, and providing health protection for key personnel if required. Although outsourcing has reduced the direct involvement of the occupational physician in planning emergency management in many organizations, particularly in the service sector, this function has not been completely replaced by external consultants because it requires a practitioner with intimate knowledge of the operations, hazards, workforce, and policies of the organization.

The well-supported occupational physician can add value to the management of catastrophic consequences in other ways. These include the following:

- Survival of key personnel in a catastrophic event
- Continuity of business following a catastrophic event
- Instant connectivity to resources for assistance in a health-related emergency
- Surveillance of the workforce and the early detection of an outbreak
- Integration of emergency response with public health agencies
- Surge capacity and capability as a resource when a local event requires mobilization of all available medical resources
- Vaccination programs and other protective measures
- Establishing on-site consequence management and mitigation programs
- Developing decontamination plans
- Providing specialized, sector-specific expertise to emergency mangers
- Participation in teams evaluating and assessing imminent hazards: chemical, biological, physical, mechanical, and psychological
- Advising on effective personal protective equipment (PPE)
- Liaison with the LEPC, prehospital care, and hospitals
- Continuing education and training on site and in the community of indigenous risks inherent to the operation
- Access to SDS (safety data sheet) information on chemical hazards
- Lead any after-action discussion to effect process and system improvement
- Fitness-for-duty evaluation of key response personnel in advance of deployment, to ensure readiness and safety (see Chapter 31)
- Respirator fitness testing (conforming to regulations of the Occupational Safety and Health Administration) in advance of deployment, for response personnel facing an airborne hazard (see Chapter 31).

To perform these duties effectively requires committed time for preparedness activities and an OHS that is structured and whose providers are trained to play such a role in time of crisis. However, it is costly and inefficient, even for large corporations, to dedicate a full staff

and support structure for the management of an event that may or may not materialize. This is why adaptation of the existing OHS makes sense for many employers, especially those in critical or hazardous industries.[3]

Adaptation of the OHS also lends itself to an "all-threats" approach, since the occupational health staff is already intimately involved with hazards in the community.[12] Focusing too narrowly on one particular threat degrades the quality of response to all threats. This degradation in capacity and capability due to over-emphasis was one of the chief concerns among the public health community in the years immediately following 2001, when emergency management was focused too narrowly on terrorism preparedness and the nation's public health capacity and capability was still grossly underfunded and its infrastructure overly centralized and dependent on the Centers for Disease Control and Prevention. Later in the decade, a spate of natural disasters featuring the incompetent response to Hurricane Katrina in 2005 made the wisdom of an all-threats approach to emergency management abundantly clear.

It should also be noted that focusing narrowly on one particular threat also degrades the quality of response to the threat getting the most attention.[11] A historical example is the response to bioterrorism, which consumed the nation's attention from about 1999 to 2004, for good reason but, not to minimize the tragedy of those that occurred, with very few actual incidents. A purpose-built system to detect and deal with a bioterror threat, alone and in isolation, was the initial knee-jerk response, but such an approach would have almost certainly been doomed to failure. Timely and fluent response requires practice and unexpected and unpredictable tests of the system. Bioterrorism events are very rare, but a public health department responds weekly and (in large communities) daily to outbreaks of infectious disease of one type or another, from simple food poisoning to urgent events that simulate plausible scenarios for a bioterror attack because they resemble scenarios following intentional introduction of a pathogen: the SARS epidemic of 2002, the West Nile Virus outbreak of 2002-2003, the H1N1 pandemic influenza epidemic of 2009, and current outbreaks and numerous serious outbreaks on a local level, such as dengue in Florida. It is now realized and accepted in government and homeland security circles, not just in the public health community, that a competent response to bioterrorism, an extremely rare event, requires competence in responding to these other infectious disease outbreaks. Further, development of this broader competence has led to greater capacity to plan and capability to respond to much more likely threats, such as pandemic influenza. As true as this demonstrably was for infectious threats, it is equally true for chemical hazards, radiation threats, and physical hazards, all of which are already in the mandate of the OHS and within the documented competencies of OM as a field.[5,14]

Incorporating emergency management into the mission of the OHS builds the efficiencies and redundancies required for a proper community response. The same resources used for tracking employees' health can be used for surveillance to detect potential disease outbreaks due to bioterrorism. The technology of hazard identification and measurement can be applied to detect chemical or radiation threats. The medical staff on duty primarily to monitor health and to provide timely clinical care can provide surge capability in time of crisis. Health protection for senior executives, and the personal knowledge that entails, can provide the detailed knowledge of health needs required to keep key personnel on the job and safe, especially when they are moved to new locations or are operating under conditions of stress and potential risk. The skills that are normally applied to ensure a safe workplace can be used to determine when it is acceptable to return to work or to venture into a facility that has been contaminated or damaged. Planning for foreseeable industrial disasters can inform and refine the response to unforeseen threats, given that sophisticated disaster planning is a matter of identifying resources and contingencies, not deriving detailed plans for single-threat incidents.

Perhaps most attractive to cost-conscious managers, investment in expanding the emergency management capacity within an OHS is not "lost" if an event never occurs. The same health management systems that support the traditional OHSs that industry and government employers require will be enhanced and available for use in emergencies. This may lead to cost savings, increased productivity, and reduced liability as added value. Conscious of their responsibility, and aware of their own position on the firing line along with the employees and executives they protect, OPs have been preparing themselves for an expanded role in emergency management. The principal specialty organization, the American College of Occupational and Environmental Medicine (ACOEM), has for some time offered training in topics relevant to emergency management. In 1999, the ACOEM began providing continuing education on the characteristics of weapons of mass destruction. Offerings have included emerging infections (particularly using the model of SARS), tabletop exercises to train participants in emergency management, health protection of first responders, and consequence management for disasters and mass casualties. Immediately following the tragedy of 9/11, an ACOEM task force produced a guide to the management of mental health issues among survivors of mass assaults, disseminated it to all members and posted it on the college website: all within four days. This achievement was unique and widely admired at the time among medical specialty organizations.

Informational Sharing and Analysis Centers (ISACs, previously "Information Sharing And Coordination") are organizations set up and managed outside the government by the owners, operators, key employers and institutions in industries and sectors recognized as critical infrastructure for continuity of essential services, vital supplies, and the national economy. ISACs have official status with the Department of Homeland Security and are intended to coordinate the planning response of critical sectors of the U.S. economy and society. They have been formed, for example, in industry sectors such as critical utilities (such as water supply), finance, health care, and transportation.

ACOEM also participated in a number of initiatives related to the interface between critical industries and the Department of Homeland Security. In 2003, leaders within the college developed the Occupational Health Coordinating Group (OH-CG) within what became the Healthcare and Public Health Coordinating Center. The OH-CG was the first health sector element to be created within the health sector's ISAC and was, for over a year, the only functioning ISAC component in the entire health sector. Because occupational health is cross-cutting across industries, the vision was for OH-CG to serve as a resource for other critical sectors rather than to focus on the health sector itself. However this proved to be nearly impossible because the OH-CG was embedded in an ISAC interested in acute delivery of health care and the supply chain, not protection for workers across critical sectors. As a result, from the beginning, the OH-CG was effectively marginalized, and it lacked the mandate or leverage to reach out to other critical sectors. Eventually, the OH-GC became unsustainable, although ACOEM itself continues to have contact with the ISAC.

The OH-CG, while it was in operation, sponsored the development of the Occupational Health Disaster and Emergency Network (OHDEN), a prototype platform for supporting worker protection during a disaster-scale emergency. It was initiated in 2004, and its efforts were supported for several years directly by ACOEM. OHDEN was a web-based system for sharing information and templates for employee tracking, disaster response, and hazard information. Its mission was to provide occupational health professionals with what they need when they need it in time of crisis, through channels that do not depend on any one mode of communication. OHDEN's first "proof of concept" came before it was really ready, when it briefly "went live" immediately following Hurricane Katrina in 2005 and was able to broker the timely sharing of information on guidelines for fitness-for-duty and return to work for employees in disaster-struck areas. A second test came in 2006 when its open website (now taken down) disseminated best practices in corporate policies related to pandemic influenza. Both "dry runs" were judged successful at the time, with evidence that the information was actually used. Unfortunately, despite efforts, no external funding to support OHDEN was forthcoming, and it was too large a project to be financed by ACOEM acting alone. Although OHDEN no longer exists, it demonstrated clearly that such a platform was feasible; it could be made efficient and cost-effective and would add value to disaster management.

Lacking a large-scale network providing a platform and templates for operationalizing worker protection in disaster management, employers have to build their capacity individually. How might an organization prepare its occupational health department to respond to a disaster?[3] The first requirement is a well-organized and effective occupational health team.[3] Teamwork in an emergency comes from training and planning before the event, but also from regular personal contact, trust, and practiced cooperation. A team that functions well in the complex duties of an OHS, and one that already knows the operations, workforce, and facilities is more likely to function well in an emergency, compared with an outside provider who may not be around in a crisis and probably has other clients and obligations.

Another part of the answer is to build redundant information and communication systems that can quickly retrieve critical information on hazards, disease or injury patterns, and individual health records in an adverse environment. Occupational health systems may require upgrading to do this effectively, but the technology is readily available. Partnerships within the LEPC, local industry, and other similar facilities not only reduce the initial and ongoing cost but also enable more efficient planning, training, and response.

Acquiring the necessary expertise is an obvious first step. The occupational health staff may require special training to take on the additional functions, but this is not much of a stretch from current duties. County emergency managers are eager to share training opportunities through grants and other programs within the public domain. On-site training and response in coordination with local prehospital care utilizing strategies of consequence management and mitigation, education, decontamination, and PPE will support efforts by the Occupational Safety and Health Administration (OSHA) to protect workers and may reduce liability exposure fur the organization's insurers. The expense for preparedness may be justified by potential reductions in insurance premiums, as well as reduction of loss in the event of an emergency.

Establishing networks and agreements for mutual assistance may be critical. Here the occupational health staff can coordinate arrangements with local hospitals, specialist practitioners, public health agencies, and first responders in advance and maintain personal relationships required for smooth operation in the event of a crisis. The first step is to forge an active participant's role in the LEPC. Some counties have a more active, dynamic, and responsive LEPC than others. An OHS for a large organization has the opportunity to lead and to become the backbone of emergency management in the community.

Facilities planning may be required, taking into account the characteristics of the site, for evacuation, securing the premises but preserving access for ambulances and first responders, defining areas of the plant for operational response (e.g., for staging rescue operations, triage, stabilizing casualties, decontamination, and "incident command" activities). Even locations without special hazards may benefit from such contingency planning in the event of an external threat. For example, the first anthrax assault was in the office of a newspaper, not normally a high-risk location but a logical target for an attack on media, and one that placed workers at risk in their workplace setting, as did the subsequent assaults on television media and congressional offices.

Surge capability may be provided under various contingencies, whether to call in help for managing mass casualties on sites (especially if local hospitals are not functioning or cannot be reached), to assist other units in a mutual assistance pact, or to perform services such as mass immunizations. On-site decontamination may have to be continued at the hospital or a second alternate care location away from the industrial incident. Surge capability operations may be created away from the hospital under the direction of the LEPC, county emergency manager or hospital. This may include separate health care mutual aid agreements specific for the incident, secondary triage and treatment, through the use of vendor agreements or prepositioned equipment and supplies, met by trained physicians and other health care providers. This strategy will enable the hospital and community health care delivery system to operate at near standard operations during the industrial incident. Any facility that has potable water, electricity, and shelter may serve. Pre-existing arrangements for accessing these sites should be spelled out under mutual aid agreements, vendor contracts, memoranda of understanding, or special circumstances agreements negotiated in advance between the County Emergency Management Office, the hospital or the local employer. Documentation of expenditures is a critical function, just as it is in the incident command structure, in order to reimburse all nonvolunteers and contracts executed in the response.

Certain routine functions can be anticipated and planned, for example, if anthrax or some other threat is suspected in the mailroom, procedures can be put in place in advance to protect employees, limit disruption and rapidly evaluate evolving situations. In the case of anthrax, these are quite simple and can be accomplished in a proactive manner, as was done by DST Output, the nation's largest direct mail operation, on the advice of its medical director. This last function is particularly important to deter inevitable hoaxes and to prevent disruptions to business from ill-defined or unknown hazards. For example, the common scenario of an unknown "white powder" appearing on a loading dock or in an office can shut down operations for a day or more until a toxic substance is ruled out. Having the capability on hand to show that it is harmless saves time and anxiety.

Confronted with a true emergency, most people behave in an adaptive, rational manner that helps them to get through the crisis and to mitigate personal damage or injury. Some are capable of helping others in an emergency.[15] This response appears to be shaped at least in part by whether the emergency arises from a natural disaster or a "technological" event (an incident arising from human agency). The perception of an intentional assault may also shape the psychological response for some people. Some people in situations of perceived catastrophic risk behave irrationally, however, and demonstrate psychogenic symptoms and maladaptive behavior.[16] Dealing with anxiety-promoting perceptions and psychogenic symptoms among employees that arise from rumors or incidental illness occurring at the worksite requires skill in rapid assessment and in risk communication, but it can save an enterprise from devastating loss of confidence and the potential loss from employees who may refuse to come to work. Distinguishing between human drama and a true emergency arising from a nonobvious cause is also a challenge requiring specialized expertise that is within the scope of the occupational physician.

An enterprise may be in a position to control its liability and potential loss from claims following a disaster by developing a flexible, effective emergency management capability within its OHS. In addition to reducing actual loss through planning and effective consequence management, which is most important, such an enterprise would also be able to show after the fact that it had done its due diligence in anticipating and preparing for plausible threats. This could reduce its exposure for punitive awards or claims based on negligence or omission. Legal opinions on this may vary, but it seems reasonable that a company that is seen to be prepared is less likely to be accused after the fact of ignoring a foreseeable threat.

In the classic business model followed during times of business as usual, the priorities of corporate management are shareholder value and profitability, continuity of production and operations, and loss control and risk management, in that order. For government agencies, there is a similar set of priorities with the mission of the agency coming first. However, in times of crisis, survival of the enterprise and protection of people take precedence. In the past, OM and OHSs have always been perceived as support functions, facilitating management priorities, but not as a core business priority. In the new era of threats to survival and business continuity, the OHS and the physicians in them may play a role in the survival of the enterprise and its people. A wise organization, faced with an extraordinary threat, may look within to build its salvation on a functioning system that is already serving its interests.

REFERENCES

1. Guérrise P. Basic principles of disaster medical management. *Acta Anaesthesiol Belg.* 2005;56:396–401.
2. Morgan O, Murray V, Snashall D. Occupational medicine, public health, and disasters: a shared agenda. *Occup Environ Med.* 2008;65:367–368.
3. Guidotti TL. Emergency management at the enterprise level. In: Guidotti TL, ed. *Occupational Health Services: A Practical Approach.* 2nd ed. London (UK): Routledge; 2013:389–403.
4. McLellan RK, Deitchman SD. Role of the occupational and environmental medicine physician. In: Upfal MJ, Krieger GR, Phillips SD, Guidotti TL, Weissman D, eds. *Terrorism: Biological, Chemical, and Nuclear.* 2003:181–190. Clinics in Occupational and Environmental Medicine; 2(2).
5. Emmett EA. What is the strategic value of occupational and environmental medicine? Observations from the United States and Australia. *J Occup Environ Med.* 1996;38(11):1124–1134.
6. McLellan RK, Guidotti TL. *Role of the occupational and environmental medicine physicians in emergency preparedness and response. Policy Statement. American College of Occupational and Environmental Medicine.* Available at, 26 May 2010. http://www.acoem.org/OEMPhysicians_EmergencyPreparedness.aspx, Accessed 1 February 2014.
7. Bender J, Joos-Vandewalle P. Global occupational health. In: Guidotti TL, ed. *Occupational Health Services: A Practical Approach.* 2nd ed. London (UK): Routledge; 2013:89–100.
8. Bender J, Joos-Vandewalle P. Corporate and in-house occupational health services. In: Guidotti TL, ed. *Occupational Health Services: A Practical Approach.* 2nd ed. London (UK): Routledge; 2013:69–88.
9. Hudson TW, Roberts M. Corporate response to terrorism. In: Upfal MJ, Krieger GR, Phillips SD, Guidotti TL, Weissman D, eds. Terrorism: Biological, Chemical, and Nuclear. 2003:389–404. Clinics in Occupational and Environmental Medicine; 2(2).
10. Guidotti TL. Managing incidents involving hazardous substances. *Am J Prev Med.* 1986;2:14–154.
11. Guidotti TL. Why do public health practitioners hesitate? *J Homeland Security & Emergency Management (on-line).* 2004;1(4). art. 403. URL, http://www.bepress.com/jhsem/vol2/iss3/4.
12. Landesman LY. *Public Health Management of Disasters: the Practice Guide.* Washington DC: American Public Health Association; 2001, p. 145.
13. US Environmental Protection Agencies. Local Emergency Planning Committees. Available at, http://www2.epa.gov/epcra-tier-i-and-tier-ii-reporting/local-emergency-planning-committees. Accessed 16 January 2014.

14. Guidotti TL, Hoffman H. Terrorism and the civilian response. In: Upfal MJ, Krieger GR, Phillips SD, Guidotti TL, Weissman D, eds. *Terrorism: Biological, Chemical, and Nuclear*. 2003:169–180. Clinics in Occupational and Environmental Medicine; 2(2).

15. Auf der Heide E. Common misconceptions about disasters: panic, the "disaster syndrome," and looting. In: O'Leary M, ed. *The First 72 Hours: A Community Approach to Disaster Preparedness*. Lincoln NB: iUniverse Publishing; 2004:340–379.

16. Guidotti TL, Alexander RW, Fedoruk MJ. Epidemiologic features that may distinguish between building-associated illness outbreaks due to chemical exposure or psychogenic origin. *J Occup Med*. 1987;29:148–150.

31 CHAPTER

Worker Health and Safety in Disaster Response

Clifford S. Mitchell, Brian J. Maguire, and Tee L. Guidotti

This chapter addresses worker safety in disaster response, including evaluation and management of workers involved in a disaster, medical surveillance, legal and regulatory requirements related to worker exposures, and specific issues for particular worker populations. Protection of worker safety and health during and after a disaster requires careful planning, training, and integration of occupational medicine, nursing, industrial hygiene, safety, and environmental functions. Major disasters, including the tsunami and reactor incident in Fukushima, Japan, in 2011; the Haitian earthquake response in 2010; Hurricane Katrina in 2005; continuing lessons from the attacks of September 11, 2001; and the anthrax attacks that same year, have demonstrated the importance of integrating emergency preparedness with other aspects of occupational safety and health.

Much of what has been learned about illness and injury among workers involved in disaster response has been due to the comprehensive surveillance and treatment programs established for workers involved in the World Trade Center (WTC) attacks of 2001. More than 200 scholarly publications have resulted from these programs because the fire department of New York had a well-designed surveillance program that it was able to adapt. This program demonstrates the value of creating registries, having baseline information in order to capture the exposure and health outcome experience of workers, and putting such comprehensive programs in place in advance for workers when major disasters occur. However, it should be recognized that the specific experience of the WTC disaster was unique, and certain aspects of the event, such as respiratory risk that followed inhalation of the unusual dust generated by the event, might not occur in other settings.[1] In addition, the military has had long experience with large-scale disaster response, and many of the lessons from that experience can be translated directly to the civilian environment.[2]

PLANNING AND TRAINING

Other chapters in this textbook discuss pre-event planning for a disaster, including the need for mutual assistance networks, facility planning and surge capacity, and consideration toward potential threat agents. However, it is equally important to consider workforce preparation and training, not only for first and secondary responders, but also for others who might potentially be involved in disaster response, including skilled support personnel and other categories of workers.[3] All workers ought to receive pre-event training and "real-life" drills in certain basic aspects of disaster response, including the following:

- Egress and evacuation
- Use of personal protective equipment
- Recognition of threats/hazards
- Activation of the emergency response system
- Incident command
- Their specific functional role in an emergency

Certain workers may need additional training, depending on their jobs. Some of these requirements are described in the U.S. Occupational Safety and Health Administration (OSHA) standard for Hazardous Waste Operations and Emergency Response Standard (HAZWOPER).[4] The HAZWOPER standard describes worker safety requirements for hazardous waste or emergency response sites that could involve chemical, biological, nuclear, radiological, or other hazards. OSHA and other federal agencies involved in worker safety and health—the National Institute of Occupational Safety and Health (NIOSH) and the National Institute for Environmental Health Sciences (NIEHS)—have spent considerable effort developing training programs for workers involved in disaster response who need basic awareness training, those at the "operations level," those workers known as hazardous materials technicians (workers involved in stopping the release of hazards), workers with specific knowledge of the hazards involved, and the on-scene incident commanders.[5]

Another aspect of pre-event planning involves personal protective equipment (PPE). Selection of PPE involves collaboration among industrial hygiene, safety, occupational medicine and nursing, and those involved in evaluating the potential risks and agents involved. OSHA and NIOSH have jointly issued guidance for selection of PPE against chemical, biological, radiological, and nuclear (CBRN) hazards.[6]

MANAGEMENT OF WORKERS INVOLVED IN DISASTER RESPONSE

During the disaster response, workers should receive limited briefings and training, sufficient to ensure that they are aware of the specific hazards they face on the site, that they are able to use their PPE appropriately, and that they understand the specific command structure and communications systems in place at the site.

The medical management of acutely exposed individuals is treated elsewhere in this textbook. There are, however, specific considerations for the management of workers who may be involved in disaster response, particularly if they have been potentially exposed to hazardous agents. These include: use of biological monitoring for acute exposures, surveillance for illness and injury following exposures, mental health considerations, and reporting requirements for specific exposures.

In many cases workers involved in disaster response will receive baseline or pre-event medical evaluations, including histories, clinical examinations, and laboratory tests (particularly baseline liver and renal function, and hematologic parameters), as well as pulmonary function tests, chest roentgenograms, electrocardiograms, and other tests. The selection of a particular test is based on the likelihood of exposure to, and toxicologic properties of, the possible agents, and medical judgment about the utility of the test as a screening test for a particular disease or injury.

Workers involved in disasters where exposures to hazardous substances may occur should be evaluated as soon as possible after the incident. The role of the evaluation is to: (1) obtain as complete a picture as possible of the exposure; (2) estimate the potential for an internal dose; (3) determine which, if any, biological measures of exposure may be appropriate; (4) treat for acute exposures as needed; and (5) determine the need for follow-up, including surveillance. Medical surveillance requirements will depend on the agent(s) involved, as well as the exposed population.[7] Some substances, such as lead or asbestos, may have specific regulatory requirements for postexposure surveillance related to occupational exposure, but in many cases it will be up to the health care provider to determine surveillance recommendations on a case-by-case basis.

Health care personnel should coordinate closely with industrial hygiene, safety, and environmental personnel to understand as completely as possible the nature and extent of exposure. Intraevent and post-event sampling should be evaluated in selecting appropriate biological exposure indicators. If the exposures occurred at an industrial location, additional information may be available through the company's environmental health and safety office, or through the company's public reports submitted in compliance with the Emergency Planning and Community Right to Know Act.[8] Standard references such as the American Conference of Governmental Industrial Hygienists' *Threshold Limit Values and Biological Exposure Indices* and numerous online references may be consulted in choosing appropriate surveillance tests. Follow-up studies of cleanup workers at the WTC demonstrate the importance of looking systematically for symptoms as well as biological indicators of exposure.[9]

Mental health issues are a critical component of worker safety and health management in disasters. Numerous studies have addressed the mental health consequences of disasters, and mental health professionals should participate in both pre-event planning and post-event management of workers involved in disaster response. There is still a need for considerable research related to the effectiveness of various mental health interventions employed in disaster management.[10] During the disaster, in addition to monitoring worker stress, consideration should be given to work-hour limitations.[11] In addition, after the disaster, both emergency responders and those who worked at the location may require considerable preparation prior to returning to their regular duties.[12] In the follow-up of the WTC event of 2001, first responders with posttraumatic stress disorder (PTSD) were more likely to have lower respiratory tract symptoms, and those responders with PTSD had more intense PTSD and more mental health problems if they also had lower respiratory tract symptoms.[13]

Although rarely immediate concerns in the post-event period, both occupational disease reporting and workers' compensation are considerations for workers who have been involved in disaster response. OSHA regulations require that employers report occupational illness and injury, and for workers in a disaster they may still ultimately be covered by these regulations if the workers are responding as a part of their job.[14] Similarly, many states have surveillance reporting requirements for occupational diseases, and in some cases these could also apply to disaster response workers. Finally, workers who become injured or ill in the process of responding to a disaster may be entitled to workers' compensation.

OCCUPATIONS INVOLVED IN DISASTER RESPONSE

This section discusses the health and safety of occupational groups that are predictably involved in disaster response: first responders, secondary responders, and skilled support personnel. Health and safety issues of health care personnel are addressed throughout this book. The experience of September 11, 2001, showed that many individuals and volunteers may also be involved in disaster response, and their health needs should also be considered in the medical response; however, the groups discussed below are in many cases expected to put themselves in situations where they are likely to be exposed to potentially life-threatening hazards.

First Responders

First responders are primarily police, fire, and emergency medical services (EMS) personnel, but the term is also often used to include other emergency services personnel (e.g., State Emergency Services [SES] in Australia); health care personnel (who are first to receive the victims in the emergency department); and public health professionals who prevent disease outbreaks, conduct outbreak investigations, and inspections. This chapter focuses on the health and safety of workers who are involved in the initial and prehospital response to a disaster: first responders (firefighters, police, and paramedics); secondary responders; and skilled support personnel, such as heavy equipment operators. These first responders are deployed in a forward position and are expected to put themselves in situations where they may be exposed to potentially life-threatening hazards.[15]

The overriding priority of first responders is to protect the victims and to secure the location. They rescue or otherwise protect others who are not able to save themselves. Protecting property from destruction or damage is a secondary objective, to be attempted if the personal risk is acceptable. In order to achieve these priorities, first responders allow themselves to be exposed to hazards, resulting in risks that would be unacceptable in other occupations. In order for this exceptionally high risk to be acceptable, the risk is managed by a combination of hazard controls (equipment), personal protection (e.g., self-contained breathing apparatus [SCBA] and "turnout gear"), administrative controls (two-officer rules and backup calls), risk assessment (determining the risk to victims and to responders of the incident and various options for controlling it), training, and fitness-for-duty standards.

The capacity to do the work of first response is essential. Without the requisite physical and mental capacity, the first responder will fail in his or her role in the mission and will become a casualty themselves, and therefore impose a burden impeding the response. Occupational safety and acute health protection then preserves the capacity of the individual to do his or her essential job and prevents degradation of the group capacity to achieve the mission; it also prevents the responder from becoming a casualty requiring care.[16] Occupational health protection against chronic health effects and disability, and the provision of fair compensation for occupational disease and disability rising from work, provides assurance that the risk the responder has assumed will be mitigated, if there is an untoward result.

Fitness-for-duty standards are medical criteria for screening workers to ensure their physical capacity to do a specific job, with or without accommodation (such as eyeglasses for driving). For first responders, fitness-for-duty standards may include tests of vision, strength, coordination, stamina (for firefighters, treadmill cardiac stress testing), and evaluation for disorders that may affect readiness or impair judgment (for example, insulin-dependent diabetes and the risk of hypoglycemia).[17] Fitness-for-duty evaluations must conform to applicable persons with disabilities acts, such as the Americans with Disabilities Act, to the extent that disability can be accommodated. However, medical standards for public safety personnel are usually higher and more inflexible than in other employment sectors. This is because public safety personnel must be able to operate at peak capacity under adverse conditions for prolonged periods, and do so without degrading performance or endangering the public safety (e.g., if carrying a firearm). In order to protect their jobs during periods of short-term partial disability, public safety personnel often have elaborate temporary assignment plans or informal "light duty" options as a resort if they are temporarily unfit for full duty. Recommended medical standards have been formulated by national standards organizations such as the National Fire Prevention Association (for firefighters),[18] professional societies such as the American College of Occupational and Environmental Medicine (for law enforcement officers [LEOs]),[19] and in some cases by private organizations.[20] Government agencies have also formulated their own medical standards, for example, California's Commission on Peace Officer Standards and Training.[21] These standards are adopted, in whole or in part, and operationalized by the agencies involved, given the resources available locally.

In addition to the public safety professionals, many private individuals and volunteers may also be involved in disaster response but may have different levels of capacity and preparation. For example, volunteer firefighters may not be held to the same medical standards as paid firefighters. The health protection of volunteers should also be considered in the medical response. In addition to their own health and safety, volunteer responders are also likely to be facing the same consequences as the rest of the community in a large-scale disaster. They may be blocked from reaching the scene by the same traffic obstacles or detours and may struggle to secure their own families in an area-wide emergency. Often, volunteers are used as a reserve to fill in the gaps in coverage left when paid crews are deployed to the scene. For example, volunteer firefighters may take over municipal firefighting duties while the paid fire service is occupied with a multialarm, multiple-station response. Because volunteers have less frequent call-ups and usually do not adhere to the same fitness standards as the regular paid service, they may be at higher risk for injury and health risks while deployed. Occupational health protection should be the same for volunteers as for regular line officers, and during the response their integration should be immediate, well practiced, and seamless.

First responders are generally the second to arrive on the scene, after concerned passersby and neighbors who rush to provide immediate assistance. In an area-wide disaster, the first responders may live in the communities affected. The occupational risks of first responders include the same hazards that threaten the victims, with the addition of the occupational hazards of the job. Because they often arrive before the site has been secured, decontaminated, or thoroughly searched, first responders may themselves face threatening situations on arrival. For example, the first arrivals at the site of a terrorist bombing must face the real possibility of a second explosive device intended for them. Even after the site is secured, first responders are confronted with events and circumstances outside the usual experience of human beings in their daily lives.

Although each of the occupations that constitute first responders has its own set of hazards, risks, and traditions, first responders share several features in common, including

- an awareness of personal danger, often accompanied by coping mechanisms that may include denial;
- long periods of relative quiet or routine interrupted abruptly by periods of intense activity, often accompanied by psychological stress;
- rigid codes of behavior and high expectations for performance, often accompanied by complicated job responsibilities and guidelines and high penalties for failure;
- a strong ethic of teamwork and camaraderie, always with a strong sense of mutual reliance, reinforced with social penalties for letting down one's co-workers; and
- a rigid hierarchy or "chain of command," often paramilitary, which is necessary in order to reduce uncertainty and to make sure that procedures are followed correctly.

Firefighters

During a disaster, firefighters may be exposed to unusual hazards in addition to the more conventional risks of fighting fires. Fires are often part of the disaster, of course, but the skills and training of firefighting also apply to rescue, extrication, identification of hazardous materials, fire prevention, and, for an increasing number of fire departments in the United States, EMS. Versatility is required. In addition to traditional fire and rescue, firefighting skills and technology may be called into play in unusual ways when circumstances require.

There are four common varieties of firefighters and several specialized classifications. Municipal firefighters respond to calls in populated areas and encounter both conventional structural fires and exceptional incidents in industrial settings that present a high risk for chemical exposure; municipal firefighters typically experience at least one or two of these over the course of a career. Woodland firefighters respond to fires in open areas, such as forests and range; they deploy as teams, and when things go terribly wrong, casualties are multiple and usually fatal. Industrial firefighters may be full time at a particular location or for a particular employer but are often operations workers cross-trained to respond to emergencies in a particular setting, such as an oil refinery; mine rescue is a highly prestigious subset of these responders. Aviation firefighters deal with structural fires on the ground and with aviation emergencies at civilian airports and in the military; municipal fire departments usually have aviation units permanently deployed at airports in their service area but not at smaller air fields serving general aviation. Within the fire service, firefighters may receive special training in hazardous materials recognition and assessment (HazMat) that places them at a different risk profile than other firefighters. In many major urban fire departments today, a large proportion of firefighters are cross-trained as emergency medical technicians (EMTs) and can work in either capacity.

Occupational hazards experienced by firefighters may be categorized as physical (mostly unsafe conditions, thermal stress, and ergonomic stress),[22] chemical,[23] and psychological.[24] Firefighters responding as EMTs may also face biological hazards. The level of exposure to hazards during knockdown and overhaul depends on what is burning, the combustion characteristics of the fire, the burning structure, the presence of nonfuel chemicals, the measures taken to control the fire, the presence of victims requiring rescue, and the position or line of duty held by the firefighter while fighting the fire. The hazards and levels of exposure experienced by the first firefighter to enter a burning building and engage in fire suppression, called "knockdown," is different from those of the firefighters who enter later to search for smoldering fuel that could flare up, a process called "overhaul." In general, the former is exposed to greater risk of trauma and the latter is exposed to more hazardous chemicals by inhalation.[25]

The energy requirements for firefighting are high and complicated by the severe conditions encountered in many inside fires.[26] The metabolic demands of coping with retained body heat, heat from the fire, and fluid loss through sweating add to the demands of physical exertion. Firefighters adjust their levels of exertion in a characteristic pattern during simulated fire conditions, as reflected by heart rate. Initially, their heart rate increases rapidly to 70% to 80% of maximal within the first minute. As firefighting progresses, they maintain their heart rates at 85% to 100% of maximal.[27]

During firefighting, core body temperature and heart rate follow a cycle over a period of minutes: they both increase slightly in response to work in preparation for entry, then both increase more as a result of environmental heat exposure, and subsequently increase more steeply as a result of high workloads under conditions of heat stress. After 20 to 25 minutes, the usual length of time allowed for interior work by the SCBA used by firefighters, the physiological stress remains within limits tolerable by a healthy individual. However, in extended firefighting involving multiple reentries, there is insufficient time between SCBA air bottle changes to cool off, leading to a cumulative rise in core temperature and an increasing risk of heat stress.[28]

Firefighters exert themselves to maximal levels while fighting fires. The most demanding activity is building search and victim rescue[29] by the "lead hand" (first firefighter to enter the building), resulting in the highest average heart rate of 153 beats per minute and highest rise in rectal temperature, 1.3 °C. Serving as "secondary help" (entering the building at a later time to fight the fire or to conduct additional searches and rescues) is the next most demanding, followed by exterior firefighting, and serving as crew captain (directing the firefighting, usually at some distance from the fire). Other demanding tasks, in decreasing order of energy costs, are climbing ladders, dragging hose, carrying a traveling ladder, and raising a ladder.

Risk varies with the activity. From the first alarm, firefighters are at transiently elevated risk of cardiovascular events with a relative risk (compared to routine duties) over three, and highly statistically significant. During fire suppression, the increased risk of cardiac events rises to 32 times the risk while performing nonstrenuous routine activities, a reflection that firefighters are under stress despite their medical standards and fitness requirements.[30,31]

Injuries associated with firefighting are predictable: burns, falls, and being struck by falling objects. Injuries can be minimized by intensive training, job experience, strict preplacement screening to ensure work capacity, competency on task, and physical fitness. However, the nature of the job is such that firefighters face dangerous situations by miscalculation, circumstance, and especially during rescues. The structure that a firefighter enters is not only on fire but often weakened structurally. Walls, ceilings, and floors may collapse abruptly and trap firefighters or cause them to fall. Exposed wires may present a risk of electrocution. Holding the nozzle runs a risk of severe scald burns from hot water. Turnout gear is designed for protection against burns and radiant heat, and so burn injuries tend to be the result of more complicated factors, such as basement fires, recent injury prior to the incident, and training outside the fire department of present employment. Falls tend to be associated with SCBA use, ladder work, and assignment to truck companies.[32]

Obviously, burns are a leading class of injury to firefighters, although standard turnout gear is very effective in minimizing the risk of burns. "Flashovers" are explosive eruptions of flame in a confined space that occur as a result of the sudden ignition of flammable gas products driven out of burning or hot materials and combined with superheated air. Fire situations that lead to flashovers may engulf the firefighter or cut off escape routes. Hot air by itself is not usually a great hazard to the firefighter. Dry air does not have much capacity to retain heat. Steam or hot, wet air can cause serious burns because much more heat energy can be stored in water vapor than in dry air. Fortunately, steam burns are not common. Radiant heat is often intense in a fire situation. Burns may occur from radiant heat alone. Firefighters may also show skin changes characteristic of prolonged exposure to heat.[33]

Improvement in turnout gear and the introduction of SCBAs and other protective equipment within the last 20 years have created much safer working conditions for the firefighter. However, the added weight of the equipment increases the physical exertion required and may throw the firefighter off balance in some situations. The firefighter's typical turnout gear may weigh 23 kg and imposes a high energy cost. The protective clothing also becomes much heavier when it gets wet. A 20% decrement has been found in work performance imposed by carrying SCBAs, a substantial restraint under extreme and dangerous conditions.

Under fire conditions, these physical demands are complicated by the metabolic demands of coping with heat and loss of fluids.[34] The combined effect of internally generated heat during work and of external heat from the fire may result in markedly increased body temperatures that climb to unusually high levels in an intense firefighting situation. Half-hour interval breaks to change SCBAs are not enough to arrest this climb in temperature, which can reach dangerous levels in prolonged firefighting. Although essential, personal protection imposes a considerable additional energy burden on the firefighter, particularly SCBAs.

Heat stress during firefighting may come from hot air, radiant heat, contact with hot surfaces, or endogenous heat that is produced by the body during exercise but which cannot be cooled during the fire. Heat stress is compounded by the same insulating properties of turnout gear that provide protection and by physical exertion, which result in heat production within the body. Heat may result in heat exhaustion, with the risk of dehydration, heat stroke, and cardiovascular collapse.

Ordinary firefighting may be associated with short-term changes similar to asthma, resolving over days, but does not appear to result in an increased lifetime risk of dying from chronic lung disease. However, unusual exposures, such as intense exposure to the fumes of burning plastics, can cause severe lung toxicity, reactive airways disease (where none existed before), and even permanent disability. The risk is substantially reduced with appropriate use of SCBAs.[35–40]

Over 50% of fire-related fatalities are the result of exposure to smoke, rather than burns. One of the major contributing factors to mortality and morbidity in fires is hypoxia because of oxygen depletion in the affected atmosphere, leading to loss of physical performance, confusion, and inability to escape. The constituents of smoke, singly and in combination, are also highly toxic. The toxicity of smoke depends primarily on the fuel (synthetic materials produce more toxic smoke, especially where there is a rich chlorine source), the heat of the fire (lower temperatures produce more toxic components), and whether or how much oxygen is available for combustion (rich fuel mixtures tend to produce more polycyclic aromatic hydrocarbons and particulate matter). Only carbon monoxide and hydrogen cyanide are commonly produced in lethal concentrations during structural fires. Depending on the fuel, firefighters may also be exposed to high levels of nitrogen dioxide, sulfur dioxide, hydrogen chloride, and irritating chemicals such as aldehydes. SCBAs substantially reduce exposure to these short-term hazards.[41–44]

Cancer risk is also elevated among firefighters for certain cancers, particularly those associated with inhaled carcinogens.[45] Firefighters are regularly exposed to carcinogenic hazards, including polycyclic aromatic hydrocarbons and nitroarenes, 1,3-butadiene, benzene, formaldehyde, polyhalogenated compounds (trichloroethylene, polybrominated fire retardants, polychlorinated biphenyl compounds, dioxins, and furans), and asbestos. SCBAs substantially reduce exposure to these cancer hazards.

SCBAs are an effective personal protection device that prevents exposure to the products of combustion when used properly.[46–51] Fire services routinely require the use of SCBAs during overhaul but individual firefighters often ignore the requirement and wear it only during knockdown. This is in part because SCBAs, while much improved, are uncomfortable, heavy, bulky, elevate the firefighter's center of gravity, impede communication, and obscure vision; necessary as they are, they are not something one would choose to wear in an environment with unstable footing and low visibility. Firefighters tend to judge the level of hazard they face by the intensity of smoke and decide whether to use a SCBA solely on the basis of what they see. This may be very misleading, especially after the flames are extinguished. There is no apparent correlation between the intensity of smoke and the amount of carbon monoxide or cyanide in the air.[52]

The psychogenic responses of firefighters to stress associated with catastrophic situations are probably similar to that of other public safety occupations but generally better characterized in the literature.[53–57] Losing a victim during attempted rescue is particularly difficult for a firefighter, but during a disaster such losses may be inevitable. It is clear that PTSD is not the only or even the most common response to shocking events, although it has been the focus of attention. Depression and self-medication with alcohol are probably more common, and most common of all may be somatization, as suggested by studies that show a high frequency of multiple health complaints without evidence of disease among responders to horrific events.[58–62] Although it continues to have advocates, critical incident stress debriefing, once thought to be effective in preventing PTSD and other dysfunctional responses, has been abandoned in favor of "psychological first aid" and ready access to psychological support for firefighters who self-refer.[63–67]

Police

In a disaster, police will have several functions: (1) establishing and maintaining order at the scene; (2) protecting the safety of the population at risk in the vicinity of the disaster; (3) protecting the safety of other responders; (4) maintaining the integrity of the scene if a criminal investigation is involved; and (5) in many cases, rescue assistance. In a disaster, one of the most important functions of the police is to maintain the security of the disaster scene from well-meaning volunteers who may inadvertently put themselves and others at risk. Although they are frequently first or second on the scene, police officers may not necessarily have access to the same level of PPE as other first responders, and the nature of their work can make it more difficult to consistently use PPE. The nature of the police force is such that in some cases, it may be challenging to ensure that all potentially exposed police officers participate in post-event medical management and follow-up.

Police, who are also known as LEOs (a term that also includes other protective services, such as correctional officers), have a number of potentially significant exposures, including injuries (both violent and from physical activity); hazardous air pollutants, including lead, noise, radio frequency radiation from radar; and psychological stressors, including violent trauma, shift work, and sleep disruption. There are relatively few studies of cancer risks among police officers, and those that exist do not indicate a consistent pattern of increased risk, though some association has been noted for thyroid, skin, and possibly male breast cancer.[68]

In the wake of the September 11, 2001, attacks, the rates of injury for police workers were comparable to those of other emergency responders.[69] Other studies have reported inconsistent results in comparing firefighters to police with respect to exposures or symptoms.[70] Police frequently have exposures that are similar to other emergency responders, even though they may not always be equipped with the same degree of PPE.

LEOs are often engaged in difficult situations that may involve physical exertion (e.g., in restraining suspects) and that presents risks to the public (e.g., when carrying a gun if the officer is disoriented or cannot see well, or is overwhelmed and loses control of the weapon). Their health status and functional capacity is therefore a matter of public safety; LEO positions are considered "safety-sensitive." A national set of evidence or expert consensus-based guidelines (when evidence is not sufficient) for the screening and health surveillance of LEOs has been developed by the American College of Occupational and Environmental Medicine and is available online, where it is updated as a

subscription service.[71] These guidelines specify levels of capacity required to perform LEO duties, to qualify an officer to carry a weapon (including conditions that may affect judgment and aim), and for prevention of conditions that could result in sudden incapacity, for example during an altercation or pursuit.

Emergency Medical Services Personnel

EMS personnel include paramedics, EMTs, and other prehospital care providers. These personnel treat an estimated 30 million patients a year in the United States.[72,73] In addition, they are first responders to natural and human-made disasters and are a crucial component of the nation's disaster response system.[74–76] Although prehospital care personnel have been operating in the United States for over a century, it is only recently that the full range of risks associated with this work have begun to be investigated. Research has shown that the occupational fatality rate for this group is more than twice the national average and comparable to the rates for police and firefighters.[77] The rate of nonfatal occupational injuries and illnesses may be more than five times the national average.[78–81] The risks are largely associated with transportation events, lifting, and violence.[82] Similar risks have been found among paramedics in Australia.[83] Because these risks are only now being recognized, EMS personnel and managers, as well as town council members and mayors, are largely unaware of the extent of the dangers associated with the work.

Historically, the role of EMS was to provide on-scene treatment and then rapid transportation to a hospital.[84] This role has been evolving in recent years as EMS agencies become more involved, not only in disaster preparation and response but also in community health. One agency, for example, instituted a program that reduced the county pediatric drowning rate by 50%.[85] EMS agencies nationwide are becoming more involved in a variety of community health initiatives.[86–88]

The National Highway Traffic Safety Administration (NHTSA) estimated that there were almost 20,000 EMS agencies in the United States in 2011. They examined almost 16,000 of them and found the operators were 40% fire departments, 25% private (nonhospital), 21% government (nonfire), 6% hospital based, and 1% tribal.

Maguire found an estimated 900,000 EMS workers in the United States; approximately 175,000 are full-time workers and 154,000 are paramedics. NHTSA found a similar number of personnel. NHTSA noted that volunteers provide much of the nation's EMS and that there are over 40 different levels of prehospital providers in the United States.[89] However, most EMS workers can be divided into two primary job classifications: basic life support personnel, such as EMTs, and advanced life support personnel, such as paramedics. Training requirements for these personnel vary by state, but in general, EMTs have a few hundred hours of training and paramedics have over a thousand hours above the EMT level. Protocols vary by state and local jurisdiction.

On a day-to-day basis, the risks faced by EMS workers include musculoskeletal injuries from carrying patients, assaults, needlesticks, and transportation-related injuries (e.g., from ambulance collisions, helicopter crashes, and by being struck by moving vehicles on the scene of a call). The EMS worker may have to carry a heavy patient down (or up) multiple flights of stairs or over slippery surfaces. EMS workers respond to calls in areas that have high crime rates and enter homes where the occupants are under great stress. The risk of needlestick injury may be increased when patients require immediate treatment in areas with poor lighting or in the back of a moving ambulance. Transportation incidents have been shown to cause the largest proportion of fatal injuries; they also account for many of the most serious nonfatal injuries.[90–96]

Psychological stress may be a significant risk factor for EMS personnel, but the short- and long-term effects are not yet well understood. Nor is it known how EMS work may affect chronic conditions.

Anecdotal information indicates that EMS workers tend to be young and have a high turnover rate. Therefore, there are no data on how EMS work may affect the workers' risk of cardiovascular disease, cancer, or other conditions. In addition, little is known about the general health of the EMS workforce. Although police and firefighting agencies typically have strenuous physical standards and requirements for recruitment and continued employment, EMS agencies may have few, if any, such policies.

The availability of PPE is believed to vary widely by agency and jurisdiction. Although all EMS workers likely have ready access to surgical gloves and masks, anecdotal information suggests that many workers do not have access to helmets, rescue gloves, turnout gear, or heavy boots. This paucity of resources may exacerbate the risks faced by EMS workers during disasters.

Smith et al. found that paramedics may be reluctant to respond to a disaster if insufficiently prepared.[97] Specialized training may double the responder's willingness to respond.[98] Factors that may contribute to increased occupational health risks among EMS workers during disasters include inadequate disaster-related training, lack of disaster preparation among EMS supervisors, poor coordination and communication with other public safety personnel, and inadequate equipment.

Little is known about the specific occupational health effects of disaster responses and operations on EMS workers, but this occupation is becoming more widely recognized as having among the highest rates of nonfatal injuries and illnesses on a day-to-day basis. It is reasonable to presume that such workers would be at even greater risk of injury during a disaster event.

Secondary Responders and Skilled Support Personnel

Two other categories of workers who are often deployed early in disaster response have been termed "secondary responders" and "skilled support personnel." Secondary responders include a broad range of workers, including certain emergency public health and medical personnel, HazMat personnel, crime scene technicians, urban search and rescue personnel, mortuary personnel, radiation safety experts, structural engineers, construction workers, and others who may be involved in all aspects of the disaster response. Skilled support personnel are defined in the HAZWOPER standard as workers who are operators of certain heavy equipment, such as hoisting equipment and cranes, earth moving, or digging equipment, and who may also be exposed to hazards on site.

Although there are few studies of the exposures or health consequences experienced by secondary responders and skilled support personnel in a disaster, experience suggests they may be at risk for significant exposures, particularly because in some cases these workers receive less training and have less access to PPE than first responders. Workers involved in post-Hurricane Katrina restoration in New Orleans, for example, showed nonsignificant but elevated prevalence rate ratios of new onset asthma and pneumonia, and significantly elevated prevalence rate ratios of sinus symptoms, fever, and cough.[99]

The WTC attack of 2001 can provide some insight into the risks faced by EMS and other emergency personnel during large-scale disasters. The hundreds of occupational fatalities following the attacks of September 11, 2001, have been well documented. Berríos-Torres et al. describe the WTC rescue workers' nonfatal injuries and illnesses during the months of September and October 2001.[69] Of the over 5000 incidents, the most prevalent case types were 19% musculoskeletal, 16% respiratory, and 13% eye. Fifty-two of the workers were admitted to hospital.

In summary, little is currently known about the specific risks faced by emergency services personnel during disasters. Research to identify these risks is critical so that effective interventions can be developed and tested.

It is also critical that these workers receive adequate training and real-life drills prior to a disaster; such training must include safety awareness and safety preparation, including the use of PPE. Finally, personnel must participate in post-event medical evaluations, counseling, and surveillance activities so that long-term effects can be minimized.

REFERENCES

1. Ekenga CC, Friedman-Jimenez G. Epidemiology of respiratory health outcomes among World Trade Center disaster workers: review of the literature 10 years after the September 11, 2001 terrorist attacks. *Dis Med Pub Health Preparedness*. 2011;5:S189–S196.
2. Decker JA, DeBord DG, Bernard B, et al. Recommendations for biomonitoring of emergency responders: focus on occupational health investigations and occupational health research. *Mil Med*. 2013;178(1): 68–75.
3. Mitchell CS, Doyle ML, Moran JB, et al. Worker training for new threats: a proposed framework. *Am J Industr Med*. 2004;46(5):423–431.
4. CFR 1910.120 and 1926.65.
5. U.S. Department of Labor, Occupational Safety and Health Administration, Directorate of Training and Education. *Outreach Training Program: Disaster Site Worker Procedures*. Revised April 2011. Available at: https://www.osha.gov/dte/outreach/disaster/disaster_procedures.html (accessed 03.03.14).
6. U.S. Department of Labor, Occupational Safety and Health Administration. *OSHA/NIOSH Interim Guidance (204). Chemical-Biological-Radiological-Nuclear (CBRN) Personal Protective Equipment Selection Matrix for Emergency Responders*. Available at: https://www.osha.gov/SLTC/emergencypreparedness/cbrnmatrix/index.html (accessed 03.03.14).
7. Svendsen ER, Runkle JR, Dhara VR, et al. Epidemiologic methods lessons learned from environmental public health disasters: Chernobyl, the World Trade Center, Bhopal, and Graniteville, South Carolina. *Int J Environ Res Public Health*. 2012;9(8):2894–2909.
8. CFR 350–372.
9. Landrigan PJ, Lioy PJ, Thurston G, et al. NIEHS World Trade Center Working Group. Health and environmental consequences of the world trade center disaster. *Environ Health Perspect*. 2004;112(6):731–739.
10. Wells JD, Egerton WE, Cummings LA, et al. The U.S. Army Center for Health Promotion and Preventive Medicine response to the Pentagon attack: a multipronged prevention-based approach. *Mil Med*. 2002;167(9 suppl):64–67.
11. Berkowitz MR. Occupational and public health considerations for work-hour limitations policy regarding public health workers during response to natural and human-caused disasters. *Am J Disaster Med*. 2012 Summer; 7(3):189–198.
12. U.S. General Accounting Office. *U.S. Postal Service: Clear Communication with Employees Needed before Reopening the Brentwood Facility*. Statement of Bernard L. Ungar and Keith Rhodes before the Committee on Government Reform, U.S. House of Representatives. GAO-04-205 T. Washington, DC, October 23, 2003.
13. Friedman SM, Farfel MR, Maslow CB, Cone JE, Brackbill RM, Stellman SD. Comorbid persistent lower respiratory symptoms and posttraumatic stress disorder 5–6 years post-9/11 in responders enrolled in the World Trade Center Health Registry. *Am J Ind Med*. 2013;56(11):1251–1261. http://dx.doi.org/10.1002/ajim.22217.
14. CFR 1904.
15. Guidotti TL. Emergency services. In: Stellman JM, ed. *Encyclopaedia of Occupational Health and Safety*. 4th ed. Geneva: International Labour Organization; 1998:95.1–95.22.
16. Emergency response resources. 2014 (accessed 18.01.14).
17. Kales SN, Christiinao DC. Fitness for duty evaluations of firefighters—Reply. *J Occup Environ Med*. 1999;41:214–215.
18. *Standard on Comprehensive Occupational Medical Program for Fire Departments*. NFPA; 2013 (accessed 18.03.14).
19. *Medical Evaluation of Law Enforcement Officers*. ACOEM; 2013 (accessed 18.01.14).

20. *Medical Screening Guidelines for Law Enforcement Officers.* Med-Tox Health Services; 2013, 18 January 2014.

21. *POST: Commission on Peace Officer Standards and Training;* 2014 (accessed 18.01.14).

22. Guidotti TL. Human factors in firefighting: ergonomic-, cardiopulmonary-, and psychogenic stress-related issues. *Int Arch Occup Environ Health.* 1992;64:1–12.

23. Guidotti TL, Clough VM. Occupational health concerns of firefighting. *Annu Rev Public Health.* 1992;13:151–171.

24. Guidotti TL. Firefighters. In: G F , ed. *Encyclopedia of Stress.* San Diego: Academic Press; 2007:64–67.

25. Baxter CS, Ross CS, Fabian T, et al. Ultrafine particle exposure during fire suppression—is it an important contributory factor for coronary heart disease in firefighters? *J Occup Environ Med.* 2010;52(8):791–796.

26. Holmer I, Gavhed D. Classification of metabolic and respiratory demands in fire fighting activity with extreme workloads. *Appl Ergon.* 2007;38:45–52.

27. Herrera JAF, Cohen FEM, Simon ESA. Physical workload during firefighting in Chilean volunteers. *Work.* 2012;41:432–436.

28. Rodriguez-Marroyo JA, Lopez-Satue J, Pernia R, et al. Physiological work demands of Spanish wildland firefighters during wildfire suppression. *Int Arch Occup Environ Health.* 2012;85:221–228.

29. Richmond VL, Rayson MP, Wilkinson DM, Carter JM, Blacker SD. Physical demands of firefighter search and rescue in ambient environmental conditions. *Ergonomics.* 2008;51:1023–1031.

30. Kales SN, Soteriades ES, Christophi CA, Christiani DC. Emergency duties and deaths from heart disease among firefighters in the United States. *N Engl J Med.* 2007;356:1207–1215.

31. Kales SN, Soteriades ES, Christoudias SG, Christiani DC. Firefighters and on-duty deaths from coronary heart disease: a case control study. *Environ Health.* 2003;2:14.

32. Heinemann EF, Shy CM, Checkoway H. Injuries on the fireground: risk factors for traumatic injuries among professional fire fighters. *Am J Ind Med.* 1989;15(3):267–282.

33. Wolfe CM, Green WH, Cognetta AB Jr, Hatfield HK. Heat-induced squamous cell carcinoma of the lower extremities in a wildlands firefighter. *J Am Acad Dermatol.* 2012;67(6):e272–e273.

34. McLellan TM, Selkirk GA. The management of heat stress for the firefighter: a review of work conducted on behalf of the Toronto Fire Service. *Ind Health.* 2006;44:414–426.

35. Jung TH. Respiratory diseases in firefighters and fire exposers. *J Korean Med Assoc.* 2008;51:1087–1096.

36. Greven F, Kerstjens HAM, Duijm F, Eppinga P, de Meer G, Heederik D. Respiratory effects in the aftermath of a major fire in a chemical waste depot. *Scand J Work Environ Health.* 2009;35:368–375.

37. Greven F, Krop E, Spithoven J, Rooyackers J, Kerstjens H, Heederik D. Lung function, bronchial hyperresponsiveness, and atopy among firefighters. *Scand J Work Environ Health.* 2011;37:325–331.

38. Greven FE, Krop EJ, Spithoven JJ, et al. Acute respiratory effects in firefighters. *Am J Ind Med.* 2012;55:54–62.

39. Greven FE, Rooyackers JM, Kerstjens HA, Heederik DJ. Respiratory symptoms in firefighters. *Am J Ind Med.* 2011;54:350–355.

40. Greenberger PA, Grammer LC. Pulmonary disorders, including vocal cord dysfunction. *J Allergy Clin Immunol.* 2010;125:S248–S254.

41. Guidotti T. Acute cyanide poisoning in prehospital care: new challenges, new tools for intervention. *Prehosp Disaster Med.* 2006;21:s40–s48.

42. Purser D. Behavioural impairment in smoke environments. *Toxicology.* 1996;115:25–40.

43. Walsh DW, Eckstein M. Hydrogen cyanide in fire smoke: an underappreciated threat. *Emerg Med Serv.* 2004;33:160–163.

44. Austin CC, Wang D, Ecobichon DJ, Dussault G. Characterization of volatile organic compounds in smoke at municipal structural fires. *J Toxicol Environ Health A.* 2001;63:437–458.

45. Guidotti TL. Evaluating causality for occupational cancers: the example of firefighters. *Occup Med (Lond).* 2007;57:466–471.

46. Guidotti TL. Evaluating causality for occupational cancers: the example of firefighters. *Occup Med (Lond).* 2007;57:466–471.

47. Cone DC, Van Gelder CM, MacMillan D. Fireground use of an emergency escape respirator. *Prehosp Emerg Care.* 2010;14:433–438.

48. Park K, Hur P, Rosengren KS, Horn GP, Hsiao-Wecksler ET. Effect of load carriage on gait due to firefighting air bottle configuration. *Ergonomics.* 2010;53:882–891.

49. Punakallio A, Lusa S, Luukkonen R. Protective equipment affects balance abilities differently in younger and older firefighters. *Aviat Space Environ Med.* 2003;74:1151–1156.

50. Williams-Bell FM, Boisseau G, McGill J, Kostiuk A, Hughson RL. Air management and physiological responses during simulated firefighting tasks in a high-rise structure. *Appl Ergon.* 2010;41:251–259.

51. Williams-Bell FM, Villar R, Sharratt MT, Hughson RL. Physiological demands and "Air Management" for firefighters breathing from an SCBA during simulated high rise firefighting tasks. *Med Sci Sports Exerc.* 2009;41:653–662.

52. Alarie Y. Toxicity of fire smoke. *Crit Rev Toxicol.* 2002;32(4):259–289.

53. Berger W, Coutinho ES, Figueira I, et al. Rescuers at risk: a systematic review and meta-regression analysis of the worldwide current prevalence and correlates of PTSD in rescue workers. *Soc Psychiatry Psychiatr Epidemiol.* 2012;47:1001–1011.

54. Berninger A, Webber MP, Niles JK, et al. Longitudinal study of probable post-traumatic stress disorder in firefighters exposed to the World Trade Center disaster. *Am J Ind Med.* 2010;53:1177–1185.

55. Bryant RA, Guthrie RM. Maladaptive appraisals as a risk factor for posttraumatic stress: a study of trainee firefighters. *Psychol Sci.* 2005;16:749–752.

56. Chamberlin MJA, Green HJ. Stress and coping strategies among firefighters and recruits. *J Loss Trauma.* 2010;15:548–560.

57. Harris MB, Baloglu M, Stacks JR. Mental health of trauma-exposed firefighters and critical incident stress debriefing. *J Loss Trauma.* 2002;7:223–238.

58. McFarlane AC, Williamson P, Barton CA. The impact of traumatic stressors in civilian occupational settings. *J Public Health Policy.* 2009;30:311–327.

59. Regehr C, LeBlanc V. *Stress and trauma in the emergency services.* Northampton, MA: Edward Elgar Publishing; 2011.

60. Slottje P, Bijlsma JA, Smidt N, et al. Epidemiologic study of the autoimmune health effects of a cargo aircraft disaster. *Arch Intern Med.* 2005;165: 2278–2285.

61. Slottje P, Smidt N, Twisk JWR, et al. Attribution of physical complaints to the air disaster in Amsterdam by exposed rescue workers: an epidemiological study using historic cohorts. *BMC Public Health.* 2006;6.

62. Slottje P, Twisk JWR, Smidt N, et al. Health-related quality of life of firefighters and police officers 8.5 years after the air disaster in Amsterdam: Erratum. *Qual Life Res.* 2007;16:909.

63. Everly GS Jr, Barnett DJ, Links JM. The Johns Hopkins model of psychological first aid (RAPID-PFA): curriculum development and content validation. *Int J Emerg Ment Health.* 2012;14:95–103.

64. Hawker DM, Durkin J, Hawker DS. To debrief or not to debrief our heroes: that is the question. *Clin Psychol Psychother.* 2011;18:453–463.

65. Mansdorf IJ. Psychological interventions following terrorist attacks. *Br Med Bull.* 2008;88:7–22.

66. Pekevski J. First responders and psychological first aid. *J Emerg Manag (Weston, Mass).* 2013;11:39–48.

67. Regel S. Post-trauma support in the workplace: the current status and practice of critical incident stress management (CISM) and psychological debriefing (PD) within organizations in the UK. *Occup Med (Lond).* 2007;57:411–416.

68. Wirth M, Vena JE, Smith EK, Bauer SE, Violanti J, Burch J. The epidemiology of cancer among police officers. *Am J Ind Med.* 2013;56:439–453.

69. Berríos-Torres SI, Greenko JA, Phillips M, Miller JR, Treadwell T, Ikeda RM. World Trade Center rescue worker injury and illness surveillance, New York, 2001. *Am J Prev Med.* 2003;25(2):79–87.

70. Amster ED, Fertig SS, Baharal U, et al. Occupational exposures and symptoms among firefighters and police during the carmel forest fire: the Carmel cohort study. *Isr Med Assoc J.* 2013;15(6):288–292.

71. Section on Public Safety Medicine, American College of Occupational and Environmental Medicine. *ACOEM Guidance for the Evaluation of Law Enforcement Officers.* Chicago IL: American College of Occupational and Environmental Medicine; 2014. Available at, http://www.acoem.org/leoguidelines.aspx (accessed 19.04.14).

72. Maguire BJ, Walz BJ. Current emergency medical services workforce issues in the United States. *J Emerg Manag.* 2004;2(3):17–26.

73. National Highway Traffic Safety Administration. *National EMS Assessment (Final Draft);* 2011. Available from, http://ems.gov/pdf/2011/National_EMS_Assessment_Final_Draft_12202011.pdf (accessed 29.08.13).

74. Maguire BJ, Dean S, Bissell RA, Walz BJ, Bumbak AK. Epidemic and bioterrorism preparation among emergency medical services systems. *Prehosp Disaster Med.* 2007;22(3):237–242.

75. Ruback JR, Wells S, Maguire BJ. New methods of planning and response coordination. In: Bissell RA, ed. *Preparedness and Response for Catastrophic Disasters.* CRC Press; 2013.

76. Walz BJ, Bissell RA, Maguire B, Judge JA 2nd. Vaccine administration by paramedics: a model for bioterrorism and disaster response preparation. *Prehosp Disaster Med.* 2003;18(4):321–326.

77. Maguire BJ, Hunting KL, Smith GS, Levick NR. Occupational fatalities in EMS: a hidden crisis. *Ann Emerg Med.* 2002;40(6):625–632.

78. Gershon RRM, Vlahov D, Kelen G, Conrad B, Murphy L. Review of accidents/injuries among emergency medical services workers in Baltimore, Maryland. *Prehosp Disaster Med.* 1995;10(1):14–18.

79. Schwartz RJ, Benson L, Jacobs LM. The prevalence of occupational injuries in EMTs in New England. *Prehosp Disaster Med.* 1993;8(1):45–50.

80. Maguire BJ, Hunting KL, Guidotti TL, Smith GS. *The Epidemiology of Occupational Injuries and Illnesses among Emergency Medical Services Personnel.* ProQuest; 2004.

81. Maguire BJ, Hunting KL, Guidotti TL, Smith GS. Occupational Injuries among Emergency Medical Services Personnel. *Prehosp Emerg Care.* 2005;9(4):405–411.

82. Maguire BJ, Smith S. Injuries and fatalities among emergency medical technicians and paramedics in the United States. *Prehosp Disaster Med.* 2013;28(4):1–7.

83. Maguire BJ, O'Meara P, Brightwell R, O'Neill BJ, FitzGerald G. Occupational injury risk among Australian paramedics: an analysis of national data. *Med J Aust.* 2014;200(8):477–480.

84. Walz BJ, ed. *Introduction to EMS Systems.* Albany: Delmar Publishing; 2001.

85. Harrawood D, Gunderson MR, Fravel S, Cartwright K, Ryan JL. Drowning prevention. A case study in EMS epidemiology. *J Emerg Med Ser.* 1994;19(6):34–38, 40–41.

86. Kinnane JM, Garrison HG, Coben JH, et al. Injury prevention: is there a role for out-of-hospital emergency medical services? *Acad Emerg Med.* 1997;4(4):306–312.

87. Yancey AH 2nd, Martinez R, Kellermann AL. Injury prevention and emergency medical services: the "Accidents Aren't" program. *Prehosp Emerg Care.* 2002;6(2):204–209.

88. Stirling C, O'Meara P, Pedler D, Tourle V, Walker JH. Engaging rural communities in health care through a paramedic expanded scope of practice. *Rural Remote Health.* 2007;7(4).

89. U.S. Department of Transportation, National Highway Traffic Safety Administration. Human resources. In: *EMS Agenda for the Future.* August 1996. DOT HS 808 441, NTS-42. Available at, http://www.nhtsa.dot.gov/people/injury/ems/agenda/emsman.html#HUMAN (accessed 08.06.04).

90. Maguire BJ, Porco FV. EMS and vehicle safety. *Emerg Med Serv.* 1997;26(11):39–43.

91. Maguire BJ. Ambulance safety in the U.S. *J Emerg Manag.* 2003;1(1):15–18.

92. Maguire BJ. Preventing ambulance collision injuries among EMS providers: part 1. *EMS Manager and Supervisor.* 2003;5(2):4.

93. Maguire BJ. Preventing ambulance collision injuries among EMS providers: part 2. *EMS Manager and Supervisor.* 2003;5(3):4–7.

94. Maguire BJ. Transportation-related injuries and fatalities among emergency medical technicians and paramedics. *Prehosp Disaster Med.* 2011;26(5):346–352.

95. Maguire BJ. Ambulance safety. In: Cone DC, ed. *Emergency Medical Services: Clinical Practice & Systems Oversight NAEMSP;* 2014, Accepted for publication—Wiley Pub.

96. Becker LR, Zaloshnja E, Levick N, Li G, Miller TR. Relative risk of injury and death in ambulances and other emergency vehicles. *Accid Anal Prev.* 2003;35(6):941–948.

97. Smith E, Morgans A, Qureshi K, Burkle F, Archer F. Paramedics' perceptions of risk and willingness to work during disasters. *Aust J Emerg Manag.* 2008;23(2):14.

98. DiMaggio C, Markenson D, T Loo G, Redlener I. The willingness of US Emergency Medical Technicians to respond to terrorist incidents. *Biosecur Bioterror.* 2005;3(4):331–337.

99. Rando RJ, Lefante JJ, Freyder LM, Jones RN. *J Environ Public Health.* 2012;1–8.

Disaster Preparedness*

Mark E. Keim

To start early is easy going, to start late is breakneck
—*Maori proverb*

DEFINITION

Disaster Terminology

In order to communicate effectively about disasters as an empirical endeavor, clear definitions of the specific terms must be used on a consistent basis. This chapter will, therefore, apply a standard nomenclature for disaster terminology. For clarity, key terms are emphasized in italics (when first used) and defined in Box 32-1.

A *disaster* is "a serious disruption of the functioning of a community or a society causing widespread human, material, economic or environmental losses that exceed the ability of the affected community or society to cope using its own resources."[1]

Disaster consequences may include loss of life, injury, disease, and other negative effects on human physical, mental and social well-being, together with damage to property, destruction of assets, loss of services, social and economic disruption, and environmental degradation.[1] The severity of these consequences is referred to as disaster impact. Disasters occur as a result of the combination of population exposure to a hazard; the conditions of human vulnerability that are present; and insufficient capacity or measures to reduce or cope with the potential negative consequences.

All disasters are said to follow a cyclical pattern known as the disaster life cycle, which includes five stages: prevention, mitigation, preparedness, response, and recovery.[2,3] These phases often overlap each other in time and in scope. The emphasis on a "life-cycle" approach to risk management is important in the case of disasters.[4]

Disaster Risk Management

Disaster risk management is a comprehensive all-hazard approach that entails developing and implementing strategies for each phase of the disaster life cycle. Disaster risk management includes both predisaster risk reduction (prevention, mitigation, and preparedness), as well as postdisaster retention of residual risk (response and recovery).[5]

The underlying drive of disaster management is to reduce risk to both human life and systems important to livelihood.[6]

Box 32-1 defines other key terms in disaster risk management.[1,7,8]

---

*The material in this chapter reflects solely the views of the author. It does not necessarily reflect the policies or recommendations of the Centers for Disease Control and Prevention or the U.S. Department of Health and Human Services.

Preparedness

Recently the overall approach to emergencies and disasters among nations has shifted from postimpact activities to a more systematic and comprehensive process of risk management that also emphasizes the importance of preimpact activities, including prevention, mitigation, and preparedness.[9,10]

Preparedness is considered one of the three components of disaster risk reduction because (like prevention and mitigation) it represents activities performed before the disaster. However, preparedness may also be contrasted with these other two elements of disaster risk reduction, in that prevention and mitigation focus primarily on reducing the *causes* of exposure to disaster hazards, while preparedness focuses on reducing the *effects* of those exposures on the population.

As preparedness increases, the ability of the society to absorb the event and thus lessen adverse outcomes is augmented as a dependent variable of the preparedness.[11] By increasing preparedness, we increase resilience, and thus lessen the risk of disasters. In addition, effective disaster-risk-reduction activities strengthen the buffering capacity of a population to respond to those everyday emergencies found in all societies (thus minimizing the change in an essential function for a given change in available resources).[11]

HISTORICAL PERSPECTIVE

Events of the past three decades have given birth to an understanding of the importance of disaster preparedness. The Guatemala earthquake of 1976 killed 23,000 people and led to the publication of multiple articles analyzing aspects of the international response.[12,13] Post-Event analyses of this and other subsequent large-scale disasters reveals a strong case for multihazard disaster preparedness. During the 1980s, new concepts based on the notions of hazards and vulnerabilities evolved. Governments of industrialized nations began to abandon their disaster relief approaches to better reflect the importance of preparedness. This growing awareness was bolstered by a growing body of disaster research; an increasing professionalism in the field that grew to include academic coursework, the development of manuals and standardized tools, a growing response fatigue among donor nations and organizations, and an economic appreciation of the cost-effectiveness of prevention and preparedness as weighed against extremely expensive response efforts. The growing burden of disasters on global health was becoming all too clear. During the following 20-year period (1990-2010), natural disasters alone killed 3 million people worldwide, affected 800 million lives, and resulted in property damage exceeding $23 billion.[14,15] In response to this growing threat, the United Nations General Assembly declared the 1990s to be the International Decade of Natural Disaster Reduction (IDNDR) and called for a global effort to reduce the suffering and losses.

BOX 32-1 Definitions of Key Terms

Absorptive capacity: A limit to the rate or quantity of impact that can be absorbed (or adapted to) without exceeding the threshold of disaster declaration

All-hazard approach: Developing and implementing emergency management strategies for the full range of likely emergencies or disasters, including both natural and technological (which also includes conflict-related hazards of terrorism and warfare)

Capability: The ability to achieve a desired operational effect under specified standards and conditions through combinations of means and ways to perform a set of tasks

Capacity: The combination of all the strengths, attributes, and resources available within a community, society, or organization that can be used to achieve agreed goals

Consequences: The result or effect when a vulnerable asset is exposed to a disaster hazard

Disaster: A serious disruption of the functioning of a community or a society, involving widespread human, material, economic, or environmental losses and impacts, which exceed the ability of the affected community or society to cope using its own resources

Disaster risk: The potential disaster losses, in lives, health status, livelihoods, assets, and services, which could occur to a particular community or a society over some specified future period

Disaster risk management: The systematic process of using administrative directives, organizations, and operational skills and capacities to implement strategies, policies, and improved coping capacities in order to lessen the adverse impacts of hazards and the possibility of disaster

Disaster risk reduction: The concept and practice of reducing disaster risks through systematic efforts to analyze and manage the causal factors of disasters, including through reduced exposure to hazards, lessened vulnerability of people and property, wise management of land and the environment, and improved preparedness for adverse events

Early warning system: The set of capacities needed to generate and disseminate timely and meaningful warning information to enable individuals, communities, and organizations threatened by a hazard to prepare and to act appropriately and in sufficient time to reduce the possibility of harm or loss

Exposure: People, property, systems, or other elements present in hazard zones that are thereby subject to potential losses

Hazard: A dangerous phenomenon, substance, human activity, or condition that may cause loss of life, injury, or other health impacts, property damage, loss of livelihoods and services, social and economic disruption, or environmental damage

Impact: A measure of the severity of consequences caused by disaster hazards

Mitigation: The lessening or limitation of the adverse impacts of hazards and related disasters

Natural hazard: Natural process or phenomenon that may cause loss of life, injury, or other health impacts, property damage, loss of livelihoods and services, social and economic disruption, or environmental damage

Preparedness: The knowledge and capacities developed by governments, professional response, and recovery organizations, communities, and individuals to effectively anticipate, respond to, and recover from, the impacts of likely, imminent, or current hazard events or conditions

Prevention: The outright avoidance of adverse impacts of hazards and related disasters

Recovery: The restoration and improvement where appropriate, of facilities, livelihoods, and living conditions of disaster-affected communities, including efforts to reduce disaster risk factors.

Residual risk: The risk that remains in unmanaged form, even when effective disaster-risk-reduction measures are in place, for which emergency response and recovery capacities must be maintained

Resilience: The ability of a system, community, or society exposed to hazards to resist, absorb, accommodate, and recover from the effects of a hazard in a timely and efficient manner, including through the preservation and restoration of its essential basic structures and functions

Response: The provision of emergency services and public assistance during or immediately after a disaster in order to save lives, reduce health impacts, ensure public safety, and meet the basic subsistence needs of the people affected

Risk: The probability of harmful consequences or expected losses (deaths, injuries, property, livelihoods, economic activity disrupted, or environment damage) resulting from interactions between natural or human-induced hazards and vulnerable conditions

Risk assessment: A methodology to determine the nature and extent of risk by analyzing potential hazards and evaluating existing conditions of vulnerability that together could potentially harm exposed people, property, services, livelihoods, and the environment on which they depend.

Risk management: The systematic approach and practice of managing uncertainty to minimize potential harm and loss

Sustainable development: Development that meets the needs of the present without compromising the ability of future generations to meet their own needs

Technological hazard: A hazard originating from technological or industrial conditions, including accidents, dangerous procedures, infrastructure failures, or specific human activities, that may cause loss of life, injury, illness, or other health impacts; property damage; loss of livelihoods and services; social and economic disruption; or environmental damage

Vulnerability: The characteristics and circumstances of a community, system, or asset that make it susceptible to the damaging effects of a hazard

---

In May 1994, one major achievement of the UN IDNDR was the hosting of the 1994 World Conference on Natural Disaster Reduction, which resulted in the Yokohama Strategy and Plan of Action for a Safer World: Guidelines for Natural Disaster Prevention, Preparedness, and Mitigation.[15] One of the strategies within the Yokohama Plan of Action stated that: "[the world] Will develop and strengthen national capacities and capabilities and, where appropriate, national legislation for natural and other disaster prevention, mitigation and preparedness, including the mobilization of non-governmental organization and participation of local communities."[15]

The Yokohama Strategy and Plan of Action affirmed that, "Disaster prevention, mitigation and preparedness are better than disaster response in achieving the goals and objectives of the Decade. Disaster response alone is not sufficient, as it yields only temporary results at a very high cost. We have followed this limited approach for too long. This has been further demonstrated by the recent focus on response to complex emergencies, which, although compelling, should not divert from pursuing a comprehensive approach. Prevention contributes to lasting improvement in safety and is essential to integrated disaster management."[15]

The Johannesburg World Summit for Sustainable Development (WSSD) plan of implementation further stated that, "An integrated, multihazard, inclusive approach to address vulnerability, risk assessment and disaster management, including prevention, mitigation, preparedness, response and recovery, is an essential element of a safer world in the twenty-first century."[16]

The United Nations General Assembly resolution on natural disasters and vulnerability then took into account the outcomes of the WSSD and the role of the International Strategy for Disaster Reduction and coordinated a review of the Yokohama Strategy and Plan of Action as requisite to the Second World Conference on Disaster Reduction held in 2005.[17]

Through its resolution A/RES/58/214, the United Nations General Assembly convened a World Conference on Disaster Reduction (WCDR), in Kobe, Hyogo, Japan, during January 2005.[17]

The conference provided a unique opportunity to promote a strategic and systematic approach to reducing vulnerabilities and risks to hazards. It underscored the need for, and identified ways of, building the resilience of nations and communities to disasters.

One of the key outcomes of the WCDR included the Hyogo Declaration, a joint statement recognizing "that a culture of disaster prevention and resilience, and associated pre-disaster strategies, which are sound investments, must be fostered at all levels, ranging from the individual to the international levels."[18]

Another key outcome of the WCDR was the 2005-2015 Hyogo Framework for Action (HFA).[19]

The HFA suggested five specific priorities for action:

1. Making disaster risk reduction a priority
2. Improving risk information and early warning
3. Building a culture of safety and resilience
4. Reducing the risks in key sectors
5. Strengthening preparedness for response

In 2003, as a result of catastrophic terrorist attacks, including the World Trade Center attack and the anthrax letter mailings, Homeland Security Presidential Directive 8 (HSPD-8) otherwise known as the National Preparedness Directive was released. This directive established policies to strengthen the preparedness of the United States to prevent and respond to threatened or actual domestic terrorist attacks, major disasters, and other emergencies by requiring a national domestic all-hazards preparedness goal, establishing mechanisms for improved delivery of federal preparedness assistance to state and local governments, and outlining actions to strengthen preparedness capabilities of federal, state, and local entities.[20]

This emphasis led to the emergence of health security as a new legislative focus as Congress recognized the need to expand the resiliency of the public health system to respond to national security threats. The Pandemic and All-Hazards Preparedness Act (PAHPA) of 2006 was passed, specifically including health security. The PAHPA broadened the previous focus on bioterrorism to a more comprehensive, all-hazards approach that acknowledged the growing concern of emerging or reemerging infectious diseases and natural disasters, in addition to intentional threats from chemical, nuclear, or radiological incidents. In turn, the U.S. Department of Health and Human Services released its National Health Security Strategy.[21]

In 2011, the White House released Presidential Policy Directive 8: National Preparedness (PPD-8). The directive was aimed at strengthening the security and resilience of the United States through *systematic* preparation for the threats that pose the greatest risk to the security of the nation, including acts of terrorism, cyber-attacks, pandemics, and catastrophic natural disasters. PPD-8 directed the development of a National Preparedness Goal that identifies the core capabilities necessary for preparedness and a National Preparedness System to guide activities that will enable the nation to achieve the goal. PPD-8 also called development of an annual National Preparedness Report based upon the National Preparedness Goal.[22]

CURRENT PRACTICE

The Approach to Disaster Preparedness

"Emergency preparedness is a program of long-term development activities whose goals are to strengthen the overall capacity and capability of a country to manage all types of emergencies and bring about an orderly transition from relief through recovery and back to sustained development."[13]

To be most effective, disaster preparedness programs should be one component of an overall disaster-risk-management strategy and should not be implemented as an isolated project. Disaster preparedness should be guided by a range of principles in order to adequately protect communities, property, and the environment. To be most effective the approach must be[23,24]:

- Comprehensive
- "All hazard"
- Multisectoral and intersectoral
- Community based and user friendly
- Culturally sensitive and specific

The all-hazard approach concerns developing and implementing emergency management strategies for the full range of likely emergencies or disasters, including both natural and technological (which also includes conflict-related hazards of terrorism and warfare).[24]

The multisectoral and intersectoral approach means that all organizations, including government, private and community, and traditional, as well as informal leadership, should be involved in disaster preparedness. If this approach is not used, emergency management is likely to be fragmented and inefficient. The multisectoral and intersectoral approach will also help to link emergency management to sustainable development, through the institutionalization of risk reduction and the use of its principles in long-term development projects.

The concept of preparedness at the community level is based upon the premise that the members, resources, organizations, and administrative structures of a community should all form the foundation of any emergency preparedness program. As the saying goes, "All disasters are local," meaning all disaster responses start at the local level.

These combined approaches will also help to link risk reduction to sustainable development, through the institutionalization of emergency management and the use of its principles in development projects. The resulting program becomes the responsibility of all and is undertaken at all administrative levels of both government and nongovernment organizations. The program concentrates not only on disasters but also on sustainable development of the society as a whole. These elements should be created at community, provincial, and national levels. An inherent capacity for risk reduction at each of these levels is a precondition for effective response and recovery when an emergency or disaster strikes. Without these capacities, any link from recovery to development will not be sustainable.

Health Objectives of Disaster Preparedness

Objectives of preparedness for health emergencies have been offered as follows[14]:

- Prevent morbidity and mortality
- Provide care for casualties
- Manage adverse climatic and environmental conditions
- Ensure restoration of normal health
- Reestablish health services
- Protect staff
- Protect public health and medical assets

The actions required to meet these needs can be grouped in four categories[14]:

1. *Preventive measures:* for example, building codes and floodplain management
2. *Protective measures:* for example, early warning and community education
3. *Life saving measures:* for example, rescue and relief
4. *Rehabilitation:* for example, resettlement and rebuilding

Key Elements of Disaster Preparedness

Even though the terms *preparedness* and *planning* are sometimes used interchangeably or redundantly, *planning* constitutes only one component of a comprehensive program of disaster preparedness. Box 32-2 lists the typical elements of an emergency preparedness program.[13,25-27]

BOX 32-2 Elements of an Emergency Preparedness Program

- Risk assessment
- Emergency planning
- Training and education
- Warning systems
- Specialized communication systems
- Information databases and knowledge management systems
- Resource management systems
- Resource stocks
- Emergency exercises
- Population protection systems
- Incident management systems
- Policy development
- Monitoring and evaluation

A Capability-Based Approach for Disaster Preparedness Programs

Populations at risk for disasters may face many vastly different hazards and threats within a nearly infinite set of unpredictable scenarios. This unpredictability is poorly suited to scenario-based approaches to risk management (i.e., risk management that focuses only on specific prioritized hazards).[7] Even though the hazards that cause disasters may vary greatly, the potential public health consequences and subsequent public health and medical needs of the population do not.[9,28] For example, warfare, chemical releases, floods, hurricanes, and earthquakes all displace people from their homes. All of these various disaster hazards require the same public health capability of shelter with only minor adjustments for the impact (severity according to hazard rapidity of onset, scale, duration, location, and intensity). Regardless of the hazard, disasters cause what are categorized into 15 public health consequences, which are addressed by 32 categories of public health and medical capabilities.[9] Tables 32-1 and 32-2 list the public health consequences most commonly associated with major natural and technological disasters, respectively.[8] Note that for most of the disaster hazards represented

TABLE 32-1 The Relative Public Health Impact Caused by Select Natural Disasters[8]

PUBLIC HEALTH CONSEQUENCE	INFECTIOUS	ENVIRONMENTAL					
	EPIDEMICS	FLOOD	HEAT WAVE	STORM	TROPICAL CYCLONE	DROUGHT	WILDFIRE
Number of deaths	Can be many	Few, but many in poor nations	Can be many (especially in large urban areas)	Few	Few, but many in poor nations	Few, but many in poor nations	Few
Severe injuries	Insignificant	Few	Can be many (heat illness)	Few	Few	Unlikely	Few
Loss of clean water	Insignificant	Focal to widespread	Insignificant	Focal	Focal to widespread	Widespread	Focal
Loss of shelter	Insignificant	Focal to widespread	Insignificant	Focal	Focal to widespread	Focal to widespread	Focal
Loss of personal/ household goods	Insignificant	Focal to widespread	Insignificant	Focal	Focal to widespread	Focal to widespread	Focal
Major population movements	Insignificant	Focal to widespread	Insignificant	Focal	Focal to widespread	Focal to widespread	Focal
Loss of routine hygiene	Insignificant	Focal to widespread	Insignificant	Focal	Focal to widespread	Widespread	Focal
Loss of sanitation	Insignificant	Focal to widespread	Insignificant	Focal	Focal to widespread	Focal	Focal
Disruption of solid waste management	Insignificant	Focal to widespread	Insignificant	Focal	Focal to widespread	Focal	Focal
Public concern for safety	Moderate	Moderate to High	Low to moderate	Low to moderate	High	Low to moderate	Moderate to High
Increased pests	Insignificant	Focal to widespread	Insignificant	Focal	Focal to widespread	Focal to widespread	Unlikely
Loss or damage of health care system	Insignificant	Focal to widespread	Insignificant	Focal	Focal to widespread	Focal	Focal to widespread
Worsening of chronic illnesses	Focal to widespread	Focal to widespread	Focal to widespread	Focal	Focal to widespread	Widespread	Focal to widespread
Loss of electrical power	Insignificant	Focal to widespread	Occasionally focal	Focal	Focal to widespread	Focal	Unlikely
Toxic exposures	Insignificant	Widespread for CO poisoning	Insignificant	Focal for CO poisoning	Widespread for CO poisoning	Focal	Widespread for air
Food scarcity	Insignificant	Focal to widespread	Insignificant	Insignificant	Common in low-lying coastal areas	Widespread in poor nations	Focal

TABLE 32-2   The Relative Public Health Impact Caused by Select Technological Disasters[8]

	TERROARISM/CONFLICT				
	INDUSTRIAL				
	TOXICOLOGICAL	**THERMAL**		**MECHANICAL**	
PUBLIC HEALTH CONSEQUENCE	**HAZARDOUS MATERIAL RELEASE**	**URBAN FIRE**	**EXPLOSIONS/ BOMBINGS**	**TRANSPORT CRASH**	**STRUCTURAL FAILURE**
Deaths	Moderate to many	Few to moderate	Moderate to many	Few to moderate	Moderate to many
Severe injuries	Moderate to many	Moderate to many	Moderate to many	Moderate to many	Moderate to many
Loss of clean water	Focal	Focal	Focal	Focal	Focal
Loss of shelter	Focal	Focal	Focal	Focal	Focal
Loss of personal and household goods	Focal	Focal	Focal	Focal	Focal
Major population movements	Focal	Focal	Focal	Focal	Focal
Loss of routine hygiene	Focal	Focal	Focal	Focal	Focal
Loss of sanitation	Focal	Focal	Focal	Focal	Focal
Disruption of solid waste management	Unlikely	Unlikely	Unlikely	Unlikely	Unlikely
Public concern for safety	High	High	High	High	High
Increased pests and vectors	Unlikely	Unlikely	Unlikely	Unlikely	Unlikely
Loss/damage of health care system	Focal	Focal	Focal	Focal	Focal
Worsening of existing chronic illnesses	Focal to widespread	Focal to widespread	Focal	Focal	Focal
Loss of electricity	Focal	Focal	Focal	Focal	Focal
Toxic exposures	Focal to widespread	Focal to widespread	Focal	Focal	Focal
Food scarcity	Unlikely	Unlikely	Unlikely	Unlikely	Unlikely

in these tables, variation exists only for the relative degree of impact for each of the public health consequences. Thus, the all-hazard preparedness program focuses not on the specific hazard but also on addressing each of the expected public health and medical consequences.

Table 32-3 lists the public health capabilities that are necessary to address those public health consequences listed in Tables 32-1 and 32-2 that are most commonly addressed in a disaster response. Thus, an effective emergency response can be developed through implementation of a preparedness program that builds capacity for each of the capabilities listed in Table 32-3 (in most cases, regardless of the hazard). An effective disaster preparedness program applies the key elements of emergency preparedness listed in Box 32-2 toward building capacity for each of the capabilities in Table 32-3.

Capability and Capacity

By using an all-hazards approach, societies and organizations prepare for, and respond to disasters by applying their own inherent capabilities to any and all disaster risks, regardless of priority. A *capability* is defined as the "ability to achieve a desired operational effect under specified standards and conditions through combinations of means and ways to perform a set of tasks."[7] The capability-based approach to planning was originally proposed by Nobel Prize-winning economists Amartya Sen and Martha Nussbaum.[29] Murphy and Gardoni have also proposed the use of a capability-based approach to measure hazard impact and to direct risk analysis[29] and hazard mitigation efforts.[30] Capability-based approaches to risk management have also been extensively applied by defense agencies, to address the challenges of uncertainty related to hazards involving asymmetrical warfare (i.e., terrorism).[31,32]

Capacity is the "combination of all the strengths, attributes and resources available within a community, society or organization that can be used to achieve agreed goals."[1] Although the two terms may be erroneously used interchangeably, it is important to differentiate capability from capacity. *Capability* is the ability to achieve a desired goal, whereas *capacity* is the measure of all the strengths, attributes, and resources available to achieve that goal. In order to measure the performance of a capability over time, capacity should be viewed as a rate (e.g., the number of lab tests performed in one day).

We may differentiate between the two by illustration. Consider whether or not a laboratory has the capability to perform a blood culture test. However, even though it does have the capability, there must also be some measure of the capacity (or rate at which these tests may be performed). The capacity for this particular capability is therefore expressed in terms of number of tests per hour or in larger magnitudes of number of tests per day. Thus, the capacity reflects not only the amount of materials available for this particular capability, but also other rate-limiting essential elements such as human resources and technical skills.

Process for Development of Disaster Preparedness Programs

Figure 32-1 illustrates the cycle followed for building and improving disaster preparedness programs. This process should be repeated, at minimum, on an annual basis. High-profile or rapidly changing events (such as large mass gatherings or high-threat environments) may require a more frequent repetitive cycle.

Box 32-3 summarizes the major phases involved in development of a capabilities-based disaster preparedness program.

TABLE 32-3   Public Health Consequences and Public Health Capabilities Associated with All Disasters

PUBLIC HEALTH CONSEQUENCES	PUBLIC HEALTH CAPABILITIES
Common to all disasters	Resource management
	Information sharing §
	Emergency operations coordination §
	Responder safety and health §/occupational health & safety
	Business continuity
	Volunteer management §
Deaths	Fatality management §/mortuary care
	Social services
	Mental health services
Illness and injuries	Health services
	Mental health services
	Injury prevention and control
	Public Health Surveillance §/epidemiological investigation
	Disease prevention and control
	Medical countermeasure dispensing §
	Medical material management & distribution §
	Public health laboratory testing §
	Medical surge §
	Nonpharmaceutical interventions (isolation, quarantine, social distancing, travel, and restriction/advisory) §
Loss of clean water	Water, sanitation, and hygiene (WASH)
	Health services (e.g., hospitals and dialysis units)
Loss of shelter	Mass care §/shelter & settlement
	Social services
	Security
Loss of personal and household goods	Replacement of personal and household goods
Loss of sanitation and routine hygiene	Sanitation, excreta disposal and hygiene promotion
	Nonpharmaceutical interventions (hygiene) §
Disruption of solid waste management	Solid waste management
Public concern for safety	Risk communication/emergency public information and warning §
	Security
Increased pests and vectors	Pest and vector control
Loss or damage of health care system	Health system and infrastructure support
	Reproductive health services
	Health services
Worsening of chronic illnesses	Health services
Food scarcity	Food safety, security, and nutrition
Standing surface water	Public works and engineering
Toxic exposures	Risk assessment and exposure modeling
	Population protection measures (evacuation/shelter in place)
	Health services
	HazMat emergency response/decontamination §
	Responder safety and health §/occupational health & safety

Entries marked as § are adapted from CDC. Public health preparedness capabilities: national standards for state and local planning. March 2011. Available at URL: http://www.cdc.gov/phpr/capabilities/Capabilities_March_2011.pdf Last accessed May 18, 2014.

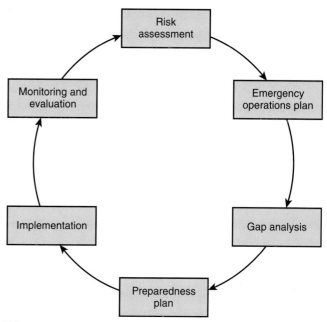

FIG 32-1 The Preparedness Program Cycle

BOX 32-3   Phases for Developing a Capabilities-Based Disaster Preparedness Program

Risk Assessment
1. Disaster risks are identified using the risk equation: $R = H \times V$
2. Public health impacts are then identified for all major disaster risks (Tables 32-2 and 32-3)

Emergency Operations Plan
1. Capabilities are then identified that will address all public health consequences expected to occur (Table 32-3)
2. Strategic objectives, operational objectives, and activities that will implement the essential capabilities are then identified and represented in an EOP (Fig. 32-2)

Gap Analysis
1. Current absorptive capacity (capabilities + capacities = absorptive capacity, AC) are assessed for each activity in the EOP and compared to those expected AC required for an adequate emergency response
2. Gaps between current AC and expected AC are identified (Fig. 32-4)

Preparedness Plan
1. Activities that will eliminate the gaps between current AC and expected AC are identified and represented in a preparedness plan (Fig. 32-4)

Implementation of the Preparedness Plan
1. Activities included in the preparedness plan are implemented
2. These activities may include projects, programs, policy, and procedures

Monitoring and Evaluation
1. Procedures are put in place to monitor and evaluate how the preparedness program is implemented and what needs to be done to improve it
2. The following four methods are used for monitoring and evaluation of preparedness programs:
   a. Project management
   b. Operational debriefing
   c. Exercises
   d. Systems analysis

Risk Assessment

Disaster risk assessment methods are used to develop plans and make operational decisions as part of a larger risk reduction strategy. Risk assessment may be based on quantitative or qualitative data, or a combination of these. Where appropriate, the confidence placed on estimates of levels of risk should be included. Assumptions made in the analysis should be clearly stated.

Ideally, risk assessment would be based on all-hazards risk modeling and a quantitative hazard analysis. Both processes are extremely costly and time-consuming to produce and are, therefore, beyond the scope of most public health disaster risk analyses. Quantitative risk analysis is based on statistical values. This requires extensive and accurate "hard data," and uses mathematical manipulation of the data to produce an accurate map of all hazards and generate tables that assign numerical values to the probability and frequency of risk, and to the population's exposure and susceptibility to risk. Unfortunately, the availability of such hard data is relatively limited for nonmaterial assets, such as the public health and safety of a population.

Risk assessment commonly uses a form of real-time Delphi method, known as the mini-Delphi method (also known as "estimate-talk-estimate").[33,34] In ideal risk management, a prioritization process is followed whereby the risks with the greatest loss and the greatest probability of occurring are handled first, and risks with lower probability of occurrence and lower loss are handled in descending order. Once hazards have been identified, their potential severity of loss and the probability of occurrence must then be assessed. In practice for public health, the process can be very difficult. "The fundamental difficulty in disaster risk assessment is determining the rate of occurrence since statistical information is not available on all kinds of past incidents."[35] Further, "evaluating the severity of the consequences (impact) is often quite difficult for immaterial assets." Thus, "best educated opinions and available statistics are the primary sources of information."[35] Nevertheless, qualitative or semiquantitative risk assessment can produce such information so that the primary risks are easy to understand and that the risk management decisions may be prioritized. The criteria for measuring disaster consequence severity (impact) may vary, but it usually addresses issues related to the following[35]:

- Number of fatalities and injuries
- Critical facilities and community lifelines
- Property and environmental damage
- Economic, social, and political disruption
- Size of the area or the number of people affected

In order to accommodate the high degree of uncertainty associated with disaster risk assessments, qualitative analysis uses descriptive scales to depict the likelihood and magnitude of risks. It may be carried out to varying degrees of complexity. It is mostly used as an initial evaluation, where the level of risk does not justify further analysis or where there are insufficient data or resources for more quantitative analysis. It often takes the form of a hazard probability/impact matrix or numerical score.

The most pertinent information sources and techniques should be used when analyzing consequences and likelihood. Sources of information may include the following[36]:

- Past records (historical data for hazard frequency and impact, population demographics, etc.)
- Practice and relevant experience
- Relevant published literature
- Results of public consultation (e.g., focus groups, public hearings)
- Experiments and prototypes
- Economic, engineering, or other models
- Specialist and expert judgment

Techniques for risk assessment may include[36]:

- Structured interviews with experts in the area of interest
- Use of multidisciplinary groups of experts
- Individual evaluations using questionnaires
- Use of models and simulations

A qualitative method for risk assessment has been widely used to quantify public health risk. The risk equation has also been applied to roughly estimate disaster risk according to the following relationship:

$$D = (H \times V) - AC$$

where D is the risk of disaster occurrence, H the probability of hazard occurrence and subsequent exposure, V the probability of population vulnerability, and AC is the absorptive capacity of the affected population (capabilities and associated capacity to respond and recover). Hazard risk (H) is calculated according the equation $H = L \times I$ (where L is the likelihood and I the impact of the hazard). Table 32-4 provides an example of criteria used to score likelihood of hazard occurrence. Table 32-5 provides an example of criteria used to score potential impact of disaster hazards.

In the case of natural hazards, historical records as well as geo-seismic and hydrometeorological analyses may be used to inform these estimates. In the case of technological hazards, formal risk analysis and threat assessments, as well as historical records may also be used. However, the predictive value of these estimates of technological risk may have a higher degree of uncertainty compared with that of natural hazards.

According to the risk equation, disaster risk may be reduced among populations at risk by removing the hazard itself; by decreasing the vulnerability; and by increasing the absorptive capacity.[10] This risk assessment begins with identification of potential hazards, followed by a prioritization of these hazards according to two criteria: likelihood and impact. Upon completion of the hazard analysis, population vulnerability is then analyzed according to set criteria. Numerous methods and tools have been developed for estimation of population vulnerability to disasters.[10,35,37]

Box 32-4 provides one example of criteria that may be considered for estimation of vulnerability.

A final risk score is then calculated using individual scores for both hazards and vulnerability. This risk score is then used to guide development of a set of prioritized risks. Absorptive capacity is then later factored into the disaster risk assessment during the gap analysis phase (Fig. 32-4).[38]

TABLE 32-4 Criteria for Scoring Likelihood of Hazard Occurrence

SCORE	DESCRIPTOR	DESCRIPTION	EXPECTED TO OCCUR
5	Almost certain	Will occur on an annual basis	Once a year or more frequently
4	Likely	Has occurred several times or more during your 10-30 yr of employment in public health	Once every 3 yr
3	Possible	Might occur once in your career	Once every 10 yr
2	Unlikely	Does occur somewhere in the nation from time to time	Once every 30 yr
1	Rare	Heard of something like this occurring elsewhere	Once every 100 yr

TABLE 32-5 Criteria for Scoring Potential Impact of Hazard

POTENTIAL IMPACT CRITERIA	SCORE = 0	SCORE = 1	SCORE = 2	SCORE = 3	SCORE = 4
Size of incident area	*None* No specific site of event	*Limited* Less than an entire municipality	*Municipal-wide* One entire municipality	*Province-wide* Entire province or multiple municipalities	*Nation-wide* Entire nation
Percentage of jurisdiction population whose health will be affected	*None* 0% of total population	*Low* Less than 25% of total population	*Moderate* 26%-50% of total population	*High* 51%-75% of total population	*Very high* 76%-100% of total population
Potential for lethality among those affected	*None* Negligible chance of being lethal	*Low* (less than 25%) chance of being lethal	*Moderate* (26%-50%) chance of being lethal	*High* (51%-75%) chance of being lethal	*Very high* (76%-100%) chance of being lethal
Potential degree of destruction of critical infrastructure or environmental ecosystem	*None* Significant destruction unlikely to occur	*Limited* Less than one municipality	*Municipal-wide* One entire municipality	*Province-wide* Entire province or multiple municipalities	*Nation-wide* Entire nation
Potential for damage to government or community reputation (Risk perception)	*None* No significant media attention	*Minor* Minor adverse local public media attention or complaints	*Moderate* Attention from media and/or heightened public concern by local community	*Major* Significant adverse national media and public complaints	*Severe* Serious public complaints and/or international coverage

BOX 32-4 Factors That Contribute to Public Health Vulnerability

- Poverty
- Age extremes (i.e., younger than 5 years old; older than 60 years old)
- Gender
- Disability
- Lack of information, education, and communication
- Lack of experience and process
- Inadequate health care
- Geographical location/isolation
- Inadequate social and organizational integration/coordination
- Malnutrition
- Inappropriate developmental policies
- Food insecurity
- Societal stratification
- Poor water and food quality
- Limited state and local resources
- Political perceptions
- Negative social interactions—administrative graft/corruption and competition
- Lack of social order
- High burden of illness/injuries
- Inadequate preparedness and mitigation

(Criteria for scoring: 0=none; 1=low; 2=median; 3=high)

Adapted from Clack Z, Keim M, Macintyre A, et al. Emergency health and risk management in sub-Saharan Africa: a lesson from the embassy bombings in Tanzania and Kenya. *Prehosp Dis Med.* 2002;17(2): 59-66.

Emergency Operations Plan

Principles of Effective Emergency Operations Planning

A *disaster plan* is an agreed set of arrangements for preparing for, responding to, and recovering from emergencies, involving the description of responsibilities, management structures, strategies, and resource and information management. Disaster planning is about protecting life, property, and the environment.

The elements of discussing, informing, learning, and negotiation that take place during the planning process are much more valuable for ensuring a well-coordinated response than any subsequent plan intended to merely document this critical decision making.

The written plan itself is only one outcome of the planning process. The planning process should produce:

- An understanding of organizational responsibilities in response and recovery
- Strengthening of emergency management networks
- Improved community participation and awareness

- Effective response and recovery strategies and systems
- A simple and flexible written plan

Effective planning allows people's needs, preferences, and values to be reflected in decisions. A basic principle of good planning is that individual, short-term decisions are coordinated in order to support strategic, long-term objectives. Planning is a social activity; that is, it involves people, and the results are affected by those whom are involved and how they participate in the process. Good planning does more than simply identify the easiest solution to a particular problem. It can be an opportunity for learning, development, and consensus building. How stakeholders are involved is a key factor in the effectiveness of a planning process. A good planning process usually begins with the most general concepts and leads to increasingly specific plans, programs, and tasks, resulting in integration between each part.[39,40]

There are several key approaches to effective emergency operations planning that have been offered in order to improve the efficiency of plan writing and to facilitate quality and timely execution of the plan.

These approaches have been described as O2C3 and include the following characteristics[39]:

- Operational-level planning
- Objective-based planning
- Capability-based planning
- Consensus-based planning
- Compliant with local, national, and international preparedness strategies, guidelines, and best practices

Operational-Level Planning

Operational plans describe short-term ways of achieving objectives and explain how (or what portion of) a strategic plan will be put into operation during a given period of time. Operational plans describe response operations as compared to the other functions within the incident command system. They are not intended to be administrative, intelligence, or logistic plans that describe support functions.

Objective-Based Planning

Objective-based planning can serve as an effective tool for making progress by ensuring that participants have a clear awareness of what they must do to achieve or help achieve an objective. Homeland Security Presidential Directive 5 (HSPD-5) established a National Incident Management System (NIMS) in the United States. Management by objectives is an essential component of NIMS communicated throughout the entire ICS organization, and it includes[41]:

- Establishing incident objectives
- Developing strategies based on incident objectives
- Developing and issuing assignments, plans, procedures, and protocols
- Establishing specific, measurable tasks for various incident management functional activities, and directing efforts to accomplish them, in support of defined strategies
- Documenting results to measure performance and facilitate corrective actions

Capability-Based Planning

Capability-based planning is also the foundation on which the U.S. Homeland Security Exercise Evaluation Program (HSEEP) and other federal preparedness initiatives are based.[42] Capabilities (or the abilities to perform a particular task) provide the common framework used for relating and comparing disparate elements of an emergency response organization.[32] The objective-based approach, when used alone, may imply a degree of certainty regarding the disaster hazard or threat that may not be attainable. This unpredictability is best met by planning to accomplish those objectives that we are actually *capable* of achieving. Homeland Security Presidential Directive 8 (HSPD-8) is the first to mandate that federal, state, local, and tribal entities, their private and nongovernmental partners, and the general public should adopt a capability-based planning approach for EOPs.[43]

Consensus-Based Planning

The U.S. Federal Emergency Management Agency (FEMA) recommends a team-based approach to writing EOPs.[28] Consensus-based decision making is a group decision-making process that seeks not only the agreement of most participants but also to resolve or mitigate the objections of the minority to achieve the most agreeable decision. *Consensus* is usually defined as meaning both general agreement and the process of getting to such agreement. Consensus-based decision making is thus concerned primarily with that process. As a decision-making process, consensus aims to be: inclusive, participatory, cooperative, egalitarian, and solution oriented. HSPD-8 charged all federal agencies involved in emergency response to participate in emergency planning on a "consensus-basis."[43]

Compliance with Local, National, and International Strategies

It is important that EOPs are compliant with local, national, and international strategies, guidelines, and best practices. On an international basis, examples of these guidelines and best practices may include Standards for Humanitarian Assistance,[44] Handbooks of Disaster Medicine,[13] or Guidelines for Pandemic Influenza Preparedness and Mitigation.[45]

In the United States, these national strategies are directed by presidential directives. Presidential directives related to emergency operations planning include HSPD-5[46] and HSPD-8.[43] In addition, specific guidelines are also available for diseases such as pandemic influenza.[47]

Plan Elements

An EOP contains a listing of response capabilities necessary to mount an effective response to all hazards. This information is best organized according to a cascading network of planning elements for each individual capability. These elements include: strategic objectives, operational objectives, activities (or tasks), responsible parties, and standard operating procedures. Table 32-6 describes each one of these plan elements.

Capabilities are derived according to the public health consequences caused by the disaster (Table 32-3). Each capability is associated with one or more strategic objectives that reflect the desired state of affairs intended to be achieved. Each strategic objective is then related to one or more operational objectives, which are, in turn, related to activities that accomplish each operational objective. Each activity is then associated with a responsible party and a standard operating procedure (SOP) for how the activity will be accomplished. This hierarchical format cascading from each capability is referred to as the acronym, "S-O-A-R-S" and is depicted in Fig. 32-2.

TABLE 32-6 Working Definitions for Plan Elements[48]

PLAN ELEMENT	WORKING DEFINITION	SIMPLE DESCRIPTION
Capability	Ability to achieve a desired operational effect under specified standards and conditions through combinations of means and ways to perform a set of tasks	Ability
Objectives	A projected state of affairs that a person or a system plans or intends to achieve	Goal
Strategic objective	A general statement of the end goal	Why
Operational objective	Specific goals that constitute the means for attaining the strategic goal	What
Activity	A set of actions that accomplish specific goals	How
Responsible parties	Individuals or groups assigned responsibility for accomplishing an activity	Who
Standard operating procedure (SOP)	A set of instructions covering those features of operations that lend themselves to a definite or standardized procedure without loss of effectiveness	When Where

Adapted from Keim M. An innovative approach to capability-based emergency operations planning. *J Disaster Health.* 2013;1(1):54-62.

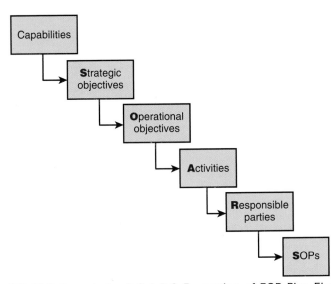

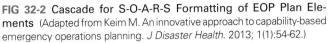

FIG 32-2 Cascade for S-O-A-R-S Formatting of EOP Plan Elements (Adapted from Keim M. An innovative approach to capability-based emergency operations planning. *J Disaster Health*. 2013; 1(1):54-62.)

Table 32-7 represents an example of how this S-O-A-R-S format would be used to depict the hierarchy of plan elements for the capability of "Water, Sanitation, and Hygiene." This example is based upon the Sphere international Standards for Humanitarian Assistance.[44]

Planning Method

A planning method is a logical and reproducible way to write a plan. Guidelines for this standardized approach should be taught to all participants of the planning workshop. Ideally, use of a training curriculum for local planners and trainers appears to impart sustainability of planning efforts using this standard approach. Figure 32-3 depicts the six major steps necessary to prepare for plan writing.

Gap Analysis

The EOP should be written within the context of currently existing capabilities and capacities. In other words, the plan should be considered as though it will be implemented on the very day that it is written. During the writing of the plan, certain deficiencies and gaps will likely become obvious. These gaps may involve a deficiency of entire capabilities, or they may involve deficiencies in capacity for capabilities that exist to an incomplete degree. For example, a hospital emergency department may or may not have the capability to treat pediatric patients. If it indeed does have this capability, then one must also consider the capacity (or rate at which a number of patients may be adequately treated in an emergency department within a given timeframe).

Once the EOP is completed, it is then necessary to perform a gap analysis. This gap analysis is intended to guide development of a preparedness plan through identification of deficiencies in capabilities and capacities in the EOP. The gap analysis begins by identifying any capabilities that may be absent from the EOP. If this capability is deemed essential to an adequate disaster response, then the preparedness plan should include a means for either internal development of this capability or rapid procurement of this capability through external assistance.

TABLE 32-7 **Example of S-O-A-R-S Plan Format for the Capability of "Water, Sanitation, and Hygiene"[44,48]**

CAPABILITY	STRATEGIC OBJECTIVE	OPERATIONAL OBJECTIVE	ACTIVITY	RESPONSIBILITY	SOP
Water, Sanitation, and Hygiene	An adequate supply of clean water is accessible to all people	A sufficient quantity of water is available to all people	Ensure that the maximum distance from any household to the nearest water point is 500 meters		
			Ensure that the average water use for drinking, cooking, and personal hygiene in any household is at least 15 liters per person per day	Public works	Etc.
		Water is of sufficient quality to be potable and used for hygiene	Ensure there is low risk of fecal contamination		
			Use a sanitary survey to indicate the risk of fecal contamination	Sanitarian	Etc.
			Ensure there are no fecal coliforms per 1000 ml at the point of delivery		
		People are able to safely collect, store, and use sufficient quantities of water	Ensure each household has at least two clean water-collecting containers of 10-20 liters		
			Ensure water-collection and storage containers have narrow necks and/or covers (or other safe means of storage, drawing, and handling)	Central supply	Etc.

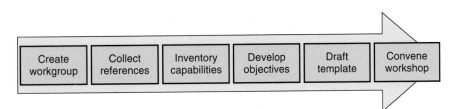

FIG 32-3 Six Major Steps Necessary to Prepare for Plan Writing (Adapted from Keim M. An innovative approach to capability-based emergency operations planning. *J Disaster Health*. 2013; 1(1):54-62.)

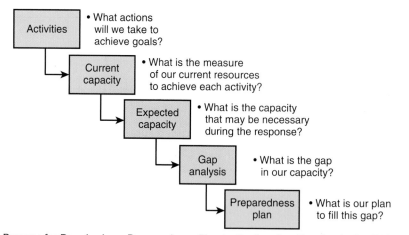

FIG 32-4 Process for Developing a Preparedness Plan by Performing Gap Analysis of EOP Activities

The next step in the gap analysis is to compare current absorptive capacity (AC) with expected AC. Current AC represents those capabilities that are now in existence and a measure of its associated capacity that could be performed within a certain timeframe (rate). Expected AC is an estimate of how much of each capability and its associated capacity will be needed for each of the public health consequences expected to be caused by a given disaster.

This process is performed for each activity identified in the EOP. Figure 32-4 depicts the process of gap analysis starting with each activity listed in the EOP and ending with a preparedness planning element intended to close this gap.

Table 32-8 provides an example of how a gap analysis is performed and preparedness project plans are developed based upon the EOP.

Implementation of Preparedness Programs

Once the gap analysis is complete, and the preparedness plan has been developed, a timeline for implementation of the preparedness program is put into place. Implementation of this program should include all of the elements identified in Table 32-6. In addition, the preparedness plan developed by the health sector will also require the partnership of other sectors such as: public safety, defense, transportation, public

works, and education, to name but a few. Key elements of preparedness programs that often require closely coordinated multisector collaboration include public policy, as well as training and education.

Policy development includes legislation that is normally developed by a national government, and will mainly relate to responsibility for emergency preparedness and special emergency powers. There is also a need for central government, provincial and community organizations, and nongovernmental organizations to develop appropriate policies.

Policy is required to ensure that common goals are pursued within and across organizations and activities. In addition, it must streamline rapid decision making, ensure that actions are legal, protect people from liability, and ensure that common practices are followed. Without agreed policies there will be poor coordination, a lack of a unified direction, and poor results. Policy can take the form of legislation, decisions by executive government, interorganizational agreements, or organizational directions.

Training and education involve training public health personnel and community responders in emergency management skills and knowledge and informing the community of the actions that may be required during emergencies and how the community can participate in emergency management.

TABLE 32-8   Example of Using Gap Analysis to Develop a Preparedness Plan Based Upon the EOP

RESPONSE PLAN		GAP ANALYSIS			PREPAREDNESS PLAN		
Capability (from the existing EOP)	Activity (from the existing EOP)	Current capability Are we *capable* of performing this activity now? (Yes or No)	Current capacity Quantify our current *capacity* to complete this activity.	Expected capacity How much would be needed in an emergency?	Gap analysis List missing capability and/or subtract essential from current capacity	Preparedness activity Identify activities that are needed to fill the gap	Checklist What steps are needed to complete the preparedness activity?
Vector control	Investigate field vector populations	Yes	200 investigations/wk	400 investigations/wk	200 investigations/wk	None	Complete exercise for 400 investigations/wk
	Ensure vector control plan is in place	Yes	2 plans	2 plans	0	None	N/A
	Instruct workers regarding vector control	Yes	50 workers are trained	100 workers	50 workers require additional training	Training for 50 workers	1. Develop training 2. Deliver training 3. Evaluate training

The objectives of training and education in emergency management are that:

- The community is empowered to participate in the development of emergency preparedness strategies.
- The community knows the appropriate actions for different types of emergencies, and the organizations it can turn to for assistance.
- Emergency management personnel are able to carry out the tasks allotted to them.

There are a number of possible training and education strategies that are suitable for different audiences and purposes. Strategy selection should be based on need, audience, purpose, available time, and available money and other resources.

Training and education strategies may include[23]:

- Workshops, seminars, formal education programs, or conferences
- Self-directed learning
- Individual tuition
- Exercises
- Pamphlets, videos, media advertisements, newsletters, or journals
- Informal or formal presentations
- Training of the public, from schoolchildren to professionals
- Public displays or public meetings
- Mentorship and temporary duty assignments

Managing the Process of Disaster Preparedness

Whether developing and implementing an entire emergency preparedness program, or conducting a key element of disaster preparedness (Box 32-2), project management methods will be required.

There are three major phases of project management: project definition, project planning, and project implementation.[49] *Project definition* concerns the aim and objectives of a project, as well as its scope and authority. *Project planning* is the process of sequencing tasks to achieve the project objectives and to ensure timely project completion and efficient use of resources. It involves: determining tasks, assigning responsibilities, developing a timetable, and determining resource allocation and timing. *Project implementation* consists of project performance, monitoring and evaluation, and taking corrective action.

In the late 1980s and early 1990s, a reformation of management theory and structure occurred in American business. Continuous quality improvement (CQI) arose out of the careful and disciplined study of traditional management approaches by a group of separate but similar thinkers.[49] Certain key features are inherent to any CQI approach, regardless of its specific application. These features include:

1. Customer focus (or, in the case of disaster management, victim focus)
2. Statistical application of knowledge of variation
3. Focus on process
4. Design and redesign
5. A redefinition of leadership

A rich body of literature has since developed regarding the implementation of CQI in a wide range of settings, in both manufacturing and service industries, including health care.[49] "CQI applications have been particularly relevant to the emergency department, given the process-based focus of quality improvement and the fact that the emergency department is a process-rich environment."[49] The same could also be said for all phases of disaster management, which are also process rich.

Monitoring and Evaluation

Monitoring and evaluation involves determining how well a disaster preparedness program is being developed and implemented, and what needs to be done to improve it. This method can be applied to all processes of a disaster preparedness program.

Four ways for monitoring and evaluating preparedness will be described here:

- Project management
- Operational debriefing
- Exercises
- Systems analysis

Project management is a means of monitoring and evaluating during the implementation phase of a project, which includes:

- Measuring the progress toward project objectives
- Analysis to determine the cause of deviations in the project
- Determining corrective actions

Operational debriefing employs the process of "after action study" or a discussion of "lessons learned" after significant or strategically important operations. These evaluation tools are generally conducted immediately after a disaster event, may not be based on statistical analysis, and are more descriptive in nature. In its simplest form, it may be a forum for discussion of what went right and what could have been done better to improve services.

Exercises are a common way of monitoring and evaluating parts of emergency preparedness programs. Exercises can be used to test aspects of emergency plans, emergency procedures, training, feasibility of coordination, communications, etc. The purpose of an exercise and the aspect of emergency preparedness to be tested must be carefully decided and fairly specific. *An exercise should not be conducted with the purpose of testing an entire emergency plan, or all aspects of training.*

Some typical types of exercise include:

- Operational exercises—where personnel and resources are actually deployed in a simulation of an emergency
- Tabletop exercises—where personnel are presented with an unfolding scenario, asked what actions would be required, and asked and how their actions would be implemented
- Syndicate exercises— where personnel are divided into syndicates to discuss and consider a given scenario, and the syndicate planning and response decisions are then discussed in an open forum.

System analysis studies the various components of a preparedness program searching for the existence of elements of the program that are assumed to be important, using objectives, checklists, and key questions for each element.[50] The national emergency profile and health policy are dealt with in general terms, whereas the element concerning technical and administrative organization is analyzed in greater detail.

DISASTER PREPAREDNESS PITFALLS

Pitfalls of Disaster Management in General

In one study of past disaster management problems and their causes, the following problems were categorized[51]:

- Inadequate appraisal of damages
- Inadequate problem ranking
- Inadequate identification, location, transportation, and utilization of resources

Among 22 U.S. disasters in this study, 93 examples of inappropriate management activities were identified. Most disaster mismanagement problems occurred because managers did not know what all of the relief activities were or how they should be accomplished.[51] Difficulties in disaster management also frequently involve breakdowns in communication and coordination.[52] The people of the Caribbean have a saying regarding the frequently recurring themes of disaster mismanagement that occurs, "Horses never step in the same hole in the road more than once . . . only people do." Many of the mistakes that we make in disaster response could easily be prevented through adequate preparedness and learning from past mistakes.

Preparedness as a Short-Term Activity Instead Long-Term Sustainable Versus Programs

"In disaster-prone countries, constant preparedness is essential."[12] To be most effective, disaster preparedness programs should be one component of an overall vulnerability reduction strategy and should not be implemented as an isolated project.[13]

Lack of Valid Assumptions and Knowledge Regarding the Disaster Phenomenon

"Proper planning and execution of disaster medical aid programs require knowledge of the types of disasters that might occur, the morbidity and mortality that might result and the consequent medical care needs."[53] Health decisions made during emergencies are often based on insufficient or unnecessary health aid, waste of health resources, or counter-effective measures.[54] In addition, the very nature of disasters adds difficulty to empirical or prospective study. These high-profile events also tend to gain a high degree of public and personal attention. The literature is, therefore, replete with inaccurate anecdotal case reporting, even though studies of disasters have identified variables that contribute to the potential for injury.[52]

Over-Reliance upon External Assistance, Mobile Field Hospitals, and Specialized Surgical Teams

Quite frequently, "families, friends and neighbors search, evacuate and extricate their own in the aftermath of a disaster,"[55] and by the time external relief teams are functional on site, a very large majority of the total dead have already died,[14,56–59] or, in the case of chemical contamination, victims often arrive at the hospital before any prehospital decontamination occurs.[59] External emergency relief is, therefore, largely expensive, wasteful, and not particularly effective.[14] These types of medical relief operations have been referred to as the "second disaster,"[60] and response measures do not always lead to the most effective means of recovery. Disasters (such as Hurricane Mitch in Central America) may additionally negate the accomplishments of a generation in human, institutional, and economic development and increase the already high dependence on external assistance and financing.[61] This does not imply that disaster relief should be abandoned, but rather that a more comprehensive and cost-effective approach to disaster risk reduction and management is needed.

Misuse of Disaster Exercises

Experience is the key to a successful disaster response. Unfortunately, disaster drills occur infrequently; they may not test the plan and the participants effectively and may create a sense of misplaced security.[52] In addition, an exercise should not be conducted with the purpose of testing an entire emergency plan, or all aspects of training.[25]

Problems in Disaster Planning

Standard disaster plans, when completed, are rarely used in operations because:

- They are cumbersome—disaster plans tend to be extremely thick, non–user friendly documents that fulfill legal regulations but do not address operational problems.
- Staff is often not trained or even aware of a developed disaster plan.
- Health disaster plans are not integrated into the overall planning process—they do not easily fit into the national plans or work on the assumption that other external players or agencies will coordinate or support public health response activities when required.
- Disaster planning that integrates governmental regulations/requirements and best practices creates plans that are difficult to operationalize.

- There is a tendency to have a single disaster plan and to send the same disaster response regardless of the particular circumstances.[25]

In addition, there are many challenges facing public health planners as they strive to perform these tasks in an efficacious and cost-efficient manner,[39,48] for example:

- Many public health officials throughout the world have limited knowledge, experience, and time for developing, evaluating, or improving the quality of EOPs.
- Plans must address a broad range of hazards and contingencies (tending toward a voluminous document) yet must also be user friendly and easily accessible during the postdisaster phase.
- Public health response activities must be well integrated with other governmental and nongovernmental agencies and institutions and be based upon scientific evidence.
- Existing models and guidance for emergency operation planning focus on plan content (or tasks) rather than the process (or management system) and lack clear indicators of performance and outcome or measures of effectiveness.

Over-Emphasis on Mass Casualty Care in Health Sector Disaster Plans

Health sector disaster planning tends to focus inordinately on mass casualty care, including surgical and critical care,[62] even though these interventions have tended to play a small role in public health.[55]

Poor Planning for Management of Human Resources

Rescue personnel are generally reluctant to ask for rest, food, and water breaks while victims are in need.[52] This results in high levels of fatigue, thus hindering effective operations, worker safety, and even patient care. Many plans and preparedness programs do not take into consideration the need for employee rest periods, occupational health measures, and critical incident stress management for disaster responders. Personnel problems can also occur associated with the inevitable onslaught of well-meaning volunteers.[52,63]

Quality Management as Applied to Disaster Preparedness

To a large extent, disaster planners have previously considered the end results of their work to be largely immeasurable. The victim's journey from impact to recovery, although subject to numerous measurements, had been considered to be largely an immeasurable process, particularly with regard to customer satisfaction, cost, outcome, and measurement.[33] This is an odd paradox in a field whose very essence concerns the nature of being able to measure quantifiable differences in public health as the course of the disaster event progresses or improves. Over the past half-century, the business administration sector has embraced a wide variety of principles directed toward quality management and efficiency (i.e., CQI, total quality management, lean management systems, and Six Sigma).[64–67]

A body of literature has developed that supports the application of principles of operations management and measures of effectiveness for evaluation and monitoring of humanitarian assistance efforts.[68,69] However, the application of quality management principles toward the goal of disaster preparedness remains remarkably underdeveloped.

Understanding the implications of variation in process is a critical skill for the disaster manager. Common cause variation refers to naturally occurring, statistically predictable variations that are inherent in all processes. By applying statistical principles one can determine the variations that are common cause in nature, which helps guide appropriate interventions to improve the system. Because of the lack of understanding of the basic principles of common cause variation, one of the most common problems is tampering with the system as a result of over-interpretation of data.[49] Special cause variation is a natural variation caused by events or circumstances that are nontypical and, therefore, not inherent in the process. Such special causes are often operator dependent (caused by variation in individuals providing service within the system). This is particularly true in cases in which different operators provide the service through a process that is inherently different from that of other providers.

THE FUTURE OF DISASTER PREPAREDNESS

The future of disaster preparedness will depend upon the maturity of disaster medicine and disaster management as an empirical science. As is the case with the practice of medicine, one universally applicable procedure or template is not applicable to all instances. The "cure" must be based upon an accurate diagnosis and appreciation of the unique needs and resources of the population involved. However, there is now a large and ever-growing body of evidence with which to guide well-informed decision making. Best practices, such as the Sphere Project minimum standards,[44] that are well implemented at the community level and that integrate all sectors may become more commonplace. Qualitative assessment and management methodologies, such as the regression analysis for quantification of risk assessment, as well as CQI[49] programs, may provide models for further objectification of disaster preparedness. A more holistic approach to disaster preparedness within the context of a comprehensive strategy of disaster risk reduction may promote sustainable development on a global scale. This will all depend upon the commitment of those now called to the task. Future generations may either admire our thoughtful investment or curse our selfish shortsightedness. The dividends of preparedness, though seldom realized today, often become tragically obvious tomorrow.

REFERENCES

1. UNISDR. *United Nations International Strategy for Disaster Reduction. Terminology on Disaster Risk Reduction.* 2009 available at URL: http://www.unisdr.org/files/7817_UNISDRTerminologyEnglish.pdf. Last Accessed 18.05.14.
2. Hogan D, Burstein J. Basic physics of disasters. In: Hogan D, Burstein J, eds. *Disaster Medicine.* Philadelphia: Lippincott, Williams & Wilkins; 2007: 5.
3. Ciottone G. *Introduction to Disaster Medicine and Emergency Management in Disaster Medicine.* Philadelphia, PA: Mosby-Elsevier; 2006, p. 4.
4. King F. The role of risk assessment in life-cycle risk management. In: *Risk Assessment and Management: Emergency Planning Perspective.* Waterloo, Canada: University of Waterloo Press; 1988:34–38.
5. Schipper L, Pelling M. Disaster risk, climate change and international development: scope for, and challenges to, integration. *Disasters.* 2006;30(1):19–38.
6. O'Brien G, O'Keefe P, Rose J, et al. Climate change and disaster management. *Disasters.* 2006;30(1):64–80.
7. Henry R. *Defense Transformation and the 2005 Quadrennial Defense Review, Parameters.* Winter; 2005-2006, 5-15.
8. Keim M. Environmental disasters. In: Frumkin H, ed. *Environmental Health: From Global to Local.* San Francisco, CA: John Wiley and Sons, Inc; 2010:843–875.
9. Keim M. Disaster preparedness. In: Ciottone G, ed. *Disaster Medicine.* Philadelphia, PA: Mosby-Elsevier; 2006.
10. Clack Z, Keim M, Macintyre A, et al. Emergency health and risk management in sub-Saharan Africa: a lesson from the embassy bombings in Tanzania and Kenya. *Prehospital Disaster Med.* 2002;17(2):59–66.
11. Sundnes K, Birnbaum M, Birnbaum E, eds. *Health Disaster Management Guidelines for Evaluation and Research in the Utstein Style.* USA: Prehospital and Disaster Medicine; 2003.
12. de Ville de Goyet C, Lechat M. Health aspects in natural disasters. *Trop Doct.* 1976;6:152–157.
13. de Boer J, Dubouloz M, eds. *Handbook of Disaster Medicine.* The Netherlands: International Society of Disaster Medicine; 2000.
14. Lechat M. *Disaster as a Public Health Problem.* Brussels: Louvain University; 1985.
15. UNISDR. United Nations International Strategy for Disaster Reduction. *Yokohama Strategy and Plan of Action for a Safer World: Guidelines for Natural Disaster Prevention, Preparedness and Mitigation.* Available at URL: http://www.unisdr.org/files/8241_doc6841contenido1.pdf. Last Accessed 18.05.14.
16. UNISDR. United Nations International Strategy for Disaster Reduction. *World Summit on Sustainable Development Plan of implementation, Johannesburg, South Africa,* Find at URL: http://www.johannesburgsummit.org/html/documents/summit_docs/2309_planfinal.htm. Accessed 08.06.04.
17. UNISDR. United Nations International Strategy for Disaster Reduction. *Second World Conference on Disaster Reduction.* Find at URL: http://www.unisdr.org/2005/wcdr/intergover/official-doc/L-docs/Final-reportconference.pdf. Last Accessed 18.05.14.
18. UNISDR. United Nations International Strategy for Disaster Reduction. *Hyogo Declaration.* Find at URL: http://www.unisdr.org/2005/wcdr/intergover/official-doc/L-docs/Hyogo-declaration-english.pdf. Last Accessed 18.05.14.
19. UNISDR. United Nations International Strategy for Disaster Reduction. *Hyogo Framework for Action 2005–2015.* Available at URL: http://www.unisdr.org/we/coordinate/hfa. Last Accessed 18.05.14.
20. White House. *Homeland Security Presidential Directive/HSPD-8.* 2003. Available at URL: http://www.fas.org/irp/offdocs/nspd/hspd-8.html. Last Accessed 18.05.14.
21. Khan AS. Public health preparedness and response in the USA since 9/11: a national health security imperative. *Lancet.* 2011;378:953–956.
22. White House. *Presidential Policy Directive/PPD-8: National Preparedness.* 2011. Available at URL: http://www.dhs.gov/presidential-policy-directive-8-national-preparedness. Last Accessed 18.05.14.
23. Natural Disaster Organisation, Disaster Concepts and Principles. *Australian Counter Disaster Handbook,* vol. 1. 1993. Canberra: 28.
24. Federal Emergency Management Agency. *State and Local Guide 101: Guide for All Hazard Emergency Operations Planning, SLG101.* Washington, DC: FEMA; 1996.
25. World Health Organization. *Health Sector Emergency Preparedness Guide.* Tazmania: The World Health Organization; 1998.
26. National Institute for Chemical Studies. *Sheltering in Place as a Public Protective Action.* Charleston: WV: EPA; 2001: 1–26.
27. White House. *Homeland Security Presidential Directive/HSPD-5. Management of Domestic Incidents.* National Incident Management System. Available at URL: http://www.fas.org/irp/offdocs/nspd/hspd-5.html. Last Accessed 18.05.14.
28. FEMA (Federal Emergency Management Agency). *CPG 101: Developing and Maintain Emergency Operations Plans.* FEMA; 2010. Available at URL: http://www.fema.gov/media-library-data/20130726-1828-25045-0014/cpg_101_comprehensive_preparedness_guide_developing_and_maintaining_emergency_operations_plans_2010.pdf. Last Accessed 18.05.14.
29. Murphy C, Gardoni P. The Role of Society in Engineering Risk Analysis. A capabilities-based approach. *Risk Anal.* 2007;26(4):1073–1083.
30. Murphy C, Gardoni P. Determining public policy and resource allocation priorities for mitigating natural hazards: a capabilities-based approach. *Sci Eng Ethics.* 2007;13:489–504.
31. NATO. *North Atlantic Treaty Organization. NATO Research and Technology Board: Panel On Studies, Analysis and Simulation (SAS).* Washington, DC: Handbook in Long Term Defense Planning; 2001, pp. 1-45.
32. Davis PK. *Analytic Architecture for Capabilities-Based Planning, Mission-System Analysis, and Transformation.* Washington, DC: RAND; 2002: 1–76. MR-1513-OSD.
33. Linstone H, Turoff M. *The Delphi Method: Techniques and Applications.* New Jersey: Institute of Technology; 1975. Available at URL: http://www.is.njit.edu/pubs/delphibook. Last Accessed 18.05.14.

34. Rowe, Wright. Expert opinions in forecasting. Role of the delphi technique. In: Armstrong, ed. *Principles of Forecasting: A Handbook of Researchers and Practitioners.* Boston: Kluwer Academic Publishers; 2001:1–86.

35. British Columbia, British Columbia Ministry of Public Safety and Solicitor General. *Hazard, Risk and Vulnerability Analysis Toolkit.* Victoria, BC: National Library of Canada; 2004. Available at URL: http://embc.gov.bc.ca/em/hrva/toolkit.pdf. Last Accessed 18.05.14.

36. Standards Australia Committee OB-007. *AS/NZS 4360:2004 Risk Management.* Sydney, Australia and Wellington, New Zealand: Standards Australia International Ltd; 2004: 2-17.

37. Shoaf K, Seligson H, Stratton S, et al. *Hazard Risk Assessment Instrument.* UCLA center for Public Health and Disasters; 2006. Available at URL: http://swperlc.ouhsc.edu/documents/HRAI_Workbook.pdf. Last Accessed 18.05.14.

38. Sun X, Keim M, Dong C, Mahany M, Xiang G. A dynamic process of health risk assessment for business continuity during the World Exposition Shanghai China 2010. *J Bus Contin Emerg Plan.* 2014;7(4).

39. Keim ME. O2C3: a unified model for emergency operations planning. *Am J Disaster Med.* 2010;5(3):169–179.

40. Christen H, Maniscalco P. *The EMS Incident Management System.* Upper Saddle River, NY: Prentice-Hall; 1998: 4–5.

41. Department of Homeland Security. *The National Incident Management System.* Washington, DC; December 2008. Available at URL, http://www.fema.gov/pdf/emergency/nims/NIMS_core.pdf. Last Accessed 18.05.14.

42. Department of Homeland Security. *The Homeland Security Exercise and Evaluation Program (HSEEP).* Washington, DC; 2013. Available at URL: https://hseep.dhs.gov/support/VolumeI.pdf. Last Accessed 18.05.14.

43. Department of Homeland Security. *National Preparedness Guidelines.* Washington, DC; September 2007. Available at URL: http://www.fema.gov/pdf/emergency/nrf/National_Preparedness_Guidelines.pdf. Last Accessed 18.05.14.

44. Anonymous. *Sphere Handbook. The Sphere Project, Humanitarian Standards in Disaster Response.* 2004. Available at URL: www.sphereproject.org/. Last Accessed 18.05.14.

45. World Health Organization. *Pandemic Influenza Preparedness and Mitigation in Refugee and Displaced Populations.* 2nd ed. May 2008. Available at URL: http://www.who.int/diseasecontrol_emergencies/HSE_EPR_DCE_2008_3rweb.pdf. Last accessed May 18, 2014.

46. Department of Homeland Security. *Homeland Security Presidential Directive 5. Management of Domestic Incidents.* February 2003. Available at URL: http://www.fas.org/irp/offdocs/nspd/hspd-5.html. Last Accessed 18.05.14.

47. US Department of Health and Human Services. *Planning and Preparedness.* Available at URL: http://www.pandemicflu.gov/. Last Accessed 21.09.12.

48. Keim M. An innovative approach to capability-based emergency operations planning. *Journal of Disaster Health.* 2013;1(1):54–62.

49. Mayer T, Salluzo R. Theory of continuous quality improvement. In: Salluzo R, Mayer T, Strauss R, et al., eds. *Emergency Department Management.* Mosby-Year Book; 1997:461–479.

50. *Guidelines for Assessing Disaster Preparedness in the Health Sector.* Washington, D.C: Pan American Health Organization; 1995.

51. Sidel V, Onel E, Geiger H, et al. Public health responses to natural and human-made disasters. In: Maxcy, Rosenthal, Last, eds. *Public Health and Preventative Medicine.* 13th ed. Norwalk, CT. USA: Appleton and Lange; 1992:1173–1186.

52. Waerckerle J. Disaster planning and response. *NEJM.* 1991;324(12):815–821.

53. Noji E. Natural disaster management. In: Auerbach P, ed. *Wilderness Medicine.* 4th ed. USA: Mosby; 2001:644–663.

54. Seaman J. Disaster epidemiology: or why most international disaster relief is ineffective. *Injury.* 1990;21:5.

55. Sapir D, Lechat M. Reducing the impact of natural disasters: why aren't we better prepared? *Health Policy Plan.* 1986;1:118.

56. de Bruycker M, Greco D, Lechat MF. The 1980 earthquake in southern Italy: rescue of trapped victims and mortality. *Bull World Health Organ.* 1983;51:1021.

57. *WHO/PAHO Guidelines for the Use of Foreign Field Hospitals in the Aftermath of Sudden-Impact Disasters.* PAHO, San Salvador, El Salvador; 2003.

58. Pluut I. *Field Hospitals in Bam, Iran.* World Health Organization. Find URL at: http://www.disaster-info.net/downloadzone/bam.htm. Accessed 08.06.04.

59. Levitin H, Siegelson H. Hazardous materials-disaster planning and response. *Disaster Med.* 1996;14(2):327–348.

60. Lechat MF. Updates in epidemiology of health effects of disasters. *Epidemiol Rev.* 1990;12:192.

61. Anonymous. Impact of Hurricane Mitch on Central America. *Epidemiol Bull.* Dec. 1998;19(4):1–13.

62. Keim M, Rhyne G. The Pacific Emergency Health Initiative: a pilot study of emergency preparedness in Oceania. *Australian Journal of Emergency Medicine.* June 2001;13:157–164.

63. Quarantelli EL. *Delivery of Emergency Medical Services in Disasters: Assumptions and Realities.* New York: Irvington; 1985.

64. Holweg M. The genealogy of lean production. *J Oper Manag.* 2007;25(2):420–437.

65. Berwick DM. Continuous improvement as an ideal in healthcare. *N Engl J Med.* 320:53–56.

66. Batalden PB, Buchanan ED. Industrial models of quality improvement. In: Goldenfield N, Nas DB, eds. *Providing Quality Care: The Challenge to Clinicians.* Philadelphia: American College of Physicians; 1989.

67. Walshe K, Harvey G, Jas P. *Connecting Knowledge and Performance in Public Services: From Knowing to Doing.* Cambridge University Press; 2010 175.

68. Burkle FM. Complex Humanitarian Emergencies: III. Measures of effectiveness. *Prehosp Disast Med.* 1995;10(1):48–56.

69. Burkle F. Measures of effectiveness in large-scale bio-terrorism events. *Prehospital Disaster Med.* 2003;18(3):258–262.

SUGGESTED READINGS

1. CDC. *Public Health Preparedness Capabilities: National Standards for State and Local Planning.* March 2011. Available at URL: http://www.cdc.gov/phpr/capabilities/Capabilities_March_2011.pdf. Last Accessed 18.05.14.

CHAPTER 33

Policy Issues in Disaster Preparedness and Response

Eric S. Weinstein and Brielle Weinstein

At the intersection of public perception, science, the duty of government to act, and the rights of the individual sits public health policy. Guiding the paths of health care providers, bureaucrats, and patients is the ethical principle of justice: to do the most good for the most people in a transparent collaboration with frequent assessments and revisions. Citations from the Bible and other ancient texts demonstrate meritorious efforts to reduce the spread of disease.[1] Scholars are quick to point out the lack of appreciation of factual scientific knowledge through centuries of political maneuvering to regulate immigration, forcefully separate innocents to protect the fearful, and hide the unfortunately afflicted from view.[2] This chapter discusses examples of public health policy in the light of individuals' rights and the (retrospective) science of disaster preparedness and response. As this science has evolved, plans that failed and plans that succeeded that have fallen under the domain of public health have supplied the material to analyze while applying guiding ethical principles. This policy has become the foundation on which governments stand as they struggle to remove populations determined to be in danger from known immediate or impending natural or human-made threats; to protect those already or potentially infected by the biological agent unleashed by a terrorist; to immediately reconfigure the local health care delivery system disrupted on a grand scale, directly contrary to established rules, regulations, and statutes; to permit our free society to function with the full enjoyment of familiar civil liberties; and to communicate as technology permits, without endangering themselves or others. In short we will cover historical and contemporary examples of pervasive and catastrophic disasters and the policies created in their wake. Through an understanding of these examples, we can begin to tackle recommendations for legislation that will honor justice and the duty to protect.

THE ETHICAL VIEW FOR THE SCIENTIST

In our free, democratic society, policy makers tasked with the authority to protect the public's health must also consider the individual's civil and political rights of liberty, privacy, association, assembly, and expression.[3] Gostin[3] writes that it is not improper to restrain the enjoyment of liberty, privacy, or property per se, but it is improper to do so unnecessarily, arbitrarily, inequitably, or brutally. This restraint can take place when government acts against a threat that is invalid or one that is not based on objective, reliable scientific knowledge. Protecting public health is difficult to do when an uncertain, evolving illness begins to affect individuals and there is limited acquisition of dynamic relevant information. Many illnesses appear the same early in the course of the illness, and it is not until later that the diagnosis can be affirmed. Consider such an illness affecting dozens, hundreds, or thousands of people spread over continents, with fear mounting and governments pressed into acting immediately. It would be the

government's burden to defend and rigorously evaluate the effectiveness of a public health measure adopted to contain and treat this mystery illness in real time. Certainly, a known illness for which research has identified the agent, vectors, susceptible hosts with evidence-based diagnostics, treatment, and cost to society can be addressed by an effective public health policy. The challenge to a public health agency is to reach this familiarity with a new syndrome or toxidrome in short order.[3] The balance between the establishment and maintenance of health and the prevention or reduction of transmission of illness with subsequent inhibition or reduction of the individual's rights should follow the doctrine of least-restrictive alternative to reduce the risk or ameliorate the harm. Legal scholars can assume this role alongside public health authorities who are not versed in the ramifications of invasiveness, the intrusion of an intervention on the individual's rights, or the scope and selection of individuals to receive an intervention. The duration of the intervention should be proportionate to the desired effect, with ongoing review to reduce untoward effects that would limit an individual's rights.[3]

This relationship of individual rights and public health places policy efforts at the crossroads of justice and autonomy. The need to properly and respectfully restrain the public will likely limit individuals' autonomy, but, at some level, it will be considered acceptable. Moreover, the policy has to do so from the outset with a carefully designed public information and education strategy and implementation with avenues to contemporaneously accept concerns put forward by scholars and citizens alike to modify actions deemed unnecessary, capricious, or onerous. Within this spectrum think of the struggle to accept the use of seatbelts and the prohibition of smoking in public areas leading to the demonstrated scientific proof of improved public health. A fair public health policy benefits those in need and burdens those who endanger the public's health. Public health policies should not discriminate against sex, ethnicity, or other demographic factors unless scientifically proven to be accurate and, if applied evenly, will achieve the intended outcome. For example if a toxic chemical release was deemed a threat to a population, then the population must be protected, which may include mass evacuation or the order for mandatory sheltering-in-place at a moment's notice, or the population that is proven to receive contaminated water through the public water supply may be given simple explicit instructions of water use regardless of the restrictions to daily living and the cost to residents and businesses.[4] A means to address perceived inequalities or lack of sensitivity to individual rights is due process. This checks-and-balances opportunity of an individual to independently determine the merits of a public health intervention in a timely manner may reduce any further effects of a misapplied policy or ineffective course of action. This unbiased informed decision can fashion redress to rectify any misapplication or unintended consequences of policies. This form of process improvement will achieve more appropriate future policy and build trust in government that permits justice to be served.[5] Unfortunately, time is of the essence when a public health agency is pressured to act against an unknown illness. Review during the course of the dynamics of the response to the threat can and should occur simultaneously to scale back any restrictions on individual rights as the science of the event is established.[6] The uninformed public must trust government to achieve compliance with public health mandates as the event unfolds before a wary media. Focused discussions in an open forum can be used to disseminate information as a systemic management tool to make it easier for the implemented public health plans to be accepted and thus achieve the intended end. Equally important will be the attraction of unknown individuals or groups to further the policy through their involvement in the process.[7] The common good for the public as a whole can be met by the involvement of the community of individuals. Transparency flushes facts, quells rumors, and dispels myths. Protection of an individual's rights can be ensured if the creation of public health policy adheres to necessity of action through proportional, nondiscriminatory, and fair means.[8]

EVACUATION ORDERS: "YOU MAY WANT TO HEED THIS ADVICE FOR YOUR OWN GOOD"

As fate yields opportunity, the writing of the first edition of this chapter began with the author under the voluntary evacuation issued for coastal South Carolina in response to the then-impending threat of Hurricane Charley (August 13, 2004).[9] New evacuation measures had been put into place after the infamous 1998 mandatory evacuation of the Charleston, South Carolina area, in advance of Hurricane Floyd. That evacuation distressed families in that some sat in traffic for 18 hours along a more-than-150-mile stretch of Interstate Highway 26 leading up to Columbia. At the time of Hurricane Floyd, roughly one seventh of the South Carolina population participated in the evacuation of the entire coastline, with Hurricane Hugo still fresh on most residents' minds.[10] The public outcry after the flawed Hurricane Floyd evacuation enabled the retrospective science of disaster medicine to produce significant changes to the entire data-gathering process that the South Carolina governor would use to declare a mandatory evacuation under state law.[11] Exercises have proven that lane reversals, new highway construction, and strategic placement of hundreds of South Carolina law enforcement officers and department of transportation workers, in concert with computer-aided scenarios, have been successful in reducing the time of evacuation by up to 10 hours, despite a surge of migration from at-risk coastal South Carolina areas.[12] Shortly after the Hurricane Floyd evacuation, honest assessments took place that led to the identification of additional data that can be used to make the executive decision to issue a mandatory evacuation order. An evacuation order can cost a state millions of dollars, disrupt local economies dependent on tourism, and further decrease an already waning public trust. In an effort to make an evacuation easier, the 2003-2004 South Carolina General Assembly voted to amend a 1976 law to allow the governor to order that traffic lanes be reversed so that all lanes in an evacuation area flow in one direction away from the evacuation area.[13] The failure to heed evacuation orders by some who could leave and the ineffective plans to evacuate those who could not leave without assistance during Hurricane Katrina in 2005 had fatal consequences, leading to numerous government agencies, academicians, and other scholars to issue recommendations across the spectrum.[14] In January 2014 as a rare ice storm approached the Atlanta metropolitan area, the lack of a timely coordinated evacuation order paralyzed highways, as schools, businesses, and governmental agencies simultaneously released their

personnel to begin the trek home. Georgia Governor Deal convened the Severe Weather Task Force and implemented immediate reforms for winter storm warnings, which was prescient, producing a smoother evacuation 2 weeks later when another ice storm hit the area.[15]

Lessons learned from Katrina, tsunamis in the Indian Ocean in 2004 and Japan in 2011, computer modeling using satellite Geospatial Information System (GIS), and other technology fueled by the climate change debate have enabled government agencies to dedicate more resources to better define the science of evacuation planning.[16,17] The 2012 Superstorm Sandy evacuation orders were adhered to in known evacuation zones in multiple states and cities, with success measured by decreased loss of life in most areas, particularly in the usual beachfront areas where evacuation is expected, and these residents left accordingly.[18] Despite advance notice using many means of communication, lives were lost in areas rarely if ever confronted with evacuation orders.[19] Emergency managers still face challenges from those who do not want to leave and are capable of leaving; those unable to leave and unable to communicate that they cannot leave; and rapidly changing storm conditions creating storm surges that exceed announced established flood zones.

AN OUTBREAK AND THE EMERGENCY MEDICAL TREATMENT AND LABOR ACT: PATIENT CARE ENSURED

The key to any containment strategy is for the local government executive to issue an emergency order or proclamation, establishing a new set of operating procedures for public health authorities, the health care delivery system, and other government agencies.[20] If an outbreak were local, the county executive or county council would issue the order or proclamation through a well-defined process. If an outbreak were to occur across counties, the governor would issue the order or proclamation. The Emergency Medical Treatment and Labor Act (EMTALA) of 1986 permits regionalization of prehospital care to afford the best possible medical care for victims of trauma; those suffering from an acute cerebrovascular accident (CVA); and patients requiring special services such as pediatrics, obstetrics, and, increasingly, psychiatry.[21] Under an executive order to mitigate the threat of a public health emergency (PHE), patients who meet predetermined criteria developed in a collaborative effort using the most accurate, timely, and, if possible, evidence-based determinations, can be directed to an established health care facility (e-HCF) or a newly created facility, which may be at an alternative site (a-HCF), and is staffed with the necessary personnel, equipment, and supplies to meet the need.[22] This plan can be accomplished ahead of time in anticipation of an outbreak of known pathogens or in the early phases of a new illness pattern detected through the triggers of syndromic surveillance. To assure that civil liberties are respected, without alarming the affected population, the lead government agency has to incorporate transparency through effective public communication using all available means that may include print, radio, television, and social media. Timeliness and accuracy is the best course to take to effect positive outcomes, especially early in the PHE, with invitation by key community leaders and learned citizens to join the process accordingly to accomplish the all-important public acceptance and participation. This will require more government staff to process solicited and unsolicited volunteers, vetting credentials for appropriate deployments. Governments have to factor-in worker fatigue and workers who become ill, as well as worker families who become ill, in the creation of all aspects of the PHE response.

Patients who enter the health care system after a telephone call to 911 (or other phone number) for emergency medical transport may be evaluated by an emergency medical technician (EMT) when the ambulance arrives. Currently, certain systems will permit an EMT-paramedic (EMT-P) evaluation for appropriateness of transport via emergency medical services (EMS). This evaluation is based on strict criteria developed by off-line medical direction that is approved by county officials with appropriate documentation and, more importantly, communication between the EMT crew, online medical control, and subsequent review of each call.[23] In a PHE, the most practical extension of this on-scene or field triage process, the PHE field evaluation team (FET), is for an EMS crew with an EMT-P, a registered nurse (RN), or a midlevel provider (physician assistant or nurse practitioner) to perform an evaluation of the patient for preset criteria. These criteria can be determined de novo, as the PHE evolves by the assembled collaborative team process or from prior known, reviewed, and learned outbreak responses. This process must include appropriate education about the outbreak; issuance of equipment, supplies, and personal protective equipment (PPE) to the first responders; and a screening process to exclude responders who may be more susceptible or less-than-adequate, placing them more at risk.[24] The patient will enter the PHE evaluation and treatment process, and anyone else at the field evaluation site must be considered a contact person and enter the PHE evaluation process. The field evaluation site must be assessed for epidemiologic concerns and adjudicated accordingly.[24] The dispatch of the FET can be accomplished through use of priority medical dispatch or a similar 911 operating system. In a PHE, a person who calls the 911 system (or another telephone number for ambulance service for those regions not yet using 911) will undergo caller interrogation specific for the symptoms and any other information that can be learned. The caller will then be given instructions on first aid for laypersons or the establishment of containment strategies pending arrival of the FET. Priority medical dispatch or a similar system can then send the FET to the scene to perform the evaluation, separate from the usual standard EMS.[25] As of May 15, 2014, major wireless service providers in the United States will make text-to-911 widely available.[26] Even though the Federal Communications Commission (FCC) still recommends a voice call over a text, this method of communication will provide 911 access to people who cannot verbally communicate due to handicap or other situation, further expanding communication with potential patients affected by the contagion.[27]

If this evaluation determines that the patient is a potential victim of a PHE, the EMS crew can transport the patient to an e-HCF or a-HCF established to evaluate and treat the presenting symptom complex. If the patient is in distress, he or she will be attended to as per standard operating procedures and then transported to the appropriate HCF.[22] The EMS crew will be told what containment strategies and procedures the designated HCF has undertaken for the patient. During the executive-declared PHE, the destination HCF may not be a standard HCF, such as the closest hospital, but it may be a "fever hospital" or an HCF specifically created for the PHE at an alternative site.[24] This location will have health care workers (HCWs) who are trained, equipped, supplied, and clothed in appropriate PPE. It may be on the grounds of the closest hospital, public health clinic, or in another building in the community, with appropriate air exchanges, water, heating and air conditioning, food preparation, restrooms, and showers to contain the PHE, thus allowing other hospitals and HCFs to attend to their usual patient loads without an influx of PHE patients.[22] In a short period, such an alternative HCF can be fully operational with prepositioned stores and vendor agreements.

Guidelines can be created, extensively reviewed from the go-forward plan, and adapted as the outbreak proceeds. If a patient meets predetermined criteria, then treatment will continue until the patient is either discharged home, perhaps with home health care or other

monitoring using available communication assets, or transferred to another HCF for long-term care or containment.[6] If the patient does not meet criteria he may receive initial care at that location and then be transported to an acute-care HCF (hospital, clinic, or physician office) for further treatment and discharge.[28] The vehicle used to transport the patient and the accompanying personnel will have to undergo containment strategies from the initial PHE HCF to the next location. EMTALA requires that the dedicated emergency department (ED) of an HCF perform a medical screening examination (MSE) for patients who present asking for a medical evaluation or when the MSE is requested by another person.[29] Patients who self-refer to the ED during a government-executive-declared PHE could receive an MSE by the hospital designated RN or midlevel provider clothed in appropriate PPE. This HCW can be screened to ensure that he or she is fit for the assignment, vaccinated accordingly, and knowledgeable of the threat at hand.[6] The patient will receive an MSE and be stabilized at the initial HCF, accepted by the physician at the PHE HCF, and transferred with the appropriate EMTALA documentation with containment strategies observed. At the HCFs, containment strategies should include training of all employees to the specific presenting symptoms and signs of the PHE, use of PPE for those who routinely meet and greet people at their work stations, and limitations on entrance locations to the public.[6] HCF-designated HCWs positioned to act as screeners can direct people entering the HCF to a receiving area for a more rigorous evaluation, separate from the ED, if they are coming to the HCF as a visitor or to conduct other business. More importantly, if a patient seeking medical attention enters the HCF though any entrance, containment strategies can commence accordingly. Signage specific for the PHE can direct patients presenting to the HCF for evaluation to containment areas designed for this initial evaluation.

It is plausible for specially trained HCWs, in tandem with personnel from law enforcement, public safety, department of transportation, or another like agency, to assist in the sorting of patients that self-refer to the HCF at roads removed from the entrance of the HCF.

To reduce drunk driving for the public good, law enforcement personnel currently set up road blocks, at which they check driver's licenses, registration, and insurance cards. They also screen for impaired drivers and passengers or vehicles suspected of being involved in illegal activities.[30] An executive PHE can extend certain powers to law enforcement to assist the public health effort to contain the illness.[31] Queues of traffic at locations safely established en route to a hospital can act as a checkpoint for screening, as previously noted, with direction of patients to the PHE HCF or their usual HCF containment area for an MSE. The vehicle and person(s) in the vehicle will undergo the epidemiologic evaluation and containment process. If the PHE HCW screening determines that a person fits the PHE symptom complex, the PHE FET can be deployed to conduct further evaluation and transport. The vehicle that carried the patient(s) will then have to be isolated, evaluated for contamination, and decontaminated accordingly.

SMALLPOX VACCINATIONS: THINK BEFORE YOU ACT

After the Centers for Disease Control and Prevention (CDC) Advisory Committee on Immunization Practices (ACIP) revised its 1991 recommendations in June 2001 to include the use of vaccinia vaccine if the smallpox (variola) virus was used as an agent of biological terrorism, or if a smallpox outbreak were to occur for another unforeseen reason, a series of events took place demonstrating how science and ethics, including the respect of individuals' rights and the role of government to protect its citizens, could alleviate fears while establishing current and future recommendations that everyone could accept.[32] What follows is a discussion of the policy development debate that lead to an effective smallpox vaccination strategy.

This plan included preexposure vaccination for first responders or treatment teams dispatched to attend to those exposed.[32] Modlin[33] was chair of the ACIP when the 2001 recommendations were released, and he later wrote a cautious editorial in March 2002 asking that policy makers weigh the best available analysis of vaccine-related morbidity and costs against the best available assessment of risk for smallpox release. Fauci[34] followed with similar caution, with a reminder of why the smallpox vaccination program was discontinued in the face of known risks, known transmissions, and known cases worldwide—there were several vaccine-related deaths each year as the risk of contracting the disease continued to decline. He concurred with the "ring-vaccination" strategy, which worked during past decades and involves isolating those suspected or confirmed of being infected with the virus and then tracing contacts and their contacts for vaccination. This minimized the risk of adverse vaccine events (AVEs) and effectively used limited vaccines and other resources, including manpower to adjudicate the plan.[34] A widespread vaccination program is estimated to produce 4600 serious AVEs and 285 deaths.[35] These numbers are unacceptable to many who are facing no known risk and no substantial proof of smallpox outside of known repositories.[36,37] Meltzer,[38] through the CDC, in December 2001, showed that the number of susceptible persons and the assumed rate of transmission are the most important variables influencing the total number of smallpox cases to be expected from an intentional release of smallpox into a community.

Non–peer-reviewed medical journals began detailing reservations about the National Smallpox Vaccination Program (NSVP) within weeks of its announcement. In preparation for the program's January 24, 2003, commencement, hospitals openly questioned the financial burden of prescreening examinations, administering the vaccines, monitoring employees for AVEs, and providing treatment if necessary to the intended 500,000 first responder HCWs. They were also concerned that the risks of such a large-scale program for an unsubstantiated rumor based on loose "what-ifs" could reduce an already short staff because vaccinated workers may have to miss work. Hospitals also noted the risk of their HCWs transmitting vaccinia to patients in their facilities and to HCW family members. Public health policy in this instance did not address the legal ramifications of compensation to inoculated HCWs who suffered an AVE, either temporary or permanent. Who should pay the HCW if he or she cannot work? Would subsequent medical costs be paid through workers' compensation or an HCW's own medical insurance?[39] The SAFETY Act for Liability Protection, part of the Homeland Security Act of 2002 (Title VII, Subtitle G), extended liability protection to the manufacturers of the vaccine, hospitals administering the vaccine, and individuals receiving the vaccine, presumably if they transmit vaccinia to another person.[40] Hospital attorneys debated what locations were protected because it appeared that hospitals themselves were protected only if their vaccination clinic was on site but not if they chose an off-site HCF such as a clinic.[41] Reports of HCW AVEs were accumulating with the commencement of the NSVP, slowing the program to a trickle. If 30% of HCWs in some facilities would have had to miss some work, the staffing nightmare could have been dangerous. In April 2003 the CDC ACIP released a supplement, Recommendations for Using Smallpox Vaccine in a Pre-Event Vaccination Program, to its 2001 smallpox vaccine recommendation, which moved the focus from each hospital establishing and maintaining at least one response team, to only having one team in the state. This revision demonstrated a healthy transparent exchange of ideas, using medical and nonmedical print media, open

forums, and committees open to all constituents: the intended vaccinee, their employer, government, and scientists.[42] The CDC ACIP released another supplement, this time excluding persons with cardiac disease or risk factors from the NSVP after reports of myopericarditis among healthy personnel who were vaccinated surfaced.[43] The dialogue between constituents has been gaining steam.

More than a year after the commencement of the NSVP, policy makers showed that they were listening to the concerns of HCW who volunteered to be vaccinated by passing the Smallpox Emergency Personnel Protection Act of 2003 (December 13, 2003).[44] Funded at $42 million, the program provides financial and medical benefits to eligible members of a smallpox emergency response plan approved by the U.S. Department of Health and Human Services (HHS) who sustain certain medical injuries caused by a smallpox vaccine. In addition, unvaccinated individuals injured after coming into contact with vaccinated members of an emergency response plan—or with a person with whom the vaccinated person had contact—may be eligible for program benefits. The program also provides benefits to survivors of eligible individuals whose death resulted from a covered injury. In response to the disconnect felt by HCWs, HHS developed the Smallpox Vaccine Injury Compensation Table published in the August 27, 2003, edition of the Federal Register.[45] The table became effective upon publication. Moving this from HHS to federal law only contributed to the loss of public faith in the program.

Bozzette and coworkers[46] posted A Model for Smallpox-Vaccination Policy on the New England Journal of Medicine's website on December 19, 2002. This stochastic model of outcomes considered a range of threats, including a hoax, and predicted the number of deaths, but not morbidity or the extent of AVEs, after the use of various measures to contain the spread of smallpox. The study brought policy implications to the forefront, specifically the benefit of isolation, while highlighting the lack of case law with concerns of denial of civil liberties.[46] Federal law gives the U.S. Public Health Service the power to detain individuals, for such time and in such a manner as may be reasonably necessary, who are believed to be infected with a communicable disease and in the contagious stage, to prevent transmission of the disease.[47] For centuries, containment strategies to combat the proliferation of smallpox, spread via large droplet respiratory transmission from face-to-face contact, have been successful. In 1988 the World Health Organization (WHO) determined that air samples taken in the vicinity of smallpox patients were rarely positive. This, coupled with the observation that most patients with uncomplicated disease are not capable of generating a strong enough cough to propel aerosols long distance, builds the clinical case for smallpox containment strategies.[48] Containment vaccination can be directed at the persons at the highest risk for disease: those who had face-to-face contact within 2 m.[49] In the end, the discussion regarding smallpox in the twenty-first century was not made earnest by an actual threat or outbreak; fortunately, time permitted science to assuage legitimate fears, as the process triumphantly yielded an ethically sound result.

LEGISLATING PUBLIC HEALTH

The Model State Emergency Health Powers Act was enacted December 21, 2001, to provide a framework for governors, legislatures, and public health officials to review their statutes and regulations, to adhere to the following principles: preparedness, surveillance, management of property, protection of persons, and communication.[50] Gostin noted that the body of public health statutes is layered on old statutes implemented in response to a public health threat decades ago and that a review for current evidence-based medicine or a review grounded in sound science are unlikely. As medical theory has expanded with technology,[51] legal appreciation of an individual's rights has also been defined without benefit of public health law keeping pace. Old legal remedies may not apply to current public health dilemmas; insufficient authority may limit effective action; and coordination between local, state, and federal authorities may be hindered by conflicting statutes that have been rendered moot through technology.[52] Coercive powers may be the only means to ensure the safety and health of the public and must not be taken lightly. Public health law gives government the authority to limit personal activities to safeguard the public health through powers bounded by necessity, effective means, proportionality, and fairness; in return, individuals forgo autonomy, liberty, or property. The Model Act itself is divided into the preemergency environment for predeclaration powers and the powers that become the governor's to use after declaration of an emergency. The declaration of a PHE must meet the following criteria: (1) an occurrence or imminent threat of an illness or public health condition that (2) is caused by bioterrorism or a new or reemerging infectious agent or biological toxin previously controlled that also (3) poses a high probability of a large number of deaths, serious or long-term disabilities, or widespread exposure to an infectious or toxic agent that poses a significant risk of substantial future harm to a large number of persons.[52]

The Model Act filters redundant statutes, removes statutes that have become irrelevant, and enhances traditional public health powers with an extensive set of conditions, principles, and requirements governing the use of personal control measures. Specific advancements include the use of home confinement or other creative less-restrictive alternatives for containment rather than compulsory isolation or quarantine and permits persons so contained to be afforded due process, appropriate medical care, activities, hygiene, and food.[52] Transparency of communication with the public to explain protective measures and access to mental health will reduce public misperceptions. With the pervasiveness of social media in society it is acceptable to include microblogs (i.e., Twitter) and social networks (i.e., Facebook) in the toolbox to communicate real-time updates. Immunity is afforded to persons exercising authority under the specific declarations of the governor.

Civil libertarians point out the evolution of public health powers with the federal government retaining authority over interstate and foreign commerce, national defense, and the expenditure of money. Even with the creation of the Department of Homeland Security, the CDC still remains the lead advisory consequence agency in a PHE. In the event of a bioterrorist outbreak, the Federal Bureau of Investigation will provide federal crisis management that is coordinated with a state crisis management agency. In most states, the lead state consequence-management agency lacks the depth required in current state law for basic public health to function appropriately. Annas[5] stated that the Model Act should respond to real problems, but the scenarios that would require use of these powers are not known and are left to the transparency of the process of a state government to recommend to the governor to use in a PHE. These powers are for all biological agents and their toxins, regardless of entry into the public. Annual influenza epidemics, by definition, are a PHE with the full depth of the government prepared to prevent a pandemic. The fear and panic after the anthrax incidents in the fall of 2001 cannot be compared to the reality of a true PHE involving the deployment of community HCWs. There is no evidence that certain containment strategies are unfounded.

Communication Policy in the Age of Social Media

Social media is a pervasive, real-time method of communication that provides a new tool for government and those affected during by a PHE. The combination of multimedia presentation, large-scale population viewing, and Global Positioning System (GPS) could make social media the ultimate mechanism to disperse information in a PHE.

According to Merriam-Webster, the term *social media* was first used in 2004, and it is currently a tool used regularly by 62% of U.S. adults.[53] Also according to Pew, 72% of Internet users looked online for health information within the past year.[54] Common platforms for information include microblogs, social networks, media sharing (i.e., YouTube), social news (i.e., Reddit), and many others.

Current policy on social media during disasters is a rapidly expanding topic for many PHE-related groups, from the Red Cross to Congress. The Red Cross, for example, has a PowerPoint presentation provided on SlideShare that takes users through everything from their "lawyer-approved" comment to a note regarding the NGO's 501(c)(3) status obliging that no Red Cross Facebook page join any religious or political advocacy groups.[55] The Air Force Public Affairs Agency has a flow chart on how to properly respond to posts, including principles of transparency, sourcing, timeliness, tone, and influence.[56] Because social media can be a powerful tool in a variety of situations, policies need to be in place to guide dispersion of information and use data mining, including GPS and tracking of epidemiologic trends. Similarly, government and disaster response agencies need to be on guard for unverified or false information or purposefully posted disinformation by malicious people or groups.

Two situations where different platforms of social media played pivotal roles in the response to PHE are Influenza A (H7N9) in China in 2013 (weibo)[57] and the Boston Marathon Bombing 2013 (Twitter).[58] The 2013 H7N9 Influenza outbreak in China was the first time that the WHO used weibo and Twitter for initial release of outbreak information. Weibo is a similar platform to Twitter in China, used by 309 million Chinese in 2013.[57] Fung and Wong suggest that by official provincial and municipal organizations dispersing information and links via weibo, they created a ripple effect of official information spreading through "retweets."[58] Information dispersed included numbers of cases confirmed, Q&A links, and locations of confirmed infections. In this situation China used weibo for epidemiologic tracking and sourcing as well as dispersion of accurate information. By using search terms *bomb**, *explos**, and *explod**, authors examining the Twitter response to the Boston bombings suggest that the social media platform provided a quicker dispersion of information than formal media outlets did, and it allowed officials to geo-localize and characterize the impact of the bombs. In this situation, the GPS feature equipped to most social media outlets allowed administrators to geo-locate precise locations of the bombings and the radius of injuries.[59]

As with any policy development, ethical considerations must be given to ensure that all groups are given equal access and protection during a PHE. Whereas most health care disparities result in ethnic and racial minorities as the underserved populations, social media appears to be more equally distributed in utilization. The diversity of users indicates that using social media as a tool to characterize a PHE or to disperse information about a PHE will speak to traditionally underserved populations. Users who are Latino, African American, between the ages of 18 and 49, or hold a college degree are also more likely to gather health information via their mobile devices, whereas women between the ages of 30 and 64 are most likely to sign up for health care alerts.[60] Obviously there are financial limitations to Internet access and literacy/language limitations to understanding the information dispersed. Privacy is another ethical beast to tackle when considering data mining for epidemiologic or geo-localization of PHE. The Code of Federal Regulations governing human subject research, 45 C.F.R. § 46.102, explains private information as individually identifiable information about behavior "that occurs in a context in which an individual can reasonably expect that no observation or recording is taking place, and information which has been provided for specific purposes by an individual and which the individual can reasonably expect will not be made public."[61] Because social media users often place their name, date of birth, workplace, GPS location, interests, religion, gender, sexual orientation, among many other defining criteria on public forms, they make data mining of their personal information well within the realms of allowed ethical and legal research. Moreover, because transparency is one of the most-valued ethical principles in online policy, explaining the sources and "publicness" of information gathered in data mining should be included in all research gained from social media.

THE DIRECTION FROM HERE

Civil libertarians and legal scholars are becoming more familiar with the science of outbreaks and other elements of public health threats. Scientists are becoming more astute in the ethical and legal ramifications of intended therapies and interventions. The synergy and collaboration between these guardians of public interest will increasingly contribute to the government's ability to formulate effective public health policy.

REFERENCES

1. Leviticus 13 Bible King James Version.
2. Sehdev PS. The origin of quarantine. *Clin Infect Dis.* 2002;2002 (35):1071–1072.
3. Gostin L. Commentary: When terrorism threatens health: how far are limitations on human rights justified. *J Law Med Ethics.* 2003;31:524–528.
4. W. Va. Gov. Tomblin Declares State of Emergency 01–09–14 @9:32 pm. Available at: http://www.governor.wv.gov/Pages/State-of-Emergency.aspx.
5. Annas G. Bioterrorism, public health, and civil liberties. *New Engl J Med.* 2002;346(17):1337–1342.
6. Dwosh H, et al. Identification and containment of an outbreak of SARS in a community hospital. *Can Med Assoc J.* 2003;168(11):1415–1420.
7. Ken Ward Jr. Tomblin meeting on chemical tank bill excluded environmentalists. http://www.wvgazette.com/News/201402040046.
8. Gostin L, Bayer R, Fairchild A. Ethical and legal challenges posed by severe acute respiratory syndrome: implications for the control of severe infectious disease threats. *JAMA.* 2003;290(24):3229–3237.
9. State of South Carolina, Office of the Governor. Gov. Sanford expands voluntary evacuation to entire SC coast [press release]. Available at: http://www.scgovernor.com/interior.asp?Site ContentId=6&pressid=119& NavId=54&ParentId=0.
10. Dow K, Cutter S. South Carolina's response to hurricane Floyd. Available at: http://www.colorado.edu/hazards/qr/qr128/qr128.html.
11. South Carolina Code of Laws. §25-1-440 (Additional powers and duties of governor during declared emergency). Available at: http://www.scstatehouse.net/code/t25c001.htm.
12. Intelligent Transportation Systems. Summary of Regional Hurricane Traffic Operations Workshops. Available at: http://www.itsdocs.fhwa.dot.gov/jpodocs/repts_te/13788.html.
13. South Carolina Legislature Online. South Carolina General Assembly 115th Session, 2003-2004. Available at: http://www.scstatehouse.net/sess115_2003-2004/prever/246_20030122.htm.
14. Emergency Preparedness and Disaster Planning White Paper. Available at: http://lra.louisiana.gov/assets/docs/searchable/reports/EmerPreparedness_1.pdf.
15. Deal implements immediate reforms for winter storm warnings. Available at: https://gov.georgia.gov/press-releases/2014-02-10/deal-implements-immediate-reforms-winter-storm-warnings.
16. Abkowitz M, Cheng P, Lepofsky M. Use of geographic information systems in managing hazardous materials shipments. *Transportation Research Board.* 1990;1261:35–43. Available at: http://trid.trb.org/view.aspx?id=348174.
17. Zerger A, Smith DI. Impediments to using GIS for real-time disaster decision support. *Computers, Environment and Urban Systems.* 2003;27 (2):123–141.
18. New York City: Hurricane Evacuation Zones. Available at: http://www.nyc.gov/html/oem/html/hazards/storms_evaczones.shtml.
19. Mayor Bloomberg Issues Order For Mandatory Evacuation of low-lying areas as Hurricane Sandy approaches. Available at: http://www.nyc.gov/portal/site/nycgov/menuitem.c0935b9a57bb4ef3daf2f1c701c789a0/index.jsp?pageID=mayor_press_release&catID=1194&doc_name=http%3A%2F%2Fwww.nyc.gov%2Fhtml%2Fom%2Fhtml%2F2012b%2Fpr377-12.html&cc=unused1978&rc=1194&ndi=1.
20. Center for Law and the Public's Health at Georgetown and Johns Hopkins Universities. The Model State Emergency Health Powers Act. Article IV. Section 401. Declaration. Available at: http://www.publichealthlaw.net/MSEHPA/MSEHPA2.pdf.
21. Emergency Medical Treatment & Labor Act (EMTALA). Available at: http://www.cms.gov/Regulations-and-Guidance/Legislation/EMTALA/index.html?redirect=/emtala/.
22. Rosenbaum S, Kamoie B. Finding a way through the hospital door: the role of EMTALA in public health emergencies. *J Law Med Ethics.* 2003;31 (4):590–601.
23. Frew S, Aranosian R. Medical-legal concerns of EMS. In: Roush W, ed. *Principles of EMS Systems.* 2nd ed. Dallas: The American College of Emergency Physicians; 1994:351.
24. McIntosh B, Hinds P, Giordano L. The role of EMS systems in public health emergencies. *Prehospital Disaster Med.* 1997;12(1):30–35.
25. Standard Practice for Emergency Medical Dispatch Management. Annual Book of ASTM Standards. 1994. Available at: http://www.google.com/url?sa=t&rct=j&q=&esrc=s&source=web&cd=6&ved=0CEgGQFjAF&url=http%3A%2F%2Fwww.nhtsa.gov%2Fpeople%2Finjury%2Fems%2Fpandemicinfluenza%2FPDFs%2FAppG.pdf&ei=HLYzU4q7Fqmks QTl2YCACw&usg=AFQjCNHur1pLe_wAO52xmIV8mo91kfxN1w& bvm=bv.63738703.
26. United States Federal Communication Commission. What You Need to Know About Text-to-911. Washington, D.C. Available at: http://www.fcc.gov/text-to-911.
27. United States Federal Communication Commission. Emergency Communications. Washington, D.C. Available at: http://www.fcc.gov/guides/emergency-communications.
28. Centers for Disease Control and Prevention. Use of quarantine to prevent transmission of SARS—Taiwan 2003. *Morb Mortal Wkly Rep.* 2003;52 (29):680–683. http://www.cdc.gov/mmwr/preview/mmwrhtml/mm5229a2.htm, Available at.
29. emtala.com. Emergency Medical Treatment and Labor Act, 42 USC § 1395dd, Stat a (Medical screening requirement). Available at: http://www.emtala.com/statute.txt.
30. Roadblock Registry. U.S. Supreme Court. Delaware v Prouse, 440 US 648 (1979). Available at: http://www.roadblock.org/federal/caseUSprouse.htm.
31. Center for Law and the Public's Health at Georgetown and Johns Hopkins Universities. Model State Emergency Health Powers Act. Article IV. Section 404. Enforcement. Available at: http://www.publichealthlaw.net/MSEHPA/MSEHPA2.pdf.
32. Rotz LD, Dotson DA, Damon IK, Becher JA. Advisory Committee on Immunization Practices. Vaccinia (smallpox) vaccine. Recommendations of the Advisory Committee on Immunization Practices (ACIP), 2001. *Morb Mortal Wkly Rep.* 2001;50(RR-10):1–25. Available at, http://www.cdc.gov/mmwr/preview/mmwrhtml/rr5010a1.htm.
33. Modlin J. A mass smallpox vaccination campaign: reasonable or irresponsible? *Eff Clin Pract.* 2002;5(2):98–99.
34. Fauci A. Smallpox vaccination policy—the need for dialogue. *New Engl J Med.* 2002;346(17):1319–1320.
35. Kemper A, Davis M, Freed G. Expected adverse events in a mass smallpox vaccination campaign. *Eff Clin Pract.* 2002;5(2):84–90.
36. Mack T. A different view of smallpox and vaccination. *New Engl J Med.* 2003;348(5):460–463.
37. Schneider C, McDonald M. "The king of terrors" revisited: the smallpox vaccination campaign and its lessons for future biopreparedness. *J Law Med Ethics.* 2003;31(4):580–589.
38. Meltzer MI, Damon I, LeDuc JW, Millar JD. Modeling potential responses to smallpox as a bioterrorist weapon. *Emerg Infect Dis.* 2001;7(6):959–969.
39. Piotrowski J. big worries. Preparing medical-response teams is easier said than done, according to healthcare providers across the nation. *Mod Healthc.* 2003;33(1):6–7, 12–13.

40. The SAFETY ACT for Liability Protection. Homeland Security Act of 2002 (Title VII, Subtitle G). https://www.dhs.gov/safety-act-liability-protection.
41. Richards E, Rathbun K, Gold J. The Smallpox Vaccination Campaign of 2003: Why Did It Fail and What Are the Lessons for Bioterrorism Preparedness? *La Law Rev.* 2004;64(4):876–883.
42. Wharton M, Strikas RA, Harpaz R, et al. Advisory Committee on Immunization Practices, Healthcare Infection Control Practices Advisory Committee. Recommendations for using smallpox vaccine in a pre-event vaccination program: supplemental recommendations of the Advisory Committee on Immunization Practices (ACIP) and the Healthcare Infection Control Practices Advisory Committee (HICPAC). *Morb Mortal Wkly Rep.* 2003;52(RR-7):1–16.
43. Supplemental recommendations on adverse events following smallpox vaccination program: recommendations of the Advisory Committee on Immunization Practices. *Morb Mortal Wkly Rep.* 2003;52(13):282–284.
44. Health Resources and Services Administration. Smallpox Emergency Personnel Protection Act of 2003. Available at: ftp://ftp.hrsa.gov/smallpoxinjury/pl10820.pdf.
45. Health Resources and Services Administration. Smallpox Vaccine Injury Compensation Program. Available at: http://www.hrsa.gov/smallpoxinjury/frn082703.htm.
46. Bozzette SA, Boer R, Bhatnagar V, et al. A model for a smallpox-vaccination policy. *Engl J Med.* 2003;348(5):416–425.
47. 42 USC chapter 6A, subchapter II, part G, §264. Available at: http://www.cdc.gov/ncidod/dq/42USC264.htm.
48. Fenner F, Henderson DA, Arita I, Jezek Z, Ladnyi ID. Smallpox and its eradication. Available at: http://www.who.int/emc/diseases/smallpox/Smallpoxeradication.html.
49. Kaplan E, Craft D, Wein L. Emergency response to a smallpox attack: the case for mass vaccination. *Proc Natl Acad Sci U S A.* 2002;99(16):10935–10940.
50. Gostin LO, Sapsin JW, Teret SP, et al. The Model State Emergency Health Powers Act: planning for and response to bioterrorism and naturally occurring infectious diseases. *JAMA.* 2002;288(5):622–628.
51. Gostin LO. *J Law Med Ethics.* 2003;31:524–528.
52. Gostin LO. *JAMA.* 2002;288(5):622–628.
53. Social Media. Merriam-Webster.com. Merriam-Webster, n.d. Web. 3 Mar. 2014. Available at: http://www.merriam-webster.com/dictionary/socialmedia.
54. Duggan, M, Smith A. Social Media Update 2013. Pew Research Centers Internet American Life Project RSS.V.P.3.0. Dec. 2013. Available at: http://www.pewinternet.org/2013/12/30/social-media-update-2013/.
55. American Red Cross. Social Media Handbook. American Red Cross. Scribd.com. October 2010. Available at: http://www.scribd.com/doc/37958422/American-Red-Cross-Social-Media-Handbook.
56. Air Force Web Posting Response Assessment. Air Force Public Affairs Agency-Emerging Technology Division. Available at: http://www.au.af.mil/pace/handbooks/web_post_response.pdf.
57. Fung IC, Fu KW, Ying Y, et al. Chinese social media reaction to the MERS-CoV and avian influenza A (H7N9) outbreaks. *Infect Dis Poverty.* 2013 Dec 20;2(1):31.
58. Cassa CA, Chunara R, Mandl K, Brownstein JS. Twitter as a sentinel in emergency situations: lessons from the Boston marathon explosions. Version 2. *PLoS Currents.* 2013 Jul 2;5[revised 2013 Jul 2].
59. Fung IC-H, Wong KK. Efficient use of social media during the avian influenza A (H7N9) emergency response. *Western Pacific Surveillance and Response Journal.* 2013;2(4).
60. Fox S, Duggan M. *Mobile health 2012. Pew research centers Internet project;* 8 Nov. 2012. Available at: http://www.pewinternet.org/2012/11/08/mobile-health-2012/.
61. Department of Health and Human Services. *Code of Federal Regulations Title 45, Pt. 46.102.* 2009.

Mutual Aid*

Brielle Weinstein, James Geiling, and Kerry Fosher

When disaster strikes suddenly, first responders gather their resources, move to the scene, and begin to execute a well-rehearsed response. Personnel, supplies, and equipment arrive at the scene and meet the requirements of the operation, and once completed they are refitted and resupplied for the next calamity. But what happens when the disaster evolves slowly over time and distance, involving many organizations across jurisdictional boundaries? Or when, given the prior scenario of a sudden-impact disaster, local resources become rapidly depleted? Victims of a disaster require a number of resources, and whether in the form of a warm bed or a hot meal these requirements may exceed the local capabilities.

Just as an individual who is baking a cake may need a cup of sugar from a neighbor, organizations responding to emergencies occasionally need the assistance of others. Mutual aid is one of the earliest and most organic forms of interagency cooperation and coordination in public safety and health services. Without prearranged mutual aid agreements, events that deplete or exhaust community resources jeopardize the health and safety of not only the victims directly affected by the disaster but also the rescuers and emergency management personnel themselves.

This chapter introduces a brief history of the federal plan to support disaster responses as it applies to working with state and local governments. The chapter also covers the basic concepts of developing mutual aid agreements, organizational examples (at the local, state, and federal levels for developing plans), pitfalls, and successful disaster responses that effectively used mutual aid.

THE MUTUAL AID CONCEPT

Response, Recovery, and Regional Capacity Building

Mutual aid can provide an organization with personnel, equipment, supplies, and pharmaceutical agents in an existing or anticipated emergency. Mutual aid agreements serve to regulate the sharing process, with the identification of what resources can be shared and under what circumstances. Agreements also address potential problems, such as the liability of sharing organizations and responders, reciprocity of credentialing and licensure, ability of the sharing organization to hold back resources to protect itself, and expectations regarding accounting and reimbursement. Logistics concerning mobilization and demobilization, transportation to and from the incident, food and shelter, and other pertinent functional aspects of the asset's deployment are addressed. The most effective mutual aid agreements apply to all phases of the disaster response.

Mutual aid agreements tend to be made between like organizations: hospitals make them with hospitals, law enforcement agencies with other law enforcement agencies, and utility companies with utility companies. Even libraries and museums have mutual aid agreements for coping with disasters.[1,2] However, agreements also are made among jurisdictions, such as state-to-state or county-to-county mutual aid, covering a range of public safety, health, and public works organizations. Mutual aid for response and recovery has become part of the decision matrix for planners in many areas of the United States.[3] As the technical base for response equipment and training expands, planners must make decisions about where to place specialized resources for the maximum sustainable value to the region.

As with the other realms of studying disaster preparedness, as a retrospective science, we will study mutual aid using multiple examples of systematic preparation and recovery. In West, Texas, a fertilizer plant explosion and fire in April 2013 displayed the well-established fire department mutual aid agreements.[4] After Hurricane (Superstorm) Sandy in 2012 the $68 billion dollar cleanup and recovery process required and led to mutual aid policy coordination between insurance companies, interstate and intrastate governments, and private organizations.[5] In this natural disaster New York City saw courageous and efficient mutual aid between hospitals: generators went down and ill patients were transferred between hospitals.[6] From scenarios like these we are able to grow the process of mutual aid, fill in gaps where agreements lack, and enhance communication between cooperating groups.

Conceptual Planning Concerns

Many regions are not able to provide exactly equal resources in every area or in each facility; mutual aid as a planning tool can build overall capacity and capability. Good agreements allow planners to consider the capability of the entire mutual aid network when choosing how to allocate resources for overall preparedness. Historically, but not always, this type of planning has taken place on an informal level. Planners tend to know what other organizations in their area have available to share when open lines of communication exist. However, in immediacy of some disasters the use of mutual aid agreements can systematize the process and make it more accountable, minimizing the chances of gaps or misunderstandings.

Most conceptual planning concerns are ultimately problems of definition, management, or sustainability. When an organization, such as a hospital, realizes it is overwhelmed, it usually requests mutual aid when somebody, preferably within the hospital's Incident Command, recognizes what "overwhelmed" means based on preset, defined parameters. Advance work to define what "almost overwhelmed" might look like in various scenarios goes a long way toward smoothing actual operations. Costly preparations are made to mitigate the effects of a hurricane only for the storm to change direction. Although most would argue that

---

*The opinions and assertions contained herein are those of the authors and are not to be construed as official or necessarily reflecting the views of the United States Marine Corps or Department of Veterans Affairs of the U.S. Government.

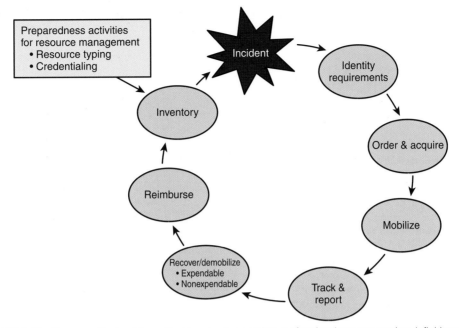

FIG 34-1 The Resource Typing Library Tool is an online catalogue of national resource typing definitions and position qualifications provided by the Federal Emergency Management Agency (FEMA) National Integration Center (NIC). (From https://www.fema.gov/national-incident-management-system/national-integration-center-resource-management.)

preparation is still the superior option over not preparing, this process can consume financial resources and manpower without deployment, making accurate prediction of when "overwhelmed" status will be reached essential. Organizations must also work to "type" their resources, categorizing assets they can share or expect to receive based on the disaster.

Resource Typing Library Tool (RTLT) (Figure 34-1) is an online catalogue of national resource typing definitions and job titles and position qualifications:

- Supporting a common language for the mobilization of resources (equipment, teams, units, and personnel) prior to, during, and after major incidents
- Providing users at all levels with access to an easily searchable database of typed definitions to identify resources for planning and incident operations, including mutual aid coordination

Resource typing definitions are provided for equipment, teams, and units. They are used to categorize, by capability, the resources requested, deployed, and used in incidents. Measurable standards identifying resource capabilities and performance levels serve as the basis for this categorization. Job titles and position qualifications are used in the inventorying and credentialing of personnel. Job titles for many personnel are cross-referenced and support the capabilities contained in resource typing definitions for teams and units. Credentialing ensures and validates the identity and attributes of individuals or members of emergency management teams through standards. There is no cost to use the RTLT, and a username or password is not required. On the World Wide Web, go to https://rtlt.ptaccenter.org.[7] Requests made under mutual aid agreements may be easier to fulfill when requestors ask for a specific capability rather than an organization. Resource Management Overview: Federal Emergency Management Agency, available at: http://www.fema.gov/resource-management[8]

Plans to manage mutual aid must include how aid is dispatched, received, managed on scene, and demobilized. Appropriate dispatch depends on the organization being able to make a considered and coherent request for resources. With the advent of technology's powerful databases, typing aid and up to the minute maintenance of surplus

and need can be maintained. Tools, such as Mutual Aid Support System (MASS), are already available for Mission Ready Packaging and mutual aid sharing.[9] The receiving organizations must also have protocols for receiving the aid and incorporating it into ongoing operations. Finally the receiving organization must understand how to demobilize human resources and return or dispose of material ones.

For many types of disasters, sustainability is a critical element of response and recovery; mutual aid can provide the resource "depth" for an organization or jurisdiction to sustain a response until state or national assistance is deployed. Problems can arise if resources are requested too quickly and are exhausted or if they are recalled before they can be useful in extending the duration of response. Some mutual aid planners now want their agreements to include discussions of response sustainability and to provide guidelines to help those on scene make sound judgments about response timeframes. Under incident management, it becomes the responsibility of the incident command structure to process assets arriving through mutual aid. The system depends on good operational guidelines to ensure that the only unpredictable element in the response is the evolving disaster itself.

Groups, such as the National Emergency Management Association and the American Hospital Association,[4] have developed model agreements for organizations, localities, and states to use when developing their own mutual aid agreements.[10] A well-known example of this standardization is the Emergency Management Assistance Compact (EMAC), a template plan for state-to-state mutual aid.[5,11] EMAC, described in more detail later in this chapter, is a national mutual aid system for states but allows some tailoring to meet local needs. For example, states in Federal Emergency Management Agency (FEMA) Region IX (HI, CA, AZ, NV, and Pacific Islands) have longer flight times with concentrated populations at larger distances, requiring mutual aid plans that would be different than others.[12]

Various templates are available online for hospitals, fire departments, municipal governments, and other groups, allowing for standardization. Time and resources saved in creating the agreement can be used for implementation and training. Standardization can also help to ensure that agreements address operational concerns consistent with national plans, such as the National Response Plan[13] and the National Incident Management System.[14] Mutual aid training is as much if not more about maintaining open lines of communication between the two agreeing groups in times of well-being as it is about preparing for the actual disaster. Coordinating aid can be best accomplished when two groups understand each other beyond a list of needed typed assets. When disaster strikes, saving time maintaining databases with technology can afford opportunity for face-to-face networking empowering partners to work with established mutual respect. A mutual aid keystone is for familiarity among partners, not just organizations but the actual people assigned the tasks of asking and sending assets.

HISTORICAL PERSPECTIVE

Although discussed in detail elsewhere in this textbook, a brief review of the national disaster response history may provide a perspective on how mutual aid agreements and processes at differing government levels have matured over time. Recent disaster response organizations in the United States at the federal level date to the early 1960s when the newly formed Federal Disaster Assistance Administration of the Department of Housing and Urban Development managed several massive disasters. For example, after the Alaska Earthquake of 1964, in which needs far exceeded available local resources, many questions arose as to the federal government's capability to appropriately respond. Review of this disaster and others in subsequent years led to the establishment of a process for presidential disaster declarations through passage of the Disaster Relief Act in 1974. This act provided the legal processes under which state governors could formally request federal assistance after disasters for support that exceeded the state's response capabilities.[15] It was in essence the first state-federal government, disaster-specific mutual aid agreement.

However, disaster response at the federal level remained fragmented. More than 100 federal agencies could be called on to respond to disasters ranging from natural events to accidents involving the transportation of hazardous materials.[9,16] In 1979 President Carter issued Executive Order 12127, which merged many disaster-related responsibilities into FEMA.[17] By 1989 with the fall of the Berlin Wall and the decline in the global threat of nuclear warfare, FEMA was funded and empowered to focus its efforts on nonnuclear disaster response as well. The current basis for federal disaster response stems from the Robert T. Stafford Disaster Relief and Emergency Assistance Act (most commonly known as the "Stafford Act"). This law gives the federal government operational guidelines and funding to execute disaster response.[11,18]

CURRENT PRACTICE

This section describes many local, state, and federal assets or policies that can be used when an organization sets out to develop a mutual aid plan. The activity level and effectiveness of organizations and policies vary, and although each possibility described in this section may not have all the answers, each provides a place to start and is part of the overall context of mutual aid. Because disaster response and mutual aid begin on the local level, we will begin by discussing local aid agreements then move to larger geographic areas' mutual aid agreements.

Local Community Assets

Community-level first responders typically serve on the front lines for disaster response, often placing their own personal safety in jeopardy in the process. Some disasters, such as biological terrorist events, may develop slowly over time and great distances, yet the first case is often identified by a local health care worker or rescuer who notes an unusual incident, such as the physician who diagnosed the incident case of anthrax in 2001.[12,19]

Disaster or emergency planning in communities has historically been developed by fire departments, in part as a result of their personnel's ongoing training and experience in managing day-to-day emergencies. In some municipal emergency operations plans (EOPs), town managers or mayors have overall responsibility; however, fire departments have typically served as both planner and operator. Close integration of the administrative lead and the fire department remains critical to the successful planning and execution of EOPs. In the West, Texas, fertilizer plant explosion in 2013, fire departments coordinated through the Texas Intrastate Fire Mutual Aid System (TIFMAS) provided manpower and resources to respond effectively in rural Texas.[20,21]

Local Emergency Planning Committees

Although since 1986 communities, by law, have had to develop a Local Emergency Planning Committee (LEPC), the events of September 11, 2001, dramatically increased the emphasis placed on these organizations to expand their disaster-planning process. Planning now must occur not only across some jurisdictional boundaries, but it also must entail other entities beyond industry, fire, and law enforcement personnel. Specifically the federal government in 1986 mandated the formation of State Emergency Response Commissions (SERCs); these SERCs were tasked to develop emergency planning districts to "... facilitate preparation and implementation of emergency plans." Within these districts, the state is to "... appoint members of a local emergency planning committee for each emergency planning district. Each committee shall include, at a minimum, representatives from each of the following groups or organizations: elected State and local officials; law enforcement, civil defense, firefighting, first aid, health, local environmental, hospital, and transportation personnel; broadcast and print media; community groups; and owners and operators of facilities subject to the requirements of this subchapter."[22] In areas where an LEPC is active, it can serve as the focal point in the community for information and discussions regarding all aspects of emergency planning as well as health and environmental risks.

U.S. Citizen Corps

The federal government created the USA Freedom Corps after September 11, 2001 in an effort to provide opportunities for citizens to serve their community and foster a culture of service, citizenship, and responsibility. Under the auspices of the Department of Homeland Security, components of the U.S. Citizen Corps are designed to be staffed by local volunteers and serve in local events.[23] The Community Emergency Response Team (CERT) program helps to train individual volunteers to be better prepared to assist their community, serving as support to first responders, directly assisting victims, and organizing volunteers who arrive on scene. They also can assist in projects designed to enhance public safety.[14,24]

The other major component of the U.S. Citizen Corps available for assistance at the local level is health care personnel who serve as part of the Medical Reserve Corps (MRC). "The MRC program coordinates the skills of practicing and retired physicians, nurses and other health professionals as well as other citizens interested in health issues, who are eager to volunteer to address their community's ongoing public health needs and to help their community during large-scale emergency situations."[25] Office of the Surgeon General within the U.S. Department of Health and Human Services oversees the program, but its components, tasks, activation, utilization, etc., are governed locally and through state Citizen Corps Councils. Local community leaders develop MRCs and outline their roles and responsibilities in disaster response. MRCs may also play a role in day-to-day public health and safety campaigns or other volunteer efforts.

Other Government Agencies

A variety of other government organizations may play a prominent role in local disaster response. Search and rescue organizations may come from state fish and game agencies, private organizations, Civil Air Patrol, and others, although federal agencies, local military, Veterans Affairs, federal law enforcement agencies, etc., may serve as first responders for some communities and hence need to clearly predetermine their roles, responsibilities, and command relationships during disaster planning.

Voluntary Organizations and Volunteers

The American Red Cross (ARC) plays an active role in the health and safety in most communities, and although it is not a government entity it has a federal mandate to assist in disasters.[26] It is a lead primary agency for Emergency Support Function #6 (Mass Care) in the National Response Plan. Staffed by both professionals and volunteers, disaster relief of the ARC is designed to meet the immediate, disaster-related needs of victims as well as emergency workers. It provides shelter, food, and health and mental health services to address basic human needs during the event and later provides services to help disaster victims and emergency workers return to some form of normalcy. Its special shelters may also be called on to assist in the care and management of hospitalized patients who are discharged because of low acuity or evacuated because of disruption of the hospital facility. The ARC normally provides care to all victims who arrive at one of its shelters for support, but pre-event mutual aid agreements and discussions can help coordinate disaster health services within a given community.[17,27]

Other relief agencies appear at disasters and play a role in supporting both victims and rescue workers. At the Pentagon disaster on September 11, 2001, the first agency to arrive was the Salvation Army (J. Geiling, personal observation).[28] The Salvation Army is a Christian-based, international organization whose mission includes "To provide support, training and resources to respond to the needs of those affected by emergencies without discrimination."[29] Additional religious or other cause-related organizations serve in part to assist their community in times of need.

Individual volunteers also tend to flock to disaster scenes, in part to assist with the rescue effort. This "convergent volunteerism" can be defined as "The arrival of unexpected or uninvited personnel wishing to render aid at the scene of a large-scale emergency incident [and who often] engage in freelancing, [that is,] operating at an emergency incident without knowledge of or direction by the on-scene command authority."[30] These volunteers are not limited to medical personnel but also can include fire and law enforcement representatives and others. Sometimes these volunteers, such as those brave civilians whose anecdotes we heard after the 2013 Boston Marathon Bombing, are on scene before emergency services. Multiple marathoners and spectators stepped in to provide immediate support after witnessing the finish line bombings.[31] In other situations they migrate to the scene, in part as a result of misinformed requests for help often by well-intended media reporters, politicians, or professionals from their specific organizations. Due to the popularity and pervasiveness of social media, one of the new tasks of emergency personnel is to monitor the information about a disaster on social media by providing quick and accurate information about the event. Incident Command may choose to use social media as an outlet to monitor the need for mutual aid as well as gather volunteers.

Challenges facing these volunteers and those tasked to oversee the response effort include volunteer safety, interference with the operations, security (especially at a crime scene), and qualifications as responders. In the immediacy of a disaster, with limited technology, active and valid certifications and licenses of responders to participate are likely to not be available to cross reference. For example, incident managers often need to deal with firefighters who self-dispatch to a scene—they may be helpful with their specific skill sets but are unproven and unknown and may pose safety hazards on scene. They may lack specific gear and equipment, and their needs may burden the overall response. Development of a National Fire Service Responder Credentialing System could help to alleviate these questions by uniformly assessing the qualifications and capabilities of fire service personnel.[32,33] Finally for large-scale disasters, sustained operations will require the expertise of professionals working later shifts in their normal place of employment; organizations' effectiveness will be depleted if their personnel report to the disaster scene as unsolicited volunteers.[19]

Volunteers will likely continue to converge on disasters because of two reasons: (1) volunteers, especially first responders, are genuinely altruistic and want to help, and (2) they often are unsure as to the exact need, so assuming any help is better than none, they migrate to the scene. People who are used to going to disasters will likely continue in their quest to provide aid. However, rapidly obtaining a needs assessment and disseminating such information may prevent unnecessary aid; this communication depends on a functioning, well-tested, interorganizational, mutual aid, redundant, two-way communication system. Internet and cell phone services may still be widely available, in which case intraorganizational email and mass texts can be used effectively per the organization's EOP. Social media outlets, such as Facebook, Twitter, and Instagram, can be used to disperse and obtain information quickly and efficiently through official EOPs to provide valid information. Key responders to disaster areas should proactively determine such roles and responsibilities, especially in scenarios that typically involve multiple organizations or jurisdictions. Convergence behavior is often not limited to the movement of personnel. Unnecessary donations of equipment, clothing, and supplies (including blood products that require significant logistical and administrative support) can also appear at a disaster scene. The management of unsolicited volunteers and this cache of supplies can, unfortunately, use critical assets otherwise needed to manage the disaster itself.[34] Public relations officers who understand the functions of social media can coordinate mutual aid public donations of material and personnel: should more aid be needed, these outlets can quickly rally public support and provide details about donation receiving sites and regulations about what can be used; should supplies or personnel be in excess, these outlets can help to curb volunteers or direct them toward a more effective service.

Local Emergency Management Plans and Mutual Aid

A review of the agencies and personnel available as well as thought given to who else may show up at a disaster are important aspects of the planning or mitigation phases of disaster response. Formalizing this information into a plan and developing mutual aid agreements optimize the chances for successful disaster relief operations. Developing a plan at the local level can be a daunting job for the individual(s) tasked (or who volunteer) to complete it. The National Response Plan outlines the basic components for a roadmap, but often state governments provide their towns with a template. For example, the 1996 state of Vermont's "Model Town Emergency Operations Plan" guides communities through purpose statements, hazard vulnerability analysis, operations, support resources, exercise and training, and other components needed to complete a town plan. Details on specific Emergency Support Functions can be found in its 13 annexes.[35] The current Appendix D offers the Mutual Aid Guideline for Police Departments and the Vermont Memorandum of Understanding (MOU) template.[22,36]

Other locations, typically large cities, may present more complicated situations—multiple agencies from a variety of jurisdictions and levels of government not only interact for daily operations but also for emergencies and disasters. The metropolitan Washington, DC, area has established a 22-member Council of Governments (COG) to help in a coordination effort for the region. Collectively with input from the state of Maryland, the Commonwealth of Virginia, the federal government, public agencies, the private sector, volunteer organizations, and local schools and universities, the COG has established a Regional Emergency Coordination Plan (RECP) to provide a vehicle for collaboration in planning, communication, information sharing, and coordination activities before, during, or after a regional emergency. The plan describes the purpose and scope, as well as the roles, responsibilities, communication, and coordination relationships among member organizations. In a manner similar to the Vermont plan, the RECP delineates its Emergency Support Functions into 16 areas, or Regional Emergency Support Functions (R-ESFs), which "identify organizations with resources and capabilities that align with a particular type of assistance or requirement frequently needed in a large-scale emergency or disaster."[37] The 16th R-ESF added since the first edition of this textbook is the necessary Volunteer and Donations Management.[38] The R-ESFs are supported by 11 Annexes including the third, "Credentialing."[39]

Mission Ready Packages are specific response and recovery capabilities that are organized, developed, trained, and exercised before an emergency or disaster. They are based on National Incident Management System (NIMS) resource typing but take the concept one step further by considering the mission limitations that might impact the mission, required support, the footprint of the space needed to stage and complete the mission, personnel assigned to the mission, and the estimated cost. Mission Ready Package templates can be developed using a blank template[40] that can be imported into the EMAC Operations System and models for Mission Ready Packages.[41] The conditions of these arrangements may be to provide reciprocal services or to receive direct financial reimbursement for labor, supplies, or equipment. Ideally the arrangements are codified in writing before an event, although they may be based on unwritten mutual understanding and may even occur after an event has taken place. FEMA's Mutual Aid Agreements for Public Assistance (Recovery Division Policy Number 9523.6) specifies criteria by which FEMA recognizes the eligibility for reimbursement of costs under the Public Assistance Program incurred by such mutual aid agreements.[24,42]

Finally even though well-defined, codified mutual aid agreements serve all parties who participate in disaster response, it is the process by which disaster planning and mutual aid arrangements develop that is most crucial to a successful disaster response. It is through the planning process that relationships among emergency response organizations, both inside and outside of the planners' jurisdiction, develop. Exchanging business cards, rehearsing plans through exercise drills, refining communications plans, and other activities during disaster preparedness all foster a sense of trust among the participating organizations, thereby improving overall interorganizational and intraorganizational communications in a disaster. It is incumbent on the agencies to maintain these relationships through personnel changes, due to staff leaving the organization, realignments, or reassignments.[27]

Hospitals

Hospital disaster preparation and incident planning have had a dramatic surge in importance since September 11, 2001. Legislation delegating hospitals as first responders also makes them eligible for funding to support the planning process, an often-quoted impediment to their preparation.[43] Individual hospital preparation and response to an incident have been reviewed in detail elsewhere.[29,44] However, outside organizations and agencies continue to expand their expectations for hospitals to be adequately prepared. Unfortunately, though, hospitals often tend to conduct their disaster preparations and training in isolation, which impairs their ability to interact with these groups when disaster strikes. As previously outlined, LEPC guidelines recommend that local hospitals participate in the community's emergency preparation. In addition to routine agreements on patient receiving and treatment, these preparations now call for expensive and underfunded capabilities, such as planning for the reception of contaminated chemical casualties. Hospitals' primary credentialing oversight comes from the Joint Commission (JC, formerly JCAHO). This body also mandates a variety of emergency preparations that, again, require additional expensive preparations. If hospitals do not receive adequate financial support and therefore are not prepared, victims of mass casualty incidents may end up riding "ambulances to nowhere."[30,45]

The JC, however, continues to refine its requirements; EM 02.02.03 preparedness activities include written agreements, MOUs, and other arrangements that are set up in advance so that resource commitments and working relationships are established before disaster strikes.[46] Another valuable reference is the 2011 Centers for Disease Control and Prevention Public Health Preparedness Capabilities: the National Standards for State and Local Planning document, which sets a priority for health care facilities (HCFs) and their strategic partners to work in conjunction with local emergency management to develop written plans and MOUs that clearly define the processes and indications to transition into and out of conventional, contingency, and crisis standards of care.[47]

Hospitals affected by disasters often become inundated with victims seeking care, who in reality need minimal medical attention. Individuals who may simply need observation during the latency period of a potential biological hazard may also overwhelm a hospital's requirements to treat the more seriously ill or injured. To prevent this increased burden, hospitals should explore mutual aid agreements with special shelters, such as those managed by the ARC or other volunteer organizations, as previously discussed. Urgent care centers, individual physician or health care worker clinics, mental health clinics, surgicenters, nursing homes, etc., may all be additional locations to provide care for low-acuity cases as well. These facilities and others may also help individuals seeking care who really only need shelter. In combination, hospitals may be able to work with these organizations to accommodate much needed surge capacity, a topic covered in detail elsewhere in this textbook.

Volunteers present a significant challenge to those planning for and managing a response. As previously discussed, well-intending volunteers tend to converge at a disaster to provide their assistance. This sense of duty also applies to health care providers who arrive at an overwhelmed or damaged hospital to assist in needed patient care activities. During disaster planning, the facility needs to decide whether volunteers will be used or in what roles they will be used, if nurse or physician volunteers will be used, and if so, how the credentials of volunteers will be verified.[48] The American College of Emergency Physicians recommends that all hospitals have a detailed process in place to allow for the emergency privileging of additional physician staff who arrive at a facility to support response efforts to a declared hospital disaster. So-called "disaster physician privileging" should ideally be completed before an event and mirror the credentials of the providers at their "home hospitals."[49,50] In the event of a disaster, immediate credentials can then be granted with proper identification. Hospitals providing these disaster credentials must also be prepared to provide professional liability coverage for physicians who provide care during a disaster in their institution and be prepared to address issues of compensation for injured workers.[51,52] The provision of disaster credentials must follow the medical staff guidelines outlined by the JC under EM 02.02.13 for Licensed Independent Practitioners (LIPs) and EM 02.02.15 for those who are not LIPs.[53] Two standards have to be met: first there has to be a disaster that triggers the EOP and second that the supply of practitioners does not meet the immediate needs of existing patients, typical future patients, and those expected to be affected by the disaster. The elements of performance for this standard include identifying the individual(s) responsible for granting such privileges, a mechanism to manage those with these credentials, and the development of a priority pathway to verify credentials within 72 hours after an event.[54] MOUs can be established with local, county, or state professional organizations' non-HCF-affiliated LIPs to precredential for a declared disaster.

Identification and credentialing are topics that can be included in mutual aid agreements to the benefit of the entire community or state. As responders and volunteers appear on scene, it is critical that security personnel are able to determine who is allowed to work and in what capacities, often without the benefit of a sophisticated understanding of licensure and credentialing. Coordinated standards for identification can increase the speed and accuracy of this process. Some national initiatives are under way, such as the fire service credentialing proposal previously described. Another initiative is the Health Resources and Services Administration (HRSA) funding for the Emergency System for the Advance Registration of Volunteer Health Professionals (ESAR-VHP) program, which is an attempt to provide standardized credentialing and identification protocols. (The basis for the ESAR-VHP initiative is U.S. Public Law 107-188, the Public Health Security and Bioterrorism Preparedness and Response Act of 2002 [section 107, Emergency system for advance registration of health professions volunteers].) (PL 107-188 is available at: http://thomas.loc.gov/.) The 2005 HRSA guidelines require awardees to develop ESAR-VHP activities in their regions. However, HCFs should seek out local initiatives and actively participate to ensure that their needs are addressed and that they are aware of the systems that are developed in their communities.[55]

Like other community-based organizations, hospitals must share resources and plans with other entities in the community. Mutual aid agreements or MOUs formalize and delineate each other's roles and responsibilities. Agreements need to include not only representatives from public safety and community industry but also those from other nearby HCFs. Developing a detailed yet functional mutual aid agreement between medical facilities can be a challenging task. Much coordination, inspection, discussion, legal review, etc., must occur before most signatories will agree to such arrangements. Fortunately several templates exist to aid the process.[56–58] These models include information, such as the purpose of the MOU, timing and method of communicating requests, documentation standards, guidance on patient transport, hospital supervision, financial and legal liabilities, and notification of next of kin and the patient's physician. It is also important that these topics be discussed not only in general principles of medical operations, but also as they apply to the evacuation of patients and the transfer of personnel, pharmaceuticals, supplies, or equipment.

Command Structure

When disaster strikes a community, local, community-level assets typically respond first. The majority of organizations in the first responder community attempt to establish command and control of the scene using principles of the Incident Command System (ICS). Discussed in detail elsewhere in this textbook, the ICS establishes a proven organizational template that can be expanded or contracted in a modular fashion to meet the demands of the event. The emergency medical services (EMS) branch of the operations section is supposed to manage medical support to the operation. Under the NIMS, which is discussed in detail elsewhere in this textbook, a medical unit is also established under the logistics section to provide medical support to the emergency responders themselves.[7] If the incident is primarily a mass casualty event involving essentially all medical assets, then the operations section chief, or even the incident commander, may be from the health sector.[45,59]

This organizational paradigm is often not followed by hospitals in their response to either an internal or external disaster; they tend to rely on their own organizational structure that has evolved to support their day-to-day operations. However, when disaster strikes, hospitals need to move toward an emergency management structure to ensure institutional and personnel safety and security, optimize patient care, and efficiently use scarce resources. As previously mentioned, the JC mandates an emergency management system that easily integrates into that of the community.

The Hospital Emergency Incident Command System (HEICS) is the standard for health care systems' disaster response originating in Orange County California in 1991. The organization of HEICS mirrors that of ICS, with five functional areas: command, operations, planning, logistics, and finance and administration. Job action sheets provide checklist tools for providers in each position to prioritize and categorize their efforts into immediate, intermediate, and extended tasks. HEICS is not a turnkey system; rather it is a process that must be adapted to each event and is supported by specific emergency management policies and procedures.[46,60] The HEICS structure focuses on management of internal disasters. As previously discussed, coordination with external agencies becomes necessary for the facility to effectively integrate itself into any community disaster response. HEICS can begin to facilitate that process by ensuring that outside groups and leaders that follow ICS principles can (ideally) find their hospital-based counterpart in the ICS structure to better coordinate the HCF disaster response.

State and federal assets that arrive on scene will similarly fall in line with their own form of an ICS, although a major event may result in the establishment of multiple incident command posts (ICPs) and agency emergency operations centers (EOCs). To manage the entire event, representative agencies may meet to form a Joint Operations Command (JOC), usually off-site to effectively provide a strategic, unified command.

State Assets

As previously discussed, most disasters begin as local events and are managed with local, community-level assets. State and federal agencies located in the vicinity may also serve as first responders without full escalation of the response outside of the community. When community resources become overwhelmed or other characteristics of the disaster mandate state or federal involvement (such as in multijurisdictional fire response or events related to terrorism), individual state emergency management organizations respond.

National Guard

Many state assets can be called on to support a state-managed disaster response. Integrating them into the state emergency management plan naturally requires detailed planning. One organization that is often overlooked, in part because of its perceived complexity, is the National Guard. At the disposal of the governor, National Guard units serve the public interest in their state in time of disaster unless they are called on for federal service. A specific asset is one of the 55 National Guard Weapons of Mass Destruction Civil Support Teams (WMD CSTs).[61] These teams, under the operational control of the adjutant general and ultimately the governor of each state, are designed to mobilize within 2 hours to augment local and regional terrorism response, principally for events known or suspected to involve weapons of mass destruction, including nuclear, chemical, or biological agents. When deployed to an event these teams report to the incident commander and provide assessment capabilities, advice, and assistance to the response effort. In essence, they supplement other fire and hazardous materials teams that may be on location, serving as a bridge until other state or federal assets arrive.[48,62]

State Emergency Response Commission

Each state develops its own disaster organizational system. However, the previously described legislation that mandated the establishment of LEPCs, also directed the establishment of SERCs. The Emergency Planning and Community Right-to-Know Act of 1986 (EPCRA) does not require a specific number of participants of the SERC nor their qualifications; thus each state and tribal land SERC varies, depending on the appointments by each governor and tribal chief executive officer. The SERC establishes local emergency planning districts, which may be a county or multiple counties of a metropolitan area. The four main duties of the SERC are to appoint, supervise, coordinate LEPC activities, to fulfill the requirements of EPCRA regarding specific reports and notifications, to make these reports and notifications available to the public, and annually review the LEPC local emergency plans.[63]

Emergency Management Assistance Compact

Disasters that cross state boundaries may be managed at the state level, without necessarily invoking the need for a federal response, under the auspices of the EMAC. Legislated in 1996 as Public Law 104-321, EMAC is a mutual aid agreement and partnership between states that exists because of the common threat from a variety of disasters; it is a legal mechanism and not an organization. Out-of-state aid organized through EMAC helps ease the movement of personnel and equipment across state borders. Requests for EMAC assistance are legally binding contracts, obligating the requesting state to reimburse all out-of-state costs and liability complaints for out-of-state personnel. Finally, EMAC permits states to both ask for assistance and to provide available resources with a minimal amount of "bureaucratic wrangling."[50,64]

Model Intrastate Mutual Aid Legislation

Produced by the National Emergency Management Association, in concert with the Department of Homeland Security, FEMA, and other emergency responders, the Model Intrastate Mutual Aid Legislation provides a robust template to expand on the mutual aid agreement legislated under EMAC. A multidisciplinary group of subject matter experts gathered in January 2004 to review a variety of mutual aid agreements from all levels of government, and on thorough review and evaluation of "best practices" developed this template. Covering 11 basic articles, "The model is meant to be a tool and resource for states and jurisdictions to utilize in developing or refining statewide mutual aid agreements. States and jurisdictions have modified the model to conform to their own state laws and authorities, or to address unique needs and circumstances. Further, the proposed articles and provisions in the model are complementary to the recommended minimum elements to be included in mutual aid agreements that are a part of the draft National Incident Management System Plan."[51,65,66]

Private Sector Resources

In 2013 the National Emergency Management Association (NEMA) recognized that a state lacked the mechanism to activate what has proven to be the majority of assets available to the state, nongovernmental, private sector, or tribal resources to fill requests for assistance through EMAC. Based on the successful deployment of these types of assets by the state of Minnesota to the North Dakota Floods (2009),

Hurricane Irene (2011), and Hurricane Sandy (2012), NEMA developed the "Intergovernmental Agreement (IGA) Nongovernmental Organizational Agreement (NGOA) Tribal Agreement (TA)." The introduction explains the premise of the EMAC with fill-in-the-blank lines for the requesting state, sending state, and the reason for the EMAC request. Clearly stated are expectations about work conditions and shift hours and that the responders should be prepared to be self-sustained for several days. Terms and conditions, employee status, liability, logistics, equipment, reimbursement, and other stipulations are in the contract.[67] The development of these types of contracts is one example of how the stream of private sector trucks headed from one state to another to repair downed power and telephone lines after an ice or other storm, tornado, or other disaster, is accomplished within hours of the event.

Federal Assets

Once the disaster response exceeds the capabilities of local, state, or interstate capabilities or the disaster results from a recognized act of terrorism, federal resources mobilize to assist the community. A large number of diverse organizations with many differing capabilities can be called on to assist; many of these are discussed in detail elsewhere in this textbook. Both in metropolitan areas and in rural areas adjacent to federal facilities these assets may appear immediately on scene, serving in a first responder capacity. However, outside of this example, federal assets mobilize in a specified manner, according to federal policy.

The 2013 edition of the National Response Framework (NRF)[65] with 14 core capabilities provides the information for the whole community to engage to achieve the National Preparedness Goal. Critical improvements over the 2008 NRF include the formal recognition of the Emergency Support Functions as coordinating structures. There are five frameworks intended to be strategic documents with tactical planning covering the preparedness missions: Prevention, Protection, Mitigation, Response, and Recovery.[66]

The Disaster Declaration Process and Federal Disaster Assistance

When disaster strikes, individual communities, states, and other organizations cooperating through mutual aid agreements respond to assist the afflicted area and its victims. As noted some federal assets may be on hand, and depending on the scenario (e.g., a terrorist event) others may preemptively deploy to the scene. Outside of these settings, the federal disaster declaration process to request federal assistance follows the guidelines outlined in the 1988 Robert T. Stafford Disaster Relief and Emergency Assistance Act. This Stafford Act requires that "all requests for declaration by the President that a major disaster exists shall be made by the Governor of the affected State."[68]

The governor's request is processed through the regional FEMA office. The first step is a preliminary damage assessment (PDA) conducted by state and federal officials. This assessment, in concert with the governor's request, must demonstrate a need beyond the capabilities of the local and state governments. The PDA normally precedes the governor's request, although it may follow for obviously catastrophic events. Pending the approval of federal assets, the governor must initiate the state's emergency plan, documenting the resources used for the state's response. Also required is an impact estimate, which is a projection of the financial cost to the public and private sectors.[69] Finally the governor must provide a needs assessment on the assistance required. Based on this information and with the governor's appeal, the president decides on the validity of the request; declaration of the event as a federal disaster activates a broad scope of federal programs and services to assist in the response, rescue, and recovery operations. Figure 34-2 presents a mutual aid flow chart.[70]

MUTUAL AID

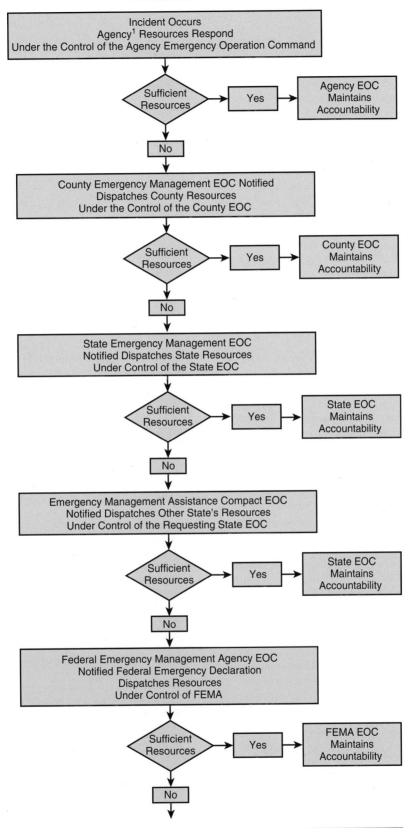

¹Agency: can be Health Care Facility, EMS, Fire, Rescue or other organization

FIG 34-2 Mutual Aid Flowchart. (Modified from Missouri State Mutual Aid. Available at: http://www.dfs .dps.mo.gov/programs/resources/mutual-aid.asp.)

OPERATIONAL PITFALLS

Too Many Contracts

Although the organizational construct for mutual aid has been studied and improved through a robust review of successful and less than successful responses by professional associations, those in the private sector eager to help, and governmental agencies that are tasked to respond promptly and efficiently, weakness remains. When the binding contract is signed by a government entity with a government or nongovernment agency, organization, or private sector source of assets, the number of contracts entered into by this partner should be considered. The agency may not be aware of the total number, depth, and breadth of obligations of their partner, thus jeopardizing the expected response of the partner. Due diligence, as with any contract, requires that both the agency and partner clearly understand expectations regardless of incident, environmental factors, or timing of the requested response. For example, a worst case scenario is a private service transport ambulance service contracting to evacuate a nursing home after the governor declares an emergency evacuation ahead of a hurricane, but the service is unavailable because they have contracted with too many nursing homes in the area and cannot get there in time. Another potential pitfall is lack of staff if there are available ambulances because the transport EMS agency's staff has primary duty obligations with their full-time positions with 911 EMS/Fire/Rescue and cannot work for their part-time transport EMS job.

Two-Hat Syndrome

As government budgets have been cut and funding for disaster-related positions have dwindled, personnel have been reduced; to help continue with necessary services, many agencies require individuals to perform a "dual-hat" mission, carrying the burden of two positions within the same agency: day-to-day operations and disaster response. People who are asked, are required, or volunteer for such duties may jeopardize response efforts in the event of a disaster with thorough lack of planning, education, maintenance of equipment and supplies, and coordination with other agencies, etc. This "two-hat syndrome" also often extends beyond the public sector. For example, asking part-time or off-duty persons to assist in relief efforts means they may not be available for other needed services that they normally perform. Agencies that have mutual aid arrangements may, in fact, be sharing personnel. These challenges are magnified during military activation of guard or reserve forces—many of these personnel also work in other public sector jobs. Surveys have determined that of all of the public service sectors, fire and rescue operations, private ambulances, and emergency management services suffer the most from this "syndrome."[71] A solution may be a computer database for agency personnel listing their obligations to effectively prioritize responsibilities and to identify conflicts to either reassign duties or eliminate obligations. Similarly an agency can detail their obligations with other agencies to highlight potential overextended obligations.

Complicated Wire Diagram—Who Is in Charge?

Finally the detailed emergency response capabilities described in this textbook all may eventually meet "on the battlefield" at the disaster scene. Defined command and control relationships, policy guidelines, regulatory edicts, mutual aid agreements, MOUs, or simple "gentlemen's agreements" outline the ideal mechanism for all parties to execute a disaster response. However, when disasters occur, the agencies that arrive to assist often come from different locations with differing and oftentimes competing ideas on management of the disaster. Mutual aid and working arrangements, even if prearranged rather than being developed on scene, often have not been rehearsed. Consequently, individuals who respond to a disaster need to have both the flexibility and the authority granted by their parent organizations to improvise on scene. This "planned improvisation" should be both expected and ideally rehearsed during disaster planning.[56,72]

The decision makers who arrive on scene also tend to come from lower levels in their organizations' hierarchy. They often fail to understand their organization's participatory role in the overall disaster response, focusing instead on their more familiar intraorganizational policies and procedures. In disaster parlance this is known as the "'Robinson Crusoe Syndrome' (i.e., 'we're the only ones on the island'). This narrow focus on one's organizational goals has been observed not only in disaster response, but in planning as well."[70] This dilemma also highlights the importance of training that focuses on interagency or interorganizational response, which unfortunately does not occur very often.

SUMMARY

Mutual aid arrangements among agencies likely to operate in a disaster clearly enhance the probability of success, giving robust and redundant response capabilities. The key to the success of the effort lies in the people—their availability, physical stamina, understanding of the disaster response milieu, and pre-event training. Only through relationships developed through the creation of mutual aid and the rehearsal of the response will the nuances of these arrangements and capabilities be delineated and repaired to meet the needs of the victims who depend on the responders and their plan. Mutual aid agreements and contracts should follow the advice of Robert Frost's 1914 poem *Mending Wall*, "good fences make good neighbors."[73]

REFERENCES

1. Inland Empire Libraries Disaster Response Network. Available at: http://www.ieldrn.org/mutual.htm.
2. Lower Hudson Conference of Historical Agencies and Museums. Available at: http://lowerhudsonconference.org/empart/Planning/Page10564/page105644.html.
3. National Emergency Management Association. If disaster strikes today, are you ready to lead? A governor's primer on all-hazards emergency management. Available at: http://www.nemaweb.org/ docs/Gov_Primer.pdf.
4. Bruce Clements, "The Texas Public Health Response to the West, Fertilizer Plant Explosion." Texas Department of State Health Services. October 8, 2013. Available at: http://www.astho.org/Preparedness/DPHP-Materials-2013/WestTexasExplosion/.
5. Smith A, Katz R. U.S. Billion-dollar Weather and Climate Disasters: Data Sources, Trends, Accuracy and Biases. *Nat Hazards*. 2013;67(2):387–410.
6. Raneri J, Diglio M, Benedetto N. How NYC REMSCO helped coordinate large-scale evacuations during superstorm Sandy. *JEMS*. May 2012;38(5):32–38.
7. Federal Emergency Management Agency (FEMA) National Integration Center (NIC). Available at: https://rtlt.ptaccenter.org/Public.
8. Resource Management Overview: Federal Emergency Management Agency. Available at: http://www.fema.gov/resource-management.
9. Central United States Earthquake Consortium. Available at: http://cusec.org/.
10. American Hospital Association. Model Hospital Mutual Aid Memorandum of Understanding. Available at: http://www.aha.org/aha/key_issues/disaster_readiness/resources/content/ModelHospitalMou.doc.
11. Emergency Management Assistance Compact. Available at: http://www.emacweb.org/.
12. FEMA Region 9. Available at: http://www.fema.gov/fema-region-ix-arizona-california-hawaii-nevada-pacific-islands.
13. U.S. Department of Homeland Security. National Response Plan. Available at: http://www.ccep.ca/responseplan.pdf.
14. U.S. Department of Homeland Security. National Incident Management System. Available at: http://www.fema.gov/nims/.

15. Federal Emergency Management Agency. Robert T. Stafford Disaster Relief and Emergency Assistance Act, as amended by Public Law 106-390, October 30, 2000. Available at: http://www.fema.gov/library/stafact.shtm.

16. Federal Emergency Management Agency. FEMA history. Available at: http://www.fema.gov/about/history.shtm.

17. Federal Emergency Management Agency. Executive Order 12127: Federal Emergency Management Agency. Available at: http://www.fema.gov/library/eo12127.shtm.

18. Roth PB, Gaffney JK. The federal response plan and disaster medical assistance teams in domestic disasters. *Emerg Med Clin North Am.* 1996;14(2):371–382.

19. Bush LM, Abrams BH, Beal A, Johnson CC. Index case of fatal inhalational anthrax due to bioterrorism in the United States. *N Engl J Med.* 2001;345 (22):1607–1610.

20. Firefighters mobilize to cover shifts for West Volunteer Fire Department. Available at: http://abc13.com/archive/9073057/.

21. Texas Intrastate Fire Mutual Aid System—Strategic Plan/Acquisition Schedule. Available at: ticc.tamu.edu/documents/incidentresponse/tifmas/texas_intrastate_fir_mutual_aid_system_acquisition_schedulefinal.pdf; January 2011.

22. 42 USC chapter 116, subchapter I, section 11001. Available at: http://www4.law.cornell.edu/uscode/42/11001.html.

23. Department of Homeland Security Citizen Corps. Available at: http://www.dhs.gov/citizen-corps.

24. Department of Homeland Security FEMA Community Emergency Response Team (CERT). Available at: http://www.ready.gov/citizen-corps.

25. Division of Civilian Volunteer Medical Reserve Corps (MRC). Available at: http://www.medicalreservecorps.gov/HomePage.

26. American Red Cross. Disaster services. Available at: http://www.redcross.org/images/MEDIA_CustomProductCatalog/m3140117_GuidetoServices.pdf. page 2.

27. American Red Cross. Disaster services. Available at: http://www.redcross.org/images/MEDIA_CustomProductCatalog/m3140117_GuidetoServices.pdf. page 5.

28. Geiling J, Foster K. Mutual aid. In: Ciottone G, ed. *Disaster Medicine.* 1st ed. Philadelphia, PA: Mosby; 2006:185.

29. Salvation Army. Relief work. Available at: http://www1.salvationarmy.org/ihq/www_sa.nsf/vw-search/E5C6EB09E25BC2A080256D4B004CEF40?opendocument.

30. Cone DC, Weir SD, Bogucki S. Convergent volunteerism. *Ann Emerg Med.* 2003;41(4):457–462.

31. Alan Duke. *Boston Marathon bombing heroes: Running to Help;* 2013. Available at: http://www.cnn.com/2013/04/16/us/boston-heroes.

32. Fire Chief. National credentials? Available at: http://www.firechief.com/preparedness/firefighting_national_credentials/.

33. National Fire Service Responder Credentialing System. Available at: http://www.usfa.fema.gov/downloads/pdf/nfa/bov/credentialing.pdf.

34. Auf der Heide E. Convergence behavior in disasters. *Ann Emerg Med.* 2003;41(4):463–466.

35. State of Vermont, Department of Public Safety. Model Town Emergency Operations Plan. Available at: http://www.higheredbcs.wiley.com/legacy/college/perry/0471920770/chap_resource/ch07/sample_munyeop.pdf.

36. Vermont Emergency Management Local Emergency Operations Plan. Available at: http://vem.vermont.gov/local_state-plans/local.

37. Metropolitan Washington Council of Governments. Regional Emergency Coordination Plan (RECP). Available at: http://www.mwcog.org/uploads/pub-documents/pF5eVI820120224112049.pdf.

38. Metropolitan Washington Council of Governments Regional Emergency Coordination Plan. Available at: http://www.mwcog.org/uploads/pub-documents/pF5eVI820120224112049.pdf. page 15.

39. Metropolitan Washington Council of Governments Regional Emergency Coordination Plan. Available at http://www.mwcog.org/uploads/pub-documents/pF5eVI820120224112049.pdf. page 4.

40. EMAC Mission Ready Package Templates. Available at: http://www.emacweb.org/index.php/mutualaidresources/emac-library/mission-ready-packages/24.

41. EMAC Operations System and Models for Mission Ready Packages. Available at: http://www.emacweb.org/index.php/mutualaidresources/emac-library/mission-ready-packages/31.

42. Federal Emergency Management Agency. Public Assistance: 9523.6 Mutual Aid Agreements for Public Assistance. Available at: http://www.fema.gov/rrr/pa/9523_6.shtm.

43. White House. Homeland Security Presidential Directive/HSPD-8. Available at: http://www.whitehouse.gov/news/releases/2003/12/print/20031217-6.html.

44. Geiling JA. Hospital preparation and response to an incident. In: Roy M, ed. *Physician's Guide to Terrorist Attack.* Totowa, NJ: Humana Press; 2004:21–38.

45. Barbera JA, Macintyre AG, DeAtely CA. *Ambulances to Nowhere: America's Critical Shortfall in Medical Preparedness for Catastrophic Terrorism.* Cambridge, MA: John F. Kennedy School of Government, Harvard University; October 2001, BCSIA Discussion Paper 2001-15, ESDP Discussion Paper ESDP-2001-07.

46. Emergency Management.tjc.2012. Available at: https://e-edition.jcrinc.com/Chapters.aspx?C=47. pages 6–8.

47. Public Health Preparedness Capabilities. *National Standards for State and Local Planning;* March 2011. Available at: http://www.cdc.gov/phpr/capabilities/DSLR_capabilities_July.pdf.

48. Burrington-Brown J. Practice brief. Disaster planning for a mass-casualty event. *J AHIMA.* 2002;73(10):64A–64C.

49. American College of Emergency Physicians. Hospital disaster planning. *Ann Emerg Med.* 2003;42(4):607–608.

50. American College of Emergency Physicians' Board of Directors. Hospital Disaster Physician Privileging Policy Approved January 2010. Available at: http://www.acep.org/Clinical–Practice-Management/Hospital-Disaster-Physician-Privileging/?__taxonomyid=471102.

51. American Hospital Association. Model hospital mutual aid memorandum of understanding. Available at: http://www.kyha.com/documents/ModelMOU.pdf.

52. Flury B, Zoppe A. Exercises in EM. *Am Stat.* 2000;54(3):207–209.

53. Emergency Management.tjc.2012. Available at: https://e-edition.jcrinc.com/Chapters.aspx?C=47. pages 12–15.

54. The Joint Commission 2010 EM and EC Update. Available at: http://www.nmhanet.org/quality/nmha-quality-education/Joint%20Commision%20EM%2020EC%20Update%20NM%2010-15-10.pdf. page 16.

55. US Dept HHS Public Health Emergency. The Emergency System for Advance Registration of Volunteer Health Professionals. Available at: http://www.phe.gov/esarvhp/pages/home.aspx.

56. New Hampshire Hospital Association and Vermont Hospital Association. Draft model language for hospital mutual aid agreements. Available at: http://www.mhalink.org/public/Disaster/files/prep-2003-13-2.pdf.

57. New Hampshire Hospital Mutual Aid Network. Memorandum of understanding. Available by permission from Bizzarro K, New Hampshire Hospital Association. Available at: http://www.nhha.org.

58. Vermont Association of Hospitals and Health Systems. Guidelines for inter-hospital mutual aid response: letter agreement. Available at: http://www.vahhs.com/lucie/mutualaid/LetterAgreement.htm.

59. Auf der Heide E. The Incident Command System. In: Disaster Response: Principles of Preparedness and Coordination. Available at: http://orgmail2.coe-dmha.org/dr/index.htm.

60. San Mateo County Health Services Agency Emergency Medical Services. HEICS, the Hospital Emergency Incident Command System. Available at: http://www.hecis.com/pdf/HEICS98a.pdf.

61. Center for Army Lessons Learned. Department of Defense Role in Incident Response, Chapter 4. December 2011. Available at: http://usacac.army.mil/cac2/call/docs/11-07/ch_4.asp.

62. 103rd Weapons of Mass Destruction Civil Support Team-General Fact Sheet. Available at: http://c21.maxwell.af.mil/wmd-cst/cst_factsheet_103rd.pdf.

63. The Role of the State Emergency Response Commission (SERC) under EPRCA. Available at: www.scemd.org.

64. Emergency Management Assistance Compact. About EMAC. Available at: http://www.emacweb.org/.

65. U.S. Department of Homeland Security. Initial National Response Plan fact sheet. Available at: http://www.dhs.gov/dhspublic/display?theme=43&content=1936.

66. FEMA Information Sheet, National Response Framework. May 2013. Available at: http://www.fema.gov/media-library-data/20130726-1914-25045-6465/final_informationsheet_response_framework_20130501.pdf.

67. National Emergency Management Association. Emergency Management Assistance Compact. Sample Agreement between State and Local, Non-Governmental or Tribal Organizations. http://www.flashcommerce.com/index.php/mutualaidresources/emac-library/12/private-sector-deployments-through-emac/278-sample-intergovernmental-agreement-between-non-governmental-and-tribal-organizations/file.

68. Federal Emergency Management Agency. A guide to the disaster declaration process and federal disaster assistance. Available at: http://www.fema.gov/rrr/dec_guid.shtm.

69. Federal Emergency Management Agency. National mutual aid and resource management initiative. Available at: http://www.fema.gov/preparedness/mutual_aid.shtm.

70. Denlinger RF, Gonzenbach K. The "two-hat syndrome": determining response capabilities and mutual aid limitations. *Perspect Prepared*. 2002;11:1–11.

71. Auf der Heide E. Principles of hospital disaster planning. In: Hogan DE, Burstein JL, eds. *Disaster Medicine*. Philadelphia, PA: Lippincott Williams & Wilkins; 2002:57–78.

72. Auf der Heide E. Disasters are different. In: Disaster Response: Principles of Preparedness and Coordination. Mosby, Incorporated, 1989. Available at: http://orgmail2.coe-dmha.org/dr/index.htm.

73. Frost, Robert. *Mending Wall*. The Poetry of Robert Frost. 1916. Available at: http://www.poets.org/poetsorg/poem/mending-wall.

CHAPTER 35

Patient Surge

Jack E. Smith II and Mark E. Gebhart

One of the fundamental objectives of any emergency preparedness program is the ability to respond to surges in demand for health care. Within the realm of health care, proactive emergency preparedness necessitates planning for large-scale emergencies that affect large numbers of persons. Occasionally these events may provide some advanced warning and gradually grow in magnitude. Examples include flooding, hurricanes, or pandemics. However, much of the time, disasters provide little to no advanced warning, as is the case with tornados, explosions, or transportation incidents.

The study of medical surge capacity as a science is relatively new, and it has mostly centered on the disciplines of disaster medicine, emergency management, public health, and the military. However, the study and measurement of surge capacity presents many challenges, and it still has yet to be clearly and precisely defined.[1] One general description of surge capacity is the "ability to manage a sudden, unexpected increase in patient volume that would otherwise severely challenge or exceed the current capacity of the health care system."[2] The Joint Commission defines *surge capacity* as "the ability to expand care capabilities in response to sudden or more prolonged demand."[3] The Health Resources and Services Administration (HRSA) defines *surge capacity* with numeric benchmarks, such as the ability to triage, treat, or reach a disposition of 50 cases per million population for burns, trauma, toxic chemical exposure, or radiation and 500 cases per million population for infectious diseases.[4] Another benchmark established by the Task Force on Mass Casualty Critical Care suggests that hospitals planning to provide emergency mass critical care (EMCC) should establish the capability to triple their typical Intensive Care Unit (ICU) census for up to 10 days without external support.[5]

Currently it is difficult for individual health care organizations and regional health care coalitions to determine exactly what steps must be taken in order to define and ensure adequate surge capacity for large-scale events or how surge plans should be tailored to the size and scope of the event.[1] Best practices in establishing surge plans, decision-triggering benchmarks, and operational procedures should be informed in part by optimal clinical outcomes in population-based care. To ensure optimal patient outcomes during the response to a large-scale mass casualty incident (MCI), surge capacity must be operationalized effectively across the community health care system, including all institutional and community-based providers.[6] Institutional-based providers include hospitals, long-term care facilities, residential behavioral health facilities, and hospice. Community-based providers include Emergency Medical Services (EMS), public health departments, public and private clinics, urgent care facilities, pharmacies, dialysis centers, outpatient surgery centers, general and specialty private medical practices, and home health agencies.

Maintaining excess capacity for patient surge runs counter to cost-efficient business practices, and hospitals of all sizes face numerous challenges to their ability to meet surge demands. Large hospitals, especially those with specialized tertiary care services, anchor the community health care system, and consistently operate at 95% to 110% capacity already, which greatly limits a hospital's ability to manage a large influx of critical patients.[7] Community health care systems in rural areas are comprised of smaller hospitals, as well as smaller or nonexistent local public health departments, and may struggle with limited resources and outside support, limited and outdated communication technology, reliance on volunteers, poorly equipped emergency medical transport units, and greater distances from other mutual aid and supportive resources.[8]

HISTORICAL PERSPECTIVE

Medical surge planning is a component of a more global Emergency Operations Plan (EOP), which in turn is developed under the auspices of a Comprehensive Emergency Management (CEM) program. The concept of CEM dictates that disaster management initiatives incorporate all four phases of emergency management (mitigation/prevention, preparedness, response, and recovery); maintain an "all-hazards" emphasis, engage, integrate, and coordinate with all stakeholders; identify and address all vulnerabilities; and be scalable to the size and scope of the event. Surge planning must consider both the facility-specific issues (hospitals, nursing homes, hospice, and behavioral health), as well as those pertaining to the community-wide health care system, including public health departments and community-based providers.

Institutional-based providers must be cognizant that whatever event is creating the surge may be affecting the community health care system as a whole. Therefore, participation of the entire emergency response system, as well as local and state offices of emergency management, can play a key role in helping to source additional resources. Coordinating with community stakeholders such as public health and emergency management during the planning phase provides for efficient flow of information, such as bed availability, the reporting of infectious disease outbreaks that may have implications for the overall community, and resource availability during the response and recovery phases. Other community-based agencies, such as mental health services, public health, and EMS agencies, may need to share important information that would be protected under the Health Insurance Portability and Accountability Act (HIPAA). Sharing clinical data, particularly data that have been redacted of all personal information, can support real-time awareness needed to help inform decision makers, particularly during epidemics.[9]

Surge triggers and crisis standards of care decisions are based on critical data points. Monitoring these key indicators that govern the change from individual-based to population-based health care is most likely to be gathered, analyzed, and shared through the community's Emergency Operations Center (EOC) during an incident. Public health should work with emergency management to ensure that appropriate data are shared to the level needed for response. Based on the typical functions of an EOC, this is the single physical location where representatives from all stakeholders within the community health care system are colocated, which facilitates the exchange of key information and the request for desired resources.[9]

CURRENT PRACTICE

Surge "Capability" Versus Surge "Capacity"

In the development of a surge plan, it is important to delineate between two terms that are often used interchangeably: *surge capability* and *surge capacity*. *Capability* is the ability to achieve a desired goal; in this case to optimize patient outcomes for the greatest number of people. *Capacity* is the measure of all the organizational strengths, attributes, and resources, such as additional beds, space, staffing, and supplies available to achieve that goal. In order to measure the hospital's surge capability, its surge capacity should be viewed as a rate or throughput (e.g., number of patients that can be triaged and treated in the first hour, 12 hours, etc.).

Consider, for example, whether or not the hospital has the ability to handle a surge of 100 patients. Even if the hospital has the flex space, extra beds, cardiac monitors, etc., its measure of surge capacity is expressed by how quickly the patients can be triaged and treated and to what level of acuity. Therefore, the overall capability is a reflection of any rate limiting factor, such as lack of staffing, specialized skills, or equipment, etc.

Homeland Security Presidential Directive 8 (HSPD-8) dictates that federal, state, local, and tribal entities and their private and nongovernmental partners should adopt a capability-based planning approach in their EOPs. Therefore, capability-based planning is the foundation for federal preparedness initiatives including the Health and Human Services (HHS) Office of the Assistant Secretary for Preparedness and Response (ASPR) Hospital Preparedness Program documents, such as the National Guidance for Health Care System Preparedness and the U.S. Homeland Security Exercise Evaluation Program (HSEEP) programs.[10]

A capabilities-based approach (or the ability to meet an objective) provides a common standard for comparing, connecting, and guiding the dissimilar elements of an organization toward the achievement of the end objective. Whereas an objective-based approach (capacity), when used alone, may inaccurately suggest a level of performance that may not be attainable. This unpredictability is best met by planning to accomplish those objectives that the organization is actually capable of achieving,[11] as demonstrated in full-scale exercises or past real-world performance.

If a new level of capability is desired, then the preparedness initiatives to attain that new capability must be developed, tested, and proven through a disaster preparedness cycle.

Figure 35-1 illustrates the cycle followed for building and improving disaster preparedness programs such as surge capacity. This process should be repeated, at least annually. High-impact or high-probability events (such as large mass gatherings or frequently occurring events) may require the cycle to be repeated more frequently.[11]

Surge plans must be flexible and scalable to meet the demands of all types and sizes of incidents. The Institute of Medicine[9] has established three basic levels of surge capacity: conventional, contingency, and crisis. Each level of surge is defined by prescribed data points of real-time situational information. This information gathered through attentive situational awareness and monitoring provides benchmarks or triggers that should prompt decision makers to declare which phase of surge the facility or community is experiencing.

The conventional level of surge would be what a facility experiences on a regular basis, perhaps during flu season or even from a multivehicle accident, and it is typically handled in-house with the staff and supplies on hand. Management strategies for conventional surge utilize

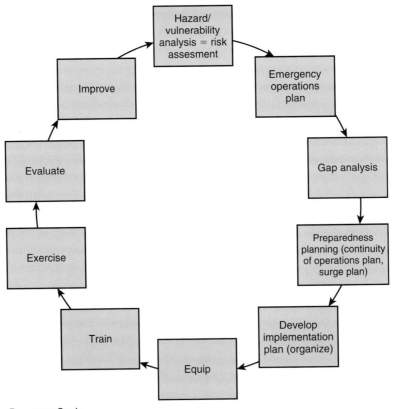

FIG 35-1 The Preparedness Program Cycle.

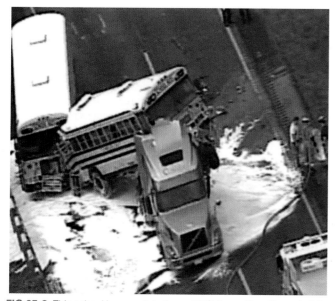

FIG 35-2 This school bus crash in August 2010 near Gray Summit, Missouri, killed two and sent 42 patients to nearby hospitals.

the physical spaces within the facility, staff, supplies, and operational processes (systems) that are typically used in normal day-to-day operations within the institution. These are the resources that are used during a major MCI. Figure 35-2 shows a typical no-notice MCI.

The contingency level of surge requires some minor changes in operations, and some resources may be replaced with equivalent alternatives, which may result in minor impacts to standards of care. Situations that require patient triage and rationing of specialized equipment, such as ventilators, fall into the contingency level. Management strategies for surge levels involve utilizing the normal spaces, staff, supplies, and systems in a manner that is not consistent with normal daily operations, in order to provide care that is functionally equivalent to usual patient care. These in-house resources may be temporarily utilized in a different manner during a major MCI or on a more sustained basis during a disaster (when the demands of the incident exceed community resources).

Crisis levels of surge require health care leaders to enact crisis standards of care and dictate a shift from individual-based care to population-based care strategies.[12] An event that is large enough in size and scope to cause a fundamental change in the community health care system and significantly changes the standards of patient care will force the community or facility into the crisis level of surge operations. The massive tornados in Joplin, Missouri, in 2011 and Moore, Oklahoma, in 2013, as well as Hurricane Katrina's impact on New Orleans and the Gulf Coast in 2005, certainly created this level of impact. Major earthquakes in urban areas, pandemics, and biological attacks also have the potential for this type of impact. Crisis levels of surge require innovative use of resources that are not consistent with usual standards of care, but do provide sufficiency of care in the context of a catastrophic disaster (i.e., provide the best possible care to the largest number of patients given the circumstances and available resources).

DEVELOPING USEFUL INDICATORS AND TRIGGERS

Surge situations by their very nature will most likely occur as part of a highly stressful situation, and both institutional and community-based health care providers will undoubtedly be affected by that stress. To provide guidance for decision makers in the middle of a crisis, surge plans should include benchmarks or triggers, to indicate when the declaration should be made as to what level of surge is currently happening. Given the number and variety of data sources, it can be challenging to identify useful benchmarks because precise numeric benchmarks are not clearly defined and easily recognized (e.g., a single case of anthrax or 10 serious patients from a vehicle crash). In many disaster situations, vague and inaccurate information, along with other real-world dynamics, may create situations that are difficult to interpret and define (e.g., an outbreak of severe gastrointestinal symptoms or unknown number of casualties from a reported tornado). Oftentimes the courses of action are not as clear-cut or significant data analysis may be required before action can be taken.

Instead of developing a cumbersome and exhaustive list of possible indicators and triggers, the Institute of Medicine[9] suggests that it may be helpful to consider the following four steps. These steps are relevant for both slow-onset and no-notice events, applicable to all types and sizes of health care facilities, and should be considered for the transition from conventional to contingency care, to crisis care, and in the return to conventional care.

1. Each facility or agency should identify key response strategies and actions necessary to respond to an incident (e.g., timely issuance of the disaster declaration if advance notice is possible or the recognition of the disaster, opening or staffing the EOC, multiagency coordination, establishment of alternate care sites, and surge capacity expansion).
2. Facility leaders should identify potential indicators that inform decisions to initiate these actions; indicators may include a wide range of data sources (i.e., bed availability, public health surveillance, or notification by EMS crews on the scene).
3. Next, decision makers should determine the trigger points or benchmarks for taking these actions. Pre-scripted triggers may be derived from certain indicators or data points. However, the data may not be sufficiently clear to support a clear decision. When pre-scripted triggers are inappropriate because the real-time information is vague or insufficient, it is important to determine and train staff on a process for identifying nonscripted triggers (i.e., who in the crisis leadership team needs to be notified/briefed, who provides the assessment and analysis of the information that is available, and who makes the decision to implement the next set of strategies).
4. Each facility or agency should utilize its emergency management or crisis leadership team to determine the tactics that should be implemented at each corresponding decision trigger point. Pre-scripted triggers or decision benchmarks should lead to appropriately pre-scripted tactics, which will support a rapid, preplanned response.

Obviously, it is impossible to predict every type of disaster scenario, but following these steps can help in identifying key sources of information that act as indicators to help determine whether or not the available information supports decisions taken to implement (trigger) specific strategies and tactics.

Decision benchmarks or triggers should be based on the key response strategies and actions that are outlined in both the facility-specific and community-wide EOPs. One primary trigger for progression from the conventional to contingency care phase would be the activation of a facility's EOP, especially if doing so enhances the patient-surge capacity that cannot be achieved in the conventional phase.[6,12,13] These types of triggers are usually tailored to the size and resources of that facility. Each facility and community should identify what the various decision benchmarks or triggers should be within their respective EOPs (e.g., on-site fire requiring evacuation within the facility, three-alarm fires in multifamily structures, second-alarm or greater EMS response, any triggers for notification of medical director or crisis leadership team, or preestablished supply consumption rates).

Regional health care coalitions that include all institutional providers, public health departments, and other community-based providers support higher levels of situational awareness, information sharing, and resource management. With preestablished lines of communication that deliver accurate, real-time situational awareness, stakeholders can be alerted when more than one coalition facility declares a disaster, when disaster victims are taken to more than three hospitals, or when staff, space, or supply shortages are anticipated. This type of real-time intelligence should also be factored in as a data point or decision trigger. The Local Emergency Planning Committee (LEPC) and Regional Health Care Coalition are both ideal venues for stakeholders to discuss, plan, exercise, and review this type of plan.

Triggers or decision benchmarks to escalate from the contingency to the crisis care phase tend to correlate to the exhaustion or overwhelming of operational resources at a level or rate that requires community-wide or regional coordination for resource allocation strategies.[9]

While it may be an individual facility that finds itself in the crisis care phase, it is critical that the regional health care coalition and emergency management Agency become involved in order to manage the resource demands regionally and ultimately ensure that as consistent a level of care as possible is provided. Another benefit to regional collaboration among stakeholders is the likelihood that most of these triggers for lack of resources will be consistent across all facilities within the region.

Establishing decision triggers or benchmarks is a process that requires a great deal of planning and coordination. Decision makers must be able to assess, analyze, and validate incoming data in order to make an informed decision. Some triggers will be based on actionable intelligence; others may be based on predictive data. Data monitoring from more than one source generally yields information that is predictive and may include monitoring of weather or epidemiologic data. Actionable data may include regional hospital bed capacity or emergency department (ED) wait times.[9]

The Components of Surge

Even though a single definition or measurement standard for surge capacity has yet to be developed, there is a general consensus on its key components; often referred to as the "4 S's" for "staff," "stuff," "space," and "systems." *Staff* refers to personnel or manpower; *stuff* consists of supplies and equipment; *space* entails both on-site areas as well as off-site alternate care facilities; and *systems* comprise integrated management policies and processes.[4,6,14]

Staff includes clinical personnel, such as nurses, physicians, pharmacists, respiratory therapists, and allied health providers, as well as nonclinical personnel, including cafeteria, housekeeping, clerical support, security officers, and physical plant engineers.[1]

Health care stuff or supplies include durable equipment, such as cardiac monitors, defibrillators, intravenous (IV) pumps, ventilators, blood glucose monitors, wheelchairs, and beds. Stuff also includes consumable supplies, such as medications, blood, oxygen, sterile dressings, IV fluids, catheters, syringes, sutures, and personal protective equipment, as well as food and water for staff, patients, and visitors.[1]

The terms "space" and "structures" are often used interchangeably. Hospitals tend to be the first structures that come to mind in health care, although institutional-based providers include extended care facilities, behavioral/mental health, and hospice facilities. Community-based providers, such as community health clinics, laboratories, outpatient surgical centers, dialysis centers, private medical practices, and public health departments, also compose the structure component of surge capacity. A more global view of "structure" also includes "buildings of opportunity" that can be utilized as alternate care facilities, such as community centers, schools, hotels, churches, or other large public assembly venues.[6]

Within the contingency level of surge, "space" can also refer to areas within the hospital that can be utilized in a different capacity to support patient triage or care (e.g., large atriums, conference rooms, hallways, and covered parking areas).

"Systems" for health care surge include integrated policies and procedures that link departments within the health care facility such as establishing the Hospital Incident Command System or opening the EOC and enacting the EOPs, Continuity of Operations plans (CoOPs), and Crisis Communications plans. Even though the term *systems* typically refers to management processes, it can also be extrapolated to include backup infrastructure systems (electric, medical gases, water, sewer, IT, communications, and security) that are critical to continuity of operations during a disaster. Additionally, systems can refer to policies and procedures that can link the health care facility with community-based providers, including public health departments, EMS, home health care, pharmacies, and physician offices.

Each level of surge operations has associated management strategies related to the 4 S's.

Staffing Strategies

Conventional staffing strategies involve the redistribution of staff that are credentialed and privileged at the institution before the event. During a disaster, staff members could be assigned in their usual area or assigned to other areas within the facility while remaining in assignments that are consistent with the typically assigned duties and scope of practice. The next step can be to utilize specialized clinicians in the roles of general care providers. For example, if all elective outpatient procedures have been canceled, those staff members can either be reassigned to other parts of the hospital or to provide general levels of care to patients now filling that area as surge space.

Contingency staffing strategies include augmentation of existing staff with outside personnel who have a similar level of credentials and are preprivileged or able to be privileged quickly from a partner hospital, staffing agencies with existing contracts, Medical Reserve Corps, and state or federal medical response teams. Contingency staffing may also include adding additional noncritical responsibilities to clinical providers. Figure 35-3 shows a Disaster Medical Assistance Team (DMAT) assisting with the evacuation of a patient.

Catastrophic incidents that overwhelm the entire community health care system will require the implementation of crisis staffing strategies. In these instances, staff are required to perform clinical duties outside their normal scope of practice in order to provide the greatest good for the greatest number of patients. This shift from individual-based care to population-based care necessitates the implementation of altered standards of care or crisis care standards. Crisis staffing strategies are stop gap measures and should be part of a preplanned and practiced systematic process to focus all of the institutional resources on lifesaving interventions and critical casualty care, while attempting to obtain additional qualified staff and initiating transfers to other facilities with higher capacity.

After 9/11 and the anthrax mailings the following month, The Joint Commission required health care facilities to establish the process to credential licensed independent practitioners in a disaster in coordination with the county or state EOC (MS.4.110, HR.1.25). In July 2013 the New York State Department of Health's Position on JCAHO Standard Regarding Disaster Privileges established a Model Disaster Privileges Policy.[15,16]

Supply Strategies

Conventional supply strategies should identify critical supplies and ensure sources of sufficient quantities of usual or equivalent materials. Increasing par levels and stockpiling are options and The Joint Commission requires at least 96 hours of all supplies be accessible. This does

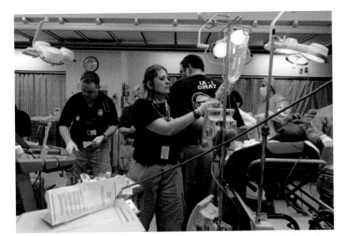

FIG 35-3 Galveston Island, Texas, September 19, 2008. Members of the Disaster Medical Assistance Team (DMAT) and medical flight crew transport a patient into a helicopter for transport to an area hospital. The DMAT was set up at the University of Texas Medical Branch as a mobile emergency following the disruption of power and services to the area caused by Hurricane Ike.

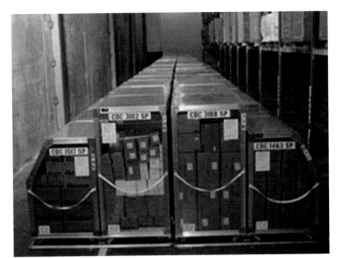

FIG 35-4 The Strategic National Stockpile of pharmaceuticals.

not mean that each hospital must maintain 96 hours of supplies on site; it is permissible that a portion of those supplies be part of a regional disaster cache.

Contingency supply strategies are implemented when standard supplies are unavailable and substitutes must be used. In contingency planning six options exist to mitigate against supply shortages:

1. *Preparedness:* stockpile necessary items or their equivalents before the event.
2. *Conservation:* use less of a resource by lowering dosage or changing utilization practices (e.g., administer oxygen only for documented oxygen saturations <90%, or use room air to nebulize albuterol instead of oxygen).
3. *Substitution:* many medications have clinically equivalent substitutes as do most consumable supplies, such as bandaging, IV supplies, etc., but not every item can be easily substituted.
4. *Adaption:* use alternative equipment or technologies to provide comparable care (e.g., using transport ventilators or anesthesia machines instead of regular ventilators).
5. *Reuse or recycle:* some supplies and equipment, such as nasogastric tubes, hemostats, scalpels, etc., can be reused after appropriate disinfection or sterilization.
6. *Reallocation:* utilizes triage strategies to prioritize the use of scarce resources (e.g., moving a ventilator from a patient that by all medical and scientific indicators is too weak to survive and reallocating it to a patient with a much higher probability of survival).

Crisis levels of surge are dire situations that require the institution of crisis standards of care, where the focus shifts from individual-based care to population-based care. These are the types of situations that were experienced in New Orleans hospitals just after the impact of Hurricane Katrina, where patients' family members were pressed into service to use handheld bag-valve ventilators on patients after electricity and battery backups failed on powered ventilators and there was no staff available to manually ventilate the patients. Other tactics utilized in crisis levels of surge include administering oxygen only to patients with O_2 saturations below 90%, not performing CPR on anyone, and reallocation of lifesaving equipment to casualties with better chances for survival. The Strategic National Stockpile of pharmaceuticals can be tapped in crisis levels of surge (Fig. 35-4).

Strategies for Expanding Space

In the conventional level of surge, strategies for creating extra space include using all available staffed beds, ensuring adequate staffing levels so that there are no unstaffed beds, adding beds to single-patient rooms, canceling elective surgeries to free up space and staff, canceling on-site clinic appointments to free up space and staff, and using reverse triage to identify patients who can be safely discharged to their home, moved to an alternate care site, or transferred to a skilled nursing facility.

Contingency space strategies include providing inpatient care in areas that have the appropriate medical infrastructure but are not typically used for this purpose. This includes using presurgical and postsurgical areas (particularly recovery beds in outpatient surgery and procedure areas, as well as the actual outpatient surgical and procedural suites for inpatient care such as endoscopy, cardiology, or radiology units). Another strategy is to temporarily utilize step-down, observation or general floor beds for higher levels of care in order to manage the initial influx of casualties until facilities that are more appropriate become available.

Crisis space strategies include using on-site nonpatient areas (such as conference rooms, hallways, and physical therapy gyms that can be quickly equipped with the necessary equipment for electrical power, oxygen supply, and vacuum) for inpatient care. Predetermined off-site areas, such as community centers, schools, and other large public assembly facilities can be used as alternate care facilities but usually require 24 to 72 hours to be set up and operational.

Systems

It is important to note that a primary institutional/agency goal should be to avoid reaching a crisis care trigger whenever possible by proactive incident management. Proactive incident management begins with developing and practicing a comprehensive EOP long before an incident ever happens. The EOP should be consistent with the National Incident Management System (NIMS) and incorporate a NIMS-compliant incident management system such as the Hospital Incident Command System (HICS). HICS and other NIMS-compliant incident command system structures provide a management framework necessary to support and coordinate operations, logistics, planning, and finance activities within the facility and throughout the region.

The EOP should also include integrated policies and procedures that link departments within the facility and provide guidance and decision benchmarks on when and how to institute the EOP, CoOP, and Crisis Communications plan, open the EOC, and establish the HICS.

Backup infrastructure systems, such as electric, medical gases, IT, water, sewer, communications, and security, are critical to the continuity of operations during a disaster. If the incident that has created the surge has also impacted the infrastructure for the facility and/or the community, these systems may be at risk for failure. One of the stark realities revealed by Hurricane Katrina was that none of the hospitals in New Orleans had planned for simultaneous complete failure of electric, water/sewer, communications, and supply chain.

Additionally, systems also include policies and procedures that can link the health care facility with community-based providers and stakeholders, such as the state and local public health and emergency management, the Centers for Disease Control and Prevention, etc. These include reporting systems for various communicable diseases, bed-availability status, ambulance-diversion status, resource needs, etc.

Strategies to Manage Demand

Developing surge capacity is a matter of managing supply and demand. The aforementioned factors are strategies to manage the supply side. Strategies to management the demand side are also referred to as surge protection or "the ability to expand the capacity of the system to triage or treat more patients in a staff-challenged environment."[17] Surge protection strategies to manage demand might include:

- Mitigating or regulating the number of patients seeking hospital services through effective community-wide planning to prevent or reduce surge. The first step is to attempt to develop a higher level of health care resiliency throughout the community by ensuring good access to public health education/prevention and access to good quality health care. A second strategy is to enhance resiliency through strategies that develop robustness by installing backup electrical generators to keep private practice clinics, public clinics, pharmacies, and other community-based providers open and operational. This reduces unnecessary surge on the hospitals by providing access to health care throughout the community. A third strategy for health care resilience is to provide a nonhospital location such as a disaster shelter that can meet the special medical needs of the disaster survivors and displaced persons (e.g., providing electric and/or oxygen concentrators for oxygen boarders, home oxygen patients who have lost electrical power). All of these resilience building strategies combine to reduce the patient surge, which reserves the fixed capacity of the hospital (number of ventilators, monitored beds, and clinical staff) for the critically ill and injured. Effective communication on a regular basis will educate the community to access these Special Needs Shelters once opened by declaration of the County or Regional Authority (see South Carolina Special Medical Needs Shelter [SCSMNS]).[17]
- Effective triage can also reduce demand by identifying those patients with a higher level of acuity who need to be in the hospital and rerouting the noncritically ill and injured to other areas in the hospital or on the grounds of the hospital designated as disaster treatment areas, long-term care facilities, and alternate care sites, or utilizing home-based health care. Constituents to develop and implement plans to route patients that self-refer to the hospital away from the ED proper should include fire, rescue, EMS, and law enforcement that may have man roadblocks with established hospital triage officers.
- Some literature suggest that higher levels of security are necessary to prevent the walking wounded, worried well, and patient families from flooding the hospital and creating demands on supplies and space. Certainly, these challenges arose in some of the New Orleans hospitals in the aftermath of Katrina. However, simply locking people out does not tend to be consistent with the mission of most health care facilities. Hospitals must remain aware of the need to provide uninterrupted medical care, and a surge in demand for medical services must take into account real need versus the perceived needs of the public. Perceived needs are those worried well and those whose baseline medical status may be inappropriate for hospital-based care, thus requiring some form of outpatient assistance. Of course, there is certainly a place for security in the hospital setting, such as in the case of preventing patients contaminated with a hazardous material from contaminating the ED; nor is it prudent to allow access to those that present a security threat. Effective triage can address the concerns of the walking wounded and worried well. In crisis situations patients' families can be disruptive especially during altered standards of care situations or evacuation of the facility. Rather than deny family access altogether, it would be much more proactive to plan on how to care for and manage that population.

Considerations for community surge include:

- Real human behaviors that encompass the worried well, oxygen boarders, anyone trying to access health care, and people seeking refuge from severe weather or maybe just looking for food or drugs; all surging on the nearest hospital.
- Providing community-based support (pharmacy access, dialysis, electricity, etc.) for those with special medical needs such as home oxygen patients, refrigeration for diabetics' insulin, dialysis patients, or anyone who is at risk of increased morbidity, which could result in unnecessary hospital visits.
- Engaging home health agencies and public health nursing to support home-based health care, states such as South Carolina have established regulations to assure proactive individual-based disaster evacuation and treatment plans (see SCSMNS).[18]
- Engaging the population at large for cooperation in personal preparedness, public health prevention strategies, compliance with official information and directions, and involvement in Community Emergency Response Teams.

All these strategies enhance the overall health and resilience of the community and enable the community-wide health care system to surge and protect the hospitals.

! PITFALLS

With regard to some of these surge capacity strategies, one point of consideration in using contingency staffing is the risk-benefit analysis of importing nonprivileged staff to provide casualty care in-house versus evacuation of casualties to another facility with better resources. Of course this requires regional coordination with other facilities who may be just as overwhelmed depending on the size and scope of the incident.

If facilities choose to participate in an off-site regional disaster stockpile in lieu of maintaining 96 hours of consumable supplies on site, consideration must be given to stock rotation of expiring supplies, the potential for formulary inconsistencies of pharmaceuticals, as well as logistical challenges. Storing supplies off-site requires logistics support to obtain and transport the supplies that may not be readily accessible in a disaster. Supplies may also be obtained from other facilities and suppliers, but this strategy has some significant limitations, including accessibility if roads are blocked and availability if other facilities are experiencing the same type of patient surge. Stockpiling is not consistent with Just-In-Time or Lean supply chain principles, but cost efficiency and supply chain resiliency can be balanced with good planning.

Even though the strategy of resource reallocation is based on the same principles of triaging patients in a population-based, crisis standard of care situation, it has some significant ethical and legal ramifications, as well as psychological implications for care givers. Not only should reallocation of resources be reserved for crisis surge operations, it also is imperative that the decision guidance for care givers be established long before the disaster and be vetted both medically and legally. Removing a ventilator or cardiac monitor from one patient in order to give it to another with a higher chance of survival or greater need may seem like a simple triage strategy. However, these issues are not always so black and white. It would be difficult enough to remove a vent from an 80-year-old chronic obstructive pulmonary disease (COPD) patient to give it to a strong 28-year-old mother of three (especially if both patients are surrounded by family). Now consider the scenario of reallocating that vent from a 3-year-old patient, who by all medical and scientific indicators is too weak to survive, to give it to a stronger 30-year-old patient with a much higher probability of survival. Anticipating worst-case scenarios is prudent crisis planning that should underscore the critical need to establish advanced planning and protocols prior to the impact of a crisis.

One other pitfall is the failure to anticipate the potential for secondary surge. Secondary surge is a cascading event or consequence resulting from a convergence of paradigms within a community. Social and physical vulnerabilities within a population, such as poverty, those with chronic health morbidities, the physically and mentally disabled, and frail elderly, along with the uninsured and underinsured, all have health needs that are created or aggravated by the disaster impacts. These vulnerabilities combined with the physical loss of community-based providers, including clinics, pharmacies, dialysis centers, counseling services, and support services, such as home delivery of meals, can further restrict access to health care and exacerbate the vulnerabilities and health conditions of these at-risk individuals.[19] Recognizing the vulnerabilities within the community and anticipating the secondary surge of patients is crucial to the long-term recovery of both the community health care system and all segments of the population.

CONCLUSION

Preparing for medical patient surge is not a process that can be distilled down into a single page of action items for quick reference as a post-disaster parade of ambulances arrives at the ED doors. Surge planning is a very complex operation that involves not only every aspect of facility operations but also many stakeholders throughout the community-wide health care system, as well.

Patient-surge operations are one component of both a facility-specific and community-wide CEM Program that encompasses:

- All four phases of emergency management (mitigation/prevention, preparedness, response, and recovery)
- An "all-hazards" approach including—
  - Severe weather (tornados, hurricanes, snow/ice storms, and flooding)
  - Geological events (earthquakes, tsunamis, and volcanos)
  - Technology failures (structural collapse, power outages, industrial explosions/toxic releases, and transportation incidents)
  - Human-made incidents both accidental and intentional (terrorism)
  - Pandemic outbreaks
- The engagement, integration, and coordination of all stakeholders, including institutional- and community-based providers, local emergency management, and public health
- Identifying and addressing all population vulnerabilities (physical and social)
- Scalability to the size and scope of the event

Surge planning must incorporate both the facility-specific issues (hospitals, nursing homes, hospice, and behavioral health), as well as those pertaining to the community-wide health care system, including public health departments and community-based providers. These issues are identified through a comprehensive hazard/vulnerability analysis and through collaboration with community stakeholders. It is paramount to successful emergency and disaster health care preparedness that leaders from institutional- and community-based providers recognize the need for community-wide collaboration and coordination.

Surge planning must also be based on pre-scripted decision benchmarks or triggers that guide and enable staff to make appropriate patient care and operational decisions during a crisis.

The final and most important points of this entire chapter are:

- It is impossible to achieve true health care resiliency throughout the community without the development of regional health care coalitions that include all primary stakeholders.
- Surge planning must integrate both the facility-specific operational issues, as well as those pertaining to the community-wide health care system, including public health departments and community-based providers.
- The entire staff must be properly trained on surge operations and the overall EOP.
- Plans are useless unless they are stressed to the point of failure through rigorous full-scale exercises—as with any aspect of providing health care, it is extremely difficult to maintain a level of proficiency in any clinical skill that is not performed on a regular basis; contingency and crisis surge operations are no different because the skills and abilities to perform proficiently under the stress of a crisis can only be maintained through regular practice and exercises.

REFERENCES

1. Adams LM. Exploring the concept of surge capacity. *OJIN Online J Issues Nurs.* March 31, 2009;14(2).
2. Hick JL, Hanfling DG, Burstein JL, et al. Health care facility and community strategies for patient care surge capacity. *Ann Emerg Med.* 2004;44:253–261.
3. The Joint Commission. *The Joint Commission Accreditation Program: Hospital Emergency Management.* 2008, Retrieved January 6, 2009 from, www.jointcommission.org/NR/rdonlyres/DCA586BD-1915-49AD-AC6E-C88F6AEA706D/0/HAP_EM.pdf.
4. Schultz CH, Koenig KL. State of research in high-consequence hospital surge capacity. *Acad Emerg Med.* 2006;13:1153–1156.
5. Rubinson L, Hick JL, Hanfling DG, Devereaux AV, Dichter JR, Christian MD, et al. Definitive care for the critically ill during a disaster: a framework for optimizing critical care surge capacity. *CHEST.* 2008;133:18S–31S.
6. Barbisch D, Koenig K. Understanding surge capacity: essential elements. *Acad Emerg Med.* 2006;13:1098–1102.
7. Katz A, Staiti AB, McKenzie KL. Preparing for the unknown, responding to the known: communities and public health preparedness. *Health Aff.* 2006;25:946–957.
8. Manley WG, Furbee PM, Coben JH, Althouse RC, et al. Realities of disaster preparedness in rural hospitals. *Disaster Manag Response.* 2006;4:80–87.
9. IOM (Institute of Medicine). *Crisis Standards of Care: A Toolkit for Indicators and Triggers.* Washington, DC: The National Academies Press; 2013.
10. Office of the Assistant Secretary for Preparedness and Response Hospital Preparedness Program. 2012 National Guidance for Healthcare System Preparedness.
11. Keim M. An innovative approach to capability-based emergency operations planning. *Disaster Health.* 2013;1(1):1–9, January/February/March 2013; Landes Bioscience.
12. Hick JL, Koenig KL, Barbisch D, Bey TA. Surge capacity concepts for health care facilities: the CO-S-TR model for initial incident assessment. *Disaster Med Public Health Prep.* 2008;2(suppl 1):S51–S57.
13. Kaji A, Koenig KL, Bey T. Surge capacity for healthcare systems: a conceptual framework. *Acad Emerg Med.* 2006;13(11):1157–1159.

14. Phillips S. Current status of surge research. *Acad Emerg Med.* 2006;13:1103–1416.
15. Greater New York Hospital Association. *Model Disaster Privileges Policy;* 2004.
16. Greater New York Hospital Association. *Letter of Notification on Disaster Privileges Policy;* 2004.
17. South Carolina Department of Health and Environmental Control. *Hurricane Plan Annex J. Special Medical Needs Shelter Management.* 2013, http://www.scemd.org/files/Plans/2013HP/Annex J - Special Medical Needs Shelter Management.pdf.
18. South Carolina Department of Health and Environmental Control. *Patient/ Client Evacuation Planning: A Tool for Emergency Preparedness;* 2013. http://www.scdhec.gov/library/D-0548.pdf.
19. Runkle J, et al. Secondary surge capacity: a framework for understanding long-term access to primary care for medically vulnerable populations in disaster recovery. *Am J Publ Health.* 2012;102(12):e24–e32.

CHAPTER **36**

Accidental versus Intentional Event

Joanne Cono and Irving "Jake" Jacoby

Not all disasters are easily recognized in their earliest stages. Although disasters caused by weather events (e.g., tornadoes, hurricanes, lightning), geologic events (e.g., earthquakes, volcanic eruptions), and some technological events (e.g., bomb explosions, nuclear reactor accidents, structural failures) are quickly attributable to a physical source, other disasters such as acts of biological, chemical, or radiological terrorism, or even some vehicular collisions or accidents, may not be readily recognized or characterized.[1] Recognizing and responding to these types of disasters require patience, a high level of awareness, clinical astuteness, and rapid epidemiological assessment and response. Disasters that manifest as physical illness in a population may go unrecognized over a period of time and not become apparent until many persons become ill or die, or the contaminating or infectious agent is identified as one that does not commonly occur or does not appear to be a plausible natural finding (such as smallpox anywhere on Earth or anthrax in Washington, DC).

When an illness is attributed to an unexpected biological, chemical, or radiological agent, information from a detailed patient clinical and epidemiological history is the most effective tool to distinguish "accidental" or "natural" outbreaks from "intentional" or "terrorism-related" outbreaks. Local and state public health authorities also will engage law enforcement agencies to begin concurrent criminal investigations, although in the United States, once a terrorist event has occurred, the Federal Bureau of Investigation (FBI) will take the lead and have ultimate responsibility for managing the event.

HISTORICAL PERSEPCTIVE

Biological, chemical or radiological terrorism is the deliberate use of any of these agents against people, animals, water sources, or agriculture to cause disease, death, destruction, or panic for political or social gains. The only factor differentiating an accidental event from a terrorist event may be the malicious intent.[2] Historically, there have been serious outbreaks that have been mistaken for intentional terrorist attacks, outbreaks for which terrorism was quickly ruled out, and an outbreak that was presumed to be a natural food-borne outbreak and was not discovered to have been an act of terrorism for nearly a year.

Two naturally occurring infectious disease outbreaks in the United States were initially feared to be the result of terrorist attacks: the Hantavirus pulmonary syndrome outbreak of 1994[3] and the West Nile virus outbreak of 1999.[4] Both were caused by newly emergent infectious diseases and required careful evaluation of both clinical and epidemiological data to assign causality. In each case, a viral pathogen was identified that was not previously endemic to the United States. Both outbreak investigations yielded reasonable alternative explanations that refuted the terrorism hypothesis.

The smallpox outbreak of 1978 in England, is an example of an accidental outbreak that today would certainly raise suspicions of a terrorist attack. The last case of naturally occurring smallpox anywhere in the world was diagnosed in Somalia in 1977, and naturally occurring smallpox had not been seen in England since 1975. Ten months after the world's last case, a 40-year-old woman in Birmingham, England, was diagnosed with smallpox.[5] She died 3 weeks later, but not before infecting her mother, who recovered, and perhaps her father, who though febrile died of a myocardial infarction within the incubation period of the disease. Prompt vaccination of contacts and isolation of febrile contacts quickly extinguished the outbreak. (Similar isolation techniques were used in the Ebola case in Dallas, Texas, in 2014, albeit without the benefit of having a vaccine available.) Public health investigators concluded that the source of the outbreak was most likely the smallpox laboratory at the University of Birmingham. The index patient was a medical photographer who worked in an office immediately above the laboratory. Matching strains of smallpox confirmed the source, although the route of virus transmission is less certain. This was the last outbreak of smallpox in the world. In May 1980, the World Health Assembly declared smallpox to be eradicated from the planet. Any smallpox outbreaks that occur posteradication most likely will be first investigated as a terrorist event, even if a laboratory accident is suspected.

During the anthrax attacks of 2001, the first case of anthrax was initially suspected to be naturally occurring.[6-8] The index patient, a resident of Florida, traveled through rural North Carolina 3 days prior to becoming ill with inhalational anthrax, an uncommon diagnosis even in animal handlers, and an even more unusual diagnosis in an office worker. As anthrax spores are regularly found in soil, and cases can occur sporadically among persons who have been exposed to animal products such as animal skin blankets and goatskin drums that have been contaminated by soil, this particular person did not have any sources of animal exposure. When further epidemiological investigation revealed anthrax spores in the patient's workplace and a co-worker became ill with inhalational anthrax, terrorism was recognized. In this attack, 21 persons were infected via the postal system, intentionally contaminated by spores that had leaked out of envelopes going through a highspeed mail-processing machine. The envelopes had been used to mail anthrax spores to prominent Congressional and media personalities.[9] This case study illustrates the importance of considering terrorism when investigating outbreaks that occur in unusual geographic locations (e.g., anthrax in urban or suburban Florida instead of a rural area), among unusual populations (e.g., office workers with no animal contact, when typical cases are in handlers of goats and other animal skins), inhalational form of the infection (when 95% of naturally acquired cases are of the cutaneous type), and in clusters (e.g., more than one person in the same office). It also illustrates that more advanced microbiological techniques are usually required in order to process and possibly weaponize biological agents, so trained lab technicians involved in such cases may be the recipients of extra scrutiny.

A final example is that of the Salmonella outbreak in The Dalles, Oregon, in 1984. A total of 751 cases of *Salmonella typhimurium*, the largest outbreak of food-borne gastroenteritis in the United States that year, were linked to restaurant salad bars, 10 of which had been intentionally contaminated, in secret, by members of the Rajneeshee religious cult, in an attempt to affect a Wasco County election by limiting the turnout. The event was initially felt to be a food-borne outbreak. The link to the cult was only identified more than a year later when definitive evidence was found.[10,11] In this setting, a number of restaurants had less than adequate food management practices, and isolation of the same organism from multiple sites suggested a common food-borne bacterial source. In retrospect, further cases of intentional poisoning of individuals by the same group were identified.[11] The additional significance of this case is that not all terrorism or intentional transmission of infectious agents will involve organisms with high mortality, and the fact that this outbreak was from an organism commonly encountered in food-borne outbreaks in the United States may have played a role in the delay in identifying it as an intentional act of terrorism.

A review of all Centers for Disease Control (CDC) outbreak investigations around the world from 1988 to 1999 found that 44 of the 1099 investigations (4.0%) involved organisms considered to have bioterrorism potential. Intentional use of infectious agents was considered in six of these investigations.[12] In the early stages of the 2014 Ebola outbreak in West Africa, there was some concern it may have been intentional because it occurred outside of the virus's normal geographic pattern, as well as the remarkably small number of viral units needed to cause illness. As of this writing there has been no definitive evidence pointing to this being an intentional event.

CURRENT PRACTICE

Disease outbreaks have occurred and been investigated for many years. However, recent events such as the 2001 anthrax attacks in the United States and the 1994 and 1995 Sarin gas attacks in Japan make it necessary to consider terrorism when evaluating clusters of infectious and noninfectious diseases. A terrorist agent may be a very common organism, such as influenza or *Salmonella,* or may be a more exotic organism such as variola virus, Q fever, or Ebola virus, which is more easily obtainable during the current epidemic in West Africa.

Unusual clusters of illness may signal terrorist events that require prompt public health and law enforcement responses. Although most clusters of disease will have a source other than a deliberate act of criminal intent, terrorism should be considered in the differential diagnosis. The evaluation of each situation must be based on its specific context.

As noted above, today a single case of smallpox would be immediately investigated as a case of biological terrorism; however, some events may be subtler. When investigating a disease outbreak, there are a number of clues that should heighten the suspicions of the clinician and epidemiologist that a terrorist attack has occurred.[13-19] Because no list of clues can be all-inclusive, all health care providers should be alert for the possibility that a patient's condition may not have occurred through natural means.

Although terrorist attacks could ultimately affect large numbers of people, disease in a single patient may be the first clue. Disease caused by an uncommon organism, such as smallpox, anthrax, or viral hemorrhagic fever, may signal a sentinel event of bioterrorism. Suspicion may be further heightened by a less common presentation of one of these organisms. For example, whereas a small number of cases of cutaneous anthrax occur naturally each year in the United States, cases of inhalational anthrax are highly unusual. Furthermore, should a disease present in a geographic location where it is not usually seen, such as anthrax in a nonrural area or plague in the northeastern United States, further investigation into the possibility of bioterrorism is needed. Unexpected seasonal distribution of disease, such as influenza in the summer (which, however, can occur with pandemic influenza strains), or antiquated, genetically engineered, or unusual strains of infectious agents, may also be clues. Multiple unusual or unexplained diseases in the same patient may indicate that multiple organisms or substances were used in an intentional act, as could disease presenting in an atypical age group or population, such as anthrax in children or varicella-like rashes in adults. Additionally, a single case of an unusual infection may in fact be that of the perpetrator himself who may have accidentally exposed himself to the causative agent or may be an intentional carrier on a suicide mission.

When a disease strikes more than one person, additional clues may arise. Large numbers of cases of unexplained disease or death may signal bioterrorism, as may an unexplained increase in the incidence of an endemic disease that previously had a stable rate. If an unusual condition strikes a disparate population, such as respiratory illness in a large population, this may signal the release of a chemical or biological agent, as would a large number of people seeking medical care the same time, signaling they may have been present at a common site when an agent was released. Likewise, large numbers of persons presenting with similar illnesses in noncontiguous regions may be a sign that there have been simultaneous releases of an agent at multiple sites. Finally, animal illness or die-off that is temporally related with human illness or death may signify the release of an agent that affects both humans and animals. When there is no other explanation for an outbreak of illness, it may be reasonable to investigate terrorism as a possible source. Common sources of exposure to an infectious agent may include food and water that has been deliberately contaminated, respiratory illness due to proximity to a ventilation source, or the absence of illness among those in geographic proximity but not directly exposed to the contaminated food, water, or air.

Each event must be evaluated in context. Terrorism is still the least common explanation for disease, and other more frequent explanations should be evaluated and ruled out. Clues that may raise the suspicion that an intentional event has occurred can be broken down into some general categories: epidemiological, unusual variations in disease outbreaks, unusual characteristics of disease, and animal signals.

Epidemiological Clues

- A single case of an unusual disease, such as plague, smallpox, or anthrax, without an acceptable epidemiological explanation
- Illness among persons with exposure to a common ventilation source and absence of disease among persons not exposed to that ventilation source (potential intentional aerosol release of an agent)

- Large numbers of persons seeking care for a similar condition at the same time (may indicate a point source)
- Clusters of similar disease outbreaks in disparate geographic locations (potential of multiple attacks)
- Large numbers of cases of unexplained diseases or deaths

Unusual Variations in Disease Outbreaks

- Unexplained increases in an endemic illness, such as an increase in plague cases in the southwestern United States
- Disease occurring outside of its usual geographic distribution, such as plague or Hantavirus occurring in the northeastern United States
- Disease that appears to be transmitted via common exposure to an aerosol, food, or water that may have been intentionally contaminated

Unusual Characteristics of Disease or Agents

- Isolation of a genetically engineered, antiquated, or laboratory-manufactured form of an agent, which may have unusual or unexpected characteristics
- Isolation of a weapons-grade form of an agent
- Isolation of a known organism with an unusual antibiotic microbial-resistance pattern
- Unusual presentations of clinical disease, such as pneumonic plague (rather than bubonic plague usually caused by bites from infected fleas) or inhalational anthrax (rather than the more common cutaneous presentation, which is seen 95% of the time)
- Common disease with a higher than expected mortality, or decreased patient response to usual treatments
- Several conditions or clinical syndromes occurring in the same patient, which may indicate genetically engineered or artificially combined agents
- Disease or syndromes occurring in unusual populations, such as outbreaks of chickenpox-like rash in adults or anthrax among office workers
- Unusual disease outbreaks that occur across a large geographic area, suggesting the aerosol release of an agent
- Similar genetic types of a pathogen identified across disparate geographic locations or at different times in the same location

Other Species Signals

- An unusual pattern of animal disease or death preceding human disease or death, or an unusual pattern of animal disease or death that follows human disease or death; either may indicate a large-scale release of an agent, with differing susceptibilities between animals and humans
- Insect die-off or plant die-off associated with human illness may indicate an environmental chemical release in which the symptoms of human poisoning syndromes may be nonspecific
- Physical findings in the environment such as liquid droplets or puddles, powders or dusts, vapors or clouds, or unusual odors in the vicinity of human or animal cases may indicate a release of a biological, chemical, or radiological agent.

Radiological and Chemical Agents

Although these examples focus mostly on biological terrorism, the tenets presented apply to radiological and chemical events too. Covert radiological events, such as intentionally hiding a cobalt or cesium source stolen from a medical or veterinary facility, may expose many unsuspecting people.[20] With accidental exposure, involved persons again may not realize that they have been exposed, such as in the 1987 Goiania incident in Brazil in which a canister of cesium-137 was inappropriately discarded by a cancer treatment facility. One family brought home the sealed radioactive element and unwittingly exposed multiple family members, who then became ill. Neighboring families came to look at the fluorescent blue substance, some covering their skin with it. Although clinicians did not make the link to radiation exposure in this cluster of illness, the family's grandmother realized that her family became ill shortly after the radioactive canister entered their home. She surrendered the canister to health authorities, though not before an estimated 244 people in the community were exposed.[21]

With sufficient exposure, whether intentional or accidental, multiple persons may present with acute radiation syndrome, which during its prodromal phase is characterized by nausea, vomiting, and diarrhea that last for several days after exposure. This is followed by a latent phase, during which a patient feels well for a few weeks until obvious radiation illness begins.[22] This spectrum of clinical illness can easily be confused with a self-limited gastrointestinal illness, particularly if a number of people attend the same event during which the exposure occurs and then present with gastrointestinal symptoms. A thorough epidemiological investigation may rule out a common food source. A high index of suspicion for a radiation event should be maintained, especially when an infectious pathogen is not readily identifiable from clinical specimens. Patients with acute radiation syndrome may also experience cutaneous radiation syndrome, a dermatological condition consisting of erythema, pruritus, and desquamation. These cutaneous symptoms and findings, accompanied by gastrointestinal symptoms and the absence of an infectious pathogen in a cluster of patients, may indicate a radiation exposure, whether accidental or intentional. Hidden sources of exposure usually lead to diagnostic delays. Concealed sources of exposure usually lead to diagnostic delays; again, prompt epidemiological investigation of unusual cases can hasten the identification of a source, while criminal investigation is needed to determine possible intent.

Likewise, recognizing exposures to chemical agents can be challenging, even though the epidemiological clues listed above still apply. Chemical exposures may be overt and quickly recognized, as in the 1984 industrial chemical release in Bhopal, India, in which a release of methyl isocyanate killed 2500 people during the first week, and an estimated 3500 more over the following 10 years.[23] Conversely, a chemical incident may be as covert as contamination of food, water, or consumer products.[24] Some exposures may cause delayed health effects, making it more difficult to identify an exposure source or prove a cause and effect. Chemical exposures often cause nonspecific illnesses or syndromes of illness that are less familiar to many clinicians. Additionally, if chemicals are mixed, classic toxicological syndromes such as anticholinergic poisoning may not be apparent because patients may experience a broad array of symptoms rather than a single recognizable syndrome.

There are many case reports that illustrate these diagnostic and investigative challenges. In the United States, in the Tylenol tampering cases of 1982[25] and other medicine tampering cases like it,[26] otherwise healthy patients who ingested cyanide-laced over-the-counter medications became seriously ill and multiple deaths occurred. In the Tylenol incident, the first two deaths were thought to be due to stroke and myocardial infarction. But an astute clinician linked the unexplained syndromes of hypotension and acidosis in multiple family members of the first victim, and subsequent toxicological testing revealed the presence of cyanide. This case report demonstrates the importance of considering chemical exposures when a cluster of patients presents with illness that is sudden, unexpected, and without a prodrome. When clinical information does not indicate a naturally occurring disease, toxicology screening for poisoning is a reasonable next step (however, a comprehensive toxicological screen may take days to perform and may still miss the offending toxin).

Similarly, unexplained deaths or serious illness in an otherwise healthy population may indicate a chemical exposure. Over a 6-month period in 1985, 109 children were diagnosed with anuric renal failure at a single hospital in Haiti.[27] This condition had not been seen at the hospital in the prior 5 years. A trace-back investigation revealed that these children had ingested an acetaminophen syrup preparation that was locally manufactured from glycerin that was contaminated with diethylene glycol, the chemical used as automotive antifreeze. Ninety-nine of the children died. A criminal investigation ensued and determined that the poisoning was not intentional, but rather was caused by a departure from manufacturing quality control measures.

Pesticides are a group of toxic chemicals that are readily available to terrorists and also can accidentally contaminate the food supply, sickening large numbers of people in disparate geographic areas. In Oregon in 1985, a physician reported five cases of organophosphate poisoning resulting in cholinergic crises to the state Health Division. Epidemiological investigation revealed that the patients had become ill after eating watermelon. Additional cases were reported in Oregon, Washington, and California.[28] Over a 3-month period, more than 700 cases were identified in seven states, and 483 cases occurred in Canada. The outbreak was linked to aldicarb sulfoxide poisoning. Aldicarb sulfoxide is a toxic metabolite of Aldicarb, the systemic pesticide that was used on the watermelons originating from California. The rapid notification of public health authorities led to timely identification of the poison, although the outbreak was protracted due to the far-reaching shipping network of the global food supply. The contamination was not found to be intentional. Aldicarb was banned by the Food and Drug Administration (FDA) in 2010 and is being phased out over a 7-year period. But this will not dissuade terrorist organizations or lone-wolf renegades from using it.

In another pesticide-related case in Michigan in 2003, 92 people became ill and 1700 pounds of ground beef were recalled due to nicotine-based pesticide contamination.[29] However, in this case, the epidemiological investigation identified a single supermarket source of the contaminated meat, and the concurrent criminal investigation led to the arrest of a supermarket employee who intentionally contaminated 200 pounds of ground beef with Black Leaf 40 insecticide, which contains nicotine.

These pesticide contamination case studies illustrate the following: (1) clinicians should consider chemical poisoning in outbreaks of unexpected serious illnesses; (2) prompt reporting to authorities can lead to more rapid initiation of public health response and investigation by linking distant outbreaks to a common source; and (3) accidental and criminal events may involve the same clinical appearance of illness but can be distinguished by epidemiological and criminal investigations.

⚠ PITFALLS

There is no one algorithm that can determine whether a biological, chemical, or radiological disaster is naturally occurring, accidental, or intentional. Situations in which multiple agents have been used may be more difficult to recognize and may pose a greater diagnostic challenge, but once identified may be more easily characterized as intentional. Certain terrorist events will remain difficult to detect; however, through careful evaluation of all epidemiological clues and a thorough outbreak investigation, it is possible to make educated decisions that will permit the public health and law enforcement emergency responses necessary to limit the damage caused by an intentional disaster and prevent further morbidity and mortality. In many historical cases the fast thinking of astute clinicians can be credited to the initiation of large-scale investigations.

REFERENCES

1. Landesman LY. Public health response to emerging infections and bioterrorism. In: *Public Health Management of Disasters: The Practice Guide.* Washington, DC: American Public Health Association; 2001:121–138.
2. Keim M. Intentional chemical disasters. In: Hogan D, Burstein J, eds. *Disaster Medicine.* Philadelphia, PA: Lippincott Williams & Wilkins; 2002.
3. Centers for Disease Control and Prevention. Outbreak of acute illness: Southwestern United States, 1993. *MMWR Morb Mortal Wkly Rep.* 1993;42:421–424.
4. Nash D, Mostashari F, Fine A. Outbreak of West Nile infection, New York City area. *N Engl J Med.* 2001;344(24):1858–1859.
5. Fenner F, Henderson DA, Arita I, Jezek Z, Ladnyi ID. *Smallpox and Its Eradication.* Geneva: WHO; 1980.
6. Centers for Disease Control and Prevention. Update: investigation of anthrax associated with intentional exposure and interim public health guidelines, October 2001. *MMWR Morb Mortal Wkly Rep.* 2001;50 (41):889–892.
7. Maillard JM, Fischer M, McKee KT, Turner LF, Cline JS. First case of bioterrorism-related inhalational anthrax, Florida, 2001: North Carolina Investigation. *Emerg Infect Dis.* 2002;8:1035–1038.
8. Traeger MS, Wersma ST, Rosenstein NE, et al. First case of bioterrorism-related inhalational anthrax in the United States, Palm Beach County, Florida, 2001. *Emerg Infect Dis.* 2002;8:1029–1034.
9. Jernigan JA, Raghunathan PL, Bell BP, et al. Investigation of Bioterrorism-related anthrax, United States, 2001: Epidemiologic findings. *Emerg Infect Dis.* 2002;8(10):1019–1028.
10. Torok TJ, Tauxa RV, Wise RP, et al. A large community outbreak of Salmonellosis caused by intentional contamination of restaurant salad bars. *JAMA.* 1997;278(5):389–395.
11. Carus WS. The Rajneeshees (1984). In: Tucker JB, ed. *Toxic Terror: Assessing Terrorist Use of Chemical and Biological Weapons.* Cambridge, MA: MIT Press; 2000:115–137. [chapter 8].
12. Ashford DA, Kaiser RM, Bales ME, et al. Planning against biological terrorism: lessons from outbreak investigations. *Emerg Infect Dis.* 2003;9 (5):515–519.
13. Treadwell TA, Koo D, Kuker K, Khan AS. Epidemiologic clues to bioterrorism. *Public Health Rep.* 2003;118:92–98.
14. Centers for Disease Control and Prevention. Recognition of illness associated with the intentional release of a biological agent. *MMWR Morb Mortal Wkly Rep.* 2001;50:893–897.
15. Cono J. Recognizing bioterrorism. In: *Bioterrorism Reference for Pediatricians.* American Academy of Pediatrics, 2006. [chapter 8].
16. Henretig FM, Cieslak TJ, Eitzen EM. Biological and chemical terrorism. *J Pediatr.* 2002;141:311–326.
17. Buehler JW, Berkelman RL, Hartley DM, et al. Syndromic surveillance and bioterrorism-related epidemics. *Emerg Infect Dis.* 2003;9:1197–1204.
18. Grunow R, Finke EJ. A procedure for differentiating between the intentional release of biological warfare agents and natural outbreaks of disease: its use in analyzing the tularemia outbreak in Kosovo in 1999 and 2000. *Clin Microbiol Infect.* 2002;8:510–521.
19. Pavlin JA. Epidemiology of bioterrorism. *Emerg Infect Dis.* 1999;5:528–530.
20. Smith JM. *Clinician outreach and communication activity conference call summaries and slides: radiation emergencies. Centers for Disease Control and Prevention;* February 24, 2004. Available at: http://www.bt.cdc.gov/coca/summaries/radiation022404.asp.
21. Neifert A. Case study: accidental leakage of cesium-137 in Goiania, Brazil in 1987. Huntsville, AL: Camber Corporation. Available at: http://nbc-med.org/sitecontent/medref/online/ref/casestudies/csgoiania.html.
22. Mettler FA, Voelz GL. Current concepts: Major radiation exposure—what to expect and how to respond. *N Engl J Med.* 2002;346(20):1554–1561.
23. Dhara VR, Dhara R. The Union Carbide disaster in Bhopal: a review of health effects. *Arch Environ Health.* 2002;57(5):391–404.
24. Centers for Disease Control and Prevention. Recognition of illness associated with chemical exposure. Broadcast transcript, August 6, 2004. Available at: http://phppo.cdc.gov/phtn/webcast/chemical-exp/8-6editedscript.htm.

25. Wolnik KA, Fricke FL, Bonnin E, Gaston CM, Satzger RD. The Tylenol tampering incident: tracing the source. *Anal Chem.* 1984;56:466A–470A, 474A.

26. Centers for Disease Control and Prevention. Epidemiologic notes and reports: cyanide poisonings associated with over-the-counter medication—Washington State, 1991. *MMWR Morb Mortal Wkly Rep.* 1991;40 (10):167–168.

27. Centers for Disease Control and Prevention. Fatalities associated with ingestion of diethylene glycol-contaminated glycerin used to manufacture acetaminophen syrup: Haiti, November 1995-June 1996. *MMWR Morb Mortal Wkly Rep.* 1996;45(30):649–650.

28. Centers for Disease Control and Prevention. Epidemiologic notes and reports: Aldicarb food poisoning from contaminated melons—California. *MMWR Morb Mortal Wkly Rep.* 1986;35(16):254–258.

29. Centers for Disease Control and Prevention. Nicotine poisoning after ingestion of contaminated ground beef: Michigan, 2003. *MMWR Morb Mortal Wkly Rep.* 2003;52(18):413–416.

Crisis Leadership in Public Health Emergencies*

Scott Deitchman

A *crisis* is "a serious threat to the basic structures or fundamental values and norms of the social system, which, under time pressure and highly uncertain circumstances, necessitates making critical decisions."[1] Public health crises include natural disasters such as earthquakes and hurricanes, biological terrorism, influenza pandemics, chemical releases, and radiological emergencies. Under circumstances of extreme stress, all leaders must meet challenges that include recognizing the crisis, making decisions rapidly despite limited and fragmented information, providing effective communications, and balancing centralization with delegation.[1] Individuals leading public health responses to crises serve as crisis leaders.

HISTORICAL PERSPECTIVE

Professions that involve leading emergency responses often include formal training in leadership. In the United States, leadership training is provided to senior leadership in wildland firefighting, whereas the military services teach leadership through progressive training, education, and experiences.[2,3] Public health leadership training, in contrast, focuses on managing organizations that provide traditional public health functions, including epidemiology and laboratory investigations, sanitation, and immunization.[4] Although tabletop exercises have illustrated the importance of public health leadership, preparing public health officials to lead those responses has not received comparable attention.[5]

This shortfall was illustrated in the Top Officials (TOPOFF) 2000, a congressionally mandated national exercise to assess the nation's response to simultaneous terrorist threats and acts across several regions in the United States. One component was a simulated bioterrorism attack in Denver using plague. Observers noted failures in crisis leadership, including reliance on massive, interminable conference calls, inability to make critical decisions, and failure to avoid leader exhaustion.[6] The subsequent 2001 anthrax attacks also showed that traditional public health decision-making processes were not adequate for complex, fast-moving emergencies.[7] The U.S. Government Accountability Office (GAO) found that the Centers for Disease Control and Prevention (CDC), which led the public health response, was hampered because at that time the agency's leadership lacked formal protocols for making timely crisis-management decisions (although the agency has since implemented a robust emergency-management infrastructure and exercise program).[8,9]

---

*The findings and conclusions in this chapter are those of the author and do not necessarily represent the views of the Centers for Disease Control and Prevention or the Agency for Toxic Substances and Disease Registry.

Public health educators and practitioners have defined competencies for public health emergency leadership as familiarity with public health roles, command systems, and emergency response plans.[10,11] Current assessments of public health emergency leadership in exercises focus on completion of tasks (identify activities to be performed, interact with relevant officials, identify one's authorities, gather necessary resources, assist special needs populations, etc.) and scientific competencies involving knowledge of threats and hazards, clinical care, and epidemiologic investigation.[12–15] Although the Incident Command System (ICS) has been adapted for use in public health programs, ICS training curricula in public health settings typically focus on ICS organization and roles rather than leadership challenges faced by public health incident leaders.[16]

CURRENT PRACTICE

The practice of leadership in public health emergencies can be informed by assessing crisis leadership attributes in other professions including aviation, military, police and fire services, nuclear power plant operations, and mining.

Aircrew Captains

Simulator-based research of aircrew performance during aviation emergencies has shown that crew-leader personality affects crew performance, particularly in critical, high-workload situations. Crews led by successful crisis leaders made fewer errors and were more likely to successfully resolve the emergency. Aircrews led by captains with a constellation of traits nicknamed "the right stuff" (including self-confidence, striving for excellence, and interpersonal warmth) also reported less stress compared with crew members led by other personality types.[17,18]

Crew Resource Management (CRM) originally was developed in aviation to reduce crew error and better use human resources among the flight deck crew.[19] The traits identified in successful aircraft captains using CRM include decisiveness, the ability to maintain awareness of the situation, and willingness to receive input from other crew members. CRM has been successfully adapted to the medical setting and used in emergency departments, operating rooms, and by delivery staff. Adaptation of CRM principles and tactics to public health crisis leadership is possible through training and simulated exercises.

Military *In Extremis* Leaders

The concept of *in extremis* leadership was developed by Colonel Thomas Kolditz of the United States Military Academy (West Point) to describe leadership when team and leader face immediate risk of death or injury. *In extremis* leaders are found in military combat units and among police and firefighters. The danger in these professions attracts leaders motivated by challenge and a willingness to share their followers' risk. Followers demand competence of *in extremis* leaders, but, in return, they develop trust in and loyalty to their leader and each other.[20]

First Responder Incident Commanders

ICS leaders are termed *incident commanders.* Key attributes of incident commanders in police and firefighting are decisiveness and the ability to conduct accurate situational assessments and execute either predefined or new courses of action as appropriate. Incident commanders coordinate across organizational and disciplinary boundaries, delegate responsibility, set priorities, and manage their own stress levels to avoid performance degradation.[21]

Nuclear Power Plant Emergency Team Leaders

A study of emergency response personnel at nuclear power plants in the United Kingdom identified key nontechnical skills for various response positions. Identified nontechnical skills among "decision makers" who set strategic-response goals included decision making, communication, situation awareness and anticipation, promoting effective teamwork, managing team stress, and displaying leadership that can be either directional or consultative depending on the situational need.[22]

Underground Mine Fire Survivors

Among miners surviving underground fires, leaders tended to notice details and be alert to their environment, which are traits likely to facilitate survival. They were decisive yet open to input from others and were flexible and willing to change decisions as circumstances evolved. They had a calming effect on other miners and inspired confidence. Competence appears to be important, particularly in the emergence of ad hoc leaders in mining emergencies. In some emergencies, an individual who was not in authority before the disaster emerged as a leader after demonstrating competence by providing consultation to the pre-disaster authority figure.[23]

COMMON ATTRIBUTES OF CRISIS LEADERS

Table 37-1 summarizes the referenced behaviors and attributes of successful crisis leaders. The disciplines surveyed for this assessment vary widely in their professional demands, training, and practice environment. An aircraft captain may supervise a crew of only two or three on the flight deck, whereas the incident commander at a large fire may oversee hundreds. Military leaders and commanders of first response organizations receive formal training in incident leadership, whereas the ad hoc leader of trapped miners may have no prior leadership role in the mine.

Nonetheless, Table 37-1 illustrates that certain traits consistently appear in the behaviors of crisis leaders across multiple settings. These traits include competence, decisiveness, situational awareness, coordination, communication, and ability to inspire trust. This commonality suggests these traits can be applied to crisis leadership in other disciplines, including public health. Surprisingly, competence does not appear in every profession-specific list, suggesting professional competence is an implied and fundamental prerequisite for crisis leaders. The CRM experience, however, indicates that competence must be complemented by skills in coordination and the management of human resources.[24]

Crisis Leadership in Public Health Emergencies

The author compared the attributes of crisis leadership presented in Table 37-1 with recent experiences in responses to public health emergencies to develop proposed attributes of public health crisis leadership. Although other traits may apply, these attributes help define initial competencies for training public health crisis leaders and for identifying individuals to serve in leadership roles during public health crises. The proposed attributes of public health crisis leadership are listed in the following:

1. *Competence in public health science:* Competence is needed to ensure that response decisions are made on the basis of sound professional judgment. Competence also is required to earn the trust of other public health professionals, collaborators in other organizations, and the public. The skills previously defined for public health emergency response and emergency leadership identify necessary scientific and technical competencies.[12–16] No leader can be an expert in all aspects of public health, but the crisis leader must sufficiently understand these disciplines to critically evaluate the information and recommendations being provided to make informed incident-management decisions.

2. *Decisiveness:* The ultimate responsibility for decisions made during the response rests with the crisis leader. However, the leader actively seeks information from diverse sources to inform those decisions. In all cases, the intent is to ensure that response decisions are both as timely and broadly informed as possible.

3. *Situational awareness:* The leader must maintain an as-clear-as-possible understanding of the current situation to make appropriate decisions. Sources of information include the National Incident Management System (NIMS) reporting and planning functions, informal reporting by staff, and outreach to counterparts in other organizations. Situational awareness also includes integrating and interpreting the information to identify strategic priorities, and conveying that perspective back to the response team.

   The crisis leader actually has a bidirectional responsibility for interpreting the situation to superiors and subordinates. Public health crisis leaders frequently report to elected or appointed officials, and, indeed, the elected head of government has final authority in the response.[25] The crisis leader is the primary liaison between the response staff and those officials and must integrate the demands of the response with the officials' guidance.[26] The leader presents his or her strategic assessment to his or her own leaders to inform the assessment and actions of that higher echelon.

4. *Coordination:* The leader coordinates the response. The use of ICS tools facilitates this coordination, but the leader must promote coordination both within and across organizations, a competency described as "meta-leadership."[27] This frequently requires reaching across disciplines, in both public health and non-health response organizations, to support the broadest collaboration possible.

5. *Communication:* The public health leader promotes communication, both within the leader's own organization and across other organizations and disciplines. Consistent with the CRM goal of promoting input from team members, the leader must create an atmosphere in which staff can air disagreements and, if necessary, present the leader with difficult challenges or bad news.[28]

6. *Inspires trust:* The crisis leader will instill in the team a sense of confidence and trust in both their comrades and their leaders, often in the midst of the most difficult circumstances. The crisis leader is also responsible for the welfare of the team, and must remain sensitive to the pressures being experienced by other team members who need appropriate rest, sustenance, and emotional support.[29]

⚠ PITFALLS AND SOULUTIONS

Past crises demonstrate that traditional public health leadership training, blending management skills with public health science knowledge, is necessary but not sufficient preparation for public health crisis leadership.[30] Public health tends to be a collaborative, democratic

TABLE 37-1 Attributes of Crisis Leadership in Different Disciplines*

ATTRIBUTES/DISCIPLINES	DECISIVE/CONFIDENT	COMPETENT	AWARE OF SITUATION	ACCEPTS INFORMATION FROM OTHERS	EMOTIONAL AWARENESS	COORDINATES & COMMUNICATES	OTHER (TRAITS IN THESE COLUMNS ARE NOT GROUPED BY SIMILARITY)
Aviation: the "right stuff"[18,19]	Self-confidence				Displays interpersonal warmth & sensitivity		Preference for challenging tasks; Being active; Strives for excellence; Competitiveness
Aviation: crew resource management[20]	Makes decisions systematically		Maintains situational awareness; Regulates information flow	Accepts crew input		Coordinates; Promotes communication	
In extremis leadership[21]		Competent			Inspires and builds trust; Inspires & displays loyalty		Shares values-based lifestyle; Shares risk
Incident commanders[22]	Makes decisions		Assesses situation (awareness & interpretation); Monitors response	Assesses situation (awareness & interpretation)		Coordinates team; Communicates	Manage stress; Delegates; Prioritizes
Nuclear power plant emergency response leaders[23]	Decision making		Maintains awareness of situation and anticipates	Consultative leadership ("in slower paced situations")		Promotes communication within & in/out of plant	Manage own and team's stress
Leaders in mining disasters[24]	Decisive but flexible	Competent, knowledgeable	Aware of environment	Accepts input from others	Inspires confidence and trust; Calming		
Proposed public health crisis leadership attributes	Decisive	Competent	Maintains situational awareness	Interprets data to provide a situational assessment	Displays warmth, sensitivity; Inspires trust	Coordinates & communicates; Meta-leadership	

*Individual professional disciplines are listed in rows. Where possible, similar traits described in multiple professions are grouped together in the appropriate column. Traits described for only one discipline are listed in the "Other" column and are not grouped by similarity.

process, considering all stakeholder perspectives and then building consensus.[7] During an emergency, this model does not meet the need to make decisions quickly despite incomplete information. The long, indecisive conference calls of TOPOFF 2000 illustrate the difficulty during a crisis of relying on traditional tools to reach consensus. This has prompted suggestion that public health decision making in a crisis should follow a more "autocratic" than "democratic" model.[31] CRM deals with this issue by clearly assigning a leader, empowering "crew members" to speak their mind, and having a "two challenge rule," where anyone can challenge a decision but only twice. After that the leader's decision is final.

There is, however, risk in promoting autocracy. Lessons from aviation CRM indicate that autocratic leaders risk missing crucial information provided by team members. This may be characteristic of the settings in which team members contribute diverse expertise, which is certainly the situation in public health, and it suggests that effective crisis management should not employ a rigid command and control hierarchy. Instead, examination of other disciplines reveals that leadership that promotes exchange of information, clarifies communication, and maintains an open atmosphere even while directing activities toward timely decisions is a more useful approach.[32]

The importance of open communication, even during a fast-moving crisis, was cogently observed by United Airlines Captain Al Haynes, who in 1989 led the crew of Flight 232 that landed a DC-10 crippled by the failure of one of its engines and the immediate loss of the plane's hydraulic controls. No training or procedure manual existed for this unprecedented double-failure scenario. Captain Haynes credited his team's use of CRM (then called CLR, Crew Leadership Resource training), commenting: "Why would I know more about getting that airplane on the ground under those conditions than the other three [flight crew members]. So if I hadn't used CLR, if we had not let everybody put their input in, it's a cinch we wouldn't have made it."[33]

Even though team performance in public health emergencies has not been studied to the extent seen in other disciplines, the author's experience as a public health incident manager is consistent with leadership models such as CRM that emphasize team input. Public health crisis leaders similarly must bridge extremes of unlimited democracy and rigid autocracy. Leading a public health emergency response involves reviewing data, soliciting opinions from diverse subject-matter experts, carefully channeling debate, and avoiding digressions, bringing discussions to a timely decision and executing those decisions.

By defining the attributes of successful crisis leaders, the concepts of crisis leadership can be taught to those who will lead public health responses to future crises. As White House officials observed after Hurricane Katrina, "At all levels of government, we must build a leadership corps that is fully educated, trained, and . . . populated by leaders who are prepared to exhibit innovation and take the initiative during extremely trying circumstances."[34] Crisis leadership skills will better equip public health response leaders to meet that challenge.

Acknowledgment

The material in this chapter is drawn from a previously published work, the content of which is in the public domain.

REFERENCES

1. Rosenthal U, Charles MT, t'Hart P cited in Boin A. Lessons from crisis research. *Int Stud Rev.* 2004;6(1):165–194. doi:10.1111/j.1521-9488.2004.393_2.x.
2. Wildland Fire Leadership: L-courses at a glance. http://www.fireleadership.gov/courses/courses.html; Accessed 27.05.14.
3. Kolditz T. *Why the Military Produces Great Leaders.* Harvard Business Review Blog Network; 2009. Available at, http://blogs.hbr.org/2009/02/why-the-military-produces-grea/Accessed 27.05.14.
4. Calhoun JG, Ramiah K, Weist EM, et al. Development of a core competency model for the master of public health degree. *Am J Public Health.* 2008;98:1598–1607.
5. Lurie N, Wasserman J, Nelson CD. Public health preparedness: evolution or revolution? *Health Aff.* 2006;25:935–945.
6. Inglesby TV, Grossman R, O'Toole T. A plague on your city: observations from TOPOFF. *Clin Infect Dis.* 2001;32:436–445.
7. Gursky E, Inglesby TV, O'Toole T. Anthrax 2001: observations on the medical and public health response. *Biosecur Bioterror.* 2003;1(2):97–110.
8. General Accounting Office. *Centers for Disease Control and Prevention: Agency Leadership Taking Steps to Improve Management and Planning, But Challenges Remain (GAO-04-219).* Washington, DC: General Accounting Office; 2004, 18.
9. Leidel L, Groseclose SL, Burney B, Navin P, Wooster M. CDC's emergency management program activities—worldwide, 2003–2012. *MMWR Morb Mortal Wkly Rep.* 2013;62(35):709–720.
10. *Bioterrorism & Emergency Readiness: Competencies for All Public Health Workers.* New York: Columbia University School of Nursing Center for Health Policy; 2002, Supported by the Centers for Disease Control and Prevention/Association of Teachers of Preventive Medicine Cooperative Agreement #TS 0740. Pages 6–8.
11. Gebbie K, Merrill J. Public health worker competencies for emergency response. *J Public Health Manag Pract.* 2002;8:73–81.
12. Savoia E, Testa MA, Biddinger PD, et al. Assessing public health capabilities during emergency preparedness tabletop exercises: reliability and validity of a measurement tool. *Public Health Rep.* 2009;124:138–148.
13. Markenson D, DiMaggio C, Redlener I. Preparing health professions students for terrorism, disaster, and public health emergencies: core competencies. *Acad Med.* 2005;80:517–526.
14. Subbarao I, Lyznicki JM, Hsu EB, et al. A consensus-based educational framework and competency set for the discipline of disaster medicine and public health preparedness. *Disaster Med Public Health Prep.* 2008;2:57–68.
15. James JJ, Benjamin GC, Burkle FM, et al. Disaster medicine and public health preparedness: a discipline for all health professionals. *Disaster Med Public Health Prep.* 2010;4(2):102–107.
16. Kohn S, Barnett DH, Galastri C, et al. Public health-specific national incident management system trainings: building a system for preparedness. *Public Health Rep.* 2010;125(suppl 5):43–50.
17. Chidchester TR, Kanki BG, Foushee HC, et al. *Personality Factors in Flight Operations: Volume I. Leader Characteristics and Crew Performance in a Full-Mission Air Transport Simulation.* NASA Technical Memorandum 102259, April 1990.
18. Bowles S, Ursin H, Picano J. Aircrew perceived stress: examining crew performance, crew position, and captains personality. *Aviat Space Environ Med.* 2000;71(11):1093–1097.
19. Helmreich RL, Merritt AC, Wilhelm JA. The evolution of crew resource management training in commercial aviation. *Int J Aviat Psychol.* 1999;9(1):19–32.
20. Kolditz T. The in extremis leader. In: *Leader to Leader, Supplement "Leadership Breakthroughs from West Point"*:6–18.
21. Crichton M, Flin R. Command decision making. In: Flin R, Arbuthnot K, eds. *Incident Command: Tales from the Hot Seat.* Aldershot: Ashgate Publishing Ltd; 2002:201–238.
22. Crichton MT, Flin R. Identifying and training non-technical skills of nuclear emergency response teams. *Ann Nucl Energ.* 2004;1317–1330.
23. Vaught C, Brnich MJ, Mallet LG, et al. *Behavioral and Organizational Dimensions of Underground Mine Fires.* Pittsburg PA: US Department of Health and Human Services, Centers for Disease Control and Prevention, National Institute for Occupational Safety and Health; 2000, Pages 166–193.
24. Safety Regulation Group. *Flight crew training: Cockpit Resource Management (CRM) and Line Oriented Flight Training (LOFT) (CAP 720).* Hounslow, Middlesex: Civil Aviation Authority; 2002.
25. Labadie J. Problems in local emergency managements. *Environ Manage.* 1984;8:489–494.

26. Somer S, Svara J. Assessing and managing environmental risk: connecting local government management with emergency management. *Public Adm Rev.* 2009;69:181–193.

27. Marcus LJ, Dorn BC, Henderson JM. Meta-leadership and national emergency preparedness: a model to build government connectivity. *Biosecur Bioterror.* 2006;4(2):128–134.

28. Drechsler D, Allen CD. Why senior military leaders fail. *Armed Forces J.* 2009;(July):34–37, 44–45.

29. Heifetz RA, Linsky M. *Leadership on the Line.* Boston: Harvard Business School Press; 2002 227.

30. Leonard HB, Howitt AM. 'Routine' or 'crisis'—the search for excellence. *Crisis Response.* 2008;4(3):32–33.

31. Kizer KW. Lessons learned in public health emergency management: personal reflections. *Prehosp Disaster Med.* 2000;15(4):209–214.

32. Driskell JE, Adams RJ. *Crew Resource Management: An Introductory Handbook.* DOT/FAA/RD-92/26, Department of Transportation: Federal Aviation Administration; 1992.

33. Haynes A. *The crash of United Flight 232.* Edwards CA: NASA Ames Research Center, Dryden Flight Research Facility; 1991. http://clear-prop.org/aviation/haynes.html, Accessed 28.11.11.

34. *The Federal Response to Hurricane Katrina: Lessons Learned.* Washington, DC: White House; 2006, 72.

CHAPTER 38

The Incident Command System

Michael A. Loesch and Mary Jo Giordano

On a day-to-day basis most organizations function independently of one another. They are able to carry on with their routine activities and operate without the assistance of other agencies, jurisdictions, and/or disciplines. When an area is affected by an emergency or a disaster, however, entities come together in a system that allows them to both continue their normal operations and support emergency operations. Representatives of these entities will also be required to coordinate with the overall command and management of the operation. The Incident Command System (ICS), which has an extensive history in fire service, is a scalable product of years of experience and lessons learned from large-scale national events to small, single-jurisdictional events. The goal of ICS is to provide accurate information, strict accountability, and planning by using a management system based on manageable scope of control, for any incident,[1] for all parties involved, including health care and hospitals. The principles of the ICS are rooted in the command and control of personnel and equipment and the coordination of objectives during the response to an emergency or disaster. ICS does not provide agencies with the techniques needed to achieve their objectives, but rather an organizational structure to reduce duplication of efforts and provide a safe and efficient working environment.

The National Incident Management System (NIMS) is synonymous with ICS; to be NIMS compliant, the mandated entities must utilize the ICS structure.[2] NIMS was implemented as part of Homeland Security Presidential Directive 5 (HSPD-5) in February 2003. This directive enables federal, state, local, tribal, and local governments, nongovernmental organizations, and the private sector with a nationwide template for the response to emergency and disaster situations. HSPD-5 also requires all federal departments and agencies to adopt NIMS and to utilize it and its components for incident planning, response, and recovery.[3] Additionally, state, tribal, and local organizations must adopt NIMS as a condition for federal preparedness assistance.[3] Hospitals and health care systems participating in the National Hospital Preparedness Program (HPP) must also adopt NIMS throughout their organizations.[4] The Hospital Incident Command System (HICS) fulfills this requirement (see Chapter 6).

HISTORICAL PERSPECTIVE

In the fall of 1970, Southern California was devastated by a number of wild-land fires that burned more than 6 million acres. The fires burned for 13 days and resulted in the loss of 772 structures and 16 lives.[5] Analysis of the overall emergency response indicated numerous issues regarding coordination and management. As a result of this devastating event, Congress funded a consortium of state, county, and city fire departments, led by the U.S. Forest Service, known as the Firefighting Resources of California Organized for Potential Emergencies (FIRESCOPE), to investigate and address the underlying causes from this event. FIRESCOPE identified several recurring problems involving multiagency response that included nonstandardized terminology, nonintegrated communications, a lack of a consolidated action plan, and an inability to expand and contract resources and management as required by the situation.[5] In an effort to address these major findings, FIRESCOPE developed the original ICS model for incident management.

The National Wildfire Coordinating Group (NWCG) conducted an analysis of the FIRESCOPE ICS model for a possible national application and by the 1980s FIRESCOPE ICS was revised and adopted as the National Interagency Incident Management System (NIIMS). FIRESCOPE and NWCG coordinated to update and maintain a comprehensive Incident Command System Operational Systems Description, which served as the basis for the NIMS ICS utilized today.[6]

CURRENT PRACTICE

All disasters or emergencies differ. It is therefore imperative that an emergency management tool be flexible, to allow users to modify their response activities to meet the needs of different circumstances without losing compatibility with the overall response. Such flexibility allows ICS to be effective regardless of the complexity of the incident. By implementing ICS in small-scale response activities, users are able to become comfortable with the system and develop best practices and lessons learned for their organization and jurisdiction. These situations will directly apply to the application of ICS during larger incidents.

ICS is a collection of basic management tools that collectively addresses the common deficiencies that occur during a response. The system allows users to have a plan for each component that requires preplanning and training. There are 14 management characteristics taught by the Department of Homeland Security that are the focus of the Federal Emergency Management Agency's (FEMA's) baseline and advanced ICS training.[7]

The 14 essential ICS features follow:
- *Common terminology:* This phrase applies to the use of plain language for organizational functions, incident facilities, resource descriptions, and position titles. When incidents involve multiple agencies and jurisdictions it is imperative to use common terminology to reduce miscommunication. This concept also includes radio transmissions, which means that 10-codes, agency-specific codes, and acronyms should not be used.
- *Modular organization:* The ICS structure is staffed based on the size and complexity of the incident, including specifics related to the hazardous environment created by the incident.

- *Management by objectives:* The command staff members of the ICS structure are responsible for developing the overall objectives for an incident. Plans, procedures, and protocols for the incident are developed based upon these objectives. Objectives will affect the organization and span of control of the incident.
- *Reliance on an incident action plan (IAP):* The IAP provides a format for communicating incident objectives and operational and support activities. IAPs are broken into different form numbers to maintain consistency.
- *Chain of command and unity of command: Chain of command* refers to the organized structure within the ICS organization. *Unity of command* refers to an individual's direct supervisor at the incident scene. It may occur that one's day-to-day supervisor is not the on-scene supervisor. Chain of command and unity of command are in place to provide the structure needed to perform the incident objectives and maintain management of personnel.
- *Unified command:* For incidents that involve multiple agencies and jurisdictions it is important that all function collectively while maintaining their individual authority, responsibility, and accountability—unified command allows for this coordination.
- *Manageable span of control:* Span of control optimizes the effectiveness of an organization by controlling the number of individuals under a single supervisor. The recommended range is three to seven subordinates, with five being optimum.
- *Predesigned incident locations and facilities:* In line with common terminology requirements, incident locations and facilities have predetermined names and functions, such as bases, camps, and staging areas.
- *Resource management:* This refers to the process for categorizing, ordering, dispatching, tracking, and recovering resources. It is important to track resources from the start of the incident, for accountability and accurate tracking, for possible reimbursement.
- *Information and intelligence management:* This is the process of gathering, sharing, and managing incident-related information and intelligence. Information and intelligence can come from multiple sources, and special care should be given to how and to whom that information is disseminated.
- *Integrated communications:* As multiple organizations come together they may not all have the appropriate communications channels to communicate with the rest of the structure. It is important to plan integrated communications in advance, so enough resources can be obtained and a comprehensive communication plan can be developed. Communication systems should include redundancy in case a system were to fail.
- *Transfer of command:* As the response operations continue, personnel will change. When this occurs it is important to brief the outgoing and incoming staff in order to continue safe and effective operations.
- *Accountability:* This not only occurs at the incident site, it should also occur at all jurisdictional and departmental levels. Accountability includes five major principles, three of which are part of the original 14 ICS essentials: resource check-in or check-out, an IAP, unity of command, span of control, and resource tracking.
- *Deployment:* Finally, it is crucial that personnel and equipment do not self-dispatch. Resources should only respond when they are requested.

Notice that none of the tools focuses on the tactical response to an emergency or disaster. It is assumed that responding agencies have the proper training and capability to perform their duties. For example, in a mass casualty event, a primary objective would be to perform triage; ICS provides the core management capabilities and the system depends on the skill and knowledge of the responders to perform the assigned objective(s). It is imperative that individuals continue their education

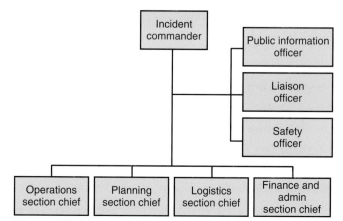

FIG 38-1 ICS Diagram.

on ICS to grasp the overall concept and to be able to implement it into their organization.

The 14 characteristics are organized under the umbrella of the ICS structure. The ICS structure consists of five major management functions: command, operations, planning, logistics, and finance and administration (Fig. 38-1). These five components, typically referred to as the incident management team, are present at all incident responses, from a routine emergency to a major disaster. The components are staffed and managed based on the type, size, scope, and complexity of the incident. For most small-scale, single-jurisdictional responses, the components may be managed by a single incident commander (IC). As the incident scale expands it may become necessary to establish each component separately and have support positions within those functions.[8] Regardless of the function, all positions have a common set of responsibilities, as well as position-specific responsibilities.

Command Function

Command activities are typically administered by a single IC. The IC is responsible for overall direction and guidance to the support staff. The priority of the IC is to "analyze the overall requirements of the incident and determine the most appropriate direction for the management team to follow during the response."[9] Some of the major responsibilities for the IC include the following:

- Establishing the incident priorities
- Determining the incident objectives and general direction for managing the incident
- Ensuring scene security
- Approving and authorizing the implementation of an IAP
- Coordinating with key stakeholders
- Ensuring the proper development and release of information

Based on the complexity of the incident, the IC should delegate authority for performing command activities. The specific activities are separated into three command staff positions: public information officer (PIO), safety officer, and liaison officer.

- The PIO is responsible for developing and releasing information to the news media, incident personnel, and other appropriate agencies and organizations.
- The safety officer is to develop and recommend measures for ensuring personnel safety. If required the safety officer has the authority to suspend, alter, delay, or terminate operations.
- The liaison officer functions as the point of contact to and from other agency representatives.

By delegating these functions to support staff, the IC can focus on life safety, incident stabilization, and property conservation.

As an incident becomes more complex the IC will delegate authority to the general staff: operations, planning, logistics, and finance and administration. Each of these functions includes a section chief and designated support staff.

General Staff Operations

The operations section consists of staff members whose primary responsibilities are to manage all tactical operations related to the incident. The operations section is typically the largest section of an incident response, because the tactical objectives being completed fall under this section. The operations section can be overseen by the IC or typically a designated operations section chief during large incidents. The operations section chief should not be involved in the tactical objectives themselves; rather they maintain a management level to oversee those resources. All tactical objectives are directed by the IAP. The operations section chief's primary responsibility is to operationalize the objectives through planning and coordination with the other functions of the ICS structure.

General Staff Planning

Under the planning section individuals are responsible for the overall accountability of the incident. This includes collection of scene information and documentation, tracking of resources, and demobilization of resources. The development of the IAP is coordinated by the planning section. The planning section does not have a tactical response function at the incident. If required, a planning section chief will be designated to coordinate the planning section.

General Staff Logistics

The logistics section is responsible for the logistical support of the incident facilities, services, and materials. Logistics staff does not provide support to civilians; rather it is dedicated to obtaining the necessary resources to assist the operations section with achieving the objectives. Additionally, logistics will coordinate support resources for incident facilities such as bases and camps, including technology support, food, and medical care for responders. If required, a logistics section chief will be designated to coordinate the logistics section.

General Staff Finance and Administration

The finance section manages the overall financial aspects of the incident. The designated finance section chief, if applicable, coordinates all procurements, compensation claims, and resource costs.

In order to effectively manage a response the aforementioned groups must work collectively through a standardized planning process. This process is the "template for strategic, operational and tactical planning that includes all steps an Incident Commander (IC) and other members of the Command and General Staffs should take to develop and disseminate an Incident Action Plan."[10] It is important to note that once the initial response has occurred, the incident management team begins preparing for the next operational period. Therefore it is the responsibility of the operations section supervisors and leaders to continue the assigned tactical objectives while the incident management team plans for the next operational period.

A properly operating planning process should provide the following[10]:

- Current information that accurately describes the incident situation and resource status
- Predictions of the probable course of events
- Alternative strategies to attain critical incident objectives
- A realistic IAP for the next operational period

This process is often referred to as the planning "P" (Fig. 38-2). This planning cycle consists of nine meetings with specific items to be addressed and prepared for. At the end of the planning cycle the IAP is approved and then executed, beginning a new operational

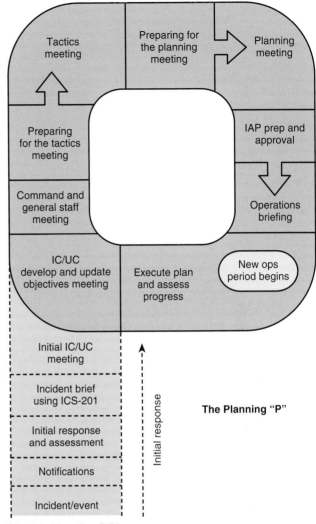

FIG 38-2 Planning P Diagram.

period. This planning cycle continues throughout the duration of an incident, even throughout the recovery phase.

The ICS system and the 14 management characteristics are not something that can be executed without proper training. It is therefore important that individuals with the responsibility to be a part of the ICS system, from the command to the operational level, have an understanding of the system and its process. The NIMS ICS training consists of two levels of training: baseline and advanced. Baseline training includes ICS-700 NIMS, An Introduction and ICS-100 Introduction to Incident Command System. ICS-100 also consists of organization-specific training for law enforcement, public works, and health care and hospitals. These organization-specific courses take the fundamentals of ICS and apply them to the dynamics of each organization. Advanced training is typically conducted in a classroom setting. It provides enhanced hands-on training of the command and general staff positions. In order to achieve a level of understanding of ICS, FEMA offers free training through the FEMA Independent Study Program (http://training.fema.gov/IS/NIMS.aspx). This program provides basic ICS training along with position-specific and awareness training in many different facets of emergency preparedness, response, recovery, and mitigation. This standardized training ensures that individuals are trained at the same level with an understanding of the same core principles.

⚠ PITFALLS

The ICS system is a strong foundation that will assist agencies, jurisdictions, and/or municipalities in properly managing an incident. However, there are areas in which the system will fail if the incident management team and responders undermine the management process. Any pitfalls of the system should be seen as an area for improvement and addressed prior to the next incident. The following are some examples of situations that occur across the board that should be noted as to avoid repeating.

- For many departments and organizations the application of ICS is not used on a regular or day-to-day basis. It therefore does not become second nature to assimilate into the roles and responsibilities as they are established by the system. Additionally, it is often difficult for individuals to relinquish their authority to act in a subordinate position within the structure. For example, during a full-scale exercise a participant assigned as the liaison officer was not familiar with the roles and responsibilities for that position. This in turn caused a failure in communication between the requesting agency and the IC. The participant's knowledge of day-to-day operations was exceptional; however, that knowledge did not transfer over into the liaison position because of a lack of proper ICS training. One solution to overcoming such obstacles is to dedicate individuals to specific positions within the ICS system and have them trained and exercised in those specific positions. This, however, will require there be many layers of trained individuals for a single role, accounting for different shifts and vacations.

- ICS is set up with a clear chain of command. Not following the proper reporting procedures established by the system can and will lead to a breakdown in communication, conflicting orders, reporting errors, and loss of personnel and/or resources. During a recent international response, an objective, set forth by the incident management team, was to provide medical care to each of the 100-plus community centers within the impacted area. However, the medical response teams in the field did not properly report back to the incident management team on which locations or what type of treatment they had provided during their operational period. As an initial result, some locations received multiple visits by different teams and other locations were not visited for several days, which caused a delay in care and duplication of effort.

- If an incident is not properly managed, well-meaning responders may have the tendency to self-dispatch. Additionally, individuals may arrive at your incident scene without being requested. Both of these situations can lead to undermining the overall objectives of the response and cause a delay in tactics. Self-dispatching also leads to a lack of accountability, as well as compromising the safety of responders and patients. On-scene personnel should follow the objectives and tactics set forth by the incident management team, and individuals should never self-dispatch to an incident scene.

- As incidents extend into multiple operational periods the documentation and tracking of resources becomes demanding and extensive. It is important that all documentation be retained, such as the IAP and resource request forms, to maintain accountability. If the ICS system is properly followed, this information will be collected by individuals in the planning and finance and administration sections. This documentation will also provide support for potential reimbursement from a disaster declaration. It is important to note that responders or equipment that is not properly documented will not be eligible for reimbursement. Therefore the local government or agency would be responsible for the costs and any damage incurred during the operation.

- ICS is taught in a utopic setting where all the functions work seamlessly and there are minimal hindrances. Because it is so difficult to train on the unknown, ICS training focuses on the responsibilities of the management of the event. In reality, lines of communication may be lost, you may have no power, or the resources you were depending on may be unavailable. During a large-scale event at a major sporting venue the planning called for a large number of public safety resources. However, because of the time and day of the event the resources were not available. Therefore the planning team was forced to modify their objectives in order to meet the available resources. It is important to train to properly manage the situation that you are presented with and work through the limitations.

ICS provides an all-hazards response management system for both small-scale incidents and large incidents that involve multiple organizations and jurisdictions. ICS allows the entities involved with a response to manage the political, economic, social, environmental, and cost implications related to the incident. With a management system in place, individuals using ICS can focus on the development of strategies to address life safety, incident stabilization, accountability, and property preservation.

Statistically, many incidents will not require the structure to expand to activation of the general staff positions. It is therefore important to train and exercise the planning cycle, in order to become familiar with the system.

REFERENCES

1. *"Part 1: What is ICS?"* ICS-402 Incident Command System (ICS) Overview for Executives/Senior Officials. Washington, DC: Department; 2013, 18. Print.
2. "Incident Command System | FEMA.gov." Incident Command System | FEMA.gov. N.p., n.d. Web. 11 Mar. 2014. http://www.fema.gov/incident-command-system.
3. "National Incident Management System Implementation & Compliance Guidance for Stakeholders | FEMA.gov." National Incident Management System Implementation & Compliance Guidance for Stakeholders | FEMA.gov. N.p., n.d. Web. 11 Mar. 2014. http://www.fema.gov/implementation-and-compliance-guidance-stakeholders.
4. "NIMS Implementation Activities For Hospitals And Healthcare Systems." FEMA, 12 Sept. 2006. Web. 11 Mar. 2014. http://www.fema.gov/pdf/emergency/nims/imp_hos_fs.pdf.
5. *Exemplary Practices in Emergency Management: The California FIRESCOPE Program.* Emmitsburg, MD: Emergency Management Institute; 1987, Print.
6. "NIMS and the Incident Command System." N.p., n.d. Web. 11 Mar. 2014. http://www.fema.gov/txt/nims/nims_ics_position_paper.txt.
7. *"Unit 2: ICS Fundamentals Review."* ICS-300 - Intermediate ICS for Expanding Incidents. Washington, DC: Department; 2012, 2.3-2.4. Print.
8. "Incident Command System." *National Incident Management System Incident Command System Emergency Responder Field Operations Guide.* Washington, DC: Department; 2010, 2-2. Print.
9. *"Command Staff."* National Incident Management System Incident Command System Emergency Responder Field Operations Guide. Washington, DC: Department; 2010, 5-2. Print.
10. *"Operational Planning Cycle."* National Incident Management System Incident Command System Emergency Responder Field Operations Guide. Washington, DC: Department; 2010, 4-2. Print.

CHAPTER 39

Scene Safety and Situational Awareness in Disaster Response

Robert L. Freitas

Emergency medical service(s) (EMS) personnel receive training in scene operations and safety during the didactic portion of their training. The training covers the events and concerns in normal EMS response, such as motor vehicle accidents, acts of violence, and electrical hazards, to name a few. Despite this training, prehospital personnel are still injured or killed in the line of duty every year. A study in the *Annals of Emergency Medicine*[1] places the fatality rate of EMS workers at 12.7 fatalities per 100,000 workers, compared with 5.0 fatalities per 100,000 workers for the general population. Because of poor data collection, less is known about EMS injury rates compared with those of other public safety personnel, although a study by the Rand Corporation that examined injury rates for all public safety personnel does address the subject.[2] Ten emergency medical technicians (EMTs) and paramedics were killed at the September 11, 2001, World Trade Center (WTC) disaster, and at least 116 were injured.[3]

Responding to a disaster presents a unique set of circumstances usually not found in normal daily work situations. Depending on the type of disaster, this could include secondary collapse of structures, operating in unfamiliar surroundings, exposure to smoke and dust, fatigue and dehydration, lack of or disregard for safety equipment, and a host of other hazards. Disasters that result from acts of terrorism present unique challenges in that terrorists may actually want to injure first responders and medical personnel. Both volunteer in-hospital personnel who respond to a disaster because of its proximity to a work site and EMS personnel called to respond to a disaster must be cognizant of the hazards and risks associated with such a response and be prepared to take measures to mitigate those risks. Responders who get injured or incapacitated add to the burden of other public safety personnel who must treat them as well as those injured in the original incident. Medical responders who become injured reduce available resources to the original victims.

HISTORICAL PERSPECTIVE

Health care personnel, both prehospital and hospital-based, have routinely responded to disasters with little regard for their own safety. One only has to look at the media coverage surrounding the 2013 Boston Marathon Bombings to understand the risks the hospital personnel faced, thinking they were going to be treating running-related injuries instead of the blast injuries associated with two lethal shrapnel bombs detonated near their aid stations at the finish line of the race.[4] If the second bomb had detonated 10 minutes later, when the area was covered with health care personnel treating victims from the first bomb, there is little doubt there would have been casualties from among their ranks. The body of literature on disaster medicine and management both in the United States and internationally is considerable, but little of this literature deals with the safety of emergency medical responders.

Formal prehospital care has been evolving for four decades, with better training programs, teaching methods, and protocols; however, safety training and equipment for in-hospital medical responders have lagged behind. The formal Incident Command System (ICS), even though in use since the 1970s for some fire services, has only recently become a true component of health care operations. EMS agencies have been slowly adopting the ICS during the last 10 years, and the hospital community conducts formal training, as mandated by The Joint Commission and reinforced by the National Incident Management System codifying a hospital's role in disaster operations.[5,6] Within the ICS and reporting directly to the incident commander is the incident safety officer (ISO), who has final authority over all operations in regard to responder safety. However, historically this organizational structure has not always been effective, especially when it comes to disasters. In large disasters, a single safety officer often does not have enough resources to control the large number of responders, including volunteers, who arrive wholly unprepared for the tasks ahead. In the WTC terrorist attack on 9/11, it was observed that "physicians dressed only in scrubs, clogs, and surgical masks attempted to negotiate the jagged metal debris to carry out their well-meaning medical interventions."[7] In some situations, firefighters gave up their own personal protective equipment (PPE) to protect the volunteers.[8]

Many hospitals have had "crash boxes" of essential medical and surgical equipment for out-of-hospital response for years, but rarely has the equipment included safety gear other than a vest and hard hat. Clinical personnel from hospitals have routinely responded to disasters—and still do as witnessed during the Boston Marathon attacks—with little or no safety training and even less PPE appropriate for the type of incident. In the 1995 bombing of the Murrah Federal Building in Oklahoma City, a volunteer nurse dressed only in jeans and a sweatshirt suffered a fatal head injury from falling debris.[6] With the vast volume of literature that has come out after the 9/11 attacks, a true understanding of the problem of keeping responders safe has now come to light.

CURRENT PRACTICE

The current practice of scene safety for disaster response is still evolving, largely in response to review of the 9/11 disaster. The Rand Corporation, in concert with the National Institute for Occupational Safety and Health (NIOSH), has published several reports that attempt to broaden the knowledge base of this problem. Rand and NIOSH undertook more research into the problem, publishing *Emergency Responder Injuries and Fatalities*,[2] which highlights the types and causes of injuries to public safety personnel while also citing the lack of adequate methods for tracking EMS personnel in injury data. They offer suggestions on how to capture better data on EMS injuries and fatalities. Three other volumes look at the problems faced with protecting public safety

BOX 39-1   Risks and Hazards Associated with Disaster Response

- Large geographic scale
- Unfamiliar environments and surroundings
- Falling debris
- Secondary collapse of damaged buildings
- Exposure to hazardous materials
- Excessive noise from machinery and equipment
- Adverse weather
- Inadequate PPE
- Debris fields, causing fall or trip hazards
- Convergent volunteers
- Secondary explosive devices planted by terrorists
- Secondary events following natural disasters (tsunami or firestorm following earthquake; levee break following hurricane)
- Prolonged duration, causing excessive fatigue, lack of sleep, and inadequate food and hydration

personnel when they respond to disasters and offer solutions to better protect those personnel.[9-11]

Still, more effort needs to be expended in understanding how disaster response is different from situations normally encountered by both EMS and hospital personnel. Auf der Heide[12] argues that the difference between the normal mission of emergency response and disaster response is not just one of magnitude managed by bringing into play larger numbers of people and equipment, but rather the interplay of a variety of factors. In normal response situations, responders might be exposed to a minimal number of hazards or risks, usually for a very short period. In contrast, in disaster operations, responders may be exposed to multiple hazards and risks for prolonged periods and often without adequate rest (Box 39-1).

Large Geographic Scale and Unfamiliar Surroundings

In most emergency medical responses, activities are confined to a small area. Responders can readily identify hazards, see who else is responding, quickly estimate the extent of the emergency, and get a sense of how many victims there are. In disasters, especially natural disasters, the geographic scale of the disaster may be overwhelming. The destruction from Hurricane Andrew in Florida and Louisiana in 1992 covered more than 1000 square miles.[11] In late 2004, a tsunami in southeast Asia spanned a vast area over three continents. The disaster area from Hurricane Katrina in the southeastern United States in 2005 covered an area of 90,000 square miles over three states. Because of the possible large geographic scale and the loss of familiar surroundings that can occur during a disaster response, it may be difficult to request assistance if responders are not certain of their surroundings. They may be unable to see hazards that could affect them but are not in their immediate field of vision. The large geographic scale may also mean that responders are on-scene for many hours, days, or even weeks as they work to ameliorate the effects.

It is reported that after the 9/11 terrorist attacks in the United States at least "six federal and municipal fire and EMS departments, three private ambulance services and a number of volunteer fire departments and ambulance squads responded to the Pentagon" and that an ambulance as far away as Texas responded to the WTC disaster.[3,8] Even though these efforts can be commended, responders unfamiliar with the local surroundings can present safety problems. Finding the way to a staging area or to the scene of a disaster will take more effort for personnel responding from long distances than it will for local units. Responders unfamiliar with the area can inadvertently end up in

locations that might contain hazardous materials, as happened during the Hurricane Andrew response.[11] Even local responders can have difficulty navigating unfamiliar surroundings if local landmarks and signs have been destroyed and traffic signals are not functioning because of power outages, which also occurred during the Hurricane Andrew response.[9] Complicate this with the fact that during the initial stages of a disaster, the public may be evacuating the area, causing highway congestion that can contribute to motor vehicle accidents.[11] Responders unfamiliar with the area may not be aware of alternative routes to arrive at their assigned destination if roads are blocked or cannot be navigated because of damage or debris. Hospital personnel who respond to disaster sites are generally not familiar with operating in situations with little light, limited resources, and multiple hazards. Escape routes and safe areas may be difficult to find for those not accustomed to operating in a particular area. Electrical hazards, a problem even when responders are familiar with the area, become more of a problem in unfamiliar surroundings when responders who are trying to orient themselves might not be as vigilant as they normally would be and could walk or drive into hazards, such as live electrical wires. It is essential for responders to ensure that they know where they are going, how to find alternative routes if original routes are blocked, and how to contact coordinating agencies if they become lost. Global positioning systems offer hope in allowing response units to navigate unfamiliar territory. It may be difficult to obtain maps in the early phases of a disaster, but having a map of the area is advisable, even if it is hand-drawn.

Falling or Flying Debris

Debris from buildings damaged during the initial disaster impact or debris that is dislodged by rescue operations can be a problem. Medical personnel on-scene who are focused on treating patients may not be aware of hazards overhead, and noise from equipment operating at the site can mask the sound of the debris as it falls. Appropriate head and eye protection is critical for all personnel at the scene. The typical eye protection provided to health care workers for body fluid splashes offers little protection in a dusty or smoky environment, as was found during the 9/11 response actions; more than 1000 eye injuries were reported during the first 10 weeks of response operations.[9]

Secondary Collapse of Damaged Buildings

Buildings that survive the initial shock in earthquakes can collapse because of aftershocks or from rescue efforts. WTC Building 7 did not collapse until after 5 PM on 9/11, almost 8 hours after the first plane struck one of the towers.[8] Responders who plan to set up triage or treatment stations in buildings should first ensure that the buildings have been deemed safe by building engineers or ISOs and are at a safe enough distance from other damaged buildings in the event of collapse. Escape routes and safe zones should be determined when operating in the vicinity of damaged buildings.

Exposure to Hazardous Materials

There is always a risk of unintentional hazardous materials exposure at every disaster site. Intentional hazardous substance exposure through terrorism is covered in other chapters of this text, but hazardous materials are ubiquitous and can be found in hospitals, laboratories, railways, universities, and transportation centers, to name a few. During earthquakes, underground pipelines or aboveground storage tanks may be damaged, leaking hazardous, often flammable materials into the environment.[13] Buildings damaged during explosions or earthquakes may have leaking fuel tanks, or chemicals used in manufacturing processes may leak or mix together to form new, more toxic compounds.

Exposure to smoke, dust, and other airborne contaminants represents a major problem in disasters where there are large fires or when buildings collapse. NIOSH continues to study the effects of smoke and dust on rescue workers from the 9/11 attacks. Shortly after the attack, NIOSH found that 60% of a subset (1138) of study participants who were evaluated on July 16 and December 31, 2002, suffered from new-onset lower respiratory symptoms, while 74% reported new-onset upper respiratory symptoms.[14] New York City reported that twice as many EMS workers who were at the scene of the 9/11 attacks have below-normal pulmonary function tests for their ages 6 to 7 years after the exposure, even among those who never smoked. Among smokers, the decline in pulmonary function is even more pronounced.[15] Proper PPE must be available and its use mandated on-scene by the ISO, and all disaster responders should have at least hazardous materials awareness training before venturing into disaster scenes. When in doubt about a situation, wait for special operations teams who have testing devices that can determine whether the scene is safe for operations.

Excessive Noise from Machinery and Equipment

Depending on the nature of the disaster, heavy equipment may be needed to facilitate the response. This equipment may create excessive noise either through the exhaust or from moving debris. This noise makes communication with other medical team members difficult and may make it difficult to hear warning signals indicating aftershocks, secondary explosions, etc. Although wearing hearing protection is advisable, it creates similar limitations. Hearing protection is also usually designed for blocking high-frequency noises and not the low-frequency noises associated with heavy equipment.[9] In addition, it is difficult to hear radios and other communications devices while wearing the protectors.

Adverse Weather

Because health care workers generally dress for their immediate shift, they may be unprepared to deal with the prolonged nature of disasters. EMS workers accustomed to short-sleeve uniform shirts for daytime wear in the summer might find themselves getting chilled by evening, and hospital personnel who respond in hospital garb might be unprepared for sudden rainstorms. Responders to the Oklahoma City bombing had to deal with temperatures that fluctuated from 80 to 40 °F, strong winds, rain, and lightning.[15] Health care workers both in and out of the hospital who might be called on to respond to disasters should have clothing appropriate for a wide range of weather conditions, including cold-weather gear and raingear.

Inadequate Personal Protective Equipment

EMS and hospital workers are commonly not well prepared and inadequately trained for disaster response when it comes to using PPE. Administrators' budgets are often thought to be too lean to spend money on something that happens infrequently and requires a large outlay of funds and training time.[10] It is also suggested that because there is no central federal authority responsible for monitoring PPE for medical response personnel, unlike firefighters and the National Fire Protection Agency (NFPA), funding from government sources for PPE is lower.[10] Even NFPA's *Standard on Protective Clothing for Emergency Medical Operations*[16] only deals with exposures from body fluids and not the types of hazards likely to be encountered in disaster operations. Experiences from recent disasters indicate that even with good PPE, the multihazard nature of disasters makes it difficult to have the right equipment all of the time.[9] In a disaster environment, PPE must not only protect the wearer from blood-borne pathogens but also offer protection from other disaster-specific hazards. In addition, because of the extended nature of disaster response, agencies must

be able to replenish PPE as it wears out, becomes wet, or breaks down from exposure to chemicals. The duration of effectiveness of filtration canisters on respirators is related to the particulate load, and thus canister replacements may be necessary more frequently than posted during heavy use periods.

The multiagency response aspect of disasters can also make the sharing of equipment difficult. With multiple standards for PPE across public safety entities, the chance of cross-agency compatibility of PPE is small. PPE that might be adequate for firefighting is generally not acceptable for the treatment phase of patient care, although it might be appropriate for the patient access phase. Having access to bunker gear is not the answer either, as experiences have indicated that too often bunker gear is too heavy and cumbersome for the prolonged response required to deal with disasters.

Eyewear designed to prevent exposure to body fluids is not adequate when removing patients from rubble piles in high-dust environments. Face shields or glasses designed to offer splash protection may not be appropriate in situations in which dust or smoke can penetrate the sides of the glasses or shields. Safety goggles of the kind used in construction may be more appropriate, although they may be uncomfortable for prolonged periods, may fog, and can hinder peripheral vision.[9] Resources should be available for rinsing off glasses because dust and dirt particles can lead to scratched lenses, hindering visibility. Many medical responders are not issued hand protection that complies with Occupational Safety and Health Administration (OSHA) standards for protection from "absorption of harmful substances; severe cuts or lacerations; severe abrasions; punctures, chemical burns; and harmful temperature extremes."[17] Gloves designed to protect against bloodborne pathogens, even though appropriate for general patient care, should be worn underneath a more durable glove when operating in the multihazard environment often encountered in disaster situations; leather is not advised because it absorbs water and cannot be decontaminated. A glove that resists wear, cuts, and punctures but is pliable enough to provide treatment is necessary.

Relying on other agencies or resources to provide adequate equipment is not advised. The different agencies responding to disasters use a variety of brands and models of equipment, making compatibility with respirators, face masks, and cartridge filters not guaranteed. Responders should not use equipment offered by others without at least some training in its use (Box 39-2).

Debris Fields Causing Fall or Trip Hazards

Most disasters, with the exception of chemical and biological exposures, will cause debris, often over large areas. Hurricanes may leave huge

---

BOX 39-2 Level D PPE for Disaster Response under Hazardous Conditions

- Long-sleeve shirts
- Protective head gear to protect against falling debris or walking into objects
- Waterproof boots when there is the potential of rolling or falling objects or objects piercing the sole (steel toe boots may cause blistering after prolonged wear)
- Gloves that protect responders' hands from absorption of harmful substances, cuts, lacerations and punctures, and burns
- Eyewear with detachable side protection when there is exposure to dust or other harmful particles
- Battery-operated or rechargeable hand light if the charging unit is with the responder
- Foul weather gear
- Cold weather gear

debris fields. Hurricane Andrew destroyed or damaged more than 157,000 homes and caused an estimated $26 billion in damage, leaving behind a huge swath of destruction.[18] This caused a huge debris field that had to be carefully negotiated by rescue workers. In the aftermath of the Murrah Federal Building bombing, debris was piled 35 feet deep.[11] Debris may consist of wiring, pipes, pieces of concrete, and other building materials; is sharp; and may wear down protective clothing. The southeast Asia tsunami left debris fields kilometers deep along the coastline of the vast area it affected. Debris may need to be cleared to gain access to patients or set up treatment areas. Wind may cause debris to be blown about long after the initial disaster. Being on the lookout for responding apparatus or overhead hazards may cause responders to not look where they are going, resulting in injuries from trips and falls. It is imperative for responders to have a good light at all times, even if the initial response is during the day. Trying to navigate through debris after dark is a perilous operation, even with a light. Furthermore, it may be necessary to enter buildings that have lost power during the day. The penlights used in hospitals are not adequate for this purpose. Lights with disposable batteries or those that can be recharged if the responder has the charging device on hand are recommended. Units without rechargers will only be useful as long as they can be charged. The prolonged nature of disasters may preclude the responder from having the ability to retrieve the charging device.

Convergent Volunteers

Part of the health care ethos is the spirit of volunteerism. This is especially true in disasters. Responders want to help those in need, whether this is done in an organized fashion through disaster medical assistance teams (DMATs) or Salvation Army or Red Cross volunteers, or through individuals who respond to the scene, often without any training or equipment. Even those who are well trained, but are unfamiliar with local conditions and do not have equipment they are familiar with run the risk of injury. One of the fatalities from the West, Texas, explosion of 2013 was an off-duty Dallas firefighter who happened to be in West and went to the scene to help.[19]

Responding agencies may have different protocols, equipment, and staffing configurations. Most of the official volunteer agencies at a disaster scene will be there following a request for a response. Even though they may present logistical challenges, most usually do not present safety challenges. Failure to communicate between those on official response to the scene and freelancers causes a breakdown in the ICS and may cause resources to be used in a haphazard manner, potentially endangering responders. Such spontaneous volunteers generally will not have radio communications with command centers or other responders, causing inadequate resource utilization. The response to an airliner crash in 1988 at the Dallas-Fort Worth airport demonstrated this point. Freelancing response units unfamiliar with the airport disaster plan set up a triage site outside the airport, causing responders to continue to look for patients and victims at the crash site who had already been evacuated.[8] Accountability for the safety of all on scene also suffers when ISOs are unaware of all personnel operating on the scene. Accounting for all responders on-scene is also important in the event of post-incident monitoring for hazardous exposures, as in the 9/11 disaster. There is evidence to suggest that most of the convergent volunteer organizations that respond as freelancers come without proper equipment, either pulling equipment out of the hospital that might be needed there or using equipment from other responders on-scene, neither of which is an optimal situation.[10]

Volunteers cannot always be counted on to complete tasks, especially if they have not received proper training on how to do the task and are unfamiliar with the terminology used by other responders.[12] Directions to volunteers should always be clear and easy to understand. In addition, the person issuing the directions should be certain the volunteer understands the task. For in-hospital personnel interested in responding to disasters outside the hospital, joining a professional group within a disaster section or other volunteer disaster medical organizations, such as the National Disaster Medical Service, is beneficial.[20] These organizations provide training and decrease the chance that volunteer responders will be unprepared and create liability for others. Because volunteers at disasters are a fact of life, coordinating agencies should develop clear strategies for dealing with them and for integrating them into the response, delegating an individual in advance to have responsibility for managing the volunteers.[12]

Secondary Explosive Devices Planted by Terrorists

Every disaster or incident resulting from terrorism has the risk of secondary devices that can cause injury to medical personnel already on-scene. Two Atlanta area bombings in 1997, although not classified as disasters, are noteworthy for having secondary explosive devices: one at a family planning center where the secondary device exploded 1 hour after the first device exploded, injuring four public safety personnel through shrapnel and blast effects, and another at a lounge where the secondary device failed to explode (if it had, it would have injured responders in the vicinity).[21] In the 9/11 attacks, the second plane struck the south tower approximately 15 minutes after the north tower had been struck by the first plane; many responders were already on-scene by the time the second plane struck.[9] Responders must always exercise caution and search for secondary devices in terrorism attacks, being on the lookout for strange packages, vehicles, or people in the disaster area who clearly have no readily identifiable purpose there. A plan for retreat or an understanding of where safe zones are is essential during operations. Rapid clearing of the injured is a tactic used at terrorist bombing sites in Israel.

Fatigue, Lack of Sleep, and Inadequate Food and Hydration

Because of the long-term nature of disaster response, it is easy to get fatigued, not get adequate sleep, and not take the time to eat or drink appropriate amounts of fluids. The Rand research indicates that responders have a tendency to do what their leaders do, and if the leaders do not take adequate time for rest and rehabilitation, neither will their subordinates.[11] Disasters commonly require calling in off-duty personnel to take over operations when initial responders become fatigued.[12] Research on shift work has demonstrated that anyone awake for more than 18 consecutive hours may show physical impairment similar to someone with a blood alcohol level of 0.05%, and those awake for more than 24 hours may demonstrate performance similar to someone with a blood alcohol level of 0.096%. Based on this research, it is recommended that all responders, including senior personnel, work no more than one 12-hour shift daily.[20] This may need to be adjusted down, depending on the working conditions. Having adequate food and drink nearby consistent with personal dietary habits is also important.

SCENE SAFETY AT THE DISASTER SITE

According to Garrison, "Avoiding danger is counterintuitive to rescuers."[22] Eliminating all hazards and risks associated with disaster medical response is impossible, and most EMS personnel know the job is dangerous at times. As can be seen in Box 39-1, disasters are complex situations, and each one is different. Therefore the challenge in disaster response is to manage the risks by having an appropriate mechanism for understanding the dynamic nature of disaster operations. Managing risks is best done by using the safety management cycle (Figure 39-1). This involves three functions that must be performed continuously throughout the incident: (1) gather information about

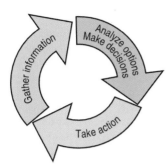

FIG 39-1 Safety Management Cycle. (Redrawn from Jackson B, Baker J, Ridgely M, et al. *Protecting Emergency Responders, Vol 3: Safety Management in Disaster and Terrorism Response.* Santa Monica, CA: The Rand Corporation, Science and Technology Policy Institute [for the National Institute for Occupational Safety and Health]; 2004.)

the current situation, (2) analyze the available options and come up with decisions, and (3) implement decisions.[11] Gathering information at disaster sites is a challenge. The sharing of information across agencies is key to protecting those on-scene. The number of organizations responding to disasters, especially disasters caused by terrorism, is enormous, with one report citing 159 public-sector agencies responding to the 9/11 disaster and another 290 organizations involved in the response.[23] Many of the different agencies involved in a typical response focus solely on their own organizational tasks and do not see how their activities fit into the big pictures. Auf der Heide[12] describes this as the "Robinson Crusoe syndrome," causing responders to believe "we're the only ones on the island." Many of these agencies may possess needed information on the hazards already encountered and hazards already mitigated, may have special expertise in disaster activities or risk assessment, and may possess information on the locations of victims or resources needed by other groups, etc. Use of the ICS, covered in Chapter 38, is essential. It is this author's belief that in disaster activities, there is no single activity that can have a greater impact on scene safety than a properly functioning ICS in which all agencies share information. Of equal importance, the incident commander must share all the appropriate information with those on-scene.

Because of the large geographic scale of many disasters, the ISO may not have an accurate picture of all the hazards present, especially if communication between all of the responding agencies is limited, a common problem in most disaster situations. Medical organizations that routinely respond to disasters are encouraged to have their own safety officers or have one of their members appointed as an assistant ISO and to set up communications channels to the ISO. According to the NFPA's *Standard for Fire Department Safety Officer,*[24] the role of the safety officer is to determine when activities are unsafe or involve significant hazards and then exercise the authority to immediately "alter, suspend, or terminate those activities." When the ISO determines that hazards or activities do not represent an immediate danger, the ISO "takes appropriate action through the incident commander to mitigate or eliminate the hazards."

Although a rare situation, the escape of wild animals from zoos and private collections may occur following an earthquake or from the intentional release of animals from captivity.[25] Specific teams designed to respond to such incidents may not be readily available, and the ISO should be involved in informing area responders of the risks and tactics to use to stay safe. Following large-scale disasters, or on humanitarian missions overseas, it is important to have an assessment made of potential animal risks, including knowledge of local venomous snake and arachnid populations. Snakes often seek shelter from floods and may be a hazard that responders should be made aware of. A hazard vulnerability analysis of risks in disaster areas should be part of the preparedness and planning process which involves the safety officer.

Once the information has been gathered, the next step is to look at the options available and make a decision, taking into account as many variables as are known. For example, in the initial response of medical personnel to the scene of a disaster, patients requiring rescue may be present. Many victims may also present for treatment who are either self-rescued or rescued by other victims. Taking the time to analyze the options may make responders realize that there are trained search and rescue personnel nearby and the available resources may be better used in setting up a treatment site first and leaving the rescue to personnel appropriately trained and equipped for the task. Once the decision is made, the next task is to follow through on the decision by taking action. The decision for any action related to safety must be communicated to all those within the immediate span of control and also up the chain of command to the incident commander. It is of great importance to know who is on-scene and how to communicate to them. As happens in many disasters, off-duty personnel will respond from home and therefore may not have adequate communications equipment (e.g., portable radios, pagers). Knowing where they are at a given moment may be a difficult task. If electronic communications are not possible, the use of runners may be an option and is often a good use of volunteers if communications relayed by them are clear and concise.

Crew Resource Management for Safety

If a decision is made regarding safety, there must be an understanding in advance that good safety practices are not optional and that the action to be taken is mandatory for all within the scope of the organization. The ISO might ultimately make a safety decision, but reasonable input and discussion should take place with those involved on-scene. Crew resource management (CRM) for safety practices has been in existence for approximately 25 years. Originally called cockpit resource management, it came out of an examination by NASA of air crashes and the role that human error played in them. It has since been adopted for use in medicine, both in the training of emergency department, labor and delivery, and operating room staffs and air-medical operations.[26] The primary tenets of the training are to discuss how errors are caused and how operating in high-stress environments with heavy workloads, fatigue, and dealing with emergency situations all contribute to errors. The principles of the training include seeking information by asking questions, advocating positions, communicating actions, and discussing and resolving conflicts. CRM is not something taught en route to or on-scene at a disaster; it is put into place during the preplanning and preparations phases of the disaster and may present a challenge to the medical community if not discussed in advance. For example, the medical director of an EMS agency must understand that a decision regarding safety applies to him or her as well, even if the decision is made by a safety officer who is a basic EMT.

Obviously, safety concerns or mandates must be reasonable for the current conditions; mandating the wearing of safety helmets in a treatment center where there is little risk of falling debris would not make much sense. The same mandate in an active incident area, where there is a chance of falling debris, would clearly be within the bounds of the safety officer's mandate. CRM also teaches that the same medical director should feel comfortable telling the ISO that he or she has noticed a crack in the building foundation and inquiring without risk of being ostracized whether it is safe for the treatment team to be there. As has been stressed here, disaster operations are not a static event; the hazards present 8 hours ago may have been dealt with or were determined to be unfounded, but those responsible for safety must constantly reassess the situation and gather new information, analyze the current options, and make new decisions, all of which may result in taking new actions. This safety management cycle must be repeated throughout the event until the incident is considered closed. Good pre-planning and preparations before the actual response, with training that includes scene safety procedures, will reduce injuries.

Response to Disasters

Initial notification of a disaster may come in many ways—some informal, others formal. Hospitals may become aware of a disaster when the first patients arrive at the emergency department door. Public safety agencies may find out through a flood of phone calls to the public safety answering point (PSAP) or if the disaster directly affects the building they are located in, for instance if the dispatch building trembles from an earthquake. For many, the initial notification may be through media outlets; others will be directed to the scene via official dispatches. Once the decision is made that a response to the disaster is indicated, based on an official request of some sort for assistance, the first thoughts of the medical responder should be personal safety, and this should generate some questions:

- "What PPE will I likely need, and if I don't have it, where will I get it?" Expecting others to provide adequate PPE once you arrive on-scene, unless this has been prearranged, is a dangerous thought. The PPE that awaits you may be equipment you are unfamiliar with or the wrong size. At a minimum, responders should be equipped with appropriate level D gear, including a safety helmet, adequate footwear, easily visible identification (e.g., reflective vests with skill level clearly stated on it), safety gloves, eye protection, a hand light, and equipment for bodily substance isolation precautions.
- "What hazards are likely to be present at the location?" If responding to an industrial site, the presence of hazardous materials must always be suspected, and different PPE or a different approach to the scene might be needed. If responding to an explosion, the concern over terrorism or secondary explosions must always be considered. Responses near water might require the use of personal flotation devices for responders. Practice an all-hazards approach with the expectation that there will be hazards on-scene and be prepared to mitigate them.
- "Where am I going, and how do I get there?" If the incident is very large, such as Hurricane Andrew was, responders may be called in from great distances. On occasion, specialized resources (e.g., a surgical team) may get an escort directly to the scene. Badly needed specialized resources do not want to spend hours lost looking for an appropriate rendezvous point or the active incident, and the people on-scene may not have the time to wait. Know where you are going; if you do not, request an escort. Have maps, but keep in mind that local landmarks may have been destroyed. Take the time to download directions from an online map service; it is better to take 5 minutes to get detailed directions than to spend time trying to find the final destination. The use of GPS devices can be helpful, especially if roads are destroyed or street signs are missing.
- "Who will I report to when I get there?" If the ICS has not been established yet, then it may be more important to understand that as the first arriving unit, you will be expected to size up the scene and report the situation to the communications center instead of providing treatment to the first patients encountered. If the ICS has been set up, it is important to know who you are reporting to and where to find them, and to let them know you have arrived. Updates on your situation are recommended every 30 minutes, unless other rules are in effect.

Scene Size-Up

Once the actual response is under way and regardless of whether response time is expected to be 30 minutes or 30 hours, try to get an update, if possible, of the current conditions on-scene. As responders approach the scene, they should begin determining the scope of the situation and continue to do so until preparing to depart the scene after disaster operations are completed. In the initial early minutes of the response, communications center personnel may be too busy receiving calls and dispatching units to be of much help, but even information being relayed to other units may be useful (e.g., traffic congestion or the presence of hazards). Responders must be vigilant for bystanders and victims fleeing the scene or curious onlookers running toward it. Once near the scene, responders must look and listen for other emergency responders, because some who are heading to the scene may be unaware of your presence or where they are going. Responders should look for signs of power outages, which could indicate downed power lines, and look for smoke or fumes.[27,28] If being transported to the scene by someone from another agency, the responder should not assume that the person operating the vehicle has more knowledge about scene safety than himself or herself; throughout disaster operations, one must take responsibility for one's own safety.

As the responder gets closer to the scene, the presence of odors may indicate chemicals, fire, or other hazardous materials. One must quickly make an assessment whether hazardous materials are evident and if they pose a direct hazard, either as a byproduct or the direct cause of the disaster, so that the responder does not end up as a victim.[28] The U.S. Department of Transportation's *2012 Emergency Response Guidebook*[29] is a good field resource for responders who believe there is a danger of hazardous materials present.

As mentioned, downed power lines are a common and deadly hazard. If the power is out and you observe damaged poles, count the number of wires at the damaged poles and then at the next undamaged pole down the line. If the number of lines atop the damaged pole is the same, there is a good chance the lines are intact.[29] On arrival at the actual disaster scene, even before the vehicle comes to a stop, a decision will need to be made about where to park the vehicle. Vehicles should park upwind and uphill if possible to avoid toxic fumes or smoke. Scanning for the direction that flags or smoke are blowing will help determine wind direction. Typically, emergency vehicles will try to get as close to the area as possible. Events at the 9/11 disaster indicate that this may not be the wisest approach. One witness reported seeing a row of 15 ambulances that "... were crushed, completely gutted by falling debris."[3] If a vehicle is not likely to be needed for emergency transport of patients and if it does not have needed supplies, PPE, or communications equipment, it should be relocated safely away from the scene. If it does have needed equipment, consider offloading the equipment and moving the vehicle to a safe location. Other vehicles may also be vying for the same space you are occupying and may be more urgently needed; an example would be an aerial ladder truck for rescue efforts. If there are burning vehicles, response units should park no closer than 100 feet from any of them to minimize explosion hazards or the risk of being exposed to leaking fuel.[28]

Lookouts, Communications, Escape Routes, and Safety Zones

Wildland firefighters and urban search and rescue technicians use an easy-to-remember system that can be adapted for disaster operations, known as LCES (lookouts, communications, escape routes, and safety zones).[13,30] Being a lookout is normally the function of the ISO, but because of the scope of a disaster, the ISO may not be in proximity to all operations or all responders may not have communications with the ISO. If hazards are present, it is important to have an individual who has good visual access to the operations and is not involved in patient care as a lookout, or site-specific safety officer. This person should be free to watch over the operation, identify hazards or potential hazards, and, if appropriate, mitigate them. He or she must be readily identified, either by his or her location or by wearing a vest identifying the person as a lookout or safety officer.

Communications should be established on arrival, not only with the incident commander but also with dispatch centers. On arrival, an exact location should be established for responding teams. This may be difficult if street signs have been destroyed, but it is imperative for all assets to have known locations. Using easily identifiable landmarks, such as buildings in the area, can be of assistance. For example, stating "we are on the south side of the lake" is not an exact location, but it can be useful. GPS devices can be of great assistance in establishing location.

Radios may not be functioning, may be overloaded with emergency traffic, or may not have common frequencies, and the use of runners may be necessary. The lookout or communications person should be alert for other forms of communications that may be used at disaster sites. Search and rescue technicians use an emergency alerting system that consists of an air horn or siren to be used in the event of emergencies:

- Three short blasts of one second each is an indication to evacuate
- One long, 3-second blast means to cease operations or work noiselessly
- One long blast and one short blast means to resume operations

Depending on the nature of the disaster, it may be important to determine escape routes in advance of need. During rescue operations at the Oklahoma City bombing, there were three bomb scares that caused evacuation of the treatment areas.[31] Personnel or vehicles may become trapped in a location by other responders and may need to relocate. On occasion, the shortest route to safety may not be the most direct, as in the case of a building collapse in which the shortest route to safety may direct one into the collapse zone. Clearly, in such an event a more circuitous route may be the safest.

The establishment of safe zones may be important in disasters where the risk of ongoing hazards is great. The safe zone is an area determined to be relatively safe from hazards. It might be an area removed from collapsed or damaged buildings, an area remote from hot or warm zones in hazardous materials incidents, or an area where additional measures have been taken to increase building structural integrity. If team members are evacuated to the safe zone, a head count should be the first task done to ensure that all members are accounted for.

⚠ PITFALLS

Much has been learned about responder safety since 9/11. The Rand/NIOSH collaboration has brought great resources to emergency managers for keeping all responders safer.[2,9–11] Measures are being put into place to keep better data about medical responder injuries at all incidents, but there are still pitfalls in all of this. Disaster medical services are provided by many organizations, often following different standards. The federal government should determine a standard of safety for emergency medical response, as has been done with firefighting through the NFPA. Research is essential; journal articles and educational materials help keep the subject in the spotlight. The Rand studies illustrate the problem with designing PPE that allows medical responders to do their jobs safely. Complacency is the major pitfall to all of this, and if it does not turn into action, medical responders will still face injury or death while responding to disasters. Standards, PPE, and training must be implemented while disasters such as 9/11 and the southeast Asia tsunami are still fresh in our minds.

REFERENCES

1. Maguire BJ, Hunting KL, Smith GS, Levick NR. Occupational fatalities in emergency medical services: a hidden crisis. *Ann Emerg Med.* 2002;40:625–632.
2. Houser AN, Jackson BA, Bartis JT, Peterson DJ. *Emergency Responder Injuries and Fatalities: An Analysis of Surveillance Data.* Santa Monica, CA: The Rand Corporation; 2004.
3. 9/11 attack on America: united we respond. *EMS Insider.* 2001;28:1–8.
4. Winter M, Moore DL, Davis S, Strauss G. At least 3 dead, 141 injured in Boston Marathon Blast. Available at: www.usatoday.com/story/news/nation/2103/04/15/explosions-finish-line-boston-marathon/2085193.
5. Joint Commission on Accreditation of Healthcare Organizations. *Guide to Emergency Management Planning in Health Care.* Oakbrook Terrace, IL: Joint Commission Resources; 2002.
6. Federal Emergency Management Agency. *National Incident Management System. NIMS Implementation Activities for Hospitals and Healthcare Systems Implementation FAQs.* Available at: www.fema.gov/pdf/emergency/nims/hospital-faq.pdf.
7. Martinez C, Gonzalez D. The World Trade Center attack. Doctors in the fire and police services. *Crit Care.* 2001;5(6):304–306.
8. Thompson S, Green WG, Lapetina J. Improving disaster response efforts with decision support systems. *Int J Emerg Manag.* 2006;3(4).
9. Jackson B, Peterson DJ, Bartis J, et al. *Protecting Emergency Responders: Lessons Learned from Terrorist Attacks.* Santa Monica, CA: The Rand Corporation; 2002.
10. Latourrette T, Peterson DJ, Bartis J, Jackson BA, Houser A. *Protecting Emergency Responders, Vol 2: Community Views of Safety and Health Risks and Personal Protection Needs.* Santa Monica, CA: The Rand Corporation; 2003.
11. Jackson B, Baker J, Ridgely M, Bartis JT, Linn HI. *Protecting Emergency Responders, Vol 3: Safety Management in Disaster and Terrorism Response.* Santa Monica, CA: The Rand Corporation; 2004.
12. Auf der Heide E. Disasters are different. In: Auf der Heide E, ed. *Disaster Response: Principles of Preparation and Coordination.* St Louis, MO: Mosby; 1989.
13. Federal Emergency Management Agency, US&R. Structural collapse technician course—student manual. Available at: http://www.fema.gov/usr/sctc.shtm.
14. Centers for Disease Control and Prevention (CDC). Physical health status of World Trade Center rescue and recovery workers and volunteers—New York City, July 2002–August 2004. *MMWR Morb Mortal Wkly Rep.* 2004;53 (35):807–812.
15. New York City Department of Health. *What We Know Now About the Health Effects of 9/11.* Available at: www.nyc.gov/html/doh/wtc/html/know/know.shtml.
16. National Fire Protection Association. *NFPA 1999: Standard on Protective Clothing for Emergency Medical Operations.* Quincy, MA: National Fire Protection Association; 2003.
17. US Department of Labor, Occupational Safety and Health Administration. *Inspection guidelines for 29 CFR 1910. Subpart 1, the revised Personal Protective Equipment Standards for General Industry.* Available at: http://www.osha.gov/pls/oshaweb/owadisp.show_document?p_table=DIRECTIVES&p_id=1790.
18. National Weather Service Forecast Office. Hurricane Andrew. Available at: www.srh.noaa.gov/mfl/n=andrew.
19. Goldstein S. Off-duty firefighter killed in West, Texas, fertilizer explosion committed to helping family says. *New York Daily News.* Available at: www.nydailynews.com/news/national/off-duty-firefighter-killed-west-fertilizer-explosion-remembered-article-1.1324593.
20. Falleti MG, Maruff P, Collie A, et al. Qualitative similarities in cognitive impairment associated with 24h of sustained wakefulness and a blood alcohol concentration of 0.05%. *J Sleep Res.* 2003;12(4):265–274.
21. *Eric Rudolph charged in Centennial Park bombing [press release].* Washington, DC: US Department of Justice; October 14, 1998.

22. Garrison H. Keeping rescuers safe. *Ann Emerg Med*. 2002;40(6):633–635.

23. Lyman F. *Messages in the Dust: What Are the Lessons of the Environmental Health Response to the Terrorist Attacks of September 11?* National Environmental Health Association: Washington, DC; 2003.

24. National Fire Protection Association. *NFPA 1521: Standard for Fire Department Safety Officer*. Quincy, MA: National Fire Protection Association; 2002.

25. Miller M. *Dangerous wild animal response team prepares state-mandated plan*. Emergency Management. McClatchy News, February 3, 2014. Available at: http://www.emergencymgmt.com/disaster/dangerous-wild-animal-response-team-ohio.html.

26. Agency for Healthcare Research and Quality. *Making Health Care Safer: A Critical Analysis of Patient Safety Practices. Evidence Report, Technology Assessment No. 43*. Available at: http://www.ahrq.gov/clinic/ptsafety.

27. Borak J, Callan M, Abbott W. *Hazardous Materials Exposure*. Englewood Cliffs, NJ: Brady; 1991, 8.

28. Limmer D, O'Keefe M. *Emergency Care*. 10th ed. Upper Saddle River, NJ: Brady; 2005, 180–184.

29. US Department of Transportation Research and Special Projects Administration. *2012 Emergency Response Guidebook*. Neenah, WI: JJ Keller; 2012.

30. Department of Agriculture, Fire and Aviation Management Division. *LCES: Lookouts-Communications-Escape Routes-Safety Zones*. Available at: http://www.fs.fed.us/fire/safety/lces/lces.html.

31. Smith C, ed. In: FEMA urban search and rescue (USAR) summaries. *Alfred P. Murrah Federal Building Bombing, April 19, 1995, Final Report*. Stillwater, OK: Fire Protection; 1996.

CHAPTER 40

Needs Assessment

Erica L. Nelson

In disasters the most effective efforts to minimize mortality are based on very specific, precisely targeted interventions against demonstrated causes of death.[1,2] Historically, however, humanitarian aid was dictated by charity, politics, and well-intentioned assumptions, and not until the introduction of epidemiology to disaster response and the advent of needs assessment did evidence-based humanitarian aid come to the fore. Ideally needs assessment is a rapid, multifocal, cross-sectoral evaluation of the sequelae of disasters that provides accurate data on morbidity, mortality, disease burden, and the impact on medical, transportation, communication, water, electricity, and other lifeline infrastructures. These data, presented in such a way to elucidate the magnitude and geographic densities of need, are meant to alert the relief community and bring about efficient and appropriate humanitarian responses.

By necessity, postdisaster needs assessment must be performed even as emergency services are being provided.[3] To address the conundrum of obtaining accurate data in extremely adverse and time-sensitive conditions, needs assessments must be coordinated across multiple levels, including local, state, federal, and international organizations; utilize various methodologies; and require horizontal processing and ongoing reevaluation. However, while the field has evolved significantly from its origins in epidemiology to a heterogeneous practice that incorporates not only the World Health Organization (WHO) Standardized Protocol but also innovative methods, such as geospatial information systems (GIS), operations research, and even crowd-sourcing, needs assessment continues to face multiple challenges in obtaining accurate, precise, timely, and compelling data. It is the goal of this chapter to introduce the history and rationale behind, components of, and challenges to postdisaster rapid needs assessment.

HISTORICAL PERSPECTIVE

Prior to the advent of needs assessment, charity, politics, and well-intentioned assumptions dictated relief efforts regardless of the needs of the disaster-affected community. Consequently, humanitarian aid initiatives were woefully ad hoc, inappropriate, and inefficient.[4]

The first practical application of epidemiology in postdisaster relief may have been on the cusp of the 1960s-1970s in response to the Nigerian Civil War (also known as the Biafran War), wherein the U.S. Centers for Disease Control and Prevention (CDC), in efforts with preventative epidemiologists, piloted new techniques for survey conduction and rapid assessment of nutritional states.[4,5] However, widespread implementation lagged behind. Directors of major relief organizations doubled as managers and planners, often lacking sufficient public health foundations to successfully respond to major humanitarian crises.

The need for a more data-driven, epidemiological approach to disaster relief was evident. As agencies faced humanitarian emergencies such as the 1970 cyclone in Bangladesh, the earthquakes in Guatemala and

Naples, and the devastating famines in Africa's Sahel region, quantitative, population-based assessments evolved.[5] While this allowed analysts to describe how mortality and morbidity varied across population groups and demonstrated the dynamic nature of postdisaster needs, significant barriers to standardized epidemiological methods, such as lack of security and the breakdown of surveillance systems, often undermined the accuracy of the assessment. In response to these concerns, the humanitarian aid community created key indicators of mortality and malnutrition that acted as early indicators of crisis and subsequent triggering mechanisms for the relief community. The Standardized Monitoring and Assessment of Relief and Transitions (SMART) method was introduced,[5] and by the 1990s appropriate responses resultant from epidemiological research and targeting strategies led to decreased morbidity and mortality, and interest in the public health of disasters heightened.

This was evidenced in the United States after Hurricane Andrew struck Florida in 1992.[6] In response to the CDC's request for a rapid needs assessment evaluating the extent of the storm's effects, cluster sampling of residents took place, identifying population demographics and the number of sick and injured, and accumulating data regarding access to clean water and food, toilet facilities, and infrastructure damage. Similar efforts were made in 1995 following Hurricanes Marilyn in the U.S. Virgin Islands and Hurricane Opal in Pensacola, FL.[7] These data were used to direct aid initiatives and assure the populace that community-driven priorities were addressed. By disseminating information about the availability of health care, food, and water, along with preventive messages regarding food spoilage, water treatment, and vector control, rumors regarding epidemics were controlled and secondary injuries and illnesses were limited.

CURRENT PRACTICE

Purpose

Rapid, postdisaster needs assessment, as it operates today, seeks to collect precise and accurate subjective and objective data that measure the damage done to and the critical needs of the affected community. The main purpose of a rapid assessment is, through the evaluation of disease burden and infrastructure fracturing, to identify the magnitude of the crisis; the location, boundaries, and density of the problem; and the immediate humanitarian priorities.[1] Optimally, needs assessments should be largely standardized and efficient, aspire to the humanitarian ethic of neutrality, and provide accurate and precise information. Evaluations should occur during or immediately after the emergency phase, with ongoing reevaluation during the response, rehabilitation, and recovery phases.

Integral components of needs assessments are as follows: (1) confirm the emergency; (2) describe the type, impact, and possible evolution of the disaster; (3) measure the present and potential health impacts; (4) alert the international community to the gravity of the situation; (5)

assess the adequacy of the current response capacity; and (6) recommend immediate humanitarian actions.[8,9] Although each particular disaster necessitates a unique needs assessment, the WHO has designed a standardized rapid health assessment protocol for common emergencies. In general, the major steps of this protocol include description of purpose, preparedness, planning, conducting the assessment, analysis of data, and presentation of results. While the purpose and priorities of a needs assessment were addressed above, the other steps will be described below.

Preparedness

Successful disaster response hinges on disaster preparedness. Thus, it is imperative that governments, health systems, and international organizations have at least a basic infrastructure in place to be able to immediately implement an appropriate rapid assessment and response. According to the WHO rapid health assessments protocol, preparedness requires (1) establishing baseline data, (2) emergency planning, (3) training of staff, and (4) monitoring and evaluation.[8] A system to establish baseline data, including population demographics, vulnerability assessment, and preexisting burden of disease, facilitates the anticipation of needs after disasters and allows for a preliminary response system that can be deployed quickly when emergencies arise. The WHO protocol recommends creating a "preparedness checklist," including the following questions that evaluate preexisting disaster response infrastructure, essential information to have when considering postdisaster resources:

- Does a national health policy exist regarding emergency preparedness, response, and recovery?
- Who is the person in the health ministry in charge of emergency preparedness?
- What type of coordination exists between the health sector, civil defense, and other key government ministries?
- What type of coordination exists between ministries of health, the UN, and nongovernmental organizations (NGOs)?
- What operational plans exist for disasters?
- Do national and local health plans exist for disaster management?
- Are surveillance measures in place that can detect early signs of disasters?
- Have environmental health services taken preparedness steps?
- Have facilities and areas been identified to serve as shelter sites?
- What training activities exist for disaster preparedness? Who is involved? Have disaster drills been administered?
- What resources exist to facilitate rapid response to disaster (e.g., emergency budget, supplies)?
- Does a system exist for updating information on key human and material resources needed in a disaster?

By acknowledging and anticipating humanitarian emergencies through preparedness programs and establishing databases of baseline demographics, infrastructure, and resources, not only will needs assessments be improved but so too will the majority of postdisaster humanitarian responses. It must be stressed that any databases established must be regularly revisited and updated.

Planning

Preparation for conducting needs assessment requires addressing crucial logistical and ideological issues, including determining who is to perform the surveillance, who receives the data, and what data are collected; creating appropriate time lines; establishing quality assurance protocols; and determining task delegation and predeployment logistics.

Ideally, rapid needs assessment is performed by an interdisciplinary team garnered from local NGOs, governmental organizations, and international agencies that includes epidemiologists, public health professionals, engineers, and statisticians. As is feasible, authority

and responsibility should be shared among members of the affected community and country as well as international personnel. Teams should include members and leaders that have familiarity not only with the type of disaster but also with the region and population, possess epidemiological and technical skills, and have decision-making capacity in the face of sparse data. While there is quite the polemic regarding the need for neutrality in humanitarian responses, sociopolitical affiliations should be carefully considered when selecting needs assessment personnel. Identification of the agency to perform or lead the rapid surveillance is crucial, and the coordination of multiple organizations intending to work within the same fora is paramount.

A critical aspect of performing needs assessment is directing the data to the appropriate audience. The main recipient, of course, will be the agency that sponsors the survey. However, it is imperative to acknowledge that such information should be dispersed as widely as possible. Such a diverse audience that includes survivors, NGOs, United Nation agencies, donor governments, and the media will require the ability to cater to differing informational needs, lexicons, and presentation styles.

The specific information gathered during the immediate emergency phase of the disaster should include (1) baseline data, including information on demographics, lifeline services, and sociopolitical conflict; (2) data intrinsic to the crisis; (3) logistical data; and (4) information about surviving resources. The following are examples of what should be included[1]:

1. Intrinsic to the crisis
   - Boundaries of the affected area and the density of impact
   - Time line of the crisis
   - Major threats to survival
   - Information regarding severely affected or isolated populations and disaggregated data based on sex and age
   - Prioritized search and rescue areas
   - Assessment of lifeline services; that is, access to water, power, sewage, etc.
2. Logistical
   - Damage to transportation infrastructure or other mobility issues en route to affected areas
   - Damage to broadcasting systems
   - Need for establishing or restoring communication infrastructure
   - Assessment of the damage to air traffic centers
3. Surviving resources
   - Assessment of health care facility damage and capacity
   - Review and itemization of government stockpiles of in-kind resources
   - Information regarding existing NGOs, governmental organizations (GOs), international organizations (IOs), and community service organizations (CSOs) that are currently operating and characterization of the recipient population and capacity

In humanitarian emergencies, there are differing time lines corresponding to different crises. Generally, four main phases of humanitarian crises and corresponding roles for needs assessment have been identified, with Phase 0 being reserved for coordinated preparedness assessment[9]:

- *Phase 1 (72 hours):* Initial assessment aimed at estimating the scale and severity of the impact, locating affected populations, and informing initial response decisions and Phase-2 rapid assessments
- *Phase 2 (weeks 1 to 2):* Multicluster or sector initial rapid assessment (MIRA) intended to inform initial planning of the humanitarian response, highlight priority actions, define the focus for follow-up in-depth assessments, and establish the baseline for monitoring
- *Phase 3 (weeks 3 to 4):* Single-cluster or sector coordinated in-depth assessments, harmonized across clusters or sectors to

analyze the situation and trends, adjust the ongoing response, inform detailed planning for humanitarian relief or early recovery, and establish baselines for operational and strategic performance monitoring

- *Phase 4 (weeks 5+):* Continued single-cluster or sector coordinated in-depth assessments with early recovery consideration, harmonized across clusters or sectors in order to analyze the situation and trends, inform the phasing out of life-sustaining activities and detailed planning for humanitarian relief and recovery, and feed into performance monitoring

This can be juxtaposed to a time line of needs assessment after *sudden-impact* disasters[8]:

- *Phase 1 (24 hours):* Local response usually occurs with simultaneous assessment and response, and medical measures are often implemented with incomplete information. Preliminary morbidity and mortality data are difficult to obtain but needed within the 24 hours following impact to guide requests for assistance.
- *Phase 2 (48 hours):* Assessments should focus on needs for medical response in the less accessible areas, shortages in primary health care resources, and secondary needs (i.e., shelter, food, and water). At this stage, the need for additional national and international resources should be evaluated.
- *Phase 3 (days 3 to 5):* Surveillance data should be collected regarding environmental health, food, special protection and shelter for vulnerable groups, and information key to reestablishing primary health care systems and facilities.
- *Phase 4 (days 5+):* Evaluation should focus on those data that inform response and recovery operations, assessing preexisting surveillance systems and health care infrastructure and health trends.

After the large questions of who, what, and when have been answered, final preparation includes establishing a quality assurance system, which allows gaps in data to be identified and information to be validated and creates time lines for reassessment. Intraorganizational and interorganizational roles should be confirmed and deliverables defined, and administrative assignments should be delegated. Logistics, such as travel clearance, transportation, safety protocols, and developing communications systems, must also be addressed before conducting the assessment.

Conducting the Assessment

In order to improve the likelihood of obtaining accurate data, rapid needs assessment must be systematic, despite having to conduct such surveillance during the chaos of a disaster. Generally accepted types of data collection include (1) review of existing data, (2) inspection of the affected area, (3) key informant interviews, and (4) rapid surveys.

While inspection of the area can be done by air or ground, aerial assessments are most helpful in determining the boundaries of the affected area and the conditions of the infrastructure and environment. Aerial surveillance provides geospatial and infrastructure data, but group assessments can provide a better sense of shelter and food availability and potential hazards and a gross sense of the type of population affected. Vital to needs assessment is the establishment of a reliable denominator, since rates depend on a moderately accurate estimate of the population at risk. Aerial inspection (e.g., house counts), along with group assessments (e.g., average family size), can augment any preexisting baseline data to create an initial denominator.[4]

Key informant interviews should include members from each sector of the affected community, including community leaders, local government officials, health workers, and personnel from community service organizations and other emergency response groups. These interviews can shed light on variables such as the following:

- Perception of the event
- Previous condition of the area
- Size of the affected community
- Estimated morbidity and mortality rates
- Existing food supplies and needs (e.g., approximately 1900 to 2100 kcal per person per day)
- Supply and quality of water (e.g., generally 15 L of clean water per person per day)
- Adequacy of sanitation (e.g., 1 latrine per 20 people)
- Existing fuel and communication links
- Existing resources in the community
- Adequacy of security and/or the prevalence of violence
- Impression of any existing conflict, specific contentious issues, tensions between community factions, etc.
- Cultural norms and mores that might affect relief efforts

Although key informant interviews can rapidly provide information, surveyors should always be cognizant that such data are likely to be exaggerated and/or biased.[8,10]

Aside from inspection of the area and key information interviews, surveys are central to accurate situational assessments and should be utilized when information cannot be obtained from alternate sources. A few of the common rapid surveillance methods after disasters include sentinel surveillance, surveys by specialist teams, and detailed critical sector assessments.

Sentinel Surveillance

Sentinel surveillance involves creating a reporting system that detects early signs of preidentified problems at certain sites. This method allows for a triggering mechanism to alert humanitarian responders during early warning phases.

Surveys by Specialist Teams (Sampling Methods)

Well-designed surveys from reliable samples allow surveyors to confidently generalize findings and apply them to a larger population. A few of the multiple methods for sampling follow:

- *Simple random sampling:* when every member of the population at risk is equally likely to be selected and such selection has no effect on other selections
- *Systematic random sampling:* choosing every 20th subject, for example, on a list. This is potentially inaccurate if the list is nonrandom or incomplete.
- *Stratified random sampling:* dividing the population into strata, randomly selecting subjects, and then combining them to give an overall sample
- *Cluster sampling:* Samples are restricted to a limited number of geographical areas, called clusters. For each geographic area selected, samples are random and then combined to give an overall sample.

SMART, as an example, is a rapid cluster sampling method that is now widely used.[5] The population is divided into groups, and a sample is randomly selected for assessment to provide statistically adequate estimates. Whereas these methods are more easily implementable and provide real-time estimation in unsecure and inaccessible settings, cluster sampling has a lower level of precision than random sampling and subsequently constrains the external generalizability of key variables such as mortality.

Detailed Critical Sector Assessments by Specialists

Critical sector surveillance is appropriately named, necessary not only for health and health infrastructure evaluation but also for assessing critical resources such as water and electricity, and it often can be performed by staff from within or outside of these systems.[1]

The impact of a disaster on the health of a population entails assessing injuries, illnesses, death rates, and missing persons. Rapid assessment of primary injuries should estimate the number of persons injured and the severity, types, and sites of injury. Primary injuries are those that are the result of the disaster itself, whereas secondary injuries occur during the postimpact phase of a disaster, such as injuries related to the cleanup. Identifying where survivors seek care for such injuries not only is valuable data in itself but also provides one major source of information.

Although communicable diseases are relatively rare in the acute phase following a disaster, surveyors should identify pathogens already present and that are likely to spread in the context of poor sanitation and the population massing that occurs at shelters and evacuation centers. A preliminary disease control plan should be derived from these data.

In crises, mortality is usually limited to reports of bodies recovered, but such passive information can be supplemented by designating burial sites and maintaining burial counts.[8] Data should include age- and sex-specific death rates, causes, and risk factors. In humanitarian crises, crude mortality rates (CMRs) should be reported as per 10,000 per day, with death rates approximately 0.4 to 0.6 per 10,000. Rates exceeding 1.0 are considered elevated, and rates over 2.0 are deemed critical.[10] When evaluating CMRs, one must take into account the unique crisis time line; rapid-onset disasters will have more front-end mortality.

The severity of a disaster is also closely associated with the number of persons missing. Though it can be difficult to obtain precise numbers, preliminary data can be derived from families and search and rescue teams.

Perhaps as crucial as characterizing the impact of the disaster on health is defining its effect on the health care infrastructure. Surveillance efforts should collect any data that help determine which facilities are still functioning and which resources are needed to restore and/or supplement existent services. Questions should address the type and location of facilities, post-event structural integrity, capacity, injuries and death of staff and personnel, and any resource limitations. If possible, data collected should include patient injury types, any need to evacuate patients for specialized care, and the types of medicines and other supplies most urgently needed.

As aforementioned, surveyors should also examine the integrity of the postimpact environmental situation. Analysis of the water supply, sanitation, shelter, transportation, communication, and electricity is crucial. An adequate supply of water is of paramount importance, so particular attention should be made to estimate the size of communities without water, potentially contaminated resources, and the magnitude of the damage to supplies.

New Innovations

With the evolution of information technologies and the Internet and the explosion in mobile device availability and usage, humanitarian response and needs assessment has at its fingertips new, powerful, real-time tools to track populations and postdisaster needs. Crisis mapping, which utilizes mobile platforms, computational and statistical models, geospatial technologies, and subsequent analytics, not only provides a wealth of data but also conveys agency to those most affected by the disaster.

Mobile communications have the potential to radically affect needs assessments.[11] Crowdsourcing, the practice of obtaining services, ideas, or content by soliciting populations through an online or mobile community, has been used to identify developing conflicts, disease outbreaks, and densities of need throughout health and lifeline sectors. Open-source platforms, such as Ushahidi, provide software for information collection, visualization, and interactive mapping. These technologies have been utilized most recently in the crises in Sudan and after the 2010 Haitian earthquake.[12,13] Initiatives that implement SMS reporting by crisis-affected populations have been shown to provide incredible volume, speed, and accuracy of information that has later been incorporated into GIS to inform humanitarian organizations regarding needs, ongoing responses, gaps in resources, and redundancies of initiatives. SIM card positioning has provided accurate geospatial data that have yielded information about crisis variables ranging from population outflows to cholera outbreaks.[12] Utilizing this model, efforts of agencies have been redistributed to those most affected by the disaster, with surveyors on the ground along with public health officials verifying data. Whereas these technologies are rife with potential, their widespread integration into needs assessment is hindered by the challenges of information bottlenecks; delays; inaccuracies; difficulties with technological dissemination, standardization, and organizational buy-in; and the need for powerful integrative programs.[11]

In so implementing any of these survey methodologies, it is imperative to collect sex- and age-disaggregated data (SADD), even in the initial phases of assessment and response.[14] Almost all of the major humanitarian standards, handbooks, and guidelines require the inclusion of SADD into assessments, and all organizations operating under WHO Health Clusters are mandated to ensure gender equality in their humanitarian response. However, in practice, there is a lack of understanding of and conviction in the merits of SADD and a skepticism regarding what can realistically be collected during the first phases of response, and thus employment of disaggregation is unfortunately rather limited and delayed until later stages.

Analyzing and Presenting Data

Throughout all phases of disaster response, it is critical to have the right data, at the right time, displayed in a fitting manner that compels the relief community to respond with appropriate action. Data should be as specific as possible, with SADD emphasized to facilitate the design of appropriate interventions.[14] Data analysis should thus be performed with standardized techniques that allow for interdisaster comparisons.

The complexity of data collection and analysis that are to culminate in efficient disaster management has highlighted the need to introduce innovative tools, such as GIS and operations research that assist in decision-making processes. Operational research (OR) is a burgeoning scientific field that offers decision support by identifying the optimum design and operations of a system under specific constraints, such as scarce and dynamic resources.[15] Through diverse techniques, including mathematical programming, probability and statistics, simulation, decision theory, and multiattribute utility theory, OR can utilize needs assessment data to comment upon the ideal location of emergency facilities, distribution schema, evacuation routes, inventory planning, infrastructure assessment, and postrecovery reconstruction. GIS able to spatially portray not only predisaster baseline data but also real-time early warning data, disaggregated needs data, and the evolving humanitarian response, is now integral to the analysis and presentation of needs assessments and is a significant part of crisis mapping.[16]

Presenting needs assessment data, postanalysis, should emphasize fidelity to the evidence but cater to the varying informational requirements and lexicons of diverse audiences, for example, implementing agencies versus donors. Per the WHO Standardized Protocol, a basic outline for a standardized presentation is as follows[8]:

1. Reason for the emergency
2. Area affected
3. Description of the affected community at baseline

4. Impact of the disaster (mortality, injuries, financial losses, and disaggregation of these data)
5. Existing resources and infrastructure
6. Additional requirements, longitudinally
7. Clearly stated priorities for the response organization.

Results should be widely distributed so that information can be verified and/or complemented and organizations without needs assessment programs or initiatives can utilize the data to design appropriate interventions.

⚠ PITFALLS

While the existence and evolution of needs assessments have, no doubt, positively influenced postdisaster relief practices, there are significant challenges that continue to stand as barriers to accurate, appropriate, and timely needs assessment reporting.

One of the most prominent challenges of needs assessment is the question of "who": which organizations possess the appropriate infrastructure and the appropriately skilled personnel, how are aid organizations performing parallel evaluations to coordinate, is there an ideal way to delegate evaluation responsibilities, and which organization is the most credible and best suited to disseminate the information.[17] Addressing these questions requires untangling politics, economics, hubris, bureaucratic complexities, and miscommunication and frequently leads to delayed reporting. This was seen in Haiti after the 2010 earthquake, wherein the initial needs assessment was officially reported on day 45, as opposed to day 12, which is the generally accepted standard.[5] Subsequently, although not entirely secondary to a delayed evaluative report, humanitarian relief projects, such as trauma response by foreign field hospitals, were uncoordinated and often too tardy for clinical efficacy (taking 10.2 days to respond, rather than 1 to 5 days).

Needs assessment is also riddled with logistical pitfalls. These include addressing inaccurate or often absent "predisaster" baselines for population, health, and infrastructure demographics; assuring appropriate timing of needs assessment and reporting; obtaining informed consent; maintaining confidentiality and information security[5]; and acquiring the access needed to perform such evaluations. In postdisaster environments, and even more so in complex humanitarian emergencies, access is hindered by political, military, and logistical barriers, be they washed-out roads and inhospitable terrain or hostile interference from local authorities and the militarization of humanitarian space. These barriers are multifactorial and dynamic and must be addressed by personnel who have experience beyond medicine, public health, or epidemiology.

Furthermore, the pitfalls of any data collection and analysis, even in its simplest form, are extensive. In this case, as in many other contexts, poor data are worse than no data at all. But in postdisaster environments, data are usually collected rapidly under extremely adverse conditions, and sources of information must be integrated.[18] In general, sample bias is a large and ubiquitous problem in disaster needs assessment. Sample sizes are frequently too small and nonrandom. Data more easily obtained by accessing health facility records can be misrepresentative, as those that need the most care may not be the population able to visit health care facilities.[4] Similarly, assessments focused on the "most affected areas" provide equally fallacious data, as sampling from these densely affected areas may artificially inflate mortality and morbidity, overlook alternatively affected populations, and misrepresent needs that cannot be easily generalizable.

Given the constraints of time, pressure, limited initial resources, and a lack of data-validation methods, it is likely that more accurate data will be collected during later phases, such as rehabilitation and/or recovery. Thus, agencies must recognize that a one-time, nondynamic assessment is inadequate to create an appropriate response to an ever-changing disaster environment.[19] Consequently, those reviewing and implementing initiatives from the information must understand the data-gathering methodologies, their inherent limitations, and sources of bias.

Lastly, it should be acknowledged that postdisaster needs assessment programs suffer from ideological challenges that are rather ubiquitous throughout humanitarian and development fields and yet remain insidious. Sociopolitical minutiae and cultural mores must be understood and respected, especially in the tumult of disaster, death, and communities in conflict.[5] Determining the role of neutrality in needs assessments design, logistics, and presentation is requisite, for without conscious effort, either actual or perceptual bias is likely to occur. Disaster assessments and relief efforts should always respect existing infrastructure and community organizations, keeping recovery, rehabilitation, and development in their sights despite the initial acuity.

Notwithstanding the challenges they face, standardized disaster surveillance algorithms have great potential to rapidly identify the acute needs of populations in the midst of disasters and to direct resources to areas most in need during the response and recovery phases.[20] The evolving fields of crisis mapping, operations research, and humanitarian aid theory have the extraordinary potential for addressing many of these pitfalls and furthering evaluative practices. Fundamentally, postdisaster needs assessments provide a medium for advocacy that ensures that the response to a disaster is not just what pleases donor or political constituents, but addresses the real problems of the affected community and thereby directly contributes to the prevention of morbidity and mortality.[17]

REFERENCES

1. Stephenson RS. *Disaster Assessment. Disaster Management Training Programme.* 2nd ed. United Nations Development Programme/Office of the United Nations Disaster Relief Coordinator; 1994.
2. Gregg M. Surveillance and epidemiology. In: *The Public Health Consequences of Disasters 1989. CDC Monograph.* Atlanta: US Department of Health and Human Services; September 1989.
3. Briggs S, ed. *Advanced Disaster Medical Response Manual for Providers.* Boston: Harvard Medical International Trauma and Disaster Institute; 2003.
4. Guha-Sapir D. Rapid assessment of health needs in mass emergencies: review of current concepts and methods. *World Health Stat Q.* 1991; 44(3):171–181.
5. Leaning J, Guha-Sapir D. Natural disasters, armed conflict, and public health. *N Engl J Med.* 2013;369(19):1836–1842.
6. CDC. Rapid needs health assessment following Hurricane Andrew—1992. *MMWR.* 1992;41(37):685–688.
7. CDC. Injury and illness/Rapid health needs assessment following Hurricane Marilyn and Hurricane Opal—1995. *MMWR.* 1996;45(4):81–85.
8. World Health Organization. *Rapid Health Assessment Protocols for Emergencies.* Geneva: WHO; 1999.
9. Inter-Agency Standing Committee. *Operational Guidance for Coordinated Assessments in Humanitarian Crises.* Geneva: IASC; 2012.
10. Leaning J, Briggs S, Chen L. *Humanitarian Crises.* Cambridge, MA: Harvard University Press; 1999.
11. Greenough P, Bateman L, Sorensen B, et al. Innovations in Humanitarian Technologies Working Group—Report of the Proceeding Humanitarian Action Summit 2011. *Prehosp Disaster Med.* 2011;26(6):428–468.
12. Bengtsson L, Lu X, Thorson A, et al. Improved response to disasters and outbreaks by tracking population movements with mobile phone network data: a post-earthquake geospatial study in Haiti. *PLoS Med.* 2011;8(8): e1001083.

13. Munro R. Crowdsourcing and the crisis-affected community. *Information Retrieval.* 2013;16(2):210–266.

14. Mazurana D, Benelli P, Walker P. How sex- and age-disaggregated data and gender and generational analyses can improve humanitarian response. *Disaster.* 2013;37(S1):S68–S82.

15. Albores P, Rodriguez O, Roy P. Operational Research: Key for Successful Disaster Management. *YOR18 Biennial Conferences Keynote Papers and Extended Abstracts.* 2013;47–59.

16. Johnson R. *GIS Technology for Disasters and Emergency Management: An ESRI White Paper.* Redlands: ESRI; 2000.

17. O'Toole M. Medical and public health needs: the role of the rapid assessment. Presented at: Proceedings of the First Harvard Symposium on Complex Humanitarian Disasters; April 10-11, 1995; Boston.

18. Noji E, ed. *The Public Health Consequences of Disasters.* New York: Oxford University Press; 1997.

19. Auf der Heide E. *Disaster Response: Principles of Preparation and Coordination.* St. Louis: Mosby; 1989.

20. Lillibridge SR. Disaster assessment: the emergency health evaluation of a population affected by a disaster. *Ann Emerg Med.* November 1993;22:1715–1720.

CHAPTER 41

Operations and Logistics

James J. Rifino

Disaster management is most effective when responding agencies are well trained, well practiced, and familiar with the hierarchy needed for disaster response. Before a major incident, responding organizations and personnel must be organized under a defined leadership structure to effectively coordinate and carry out the tasks needed to properly mitigate the event. One of the hallmarks of a developed country from the emergency response perspective is its ability to effectively respond to and manage a complex disaster event in an organized fashion.[1,2]

By definition, the Incident Command System (ICS) is a management system designed to enable effective and efficient domestic incident management by integrating a combination of facilities, equipment, personnel, procedures, and communications operating within a common organizational structure. ICS is normally structured to facilitate activities in five major functional areas: Command (directed by the Incident Commander [IC]), Planning (collects and disseminates information about the incident and advises about resources), Finance and Administrative (critical for tracking incident costs and reimbursement accounting), Operations, and Logistics. These functions task individuals with different responsibilities crucial for disaster response and recovery. They can also be applied routinely for local and regional incidents, not just disasters.

The Operations section is responsible for carrying out the response activities described in the Incident Action Plan (IAP). This includes directing and coordinating all operations, assisting in the development of response goals and objectives, requesting and releasing resources, and providing situation and resource status updates. The Logistics section is responsible for services and support necessary to sustain the tactical objectives of the Operations section. This includes facilities, services, materials, and personnel to operate the requested equipment for the incident. This function is most significant with respect to long-term or extended operations when more resources are required. Operations and Logistics are two completely separate functions and functional entities, but an efficient and effective Operations section at a major incident is partly dependent on a well-organized and properly functioning Logistics section.

HISTORICAL PERSPECTIVE

History has documented disasters on many levels all around the world. Some of the larger disasters were the result of infection (North American Smallpox Epidemic of 1775, Black Death of 1348 to 1351, Spanish Influenza in 1918) as well as natural disasters (Great Earthquake of 1202, Aleppo Earthquake of 1138, volcanic eruptions in Greece and the Pacific). These horrific events killed millions around the world. Documentation of "disaster preparation" and "disaster response" internationally was very poor, essentially nonexistent. In the United States, we have documentation of a series of fires in the city of Portsmouth, New Hampshire, in 1803. After the devastating fires demolished the area and injured many, the Seventh U.S. Congress passed the Congressional Act of 1803, which provided relief for Portsmouth merchants by extending the time they had for remitting tariffs on imported goods. This is widely considered the first piece of legislation passed by the federal government that provided relief after a disaster.[3,4] In 1900 Congress granted a charter to the American Red Cross, which had provided disaster relief following the Johnstown Flood in Pennsylvania in 1889. The charter included the mandate to "carry on a system of national and international relief in time of peace and to apply the same in mitigating the sufferings caused by pestilence, famine, fire, floods, and other great national calamities." This was the so-called American Amendment calling for peacetime disaster relief.[5] For the next several decades, disaster relief was expected to be delivered by charitable organizations. Military assistance, however, was provided following the San Francisco Earthquake in 1908.

The next documented federal action came in 1932, when President Herbert Hoover commissioned the Reconstruction Finance Corporation (RFC). This federal assistance lent money to banks and institutions, with the goal of stimulating the economy and is considered the first organized federal disaster response agency.[6] Over the last half of the twentieth century, the U.S. federal government continued to grow, while disastrous events stimulated the growth of the idea of "disaster response" and "disaster preparedness" largely as a result of the effects of war, hurricanes, earthquakes, and wildfires. It is important to state that, like most laws in the United States, provisions for disaster response have been more reactive rather than proactive.

Disaster response in the United States is largely legislated at the federal level, but it is also legislated at the state and local levels. Local resources and personnel are ultimately responsible for coordinating and deploying resources needed after an incident. All disasters are "local," and most jurisdictions across the United States authorize and recognize the Fire Chief (or designee) as the IC of any incident involving imminent danger to life or property. The exception to this is any situation that is more of a law enforcement issue (e.g., sniper, hostage situation). It is the IC who has overall authority for any disaster operation, unless he transfers command to another individual.

The IC must assess every situation and determine the scope of resources needed. If local resources are insufficient to manage the incident, additional manpower and equipment and supplies are typically requested from neighboring communities (a concept known as "mutual aid"). This may or may not be based on a formal agreement between individual agencies and/or political jurisdictions. For any major incident, local resources need to rely on each other as national resources typically take a few days to organize and deploy. In more progressive fire-rescue systems, mutual aid resources are dispatched according to a predefined algorithm or plan, and this concept is known as "automatic aid." The difference is that "mutual aid" is requested once the scene is assessed and it is determined that there is a lack of resources. "Automatic aid" is requested by the service upon dispatch to a situation that is recognized immediately as requiring additional assistance not available at the time of the call (e.g., calling for a ladder truck from a neighboring town for a fire in a tall building).

If regional resources do not satisfy the needs of a disaster response, the traditional next step has been to request aid from the state emergency management agency. Governors can declare a state of emergency, thereby allowing for access to necessary materials, equipment, and financial resources. The state governor may also activate the National Guard. In the last 10 to 15 years, many states have developed specialty response teams capable of mobilizing in response to a disaster. These include urban search and rescue (US&R) teams, hazardous materials (HazMat) teams, weapons of mass destruction (WMD) task forces, emergency medical service(s) (EMS) and ambulance strike teams, and similar entities. In 1996, Congress enacted the Emergency Management Assistance Compact, a mutual aid agreement that allows human and material resources to cross state lines and operate in a declared disaster situation in a "state-to-state" assistance operation when requested through the proper channels and approved by the governor of the affected state. Because disaster preparedness and response evolved out of the military in the United States, many of the Logistics and Operations processes today have roots in military practice.

Throughout Europe, the European Commission coordinates emergency relief and assistance in the wake of all disasters. Floods and fires are quite common in the summer months, although all disasters are monitored for and an appropriate response is expected. The Monitoring and Information Centre (MIC) within the European Commission is a centrally based center in Brussels that monitors emergencies worldwide and coordinates European resources for relief operations. The MIC acts as a communication hub between countries after a disaster occurs, whether natural or human-made. Upon receiving a request for help, duty officers alert potential donor nations and match offers of aid to the needs on the ground. In addition to rounding up equipment and supplies, the MIC dispatches field experts to disaster sites.[7]

Asian Disaster Preparedness Center (ADPC) is an organization that helps to reduce the impact of disasters on communities and countries in Asia and the Pacific, the most hazard-prone region in the world. Established in 1986, ADPC is an independent nongovernmental organization (NGO) that promotes disaster awareness and the development of mitigation and management policies in advance of a disaster. With headquarters located in Bangkok, ADPC also has country offices in Bangladesh, the Lao People's Democratic Republic (Lao PDR), and Myanmar. ADPC raises awareness, helps establish and strengthen sustainable institutional mechanisms, enhances knowledge and skills, and facilitates the exchange of information, experience, and expertise. The organization also deploys disaster risk management (DRM) information and systems to reduce local, national, and regional risk across this large region.[8]

Australia has a system very similar to the United States. The states and territories have primary responsibility for life and property within their borders, and they must rely on their own plans and arrangements to respond to natural or human-made emergencies that threaten life or property. When a jurisdiction deems that their resources will not be able to effectively manage an incident it can ask for help from the Australian Government. This request is delivered through the Australian Government Disaster Response Plan (COMDISPLAN). Emergency Management Australia (EMA) receives the request for assistance and responds through the Australian Government Crisis Coordination Centre (CCC).

CURRENT PRACTICE

Operations

Most disaster response begins with an immediate response from bystanders on the scene. Some will immediately act, and others will run. Most people, if able, call for help (911, 112, 118, 119, 999, etc.). Police, fire, and EMS personnel are usually the first responders to the incident or disaster. Those first on-scene will undoubtedly be overwhelmed, but these important rescuers need to sweep the scene for safety, assess the scope or extent of the situation, identify the number of victims, determine and summon additional resources needed, and then assess for the need for immediate lifesaving techniques. Disaster mitigation very often starts with the very first arriving group to the incident. Triage priorities change during any mass casualty incident (MCI), and personnel must be well versed and well trained with the concepts of disaster management and triage of multiple casualties. An initial command area, known as the emergency operations center (EOC), will need to be designated and set up in an appropriate area, followed by an assessment of short- and long-term additional resources needed from local, state, and federal partners. This will simultaneously include organizing an ICS.

Disaster operations vary in size and complexity depending on the nature and duration of the event, as well as resources needed to stabilize the incident. The operations section is responsible for managing all operations directed toward reducing the immediate hazard at the incident site, save lives and property, establish situation control, and restore the area to normal conditions (Figure 41-1). This section establishes a methodical strategy and the actions needed to accomplish the goals and objectives set by Command (IC, Safety Officer, Public Information Officer, Senior Liaison, and Senior Advisors) to achieve response objectives. Common tactical resources required at a disaster incident include fire suppression, public health, public works, technical rescue, hazardous materials containment, and EMS. The incident itself will define the type and quantity of resources needed to attain the objectives set by command personnel. A hurricane, tropical storm, tornado, or earthquake may often require a national response and will have specific concerns and issues, but an act of war or terrorism will require other additional resources to be deployed.

The ICS is the national standard for providing guidance and organization with respect to the assets needed to respond to an incident and the process of the response through all stages of the event, no matter the size or complexity. The ICS introduces a number of concepts, including "Span of Control" and "Unified Command" (all discussed elsewhere in this book). It is a flexible management structure, allowing for expansion and contraction of all sectors based on the dynamics of the incident. In

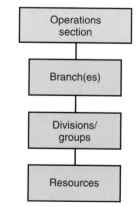

FIG 41-1 Operations Functions.

late 2004, the Department of Homeland Security (DHS) released the National Incident Management System (NIMS) as a template to complement the ICS. NIMS is an essential foundation of the National Preparedness System (NPS). Per the Federal Emergency Management Agency (FEMA), NIMS is a "systematic, proactive approach to guide departments and agencies at all levels of government, nongovernmental organizations, and the private sector to work together seamlessly and manage incidents involving all threats and hazards—regardless of cause, size, location, or complexity."[9] It provides a common approach for managing all incidents consistently while allowing for flexibility. It is strongly encouraged and recommended that all agencies practice the basics on a daily basis with small incidents, so that a response to a larger incident is more seamless and practiced when it occurs.

The Operations Section Chief is the individual designated by the IC to manage and command the Operations section. He is ultimately responsible for developing and implementing strategies and tactics to meet the incident objectives set by the IC and the IAP. This plan details the objectives of the mission and how they will be met. An IAP should be written for every operational period during the disaster. Tactical decision making (i.e., how, when, and where to deploy certain resources to mitigate a disaster) is also the responsibility of the Operations Section Chief. The ability to make these decisions in a competent fashion, however, is predicated on a continual flow of information both from the field and from the command sector. If an incident spans more than one operational period (usually one work cycle), the operations chief may assign a deputy to work the opposite shift to ensure adequate time for nourishment and rest. An Operations Section Chief should be designated for each operational period.

There are several goals that the Operations Chief must accomplish during the initial stages of the response to a disaster. In addition to managing all incident tactical activities and implementing an IAP, the Operations Chief must decide how much to expand his or her organizational structure to match the size and scope of the incident, and the numbers of personnel needed for assigned operations (span of control). Supervisory personnel should be titled and placed in charge of subsidiaries within the operations section by who is most qualified to perform the task rather than on a person's rank or predisaster title. Span of control within the Operations Section is recommended to be 1:5, but may be as high as 1:10 in larger scale incidents. If this is exceeded, branches need to be established with the same concept. The Operations Chief must decide, in conjunction with the IC and Safety Officer, what degree of risk he or she is willing to assume when sending emergency responders into an unstable environment to perform search, rescue, evacuation, medical care, and mitigation activities related to the disaster event. The Operations Chief must maintain an effective line of communication with the various components within the section as well as with the other ICS sections and the IC. Finally, the Operations Chief must understand the concept of flexibility when making decisions. Disaster events may appear static to the civilian population, but emergency responders understand that these events are dynamic in nature. Changing environmental conditions, secondary hazards, fatigue, resource availability, psychological stressors, and many other factors contribute to ever-changing disaster conditions, and these conditions require adaptability and flexibility in decision-making.

Thankfully, there is usually no reason to expand the operations section of the ICS for the great majority of local incidents. An event that the DHS labels an "incident of national significance," however, may necessitate creation of divisions, groups, branches, task forces, and strike teams. These entities represent functional and geographic separation of duties. A good example of this was demonstrated after the 9/11 disaster. The fire department of the City of New York (FDNY) retained command and control of the entire incident and eventually developed a

"unified command structure" according to principles of the ICS. The terrorist attack claimed many lives and resulted in a disaster site that spanned 16 acres. This required a large-scale expansion of the Operations section. Divisions were created according to street names that bordered the scene. Groups included functional components such as technical rescue, fire suppression, and EMS. Branches of each group were composed of personnel attached to a specific type of resource, such as the US&R branch. Within the US&R were individual US&R task forces. EMS strike teams from FDNY and surrounding mutual aid organizations were deployed in support of US&R task forces and other specialized resources. Health and medical resources to support rescue and recovery workers on site were provided by the National Disaster Medical System (NDMS) under FEMA's Emergency Support Function (ESF) #8, using disaster medical assistance teams (DMATs).

A variety of federal resources are available to assist local ICs in planning for and handling large-scale disasters and their aftermath. Recognizing that government resources cannot meet the needs of those affected by catastrophic events, the National Response Framework (NRF) was developed to prepare communities. Updated in 2013, it provides context for how the entire community works together as well as the response efforts related to other parts of national preparedness. The NRF uses the comprehensive framework of NIMS and provides mechanisms for expedited and proactive federal support. It is a more operational incident management and resource allocation plan. The NRF aligns federal coordination structures, capabilities, and resources into a unified, all-discipline and all-hazards approach to domestic incident management. The priorities of the NRF include saving lives and protecting the health and safety of all at the incident, ensuring security of the homeland, prevention of imminent incidents, protecting and restoring critical infrastructure, and facilitating the recovery of individuals as well as families, businesses, governments, and the environment.

Regarding federal assets and personnel, there are multiple emergency response resources deployable through the DHS. US&R task forces specialize in the response to collapse of reinforced concrete buildings, and other infrastructure and their primary mission is to rescue persons trapped in confined spaces regardless of the etiology of the event. They are dispatched under ESF #9 (Search and Rescue). (As noted above, health and medical operations are deployed under ESF #8.) The NDMS is now located in the U.S. Department of Health and Human Services, under the purview of the Assistant Secretary for Preparedness and Response (ASPR) and the Office of Emergency Management (OEM). DMATs are multidisciplinary teams of health care professionals that can provide medical care for prolonged periods in a variety of formats, when local infrastructure is incapacitated. Disaster mortuary operations response teams (DMORTs) can assist or augment local medical examiners in victim identification and mortuary services, while national veterinary response teams (NVRTs) can provide assistance when animal issues arise.[10]

Logistics

The Logistics section supports Command and Operations. This section performs technical activities to maintain the function of operational facilities and processes. Typical logistics functions during a disaster revolve around providing all the support needs for the incident, including finding and ordering supplies and other resources; searching out and setting up facilities (dining hall, incident command, etc.); arranging transportation for personnel and supplies; equipment maintenance; maintaining fuel, medical, and pharmaceutical supplies; food services; communications equipment or hardware and capabilities; and medical services for incident personnel. The size, duration, and specific needs of an incident dictate whether a separate logistics functional element must be created within the ICS. Most disasters, by definition, meet the criteria that any IC would use to establish a logistics section. Essentially, the Logistics section's function is to figure out how to obtain what is needed and get it to where it is needed in a timely fashion. This is one of the most challenging sections, as resources are rarely preestablished. Physical space that is structurally sound can be very challenging to find, and manpower may be an issue depending on the scale of the event.

The Logistics Section Chief manages and commands this section. He or she has a list of tasks including briefing the IC, determining which facilities can be used, notifying resource units when they are activated, assessing the Incident Communications Plan, providing input with regard to preparation of the IAP, ensuring coordination between Logistics and other Command and general staff, attending planning meetings, ensuring the safety and welfare of Logistics personnel, and ensuring proper documentation with respect to Logistics tasks. If an incident spans more than one operational period (usually one work cycle), the logistics chief may assign a deputy to work the opposite shift to ensure adequate time for nourishment and rest.

The section is typically divided into two branches (Figure 41-2): Service and Support. units located within the Service branch require human interaction and include Communications, Medical, and Food. The Support branch is composed of functions that typically do not involve human interaction and include Supplies, Facilities, and Ground Support.

The Communications unit is responsible for installing, maintaining, tracking, and testing all communications equipment. This unit is responsible for planning the radio frequencies, establishing networks, setting up on-scene telephone and public address equipment, and providing all communication links. This is possibly one of the most important units, as efficient communication is the key to response and mitigation. This unit also supervises and operates the incident communications center, as well as prepares a communications plan.

The Medical unit located within the Service branch warrants special attention. It is often confused with the delivery of routine EMS at a large-scale incident. Emergency medical functions fall within two distinct categories in the ICS. EMS is typically a branch within the Operations section, and the responsibility of the EMS branch is to provide emergency medical care and treatment to victims of the disaster. The Medical unit of the Logistics section is designed only to provide emergency medical evaluation and treatment to disaster responders and incident personnel. This unit is also responsible for developing the

Incident Medical Plan for incident personnel, providing basic public health medical needs (vaccines, prophylaxis, mental health), transporting incident personnel if injured, and coordinating mortuary affairs for incident personnel fatalities. The Incident Medical Plan needs to include potentially hazardous areas or conditions, off-site medical assistance facilities, procedures for handling complex medical emergencies, and information on medical assistance capabilities at incident locations.

The Food unit is responsible for planning menus, ordering food, providing cooking facilities, maintaining food service areas, and managing food security and safety. This unit is especially important for extended incidents. This unit is often assisted by NGOs such as the Red Cross, who may provide personnel or other assistance. If this is the case, the Operations Section Chief and IC need to be involved to ensure operational continuity.

The Supply unit orders, receives, processes, stores, inventories, and distributes all supplies. It also handles all tool operations and is responsible for projecting resource needs based on the IAP. The Facilities unit sets up, maintains, and demobilizes facilities including the Incident Command Post, Incident Base, camps, food and hydration areas, sleeping quarters, sanitation areas and showers, lighting, and staging areas. It is also responsible for ordering lighting units, fire extinguishers for tents, and portable toilets. The Ground Support unit maintains vehicles, all ground support equipment, fuel supplies for the mobile equipment, provides transportation supporting the operation, and develops the Traffic Plan.

There are numerous examples of large, devastating disasters that resulted in high mortality around the world. Many of the issues with regards to rescue and medical assistance were a result of a severe deficiency with respect to Logistics. The United Nations called the 2004 Indian Ocean 9.0-magnitude earthquake and resulting tsunami a "logistics nightmare." The tsunami killed more than 230,000 people, left 1.7 million people homeless, and traveled 375 miles in just 75 minutes. The response to the tsunami disaster was quite complicated, but was also significant. NGOs and governments from all over the world sent supplies to the area. Early in the response, flights to an airport in Indonesia were suspended because there were too many airplanes already on the ground, unable to unload their cargo because of lack of space at the airport. Ground transportation was ineffective and in short supply, and washouts of the roadways made delivery of the supplies difficult.[11] Ironically, the biggest ongoing logistical challenge in the response to the Southeast Asia tsunami was how to distribute the abundance of supplies and funding.

Similar issues with logistics were seen in Haiti in 2010 after a 7.0-magnitude earthquake resulted in the deaths of 230,000 people and essentially displaced 2.3 million people. The infrastructure there could not handle the international response, and many issues persisted for years. In the United States, Hurricane Katrina struck the Gulf Coast in 2005, causing levee breaks that devastated New Orleans. It had quickly strengthened from a category 1 hurricane to a category 5 hurricane after it crossed Florida, and struck as a category 4 hurricane. A White House document from the office of President George W. Bush called *The Federal Response to Hurricane Katrina: Lessons Learned* noted the following: "The Department of Homeland Security, in coordination with State and local governments and the private sector, should develop a modern, flexible, and transparent logistics system. This system should be based on established contracts for stockpiling commodities at the local level for emergencies and the provision of goods and services during emergencies. The Federal government must develop the capacity to conduct large-scale logistical operations that supplement and, if necessary, replace State and local logistical systems by leveraging resources within both the public sector and the private sector."[12]

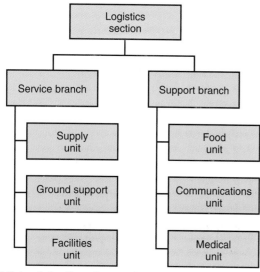

FIG 41-2 Logistics Functions.

! PITFALLS

There are many systems internationally for the management of large-scale disasters. The basics of disaster management remain the same, but the application of these concepts to the incident often illuminates the shortfalls and issues with all systems. Most problems are predictable and recur at every major disaster to some degree, but there are some common factors that are associated with ineffective disaster management (Box 41-1). ICs and Section Chiefs must be flexible in decision making and delegate authority when necessary. They must adapt to changes in incident conditions; maintaining mission priorities is essential. Regardless of the amount of training and preparation, there are still predictable obstacles to overcome during any disaster response. Personnel from different agencies are usually not accustomed to working with each other, and terrorist events will especially create a level of distrust and anxiety when interacting with others one is not familiar with. Communications systems are commonly very different among responding agencies, and communication is the key to facilitating any response. Tactical objectives, resource familiarity, personalities, and political motivations are all additional factors that can make a response less effective.

While it seems obvious for every local government to have a discussion around emergency preparedness, there is still an overwhelming false comfort that the cavalry (federal government) will show up in a timely manner. The truth is that federal assistance will usually take up to 72 hours to organize and deploy. This leaves many communities on their own for the first 72 hours as they respond and begin recovery. Most communities have developed fairly comprehensive emergency management plans to address the hazards in their region, but they lack key personnel from the public health and medical sectors and they fail to define everyone's roles in advance of a major incident. They also usually have one plan and no back-up plan. For example, they may designate a school for a shelter, without taking into account that the school may also be affected, necessitating multiple back-up alternatives.

There are a number of resources for planning from many reliable sources. FEMA has a website dedicated to preparedness. The World Health Organization (WHO) has resources as well, and the Centers for Disease Control and Prevention (CDC) also has resources readily available with regard to managing MCIs. Dr. Joe Barbera and Dr. Anthony MacIntyre at George Washington University have designed a comprehensive model for the management of MCIs as well as more routine emergency incidents that have predominantly a health and medical focus. The Medical and Health Incident Management (MaHIM) system describes an "overarching system for organizing and managing the many diverse medical and public health entities involved in mass casualty response." It is based on principles of public health and emergency management and attempts to delineate the community approach to problem-solving and emergency response in the setting of a MCI rather than the individual response of an EMS service, hospital, or public health department.[13] The value of having an area Medical Operations Center (MOC) was demonstrated during the 2007 wildfires in San Diego County, California; its roles and involvement in evacuation of three hospitals and multiple nursing home patients and their later repatriations have been well documented.[14] Health care and hospital workers should be familiar with the Operations section of the Hospital Incident Command System (HICS), which complies with the NRF.

Finally, EMS is different all over the world, and the concept of prehospital emergency care is still foreign to many communities, countries, and governments. An effective disaster response works best when prehospital personnel are trained, prepared, and ready to go. Skilled prehospital providers are the key to mitigating and recovering from a large-scale incident. Internationally, we must work to educate communities about the importance of EMS and the absolute need to fund such initiatives.

CONCLUSION

The concepts of "Operations" and "Logistics" are common ideas internationally, although initiated differently in different countries. Around the world, disaster experts are talking about the operational and logistical issues we all face within our regions. Some countries are rich in resources and others are very poor in resources. With the Internet and "breaking news" on television we hear of catastrophes shortly after they occur; international responses are not only planned, but also immediately initiated. Eventually we are going to need to speak a similar language internationally, conform to the same rules of conduct, credential our people to ensure the safety of the victims as well as our humanitarian responders, and educate each other with regard to our resources and needs ahead of time. Coordination and credentialing of emergency responders, development of a command structure, tracking of resources, and maintenance of functional communications systems remain challenges that will be encountered at every disaster event. Anticipation of pitfalls in disaster response and logistics support and development of adequate contingency planning may be the most important lessons to teach to those who will fill command and leadership positions at a disaster incident.[15] It is time we start speaking the same language, remove the barriers, and help each other prepare, educate, respond, and recover after a devastating event.

BOX 41-1   Partial List of Factors Associated with Inefficient or Ineffective Disaster Operations

- Lack of accountability, including inadequate supervision and ambiguous or absent chains of command
- Poor communications due to inefficient uses of available communications, failure of and lack of redundancy in communications systems, and conflicting codes and terminology
- Lack of an orderly, systematic planning process
- No common, flexible predetermined management structure to enable delegation of responsibilities and manage workloads efficiently
- No predefined methods to integrate interagency requirements into the management structure and planning process effectively
- Inability to control access to the disaster site, to manage a large influx of unsolicited disaster volunteers, and to curb "freelancing" among emergency response personnel
- Difficulty in coordinating, tracking, and documenting human and materials resources

---

REFERENCES

1. Lewis CP, Aghababian RV. Disaster planning, part I. Overview of hospital and emergency department planning for internal and external disasters. *Emerg Med Clin North Am.* 1996;14(2):439–452.
2. Dara SI, Ashton RW, Farmer JC, Carlton PK, Jr. Worldwide disaster medical response: an historical perspective. *Crit Care Med.* 2005;33(1 Suppl):S2–S6.
3. Wikipedia Free Encyclopedia. Federal emergency management agency. Available at: http://en.wikipedia.org/wiki/Federal_Emergency_Management_Agency#Prior_to_1930.
4. History of Federal Domestic Disaster Aid Before the Civil War, Biot Report #379: July 24, 2006. Suburban Emergency Management Project.

5. American Red Cross. Our federal charter. Available at: http://www.redcross.org/about-us/history/federal-charter#obtaining-charter.

6. Wikipedia Free Encyclopedia. Reconstruction finance corporation. Available at: http://en.wikipedia.org/wiki/Reconstruction_Finance_Corporation.

7. European Commission. Disaster response news. Available at: http://ec.europa.eu/news/environment/100813_en.htm.

8. Asian Disaster Preparedness Center. Available at: http://www.adpc.net/igo.

9. Federal Emergency Management Agency. Available at: http://www.fema.gov/about-agency.

10. Roth PB, Gaffney JK. The federal response plan and disaster medical assistance teams in domestic disaster. *Emerg Med Clin North Am.* 1996;14(2):371–382.

11. VanRooyen M. After the tsunami—facing the public health challenges. *N Engl J Med.* 2005;352(5):435–438.

12. The White House, President George W. Bush. *The Federal Response to Hurricane Katrina: Lessons Learned.* Available at: http://www.au.af.mil/au/awc/awcgate/whitehouse/katrina/katrina-lesns-chap5.pdf.

13. Barbera JA, Macintyre AG. *Medical and Health Incident Management (MaHIM) System: A Comprehensive Functional System Description for Mass Casualty Medical and Health Incident Management.* Washington, DC: Institute for Crisis, Disaster, and Risk Management, The George Washington University; 2002.

14. Chapter 3. Medical operations. In: *2007 San Diego County Firestorms: After Action Report.* Office of Emergency Services, County of San Diego; February 2007:51–55. Available at: http://www.sandiegocounty.gov/content/dam/sdc/oes/docs/2007_SanDiego_Fire_AAR_Main_Document_FINAL.pdf.

15. Auf der Heide E. Disaster planning, part II. Disaster problems, issues, and challenges identified in the research literature. *Emerg Med Clin North Am.* 1996;14(2):453–480.

CHAPTER 42

Disaster Communications*

Gerard DeMers and Irving "Jake" Jacoby

Disaster communications entail using processes and technology to relay timely, pertinent, and accurate information for communities, responding agencies, transport assets, and receiving facilities. Misinformation can derail coordination efforts and delay assessment of damage, misallocate appropriate resources, delay arrival of life-saving interventions, create mistrust among victims, and may impact appropriate funding, at a minimum. Communication procedures and infrastructure must be established and tested to ensure that they perform successfully across the disaster cycle of preparedness, response, recovery and mitigation (Box 42-1). Building capacity and disaster resilience requires active community education to develop a continuous state of preparedness, which relies on communication (in both the delivery and quality of accessible public information). From early warning notification to full-scale response operations, preparations for proper communications should begin before the disaster occurs by anticipating and exploring potential system-based needs. An effective communication system is integral to the success of disaster management, yet communication is routinely identified as a problem area during training exercises and in real-world events where it is needed most.[1,2] Emergency management and incident response depends on flexible communications and information systems that provide a common operating picture for personnel and agencies. Systems concepts and principles should incorporate interoperability, reliability, scalability, portability, resiliency, and redundancy.[3]

Access to information and media technology has evolved significantly over the last two decades, with ubiquitous smartphones and social media changing the flow of information and how society communicates. Social media have become an integral part of relaying information regarding disasters to provide situational awareness, locate loved ones, notify authorities through crowdsourcing of local conditions, and provide support.[4] Social media's role in disasters is discussed further in Chapter 41.

HISTORICAL PERSPECTIVE

In the past, the U.S. government's response to disasters involved dozens of federal agencies handling various individual components. Communications planning was rarely addressed explicitly. Instead, often the assumption was that the existing communications infrastructure would be sufficient.

*The views expressed herein are those of the authors and do not necessarily reflect the official policy or position of the Department of the Navy, Department of Defense, or the U.S. Government; or the U.S. Department of Health and Human Services, ASPR, or the National Disaster Medical System.

In 1979 President Jimmy Carter created the Federal Emergency Management Agency (FEMA) to coordinate domestic disaster response. Although FEMA represented a consolidation of response efforts, communications planning initially was not directly addressed. Furthermore, disaster management remained largely focused on natural catastrophes, such as hurricanes and earthquakes, or unintentional human-made events, including oil spills and radiation leaks.[1] Following the explosion that leveled the Alfred P. Murrah Federal Building in Oklahoma City on April 19, 1995, it became evident that reliance on call-forwarding of emergency medical service (EMS) dispatches from a police- or fire-based 911 phone system would fail when local phone lines were overwhelmed by numbers of calls that exceeded capacity.[5] The importance of disaster planning and response with local commercial providers of landline and cellular communications services was exemplified by the Oklahoma City response.

With the terrorist attacks of September 11, 2001, the United States experienced unprecedented challenges in domestic disaster management, including a substantial strain on its communications systems. Within minutes of the first plane hitting the World Trade Center, the New York City Police Department established command central in a conference room at Bellevue Hospital's emergency department and began coordinating with EMS. As the media and public picked up on events, telephone lines became jammed and connections were unreliable. Additionally, the Emergency Operations Center that had been designed to handle large-scale disasters affecting New York City was evacuated and most of its structures were destroyed; it had been located at 7 World Trade Center.[2] Communications within the emergency department grew difficult as misinformation regarding the attacks circulated. Police and administrators were able to correspond through direct conversation, radios, and pagers; however, cell phones and landlines remained unreliable. Amateur radio played a large role in facilitating communications among affected emergency departments and New York City administrative departments.[6] Even days into the response, National Disaster Medical System (NDMS) teams experienced frequent bomb scares and evacuation notices in response to terrorist threats. The issues surrounding false information with regard to the policies on the use of personal protective equipment (PPE) also exemplify a failure in communications.

In the wake of 9/11, many changes have taken place in U.S. disaster management. The Department of Homeland Security was established, bringing FEMA under its auspices. With this reorganization, the conception of disasters has been expanded to focus on intentional terrorist acts, and greater attention has been paid to establishing and protecting emergency communications infrastructure.[3]

At the level of operational communications responses, case studies of other specific historical events have played a major role in learning lessons from actual events. After Hurricane Katrina struck New Orleans in

BOX 42-1 Communications Roles through Disaster Cycles

Preparedness	• Relay education for effective disaster risk reduction and develop preparedness among communities
Response	• Platform for effective command structure within and between responding agencies
	• Collaboration between various agencies and the community
	• Mass media coverage
	• Official and unofficial channels for updates
Recovery	• Accurately relay damage impact
	• Coordinate funding
Mitigation	• Disseminate lessons

TABLE 42-1 Federal Agencies ESF #2 Communications Roles

AGENCY	ROLE (PRIMARY OR SUPPORT)
Department of Agriculture	Support
Department of Defense	Support
Department of Commerce	Support
Department of Homeland Security (FEMA)	Primary (coordinator)
Department of Interior	Support
General Services Administration	Support
Federal Communications Commission	Support

ESF, Emergency support functions; *FEMA,* Federal Emergency Management Agency.

2005, leading to levee breaks and flooding of the city, emergency communications systems were completely destroyed, including power stations, Internet servers, cell phone towers, and 911 services, leading to loss of command and control of the entire disaster response.[7] Additional problems resulted when military assets were not interoperational with civilian communications assets because of security issues.

The 2007 Virginia Tech Massacre, when a student killed two fellow students in a campus dorm at 7 AM, then proceeded to murder 30 others 2 hours later, revealed the need for higher education institutions to communicate information about potential threats quickly and efficiently to everyone who needs to know, as soon as possible.[8] Such communication is mandated by the Clery Act of 1990, as amended on numerous occasions, and includes informing the campus community about a "significant emergency or dangerous situation involving an immediate threat to the health or safety of students or employees occurring on the campus."[9,10]

CURRENT PRACTICE

The National Incident Management System (NIMS) was approved in 2004 as a means to coordinate first responder disaster management between federal, state, and local levels using a military model of command and control.[11] The amended Homeland Security Act of 2006 mandated the creation of an overarching strategy to address emergency communications shortfalls. The Department of Homeland Security's Office of Emergency Communications (OEC) developed the National Emergency Communications Plan (NECP) in 2008 to provide a disaster communication framework for the United States. The NECP outlines a strategy to identify agencies' communication processes, capabilities, and potential obstacles to the deployment of interoperable systems. The plan offers short- and long-term solutions for ensuring interoperability and continuity of communications infrastructure coordination among federal, state, local, and tribal governments. Provision of goals, timeframes, and benchmarks for current and future emergency communications systems is made through the NECP to achieve a baseline level of national standards for interoperable communications.[12]

A declaration of disaster will activate Emergency Support Functions (ESF) where federal agencies provide or support an impacted region. ESF #2 pertains to communications, and the lead and supporting agencies are listed in Table 42-1. Federal agencies are tasked during a disaster to assist with coordination with telecommunications and information technology industries; protect, restore, and repair communications and informational technology infrastructure; and provide oversight of communications within the federal incident management and response structures.[13]

Best practices in disaster settings involve the NIMS Incident Command System (ICS) structure where communication chains are well defined. ICS encourages the use of common communications plans, interoperable equipment, processes, standards, and system designs.[14] The ICS informational flow framework consists of processes, procedures, and systems to communicate timely, accurate, and accessible information promoting situational awareness for all involved stakeholders. Provision of public information must be coordinated and integrated across jurisdictions and organizations to include affected government agencies, the private sector, and others. ICS meets this objective through the Public Information Officer (PIO), the Joint Information System (JIS) and the Joint Information Center (JIC).[15] The JIC integrates critical incident information and provides crisis communications along with public affairs functions through the JIS to ensure timely, accurate, accessible, and consistent communication.

FEMA has multiple communication components involving early warning and notification to support destroyed communications infrastructure. The Integrated Public Alert and Warning System (IPAWS) provides public safety officials with a widespread method to alert and warn the nation's community about crises using the Emergency Alert System (EAS), Wireless Emergency Alerts (WEA), the National Oceanic and Atmospheric Administration (NOAA) Weather Radio, and other public alerting systems from a single interface.[16] FEMA has established Mobile Emergency Response Support (MERS) systems to provide support in disaster-affected regions throughout the United States. In this system, the country is divided into 10 regions. Mobile units are located in each region and can provide assistance in the form of telecommunications with satellite, line of sight microwave, and radio (high frequency [HF], ultrahigh frequency [UHF], and very high frequency [VHF]) communications as well as generators in the event of power failure. HF radio is used to communicate with federal, state, and local emergency centers via the FEMA National Radio Network and FEMA Regional Radio Network. VHF and UHF can be used for local radio communications.[16]

The Government Emergency Telecommunications Service (GETS) supports national leadership; federal, state, local, tribal and territorial governments; and other authorized national security and emergency preparedness users. It is intended for use when entire networks of phone lines are so congested as to be near useless, reducing the chances of successful calls being connected. The system is designed in conjunction with the leading providers of public telephone service to label calls being made through the system as higher priority than routine calls, increasing the chances that such calls can be completed.[17]

There are many resources available to reinforce health systems communications. The Centers for Disease Control and Prevention (CDC) has established the Health Alert Networks, which aim to ensure high-speed Internet access for local health officials, increase capacity for secure communications, improve early warning broadcast alert systems, and optimize general organizational capacity of local systems.[18]

In addition to these established systems, Radio Amateur Civil Emergency Services (RACES) provides certified volunteer personnel to perform many tasks related to augmentation of disaster communications.[19] This public service is intended to assist government agencies and health care facilities in times of extraordinary need by providing or supplementing communications during emergencies where public communication infrastructure has sustained damage.

Accessing and reporting emergencies in North America for disaster and nondisaster events involve a complex system with multiple formats for dispatching local emergency response agencies. In most situations, a 911 telephone call is routed through a dispatch center, also known as a public safety answering point (PSAP), before being referred to the responding agency or agencies including fire, police, and EMS.[20] These systems may be able to localize calls from landline or wireless sources and provide a physical address if enhanced 911 services are available. Resources are dispatched to the scene following local protocols as the situation dictates. Computer-aided dispatch (CAD) provides the priority dispatcher with in-service responder status updates to handle calls-for-service as efficiently as feasible via geolocation of nearby units. Field units may be notified of call details over two-way radios on designated emergency frequencies and may receive text messages with dispatch details through pagers or wireless text services like Short Message Service (SMS).[20]

Dispatch centers may also relay emergency information to the surrounding populace via reverse 911 messages. A recorded message or SMS can be sent out simultaneously to all phones in a preprogrammed area. Notifications including evacuation announcements and routes, shelter information, and potential hazards warnings may be pushed to impacted communities. Reverse 911 warnings have been shown to outperform other evacuation warning sources, as indicated by the high influence and successful hit rate. Individuals who received reverse 911 warnings also were significantly more likely to evacuate, as did those who received warnings from more than one source.[21]

Ambulances en route from the scene may contact base stations or hospitals to notify them of potential inbound patients. In most areas, this point-to-point radio communication is based on VHF band (30 to 300 MHz) and UHF band (300 to 3000 MHz) transmissions that are broadcast via radio towers located at specific sites throughout a service region. UHF and VHF systems both vary widely in functionality, capability, and range. Transmission is affected by intentional and unintentional interference, which can lead to loss of relayed information. Catastrophes such as earthquakes and tsunamis can destroy relay towers or repeaters, the mainstay of VHF/UHF communications to increase range of signal. Obstructions, severe weather, natural disasters, power outages, and military attacks can also render them ineffectual. To allow for the efficient transmission of airwaves, radio towers require a degree of unobstructed space; this lack of obstruction makes them difficult to protect. Even though this type of infrastructure presents a vulnerability, strategic duplication of radio towers may serve as a buffer in the event of distress. Not all radio devices possess encryption functions for transmitted messages.[22]

Local and nearby prehospital and hospital assets would be placed in an emergency operating status upon activation of community mass casualty incident (MCI) or disaster protocols. Medical facility plans are initiated from the moment of disaster notification, based on the potential patients that may present. Response plans are based on the Hospital Incident Command System (HICS) with a recall of employees to support a potential surge of victims. Predetermined rosters with demographic information for hospital staff may be utilized to manually phone, or more efficiently, utilize automated SMS paging of required employees during emergency operations.[22] In addition to establishing a hierarchy, HICS is also essential to clarify the means by which information will be relayed. An emergency operations center (EOC) is activated to coordinate hospital command functions and provide communication links within a facility and to outside agencies and institutions.[23,24]

The Incident Commander (IC) will assign roles to senior staff present. Areas to be addressed should include the following:
- Media communications
- Interfacility communications
- Intrafacility and interdepartmental communications
- Emergency department medical care
- Transfer of stabilized patients out of the emergency department
- Communications between the emergency department and the hospital command center

One person is often assigned to supervise and coordinate each of these tasks. In many cases, hospitals already have public relations staff members who handle media communications so that the main focus of practitioners can remain on patient care. Additionally, the local IC must be able to maintain two-way communication with the disaster site. Information that should be prioritized in such communications includes emergency department capacity, hospital capacity, and potential hazards. A robust intrahospital communications system is beneficial to normal hospital operations in the absence of disaster. These systems may be used to facilitate movement of patients in the hospital and assist in coordinating tasks that could increase overall efficiency of operations.

Accurate communications regarding the status of events can serve to minimize confusion. Even though effective communication should be a goal in any workplace, it is crucial in disaster management. All pathways of communication should be designed to function both up and down the chain of command. Nurses, residents, and physicians should be able to discuss trends or concerns regarding patients with their supervisors, who can then relay these details to superiors to avoid loss of valuable information. Within a hospital, there are several means to alert personnel of potential disasters, plan activation, and status updates. Overhead announcements are often possible, but text paging is a simpler and arguably better means of communicating this information. A list of key personnel is distributed to page operators, and in the event of a disaster, a single SMS message can be sent to all parties via a group page. This is an approach that requires advance discussion and preparation but one that can save considerable time and minimize confusion. Text paging may also be an effective means of communication within individual departments.[25]

Interfacility communications may provide relief when a disaster overwhelms a medical facility. E-mail, telephone, and radio communications are excellent means by which hospitals can maintain contact and ensure that patient care is optimally coordinated. For example, if two hospitals are fairly close in location, specific patients may be directed to the site that is best equipped to manage their presenting concerns. In another scenario, if evidence of potential hazards to caretakers becomes apparent at one facility, it is essential that other facilities at risk be notified.

Communication of resource needs, shortfalls, and availabilities can be facilitated among the hospitals in a community through use of web-based communications tools. Representation of medical needs of communities can occur through the use of a county-based Medical Operations Center, which can report medical needs and situations directly to a county EOC.

A novel disaster communications system was created in the wake of the Station nightclub fire incident in Rhode Island, with grant support from the federal government. A mobile self-contained communications box was created with generator power and satellite communications capabilities that could be interfaced into a hospital's communications system to provide temporary telephone, data, and radio communications. These units were dispersed to all acute care hospitals in the state and tested regularly. However, these units are expensive and require ongoing funding to maintain. These and other systems which are not routinely used and devoted to disaster operations are subject to failure when the sinusoidal disaster funding cycles hit a nadir.

Finally, testing the plan and communication systems with local and interagency exercises at regular intervals ensures competency among users. It is even desirable to incorporate as much of disaster communications systems as possible into routine daily operations.

! PITFALLS

Despite many technological avenues available to relay information, disasters may drastically impact communication infrastructure in an affected community by damaging wireless or radio towers, causing sustained power outages, and overwhelming networks burdened with too many users. Devastation of the communications infrastructure leaves responding agencies and local populations without the ability to coordinate, dispatch medical resources, or relay critical updates.[1] Mitigation strategies to preserve communications in affected areas include developing redundant cellular and radio towers, having on hand backup power supplies such as generators, encouraging the populace to have backup battery-operated radios to receive local updates, promoting texting in lieu of calling which requires less bandwidth, and limiting unnecessary radio traffic.

Additional communication pitfalls include the following:

- The majority of the nation's emergency access is through a legacy 911 system, which is based on 1960s technology. The legacy 911 system does not work with the text messages, data, images, or videos that are now standard use for personal communications and can increase capability through real-time situational awareness on the ground. Reverse 911 is currently not an automatic service, as it requires individuals to voluntarily sign up to receive notices.
- Lack of interoperability of systems and equipment among agencies still exists. A system that works perfectly in one setting but cannot interact successfully with neighboring areas and outside agencies is likely to be of limited use. Local systems should be able to easily integrate into a larger scheme of communications when needs exceed local capabilities.
- Risk communication to populations through news media coverage may be inaccurate or misleading and based on information provided from unofficial sources, without appropriate situational awareness. Validation of information sources is needed to avoid the "fog of war" in disaster settings.
- Hospitals in an emergency operations status are dependent on recall of employees for sustained operations. Recall systems are not a satisfactory solution because of inaccurate or outdated recall lists, inability to contact personnel due to devices not being on or not with individuals, or simply missing the message. Multiple sources of recall may be needed. Periodic testing of the recall system and frequent updates to databases should reduce noncontact of critical personnel.
- Social media and mobile technologies have not been fully integrated into disaster operation plans, and their role and extent of use are not standardized.

SUMMARY

The most important principles of communications related to disaster management are preparation, efficiency, and backup plans. Preparation will ensure that disaster federal management workers know their responsibilities and how to complete them. Efficient communications systems at each facility will optimize the use of technology and help to maintain an effective chain of command. Finally, establishing backup plans will ensure that response workers can carry out their tasks, even in the midst of unpredictable concerns that are so often part of both natural and human-made disasters. In essence, the more focus that is given to communications before a disaster, the better workers will be able to carry out their roles in the event that a disaster occurs.

REFERENCES

1. Donahue A, Tuohy R. Lessons we don't learn: a study of the lessons of disasters, why we repeat them, and how we can learn them. *Homeland Security Affairs*. 2006;2(2). Available at: http://www.hsaj.org/?article=2.2.4.
2. Palttala P, Boano C, Lund R, Vos M. Communication gaps in disaster management: perceptions by experts from governmental and non-governmental organizations. *J Contingencies Crisis Man*. 2012;20(1):2–12.
3. FEMA. Communications & Information Management. Available at: http://www.fema.gov/communications-information-management.
4. Maron DF. How social media is changing disaster response. *Sci Am*. June 7, 2013. Available at: http://www.scientificamerican.com/article/how-social-media-is-changing-disaster-response. Accessed July 30, 2014.
5. Communications. *Final Report: The City of Oklahoma City Alfred P. Murrah Federal Building Bombing*. Stillwater, OK: Fire Protection Publications; 1996:353–364.
6. Amateur Radio Emergency Communications Services. New York City ARECS members and the attacks of September 11, 2001. Available at: http://www.nyc-arecs.org/911.html. Accessed July 30, 2014.
7. Miller R. Hurricane Katrina: Communications & Infrastructure Impacts. Available at: http://www.carlisle.army.mil/DIME/documents/Hurricane%20katrina%20Communications%20&%20Infrastructure%20Impacts.pdf. Accessed July 30, 2014.
8. Davies GK. *Connecting the dots: lessons from the Virginia Tech shootings*. Mag High Learn: Change; Jan-Feb 2008. Available at: http://www.changemag.org/Archives/Back%20Issues/January-February%202008/full-connecting-the-dots.html. Accessed July 30, 2014.
9. Clery Center for Security on Campus. Summary of the Jeanne Clery Act. Available at: http://clerycenter.org/summary-jeanne-clery-act. Accessed July 26, 2014.
10. Federal Student Aid vs Virginia Polytechnic Institute and State University. Docket #11-30-SF Federal Student Aid Proceeding, Decision of the Secretary and Order of Remand. Available at: http://s3.documentcloud.org/documents/813630/department-of-educations-decision-on-va-tech.pdf. Accessed July 30, 2014.
11. US Department of Homeland Security. National incident management system. Available at: http://www.dhs.gov/interweb/assetlibrary/NIMS-90-web.pdf. Accessed July 30, 2014.
12. Department of Homeland Security. National Emergency Communications Plan, July 2008. Available at: https://www.dhs.gov/xlibrary/assets/national_emergency_communications_plan.pdf. Accessed July 30, 2014.
13. FEMA. *Emergency Support Function Annexes: Introduction*. Available at: http://www.fema.gov/media-library-data/20130726-1825-25045-0604/emergency_support_function_annexes_introduction_2008_.pdf. Accessed July 30, 2014.
14. FEMA. ICS review material. Available at: http://www.training.fema.gov/EMIWeb/IS/ICSResource/assets/reviewMaterials.pdf. Accessed July 30, 2014.
15. FEMA. Public information. http://www.fema.gov/public-information. Accessed July 30, 2014.
16. FEMA. Integrated public alert & warning system. http://www.fema.gov/integrated-public-alert-warning-system. Accessed July 30, 2014.

17. Department of Homeland Security. Government emergency telecommunications service. Available at: http://www.dhs.gov/government-emergency-telecommunications-service-gets. Accessed July 30, 2014.

18. Centers for Disease Control. Health alert network (HAN). Available at: http://www.bt.cdc.gov/han/. Accessed July 30, 2014.

19. Radio Amateur Civil Emergency Service (RACES). http://www.qsl.net/races/. Accessed July 30, 2014.

20. Next Generation (NG911) System Initiative: 911 Proof of Concept Test Report. Intelligent Transportation Systems, U.S. Dept of Transportation. Available at: http://www.its.dot.gov/ng911/pdf/NG911_POCTesTReport091708.pdf. Accessed August 4, 2014.

21. Strawderman L, Salehi A, Babski-Reeves K, Thornton-Neaves T, Cosby A. Reverse 911 as a complementary evacuation warning system. *Nat Hazards Rev.* 2012;13(1):65–73.

22. Stephenson R, Anderson P. Disasters and the information technology revolution. *Disasters.* 1997;21(4):305–334.

23. Perry RW. Incident management systems in disaster management. *Disaster Prev Manag.* 2003;12(5):405–412.

24. Perry RW, Lindel MK. Preparedness for emergency response: guidelines for the emergency planning process. *Disasters.* 2003;27(4):336–350.

25. Epstein RH, Ekbatani A, Kaplan J, Shechter R, Grunwald Z. Development of a staff recall system for mass casualty incidents using cell phone text messaging. *Anesth Analg.* 2010;110(3):871–878.

43 | CHAPTER

Mobile Disaster Applications

David T. Chiu, Larry A. Nathanson, and Steven Horng

Patient care in disaster situations is fraught with challenges as varied as the types of disasters that occur. Natural and human-made disasters not only create large numbers of casualties but can also wreak havoc on the infrastructure that modern providers rely on, including the power grid, cell towers, and Internet access. Ubiquitous access to consumer mobile devices, such as smartphones, tablets, and wearable devices, has spurred innovative solutions to the challenges in communication, coordination, and documentation that medical teams encounter during disaster events. Challenges faced by medical professionals during disaster situations include power outages, cell service outages, patient identification, patient tracking, family reunification, emergency medical service(s) (EMS) deployment and resource allocation, health records, loss of electronic medical records, and hospital communications. We present "mobile disaster applications" as a collective term for solutions used in disaster scenarios that help rescue and health care workers overcome these types of challenges.

FORM FACTORS

Commercially available consumer electronic devices such as cell phones can be useful in disasters. A smartphone (e.g., Apple iPhone, Samsung Galaxy S4, Blackberry) with cellular data or Wi-Fi connectivity combined with a camera can be a powerful solution that is inexpensive, readily available, and allows disaster workers to "bring your own device." Their small size makes them easy to carry and be easily available. However, the screen size of most smartphones is relatively small, making it difficult to visualize large amounts of data on-screen at once. This can limit the amount of information that disaster workers can process at one time and makes data entry more cumbersome, particularly for those wearing personal protective equipment.

Tablet computers (e.g., Apple iPad, Samsung Galaxy Tab, Microsoft Surface) solve the issue of small screen size and often offer longer battery life; the tradeoff however is decreased portability and increased difficulty in handling. These problems are not inconsequential, as disaster workers in the field often require both hands to accomplish many tasks and may find limited options for storing their device while maneuvering among patients and providing care. Whereas a smartphone can be dropped into a pocket, tablet computers are harder to carry and more likely to be dropped and/or misplaced. Most consumer electronic devices are not designed for the types of physical challenges that can be found during a mass casualty incident (MCI), including shock, vibration, dust, humidity, water, chemical exposure, and extremes of temperature. Rugged cases are available that meet standards (such as MIL-STD-810G) for imperviousness to such threats. These cases can be cumbersome and add additional weight; these problems must be balanced against the extreme difficulty of repairing or replacing broken components in austere conditions.

A novel class of wearable technologies (e.g., Google Glass, Sony SmartEyeglass) may provide a compromise as they provide many of the functions of a smartphone and can be worn, allowing the user full use of their hands. This form factor has unique features that have tremendous potential for emergency field use. The device can stream live video from the user's point of view so that incident commanders can quickly gain situational awareness in advance of arriving on the scene. The screen is located in the user's peripheral visual field and can provide critical scene safety information or detailed information on the location and conditions of victims in need of rescue. This class of device has tremendous potential, but is currently hampered by limited battery life and heavy dependence on networked resources.

THIN VERSUS THICK CLIENT

When choosing or designing an application for field use, one of the most important initial decisions is whether to use a so-called thin client or a thick client model. Thin client devices relegate the bulk of data processing to a centralized server, using the local device primarily to display information to the user. This is contrasted with thick client devices, which process the data locally on the user's device. The difference is not always completely dichotomous, and it is possible to have an application that draws on the features and benefits of both models.

Each approach has its advantages and disadvantages. Thin client applications typically allow the user to view the output of a program that is running on a remote computer, using communication networks to present the information. This approach requires less powerful hardware and can result in smaller form factors, inexpensive devices, decreased power consumption, and longer battery life. In such models, most logic and data processing occurs on the server, which greatly simplifies maintenance and software updates. One update on the server can instantly improve the functionality for large numbers of users. This type of rapid iterative development can be essential in disasters, as application requirements can change quickly as the situation unfolds and details emerge. Changes can be made both quickly and frequently without having to update individual devices or adding tasks to responders who may already be maximally extended. Most modern web applications are built using the thin client model, resulting in a large reservoir of talent from the web-based software community. However, thin client models are highly dependent on reliable and fast communication channels, most commonly Wi-Fi, cellular data (i.e., 3G, 4G, LTE), or satellite communications. Interruptions in this connectivity (such as damage to cellular infrastructure) can lead to near complete loss of functionality.

Thick client models are more immune to disruptions of infrastructure and can utilize slower and less reliable methods of communication. They do not rely upon a central server for basic functionality and can allow users to continue working, viewing, and entering data while the device is not connected. When connectivity resumes, these systems can upload any data entered and download available updates. Less dependence on communication channels can be advantageous as these networks are doubly threatened. Direct impact from the event often damages the underlying infrastructure; also, the demand on the communication networks increases sharply as the general population engages in health and welfare checks on friends and family in the aftermath. This independence, however, comes at a cost. Devices for thick client models often need more storage, memory, and computing power, which can increase cost and weight and consume more power. Also, data that sit unsynchronized between servers and devices quickly become stale and less actionable. Software on these devices must be updated often, and more effort is required to maintain the devices and address disparate versions that users might be running.

There is no solution that is ideal for all situations. The correct choice depends on the unique characteristics of the scene and the availability of connectivity and can rapidly change as things progress.

PATIENT IDENTIFICATION

As search and rescue teams locate increasing numbers of injured victims, the challenge of tracking these patients becomes difficult. If patients are fortunate enough to be conscious and able to supply their identification information or have identification on them, an immediate issue that arises is how to standardize the identification process among different hospitals or treatment centers, both to track the patient, but also to monitor and allocate resources.

In MCIs such as the Indian Ocean tsunami of 2008 or the Haiti earthquake of 2010, thousands of patients and tens of thousands of bodies required identification. This process can be time-intensive and laborious. Prior to the proliferation of mobile devices, photos taken either on film or digital media required printing and posting on massive physical bulletin boards so that family and friends could attempt to identify the patient. This method requires family members or friends to be geographically located near the disaster. Also, there can be significant delays between capturing, transmitting, printing, and posting physical photos.

With the proliferation of Web 2.0 services and mobile computing, photos can be snapped on tablets and smartphones and then posted on designated websites where identification can then be crowdsourced. This can also work in the reverse direction with family members and friends posting pictures of people who are missing onto similar websites. During disasters, organizations including Google and the National Library of Medicine have set up so-called People Finder websites to help with patient identification and family reunification. Many of these sites use the People Finder Interchange Format (PFIF), which provides a standardized method of storing information and exchanging it between sites. Google's solution has been used for over 10 disasters to date and includes over 600,000 names. However, the utility has been varied, with a notable failure after the 2010 Pakistan floods when the local population had no Internet access.

PATIENT TRACKING

Another major challenge in disaster situations is tracking the patients who are receiving care, from their initial rescue through the acute and recovery phases. Identifying a patient's location after transport from the field can be difficult even when the identity of a patient is known. Different disaster situations require different methods of addressing these challenges. In an MCI where the affected geographic area is limited with one dedicated triage area, such as with a school shooting, the focus shifts to how to get a correctly identified patient from the disaster area to the on-site triage area to the definitive medical care center. Contrast that with a broad natural disaster where the affected area is thousands of square miles with casualties scattered over multiple countries or states. Both scenarios deal with multiple transports to multiple possible locations, which makes keeping track of which facility each patient went to difficult.

Most devices also have global positioning satellite abilities allowing for real time localization. Since most cell phones have built-in cameras, geographical positioning system (GPS), and networking, applications can be created that use these different modalities to help locate and track patients in conjunction with a Geographic information system (GIS).

CELL SERVICE AND INTERNET DISRUPTION

The most obvious problem that arises from disruption of cell service is loss of communication among disaster victims and responders. Whether the communication is to victims from response teams, victims to family members, or vice versa, disasters will cause mass communication disruption. Another challenge is dissemination of information by the disaster management team to the masses.

Beyond the destruction of the mobile network infrastructure, another big issue is network overloading. This problem has been repeatedly seen in disasters where there was no widespread power loss. As victims of the disaster attempt to reach family as well as gather information and garner emergency management recommendations, mobile networks become overloaded, resulting in frequent dropped calls or loss of service.

After a disaster, restoration and preservation of cellular networks are priorities. In recent MCIs, emphasis has been placed on using Short Message Service (SMS) text messaging and social networks to disseminate information and to reassure family members. After the initial blasts of the 2013 Boston Marathon Bombing, authorities urged the public to contact loved ones through Facebook, Twitter, and E-mail. They also urged runners, spectators, and anyone else involved to stay off cellular networks so that police and first responders could access this resource.

Use of social networking and other Web 2.0 modalities is only useful in a society that has adopted regular use of such services. Urging the public to use applications and technology that they have not previously been exposed to would be ineffective during disasters. However, if the community affected already does use social networking technologies, these can be very effective in disseminating information to the masses easily. Furthermore, they can allow one individual to assure multiple friends and family members of their safety, thereby exponentially decreasing the number of calls that previously would have been necessary.

The limitation, beyond the widespread adoption of these applications in daily life, is the ubiquity or lack thereof of smartphones and other web-enabled portable devices. One major difference in communication methods between the 9/11 World Trade Center attacks and the 2013 Boston Marathon Bombing was the availability of mobile devices. In 2001 the iPhone had not yet been created. By 2013, when the bombings occurred, smartphone and tablet ownership was commonplace in Boston. Many of those running who had access to their phones would post on Facebook and Twitter that they were unharmed. Contrast that with 9/11 where many did not know the condition and whereabouts of family members until hours or days later.

Whereas smartphone and similar technologies equipped with social networking sites are clearly beneficial in some disaster events, a plain cell phone with SMS capabilities can also prove to be useful. As previously described, the saturation of cell phone towers with data-intensive calls can be abated by the use of text messages demanding much less data. Messages can also be cataloged and saved, allowing important information to be recorded for review at a later time, whereas telephone conversations can pass information without any record.

RESOURCE MANAGEMENT

Frequently it is assumed that scarcity of resources is the biggest issue that faces incident commanders at disaster situations. This is not always true. The problem sometimes is not a scarcity of resources, but the distribution of resources. Once again, there must be an emphasis on having real-time, up-to-date information about what personnel are available, which receiving facilities have capacity, and what medical resources are available for distribution. In past disasters, much of this information was kept on white boards. The potential for error was large, and often the information was not accurate. Current technology is evolving toward use of web-based disaster management systems such as WebEOC, which allows restricted information to be communicated between facilities, incident command centers at hospitals, and emergency operations centers (EOCs) in local communities, as well as facilitates sharing of resources, personnel, and accountability information. Such a system allows implementation of a web-based tracking system for hospital availability, emergency department status, quantity and severity of patients at each hospital, EMS and other personnel availability, and medical supplies currently available to be distributed.

FEMA's Disaster Reporter application is a thick client application that allows the public to crowdsource and share geotagged images of disasters to provide more timely and accurate situational awareness to emergency responders, decision makers, and the general public. These can be used not only to identify areas in need, but also appropriately allocate needed resources.

There are several open source initiatives like Ushahidi that also provide mobile tools to crowdsource disaster intelligence from the public. Initially created in the aftermath of the disputed 2007 Kenyan election, it uses mashups of crowdsourced intelligence and geomapping to not only record disasters as they unfold, but provide insights that only a consolidated, synthesized view could provide.

❗ PITFALLS

Widespread availability of cameras on smartphones can lead to transmission of photographs that may violate the privacy of individuals who are victims at disaster sites. Without supervision, photographs may be distributed that may be unsuitable for dissemination.

Following an initial terrorist attack, information about the site might be transmitted that reveals security information which could be beneficial to terrorists still operating in the area. Each responding organization should have specific policies and procedures to alert their responders about how to treat such information during the response phase. Just as cameras and photography can be restricted or prohibited by government agencies at military bases, border areas, and around ports, so too such policies and guidelines should be attempted and disseminated to the public to prevent inappropriate transmission of information from a secured area.

SUMMARY

The evolution of new technologies like social networking and mobile online devices has resulted in more efficient ways of communication, patient identification, and family reunification. As our society integrates technology and health care more and more, it becomes increasingly important to have systems in place that can handle a rapid influx of patients, or to have a system in place should the need arise to deploy an information system rapidly in an infrastructure-poor disaster scenario.

SUGGESTED READINGS

1. Chan TC, Killeen J, Griswold W, Lenert L. Information technology and emergency medical care during disasters. *Acad Emerg Med.* 2004;11:1229–1236.
2. Chan TC, Buono CJ, Killeen JP, Griswold WG, Huang R, Lenert L. Tablet computing for disaster scene managers. *AMIA Annu Symp Proc.* 2006;875.
3. Fry EA, Lenert LA. MASCAL: RFID tracking of patients, staff and equipment to enhance hospital response to mass casualty events. *AMIA Annu Symp Proc.* 2005;261–265.
4. Killeen JP, Chan TC, Buono C, Griswold WG, Lenert LA. A wireless first responder handheld device for rapid triage, patient assessment and documentation during mass casualty incidents. *AMIA Annu Symp Proc.* 2006;429–433.
5. Levy G, Blumberg N, Kreiss Y, Ash N, Merin O. Application of information technology within a field hospital deployment following the January 2010 Haiti earthquake disaster. *J Am Med Inform Assoc.* 2010;17(6):626–630.
6. Paul SA, Reddy M, Abraham J, DeFlitch C. The usefulness of information and communication technologies in crisis response. *AMIA Annu Symp Proc.* 2008;6:561–565.
7. Troy DA, Carson A, Vanderbeek J, Hutton A. Enhancing community-based disaster preparedness with information technology. *Disasters.* 2008;32:149–165.

CHAPTER 44

The Role of Social Media in Disasters

Stephen P. Wood

Effective communication is vital during any mass casualty or disaster event.[1] A variety of communication modalities are used in these scenarios, including hard-wired telephones, handheld radios, cellular phones, and text messaging. Social media is a developing platform that allows real-time communication among a network of individuals.[2] It is a construct that utilizes a variety of formats, including web and text, and has been increasingly utilized in disaster communications.[3] Social media is a platform that allows peer-to-network communication using a variety of formats, including social sites such as Facebook, Twitter, and Instagram, collaborative projects such as Wikipedia, gaming sites such as World of Warcraft, content sites such as YouTube, and search engines (Google), among others.[3,4] These web-based formats allow users to develop virtual networks and share information, photographs, videos, and web-links. Moreover, they can be utilized for real-time surveillance and just-in-time education, and activities including interactive gaming. Social media has significant potential in the rapid dissemination of critical information during disasters, and it may replace historical methods such as the emergency broadcast system.[3] Social media use will increase among both providers and victims of disasters, with advancing technology and the spread of smart, hand-held communication devices. The development, defining, and refining of disaster-specific uses for social media platforms is an imperative for disaster and relief workers moving forward.

HISTORICAL PERSPECTIVE

While the concept of networked communication has existed for many years, the specific use of social media in disaster response became prominent after the earthquake in Haiti in 2010.[3] Several platforms including Facebook, Google Maps, and texting provided up-to-the-minute information, mapping resources, funding streams, and communication networks during and in the wake of this disaster.[3] The use of social media has become even more widespread since then. There were approximately 20 million users of the platform Twitter, a networking program that utilizes short, 140 character messages called tweets, after Hurricane Sandy struck the Eastern seaboard in 2012.[5] After Typhoon Haiyan, considered the strongest landfall storm on record, hit the Philippines in 2013, volunteers called micromappers combed through hundreds of thousands of Twitter tweets, and helped to categorize data, such as requests for aid, medical needs, or infrastructure damage.[6]

CURRENT PRACTICE

Social media has become an acceptable, widely used method for disseminating information during crisis and disaster. The use of social media has spread from the individual user to local and state agencies, local law enforcement, as well as large organizations such as the Centers for Disease Control and Prevention (CDC), the Federal Emergency Management Agency (FEMA), and the Red Cross. Simple applications such as Bluelight and other personal safety applications allow members to send a prepared, single text as to their safety and location to a wide network of predetermined individuals with just the press of a button.[7] Peer-to-peer networking has become integral to communications during disasters, providing support, funds, and safety advice.[3,8,9] Mapping has been an integral part of the use of social media. "Geotagging" refers to the use of global positioning systems (GPS) technology to identify the origins of a social media post.[10,11] This can help to identify areas most in need of deliverables, the location of aid tents or other resources, or even where there is military action or violence. This can also be utilized to locate family members, friends, and caregivers, as well as aid organizations, security forces, and others in time of crisis.

Social media has some advantages over traditional communications in that it can reach a broad, preselected audience, is broadcast in real time, and utilizes text, photographs, and video to convey information. Geotagging allows for identification of user location, which could be a useful tool for rescue, hotspot identification, or as a means to identify aid sites, food, water, and medical care. The "Wikipedia Effect" allows for an interactive process for rumor control and for users to continually edit and correct information in real time,[5] which means that users will continually evaluate and edit the posted material for accuracy: this is the format utilized by the popular web-based encyclopedia Wikipedia. In contrast to public service messages, the content is in real time, and it is constantly changed and updated as the situation warrants. Social media is not limited to the integrity of phone lines; it can reach a broader audience simultaneously, as compared with handheld radios. Social media can also be far reaching; anyone with an account to a specific social media outlet can receive news of an event happening across the world, unless the local government has blocked this service.

There are several disadvantages to the use of social media as well. It requires active Internet availability; preselected virtual networks must typically be established; and users can manipulate data without any verification of accuracy. The availability of Internet connection is integral to the use of social media in disasters. The "street-light" effect is an observational bias that results from using the easiest method to gather data.[12] This concept was coined using the example of a gentleman looking for a lost coin under the nearest streetlamp, which provided good lighting, despite having lost the coin a few blocks away; applied to social media, this refers to the fact that postings and information will come from areas that have active Internet and not necessarily the most geographically desperate areas of need.[12] Internet availability in some of the most impoverished nations is lacking, and this is a significant limitation. Even with urbanization, remote areas that are susceptible to strife, crisis, and disaster may not possess the resources to link into social media outlets. Some governments limit or block the use of social media for political purposes, which may be a pitfall for use of this medium for crisis communication. However, recent events in Turkey, where such restrictions were applied, show that resourceful citizens can bypass most restrictions, using proxy servers and other technological methods.

Synthesizing all of the information available can be difficult for consumers. There may be multiple sites or "hashtags," electronic tags that identify a specific topic, which makes synthesizing data difficult for users.[5] Hashtags are a means of categorizing data to make synthesis easier, but if there is not uniform hashtag nomenclature, information can be lost. A good example of this occurred during the Boston Marathon Bombing on April 15, 2013. A multitude of hashtags were used, which made synthesis of important information difficult.[5] Postings on social media sites can degenerate into political and religious arguments that add little to the response and relief efforts, and can create distrust. A review of the postings on a Hurricane Sandy website in 2013 revealed that the most common posts were discussions on government and religion, while safety tips ranked the lowest.[13] Similar issues were seen with student use of social media in the Virginia Tech shootings in 2007.[14] Users can post misinformation without any oversight, and there is no guarantee as to the expertise of the poster providing advice. Monetary scams can also occur with donations intended for providing aid going to untrustworthy or fake sources.

Social media is in its infancy as a means of communication in crisis and disaster. It will continue to develop and mature as technology advances, urbanization centralizes populations, and access to the Internet becomes more far reaching. Methods of oversight will need to be developed to ensure that information is current and accurate. Protocols for identifying geotagged hotspots will need to be developed to identify areas most in need, as well as to guide rescue and relief efforts. Processing and categorizing posts and messages will require significant effort to standardize the immense amount of data created by social media platforms. Last, research efforts will need to continually assess the utility and use of social media platforms in disaster response.

! PITFALLS

- Social media sites do not typically have oversight for editing content, and information can be inaccurate and unsafe.
- Technology may be lacking in areas most prone to crisis and disaster.
- Misinterpretation of geotagged data may delay or misappropriate rescue and relief efforts.
- Unsupervised posting of photographs of disaster sites or disaster victims by responders may compromise scene security or patient

confidentiality. Accordingly social media guidelines[15] should be distributed to disaster responders as part of their initial orientation so as to preclude such events from occurring.

REFERENCES

1. Federal Emergency Management Agency. Available at: http://www.fema .gov/disaster-emergency-communications.
2. Kaplan A, Haenlein M. Users of the world, unite! The challenges and opportunities of social media. *Bus Horiz*. 2010;53(1):61.
3. Keim ME, Noji E. Emergent use of social media: a new age of opportunity for disaster resilience. *Am J Disaster Med*. 2011;6(1):47–54.
4. *The Complete Guide to Social Media from The Social Media Guys*. Available at: http://rucreativebloggingfa13.files.wordpress.com/2013/09/ completeguidetosocialmedia.pdf.
5. Maron D. How social media is changing disaster response. *Scientific American*. 2013; Available at, http://www.scientificamerican.com/ article.cfm?id=how-social-media-is-changing-disaster-response.
6. Gilbert-Knight A. Social media, crisis mapping and the new frontier in disaster response. *The Guardian*. 2013; Available at, http:// micromappers.com/.
7. Foster S. Personal safety apps: the next generation of blue light phones. *Campus Safety*. 2011; Available at, http://www.campussafetymagazine.com/ Blog/Campus-Command-Post/story/2011/09/Personal-Safety-Apps-The- Next-Generation-of-Blue-Light-Phones.aspx.
8. Lobb A, Mock N, Hutchinson P. Traditional and social media coverage and charitable giving following the 2010 earthquake in Haiti. *Prehosp Disaster Med*. 2012;27(4):319–324.
9. Sawchak A. Social media's role in disaster response improves overall organizational resiliency. *Forbes*. 2013; Available at, http://www.forbes.com/ sites/sungardas/2013/10/29/social-medias-role-in-disaster-response- improves-overall-organizational-resiliency/.
10. Anonymous. *Geotagged Photos Facilitate Requests for Federal Aid after Disasters*; 2010. Available at, http://www.pobonline.com/articles/94046- geotagged-photos-facilitate-requests-for-federal-aid-after-disasters.
11. Disaster mapping. Available at: http://citizencyberlab.eu/portfolio/geotag- libya/.
12. Meier P. *Social Media, Disaster Response and the Streetlight Effect*; 2013. Available at, http://irevolution.net/2013/11/07/social-media-disaster- response-and-the-streetlight-effect/.
13. Wood SP. SAEM Regional Conference Poster Presentation. The utility of social media in disseminating information during disasters: The Hurricane Sandy experience. 2013. Presented at Brown University, April 3, 2013.
14. Guth DW. After Virginia Tech: an analysis of Internet and social media use in campus emergency preparedness. *J Emerg Manag*. 2013;11(4):303–312.
15. Virginia Board of Nursing Guidance on the Use of Social Media. Available at: http://www.dhp.virginia.gov/nursing/guidelines/90-48_SocialMedia.doc.

CHAPTER 45

Volunteers and Donations

Andrew M. Milsten

Offering help to people in need is a basic human instinct. During the war in Yugoslavia (1999), thousands of people were able to survive because of donations from foreign governments and private individuals or organizations.[1] Donations and volunteerism can be a help or hindrance, though, depending on whether the right amount of goods, people, and materials are sent to the disaster region. There is a common misperception that when a disaster occurs, people should send everything they have as rapidly as possible. Misperceptions such as this can result in large amounts of wasted human and nonhuman resources. There are two types of donations: in cash and in kind. Cash donations are often ideal because of flexibility, ease of coordination, and because cash allows materials to be purchased through normal channels while supporting the local economy.

The Internet and social media have become efficient methods for obtaining cash donations. During the South Asia Tsunami disaster (2004-2005), large amounts of money were donated rapidly through the Internet, with sites such as Amazon.com collecting upward of $3 million within days of the event.[2] Lobb et al. examined the relationship between media coverage during the 2010 Haiti Earthquake disaster and charitable donations during 4 weeks after the event.[3] Traditional media coverage quickly spiked after the earthquake and then waned over the next 3 weeks, with charitable contributions following this trend. Social media outlets such as Twitter also followed this trend, although they tended to dissipate more quickly. The authors found that Facebook could provide a medium for longer-term engagement. There was a positive correlation with media coverage and donations: "every 10% increase in Twitter messages relative to the peak percentage was associated with an additional US $236,540 in contributions, whereas each additional ABC News story was associated with an additional US $963,800 in contributions." Finally, text messages also were found to be a useful way to gather donations.

The downside to cash donations is that they are susceptible to misuse.[1] Nonetheless, the importance of cash donations cannot be underestimated. Multiple recent disasters show that donors are responding. Médecins Sans Frontières reported that donors gave $150 million for emergency aid after the 2004 Indian Ocean earthquake and tsunami. Within 2 weeks of the tsunami, MSF instructed donors that they had received enough money for tsunami relief and redirected donations to other global emergencies.[4,5]

Donations in kind are less standardized, but while often being immensely helpful, they can cause problems unknown to the donor.[1] In this chapter disaster volunteerism and in-kind drug and blood donations will be examined. It is interesting to note that in-kind donations of materials other than drugs and blood can be important in certain situations. Dzwonczyk and Riha looked at medical equipment donations after the 2010 Haiti earthquake.[6] They inventoried and assessed 951 pieces of clinical medical equipment at seven public Port-au-Prince area hospitals (of which 86% had been donated to these hospitals before the earthquake). They found 28% of the equipment was working and being used; 28% was working and not in use (because of lack of parts and supplies or lack of a location in which to use them, such as an operating room); 30% was not working, but repairable; and 14% was neither working nor repairable. The authors concluded that failure to follow the 2000 World Health Organization (WHO) guidelines for equipment donation lead to these equipment issues.

Overall, coordination of in-cash and in-kind donations remains a challenge. Donations after the 2004 Indian Ocean Earthquake and Tsunami are a good example of these challenges. The worldwide response was estimated at $13 billion, the largest relief effort in history. The United Nations raised $2.5 billion (much of which came from individuals), whereas American companies raised $273 million in-cash and $140 million in-kind donations. However, some companies wanted to do more than just send money or supplies; there was a desire to send communications, managerial, logistical, and IT support. No coordination enabled this to occur. On the ground, the local authorities were already swamped with unsolicited donations. For example, "Sri Lanka's Colombo airport reported that within two weeks of the tsunami, 288 freighter flights had arrived without airway bills to drop off humanitarian cargo ... a large number brought unsolicited and inappropriate items (such as used Western clothes, baked beans, and carbonated beverages), which piled up at the airport, clogged warehouses, and remained unclaimed for months. Worse yet, these prepaid flights refueled and then returned empty, when they could have carried commercial cargo. As a result, the airport ran out of fuel for the scheduled flights." What did work, though, was using corporate partnerships that had already existed in that region. "Coca-Cola, for example, has for years maintained relationships with the Red Cross and other aid agencies in many countries. Working with local subsidiaries, Coca-Cola converted its soft-drink production lines to bottle huge quantities of drinking water and used its own distribution network to deliver it to relief sites."[7]

DRUG DONATIONS

During times of crisis, many different entities provide drug donations, including private individuals or companies, nongovernmental organizations (NGO), international agencies such as the UN, and foreign governments.[8] The literature on this subject, which focuses on disasters, as well as complex humanitarian emergencies such as refugee situations, indicates that many disaster-stricken regions become dependent on foreign medical aid for both acute emergencies and long-term aid.[8,9] Drug donation is a complex issue, however, and even though such donations can help disaster-stricken countries retain their treatment quality and meet health care needs, there are numerous negative outcomes that can occur as well. For example, the common misperception that it is better to send any drug than none at all results in often-inappropriate medical materials arriving in the recipient country.[10] Despite the donors' good intentions, donated drugs and goods are often inappropriate to treat local diseases (e.g., Zaire 1994, commercial soft drinks were sent to treat cholera).[11-13] In addition, a practice known as "drug dumping" often results in large quantities of useless drugs arriving in the disaster-struck region.[14,15] *Drug dumping*, a term meaning the donation of defective products, has been studied both in terms of quantity and quality (e.g., amount, appropriateness, and usability).[8,16]

HISTORICAL PERSPECTIVE: DRUG DONTATIONS

Standardization and management of medical donations has been an issue for years. It was the domain of the Red Cross Movement until 1957. Following World War II, national and international organizations focused on this issue. It was not until after the Gulf War, however, that emergency relief deficiency came under the scrutiny of the UN.[17]

Starting in 1976, reports began appearing about the deleterious effects large amounts of inappropriate donated drugs can have on a recipient country. In 1996 the UN designated WHO the coordinator of health-related international agency work.[17] WHO took several actions to facilitate this mission in Bosnia, including establishing inter-agency coordination committees, assessing needs, coordinating drug supplies, disseminating drug lists and guidelines, and promoting the use of essential drug kits.[18] Despite WHO's efforts, drug donations to Bosnia and Herzegovina were criticized for being of low quality. Frequently the donated drugs had expired, adding to the postwar chaos; drugs were unequally distributed, because NGO were allowed to deliver materials to an area that had recently received similar materials from a different NGO. The influence of the media was often inappropriate, and it could sway what donors gave and how much.[1,8,19-21] Some authors felt these criticisms were "elitist," and noted that, for example, drug expiration dates are extremely conservative and that a possible solution to the problem of expired drugs could be to "perhaps double the usual dose."

These authors also noted that human suffering would be worsened by not using donated drugs.[22] Nevertheless, using expired drugs has generally not been acceptable because of problems related to toxic metabolites and unknown efficacy, for example, which opens the door to bad donation practices and may lead to a loss of credibility for the donors. Moreover, the practice violates the Basel Convention, which regulates the transnational movement of hazardous waste (including unused drugs) and its disposal, and requires the owner, receiver, and transporter of any chemical that could be toxic, poisonous, or eco-toxic to get clearance from the relevant authority in charge of the Basel Convention.[1,8,11,23]

Examples of inappropriate donation practices are shown in Table 45-1. During the war in Sudan, in 1985, inappropriate pharmaceutical donations included contact lens solution, appetite stimulants, cholesterol lowering drugs, and expired antibiotics.[10] In Lithuania (1993), 11 women were temporarily blinded after taking a drug donated by Cartias (closantel, a veterinary anthelmintic) that was mistakenly given to treat endometriosis because of poor labeling.[10,24] In Georgia (1995) 20 tons of expired silver sulphadiazine were received, and Eritrea (1994) received seven truckloads of expired aspirin, a container of unsolicited cardiovascular drugs with 2 months to expire, and 30,000 bottles of expired amino acid infusion (that could not be disposed of because of the smell).[10,25] Other examples of completely nonsensical donations—although not drug donations per se—include bikinis sent to Gujarat (after the earthquake), crates of Double-D bras sent to Kobe (after the earthquake), breast implants sent to a hospital in Malawi, and ski jackets sent to Sri Lanka.[24,26]

U.S. pharmaceutical companies often are saddled with a negative image for their poor donation practices, which may be somewhat justified. For example, Eli Lilly donated six million poorly labeled Ceclor CD tablets, even though the tablets were nearing expiration and had not received Food and Drug Administration (FDA) approval for sale in the United States.[24] There are worthwhile long-term sustainable U.S. pharmaceutical programs, however, including the Merck Mectizan Donation Program (providing free drugs to treat river blindness since 1988), Aventis's partnership with WHO, Roche's policy to make HIV

TABLE 45-1	Examples of Drug Dumping			
YEAR	LOCATION	AMOUNT DONATED (METRIC TONS*)	INAPPROPRIATE AMOUNT	NOTES
1976[9]	Guatemala (earthquake)	100 (7000 cartons)	90% unsorted	1120 hours of sorting time
1984-1985[27]	Ethiopia (famine)	Not listed	Not listed	US $500,000 worth of inappropriate drugs were destroyed
1985[28]	Mexico (earthquake)	1088 Drugs: 31% Food: 14% Supplies, clothes, and blankets: 24%		Heavy machinery 6%-14% (most needed)
1985-1987[11]	Sudan (famine)	Not listed	8 million chloroquine and 500,000 piperazine were expired	380,000 Citramon tablets were banned. Vitamins and baby food were not registered
1989[5,29]	Armenia (earthquake)	5000 Drugs: 65% IV: 20% Consumables:15%	70% Expired: 8% Frozen: 4% Unsorted: 18% Useless: 11% Unidentifiable: 12%	Poorly labeled antibiotics (238 names in 21 languages) Sorting time was 6 mo with 50 people
1992-1996[3]	Bosnia and Herzegovina	27,800-34,800	50%-60%	
1994-1997[23]	Armenia, Haiti, and United Republic of Tanzania	16,500 shipments (no weight listed)	10%-42%	6% expired
2000[19]	Venezuela (floods)	Not listed	70%	$16,000 spent to sort drugs

*1 metric ton = 2204.6 pounds; 1 ton is approximately 40 cubic feet.

protease inhibitors (nelfinavir and saquinavir) available to the developing countries at much reduced costs, and the medical NGO Médecins Sans Frontières that distributes medicines for African sleeping sickness.[24,29]

In 1999 WHO identified six specific problems associated with drug donations, leading to the development of "good practice" guidelines.[20,30,31] The problems identified by WHO were: the donation of drugs irrelevant to the recipient country's situation, unsorted and poorly labeled drugs, low-quality drugs (e.g., expired drugs and returns), ignorance of local administrative procedures, high custom charges to the recipient (because of high declared drug value), and donation of incorrect quantities (too much of some drugs and too little of others).[10,30,32] Many authors agree with the assessment by WHO and add other factors to consider.[20] For instance, Berckmans noted three categories of donations that were sent to Bosnia and Herzegovina: those that conformed to WHO's interagency guidelines for drug donations, miscellaneous medicines (e.g., unsorted drugs and free samples), and large quantities of donated drugs that were useless or unusable (e.g., plaster tape from 1961 and World War II supplies).[8] During the 1985 war in Sudan, the country received drugs that were in small packets and in partly used open blister packets.[9] Another problem with donations to Sudan was that local doctors often were unfamiliar with newly introduced drugs. Further, once the stock of new drugs ran out, patients wished to continue the often more expensive drug, which led to treatment interruptions.[9] In Croatia (1990-1994), it was found that drug donations led to "changes in therapeutic principles," as well as changes in prescribing patterns and organized drug acquisition at the University Hospital Center of Rijeka (e.g., decreased use of cotrimoxazole, ampicillin, and cephalexin and increased use of amoxicillin +clavulanic acid, gentamicin, and cefuroxime).[15] Médecins Sans Frontières also notes that the practice and culture of corporate drug donations does not encourage local production of generic drugs and may hinder the recipient countries' attempts at a sustainable cost-recovery program.[24] Finally, Hogerzeil points out that donation of excessive quantities leads to stockpiling, pilfering, and black market sales.[10,33]

There are many reasons to donate medical materials to a disaster-stricken region, and most donations are well intentioned.[11,18] However, there are several nonaltruistic reasons for donating drugs, such as avoiding drug destruction costs, seeking publicity, disposing of surplus or wasted medicines, political pressure to take action (drug donations "film well"), tax benefits for donor companies and private voluntary organizations (PVO), and stimulating the market for certain products (brand recognition in a potential new market).[8,11,20,24,32] Whether these motivations are viewed as morally corrupt and self-serving or as well intentioned but gone awry depends on perspective, and it constitutes a debate beyond the scope of this chapter.

Whatever the reasons behind it, there are definite consequences to drug dumping, and the resource-strapped recipient country usually suffers them. It is difficult to store, sort, organize, and handle large quantities of donated medical supplies. Researchers studying the situation in Bosnia and Herzegovina had difficulty locating unused medical supplies because the warehouses were subject to restricted access, and their whereabouts were often unknown.[8] There can also be high destruction costs associated with donated unusable drugs: 1 ton of drugs in Bosnia and Herzegovina cost $2000 U.S. dollars to destroy, costing the recipient country a total of $34 million dollars and requiring the construction of incinerator plants—a situation that occurred in Macedonia and Armenia as well.[8,11,31,34] In cases where the drugs are inappropriate to the situation but are usable, the drugs could be shipped to another country rather than be destroyed; however, shipment can cost $2 to $4 million per 1000 metric ton.[31] Other less-tangible destruction costs include health and environmental hazards, as well as storage, handling, and transportation costs, which are often greater than the donated drugs.[8,10] In the wake of the South Asia

Tsunami disaster (2004-2005), there were concerns about empty water bottles littering the environment, as well as medicines no longer needed (morphine) being loose and uncontrolled in Sri Lanka.[26] WHO has developed guidelines for the safe disposal of drugs, including the use of sanitary landfills, encapsulation, inertization, discharge to a sewer, high temperature (1200 °C) incinerators, and chemical waste treatment centers.[11,18,31,34]

The Armenian earthquake situation vividly demonstrates the local costs associated with poor donation practices. In December 1988, Armenia was rocked by an earthquake (6.9 M) in an area populated by 700,000 people. Deaths were estimated between 24,000 and 60,000 people. Three days after the earthquake, international relief from 74 countries arrived, including 5000 tons of medical materials (valued at $55 million U.S.), money, and human resources.[34] Local resources in the ill-prepared region were depleted, and disorganization reigned. The Armenian airport handled 150 landings a day, where unaccompanied shipments were dropped onto the airstrip and left behind. Armenian personnel were quickly overwhelmed as they attempted to locate specific supplies amid the sea of donations and deliver medical materials to the field. It took a month to set up an efficient donation management strategy.[34] Pharmacists spent two thirds of their time searching for appropriate drugs, and it took 50 people 6 months to sort the donations (mostly nonmedical personnel using pharmaceutical textbooks and cross-indexes to decipher the donated drugs).[10,34] There were also problems handling large heavy packages, finding adequate storage space (32 new storage buildings were constructed holding 70% of donations, while the rest were shipped to Moscow), and disposing of drugs destroyed by cold temperatures (4%).[34]

CURRENT PRACTICE: DRUG DONATIONS

Suggested solutions to problems associated with drug donations are based primarily on basic disaster planning techniques, such as preparing for anticipated needs, recognizing that each disaster is different and priorities change, and performing realistic needs analyses.[35,36] Many have advocated for better communication of needs and the exchange of information that is more reliable between recipient countries and donors.[10,11,18] Mitigation planning should be done by countries to help strengthen legislative policies toward donors, centralize drug donations and emergency aid (using principles of good pharmacy practice), put registration and quality-assurance procedures in place, and develop a national essential drug list.[8,10,30]

The Pan American Health Organization (PAHO) and WHO's Supply Management System (SUMA, 1992) is a good example of an information management tool that could help disaster-stricken countries deal with donations more effectively. To help disaster managers to sort through large amounts of donations, the SUMA system uses simple tracking software. SUMA works by prioritizing and collecting data at donation entry points (airport, seaport, or border) and categorizing these items. Other SUMA team members gather data at warehouses and distribution centers and then electronically send this information to the central area. From this area, customized reports detailing donation activity and status can be generated.[37]

WHO has taken the lead on setting standards for good donation practices, with the guidelines promulgated in 1999.[31] WHO started work on these guidelines in 1990 and finished them through an international consultative process involving more than 100 agencies.[10] WHO's guidelines provide core donation principles and contain four categories (Box 45-1 and Table 45-2).[10,19,30,27,38,39] WHO also maintains a list of essential drugs (the Model List, revised in 2003) and encourages each country to produce its own national drug list (focusing on safety, appropriateness, efficacy, and cost-effectiveness).[11,40]

BOX 45-1   WHO Guidelines: Core Principles for Drug Donation

- Maximum benefit to the recipient
- Respect for the wishes and authority of the recipient
- No double standards in drug quality
- Effective communication between donor and recipient

Although WHO's guidelines have not been followed on a consistent basis, such as in Albania, Rwanda, and Somalia, their acceptance appears to be growing, leading to a large change in donation practices.[25,31,27] As Autier points out, however, just developing guidelines is not sufficient for effective coordination. For example, guidelines alone cannot resolve the problems associated with massive quantities of unsolicited donations, weak monitoring systems, high costs of dealing with useless drugs, training gaps, poor coordination, unclear responsibilities, local and traditional values not being respected, dependency on donated goods, and involvement of military personnel unfamiliar with humanitarian work (during the Kosovo crisis in 1999, NATO military staff were unaware of standard humanitarian distribution procedures).[41] Ideally, donation management and coordination would be carried out by small teams of experts, familiar with disasters and able to continually adjust donation demands for community health needs. Organizations with minimal bureaucracy are best suited for this task, especially if they are willing to apply some donated monies earmarked for material purchases (such as drugs) to setting up a coordination system.[23]

WHO also developed the emergency health kit, a standardized kit containing sufficient drugs and medical supplies for 10,000 people, designed for immediate release to a refugee situation.[10,42,28] Both the United Nations Children's Fund (UNICEF) and the International Dispensaries Association stock emergency health kits.[9] The emergency health kits were put together as a short-term use (3 months) commodity that could be utilized while more specific needs assessments are being accomplished and purchases are organized within the country.[42] The kits are prepackaged (easing logistics), and they include suggested treatment schedules, equipment, and two drug lists ("A" has 25 drugs for use by minimally trained health workers; "B" has 31 drugs for prescribing physicians). The emergency health kit evolved after 1990; it was updated in 1998 and was requisitioned and used more than once within the same disaster, which prompted fears of dependency on international suppliers. To combat dependency on the kit, WHO promotes development of country-specific emergency drug lists and supplies based on local disease patterns. Emergency health kits were designed for use during the emergency phase of drought, famine, or war. The kits were not recommended for use in acute onset disasters such as hurricanes or earthquakes (where immediate assistance within 24 to 48 hours exists and health needs widely vary), in situations where the cost of transportation was more than the kit itself, or in countries that have a national emergency formulary. The kit has proven useful; however, the list of drugs it contained has been the most valuable component.[42]

There have been other ideas and regulations put forth to help encourage good donation practices and to eliminate the undesirable practice of drug dumping. The ideas are wide ranging, but the focus is primarily on holding donors accused of dumping accountable for their actions and providing quality-assurance monitoring.[43] Snell notes that donors and "relief agencies need to educate the public about donations and maintain a commitment to high standards of excellence through consultation with media and policy makers."[11] Hillstrom

TABLE 45-2   WHO Donation Guidelines (1999)*

Selection of drugs	• All drug donations should be based on an expressed need and be relevant to the disease pattern in the recipient country. Drugs should not be sent without prior consent by the recipient.
	• All donated drugs or their generic equivalents should be approved for use in the recipient country and appear on the national list of essential drugs, or, if a national list is not available, on the WHO Model List of Essential Drugs, unless specifically requested otherwise by the recipient.
	• The presentation, strength, and formulation of donated drugs, as much as possible, should be similar to those of drugs commonly used in the recipient country.
Quality assurance and shelf life	• All donated drugs should be obtained from a reliable source and comply with quality standards in both donor and recipient country. The WHO Certification Scheme on the Quality of Pharmaceutical Products Moving in International Commerce 7 should be used.
	• No drugs should be donated that have been issued to patients and then returned to a pharmacy or elsewhere, or were given to health professionals as free samples.
	• After arrival in the recipient country, all donated drugs should have a remaining shelf life of at least 1 yr.
Presentation, packing, and labeling	• All drugs should be labeled in a language that is easily understood by health professionals in the recipient country; the label on each individual container should at least contain the INN or generic name, batch number, dosage form, strength, name of manufacturer, quantity in the container, storage conditions, and expiry date.
	• As much as possible, donated drugs should be presented in larger quantity units and hospital packs.
	• All drug donations should be packed in accordance with international shipping regulations, and be accompanied by a detailed packing list, which specifies the contents of each numbered carton by INN, dosage form, quantity, batch number, expiry date, volume, weight, and any special storage conditions. The weight per carton should not exceed 50 kg. Drugs should not be mixed with other supplies in the same carton.
Information and management	• Recipients should be informed of all drug donations that are being considered, prepared, or actually under way.
	• In the recipient country the declared value of a drug donation should be based upon the wholesale price of its generic equivalent in the recipient country, or, if such information is not available, on the wholesale world-market price for its generic equivalent.
	• Costs of international and local transport, warehousing, port clearance, and appropriate storage and handling should be paid by the donor agency, unless specifically agreed otherwise with the recipient in advance.

*INN, International Nonproprietary Name.
From the WHO. *Guidelines for Drug Donations—Revised 1999.* 2nd ed. Available at: http://www.who.int/medicines/library/par/who-edm-par-1999-4/who-edm-par-99-4.shtml.

suggests allowing donations to be used only for care of the ill, needy, or infants, and not allowing donations to be transferred in exchange for money.[32] Further, donations should comply with WHO's guidelines, include proper documentation, and be valued at reasonable market rates to avoid donations made solely for tax deductions.[32,44] Thomas recommends that any U.K. pharmaceutical company taking a deduction in its tax bill for donations should list the donation in its annual accounts (published publicly).[24] Thomas also suggests a change in the laws that would give the tax credit to the recipient country and not allow any donations that fall outside of WHO guidelines to receive benefits.[24] Britain (2002) announced a series of measures that would ease access to essential medicines for many poor people living in developing countries. These measures include funding research into new treatments for the three "target" diseases identified by the UN (malaria, TB, and AIDS), as well as legislation encouraging donations of medicines by U.K.-based pharmaceutical companies.[24] WHO recommends that donors pay attention to logistical issues, such as proper documentation, looking into applicable local laws, considering warehouse costs and weather, and obtaining better information from the recipient.[1] Other WHO suggestions include allocating resources at the beginning of an emergency situation for coordinating donations, creating collection centers, setting donation and national drug policies, and educating the public.[1,44]

Bero et al. reviewed the literature from 2000 to 2008 concerning WHO drug donation compliance and found that most drug donation issues stemmed from donations during emergencies. For the most part, WHO drug donation guidelines do not require major change, but stricter enforcement is needed. The authors point out several interventions that could make the whole system run more smoothly. These include better monitoring and coordination of incoming medicines with fieldwork and real-time monitoring. They suggest surveillance of the donated drugs with an independent registry for coordination (e.g., the Donations of Medicines Eligibility Program, launched by the Canadian International Development Agency [CIDA] in 2008).[45] Coordination of drug donations is made more complex and vulnerable to inefficiency because there are multiple agencies working to give medicines in a time of crisis, such as governmental organizations, NGOs, ministries of health, manufacturers, and donor agencies.[46] It is important for individual countries to formulate their own national drug donation guidelines to avoid receiving unnecessary medicines. This list should also include financial and human resources that would cover logistical and financial issues arising from donations.[45]

Recurring issues with disaster-related donations were found consistently. These included failing to meet the needs of the country; many unsolicited, unnecessary, or insufficient drug donations; inability to reject unsolicited donations; incomplete coordination among donors, leading to duplications; donation of expired medicines, those with short shelf lives and improperly labeled drugs; and excessive, unorganized donations that lead both to local aid workers being overwhelmed and increased costs (hiring workers, storage, transportation, processing, and eventual disposal. In Aceh, Indonesia, the government spent > $3 million U.S. to dispose of drugs); excessive donations also led to space issues, where these drugs would take up space that could have been used as a shelter.[45,46] Further, excessive donations can lead to downstream harm to the local pharmaceutical economy as the market becomes saturated. The issue of excessive donations and issues of storage space limitations was believed to have caused harm in Sri Lanka. "There is evidence suggesting that in Sri Lanka improper storage of an anaesthetic agent left over from a donation in 2005 led to contamination with *Aspergillus fumigatus* and to the death of three pregnant women who contracted nosocomial meningitis after receiving spinal anaesthesia for Caesarean sections."[45]

BLOOD DONATIONS

Blood donations are "part of the altruistic response of the general public."[47] After a disaster, people donate blood because of an awareness of the need for blood in the community, a sense of social obligation or duty, personal social pressure, the need to replace blood used by a friend or relative, and to increase self-esteem.[48] These reasons seem to outweigh the reasons people do not donate, such as fear, inconvenience, perceived medical disqualification, being too busy, not being asked, and apathy.[48] As people are inspired to donate blood after a disaster, the number of first-time donors increases. This effect does not persist, though, and the return donation rates for first-time donors remains around 30%.[49]

Staggering amounts of blood are donated after a disaster.[50] Within 5 days after the 1989 San Francisco Earthquakes, donations were up 200% from baseline (in affected and unaffected cities).[47] After the 9/11 terrorist attacks (in 2001), blood donations increased 1.3- to 2.5-fold. Mass appeal and blood drives led to the collection of 572,000 units, with enough blood to serve the situational needs collected by the second day. The overwhelming response included 12,000 phone calls (to blood banks) and 5000 units donated in 24 hours, 1800 units of blood escorted by police into the area, and the public lining up for hours and organizing themselves by blood type.[51] Although flights were grounded, the American Red Cross activated its aviation incident response team and mobilized 50,000 units of blood from around the country to be shipped by military transport.[48,51]

Further reports from American Blood Centers (75 centers collecting half of the volunteer blood supply in the United States) noted 259,000 people donating during the 4 days after the attacks (increase 3 times the normal level).[52] Moreover, the Red Cross reported 615,995 donations at 36 sites (double the normal level).[52] So much blood was donated outside of hospitals, that 208,000 units of blood were discarded in the weeks after 9/11 (5 times the normal amount discarded), and in the end, only 206 units of blood were used for individuals injured in the attacks.[53]

DISASTER VOLUNTEERISM

Volunteer numbers also surge after disasters. With proper management and direction, volunteers can accomplish a lot; otherwise, they may hinder the response and become a logistical problem.[35] Some authors believe that "what the public does (individually and collectively) will make the biggest difference in the outcome of a disaster," and that volunteers can be integrated into the disaster response.[54,55] Others note, however, that "freelancing" medical personnel and "convergent volunteerism" are system problems that are disruptive to disaster management.[54,56] Convergent volunteerism has been defined as the unexpected or uninvited arrival of personnel wishing to render aid at the scene, who then engage in freelancing (operating at an emergency incident scene without the knowledge of the command authority).[56] Most volunteer convergence occurs for two reasons; first, officials overestimate the damage and issue requests from the scene to "send everything you've got," and, second, the immediate shortfall of official responders is filled by bystanders.

The American College of Emergency Physicians (ACEP) and the National Association of EMS Physicians (NAEMSP) weighed in on this issue with a joint statement where unsolicited medical personnel who respond to a disaster scene require organization under the established Incident Command System (ICS) medical unit. Further, these organizations state, "volunteer medical personnel (physicians, nurses, emergency medical technicians, etc.) should not respond to a disaster scene unless officially requested by the jurisdiction's established ICS. All personnel must understand the authority and resources of local EMS and health care systems, the importance of staffing their facilities as their primary responsibility, and the dangerous conditions associated with on-site operations."[57]

Certainly, most disasters can benefit from volunteers. Civilian volunteer organizations such as the Red Cross, Voluntary Organizations Active in Disasters (VOAD), and the New York City (NYC) Mayor's Voluntary Action Center allow people to get involved and be helpful where needed.[58] NYC has civilian volunteer managers who are experts in this field but were underused during the initial phases of 9/11.[58] Aside from large civilian volunteer organizations, most volunteers in disasters do so because of timing, situation, and a desire to help others. Spontaneous volunteers are particularly important for early search and rescue. During the Nimitz Freeway collapse (Loma Prieta Earthquake), 50 people were rescued; 49 by bystanders. These volunteers fashioned backboards out of road signs and then waited hours for emergency medical services (EMS) to arrive.[55] Bystanders frequently conduct immediate uncoordinated search and rescue (mostly during large multisite disasters where EMS is disrupted) and will leave once they feel adequate EMS services have arrived.[54,55,59,60] Because bystanders and victims accomplish most immediate search and rescue, it seems wise to plan around this, instead of completely discouraging it. Emergency responders can be trained to direct and coordinate these efforts—especially because it is the spontaneous volunteers who often know who is missing and where they were last seen. During the 1998 Swissair crash, local firefighters and anglers were organized into search and rescue boat groups ("recovery volunteers"), while other local residents ("instrumental volunteers") performed supportive roles. Unfortunately, and not for lack of effort or organization, they found no survivors, only wreckage and human remains. The volunteers were given inadequate support (46% to 71% of volunteers suffered from posttraumatic stress disorder).[61]

Nevertheless, volunteers can become a liability at disasters when they hinder logistics, cross roles, compromise safety and control, and do not follow proper incident command structure or medical oversight.[62] Anecdotally from 9/11, there are stories of surgical medical students wearing scrubs and carrying sterile thoracotomy kits around the World Trade Center (WTC) collapse zone. Clearly, though well intentioned, these types of efforts are ill conceived and have substantial risks with minimal benefits.[56] For example, a nurse who attempted to offer assistance without proper on-scene protective gear at the Oklahoma City Murrah Building Bombing was killed by falling debris.[63] In addition to the concern about safety and training, there is also the issue of medical malpractice liability coverage. The Emergency Management Assistance Compact (EMAC) allows medical volunteers to function in an official disaster capacity with tort liability and worker's compensation coverage. Congress ratified EMAC in 1996, and all 50 states and three territories have adopted it.[64]

How nonmedical volunteers fit into to the disaster response, stay safe, and remain culturally sensitive are all questions. Nelan and Grineski conducted a survey of nonmedical volunteers to the 2010 Haiti Earthquake. They surveyed 660 individuals who worked with a U.S.-based NGO and had a 16% response rate. Despite this low response rate, they were able to garner some interesting information about volunteer behaviors. Most volunteers were young, single, highly educated females, with prior volunteer experience, and were from household incomes below $30,000 a year. Most volunteers were decently protected with 61% taking antimalarial pills and most using sunscreen with bug repellent (females more so than male volunteers). Risky behavior among nonmedical volunteers was an area of some concern with 25% having unprotected sexual relations; 30% using tobacco products; 87% consuming alcohol (including 27% who drank moonshine); and

leading a lifestyle after work described as "disaster junkie culture."[65] Barsky and colleagues examined how unsolicited nonmedical volunteers interacted with the Federal Emergency Management Agency (FEMA) urban search and rescue teams. These urban search and rescue (USAR) teams overall felt that volunteers are a resource that needs channeling. The volunteers are evaluated by USAR personnel by their legitimacy, utility, and liability, and they are considered useful for certain important on-scene tasks, such as a bucket brigade.[66]

HISTORICAL PERSPECTIVE: VOLUNTEERISM

Volunteers have been referred to as the "silver lining" in the cloud of disasters, and seen as heroes with a badge of honor. Feelings of patriotism, courageousness, spirituality, sense of duty, and even guilt compel people to volunteer.[58,67,68] Volunteerism benefits the community, as well as the individual donating his or her efforts, by allowing the individual to do something "constructive and communal for his or her own mental health, as an outlet for rage, and to overcome the sense of powerlessness."[58] Generally, volunteers tend to be people who believe in the good intentions and honesty of others; they are agreeable, altruistic, and sympathetic.[69] Further, a study by Elshaug found that volunteers were easygoing, active, energetic, and able to concentrate on the task at hand.[69]

Understanding the public's disaster response is important for realistic disaster planning.[54,55] Studies of public behavior during disasters have shown that panic is extremely rare in these situations. Certain situations, though, such as being trapped in a burning building, can lead to panic (Coconut Grove Night Club Fire of 1942), but again this is rare. Extensive studies of over 900 building fires (including the WTC attacks in 1993 and 2001 and the Beverly Hills Supper Club Fire) failed to find any panic.[70,71]

What role volunteers play during a disaster is another question. The literature deals primarily with convergent volunteerism by medical, fire, law enforcement, and civilian personnel.[56] Bissell put forth some general rules for individual roles in disaster situations, including that physician intervention should be at the triage area (except entrapment situations), that only specially trained physicians and nurses should work in the field environment, and that a physician's primary role is at the hospital.[60] Most physicians are not trained to work in austere environments, such as a California bus accident where on-scene volunteer physicians and nurses contributed to a chaotic scene by "performing poorly" (such as not knowing basic CPR).[56,72] Physician roles can become even more confused when individuals with various academic training levels are on scene (medical student, resident, and attending) and most of the rescue personnel do not understand the difference between them and cannot verify credentials. Medical personnel perform best when they do tasks similar to their day-to-day activities.[35,63,73]

Convergent volunteers often tend to be viewed as an unwanted nuisance by disaster planners, whose conception of a disaster response often focuses exclusively on the activities of authorized agencies.[55] Some, for example, have complained that convergent volunteers create problems with protocol adherence, crowd control, security, safety, patient tracking and liability, and accountability, and that they have to be provided with food, shelter, and sanitary facilities.[56,74] However, field disaster research studies have shown that most initial search and rescue, casualty care, and transportation in disasters is not carried out by police, fire, or EMS, according to a disaster plan. Rather, it is carried out on an ad hoc basis by untrained citizens (family members, coworkers, neighbors, and persons who just happen to be in the area).[55,75]

This often occurs because early in the disaster response, there are not enough authorized and trained people available to do the job, when and where it needs to be done. In that case, bystanders, the victims themselves, and other persons fill in the gap. Sometimes, some simple measures by the first arriving police, fire, or EMS units can help to guide and channel the efforts of bystander volunteers and make their efforts more effective. For example, after a tornado struck Waco, Texas, in 1953, initial search and rescue was uncoordinated and inefficient. However, military workers subsequently brought organization to the rescue efforts by incorporating civilian volunteers into their teams. Most of these teams were composed of 15 men under a leader and an assistant leader, along with another person carrying a walkie-talkie to keep in contact with headquarters and other nearby teams. Signs were put up showing each team's area of operation.[76] Disaster plans should include provisions indicating who is responsible for coordinating spontaneous volunteers working at the scene. Disaster training and drills should also address this responsibility.

Volunteer convergence at hospitals can lead to problems with safety and quality care.[77] Hospitals have to comply with the Joint Commission's standards for emergency credentialing of physicians and nurses. Acceptable sources of identification include a current picture hospital ID card, a current license to practice with picture ID, DMAT membership, or verification of the volunteer's identity by a current member of the hospital staff.[77] A volunteer's licensure and competency should be verified through a set process, including shadowing a staff physician.[77]

CURRENT PRACTICE: VOLUNTEERISM

The effectiveness of physician volunteers may be enhanced to be integrated into a planned response (e.g., one coordinated by the local medical society, Metropolitan Medical Response System, or Medical Reserve Corps). Knowledge of the ICS is also a useful asset.[35] This type of integration worked in the wake of the 1995 Murrah Building Bombing, the 1985 Mexico Earthquake, the 1953 Waco Tornado, and the 1994 Northridge Earthquake (where volunteering nurses were integrated into the Visiting Nurse Association through the local emergency medical services agency).[50,55,74,78] Physicians who become involved with patient care outside of the hospital should try not to deter EMS personnel from following their protocols, unless there is a compelling reason to do so, and after consulting with their base station physician, if it is possible.[56] Medical personnel should ignore overly hyped media reports and understand credible calls for help and the normal channels they go through.[54] On the other side, the government officials or news media that are calling for volunteers or donations should check with the intended recipients to see what kind of help is really needed. Further, government officials should inform the news media proactively when volunteers or donations are not needed.[55]

Various guides, such as those produced by the states of California and Florida, discuss ways of handling volunteer convergence among the public.[79,80] Some authors report that the public is "treated as an unwanted nuisance by professionals," and the yellow tape perimeter acts as physical and psychological barrier.[55] Instead of pushing the public into a secondary role, Glass suggests getting the public involved through announcements, forming partnerships, and mobilizing local organizations. Because it is a virtual certainty that untrained members of the public will become involved in casualty care in widespread disasters, it is important to provide them information on how they can protect themselves and help others. This can be provided before an event and can be supplemented by real-time information during a disaster. Examples include how to shelter-in-place; how to decontaminate exposed persons; how to shut off gas and electricity; where to obtain antidotes, potassium iodide, or prophylactic antibiotics; and what hospitals and medical facilities are open and least crowded and where they are located.

Further, disaster personnel should enlist the media as an ally, as was done during Hurricane Andrew, when a Homestead, Florida, area AM radio announcer was credited with saving many lives by instructing people to get into their bathtubs and cover themselves with mattresses.[55] In addition, it is important to educate volunteers, perform community-wide rapid needs assessment, set up statewide medical mutual aid radio systems, and announce what type of donations and volunteers are needed.[54] The Joint Commission recommends promoting community emergency preparedness plans. This comprises enlisting the community in local response preparations, encouraging an emergency preparedness focus, developing emergency planning and preparedness templates, preserving local health care, and establishing leadership and sustainment.[81] The development of local Community Emergency Response Teams (CERTs)[82] in many U.S. communities has resulted in many individuals being trained in how to respond in their immediate neighborhoods to earthquakes and other mass casualty situations, before first responders arrive, and such programs supply a hard hat and other basic gear to participants, along with experience in triage exercises and basic shoring techniques.

The Emergency System for Advanced Registration of Volunteer Health Professionals (ESAR-VHP) is a program of the U.S. Department of Health and Human Services that consists of a national network of state-based registries to allow medical professionals the opportunity to preregister and get their licenses and credentials verified before a disaster happens.[83] They then provide a pool of potential volunteers who can be called upon by the states for a variety of needs.

REFERENCES

1. WHO. *Private Donations: An Ounce of Prevention is Worth a Pound of Cure;* 1994. Available at: http://apps.who.int/medicinedocs/documents/s21258en/s21258en.pdf. Accessed January 23, 2015.
2. Markon J, Smith L. Internet sparks outpouring of instant donations. *Wash Post.* 2004;A1, A23.
3. Lobb A, Mock N, Hutchinson PL. Traditional and social media coverage and charitable giving following the 2010 earthquake in Haiti. *Prehosp Disaster Med.* 2012;27(4):319–324.
4. Eggertson L. Tsunami donations help worldwide. *CMAJ.* 2006;174(3):299.
5. Butler D. Agencies fear global crises will lose out to tsunami donations. *Nature.* 2005;433:94.
6. Dzwonczyk R, Riha C. Medical equipment donations in Haiti: flaws in the donation process. *Rev Panam Salud Publica.* 2012;31(4):345–348.
7. Thomas A, Fritz L. Disaster relief, inc. *Harv Bus Rev.* 2006;84(11):114–122, 158.
8. Berckmans P, Dawans V, Schmets G, Vandenbergh D, Autier P. Inappropriate drug-donation practices in Bosnia and Herzegovina, 1992 to 1996. *N Engl J Med.* 1997;337(25):842–845.
9. Khare AK. Drug donations to developing countries. *World Hosp Health Serv.* 2001;37(1):18–19, 33–34.
10. Hogerzeil HV, Couper MR, Gray R. Guidelines for drug donations. *BMJ.* 1997;314(7082):737–740.
11. Snell B. Inappropriate drug donations: the need for reforms. *Lancet.* 2001;358(9281):578–580.
12. Smego Jr RA, Gebrian B. Donation of medicines to developing countries. *Clin Infect Dis.* 1994;18(5):847–848.
13. WHO. Getting the best from drug donations. *Essent Drugs Mon.* 1996. Available at: http://apps.who.int/medicinedocs/documents/s16516e/s16516e.pdf. Accessed January 23, 2015.
14. Lacy E. Pharmaceuticals in disasters. In: Hogan DE, Burstein JL, eds. *Disaster Medicine.* Philadelphia, PA: Lippincott Williams & Wilkins; 2002:34–40.
15. Vlahovic Palcevski V, Vitezic D, Palcevski G. Antibiotics utilization during the war period: influence of drug donations. *Eur J Epidemiol.* 1997;13(8):859–862.

16. Ali HM, Homeida MM, Abdeen MA. "Drug dumping" in donations to Sudan. *Lancet.* 1988;1(8584):538–539.

17. Gray R. Standardization of health relief items needed in the early phase of emergencies. *World Health Stat Q.* 1996;49(3–4):218–220.

18. Forte GB, Alderslade R. Inappropriate drug-donation practices in Bosnia and Herzegovina. *N Engl J Med.* 1998;338(20):1473, author reply 1473–1474.

19. Bonn D. Call made for application of drug-donation guidelines. *Lancet.* 1999;353(9170):2131.

20. Saunders P. Donations of useless medicines to Kosovo contributes to chaos. *BMJ.* 1999;319(7201):11.

21. Kent D, Glatzer M. Inappropriate drug-donation practices in Bosnia and Herzegovina. *N Engl J Med.* 1998;338(20):1472, author reply 1473–1474.

22. Hoehn JB. Inappropriate drug-donation practices in Bosnia and Herzegovina. *N Engl J Med.* 1998;338(20):1472–1473, author reply 1473–1474.

23. Autier P. Inappropriate drug-donation practices in Bosnia and Herzegovina. *N Engl J Med.* 1998;338(20):1472, author reply 1473–1474.

24. Thomas M. *Drug Donations: Corporate Charity or Taxpayer Subsidy?* London: War on Want; 2002, 28.

25. Schouten E. Drug donations must be strictly regulated. Georgia has tight guidelines. *BMJ.* 1995;311(7006):684.

26. Barta P, Bellman E. Sri Lanka is grateful, but what to do with ski parkas? Well-meaning donors send heaps of useless stuff: pajama tops, no bottoms. *Wall Street J.* 2005;A1.

27. Ahmad K. WHO releases stricter guidelines on emergency drug donations. *Lancet.* 1999;354(9182):928.

28. WHO. *The New Emergency Health Kit.* 1998, Available at: http://www.who.int/disasters/tg.cfm?doctypeID=12. Accessed October 31, 2014.

29. *Roche Drug Donation Policy.* Available at: http://www.roche.com/pages/downloads/sustain/pdf/drug_don_pol.pdf. Accessed January 23, 2015.

30. Reich MR, et al. Pharmaceutical donations by the USA: an assessment of relevance and time-to-expiry. *Bull World Health Organ.* 1999;77(8):675–680.

31. WHO. *WHO Calls for Good Drug Donation Practice During Emergencies as It Issues New Guidelines;* 1999. Available at: http://www.who.int/hac/techguidance/guidelines_for_drug_donations.pdf. Accessed January 23, 2015.

32. Hillstrom S. *Charitable Donations of Drugs by Corporations;* 2000. Available at: http://www.drugdonations.com.

33. Aplenc R. Inappropriate drug-donation practices in Bosnia and Herzegovina. *N Engl J Med.* 1998;338(20):1472, author reply 1473–1474.

34. Autier P, Férir MC, Hairapetien A, et al. Drug supply in the aftermath of the 1988 Armenian earthquake. *Lancet.* 1990;335(8702):1388–1390.

35. Waeckerle JF. Disaster planning and response. *N Engl J Med.* 1991;324(12):815–821.

36. Rottman SJ. Priorities in medical responses to disasters. *Prehospital Disaster Med.* 1989;5(1):64–66.

37. *Humanitarian Supply Management System.* Available at: http://www.disaster-info.net/SUMA/english/. Accessed January 23, 2015.

38. d'Alessio R. *Drug Donations.* Pan American Health Organization. Available at: http://www.paho.org/english/PED/te_ddon.htm.

39. WHO. *Guidelines for Drug Donations—Revised 1999;* 1999. Available at: http://www.who.int/medicines/library/par/who-edm-par-1999-4/who-edm-par-99-4.shtml.

40. WHO. *The WHO Model List of Essential Medicines;* 2003. Available at: http://www.who.int/medicines/publications/essentialmedicines/en/. Accessed January 23, 2015.

41. Borrel A, Taylor A, McGrath M, et al. From policy to practice: challenges in infant feeding in emergencies during the Balkan crisis. *Disasters.* 2001;25(2):149–163.

42. Simmonds S, Mamdani M. Essential drug lists and health relief management. *Trop Doct.* 1988;18(4):155–158.

43. WHO. *WHO Medicines Strategy 2004–2007: Countries at the Core;* 2004. Available at: http://apps.who.int/medicinedocs/en/d/Js5416e/. Accessed January 23, 2015.

44. WHO. *Managing Drug supply, in Essential Drugs Monitor;* 1998. Available at: http://apps.who.int/medicinedocs/pdf/whozip10e/whozip10e.pdf. Accessed January 23, 2015.

45. Bero L, Carson B, Moller H, Hill S. To give is better than to receive: compliance with WHO guidelines for drug donations during 2000–2008. *Bull World Health Organ.* 2010;88(12):922–929.

46. Pinheiro CP. Drug donations: what lies beneath. *Bull World Health Organ.* 2008;86(8):580-A.

47. Busch MP, Guiltinan A, Skettino S, Cordell R, Zeger G, Kleinman S. Safety of blood donations following a natural disaster. *Transfusion.* 1991;31(8):719–723.

48. Glynn SA, Busch MP, Schreiber GB, et al. Effect of a national disaster on blood supply and safety: the September 11 experience. *JAMA.* 2003;289(17):2246–2253.

49. Tran S, Lewalski EA, Dwyre DM, et al. Does donating blood for the first time during a national emergency create a better commitment to donating again? *Vox Sang.* 2010;98(3 Pt 1):e219–e224.

50. Zeballos JL. Health aspects of the Mexico earthquake—19th September 1985. *Disasters.* 1986;10(2):141–149.

51. Becker C, Galloro V. An overwhelming response. Within hours of the disaster, medical supplies were on their way to N.Y., D.C. *Mod Healthc.* 2001;31(38):18–19.

52. Villarosa L. Out to do good, some first-time blood donors get bad news. *New York Times.* 2001;B6.

53. Meckler L. Five times more blood discarded than is usual. *Standard-Times.* 2002;A7.

54. Auf der Heide E. Convergence behavior in disasters. *Ann Emerg Med.* 2003;41(4):463–466.

55. Glass TA. Understanding public response to disasters. *Public Health Rep.* 2001;116(suppl 2):69–73.

56. Cone DC, Weir SD, Bogucki S. Convergent volunteerism. *Ann Emerg Med.* 2003;41(4):457–462.

57. Asaeda G, Cherson A, Richmond N, Clair J, Guttenberg M. National Association of EMS Physicians. American College of Emergency Physicians: Unsolicited medical personnel volunteering at disaster scenes: a joint position paper from the National Association of EMS Physicians and the American College of Emergency Physicians. *Prehosp Emerg Care.* 2003;7(1):147–148.

58. Ellis SJ. *A Volunteerism Perspective on the Days after the 11th of September;* 2001. Available at: http://www.energizeinc.com/hot/01oct.html. Accessed March 17, 2014.

59. Barbera JA, Lozano Jr M. Urban search and rescue medical teams: FEMA Task Force System. *Prehospital Disaster Med.* 1993;8(4):349–355.

60. Bissell RA, Becker BM, Burkle Jr FM. Health care personnel in disaster response. Reversible roles or territorial imperatives? *Emerg Med Clin North Am.* 1996;14(2):267–288.

61. Mitchell TL, Griffin K, Stewart SH, Loba P. 'We Will Never Ever Forget': the Swissair flight 111 disaster and its impact on volunteers and communities. *J Health Psychol.* 2004;9(2):245–262.

62. Cook L. The world trade center attack. The paramedic response: an insider's view. *Crit Care.* 2001;5(6):301–303.

63. Martinez C, Gonzalez D. The World Trade Center attack. Doctors in the fire and police services. *Crit Care.* 2001;5(6):304–306.

64. Lopez W, Kershner SP, Penn MS. EMAC volunteers: liability and workers' compensation. *Biosecur Bioterror.* 2013;11(3). http://www.ncbi.nlm.nih.gov/pubmed/24041195.

65. Nelan M, Grineski SE. Responding to Haiti's earthquake: international volunteers' health behaviors and community relationships. *Int J Mass Emerg Disasters.* 2013;31(2):293–314.

66. Barsky LE, Trainor JE, Torres MR, Aguirre BE. Managing volunteers: FEMA's urban search and rescue programme and interactions with unaffiliated responders in disaster response. *Disasters.* 2007;31(4):495–507.

67. Ruderman SR. Convergent volunteerism. *Ann Emerg Med.* 2003;42(6):847.

68. Adelman DS. Reaction to disaster volunteering not what I expected. *Nurse Educ.* 2002;27(1):5.

69. Elshaug C, Metzer J. Personality attributes of volunteers and paid workers engaged in similar occupational tasks. *J Soc Psychol.* 2001;141(6):752–763.

70. Noji EK. The nature of disaster: general characteristics and public health effects. In: Noji EK, ed. *The Public Health Consequences of Disasters.* New York, NY: Oxford University Press; 1997:3–20.

71. Auf der Heide E. Common misconceptions in disasters: panic, the "disaster syndrome," and looting. In: O'Leary M, ed. *The First 72 Hours: A*

Community Approach to Disaster Preparedness. Lincoln (Nebraska): iUniverse; 2004:340–380.

72. Lewis FR, Trunkey DD, Steele MR. Autopsy of a disaster: the Martinez bus accident. *J Trauma.* 1980;20(10):861–866.

73. Wegner D, James TF. The convergence of volunteers in a consensus crises: the case of the 1985 Mexico City Earthquake. In: Dynes RR, Tierney KJ, eds. *Disasters, Collective Behavior, and Social Organization.* Newark: University of Delaware Press; 1994:229–243.

74. Team OCDM. *Final Report: Alfred P. Murrah Federal Building Bombing, April 19, 1995.* Stillwater, OK: Fire Protection Publications; 1996, B-114, C-246.

75. Auf der Heide E. Principles of hospital disaster planning. In: Hogan D, Burnstein JL, eds. *Disaster Medicine.* Philadelphia, PA: Lippincott Williams & Wilkins; 2002:57–89.

76. Moore HE. *Tornados over Texas: A Study of Waco and San Angelo in Disaster.* Austin, TX: University of Texas Press; 1958.

77. Downs K, Jefferies C, Klass M. Credential volunteers during disasters. *Hosp Peer Rev.* 2003;28(8):108–110.

78. Stratton SJ, Hastings VP, Isbell D, et al. The 1994 Northridge earthquake disaster response: the local emergency medical services agency experience. *Prehospital Disaster Med.* 1996;11(3):172–179.

79. State of California, Governor's Office of Emergency Services. *They Will Come: Post-Disaster Volunteers and Local Governments;* 2001. Available at: http://www.calema.ca.gov/. Accessed January 23, 2015.

80. *Unaffiliated Volunteers in Response and Recovery.* Volunteer Florida, The Governor's Commission on Volunteerism & Community Service. Available at: www.fccs.org. Accessed March 17, 2014.

81. Introduction to health care at the crossroads: strategies for creating and sustaining community-wide emergency preparedness systems. *JCAHO Press Kits,* JCAHO. Available at: http://www.jointcommission.org/assets/1/18/emergency_preparedness.pdf. Accessed January 23, 2015.

82. Community Emergency Response Teams. Available at: http://www.fema.gov/community-emergency-response-teams. Accessed March 17, 2014.

83. Emergency System for Advanced Registration of Volunteer Healthcare Professionals. Available at: http://www.phe.gov/esarvhp/pages/about.aspx. Accessed March 17, 2014.

Personal Protective Equipment

Andrew J. Eyre, John L. Hick, and Craig D. Thorne

PPE, for personal protective equipment, has become a rather common acronym in the lexicon of health care providers. The acronym has been common in fire services, emergency medical services (EMS), and the military for quite some time. Essentially, PPE helps to ensure that individuals are safe from physical hazards that they may encounter in their work environment. PPE may be used to protect workers from general environmental threats (e.g., temperature extremes and noise), specific work-related threats (e.g., industrial equipment and falls from elevated work areas), or threats faced in an emergency situation (e.g., hazardous chemical and infectious agents). No equipment is appropriate for all individuals and threats: rather, equipment must be selected and properly used according to the setting of use and the level of risk.

The critical problem with most PPE, particularly in regard to chemically protective suits and respirators, is that with higher levels of protection come not only higher prices and required training levels but also a higher physiological and physical burden to the user. Thus a structured approach to assessment of risk and selection of proper equipment is important to achieve a reasonable level of protection in relation to the hazard.

In this chapter we review the concepts of PPE, including recent lessons learned, types of respirators, key regulations, and issues in the selection of PPE for emergency medical care and decontamination operations.

HISTORICAL PERSPECTIVE

Previously PPE for medical providers received little attention short of the "standard precautions" of gloves, with the addition of simple masks, eye protection, and barrier precautions, as needed for respiratory and contact precautions. A number of events have highlighted the importance of PPE for first responders and health care workers. The 2003 Severe Acute Respiratory Syndrome (SARS) Epidemic, the 2009 H1N1 Influenza Pandemic, the 1995 Tokyo Subway Sarin Attack, the 1995 Murrah Federal Building Bombing in Oklahoma City, and the terrorist attacks of September 2001 are some examples of situations in which the lack of proper PPE or the improper use of it resulted in adverse health effects for health care providers. Such events and adverse outcomes have focused attention on PPE as a critical issue in routine emergency department operations and disaster response.

In March 1995, a crude form of the nerve agent sarin was released in the Tokyo subway system on separate cars bound for a common downtown station. This attack resulted in 12 deaths and more than 4000 persons presenting to the hospital for medical evaluation. None of the casualties was decontaminated before treatment or transport. Retrospectively, 135 prehospital and 100 hospital personnel reported symptoms consistent with nerve agent exposure. Fortunately, none required

emergency treatment.[1] Eleven physicians caring for the sickest victims (including one in cardiac arrest and one in respiratory arrest) were most affected, and six of them required treatment with specific antidote. All recovered fully and did not have to cease their patient care efforts because of symptoms.[2] Approximately 80% of victims self-referred to hospitals, which is consistent with U.S. experiences, indicating that few victims of chemical contamination events undergo decontamination before arrival at a medical facility.[3,4] This has caused most jurisdictions to reconsider historical plans that contaminated patients would not be in contact with medical care personnel until they were "clean." EMS and hospital personnel need to be prepared for contaminated patients presenting directly to them and recognize that in certain situations PPE may be required to safely provide care.

SARS posed unique risks and challenges to health care workers. This novel viral agent with incompletely defined transmission characteristics was controlled in 2002, with aggressive quarantine measures and use of PPE. In the first wave of SARS in Toronto, 79.2% of all cases were acquired in a health care setting.[5] Aggressive use of PPE, including N95 masks, barrier precautions, and gloves, was generally effective at preventing spread, although during one difficult and prolonged intubation attempt, at least 6 providers contracted SARS from a patient, despite complying with PPE recommendations.[6] This case led to recommendations that higher levels of PPE may be required during procedures that are likely to generate aerosols or provoke coughing, such as intubation, airway suctioning, positive pressure ventilation, and nebulized treatments.[7] Many of the lessons learned from the SARS epidemic, including the importance of appropriate respiratory PPE and compliance programs, were later applied to the 2009 H1N1 Influenza Pandemic. Even so, H1N1 took a toll on health care workers, and analysis of both of these events has led to future improvements for disaster preparedness.[8–12]

The National Institute for Occupational Safety and Health (NIOSH) and the RAND Corporation produced a comprehensive "lessons learned" report, summarizing issues from the 2001 terrorist bombings at the World Trade Center (WTC), anthrax incidents, and the 1995 Oklahoma City Murrah Federal Building Bombing. The report, titled Protecting Emergency Responders: Lessons Learned from Terrorist Attacks, describes in detail many of the challenges responders faced (Box 46-1).[13]

It is clear from the WTC events that a large number of jurisdictions responding, conflicting messages regarding use of PPE and safety of the environment, unavailability of appropriate PPE, poor design characteristics of current PPE models, and lack of a plan to implement respiratory precautions can complicate a response and potentially place providers at risk. WTC responders continue to suffer respiratory symptoms attributable to exposures at "ground zero."[14]

BOX 46-1   Historical Hazards Faced by Responders to Terrorism Events

- Physical hazards including fires, burning jet fuel and explosions, rubble piles with sharp rebar and heated metal, falling debris (which resulted in the death of a nurse in Oklahoma City), hazardous materials, electrical hazards, structures prone to collapse, heat stress, exhaustion, and respiratory irritants
- Heat-related seizures while wearing chemically protective suits
- Eye injuries (usually related to particulate exposure), which accounted for 12% of all WTC disaster response worker injuries
- Potential for secondary hazards, including explosive devices and chemical, biological, and radioactive agents
- PPE shortcomings:
  - Heavy helmets hindered performance
  - SCBA was heavy and cumbersome
  - SCBA face pieces fogged (reducing visibility), and the equipment hindered verbal and radio communication
  - SCBA air bottle made it difficult to enter small spaces, and the limited air supply (up to 1 hour) necessitated leaving the operation to exchange the air bottle
  - Air tanks and/or filters were not interchangeable between teams, and teams worked under different standards
  - PAPR filters became clogged and were uncomfortable for long-duration use. Many workers instead opted to use dust masks (which offered little protection and caused nose-bridge chafing) or to wear the masks/hoods around their necks ("neck protectors")
- Use of respirators made it difficult for workers to communicate with each other, often resulting in users breaking the face seal to talk
- Turnout gear (the common protective garments used by firefighters) increased heat stress and physical fatigue
- At the WTC, the rubble pile was so hot in places that it melted the soles of workers' boots; providing wash stations to cool the boots resulted in wet feet and serious blisters for many workers; some 440 WTC disaster response workers sought treatment for blisters
- Steel-reinforced boots (soles and toes) protected against punctures by sharp objects but conducted and retained heat, which contributed to blisters and burns
- Structural firefighting gloves worked well until they got wet and hardened, reducing their dexterity
- WTC disaster response workers did not consistently protect their hands against potential hazards such as human remains and bodily fluids
- Safety glasses were readily available but often were open at the sides and did not offer adequate protection against airborne particles
- Goggles were uncomfortable, hindered peripheral vision, tended to fog, and did not fit well in conjunction with half-face respirators
- Many disaster response workers at the WTC (especially law enforcement officers) did not consistently use hearing protection, even around heavy machinery, because they needed to hear their radios and voices and listen for tapping when they were searching for survivors
- Most volunteers at the WTC, Pentagon, and Oklahoma City did not receive pre-event training on PPE and hazardous materials
- Although firefighters generally received detailed pre-event training, this was less true for law enforcement officers
- Accurate "real-time" hazard information was not readily available, especially during the anthrax incidents
- Protection from falls was available at some sites (in the form of ropes and harnesses) but was inconsistently used

---

CURRENT PRACTICE

Hazard Vulnerability Analysis

Selection of appropriate PPE begins with an analysis of the hazards that responders may encounter, as well as an assessment of responders' roles and responsibilities. Hazard vulnerability analyses (HVA) are required for community emergency planning grants and are required of health care facilities that are accredited by The Joint Commission, previously known as the Joint Commission on Accreditation of Health Care Organizations (JCAHO).[15,16] The HVA uses a numerical ranking of factors for specific threats (e.g., chemical release), including the risk of the event occurring, the current preparedness for the threat, and the risk to life. The numerical score determines the gravity of each threat to the community. Each community's HVA will reflect the unique risks that must be considered by its emergency responders. Choice of PPE may be affected by factors within the HVA, such as

- Population density of the community and surrounding area
- High- or moderate-risk terrorist targets in the community (e.g., government buildings, centers of commerce, or other symbolic sites)
- Chemical hazards posed by community industry (e.g., use of cyanide and hydrofluoric acid in the electronics industry)
- Risk of transportation incidents and major transportation routes, particularly highways and railroads
- Proximity of health care facilities, schools, or other key locations to these potential targets and industrial and transportation hazards
- Frequency of hazardous materials (HazMat) incidents in the community
- Resources available to respond to HazMat incidents (e.g., rapid access to on-site decontamination may decrease, but not eliminate, contaminated persons leaving the scene)

Defining the Agency and the Facility Role

Stakeholders in emergency response, including EMS, fire and rescue, and law enforcement agencies, emergency management teams, and health care facilities, must clearly define the responsibilities of each entity and the support and resources that each may need or offer during an emergency, particularly one involving a HazMat release.

The EMS role in a HazMat event may vary depending on jurisdictional planning and the availability of resources. Fire services personnel may or may not be able to provide treatment in a "warm zone" (i.e., the area of reduced contamination outside of the immediate release zone) depending on their training. Nonfire-based EMS personnel may require PPE to triage and treat victims in the warm zone. In the event of a mass chemical exposure, victims will likely self-refer to visible ambulances, call for emergency assistance from locations removed from the site of release, or make their way to hospitals, by-passing organized EMS and fire services altogether. This movement of contamination on the bodies of patients essentially causes a "migrating" warm zone, resulting in contamination of previously clean ("cold") areas. This migrating contamination may require protective equipment for EMS responders and hospital personnel, and appropriate plans and equipment should be in place. The roles and responsibilities of the responders, as well as the equipment required, need to be defined and drilled in advance of an incident.

Hospitals usually have relied on fire services for patient decontamination at the hospital. These resources, however, are often deployed to the scene of the event and are thus unavailable to support the hospital. Most hospitals have recognized the need for at least some internal capacity for patient decontamination and are equipping their teams with PPE appropriate for decontaminating self-referred patients and the means to decontaminate patients prior to entry into the emergency department (ED). In some instances, the hospital teams integrate with community HazMat teams, necessitating additional training and equipment as the mission then changes from a defensive decontamination response at the health care facility to an offensive response at the scene of release.

Risks to Providers

Even though HazMat releases seldom cause serious traumatic injury in the absence of concomitant explosions, the potential exists for both scene responders and hospital receivers to suffer serious consequences of exposure. The Agency for Toxic Substance and Disease Registry (ATSDR) maintains a multistate voluntary accounting of hazardous substance releases. The National Toxic Substance Incidents Program (NTSIP), which replaced the Hazardous Substances Emergency Events Surveillance (HSEES) database in 2010, currently collects data from seven states on HazMat events.[17-19] From 1993 to 2001, 44,015 events were recorded in the database: 3455 (7.8%) of the incidents caused injuries, and 74% of victims were transported to a health care facility.[4] In another analysis of HSEES data, only 5% of victims required admission to a health care facility, with the vast majority of patients presenting with self-limited respiratory symptoms.[20] In 2011, the NTSIP reported 3128 separate incidents, resulting in 62 fatalities and an additional 1115 ill or injured patients. Carbon monoxide, chemicals for illicit methamphetamine production, paints/dyes, and petroleum products were the most common offending agents. A review of these events found that 344 of the patients were employees or first responders whose illness and injuries could have been prevented with appropriate PPE.[21]

HSEES data from 2003 to 2006 shows that of 33,157 documented events, secondary contamination of facilities and providers occurred in 15 (0.05%) cases, resulting in illness in 17 providers. Of these secondary contamination victims, only two had employed any PPE when the contamination occured.[22] Even though secondary contamination events are relatively rare, they pose significant risk to health care providers and to the entire health care system because emergency departments and transport vehicles may be closed or taken out of service for

proper decontamination. Events resulting in emergency department evacuation and/or provider illness are especially serious in situations of "off-gassing," where toxic gases are released from contaminated patients and/or their clothing.[23-28] The most serious of these incidents involve patients with suicidal ingestions of organophosphate pesticides.[23-25] Exposures to these patients have caused at least one provider to require intubation and receive aggressive treatment with specific antidote because of contact with pesticide in emesis and vapors during patient resuscitation.[23] Patients who have ingested organophosphate may "off-gas" for days and present an ongoing risk to health care workers.[25] In conjunction with the information from the Tokyo Subway Sarin Attack and the chemical terrorism risk posed by these agents, it is clear that these pesticides present a substantial risk of toxicity from secondary exposures.

Limited research is available to document the degree of the off-gassing that occurs from the bodies and clothing of contaminated patients.[29,30] Clothing removal and control may be expected to remove 90% of the contaminant and thus should be a priority.[30,31] Ideally, this should take place in an open-air environment.

Chemical Protective Equipment

Providers may not initially recognize a chemical release when they arrive at a scene. Even though structural firefighting ensembles with self-contained breathing apparatus (SCBA) offer some chemical protection that may be sufficient for victim rescue,[32] the incident commander must determine what actions are appropriate for any given situation and maintain a high level of suspicion that a HazMat situation is present. Protective suits, gloves, boots, and appropriate respiratory protection must be donned as soon as possible when a chemical threat is recognized.

The Occupational Safety and Health Administration (OSHA) and Environmental Protection Agency define four basic levels of PPE for HazMat scene responses (Table 46-1 and Fig. 46-1; OSHA standard 29 CFR 1910.120, Appendix B). Generally, as the level of protection increases (Level A being the highest level), so do the weight, cost, and physiological

TABLE 46-1	Categories of PPE		
LEVEL	BRIEF DESCRIPTION	ADVANTAGES	DISADVANTAGES
A	Completely encapsulated suit and SCBA	Highest level of protection available for both contact and vapor hazards	• Expense and training requirements typically restrict use to HazMat response teams • Lack of mobility • Heat and physical stresses • Limited air supply • Fit-testing requirements
B	Encapsulating suit or junctions/seams sealed, and SAR or SCBA	High level of protection adequate for entry into unknown environments	Same as for Level A • SAR hose may pose a trip hazard or become dislodged
C	Splash suit and APR (note APR and PAPR considered equivalent in classification despite significant difference in protection)	• Significantly increased mobility • Less physical stress • Extended operation time with high levels of protection against certain chemical hazards • No fit testing required for hood type	• Not adequate for some high-concentration environments, less-than-atmospheric-oxygen environments, or high levels of splash contamination • Expense and training moderate
D	Usual work clothes	• Increased mobility • Less physical stress • Extended operation time • More fashionable	• Offer no protection against specific hazards • Expense and training minimal

From Agency for Toxic Substances and Disease Registry. Emergency Medical Services Response to Hazardous Materials Incidents. Available at: http://www.atsdr.cdc.gov/mhmi-v1-2.pdf.

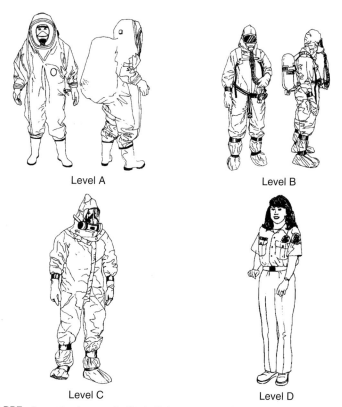

Level A

Level B

Level C

Level D

FIG 46-1 The four basic levels of PPE. From the Agency for Toxic Substances and Disease Registry. Emergency Medical Services Response to Hazardous Materials Incidents. Available at: http://www.atsdr.cdc.gov/mhmi-v1-2.pdf.

burden of the appropriate PPE. Increasing protection also generally means decreasing mobility, dexterity, and scope of vision. Inherent risks to PPE include trip and fall hazards, reduced ability to complete tasks, heat stress, anxiety, and seizures.[28,33-37] Cardiovascular demand is dramatically increased as ensemble weight and heat retention increase. PPE must be selected on the basis that it does not impose unnecessary risks to the provider while at the same time offering an appropriate margin of safety against the hazard. Because the selection of PPE usually revolves around the selection of the respiratory component, various types of respirators must be reviewed. Each respirator has an assigned protection factor that reflects the degree of protection afforded to the user. Simply put, 1/protection factor equals the amount of exposure for the wearer. For example, a provider wearing a powered air-purifying respirator (PAPR) with an assigned protection factor (APF) of 1000 is exposed to 1/1000 the level of contaminant as compared with wearing no protection.

Atmosphere-Supplying Respirators

Atmosphere-supplying respirators provide breathable, fresh air to the user, independent of the environment, via an air supply hose and/or tank, and thus offer a high level of respiratory protection. This type of respirator is required for entry into environments where the identity of and/or the potential quantity of a hazardous substance are unknown or where the quantity of oxygen in the air is unknown.

SCBA is the most common atmosphere-supplying respirator for emergency responses. It provides air via a tank, usually worn on the back. The operational time is limited by the capacity of the tank (usually less than 1 hour). Fire service personnel routinely use this form of respiratory protection, and fire-based EMS services personnel generally incorporate this PPE into their chemical protection planning. Limitations include the equipment's weight (approximately 25 to 30 pounds), cost, need for fit testing, duration of air supply, and need to refill air

bottles. Even though SCBA provides excellent protection, its limitations make it inappropriate for many situations (e.g., caring for a patient with an infectious disease, providing hospital-based decontamination, or securing a perimeter in the warm zone). SCBA has an APF of about 10,000, the highest of any type of respirator.[38,39]

Supplied-air respirators (SARs) provide air via a hose line from a nearby clean air source (e.g., compressor or hospital supply line). To meet OSHA requirements for Level B, respirators must have a tight-fitting face piece and an emergency supply of air in case of line failure or problems.[40] Loose-fitting hoods with a supplied-air source do not meet Level B standards but are used by some decontamination teams when an additional level of protection is desired because of institutional preference or local hazard profile. Advantages include a potentially unlimited supply of fresh air and longer duration of use. Limitations are primarily mobility and thus flexibility of response. These respirators are best suited to health care provider use in a decontamination room or well-defined area in which the air lines are unlikely to be tangled, stretched, or become a trip hazard. The APF of a typical tight-fitting face piece SAR is 1000, although there may be variability among models and designs (e.g., tight-fitting mask vs. loose-fitting hood).[38,39]

Air-Purifying Respirators

Air-purifying respirators (APRs) have cartridges that filter the air in the user's environment to remove particulate matter and specific chemicals that the filter is designed to capture. These filters do not affect the oxygen concentration of the ambient air and thus cannot be used in potentially oxygen-deficient environments. Only those chemicals for which the filter is designated are removed. In addition, the capacity of the filter can be exceeded by large amounts of contaminant, thus these respirators are designed for situations in which the concentration of the agent is either established to be or assumed to be below the threshold for the canister.

Nonpowered APRs use the wearer's work of breathing to pull ambient air through the filter. Examples include dust masks and military and civilian "gas masks." The APF of a nonpowered full-face piece APR is 50 when appropriate quantitative fit testing is performed.[38,39] Of note, this type of mask is used by military and tactical personnel for protection against dangerous lethal levels of nerve and other chemical agents. Advantages include low cost and long duration of use. Disadvantages include increased work of breathing and physiological stress, mask fogging, and the need for fit testing.

A PAPR uses a motor to pull air through the filter canisters, thus decreasing the work of breathing and risk of air entrainment around the respirator face piece. PAPRs are often supplied with a loose-fitting disposable or reusable hood that eliminates the need to perform fit testing and allows use by a broad range of individuals. Hooded PAPRs with "stacked" canisters that offer protection against common hazardous chemical and biological agents encountered by first responders and hospital personnel are in widespread use because of their low cost, weight, and the increased flexibility of use. Dependence on battery power, shelf life of the filters, and the need to be able to match the filter to the agent are limiting factors. The APF for a PAPR ranges from 25 to 1000, depending on the specifics of the model and how it is employed. Battery packs are usually either single use or rechargeable. Rechargeable battery packs require ongoing attention to ensure a proper charge, but they offer the flexibility of allowing PAPR reuse during a prolonged event.

Particulate filter masks such as those commonly used for patient care to protect against tuberculosis and other organisms are also considered APRs. Masks are classified N (not oil resistant), R (oil resistant), and P (oil proof). N95 refers to a filter (the entire mask) that removes 95% of a particulate challenge in the 3- to 5-μm range. N100 respirators filter 100% of the same challenge, yet simple half-face respirators offer an APF of only 10 because of the entrainment of air around the mask and other factors; therefore changing from an N95 to an N100 offers little additional protection unless a more robust mask ensemble, rather than a simple half-face mask, is used.[41,42]

Respiratory protection technologies are rapidly evolving, and respiratory program administrators should make sure they are familiar with the available options and their relative advantages and disadvantages. Regional cooperative planning and purchases may be helpful to allow for sharing of resources, including staff, during an incident.

Chemical Protective Equipment

Chemically protective suits must be tailored to the type of use. Suits for hot-zone entry, where direct contact with a hazardous material is likely, must be much more robust than suits for patient decontamination activities. Selection should be guided by National Fire Protection Association (NFPA) standards 1992 and 1994, for site-of-release response activities, and by OSHA guidelines, for hospital decontamination activities.[43,44] Chemicals commonly found in local transit, agriculture, or industrial use should also guide selection. Appropriate PPE for perimeter control and EMS warm-zone operations remain topics of debate at this time. Generally, suits should be sized far more generously than standard work clothing, to prevent tearing during squatting and other activities (e.g., an average-sized 70-kg man should plan to wear a size XXL suit). Many suit configurations are possible, and the optimal configuration will depend on the mission and other equipment in the ensemble. For example, suits without "feet" are preferred when worn with boots (to allow taping over the boot) but those with integrated bootie "feet" are preferred when pull-on "sock" type butyl booties are to be used. These integrated feet should not be used as primary footwear at any time because they have poor abrasion resistance.

Boots supplied in sizes medium, large, and extra-large rather than fitted sizes may be preferred when equipment is purchased for a group (e.g., hospital decontamination team) rather than being purchased for an individual responder (e.g., firefighter). Butyl or other rubber boots probably afford appropriate protection for warm-zone operations. Butyl "sock" type booties may be used on very low abrasion surfaces (e.g., internal hospital decontamination room) but are not generally appropriate for outside use.

Nitrile undergloves with butyl overgloves provide protection against a broad range of hazards for warm-zone activities. The U.S. Army Center for Health Promotion and Preventive Medicine (USACHPPM) recommends 14-mil thickness butyl gloves (standard examination gloves are 4 mil) as a minimum for working with patients contaminated by chemical warfare agents or toxic industrial chemicals.[44,45] Overglove selection must balance the need for abrasion resistance and chemical protection with dexterity required to perform tasks and patient care (e.g., administer intramuscular antidotes or intubate).[44,45]

Biological Protective Equipment

Very few situations require physical decontamination of patients exposed to biological agents. An exception would be patients who present after contamination with biological agents (e.g., anthrax spores) from a dissemination device. PPE for decontamination should consist of the same chemical protective suit and high level of respiratory protection, including a high-efficiency particulate (HEPA) or SAR that would be used for chemical decontamination activities. PPE for biological agents in relation to care of patients who are already infected and symptomatic is discussed in the following section.

Categories of PPE for biological agents include[46]:

- *Standard precautions:* Use of gloves and proper hand hygiene to prevent disease transmission for any potentially infectious patient. Gowns and eye protection are added only when patient care activities are likely to result in splashing or soiling.
- *Contact precautions:* Standard precautions plus use of barriers during all patient care activities to protect face, arms, and front torso to prevent contact with secretions, emesis, feces, etc. (e.g., enteric infections and many hemorrhagic fever viruses).
- *Droplet precautions:* Standard precautions with the addition of a droplet respirator (e.g., surgical mask) when working within 3 feet of the patient, to prevent transmission of infectious agents that travel by large-droplet spread; may not be protective against all droplet nuclei.
- *Airborne precautions:* Standard precautions with an N95 or higher protection respirator to prevent transmission of infectious agents that are spread by aerosols (e.g., airborne precautions are used against chickenpox, smallpox, and tuberculosis).
- *"Special pathogen precautions":* Based on the SARS experiences, a high-risk pathogen with respiratory spread probably requires greater levels of protection than previously recommended. Constant use of both contact and airborne precautions has generally been advised with the optional use of a PAPR rather than an N95 mask during "high-risk" interventions likely to generate aerosols or provoke coughing (e.g., suctioning, intubation, positive pressure ventilation).[6,7]

Patient care providers should have routine access to nonsterile examination gloves, barrier gowns that protect the arms and anterior torso, standard surgical (droplet) masks, and face shields that provide adequate splash protection (which may be integrated with the mask, a separate face shield, or goggles) according to the OSHA bloodborne pathogens standards.[47,48]

When needed, providers should have easy access to higher levels of protection. "Precaution carts" or "Bad bug bags" may be preassembled with appropriate gowns, gloves, face shields or goggles, N95 or PAPR respirators, and other supplies so that health care providers do not have to assemble the necessary components when hazards arise. Instruction sheets for donning or doffing and disinfection procedures can be included in these kits.[49,48]

Practitioners fitted for N95 respirators may use these for patient care, and others should have access to a PAPR until they can undergo fit testing for an N95 respirator. Plans to rapidly fit test additional employees during an event that might require prolonged use of airborne precautions (e.g., SARs) should be in place.

Regulations and Training

All PPE must be part of an ongoing program for respiratory protection and HazMat or decontamination responses within the agency or institution, to ensure that employees who are expected to use protective devices are competent and comfortable with the indications, use, and limitations of their equipment. Numerous regulations apply to the selection and proper use of PPE. All persons using PPE must conform to OSHA standards on respiratory protection (29 CFR 1910.134), PPE (29 CFR 1910.132), eye and face protection (29 CFR 1910.133), hand protection (29 CFR 1910.138), hazard communication (29 CFR 1910.1200), and bloodborne pathogens (29 CFR 1910.1030). State OSHA agencies may have stricter requirements than the federal standards. Most occupational or employee health services of agencies and facilities where PPE is used are very familiar with these standards and their application to employees.

The NFPA has numerous standards for training and equipping HazMat responders, including EMS personnel (e.g., NFPA standards 471, 473, 1981, 1992, 1994, and 1999). Specific guidance is also provided for urban search and rescue teams (NFPA standard 1951).[43] Responders to HazMat releases are covered by OSHA's HAZWOPER (Hazardous Waste Operations and Emergency Response) standard 29 CFR 1910.120, which is perhaps the most comprehensive standard guiding hazardous materials responses.

OSHA requires use of a minimum of Level B equipment (i.e., an atmosphere-supplying respirator and chemically protective suit with sealed seams) during a response into a contaminated environment until the concentration of the agent is shown via air monitoring to be below the threshold required for the safe use of an APR or other lesser degree of protection.[50] This requirement presents difficulty for EMS and hospital providers because the agent is often unknown at the time that medical care is provided in the warm zone (i.e., an area where the level of contamination is minimal and controlled). Particularly for hospitals, confusion existed as to what constituted appropriate protection for decontamination team members who provide medical care for contaminated patients and to what degree the HAZWOPER standard applied to community responders geographically separate from the site of release.

OSHA clarified this issue for health care facility providers in two letters of interpretation[51,52] and a comprehensive guidance document on PPE and training released in 2004.[44] In this document OSHA codifies use of PAPRs as the minimum level of respiratory protective equipment for hospitals under certain conditions:

- The facility acts as a "first receiver" for self-referred contaminated casualties, not as a responder to a release zone.
- The facility itself is not the site of the hazardous substances release.
- An HVA has been conducted to identify specific hazards to the community and facility.
- The victims must present at least 10 minutes after exposure (to allow time for some of the contaminant to evaporate or dissipate). It will usually take at least this long to get personnel into PPE at the facility.
- The victims' clothing must be rapidly removed and contained.

- Decontamination must occur in a well-ventilated area, preferably outdoors.

When these conditions are met, and absent any particular threats within the community that require higher levels of protection (such as close proximity to a specific chemical production, storage, or disposal site), the minimum level of respiratory PPE is a PAPR with a protection factor of 1000 or greater, which filters organic vapor, acid gas, particulate matter, and biological agents (at the HEPA level).[44]

HAZWOPER also defines training requirements for responders.[53] The application of these regulations to hospital decontamination teams was also clarified in recent OSHA guidance.[44] Awareness training is required for individuals involved in a HazMat response who will not be using PPE or taking actions beyond recognizing and reporting an incident (emergency department staff, law enforcement officers).[44]

At a minimum, all responders who will use chemical PPE must be trained to the operations level (8 hours minimum)[44] so that each responder can

- Understand his or her role in the response and the emergency response plan.
- Assess site safety, including risks to self.
- Select and safely use appropriate PPE.
- Understand decontamination procedures.

HazMat-awareness educational competencies must also be met by providers trained to the operations level. The awareness competencies may be included in the 8 hours of operations training or conducted separately.[44]

In addition, any personnel using respiratory protective equipment must be in compliance with OSHA's respiratory protection standard (29 CFR 120.134). Key features of this standard are

- Respirator selection procedures
- Proper use of respirators in routine and reasonably foreseeable emergency situations
- Medical clearance before use (at minimum, a screening questionnaire; see Appendix C of the standard)
- Fit testing before use and annually thereafter (see Appendix A and B1 of the standard)
- Inspecting, cleaning and disinfecting, storing, repairing, and maintaining the equipment
- Training and education on topics such as the types of respiratory hazards they might be exposed to, proper use (including donning and doffing), limitations, and maintenance

Most medical facilities and response agencies have a respiratory protection program in place. This existing foundation and the subject matter experts in occupational safety and health, infection control, or other related disciplines can assist with implementation of new technologies and protocols.

⚠ PITFALLS AND ONGOING CHALLENGES

PPE technology continues to change rapidly. Hopefully, technologies that are lighter weight, less expensive, and less heat-retaining can be developed. There is experimentally developed PPE that are easier to don and doff, and which provide improved mobility and visibility to perform procedures. In one project completed at Brown University in conjunction with the Rhode Island School of Design, engineering and industrial design students paired up to develop a new model of Level B PPE that could be donned in half the time with a single user compared to two users with traditional PPE. Even though a prototype was developed and showcased, there were no clear funding sources available to bring this design to market.[54] Technology change is occurring far more rapidly than the current approvals process and new standards that have arisen in the wake of recent events. Clear guidance on appropriate technologies for warm-zone activities is lacking at this time. This can lead to confusion and difficult choices for agencies and facilities, knowing that their PPE selection may be either too much or too little to satisfy future standards. Currently, there is no recommendation or consensus on the level of PPE that is required for hospital-based personnel, much to the consternation of hospital preparedness leaders. Some have proposed a PPE Level H to meet this need. Additional research is clearly needed regarding safe but comfortable PPE, methods of decontamination, modeling of airborne concentrations of specific agents, and PPE selection.

Further, detection technologies are needed that can provide better environmental screening for a wide range of hazardous substances and a quantitative assessment of agent concentration. Currently, incident commanders may remain confused about appropriate PPE, and this may result in PPE selection that is overly conservative (risks provider noncompliance and adverse effects from the PPE) or overly liberal (risks provider injury from the contaminant).

Finally, providers need to be educated about the consequences of not using PPE appropriately, including acute chemical effects and delayed pulmonary effects.

In general, communities and regions can help to reduce issues of PPE interoperability by planning, purchasing, and training together whenever possible, which allows for caches of materials to be deployed that are true replacements for usual materials and thus will be better accepted and require minimal training.

For too long, jurisdictions have been reluctant to share their problems, issues, and roadblocks in the area of PPE, lest the agency be seen as having problems protecting its responders. Better dialogue and sharing of best practices and lessons learned are of immense value, and better HazMat response and planning should be encouraged. The NIOSH/RAND report[13] and release of select after-action reports are welcome changes in this history.

Defining hazards in this age of potential chemical terrorism is fraught with peril because we are unable to truly assess the scope of the threat. Thus PPE must be chosen that will protect appropriately against a broad range of threats without being so restrictive that in the heat of the moment, the provider decides to forgo the PPE and is at risk of becoming a casualty of the event. Balancing cost, ease of use, and scope of protection concerns are delicate decisions with few answers at this time, particularly for those who may have long-duration job tasks in a warm-zone environment.

We can only hope that we are not forced to learn too many more harsh lessons about PPE use in the future. In the meantime, we should strive to prepare our communities by selecting appropriate protective technologies in relation to perceived threats and practicing our responses so that our personnel both are comfortable using their PPE and understand the consequences of not doing so.

REFERENCES

1. Okumura T, Suzuki K, Atsuhiro F, et al. The Tokyo subway sarin attack: disaster management, part 1: community emergency response. *Acad Emerg Med*. 1998;5:613–617.
2. Nozaki H, Hori S, Shinozama Y, et al. Secondary exposure of medical staff to sarin vapor in the emergency room. *Intensive Care Med*. 1995;21:1032–1035.
3. Okumura T, Suzuki K, Fukada A, et al. The Tokyo subway sarin attack: disaster management, part 2: hospital response. *Acad Emerg Med*. 1998;5:618–624.
4. Horton DK, Berkowitz Z, Kaye WE. Secondary contamination of emergency department personnel from hazardous materials events, 1995-2001. *Am J Emerg Med*. 2003;21:199–204.
5. Svoboda T, Henry B, Shulman L, et al. Public health measures to control the spread of the severe acute respiratory syndrome during the outbreak in Toronto. *N Engl J Med*. 2004;350:2352–2361.
6. Cluster of severe acute respiratory syndrome cases among protected healthcare workers-Toronto, Canada, April 2003. *Morb Mortal Wkly Rep*. 2003;52:433–436.
7. Centers for Disease Control and Prevention. *Public Health Guidance for Community-Level Preparedness and Response to Severe Acute Respiratory Syndrome (SARS) Version 2: Supplement I: Infection Control in the Home, Healthcare, and Community Settings*. Atlanta: Centers for Disease Control and Prevention; 2004.
8. Kuster SP, Coleman BL, Raboud J, et al. Risk factors for influenza among health care workers during 2009 pandemic, Toronto, Ontario, Canada Centers for Disease Control and Prevention. *Emerg Infect Dis*. 2013;19(4):606–615. http://dx.doi.org/10.3201/eid1904.111812.
9. Centers for Disease Control and Prevention: The 2009 H1N1 Pandemic: Summary Highlights, April 2009-2010.
10. Bhadelia N, Sonti R, McCarthy JW, et al. Impact of the 2009 influenza A (H1N1) pandemic on healthcare workers at a tertiary care center in New York City. *Infect Control*. 2013;34(8):825–831.
11. Beckman S, Materna B, Goldmacher S, et al. Evaluation of respiratory protection programs and practices in California hospitals during the 2009-2010 H1N1 influenza pandemic. *Am J Infect Control*. 2013;41(11):1024–1031.
12. Jaeger JL, Patel M, Dharan N, et al. Transmission of 2009 pandemic influenza (H1N1) virus among healthcare personnel-Southern California, 2000. *Infect Control*. 2011;32(12):1149–1157.
13. Jackson BA, Peterson DJ, Bartis JT, et al. *Protecting Emergency Responders: Lessons Learned from Terrorist Attacks*. Santa Monica, CA: RAND Corporation; 2002.
14. Physical health status of World Trade Center rescue and recovery workers and volunteers-New York City, July 2002-August 2004. *Morb Mortal Wkly Rep*. 2004;53(35):807–812.
15. Joint Commission on Accreditation of Healthcare Organizations. *The 2001 Joint Commission Accreditation Manual for Healthcare Facilities EC 1.4 and 1.6 (rev)*. Oakbrook Terrace, IL: Joint Commission on Accreditation of Healthcare Organizations; 2001.
16. Joint Commission. Standards Manual. Updated March 2014.
17. Agency for Toxic Substances and Disease Registry. Hazardous Substances Emergency Events Surveillance.
18. Duncan MA. Orr MF Evolving with the times, the new national toxic substances incidents program. *J Med Toxicol*. Dec 2010;6(4):461–463.
19. Agency for Toxic Substances & Disease Registry, National Toxic Substances Incidents Program (NTSIP), state partners. available at: http://www.atsdr.cdc.gov/ntsip/state_partners.html, Accessed 4/14/2014.
20. Burgess JL. Risk factors for adverse health events following hazardous materials incidents. *J Occup Environ Med*. 2001;43(6):558–566.
21. National Toxic Substance Incidents Program (NTSIP) Annual report 2011. Agency for Toxic Substances and Disease Registry, Atlanta, GA, 43 pp. Accessed at: http://www.atsdr.cdc.gov/ntsip/docs/ATSDR_Annual%20Report_121013_508%20compliant.pdf.
22. Horton DK, Orr M, Tsongas T, et al. Secondary contamination of medical personnel, equipment and facilities resulting from hazardous materials events, 2003-2006. *Disaster Med Public Health Prep*. 2008;2(2):104–113.
23. Centers for Disease Control and Prevention. Nosocomial poisoning associated with emergency department treatment of organophosphate toxicity-Georgia, 2000. *Morb Mortal Wkly Rep*. 2001;49(51):1156–1158.
24. Merritt NL, Anderson MJ. Malathion overdose: when one patient creates a departmental hazard. *J Emerg Nurs*. 1989;15:463–465.
25. Merril D. Prolonged toxicity of organophosphate poisoning. *Crit Care Med*. 1982;10:550–551.
26. Thanabalasingham T, Beckett MW, Murray V. Hospital response to a chemical incident: report on casualties of an ethyldichlorosilane spill. *BMJ*. 1991;302:101–102.
27. Nocera A, Levitin HW, Hilton JMN. Dangerous bodies: a case of fatal aluminum phosphide poisoning. *Med J Aust*. 2000;173:133–135.
28. Hick JL, Hanfling D, Burstein JL, et al. Personal protective equipment for healthcare facility decontamination personnel: regulations, risks, and recommendations. *Ann Emerg Med*. 2003;42:370–380.

29. Schultz M, Cisek J, Wabeke R. Simulated exposure of hospital emergency personnel to solvent vapors and respirable dust during decontamination of chemically exposed patients. *Ann Emerg Med.* 1995;26:324–329.

30. Fedele P, Georgopolous P, Shade P, et al. *Technical report: In-hospital response to external chemical emergencies: Personal protective equipment, training, site operations planning, and medical programs (final draft).* Washington, DC: Joint publication of the U.S. Army Soldier and Biological Chemical Command, Environmental and Occupational Health Sciences Institute, and Veterans Health Administration (VHA); 2003.

31. Macintyre AG, Christopher GW, Eitzen E, et al. Weapons of mass destruction events with contaminated casualties: effective planning for healthcare facilities. *JAMA.* 2000;4:261–269.

32. U.S. Army Soldier Biological and Chemical Command. *Guidelines for incident commander's use of firefighter protective ensemble with self-contained breathing apparatus for rescue operations during a terrorist chemical agent incident.* Aberdeen Proving Ground, MD: U.S. Army Soldier Biological and Chemical Command; 1999.

33. King JM, Frelin AJ. Impact of the chemical protective ensemble on the performance of basic medical tasks. *Mil Med.* 1984;149(9):496–501.

34. Hendler I, Nahtomi O, Segal E, et al. The effect of full protective gear on intubation performed by hospital medical personnel. *Mil Med.* 2000;165 (4):272–274.

35. Carter BJ, Cammermeyer M. Emergence of real casualties during simulated chemical warfare training under high heat conditions. *Mil Med.* 1985;150 (12):657–663.

36. Carr JL, Corona BM, Jackson SE, Bochovchin V. *The effect of chemical protective clothing and equipment on Army soldier performance: A critical review of the literature. Technical Memoranda 12080.* U.S. Army Human Engineering Laboratory: Aberdeen Proving Ground, MD; 1980.

37. Carter BJ, Cammermeyer M. Biopsychosocial responses of medical unit personnel wearing chemical defense ensemble in a simulated chemical warfare environment. *Mil Med.* 1985;150(5):239–249.

38. Occupational Safety and Health Administration. 29 CFR Parts 1910, 1915 1926: Assigned Protection Factors; Final Rule.

39. Occupational Safety and Health Administration. CFR29. Part 1910.1030. Bloodborne Pathogens.

40. Occupational Safety and Health Administration. *Hazardous waste operations and emergency response. Code of Federal Regulations;* 1910, 120.

41. Weber A, Willeke K, Marchioni R, et al. Aerosol penetration and leakage characteristics of masks in the health care industry. *Am J Infect Control.* 1993;21:167–173.

42. Chen CC, Willeke K. Characteristics of face seal leakage in filtering facepieces. *Am Ind Hyg Assoc J.* 1992;53(9):533–539.

43. National Fire Protection Association. Codes and Standards. Standard 1992 and 1994.

44. Occupational Safety and Health Administration. *OSHA 3249-08 N Best Practices for Hospital-Based First Receivers of Victims from Mass Casualty Incidents Involving the Release of Hazardous Substances;* 2005.

45. U.S. Army Center for Health Promotion and Preventive Medicine. Personal protective equipment guide for military medical treatment facility personnel handling casualties from weapons of mass destruction and terrorism events. Technical guide 275. Aberdeen Proving Grounds, MD: U.S. Army Center for Health Promotion and Preventive Medicine.

46. Garner JS. Guideline for isolation precautions in hospitals. The Hospital Infection Control Practices Advisory Committee. *Infect Control Hosp Epidemiol.* 1996;17(4):53–80.

47. Department of Health and Human Services. Department of Labor. Respiratory protective devices: final rules and notice. *Fed Regist.* 1995;60 (110):30336–30402.

48. Occupational Safety and Health Administration. CFR29. Part 1910.1030. Bloodborne Pathogens.

49. Minnesota Department of Health Chapter Association for Practitioners of Infection Control. Personal Protective Equipment for Smallpox and Viral Hemorrhagic Fever Patient Care.

50. Occupational Safety and Health Administration. *Hazardous waste operations and emergency response. Code of Federal Regulations;* 1910, 120 (q)(3)(iii-iv).

51. Occupational Safety and Health Administration. Standard interpretations. Training and PPE requirements for hospital staff that decontaminate victims/patients.

52. Occupational Safety and Health Administration. Standard interpretations. Respiratory protection requirements for hospital staff decontaminating chemically contaminated patients.

53. Occupational Safety and Health Administration. *Hazardous waste operations and emergency response. Code of Federal Regulations;* 1910, 120(q)(6). Available at, http://www.osha.gov/pls/oshaweb/owadisp.show _document?p_table=STANDARDS&p_id=9765.

54. Cottam M, Suner S. *The Next Generation PPE: Industrial Design meets Disaster Medicine. Biennale Internationale Design 2006 Saint-Etienne.* France: Saint-Etienne; November 22-December 3, 2006.

Role of Bystanders in Disasters

Selwyn E. Mahon and James J. Rifino

Disasters occur with or without warning, and they can be "sudden" or "sustained." With respect to disaster response, the terms *volunteer* and *bystander* are often used together, though they are seldom synonymous. When a "sudden disaster" occurs, bystanders witness the event and are among the first to respond. The word *bystander* is appropriate here referring to a person who happens to pass by or be in the proximity of an event when it occurs and often would have been a victim him- or herself but for chance. They are usually members of the general public, not part of the formal response, and have little to no formal training in disaster management, search and rescue, or advanced first aid. *Volunteers,* however, may be trained professionals in the first responder or health care communities. Their underlying knowledge and skills in medical care make them useful in disaster response and recovery. They may be associated with a disaster-response organization and be familiar with the "Incident Command System (ICS)," but they often have varied levels of experience and training in disaster response. Unlike "bystanders," volunteers are usually not the very first to arrive. Other "volunteers" may be entirely untrained in disaster response, but they may have other skills that can assist with disaster recovery. They may also spontaneously present themselves to a disaster site after the event has occurred.

According to the U.S. Federal Emergency Management Agency (FEMA), 95% of all emergencies result in the victim or a bystander providing immediate assistance first.[1] In his testimony discussing government disaster response after Hurricane Katrina, FEMA Administrator Craig Fugate was quoted as saying, "Neighbors are almost always the most effective and most immediate first responders."[2] All evidence and discussions suggest that emergency managers should reexamine the role of the "bystander" in disaster response and include these very important assets in the planning, response and training for disaster response. It is clear that health, safety, and security are everyone's responsibility and should not be left to professionals alone.

HISTORICAL PERSPECTIVE

Historically, bystanders have been the first providers during disaster incidents worldwide. They have been thought to be effective in disaster response. For obvious reasons, it is very difficult to obtain data for such incidents. There are clear data, however, with respect to everyday life-threatening events, and these data demonstrate bystander effectiveness. "Bystander CPR" has become a part of many communities and has been scientifically proven to be effective. The data clearly show that survival rates are much higher when a bystander immediately initiates CPR after an individual sustains cardiac arrest, compared with survival rates when no bystander CPR was initiated.[3–5] These conclusions have been repeated in numerous studies throughout many different communities. In addition, there are data with respect to automated external defibrillators (AEDs), which have become part of our culture and

can be found in most airports, gyms, sports arenas, police cars, and many public areas. The placement of AEDs throughout these high-traffic areas has provided bystanders with an effective tool capable of assessing for "shockable" arrhythmias and treating them. Studies have demonstrated that this intervention increased survival with intact neurological function from 14.3% to 49.6%.[6] The Heimlich maneuver, taught as a module in CPR training programs, has been performed by many bystanders throughout the world and has alleviated airway obstructions that could otherwise result in death.

Throughout history, bystanders have been recognized for completing the majority of rescues following documented disasters, and they have been credited with increased survival rates. There are numerous documented examples:

1. *June 17, 1978:* The showboat *Whippoorwill* was struck by a tornado in Kansas, causing the boat to capsize. Out of the 58 passengers and crew, 16 people perished from drowning. Nearby recreational boaters acted as "search and rescue" and were responsible for all of the lives saved.[7]

2. *July 16, 1979:* Following a tornado in Cheyenne, Wyoming, an estimated 29% of the total search-and-rescue effort was completed by individuals not affiliated with any emergency organization.[8]

3. *July 7, 2005:* Following the London bombings, bystanders performed most of the triage at the Edgeware Road site, one of the four main triage sites, as overwhelmed emergency responders were busy at the other major triage sites.[9]

4. *April 22, 1992:* A series of 10 gasoline vapor explosions occurred in the sewers in Guadalajara, Mexico, killing 252 people and injuring nearly 500 more. Bystanders (with no formal training) formed search-and-rescue teams, using car jacks to lift rubble and garden hoses to siphon air to their entrapped neighbors.[10]

5. *March 20, 1995:* following the sarin gas attacks in the underground system in Tokyo, numerous accounts of bystanders and mildly injured passengers assisting more seriously poisoned passengers to hospitals were documented.[11]

6. *September 11, 2001:* New York City was one of a number of sites attacked by terrorists. As buildings burned and rubble fell, many bystanders helped others evacuate the World Trade Center areas before the buildings collapsed. Some perished as a result of their heroic efforts, as was the case with equity trader Welles Crowther. As with many of the other bystanders who saved thousands of lives that day, he was credited with saving the lives of at least 18 people.[12] Throughout the world that day, more than 250 international flights inbound to the United States were ordered to be grounded. As a result, more than 43,000 passengers and crew were diverted and forced to land at 15 Canadian airports. In each of these cities, armies of bystanders and volunteers assisted the stranded passengers and crews with food and shelter.[13]

7. *January 12, 2010:* Haiti was struck by a devastating major earthquake. A survey of people who were victims of the earthquake showed that more than 90% were either "self-rescued" or rescued by bystanders.[14]

8. *April 15, 2013:* Lone terrorists used homemade bombs at two different sites close to the finish line of the Boston Marathon. Bystanders used shirts and belts as tourniquets and applied direct pressure to staunch bleeding. They assisted victims to the first aid tents and comforted those around them. Those with medical training began triaging victims. They are credited with saving many lives that day.[15]

These and other accounts highlight the importance of bystanders with respect to disaster response and decreased mortality. The roles are endless and can successfully include critical search and rescue, extrication, water rescue, immediate lifesaving first aid, hemorrhage control, splinting of suspected fractures, triage and transportation of victims to definitive care centers, comforting victims and their relatives, and the provision of food and shelter.

CURRENT PRACTICE

Disaster response usually begins after bystanders, witnesses, or victims alert the response agencies. In the United States, Canada, and the Cayman Islands, response agencies are notified via the 911 system. Throughout the European Union, Russia, Ukraine, and Switzerland, activation is by the 112 system. In some Caribbean countries and countries with British influence, 999 is used for activation. In Mexico, separate numbers are used for Police (#066), Fire (#068), and emergency medical services (EMS) emergencies (#065). Immediate disaster response is initiated at the local level. When needs exceed resources, official requests can be made to adjacent local communities or jurisdictions for mutual aid response. As the size of a disaster and needs increase, assistance can be requested from city, county, regional, state, and, ultimately, federal resources. If the initial disaster occurs on federal property, such as the Murrah Federal Building Bombing in Oklahoma City, federal officials would be more directly and immediately involved.

Sudden onset disasters (earthquakes, building collapses, and explosions) usually result in uninjured or minimally injured bystanders stepping forward and initiating evacuation, scene control, hemorrhage control, search and rescue, CPR, and many other roles. It is usually not possible to predict the timing of an event, its location, or the presence of bystanders. This makes planning for bystander action difficult, and therefore a confusing issue, with reliance on bystanders as a part of the formal response. For disaster incidents occurring in remote locations, however, the response time of professional rescuers is likely to be delayed, often by hours, and bystander action is critical for survival. For example, a towboat outside of Mobile, Alabama, in 1993 struck the Big Bayou Canot Bridge, displacing it and the attached rails. The oncoming Amtrak train, the *Sunset Limited*, struck the deformed rails, derailed, fell into the swamp, and caught fire. Because of the remote location and heavy fog, it took the Coast Guard 1 hour and 40 minutes to arrive, and the first rescue helicopter arrived an hour after that. By then, 28 individuals were rescued by the crews of the towboat and a second boat.[16]

By all historical accounts, bystanders have various levels of training in first aid, CPR, and disaster response. It is thought that those who are trained can contribute more effectively. It is therefore in the best interest of the public that individuals are trained in such basic skills. This seems like a daunting task, but it is not without precedent. In 2009, 40% of cardiac arrest patients received bystander CPR, up from 28% in 2005.[17] Programs teaching Basic Life Support (BLS) and CPR are common, so that people who witness a cardiac arrest can initiate assistance quickly, prior to the arrival of first responders. Public access

defibrillation enhances survival as well. Using CPR training of the lay public as a model demonstrates that other skills training of the public could benefit victims injured in disasters. In the setting of disasters, it is unlikely that first responders will be able to respond to all 911 calls associated with a major disaster, and response times in remote locations will be long. Individuals can initiate search and rescue, hemorrhage control, and advanced first aid in their absence. This realization formed the basis for the development of such programs as the Community Emergency Response Teams (CERTs) in earthquake-prone Southern California. The training conducted as part of CERT also promotes safety in earthquake zones, to prevent further injury. The use of simple shoring techniques for urban search and rescue and victim extrication, hard hats, and instruction in triage principles have been found to be effective. It is important to note that not all experts see the importance of utilizing laypersons in disaster response, and some continue to separate these people from incidents. Experts have presented data and descriptions of many actual disaster situations and have discussed the pros and cons to both management styles. As the debate ensues, one thing is apparent: the usually large number of people immediately available for rescue at many scenes is an untapped resource. Any efficient and organized use of this immediate workforce is clearly beneficial.

Internationally, disasters are frequent, whether natural or human-made. Hurricanes, earthquakes, tsunamis, tornadoes, and other weather-related catastrophes seem more prevalent, and there is an expectation of the growing public for a proper response. There is also an interest and thirst for knowledge with respect to disaster management. We have entered a worrisome new world of human-made disasters over the last few decades. With the current "War on Terror," attacks must be on everyone's mind and not just the planners of such events as mass gatherings. The 2013 Boston Marathon Bombing clearly showed this. In addition to the well-drilled EMS and police agencies attending such incidents, the importance of bystander actions were never more apparent. The blast and ballistic injuries resulted in significant life-threatening hemorrhage, and the swift use of tourniquets (proven by the military to drastically reduce the number of preventable deaths from battlefield gunshot and blast injuries) by bystanders was lifesaving. Despite multiple explosions, many bystanders also assisted injured runners and observers to the medical tents, thereby saving lives.[18] Another example of layperson training can be found in Ghana. This country does not have an EMS system, so the ever-present taxi cab and truck drivers were trained in initial first aid, splinting, airway management, and hemorrhage control.[19] They now account for the transportation of many, if not most, trauma victims to hospitals in that country.

According to FEMA, the National Response Framework utilized in the United States provides context for how the entire community works together after a catastrophic event. The response effort cannot be from the government alone, and it is the residents of the affected communities that come together to help in the most-expedient way. The National Response Framework is organized into five disaster-preparedness mission areas: prevention, protection, mitigation, response, and recovery. Bystanders and people of the community need to be a part of each of these phases and must be prepared through training and discussion. In the United States, it is recognized that bystanders often assume the role of the true first responders. Thus there are efforts to improve their capabilities with the hope that this would lead to better response to any catastrophic event. On local levels, however, bystanders are often forgotten in many emergency-management plans and drills. It is well documented and understood that disaster situations often overwhelm Fire, Police, and EMS personnel. Despite this, few emergency plans include the use of bystanders as initial assets in a disaster. They also fail to recognize bystanders in the roles as already discussed. Disaster response has a few goals including decreasing morbidity and mortality, minimizing loss of property, and promoting recovery. Achieving these goals often requires efficient use of all available resources, including bystanders and volunteers. Coordination of bystanders, often accompanied by spontaneous volunteers, will have an effect on the efficiency of this response. Involvement of the community in their own disaster response also promotes the resiliency of the community. In one interview survey, volunteers and nongovernmental organizations (NGOs) were described as adhesives for connecting people together or connecting various activities together, and as catalysts for reconnecting the affected area with the rest of the world. The article also stated, "As various people and activities became connected, new relationships came into being. Relationships thus formed while dealing with a disaster together may have commercial and cultural significance and might help the affected area recover."[20]

Bystanders are usually present, and they play some part in disaster response, regardless of any invitation. Their presence at the scene can have positive or negative effects, depending on how they are utilized. Bystanders and volunteers at the site of an incident often remain unused and idle, despite their motivation to help. Upon arrival of Police and EMS to any incident, the usual protocol is to set up a perimeter with yellow tape. Although designed to keep the public out, this may effectively block further assistance of willing bystanders or highly trained volunteers at a scene. Valid reasons for this include: decreased risk of injury to bystanders, decreased legal and forensic ramifications, inability to verify credentials, risk of looting of victim personal property if the scene is not controlled, and prevention of imposters who can harm the victims. This last point includes prevention of secondary devices on a scene intent to harm rescue workers. Realistically, bystanders and volunteers will initiate their own missions, which are often parallel, redundant, and obtrusive to public safety responders if they are not properly utilized. In some instances, collective behavior emerges, with victims forming their own spontaneous work groups, with rules, guidelines, and spontaneous leadership.[21] In Oklahoma City following the federal building bombing, multiple triage sites were initially set up, on different sides of the building, each unaware of the others' existence.

Realistically, any government response will be limited and delayed for many individuals. This is usually a matter of resource allocation, access to the incident, and the scale of the event. First responders are therefore family, friends, neighbors, and "Good Samaritans." In any incident, the greatest opportunity to save lives is in the first couple of minutes or hours, usually prior to the arrival of the organized local response. It is important to remember that a federal response usually takes up to 72 hours to fully organize and to access the affected area. Therefore bystanders play a major role in limiting avoidable and unnecessary deaths.[22] Avoidable deaths are moderate injuries that, without treatment, cause death within hours, such as continuous

bleeding from an open wound. Saving the lives of these victims is possible through early detection, first aid, and rapid evacuation to a medical facility. Statistically, most of these injured patients are saved from the rubble by themselves, family members, neighbors, and other bystanders. Few are saved by professional search-and-rescue forces.[23–27] "Unnecessary" deaths are victims who become trapped in a confined space under rubble, suffering from minimal injuries or no injuries. If not detected in time, these victims can die from dehydration, heatstroke, frostbite, inhalation of smoke, earthquake aftershocks, and dust or hazardous materials, or they become trampled and crushed while attempts to remove rubble by bulldozers and heavy equipment machines are used. Thus, in the aftermath of an earthquake, many trapped victims may not be pulled out of the rubble and thus gradually die an "unnecessary" death, according to Angus et al. and Ashkenazi.[14] Their findings indicate that the main reason is the sluggish arrival of search-and-rescue teams with domestic and international rescue forces reaching the disaster area too late. In earthquakes, this is the largest population that can be saved if there were sufficient manpower to locate and remove these victims from the rubble. Advocacy for bystander incorporation into response plans for disasters requires that we ask if bystanders will be reliable partners in such a situation. Can their lack of formal training be overcome? Will their involvement in disaster response expose the public and bystanders to unnecessary risk and injury and create increased liability to bystanders? Last, is there consensus in the government and the first responder community on the use of volunteers in disaster response? Through research, change in legislative policy, public education, and proper coordination with officials involved in local disaster planning, the integration of bystanders in disaster response can lead to improved outcomes in disaster response, resulting in decreased morbidity and mortality associated with any catastrophic event. We must not only educate the public to become active partners in a disaster response but also train first responders to organize, manage, and harness the talents of bystanders (Box 47-1).

⚠ PITFALLS

Bystanders are unknown entities in disaster response, and their dependability and reliability in these events remains unknown. There has been some research into the behavior of bystanders in response to emergencies. For years, those who oppose the use of bystanders have cited a phenomenon referred as the "bystander effect" as a reason to doubt their reliability. The term *bystander effect* refers to the observance that the greater the number of people present, the less likely people are to help a person in distress. When an emergency situation occurs, observers are more likely to take action if there are few or no other witnesses. Rebecca Solnit[28] researched the behavior of bystanders following disasters (1906 San Francisco Earthquake through the 2006 Hurricane Katrina). Her work revealed that, in the aftermath of each of these incidents, bystanders came together to assist one another,

---

BOX 47-1   Role of Bystander in Disasters

- During the event, find a safe location so that you do not become a casualty.
- Alert the response system that there is an event.
- When the scene is safe, try to assess and provide as many situation details as possible to the emergency call center.
- Remove as many victims from entrapment as possible.
- Provide aid based on your level of training and personal skills.
- Do no harm.
- On arrival of the official response team, report all information to the on-scene incident leader or manager.

- The official responders will institute an incident command structure that identifies who will assign tasks and to whom each participant in the incident must report. If you continue in the incident, you will be expected to participate in this system.
- Be flexible as the situation may require you to do tasks unrelated to your current profession or expertise.
- Participate in training exercises and preparedness education so that you may be more effective in an incident.

behaving cooperatively and working for the common good. This, in fact, is what was witnessed in Haiti.[29] These case examples provide valuable lessons for those who plan and execute emergency responses.

Bystanders can be directly responsible for obstructing the scene of terror events and disasters as they are drawn to the scene out of curiosity and/or the desire to offer assistance. Bystanders who are not injured usually try to assist in any way possible. While some are trying to flee the scene, others are trying to enter, often leading to significant difficulty and delay of the EMS professionals responding to the call. It is not unusual that streets are filled with responding vehicles while people jam the streets to the point where no one can enter or exit. This leaves critical victims without a way to exit the scene to definitive care. It is clear that the professionals often have the skill and knowledge of the command structure needed to properly manage the scene, but bystanders tend to have no knowledge of the structure and therefore can impede the process. In the Dizengoff Center Shopping Mall suicide bomber attack in Tel Aviv, Israel, in 1996, it is documented that bystanders stayed in place to help rather than leave the scene as instructed. It was specifically noted that EMS personnel were able to control the scene better when they included the bystanders in the rescue process, utilizing them in a number of ways, including as stretcher-bearers to evacuate casualties to the ambulances. They also turned out to be very helpful in directing traffic away from the scene.[29] Bystanders, however, can also disrupt the flow of reliable information and create rumors as information is passed on that is not correct. If not dealt with effectively, bystanders and survivors of the event can contribute significantly to the chaos and have the potential to magnify its consequences.[29] Leadership on scene, clearly defining expectations and giving direct orders with defined tasks, has been found to be the key ingredient in managing bystanders on scene in the most-effective way. Without this defined leadership, individuals who are not considered part of a structured response may be seen as intrusive and conflicting to the EMS personnel as they arrive and, further, as potential liabilities. Training of EMS personnel to manage bystanders is of the utmost importance. With increasing use of social media and instant TV coverage of an event, the public has become intolerant of any delays in disaster response and relief. The development and widespread use of cameras in smartphones allows the bystander to record any event and post it online, thus giving the world an instant eye at the event itself.

Bystanders are usually not formally trained to respond to disasters, and they often have little training in First Aid or the ICS. This complicates the use of bystanders and spontaneous volunteers by public safety responders. Disaster response is obviously more effective when some form of ICS is adopted, but untrained bystanders often need explicit instructions and resources to ensure that they adhere to the chain of command and not wander off on their own missions. In the chaos of multiple agency responses, bystanders are often seen as a nuisance to the organized responders. Bystanders must be able to attach to a unit that is incorporated in the response and should be self-sufficient. The public should receive comprehensive training that includes basic disaster-response training and awareness of ICS so that their participation in these events can be more effective. For those in the United States, they should be encouraged to join a CERT team if one is available in their community, or a unit of the Medical Reserve Corps if they are a medical professional. For those living internationally, they should find the local equivalents of these teams or lead the charge in developing such a team if it does not exist locally. Emergency managers and planners all over the world need to encourage community involvement in training and exercises. Depending on the bystander's level of training, a culture of civic responsibility and preparedness should be fostered by all preparedness agencies. Just-in-time

training paradigms should also be developed and disseminated to first responders to use as a management tool for bystander utilization. Although mitigation and preparedness save more lives in disasters, "maximum lives saved" is associated with bystander actions as a part of the response. Empowering bystanders with knowledge in disaster response will give them the confidence to act when confronted with an event. Bystanders should train and exercise with government organizations and NGOs that prepare and respond to disasters. Disaster planners need to consider bystanders in their plans and have training campaigns similar to Public Access Defibrillation programs, shown to be effective in decreasing mortality caused by sudden cardiac arrest within the community. In the United States, the nationwide "If You See Something, Say Something" public awareness campaign, originally used by New York's Metropolitan Transportation Authority and now promoted by the U.S. Department of Homeland Security,[30] is described as "a simple and effective program to raise public awareness of indicators of terrorism and terrorism-related crime, and to emphasize the importance of reporting suspicious activity or packages to the proper local law enforcement authorities." Civilian response to this program has resulted in early neutralization of terrorist attempts and demonstrated the positive role that the public can play in emergencies.

Bystanders have no moral or legal responsibility to respond in many states and countries. Most bystanders are not registered as responders for disasters, and there is little time or ability during a disaster to document individuals who responded to the events. Thus their actions and involvement are often undocumented, and there is little accountability, whether heroic or not. Bystanders confronted by the damage and injuries around them have been shown to be willing to take responsibility and put themselves in physical danger to rescue victims. In the bombing of the Alfred P. Murrah Federal Building in Oklahoma City on April 19, 1995, nurse Rebecca Anderson was running toward the building to render assistance when she was thought to have been struck on the head by falling debris. She never made it to the building and died in a hospital four days later from an intracranial bleed.[31] This unfortunate incident highlights that untrained and unprepared bystanders and victims of any event face potential harm from an unsafe scene. Preparedness of first responders needs to include training with and use of personal protective equipment (hard hats, steel-toed boots, dust masks/respirators, etc.), and the importance of having this equipment readily available at the time of a disaster. There is also the potential for abuse and harm to the public because without security there is no protection from predators disguised as volunteers. Bystanders may be exposed to risk, but the public may be exposed to additional risk and injuries created by untrained or overeager bystanders. In the United States, coverage for liability, as well as injury for volunteers helping in disasters, differs significantly. Many states have no workers' compensation coverage for volunteers injured while responding, and most "Good Samaritan" statutes are limited to providing some degree of legal immunity at an emergency scene. Most of these laws are not comprehensive enough to cover volunteer providers acting during declared public health emergencies. Further legislation is needed to cover people caring for others in the immediate scenario, as well as the later stages of a disaster as conditions slowly return to normal. Over time, it is likely that federal legislation will need to be enacted to protect "Good Samaritans" during disaster responses.

The United States is not unique in its attempt to deal with legislation aimed at protecting those who assist a victim during a medical emergency. A number of countries have enacted national legislation to establish a single policy for such circumstances. Australia, Belgium, Finland, France, Germany, Italy, Portugal, and Spain have criminal penalties for failing to come to the aid of another person.[32]

When it comes to their roles in disasters, members of the general public are often confused. Some disaster experts have recommended that bystanders and members of the public be encouraged to participate in all phases of the emergency-management cycle: mitigation, planning, preparedness, response, and recovery. Despite a strong desire to help out, bystanders who are present at a disaster site can actually impede rescue and recovery efforts if they are unaffiliated and untrained in disaster operations. There have been significant government campaigns focused on citizen preparedness and urging individuals to plan on being self-sufficient for 72 hours after a disaster. These campaigns recommend that families have an emergency plan that includes stockpiling water, food, and personal medications, and arranging for meeting places of family members when they are displaced. Even though personal preparedness is a great beginning, community disaster preparedness should also be the goal.

Search, rescue, and medical teams may be rapidly deployed to extricate trapped victims and treat the wounded in disasters, but they cannot go everywhere and save everyone at the same time. It can take upward of 24 hours or more to bring in resources from out of the area. The time it takes for help to be administered to a victim often determines who lives and who dies. Officials and emergency managers must develop a more-sophisticated understanding of bystander capabilities, motivation, and expectation so that these true first responders can be incorporated into plans when appropriate.

An understanding of bystanders and the positive effect they can have is essential to planning an effective response to a disaster. Emergency response planners may do well to scrutinize their own assumptions about bystanders and how they can be integrated into a disaster scenario. Research shows that bystanders can be fully capable in disaster response.[14] Bystanders are being recognized as a critical addition in the conversation of local preparedness. As government officials and the public start demanding better preparedness for natural disasters (tornadoes, hurricanes, ice storms, landslides, and forest fires) and human-made disasters caused by weapons of mass destruction (WMD) and terrorist attacks, the discussion is starting to include training the layperson prior to an incident. This is no small undertaking. Volunteers for disaster simulation are always needed to help with exercises and participate as victims. These individuals are not just bodies for use during the drill. They should be thought of as conveyors of important information to other laypersons and possible rescuers on scene after an attack or sudden violent storm. Bystanders should be trained and empowered so that their integration into a response supports rather than undermines the parallel activities of first responders. Research is greatly needed with respect to the educational didactics, practical skills, and most appropriate organizational structure for bystander response. Empirical data with respect to bystander response actions, both productive and counterproductive, are needed. Such research will help us all maximize the use of bystanders and develop the most-effective structure for the most-expedient response.

Because it is not possible to predict where or when an attack or natural disaster will occur, it is difficult to train everyone in the world about preparation and protocol. In addition, it is not possible to predict who will jump in to help versus who will run away from the situation. What is known, however, is that there is a need to better understand the role of the bystander and include the bystander in the plan and response effort. The Centers for Disease Control and Prevention (CDC) describes the term *acute injury care* as, "The care of the acutely injured is a public health issue that involves bystanders and community members, health care professionals, and health care systems. It encompasses prehospital emergency medical services; emergency department assessment, treatment, and stabilization; and in-hospital care surgery and medical management among all age groups."

Incorporating bystanders in the definition is important, as this starts the groundwork for the education process and discussion of how to fully educate laypersons on a local level. Gregg Lord, former Director of the Emergency Care Coordination Center of the U.S. DHHS, wrote

> *When prepared with the basics, however, people generally jump in and help if they feel they have some skills to help. At the core, education of the average citizen will alleviate many of the impediments to bystanders acting, and there are issues that many emergency planners, response organizations and hospitals can help fix. By supporting first aid and CPR education for members of your community, you can give them the skills that they need to help someone in an emergency. You're also letting your community know that they can and should be a part of an effective emergency response and that you want them to help protect their loved ones and their communities.*[33]

This outlines the many educational steps needed for community leaders to begin the process of emergency management within their own community. In addition to a monetary commitment for the education itself, expertise is needed to conduct the education. The message should be uniform and consistent. Government, voluntary agencies, and private sector representatives should join together to create multimedia public education campaigns on how to be an effective disaster volunteer. The public also needs to be educated of the fact that untrained bystanders (family members, neighbors, and the general public) are often the first at the scene offering assistance and transportation. This is in contrast to the misperception that well-trained professionals will be among the first to respond and care for victims in a disaster situation. Dr. Rick Hunt, director of the Division of Injury Response at the CDC National Center for Injury Prevention and Control, called the train bombings in Madrid in 2004 "an inflection point," as there were more than 2000 casualties. He pointed out the importance of bystanders to the response: "Look at photos of the Madrid bombings. How many uniforms do you see? The public must be prepared because they will be the ones with immediate access to the injured."[34]

REFERENCES

1. https://www.fema.gov/frequently-asked-questions-teens. Updated July 2014.
2. Fugate C. *Post Katrina: What It Takes to Cut the Bureaucracy and Assure a More Rapid Response.* July 27, 2009, Washington DC, http://www.fema.gov/pdf/about/testimony/072709_fugate.pdf.
3. Gallagher EJ, Lombardi G, Gennis P. Effectiveness of bystander cardiopulmonary resuscitation and survival following out-of-hospital cardiac arrest. *JAMA.* 1995;274(24):1922–1925. http://dx.doi.org/10.1001/jama.1995.03530240032036.
4. Ritter G, Wolfe RA, Goldstein S, et al. The effect of bystander CPR on survival of out-of-hospital cardiac arrest victims. *Am Heart J.* 1985;110(5):932–937.
5. Cummins RO, Eisenberg MS, Hallstrom AP, Litwin PE. Survival of out-of-hospital cardiac arrest with early initiation of cardiopulmonary resuscitation. *Am J Emerg Med.* 1985;3(2):114–119. http://dx.doi.org/10.1016/0735-6757(85)90032-4.
6. Berdowski J, Blom MT, Bardai A, Tan HL, Tijssen JGP, Koster RW. Impact of onsite or dispatched automated external defibrillator use on survival after out-of-hospital cardiac arrest. *Circulation.* 2011;124:2225–2232.
7. Auf der Heide E. *Disaster Response: Principles of Preparation and Coordination.* St. Louis, MO: The C.V. Mosby Co; 1989, p. 114.
8. Drabek TE, et al. *Managing Multiorganizational Emergency Responses: Emergent Search and Rescue Networks in Natural Disaster and Remote Area Settings.* Natural Hazards Information Center, Boulder, CO: University of Colorado, Boulder; 1981.

9. Aylwin CJ, Konig TC, Brennan NW, et al. Reduction in critical mortality in urban mass casualty incidents: analysis of triage, surge, and resource use after the London bombings on July 7, 2005. *Lancet.* 2006;368:2219–2225.

10. Glass TA. Emergency, catastrophe and disaster: a typology with implications for terrorism response. In: Wessely S, Krasnov YN, eds. *Psychological Responses to the New Terrorism: A NATO-Russia Dialogue.* IOS Press; 2005:25–36.

11. Murakami H. *Underground: The Tokyo Gas Attack and the Japanese Psyche. Translated from the Japanese.* New York: Vintage International; 2001, 366 p.

12. Welles Crowther "The Man in the Red Bandanna" posthumously named Honorary Firefighter. http://www.nyc.gov/html/fdny/html/events/2006/121506a.shtml; Accessed 09.10.14.

13. Defede J. *The Day the World Came to Town: 9/11 in Gander, Newfoundland.* New York: Harper Collins Publishing; 2002:6–7.

14. Ashkenazi I, McNulty E, Marcus LJ, Dorn BC. The role of bystanders in mass casualty events: lessons from the 2010 Haiti earthquake. *J Def Stud Resour Manag.* 2012;1:2.

15. Kellerman AL, Peleg K. Lessons from Boston. *N Engl J Med.* 2013;368: 1956–1957. http://dx.doi.org/10.1056/NEJMp1305304, Accessed 24.09.14.

16. *Technical Rescue Incident Report: The Derailment of the Sunset Limited: Sept. 22, 1993, Bayou Canot, Alabama.* United States Fire Administration. Available at: http://www.usfa.fema.gov/downloads/pdf/publications/fa-163b.pdf.

17. Bobrow BJ, Spaite DW, Berg RA, et al. Chest compression-only CPR by lay rescuers and survival from out-of-hospital cardiac arrest. *JAMA.* 304 (13):447–1454. doi:10.1001/jama.2010.1392.

18. Jarrett E. Bystanders who didn't stand by. Accessed at: http://www.phe.gov/ASPRBlog/Lists/Posts/Post.aspx?ID=51].

19. Mock CN, Tiska M, Adu-Ampofo M, Boakye G. Improvements in prehospital trauma care in an African country with no formal emergency medical services. *J Trauma Inj Infect Crit Care.* 2002;53(1):90–97.

20. Suzuki I. Roles of volunteers in disaster prevention: implications of questionnaire and interview surveys. In: Ikeda S, Fukuzono T, Sato T, eds. *A Better Integrated Management of Disaster Risks: Toward Resilient Society to Emerging Disaster Risks in Mega-Cities.* Terrapub and NIED; 2006:153–163. Accessed at, http://www.terrapub.co.jp/e-library/nied/pdf/153.pdf.

21. Glass TA. Understanding public response to disasters. *Public Health Rep.* 2001;116(suppl 2):69–73. http://www.ncbi.nlm.nih.gov/pmc/articles/PMC1497258/pdf/11880676.pdf.

22. Ashkenazi I, McNulty E, Marcus LJ, Dorn BC. The role of bystanders in mass casualty events: lessons from the 2010 Haiti earthquake. *J Def Stud Resour Manag.* 2012;1:2.

23. Ashkenazi I. Predictable surprise—the 2008 Sichuan earthquake. *Harefuah.* 2008;147:578–586, 664.

24. Ashkenazi I. Do bystanders fail to act in emergencies? The Haiti Earthquake. *Israeli Military Medicine.* 2010;7:90–95.

25. Ashkenazi I, Shemer J. Tsunami: the death waves. *Harefuah.* 2005;144:154–159, 232.

26. de Ville de Goyet C. Stop propagating disaster myths. *Lancet.* 2000;356:762–764.

27. MacIntyre AG, Barbera JA, Petinaux BP. Survival interval in earthquake entrapments: research findings reinforced in the 2010 Haiti earthquake response. *Disaster Med Public Health Prep.* 2010;5:13–22.

28. Solnit R. *A Paradise Built in Hell: The Extraordinary Communities That Arise in Disaster.* New York: Viking; 2009.

29. Cole LA, Connell ND, Adini B. *Local Planning for Terror and Disaster: From Bioterrorism to Earthquakes. The Role of the On-Scene Bystander and Survivor.* October 2012, 165–167.

30. *"If You See Something, Say Something" Campaign.* U.S. Dept of Homeland Security. Accessed at: http://www.dhs.gov/if-you-see-something-say-something.

31. Linenthal ET. *The Unfinished Bombing—Oklahoma City in American Memory.* Oxford: New York, NY; 2001.

32. Howie WO, Howie BA, McMullen PC. To assist or not assist: good Samaritan considerations for nurse practitioners. *J Nurse Pract.* 2012;8 (9):688–692.

33. U.S. DHSS Public Health Emergency ASPR blog. http://www.phe.gov/ASPRBlog/Lists/Posts/Post.aspx?ID=64.

34. American Trauma Society webpage: Trauma Resources, Bystander Care. http://www.amtrauma.org/resources/bystander-care/index.aspx.

48 CHAPTER

Surveillance

P. Gregg Greenough and Mandana Mehta

The World Health Organization (WHO) defines *surveillance* as "the ongoing systematic collection, analysis, and interpretation of data in order to plan, implement and evaluate public health interventions."[1] There are three key elements to surveillance: (1) the continuous, cyclical collection of data in a systematic manner; (2) the timely analysis and interpretation of these data, and (3) the linkage of this information to operational activities and policies.[2] These three elements share a symbiotic relationship, and each one is of little value without the other two. Together they provide a unique tool to track trends in overall population health and identify emerging public health concerns. Surveillance differs from other data gathering mechanisms used during disasters, such as rapid assessments and field surveys, which typically are cross sectional and provide a "snapshot" of particular health needs and outcome variables.

Disasters create circumstances in which general-population health is difficult to sustain and epidemics can easily arise. In this context, robust surveillance provides the only reliable means of monitoring public health, managing the burden of disease on health care systems, identifying emerging diseases with epidemic potential, and evaluating successes or failures in policy, programming, and disaster management.

HISTORICAL PERSPECTIVE

Surveillance has been practiced in some form since the 1348 bubonic plague epidemic.[3] However, in the seventeenth century, Leiniz in Germany and Graunt in England advanced the notion of applying numerical value to disease and tracking death counts. At the same time, Sydenham developed a classification for diseases, providing a uniform recognition of disease definitions and the basis upon which statistical analyses could be understood. By the nineteenth century, efforts were being made to nationalize health information, collect vital statistics, perform analyses, and initiate a reporting mechanism. Chadwick in England and Shattuck in Massachusetts noted the links between poverty and disease and promoted the idea of adding socioeconomic information, as well as geographic and occupational information, to death notices.[4] By the turn of the century, all U.S. states and most European countries mandated the reporting of specific infectious diseases. In the United States the Great 1918 Influenza Pandemic prompted a national mortality reporting requirement.[5]

Events occurring during the 1950s and 1960s helped to hone the definition of the term *surveillance* and to elucidate its role in public health practice. Langmuir at the U.S. Centers for Disease Control and Prevention (CDC) emphasized the need for the systematic collection of pertinent data and its timely analysis and dissemination to policy makers. Meanwhile, Raska at the WHO stressed that surveillance should apply not only to the control of communicable diseases but also to their prevention. In 1968 the World Health Assembly broadened the role of surveillance beyond the realm of communicable diseases. Since

then, surveillance has been applied to lead poisoning, injury, substance misuse, congenital malformations, behavioral risk factors, and disasters, along with a comprehensive list of other public health issues.

The routine use of surveillance in humanitarian relief response followed the massive population displacement into Goma, Zaire, in 1994. When over one million people rapidly moved onto uninhabitable land with inadequate public health infrastructure, an epidemic of cholera, followed soon after by dysentery, swept through their camps, killing 50,000. The crude mortality rates recorded by the humanitarian community during the first month of the epidemic were among some of the highest in recent history: between 19.5 and 31.2 deaths per 10,000 population per day, far above the emergency threshold of 1 death per 10,000 per day.[6] The crisis led to an initiative to develop standards of practice in field operations: in 1996 a group of experts from 228 humanitarian organizations inaugurated the Sphere Project, a consensus-driven document elaborating minimum technical and ethical standards in all sectors of humanitarian aid work. The resulting Sphere Handbook emphasizes that "the design and development of health services should be guided by the collection, analysis, interpretation, and use of relevant public health data."[7]

Likewise, the contemporaneous Médicins sans Frontières refugee health handbook identified surveillance as one of the top-ten priorities in an emergency and "an integral part of all relief activities."[8]

The cholera epidemic that followed the 2010 Haiti Earthquake focused attention on postdisaster surveillance. Prior to the earthquake, the Haitian Ministry of Health tracked only six indicators, all communicable diseases (acute hemorrhagic fever, acute flaccid paralysis, suspected bacterial meningitis, suspected diphtheria, suspected measles, and bite by animal suspected of having rabies). Within weeks following the event, a national sentinel surveillance system had expanded to 25 indicators, including watery diarrhea, bloody diarrhea, tuberculosis, and tetanus, as well as earthquake-related noncommunicable diseases, such as renal failure (from crush injuries), trauma and fractures, mental health, infected wounds, and concussion, among others.[9] When cholera not endemic to the country emerged 9 months later, a rapidly scalable cholera-specific surveillance system was needed to capture daily cases in all areas of the country. The implementation of Haiti's National Cholera Surveillance System was built on the rigorous postdisaster national system that by then also critically included the displaced populations.[10]

The role of ongoing, pertinent health information that is iterative and available to those who must intervene in the context of humanitarian crises is now a widely accepted and essential component of disaster response and rehabilitation.

CURRENT PRACTICE

During and immediately after a disaster, health information systems and national surveillance systems may be underperforming, being either overwhelmed quickly and disabled or destroyed. To provide timely data on the primary needs of a disaster-affected population in the early days of the emergency, the WHO, in 2012, published guidance on the establishment of an Early Warning Alert and Response Network (EWARN).[11] The first steps are to identify the EWARN network (responsible for collecting and analyzing data and disseminating information to relevant organizations) and to establish objectives for the surveillance system. The WHO outlines six objectives of surveillance applicable in emergencies: (1) identify public health priorities, (2) monitor the severity of the emergency by collecting and analyzing mortality and morbidity data, (3) detect outbreaks and monitor the response to these, (4) track trends in incidence and case fatality from major disease, (5) monitor the effects of specific health interventions, and (6) provide information to the Ministry of Health and other implicated organizations in the affected area to assist in planning and implementing health programs and mobilizing resources.[12] To achieve these objectives, the surveillance system should be simple and clear in its focus, easily understood by all who receive its directions, and flexible enough to respond to new health problems and program activities.

The next step is to define the population of interest and its relationship to the health sector in the disaster area. What is the demographic makeup of the population (age, sex, ethnicity, etc.)? Where do people live before and after the disaster? Where do people access health services, if at all? Where do health events occur? What are the barriers to universal health coverage? What is the structure and capability of the national health information system and which governmental, nongovernmental (NGOs), and international agencies are working in the health sector?

To answer these questions, surveillance systems track *indicators*, primarily quantitative measures that describe the overall health of the population and the process and outcome of health services. These give an indication of the efficacy and efficiency of a program, system, or organization. Their inherent value in a surveillance system is their ability to be tracked over time and to be compared with a baseline. Mortality, morbidity, and nutrition rates are the most common quantitative indicators followed during the emergency phase.

A surveillance methodology is built based on the initial rapid assessments made during the first phase of the emergency response. The outputs of those assessments should focus on the health problems that produce the highest morbidity and mortality rates, especially if the population affected is displaced. Mortality rates are the most important indicator for identifying a population under stress. Most commonly, the crude mortality rate (CMR) is used in emergencies to track the effects of disaster-generated communicable diseases or injuries. The practical initial quantitative baseline data captured at the onset of the disaster are the following:

- *Population size:* specifically the total population affected, disaggregated by age and gender (common at-risk groups include women and children less than 5 years old), in-migration and out-migration as a result of the disaster or conflict
- CMR, in units of deaths per 10,000 persons per day
- Mortality rate for children under 5 years old (U5MR), in units of deaths of children under 5 years per 10,000 population of children under 5 years per day
- Case fatality rates (CFRs), the percentage of persons diagnosed as having a specified disease who die because of that disease within a given period
- Nutritional status, specifically weight-for-height ratios of children aged 6 to 59 months, expressed as a percentage of population with a Z-score less than −2 (moderate global acute malnutrition) and less than −3 (severe global acute malnutrition)

In the emergency phase, surveillance activities should specifically focus on those diseases most likely to cause death or significant morbidity, namely diarrheal illnesses (especially in a malnourished, displaced population), acute respiratory infections, measles, and meningitis. As the emergency evolves into the postdisaster phase, other communicable and noncommunicable diseases are added to surveillance monitoring, and, depending on context, may include HIV/AIDS, tuberculosis, sexually transmitted diseases, chronic diseases, injury, immunization coverage (e.g., the Expanded Program on Immunization), and health care access. Surveillance for the displaced, disaster-affected population should eventually be integrated into the national health information system of the country, which is discussed later in this chapter.

Initial sector-specific indicators will identify population needs in relation to critical services, specifically water, sanitation, and hygiene (WASH), food, and health services. Early critical sector indicators, expressed as ratios of populations, include the following:

- Access to sanitation services and adequate access to potable water
- Access to health care services
- Capacity or level of function of health care services (numbers of providers for the population)
- Health care infrastructure (functioning hospitals and clinics)
- Food security (physical and economic access to food)

As the disaster response becomes established and transitions into the postdisaster phase, qualitative indicators that examine the relief effort will guide resources and programming. These may include the following:

- Factors that affect the ability of the population to access health care services
- Quality of services (degree to which services received are adequate for population needs)
- Equity in distribution of health resources (may explain why one subgroup of the population fares worse than another)
- Main program activities (for individuals or groups of relief agencies involved in the delivery of care)

In terms of program performance, field epidemiologists recommend that indicators have SMART attributes: in other words, they should be "*s*pecific, *m*easurable, *a*ccurate, *r*ealistic and *t*ime-bound."[13] Indicators must also be sensitive enough to assess the effect of interventions on health problems and determine whether the effort is having a tangible effect on the population or whether new strategies are needed. Once the emergency phase is over, the WHO emphasizes the importance of "re-integrating EWARN back into the national surveillance system."[14]

Data Collection

Methods for data collection depend on the type of surveillance used and the preexisting status of national health information gathering systems. *Active* surveillance involves a proactive seeking out of cases through some type of sampling mechanism in defined regions; this type of surveillance is used more frequently during the emergency phase and usually relies on direct reporting from households or, more commonly, health facilities. *Passive* surveillance systems rely on reports from the data sources, typically, as cases present themselves to health facilities. Passive systems are more suited to long-term, ongoing surveillance during the postemergency phase, once health systems and national surveillance programs have been restored. Both have practical pros and cons. Although active surveillance produces data that are more accurate, it is far more labor intensive and thus more costly to implement. However, the need for accurate mortality rates and incidence of critical diseases justifies the cost and effort during the first phase of the emergency. Passive systems by definition represent a self-selected sample and may not reflect accurately a health issue within the greater population. Because passive systems are less costly and require less training, they are more practical for long-term surveillance. In either case, the surveillance system must have high sensitivity in detecting disease (i.e., the ability to detect "true" cases of illness or injury).[15] Another frequently used method of surveillance is *sentinel surveillance*, in which selected data collection points (e.g., designated health facilities within the system and in strategic geographic locations) are tasked with identifying and reporting specific diseases or health events. Designated segments of the population or particular locales in the disaster-affected population may be specially chosen for monitoring certain indicators (e.g., the parameter weight-for-height in children aged 6 to 59 months). Sentinel health events refer to conditions with the potential to affect the health stability of the population, often a warning signal that the current level of preventive and curative care needs attention. The occurrence of one of these events should prompt immediate action. One case of meningitis in an overcrowded camp for displaced persons demands an instantaneous response from health agencies to avert an epidemic catastrophe.

Data collection tools, especially in the emergency phase, should be short, easy to use, and readily understandable. Moreover, they should remain consistent over time. These tools are designed to collect only the minimal, most-essential information in a clear and unambiguous fashion. The use of simple, uniform case definitions for communicable diseases is critical. Such definitions can be found on the websites of both the Centers for Disease Control and Prevention (CDC) and the WHO. All health providers involved in surveillance should know, for instance, that a generalized rash for more than 3-days duration *and* a temperature greater than 38 °C *and* one or more symptoms of cough, rhinorrhea, or red eyes define a case of measles. Common diarrhea is classified as three or more liquid stools per day. In countries where malaria is endemic, a temperature greater than 38.5 °C in the absence of other infection is indeed malaria for data purposes. From these simple yet sensitive definitions, trends can be established and monitored. Epi Info software, available free of charge from the CDC website, assists in both generating data forms and analyzing data.

Data sources are most often health facilities, specifically the health care providers who daily record hospital emergency departments and clinic visits. In a displaced population living in temporary camps, registration systems provide demographic data. Household surveillance may be necessary to identify basic needs. Other sources of demographic and health data include vaccination cards (often carried by mothers), burial records, networks of community health workers, and distribution lists of nongovernmental agencies responsible for other sectors of the disaster response. Nontraditional sources of information should also be remembered, including police, fire, aid agencies, pharmacies, gravediggers, and others.[16] With the global spread of Internet access, mobile communications, and social media, digital communications are proving valuable assets to public health informatics supporting surveillance data collection and analysis.[17]

Surveillance systems should be judged by their simplicity. Data collection should be an easy process with a logical format. Indicators should represent communicable and noncommunicable diseases of the population of concern that are relevant to both the disaster and the phase of the emergency (e.g., diarrhea is more likely to be a problem than hookworm infestation in an emergency). Data outputs should be produced in a timely fashion to identify outbreaks and be reliable (using standardized case definitions, for example). Data collection must occur in an ongoing way at regular intervals but be flexible enough to adapt to new health problems or sudden program changes.

Analysis, Interpretation, and Dissemination

During the emergency phase, data should be collected daily and reported weekly to all government and nongovernment relief agencies working in the health sector. Such reports are often collated by the United Nations Office for the Coordination of Humanitarian Affairs (OCHA) and published on their website (www.unocha.org), as well as ReliefWeb (www.reliefweb.int). In the postemergency phase, most likely, data will be collected daily but analyzed monthly. During all phases, surveillance data should be sent in either paper or digital form to a central location at the field level for analysis. Most countries have some type of ongoing surveillance system, with personnel tasked for inputting new data, rapidly analyzing it, and tracking disease burden. Usually this is a component of a broader health information system housed within a Ministry of Health with an established means for data analysis (in the United States, state and local public health offices and the CDC). A country's health information system, assuming it remains intact after the disaster, should provide baseline predisaster health information on communicable and noncommunicable diseases. This information provides important contextual information, such as seasonal variability of endemic diseases and the burden of chronic diseases and periodic health trends, information that is useful for program planning and conducting comparisons with newly acquired postdisaster data. In the event where a national surveillance and health information system is rendered disabled from the disaster, the WHO's EWARN and the CDC provide technical analytical assistance working with the affected country's health ministry and participating health NGOs to establish emergency-phase surveillance and to support ongoing postemergency-phase surveillance and its transition to a formalized health information system.

The analysis of surveillance data should focus on the clustering of events over time, within specific subgroups of the population, emphasizing trends in time, place, and person.[18] The interpretation should highlight the needs and priorities and, where possible, be referenced against "normal" values or indicator thresholds. What matters most is how indicators change over time and how these changes may be linked to programming. Finally, the flow of surveillance data must ensure that those persons responsible for program planning and implementation receive the information in an actionable format. The use of geographic information system (GIS) software for mapping and geopatial graphic analysis makes interpretation more meaningful to stakeholders.

If an alert threshold is crossed during data collection or analysis or if the analysis demonstrates an increasing trend, an alert verification goes out to point persons within the health information system at the regional and national levels (designated by the EWARN framework), to initiate an outbreak investigation and control measures. The 2005 International Health Regulations (IHR) provide a framework for WHO epidemic alert and rapid-response activities in collaboration with national EWARN systems.[19]

⚠ PITFALLS

A surveillance system must have high sensitivity, that is, the ability to detect true cases of a particular disease. One of the greatest enemies of effective surveillance is underreporting by data reporters. Underreporting may happen for a number of reasons. First, surveillance depends on a flow of information. During a disaster, established systems of information flow are easily disrupted (e.g., a health center is destroyed; the population migrates; or communications and transportation networks are damaged). In addition—and this is true especially of passive systems—health providers may lack interest, not see the value of an iterative data collection process, or feel overworked and under time constraints because of increased patient loads and therefore may not engage in data reporting. Lack of interest often arises when health providers are not included in the cycle of information flow and do not receive the data analyses and resulting guidelines. Without this information, they are unable to appreciate the beneficial results of surveillance on the health of the population. Underreporting for any of these reasons undermines the strength of a surveillance system.

Another potential cause for concern is the source of the information. Relying on facility-based data on a population with inadequate access to formal health care cannot represent the needs of said population accurately.[20] Thus emergent health concerns arising out of the community may not be reliably captured in time to prevent an outbreak.

Finally, the other obstacle to good surveillance is the lack of capacity for meaningful analysis and interpretation in many disaster and conflict-affected areas. Despite readily accessible tools, such as Epi Info, and the presence of computer-savvy technical staff able to manage data, there is often a need for personnel with public health acumen to interact with the data and explain its significance to disaster program managers and other key stakeholders. Without an appreciation of the importance and strategic use of such data, the value of surveillance is significantly reduced. More resources should be allocated to building the capacity of local personnel to make use of the information generated by surveillance.

REFERENCES

1. World Health Organization. Communicable Disease Surveillance and Response. Available at: http://www.who.int/csr/en/.
2. M'ikanatha NM, Lynfield R, Julian KG, et al. Infectious disease surveillance: a cornerstone for prevention and control. In: M'ikanatha NM, Lynfield R, Van Beneden CA, et al. *Infectious Disease Surveillance*. Oxford: Blackwell; 2007:3–17.
3. Choi BCK. *The Past, Present and Future of Public Health Surveillance*. *Scientifica;* 2012. Available at: http://dx.doi.org/10.6064/2012/875253.
4. Declich S, Carter AO. Public health surveillance: historical origins, methods and evaluation. *Bull World Health Organ.* 1994;7(2):285–304.
5. Thacker SB. Historical Development. In: Teutsch SM, Churchill RE, et al. eds. *Principles and Practice of Public Health Surveillance*. New York, NY: Oxford University Press; 2000:1–16.
6. Goma Epidemiology Group. Public health impact of Rwandan refugee crisis: what happened in Goma, Zaire, in July, 1994? *Lancet.* 1995;345 (8946):339–344.
7. The Sphere Project. *Humanitarian Charter and Minimum Standards in Humanitarian Response. Rugby*. Practical Action Publishing; 2011. 270.
8. Médicins sans Frontières. *Refugee Health: An Approach to Emergency Situations*. London: Pan Macmillan; 1997.
9. US Centers for Disease Control and Prevention. Launching a national surveillance system after an earthquake—Haiti, 2010. *MMWR Morb Mortal Wkly Rep.* 2010;59(30):933–938.
10. Barzilay EJ, Schaad N, Magloire R, et al. Cholera surveillance during the Haiti epidemic—the first 2 years. *N Engl J Med.* 2013;368(7):599–609.
11. World Health Organization. WHO Guidelines for EWARN Implementation. In: *Outbreak Surveillance and Response in Humanitarian Emergencies*. Geneva: World Health Organization; 2012.
12. World Health Organization. Surveillance. In: Connolly MA, ed. *Communicable Disease Control in Emergencies*. Geneva: World Health Organization; 2005.
13. Bradt DA, Drummond CM. Rapid epidemiological assessment of health status in displaced populations—an evolution toward a standardized minimum essential data set. *Prehosp Disaster Med.* 2003;17(4):178–185.
14. World Health Organization. WHO Guidelines for EWARN Implementation. In: *Outbreak Surveillance and Response in Humanitarian Emergencies*. Geneva: World Health Organization; 2012.
15. Wetterhall SE, Noji EK. Noji EK, ed. *The Public Health Consequences of Disasters*. New York, NY: Oxford University Press; 1997:37–64.
16. Johns Hopkins Bloomberg School of Public Health. Epidemiology and surveillance. In: Burnham G, ed. *The Johns Hopkins and Red Cross Red Crescent Public Health Guide for Emergencies;* 2008. Available at: http://www.jhsph.edu/research/centers-and-institutes/center-for-refugee-and-disaster-response/publications_tools/publications/_CRDR_ICRC_Public_Health_Guide_Book/Forward.pdf.
17. Savel TG, Foldy S. The role of public health informatics in enhancing public health surveillance. *MMWR Morb Mortal Wkly Rep.* 2012;61(3):S20–S24.
18. Rowley E, Robinson WC. Surveillance and registration systems. In: Robinson WC, ed. *Demographic Assessment in Disasters: A Guide for Practitioners*. Baltimore Center for International Emergency Disaster and Refugee Studies. Johns Hopkins Bloomberg School of Public Health; 2002.
19. World Health Organization. *International Health Regulations*. 2nd ed. Geneva: World Health Organization; 2005.
20. Roberts L, Hofmann CA. Assessing the impact of humanitarian assistance in the health sector. *Emerg Themes Epidemiol.* 2004;1(3):1–9.

Available at: http://www.spherehandbook.org/en/health-systems-standard-5-health-information-management.

Geographic Information Systems in Crises

Erica L. Nelson and P. Gregg Greenough

The technical term *geographic information system* (GIS) describes a relational computer system that captures, stores, manages, retrieves, analyzes, and displays geographic data. Practically understood, a GIS allows users to understand the "where" dimensions of their work and to relate place to information about that place, especially information about population. *Everything happens in space and time* is a fundamental principle of disaster response and of epidemiology, the population-based science that is part of public health practices. GIS provides a way to visualize how populations are dispersed, how they migrate, how they are affected by their environment, how they affect their environment, and their relationship to all manner of critical variables, outcomes, and risk factors.

At its core, GIS consists of hardware, software, and management systems that rely on an array of computing technologies for capturing and processing geographic data. As such, it is a valuable mapping and analysis system. Geospatial technologies that capture data include global positioning systems (GPSs), remote sensing, and map scanning and digitization. Most people are familiar with the portable GPS receivers that capture locations of latitude and longitude from orbiting satellites and Earth-bound satellite sensors. Remote sensing refers to data gathered away from the Earth's surface. Remote sensing involves sensors linked to platforms and includes modalities such as aerial photography (cameras on aircraft or unmanned aerial vehicles) and satellite imaging with digital image processing (cameras, digital scanners, light detection and ranging [LIDAR]). Optical lasers and other reading devices can also scan maps into digital formats or convert map features into geospatial data.

Geospatial data by definition are observations and measurements linked to locations on the surface of the Earth and are graphically represented as two models: the raster model, which is represented as pixels or cells; and the vector model, which include points, lines, networks, and polygons (areas with vectored boundaries). The former contains continuous data with values that convey units of space on the Earth's surface (such as land use, elevation, or population) and can vary in size, determining the degree of resolution; the latter has a single class of objects with similar dimensions. The vector model tends to be more geographically accurate and lends itself to common mapping and operational graphing queries for items such as transportation lines, area boundaries, points of interest, etc. Spatial features also include attributes, additional information about a data feature in tabular form. For example, a field hospital is a spatial feature, identified by a spatial locator (coordinate) represented by a point (in a vector layer), with tabulated attributable information items such as number of personnel, types of services and specialties, number of beds, among others.

Once digitalized spatial data are acquired, computer graphics software can create maps with an array of attributes and variables.

Exploring geography through digital means enables mapping, and mapping provides a visual tool for targeted interventions and efficient response: for disaster managers and responders, a map of "who is doing what and where" is an invaluable tool. With current graphic technologies, mapping is interactive and functional, especially as conditions on the ground rapidly change and the dynamics of the response efforts need to be plotted in real time.

Most importantly, GIS is a relational database. Geographical data are referenced to places on the Earth's surface as coordinates of latitude, longitude, and elevation; it is these coordinates that link a variety of raster and vector data layers together. Any place on Earth, as long as it has a geo-reference, can be spatially represented. Thus any variable that can be *geo-located* with these relational spatial coordinates—health facilities, population demographics, transit lines, power stations, socioeconomic metrics, phone calls and communications networks, Earth features such as topography, climate, vegetation, soils, variables linked to natural hazards, among many other examples—can be linked spatially and often temporally, not only providing a graphic visualization of place and links to attributes, but also opening up possibilities for spatial analytics.

Spatial analysis, a toolkit afforded to GIS software (ArcGIS and QuantumGIS), allows one to investigate geographic patterns in spatial data and the relationships between features and, if needed, to apply inferential statistics to determine the relevance of spatial relationships, trends, and patterns; to see if "what is next to what" and "what is connected to what" have significance. The concepts of "nearness" and "relatedness" have at their core geographic significance, and the relationships among things that are near can generate complex spatiotemporal phenomena. Yet nearness does not necessarily imply causation. Spatial analytics affords the opportunity to take spatial characteristics into account to make those determinations. The concept of spatial autocorrelation is the name given to the degree to which one object is similar to other near objects and helps determine if objects are spatially independent from each other; this correlative statistic may be positive (similar values cluster together spatially, such as an emerging epidemic), negative (dissimilar objects cluster together spatially), or something in between. Flow-through networks to maximize time and efficiency, impacts of distances on health, impacts of typology on health services delivery, potential environmental hazards, and risk of death or injury are all examples in which spatial features are the critical element of analysis. In multivariate health outcomes studies, spatial features may need to be included in the regression if one is, for example, to fully appreciate the geographic variation of health outcomes in exposed and unexposed groups. Spatial statistics help see spatial variation in the relationships between factors contributing to disease and health outcomes. Once spatial effects are established, they can be used in risk modeling (Box 49-1).

HISTORICAL PERSPECTIVE

Intuitively, geography has always played a role in disaster response, even if originally used in the form of stagnant logistical tools to inform organizations about where to target programs and how to shuttle resources. With the incorporation of epidemiological methods and the evolution of computer and communication systems, GIS has progressed beyond the use of often incomplete, outdated maps to a complex and interdisciplinary field that includes advanced mapping and data collection techniques, crowd-sourcing, participatory mapping and needs assessment, hazard modeling, operations research, and programmatic decision support, all of which inform the many phases of disaster management and subsequently disaster medicine.

Aerial Photography, Satellite Imaging, and Remote Sensing

After centuries of parchment and compasses, cartography transformed significantly during the twentieth century with the advent of aerial photography, satellite imaging, remote sensing, and advanced mapping software. But not until the 1990s did this advancement revolutionize the field of disaster management. In response to the Japanese earthquakes in Hokkaido and Kobe that took place in 1993 and 1995, respectively, along with the Northridge California Earthquake in 1994, governmental organizations used aerial photography and satellite imaging to delineate damage zones and characterize infrastructural casualties. In 2001, after the attacks on the World Trade Center, light detection and ranging imagery (LIDAR), satellite imagery, and handheld GIS-linked devices were used to support rescue and recovery operations.[1]

As humanitarian programmatic design evolved, operatives needed more than geographic information to advance disaster response initiatives, so GIS platforms began to incorporate thematic overlays into mapping. In response to the 2004 Indian Ocean Tsunami, the United Nations (UN) Environmental Programme reported critical gaps in geographic, infrastructural, and disaster impact information. Preexisting maps maintained by the Indonesian national mapping agency were lacking accurate and timely data regarding infrastructure; there was a lack of vulnerability and risk assessment mapping and environmental baseline data, and minimal field assessments hindered any appropriate response. Acknowledging this dearth, the UN Humanitarian Information Center, using ArcGIS, augmented old topographic maps with satellite imagery and then applied thematic layers to indicate damage assessments, displaced populations, injured peoples, and organizational distribution. During this campaign, GIS was used to create potable water, food, and medical supply chains; assess village mapping and inform community planning; determine field hospital and mobile health clinic locales, and monitor for communicable diseases.[2]

Expanding Agency: Crowd-Sourcing, Participatory Mapping, and Collective Intelligence

Conventionally, humanitarian programs and their GIS counterparts have been led by centralized, top-down teams that grapple with vast amounts of information and disseminate culled data and subsequent analyses with a significant amount of discrimination in terms of what is graphically presented. Recent developments in web-mapping, mobile technologies, and open platforms have led to "a kind of collective intelligence"[3] that decentralizes disaster response, empowers affected communities, and capitalizes upon the vast capacities of a technologically savvy, cosmopolitan population. Forays into open participation occurred as early as 2001, when volunteers were deployed from the Emergency Mapping and Data Center in Manhattan to gather much of the early GIS data after the 9/11 attacks, and in 2004, with the creation of the Chuetsu Earthquake disaster and recovery GIS open website project.[1] Amidst the aftermath of the violence following the 2007 Kenyan elections, Ushahidi launched a crowd-sourced, open-platform initiative that collected eyewitness reports of violence via E-mail and Short Message Service (SMS) texts and overlaid them onto Google Maps.

But in 2010, following the Haitian earthquake, community-sourced information and open participation truly came to the fore. Volunteer and technical communities (V&TCs) emerged, utilizing the input of affected populations to provide real-time, ground-level data. The voice of the community, empowered by more than 3 million Haitian cell phone users,[4] was incorporated to rebuild maps through OpenStreetMap, identify health facilities, and, via SMS texting, to augment needs assessments surveys. Internet collaborations between V&TCs emerged for aggregation and analysis of this overwhelming amount of data. Since that time, open participation in mapping, needs assessment, and data analysis continues to blossom, with disaster response efforts ranging from the Ushahidi Missouri River Floods project in 2011 to Crisis-Mapping of the 2010 Chilean earthquake and the employment of OpenStreet map by the UN High Commissioner for Refugees (UNHCR) in the Zaatari refugee camp in Jordan following the Syrian conflict.

Hazard Modeling, Operations Research, and Geographic Information System for Decision Support

One of the first uses of GIS for hazard modeling and disaster preparedness was the Sea, Lake and Overland Surges from Hurricanes (SLOSH) program.[5] First developed in the late 1960s, SLOSH was originally created for the purpose of forecasting weather, but it soon became apparent that SLOSH's hydrologic modeling could be used as hazard analysis to delineate communities susceptible to surge flooding and to design preparedness programs. In 2005, after decades of permutation, these data, initially disseminated to organizations via print maps, were now presented in graphical, often animated form via the SLOSH Display Program to the Federal Emergency Management Agency (FEMA), the Army Corps of Engineers, and state and local emergency managers during Hurricane Katrina. Similar hazard models have been developed for identifying populations vulnerable to natural disasters such as earthquakes,[6] floods, wildfires,[7] and landslides and have been integral to international disaster risk assessments, as illustrated through the Natural Disaster Hotspots project and the UN Development Programme (UNDP)'s Disaster Risk Index.[8] Incorporation of preexisting community health demographics into hazard modeling has led to a richer understanding of the postdisaster medical needs of an affected community—invaluable knowledge that undoubtedly fosters a more comprehensive and competent disaster preparedness plan.[9] Further interdisciplinary efforts wedding hazard modeling and operational research (OR) have bred powerful decision support tools that address evacuation routing,[6] optimal resource allocation to emergency shelters and clinics, and supply chain and distribution schema.[10]

Notwithstanding these exponential advancements made in the field of GIS and its incorporation into disaster response, there continue to be challenges surrounding uptake, interoperability, data-verification and security, residual logistical obstacles, and information sharing. While these pitfalls are indeed formidable, as discussed in the following, technology does nothing but evolve, and its role in disaster response will undoubtedly continue to burgeon.

CURRENT PRACTICE

The foundation of all disaster response is preparedness. Disasters originate from diverse geophysical, climatological, technological, biological, and sociopolitical variables that impact populations not only by the magnitude of the disaster itself, but also through breakdowns of the infrastructural foundations and inherent vulnerabilities of the affected population. In order to amass appropriate food and water resources, medical inventories, volunteer and nonvolunteer response personnel, and equipment and to create warning, evacuation, search and rescue, and other response and recovery plans, effective preparedness requires an accurate understanding of both the potential hazards and the pre-existent demographic, infrastructural, sociopolitical, economic, and medical realities of the communities they affect.

Hazard modeling imports multivariate geospatial, climatological, meteorological, temporal, and infrastructural data into a computational model or simulation, frequently superimposed upon a GIS platform, to determine the likelihood and potential magnitude of disaster impacts. Explicitly, modeling can be used to predict flood inundation, coastal surge heights, seismic vulnerability, landslide and liquefaction susceptibility, smoke plume distribution, and infectious disease transmission. Vulnerability—the capacity to anticipate, cope with, resist, and recover from a hazard[11]—can also be mapped. And when hazard predictions and vulnerability demographics are synthesized, risk, defined as the "probability of harmful consequences, or expected losses (i.e., deaths, injuries, property, livelihoods, economic activity disrupted or environment damaged) resulting from interactions between hazards and vulnerable conditions,"[8] can be estimated. Quantitative methods, including complex analytic and measurement methods, causal inference, structural equation modeling, and decision theory are commonly used in public health research to create these predictions.[12] Predictably, organizations and governments are increasingly leveraging resultant information to advocate for resources, identify and prioritize mitigation activities, plan evacuation routes, strengthen medical response infrastructures, and create better, flexible disaster management frameworks.

During the emergency phase of a crisis, GIS continues to play a significant role in capturing rapid assessment mapping data and estimating populations. High-resolution satellite images are more immediately and readily available than in the past. The UN Institute for Training and Research (UNITAR) Operational Satellite Applications Programme (UNOSAT) in particular supports the UN agencies that anchor the humanitarian cluster system with satellite imagery and geospatial data. UN field operations have personnel trained in harnessing the cartographic power of GIS, digitizing georeferenced data, and overlaying raster and vector layers for gap and network analyses. And as the communities of the world have become saturated with mobile communications (wealth ceasing to be a meaningful factor), the ability to send vital information to a platform equipped with GIS analytic capacity is nearly ubiquitous. GIS-facile humanitarian nongovernmental organizations (NGOs) whose sole role is to support information and communication technologies have emerged in the field alongside the traditional conveyers of water, sanitation, health, food, and shelter.

What is far less common, however, is the use of GIS for geospatial analysis and inferential statistical applications. This stems from a variety of reasons. The emergency response phase is a more frenzied one and the focus necessarily needs to be on rapid "who is doing what where" information that naturally requires more mapping than a complex population study. There is a dearth of readily available geolocated population data in much of the world, as most recent censuses are remote in time if they have been done at all. Finally, technical training on the use of GIS statistical software is less pervasive among field personnel whose focus, and rightly so, tends to be on operations.

Presently, the use of GIS in the response and recovery phases of disaster management is as diverse as its role in preparedness, and for rapid needs assessments ranges from mapping the impact of the disaster and cataloging destroyed infrastructure to identifying displaced populations to computer-aided dispatch to logistical decision support mechanisms and web-based coordination dashboards. This use is largely intercalated with other developing mobile, dispatch, modeling, and computational technologies and continues to evolve in its accuracy and efficacy, yet remains inextricable.

Computer-aided dispatch (CAD), a system that identifies the most appropriate and available resources required to respond to a specific need, integrates GIS-linked data to reduce response times, increase responder safety, and enhance situational awareness. Within CAD, GIS technology is used to store and analyze specifically referenced data that provides more efficient interpretation of geospatial and infrastructural information and enhances CAD functionality via thematic layers, advanced analytics, and data visualization. In order to realize its significant potential, georeferenced data should not only include street, address, and infrastructure layers, but also information regarding incident distribution and boundaries, mobile and immobile resource availability, and real-time response unit information. Advanced vehicle locating (AVL), a component of CAD, superimposes the real-time tracking of response units, along with status monitoring (i.e., en route, on location, out of service, etc.) onto maps that demarcate disaster boundaries. Reducing appropriate response time also requires a sophisticated understanding of resource capacity, and CAD programs are enabled to query such details as personnel rosters and available fire and rescue apparatus.[13]

An added benefit of CAD is the ability for responders to interface with the application remotely. They, too, should have access to a visual, real-time representation of the geographic basics surrounding the incident-affected area, assigned response locales, and alternate response unit locations and capacities. GIS applications that include infrastructural resources, such as fire hydrants, water mains, and electricity outlets, and routing options that take into account traffic, barriers, and hazard conditions, including disaster-specific meteorological phenomena such as fire plume notifications, lend responders a situational awareness that both protects the disaster response workforce and garners a more efficient response.[13]

OR is a burgeoning field increasingly used to optimize humanitarian response logistics ranging from resource distribution to transportation and evacuation routing. Several techniques, including mathematical programming, probability and statistics, simulation, stochastic programming, fuzzy set theory, decision theory, queuing theory, system dynamics, and constraints programming, are currently being used to improve disaster response efforts through decision support mechanisms.[10,14] The power of OR is greatly augmented when these optimization tools are combined with the geographic potentials of GIS: we can now address multivariate questions that were deemed too complex to be previously modeled.[10,15]

Practically, OR scientists use certain techniques to create optimization models either before or after disaster occurrence, thereby providing decision support regarding predisaster operations (e.g., facility location, stock prepositioning and evacuation planning) or postdisaster response (e.g., relief distribution and casualty transportation).[16] While the following examples are not intended as a comprehensive account, a detailed explanation, or even explicit endorsement of certain

OR-produced decision support tools, these specific cases demonstrate well the breadth of current practice.

First is the use of maximal covering location models (or variants thereof) that consolidate facility location and inventory decisions by capturing variables such as budgetary constraints and capacity restrictions to determine the number and location of distribution centers in a relief network and the amount of supplies to be stocked.[17] Alternative techniques, utilizing stochastic optimization, are being used to approach the question of medical supply chain in a variety of disaster types and magnitudes.[18] By concatenating historic disaster-specific information, a preliminary framework is created to address loading and routing of vehicles to transport medical supplies and can be modified given up-to-date disaster field information. Additional multiobjective modeling has been created to integrate with GIS, such as web-based decision support systems to assist fire departments and emergency medical services (EMS) in the design of evacuation plans for urban areas. This modeling system includes the number and locations of rescue facilities as well as primary and secondary routes to these locations and multicriteria tools to help with prioritizing routes. Often presented through case studies involving one disaster type, these decision support tools, like the multitude of alternate OR algorithms, can be modified via historical and GIS data to address other disasters.[15]

GIS, while more and more integral to the logistics of disaster management, also allows for more effective reporting of humanitarian aid. The visual representation of disaster management efforts superimposed on disaster impact maps has not only facilitated interagency discourse and coordination, but also made public awareness and donor communication more efficient. HumanitarianResponse.info, managed by the UN Office for the Coordination of Humanitarian Affairs (OCHA) and the On-Site Operations Coordination Centre (OSOCC), is one such platform that uses GIS to assist in the coordination of disaster-specific operational information and related activities. Updated to version HR2.0 in 2014, this web-based GIS-linked dashboard includes global information management tools, cross-emergency searches, humanitarian responder check-in or check-out, interactive mapping, SMS notifications and email group integration, data cleaning tools, ReliefWeb, and cluster site search integration. Maps and infographics can be searched with the application of multiple filters including map type, organization, cluster or sector, locations, themes, and funding methods. These visualizations are frequently adopted in coordination efforts and donor presentations.

While web-based interfaces that use GIS to report humanitarian aid continue to flourish, notably the Sahana Free and Open Source Disaster Management System, OSOCC, and the aforementioned Humanitarian-Response projects, these dashboards have yet to be amalgamated into a globally used forum. And despite the undoubted benefit that the integration of GIS has brought to the disaster management community, it has large obstacles to address if it is to realize its true potential in disaster response.

Unmanned aerial vehicles (UAVs) or drones, which have infiltrated the market and proliferated in the hands of hobbyists, will likely have an impact on improving disaster response operations. One of the many uses of this technology in disaster operations will be to interface with GIS systems to provide granular real-time data to disaster workers and planners. Many companies and agencies are exploring applications for this technology in disaster operations.

⚠ PITFALLS

GIS has undeniably advanced the field of humanitarian aid and has significant potential for further revolutionizing disaster medicine. Notwithstanding, there exist formidable political, organizational, methodological, and technological challenges to the effective incorporation and utilization of such a rapidly evolving toolkit.

Critical to the development and optimization of GIS in the field of humanitarian aid is the global awareness needed in regards to adopting GIS technologies and in creating a functional collaboration between geospatial experts, technologists, governments, affected communities, and humanitarian responders. However, as with most technological trends, the adoption of such tools has yet to reach the majority, and its utilization is varied in form and extent. Concerns regarding the feasibility or affordability of GIS and/or mobile technologies in austere environments often prevents field uptake and lengthens the gap between the capabilities of innovative technology and practical implementation.[19] A shared understanding of the semantics, procedures, capacities, and limitations of current GIS strategies has yet to be realized and has led to incidents of duplication, miscommunication, inappropriate utilization, infeasible expectations, subsequent failures and, ultimately, disregard of this powerful tool.

Integral to any data exchange is a shared technological lexicon that incorporates open standards, public application programming interfaces (APIs), common operational datasets (CODs), and a global data dictionary. While examples of these shared languages and platforms are expanding in the humanitarian space, as is exemplified by the use of open source platforms like Ushahidi and the use of Open Geospatial Consortium, Extensible Markup Language (XML), and Keyhole Markup Language (KML) standards, the majority of operators in the field continue to use proprietary, desktop-based applications that lack interoperability. UN-developed common operational datasets have done a good deal to facilitate communication between data streams, but a lack of universality and specificity surrounding a data dictionary, codification of data, varied approaches to structured verses, unstructured data, and even commonality regarding georeferenced labeling continues to jeopardize interagency sharing and can create significant data fragmentation.

Beyond the construction of a shared, interdigitizing technological language, the humanitarian community must also address the more pragmatic obstacles facing GIS. Data delay, insecurity, and telecommunications failures are all expected obstacles when operating in austere environments, some developing nations, and postdisaster environments. Disaster response relies upon accurate and up-to-the-minute data. And while GIS has great potential to provide expedient data, mundane details such as language translation, lack of cellular phone adoption, undependable electricity and cellular service, and even broken satellite antennae can easily retard collection and dissemination. In response to the Haitian earthquake, exceptional web-based maps were generated by Ushahidi and OpenStreetMap that provided invaluable data about road blockages, food and water distribution points, and multiple other indicators. But these were often unavailable to responders on the ground. A logistical "falling back to paper" mode demonstrates one of the biggest challenges faced by the GIS community.[1] After the Haiti earthquake, there was a thrum of excitement regarding the integration of telecommunication and GIS technologies, but different logistical realities prevented comparable deployment after the 2010 floods in Pakistan.[3] Closed information streams—those sanctioned by not only cultural mores, public pressures, and governments but also by the international humanitarian system, insular NGOs, and the Disaster Space Charter—are not challenges unique to GIS, but need to be addressed for coordinated efforts to evolve.[3,20]

A valid rationalization for closed information systems, such as the proprietary systems used by the UN Cluster System, focuses on concerns regarding cyber-security, intellectual property, and individual protection. Admitting that the argument weighing intellectual property and information fragmentation in humanitarian response could be a protracted one, it is still imperative to acknowledge the compounded ethical and security dilemmas posed by geospatially labeled data. Any personal identifying information, even if not georeferenced, is critically safeguarded in the medical field. In postdisaster communities, populations are already highly vulnerable and need to be protected from insecure data collection, sharing, and exploitive data-mining situations. Furthermore, in complex humanitarian emergencies, where conflict threatens the security of both response personnel and beneficiary communities, geospatially linked data poses even more of a potential hazard if not securely collected and stored. The crucial challenge to GIS and disaster medicine, then, is establishing a standardized mechanism to maintain data security in order to garner trust and necessary collaboration.

Finally, assuming all the aforementioned pitfalls are addressed, simply providing more data through GIS and mobile technologies is not a panacea for disaster response. Raw data produced from crowd-sourcing methods, aerial surveillance, and hazard modeling are invaluable, but must still be vetted and are not a replacement for formal technical assessments.[21] And currently, much of the existing disaster response infrastructure lacks the capacity to reliably validate and analyze the velocity and volume provided by such innumerable sources. GIS-produced maps can provide powerful visualization for decision making, but must still be contextualized and compared to baseline data. To address this, resources must be allocated to trusted and secure networks that can empower affected populations to provide true and constructive information, filter and substantiate reports, and thereby assure the veracity and quality of data necessary for effective disaster response. Incident command and cluster leads, along with program directors, must understand the backdrop onto which GIS data are projected. Furthermore, the humanitarian and data science communities must support not only interdisciplinary working groups to discuss the roles and standards of GIS and mobile technologies, but also the research, monitoring, and evaluation that must take place to determine best practices and the true impact of GIS on disaster response.

Assuredly, these conversations are being held, as is epitomized by the formation of the Working Group on Applied Technologies that operates under the auspices of the Humanitarian Action Summit. Dissemination mechanisms have grown from the creation of the Center for Research on the Epidemiology of Disasters' Emergency Events Database (EM-DAT),[22] established in 1988, to data portals and online dashboards. Online initiatives, such as the MIT/Harvard Data Portal, the Global Disaster Alert and Coordination System (GDAC)'s Virtual OSOCC, as well as the Sahana Free and Open Source Disaster Management System, have significantly changed disaster response communication and coordination modalities. With such robust collaborative tools being adopted by the humanitarian community and the growing inclusion of interdisciplinary, multilevel, local, and global actors, GIS and mobile technologies will indeed evolve to address these challenges and their role will grow to not only advance disaster response, but also empower disaster-affected communities.

REFERENCES

1. Kawasaki A, Berman ML, Guan W. The growing role of web-based geospatial technology in disaster response and support. *Disasters*. 2013;37 (2):201–221.
2. ESRI. *GIS for Disaster Recovery*. Redlands, CA: ESRI; 2007.
3. Harvard Humanitarian Initiative. *Disaster Relief 2.0: The Future of Information Sharing in Humanitarian Emergencies*. Washington, DC and Berkshire, UK: UN Foundation & Vodafone Foundation Technology Partnership; 2011.
4. Greenough PG, Bateman L, Sorensen BS, Foran M. Innovations in humanitarian Technologies Working Group: report of the proceedings, Humanitarian Action Summit 2011. *Prehospital Disaster Med*. 2011;26 (6):482–486.
5. Glahn B, Taylor A, Kurkowski N, Shaffer W. The role of the SLOSH model in National Weather Service storm surge forecasting. *Natl Weather Digest*. 2009;33(1):3–14.
6. Zlatanova S, Peters R, Dilo A, Scholten H, eds. *Intelligent Systems for Crisis Management: Geo-information for Disaster Management*. Berlin: Springer-Verlag; 2013.
7. Reddick C. Information technology and emergency management: preparedness and planning in US states. *Disasters*. 2011;35(1):45–61.
8. El Morjani ZE, Ebener S, Boos J, Ghaffar E, Musani A. Modelling the spatial distribution of five hazards in the context of the WHO/EMRO Atlas of Disaster Risk as a step towards the reduction of the health impact related to disasters. *Int J Health Geogr*. 2007;6(8):1–28.
9. Wilson JL, Little R, Novick L. Estimating medically fragile population in storm surge zones: a geographic information system application. *J Emerg Manag*. 2013;11(1):9–24.
10. Kucukkoc I. *YOR18 Biennial Conferences Keynote Papers and Extended Abstracts*. Exeter: University of Exeter; 2013.
11. Wisner B, Blaikie P, Cannon T, Davis I. *At Risk: Natural Hazards, People's Vulnerability and Disasters*. 2nd ed. London: Routledge; 2004.
12. Testa M, Pettigrew ML, Savoia E. Measurement, geospatial, and mechanistic models of public health hazard vulnerability and jurisdictional risk. *J Public Health Manag Pract*. 2014;20:s61–s68.
13. ESRI. *Geospatial Computer-Aided Dispatch*. Redlands, CA: ESRI; 2007.
14. Altay N, Green W. OR/MS research in disaster operations management. *Eur J Oper Res*. 2006;175:475–493.
15. Alçada-Almeida L, Tralhão L, Santos L, Coutinho-Rodrigues J. A multiobjective approach to locate emergency shelters and identify evacuation routes in urban areas. *Geogr Anal*. 2009;41(1):9–29.
16. Caunhye AM, Nie X, Pokharel S. Optimization models in emergency logistics: a literature review. *Socioecon Plann Sci*. 2012;46(1):4–13.
17. Balcik B, Beamon BM. Facility location in humanitarian relief. *Int J Logist Res App*. 2008;11(2):101–121.
18. Mete HO, Zabinsky ZB. Stochastic optimization of medical supply location and distribution in disaster management. *Int J Prod Econ*. 2010;126 (1):76–84.
19. Greenough PG, Chan JL, Meier P, Bateman L, Dutta S. Applied technologies in humanitarian assistance: report of the 2009 Applied Technology Working Group. *Prehospital Disaster Med*. 2009;24(2):s206–s209.
20. Morton M, Levy J. Challenges in disaster data collection during recent disasters. *Prehospital Disaster Med*. 2011;26(3):196–201.
21. Kerle N. Disaster mapping by citizens is limited. *Nature*. 2015;517:438.
22. Benjamin E, Bassily-Marcus A, Babu E, Silver L, Martin M. Principles and practice of disaster relief: lessons from Haiti. *Mt Sinai J Med*. 2011;78 (3):306–318.
23. Cromley EK, McLafferty SL. *GIS and Public Health*. 2nd ed. New York, NY: The Guilford Press; 2012.

CHAPTER 50

Management of Mass Fatalities

Jack E. Smith II

Management of large numbers of fatalities is one of the most difficult aspects of disaster response. Natural disasters, in particular, can cause large numbers of deaths, as underscored by the massive loss of life (283,000) from the South Asian tsunami in 2004,[1] the 2005 earthquake in the Kashmir region of northern Pakistan and India (86,000 dead)[2], and the Haitian earthquake in 2010 (310,000 dead).[3]

As population vulnerabilities increase across the globe and the density of the populace and coastal habitation rates increase, modern disasters have a higher potential for creating large numbers of fatalities; this is so domestically as well. The evolution of current emergency management concepts is placing an increased emphasis on the effective management of mass fatalities, and it can no longer be an afterthought in the planning and operational response to such events. Within the United States, the estimated number of fatalities during another pandemic influenza outbreak is estimated to be between 3 million and 5 million people.[4] As with any disaster-related surge, local authorities including the ME/C, law enforcement, public health, and funeral directors, as well as hospitals, nursing homes, and hospice care organizations, will be required to manage this surge in addition to the normal case load of day-to-day deaths.

The objective of this chapter is not to provide a conceptual academic discussion on concepts or controversial topics surrounding the management of a mass fatality event. Rather, the chapter is written to be a desk reference for planning strategies and tactics to address the historical challenges faced in past mass-fatality events.

HISTORICAL PERSPECTIVE

In order to develop an accurate perspective of the term *mass fatality*, it is important to first define the paradigm in which we are working. The discipline of emergency management embodies a concept known as *comprehensive emergency management* (CEM), which dictates that disaster management initiatives incorporate all four phases of emergency management: mitigation or prevention, preparedness, response, and recovery. In addition, disaster management initiatives must maintain an "all-hazards" emphasis; engage, integrate, and coordinate with all stakeholders; identify and address all vulnerabilities; and be scalable to the size and scope of the event. With regard to mass fatality management (MFM), the all-hazards approach has important operational implications. No-notice or short-notice events such as earthquakes or tornados create a sudden surge of fatalities, whereas slower-evolving events, such as a biological attack or pandemic, develop over time and yet have the potential for greater numbers of fatalities. Explosions and aircraft disasters often produce highly fragmented human remains that may be difficult to recover, which greatly complicate the process of identification and reunification with next of kin, whereas remains that are contaminated with hazardous chemicals, radiation, or communicable diseases create other management challenges or decontamination and health risks to responders. Additionally, the meticulous criminal investigation and evidence collection requirements of law enforcement make the prospect of managing large numbers of deceased individuals a highly complex operation.

Although generally viewed as a second-tier response consideration after the immediate threats to life safety have been addressed, the appropriate handling, identification, and disposition of the deceased are still critical factors in the competent response to a mass fatality incident (MFI).

MFM plans must also provide adequate flexibility in order to address the unpredictable size and scope of different incidents. There are, quite literally, dozens of different definitions for the term *disaster*. However, the Federal Emergency Management Agency (FEMA), American College of Emergency Physicians (ACEP), National Disaster Life Support Foundation (NDLSF), and many other sources have developed some consensus in incorporating the concept of a destructive event that overwhelms the ability of a community to respond to and recover from the effects of that event.[5-7] The key point of emphasis here is that a disaster is an event that overwhelms local resources and capabilities. This definition is intentionally flexible enough to be applied across all communities regardless of size and resource availability. As an example, a bus crash in a metropolitan area may produce a significant number of casualties but will not have the same overwhelming effects on the community that the same incident would have on a small rural community with far fewer emergency response resources.

Often, the terms *disaster* and *catastrophe* are used interchangeably, but there is an important distinction between the two. Quarantelli[8] defines a *catastrophic disaster* by these four attributes:

1. The majority of the entire community's infrastructure is impacted.
2. Local responders, health care providers, and officials are unable to perform their usual roles throughout most of the response and/or recovery phase because many of them are among the casualties.
3. Most or all routine community functions (public services, health care, business and industry, and education) are immediately and simultaneously interrupted or destroyed.
4. All surrounding communities are similarly affected; eliminating mutual aid assistance from the surrounding region.

Disasters overwhelm a community's ability to respond and recover, whereas catastrophes create exponentially larger effects. The aforementioned disasters would more accurately be classified as catastrophic events. These distinctions are important to emergency planners because developing a MFM plan to manage 150 bodies from a tornado or an airline disaster is completely different from a plan to manage 10,000 bodies from a pandemic outbreak or that are contaminated with radiation from a radiologic dispersion device (e.g., "dirty bomb").

Another important consideration in developing a MFM plan is whether the plan is facility specific or community based. Many documents on MFM planning fail to make this distinction. Even though a hospital MFM plan, for example, may not need to be concerned with search and recovery of human remains in the field, it is critical that all planners recognize the necessity to engage the wide array of stakeholders that will be involved in response to an MFI.

All strategic disaster planning must be based on evidence-based facts, if available, and assumptions as well as current best practice.

In the 3 decades 1980-2010 there were 640 natural disasters within the United States, which killed a total of 12,366 people.[9] Commercial airlines disasters for the period 1959-2012 have accounted for 6574 fatalities in North America.[10] All of these mass fatality events within the United States have been managed with the surge strategies outlined in this chapter with the exception of temporary interment or mass graves. Even though this proves our capability at some level to manage an MFI through the utilization of national resources, nowhere in the United States has anyone ever had to attempt to manage a truly catastrophic MFI with only local or regional resources. Even the terrorist attacks on September 11, 2001, which created nearly 3000 highly fragmented remains, were confined to three fairly localized areas, and the size and scope of each incident site did not overwhelm the capabilities of our nationwide resources.

What we have never experienced within the United States is the need to manage an MFI of even 10,000 bodies—let alone several hundred thousand, as has been the case in incidents around the globe. In recent history, we have never had to resort to mass burials in the United States, the very concept of which is highly controversial in our society. The challenge becomes getting emergency managers and disaster planners to even begin to comprehend and think beyond the 50 to 100 body event, up to and including plans on the catastrophic scale.

CURRENT PRACTICE

Current practice for MFM spans a wide spectrum that typically correlates to the capability of the respective facility, community, or state to manage any other aspect of disaster response or recovery. MFM plans can range from those that are very detailed down to one sentence plans that quite literally direct the reader to contact the coroner in the nearest major metropolitan area or the state emergency management agency. The major MFIs around the globe over the past 10 years in addition to the H1N1 influenza outbreak of 2009 have made most disaster planners realize the necessity of having a proactive and comprehensive plan in place.

Facts on the proper handling of dead bodies have been identified by Morgan et al., in their 2009 work for the Pan American Health Organization and World Health Organization (WHO), titled *Management of Dead Bodies after Disasters: A Field Manual for First Responders.*

- Dead bodies do not cause epidemics or pose public health risks after natural disasters.
- The risk to the public is negligible if they do not touch dead bodies.
- The surviving population is much more likely to spread disease.
- There is the potential (but as yet undocumented) risk of drinking water supplies contaminated by fecal material released from dead bodies.
- Most disaster-related fatalities are the result of some traumatic mechanism of injury, not by disease.
- Most disaster victims are not likely to be sick with epidemic-causing infections (i.e., Ebola, cholera, typhoid, and anthrax). However, those that are must be handled with appropriate infection control procedures.

- A few victims will have chronic blood infections (hepatitis or HIV), tuberculosis, or diarrheal disease.
- Most infectious organisms do not survive beyond 48 hours in a dead body. An exception is HIV, which has been found 6 days postmortem. The Ebola Marburg virus has been known to survive up to 5 days on contaminated surfaces,[11] but to date no research has been done on human remains.
- Individuals handling human remains have a small risk through contact with blood and feces (bodies often leak feces after death) from Hepatitis B and C, HIV, tuberculosis, and diarrheal disease. Workers should also be cognizant of the hazards posed by highly fragmented remains as body fluids can be dripping from trees (e.g., airline disaster), soaked into surrounding soil, or become an inhalation hazard with airborne dust in collapsed buildings. Additionally, as seen in the 2014 Ebola outbreak, cultural burial practices combined with poor understanding of viral transmission greatly exacerbated the propagation of the disease through direct contact with infected corpses.[12]
- Body recovery teams that work in hazardous environments (e.g., collapsed buildings and debris) may also be at risk of injury and tetanus (transmitted via soil).[13]
- Considerations for MFM planning are based on the following assumptions identified in 2006 by the U.S. Northern Command and Department of Health and Human Services Fatality Management Pandemic Influenza Working Group[4]:
  - Most catastrophic MFIs are single events that create the majority of the fatalities outside the hospital setting.
  - However, a virulent communicable disease outbreak such as pandemic influenza, hemorrhagic fever, or a biological attack will create a surge of mass fatalities within the hospital setting as well.
  - Further, a pandemic or biological attack is an ongoing event that will develop over a period of weeks and months; therefore body recovery will need to be a continual process both within the hospital and throughout the community.
  - In order to streamline this process, planners will have to establish multiple centralized locations throughout the local area for the collection, storage, and processing of bodies until the event abates to the point that normal operations can accommodate the surge in deaths.
  - A pandemic or biological event will affect the entire nation and strain the capabilities of every local community. Local and state authorities will have insufficient personnel, supplies, equipment, and storage capacity to handle the demand, and it is unlikely that mutual aid resources from surrounding jurisdictions will be available.
  - Therefore institutional-based providers, such as hospitals, nursing homes, home care and hospice care organizations, along with local public health departments, will be forced to rely on local resources from existing public and private agencies.
  - Every jurisdiction will require similar types of critical resources, including personnel, equipment, supplies, and storage capacity to manage the surge in the number of decedents. Further, current business and industry practices utilizing just-in-time (JIT) inventory and Lean supply chain strategies reduce overall community access to supplies and lower resilience to disaster impacts and will be unable to meet the spike in demand for these critical resources unless they have access to local or national supply stockpiles.
  - One of the primary strategies for containing the spread of disease is quarantining entire communities and closing state borders. Even though such actions provide limited proven disease containment value, they most certainly will impede the accessibility to critical resources.

- Escalating death rates combined with social distancing and quarantine strategies will also affect the overall supply chain, causing shortages of water, food, medicine, and gasoline. These shortages will not only affect the entire population but will further hamper the delivery of public services as well. Public agencies may need to develop creative strategies to reduce their demand for gasoline and diesel fuel; both of which are projected to be the most difficult to obtain. Additionally, health care institutions should establish contingencies plans to ensure supply chain resiliency.
- Additionally, public utility infrastructure including electricity, natural gas, water, and sewer may experience interruptions.
- In jurisdictions that consider communicable disease fatalities to not be a ME/C case, the public health department may authorize the ME/C to take jurisdiction of the bodies.
- The surge in fatalities will also overwhelm the death care industry as well. Funeral homes, coffin manufacturers, crematoria, and cemeteries will be unable to process remains in the traditional manner because of the increased number of cases. This will necessitate the establishment of temporary massive storage capacity until bodies can be properly processed for final disposition, in the absence of mass burial strategies.
- Pandemic-related deaths will primarily fall into two major categories: attended and unattended. The process to identify remains from attended deaths will be relatively straightforward. However, unattended deaths will require verification of identity, issuing a death certificate, and notifying the next of kin, which will be both labor intensive and time consuming.
- The resultant delays in issuing death certificates for both attended and unattended deaths will place substantial pressure on the ME/C so that the next of kin can manage the decedent's estate.[4]

Localized mass fatality disasters may overwhelm local and state resources, but mutual aid resources should still be available through the state-to-state Emergency Management Assistance Compact (EMAC),[14] as well as the federal government. However, catastrophic nationwide events such as a pandemic or biological attack may overwhelm all resources, thus eliminating the potential for outside assistance.

One of the primary challenges in managing an MFI is the work necessary to positively identify each deceased victim. These procedures are collectively referred to as disaster victim identification (DVI). Positive identification of human remains is required for legal requirements necessary to settle the victim's estate, as well as for the psychological well-being of the families of victims. The goal of DVI is to identify all victims by gathering and cataloguing all corresponding ante mortem and postmortem data.

In catastrophic events mortuary and morgue resources will be scarce and fatality processing throughput (e.g., identification, processing, and final disposition) will be limited; all existing resources should be focused on performing only the highest priority functions. These critical functions include body recovery, abbreviated processing, temporary storage, and tracking. With scarce resources the capability may not exist to perform even these critical functions simultaneously, necessitating the use of a sequential approach to managing remains.

Obviously, body recovery will be ongoing throughout the response phase of the event. Identifying those deaths that are likely the result of the pandemic makes the victim identification process more efficient and reduces the case load for ME/C. Those deaths that are attended by family members or health care providers will have a known identity and may have a signed death certificate. Unattended deaths will require the ME/C to further process remains in order to determine victim identification, issue the death certificate, track personal effects, and notify the next of kin.

These complications will be the rate-limiting factors that will overwhelm the ME/C and hinder the process of getting remains to the point of final disposition. Working on the assumption of no available outside resources, there will be no way of expanding the throughput to expedite the processing of remains. Because the processing capability (supply) is virtually fixed, then the only strategy for meeting the increased demand is to manage the demand. This can be accomplished by establishing multiple collection points and temporary morgues throughout the community to provide the capability of holding remains until they can be managed through a centralized process in the ME/C office.

Bodies can be stored for up to 6 months in refrigerated storage, which may provide the ME/C and funeral directors enough time to process all bodies in accordance with jurisdictional standards and traditional public expectations. Performing fatality management operations sequentially allows officials to leverage limited resources to employ best management practices during a worst-case scenario, to ensure that bodies will be properly identified and handled with dignity.

Although this sequential strategy of processing and releasing bodies back to the next of kin will be protracted, public expectations can be managed through proactive crisis communication planning that is well coordinated among state and local emergency management, public health, and public administration offices. The stress of delayed processing and reunification with next of kin will challenge the public trust in the government's ability to manage the event; however, the crisis will be greatly magnified if bodies are handled haphazardly and the accuracy of identification is compromised.[4]

In sudden onset, single point MFIs, local ME/C offices can call on state and federal mortuary surge assets. A component of the National Disaster Medical System (NDMS) under the Department of Health and Human Services (DHHS), Disaster Mortuary Operational Response Teams (DMORTs) are federal resources that are composed of volunteer medical and forensic specialists who have specific training and skills in victim identification, mortuary services, and forensic pathology and anthropology methods (Fig. 50-1). Florida, Indiana, Michigan, and Ohio are among the handful of states that have robust state level disaster mortuary teams patterned after the federal DMORTs. These disaster mortuary teams provide the resources and forensic specialists, including fingerprinting, radiographic, and forensic dental identification, necessary to set up and operate a Disaster Portable Morgue Unit (DPMU) for the identification of disaster victims and reunification with next of kin (Figs. 50-2 through 50-5).

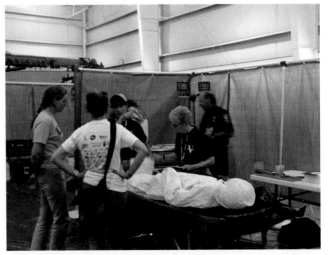

FIG 50-1 Members of a Federal DMORT Explain Their Procedures During an Exercise. (Photo by Bob Shank, Jr.)

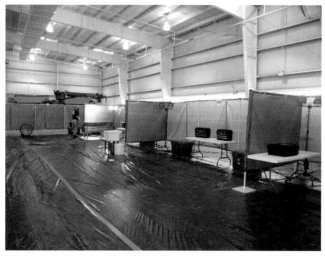

FIG 50-2 A Disaster Portable Morgue Set Up in a Building of Opportunity. (Photo by Bob Shank, Jr.)

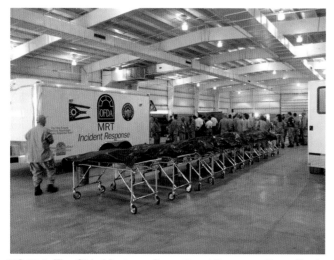

FIG 50-3 The Ohio Mortuary Operational Response Team Participating in the Talon Shield Full Scale Exercise at the Ohio National Guard's Camp Ravenna Joint Military Training Center in August 2010. (Photo by Bob Shank, Jr.)

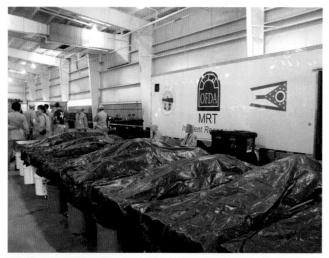

FIG 50-4 The Ohio Mortuary Operational Response Team Participating in the Talon Shield Full Scale Exercise at the Ohio National Guard's Camp Ravenna Joint Military Training Center in August 2010. (Photo by Bob Shank, Jr.)

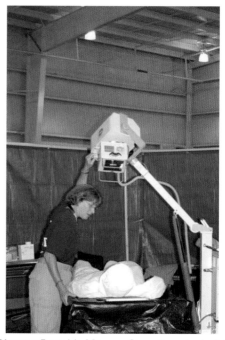

FIG 50-5 Disaster Portable Morgue Operations Include Radiological Capabilities for PostMortem Identification. (Photo by Bob Shank, Jr.)

Considerations for MFM usually focus on acute events; however, at the state and community level, MFM also encompasses other issues involving identification of human remains. The most common example of this is the destruction of cemeteries along the Gulf Coast during hurricanes. The high water table and aboveground burial practices result in coffins being displaced and washed inland 20 to 30 miles in some cases. DMORT teams have assisted in recovery and reidentification of many coffins. In fact, coffins are now identified with a brass tag, which greatly streamlines the process of identification and reinterment (some have been through the process three to four times).

Another nonacute MFM incident involving DMORT was the 2002 Crematory Scandal in Noble, Georgia, where several hundred bodies had been dumped in the woods and surrounding buildings instead of being properly cremated. Federal DMORT was deployed to the scene to work with the Walker County coroner to recover and identify the remains.[15]

The Army National Guard's Homeland Response Force supports 17 teams that are trained and equipped to respond to incidents involving chemical, biological, radiological, nuclear, and high-yield explosives (CBRNE). Each CBRNE-Enhanced Response Force Package (CERFP) team consists of 186 soldiers and airmen and includes a command and control section, a hazardous materials decontamination unit, a medical section, a casualty search and extraction unit, and a fatalities search and recovery element.[16]

However, state and local planners must realize that in the event of a nationwide catastrophic MFI such as a pandemic these resources will be equally affected by the event and quickly overwhelmed, and each local community will be forced to rely on their own resources.

In catastrophic MFIs normal transportation resources will be overwhelmed. Planners should anticipate the need to use nontraditional means of transportation, such as buses, trucks, and vans and employ nontraditional drivers and handlers. Authorities should preidentify potential pools of suitable drivers and handlers and be prepared to provide JIT training regarding their transportation and handling duties. Planners should also develop a highly efficient methodology for the transport of remains from recovery through final disposition in order to conserve manpower effort and fuel.[4]

In catastrophic MFIs local ME/C offices will become quickly overwhelmed, and even the expeditious recovery of bodies from throughout the community will be delayed. To accommodate this surge, local ME/C and emergency management offices should consider establishing local collection points and temporary morgues throughout the community, to provide family members a place to transport their deceased loved one to. Setting up centralized temporary collection points and temporary morgue sites throughout the community will minimize the number of people traveling to faraway locations, prevent large crowds from gathering during a public isolation period, and help workers achieve a more effective span of control to manage the large influx of human remains.[4]

Local ME/C morgues, hospitals, and funeral homes do not maintain extensive excess storage capabilities, and most typically operate at around 90% capacity.

For those agencies that have developed a MFM surge-capacity plan, it typically only identifies one alternate means of expanding their storage capability. Many emergency managers and public health officials are beginning to realize that any significant MFI will quickly overwhelm the community's storage capability, and it is likely that in catastrophic events, human remains may need to be stored for an extended period until the local ME/C is able to process the remains and issue a death certificate.

Temporary refrigerated storage (between 37 and 42 °F) provides the best temporary storage option. Bodies can be stored for up to 6 months in refrigerated storage. Refrigerated-storage options include prepurchased temporary refrigerated morgues, cooling systems for remains pouches, racking systems, and nontraditional holding facilities, including cold-storage warehouses, refrigerated vans, hangars, and refrigerated rail cars. This strategy may provide the ME/C and funeral directors enough time to process all bodies in accordance with jurisdictional standards and traditional public expectations and allows officials to balance the demand side of the surge with the limited processing capacity (supply) and still employ best management practices.

If the surge of fatalities completely overwhelms all refrigerated-storage resources, the emergency management and ME/C offices may be forced to utilize nontraditional methods of temporary storage, such as temporary interment.[4]

Temporary interment provides a good option for immediate storage, where no other method is available or where longer-term temporary storage is needed. The temperature underground is lower than at the surface, thereby providing some level of natural refrigeration. As part of the crisis communication plan, local authorities must be prepared to inform the public regarding long-term temporary interment. It is also important to note the possibility that the temporary interment site may in fact become the final resting location for many of the deceased, so the location should be selected with great care.[13]

Local emergency management and ME/C planners should collaboratively identify and acquire morgue surge equipment and MFM supplies including temporary interment (burial) supplies.

As part of their continuity of operations and emergency operations planning, local authorities should prescript active and dormant contracts with local private-sector resources to obtain crucial storage supplies and other services. Preplanning, identifying and/or purchasing resources, and balancing local jurisdictional requirements with local available assets will assist emergency managers and the ME/C in obtaining those resources during a catastrophic MFI.

In catastrophic events where local capabilities are expected to be overwhelmed, local ME/C offices and public health departments should develop a crisis communication plan to coordinate the dissemination of public information through the local emergency management office.

This information should include the location of collection points and temporary morgues, need for personal protection for handling a body, type of identification procedures and reunification plan the ME/C may employ, and official plan for final disposition of all remains. In the end, the message to the public must be that the authorities may be forced to implement alternate processing methods, which may lengthen the time frame but ultimately will maintain the dignity of the deceased and strive to keep family members informed.

Local health care institutions should develop their MFM plans in conjunction with all community stakeholders to ensure effective coordination and prevent duplicating reliance on the same scarce resources.

In catastrophic MFIs bodies should be classified by the cause and manner of death. In the case of a pandemic or biological event, these cases should be segregated from ME/C cases that require further investigation or autopsy. Remains should be further segregated between attended cases that can be processed quickly (those with a known identity and signed death certificate) from unattended cases wherein the victim's identification is not known and there are subsequent delays in obtaining a signed death certificate.

Once remains are sorted by case type, they should be stored in different containers and locations at each collection point and morgue to simplify the process and ensure that only remains with a positive identification and a death certificate are processed for final disposition.

Creating an organized, segregated storage method that simplifies how remains are processed will reduce the amount of time most family members will wait for final disposition to occur, and provide the public a higher level of confidence that government agencies are managing the MFI competently.

Responding to and managing an MFI creates high levels of psychological stress on health care, rescue, and mortuary workers. Postdisaster mental health research provides some evidence to suggest that training and experience levels may not correlate with adequate emotional and psychological resilience. Responders and health care workers as a demographic seem to have the same levels of variability with regard to emotional reactions and psychological vulnerabilities as other segments of the population.[17,18] It is imperative that emergency managers and health care and response leadership proactively provide for the stress debriefing and mental health recovery of those workers involved, especially those tasked with handling and identifying the remains of disaster fatalities.

⚠ PITFALLS

Mismanagement of a disaster begins with the failure to adequately plan and prepare. The consequences of poor disaster response and recovery not only include extended human suffering, greater social and economic losses for the survivors, and increased mental distress and legal complications for relatives of the victims but also political ramifications for both elected officials and government leaders as well.

There are a number of potential pitfalls of which planners must be aware, but thankfully these are not hidden. The application of standard CEM and crisis management principles apply to MFM, just as they do to any other aspect of emergency or disaster management. The primary pitfall that results in the failure to plan and prepare for any type of disaster is rooted in the lack of vision or failure to recognize the risk (probability of occurrence × potential impact).

Leaders at the organizational, community, and state levels must recognize that a pandemic or biological event has the potential to affect the entire nation and strain the capabilities of every local community. In a catastrophic MFI, local and state authorities will have insufficient personnel, supplies, equipment, and storage capacity to handle the demand, and it is unlikely that mutual aid resources from surrounding jurisdictions will be available. Therefore institutional-based providers, such as hospitals, nursing homes, and hospice care organizations, along with local public health departments, will be forced to rely on local resources from existing public and private agencies. As with any aspect of CEM, planners must engage stakeholder organizations to ensure proper coordination of logistics and supply planning and to eliminate the potential of every individual agency counting on the same scarce resources as the critical backup in their plan.

In this type of event every jurisdiction will require similar types of critical resources, including personnel, equipment, supplies, and storage capacity to manage the surge in the number of decedents. Further, current business and industry practices utilizing JIT inventory and Lean supply chain strategies reduce overall community resilience to disaster impacts and will be unable to meet the spike in demand for these critical resources. In the aftermath of Hurricane Katrina, FEMA nearly exhausted the entire nationwide supply of remains pouches as they attempted to support logistical demand forecasts of 25,000. The fact that the entire nationwide supply of remains pouches will be wiped out after the first 25,000 fatalities should give planners an idea of how quickly a nationwide pandemic or truly catastrophic MFI will overwhelm MFM capabilities at the local, state, and federal levels.

Another potential pitfall is applying the same type of MFM strategies that are typically used for the 100 to 200 decedent event to manage 1000 to 10,000 decedents. Surge capacity for living patients must provide additional throughput capacity, higher levels of critical care, and be provided simultaneously in order to provide the greatest good to the greatest number of patients. MFM need not be under the same time constraints or demand for capacity.

Even though the strategy of refrigerated storage and sequential processing and releasing of bodies back to the next of kin will be protracted, public expectations can be managed through proactive crisis communication planning that is well coordinated between state and local emergency management, public health, and public administration offices. Although the stress of delayed processing and reunification with next of kin will challenge the public trust in the government's ability to manage the event, the crisis will be greatly magnified if bodies are handled haphazardly and the accuracy of identification is compromised.

One complicating issue of employing this strategy is that some religious and ethnic practices require a person to be buried within 24 hours of death. Recognizing that the various faiths and ethnic groups within the community are in fact stakeholders and then engaging them in this planning process is key to crafting a plan that addresses their concerns and manages their expectations in the event of an MFI.

Other pitfalls of the long-term refrigerated-storage option include limited fuel to power cooling units, limited maintenance personnel to repair broken units, and limited availability of refrigeration units (as the entire nation will need this same resource).

Other refrigerated-storage options include prepurchased temporary refrigerated morgues, cooling systems for remains pouches, racking systems, and nontraditional holding facilities, including cold-storage warehouses, refrigerated vans, hangars, and refrigerated rail cars. However, these alternative resources require additional considerations. For example, most refrigerated semi-trailers, rail cars, and warehouses are used for hauling and storing grocery items, and will be deemed unfit for such use after being used as temporary morgues. Therefore agencies planning on using these resources should plan on being required to purchase transportation units at time of use. Further, retail food chains are very sensitive about their brand being associated with dead bodies, and they will require the covering or removal of all company logos. Planners must also be aware that as our society considers stacking human remains to be highly disrespectful and that stacking will permanently distort the face, a 53-foot semi-trailer can only hold 30 bodies unless rack storage systems are installed inside.

Cold-storage warehouses that are typically part of the regional grocery supply chain may provide storage capacity for several thousand bodies, but planners must be aware of the potential effects on food supplies in an already strained supply chain system and should anticipate major issues for financial compensation and decontamination of cold-storage warehouses. Sometimes ice and dry ice are considered for cold storage, but both are logistically challenging to support long term.

Sound crisis communication strategies that support an accurate and consistent flow of public information go a long way in assuaging the fears that dead bodies pose extreme public health risks. What makes this erroneous information so influential is that it is in fact promoted by some medical and disaster professionals and the media. With the "officials" publicizing this incorrect information, it can create undue panic throughout the public, as well as political pressure on authorities to use unnecessary measures such as rapid mass burials and spraying "disinfectants."

Conversely, victims of deadly communicable diseases such as Ebola do in fact present a significant public health hazard, as they can be infectious for 4 to 5 days after death.[11] In these cases handling remains in accordance with Centers for Disease Control and Prevention (CDC) and WHO guidelines, along with rapid burial, is the best strategy to limit further disease transmission.[19]

Even though the concept of temporary interment provides a good option for immediate storage where no other method is available or where longer-term temporary storage may be needed, it is still a strategy that most likely will evoke controversy and public dispute. As with any disaster response and recovery strategy, local authorities must have a coherent crisis communication strategy that clearly and transparently communicates the points of a long-term temporary interment to the public. Proactive leaders that have engaged community stakeholders in the development of this plan long before the disaster hits will be much more effective in communicating the plan and efficient in enacting the plan, compared with those who are trying to manage it on the fly in the midst of a crisis with no plan at all.

To help ensure future relocation and recovery of bodies, temporary burial sites should be properly identified. Burial should be at least 5-feet deep and at least 600 feet from drinking water sources. Remains should be placed in the trench with 1-foot spacing and not stacked. Each body should be clearly identified with corresponding location markers at ground level.[13] Incorporating these tactics to demonstrate best practices in the management of mass fatalities helps supplant the images of bodies being dumped like trash into a landfill, by showing dignity to the deceased, and providing respect and closure for the families.

Disasters that occur as single point, sudden onset events, such as earthquakes, hurricanes, explosions, or airline disasters, have the potential to create a sudden surge of mass fatalities that will likely overwhelm local and regional response capabilities. Catastrophic MFIs such as massive tsunamis or pandemic outbreaks will create an exponentially larger surge of fatalities that may either present as a sudden surge or exhibit a more protracted development profile over time. It is imperative that emergency management planners in specific facilities, as well as at the community and state level, apply the concepts of CEM to MFM, as they do for all other aspects of disaster preparedness, response, and recovery.

CEM supports engaging all stakeholders in an integrated, coordinated approach to planning and preparedness that ensures the capability to effectively manage large numbers of fatalities. For localized disasters, additional MFM resources are available from a handful of states, including Florida, Michigan, and Ohio, as well as the Army National Guard CERFP teams and the federal government through the

NDMS. Prudent planners will embrace FEMA's "Whole Community" concept and develop public and private partnerships to provide local MFM capability in the event that outside assistance is unavailable.

After the immediate threats to life safety have been addressed, the appropriate handling, identification, and disposition of the deceased are still critical factors in the competent response to an MFI.

Crisis communication planning will ensure an informative and consistent message to the public that will assist in managing expectations and engender confidence that the event is being managed in a competent fashion. Leaders must be aware of the physical health and safety, as well as mental health risks, to those personnel managing disaster fatalities, and proactively provide the necessary protective equipment and recovery therapy as needed.

REFERENCES

1. Tsunami death toll passes 283,000. January 28, 2005 Sidney Morning Herald. http://www.smh.com.au/news/Asia-Tsunami/Tsunami-death-toll-passes-283000/2005/01/27/1106415737181.html Accessed April 27, 2014.

2. October 8, 2005 Kashmir Pakistan Earthquake. National Oceanic and Atmospheric Administration-National Geophysical Data Center. http://ngdc.noaa.gov/hazardimages/event/show/27 Accessed April 27, 2014.

3. Haiti raises quake death toll on anniversary. CBC News Posted: Jan 12, 2011. http://www.cbc.ca/news/world/haiti-raises-quake-death-toll-on-anniversary-1.1011363 Accessed April 27, 2014.

4. U.S. Northern Command and Department of Health and Human Services Fatality Management Pandemic Influenza Working Group Conference, White Paper: The Provision of Family Assistance and Behavioral Health Services in the Management of Mass Fatalities Resulting from a Pandemic Influenza in the United States, September 2006 available at Joint Task Force Civil Support. http://www.jtfcs.northcom.mil.

5. U.S. National Library of Medicine, National Institutes of Health. http://www.ncbi.nlm.nih.gov/pmc/articles/PMC1291330/ Accessed April 27, 2014.

6. Dombrowski, J. Disaster Life Support. American Medical Association Journal of Ethics. http://virtualmentor.ama-assn.org/2004/05/cprl1-0405.html Accessed April 27, 2014.

7. Blanchard, W. Guide to emergency management and related terms, definitions, concepts, acronyms, organizations, programs, guidance, executive orders, & legislation. 10/27/08 FEMA. http://training.fema.gov/EMIWeb/edu/docs/terms%20and%20definitions/Terms%20and%20Definitions.pdf Accessed April 27, 2014.

8. Quarantelli EL. Emergencies, disaster and catastrophes are different phenomena. University of Delaware; 2000.

9. USA Disaster Statistics. http://www.preventionweb.net/english/countries/statistics/?cid=185.

10. Boeing Airlines. Statistical Summary of Commercial Jet Airplane Accidents Worldwide Operations. 1959–2012. http://www.boeing.com/news/techissues/pdf/statsum.pdf.

11. Belanov EF, Muntianov VP, Kriuk V, et al. Survival of Marburg virus infectivity on contaminated surfaces and in aerosols. Vopr Virusol. 1995;41(1):32–34.

12. Haglage A. Kissing the corpses in ebola country. The Daily Beast; August 8, 2014. http://www.thedailybeast.com/articles/2014/08/13/kissing-the-corpses-in-ebola-country.html.

13. Morgan O, Tidball-Binz M, van Alphen D. Management of Dead Bodies after Disasters: A Field Manual for First Responders. Washington, DC: Pan American Health Organization/World Health Organization; 2009.

14. Emergency Management Assistance Compact. At: http://www.emacweb.org Accessed 5/19/14.

15. Ledger, M. Tri-State Crematory: Government leaders recall how it happened. Northwest Georgia News. Posted: Sunday, February 19, 2012. http://www.northwestgeorgianews.com/rome/tri-state-crematory-government-leaders-recall-how-it-happened/article_b58a857d-5044-5cf4-ab06-14fcd5c7b50e.html.

16. Army National Guard CERFP Teams. http://www.arng.army.mil/news/publications/fs/2010/Subject_papers/National%20Guard%20CERFP%20Teams.pdf.

17. Keller RT, Bobo WV. Handling human remains following the terrorist attack on the Pentagon: experiences of 10 uniformed healthcare workers. Mil Med. 2002;167(4):8–11.

18. Taylor AJ, Frazer AG. The stress of post-disaster body handling and victim identification work. J Human Stress. 1982;6:4112.

19. INTERIM version 1.2 Ebola and Marburg virus disease epidemics: preparedness, alert, control, and evaluation. WHO, Geneva, Switzerland, August 2014. http://apps.who.int/iris/bitstream/10665/130160/1/WHO_HSE_PED_CED_2014.05_eng.pdf?ua=1.

Disaster Management of Animals

Robert J. Tashjian and James M. Burke

The management of animals is an important part of any field response to disasters. Whether it is the management of displaced, injured, or ill animals after a natural disaster or the care of search and rescue animals as part of the response team, animal care remains an integral piece of the disaster-preparedness and response system. The current geopolitical climate has forced the United States to explore contingency plans for future environmental disasters. Although most of the research along these lines is focused on human safety, the animal and agricultural aspects of disaster management also need to be explored. Because natural disasters are a more-frequent risk to animal populations than possible biological or terrorist threats are, the protection of these resources demands proper consideration.

U.S. agriculture, a $100 billion business, is an important nutritional source, and it helps sustain the country's economic growth and military readiness.[1] However, concentrating animals into larger facilities to provide abundant food sources increases agricultural risk, especially in the event of a biological disaster or terrorist threat. In addition, the large numbers of companion animals in urban areas should be considered during an evacuation, because most disaster shelter facilities do not accept animals. Overall, a large number of animals—both livestock and pets—are likely to need care during a disaster.

Analysis of past disasters highlights some mistakes, but lessons may be learned from them. Large-scale natural disasters, such as Hurricanes Andrew and Floyd in 1999, may be viewed as test scenarios from which future contingencies can be developed. Evaluating the mobilization, transportation, and housing of displaced companion animals and livestock helps prepare pet owners and animal producers for future events. Not all contingency factors can be addressed in every disaster plan, and, for this reason, a flexible, well-thought-out plan is necessary.

Animals, their behavior patterns, and their habitats can also be affected by natural disaster. The Lushan Earthquake that occurred in Southern China in 2013 dramatically disrupted the giant panda natural habitat, resulting in pandas being killed, as well as behavioral changes in surviving animals. Such disruptions can cause decreases in populations by both direct (death of animals) and indirect (disruptions of reproductive behaviors and raising of young) ways.[2]

According to the National Academies Board on Agriculture and Natural Resources' report, "Countering Agricultural Bioterrorism," not only is America vulnerable to terrorist attacks against agriculture, but insufficient plans are in place to defend against such attacks.[3] The crippling effects of the foot-and-mouth disease epidemic of 2001 illustrate the local economic disruption and global effects such events entail.[4] Even though biological attacks are not likely to cause widespread famine, they could have a direct effect on the national economy, public health, and the public's confidence in the food system. Plans need to be drafted now to provide a framework in which a safe, continuous supply of food can be guaranteed, epidemic disease outbreaks can be prevented, and proper care for injured animals can be ensured.

HISTORICAL PERSPECTIVE

As some of history's most recent disasters show, animal health care, veterinary infection control, control of stray animals, and the revival of veterinary infrastructures are the primary areas that need to be addressed in effective implemental models developed for the future.

On August 24, 1992, Hurricane Andrew ripped through Southern Florida, leaving thousands of animals injured, abandoned, or dead. Relief efforts were hampered because organizations and volunteer groups lacked a central command structure. These groups, though well intentioned, were unable to coordinate the necessary supplies and medical resources in a cohesive effort to help those areas most devastated by the hurricane.

On September 16, 1999, Hurricane Floyd devastated North Carolina, affecting poultry, pork, and cattle production, as well as horses, cats, dogs, and other pets. North Carolina residents, because of the unsubstantiated, predicted dangers in previous media-hyped disasters, ignored calls for evacuation. The lack of pet-friendly evacuation shelters, in addition to the lack of public preparedness, contributed to evacuation failures. Such failures endanger not only animals but their human owners as well. North Carolina State University's College of Veterinary Medicine was able to reestablish a veterinary infrastructure, contributing to the success of the disaster-management operation. With its large number of trained personnel, resources, and medical supplies, the college was able to immediately take charge of animal care and control issues and organize volunteers. In addition to a large number of volunteers, enormous amounts of food and medical supplies were donated, and transportation was made available to help agencies contend with the disaster.

During the Hurricane Floyd disaster, medical care for animals was administered through a three-tier system. Tier 1 consisted primarily of vaccinations for cats. Tier 2 included heartworm infection and other diagnostic testing. Tier 3 treatments included surgical and medical stabilization of injuries.[4]

On April 25, 1994, a tornado struck West Lafayette, Indiana, destroying 67 homes and 60 mobile homes. The civic response to this incident is an example of a lack of evacuation procedures. It resulted in massive pet abandonment by individuals in an urban location. Pet abandonment is a consequence of unplanned or poorly executed evacuations. Human-animal bonds are strong, and, during a disaster, such bonds may influence peoples' decisions to reenter a disaster area to retrieve a family pet. Such decisions may pose significant risks not only to individuals and families but also to emergency personnel, who may need to become involved in rescue efforts.[5] Statistically, owners who regularly visit their veterinarians are less likely than those who do not to lose their pets during evacuations. Individuals with weak or poor human-animal bonds, who have low levels of disaster preparedness, or who own many animals are more prone to leave their animals behind during a disaster.[6] Although pet abandonment is common during disasters, in a national survey, the proportion of animals abandoned during disasters was similar to the proportion of animals relinquished to 12 U.S. animal shelters.[6] Pet evacuation failures generally result from low levels of pet care. Promoting responsible pet ownership that includes planning for emergencies, both natural and human-made, is a logical strategy to make owners more responsible for the evacuation of their pets.

On March 4, 1996, a train derailed near Weyauwega, Wisconsin, causing a fire to erupt in the train's propane-filled cars. Local residents were asked to evacuate because of fears of a major explosion. Risk factors influencing the failure of owners to evacuate the area's cats and dogs included a weak human-animal bond, logistical challenges, and generally low levels of disaster preparedness. During the Weyauwega disaster, 15% of all pet owners were at work and were unable to evacuate their pets. The most common reasons for failing to evacuate pets included owners thinking that they would not be gone long and that the evacuated areas were safe for pets.[7] Outdoor cats were at higher risk of evacuation failure because they are more difficult to catch and transport. The higher incidence of the failure to evacuate cats compared with the failure to evacuate dogs likely reflects the greater ease with which dogs can be caught, restrained, and transported. It could also reflect the assumption that cats can "fend for themselves" if left outdoors. Interestingly, households with a high number of cats are more likely to leave a dog behind during evacuation procedures.[7]

In November 1990, Western Washington experienced severe flooding. Dairy farmers who were surveyed were asked to evaluate the amount of equipment and personnel available to evacuate cattle, numbers of cattle evacuated, time required for evacuations, and destination and care of the animals. Financial loss from cattle deaths, illnesses, and halts in production was estimated at $2,786,629.[8] Help for evacuation was readily available from family members, employees, and friends. Because of adequate notice, 5000 animals were evacuated in 20 hours. Evacuated cattle were housed at neighbors' farms, at friends' homes, on high ground, and at a vacant dairy. Not one cow went more than 2 days without fresh water or normal rations. Unfortunately, however, most of the farmers did not plan in advance on where to evacuate and how to care for their animals. In hindsight, farmers said they could have sheltered all of their animals if necessary. Overall, however, it was adequate time that led to the successful evacuation of a large number of animals to safe locations. On shorter notice, such a successful evacuation may not have been achievable.

Whereas evacuating a large number of cattle is very difficult, horses are easier to find and transport. Horse owners typically treat their animals differently than owners treat general livestock, and they usually have been able to move most, if not all, of their horses within 90 minutes. Data suggest that both the relatively small number of horses kept on a farm and the high emotional bond between owners and horses increase the chances of horses being evacuated in a timely manner. According to horse owners in Madison County, Kentucky, 100% of the horse population could be evacuated if a 12-hour evacuation notice were given.[9]

CURRENT PRACTICE

The first priority in disaster relief is protecting and saving human lives. Animals have traditionally been viewed by emergency management officials as property, and therefore they receive much less attention than humans. Animal owners, however, consider animals either as an important source of income or as part of the family. Animal management during natural disasters is best accomplished with a plan created by state and local officials that provides a detailed framework in which to implement care during evacuations. The objectives of such a plan should be to bring some type of logistical structure to the chaos that occurs during and after a disaster. As part of such a plan, it is essential that veterinarians understand disaster preparedness so that they can integrate themselves more effectively into national, state, and local disaster-management systems.

The first step in an adequate disaster plan is denoting a clear chain of command that includes the delegation of responsibility. Without such a framework, independent groups may unintentionally direct resources away from needed areas. State veterinary agencies and practitioners will need to take responsibility for assuming leadership roles to organize animal professionals and lay volunteers. These roles may include developing liaisons with representatives from the Department of Homeland Security (DHS), Department of Health and Human Services (DHHS), the American Red Cross, the National Urban Search and Rescue Response System, and the U.S. Army Veterinary Core at the Department of Defense. The U.S. Army Veterinary Core is activated at the request of a state's governor via the president of the United States. DHHS provides National Veterinary Response Teams (NVRTs), formally named Veterinary Medical Assistant Teams (VMATs), to assist local authorities during a federal emergency. NVRTs provide care to injured animals and assist with preventative measures to maintain human health and safety. In addition, NVRTs also provide support for assessment and monitoring of zoonotic diseases and their risk for transmission. It is well established that some diseases can jump species, from animal to human (zoonosis). Moreover, a number of the most virulent and dangerous diseases the world has seen came from animals. These include human immunodeficiency virus (HIV), avian and swine flu, and the recent Ebola outbreak of 2014. The NVRTs can be deployed to assist in the management of animals with potential for zoonotic spread of disease. In addition, the U.S. Department of Agriculture is responsible for assessing food supply safety issues during disaster situations, including disease outbreaks.[10]

NVRTs also care for the search and rescue and law enforcement animals that may also deploy to a disaster scene. Like humans, animals can be injured, stressed, or worked to exhaustion in a natural or human-made disaster response. Care for these animals is a crucial part of maintaining their effectiveness in a disaster zone. Adequate food and water should be provided. Moreover, the immediate care of injury and illness, as well as scheduled rest and sleep periods, are vital to their ongoing well-being of animals and mission-critical tasks.

Once a command structure is in place, pet owners need to identify the types of disasters for which they are at risk. To assist pet owners in this process, it is recommended that veterinarians promote the creation of individual household disaster plans. Farms and large agricultural centers with a large number of animals will need to provide an equally detailed evacuation plan that ensures the appropriate feeding, sheltering, and burial of livestock.

NVRTs should be called into emergency situations to augment state and local veterinary resources until a self-sufficient response solution is reached in the disaster area. NVRTs should be available immediately after a disaster, slowly tapering off as local needs decrease and local resources expand to meet the needs of the victim population. NVRTs consist of two or more veterinarians, four or more veterinary technicians, and one to three logistical support personnel.[10] The director of the Offices of Emergency Response within DHHS and the American Veterinary Medical Association should activate NVRT intervention in an emergency. With necessary medical equipment and supplies at their disposal, these teams will operate as mobile units in disaster areas, responding to advice from regional veterinary activities commanders.[11]

Identifying potential problems in a disaster begins with the process of eliminating any mitigating hazards that may be present on a farm or in an area with animals. Alternative housing and shelter locations, clean food and water access, and accessible transportation must be designated before successful egress can occur. Repairs to barns and buildings will help to decrease the number of potential dangers during evacuation procedures. Most farms have the workforce and resources to move a large number of animals.[8] Farm cats and dogs should be placed in a disaster-proof location or, because they generally stay close to their homes, turned loose. If shelter cannot be found for aggressive animals, euthanasia is the most humane method of treatment.

Animals that are important to agricultural production or have sentimental value need to be identified ahead of time so they can be transported rapidly. Large-animal transports may present a problem to human evacuation, clogging already busy exit routes; therefore alternative evacuation routes need to be considered in advance. In the event that animal evacuation is not possible, sources of shelter, food, and water will need to be designated, and a plan that addresses how best to reenter the disaster area to attend to the animals must be in place.

It is important that local kennels and pet shelters are able to accommodate the influx of small animals during a disaster. Veterinarians are the best channels for communicating with local pet owners about the safe evacuation of their pets. The American Red Cross, although it does not shelter animals, should also be able to provide information, in coordination with local animal shelters, on how to care for pets in evacuation areas.

Veterinarians play an important role during disasters. Their primary responsibilities include control of disease factors and disease transmission, herd management, animal health care, animal control, disaster assessment, and search and rescue operations. Even though it is important that veterinarians have the resources available to locate and call on appropriate experts during a disaster, they also will need to address the proper sheltering of animals, provide advice to animal owners on nutritional requirements, tend to the proper disposal of carcasses, provide housing to animals, manage food safety, and care for sick and injured animals. Veterinarians should have detailed maps of animal centers in their areas, such as veterinary hospitals, boarding kennels, fairgrounds, racetracks, and other evacuation locations, including slaughterhouse facilities. Veterinarians should also organize therapeutic intervention methods, systems, procedures, and processes to prevent potential illnesses.

A large number of animal habitats around industrial livestock production facilities and home farms may be destroyed during a disaster, jeopardizing vital food stores. Diseases, exacerbated by impaired food and water supplies, could lead to outbreaks of food poisoning, typhoid, cholera, infectious hepatitis, and gastroenteritis. Removal of fences and enclosures results in the release of animals that subsequently roam unrestricted, increasing their interaction with wildlife, domestic animals, and human populations, providing vectors for potential disease transmission.[12] In addition, veterinarians with training in food and meat hygiene should decide which foods (e.g., milk or meat products) are potentially unsafe and which are acceptable for human consumption in the given disaster circumstances.

The American Veterinary Medical Association has created a disaster-preparedness series, which is included on its website, designed to educate both pet owners and the large industrial animal producers on the natural and technological aspects of disaster preparation.[13] The University of California-Davis Veterinary School also provides

---

BOX 51-1   Methods of Large- and Small-Animal Identification

EQUINE AND LIVESTOCK	SMALL ANIMAL
Microchip	Collar tag
Ear tag	Microchip
Halter tag	Tattoo
Neck chain	Temporary neck band
Ear notches	
Leg bands	
Brand	
Mane clips	
Livestock crayon	

---

online information for facilities planning to offer animal care during evacuations. Animal care operations can find additional printable forms online to help organize the influx of evacuated animals.

Disasters may occur when owners are away from home. In such instances, stickers placed around the homeowner's property in advance can aid rescue personnel. These stickers should contain information pertaining to the types of animals located on the property, the location of the animals, their possible hiding spots, and the location of evacuation supplies. Owners should designate a neighbor familiar with their animals and evacuation plans to be responsible for the animals in the event that they are not at home when a disaster occurs. Identification tags, including rabies and license tags, will help reunite owners with their pets after a disaster. Identification should include the owner's name, home address, phone number, and an out-of-state phone number of someone who can be contacted in the event of an emergency. Suggested methods for identifying large and small animals are included in Box 51-1.

During an evacuation, it is best to separate animals into individual evacuation areas, based on household location and species, to decrease disease transmission. Large-animal evacuations are more difficult to manage than small-animal evacuations. Specifically, animals unfamiliar with trailers provide a unique handling and capture challenge. A key recommendation for evacuating larger animals is to acclimate the animals to transportation equipment and the evacuation process in advance.

The evacuation of exotic animals, such as birds, amphibians, and reptiles, can be equally challenging. Birds are best transported in small, securely covered containers to prevent injury. Cages should be covered and placed in quiet locations to decrease the stress of evacuation. Amphibians can be transported in watertight plastic bags and plastic containers, one species per container. Small pet reptiles can be transported effectively in pillowcases, sacks, or transfer carriers. Using the same water that an amphibian inhabited before the evacuation will help minimize physiological stress. All exotic animals should be provided with clean food and water every day, including dietary supplements unique to that animal. Once animals arrive at evacuation facilities, special care must be taken to monitor water and air temperature, humidity, and lighting.

After intake areas at evacuation sites are established (Box 51-2), animals need to be secured in cages or on leashes and properly identified. Identification includes taking a picture of the animal with the owner, if the owner is available. Intake information should include a unique number for the animal and its date of birth, sex, and breed. Bite alert badges, if relevant, should be placed on cages or on the animals' collars. Unless the animal is injured and needs to see a veterinarian, shelter

BOX 51-2 Potential Evacuation Sites

- Veterinary hospitals
- Fairgrounds
- Racetracks
- Boarding kennels
- Animal shelters

personnel should then take the animals to their perspective housing areas. Injured animals should be taken to a triage area. Intake for dead animals (including strays) should be handled in much the same manner, except that carcasses should be placed in properly designated areas or disposable containers.

The treatment of injuries and infectious diseases needs to occur before an animal is transferred to an intake area and placed among other evacuated animals. Triage sites are to be used as temporary holding facilities where veterinarians can determine whether an animal is stable enough to be transferred to a housing facility. Animals determined to be in life-threatening situations with reasonable prognosis of a full recovery should be triaged to one area, animals with non–life-threatening injuries should be triaged to a second area, and uninjured animals should be transferred to a third area.

Information on housed animals should include the following:

1. What food and what quantity of food the animal should be fed (Table 51-1)
2. Whether, and how much, the animal is eating
3. Whether the animal is drinking its water
4. Whether the animal is defecating in the cage, and whether stools appear normal
5. Whether the animal appears mentally or physically well

Sheltered animals need to be walked for a total of 3 hours per day, no longer than 15 minutes per walk. Information regarding larger animals needs to be noted, such as their movements or lactations. Abnormalities or unusual behavior occurring in either large or small animals, when properly recorded, will alert veterinary and housing personnel of a potentially sick animal. It is also important to understand and address the effects of disaster on research animals in order to ensure the continuation of their humane treatment. Steps should be taken before the disaster strikes to mitigate against disruption of their food, water, or shelter.[13]

Once a disaster is declared over, all animal habitats used before the disaster need to be cleaned and cleared of potential hazards before animals are released back into those environments. Areas surrounding buildings and facilities need to be cleared of any sharp objects, dangerous materials, and wildlife. Large animals should be released into safe, enclosed outdoor areas. Because small animals may encounter dangerous wildlife and other debris if allowed outside unsupervised and unrestrained, they should be released indoors. Animals that may have been left behind without food sources should be reintroduced

TABLE 51-1 Housed Animals' Food and Water Requirements

ANIMAL	WATER PER DAY	FEED PER DAY
Cat or dog	1-3 quarts per animal	Varies
Cows or horses	7-9 gallons	8-20 lb hay
Poultry	0.5-1.5 gallons per 10 birds	2-4 lb per 10 birds
Sheep or swine	1-4 gallons	3-8 lb hay or grain

Adapted from USDA Animal Welfare Information Center Newsletter. Available at: http://www.nal.usda.gov/awic/pubs/awicdocs.htm.

to food in small servings, gradually working up to full portions. Uninterrupted rest and sleep will help the animals to recover from trauma or stress.[14]

! PITFALLS

Traditionally, veterinary public and animal health concerns in disaster management have focused primarily on food safety and supply, injury, and treating infectious diseases. Data, however, suggest that it is equally important to focus on the animals left behind by their owners. In preparation for future events, the evacuation of pets along with human household members must be prioritized.

In surveys of previous disasters, most pet owners proved self-reliant, requiring no public services. Such self-reliance should be encouraged. Unfortunately, however, owners who evacuate pets can hinder the efforts of emergency management officers, who are primarily focused on evacuating people. In New York City, after a scaffolding collapse, emergency management personnel initially told people to leave their animals, and several days passed before pet owners were allowed to tend to their animals. Later, emergency management officials were prosecuted for preventing pet rescue.[6] Better coordination with local animal health officials may prevent such problems.

Thirty percent of respondents in one city suggested that they would not evacuate with their pets in an emergency because they would not be able to catch or transport them.[14] Pet evacuation failures occur independently of geographic location and weather conditions at the time of the disaster. Sociodemographic risk factors of pet abandonment, however, are usually present before disasters strike. They include low pet attachment, dogs living outdoors, and owners not having carriers for cats. Therefore, to promote solid animal evacuation practices, animal owners require education by local animal health personnel. In addition, emergency medical systems somewhat promote negligence by pet owners by forcing them to keep their pets at home during an emergency. Further, local emergency shelters do not provide suitable housing for people and their animals. In some instances, individuals abandon evacuation shelters because they are afraid their pets will be jeopardized. Most shelters do not provide any means of animal support because they do not want, or cannot afford, the liability involved in housing both humans and pets. One solution would be to create pet-friendly shelters, where humans can evacuate with their animals. Unfortunately, at present, the American Red Cross only has rooms and resources to manage the large number of displaced people and not their pets.[5]

Farms, which usually have large numbers of animals of different species, present unique evacuation planning problems. Most farmers are middle-aged, well-educated individuals living in rural areas. These individuals tend to be somewhat skeptical about evacuation orders delivered through radio and television and instead rely heavily on themselves and their neighbors for information. In one survey, farmers prioritized their evacuation plans by placing family safety first, farm and home security second, and animal concerns third.[14] If cattle needed to remain on the farm, most farmers suggested that 3 days of feed and water would be available. A majority of the farmers surveyed agreed that within 2 weeks, additional feed and water would be needed.[15] Further complicating matters, few areas in disaster situations are big enough to accommodate a large number of animals from multiple farms. Therefore preplanned evacuation areas to corral valuable herd animals need to be identified in advance. Farms can use numerous individuals, family members, employees, and friends to help transport herds of livestock, provided that adequate notice is given. The sheer amount of work necessary to transport agricultural animals necessitates a larger time frame, allowing greater compliance and removal of animals to safety.[8] The difficulty of gathering a large number of animals, both agricultural and domestic, suggests that animal-control personnel need to be more centrally included in evacuation planning and assistance teams.

REFERENCES

1. Adams J. The role of national animal health emergency planning. *Ann N Y Acad Sci.* 1999;894:73–75.
2. Zhang Z, Yuan S, Qi D, Zhang M. The Lushan earthquake and the giant panda: impacts and conservation. *Integr Zool.* 2014 Jun;9(3):376–378.
3. Moon H, Kirk-Baer C, Ascher M, et al. US agriculture is vulnerable to bioterrorism. *J Am Med Vet Assoc.* 2001;218:96–104.
4. Gibbs P. The foot-and-mouth disease epidemic of 2001 in the UK: implications for the USA and "war on terror." *J Vet Med Educ.* 2003;30:121–131.
5. Heath S, Champion M. Human health concerns from pet ownership after a tornado. *Prehospital Disaster Med.* 1996;11(1):79–81.
6. Heath S, Beck A, Kass P, et al. Risk factors for pet evacuation failure after a slow-onset disaster. *J Am Med Vet Assoc.* 2001;218(12):1905–1909.
7. Heath S, Voeks S, Glickman L. Epidemiologic features of pet evacuation failure in a rapid-onset disaster. *J Am Med Vet Assoc.* 2001;218:1898–1904.
8. Linnabary R, New J. Results of a survey of emergency evacuation of dairy cattle. *J Am Med Vet Assoc.* 1993;202:1238–1242.
9. Linnabary R, New J, Vogt B, et al. Emergency evacuation of horses—a Madison County, Kentucky survey. *J Equine Vet Sci.* 1993;13:153–158.
10. Heath S, Dorn R, Linnabary R, et al. Integration of veterinarians into the official response to disasters. *J Am Med Vet Assoc.* 1997;210:349–352.
11. Anderson R, Tennyson A. AVMA emergency preparedness planning. *J Am Med Vet Assoc.* 1993;203:1008–1010.
12. Moore R, Davis Y, Kaczmarek R. The role of the veterinarian in hurricanes and other natural disasters. *Ann N Y Acad Sci.* 1992;653:367–375.
13. Durkee SJ. Planning for the continued humane treatment of animals during disaster response. *Lab Anim (NY).* 2013 Oct;42(10):F8–F12.
14. American Veterinary Medical Association. *Saving the Whole Family. Disaster Preparedness Series.* Schaumburg, IL: American Veterinary Medical Association; 2004.
15. Linnabary R. Attitudinal survey of Tennessee beef producers regarding evacuation during an emergency. *J Am Med Vet Assoc.* 1991;199:1022–1026.

CHAPTER 52

Urban Search and Rescue

Michelangelo Bortolin and Gregory R. Ciottone

An Urban Search and Rescue (US&R) team is a specialized group of individuals with appropriate equipment, skills, and training that may be called into action during the disaster response phase. A US&R team or task force (TF) plays a crucial role in any situation where victims are trapped under debris or in confined areas. The US&R team's tasks and duties are localization of victims, victim extrication, and provision of initial medical treatment to victims during extrication operations. In many cases, both human-made and natural disasters involve collapsing buildings and entrapped casualties. These disasters include tsunamis, hurricanes, earthquakes, explosions, terrorist attacks, typhoons, avalanches, and mudslides, as well as confined spaces including mines, caves, wells, and trenches. US&R operations may be conducted over short or extended timelines, depending on the type of incident and the specific situation. One extreme example of extended operations is the mudslide in Oregon in March 2014 that killed more than 40 people and required more than a month of operations by US&R teams.

It is essential for any disaster responder to have a basic understanding of the role of US&R in an overall incident response where there may be trapped or confined victims because, during disaster medicine operations, significant overlap in geography and roles may occur between routine disaster response and the US&R TF operations. Disaster medicine physicians, paramedics, and other medical providers may be asked to provide medical support for specific US&R missions or may provide patient care to the victims rescued by US&R personnel, although such responders should not be put in harm's way without proper training and equipment. In addition, first responders and firefighters may be asked to provide additional workforce for search operations, for victims in widespread disasters such as tornados or hurricanes.

HISTORICAL PERSPECTIVE

Search and rescue operations have been part of disaster response since ancient times. The first existing literature regarding this topic is perhaps contained in a piece written by Pliny the Younger, where he described how his uncle, Pliny the Elder, died (AD 79) during the Vesuvius eruption while he was attempting to rescue his friends from that ongoing disaster. A more recent example would be after the Haiti Earthquake of 2010 or New Zealand Urban Search and Rescue (NZUSAR). NZUSAR was originally established as a Coast Guard organization in the 1890s, in response to multiple failed ship-rescue operations. In the United States, the first specific US&R teams were founded and developed in the 1980s, by the Fairfax County Fire & Rescue Department and the Metro-Dade County Fire Department. The tasks of the teams were to respond to disasters (most often hurricanes) by providing heavy rescue and search capability and medical care and to communicate a damage assessment while doing so. In addition, they provided support in the research of search and rescue operations, attempting to improve the field as a whole. Under an agreement with the Office of Foreign Disaster Assistance (OFDA) of the U.S. State Department, these US&R responders have been deployed to respond in several international disasters, including earthquakes (1985 Mexico City, 1986 El Salvador, and 1988 Armenia) and hurricanes (1988 Jamaica and 1989 Eastern Caribbean).[1] In 1988 the very well-known Robert T. Stafford Disaster Relief and Emergency Assistance Act (Stafford Act) codified the role of all agencies of the Federal Government in provision of assistance to state and local governments during and following a disaster. The Stafford Act also established a formal search and rescue component to federal disaster response, and, in 1989, the Federal Emergency Management Agency (FEMA) formally created the National US&R Response System to satisfy provisions of the Stafford Act. Twenty-five US&R teams from 19 states were created within this system. In 1991 the US&R teams were incorporated as part of the Federal Response Plan (FRP). US&R is now incorporated in the National Response Framework (NRF), an update to the FRP, in the Emergency Support Function (ESF) #9 (Box 52-1). At present, 28 teams are sponsored by FEMA and the Department of Homeland Security (DHS).[2] Multiple other nonfederal US&R teams sponsored by state and municipal authorities provide primarily local response. (In Oklahoma, e.g., the state sponsors an equivalent US&R team [OK-TF1] that is equipped, trained, and staffed to federal standards and has responded both in-state and to contiguous states for multiple disasters.)

CURRENT PRACTICE

Urban Search and Rescue Task Force Composition and Deployment

As stated previously, there are 28 FEMA-sponsored US&R teams in the United States (Table 52-1), and additional US&R teams have been sponsored by states and large municipalities, such as Oklahoma's US&R TF1. The TF teams are geographically distributed across the United States in a manner to best assure that a FEMA-sponsored TF team could be on the site of a disaster after only a few hours from when it is initially called for. In accordance with the overall federal direction of disaster response,

BOX 52-1	Emergency Support Functions
ESF 1	Transportation
ESF 2	Communications
ESF 3	Public works and engineering
ESF 4	Firefighting
ESF 5	Emergency management
ESF 6	Mass care, housing, and human services
ESF 7	Resource support
ESF 8	Public health and medical services
ESF 9	Urban search and rescue
ESF 10	Oil and hazardous materials response
ESF 11	Agriculture and natural resources
ESF 12	Energy
ESF 13	Public safety and security
ESF 14	Long-term community recovery and mitigation
ESF 15	External affairs

TABLE 52-1 Distribution by State of Urban Search and Rescue Task Forces

NO. OF US&R TFS	STATE
1	Arizona
8	California
1	Colorado
2	Florida
1	Indiana
1	Maryland
1	Massachusetts
1	Missouri
1	Nebraska
1	Nevada
1	New Mexico
1	New York
1	Ohio
1	Pennsylvania
1	Tennessee
1	Texas
1	Utah
2	Virginia
1	Washington

the primary mission objectives of a US&R TF in the response phase are to save lives, protect property and the environment, stabilize the incident, and provide for basic human needs.[3] Specifically, when called upon, US&R teams locate, extricate, and give immediate medical care to casualties found under collapsed buildings and in other confined spaces. Their activities are required in response to multiple kinds of disasters, such as earthquakes, hurricanes, tornados, and floods, among others. Their activities are noted among the most challenging and dangerous in disaster response.[4] US&R teams are also trained in trench rescue; however, most trench rescues are local events involving limited numbers of casualties. Therefore federal teams are rarely involved.

In a disaster, FEMA will typically deploy the three closest TFs to the event, supplementing any state and municipal US&R teams that may also be deployed at the disaster. Each TF consists of at least 62 active members and each is given 6 hours to assemble, deploying members at their departure point when activated. US&R members include firefighters, health care professionals, hazardous-material specialists, rescue specialists, structural engineers, and canine search teams. Many

US&R organizations have multiple teams to ensure full staffing. For example, Oklahoma TF1 US&R has red, blue, and white teams, with response duties on a daily rotation. Each team and each member is equipped and trained to be self-sufficient for the first 72 hours. US&R TFs have six components, as follows:

- "Search"—locating casualties and victims in the collapsed buildings or destroyed structures—this component consists of canine search teams and technical teams with fiber-optic cameras (eyes), electronic listening devices (ears), potential ground-penetrating radar, and even "sniffers" for electronic odor detection.
- "Rescue"—removing entrapped victims or victims in a confined space—the rescue group has equipment to stabilize structures, ensure the safety of rescuers and victims, and extricate victims from surrounding damaged structures.
- "Technical"—providing technical support for the TF—this component is provided by the medical director and the structural engineers who monitor for the possibility of noxious substances and other health threats, as well as structural instability and recommend mitigation and response strategies.
- "Logistical"—providing logistical support for the group—the logistics group provides and repairs all of the specialized equipment needed, as well as the supplies for the accommodations, food, and water for the TF members.[5]
- "Medical"—providing medical treatment for victims before, during, and after rescue at the disaster site—medical teams are typically composed of two TF physicians and four Medical Specialists.[6] The TF medical equipment carried includes medications, fluids, devices to allow intubation and ventilation, defibrillators, burn and amputation sets, and emergency surgical and suture kits. During the operation, the medical section is also responsible for the well-being and medical care of the other TF team members.
- "Command"—providing overall leadership and direction, as well as supporting communications—the command group is responsible for overall decision making within the Incident Command System (ICS) framework. The communications section of the TF is managed by the command group and is responsible for communications with local emergency medical service(s) (EMS) providers, hospitals, fire, and police. They may also be able to set up satellite access and wide-area wireless network systems.

Search and Rescue Operations

Injuries and fatalities are a major and persistent threat during search and rescue operations, as rescuers are operating in a hazardous environment and are at the same risk of sustaining injuries as the disaster victims are. Therefore it is important that every TF member receives sufficient, proper training and education regarding current and possible hazards, wears appropriate personal protection equipment (PPE), and always enters and works in a building or a confined space with a partner or supervised by another member (the "two person rule"). Appropriate PPE may include a mask or respirator, helmet, glass, gloves, clothing protecting against chemical and fires, and safety shoes, among other equipment. The accountability for team members is also essential during search and rescue operations. All team members must check in and out of response areas. Typically, team members are issued multiple ID cards, and the team leader uses another ID card to check the team member in and out of the specific response area and to identify the partner paired with the team member. The S&R TF command group and physicians in the team have the general responsibility to ensure that each team member has appropriate PPE, adequate hydration, and sufficient rest to perform his or her duties properly.

When first arriving on a disaster scene, the TF command group will evaluate the situation including safety considerations, environmental assessments, weather updates, and tasks assigned by the ICS, and then decide on the tactical plan and assign tasks for the work site. The search and rescue operations are subdivided into the following five phases:

1. Assessment of the disaster area
2. Removal of all surface victims as quickly and safely as possible
3. Search and rescue of victims from accessible void spaces
4. Selected debris removal to locate and rescue victims
5. General debris removal to render the scene safe for further operations.[7]

The assessment phase involves survey of the operational area to identify and evaluate the buildings involved and to consider their configuration and structural features (occupancy and void locations). During this first step, responders consider the size of the area involved in the operations, the possible hazards to victims and rescuers, the best access and escape routes, and the type of materials and equipment the TF needs to pursue the operations. The assessment phase also may involve structural engineers who provide building reconnaissance and evaluations, including structural triage, assessment, and marking of both safe ingress and clearly dangerous areas. The assessment phase often includes the rapid reconnaissance of the area and localization of victims, which begin with verbally calling out to locate awake and alert victims. When nonambulatory casualties are located, the rescuer can safely remove light debris and free minimally entrapped casualties. When multiple casualties are found, triage may or may not be needed. If the casualties are in close proximity and outnumber the medical providers, triage of the casualties will likely be necessary. However, when the extrication process is slow because of heavy structural damage or large amounts of overburden, triage may not be needed because the casualties are evacuated one by one. As casualties are evaluated and extricated, the medical provider plans for further treatment and subsequent medical evacuation.

After the rapid operations to locate and extricate easily found victims conclude, the team then begins a more detailed and systematic research to check every building and area where victims may be trapped. For casualties who are not easily found, dogs, cameras, or other more sophisticated devices are often employed to explore any space that could be created during the collapse. Dogs can be very useful to identify unconscious victims and can fit in much smaller spaces than humans can. Humans may also use acoustic and seismic listening devices, fiber-optic equipment, or thermal imaging to identify victims. For these casualties, access and extrication are determined by the mechanism of rescuer access and the machinery required for evacuation of each specific casualty. Access to and extrication of victims can require hours of work to build a retrieval system and ensure safety for both victims and rescuers during the operations.

During the search phase, it is frequently suggested to interrupt the research activities for a while and periodically call out and listen for possible answers or noises coming from entrapped victims.

The medical care of entangled and/or entrapped victims has had several developments over the years. It is known that casualties under debris can be found alive, having survived the event after days, but rarely after weeks. In some situations, the rescue and medical support for entrapped people can even take months. An extreme example is the Copiapò Mining Accident in 2010, when 33 miners remained trapped for 69 days and remained in a void space of 540 square feet, at around 2300 feet (700 m), underground about 3 miles (5 km) from the mine's entrance.

The physician must be prepared and trained to treat casualties in different types of incidents with different types of injuries, often while the victims are still entrapped. Each casualty must be assessed and treated based on the unique circumstances to which he or she has been exposed. For the entrapped victim, the physician must carefully consider the risks and potential benefits of every maneuver or medical care provided, determine the value of all equipment needed (transport to the patient's side may be convoluted and dangerous), and consider how to improvise equipment on scene. The physician must consider that everything that the provider accomplishes (i.e., orotracheal intubation) must be managed for the entire duration of the rescue operation, including transportation out of the immediate disaster area. This medical care should not delay the extrication, unless there is a life-threatening condition that requires immediate action.

The first step is the initial medical care to evaluate the victim's level of consciousness and assure integrity of airway and breathing. If there is airway and/or breathing compromise, it is necessary to obtain a definitive airway. Depending on how the victims are trapped and what kind of access there is to the victims, the rescuer may need to use unusual airway techniques, such as blind nasal intubation, digital intubation, or cricothyrotomy in suboptimal conditions. As per usual trauma protocols, the cervical spine must be stabilized and the back immobilized during extrication, as soon as possible. Next, the medical providers should assess for potential major hemorrhage and look for burns, hypovolemia, dehydration, and thermoregulatory problems. If patient access and circumstances permit, intravenous access should be obtained to provide fluid replacement and, if necessary, to start the administration of medications. Analgesics are indicated both for pain relief and to ease the extrication operation. If attempts to obtain IV access are unsuccessful, intraosseous vascular (IO) access may be considered; IO access is a reliable bridging method to gain vascular access in patients under resuscitation with difficult peripheral veins. Moreover, IO access is more efficacious with a higher success rate on first attempt and a lower procedure time compared with central venous catheterization (CVC) and without other complications such as infection, bleeding, or pneumothorax.[8]

It is fundamental to consider the amount of time required to extricate victims. Buried victims can develop acute crush syndrome, dehydration, hypoglycemia, and hypothermia or hyperthermia. To avoid worsening these conditions and the initial injuries, rapid extrication is essential. It is also crucial, of course, to treat any ongoing external bleeding. Although tourniquets can be appropriate for field management of rapid exsanguination, the rescuer must realize that the victim sought by US&R may require hours of extrication time and limb ischemia from a tourniquet may impair limb salvage. Tourniquets should be used only as a last resort when all other methods of controlling external bleeding have failed.[9]

The US&R medical teams must check status and vital signs frequently during the extrication. Even with a conscious patient, the risk of medical deterioration is high, so ongoing reassessment of the victim's condition is crucial.[10,11] In case of development of respiratory problems, it is essential to provide prompt and aggressive treatment. The patient should be kept dry, with eye protection as needed, and warm.

Victims can be exposed to several different conditions: heat or cold, burns, chemical or electrical burns, poisoning. If possible, any wet clothing should be removed, and assurance provided that the patient's body temperature is being maintained within the normal range, with warm and dry skin, to prevent subsequent hypothermia.

Confined Space Medicine

Confined spaces with potentially life-threatening gases or lack of oxygen present perhaps the most dangerous environments for rescuers. Data regarding confined space rescue show that up 60% of the fatalities occurring during the process of disaster response in this very dangerous environment actually are rescuer fatalities.[12] It is important to consider that confined spaces can increase the risk of explosions caused by inflammable gas and also increase the inhaled concentration of other agents. For example, silos or pits containing animal slurries can release hydrogen sulfide, which has flammable and explosive features, and is highly toxic, affecting the nervous system and able to cause unconsciousness rapidly after exposure.[13] The practice of medicine in these confined spaces is always demanding and stressful, and it requires close attention. Therefore, the rescuers must always check and size up the scene carefully to provide safety, assess the situation, and arrange for precautions. Confined spaces are prone to extreme conditions in terms of temperature and humidity, and it is important to evaluate the casualty's circulation and perfusion. Even though the general approach to the patient is the same as any other emergency, the limited space, environmental conditions, and time to extricate and recover the victim make operations in confined spaces very challenging.

Crush Injury and Crush Syndrome

Crush injury and crush syndrome are typical medical conditions that US&R medical teams find frequently during the rescue of trapped victims. Second only to direct trauma impact, crush syndrome is the second most frequent cause of death after mass disasters.[14] It often appears in victims trapped under the rubble of a building collapse.

Crush injury is defined as compression of extremities or other parts of the body that causes muscle swelling and/or neurologic disturbances in the affected areas of the body,[15] usually the extremities. *Crush syndrome* is the systemic manifestation of breakdown of muscle cells caused by the compression, provoking the releasing of cell components (creatine kinase, lactic acid, myoglobin, and potassium) into the extracellular fluid. This causes hypovolemia, hyperkalemia, metabolic acidosis, renal hypoperfusion, and ischemia resulting in acute renal failure (ARF).[16]

The likelihood of developing acute crush syndrome is directly related to the compression time (at least 1 hour, generally after 4 to 6 hours). Therefore victims should be extricated as quickly as possible. However, extrication must be performed carefully to try to avoid a complication often called "smiling death" or "the grateful dead syndrome," because the casualty may smile when freed only to die shortly thereafter.[17] This complication occurs because the trapped victim may have had severe extremity compression, which does not allow extremity perfusion. During this period of limited or absent perfusion, dangerous electrolyte disturbances and toxic metabolites can accumulate in the tissues, only to suddenly distribute centrally when the trapped person is freed. This abrupt release of potassium and other intracellular electrolytes can induce malignant cardiac dysrhythmias soon after the extrication.

These complications are potentially manageable or preventable with aggressive therapy consisting of adequate IV fluid hydration given during the extrication operations.

After a long extrication time, it is necessary to evaluate the hydration status, urine output, and urine pH (better pH greater than 6.5) and check electrolytic abnormalities. The administration of a large amount of intravenous crystalloid is crucial to dilute the myoglobin and preserve the renal perfusion. If the patient has decreased urine output, the first therapy should be an appropriate fluid challenge. After hydration is assured, the medical provider may consider mannitol and the use of furosemide.[18] To promote urine alkalization and prevent myoglobin precipitation with intratubular cast formation it is often suggested to give bicarbonate, which also acts to reduce hyperkalemia. If the patient develops renal failure, hemodialysis may be needed.

During the extrication of these patients, it is appropriate to identify in advance a hemodialysis facility that can accommodate the patient once freed. If possible, the transportation should be minimal: the duration of the sustained crush injury and time until appropriate in-hospital treatment of the patient with crush injury increase morbidity and mortality. The medical provider must evaluate the risks and benefits of any long-distance transportation of the patient with crush syndrome.[19]

When the compression involves the thorax, by direct chest pressure from debris, traumatic asphyxia (also called Perthes syndrome), can occur. Traumatic asphyxia can be caused by any compression of the thorax or upper abdomen. The patient has limited chest excursion, which limits both oxygen intake and carbon dioxide exhalation. The direct pressure increases intrathoracic pressure and decreases the cardiac pump function. This syndrome is associated with subconjunctival hemorrhage, craniocervical cyanosis, petechiae, and neurologic symptoms.

⚠ PITFALLS

- US&R settings are dangerous, and not all dangers are immediately obvious to untrained rescuers. All responders involved in rescue situations must ensure that they have access to appropriately trained experts who can assess for all potential scene hazards.
- Because of the danger of US&R scenes, personnel operating in them should have adequate education about US&R operations and sufficient supply of and training with proper PPE, and they should operate under strict safety rules to avoid adding to the casualty tolls of the event.
- Medical providers working in US&R scenes and/or receiving victims from such scenes must know the pathophysiology of crush syndrome so that it may be properly anticipated and treated.

REFERENCES

1. Miami Dade County - Urban Search and Rescue (US&R). Available at http://www.miamidade.gov/fire/about-special-urban-search.asp. Accessed 27th April 2015.
2. Department of Homeland Security—FEMA. In: *National Urban Search And Rescue Teams Deployed.* Available at https://www.fema.gov/news-release/2005/09/03/national-urban-search-and-rescue-teams-deployed. Accessed 27 April 2015.
3. Department of Homeland Security—FEMA. In: *National Response Framework,* Second Edition. May 2013, p.5.
4. Barbera JA, Macintyre A. Urban search and rescue. *Emerg Med Clin North Am.* 1996;14(2):399–412.
5. Department of Homeland Security—FEMA. In: *Task Force Equipment.* Available at http://www.fema.gov/task-force-equipment. Accessed 27 April 2015.
6. Department of Homeland Security—FEMA. In: *Urban and Search Rescue 2003-2004 Task Force Cache List,* p.4.
7. Department of Homeland Security — FEMA, In: *National Urban Search & Rescue (US&R) Response System Rescue Field Operation Guide,* 2006 , p. 5-1. Available at http://www.fema.gov/pdf/emergency/usr/usr_23_20080205_rog.pdf. Accessed 27 April 2015.
8. Leidel BA, Kirchhoff C, Bogner V, Braunstein V, Biberthaler P, Kanz KG. Comparison of intraosseous versus central venous vascular access in adults under resuscitation in the emergency department with inaccessible peripheral veins. *Resuscitation.* 2012;83(1):40–45. http://dx.doi.org/10.1016/j.resuscitation.2011.08.017 [Epub 2011 Sep 3].
9. Australian Resuscitation Council, In: *The ARC Guidelines, Guideline 9.1.1. Principles of Control of Bleeding for First Aiders,* 2008, p. 2. Available http://resus.org.au/guidelines/. Accessed 27 April 2015.
10. Centers for Disease Control and Prevention (CDC), In: *Mass Trauma - Explosions and Blast Injuries, A Primer for Clinicians.* Available at http://www.cdc.gov/masstrauma/preparedness/primer.pdf. Accessed 27th April 2015.
11. Australian Resuscitation Council, In: *The ARC Guidelines, Guideline 9.1.7 - Emergency Management of a Crushed Victim,* 2013, p. 2. Available at http://resus.org.au/guidelines/. Accessed 27th April 2015.
12. United States Department of Labor, Occupational Safety & Health Administration "Confined Space Rescue Awareness - An Overview of Confined Space Rescue" PowerPoint presentation. slide 9.
13. Health and Safety Authority "Code of Practice for Working in Confined Spaces", p. 11. Available at http://www.hsa.ie/eng/Publications_and_Forms/Publications/Codes_of_Practice/COP_Confined_Space_Document.pdf. Accessed the 27th April 2015.

14. Sever MS, Vanholder R. Management of crush syndrome casualties after disasters. *Rambam Maimonides Med J.* 2011;2(2):e0039. http://dx.doi.org/10.5041/RMMJ.10039.

15. American College of Emergency Physician, In Bombings: Injury Patterns and Care. Available at http://www.acep.org/blastinjury/. Accessed 27th April 2015.

16. Genthon A, Wilcox SR. Crush syndrome: a case report and review of the literature. *J Emerg Med.* 2014;46(2):313–319. http://dx.doi.org/10.1016/j.jemermed.2013.08.052 [Epub 2013 Nov 5].

17. Hogan DL, Burstein JL. *Disaster Medicine.* 2nd ed Philadelphia, PA: Lippincott Williams & Wilkins; 2007, 80.

18. Huerta-Alardín AL, Varon J, Marik PE. Bench-to-bedside review: rhabdomyolysis—an overview for clinicians. *Crit Care.* 2005;9(2):158–169 [Epub 2004 Oct 20].

19. Sever MS, Erek E, Vanholder R, et al. Clinical findings in the renal victims of a catastrophic disaster. *Nephrol Dial Transplant.* 2002;7(11):1942–1949.

Medical Care in Remote Areas

Ashley L. Greiner

In the medical context, the term *remote areas* is defined as "locations that are geographically, professionally, and personally isolating, with limited sophistication of medical and logistic support, limited access to peers, [and/or] in extreme climatic, political, or cross-cultural environments."[1] Despite the trend of increasing urbanization and centralization of medical centers, in the United States, where almost 59 million live in rural areas, there is a persistent need to improve health care access and services to these remote populations.[2] Elsewhere in the world, the features of remote areas can be even more extreme, where areas are so remote that evacuation times to comprehensive medical care are measured in days or more. In both contexts, limitations in health care access and quality highlight the importance of not only planning to meet the unique needs of remote populations but also training professionals to operate successfully in such contexts.

HISTORICAL PERSPECTIVE

Historically, medical care has followed the movement of society as it has shifted from agrarian to more urban environments. The history of the evolution of medical care in remote areas is unique to each country, dependent on the specific political and economic forces in play. In the United States, there have been five eras, as described by Rosenblatt and Moscovice, that characterize the evolution of rural and/or remote health services in the United States.[3] The period of colonization to industrialization (1620-1850) was characterized by health care delivery by nonphysicians: midwives, clergy, and men who "moonlighted" during their off-hours. The pre-Flexner era was marked by general practitioners providing care without necessarily undergoing standardized medical education or training. The Flexner era (1910-1940), named after the Flexner Report, revolutionized the practice of medicine by formalizing the education required to practice medicine in the United States.[4] As a result, the number of poorly trained general practitioners significantly declined, as many were no longer considered qualified. Around this time, however, a new stigma also emerged associated with general practitioners who were not pursuing a career in a medical "specialty" in an urban setting. This created a significant health care access disparity leading to the era during the War on Poverty (1940-1970), which was characterized by the federal government's effort to increase hospital and medical care access, especially in more remote, rural areas of the United States. The last period that they describe is our current era, the "Technological Era" (1970-present).[3]

In addition to hospital and clinic-based programs focused on preventive and routine medical care, the establishment of the emergency medical technician (EMT) in 1966 by the National Highway Safety Act significantly improved and increased access to emergency medical care outside of the hospital and clinic throughout the United States. With the advent of the EMT trained to a specifically defined curriculum, people in remote regions in the United States began to have access to trained medical professionals who were able to provide initial medical stabilization without a physician physically present. Over the last 50 years, subsequent changes in prehospital care have led to an expanded system in the United States known as the emergency medical service(s) (EMS) system.

Similar changes have also occurred elsewhere in the world. In the 1970s, select European countries chose to employ an emergency medical care model known as the Franco-German model, which did not use EMTs but rather projected emergency medical care outside of the hospital setting, with physicians in the field. The focus was to provide definitive treatment in the field and avoid hospital transfer, in contrast to the U.S. system's practice of stabilizing and transporting to the nearest facility.[5]

CURRENT PRACTICE

Health care access in remote settings is dependent on not only the existence of appropriate medical facilities and infrastructure but also the distribution of physicians and other trained medical specialists in the area. In the United States, only about 10% of physicians practice in rural environments, despite that almost a quarter of the population lives in rural areas.[6] This lack of access to trained medical professionals, sometimes for even preventive medical care, in these environments has led to a higher prevalence of chronic medical problems, such as cerebrovascular disease and hypertension, in remote areas in the United States.[6] In developing regions of the world, rural areas demonstrate higher rates of malnutrition in children compared with urban areas.[7] This lack of access to preventive care in remote regions is even highlighted during humanitarian emergencies, when in addition to the acute medical issues, many chronic medical conditions come to the forefront.[8]

In an attempt to close this health care gap and address the medical issues afflicting remote populations, there has been a movement to recruit nonphysician medical professionals to provide basic care in these regions. More specifically, this movement has included the incorporation of physician assistants (PAs) and nurse practitioners (NPs).[9,10] This movement has resulted in the evolution of health care teams that can be a mixture of physicians, PAs, NPs, nurses, rescue workers, and/or EMS providers. Thus the roles of each team providing care are often dynamic, with adaptability being a key characteristic for the optimization of care in remote environments.

Beyond the chronic medical issues seen in this population, there is an increased rate of morbidity and mortality associated with accidents and trauma in remote regions. Accidents leading to serious injury or death account for 60% of total rural accidents versus only 48% of urban accidents in the United States. It has been proposed that this discrepancy is likely secondary to delays between the time of the accident and the first receipt of medical care (18 minutes in rural areas versus 8 minutes in urban areas).[6] Sometimes, this increased length of time to care is due to not only the physical distance but also the environmental challenges in accessing these remote locations (i.e., terrain, weather, road conditions, etc.).

Related to issues of access, the EMS system in the United States has developed subspecialty capabilities including the development of wilderness EMS training. Other similar emergency systems have been adopted around the world. However, many developing countries do not have an established EMS system or, if a system exists, it is often only in its infancy.

Preplanned large-scale events in remote areas, such as the Burning Man festival, which occurs every year in the Nevada desert and in 2013 hosted 65,000 visitors, produce special challenges for the provision of medical care to large crowds in remote areas. The medical response to the 1969 Woodstock Festival highlighted the severe difficulty in accessing populations remotely, especially during mass gatherings. The unexpected volume rendered the prearranged and existing medical system impractical. In response, more providers were emergently mobilized; schools were converted into triage centers; and an employee tent was transformed into a field hospital.[11] Unfortunately, the mass of people obstructing the roads also limited the use of ambulances to transport injured and sick patients to area hospitals, and there were significant problems with the delivery of medical supplies to the site, requiring that helicopters be employed.[11] Thankfully, because of on-site improvisations, the morbidity and mortality rates were relatively low, although the event still serves as a monument to the importance of evidence-based preplanning.

Mobile or deployable clinics have also been used both in the United States and globally, to address the difficulties in delivering care to remote regions. The forms of various mobile clinics can be quite diverse, and they can be configured to tackle a number of different medical issues, from routine medical care to vaccination campaigns to the provision of surgical services.[12] Mobile clinics are often employed in disaster settings for both frontline care and as tertiary care. For example, in the November 2013 Philippines' Typhoon Haiyan disaster response, in addition to the mobile clinics and operating theaters installed on the ground, China's "Peace Ark" ship, a fully staffed and equipped 300-bed hospital, with 20 ICUs and eight operating theaters, was available offshore for tertiary care. The United States Navy's hospital ships, the USNS *Comfort* and USNS *Mercy*, have often served in a similar role in events such as the Indonesian Tsunami and Hurricane Katrina.

Similar in concept to these mobile clinics is the military's MASH, the 60-bed Mobile Army Surgical Hospital deployed during the Korean War to provide more advanced care to injured soldiers as close as possible to the battlefield. (Because of the popularity of the movie and TV series *M*A*S*H*, colloquial use often refers to any small mobile military field hospital, and multiple similar military variants now exist.) During the Burning Man festival, previously mentioned, three small portable medical care facilities, termed MASH units, are deployed and staffed by volunteers.

Medical care can also be delivered to remote areas not only through mobile clinics but also by using telecommunication technologies, often known as telehealth or telemedicine. Telemedicine has recently been employed as a tool to reach patients in remote areas, for a wide variety of reasons, including provision of primary care, as well as for immediate access to emergency specialty care, such as with acute stroke and trauma surgery consultation.[13,14] In an attempt to close the geographic gap and better address the health needs of remote communities, telemedicine has improved not only health care access but also the quality of care delivered for both chronic and more recently, more acute conditions. Widespread adoption of radiological services through telecommunication is evident in rural communities throughout the United States, and this success could be translated internationally.[15] These services have continued to expand to include more specialized care, such as neurology for stroke evaluation. More recently, beyond the clinical consultation aspect of telemedicine, the tool has also been employed for training sessions and continuing medical education for personnel in remote regions.[16]

It is important to note that telemedicine requires the presence of certain infrastructure (i.e., electricity, Internet, satellite connectivity, etc.) to be a feasible method of providing medical care. Therefore, in areas of extreme austerity and remoteness, or even in complex environments such as disaster settings, telemedicine has been more challenging to implement.

Expedition and wilderness medicine specialists have unique challenges when providing medical care in remote settings. These specialists need not only a wide knowledge base to be able to care for those in distress but also the ability to be able to depend solely on the resources they carry with them. Similarly, disaster medical teams working in remote areas or in areas with widespread infrastructure destruction may be limited in the care they can provide to the materials and supplies that they bring with them to the event. In such settings, the objectives may often be only to triage and stabilize the patients for transportation to the nearest facility for definitive medical care, even the nearest facility may be days away. Therefore teams require a skill set to be able to address ongoing medical concerns during the period of evacuation as well.

It is important to note that rural and/or remote populations may also be demographically different from their urban, metropolitan counterparts in terms of age, gender, and educational and occupational backgrounds, among other factors. Remote areas often have different proportions of children, pregnant women, people with disabilities, and the elderly than those found in urban centers, and all of these groups might require differing levels and types of resource availability.[17-19] Moreover, the demographics and health risks of a region can actually evolve rapidly, particularly with a period of significant worker migration or immigration. This was recently evident in North Dakota, where there was a massive influx of oil workers into a relatively remote region of the state because of economic change. The existing health care infrastructure was overwhelmed by not only the rapid increase in population size but also the unique health needs of the incoming population. For example, with this change in regional population demographics, there was a sudden and significant increase in sexually transmitted diseases, requiring local and state health departments to implement vaccination campaigns, increase clinic availability, and start educational programming.[20] The advanced determination of the most suitable medical equipment, essential medications, and knowledge of appropriate specialty health care facilities if transfer is needed is critical to providing care in remote regions.

Cultural norms also must be considered when planning to respond to an area's medical concerns. Specifically, understanding how medical problems are typically approached in a community is important. In some remote areas, people exhibit an increased dependence on family and social support[21,22] and might be hesitant to seek formal medical care, delaying definitive treatment.[23] Additionally, some communities might have certain preconceived notions and perceptions of "Western Medicine," and this should be considered when trying to provide effective care.[24,25] For example, the reasons for the 2013 reemergence of polio in Syria's complex humanitarian emergency was multifactorial in nature, but it appears to have been exacerbated in part by a false rumor spread by certain Muslim groups that the medication was a Western attempt to create "a poison meant to sterilize Muslim women."[26] In an effort to mitigate this belief, the World Health Organization worked with notable Islamic scholars to campaign the message that those who opposed the vaccination process were "un-Islamic."[27] Therefore, in addition to the challenge of vaccinating in remote regions of Syria from a logistical standpoint, cultural challenges also must be addressed to be an effective response.

⚠ PITFALLS

A number of obstacles in the implementation of current interventions for health care delivery to remote areas exist. Although each country has a unique set of barriers based on their current context, lack of infrastructure is a common hindrance identified. This can include roads, EMS networks, hospital or medical facilities, and technology. Without roads, a mobile clinic's delivery of health care can be significantly impeded. Without suitable tertiary care centers, neither EMS nor primary clinics may be able to access definitive or specialty care. Without effective communication and technology systems, the population may not have access to contact EMS or access advanced telemedicine networks.

In addition, barriers to providing sufficient and appropriate care can include inadequate access to adequately trained medical staff in remote areas. In order to close the health care access gap, medical systems must support the education of physician and nonphysician medical providers who are willing and able to work in such areas. For example, in response to the projected increase in the physician shortage in the United States over the next 10 years, there have been a number of measures to incentivize doctors to enter the field of primary care, starting with their education.[28,29] Providing health care in remote settings further requires an understanding of the unique characteristics of the population one is serving, the medical problems unique to that environment, and the ability to triage and remain adaptable to ever-changing surroundings. Therefore, as educational curricula are established, there should be a focus on developing the unique knowledge base and skill set required to provide medical care effectively in remote settings.[30]

REFERENCES

1. Smith JD, Margolis SA, Ayton J, et al. Defining remote medical practice. A consensus viewpoint of medical practitioners working and teaching in remote practice. *Med J Aust.* 2008;188(3):159–161.
2. United States Census Bureau. 2010 Census Urban and Rural Classification and Urban Area Criteria 2010. Available at: http://www.census.gov/geo/reference/ua/urban-rural-2010.html.
3. Rosenblatt RA, Moscovice IS. Rural Health Care. New York, NY: Wiley; 1982.
4. Flexner A. Medical Education in the United States and Canada. Bulletin Number 4. Standford: The Carnegie Foundation for the Advancement of Teaching; 1910.
5. Dick WF. Anglo-American vs. Franco-German emergency medical services system. *Prehospital Disaster Med.* 2003;18(1):29–35, discussion 35–37.
6. Gamm LD, Hutchison LL, Dabney BJ, Dorsey AM, et al. *Rural Healthy People 2010: A Companion Document to Healthy People 2010.* volume 1. College Station, Texas: The Texas A&M University System Health Science Center, School of Rural Public Health, Southwest Rural Health Research Center.
7. Strasser R. Rural health around the world: challenges and solutions. *Fam Pract.* 2013;20(4):457–463.
8. The Sphere Project. *The Sphere Handbook: Humanitarian Charter and Minimum Standards in Humanitarian Response.* United Kingdom: Belmont Press; 2011. Available at: http://www.ifrc.org/docs/idrl/I1027EN.pdf.
9. Grumbach K, Hart LG, Mertz E, Coffman J, Palazzo L. Who is caring for the underserved? A comparison of primary care physicians and nonphysician clinicians in California and Washington. *Ann Fam Med.* 2003;1(2):97–104.
10. Institute of Medicine. The Future of Nursing: Leading Change, Advancing Health. Washington, DC: National Academies Press; 2011.
11. Doyle M. Statement on the Historical and Cultural Significance of the 1969 Woodstock Festival Site. Preliminary Draft Generic Environmental Impact Statement—Appendix B. [Report] For Allee King Rosen and Fleming, Inc., on behalf of the Gerry Foundation, Inc. Bethel Performing Arts Center, New York 2001. Available at: http://www.woodstockpreservation.org/SigStatement/FinalSigState.pdf.
12. Du Mortier S, Coninx R. Mobile Health Units: Methodological Approach; 2006. Available at: www.icrc.org/eng/assets/files/other/icrc_002_0886.pdf.
13. Latifi R, Weinstein RS, Porter JM, et al. Telemedicine and telepresence for trauma and emergency care management. Trauma surgery telemedicine. *Scand J Surg.* 2007;96(4):281–289.
14. Wamala DS, Augustine K. A meta-analysis of telemedicine success in Africa. *J Pathol Inform.* 2013;4:6.
15. Moore AV, Allen B, Campbell SC, et al. *Report of the ACR Task Force on International Teleradiology. American College of Radiology,* 2003. Available at: http://www.acr.org/Membership/Legal-Business-Practices/Telemedicine-Teleradiology/Report-of-the-ACR-Task-Force-on-International-Teleradiology.
16. Hassol A, Irvin C, Gaumer G, Puskin D, Mintzer C, Grigsby J. Rural applications of telemedicine. *Telemed J.* 1997;3(3):215–225.
17. Karunakara U, Stevenson F. Ending neglect of older people in the response to humanitarian emergencies. *PLoS Med.* 2012;9(12):e1001357.
18. *Inter-Agency Field Manual on Reproductive Health in Humanitarian Settings. Inter-Agency Working Group on Reproductive Health in Crisis.* World Health Organization; 2010. Available at: http://www.who.int/reproductivehealth/publications/emergencies/field_manual_rh_humanitarian_settings.pdf.
19. Manual for the Health Care of Children in Humanitarian Emergencies. World Health Organization; 2008. Available at: http://whqlibdoc.who.int/publications/2008/9789241596879_eng.pdf.
20. Dwelle T. *North Dakota's Oil Boom Results in Population Growth Across the State and Public Health Challenges. Association of State and Territorial Health Officials Infectious Disease;* 2013. Available at: http://www.astho.org/Programs/Infectious-Disease/North-Dakota's-Oil-Boom-Results-in-Population-Growth-Across-the-State-and-Public-Health-Challenges/.
21. Amato PR. Urban-Rural differences in helping friends and family members. *Soc Psychol Quart.* 1993;56(4):249–262.
22. Beggs JJ, Haines VA, Hurlbert JS. Revisiting the rural-urban contrast: personal networks in nonmetropolitan and metropolitan settings. *Rural Sociol.* 1996;61(2):306–325.
23. Strasser R. Rural health around the world: challenges and solutions. *Fam Pract.* 2003;20:457–463.
24. Scrimgeour M, Scrimgeour D. Health Care Access for Aboriginal and Torres Strait Islander. People Living in Urban Areas, and Related Research Issues: A Review of the Literature. Darwin: Cooperative Research Centre for Aboriginal Health; 2007.
25. Koss-Chioino J, Leatherman TL, Greenway C. Medical Pluralism in the Andes. New York, NY: Routledge; 2003.
26. Teepu IA. Islamic Law and Suspicion Fuel Polio Resurgence. *USA TODAY;* November 30, 2013. Available at: http://www.usatoday.com/story/news/world/2013/11/30/pakistan-polio-resurgence/3591683/.
27. Sindi WA. Islamic scholars call for access to vaccinate children. *World Health Organization;* 2014. Available at: http://www.emro.who.int/polio/information-resources/iag-polio-meeting-adopts-plan.html.
28. Petterson SM, Liaw WR, Phillips RL, Rabin DL, Meyers DS, Bazemore AW. Projecting US primary care physician workforce needs: 2010-2025. *Ann Fam Med.* 2012;10:503–509.
29. AAMC Center for Workforce Studies, June 2010 Analysis. Available at: https://www.aamc.org/download/286592/data/.
30. Strasser R, Neusy A. Context counts: training health workers in and for rural and remote areas. *Bull World Health Organ.* 2010;88:777–782.

SUGGESTED READINGS

1. Razzak JA, Kellermann AL. Emergency medical care in developing countries: is it worthwhile? *Bull World Health Organ.* 2002;80(11):900–905.
2. VanRooyen MJ. Development of prehospital emergency medical services: strategies for system assessment and planning. *Pac Health Dialog.* 2002;9(1):86–92.

CHAPTER 54

Triage

Elizabeth Foley and Andrew T. Reisner

The train was cut open like a can of tuna. We didn't know who to treat first. There was a lot of blood, a lot of blood.

—*Enrique Sanchez, Madrid Emergency Medical Services, of simultaneous commuter train bombings, March 2004[1]*

Triage is the utilitarian sorting of patients into categories of priority to allocate limited resources rationally; it is, proverbially, to do "the greatest good for the greatest number." Triage systems are used to determine the order in which patients will receive treatment and transport based on their condition, prognosis, and the availability of resources. Triage typically fails in one of two basic ways: undertriage and overtriage. Undertriage represents a failure to identify the casualties who could benefit from scarce medical resources, such as the serious casualty whose life would be saved with rapid evacuation and prompt emergency surgery. In terms of test characteristics, undertriage means poor sensitivity to those who would benefit from the medical resources available, whereas overtriage occurs when casualties who, relatively speaking, do not benefit from a scarce resource, nonetheless receive that resource. Overtriage signifies a sorting system with low specificity and overloads of scarce resources. Noncritical patients who receive immediate care even though they could safely wait (at the expense of more serious, savable casualties) constitute one form of overtriage. It can also occur when expectant patients, with little chance of survival, are provided with precious medical resources.

Triage following disaster is not a single processing step; rather, triage underlies all aspects of the response, including on-site rescue, evacuation, receiving hospital activities, decontamination, and so on. Because the resources available, the clinical conditions of casualties, and the information available all change throughout the time-course of the response, response priorities do as well; triage is a dynamic process.

It has been suggested that disaster responses should match normative practice as much as practically possible,[2,3] and that, of course, would apply to triage methods. However, normative practice could pose a liability for massive disasters, in which a set of reflexes could interfere with the truly rational allocation of resources. This trade-off is discussed throughout the chapter. As noted in the following section, many recent disaster responses have been characterized by a general lack of meaningful triage.

HISTORICAL PERSPECTIVE

The roots of disaster triage stretch back at least to eighteenth-century military casualty care. Baron Larré, a surgeon with Napoleon's army, established a system under which wounded soldiers received initial treatment in the field before being transported to hospitals. In 1846, British naval physician John Wilson first proposed that treatment be deferred for casualties with either minor or likely fatal injuries, so that treatment could be provided to the severely injured, who were most likely to benefit.[4] Military triage evolved sporadically, but, by World War II, a hierarchical structure for combat casualty care had been developed. During World War II, the average time from injury to definitive care was 12 to 18 hours. By the Vietnam War, improved triage and air-ambulance capabilities reduced this time to less than 2 hours.[5] The early military history of triage was well reviewed by Kennedy.[4]

In the 1980s, civilian prehospital systems became interested in trauma triage for the individual trauma casualty. West et al.[6] showed that serious trauma casualties had superior outcomes when cared for at specialized trauma centers. There were investigations of prehospital criteria for differentiating between individual casualties that should be taken to major trauma centers and those that could receive care safely at community medical centers (to avoid overburdening trauma centers with nonserious casualties). Trauma registries enabled the development and validation of various field triage decision rules, although such criteria have proven problematic (see the Triage Scoring System section). Such civilian trauma scoring in turn influenced modern military triage. In the 1991 Persian Gulf War, Burkle et al.[7] explored the use of Champion's Revised Trauma Score[8] for triage of combat casualties. Triage classification schemes for military and civilian mass casualties, to a large extent, have converged. Both military (e.g., NATO) and civilian (e.g., color coding) triage systems make use of comparable levels of acuity, and the Trauma Sieve and START, which are similar triage decision systems, have been used by both civilian emergency medical service(s) (EMS) as well as British Army soldiers.[9]

Regarding civilian triage, the past several decades have seen a litany of tragic events in industrialized countries, including bombings, fires, shootings, and plane crashes.[10] These events show a consistency of scale, with immediately surviving casualties numbering in the dozens or hundreds. Unfortunately, many retrospective reports continued to note unsatisfactory execution of triage, particularly prehospital triage, for these events. In the mid-1980s, Vayer et al.[3] cited Butman's analysis of 51 mass-casualty incidents (MCI) that identified a universal failure to execute proper triage. Inadequate prehospital triage continues to be reported following MCIs: an aircraft crash in Singapore in 2000,[11] the Tokyo sarin attacks,[12] and the Gothenburg Fire Disaster.[13] Typically, documentation of prehospital triage during an MCI is quite poor; therefore, retrospective analysis of field triage is simply not feasible, as was the case for the Oklahoma City Bombing.[14]

The urban community in a developed country may very well possess the resources necessary to treat dozens or even hundreds of casualties, provided the resources are mobilized and the patients in need of immediate care are identified in a timely fashion. Yet even in these settings, suboptimal use of available community resources is the rule rather than the exception; for instance, most casualties self-transport to the closest hospital and leave distant facilities underused.[15] Community resources, such as urgent care centers and outpatient clinics, capable of treating the majority of casualties with relatively minor injuries, are almost always underused. Almogy et al.,[16] reporting on the Israeli response to the Jerusalem Sbarro Pizzeria Bombing in 2001, observed: "in these circumstances (e.g., a MCI such as a suicide bombing), ordinary hospital resources are heavily burdened, yet delivery of efficient medical treatment is possible by recruitment of all available personnel and resources."

In contrast to the many reports of poor triage after disasters, exemplary responses to MCIs have stemmed from exemplary mobilization of resources. After the bombing at the Atlanta Centennial Olympics, 30 EMS units evacuated all 111 casualties to area hospitals within 32 minutes. The vast majority of serious casualties were taken to Grady Memorial Hospital, where, "at one point, there were more physicians than victims in the emergency care center."[17] Those casualties all had good or excellent outcomes. After the Jerusalem Sbarro Pizzeria Bombing, the prehospital response was largely "scoop and run." The Ein Kerem Campus, receiving 132 surviving casualties, performed two emergency department (ED) thoracotomies, with no apparent shortage of resources available for those less-critical casualties.[16] After the 2013 Boston Marathon Bombings, all 30 "red-tagged" patients, the most critically ill, were transported to area hospitals within[18] minutes, and all survived.[18] Almogy's dictum pertains to most recent disasters in developed countries, which have been limited to dozens or hundreds of casualties. Popular field triage systems (see the Triage Scoring Systems section) are most appropriate for this scale of events.

Such triage systems, however, are less applicable to disasters of enormous scale. The greater the scope of the disaster, both in terms of geographic area and number of casualties, the more challenging triage becomes. Including the 1918 Influenza Pandemic and Hurricane Katrina, in 2005, there have been only nine nonmilitary disasters in the entire history of the United States that resulted in more than 1000 deaths. Internationally, massive disasters have produced tens or hundreds of thousands of dead and injured, such as earthquakes in Tangshan (1976), Armenia (1988), Hanshin-Awaji (1995), and Iran (2003), as well as the Indian Ocean Tsunami (2004) and the Tohoku Earthquake and Tsunami in Japan (2011). Field triage systems tend to be sensitive and not specific, leading to overtriage, and they may be too unwieldy to triage massive numbers of casualties spread over a wide area. Additionally, they are tailored to traumatic pathology, but broad medical pathology (e.g., infectious disease and metabolic disarray) occurs in the aftermath of these massive disasters, and baseline medical emergencies (e.g., myocardial infarctions and ectopic pregnancies) continue to occur unabated.

To the extent that one seeks historical guidance when planning for the future, the emphasis that should be given to preparing for enormous-scale disasters in the United States is unknowable. Such events are rare, and we have little experience to guide us. Traditionally it has been difficult to find the resources-funding, time, and materials to develop and maintain preparedness. Some respected authorities have suggested that too much attention has been paid to the unprecedented scenario of weapons of mass destruction (WMD). Frykberg[10] wrote: "We must resist our current tendency to become overly enamored with the 'weapons of mass destruction' of biologic, chemical, and radiologic attacks, in terms of funding priorities and resource allocations that are wholly disproportionate to the clear reality of the terrorist bombing threat." Even though history has shown that smaller, more mundane MCIs are more likely, there remains concern for a nuclear attack on U.S. soil. One WMDs event could dwarf the sum of preceding MCIs in morbidity and mortality, and it seems prudent to prepare for this possibility and the unique challenges it would create for disaster triage.

Natural disasters of enormous scale, even though uncommon in the United States, are also a threat. The New Madrid seismic zone, located in the Southern and Midwestern United States, produced several earthquakes of magnitude 7.0-8.0 in 1811 and 1812. Damage was not significant at the time because there were few settlements in the region, but a 2009 report published by the Mid-America Earthquake Center predicted that another earthquake of similar magnitude would result in approximately 86,000 casualties across eight states.[19] The U.S. Geological Survey estimates a 7% to 10% probability of an earthquake of this magnitude within the next 50 years.[20] Even though the extent to which preparedness can and should be maintained for massive disasters is unclear, it would be unwise to disregard the real possibility of such an event.

CURRENT PRACTICE

This section offers a technical framework for triage following a disaster. The issues discussed here are important to consider for disaster planning and training (and real-time execution), but the reader must always bear in mind the sobering limitations of triage systems detailed in the previous section. All the same, triage should be carried out to the extent possible at the scene and at every facility and site providing disaster care. Box 54-1 lists considerations that should be made in advance of any disaster. Box 54-2 lists details that need to be determined in real time after a rapid survey of the disaster and the scope of casualties. Triage training is specifically discussed at the end of the chapter.

What Triage Classification Will Be Used?

There are several issues to consider for planning a disaster response. First, will a multiple-level triage classification system be used? As noted in the previous section, there are precedents for responses to MCIs with

---

BOX 54-1 Triage Plan Preparation (to Be Determined Before Any Disaster)

- What triage classification will be used, if any (e.g., four or five levels of severity)?
- Will a formal triage scoring system be used?
- What on-site/hospital documentation will be used?

BOX 54-2 Triage Plan Details (Requires Survey of Specific Disaster Site)

- Who will be the triage officer(s)?
- Who will collect vital signs for the triage officer(s)?
- Physically, where will casualties from each triage category be treated (and who will staff each area)?
- What overtriage and undertriage rates are acceptable?
- What level of casualty gets "black-tagged"?
- Assuming 10 patients in 20 minutes per triage officer,[17] are there enough officers?
- Are there enough other personnel to keep up with the triage team (e.g., litter bearers and care providers); if not, is the triage team too big?
- Are resources being used appropriately, including (1) on-site medical interventions, (2) evacuation resources, and (3) hospital-based resources (e.g., ED care and OR)?
- After initial triage, who reevaluates the casualties, and how often?
- Have all details of the triage plan been reevaluated on an ongoing basis?
- Has an updated triage plan been communicated to all active rescuers, including victims and participating bystanders, as is appropriate?

over 100 casualties that consist of prehospital "scoop and run." Then, rather than a rigid triage scheme outside of normative practice, casualties were, in essence, sorted into one of two categories, using clinical judgment: OR or no OR[14,16] These events were notable for a lack of clinically significant bottlenecks in field evacuation and hospital capacity, thus reducing the importance of triage.

In planning for a disaster, it hardly seems prudent to assume such ample evacuative and hospital-based resources would be available, but it does speak to the importance of mobilizing maximum resources. This is the impetus for a formalized formal triage scheme, such as a four- or five-level classification system. In the common four-level system, such as the well-known civilian START system,[21] the categories are: (1) those who will get immediate priority (color-coded red), (2) those casualties who must wait (color-coded yellow), (3) those with the least severe injuries (often referred to as "walking well," color-coded green), and (4) those casualties whose prognosis is so poor that there is no justification for spending limited resources on them (color-coded black). Military triage hierarchies have a similar four- or five-level structure, although the nomenclature is different. For instance, color-code green is equivalent to NATO Level T3. People responding to international disasters should be aware of all of the triage classifications used by the host country and by the other responding agencies. A slightly more complicated five-level system makes a distinction between patients who will not survive (color-coded black) and those too gravely injured to receive limited resources (sometimes color-coded blue). Nevertheless, if enough resources become available, blue-coded casualties can then receive care. It has been argued that the option for an intermediate level such as blue may actually produce superior triage decision making. Given a stark choice between red or black for gravely injured patients who are not yet dead, it might be emotionally difficult for responders to apply a black tag, even though resources would be wasted on the casualty with a very poor prognosis.

When a tiered triage system is to be used, the most complicated issue is selecting the formal criteria to use for assigning each acuity level. This is discussed in detail in the sections "Will a Formal Triage Scoring System Be Used?" and "Are Normative Overtriage and Undertriage Rates Acceptable?" Most triage plans assume, and rightly so, that a casualty who can ambulate (i.e., the "walking wounded") is truly low risk. In a review of nearly 30,000 routine civilian trauma casualties, Meredith[22] found that the ability to follow commands (i.e., Glasgow Coma Scale [GCS] motor = 6) upon arrival to an ED is an outstanding positive predictor of patient survival. Still, these casualties do require medical attention at some point; head or extremity hemorrhage, open fractures, or penetrating abdominal trauma are injuries that might be present in ambulating patients, which are manageable conditions that become dangerous if not treated within an appropriate timeframe. In Meredith's study, the patients with GCS motor of 6 and outstanding prognoses received normative medical care, not indefinite neglect.

Will a Formal Triage Scoring System Be Used?

A formal scoring system can help categorize casualties by objective criteria. Reliance on EMS subjective assessments of severity has been studied as an independent predictor of acuity in routine trauma patients (e.g., not disaster casualties). EMS judgment has been found to be better,[23] equal,[24,25] and worse[26,27] than formal triage scoring. There is evidence that EMS judgment complements objective triage scoring.[24,26,27] Prehospital triage systems are tailored to traumatic pathology, not squeezing chest pain or focal pain at McBurney's point; EMS providers can easily recognize that patients with these signs and symptoms require urgent care. The GCS, published in 1974, offered a historic means of stratifying prognosis after head injury.[28] Triage scores for individual trauma patients (see the Historical Perspective section) arose from the need to decide if individual trauma casualties should be transported to specialized trauma centers. The best known are Champion's Trauma Score and Revised Trauma Score (RTS). The original Trauma Score used capillary refill and respiratory expansion, which were felt to be too unreliable. The RTS uses GCS, systolic blood pressure, and respiratory rate, and it yields a score between 0 and 12.[8,29] An RTS of 12 predicts mortality of less than 1% (when given routine clinical care). Mortality of roughly 50% is predicted by an RTS of 5. In general, the use of physiologic criteria tends to be specific but not as sensitive for predicting critical injury. Other notable triage scores include the contract research and manufacturing services (CRAMS) and Triage Index, which have also shown suboptimal test characteristics.[30-35] The advantage of a scoring system is that no particular physiologic state preordains a specific triage category; rather, scores for "black" and "red" and "yellow" can be established in real time, based on the perceived balance of casualties and medical resources. Triage scoring offers a flexible, sophisticated approach to triage. However, in the chaos and uncertainty of a disaster—a high-acuity, low-probability event—"sophisticated" can become "complicated," and "flexible" can become "uncertain." If formal triage scoring is used, emergency responders must be extremely facile with its use. For triage of pediatric casualties, neurologic, cardiovascular, and respiratory triage criteria should be different from those for adults because of the differences in physiology and recuperative capabilities. The differences motivated the development of specialized pediatric triage criteria, including the pediatric trauma score[36,37] and pediatric triage tape.[38] The former instrument did not prove superior to adult triage scoring systems,[39-41] and the latter has not been extensively validated.

A far simpler alternative to triage scoring is a triage algorithm, such as the START system. This system, for example, assigns "red" based on a rigid set of criteria (if airway is compromised; if minute respiratory rate is over 30; if capillary refill is over 2 seconds; or if simple commands cannot be followed).[21] The Triage Sieve is another similar example of an inflexible assignation algorithm; it includes an upper and lower limit for "red" respiratory rate, as well as a fixed upper limit for heart rate (unlike START, it does not use capillary refill).[42] The advantage of such rigid systems is the simplicity to teach and learn, and the appropriateness for typical MCIs with dozens or hundreds of casualties. The disadvantage, the inflexibility, is discussed further in the Acceptable Overtriage and Undertriage Rate section. More complex triage systems have also been developed, such as the Sacco Triage Method (STM). The system uses mathematical modeling to predict patient survival and to prioritize triage and transport to maximize the number of survivors based on available resources.[43] In a retrospective review of trauma registry patients, STM was shown to predict mortality more accurately compared with other triage systems, but whether this system identifies patients that would most benefit from expedited care is unclear.[44] It should also be noted that STM requires proprietary software and assumes an operational incident command system.[45]

In 2011, the Centers for Disease Control and Prevention (CDC) sponsored a project to review existing triage systems and develop a national standard for mass-casualty triage. The group concluded that there was insufficient evidence to compare systems rigorously or to identify a superior system. Combining features of known triage systems, they developed a new, algorithmic system, called SALT triage (Sort, Assess, Lifesaving Interventions, Treatment and/or Transport). The algorithm uses the ability to ambulate or follow commands to globally sort patients and prioritize assessment, and it emphasizes the rapid performance of simple, potentially lifesaving interventions such as hemorrhage control and chest decompression. Ultimately, patients are assigned 1 of 5 categories and transported or treated accordingly: immediate, expectant, delayed, minimal, or dead.[46] While SALT was designed in consideration of the best available evidence, it, like other triage systems, is largely consensus-based, and further research is required to determine if it is effective.

What On-Site/Hospital Documentation Will Be Used?

The triage tag, a minimal document that can be attached to each casualty, might be the only practical method of communicating findings, interventions, and so on, as countless casualties are passed through a chain of emergency care. However, it has been argued that triage tags are impractical to use, and geographic triage (see later) can obviate the need for tags.[3] In a disaster, hundreds or thousands of tags for each triage category must be immediately available to the responders, who need to be exceptionally familiar with the tags to use them properly under trying circumstances, and frenzied casualties may not take proper care of the tags. After an enormous disaster (thousands of casualties), tags might be especially challenging to use properly, although they could also be especially useful.

Consideration of the use of triage tags requires some research on the part of the customer, since there are over 120 triage label systems in use internationally.[42] Hogan and Burstein[47] suggested the following criteria for the optimal triage tag: (1) It must attach securely to each casualty's body, (2) it must be easy to write on, (3) it must be weather-proof, and (4) it should permit the documentation of the patient's name, gender, injuries, interventions, care-provider IDs, casualty triage score, and an easily visible overall triage category. It must also permit changes to be made, because triage is always dynamic. One unfortunate potential limitation for such a tag is the presence of contamination that may limit the ability of the triage tag to persist through hospital-based decontamination efforts if the patient is not decontaminated prior to transport.

Who Will Be the Triage Officer(s)?

There must be a major first-pass decision to establish which casualties can wait, which are top priority, which are expectant, etc. This can occur in the field and/or receiving hospital, but the designated triage officer needs a deep understanding of emergency medical treatments, what outcomes are likely for various casualties, and what resources are necessary for treatments. It may be advantageous to have a physician in this role, but in all cases the person performing this role should be among the most-experienced clinicians available because of the vital importance of triage with respect to resource utilization. In Israel, the role is taken by the surgeon-in-charge, because the emergency care bottleneck following a suicide bombing MCI typically occurs in determining operative priority after rapid evacuation to a receiving hospital.[16] Among multiple important traits, a triage officer needs the experience, disposition, and judgment to act as an able leader under incredible pressure.[47,48]

Who Will Collect Vital Signs for the Triage Officer(s)?

The measurement of vital signs should be delegated to assistants to the triage officer. Unfortunately, even in routine clinical conditions, vital sign measurements are confounded by human error and poor technique. Retraining improves the accuracy of vital signs; this is important, because during the chaos and stress of an MCI, an accurate set of vital signs determines the fate of an individual (e.g., placement in a triage category).

Physically, Where Will Casualties from Each Triage Category Be Cared for (and Who Will Staff Each Area)?

Geographic triage means assigning casualties to different physical locations based on severity. Initially, casualties can be brought to a collection point. From there, the triage officer can determine the appropriate triage category (e.g., red, yellow, black, and possibly blue), and then the

casualty can be moved to a triage category-specific collection point for further on-site treatment and/or transportation. The walking wounded (green) are readily separated from more seriously injured casualties through good crowd communication and control; most of these casualties could be taken care of in an urgent care center, clinic, or private physician offices, and having some mechanism for directing these casualties away from larger medical centers may be valuable. Briggs[49] suggests the following are desirable characteristics for on-site triage and treatment locations: (1) proximity to the disaster site, (2) safety from hazards, (3) location upwind when contamination is an issue, (4) protection from climactic conditions, (5) easy visibility, and (6) convenient access for air and land evacuation. Vayer[3] cited a number of MCIs, including the Hyatt Regency Skywalk Collapse and the IBM shooting incident, in which a collection point for triage was useful. However, in other situations, no ideal location may be available and an on-site collection point may be of mixed utility. Quarantelli,[50] in a classic study of EMS in 29 U.S. disasters, noted that most casualties are not transported by a properly staffed ambulance, but by private cars, buses, taxis, and even on foot. Field triage and first aid stations are often bypassed, either because their location or existence is unknown or because they are considered an inferior level of care compared with hospitals. Following the Centennial Olympics Bombing, ample EMS resources allowed rapid, complete evacuation of casualties, so on-site geographic triage was unnecessary.[17] In small or large disasters, it may be preferable for the triage officers and litter bearers to circulate and directly move casualties from the scene to appropriate treatment locations, eliminating any collection point. In extremely large disasters, several collection areas might be useful.

It is important to consider the manner and degree to which geographic separation will be enforced. The bigger the disaster, the more crowd control is an issue. For receiving hospitals, crowd control must be a priority; an unstructured influx of casualties should be anticipated, with most casualties ending up at the closest hospitals. Following the Tokyo Subway sarin attack, the St. Luke's ED was deluged with 500 patients in the first hour alone.[51] At the scene, crowd control is a more complicated issue. Einav[52] described how Jerusalem EMS evacuates casualties so rapidly that only minimal medical interventions are performed, and no crowd control at all is attempted. Crowd control requires emergency resources and may eliminate the assistance by untrained local citizens, who often constitute the majority of the response resources after disasters. Regarding crowd control on scene, Vayer[3] suggested that "if patients are medically and emotionally stable and choose to leave, they should be allowed to do so."

What Overtriage and Undertriage Rates Are Acceptable, and What Level of Casualty Gets "Black-Tagged"?

Investigations of trauma triage rules (the prehospital decision of whether or not a patient's severity warrants transport to a specialized trauma center) suggest that overtriage of 50% to 60% is necessary to achieve undertriage rates around 10%.[4,26,27,32,47,53] It has also been noted that the four-tiered START triage algorithm leads to substantial overtriage of disaster casualties.[9,47] This might be acceptable in a response to an MCI with a few hundred surviving casualties. Consider Table 54-1: after a hypothetical terrorist bombing with 100 to 200 surviving casualties, conventional triage practice might overtriage 50% of the intermediate "true yellow," increasing the number of total red. Would it be worth attempting a dramatic departure from normative triage to attempt to reduce the 10 or 20 "false reds"? Routine rates for trauma overtriage and undertriage may be tenable for incidents on this scale. It is worth examining other scenarios that suggest how overtriage and undertriage goals must be adapted to the scale of the

TABLE 54-1 Spectrum of Casualties for Different Scales of Disasters (Hypothetical)

SURVIVING CASUALTIES	TRUE GREEN −60%*	TRUE RED −20%*	TRUE YELLOW −20%*	TOTAL RED TRUE RED + 50% OVER TRIAGE OF TRUE YELLOW†	EXPECTANT −2%
100	60	20	20	30	NA
200	120	40	40	60	NA
1000	600	200	200	300	20
2000	1200	400	400	600	40

*Based on typical distributions of injury severity[54] for illustrative purpose only.
†Based on typical rates of overtriage of less severely injured casualties, see text for details.

disaster. An event with 1000 to 2000 surviving casualties would yield 100 to 200 "false reds" in addition to the 200 to 400 "true-reds" if triage criteria were not appropriately adjusted (Table 54-1). Such numbers of red critical casualties would likely overwhelm even a large urban area's facilities; therefore the rate of overtriage should be lowered even if that means increasing rates of undertriage (this is the classic sensitivity/specificity trade-off embodied by receiver-operator curves). There are many options of how to define "black" casualties, who are considered so sick (e.g., pulseless and apneic) that resources are wasted on them: an Israeli EMS protocol for MCIs is more specific, considering as dead those with amputated body parts who are not showing signs of movement, as well as those who are pulseless with dilated pupils.[16] In published reports, there is mixed evidence that the overtriage of excessively sick casualties (e.g., the failure to apply a black tag to unsavable survivors) has been an issue. One retrospective analysis of seven separate terrorist bombings noted a correlation between high mortality rates for hospitalized casualties with critical injuries and the fraction of casualties hospitalized without critical injuries.[54] One explanation would be that overtriage of noncritical casualties cost the truly critical casualties the medical attention they required. However, the paper did not describe other characteristics of the casualties, such as the age of victims, the distribution of injury severity, and the incidence of head injury. These factors might suggest alternative explanations. Historically, resuscitation of moribund casualties following MCIs offers dismal outcomes,[14,55,56] and such heroic measures are generally discouraged. Failure to triage the unsavable as "black" (a form of overtriage) will produce "false reds," who will pointlessly be given precious medical resources (Table 54-1). Indeed, in designing a response to an earthquake with many thousands of casualties, it has been suggested that casualties with a likelihood of survival less than 50% may need to be "black-tagged."[57] If so, an RTS of 5 or less would be an appropriate criterion.[8]

Undertriage of the critically injured may be just as much of a problem, historically. Following the Oklahoma City Bombing, 100% of the 72 casualties admitted to hospitals survived.[14] Only 3 of the 167 fatalities were even transported from the scene, and those 3 were dead on arrival to the ED. Is it possible that there had been savable casualties at the scene who never received needed care in time? It is important to not reflexively deprive serious casualties of the intensive care they may need when resources are available. Pepe and Kvetan[2] propose a scenario in which "there are 40 patients, 39 of whom are 'walking wounded' and one patient . . . is in a state of cardiopulmonary arrest." In such circumstances, standard resuscitation, or at least a "quick look" with a defibrillator, may be appropriate for patients who are moribund. Indeed, for both the Centennial Olympics Bombing[17] and the Israeli Sbarro Bombing,[58] the balance between the spectrum of casualties and the available medical resources was sufficient that CPR and ED thoracotomies were attempted, respectively.

Ideally, triage criteria would be calibrated, using a severity score such as the RTS, to balance the scope of resources available with the scope of casualties. An ideal method would further consider not only mortality, but other issues such as functional outcomes or years-of-life saved. Realistically, however, it does not make sense to expect that the triage method can be tailored so carefully to a given disaster in real time. Most disaster experiences suggest tremendous uncertainty exists about the extent of the casualties during the initial response[10,58]; when extrications are necessary, the sickest patients are usually last to arrive.[3,14] The "fog of war" complicates the initial responses to any disaster. At the same time, it seems prudent to prepare different triage plans for different scales of disaster.

Assuming 10 Patients in 20 Minutes per Triage Officer,[21] Are There Enough Officers? Are There Enough Other Personnel to Keep Up with the Triage Team (e.g., Litter Bearers and Care Providers), If Not, Is the Triage Team Too Big?

In general, the litter bearers, triage officers, and other care providers will not always operate in perfect synchronicity, since there will be irregular holdups for various activities. Responders may need to briefly change roles during operations (i.e., a triage officer may hold pressure on a compressible site of hemorrhage for a few moments until someone else becomes available to take over). If any specific activity becomes truly rate limiting (triage, stretcher transport, etc.), personnel should be reassigned to balance the response. Moreover, if extrication from the site is the rate-limiting step, triage can be moved to the site itself, so that extrication efforts themselves are triaged, with consideration given to both medical severity and the difficulty of extrication.

Are Resources Being Used Appropriately, Including On-Site Medical Interventions, Evacuation Resources, and Hospital-Based Resources (e.g., Emergency Department Care and Operating Room)?

This chapter on triage refers to "response resources" and "emergency care" in rather abstract terms. Detailed discussion gets into the excessively broad subject of trauma management and critical care. Yet, to understand and perform triage, one must understand the costs (in terms of time and materials) and benefits of emergency care. For instance, placing a tourniquet to control extremity hemorrhage or dressing an open chest wound should be high priority for any responder, since such simple measures can save a life. Other critical interventions that can be performed on-site if resources permit include needle decompression of a tension pneumothorax, nasopharyngeal airway placement, splinting, and applying a hemostatic dressing. If the balance of responder resources to casualties is permitting, on-site intervention may even include some resuscitation, although attempting such heroic interventions always runs the risk of using up precious resources. When neither evacuation nor hospital resources are bottlenecked, on-site interventions should be kept to a minimum. For those casualties evacuated by ambulance, consideration might be given to bypassing the closest hospitals. In addition, casualties transporting themselves to the hospital could be advised which hospitals are not getting very many patients and therefore will have shorter waiting times. When evacuation from the scene is a bottleneck, common sense dictates that evacuation priority is for patients who would most benefit from timely hospital care. Suspected abdominal hemorrhage thus precedes compressible extremity hemorrhage, because the former requires an operating room, whereas the latter can be treated initially in the field. A lucid but hypotensive patient with penetrating abdominal trauma should precede one with a penetrating head injury with altered mental status, since the former has a better prognosis if prompt operative care is provided. At the receiving hospital, too, resources must be triaged. Many authors suggest that the most-experienced surgeon direct in-hospital triage, as he or she can best estimate the resources each patient will require, such as blood products and operating room time. One of the important and often overlooked issues in triage is redistributing the patient load. Receiving hospitals may redirect appropriate casualties to remote hospitals with available capacity. Some have argued for turning the closest hospital into a triage center and redistributing the casualties to other facilities from there. However, federal patient transfer regulations (EMTALA) make this challenging.

After Casualties' Initial Triage, Who Reevaluates the Patient, and How Often? After Each Reassessment, Has the Triage Plan Been Communicated to All Active Rescuers, Including Victims and Participating Bystanders, as Is Appropriate?

A patient's apparent clinical condition will evolve, as will the available resources. After an initial triage, a formal mechanism for ongoing reevaluation of casualties is necessary for all triage categories (with the possible exception of black). These clinical reevaluations can also establish treatment priorities within various triage groups, because, for instance, red casualties will have intracategory variation in terms of severity and the specific management they require. In some cases, conditions will worsen, and a yellow designation may become red (e.g., evolution of blast lung injury) or a red designation may become black (e.g., hypovolemic arrest). In other circumstances, new resources may permit more aggressive care, and a blue or even black designation may be upgraded to red (discussed in the What Triage Classification Will Be Used? section). Even some of the walking wounded may have conditions that require timely intervention, in case an excellent prognosis is threatened. To effectively retriage requires updated knowledge of the spectrum of casualties and the resources available; there should be a formal mechanism for such updates.

Focus: Training/Planning Specific Issues

This chapter described options for disaster triage. From a training perspective, the bottom line is this: more sophisticated systems may enable optimal triage, but one must fully commit to training and mastery of any system for it to be of value in the chaotic aftermath of a disaster. Therefore, a system such as START, with its straightforward four levels and rigid criteria for each category, may be better than a fully improvisational approach that relies on clinical judgments, but not unless it is mastered in training. A five-level system may offer even better triage than a four-tiered system,[4] but it is all the more complicated to learn and execute and, therefore, may be less likely to be used in practice.

Triage tags may offer better record-keeping and patient care, but they will prove simply burdensome if they are unfamiliar to the caregivers dealing with a major crisis. Finally, formal trauma scoring, such as Champion's RTS, might enable the most sophisticated triage, but not if the responders are struggling to properly compute the revised trauma score.

One suggestion for planning a triage response to a disaster is this: select the most flexible methodology of which your training resources will permit mastery. Rehearsal is crucial, so that the principle of "normative practice" (see the opening paragraphs in this chapter) can be followed in an actual disaster. Authors have suggested the need for weekly practice for proper maintenance of disaster-response skills (e.g., "Triage Tuesday").[3,47] Many triage systems rely on measured vital signs, but, as noted, vital signs are often measured poorly, even under normal clinical conditions; retraining such skills can be very useful. Formal triage scoring, such as the RTS, can also be used in designing simulations so that the survival rate of the hypothetical casualties can be computed and the performance of triage during the exercise can be evaluated objectively. Finally, simple table-top simulations may be useful as an inexpensive, undemanding complement to full-scale rehearsals.

⚠ PITFALLS

- Ineffective triage after unexpected disasters has been the historical norm.
- Effective responses have required exceptional mobilization of prehospital and hospital resources, making triage easier.
- In developed countries, disaster casualties typically number in the dozens to hundreds.
- Assuming that a single triage plan will be suitable for disasters of all scales and conditions.
- Assuming that the majority of health care emergencies following large disasters will be traumatic in nature.
- Failing to appreciate the enormous amount of training required for any triage plan that deviates from normative health delivery practice.
- Failing to appreciate trade-offs between utility and complexity (four- vs. five-level triage, rigid "cookie cutter" triage criteria versus flexible criteria using severity scores, triage tags versus geographic triage, etc.).
- Not realizing that vital sign measurement technique must be addressed in training.
- Failing to select appropriate, safe locations on scene and to plan for crowd control.
- Failure to reevaluate and reassign patients and to relate updates to responders as their condition changes in real time.

REFERENCES

1. Trotta D. Bomb kills 173 on packed Madrid trains. *Sydney Morning Herald*. 12 March 2004.
2. Pepe PE, Kvetan V. Field management and critical care in mass disasters. *Crit Care Clin*. 1991;7(2):401–420.
3. Vayer JS, Ten Eyck RP, Cowan ML. New concepts in triage. *Ann Emerg Med*. 1986;15(8):927–930.
4. Kennedy K, Aghababian RV, Gans L, Lewis CP. Triage: techniques and applications in decision making. *Ann Emerg Med*. 1996;28(2):136–144.
5. Eiseman B. Combat casualty management in Vietnam. *J Trauma*. 1967;7(1):53–63.
6. West JG, Trunkey DD, Lim RC. Systems of trauma care. A study of two counties. *Arch Surg*. 1979;114(4):455–460.
7. Burkle FM Jr, Newland C, Orebaugh S, Blood CG. Emergency medicine in the Persian Gulf War-Part 2. Triage methodology and lessons learned. *Ann Emerg Med*. 1994;23(4):748–754.

8. Champion HR, Sacco WJ, Copes WS, et al. A revision of the trauma score. *J Trauma.* 1989;29(5):623–629.

9. Hodgetts TJ. *Triage: A Position Statement.* European Union Core Group on Disaster Medicine; 2002, 1–15.

10. Frykberg ER. Principles of mass casualty management following terrorist disasters. *Ann Surg.* 2004;239(3):319–321.

11. Lee WH, Chiu TF, Ng CJ, Chen JC. Emergency medical preparedness and response to a Singapore airliner crash. *Acad Emerg Med.* 2002;9(3):194–198.

12. Okumura T, Suzuki K, Fukuda A, et al. The Tokyo subway sarin attack: disaster management, Part 1: Community emergency response. *Acad Emerg Med.* 1998;5(6):613–617.

13. Gewalli F, Fogdestam I. Triage and initial treatment of burns in the Gothenburg fire disaster 1998. On-call plastic surgeons' experiences and lessons learned. *Scand J Plast Reconstr Surg Hand Surg.* 2003;37(3):134–139.

14. Hogan DE, Waeckerle JF, Dire DJ, Lillibridge SR. Emergency department impact of the Oklahoma City terrorist bombing. *Ann Emerg Med.* 1999; 34(2):160–167.

15. Auf der Heide E. *Disaster Response: Principles of Preparation and Coordination.* St. Louis: Mosby; 1989.

16. Almogy G, Belzberg H, Mintz Y, et al. Suicide bombing attacks: update and modifications to the protocol. *Ann Surg.* 2004;239(3):295–303.

17. Feliciano DV, Anderson GV Jr, Rozycki GS, et al. Management of casualties from the bombing at the Centennial Olympics. *Am J Surg.* 1998;176(6): 538–543.

18. Biddinger PD, Baggish A, Harrington L, et al. Be prepared—the Boston Marathon and mass-casualty events. *N Engl J Med.* 2013;368(21): 1958–1960.

19. Elnashai AS, Cleveland LJ, Jefferson T, et al. *Impact of New Madrid Seismic Zone Earthquakes on the Central USA.* Mid-American Earthquake Center Report, Urbana, IL: University of Illinois at Urbana-Champaign; 2009.

20. Frankel AD, Applegate D, Tuttle MP, et al. Earthquake hazard in the New Madrid Seismic Zone remains a concern: U.S. Geological Survey Fact Sheet 2009–3071.

21. Super G. *START: A Triage Training Module.* Newport Beach, CA: Hoag Memorial Hospital Presbyterian; 1984.

22. Meredith W, Rutledge R, Hansen AR, et al. Field triage of trauma patients based upon the ability to follow commands: a study in 29,573 injured patients. *J Trauma.* 1995;38(1):129–135.

23. Ornato J, Mlinek EJ Jr, Craren EJ, Nelson N. Ineffectiveness of the trauma score and the CRAMS scale for accurately triaging patients to trauma centers. *Ann Emerg Med.* 1985;14(11):1061–1064.

24. Hedges JR, Feero S, Moore B, et al. Comparison of prehospital trauma triage instruments in a semirural population. *J Emerg Med.* 1987;5(3): 197–208.

25. Emerman CL, Shade B, Kubincanek J. A comparison of EMT judgment and prehospital trauma triage instruments. *J Trauma.* 1991;31(10):1369–1375.

26. Esposito TJ, Offner PJ, Jurkovich GJ, et al. Do prehospital trauma center triage criteria identify major trauma victims? *Arch Surg.* 1995;130(2): 171–176.

27. Simmons E, Hedges JR, Irwin L, et al. Paramedic injury severity perception can aid trauma triage. *Ann Emerg Med.* 1995;26(4):461–468.

28. Teasdale G, Jennett B. Assessment of coma and impaired consciousness. A practical scale. *Lancet.* 1974;2(7872):81–84.

29. Champion HR, Sacco WJ, Carnazzo AJ, et al. Trauma score. *Crit Care Med.* 1981;9(9):672–676.

30. Gormican SP. CRAMS scale: field triage of trauma victims. *Ann Emerg Med.* 1982;11(3):132–135.

31. Knudson P, Frecceri CA, DeLateur SA. Improving the field triage of major trauma victims. *J Trauma.* 1988;28(5):602–606.

32. Baxt WG, Berry CC, Epperson MD, Scalzitti V. The failure of prehospital trauma prediction rules to classify trauma patients accurately. *Ann Emerg Med.* 1989;18(1):1–8.

33. Baxt WG, Jones G, Fortlage D. The trauma triage rule: a new, resource-based approach to the prehospital identification of major trauma victims. *Ann Emerg Med.* 1990;19(12):1401–1406.

34. Bever DL, Veenker CH. An illness-injury severity index for nonphysician emergency medical personnel. *EMT J.* 1979;3(1):45–49.

35. Kilberg L, Clemmer TP, Clawson J, et al. Effectiveness of implementing a trauma triage system on outcome: a prospective evaluation. *J Trauma.* 1988;28(10):1493–1498.

36. Tepas JJ 3rd, Mollitt DL, Talbert JL, Bryant M. The pediatric trauma score as a predictor of injury severity in the injured child. *J Pediatr Surg.* 1987; 22(1):14–18.

37. Tepas JJ 3rd, Ramenofsky ML, Mollitt DL, et al. The Pediatric Trauma Score as a predictor of injury severity: an objective assessment. *J Trauma.* 1988;28(4):425–429.

38. Hodgetts TJ, et al. Paediatric triage tape. *Pre-hospital Immediate Care.* 1998;2:155–159.

39. Kaufmann CR, Maier RV, Rivara FP, Carrico CJ. Evaluation of the pediatric trauma score. *JAMA.* 1990;263(1):69–72.

40. Eichelberger MR, Gotschall CS, Sacco WJ, et al. A comparison of the trauma score, the revised trauma score, and the pediatric trauma score. *Ann Emerg Med.* 1989;18(10):1053–1058.

41. Nayduch DA, Moylan J, Rutledge R, et al. Comparison of the ability of adult and pediatric trauma scores to predict pediatric outcome following major trauma. *J Trauma.* 1991;31(4):452–457, discussion 457–458.

42. Hodgetts TJ, Brett A. Triage. In: Greaves I, Porter K, eds. *Pre-Hospital Medicine.* London: Arnold Publishers; 1999.

43. Sacco WJ, Navin DM, Fiedler KE, et al. Precise formulation and evidence-based application of resource-constrained triage. *Acad Emerg Med.* 2005; 12(8):759–770.

44. Cross KP, Cicero MX. Head-to-head comparison of disaster triage methods in pediatric, adult, and geriatric patients. *Ann Emerg Med.* 2013;61(6): 668–676.e7.

45. Cone DC, MacMillan DS. Mass-casualty triage systems: a hint of science. *Acad Emerg Med.* 2005;12(8):739–741.

46. SALT mass casualty triage: concept endorsed by the American College of Emergency Physicians, American College of Surgeons Committee on Trauma, American Trauma Society, National Association of EMS Physicians, National Disaster Life Support Education Consortium, and State and Territorial Injury Prevention Directors Association. *Disaster Med Public Health Prep.* 2008;2(4):245–246.

47. Hogan DE, Burstein JL. Triage. In: *Disaster Medicine.* Philadelphia: Williams & Wilkins; 2002:10–15.

48. Burkle FM Jr. *Disaster Medicine: Application for the Immediate Management and Triage of Civilian and Military Disaster Victims.* New Hyde Park, NY: Medical Examination Publishing; 1984.

49. Briggs SM, ed. Triage. In: *Advanced Disaster Medical Response Manual for Providers.* Boston: Harvard Medical International; 2003.

50. Quarantelli EL. *Delivery of Emergency Medical Care in Disasters: Assumptions and Realities.* New York: Irvington Publishers; 1983.

51. Okumura T, Suzuki K, Fukuda A, et al. The Tokyo subway sarin attack: disaster management, Part 2: hospital response. *Acad Emerg Med.* 1998; 5(6):618–624.

52. Einav S, Feigenberg Z, Weissman C, et al. Evacuation priorities in mass casualty terror-related events: implications for contingency planning. *Ann Surg.* 2004;239(3):304–310.

53. Wesson DE, Scorpio R. Field triage—help or hindrance? *Can J Surg.* 1992; 35(1):19–21.

54. Frykberg ER, Tepas JJ 3rd. Terrorist bombings. Lessons learned from Belfast to Beirut. *Ann Surg.* 1988;208(5):569–576.

55. Boehm TM, James JJ. The medical response to the LaBelle Disco bombing in Berlin, 1986. *Mil Med.* 1988;153(5):235–238.

56. Brown MG, Marshall SG. The Enniskillen bomb: a disaster plan. *Br Med J.* 1988;297(6656):1113–1116.

57. Schulz LH, DiLorenzo RA, Koenig KL. Disaster medical direction: a medical earthquake response curriculum. *Ann Emerg Med.* 1991;20:470–471.

58. Peleg K, Aharonson-Daniel L, Stein M, et al. Gunshot and explosion injuries: characteristics, outcomes, and implications for care of terror-related injuries in Israel. *Ann Surg.* 2004;239(3):311–318.

Patient-Tracking Systems in Disasters

Charles Stewart and M. Kathleen Stewart

Communication and information management from the field to the care facilities are consistently challenging during disaster response. A critical interdependence exists among the following: accurate information from the field about the incident, medical needs at the scene, and patient numbers and types of their injuries. Care of these patients triaged and treated will affect the demand and use of resources such as ambulances, emergency departments, surgical suites, specialist needs, and intensive care units. Similarly, information on the availability of ambulances and hospital resources will alter the management and disposition of the victims at the scene.

Patient tracking is the art (and science) of determining which patient with which condition went to which destination (and where he or she is presently). This includes identification of the patient and identification of the patient's intermediate and ultimate destination(s). Ideal practice would also have the patient's medical records included with this tracking information and/or travel with the patient.

Recent acts of mass terrorism and natural disasters have called attention to the urgent need to improve response during mass-casualty incidents.[1] The risk of these mass-casualty incidents appears to be increasing as a result of population growth, industrialization (and concomitant use of high-energy chemicals and sources), and the threat of terrorism.[2] Following the initial impact of the disaster, the casualties generated by the disaster must be determined. Relatives of patients will want to know where their loved ones are being treated; law enforcement officials may want to interview survivors and suspects; and public health officials will want summaries of patient conditions, initial dispositions, and final disposition (if there is a change). To respond effectively to inquiries about the missing, victim data may have to be collected not just from hospitals but also from alternative care sites, shelters, jails, and morgues. Victim information should be collected at a central location and made available via telephone hotlines or websites distant from the impact area. In very large disasters, the numbers of inquiries about the missing can exacerbate local telephone and cellular circuit congestion and shut the services down momentarily. Hospitals may be reluctant to provide patient information to the Red Cross or local authorities because of concern about Health Insurance Portability and Accountability Act (HIPAA) regulations and patient confidentiality. However, HIPAA regulations do allow the release of information on patient names, locations, and general status for the purposes of notifying patients' next of kin. (See www.hhs.gov.ocr/hipaa.)

Nevertheless, most disaster evacuees do not stay in public shelters and often do not require hospitalization, but rather seek refuge with family, friends, and neighbors or at a motel or hotel. Therefore, in order to track these victims, they will need to be contacted via the mass media and encouraged to register via telephone hotlines or websites. Tracking of these noninjured evacuees is beyond the scope of this chapter.

HISTORICAL PERSPECTIVE

If the disaster happens in an isolated area, such as a complex multi-vehicle accident along I-80 in Wyoming, tracking of patients is comparatively easy; most (if not all) casualties will be taken to one or two facilities.[3] In such a disaster, the major casualty tracking problem generated is identification of victims who have been burned beyond recognition. In large-scale disasters and/or in disasters in urban areas, casualties may have multiple potential destinations. The patient-destination matching is complicated by the large number of patients who will take available transportation to a medical facility without involving emergency medical service(s) (EMS) workers. For example, during the response to the 9/11 World Trade Center attack, only 6.8% were transported by ambulance.[4] In addition, emergency response units from surrounding jurisdictions will often self-dispatch to the disaster.[5,6] Accordingly, they may not be aware of existing local victim-tracking system(s). Further complications include air evacuation to remote destinations, transfers to higher levels of care for patients with more complex conditions, and switch of destination during EMS transport. In response to Hurricane Katrina, for example, children were taken to different states than their parents.

In a disaster, a number of factors make it difficult or impossible to track patients from scene to final destination.
1. The number of patients generated may exceed the capacity of the local EMS system.
2. There may be multiple incident locations geographically separated.
3. Multiple EMS systems may be assigned or may self-deploy into the affected region. These providers may use differing systems for patient tracking that may or may not be intercompatible.[5,6]
4. EMS providers may transport patients to alternate care facilities when the hospital system is overwhelmed.
5. EMS providers may be diverted en route to their assigned hospital or other destination.
6. Hospital facilities may be damaged and be forced to evacuate existing patients and/or divert incoming patients, while simultaneously receiving casualties from one or more disaster scenes.
7. Patients may be transported to other cities, counties, states, or countries, depending on the magnitude of the disaster. Parents or guardians may or may not accompany the evacuee in this case.
8. Hospital medical record systems, communications, and EMS tracking systems may be inoperable because of damage or power failure.
9. With electronic systems, data from one system may be in a format that is incompatible with other systems.

CURRENT PRACTICE

Although separate from triage, the tracking process starts with triage. As patients are categorized by the triage officer and assistant triage officers, they are often tagged with a visible indicator of their priority (triage tags) or grouped with similar types of patients in a geographic area (geographic triage). Tracking can start with the recording of these patients (and as much data as time and condition permits) as they enter the medical care system. The patient-tracking officer(s) can relay the information via phone, radio, or fax, sending the information to the destination, although in practice this is often a difficult task.

There are currently two general types of tracking systems in use in the field setting: (1) manual, consisting of paper tags, cards, and charts and (2) electronic, depending on bar codes or radio frequency identification (RFID) devices and/or Wi-Fi networks.

Manual Systems: Paper Tags, Cards, and Charts

When a triage or medical documentation tag is applied to the patient, the preassigned number on the tag is the patient's first identification in the system. In some systems, this tag may be the only reported identification and documentation of medical care until the patient is taken to the hospital. (This tag may also have a bar code or an RFID to enable electronic systems.)

If the appropriate systems and supports are in place, a triage officer can rapidly prepare a patient-tracking list containing the patient's identification number, sex, apparent age, triage condition, destination, and the time the patient left the scene. The receiving hospital prepares a similar list with identification number, sex, apparent age, triage condition, disposition, and time of disposition upon arrival of those patients (Fig. 55-1). Paper tracking forms are nationally recognized and available as Hospital Incident Command System (HICS) forms 254, 255, and 260; their use is incorporated in many HICS and other incident command courses.

Several commercially available tag systems can be purchased (Fig. 55-2). These include the METTAG and the Multi-Tag. These tags are preprinted with a unique number to facilitate patient tracking during an incident. Each contains a section for patient information and a section with tear-off strips to categorize the patient's condition. Many municipal and state variants of these tags have been developed. These multiple tag and card formats may be used in the same disaster by different teams responding under cross-state mutual aid agreements. This allows the possibility of identical patient numbers for different patients, as well as creating confusion for medical providers receiving patients with different charting systems.

These tags are advocated by multiple incident training programs such as the Major Incident Medical Management and Support training program.[7,8] In these systems, either tags or a substitute (such as pieces of colored aluminum, colored chemical light sticks, or surveyor's tape in multiple colors [red, green, yellow, black, or white]) are used to tag each patient.[9-11] Other examples of medical documentation cards designed to travel with the patient include the NATO military "casualty cards" and the International Committee of the Red Cross casualty card.[12] These alternative systems often have no unique identification number for the casualty.

There are several disadvantages to the use of paper tags and cards for patient-tracking purposes.

- Application of tags takes time. There is only a single accident where triage tags have been described as being of benefit and this was limited to 22 live casualties.[13] Indeed, multiple casualties have been managed without triage tags, and significant time was thought to have been saved in the Sioux City, Iowa, DC-10 plane crash.[14] (The alternative to triage tags was a geographical system of triage and sorting.)
- Triage tags are often not weather resistant and may be destroyed or mutilated easily.[15] Water can smudge and render illegible data on triage tags.
- Triage tags provide no advance information to the destination. (The information provided is also unavailable to other sites.)
- When patient information, such as vital signs, condition, or even destination changes, it may be difficult to change the card or tag.

HOSPITAL	TRIAGE TAG NUMBER	HOSPITAL ID NUMBER	LAST NAME	FIRST NAME	SEX	AGE	STATUS	INITIALS

FIG 55-1 Sample Patient-Tracking Form.

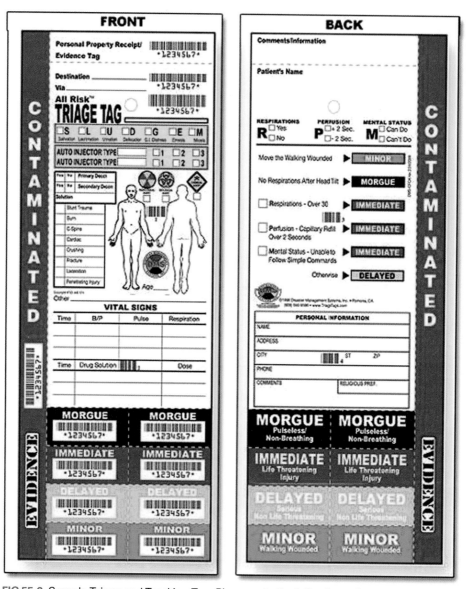

FIG 55-2 Sample Triage and Tracking Tag. Please note the following color coding in the tag: morgue—black; immediate—red; delayed—yellow; minor—green. (Courtesy of Disaster Medicine Systems, Inc., Pomona, CA.)

Tear-off triage tags allow only unidirectional changes in the patient's condition. Tear-off triage tags may be changed easily by patients or family members in an effort to upgrade the triage classification and expedite medical care or evacuation.

- There is little limited paper "real estate" space for continuation of vital signs and additional information. On the way to the hospital, the EMS provider can often obtain quite a bit of additional information, for example, comorbid factors such as diabetes and heart disease, allergies, and current medications. The usual tag does not provide space for this information to the treating physician or medical provider.
- Triage tags are often discarded at the hospital, even though they should be part of the medical record. They are often an awkward shape to put into the medical record and may not be recognized by the medical records clerks as part of the medical record. Documentation cards that are attached to the patient in some form are more likely to remain with that patient and document recent medical interventions to the receiving hospital.

- When a destination is overwhelmed and the ambulance is diverted to a different destination, the paper triage tag does not reflect a new destination back to the triage officer.
- One of the factors that complicates the use of tracking systems (e.g., triage tags) is the logical and appropriate tendency in disasters to abandon paperwork in favor of treating patients.[16]
- In some disasters, triage tags have not been available where needed.[17]
- Triage tags do have significant advantages:
- They are cheap and simple to use.
- They are widely used, so many prehospital providers are familiar with their use and layout.
- Even cross training with different tag formats is relatively rapid and simple.
- They require little financial outlay for the disaster response team prior to the accident.
- They consistently work despite degradation of power supplies and adverse weather conditions.

Electronic Systems: Bar Codes or RFID and Wi-Fi Networks

Commercial package tracking as used by FedEx and UPS allows customers to find the shipping status and location of bar-coded packages and envelopes online. These tracking programs use RFID or bar codes to allow electronic reading of the package identification and subsequent transmission of package location. Extension of this technology to triage and patient-tracking programs remedies most of the faults of the paper system and allows the hospital, EMS dispatcher, triage officer, and other appropriate parties to track the human package from triage site to final destination.[18,19] Alternative schemes with handheld collection devices to supplement basic triage tag data collection have added additional medical information and linked this to the triage tag number and the medical record.[20-23]

There are no current nationally recommended electronic systems, although data exchange standards are in development. Several victim-tracking systems have been designed to aid the reunification of family members following a large-scale disaster. The Department of Defense (DoD) and National Disaster Medical System (NDMS) in the United States uses a system developed by the U.S. Air Force, called TRAC2ES, which tracks patients transferred to partner hospitals in the DOD and/or NDMS system.[24] The American Red Cross uses a system called "Safe and Well," in a website that allows individuals on the Internet to notify others that they are safe and well.[25]

A bar code is an optical machine-readable representation of a unique alphanumeric number. Originally developed in the 1960s to identify railcars from a distance, they have become ubiquitous identification of stock numbers in many industries. Bar codes for patient tracking may be found on triage tags or bracelets that are attached to the patient. Bar code readers can be dedicated devices or even programs (apps) on smartphones or computers and are inexpensive and readily available.

RFID is a non–line-of-sight and contact-less automatic identification technology.[26] It is capable of communicating remotely, even when obscured, and without direct contact between the chip and the receiver. The identification data are stored on chips that can be attached or imbedded in products, tags, or even humans. The chip is an integrated circuit (about 0.4×0.4 mm in size) and an integrated antenna. The antenna size dictates the distance from which the chip can be interrogated by a reader. Chips may have an integral power supply or be powered by induction or radiation from the reader. An inherent strength of RFID chips is that they can provide both spatial and temporal context to the tagged subject, in addition to the unique identity code.[26-28]

By scanning a unique patient wristband, tag, or RFID at any location (disaster site, site treatment center, emergency department, hospital ward, operating suite, or ICU), the electronic system can track and provide the last known location of patients.[15,29-32] These systems have been tested in simulated disaster drills in the United States and Europe with good efficacy.[33,34] Similar systems using an RFID chip can allow remote query of the triage tag or band.[32,33] Marathon runners at large races are tracked during the race with similar technology, which can provide an accurate location of each runner during the race. The addition of a Wi-Fi network collection point would allow real-time tracking, dispatch, and diversion updates to all participating hospitals and agencies. This gives any participating agency the ability to direct family members to the last known location of the patient.[28]

Bar-coded tags or RFID with Wi-Fi networks do have some significant disadvantages, however.

- The technology requires a Wi-Fi network infrastructure to be set up at the disaster site.[18] This requires a substantial hardware and software outlay for all participating agencies and hospitals.[32] The

system may be unavailable if any electromagnetic jamming occurs, and will be destroyed by any electromagnetic pulse (EMP) effect, which is significant in the case of a nuclear weapon explosion.

- The overall security of Wi-Fi networks is open to question. Both modification of data and compromise of patient medical data can occur with Wi-Fi networks.
- Each bar code system represents a proprietary software system that may be incompatible with another similar system. This may have significance in adjoining city, county, or state governments and some mutual response agreements. As noted below, standards are being developed to mitigate this problem.
- Bar code systems require the presence of providers with scanning devices to obtain the tracking data. Keyboard entry of data can occur, but it is much slower and requires a computer with attendant power supply.[35]

Use of bar code readers or RFID and networked computers has significant advantages to all parties, including the patient:

- Information about prospective patients is readily available to the receiving hospital. (Information about final destination is available to the dispatch officer for further transportation planning.)
- Information about patients at one facility is readily available to other participating hospitals and agencies.
- Information entered travels with a casualty and can be cross-referenced to medical history, when available. Allergies, medications, and comorbid factors can be entered at participating sites, at any point in the evacuation process. This information can follow the casualty through all levels of medical treatment and be concisely printed for the patient's final chart.
- Information is not limited to a small amount of paper "real estate." This information can even include pictures of the patient and identifying personal effects.[26]
- Entry of initial data and identification of patients in a selected area are both rapid as the bar code is scanned with a reader.[32]

The disaster medicine practitioner should remember that bar codes and RFID are simply a rapid means of data entry and not the tracking system itself. They do not give the patient condition or location without the accompanying and functioning software program and associated network and hardware.

General Considerations

In the design of tracking systems, whether manual or electronic, the following factors must be considered:

1. Data entry
   a. Who will enter the data?
      i. Does data entry require specialized tools or training?
      ii. How much data can be automatically uploaded or entered to minimize data entry burdens?
   b. How will it be entered?
      i. Can the data be entered under adverse conditions such as in the back of a moving ambulance?
   c. How much data will be entered about each patient?
      i. What are critical data?
      ii. What additional elements would be desirable but not mandatory?
   d. How long will it take to enter the data?
      i. Typically providers prefer to do patient care rather than data entry, so data entry often suffers when providers feel that patient care is jeopardized.
2. Data dissemination
   a. How will the data be aggregated?
   b. How will it be disseminated?
   c. Who will get the data and how much data will be transmitted?

i. As communications degrade, data transmission rates will markedly decrease.

ii. Does the system automatically decrease data transmitted by shedding noncritical elements, retaining these in a common server as communications degrade? (Pictures are large data items and often not immediately critical elements.)

d. How will the data be protected from inappropriate access?

e. Where will the data be stored?

3. Who is the system meant for?

a. Should the system be designed only for "local use," or is it meant to collect and share with multiple communities, counties, the entire state, neighboring states, national, or even international.

4. What is the current system in place?

a. Is the current or proposed system compatible with other systems employed by EMS providers that may respond to a disaster?

5. How much will the system cost?

a. How much will equipment cost?

b. How much will training cost?

c. How much will maintenance cost?

6. How well will the system work when power supplies, communications systems, or logistical resupply is degraded?

a. What is essential to ensure the smooth functioning of the system under adverse weather considerations?

7. Will the system actually be used in a real disaster if it is substantially different from the day-to-day systems used by responders and clinicians?

THE FUTURE

The Department of Homeland Security Science and Technology Directorate is engaged in developing a suite of emergency-messaging standards to allow emergency responders to share data, despite disparate programs and program developers.[36–38] This suite of standards is the Emergency Data Exchange Language (EDXL), a subset of XML or extensible markup language, and it consists of a format for routing the message between networks, a standardized vocabulary, and a standardized message format. Currently developed protocols include an alerting protocol (Common Alerting Protocol [CAP]) for exchanging alerts and public warnings, a distribution element (DE) for routing the messages along multiple warning systems, a hospital availability exchange (HAVE) for sharing hospital capacity and resources, and resource messaging (RM) for exchanging requests and availability of equipment, supplies, personnel, and logistics. Planned modules include situation reporting (Sit-Rep) for exchanging information about the incident from multiple sources to form the basis for management and decision making, and tracking of emergency patients (TEP) for tracking and updating information on location, condition, care, and notifications of family of patients in the disaster. The current HAVE module was extensively tested during the 2010 Haiti Earthquake.[39] These proposed data exchange standards will allow programs by different software developers to communicate with each other and allow disparate units in a widespread disaster to exchange data when patients cross jurisdictional boundaries.

Both bar codes and RFID are generally unable to record information, which means that they simply have a unique identification number for the patient and do not have any further information about the specific patient data such as initial location or treatment rendered. The United States Department of Defense has been experimenting with "electronic dog tags" that both incorporate an RFID for rapid unique identification of the patient and a readily readable memory chip to contain data about patient identification, treatment, and condition. The U.S. Navy has fielded a wearable plastic tag with an imbedded electronic chip that stores individual medical data, a palm-sized scanner that electronically reads and writes to the chip, and a central server that collects the database.[40] The United States Army has a similar project using simple USB technology.[41] These smart-card "dog tags" allow data to be carried with the patient, rather than as a network. Use of small automated patient monitoring devices such as the Mobile Medical Monitor (M3) can provide automated data transmission of vital signs, linked to the patient's RFID.[42] These electronic dog tags have been successfully used for troops evacuated from battlefield in Afghanistan and Iraq through hospitals in Europe to the United States in Navy tests.

The addition of global positioning data to the electronic tracking records will assist researchers in determining the spot where a specific patient was found during the disaster for later incident reconstruction.

An interesting alternative technology for tracking patients within a hospital has been proposed by a former air traffic controller (ATC) who became a physician. The ATC tracking procedure uses a simple tactile process with informational strips representing each aircraft or patient that are held in bays representing each stage of flight to prioritize and manage aircraft (or patients). The strips can be easily reordered within the bay to reflect changing conditions of the patient.[43–45]

⚠ PITFALLS

- When there is no means of linking identification of patients or casualties with a unique identification number, tracking systems either lose all possible privacy and security or become quite difficult.
  - Is the unique patient identification number really unique? Are you sure and how can you determine that?
    - Numbering systems or tag numbers may be duplicated. This can also occur when different agencies respond to the disaster and bring nonunique numbered tags to the disaster. This will totally confuse efforts at tracking patients.
    - Surveyor's tape, light sticks, and aluminum tags do not allow the triage officer a ready system of counting patient numbers nor allow for numbered patient tracking. Another mechanism will be needed to provide this information.
    - Multiple triage tag designs may be used in the same incident, resulting in confusion for providers at all levels.[46,47] This can occur when different agencies respond to the disaster and bring their own tags. Although states may have standardized triage tags within the state, when large-scale disasters occur, bordering state EMS agencies may respond.
  - There may be insufficient quantities of tracking tags or supplies for the mass-casualty event that may occur in a large disaster. This was the case during the early phases of the Tokyo Sarin Attack and the 9/11 World Trade Center Attack and during response to the Haiti Earthquake, Hurricane Katrina, and the Japanese Earthquake and Tsunami.
- Multiple entry points exist for casualties into the system. As was apparent in the Tokyo Sarin Attack, casualties often do not wait for a triage officer and ambulance before they seek medical care. The robust tracking system must be able to account for these patients as they progress through the system.
  - How do you handle patients who show up at a clinic or alternate treatment center without EMS involvement?
  - What are you going to do about the unconscious patient who does not have identification? (Females frequently have ID only in a purse that is easily separated from the patient during adverse conditions.)
- Failure to update the tracking model to reflect a changed destination can occur, which happens when ambulances are diverted from one

facility to another. When this occurs, finding a patient can become quite difficult if multiple hospitals or receiving facilities are involved in the disaster. Manual tracking systems are often unable to accommodate these changes.

- Inability to gracefully degrade or back up an electronic system can occur. Battery life for electronic devices is limited. When power supplies and batteries run out, electronic systems will fail. Tracking officers should have a current paper back-up system readily available and should have hard-copy printouts of the current patient load prepared at set intervals. When power supplies fail, these hard-copy editions can gracefully assume the load without complete degradation of the tracking system.

- Given the difficulties ensuring that victim destinations are recorded during transport to hospitals, it is likely in many cases that these data will have to be collected retrospectively after transport has occurred.

- Placing more than minimal burdens on providers for data entry substantially increases the likelihood that tracking systems will not be used properly or at all in a disaster. Important questions revolve around how complex the data entry is and how long the EMS provider will spend doing this data entry.[35]
  - How long will it take to train the operator in data entry?
  - Can the device be used in a moving vehicle?

- Several systems discussed in this chapter use electronic communications on radio frequencies that are easily jammed or rely on the Internet for communication. Because communications in a disaster are often casualties of the disaster themselves, the wise tracking officer must plan for this contingency and have a simpler back-up system available.
  - How are you going to transition from electronic data entry or management to paper data entry or management when the electronic system degrades from communication or power failures?
  - Does the system depend on satellite communication, which is both expensive to use and not frequently found?
  - Does the system depend on cellular telephones, computer Internet interface, or Wi-Fi, which may be inoperable in a widespread disaster such as those in Haiti or Japan? (For both of these disasters, both cellular and Internet communications were inoperable for days after the disaster. Wi-Fi without Internet is very short-range communication.)

- Remember that system reliability is often inversely proportional to the sophistication of the device or system under stress.

- In large-scale disasters, data transmission rates can adversely affect tracking systems. It is important to assess how the system handles data transmission degradation, and ask if the system degrades by slowing all data or if it degrades by filtering data for critical data priority.

- Power supplies can be a critical point of failure for electronic tracking systems. Key considerations include:
  - Batteries may not be readily available if nonstandard size is required.
  - Where will the recharging of rechargeable batteries occur? How long will it take, and what is the battery life between recharge with heavy use?
  - Will special power supply filters be needed for generator power? How would you handle extended power outages such as those that occurred after Hurricane Katrina?

REFERENCES

1. Waeckerle JF. Domestic preparedness for events involving weapons of mass destruction. *JAMA*. 2000;283(2):252–254.
2. Noji EK. Disaster epidemiology. *Emerg Med Clin North Am*. May 1996;14 (2):289–300.
3. The Star-Tribune staff. Big highway accident occurs on I-80. *Casper Star-Tribune*. August 20, 2004.
4. Guttenberg MG, Asaeda G, Cherson A, et al. Utilization of ambulance resources at the World Trade Center: implications for disaster planning. *Ann Emerg Med*. 2002;40(S92)[ACEP Poster Presentation].
5. Auf der Heide E. Principles of hospital disaster planning. In: Hogan D, Burstein JL, eds. *Disaster Medicine*. Philadelphia: Lippincott, Williams & Wilkins; 2002:57–89.
6. Auf der Heide E. *Disaster Response: Principles of Preparation and Coordination*. CV Mosby: St. Louis; 1989.
7. Hodgetts TJ, Mackaway-Jones K, eds. *Major Incident Medical Management and Support, The Practical Approach*. Plymouth, UK: BMJ Publishing Group; 1995.
8. Dernacoeur K. *Disasters: Tag, You're It!* 4-5, *Spartenburg EMS Newsletter*; 2003. http://www.spartanburgems.com/Newsletter/On The Street-Jan-03 .pdf, Accessed 17 December 2013.
9. Vayer JS, Ten Eyck RP, Cowan ML. New concepts in triage. *Ann Emerg Med*. Aug 1986;15(8):927–930.
10. Mac Mahon AG. Sorting out triage in urban disasters. *S Afr Med J*. 1985;67 (14):555–556.
11. Knotts KE, Etengoff S, Barber K, Golden IJ. Casualty collection in mass-casualty incidents: a better method for finding proverbial needles in a haystack. *Prehosp Disaster Med*. Nov-Dec 2006;21(6):459–464.
12. Coupland RM, Parker PJ, Gray RC. Triage of war wounded: the experience of the International Committee of the Red Cross. *Injury*. 1992;23 (8):507–510.
13. Beyersdorf SR, Nania JN, Luna GK. Community medical response to the Fairchild mass casualty event. *Am J Surg*. May 1996;171(5):467–470.
14. Kerns DE, Anderson PB. EMS response to a major aircraft incident: Sioux City, Iowa. *Prehospital Disaster Med*. 1990;5(02):159–166.
15. Plischke M, Wolf KH, Lison T, Pretschner DP. Telemedical support of prehospital emergency care in mass casualty incidents. *Eur J Med Res*. 1999;4 (9):394–398.
16. McKinsey & Company. The McKinsey Report—Increasing FDNY's Preparedness. New York, NY: McKinsey & Company: http://www.nyc.gov/ html/fdny/html/mck_report/toc.html. Accessed 17 December 2013.
17. Orr SM, Robinson WA. The Hyatt Regency skywalk collapse: an EMS-based disaster response. *Ann Emerg Med*. Oct 1983;12(10):601–605.
18. Lenert LA, Kirsh D, Griswold WG, et al. Design and evaluation of a wireless electronic health records system for field care in mass casualty settings. *J Am Med Inform Assoc*. Nov-Dec 2011;18(6):842–852.
19. Lenert LA, Palmer DA, Chan TC, Rao R. *An Intelligent 802.11 Triage Tag for medical response to disasters*. AMIA . . . *Annual Symposium Proceedings/ AMIA Symposium*. *AMIA Symposium*. 2005, 440–444.
20. Ingrassia PL, Carenzo L, Barra FL, et al. Data collection in a live mass casualty incident simulation: automated RFID technology versus manually recorded system. *Eur J Emerg Med*. Feb 2012;19(1):35–39.
21. Buono C, Huang R, Brown S, Chan TC, Killeen J, Lenert L. *Role-tailored software systems for coordinating care at disaster sites: enhancing collaboration between the base hospitals with the field*. AMIA . . . *Annual Symposium Proceedings/AMIA Symposium*. *AMIA Symposium*. 2006, 867.
22. Alm AM, Gao T, White DM. *Pervasive patient tracking for mass casualty incident response*. AMIA . . . *Annual Symposium proceedings/AMIA Symposium*. *AMIA Symposium*. 2006, 842.
23. Killeen JP, Chan TC, Buono C, Griswold WG, Lenert LA. *A wireless first responder handheld device for rapid triage, patient assessment and documentation during mass casualty incidents*. AMIA . . . *Annual Symposium Proceedings/AMIA Symposium*. *AMIA Symposium*. 2006, 429-433.
24. Transcom Regulating and Command & Control Evacuation System (TRAC2ES). 2000. http://www.dote.osd.mil/pub/reports/FY2000/airforce/ 00trac2es.html. Accessed 13 December 2013.
25. American Red Cross. Safe and Well. 2013; https://safeandwell.communityos .org/cms/index.php. Accessed 13 December, 2013.
26. Gadh R, Prabhu BS. Radio frequency identification of Hurricane Katrina victims. *Signal Processing Magazine, IEEE*. 2006;23(2):184.
27. Fry EA, Lenert LA. *MASCAL: RFID tracking of patients, staff and equipment to enhance hospital response to mass casualty events*. AMIA . . . *Annual Symposium Proceedings/AMIA Symposium*. *AMIA Symposium*. 2005, 261–265.

28. Shamdani AN, Nicolai BJ. *Applications of RFID in Incident Management. The Seventh International Multi-Conference on Computing in the Global Information Technology.* 2012, Venice, IT.

29. Bouman JH, Schouwerwou RJ, Van der Eijk KJ, van Leusden AJ, Savelkoul TJ. Computerization of patient tracking and tracing during mass casualty incidents. *Eur J Emerg Med.* Sep 2000;7(3):211–216.

30. Noordergraaf GJ, Bouman JH, van den Brink EJ, van de Pompe C, Savelkoul TJ. Development of computer-assisted patient control for use in the hospital setting during mass casualty incidents. *Am J Emerg Med.* May 1996;14(3):257–261.

31. Hamilton J. Automated MCI, patient tracking: managing mass casualty chaos via the Internet. *JEMS.* Apr 2003;28(4):52–56.

32. Marres GM, Taal L, Bemelman M, Bouman J, Leenen LP. Online Victim Tracking and Tracing System (ViTTS) for Major Incident Casualties. *Prehosp Disaster Med.* Oct 2013;28(5):445–453.

33. Yuh-Wen C, Guan-Jie W, Tzung-Hung L, et al. *A RFID model of transferring and tracking trauma patients after a large disaster. Paper presented at: Service Operations, Logistics and Informatics, 2009.* 2009, SOLI '09. IEEE/INFORMS International Conference on; 22-24 July 2009.

34. Jokela J, Radestad M, Gryth D, et al. Increased situation awareness in major incidents—radio frequency identification (RFID) technique: a promising tool. *Prehosp Disaster Med.* Feb 2012;27(1):81–87.

35. Chan TC, Griswold WG, Buono C, et al. Impact of Wireless Electronic Medical Record System on the Quality of Patient Documentation by Emergency Field Responders during a Disaster Mass-Casualty Exercise. *Prehosp Disaster Med.* Jul-Aug 2011;26(4):268–275.

36. OASIS. *OASIS Emergency Interoperability EDXL Product Directory.* Organization for the Advancement of Structured Information Standards (OASIS); 2013.

37. Gusty D. *Emergency Data Exchange Language Overview*; 2010, http://www.fema.gov/media-library-data/20130726-1732-25045-5898/100317edxl_niembrief.pdf, Accessed 13 December 2013.

38. DHS Science and Technology Directorate. Emergency Data Exchange Language Suite of Standards. 2012. http://www.dhs.gov/sites/default/files/publications/Emergency%20Data%20Exchange%20Language%20Suite%20of%20Standards-508.pdf. Accessed 13 Dec 2013.

39. Operational Deployment of EDXL-HAVE—Recording. 2010. http://docs.oasis-open.org/emergency/edxl-tep/v1.0/edxl-tep-v1.0.html. Accessed 13 December 2013.

40. Clark D. *Smart Military Medical "Dog Tags"*; 2011. http://www.technet.pnnl.gov/sensors/electronics/projects/ES4rfT-DogTag.stm, Accessed 15 December, 2013.

41. Electronic Information Carrier (EIC). http://www.tatrc.org/projects_eic.html. Accessed 15 December, 2013.

42. Deniston WM, Konoske PJ, Pugh WM. *Mobile medical monitoring at forward areas of care (report).* Naval Health Research Center Medical Information Systems and Operations Research Department: San Diego, CA; 1998.

43. Hoskins JD, Graham RF, Robinson DR, Lutz CC, Folio LR. Mass casualty tracking with air traffic control methodologies. *J Am Coll Surg.* Jun 2009;208(6):1001–1008.

44. Graham RF, Hoskins JD, Cortijo MP, Barbee GA, Folio LR, Lutz CC. A casualty tracking system modeled after air traffic control methodology employed in a combat support hospital in Iraq. *Mil Med.* Mar 2011;176(3):244–245.

45. Hoskins JD, Graham RF, Robinson DR, Lutz CC, Folio LR. Mass casualty tracking with air traffic control methodologies. *J Am Coll Surg.* Jun 2009;208(6):1001–1008.

46. Paschen HR. High speed train crash at Eschede. *Trauma Care.* 1999;9:68–89.

47. Coping with the early stages of the M1 disaster: at the scene and on arrival at hospital. Staff of the accident and emergency departments of Derbyshire Royal Infirmary, Leicester Royal Infirmary, and Queen's Medical Centre, Nottingham. *BMJ.* Mar 11 1989;298(6674):651–654.

CHAPTER 56

Infectious Disease in a Disaster Zone

Stephanie Chow Garbern

In the wake of natural and human-made disasters, displaced populations, often living in overcrowded shelters with disrupted access to clean drinking water, proper sanitation systems, and adequate medical services, face conditions conducive to the rapid spread of infectious diseases. In some instances, morbidity and mortality from infectious disease in disaster zones may be even greater than that caused by the direct impact of the disaster itself. Recognizing, controlling, and treating infectious disease outbreaks in these settings has challenged the ingenuity of many health care workers since the beginning of human civilization and will continue to do so in the future. The purpose of this chapter is to provide a framework that physicians involved in disaster relief may use to aid the prevention, identification, and control of infectious disease in disaster zones.

The World Health Organization (WHO) defines a disaster as a catastrophic situation or event that overwhelms a community's local capacity, necessitating external assistance.[1] Some examples of human-made and natural disasters include war, industrial accidents, hurricanes, tsunamis, floods, and earthquakes. Floods are the most common natural disaster worldwide, accounting for 40% of all natural disasters.[2] Populations affected by floods are at a particularly high risk for infectious diseases because of the difficulty in obtaining clean, potable water as well as the increased prevalence of vector-borne diseases that thrive in damp, crowded conditions. With increasing globalization, victims of a disaster may turn up in emergency departments hundreds of miles from the original site.

Infectious disease outbreaks may occur days, weeks, or even months after the initial disaster. It is important to realize that the conditions experienced in disaster zones are generally not new diseases but preexisting endemic diseases that become uncontrolled after disruption in community structures, including the following[3]:

- Disruption in water supply and sewage disposal: diarrheal illnesses (e.g., cholera, shigella, and *Escherichia coli* infections)
- Displaced populations and overcrowding: respiratory infections (e.g., measles, influenza, pneumonia)
- Disruption in ecological systems: vector-borne diseases (e.g., malaria, dengue fever, typhoid fever)
- Diseases from trauma and reconstruction activities: skin and soft tissue infections (e.g., tetanus, methicillin-resistant *Staphylococcus aureus* [MRSA])[3]

The capability of a health system to tackle a potential disaster can be defined by its vulnerability, which reflects its level of exposure to risk, shock, and stress.[4] A community may be more vulnerable because of poverty, gender, age, ethnicity, comorbid conditions such as HIV/AIDS and malnutrition, or religious identity. Exposure to warfare, destruction of property, and direct attempts to undermine care to the afflicted may also make a system less functional. The ability to handle such factors may be referred to as resilience, or the ability to recover from adversity.[4] Resilience can be increased, and vulnerability lessened, with disaster preparedness planning and appropriate external support.

HISTORICAL PERSPECTIVE

History provides numerous examples of war and natural disasters resulting in widespread infection and mortality. In 31 BC, Marc Antony stationed his army, estimated at 30,000 men, on the hills above the marsh-bound city of Actium, Greece, in preparation for his invasion of Italy. Octavian, his rival, quickly encircled the city and camp on both land and sea, preventing supply wagons from entering and diverting the city's supply of freshwater. Such tactics sent the soldiers and the people of Actium into the mosquito-infested swamps to find nourishment. Within 30 days, Antony had lost more than one third of his army to disease and malnutrition, and Octavian soon became Augustus Caesar. As recently as the twentieth century, army commanders expected to lose more soldiers from infectious diseases than from combat. Although widespread infectious diseases may have been simply part of life in the preindustrialized world, we now have the knowledge and capability to prevent such epidemics. Nevertheless, hundreds of thousands still die annually because of lack of appropriate planning and sufficient resources during and after major disasters.

On January 12, 2010, Haiti, the poorest country of the Western hemisphere, experienced one of the most devastating natural disasters in recent history. A 7.0 Richter-scale earthquake whose epicenter was located in close proximity to the densely populated capital and economic center of Port-au-Prince caused over 200,000 deaths and left over 1 million people homeless.[5] Approximately 30,000 of the postquake deaths were due to infectious diseases from infected wounds, pneumonia, and diarrheal illnesses such as cholera.[5] Examples such as this are evidence of the havoc that disasters can still inflict on humanity.

Diarrheal illnesses are widespread in disaster settlements and can cause significant mortality. After the 2010 earthquake in Haiti, a cholera epidemic developed in the Artibonite department with over 100,000 cases reported and more than 1100 deaths.[6] Cholera had been virtually nonexistent in Haiti before the quake, but became epidemic 9 months afterward because of inadequate water supplies and sewage disposal.[5] The initial case fatality rate from patients during the epidemic was strikingly high at 6.4% but improved to less than 1% with subsequent increases in cholera treatment centers, oral rehydration points, and preventive education messages.[3,8] Studies of refugee settlements have estimated that up to 40% of deaths are attributable to diarrheal illnesses and account for more than 80% of deaths in children less than 2 years old.[7] In Bangladesh, a country that experiences frequent flooding, a study analyzing water samples from taps, ponds, and wells after a storm found that 33% of samples were contaminated with *Vibrio cholerae*. Reports of outbreaks of viral hepatitis A and E were also reported in communities in Banda Aceh, Indonesia, after the 2004 Indian Ocean tsunami and were attributed to inadequate sewage and sanitation systems.[3]

Acute respiratory infections (ARIs) such as viral upper respiratory infections (URIs), influenza, tuberculosis, and pneumonia also rapidly spread in enclosed, poorly ventilated, overcrowded refugee shelters after disasters. After the 2004 Indian Ocean tsunami, respiratory infections were the most common infectious disease found in refugee settlements, with 27.8% of people receiving medical care for respiratory problems during the first 2 weeks after the tsunami. The high incidence of respiratory illnesses was thought to be due to dusty living conditions and overcrowding.[3]

Skin and soft tissue infections are common, often due to contamination of traumatic wounds sustained in the immediate postdisaster period. Tetanus emerged as a serious problem after the 2004 Indian Ocean tsunami among the largely unvaccinated population in Banda Aceh, with 106 patients admitted to hospitals between December 2004 and January 2005 and an 18% case fatality rate.[9] Vibrio and MRSA infections were also reported among victims of Hurricane Katrina.[10]

Increased prevalence of vector-borne diseases after disasters has been well described in the literature. Vectors such as mosquitos, flies, lice, mites, and rodents quickly multiply in crowded settlements. In 1997, a prolonged drought struck the Australasian region of Indonesia; a retrospective investigation revealed that increased standing water and food shortages resulted in a substantial movement of highland populations with low immunity to Plasmodium falciparum to low-lying coastal regions, which led to numerous deaths due to malaria. Subsequent evaporation of stream beds and mass antimalarial drug distribution resulted in a sharp decline in mortality.[11] Moreover, during massive flooding in Brazil in 2008, 57,010 cases of dengue fever were reported, thought to be due to disruption in water supplies and solid waste management services.[12]

A study in 2012 reviewing the major natural disasters during the years 2000-2011 found that the key risk factors for communicable diseases were population displacement from nonendemic to endemic areas, overcrowding, stagnant water, insufficient or contaminated water and poor sanitation, high exposure to disease vectors, insufficient nutrient intake, low vaccination coverage, and injuries.[3]

Even industrialized nations are not impervious to infectious disease outbreaks. Hurricane Katrina hit the Gulf Coast of the United States on August 29, 2005, forcing the displacement of over 1 million people. Federal, state, and local health departments deployed medical teams and implemented infectious disease surveillance in evacuation shelters. Despite these efforts, more than 1000 cases of norovirus emerged over a period of 11 days in the Reliant Park Complex mega-shelter housing more than 27,000 people in Houston, Texas.[13] Although the norovirus outbreak was the only communicable disease outbreak reported in the aftermath of Hurricane Katrina, the outbreak serves a reminder of the difficulty of containing infectious diseases even in settings with advanced medical resources.[14]

CURRENT PRACTICE

Today's disaster response encompasses a large scope of actions to prevent and control the spread of infectious diseases. Described below are some of the key practices that must be followed to prevent and control infectious diseases in any disaster response effort. A widely used resource for relief workers is the Sphere Handbook, *Humanitarian Charter and Minimum Standards in Humanitarian Response*, which details necessary interventions in living conditions to reduce the spread of diseases caused by crowding, unsafe water, and inadequate sewage.[14] These interventions include the following:

- *Identification and maintenance of clean and adequate water supply.* Providing continuous, adequate amounts of clean water is essential to the prevention of the spread of pathogens via the fecal-oral route, such as noroviruses and *V. cholerae*. Sources of water vary, depending on the geography and resources of the region, but generally come from surface water (lakes, ponds, rivers) or groundwater (wells, springs). Early involvement of sanitation and water supply engineers is essential for identification of water sources of acceptable quality and proximity to dwellings to ensure adequate water for cooking, drinking, and basic personal hygiene. Sanitary inspection of the water source is done to assess water quality (optimally, 0 to 10 fecal coliforms per 100 mL of water) using a field test kit or a local laboratory.[15] Most commonly, water is distributed to large groups via a handpump or piped distribution method. If water treatment is needed, chlorination is the most effective method of disinfection, and water safety can be measured by determining the level of chlorination at the point of water collection or even in the bucket used for water collection (adequate levels are >1.0 mg/L of chlorine).[16] Relief efforts often dispense water collection containers to households to encourage safe water usage and storage.[14]

- *Proper sanitation and sewage disposal.* Usage of containment facilities for excreta, such as latrines, has been shown to offer the greatest protection from diarrheal illness over any other form of intervention.[16] In the immediate phase (hours to days) after a disaster, trenches or open-defecation fields located downhill from settlements and away from water sources may be used until latrines have been constructed.[16] Latrine construction is undertaken by sanitation engineers, aid workers, and community members to ensure they will be used by all members of the community. Failure to involve community members in the development of sanitation facilities will often result in people using alternative areas for fecal and solid waste disposal. increasing the risk of contamination of food and water supplies.[16] Special consideration should be given to the needs of women and girls as they face risk of assault if facilities are not placed in safe locations.[16] Per Sphere guidelines, latrines should be shared by no more than 20 people, located conveniently near dwellings (so they may be used at any time of day), and comfortable and culturally appropriate (designed by community, segregated by gender or family).[14] Pit latrines—the most commonly used type of latrine in disaster relief—must be located >30 m from any groundwater source.[16] Education is essential for the community to accept usage of latrines as well as to ensure handwashing afterward.[14]

- *Overcrowding prevention.* Overcrowding and poor ventilation lead to spread of respiratory-borne illnesses such as measles and influenza. Housing construction and settlement planning should ensure that every person has at least 3.5 m^2 of living space. Dwellings should be constructed in a way that reduces the amount of smoke exposure from cooking fires.

- *Vector control.* Assessment of populations' underlying immunity and possible exposure to vector-borne diseases should be carried out with the help of local governments and aid organizations to identify risk factors that may be mitigated. Vector control includes reduction of vector breeding environments as well as personal protection for individuals. Mosquito breeding sites such as standing pools of water can be eliminated by draining or filling.[16] Water storage containers may become vector breeding sites, so containers with lids should be provided.[14] Populations at high risk for malaria and mosquito-borne diseases may receive mosquito nets and mosquito repellants to limit exposure. Chemical insecticides are only used when environmental controls are insufficient.[16] Options include larvicides (destruction of eggs and larvae) applied to breeding sites, indoor residual spraying (spraying of long-lasting insecticide to walls of dwelling), insecticide-treated mosquito nets, and outdoor space spraying (reserved for situations in which large numbers of vectors must be eliminated quickly).[16] Proper disposal of solid waste and sewage (see above) will also reduce possible breeding sites of insects and rodents. Controlling rodent-borne diseases includes storing food in rodent-proof containers and containing solid waste so these areas do not become breeding grounds. Usage of traps and rodenticide is less effective and can be dangerous, especially in settlements with many children.[16] Control of lice and mites includes laundering the entire household's bedding in hot water, delousing with insecticides, and regularly airing bedding.[16,15] The appropriate vector control measures are undertaken with the assistance of national and international vector control experts.

- *Personal hygiene.* Education is the most important step in ensuring personal hygiene. Community members are enlisted to assist with culturally appropriate hygiene promotion, as well as educating the public on disease transmission and prevention.[16] Handwashing facilities with soap and water should be readily available and usage encouraged after using latrines, before cooking, and for prevention of the spread of respiratory illnesses. Basic hygiene provisions include at least 250 g of bathing soap and 250 g of laundry soap per person per month, as well as sanitary materials for women to use during menstruation.[14]
- *Wound care.* Wounds from injuries due to the disaster itself (lacerations, amputations) as well as those sustained during reconstruction and cleanup efforts should be addressed by trained health workers familiar with proper cleaning and dressing of wounds. Basic first aid should be readily available at easily accessible local health units. Tetanus vaccines should be administered to anyone with dirty wounds or those at high risk from working in rescue or cleanup activities.[14]

Disaster preparedness and response to infectious disease outbreaks generally occur at multiple levels—local, state, federal, and international. Local and state agencies play the main role in the response to disasters by performing situation assessment, organizing emergency medical services, obtaining fire department and law enforcement involvement, assigning and deploying resources, collecting data, and contacting federal and other agencies when assistance is needed.[17] The Federal Emergency Management Agency (FEMA) works only at the request of a state government to assist with large disasters.[17] The Centers for Disease Control and Prevention (CDC) also serves as the lead federal agency for disease surveillance and epidemic response.[18] Several departments within the CDC work together to quickly assess an outbreak and prevent its spread. The Health Alert Network (HAN) is the primary method of quickly conveying information regarding urgent public health incidents among federal, state, and local health practitioners as well as public health laboratories.[19] A rapid response team is sent to investigate, confirm the presence of infectious disease, and assist in the control of the outbreak. The Laboratory Response Network (LRN) provides laboratory testing, identification, and creation of effective treatment protocols. The National Electronic Disease Surveillance System (NEDSS) enters, updates, and electronically transmits demographic disease data to allow rapid reporting of disease trends in an effort to prevent outbreaks.[20]

The Strategic National Stockpile (SNS) program is a repository of antibiotics, antidotes, antitoxins, life support medications, and other medical and surgical supplies that may supplement and supply state and local health agencies in the event of an infectious disease outbreak.[21] The SNS may be deployed once the affected state has requested assistance from the CDC. Initial deployment consists of "push packages," which are caches of pharmaceuticals, antidotes, and medical

supplies designed to address a variety of agents and ready for delivery anywhere in the continental United States within 12 hours; however, the actual delivery time of these essential supplies may be delayed considerably by disruptions in transportation systems. Although not a first-response tool, the National Pharmaceutical Stockpile (NPS) may be needed to augment state and local agency supplies. If additional resources are needed, followup vendor-managed inventory supplies can be provided within 24 to 36 hours and can be tailored to the specific needs of the state.

As an operational organization of the United Nations, WHO acts as the directing and coordinating authority on all international health activity.[22] WHO provides immediate care anywhere in the world when disaster and infectious disease have overrun the local resources of a country. In 2003 a devastating earthquake shook the city of Bam in Iran, killing as many as 30,000 people. With most hospital and health centers destroyed and approximately 80% of all buildings damaged, local and neighboring health facilities were overwhelmed by the needs of the 100,000 residents of the Bam area. WHO completed a rapid health assessment and immediately became involved in the provision of food, clothing, sanitation, and medical supplies.[23] Their surveillance systems have also documented infectious diseases and further morbidity and mortality in the area. Weekly assessments available to the public on the WHO website allowed for identification of potential outbreaks and better allocation of resources to areas of need. Three weeks after the earthquake, there were no new outbreaks of disease and the incidence of diarrhea and other infectious diseases returned to predisaster levels.[23]

Numerous international humanitarian organizations exist to provide rapid assistance in preventing and controlling infectious disease outbreaks in disaster zones. Well-established humanitarian organizations that respond to disasters worldwide include the International Committee of the Red Cross (ICRC) and Médecins Sans Frontières (MSF). National Red Cross societies exist in 178 countries, providing local care and international aid if requested by the ICRC. The mission of the ICRC is to "protect the lives and dignity of victims of war and internal violence and to provide them with assistance."[24] MSF was established to provide international emergency medical care, with its volunteers often being deployed to the most remote and unstable parts of the world to provide care to victims of both human-made and natural disasters. They can provide medical or surgical care, nutrition, sanitation, and local health training quickly and efficiently throughout the world. MSF was awarded the Nobel Peace Prize in 1999 for its efforts in emergency medical care.[25] These and many other organizations often work together with the United Nations and WHO to provide care in complex humanitarian emergencies.

Countries with proper disaster management strategies in place are likely to be the most resilient when faced with a disaster, both during and immediately after. The Great East Japan (Tohoku) earthquake of March 2011 was one of the strongest recorded earthquakes in the history of Japan. Whereas the tremors themselves created relatively little damage, the subsequent massive tsunamis, as well as the infamous Fukushima nuclear power plant malfunction, created havoc, displacing more than 400,000 people from the northwest region of Japan.[26] There were no significant infectious disease outbreaks recorded despite this huge population displacement.[27] This result is attributable to the timely and planned response of well-trained medical and public health personnel, rapid distribution of supplies to the victims of the disaster, and an advanced disease surveillance system that enabled daily surveillance for outbreak detection in 40 large evacuation centers, as well as education on basic hygiene.[28]

Disease surveillance and the investigation of early signs of disease are essential to preventing infectious disease outbreaks from becoming epidemics. Large-scale monitoring systems must be instituted at the initiation of a disaster response to recognize infectious diseases and to identify sources of diseases. After the 2010 Haiti earthquake, MSF conducted public health surveillance through data collection on patient visits at MSF-run outpatient sentinel sites. Acute respiratory infections and diarrheal illnesses were among the most common causes for visits, but the surveillance system also was designed to generate alerts for suspicious clusters of diseases. This alert system allowed MSF to identify a cluster of acute jaundice cases as being caused by an outbreak of hepatitis A.[29]

Vaccination in disaster settings has also been used with promising results in several situations. Measles vaccinations have been shown to be a cost-effective intervention in refugee settings. A 2013 trial of distribution of a cholera vaccine in the Mae La refugee camp in Thailand housing ethnic Karen refugees from Burma showed some early success—as of 2014, no additional cases of cholera had been reported.[8] Further research into the efficacy of vaccine campaigns in other disaster zones is required to evaluate for possible roles for influenza, hepatitis, and tetanus.

The importance of informing and mobilizing the public cannot be overemphasized. Television, radio, cell phones, and the Internet can disseminate vital information from local, state, and federal agencies to large numbers of people in a short amount of time. Public health campaigns to educate people on the importance of hygiene, clean water, and routes of transmission of infections can decrease the spread of diarrheal illnesses as well as sexually transmitted infections.[7]

Infectious diseases in disaster zones are a preventable cause of significant morbidity and mortality in communities already facing devastating losses. Natural disasters may be unavoidable, but we can reduce further calamity by improving epidemic preparedness. By installing effective surveillance systems to track infectious disease incidence; ensuring basic standards of water safety, sanitation, and living conditions; and providing multidisciplinary rapid response personnel including public health workers, medical professionals, and sanitation engineers, we have shown we can effectively tackle even overwhelming challenges. As evidenced by the overwhelming worldwide humanitarian responses to the 2004 Indian Ocean tsunami and the 2010 Haiti earthquake, steady progress is being made toward controlling disease in areas where this was once considered an impossibility.

! PITFALLS

Although many local and international agencies are available to respond to disasters with strategies to quickly bring personnel and stockpiled supplies, limitations still exist. Remote locations in heavily forested or mountainous regions may lack roads or landing sites from which to deploy large-scale response services. War and civil unrest often prevent aid from reaching communities in need. Some areas may be so dangerous that international agencies will not deploy relief workers, or they may be recalled for fear of injury or death, as seen in the MSF withdrawal from Darfur, Sudan, in 2009 and from Somalia in 2013.[17,30] Some governments may even refuse help when offered because of political or personal motives. Some disaster response efforts have neglected the importance of involving sanitation and civil engineers in planning strategies for adequate water supply and sewage disposal and are then faced with problems with water shortages, contaminated water or inadequate living conditions.

Children and elderly people are often the most vulnerable after a disaster. In developing regions, children are dependent on their caretakers for both food and safety and have poor immunity to endemic diseases. The elderly may be marginalized and often have preexisting comorbidities that leave them less likely to be able to mount appropriate immune responses to infectious diseases. People who are malnourished are also less capable of mounting an adequate immune response to infectious diseases if they become infected. Such fragility requires special attention to these populations so that they do not succumb to infectious diseases after a disaster.

REFERENCES

1. World Health Organization. Emergency Health Training Programme for Africa. Available at: http://www.who.int/disasters/repo/5506.pdf.
2. Watkins RR. Gastrointestinal infections in the setting of natural disasters. *Curr Infect Dis Rep.* 2012;1:47–52.
3. Kouadio IK, Aljunid S, Kamigaki T, et al. Infectious disease following natural disasters: prevention and control measures. *Expert Rev Anti Infect Ther.* 2012;10:95–104.
4. Chambers R. Vulnerability, coping and policy. *IDS Bull.* 2006;37:33–40.
5. Pan American Health Organization. *Special report: update on the health response to the earthquake in Haiti*; February 9, 2010. Available at: http://www.paho.org/disasters/index.php?option=com_content&view=article&id=1099&Itemid=0&lang=en.
6. Abrams JY, Copeland JR, Tauxe RV, et al. Real-time modeling used for outbreak management during a cholera epidemic, Haiti, 2010–2011. *Epidemiol Infect.* 2012;1:1–10.
7. Connolly MA, Gayer M, Ryan MJ, et al. Communicable diseases in complex emergencies: impact and challenges. *Lancet.* 2004;364:1974–1983.
8. Phares CR, Ortega L. Refugee health and cholera vaccine. *Clin Infect Dis.* 2014;58(1):iv–v.
9. World Health Organization. Epidemic-prone disease surveillance and response after the tsunami in Aceh Province, Indonesia. *Wkly Epidemiol Rec.* 2005;80:160–164.
10. Ivers LC, Ryan ET. Infectious diseases of severe weather-related and flood-related natural disasters. *Curr Opin Infect Dis.* 2006;19(5):408–414.
11. Bangs MJ, Subianto DB. El Nino and associated outbreaks of severe malaria in highland populations in Irian Jaya, Indonesia: a review and epidemiological perspective. *Southeast Asia J Trop Med Public Health.* 1999;30(4):608–619.
12. World Health Organization. *Dengue/dengue hemorrhagic fever in Brazil*; 2008. Available at: www.who.int/csr/don/2008_04_10/en/index.html.
13. Yee EL, Palacio H, Atmar RL, et al. Widespread outbreak of norovirus gastroenteritis among evacuees of Hurricane Katrina residing in a large "megashelter" in Houston, Texas: lessons learned for prevention. *Clin Infect Dis.* 2007;44(8):1014–1019.
14. Sphere Project. *Sphere Handbook: Humanitarian Charter and Minimum Standards in Disaster Response*; 2011. Available at: http://www.refworld.org/docid/4ed8ae592.html.
15. USAID. *Field Operations Guide for Disaster Assessment and Response. Version 4.0.* United States Agency for International Development; September 2005. Available at: https://scms.usaid.gov/sites/default/files/documents/1866/fog_v4.pdf.
16. Anonymous. Water, sanitation and hygiene in emergencies. In: *Public Health Guide for Emergencies.* 2nd ed The Johns Hopkins and the International Federation of Red Cross and Red Crescent Societies; 2008 Available at: http://www.jhsph.edu/research/centers-and-institutes/center-for-refugee-and-disaster-response/publications_tools/publications/_CRDR_ICRC_Public_Health_Guide_Book/Forward.pdf.
17. Sudan: MSF's International Teams Withdraw from Darfur. Available at: http://www.doctorswithoutborders.org/news/article.cfm?id=3535.
18. National Center for Infectious Disease. *Protecting the nation's health in an era of globalization: CDC's global infectious disease strategy*; 2002. 1–9. Available at: http://www.cdc.gov/globalidplan/4-introduction.htm.
19. Centers for Disease Control and Prevention. Health Alert Network. Available at: http://emergency.cdc.gov/han/.

20. Centers for Disease Control and Prevention. National Notifiable Diseases Surveillance System. Available at: http://wwwn.cdc.gov/nndss/script/nedss.aspx.

21. Centers for Disease Control and Prevention. Strategic National Stockpile. Available at: http://www.cdc.gov/phpr/stockpile/stockpile.htm.

22. World Health Organization. *Basic texts: Constitution of the World Health Organization*; 2006. Available at: http://www.who.int/governance/eb/who_constitution_en.pdf.

23. World Health Organization. Rapid health assessment from Iran earthquake, 27 December 2003. Available at: http://www.who.int/disasters/repo/11635.pdf.

24. International Committee of the Red Cross. Mission statement. Available at: http://www.icrc.org/eng/resources/documents/misc/icrc-mission-190608.htm.

25. Doctors without Borders. What is Doctors without Borders/Médecins Sans Frontières? Available at: http://www.doctorswithoutborders.org/aboutus/index.cfm.

26. Takashi T, Goto M, Yoshida H, et al. Infectious diseases after the 2011 Great East Japan earthquake. *J Exper Clin Med.* 2012;4(1):20–23.

27. Ohkouchi S, Shibuya R, Yanai M, et al. Deterioration in regional health status after the acute phase of a great disaster: respiratory physicians' experiences of the Great East Japan earthquake. *Resp Invest.* 2013;51 (2):50–55.

28. Nohara M. Impact of the Great East Japan earthquake and tsunami on health, medical care and public health systems in Iwate prefecture, Japan 2011. *Western Pac Surv Resp J.* 2011;2(4):1–7.

29. Polonsky J, Luquero F, Francois G, et al. Public health surveillance sfter the 2010 Haiti earthquake: the experience of Médecins Sans Frontières. *PLOS Currents Disasters.* 2013;5.

30. MSF forced to withdraw from Somalia: an in-depth Interview. Available at: http://www.doctorswithoutborders.org/news-stories/video/msf-forced-withdraw-somalia-depth-interview.

Pharmaceuticals and Medical Equipment in Disasters

Charles Stewart and M. Kathleen Stewart

Most disasters create a predictable pattern of public health consequences, though the pattern varies according to the type of disaster.[1] The types of disasters that may be expected and the potential risks that those disasters pose to the community should be outlined in the threat assessment resulting from the Hazard Vulnerability Analysis (HVA) for the local area conducted as a routine part of disaster planning (see Chapter 22 for further information on community-based HVAs). Epidemiologic and surveillance information is critical for determining current and predicted casualties and the amounts and specific types of medical supplies or equipment required.[2] In addition to natural or technological disasters, the threat of domestic and international terrorism involving weapons of mass destruction (WMD) has become an increasing public health concern in the United States and abroad.[3]

Because local resources will not always be sufficient for certain unlikely events such as WMD attacks, or for large-scale disaster response, additional resources can be made available through effective planning with suppliers and local and regional emergency response partners, as well as through agreements with and assistance from regional, state, and federal response organizations.

Equipment and supplies essential to the response capacity of a community can be categorized as follows: direction and control, communications, mass care, and health and medical supplies. Equipment and supplies for health and medical care may be divided into two broad categories. The first category includes the drugs, medical equipment, and supplies necessary for direct patient care. This category also includes provisions for care of routine chronic and acute medical conditions in the local populace in addition to the medical and health needs created by the disaster.

Because pharmacies and medical care clinics may be destroyed, have no power, or lack staff during a disaster, health planners should expect that patients will seek medical care for chronic conditions in acute care hospitals or in any available medical relief setting.[1] If persons with chronic diseases who are medication dependent are unable to access their medications, they may no longer be simply evacuees or survivors of the event, but instead become patients requiring acute medical care. For example, the diabetic patient whose blood sugar is normally under good control, if deprived of his medications, may rapidly decompensate and suffer problems related to high blood sugar.[4,5]

The second category includes the logistical and occupational health supplies used to support emergency workers and facilities. Some examples include portable shelters such as tents, portable water containers, patient stretchers, and personal protective equipment (PPE). The emergency manager must also plan to support uninvited volunteers.

The initial HVA should identify and inventory existing resources, equipment, and supplies essential to health and disaster management.[6] This inventory will help the manager determine what additional supplies are needed, identify storage areas safe from both damage and pilferage, and ensure that perishable stocks do not exceed safe expiration dates. Appropriate management includes inventory of assets and distribution of this inventory to officers authorized to distribute the assets during time of need. Inventory logs should include potential bulk resupply sources and authorization codes, specialized equipment sources, and alternative sources for fuel, oxygen, and other expendable resources. Since transportation routes may be affected by any disaster, experienced emergency managers may include in pre-event planning alternative sources for all items. For example, supplies for southern Illinois usually come from St. Louis, but during the 1993 Midwestern floods, bridges across the Mississippi River were closed for more than 300 miles, so bulk supplies could be procured more quickly from Chicago.

Determining the quantities of medical supplies and pharmaceuticals needed during the initial disaster will depend on several factors including, but not limited to, the specific threat or disaster, availability of medical assets within the community, extent of disruption of the medical and health systems, number of potential and actual patients, clinical treatment or prophylaxis protocols, damage to roads and other transport modalities, damage to communication infrastructure, and time to the recovery phase of the disaster response. Attempts have been made to quantify pharmaceutical stockpiling or evaluate preparedness of emergency departments for a terrorist event involving a chemical nerve agent with 50 to 500 casualties.[7,8] As noted later in this chapter, similar planning can and should occur for natural disasters such as tornados, hurricanes, earthquakes, and ice storms.

In addition to planning for specific threats, the emergency manager should contact the local public health authorities to ascertain the local prevalence of chronic diseases, such as hypertension, diabetes, and chronic obstructive pulmonary disease (COPD). This information can be used to augment supplies of anticipated necessary medicines for shelters and emergency clinics. The need for medications such as antiseizure medications, antihypertensives, tetanus immunizations, and antibiotics, for instance, can be estimated from local incidence rates provided by public health authorities as well as the expected illnesses and injuries from the disaster.

Although the federal government may provide assistance including medical assets and equipment, the local area should not expect that this assistance will arrive until at least 24 hours and perhaps up to 72 hours after a formal request from the state government(s) through the President.[9] International aid often does not arrive for 72 hours or more.[1,10] International requests for field hospitals should be made to the World Health Organization (WHO)/Pan American Health Organization (PAHO).

More and more such plans include planning for vulnerable populations in the disaster area. In the past, inadequate preparation for these vulnerable populations has led to catastrophic consequences and

TABLE 57-1	Health Care Populations to Plan For
POPULATION	**NEEDS**
Victims of the disaster	Needs vary by type of disaster as injuries/illness caused by disaster may range from minor to lethal.
Vulnerable populations	Needs will vary by type of disaster and by vulnerability. Generally includes current hospital patients.
Rescue and health care workers	Rehabilitation, water, food, shelter, immunizations. Some may become victims of the disaster or aftermath.
General population	May include those with chronic illness who are not otherwise "vulnerable." Some may become victims of the disaster or aftermath.
Evacuees/displaced persons	May include vulnerable populations. May include those with chronic illness who are not otherwise "vulnerable." Some may become victims of the disaster or aftermath.

increased death tolls. Regardless of the type of disaster, the planner must recognize that current health problems will persist and may be markedly exacerbated by the ongoing disaster. Such vulnerable populations are listed in Table 57-1.

Water, food, shelter, and effective sewage disposal will be needed for everyone in the affected area.[1] Although provision of such essentials is not often considered as part of the medical response, one only has to look at the Haiti earthquake to note the medical results from their lack.

Provision of critical medical needs is the province of the resource logistics manager. Effective resource logistics management requires several basic actions:

- Determining specific resources required for each group and the amounts required in each area affected by the disaster
- Procuring appropriate amounts of resources prior to an event
- Monitoring expiration dates and rotating stock as needed
- Developing systems to procure additional resources when needed through agreements with suppliers and response partners
- Preparing to receive potentially large amounts of unrequested medical assets
- Having mechanisms to monitor inventory and track resource use and identify potential shortages before they occur
- Identifying a means to transport and distribute resources
- Identifying locations for dispensing pharmaceuticals or other medical assets
- Developing a system for dispensing the medical assets[10]

HISTORICAL PERSPECTIVE

The Homeland Security Act of 2002 and Homeland Security Presidential Directive (HSPD)-5 required the creation of the National Response Framework (NRF), which superseded both the Federal Response Plan and the National Response Plan.[11] The NRF is a guide to how the nation conducts all hazards responses. It is built upon scalable, flexible, and adaptable coordinating structures that align key roles and responsibilities across the nation, linking all levels of government, nongovernmental organizations, and the private sector.[12] It identifies specific authorities and best practices for managing incidents from the serious but purely local to large-scale terrorist attacks or catastrophic natural disasters defined under the Robert T. Stafford Disaster Relief and

Emergency Act as events that result in extraordinary levels of casualties, damage, and disruption affecting the population or environment of a community.

In 1999 Congress charged the Department of Health and Human Services (HHS) and the Centers for Disease Control and Prevention (CDC) with the establishment of the National Pharmaceutical Stockpile (NPS).[13] The mission was to provide large quantities of essential medical material to states and communities during an emergency within 12 hours of the federal decision to deploy. After the attacks in 2001, the Department of Homeland Security briefly assumed control of the stockpile and changed the name to the Strategic National Stockpile (SNS). The Department of Homeland Security gave the SNS back to the Department of Health and Human Services and the CDC. The CDC received funding under an Anti-Bioterrorism Initiative to develop the SNS into a program to assist states and communities respond to public health emergencies, primarily those resulting from chemical, biologic, and radiologic terrorist attacks.[2] The resulting SNS program is part of the NRF and ensures the availability of medicines, antidotes, medical supplies, vaccines, and medical equipment necessary for states and communities to counter the effects of biologic pathogens, chemical agents, radiologic events, and explosive devices.

The SNS program is designed to deliver medical assets to the site of a biologic or chemical national emergency within 12 hours of the federal decision to deploy medical assets. (Under the Stafford Act, state authorities must request federal assistance before it is delivered.) Medical assets available through the SNS program include antibiotics, chemical nerve agent antidotes, intravenous fluids and administration supplies, bandages, burn ointments, analgesics, antiemetics, sedatives, antiviral medications, antitoxins, and vaccines. The SNS program includes "push packages" (prepackaged assortments of these pharmaceuticals) and medical supplies that may be needed for general resupply during a disaster. The push packages do not contain drugs and equipment for general primary care problems such as hypertension or diabetes.

CURRENT PRACTICE

Terrorism

There are multiple sources for clinical recommendations with regard to the treatment of casualties from biologic, chemical, or radiologic weapons.[14–18] Recommendations regarding PPE have been hampered by limited regulatory guidance and lack of focused research on use of PPE in health care facilities. However, the current consensus appears to support the use of Level C PPE (i.e., splash suits, gloves, boots, air-purifying respirators) in most health care settings.[19,20] Hospitals and health emergency planners should maintain stockpiles of appropriate PPE and be prepared to decontaminate and care for persons in their community in response to threats identified in their HVA.

As noted, the SNS program's formulary is directed at biologic, chemical, radiologic, and explosive weapons. A 12-hour or longer response time for delivery of chemical agent antidotes is not optimal for the initial care of casualties. In addition, many hospitals carry only limited stocks of chemical nerve agent antidotes.[7,8,12,21] These antidotes have variable shelf lives; replacing them is costly and may impact a community's ability to respond. Therefore, the SNS program has executed a nationwide forward deployment of chemical nerve agent antidotes under its CHEMPACK project. Through this project, emergency medical services and hospitals will have access to chemical nerve agent antidotes for immediate use during an event. Even with this forward deployment of chemical nerve agent antidotes, it is doubtful that antidotes will be immediately available after a terrorist release of a nerve agent.

Certain biologic threat agents and public health disasters such as epidemics may require prophylaxis for persons responding to the event. Stockpiles provided through the SNS can reduce the time to prophylaxis for first responders and provide a sense of security for their welfare. Local medical stockpiling may be one option for treatments that must be given within minutes to hours after an event, often much sooner than federal assistance can arrive. Communities with specific technological risks, such as chemical storage depots or nuclear power plants, may consider stockpiling specific antidotes or treatments as part of their disaster plan.

Appropriate training for the use of all stockpiled equipment should be considered.[17] Medical personnel in charge of stockpiles used to address biologic, chemical, or radiologic agents will need to regularly review their formularies for inclusion of improved vaccines and newer treatment modalities, and for changes to a drug's approval status by the Food and Drug Administration (FDA).

Natural Disasters

The SNS is not designed to handle natural disasters such as hurricanes, earthquakes, tornados, and floods. Similar rapidly deployable stockpiles (or subsets of stockpiles) could be designed to meet the needs incurred by natural disasters likely to strike in a particular area; however, no such current rapidly deployable assets are currently configured.

The public health consequences of natural disasters should also guide emergency planners in assessing the pharmaceutical and medical equipment needs of their communities.[1,22] Several medical equipment and supply lists exist and can provide examples from which emergency planners may select and begin developing an inventory appropriate for their populations based on the threat analysis.

When planning for extremely large, or prolonged events, an available international resource is WHO's Emergency Health Kit.[23] This publication offers a standard list of essential emergency health supplies that are widely accepted internationally, calculated to meet the needs of 10,000 persons for 3 months. The kit inventory is divided into 10 identical units that each treat 1000 persons, so it is scalable to need. It is designed to meet the needs of a refugee camp and the priorities associated with austere conditions in developing nations.[23] In addition, WHO has published and developed an essential drug list of pharmaceuticals that should be available at any given time in appropriate amounts and formulations. The WHO essential drug list has been adopted by numerous international agencies that supply pharmaceuticals within their health care programs and is being used to evaluate the appropriateness of drug donations.[24–26]

A recommended list of medical supplies for health care personnel responding to victims of earthquakes has been developed by emergency medicine faculty at the University of California, Irvine Medical Center. The listed supplies can fit into backpacks kept by specially trained medical personnel in the trunks of their cars at all times.[26]

Centralized or decentralized stockpiles of medical supplies and equipment may be considered as an option for disaster preparedness. Stockpiling medical assets for natural disasters is an expensive option.[10] Not only are the costs high for initial purchase of pharmaceuticals and equipment, but the budget must include the cost of replacement for expired or worn-out items. Equipment must be maintained and quality assurance provided. Equipment may also need to be replaced as newer models become available. There may be significant logistical costs associated with maintenance, storage, and transportation of the inventory. The SNS can supply some equipment needs for disasters due to natural hazards, but only to a limited extent.

Beyond the financial concerns of stockpiling medical supplies and assets, there are multiple logistical and clinical considerations for states, communities, or hospitals. First, storage locations must be determined.

Pharmaceuticals should be stored in a secure and temperature-controlled environment. An inventory system should be incorporated that allows up-to-date information on available products and expiration dates, controls access to restricted pharmaceuticals such as narcotics, and tracks distributed products or assets. Any centralized storage system of medical assets must be combined with an efficient and secure distribution system. Preference should be given to medical assets that have longer expiration dates and require no specialized storage needs or ancillary supplies.

Clinical considerations include assessing products for duplicity of use. Products that can be used to respond to multiple agents or events can reduce the number of pharmaceuticals purchased. For example, doxycycline is approved by the FDA to treat multiple biologic agents including, anthrax, tularemia, and plague. Decisions regarding which formulations of products to stockpile should consider special populations such as children or those persons who cannot swallow pills. Appropriate sizes of medical equipment for children should be considered.[8,27]

Emergency managers may opt to arrange for anticipated necessary supplies from bulk drug/medical supply houses to be delivered on a "just-in-time" basis after a specific disaster. Examination of needs for similar disasters can guide these arrangements. These supply houses can also ensure that soon-to-expire drugs are sent to hospitals for rapid real-time use rather than discarding them months later from a stockpile. Coordination with commercial pharmacy chains may also enhance recovery efforts as these large chains have the ability to provide response packs tailored to local population needs for chronic illness maintenance drugs or provide prescription information for evacuees who use their services.

Management of Pharmaceutical Donations

After an event, multiple individuals, corporations, and governments may wish to contribute by sending possibly needed medications to the disaster area. Publicity following major disasters may lead to inappropriate donations that can create multiple secondary problems at the scene of the disaster. Recurrent problems with these donations and some possible solutions are identified in Box 57-1.[26,28–30]

Some donors assume that any medications can be used at the disaster, while others take the opportunity to "dump" soon-to-expire medications, outdated medications, or even medications that are banned or pulled from a market.[31] Such drug dumping can solve tax and disposal problems and mitigate costs of storage of medications

---

BOX 57-1   Pharmaceutical Donation Guidelines[29,34]

- No drug should be sent without a request or a clearance by the receiving government.
- No drug should be sent that is not on the WHO list of essential drugs or a similar list generated by the local government.
- No drug should be sent with an expiration date that is less than 1 year from the date sent.
- Labeling of the drug should be in the appropriate language of the local government. Labels should contain the generic name, strength, expiration date, and name of the manufacturer.
- Bulk packages should be labeled with the same information plus the total quantity of the drugs in the package.
- Bulk packages of drugs should weigh no more than 110 pounds (50 kg), so that two people can move these packages. (Usual means of transportation may be compromised by the disaster.)

for the donor, while creating massive disposal and storage problems for the recipients.[32,33]

Other donors may send appropriate drugs, but in packages that contain a mixture of unlabeled items or with labels that do not identify the drug, manufacturers, and dosage in a language that the local medical providers understand. Sorting these drugs takes substantial time and energy that would be better expended on disaster response and recovery.[34]

Poorly packaged drugs can be contaminated or ruined by environmental exposure at the disaster site. Special storage requirements should be clearly marked on the exterior of the package, and packages should be waterproof whenever possible. Drugs should be clearly marked and not shipped with other supplies needed in the disaster, if possible. Packages should be easily opened and should not be so heavy that two workers cannot move them. Heavier packages may need to be divided into smaller packages for transport over rough roads and pathways found in disaster sites.

! PITFALLS

- Problems in disaster resource management can result from insufficient information or assessment of a community's health and other needs. The health resources emergency manager should carefully review the literature from prior similar incidents and coordinate with public health authorities to ensure that adequate supplies/medications for locally prevalent chronic diseases are covered in operational plans.

- As discussed above, donations may be inappropriate. WHO has prepared general guidelines for pharmaceutical donations that include the selection of drugs, quality assurance and shelf life, packaging and labeling, and information and management of pharmaceuticals.[26,28,29] Unfortunately, there are countless examples of useless medical supplies and consumables sent to a disaster site, such as drugs labeled in a foreign language, expired drugs, or drugs not commonly used in a particular country.[10,29,35–37] Unsolicited medical supplies may arrive unsorted, unlabeled, or mislabeled. Many supplies that are sent are not intended for emergency use. Time and effort by logistics staff must be expended to determine which resources are needed and which are unusable and must be discarded. During the 1988 earthquake in Armenia, the donation of tons of pharmaceuticals and other medical supplies overwhelmed the local capacity to store and inventory the donations. At least 50% of medical assets donated to Bosnia and Herzegovina between 1992 and 1996 were considered inappropriate.[11,35,38] Inappropriate and unrequested aid can cost a community money for storage, handling, and destruction of medical assets. Finally, unrequested and inappropriate donations have occurred because donors want to receive tax deductions or avoid the costs associated with the destruction of soon-to-expire medical supplies, a practice that has been referred to as "drug dumping."[38] The cost of handling and or disposing of the drugs may exceed the actual value of the pharmaceuticals themselves.[29,37–39]

- The response/distribution time for stockpiled supplies and medications is often substantially longer than the "optimum" time quoted in plans. These delays may be due to communication of the situation report up the chain of command, decision time delays, transportation delays due to infrastructure damage or delays in implementation of local distribution mechanisms. The optimum time quoted should be at least doubled in planning.

- Responsibility for inventory control and assessing the overall response needs is often not assigned.[39] To address this problem, WHO has developed a system known as the Supply Management

Project. The purpose of this project is to assist nations in categorizing and inventorying donations supplied during relief efforts.[37] As noted above, implementation of local distribution may involve a substantial delay.

SUMMARY

The types and amounts of medical equipment and pharmaceuticals required to respond to disasters will be determined by the disaster itself, the response capability of the community, and existing resources that remain functional within the community. There is no specific list of pharmaceuticals or medical assets that will apply to all communities and cover all types of disasters.

United States federal assistance is designed to augment the community and state response to disasters. It is imperative that communities identify in advance the medical resources available for a disaster response and categorize potential needs based on the HVA. Identification of available assets before the fact will help to avoid duplication of efforts. Communities should closely coordinate the arrival of federal assistance with a distribution system that can efficiently transport critical medical assets where they are most needed. Predisaster preparations may include stockpiling of pharmaceuticals and equipment to respond to a variety of disasters as well as prearrangements with medical or pharmaceutical supply houses and commercial pharmacy chains.

Stockpiling or forward placement of pharmaceuticals may be considered when a product must be given within minutes to hours for maximum effectiveness, when supplies are limited within a community, and when hazard assessments indicate a technological risk to a community. Understanding what pharmaceuticals and medical equipment will be needed for a disaster should, at a minimum, include taking an inventory of community assets and considering the regional, state, and federal resources that may be available upon request.

REFERENCES

1. Noji EK. The public health consequences of disasters. *Prehosp Disaster Med.* 2000;15(4):147–157.
2. Rotz LD, Koo D, et al. Bioterrorism preparedness: planning for the future. In: Novack LF, ed. *Public Health Issues in Disaster Preparedness Focus on Bioterrorism.* Gaithersburg, MD: Aspen Publications; 2001:99–103.
3. Sidel VW. Weapons of mass destruction: the greatest threat to public health. *JAMA.* 1989;262(5):680–682.
4. Henderson AK, Lillibridge SR, Salinas C, Graves RW, Roth PB, Noji EK. Disaster medical assistance teams: providing health care to a community struck by Hurricane Iniki. *Ann Emerg Med.* 1994;23(4):726–730.
5. Alson R, Alexander D, Leonard RB, Stringer LW. Analysis of medical treatment at a field hospital following Hurricane Andrew, 1992. *Ann Emerg Med.* 1993;22(11):1721–1728.
6. Pesik N, Keim M. Logistical considerations for emergency response resources. *Pac Health Dialog.* 2002;9(1):97–103.
7. Wetter DC, Daniell WE, Treser CD. Hospital preparedness for victims of chemical or biological terrorism. *Am J Public Health.* 2001;91(5):710–716.
8. Henretig FM, Cieslak TJ, Madsen JM. The emergency department response to incidents of biological and chemical terrorism. In: Fleisher GR, Ludwig S, eds. *Textbook of Pediatric Emergency Medicine.* 4th ed. Philadelphia: Lippincott, Williams, and Wilkins; 2000:1763–1784.
9. Manning FJ, Goldfrank L. *Preparing for Terrorism: Tools for Evaluating the Metropolitan Medical Response System Program. Committee on Evaluation of the Metropolitan Medical Response System Program: Board on Health Sciences Policy,* Washington, DC: National Academy Press; 2003:1–332.
10. Pan American Health Organization. *Natural Disasters: Protecting the Public's Health,* vol. 575 Washington, DC: PAHO-OPS; 2000.

11. Pan American Health Organization. *Disasters Preparedness and Mitigation in the Americas.* Washington, DC: PAHO-OPS; 1984.

12. Department of Homeland Security. *National Response Framework.* Washington, DC: Department of Homeland Security; 2013.

13. CDC. *Strategic National Stockpile (SNS);* 2014. Accessed 10.01.14.

14. *Medical Management of Chemical Casualties Handbook.* 4th ed. Aberdeen Proving Ground, MD: Cemical Casualty Care Division, United States Army Medical Research Institute of Chemical Defense; 2007.

15. Henderson DA, Inglesby TV, O'Toole T, eds. *Bioterrorism: Guidelines for Medical and Public Health Management.* Chicago, Ill: American Medical Association Press; 2002:1–244.

16. Jarrett DG, ed. *Medical Management of Radiological Casualties Handbook.* Bethesda, MD: Armed Forces Radiobiology Research Institute; 1999.

17. Kortepeter M, ed. *Management of Biological Casualties Handbook.* 3rd ed. Frederick, MD: United States Army Medical Research Institute of Infectious Diseases; 1998.

18. National Academies of Science. *Distribution and Administration of Potassium Iodide in the Event of a Nuclear Incident.* Washington, DC: National Academies Press; 2004.

19. Hick JL, Hanfling D, Burstein JL, Markham J, Macintyre AG, Barbera JA. Protective equipment for health care facility decontamination personnel: regulations, risks, and recommendations. *Ann Emerg Med.* 2003;42(3):370–380.

20. Macintyre AG, Christopher GW, Eitzen E, Jr., et al. Weapons of mass destruction events with contaminated casualties: effective planning for health care facilities. *JAMA.* 2000;283(2):242–249.

21. Keim ME, Pesik N, Twum-Danso NA. Lack of hospital preparedness for chemical terrorism in a major US city: 1996–2000. *Prehosp Disaster Med.* 2003;18(3):193–199.

22. Paola Lichtenberger MD, Ian N, Miskin MD, et al. Infection control in field hospitals after a natural disaster: lessons learned after the 2010 earthquake in Haiti. *Infect Control Hosp Epidemiol.* 2010;31(9):951–957.

23. *The New Emergency Health Kit 1998. World Health Organization.* Geneva, Switzerland: WHO; 1998.

24. *Essential Medications—Children.* 4th ed. World Health Organization; 2013. *http://www.who.int/medicines/publications/essentialmedicines/en/index.html.* Accessed 26.12.13.

25. *Essential Medications.* 18th ed. World Health Organization; 2013. *http://www.who.int/medicines/publications/essentialmedicines/en/index.html.* Accessed 26.12.13.

26. Harrington RV. Pharmaceuticals in disasters. In: Hogan DE, Burnstein JL, eds. *Disaster Medicine.* 2nd ed. Philadelphia: Williams and Wilkins; 2007.

27. Schultz CH, Koenig KL, Noji EK. A medical disaster response to reduce immediate mortality after an earthquake. *N Engl J Med.* 1996;334(7):438–444.

28. Hogerzeil HV, Couper MR, Gray R. Guidelines for drug donations. *BMJ.* 1997;314(7082):737–740.

29. *Guidelines for Medicine Donations. World Health Organization.* 2nd ed. Geneva, Switzerland: WHO; 2010.

30. Carballo M, Serdarevic D. *Responding to Emergency Drug Needs: Lessons for the Future.* Geneva: ICMH; 1996.

31. Pinheiro CP. Drug donations: what lies beneath. *Bull World Health Organ.* 2008;86:580A.

32. Reich MR, Wagner A, McLaughlin T, Dumbaugh K, Derai-Cochin M. Pharmaceutical donations by the USA: an assessment of relevance and time-to-expiry. *Bull World Health Organ.* 1999;77(8).

33. Thomas M. *Drug Donations: corporate charity or taxpayer subsidy?* 2009.

34. Bero L, Carson B, Moller H, Hill S. To give is better than to receive: compliance with WHO guidelines for drug donations during 2000–2008. *Bull World Health Organ.* 2010;88(12):922–929.

35. Autier P, Ferir MC, Hairapetien A, et al. Drug supply in the aftermath of the 1988 Armenian earthquake. *Lancet.* 1990;335(8702):1388–1390.

36. de Ville de Goyet C. Stop propagating disaster myths. *Lancet.* 2000;356 (9231):762–764.

37. de Ville de Goyet C, Acosta E, Sabbat P, Pluut E. SUMA (Supply Management Project), a management tool for post-disaster relief supplies. *World Health Stat Q.* 1996;49(3–4):189–194.

38. Berckmans P, Dawans V, Schmets G, Vandenbergh D, Autier P. Inappropriate drug-donation practices in Bosnia and Herzegovina, 1992 to 1996. *N Engl J Med.* 1997;337(25):1842–1845.

39. Auf der Heide E. Resource management. In: Auf der Heide E, ed. *Disaster Response: Principles of Preparation and Coordination.* St. Lous, MO: Mosby; 1989:103–132.

SUGGESTED READINGS

1. World Health Organization. *Community Emergency Preparedness: A Manual for Managers and Policy Makers.* Geneva, Switzerland: WHO-OMS; 1999, 141–160.

2. Lillibridge SR, Noji EK, Burkle FM, Jr. Disaster assessment: the emergency health evaluation of a population affected by a disaster. *Ann Emerg Med.* 1993;22(11):1715–1720.

3. Guha-Sapir D, Lechat MF. Information systems and needs assessment in natural disasters: an approach for better disaster relief management. *Disasters.* 1986;10(3):232–237.

4. Guha-Sapir D, Van Panhuis WG, Lagoutte J. Short communication: patterns of chronic and acute diseases after natural disasters—a study from the International Committee of the Red Cross field hospital in Banda Aceh after the 2004 Indian Ocean tsunami. *Trop Med Int Health.* 2007;12(11):1338–1341.

5. World Health Organization. *Guidelines for the Use of Foreign Field Hospitals in the Aftermath of Sudden-Impact Disasters.* Washington, DC: WHO-PAHO; 2003:1–20.

6. Plutt I. *Field Hospitals Arrive in Iran following December Earthquake. Disasters: Preparedness and Mitigation in the Americas.* Geneva, Switzerland: WHO-PAHO; 2003:94.

CHAPTER 58

Displaced Populations

Amalia Voskanyan and John D. Cahill

Displaced populations have occurred throughout the history of humankind. A large population can be displaced by a number of events. These include, but are not limited to, natural disasters (e.g., floods, famine, earthquakes, hurricanes, monsoons, and volcanoes), persecution, conflict, and war. As seen in the Haiti earthquake of 2010, populations that are displaced face many difficult challenges. They are forced to leave their home, possessions, and occupations and be separated from their family and friends. These disasters can have direct effects on the physical and mental health of these populations and expose them to violence stemming from social inequalities.[1] Displaced persons experience fear of the unknown and loss of control and self-identity. These populations are vulnerable to abuse on many levels, including human rights and gender-based crimes. Although the burdens of any displaced population may be similar, generally they fall into one of two broad groups: refugees and internally displaced populations.

REFUGEES

For a person to be considered a refugee, he or she must cross a border into another country. Certain displaced persons are not considered refugees: war criminals, persons who commit acts of terrorism, criminals who have a fair trial and seek refuge to avoid incarceration, soldiers, and economic migrants (those who leave their country of their own will to better their lives). The United Nations High Commissioner for Refugees (UNHCR), through the 1951 Convention Relating to the Status of Refugees, defines a refugee as a person who "owing to a well-founded fear of being persecuted for reasons of race, religion, nationality, membership of a particular social group, or political opinion, is outside the country of his nationality, and is unable to or, owing to such fear, is unwilling to avail himself of the protection of that country."[2] UNHCR estimates that by the end of 2011, there were approximately 43.3 million refugees worldwide "due to either conflict or persecution," and the largest refugee camp in the world, Hagadera Camp in Dabaab Kenya, held approximately 138,000 people.[3] These enormous numbers reflect the ever-growing need for worldwide attention to this problem. The needs of displaced populations at such numbers are vast. In addition, it has been found that at least 1 in 5 displaced women in refugee camps is a victim of sexual predation and violence.[4] The role of UNHCR is to protect and act as an advocate for this population.

An important principle of refugee law is *nonrefoulement*, which is "a concept which prohibits States from returning a refugee or asylum-seeker to territories where there is a risk that his or her life or freedom would be threatened on account of race, religion, nationality, membership of a particular social group or political opinion."[5] This works in theory, however, either by force or voluntary action, some refugees continue to return to still unsafe situations in their homelands.

Refugee status is often considered to be a temporary matter, when in reality it can go on for years to decades. Whole new generations have been born in refugee camps, having no identification with their original country. Generally, there are three options for a refugee's destiny: to repatriate to his country, to resettle in the country where he has sought refugee status, or to be resettled to a third country.

INTERNALLY DISPLACED PERSONS

Internally displaced persons (IDPs) are those who have been forced to flee their homes to escape armed conflict, generalized violence, human rights abuses, or natural or human-made disasters. They differ from refugees in that they stay within the borders of their home country. It is estimated that the number of IDPs increased to 28.8 million in 2012, with much of that increase due to the conflict in Syria.[6] Because they exist within the borders of a potentially hostile home country, they lack the services and protections available to refugees.

PRIORITIES FOR A DISPLACED POPULATION

Although events that lead up to a movement of a large population may differ, there are certain principles that generally apply. Many different actors may be involved in these movements: governments (including multiple countries, states, or localities), military units, and nongovernmental organizations. Whenever possible, members of the local community should be involved in the decision to move. This includes government officials, professionals (e.g., public health, health care providers, engineers), and the local workforce. These groups can be an invaluable resource in understanding the population needs, potential challenges, infrastructure, and cultural issues. Box 58-1 lists the top priorities of a displaced population. The remainder of this chapter will go through the priorities of the initial management of a displaced population.

- Initial assessment
- Measles immunization
- Water and sanitation
- Food and nutrition
- Shelter and site planning
- Health care in the emergency phase
- Control of communicable diseases and epidemics
- Public health surveillance
- Human resources and training
- Coordination

INITIAL EVALUATION

There should be a clear understanding of the context and the event that led to the movement of the population being evaluated. The effects of war or genocide will require very different resources and management than those of a hurricane or earthquake. Even though the initial assessment might be difficult, one should try to consider the potential length of time that this population may be displaced. Historically, the time frame is often much longer than one would expect. Remember that there are refugees who have been displaced for decades from their original home, and two thirds of refugees are still living in camps 5 years after the initial event. The well-being and security of both the population and those responding to the situation need to be of utmost importance. Unfortunately, at times, this important concept has gone underappreciated or poorly understood. We are seeing evidence of this now in postearthquake Haiti,[7] and postconflict Sudan.[8]

It is of great value to learn the demographics of the population that has been displaced. With a better understanding of things such as work experience, education, and language skills, trauma-related psychological pathology, social relationships, and perceived quality of life can be dramatically affected.[9] This information can be obtained by initial registration of the population, census information, health records, sample surveys, and speaking with local authorities. Basic essential data include the size, sex, and age distribution of the population; family members; cultural makeup (e.g., religion and ethnicity); medical health, disease prevalence, and vaccine status; and the identification of potential vulnerable groups. The region where the population is relocating to also needs to be well understood. What resources are available to the population? Is there an adequate water supply, and to what extent can it be used? Will proper sanitation be available, and for how long? What amount of food is available locally, and what kind of stores are available? Is the land suitable for living on? What local supplies are available for constructing shelter? What medical care and provisions are available locally? How secure are all of these items? What infrastructure is available to bring in further supplies? Are there suitable roads? What size vehicle can the roads accommodate? Are there facilities to repair vehicles that encounter mechanical problems? Are there train stations in close proximity? Where is the closest landing strip, and what is the maximum size aircraft that can land there? Where is the nearest port? If goods are to be shipped in, where can they be stored, and can these items be secured? What are the options to distribute water, food, and supplies in an orderly and safe manner?

MEASLES AND TUBERCULOSIS

Refugee camps are small, close-quartered communities, often with poor sanitation and health care. This type of living condition is prone to many forms of infectious diseases, particularly organisms spread by droplets and aerosolization.[10] Many health care providers are often very surprised to learn that measles continues to be a major cause of morbidity and mortality throughout the world, and outbreaks are often seen in refugee camps.[11] The pediatric population is at highest risk, and mass vaccination should be highest priority in children from 6 months to 15 years of age.[12] Measles is an RNA paramyxovirus that is highly contagious and spread through secretions in the respiratory tract. Approximately 90% of susceptible persons will contract the disease after exposure to an infected person.[13] It should be noted that vitamin A deficiency can cause cases of measles that are more severe and complicated. All refugee populations should be vaccinated for measles, and vitamin A should be distributed when vaccinating.

Tuberculosis continues to be a concerning infectious disease, representing a leading cause of death in the developing world.[14] The disease burden seen in these areas is exacerbated and heightened by the complex nature of refugee camps, consisting of displaced populations from developing countries. Data have shown that tuberculosis morbidity and mortality correlates with the existence and quality of identification and treatment programs.[15] The data speak to the need for early establishment of screening and treatment facilities in refugee camps and displaced populations.

WATER

Clean water should be top priority in any disaster situation. It is the cornerstone of any emergency response involving refugee care. Water is not only a necessity for life but also for basic hygiene. In the initial response, the quantity of water is more important than the quality. The absolute minimum requirement of water is 5 L/person/day; this should be increased as soon as possible to reach a level of 15 to 20 L/person/day. Other things to consider about water include the source, accessibility, location, availability of carrying containers, and security considerations.

Water can be a source of disease on many different levels, as evidenced by the cholera outbreak months after the earthquake in Haiti. Even though it was most likely brought into the country by an aid worker, it flourished in the standing water and poor sanitation seen in and around the tent cities.[16] Contaminated water, as shown in Table 58-1, contributes significantly to global morbidity and mortality. Freshwater can act as the home for the intermediate hosts that cause schistosomiasis and guinea worm infection. These infections commonly occur when a person stands in water as he or she is collecting it. A lack of water or contaminated water can also contribute to trachoma, which is a major cause of blindness and skin infections. Finally, water can act as the home to insect vectors that cause malaria, dengue fever, filariasis, onchocerciasis, and African trypanosomiasis.[17] Adequate ways to filter and purify water should be made available.

SANITATION AND HYGIENE

Besides water, sanitation and hygiene are of top priority in the emergency response. These measures are the first barrier to preventing

TABLE 58-1 Waterborne Diseases from Contaminated Water Ingestion

DISEASE	MORBIDITY PER ANNUM	MORTALITY PER ANNUM
Diarrhea	1000 million	3.3 million
Typhoid	12.5 million	>125,000
Cholera	>300,000	>3000
Ascaris infection	1 billion	

TABLE 58-2 Sanitation Systems

WET	DRY
Water seal latrines	Trench
Aquaprives	Pit latrines
OXFAM Sanitation Unit	VIP latrine
	Bore holed
	Composting

the spread of fecal/oral disease. On average, humans produce 0.25 L of stool/day and 1.5 L of urine/day. One can easily see how quickly proper disposal and management of waste can become a problem. When considering a sanitation system, one needs to be culturally sensitive to the population that is being served. It is a futile effort to set up a sanitation system if no one is going to use it. Therefore it is a good idea to involve local residents in setting up a system. Environmental implications should be considered as well: what affect may it have, how long is it going to be used, and is there any potential to contaminate the water supply? Sanitation systems come in two forms, which are listed in Table 58-2.[18]

FOOD AND NUTRITION

The demand for food may lead to displacement. This may occur from a natural disaster or from the effects of conflict and war. Malnutrition is a significant cause of morbidity and mortality in many disasters. It is important not only to remember the direct complications of malnutrition and disease states (Table 58-3) but also to understand that many diseases are accelerated or made more severe secondary to malnutrition, particularly in the pediatric population, where the main causes of death are closely connected with malnutrition. The following are strongly tied to malnutrition: diarrhea, pneumonia, HIV, tuberculosis, malaria, measles, hypoglycemia, and hypothermia. As well, *Giardia*, which has been found in abundance in postdisaster areas of the developing world, including most recently Haiti, has a known correlation with malnutrition.[19]

The daily minimum nutritional requirement should be 2100 kcal/person/day. At least 10% of the calories in the general ration should be in the form of fats, and at least 12% should be derived from proteins.[20]

The caloric demand may be higher based on shelter, environment, burden of disease, and underlying nutritional status of the population. Distributing food equitably is an important aspect of feeding large populations. Ideally, this should be done in a community-based setting, in an organized and secure manner. Otherwise, food stores will not be distributed equally. Feeding centers should be established for the severely malnourished. Particular attention should be paid to the very young because of the established link between malnutrition and poor development.[21,22]

A food basket for distribution may include wheat flour, rice, sugar, vegetable oil, salt, and possibly local fish or meat. Other supplements may be included for additional nutritional benefit. It is preferable to use local food when available and to encourage the planting of vegetables. Seeds and other equipment can be distributed to the population. Cultural practices and diet also need to be considered. Utensils and fuel for cooking need to be supplied, depending on the food being distributed. Breast-feeding should be encouraged and bottle feeding avoided.

Nutritional screening of the population should be performed to assess particular needs. In general, the incidence of malnutrition in children younger than 5 years of age is used as the general indicator of malnutrition for the population. The weight-to-height index (ideally used), evidence of edema, and the mid–upper-arm circumference are means to do a nutritional survey.[23]

SHELTER

Depending on the size of the displaced population, several different options may be considered for shelter. With small populations, an attempt may be made to house them with the local population in their homes. As the size grows, this is not possible. Another shelter option is to use existing structures that are already available (e.g., schools, factories, warehouses, and public buildings). Finally, camps can be established for the population to live in. When a camp is being established, considerations on shelter and the site will be based on a number of factors, including type of disaster, size and demographics of the population, anticipated time of displacement (although this is often underappreciated), environmental health risks, terrain, accessibility, available existent structures and infrastructure, climate, security (ideally away from borders), local building materials, and cultural considerations. Table 58-4 lists some general guidelines that are used for site planning.[24]

MEDICAL CARE

Medical needs may be anticipated based on the circumstances of the event leading to the displaced population. There are some general principles in responding to the acute medical needs of a displaced population. The goals of the health care system should be to implement preventative health care practices, treat the common communicable diseases (i.e., diarrhea, respiratory tract infections, measles, and malaria), reduce the suffering from debilitating diseases, afford easy access to the necessary care for the population, deal with the majority of diseases at the basic level, and carry out public health surveillance.

TABLE 58-3 Disease States Associated with Malnutrition

DISEASE	DEFICIENCY
Anemia	Iron/vitamin B_{12}
Goiter/cretinism	Iodine
Scurvy	Vitamin C
Rickets/osteomalacia	Vitamin D
Beriberi	Vitamin B_1 (thiamine)
Pellagra	Niacin
Ariboflavinosis	Vitamin B_2 (riboflavin)
Night blindness/xerophthalmia	Vitamin A
Kwashiorkor	Protein

TABLE 58-4 Recommendations for Shelter

CONSIDERATION	SPACE
Area available per person	30 m^2
Shelter space per person	3.5 m^2
Number of people per water point	250
Number of people per latrine	20
Distance to water point	150 m, maximum
Distance to latrine	30 m
Distance between water point and latrine	100 m
Firebreaks	75 m every 300 m
Distance between two shelters	2 m, minimum

Whenever possible, local health care facilities and professionals should be used. A large population can quickly overburden the local system, and often a parallel system needs to be developed. A four-tier model for the levels of health care managing the initial acute phase has been repeatedly used with success in reducing excess mortality. The levels include a referral hospital (preferably an already functioning local hospital), a central health facility, a peripheral health facility, and home visits/assessments. A referral hospital is used for more specialized care, such as major surgery, obstetric emergencies, and more elaborate laboratory and diagnostic facilities. Patients should be referred to this facility only by one of the other tiers, preferably from the central health facility. Depending on the situation, one central health facility should be present for every 10,000 to 30,000 persons in a camp. This facility should include triage, an outpatient clinic (including minor surgical procedures), simple inpatient services (including uncomplicated deliveries), a pharmacy, and simple laboratory facilities. A peripheral health facility should be established for every 3000 to 5000 persons. Here a simple outpatient clinic or department can treat basic health needs (e.g., dehydration and dressing changes) and refer patients to a higher level of care. At all levels, public health surveillance should be conducted.[25]

Based on disease prevalence in the population or region, certain medications may be required. In general, "essential" medical kits have been developed and are available from a number of government and nongovernment organizations. Ideally, health care treatment protocols should be established for the more common illnesses. This affords easier management and better treatment when dealing with large populations. It also allows for the anticipation of necessary supplies and medications.

REFERENCES

1. Rahill GJ, Ganapati NE, et al. Shelter recovery in urban Haiti after the earthquake: the dual role of social capital. *Disasters.* 2014;38(suppl 1): S73–S93.
2. United Nations High Commissioner for Refugees. *Convention and Protocol Relating to the Status of Refugees.* Geneva: UNHCR; 1951, 16.
3. *Protecting Refugees.* Geneva: United Nations High Commissioner for Refugees; 2012, 28.
4. Vu A, Adam A, et al. The prevalence of sexual violence among female refugees in complex humanitarian emergencies: a systematic review and meta-analysis. *PLoS Curr.* 2014;18:6.
5. United Nations High Commission of Refugees. *The Scope and Content of the Principle of Non Refoulement.* Geneva: UNHCR; 2001, 5.
6. Internal Displacement Monitoring Centre, Norwegian Refugee Council, Geneva, 2013.
7. Versluis A. Formal and informal material aid following the 2010 Haiti earthquake as reported by camp dwellers. *Disasters.* 2014;38(suppl 1): S94–S109.
8. Green A. Aid groups struggle to meet South Sudan's needs. *Lancet.* 2014;383(9919):769–770.
9. Opaas M, Hatmann E. Rorschach assessment of traumatized refugees: an exploratory factor analysis. *J Pers Assess.* 2013;95(5):457–470.
10. Tabbaa D, Seimenis A. Population displacements as a risk factor for the emergence of epidemics. *Vet Ital.* 2013;49(1):19–23.
11. Polonsky JA, Ronsse A. High levels of mortality, malnutrition, and measles among recently displaced Somali refugees in Dagahaley camp, Dadaab refugee camp complex, Kenya, 2011. *Confl Health.* 2013;7(1):1.
12. Médicins Sans Frontières. The emergency phase: the ten top priorities. In: Hanquet G, ed. *Refugee Health: An Approach to Emergency Situations.* London: Macmillan; 1997:39.
13. Cook GC, Zumla A, eds. Cutaneous viral diseases, In: *Manson's Tropical Disease.* 21st ed. Philadelphia: WB Saunders; 2003:842.
14. Dielmann JL, Graves CM, et al. Global health development assistance remained steady in 2013 but did not align with recipient's disease burden. *Health Aff (Millwood).* 2014;33(5):878–886.
15. Kimbrough W, Salimba V, et al. The burden of tuberculosis in crisis-affected populations: a systematice review. *Lancet Infect Dis.* 2012;12(12):950–965.
16. Orata F, Keim P, et al. The 2010 cholera outbreak in Haiti: how science solved a controversy. *PLoS Pathog.* 2014;10(4).
17. Cahill J, ed. International emergency medicine, In: *Updates in Emergency Medicine.* New York: Kluwer Academic Publishing; 2003:131–133.
18. Eade D. *The OXFAM Handbook of Development and Relief.* Oxford, UK: OXFAM; March 1994, 22–23.
19. Ray K. Infection: modelling persistent giardiasis and malnutrition. *Nat Rev Gastroenterol Hepatol.* 2013;10(7):382.
20. Centers for Disease Control. Famine-affected, refugee, and displaced populations: recommendations for public health issues. *MMWR.* 1992;41(RR-13).
21. Prado EL, Dewey KG. Nutrition and brain development in early life. *Nutr Rev.* 2014;72(4):267–284.
22. Ali SS, Dahded, Goudar S. The impact of nutrition on child development at 3 years in a rural community of India. *Int J Prev Med.* 2014;5(4):494–499.
23. Médicins Sans Frontières. *Clinical Guidelines.* Paris: Médicins Sans Frontières; 2003.
24. United Nations High Commission of Refugees. *Handbook for Emergencies.* Geneva: UNHCR; 1982.
25. Médicins Sans Frontières. Health care in the emergency phase. In: Hanquet G, ed. *Refugee Health an Approach to Emergency Situations.* London: Macmillan; 1997:125–132.

CHAPTER 59

Rehabilitation and Reconstruction

Elizabeth S. Temin, Michelangelo Bortolin, and Alice Venier

There are four phases of emergency management as noted in the following:

1. *Preparedness:* Planning a response to a disaster.
2. *Response:* Activities that occur immediately after a disaster. These actions are designed to provide emergency assistance to victims. This phase usually lasts a few days to a few weeks.
3. *Recovery:* Returning the community to normal or near normal. This phase may last for many years.
4. *Mitigation:* Preventing or reducing the effects of a disaster. This phase should be integrated into the other three.[1]

This chapter discusses the third and least understood phase of emergency management: recovery.[2] Recovery is a multifactorial process including the physical reconstruction of homes and public buildings, transportation, and basic services infrastructure, as well as psychological mending of the community and economic recovery of lost time and resources. This stage cannot be considered in isolation because mitigation, the fourth phase, must be integrated into recovery for it to be sustainable.

In 1977, Haas and co-workers became the first group to identify and describe the recovery process.[3] They listed recovery as a sequential four-stage model of emergency, restoration, replacement, and development. Current models describe a more fluid recovery process with these stages overlapping and potentially occurring simultaneously.[4] Replacement reconstruction may occur in some locations, while at the same time debris clearance occurs elsewhere. Recovery currently focuses on the idea of sustainable development, a concept created by a United Nations Commission in 1986, which refers to recovery as a way to improve the quality of lives and durability of communities.[4,5] This concept has been defined in the World Commission on Environment and Development as "meeting the needs of the present without compromising the ability of future generations to meet their own needs."[6] In the short run, it may cost more; better materials may be used, houses and businesses may be relocated, and more stringent building codes and zone laws may be implemented. In the long run, its goal is to protect and strengthen key social and economic infrastructure before disasters strike so as to reduce the likelihood of loss of life and assets and, ultimately, improve community resilience, thus saving money.[5,7]

Out of a vast spectrum of disasters, some may yield predictability based on hazard vulnerability analysis tools, while others will remain unexpected. The process of disaster recovery can adapt currently available recovery tools to fit the specific situation. It is useful to apply a framework to aid comparisons of the similarities and differences in disasters. They can be categorized as natural or human-made, sudden onset or slow onset. Examples of natural disasters that are slow onset are droughts or epidemics such as severe acute respiratory syndrome (SARS); sudden onset examples are floods, hurricanes, and earthquakes. Examples of human-made disasters that are slow onset are wars, such as the war in Iraq, and sudden onset examples are bombings or terrorist activities such

as the September 11, 2001, attacks and the accidental Exxon Valdez oil tanker spill in 1989. The important differences are the duration of impact and severity of direct and indirect effects. Direct effects are defined as the physical destruction and lives lost as a result of the disaster. Indirect effect examples include those such as work time lost, jobs lost, and the change in spending in the community involved.

Recovery framework can also be categorized as vertically or horizontally mediated. Vertical mediation recovery refers to the hierarchy of local communities, the state government, and the federal government. Horizontal mediation refers to the network of groups within a community. Every recovery and management process needs a balance of both vertical and horizontal mediation.

HISTORICAL PERSPECTIVE

The first existing literature on reconstruction and rehabilitation dates back to 79 AD when Mount Vesuvius erupted and destroyed surrounding villages. A document by the historian Pliny details search and rescue attempts to save individuals from debris. The Emperor Titus declared a state of emergency and immediately sent his army to assist with the relief effort in Stabia, Ercolano, and Pompei. The survivors were relocated to unaffected areas to rebuild with new cities. Despite all the populations' efforts and funding from Titus, the devastated populations were unable to recover. Only decades later under Emperor Adrian, in 120 AD, was the devastated area restored.[8]

The modern concept of recovery, reconstruction, and rehabilitation began in 1755 with the Great Lisbon earthquake. Lisbon was struck by a 9.0 magnitude earthquake which caused between 10,000 and 100,000 deaths. It was one of the deadliest earthquakes in modern history. The Royal Family escaped unharmed from the catastrophe, and the Prime Minister implemented and managed a formal search and rescue initiative with regional rehabilitation efforts. After the first response phase, the King and Prime Minister Marquis de Pombal proposed plans to rebuild the city. Less than a month after the event, five plan options were proposed for the rebuilding of Lisbon and, within a year, the city was cleared of debris and reconstruction began. The event had wide-ranging effects on the population. Moreover, a disaster recovery program was established that included, among other things, rebuilding the city with more solid construction.[9,10]

A good example of reconstruction and rehabilitation was observed in 1945 after the atomic bomb was dropped on Hiroshima and Nagasaki. The bomb destroyed nearly 70% of each city's infrastructure and had a devastating effect on the population's health. Within the first few months after the bombing, it is estimated that 140,000 people died in Hiroshima, while another 70,000 died in Nagasaki. Among the long-term health effects suffered by survivors, the most deadly was leukemia, and children were the population group affected most severely.

In 1946 a plan was proposed to reconstruct the destroyed cities. However, due to a lack of financial backing, the plan made very little progress. In 1949 the Hiroshima Peace Memorial City Construction Law and the Nagasaki International Culture City Reconstruction Laws were implemented. The initiatives covered by these laws fueled the funding for reconstruction by promoting the development of foreign trade, shipbuilding, and fishing, thereby bolstering the local economy. Little more than a decade later, the cities of Hiroshima and Nagasaki were completely restored and the population had recovered to its former numbers.[11]

The 2010 Haiti Earthquake affected nearly 3 million people with a death toll estimated to be about 100,000. Many countries responded to appeals for humanitarian aid, pledging funds and dispatching rescue and medical teams, engineers, and support personnel. Six months after the earthquake as much as 98% of the rubble remained uncleared, making most of the capital impassable. In 2015, more than 5 years after the disaster, the capital is still not completely clear of debris. More than 1.6 million citizens remain displaced and live in refugee camps with no electricity, running water, or sewage disposal. A cholera epidemic, which began in October 2010, killed more than 8000 Haitians. Crime in the camps is widespread with women and children as the predominant victims. Despite the estimated 1.1 billion USD collected for the Haitian relief efforts,[12–14] the rehabilitation and reconstruction have been stagnant.[12–14]

CURRENT PRACTICE

In the United States, recovery planning started in 1803 when local resources were overwhelmed during a fire in Portsmouth, New Hampshire. The local government asked Congress for help, creating the first legislative act for federal resources. In 1950 the first permanent and general legislation, the Federal Disaster Act, came into existence. This was revolutionary because it was the first act to create a general response to all disasters. Before this, each disaster resulted in Congress passing a new localized piece of legislation. In 1978, President Jimmy Carter pulled all the distinct response groups together along with the military resources to create FEMA, the Federal Emergency Management Agency, which was formally implemented by executive orders on April 1, 1979.

The U.S. Congress passed the Stafford Act in 1988, an amended version of the Disaster Relief Act of 1974. This focused FEMA toward hazard mitigation and coordination of disaster recovery programs. The Disaster Mitigation Act of 2000 established specific requirements for hazard mitigation planning, and grants became available to allow local and state governments to use mitigation funds for predisaster planning.[6] In 2001 the actions of September 11 pushed Congress to create the Department of Homeland Security, which was the largest reorganization of federal agencies since the Great Depression.[6]

The magnitude of disaster recovery depends on the magnitude of destruction. In a small local disaster, volunteer organizations such as the Red Cross and private insurers may be enough to aid victims. When a disaster overwhelms the recovery forces of a community, that community in the United States can turn to the State government, and ultimately to FEMA, for resources. Within the first 48 hours of a disaster, assessment teams should provide an initial assessment of the damage. This includes identifying immediate needs such as food, shelter, and infrastructural deficits and requirements. Local government will conduct a preliminary damage assessment to determine whether federal aid should be requested. Once the immediate needs are identified, and if federal aid is requested, a second, more in-depth survey should be done by FEMA. This second survey should include reviewing plans of and for the displaced citizens: Do they plan to move, or rebuild in the

same spot? Public infrastructure, sewers, and storm drains should be examined. What about the town? What was there before the disaster? What currently exists? Were there any existing plans for expansion of the area that could be used for rebuilding? What are the opportunities looking at the long term?[15]

Every U.S. state maintains an Emergency Management Agency (EMA) and an Emergency Operations Plan. Their role is to establish and maintain an emergency program concerned with preparedness, response, mitigation, and recovery; to coordinate and train state and local governments; to recommend whether federal aid is needed in the case of a disaster; and to coordinate state and federal resources and act as an intermediary between local and federal groups.[6] In the past, the majority of these plans have been concerned primarily with the short-term response.[2] Recently states have been trying to adapt to a more long-term response.

When a disaster impacts a community in any part of the United States, the federal government may declare a federal disaster under the Robert T. Stafford Disaster Relief and Emergency Assistance Act, if that state is overwhelmed and state resources are not enough to provide aid.[16] In 2000 there were 45 major disaster declarations from 31 states and the District of Columbia.[17] These disasters ranged from tornados to wildfires to winter storms. Initial resources supplied included food, water, emergency generators, and the mobilization of specialized teams (e.g., search and rescue, medical assistance, damage assessment, and communications). For longer term relief, there are loans and grants to repair or replace housing and personal property, roads, and public buildings. There is also assistance for mitigation opportunities, counseling, and legal services. These services are outlined in the U.S. Federal Response Plan (FRP), which describes the policies and plans of 25 federal departments and the U.S. Red Cross.[16] The FRP can be implemented in conjunction with other specialized groups including plans for telecommunications support, the National Oil and Hazardous Substances Pollution Contingency Plan, the Federal Radiological Emergency Response Plan, and the Terrorism Incident Annex.[16] Some federal agencies have the authority to provide disaster aid even when the magnitude is not sufficient for the president to declare a federal disaster, such as the Department of Agriculture, Department of Commerce, Department of Housing and Urban Development, and the Small Business Association (SBA). The FRP employs a multiagency operations structure based on the Incident Command System (ICS). Disaster Field Offices under the Department of Homeland Security may be created along with a national emergency response team. Recovery efforts are the responsibility of logistics and administration teams within disaster field offices.

The first source of insurance for all homeowners, businesses, and towns is private insurance. If that is not adequate or not available, the next action should be to register with FEMA by the stated deadline, usually within 2 months of the disaster. After individual private insurance carriers, the SBA provides the next largest portion of aid. All those above a minimum income are referred to SBA and should apply for SBA loans.[15] The loans must be repaid, but they carry low interest rates. These loans include the following:

1. Home disaster loans to homeowners or renters to repair personal property;
2. Business physical disaster loans to businesses to repair or replace property including real estate, equipment, and inventory (not-for-profit organizations are also eligible);
3. Economic injury disaster loans to small businesses and agricultural cooperatives to replace working capital.[15]

FEMA also offers three types of assistance as noted in the following:

1. Individual and family grants: These loans are granted to persons with needs not met by private insurances, SBA, or volunteer

organizations. These grants are for basic needs only, not to return life to normal. Costs can include medical and counseling assistance, housing repair, funeral expenses, and insurance premiums.

2. Public assistance: This program gives aid to local governments for emergency services and the repair or replacement of public facilities, for example, the removal of debris, repair of infrastructure, or emergency protective measures. It is often the most costly element of recovery, and typically the cost is shared with the state in a 75%/25% split.[6]

3. Hazard mitigation grant program: These grants are used by the federal, state, and local governments to incorporate mitigation into the recovery process.[15] Actions may include acquisition of homes, public education, and retrofitting structures to better resist subsequent disasters such as floods and hurricanes. Cost will be shared between federal and state resources.[6]

Businesses have special considerations in light of a disaster. The primary objective of recovery planning is to enable an organization to survive a disaster and to continue normal business operations. To survive, the organization must ensure that critical operations can resume or continue normal processing and minimize the duration of a serious disruption to operations and resources (both information processing and other resources); a premade contingency plan is the best method of accomplishing this.[18] Specific measures may include having an alternate site of operations if the current facility is damaged, storing vital documents off-site or virtually in the Cloud, and having an alternative energy source such as a generator which is located well above the high water line and not in a basement. Larger businesses may be better able to withstand a disaster because assets and the workforce may be dispersed across a wider geographic area.[6]

A disaster is a life-altering event. Survivors share a considerable experience and come to view the world around them in new and different ways. Seeking help from the government, voluntary agencies, and insurance companies can be a frustrating prolonged process, which may only compound the feelings of helplessness. Anger and despair are common. Mental health staff may assist persons by reassuring them that this "second disaster" is a common phenomenon and that they are not alone in their frustration.[19] Some may not want to seek formal counseling, either because of the perceived stigma associated with seeking help or because they are unwilling to take time away from putting their lives back together or helping others. Very effective mental health assistance can be provided while the worker is helping survivors with concrete tasks. The "over a cup of coffee" method of informal intervention may be the best method to help. A trained effective mental health worker can use skilled but unobtrusive interviewing techniques to help a survivor sort out demands and set priorities while they are jointly sifting through disaster rubble.[19]

Although having community involvement is beneficial to the process of recovery, it is also very important for the mental health resilience of the community. Failing to involve the community can lead to resentment and fragmentation. The inhabitants may be unhappy when aid is not appropriate to the community's perceived needs, and this insult may be compounded if they are then labeled unappreciative of the federal help. When people have a hand in their own recovery, they feel empowered and will increase their involvement. This leads to a stronger community network that in turn increases the ability to provide self-help and community resilience.

⚠ PITFALLS

In general, there are two broad problems with disaster recovery: too little horizontal planning or too much dependence on vertical aid. The pitfalls occur when the horizontal and vertical planning are not balanced.

With too much dependence on vertical planning, the community does not contribute anything to the recovery process and the government organizations and nongovernmental organizations dictate the recovery plans. In the past, these groups have come in with the intention of "fixing" the situation. This is referred to as "top-down" theory.[20] In addition to not providing optimal care, this may impede self-sufficiency of these disaster-stricken areas. Assumptions may be made, including the following: (1) the victims are a burden; (2) the host government is weak and cannot manage alone; (3) foreign aid organizations do not require accountability; (4) aid for the victims reflect the defined needs of the victims (when, in fact, the aid reflects the projected need by the donor).[20] An example of this last point was when Hurricane Hugo struck Montserrat in 1989. Ninety-eight percent of all homes were affected, 50% severely and 20% completely destroyed.[20] The Peace Corps brought in large numbers of prefabricated housing to replace all the destroyed homes. Although they were able to help a lot of people numerically, the homes they provided had two-sided pitched roofs instead of the typical Caribbean four-sided roofs that were better able to withstand tropical winds. They also did not have an interior design to allow for cross ventilation. The early recipients of the homes reported this finding to the Peace Corps, but the Peace Corps was unable to change the design. Although well intentioned, the Peace Corps was predominantly meeting the need projected by the donors instead of the actual needs of the victims.[20]

Overdependence on vertical planning can also result in a lack of accountability and thus uneven recovery results. In Jamaica, after Hurricane Gilbert, the primary housing aid program was the Building Stamp Programme, which was set up by the Jamaican government, the World Bank, Canada, Germany, Japan, OPEC, and the United States. Homeowners were issued building stamps based on the extent of damages and financial need. These stamps would then be redeemed only at building supply stores who were members of the Jamaican Hardware Merchants Association for building materials, including zinc sheets, nails, and lumber. Squatters and renters were not eligible for stamps and were left without any recourse for finding aid. People who were not at home during the time of the survey were not listed as needing aid.[20] It was also found that the stamps were distributed unequally. As a result, many needy people were left without any support.

There is also a real risk of creating a "dependency syndrome" by not thinking of sustainable development when investing money and effort into the recovery process.[20] This occurs when infrastructural replacement of homes is completed in such a way that replacements are likely to be destroyed by subsequent disasters resulting in the need for continued care for each disaster. Instead of being able to learn from prior occurrences and create a more resilient town and infrastructure, the same mistakes are repeated over and over again. For example, Jamaicans used the stamps to fulfill daily needs such as mattresses and utensils and did not spend time reinforcing their homes against further hurricanes or floods. When the next hurricane hits, these people will have the same destruction to their homes as occurred with Hurricane Gilbert.[20]

With too little horizontal planning, the results may be a chaotic lack of cooperation between groups and potential leaders. Internationally, studies have shown that many community plans focus primarily on the emergency period and do not give adequate attention to recovery and reconstruction. If there is a plan, it often exists on paper only and, in the case of an actual disaster, it is not used. Many officials may not be aware that a plan exists.[4] These flaws lead to chaotic implementation of an ad hoc recovery. The community lacks the ability to work together and thus fragments and cannot unify to control its own affairs. As a result, the redevelopment is likely to be inadequate to fulfill the needs of the community. If there is aid from government and nongovernmental groups, they are sometimes uncoordinated, either duplicating actions, leaving areas without any aid, or giving aid that is inadequate for the needs of the area.[4] In Saragossa, Texas, a small isolated community devastated by a tornado in 1987, there was no local government in place at all. When a disaster advisory board was created, it was done without any input from the local inhabitants. The outcome was that the Saragossans considered themselves worse off 2 years after the tornado than they had been beforehand, both because of the quality of the rebuilt neighborhoods and because they felt they were looked on as helpless and ungrateful.[2]

Studies in the Caribbean have shown that the different power levels in an uncoordinated community may lead to powerful interest groups pressuring public authorities to rebuild first in areas in which they have the greatest interest. Poorer neighbors with weaker ties to public authorities will get delayed care.[2]

In the United States, vertical planning predominates because few communities have detailed plans in place and because they may not have the financial reserve to pay for the recovery. When a plan is in place before a disaster, it allows for a strong horizontal network. Then, when a useful vertical element is added, the results can work wonders. By 1975, recurrent floods had repeatedly decimated the town of Soldiers Grove, Wisconsin. Each time the town rebuilt. At one point they added a dam, and they planned for a levee, but were unable because of financial restrictions. They decided they would take the funds allocated for the levee and use it to plan for town relocation. Although federal funds were slow in coming, they did create a plan. In 1978, when the largest flood in the history of the area occurred, they were ready with a fully written strategy. When they were granted funds for reconstruction, they put their plan into effect. Not only did they relocate out of the flood plain to prevent reoccurrence of this destruction, but they also decided to create a town that was 75% solar powered.[5] Because they had had the luxury of time in the planning stage, they had asked each business owner where they wanted to be located and how they wanted their business to be built. As a result, the town became not only exactly what the community wanted, but also its creation instilled a great sense of pride and satisfaction in its citizens, thus creating a happier community as well.

REFERENCES

1. Drabek T, Hoetmer G. *Emergency Management: Principles and Practice of Local Government.* Washington, DC: International City Management Association; 1991.
2. Berke P, Kartez J, Wenger D. Recovery after disaster: achieving sustainable development, mitigation and equity. *Disasters.* 17(2):93-109.
3. Haas E, Kates R, Bowden M. *Reconstruction Following Disaster.* Cambridge, MA: MIT Press; 1977.
4. Petterson J. *A Review of the Literature and Programs on Local Recovery from Disaster.* University of Colorado: Natural Hazards Research and Applications Information Center, Institute of Behavioral Science; 1999.
5. Smart Communities Network. Rebuilding for the future: a guide to sustainable redevelopment of disaster-affected communities, September 1994. Available at: http://www.smartcommunities.ncat.org/articles/RFTF1.shtml.
6. Emergency Management Institute. Holistic disaster recovery: creating a more sustainable future [online course]. Available at: http://www.training.fema.gov/hiedu/aemrc/courses/completecourses/sdr.aspx.
7. World Bank Finances Emergency Recovery and Disaster Management Program for the Caribbean. News release no: 99/2035/LAC. Available at: http://reliefweb.int/report/dominica/world-bank-finances-emergency-recovery-and-disaster-management-program-caribbean.
8. Giacomelli L, Perrotta A, Scandone R, Scarpati C. *The eruption of Vesuvius of 79 AD and its impact on human environment in Pompei;* 2003. Retrieved May 2010, from: http://vulcan.fis.uniroma3.it/lavori/episodes.pdf.
9. Weber C. The Lisbon Earthquake of 1755: Representations and Reactions. *Monatshefte.* 2008;100(1):139–141. Retrieved from: https://muse.jhu.edu/.
10. Mullin JR. The reconstruction of Lisbon following the earthquake of 1755: a study in despotic planning. *Landscape Architecture & Regional Planning.* Amherst: University of Massachusetts; 1992. Retrieved from: http://scholarworks.umass.edu.
11. Sakata R, Grant EJ, Ozasa K. Long-term follow-up of atomic bomb survivors. *Maturitas.* 2012;72(2):99–103.
12. Babcock C, Theodosis C, Bills C, et al. The academic health center in complex humanitarian emergencies: lessons learned from the 2010 Haiti earthquake. *Acad Med.* 2012;87:1609–1615. http://dx.doi.org/10.1097/ACM.0b013e31826db6a2.
13. Rahill GJ, Ganapati NE, Clérismé JC, Mukherji A. Shelter recovery in urban Haiti after the earthquake: the dual role of social capital. *Disasters.* 2014;38(Suppl 1):S73–S93. http://dx.doi.org/10.1111/disa.12051.
14. Katz A. *Four Years Later, Haiti's Troubled Recovery Haunts Its Future. Grim anniversary marked by slim progress and renewed aid calls.* January 12, 2014. Retrieved from: http://world.time.com/2014/01/12/four-years-later-haitis-troubledrecovery-haunts-its-future/.
15. Minnesota Homeland Security and Emergency Management. Recovery from Disaster Handbook. Available at: https://dps.mn.gov/divisions/hsem/library/Documents/2012_EMDH_Complete_Web.pdf.
16. Department of Homeland Security. National Response Plan 2004. Available at: http://www.fas.org/irp/agency/dhs/nrp.pdf.
17. FEMA News. *FEMA Hails 2000 as Year of Major Gains in Disaster Prevention.* December 22, 2000. Available at: https://www.fema.gov/news-release/2000/12/22/fema-hails-2000-year-major-gains-disaster-prevention.
18. Disaster Recovery Journal. DRJ's Sample DR Plans and Outlines. Available at: http://www.drj.com/resources/sample-plans.html.
19. Myers D. Psychological recovery from disaster: Key concepts for delivery of mental health services. *NCP Clin Quart.* 1994;4(2):1–5.
20. Berke P, Beatley T. *After the Hurricane.* Baltimore: The Johns Hopkins University Press; 1997.

CHAPTER 60

Disaster Education and Research

Kenneth A. Williams, Leo Kobayashi, and Marc J. Shapiro

Disaster education, regardless of the audience, has two goals: prevention of disasters and mitigation of disaster effects, including improved outcome for victims and safety for responders.

Disaster education should be age appropriate and based on valid research. Education competencies and design should go hand in hand with the design and implementation of disaster research. Unfortunately, most prior disaster research is descriptive and not relevant for education planning. However, advent of new technologies may allow significant improvements in disaster research.

For the public, disaster preparedness once consisted of personal knowledge. People tended to know their limitations and had familiarity with the risks inherent in local environment, activities, and trades. Technological advances have both protected the population in developed countries and increased the risk of extraordinary catastrophe. Disaster research and education must address these changes to remain relevant.

HISTORICAL PERSPECTIVE

Various public health triumphs have mitigated epidemics and disasters. Dr. John Snow,[1] after a brilliant but straightforward epidemiological investigation, mitigated a cholera epidemic in 1855 by simply removing the handle from the contaminated pump. Hygiene, antibiotics, and field medicine saved countless other lives. However, disaster response remained largely an uncoordinated humanitarian effort until recently.

The dictum that there were "no rules" in a disaster was once an excuse for lack of planning, deficient education, and response failures. The modern approach recognizes that disasters can be prevented and effects mitigated, hence there *are* rules and expectations that can be developed from research and promulgated through education. Although disasters overwhelm local response capability, certain types of disasters recur; prevention and mitigation strategy can therefore be formulated. Prior efforts to plan for disaster response, however well intentioned, failed in relation to divergence from daily practice and lack of sufficient scope, flexibility, and resource. Unfamiliar and complex plans involving communication,[2] patient identification and documentation, and command systems that were literally only pulled from cabinets or trailers for annual drills failed in actual events. The military understands that soldiers "fight like they train," and they train frequently when they are not actually fighting. Disaster responders need to learn this lesson; disaster-response paradigms fail in proportion to their deviation from daily practice. Daily practice that is flexible and scalable to meet disaster challenges is a more effective approach. Do it every day. Do more of it on a challenging day. Then, research and education for daily practice can be linked to disaster circumstances effectively.

DEFINITIONS

Flexibility: An asset (technology, provider, or method) is flexible if it can successfully adapt to changing circumstances. For example, a disaster documentation system that requires writing on paper might not be flexible enough to work well during a dark, rainy night.

Scalability: An asset is scalable if it can, through duplication or other means, provide adequate capacity to meet varying demand. For example, a communications system is scalable if design includes an adequate number of devices and staff to provide communications during both daily operations and a disaster situation.

Preparedness: Capacity acquired through planning, education, and training, to provide a function or service. For example, a trained and experienced paramedic is prepared to provide patient care.

Readiness: Ability including willingness, availability, adequate equipment, and preparedness, to respond and provide a function or service within an expected time. For example, a team of paramedics on duty with a fully equipped ambulance is ready to respond and provide patient care.

CURRENT PRACTICE

Education

Adequate disaster education should include age-appropriate guidelines and must follow a basic format for training that allows evaluation of effectiveness. One recommended format is the establishment of clearly stated objectives (e.g., "The children will be evacuated from the school in under 5 minutes," or "The physicians will properly recognize nerve agent exposure from symptoms presented during simulation"). These objectives are next used to develop evaluation tools (e.g., a timed drill for the school, written testing, or observed performance for the physicians). Training curricula are then developed to achieve the desired objectives as measured by the evaluation tool. The students, for example, may need little more than general principles ("Follow the teacher's instructions in an emergency") and awareness that the alarm bell signals such an emergency. Therefore occasional drills may suffice to maintain the needed level of training for them. The teachers, however, require frequent education and practice to be ready for a variety of scenarios. Adults may be trained using a variety of adult learning techniques, but "just-in-time" education should be reserved for situations where response time is not critical or as a brief immediate refresher.

Target audiences for disaster education include the public, non-medical responders, and medical responders. The same principles of effective education apply. General public topics include general disaster readiness, sheltering, evacuation, and first aid. Such education can reduce panic, minimize load on evacuation or shelter systems, and mitigate illness and injury. Nonmedical responder topics vary with the type of responder but should include awareness of medical-response issues and plans. Nonmedical responders may include those who provide shelter, evacuation, security, law enforcement, administration, logistics, food and water supply, sanitation systems, transportation, and structural engineering, among many others. Most disaster response is nonmedical, and injury or illness in nonmedical responders can be mitigated through education and safe practices. Medical responders should improve their readiness through frequent training or experience, including knowledge of education provided to the public and nonmedical responders. This inclusive and coordinated approach will optimize readiness, prevention, and mitigation.

Readiness, the ability to perform on request, requires preparedness and the availability of personnel and resources. To improve readiness, an agency could work on communication essential to notify personnel of a request for service and coordinate their actions, equipment logistics, optimal performance of specific tasks, or means to increase the efficiency of performance. Each of these areas can be the subject of a variety of types of research and training and can apply to the public and nonmedical responders, as well as medical responders. For example, is a population ready to evacuate? Are the regional water suppliers ready to secure their facilities and prevent an effort to contaminate public drinking water? What is the best way to pack medical supplies in kits to optimize paramedic effectiveness? A variety of research exercises linked to training programs can improve readiness in such areas.

Communication, a common challenge in disaster response, can be improved with use of robust and redundant technology that is familiar to all users, and adequate staffing to manage that technology. Communication staff levels adequate for routine practice are inadequate for disaster situations. Flexible and scalable communications response includes both sufficiently redundant technology and the staff to operate that technology. Practical research can assist agencies in the selection and adoption of flexible communication systems likely to remain functional during disaster events. Research parameters for such systems might include features such as interagency interoperability (including linkage with remote responders from other states or agencies), simplicity and flexibility of use, sufficient power sources and operational range for anticipated events, and the ability to move data between variable system elements. Drills, technical demonstrations, and prospective data-gathering during real events are some research methods for the evaluation of communication systems, but successful daily use of systems designed to scale up for disaster response also provides useful data.

Similar to readiness, prevention may encompass public health, engineering, zoning, security, or other measures that trap errors that would otherwise, in certain circumstances, lead to disaster. In most cases, a disaster (defined as "an overwhelmingly damaging event") results in few if any immediate medical casualties. Loss of computer data, defective products, and financial crisis are a few events that can have disastrous results without illness or injury, depending on those affected. Nevertheless, "atraumatic" disasters should be considered in disaster planning, education, and research alongside casualty-producing disasters, at least for health care systems if not for all community entities. The disruption caused by a loss of computer data, by revelations of administrative scandal, or by bankruptcy of a relied-on local service can be significant and can create stress and damage comparable to an event that causes injury or illness, and may eventually result in need for medical care.

Many models of adult education can be used to train disaster responders: self-study, distance learning, direct education, hands-on learning, drills and exercises, and, most recently, simulation laboratories. The types of education must be matched to the audience and the task to be taught, and must take into account available resources. For example, although the best method of teaching personnel how to do a particular skill may be intensive hands-on experience, there may not be the time or money for large-audience training of this type or there may not be adequate actual experience available for the number of interested students. Types of education include the following:

- *Self-study:* It allows self-paced learning, either from a text or Internet source. This type of learning lends itself well to those with episodic downtime during their workdays and with time to study that may be off shift or off hours for other educational opportunities. Because it is often location and time independent, it accommodates a wide variety of learners, but the ability for discussion and feedback is somewhat limited.
- *Distance learning:* This type of learning uses live two-way video technology and is most often Internet-based. It allows many to be trained in a "live environment" where their questions and issues can be addressed by the teacher and allows group interaction. Although somewhat location independent, depending on technology, it is time dependent—learners must "log in" at the specified time.
- *Direct education:* This involves a lecturer delivering content in person to an audience. Although this type of education facilitates questions and feedback, as well as group discussion, it requires a ready pool of both expert educators and available learners that may not exist in a particular subject of interest, period, or geographic area.
- *Hands-on learning:* Particularly suited for teaching skills, such as the use of protective equipment, this training is labor and time intensive and requires the use of local expertise and small-class-size-to-instructor ratio. However, it is very effective for learning manual tasks.
- *Feedback and quality improvement:* Useful for measuring compliance, honing skills, and correcting errors, this type of education involves either direct educator presence (such as faculty mentoring a resident physician) or review of documented performance (such as medical director review of emergency medical service [EMS] charts).
- *Drills and exercises:* Effective drills and exercises combine features of hands-on learning, direct education, and feedback. The event size can vary, but it typically involves more than one learner. Technology (computer simulations, communications links between simulation centers, etc.) can facilitate very large exercises. Extensive full-scale events are expensive and time consuming but offer significant training, error trapping, and networking opportunities for the agencies and personnel involved. Drills and exercises are an excellent place to solidify training, identify future needs, and conduct some types of research.

Simulation Training

The goal of simulation is creation of an immersive environment that mirrors reality. Learners should feel like the situation is real in a successful simulation, or at least real enough for their thoughts and actions to be realistic. In many cases, such realism allows research where manikins substitute for actual patients.

Human-patient simulation is reaching a larger audience as the technology improves and becomes more accessible. Distinct from the training offered by simple cardiopulmonary resuscitation manikins or personal computer–based multimedia software, high-fidelity medical simulation features integrated life-sized "patients" with programmable, reproducible, and physiological response capabilities. Interactive communication, the ability to undergo procedural interventions, and real-time recording of events are key features. Flexibility is improved with expert manikin control, allowing adaptation to a variety of learner actions. The application of these tools and techniques to disaster-medicine education is now taking place.

Both manikin and virtual reality (VR) simulated patients have been used to train health care personnel in various fields. Detailed patient presentations in realistic treatment settings, accurate modeling of human physiology, and dynamic changes in response to interventions contribute to these educational experiences. Otherwise unachievable training is also made possible when clinical events and care settings would harbor significant risk and enormous consequences to real patients. Difficult medical resuscitation and intraoperative crisis management are representative subject areas; learners can make mistakes in a simulated environment without risk to actual patients.

Self-contained high-fidelity manikin-based systems are useful in disaster training because of the relative ease of setup and maintenance compared with VR counterparts. Expanding from their original role in anesthesia and resuscitation instruction, these manikins are being applied to disaster training in an ongoing exploration of their capabilities.[3-9] Re-creation of the physical barriers and material impediments to patient care at disaster scenes is a prime area of inquiry. For example, practicing intravenous access, medication administration, and endotracheal intubation while garbed in personal protective equipment (PPE) has been investigated using manikins.[3-13] Such training and research would be hazardous using real patients and would lack fidelity in a VR environment.

Total-immersion VR (TIVR) and associated technologies are also being applied to disaster education.[14] Featuring fully computer-generated environments and patients with multisensory interactivity (i.e., visual, auditory, and haptic), TIVR advances the "perceptual illusion of non-mediation."[15] This capacity to establish the presence of participants within the TIVR-constructed world seamlessly hints at the potential for tremendously flexible and virtually unlimited simulations for training. Early endeavors were conducted at the University of Michigan 3D Lab,[16,17] University of Missouri-Rolla,[18] and the University of Padova,[19] where researchers implemented TIVR-enhanced disaster scenarios. Additional TIVR-based disaster-medicine work is ongoing.[20-24] Lack of standardization and significant startup requirements still limit TIVR's accessibility for the time being.

Civilian and Commercial High-Fidelity Simulation Applications in Disaster and Weapons of Mass Destruction Education

With the increasing number of civilian sites featuring various forms of patient simulators, training courses have begun in earnest to delve into disaster-specific content. High-fidelity simulation is now accessible at paramedic training sites and nursing, pharmacy schools, and medical schools. The fundamentals of disaster medical response, such as situational and hazard assessment, triage, patient examination and treatment, decontamination and provider protection, and evacuation have been addressed using these assets.[25] Focused task training and exercises fostering specific cognitive processes and teamwork behaviors[26,27] have been undertaken. Research comparing approaches to complex resuscitation and research where the responder is the subject (ergonomics, effort, and fatigue, etc.) instead of the patient undergoing complex resuscitation is also facilitated by simulated environments.

Increased funding for disaster and weapons of mass destruction (WMD) training released since September 2001 has helped prehospital systems in several states experience sophisticated disaster exercises employing advanced medical simulation. These efforts in Florida, Maryland,[26] and Rhode Island[27] have been primarily based at university-affiliated academic simulation centers receiving state and/or federal support. Significant use of high-fidelity simulation technology for nuclear, biological, and chemical preparedness is most apparent internationally in the Israel Center for Medical Simulation's activities.

Their programs address the preparation of physicians, nurses, and paramedics for the casualties of nonconventional warfare.[10,11,28]

In the commercial sphere, various U.S. centers are offering courses using high-fidelity manikin patient simulators for training in WMD and hazardous materials (HazMat). Early disaster-related high-fidelity simulations in the form of Simulation Training in Emergency Preparedness courses[29] (supported by the Health Resources and Services Administration) trained hundreds of first responders and hospital personnel at the Rhode Island Hospital Medical Simulation Center in 2005-2006, along with the Texas Engineering Extension Service that provided WMD-focused prehospital operations and planning curriculum.[30] Similar courses for the EMS community contain assorted applications of patient simulation, ranging from isolated patient care duties to full-scale multimanikin disaster drills.

High-fidelity simulation applications in disaster and WMD education for military forces have become routine to assist with personnel support roles for natural calamities and/or in combat preparation duties. Consequently, many of the issues raised by terrorism and WMDs have been addressed by the military in their established training. Troops engaging in combat have been expected to encounter weaponized chemical toxins, bioweapons, explosives, and radioactive hazards. Whereas the settings in which such exposures can occur have changed, the knowledge and techniques involved in responding to them remain mostly unaltered. However, actual experience in combat theater may vary from training based on expectations. In an example of rapid cycle adaptation using simulation-based training, a program whereby returning U.S. Army Reserve medical personnel were debriefed after deployment in Iraq or Afghanistan and that knowledge used to develop training scenarios for units preparing to deploy was trialed successfully.[31] Numerous similar programs are ongoing.[32,33]

The U.S. military is developing and running training programs focused on the health care services specialist, known as a "91W," with a particular interest in chemical, biological, radioactive, nuclear, and explosive qualifications.[34] Component modules include personal computer–based Simulation Technologies for Trauma Care (STAT-Care)[35] and Nuclear Biological Chemical Casualty Training System (NBCCTS)[36] software. Advanced patient simulation within the various project efforts features prominently under the Medical Simulation Initiative. Several hundred high-fidelity manikins in on-site and distance-learning settings have been integrated into 91W training at various locations.[37-39] WMD-specific applications are being phased in. Logistical simulation of the mechanics and delivery of medical care at multiple levels in a realistic and complete battlefield environment is also progressing with the Combat Trauma Patient Simulator program.[40]

Future Directions in Simulation

Numerous simulation experts and groups are pursuing scientific validation of simulation techniques in health care education. The disordered environment of a true disaster makes prospective, controlled, and objective studies of educational content transfer difficult. Retrospective analyses may have a role, whereas surrogate markers of training efficacy and improvement in emergency preparedness could serve to demonstrate simulation utility in the interim. For example, response protocol changes developed from the Rhode Island Disaster Initiative (RIDI) Project in 2001-2003[5] were also noted in a thorough after-action report on the deadly 2003 Station Nightclub Fire, including need for flexible and scalable practices in disaster triage, treatment, and transport.[41] Many responders to the fire had participated in RIDI drills and training sessions.

Enhancement of independent disaster-response abilities can be individually assessed at "skill stations" akin to those in advanced cardiac life-support courses. Global rating scales have surfaced as potential indicators of overall learner competence in educational settings using high-fidelity simulation.[42] Such instruments, using properly defined scoring systems, should help in investigating basic disaster-response competencies in conjunction with fully immersive multiple-manikin disaster drills; investigative efforts are ongoing.[43–47]

Development and testing of tools to demonstrate improved medical-responder preparedness with proper disaster training are taking place through federally and state-funded projects. Extensively incorporated into these activities, high-fidelity simulation has already allowed objective examination of EMS providers' scene hazards assessment, triage decision making,[48–50] use of novel interventions,[51] and resuscitative actions[9] in PPE. Continued work through such ventures is aimed to establish causal associations between high-fidelity simulation training, enhanced responder readiness training, improved disaster medical response, and, ultimately, better patient outcomes.

The greatest challenges for disaster trainers are to maintain the training competencies and certifications initially acquired and to work on continual skill development in an environment where little is changing, and the next disaster may seem far away.

CATEGORIES OF RESEARCH

Disaster research can be categorized and associated with educational objectives. Categories include after-action report and case studies; aftermath epidemiology; discussion of planning, training, and mitigation techniques; trials of specific techniques or equipment; organizational or analytical schemes; and randomized controlled trials.

After-Action Report and Case Studies

A description of the first 10 cases of anthrax in the United States caused by a terrorist event[52] provides an example of the after-action report and case study. These data are useful in planning response magnitude and type. Recurring failures in response are well elucidated in this type of report and are a common theme in after-action reports. While cogently documenting the events surrounding various natural and human-made tragedies, these papers also often report shockingly similar response failures, including those involving communication, logistics, clothing, equipment, interagency cooperation, perimeter control, patient care delays, and suboptimal distribution of casualties.[53] Although various nonmedical entities, such as the Federal Aviation Administration and the National Transportation Safety Board, have implemented various regulatory and technology improvements during the past few decades, reducing the incidence of human-made disasters and mitigating their severity, medical responders often face the same challenges reported 25 years ago.

Epidemiology

The advent of widespread cellular communications coverage internationally allows for gathering epidemiological data during and after disaster events. Crowdsourcing information related to geography of events, symptoms, need for rescue or supplies, or other information might be of utility during both the response and recovery and planning phases of response.[54]

Descriptions of the delayed effects of a disaster point out needs for planners and responders who arrive after the acute incident phase. The need to reestablish infrastructure rapidly, to attend to chronic health care needs and sanitation, to distribute medications, etc., recurs in a review of these research papers. Additionally, descriptions of lingering effects, such as the description of "eye injuries" following the Tokyo Subway Sarin Attacks,[55] can be illuminating and have been cited in discussions of the need for culturally sensitive media communications and other relevant planning. Cultural diversity may alter the expression of disaster effects, but awareness that disasters have long lasting and significant effects can be important for planners and educators seeking to address these concerns.

Discussion of Planning, Training, and Mitigation Techniques

A discussion of planning, training, and mitigation techniques might include a survey and discussion related to bioterrorism training for emergency medicine residents.[56] These papers document education and planning methodologies and are useful in two ways. First, they provide a benchmark for the schemes in place that can be compared with outcome when an event occurs. If a system has a plan in effect, with specific training methods and techniques, readiness (as measured in a well-run drill or an actual event) can be compared with alternative systems. Second, these papers serve to distribute the ideas, good and bad, that others have developed. Planners should be familiar with this literature and should seek to learn from the mistakes and brilliant insights of others as they design training and response plans.

Trials of Specific Techniques or Equipment

Although rare in the disaster research literature, trials of specific techniques or equipment present various methodologies for care and use of equipment. Topics such as triage technique, categories of patient condition, patient identification tags, communications equipment, training programs in specific scenarios or problems, and command structures fall into this literature category. A weakness of many of these papers is the failure to document use of the topic item (method, equipment, etc.) in a real event or in a controlled series of drills where it can be realistically compared with an alternative. Papers that tout the utility of an item and offer only a single drill designed to display the item should be scrutinized carefully and critically.

Organizational and Analytical Schemes

Organizational and analytical schemes discuss progress in disaster management, or lack thereof, and offer schemes or suggestions to improve international coordination, planning focus, funding allocation, etc.[57] They often report the collective wisdom of a group of experts, but occasionally offer the scheme of a single person. In either case, this body of literature should be familiar to all disaster researchers and educators because a certain level of standardization and commonality in definitions and language is essential to collaborative effort. The current U.S. response scheme, which incorporates many of the lessons learned from prior disasters and focuses on flexibility and scalability, is the National Response Framework.[58] The World Association for Disaster and Emergency Medicine has developed standards and guidelines for disaster-response education and training.[59]

Randomized Controlled Trials

Although rare in disaster research, randomized controlled trials are nonetheless very important and can be accomplished using simulation-based repetitive drills. The potential to perform research on actual recurring disasters (e.g., floods, earthquakes, and certain transportation disasters) also exists, and a few researchers have attempted to gather data comparing use of techniques or equipment with some degree of randomization.

Currently, the most feasible option is the use of recurring simulation-based drills to conduct research. The RIDI, a federally funded disaster research project (1999-2004), included a series of twelve disaster drills performed in a high-fidelity multiplace simulation center, compared control groups to experimental groups across a variety of response parameters using a time-to-critical-event evaluation tool developed by the investigators.[12] The ability to reproduce a disaster drill accurately allowed the RIDI team to compare training and equipment practices between randomized responder groups. Future initiatives should move this type of research into formal research formats, such as crossover control or randomized trial models.

SUMMARY

Education and research related to disasters and disaster response are tightly linked.[60] The advent of widespread communications technology now allows near real-time data reporting from disaster scenes, including accurate location information. This technology also allows dissemination of educational information to responders, victims, and others. Advances in simulation and VR have enhanced both research and education. Successful disaster prevention mitigation and response depend on the adoption and implementation of these improvements.

REFERENCES

1. Snow J. *On the Mode of Communication of Cholera.* London: John Churchill; 1855. Available at: http://www.ph.ucla.edu/epi/snow/snowbook2.html, 38–55.
2. Yoho Jr. D. Wireless communication technology applied to disaster response. *Aviat Space Environ Med.* 1994;65(9):839–845.
3. Scott J, Miller G, Issenberg S, et al. Skill improvement during emergency response to terrorism training. *Prehosp Emerg Care.* 2006;10(4):507–514.
4. Subbarao I, Bond W, Johnson C, Hsu EB, Wasser TE. Using innovative simulation modalities for civilian-based, chemical, biological, radiological, nuclear, and explosive training in the acute management of terrorist victims: a pilot study. *Prehosp Disaster Med.* 2006;21(4):272–275.
5. Summerhill E, Mathew M, Stipho S, et al. A simulation-based biodefense and disaster preparedness curriculum for internal medicine residents. *Med Teach.* 2008;30(6):e145–e551.
6. Cicero M, Auerbach M, Zigmont J, Riera A, Ching K, Baum CR. Simulation training with structured debriefing improves residents' pediatric disaster triage performance. *Prehosp Disaster Med.* 2012;27(3):239–244.
7. Scott L, Maddux P, Schnellmann J, Hayes L, Tolley J, Wahlquist AE. High-fidelity multiactor emergency preparedness training for patient care providers. *Am J Disaster Med.* 2012;7(3):175–188.
8. Scott L, Swartzentruber D, Davis C, Maddux PT, Schnellman J, Wahlquist AE. Competency in chaos: lifesaving performance of care providers utilizing a competency-based, multi-actor emergency preparedness training curriculum. *Prehosp Disaster Med.* 2013;28(4):322–333.
9. Jose M, Dufrene C. Educational competencies and technologies for disaster preparedness in undergraduate nursing education: an integrative review. *Nurse Educ Today.* 2014;34(4):543–551.
10. Vardi A, Levin I, Berkenstadt H, et al. Simulation-based training of medical teams to manage chemical warfare casualties. *Isr Med Assoc J.* 2002;4(7):540–544.
11. Berkenstadt H, Ziv A, Barsuk D, Levine I, Cohen A, Vardi A. The use of advanced simulation in the training of anesthesiologists to treat chemical warfare casualties. *Anesth Analg.* 2003;96(6):1739–1742.
12. Williams K, Sullivan F, Suner S, et al. Rhode Island disaster initiative. *Int J Risk Assess Manag.* 2008;9(4):394–408.
13. Kobayashi L, Shapiro M, Suner S, Williams KA. Disaster medicine education: the potential role of high fidelity medical simulation in mass casualty incident training. *Med Health R I.* 2003;86(7):196–200.
14. Deleted during review.
15. Lombard M, Ditton T. At the heart of it all: the concept of presence. *J Computer-Mediated Commun.* 1997;3(2)Available at: http://www.ascusc.org/jcmc/vol3/issue2/lombard.html.
16. University of Michigan 3-D Lab. CAVE Technology Demonstration Disaster Scenario Web site. Available at: http://um3d.dc.umich.edu/index.html.
17. University of Michigan Virtual Reality Laboratory at the College of Engineering. Medical Readiness Trainer Web site. Available at: http://www-vrl.umich.edu/mrt.
18. Deleted during review.
19. Gamberini L, Cottone P, Spagnolli A, Varotto D, Mantovani G. Responding to a fire emergency in a virtual environment: different patterns of action for different situations. *Ergonomics.* 2003;46(8):842–858.
20. Vincent D, Sherstyuk A, Burgess L, Connolly KK. Teaching mass casualty triage skills using immersive three-dimensional virtual reality. *Acad Emerg Med.* 2008;15(11):1160–1165.
21. Wilkerson W, Avstreih D, Gruppen L, Beier KP, Woolliscroft J. Using immersive simulation for training first responders for mass casualty incidents. *Acad Emerg Med.* 2008;15(11):1152–1159.
22. Andreatta P, Maslowski E, Petty S, et al. Virtual reality triage training provides a viable solution for disaster-preparedness. *Acad Emerg Med.* 2010;17(8):870–876.
23. Heinrichs W, Youngblood P, Harter P, Kusumoto L, Dev P. Training healthcare personnel for mass-casualty incidents in a virtual emergency department: VED II. *Prehosp Disaster Med.* 2010;25(5):424–432.
24. Ingrassia PL, Ragazzoni L, Carenzo L, Colombo D, Ripoll Gallardo A, Della Corte F. Virtual reality and live simulation: a comparison between two simulation tools for assessing mass casualty triage skills. *Eur J Emerg Med.* 2015;22(2):121–127.
25. Suner S, Williams K, Shapiro M, et al. Effect of personal protective equipment (PPE) on rapid patient assessment and treatment during a simulated chemical weapons of mass destruction (WMD) attack. *Acad Emerg Med.* 2004;11(5):605 [Abstract].
26. Kyle R, Via D, Lowy R, Madsen JM, Marty AM, Mongan PD. A multidisciplinary approach to teach responses to weapons of mass destruction and terrorism using combined simulation modalities. *J Clin Anesth.* 2004;16(2):152–158.
27. Kobayashi L, Shapiro M, Hill A, Jay G. Creating a MESS for enhanced acute care medical education and medical error reduction: the multiple encounter simulation scenario. *Acad Emerg Med.* 2004;11(8):896 [Abstract].
28. The Chaim Sheba Medical Center at Tel Hashomer. Israel Center for Medical Simulation Web site. Available at: http://eng.sheba.co.il/main/siteNew/index.php?page=45&action=sidLink&stId=435.
29. Deleted during review.
30. Deleted during review.
31. Kobayashi L, Williams K, Morey J, et al. *TATRC Reserve Medical Component Training (RCT) Case Scenarios.* MedEdPORTAL; 2007. Available at: http://services.aamc.org/jsp/mededportal/retrieveSubmissionDetailById.do?subId=524.
32. King D, Patel M, Feinstein A, Earle SA, Topp RF, Proctor KG. Simulation training for a mass casualty incident: two-year experience at the Army Trauma Training Center. *J Trauma.* 2006;61(4):943–948.
33. Pereira B, Ryan M, Ogilvie M, et al. Predeployment mass casualty and clinical trauma training for US Army forward surgical teams. *J Craniofac Surg.* 2010;21(4):982–986.
34. Deleted during review.
35. RTI International. Simulation Technologies for Advanced Trauma Care (STATCare) Web site. Available at: http://www.rti.org/page.cfm?objectid=3F6A5676-FEF7-423F-92479553E912FB73.
36. Deleted during review.
37. Deleted during review.
38. Deleted during review.
39. Research, Development and Engineering Command (RDECOM) Web site. Available at: http://www.globalsecurity.org/military/agency/army/rdec.htm.
40. U.S. Army Program Executive Office for Simulation, Training, and Instrumentation. Combat Trauma Patient Simulator (CTSP) program Web site. Available at: http://www.peostri.army.mil/products/CTPS.
41. *The Station Club Fire: After-action Report: State, Local, and Federal Government and the Private Sector United States.* Department of Homeland Security. Office for Domestic Preparedness. Titan Corporation; 2004.
42. Gordon J, Tancredi D, Binder W, Wilkerson W, Shaffer DW, Cooper J. Assessing global performance in emergency medicine using a high-fidelity patient simulator: a pilot study. *Acad Emerg Med.* 2004;10(5):472 [Abstract].
43. Rüter A, Ortenwall P, Vikström T. Staff procedure skills in management groups during exercises in disaster medicine. *Prehosp Disaster Med.* 2007;22(4):318–321.

44. Gillett B, Peckler B, Sinert R, et al. Simulation in a disaster drill: comparison of high-fidelity simulators versus trained actors. *Acad Emerg Med.* 2008;15(11):1144–1151.

45. Ingrassia P, Prato F, Geddo A, et al. Evaluation of medical management during a mass casualty incident exercise: an objective assessment tool to enhance direct observation. *J Emerg Med.* 2010;39(5):629–636.

46. Wallace D, Gillett B, Wright B, Stetz J, Arquilla B. Randomized controlled trial of high fidelity patient simulators compared to actor patients in a pandemic influenza drill scenario. *Resuscitation.* 2010;81(7):872–876.

47. Smith M, Bentley M, Fernandez A, Gibson G, Schweikhart SB, Woods DD. Performance of experienced versus less experienced paramedics in managing challenging scenarios: a cognitive task analysis study. *Ann Emerg Med.* 2013;62(4):367–379.

48. Lerner E, Schwartz R, Coule P, Pirrallo RG. Use of SALT triage in a simulated mass-casualty incident. *Prehosp Emerg Care.* 2010;14(1):21–25.

49. Rehn M, Andersen J, Vigerust T, Krüger AJ, Lossius HM. A concept for major incident triage: full-scaled simulation feasibility study. *BMC Emerg Med.* 2010;10:17.

50. Cicero M, Riera A, Northrup V, Auerbach M, Pearson K, Baum CR. Design, validity, and reliability of a pediatric resident JumpSTART disaster triage scoring instrument. *Acad Pediatr.* 2013;13(1):48–54.

51. Vardi A, Berkenstadt H, Levin I, Bentencur A, Ziv A. Intraosseous vascular access in the treatment of chemical warfare casualties assessed by advanced simulation: proposed alteration of treatment protocol. *Anesth Analg.* 2004;98(6):1753–1758.

52. Jernigan J, Stephens D, Ashford D, et al. Bioterrorism-related inhalational anthrax: the first 10 cases reported in the United States. *Emerg Infect Dis.* 2001;7(6):933–944.

53. Williams A. *Lessons learned from transportation disasters [unpublished thesis, MPH program].* Cambridge, MA: Harvard University; 1995.

54. Goodchild M, Glennon J. Crowdsourcing geographic information for disaster response: a research frontier. *Intl J Digit Earth.* 2010;3(3):231–241.

55. Kawana N, Ishimatsu S, Kanda K. Psycho-physiological effects of the terrorist sarin attack on the Tokyo subway system. *Mil Med.* 2001;166(12 Suppl):23–26.

56. Pesik N, Keim M, Sampson TR. Do US emergency medicine residency programs provide adequate training for bioterrorism? *Ann Emerg Med.* 1999;34(2):173–176.

57. Sundnes K, Adler J, Birnbaum M, et al. Health disaster management: guidelines for evaluation and research in the Utstein style: executive summary. *Prehospital Disaster Med.* 1996;11(2):82–90.

58. Available at: http://www.fema.gov/national-response-framework.

59. Seynaeve G, Archer F, Fisher J, et al. International standards and guidelines on education and training for the multi-disciplinary health response to major events that threaten the health status of a community. Education Committee Working Group, World Association for Disaster and Emergency Medicine. *Prehosp Disaster Med.* 2004;19(2):S17–S30.

60. Hubloue I, Debacker M. Education and research in disaster medicine and management: inextricably bound up with each other. *Eur J Emerg Med.* 2010;17(3):129–130.

Practical Applications of Disaster Epidemiology

P. Gregg Greenough and Frederick M. Burkle Jr.

All disasters—whether natural or human generated—have their own unique epidemiology and patterns of health outcomes on the populations they afflict. Commonly defined, epidemiology is the study of the distribution and determinants of health-related states or events in specified populations of interest, and the application of that study to managing and controlling health problems. The science of epidemiology illuminates how specific disasters generate specific expected and sometimes unexpected patterns of morbidity, mortality, and health system damage within a population and civil society. By applying epidemiological methods to crisis-affected populations, the disaster response community has embraced an evidence base for its work and, in so doing, opened the door to more data-driven response strategies and impact measures.

Disaster epidemiology has a role in every phase of the disaster cycle, from the development of prevention strategies during the preparedness phase to needs assessments during the emergency phase to the measurement of disaster response during the postimpact and reconstruction phase. Cognizance of public health effects from given disasters guides preparedness and mitigation efforts. For instance, an earthquake in a dense urban zone will likely damage health system infrastructure at a time when large numbers of the population will seek care for fractures, closed-head injuries, lacerations, and soft-tissue injuries. Often these are multiple and spatially aggregated in places where the health delivery system is destroyed.[1] Within days, a significant number will develop wound infections and renal failure from crush injuries. Surgical services will be stressed providing wound debridement, orthopedic reduction and fixations, and multiple revisions. Long-term mental health issues and physical disabilities will arise, with the potential to disrupt a society's economy and subsequent ability to repair itself.[2] Advanced understanding of a specific disaster's epidemiology at all phases can guide disaster managers and relief organizations in planning for an effective response and directing critical resources. More importantly, disaster epidemiology–guided mitigation efforts can reduce the death, disease, and injury burden potentiated by a given disaster.

HISTORICAL PERSPECTIVE

The practical applications of disaster epidemiology grew from potent natural disasters of the 1970s and 1980s.[3–6] These events demonstrated that epidemiological methods could measure and minimize risk, assess the relief effort, describe patterns of morbidity and mortality, and suggest prevention and intervention strategies. The field evolved more fully and became better organized during the 1990 International Decade for Natural Response Reduction, as the international disaster response community, consisting of multilateral organizations and nongovernmental organizations (NGOs), embraced the contribution of disaster epidemiology in providing an evidence-based understanding of response efforts; this led, in part, to the development of standards in humanitarian practice. By the late 1990s, the Sphere Project was born. The consensus-driven initiative, now in its fourth iteration, draws on both empirical evidence and aggregated experience informed by disaster and conflict epidemiology in determining minimum standards in the health, food, nutrition, shelter, water, and sanitation response sectors.[7] Similarly, the Active Learning Network for Accountability and Performance in Humanitarian Action (ALNAP) was established to improve performance, enhance education, and inculcate accountability within the humanitarian enterprise and, in so doing, has adopted qualitative and quantitative epidemiological tools as a means of professionalizing humanitarian response work.

During this time, the Center for Research on the Epidemiology of Disasters (CRED) established a database to track health outcomes in disasters. EM-DAT, the international Emergency Events Database, has archived and tracked more than 18,000 major disasters since 1900. This wealth of data allows donors, disaster managers, disaster researchers, and key policy makers to study comparisons across types of hazards, geopolitical contexts, and vulnerability and resilience factors.

Since the late 1990s, epidemiological methods have also been applied to conflict-affected populations to estimate both direct mortality and indirect mortality. Direct mortality stems from both the conflict's immediate violence and its incapacitating effect on the health delivery system, such as in Kosovo and Iraq.[8] For instance, in Kosovo, despite the expected levels of deaths due to violence, death from chronic diseases was significant, owing to the affected population's health demographic, its health profile, and its disconnect from a health system broken by violence, insecurity, and migration. Indirect and excess mortality from preventable and readily treatable causes results from the breakdown of the public health infrastructure due to the conflict, as has been the case in prolonged but less condensed conflicts, such as that in the Democratic Republic of the Congo.[9] In conflict settings as in other population crises, an epidemiological focus guides humanitarian public health responses to populations in dire need and targets political and aid policy makers and human rights advocates.[10]

CURRENT PRACTICE

Disaster epidemiology plays a role in all phases of disaster response. Evidence-based decision-making promises to protect vulnerable populations from significant morbidity and mortality if such studies are: conducted in a proactive and timely fashion, well designed to address critical questions for disaster preparedness and response, disseminated to all critical stakeholders, and brought into the preparedness and response discourse. The following types of epidemiological applications are most common in the preparedness, emergency, and response and recovery phases.

Vulnerability Analyses

The key purpose of these analyses is to identify populations at risk from all hazards in an effort to implement preparedness and mitigation strategies, as well as establish a baseline from which recovery efforts can be measured. In addition to disaster managers, a variety of stakeholders concerned with risk and vulnerability, including urban planners and insurance actuaries, rely on these studies. A more detailed discussion can be found elsewhere in this text; the brief mention here is to emphasize the relevance of a population-based science.

Vulnerability is defined as the characteristics and circumstances of a community, system, or asset that make it susceptible to the damaging effects of a hazard; hazards are dangerous phenomena, substances, human activities, or conditions that may cause loss of life, injury, or other health impacts, property damage, loss of livelihoods and services, social and economic disruption, or environmental damage.[11] In epidemiological terms, vulnerability is the physical, social, economic, and environmental factors within a population that puts it at risk from a given hazard. The population's social sensitivity and adaptive capacity are functions of the potential public health effects of a hazard on a population.

An understanding of population vulnerability in relation to a hazard allows epidemiologists to model risk and potential outcomes, and further delineate the factors that may worsen or mitigate outcomes. For instance, retrospective analyses undertaken in postdisaster phases have identified vulnerable groups and risk factors associated with certain hazards: with extreme heat, individuals with cardiovascular disease and the elderly;[12] with earthquakes, those with mental disorders and moderate physical disabilities;[13] and with a variety of disasters, socioeconomic inequities,[14,15] to name a few. Population-based methods are being explored to understand disaster impacts in the interdisciplinary area of human-environment (coupled human and natural systems) research.[16]

Local factors in the human-environment system that affect the population's ability to absorb the shock of a hazard may include, among others, the degree of foliage degradation and deforestation; the degree of urbanization, density, and land use and development; patterns of employment and livelihoods; the quality and extent of transportation and communications networks; the quality of construction; and the quality and availability of health services delivery. On a national level, factors such as climate change risks, debt-relief policies, zoning policies, the quality of construction codes, the degree of government stability, and the adherence to the rule of law all directly contribute to a population's vulnerability and reflect critical variables in interdisciplinary population-based public health disaster impact studies.

A population's perception of risk and its vulnerability in relation to a hazard calls for qualitative epidemiological studies to better understand how disaster managers can customize their planning initiatives and assist their populations with more effective preparedness and response. This is in addition to readily quantifiable risk analysis and modeling. The public's perception of risk and that of public officials have multiple dimensions and complexities, driven by subjectivity and warranting a qualitative approach. Examples include identifying the constraints of integrating climate change adaptation policies into disaster risk reduction strategies[17]; understanding public responses to chemical, biological, radiological, or nuclear events[18]; or coming to consensus on indicators of community postdisaster recovery.[19] Such methods provide the ability to get at the underlying thought processes of all stakeholders and engage multiple disciplines in the discourse.

Rapid Needs Assessments

Rapid assessments seek to determine the magnitude of a crisis, the degree of impact on the population, the status of sector-specific population needs (food, water, sanitation, shelter, health care), vulnerable populations at particular risk, and the state of the disaster response.

This requires public health providers to be on the ground characterizing and quantifying the affected population: identifying existing and potential pubic health problems; measuring present and potential impact, especially health and nutritional needs; assessing resources needed, including the availability and capacity of a local response; aiding in planning and guiding an appropriate level of external response; identifying vulnerable groups; and providing baseline data from which the public health system can be restored. Interviewing health workers, reviewing clinic records, or directly observing displaced and nondisplaced settlements and households within settlements are field techniques commonly used to collect data.

Epidemiological data can be gathered through a variety of quantitative, qualitative, and mixed-methods study designs. The critical point is to gain familiarity with the various methods and their appropriate applications. Crises tend to limit the purity of traditional study designs: insecurity, lack of baseline population data for sampling frames, and the need for rapid analysis and dissemination factor into the difficulty of gathering primary population data in these settings. Despite these limitations, crisis epidemiologists have built on a body of literature and devised commonly accepted methodologies for deriving and tracking critical *indicators*—the qualitative or quantitative criteria used to correlate or predict the value or measure of a program, system, or organization.[20] Such tools inform and guide decision making during the crisis and beyond.

The interagency Standardized Monitoring and Assessment of Relief and Transitions (SMART) initiative has assisted humanitarian practitioners in developing field methodologies to generate and track two key crisis indicators: the nutritional status of children under the age of 5 years and the mortality rate of the population.[21] These two quantitative indicators assess the magnitude and severity of a crisis and are critical in determining if conditions are improving and, by proxy, whether interventions are having an effect.

Mortality rates express the number of deaths within a population of interest per unit of time. Two mortality rates of particular interest in crises are the crude mortality rate (CMR) and the under-age-5 mortality rate (U5MR). The CMR is calculated for an entire population, whereas U5MR signifies a specific vulnerable group (the number of deaths of children under 5 years of age population in a defined time). In a sense, the U5MR is the more sensitive of the two indicators: if mortality rises in the under-5 age group, it portends a rise in overall mortality. Doubling of either or both of these mortality rates from their respective precrisis baselines signals a public health emergency that should alert crisis responders.

The CMR is given by the equation

$$CMR = \frac{\text{Number of deaths in a time period}}{\text{Total population at midperiod}} \times \frac{K}{\text{Number of days in time period}}$$

where K is a uniform constant by which rates or proportions can be multiplied for purposes of comparison and easy understanding, usually a multiple of 10, such as 1000, 10,000, or 100,000. CMRs are expressed during the emergency phase as deaths per 10,000 people per day, the latter unit used to capture a significant number of deaths in short periods of time if the intensity of mortality is high. As the health crisis of an impact passes into a more stable recovery period, the crude death rate is more commonly used, expressed as deaths per 1000 population per year.

Similarly, age-specific death rates such as the U5MR are used in emergencies to identify subgroups particularly at risk during a disaster and help clarify the mortality nested within the CMR. Similar to the CMR calculation, the U5MR uses the number of deaths in children younger than 5 years of age over a time interval divided by the total population of children younger than 5 years of age at the middle of the specified time period:

$$U5MR = \frac{\begin{array}{c}\text{Number of deaths under-age-5 years}\\\text{in a time period}\end{array}}{\begin{array}{c}\text{Total under-age-5 years}\\\text{population at midperiod}\end{array}} \times \frac{K}{\text{Number of days in time period}}$$

Like the CMR, this is expressed in terms of under-age-5 deaths per 10,000 population of under-age-5 children per day during the emergency phase, or per 1000 population of under-age-5 children per 1000 per month in the postemergency phase.

Numerators (the number of deaths) and denominators (the total population of interest at the midpoint of some time frame) are necessary to calculate a rate. To capture the number of deaths with any degree of accuracy, a system that dutifully records and time-stamps deaths must be in place. Often in crises, this component of the health information system fails, and disaster response agencies must aggregate the number of deaths from a variety of sources, including health facilities (if they are still functioning), relief agencies working in specific sectors, makeshift gravesites, rapid household surveys, and the like. Population estimates for the denominators may also present a challenge during crises: mass displacement, outdated population censuses, or inadequate vital registration systems make determining absolute numbers difficult to obtain, especially population figures disaggregated by age, as would be needed to calculate the U5MR. In such settings, rapid assessments will include activities that estimate the population and may necessitate various means of population reconnaissance. On-the-ground counts using GPS supported by remote sensing, registration systems that catalog displaced populations (as in refugee settlements), or compiled distribution lists from operational UN agencies tasked with sector support, such as the World Food Programme, can be used to triangulate population figures in lieu of an actual census.

Mortality information from the emergency phase assessments may also include cause-specific mortality, the causes of death that occur during an emergency over time. Aside from the mortal injury caused by the disaster or conflict itself, excess mortality from communicable and noncommunicable diseases can be tracked and, in so doing, gives an epidemiological picture of the affected country. Noncommunicable disease deaths are often seen in developed countries in which the affected population is dissociated from its health system due to insecurity, the breakdown of the health system, physical displacement, or some combination of these. Deaths from communicable diseases, frequent in developing-world settings, can be rapidly and efficiently chronicled by using standard and simple case definitions as opposed to laboratory confirmations. Classified cases are the numerator for the cause-specific mortality rate:

$$\text{Cause-specific MR} = \frac{\begin{array}{c}\text{Number of deaths from specific}\\\text{cause in a time period}\end{array}}{\text{Total population at midperiod}} \times \frac{K}{\text{Number of days in time period}}$$

Diarrheal disease, measles, acute respiratory infections, malaria, and meningitis are common communicable diseases triggered by the breakdown of the public health infrastructure of a disaster-affected country, and they have historically contributed significant cause-specific mortality. They must be identified in rapid assessments and emergency surveillance systems. Cause-specific mortality rates can

target interventions. For instance, if the incidence of deaths from diarrhea is high, then an operational focus on water, sanitation, and hygiene will be important.

Malnutrition is an important cause of mortality in crises, and for that reason the nutritional status of the under-5 population is part of rapid assessment and ongoing surveillance. During emergencies in which general access to macronutrients is reduced, adults and older children have more capacity to access reserve sources of energy compared with young children. Thus malnutrition in this most vulnerable group is a sensitive indicator of nutrition in the greater population. Wasting, an indicator of acute malnutrition, is defined as the ratio of a child's weight to height and is expressed as a Z-score. The Z-score is the difference between an individual child's weight-for-height and the median weight of a healthy reference population (based on WHO Child Growth Standards)[22] of similar height, divided by the standard deviation of the reference population:

$$\text{Z-score} = \frac{\begin{array}{c}\text{Measured weight}\\\text{for a given height}\end{array} - \begin{array}{c}\text{Median weight of reference}\\\text{for same height}\end{array}}{\text{Standard deviation of the reference population}}$$

The Z-score describes how many standard deviations an undernourished child's weight-for-height is below the median of a reference population. Less than -2 Z but ≥ -3 Z and < -3 Z refer to moderate acute malnutrition and severe acute malnutrition, respectively. Because it reflects recent population dynamics—most often variables associated with access to not only adequate food, but also adequate water, sanitation, and health services—the rise of acute malnutrition in a population should prompt an investigation as to cause as well as inform the response. More in-depth surveys can address the former (see the following discussion); the initiating of therapeutic feeding strategies defines the latter.

Whereas mortality and undernutrition are universally understood and tracked by disaster responders and humanitarian organizations, other health qualitative and quantitative indicators, such as immunization coverage, the function of the health delivery systems, the provision of a variety of health programs such as reproductive health, and the emergence of diseases with outbreak potential, are among a variety of tracked indicators as the emergency response evolves. Other sectors that affect public health—water and sanitation, shelter, and food in particular—also track key indicators gathered through rapid assessments. A repository of commonly accepted, consensus-derived multisector operational indicators can be found at Sphereproject.org.[7]

Surveys

Changes and irregularities in indicators found during rapid assessments or surveillance activities during emergencies may prompt a more in-depth population-based study to determine the causes or implications of the impact. For instance, properly powered studies can determine the incidence and prevalence of a disease or injury. *Incidence* refers to the number of new cases of a disease that occur during a specific time period; *prevalence* is the number of cases present in the population at the time of assessment. Such studies require a sampling methodology and rely on observations, interviews, or questionnaires to yield defined outcome variables. Those data undergo a formal analysis and interpretation that relate *independent variables* with a *dependent variable*. In general, a survey should be considered when greater precision is needed to make informed decisions during any phase of the disaster cycle.

In quantitative epidemiology, a *sample* is that subset of a population that represents the population well enough to make inferences about the findings in relation to the population. A sample may be one of two types: probability- or nonprobability-based. The former uses random selection to minimize inherent bias and to ensure that everyone in the population of interest has an equal, nonzero chance of being selected; the latter implies that respondents are chosen subjectively by the researcher and, as such, engenders inherent selection biases. If, for instance, a ministry of health wanted to know the burden of crush injury after an earthquake to determine the need for intravenous fluids and hemodialysis, it could draw samples from health facilities. However, this nonprobability sampling technique—a type of convenience sample—would miss those in the population with crush injury sufficient enough to prevent them from accessing health facilities. Nonprobability sampling prevents the ability to measure the uncertainty of the sample outcomes in relation to the population.

In comparison, deriving a probability sample requires a *sampling frame*, which involves a full list of persons or households in the population of interest from which a sample is drawn. In areas where no such lists exist, epidemiologists can create sampling units, as in cluster sampling, from which random sampling can still be done. This requires reasonably accurate population estimates and knowledge of its geographic distribution. The benefit of employing a probability-based sampling method is that inferential statistics can be used to make conclusive statements about the population with a given level of calculated certainty as well as analyze the effects of different variables on an outcome measure. Invariably, randomized population-based surveys, given their breadth and depth, are more expensive (and may be prohibitive in the setting of low-income resources), demand time (when often an answer is needed immediately), and require a certain level of skill and training (not always readily available in low-income country disasters). Nonprobability-based samples, not being random, do not require generating a sampling frame and as such tend to be easier and faster to accomplish. Each offers benefits and has limitations.

Because of the degree of time and effort needed to undertake a survey, most quantitative epidemiological studies are "one-off" events, and for that reason tend to be cross-sectional or retrospective in scope. As the emergency phase transitions to recovery and development, and time and finances allow, the use of surveys to investigate nuanced health outcomes in the population becomes more common.

Qualitative Assessments

Whereas this chapter has largely focused on quantitative data in rapid assessments and surveys, qualitative and mixed methods also play a critical role in disaster epidemiology. For rapid assessments or surveys, qualitative approaches provide insight into the context of health events and better elucidate the question "why?" It is vitally important that voices from the affected population are heard and their perceptions, attitudes, bases for behaviors, intentions, and priorities are systematically captured and analyzed. This approach is necessarily an ethnographic one, appreciating the cultural, religious, gender, socioeconomic, and political influences within a population of interest.

Sampling for qualitative studies tends to be purposive and nonrandom; respondents are selected for specific reasons. Individuals or groups may be chosen for their socioeconomic background, educational level, gender, age, or other relevant classes, based on the areas of inquiry, such as their ability to identify root causes of an issue or concern in the disaster preparedness and response context. Because of the focused subjective nature of the inquiry, sample sizes are smaller than those needed for a randomized study, and data collection can be done quickly if needed. Qualitative formats include direct observation, key informant interviews, semistructured interviews, focus group discussions, and participatory appraisals. Assessment teams take a listener and observer role and rely on inductive reasoning to probe thematic

areas. As narratives develop from these formats, patterns and themes emerge. The analysis of these nongeneralizable subjective data involves coding key words and phrases to illustrate these patterns. Discerning when to most effectively use qualitative, quantitative, or a combination of methods in rapid needs assessments and surveys will help provide the most complete and useful information.[23]

⚠ PITFALLS

Every epidemiological method has its drawbacks. Most vulnerability analyses fail to take into account all the factors that contribute to the structure of the human environment, particularly the knowledge, attitudes, and behaviors of the population at risk. Rapid needs assessments continue to suffer from a lack of common indicators that can be linked in standard formats and commonly shared among response agencies. Mortality rates may be inappropriately underestimated or overestimated if population estimates are not accurate or if mortality events are clustered in time and place. Respondents may readily introduce selection biases in nonrandomized quantitative or qualitative surveys. Depending on perceived incentives or disincentives, respondents may exaggerate the needs of the community (if the interviewer has access to outside resources) or minimize the needs of the community (if the interviewer is seen as an outsider and garners mistrust). Since all epidemiological methods have benefits and pitfalls, it is imperative that they are used correctly, with thoughtful consideration to the population's needs, the space and time context, and the potential biases that may be introduced.

REFERENCES

1. Lu-Ping Z, Rodriguez-Llanes JM, Qi W, et al. Multiple injuries after earthquakes: a retrospective analysis on 1,871 injured patients from the 2008 Wenchuan earthquake. *Crit Care.* 2012;16:R87.
2. Sudaryo MK, Besral, Endarti AT, et al. Injury, disability and quality of life after the 2009 earthquake in Padang, Indonesia: a prospective cohort study of adult survivors. *Glob Health Action.* 2012;5:11816.
3. Binder S, Sanderson SM. The role of the epidemiologist in natural disasters. *Ann Emerg Med.* 1987;16:1081–1084.
4. Sommer A, Mosley WH. East Bengal cyclone of 1970: epidemiological approach to disaster assessment. *Lancet.* 1972;1(7759):1029–1036.
5. deVille deGoyet C, del Cid E, Romero A, et al. Earthquake in Guatemala: epidemiologic evaluation of the relief effort. *Bull Pan Am Health Organ.* 1976;10(2):95–109.
6. Armenian HK, Melkonian A, Noji E, et al. Deaths and injuries due to the earthquake in Armenia: a cohort approach. *Int J Epidemiol.* 1997;26:806–813.
7. The Sphere Project. The Sphere Project: Humanitarian Charter and Minimum Standards in Humanitarian Response. 2011. Available at: http://www.sphereproject.org.
8. Spiegel PB, Salama P. War and mortality in Kosovo, 1998-1999: an epidemiological testimony. *Lancet.* 2000;355:2204–2209.
9. Coghlan B, Brennan RJ, Ngoy P, et al. Mortality in the Democratic Republic of Congo: a nationwide survey. *Lancet.* 2006;367:44–51.
10. McDonnell SM, Bolton P, Sunderland N, et al. The role of the applied epidemiologist in armed conflict. *Emerg Themes Epidemiol.* 2004;1:4.
11. United Nations International Strategy for Disaster Reduction. UNISDR Terminology on Disaster Risk Reduction, 2009. Available at: http://www.unisdr.org/files/7817_UNISDRTerminologyEnglish.pdf.
12. Kovats RS, Hajat S. Heat stress and public health: a review. *Annu Rev Public Health.* 2008;29:41–55.
13. Chou YJ, Huang N, Lee CH, et al. Who is at risk of death in an earthquake? *Am J Epidemiol.* 2004;160(7):688–695.
14. Heinz Center for Science, Economics and the Environment. Human Links to Coastal Disasters. Washington, 2002.

15. Myers CA, Slack T, Singelmann J. Social vulnerability and migration in the wake of disaster: the case of Hurricanes Katrina and Rita. *Popul Environ.* 2008;29:271–291.

16. Gray C, Frankenberg E, Gillespie T, et al. Studying displacement after a disaster using large-scale survey methods: Sumatra after the 2004 tsunami. *Ann Assoc Am Geogr.* 2014;104:594–612.

17. Rivera C. Integrating climate change adaptation into disaster risk reduction in urban contexts: perception and practice. *PLoS Curr.* 2014;6. http://dx.doi.org/10.1371/currents.dis.7bfa59d37f7f59abc238462d53fbb41f.

18. Krieger K, Amlot R, Rogers MB. Understanding public responses to chemical, biological, radiological, and nuclear incidents—driving factors, emerging themes, and research gaps. *Environ Int.* 2014;72:66–74.

19. Jordan E. *Pathways to Community Recovery: A Qualitative Comparative Analysis of Post-Disaster Outcomes. PhD Thesis.* University of Colorado; 2012. Available at: https://mcedc.colorado.edu/sites/default/files/Jordan_Dissertation.pdf.

20. Spiegel PB, Burkle FM, Dey CC, et al. Developing public health indicators in complex emergency response. *Prehospital Disaster Med.* 2001;16 (4):281–285.

21. US Agency for International Development. Measuring Mortality, Nutritional Status, and Food Security in Crisis Situations: SMART Methodology, 2006.

22. World Health Organization and UNICEF. *WHO Child Growth Standards and the Identification of Severe Acute Malnutrition in Infants and Children. Geneva and New York.* 2011, Available at: http://apps.who.int/iris/bitstream/10665/44129/1/9789241598163_eng.pdf.

23. The Assessment Capacities Project. *Qualitative and Quantitative Research Techniques for Humanitarian Needs Assessment: An Introductory Brief.* May 2012, Available at: http://www.acaps.org/resourcescats/downloader/qualitative_and_quantitative_research_techniques/104.

Measures of Effectiveness in Disaster Management

P. Gregg Greenough and Frederick M. Burkle Jr.

Measures of effectiveness (MOEs) define quantitative and qualitative management tools that provide means for measuring the effectiveness, performance, and outcome of an operation, strategy, or project.[1] They allude to a set of parameters that ultimately determine the degree to which an operation has been a success or failure relative to the operation's objectives. MOEs define needs and objectives and the seeking and selection of solutions to address those objectives. *Measure* implies a metric or standard; *effectiveness* suggests how well something is done or whether the intended objectives were met. Disaster management operations rely on indicators as the fundamental units measured against an agreed set of criteria for critical operations performance and impact in relationship to operational goals. Indicators, whether quantitative or qualitative, usually have limits or a range of values. These are integrated into the evaluative design process at the outset.

MOEs should be differentiated from more granular metrics such as measures of performance (MOPs), which are bundled sets of rates, averages, counts, or percentages—parameters that determine a system's or operation's level of performance against a benchmark.[2] The MOEs assess the impact of those performance levels and are necessarily more complex, often cross-referencing MOPs for a given operational objective. The term *monitoring* is the ongoing, systematic collection, analysis, and use of data during the course of a project. *Evaluation* is the periodic review of program activity, outcome, and impact, with an emphasis on lessons learned.[3]

Systems interact with their surrounding environments. Disaster response systems and the variety of organizations that compose and support them, operate in dynamic climates that evolve in both deterministic and stochastic patterns. These patterns are represented by numerous ever-changing variables. As systems provide solutions to problems (e.g., disaster response systems respond to public crises), organizations rely on operational procedures as solutions to those problems. MOEs measure how well a system's objectives are being met in applying solutions to problems; in a disaster, the efforts to mitigate against further loss of life and to restore order similarly require a measure of response effectiveness and impact.

HISTORICAL PERSPECTIVE

The term MOE was first applied by Morse and Kimball to operational research on weapons systems and strategies used in World War II.[4] In the 1990s systems engineering and industry adapted the term to the performance of products and to the ability of solutions to manage problems. It encouraged building consensus among stakeholders—those affected by products and solutions—on selecting the MOE metric and determining the nature of the MOE and whether a performance, product, or solution was functionally successful and met their needs.[5]

Systems engineers adapted MOEs to understand how organizations work, perform, and deliver, specifically on measures of solution to problems experienced in a variety of industries. The concept has subsequently been modified to address strategic problems posed to militaries and public agencies. In the 1990s, as humanitarian and disaster relief agencies strove to professionalize their operations through evidence-based research and donor accountability initiatives, the idea of MOEs took hold likewise across the multiple sectors involved in crisis response (food, health, water, sanitation, shelter, etc.). For instance, the health sector embraced critical consensus-driven mortality, morbidity, and nutritional indicators that gauged the mission's success or failure on the affected population. With humanitarian assistance projects, MOEs have measured access, influence, sectoral impacts, and local capacity building.

CURRENT PRACTICE

MOEs should represent the needs and concerns of the stakeholders defining the operational problem; in the setting of disaster response operations, these would include beneficiaries and local populations, multilateral organizations, nongovernmental organizations (NGOs), and officials of the affected country. Engaging these critical stakeholders engenders consensus agreement and clarity and facilitates communication between them in real time to see if goals are being met and where operations should be improved. When disaster organizations agree to share information and work with stakeholders for a common goal, MOEs become a priority in management, evaluation, and monitoring for all concerned, especially the beneficiaries of relief and development. Only with transparency can stakeholders feel confident and organizations be held accountable. These measures can promote unification of medical assistance, allow for comparison of responses, and bring accountability to postdisaster acute-phase medical care.

The key to understanding MOEs and the process by which they are generated in disaster response lies in (1) the recognition of which indicators are considered essential measures of sector performance, (2) the assessment of the applicability and reliability of these essential indicators in whether they meet usefulness criteria, and (3) the ability of these essential indicators to provide the coordinating language of the timeline or critical pathway specific to the disaster event (Fig. 62-1).

MOEs should be timely, consistently measureable, standardized and readily understood by all stakeholders, sensitive, easily shared, consistently measureable, verifiable, and credibly appropriate for the project or operation. Common language and standard terminology allow participants to know what others are doing, elaborate a timeline, and provide a rationale for certain operational decisions. As tools for communication, MOEs minimize confusion and risk and have the added

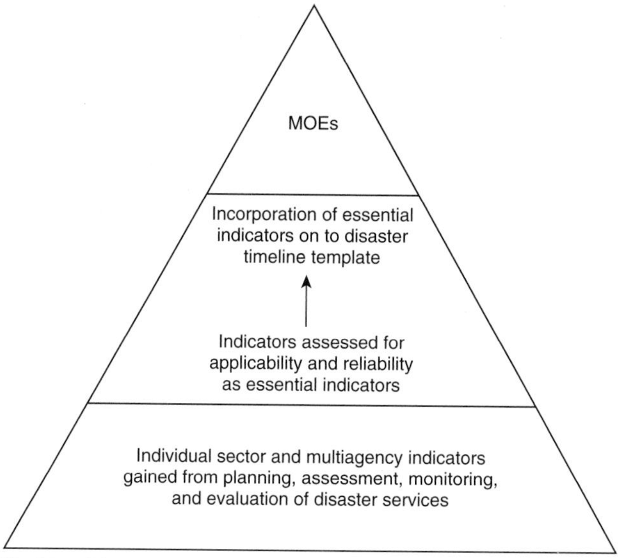
MOEs
Incorporation of essential indicators on to disaster timeline template
Indicators assessed for applicability and reliability as essential indicators
Individual sector and multiagency indicators gained from planning, assessment, monitoring, and evaluation of disaster services

FIG 62-1 Measures of Effectiveness Are Based on Essential Indicators.

benefit of affording feedback to disaster responders. If defined well, MOEs will reflect factors known to affect outcome (sensitivity) and change with progress toward meeting operational objectives. MOEs in disaster management are based on the assumption that the majority of disasters and their management have predictable timeline events. As such they will also have predictive value as they are derived from similar missions in previous disasters and synthesized from lessons learned. When addressing impacts of performance, MOEs should be timely in such a way as to allow participants to act, prompt their decision making, make corrections, and link early actions taken to long-term impact.

Although MOEs tend to be quantifiable in nature, qualitative or semiqualitative indicators and descriptors can add a reliable measure of social, cultural, behavioral, and mental health disaster-related services. Using a consensus methodology, a group of disaster experts representing a range of institutions identified 37 quantitative and qualitative MOEs as a tool for rapid evaluation of a medical response during the first two weeks following a natural disaster.[6] These performance targets, while yet to be implemented and validated, illustrate the need for prioritized, easily communicated objective markers that can be readily deployed and that do not require an extensive data gathering mechanism.

Throughout disaster operations MOEs should be regularly analyzed, tracked, and reported within an organization and to others coordinating the overall disaster response. In disaster operations that require a global humanitarian response, the UN Office for the Coordination of Humanitarian Affairs (UNOCHA) maintains responsibility for the management of information across multiple sectors, including health.[7] By determining trends and endpoints, MOEs bring agencies, organizations, and stakeholders together. The analysis should take into account that MOEs are subject to variance, the deviation from predicted or expected outcomes. If expected requirements are not met across the management timeline, this becomes a *negative variance* that must be investigated for causal factors and solved as soon as possible. There may be an unexpected improvement or acceleration of the disaster response timeline that becomes a *positive variance*, which may eventually alter the way time-dependent management will be defined for future disasters.

When entrance and exit criteria are mutually agreed upon, MOEs help avoid mission creep and encourage mission shifting as needed. For its civil reconstruction projects in Afghanistan and Iraq, the U.S. Department of Defense's Overseas Humanitarian, Disaster and Civic Aid Program has explored the routine use of MOEs in such as way as to align them with similar efforts by other multilateral organizations and NGOs.[8] Such initiatives ensure capacity building and sustainability.

! PITFALLS

The main pitfalls of MOEs are organizational ones that lead to lack of interagency cooperation. In the heat of a disaster event they are often neglected or forgotten. It takes effort for a centrally acting information management agency such as UNOCHA to coordinate multiple agency and organizational compliance and stakeholder participation. The inherent verticality of disaster response agencies and organizations prohibits the horizontal cooperation needed to get MOEs operational and consistently tracked, analyzed, and reported.

Disaster operational agencies themselves often mistake the focus of assessing effectiveness of mission (MOEs) with one of accomplishing supporting tasks (MOPs). They may neglect to implement MOEs within a project's or operation's framework at the onset. They often misdirect their focus on methodologies rather than operational issues and goals. New disaster contexts may require new MOEs customized to meet new response parameters, and relying on previously valid MOEs may not be enough to address new challenges.

REFERENCES

1. Burkle FM. Complex humanitarian emergencies III: measures of effectiveness. *Prehospital DIsaster Med.* 2003;18(3):258–262.
2. Technology Digest. *Measures of Effectiveness in Government Organizations.* Technology Digest white paper; August 2008.
3. Office of Foreign Disaster Assistance. *Foreign Operations Guide,* version 4.0. September 2005.
4. Roche JG, Watts BD. Choosing analytic measures. *J Strategic Stud.* 1991;14:169–201.
5. Sproles N. Coming to grips with measures of effectiveness. *Systems Eng.* 2000;3(1):50–58.
6. Daftary RK, Cruz AT, Reaves EJ, et al. Making disaster care count: consensus formulation of measures of effectiveness for natural disaster acute phase medical response. *Prehosp Disaster Med.* 2014;29(5):461–467.
7. United Nations. How are disaster relief efforts organized? Cluster approach and key actors. Available at: https://business.un.org/en/documents/6852.
8. Bonventre E. Monitoring and evaluation of Department of Defense humanitarian assistance programs. *Military Review.* Jan-Feb 2008;68–72.

63 | CHAPTER

Lessons Learned as a Result of Terrorist Attacks*

Mark E. Keim and Scott Deitchman

The threat of terrorism is a high-priority national security and law enforcement concern in the United States. Modern policy on combating terrorism against the United States has been evolving over the past 30 years. A series of Presidential Decision Directives (PDDs), along with implementing guidance, executive orders, interagency agreements, and legislation, now provide the basis for counterterrorism programs and activities in more than 40 federal agencies, bureaus, and offices. Unfortunately, public policy and societal reactions regarding disasters do not always translate into effective outcomes of "lessons learned."

Terrorism itself has been an age-old threat to the public health and security of many populations throughout the world. Since the 1980s, terrorist attacks against the United States have led to legislative, regulatory, organizational, and programmatic actions associated with comprehensive and ambitious expectations. Further study is needed before we can conclude the extent to which these major changes will have a lasting and significant effect upon the practice of disaster medicine as a health science.

Nevertheless, two major accomplishments have been realized since the terrorist attacks of 2001: (1) National capacity of emergency management appears to have been increased and (2) awareness and possibly even commitment to the issue of emergency preparedness appears to be greater.[1] This chapter will identify recent terrorist events that have had a significant effect upon U.S. society and public policy.

HISTORICAL PERSPECTIVE

U.S. domestic emergency management policy has evolved over the past 70 years. Since the 1990s, terrorist events have taken an increasingly important role in shaping larger response strategies related to U.S. emergency management policy, the implementation of the incident management system, and the development of comprehensive disaster mitigation strategies. One must first understand the fundamentals of these three major historical developments to appreciate fully the lessons learned and residual pitfalls.

---

*The material in this chapter reflects solely the views of the author. It does not necessarily reflect the policies or recommendations of the Centers for Disease Control and Prevention or the U.S. Department of Health and Human Services.

The Development of Current U.S. Emergency Management Policy

Modern emergency management policy in the United States began with the "Unlimited National Emergency" (Proclamation 2487 of May 27, 1941), immediately prior to World War II. Over three decades later, out of concern for a catastrophic earthquake predicted to occur in the central United States, the Earthquake Hazards Reduction Act of 1977 mandated the development of a Federal Response Plan for a Catastrophic Earthquake. In July 1979 Executive Order 12148 delegated authority to the Federal Emergency Management Agency (FEMA) to establish federal policies and to coordinate civil defense, as well as civil emergency planning, management, mitigation, and assistance functions, of executive agencies. Then, FEMA was also assigned the lead responsibility for response to consequences of terrorism. The Robert T. Stafford Disaster Relief Act, P.L. 100-707 was enacted in 1986 to formalize a coordinated federal policy that included development of a Federal Response Plan. In 1990 FEMA issued the Federal Response Plan to establish a process for coordinated delivery of federal disaster assistance. Acting upon lessons learned during the Hurricane Andrew response in 1992, Congress adopted a formal "all-hazards approach" to emergency management in the National Defense Authorization Act of 1994, PL 103-160.

In June 1995 President Clinton issued PDD-39, the central blueprint for the U.S. counterterrorism strategy. PDD-39 elaborated a strategy for combating terrorism consisting of three main elements: (1) reducing vulnerabilities and preventing and deterring terrorist acts before they occur; (2) responding to terrorist acts that occur, including managing crises and apprehending and punishing terrorist perpetrators; and (3) managing the consequences of terrorist attacks. All three elements of the strategy apply to terrorism involving weapons of mass destruction (WMD).[2] Emergency managers will recognize these elements as phases of the risk-reduction cycle, including disaster prevention, mitigation, and response.

The Defense against WMD Act of 1996, P.L. 104-201 (also known as the Nunn-Lugar-Domenici Act), September 23, 1996, drew upon the convergence of federal assets at the Atlanta 1996 Olympic Science and Technology Center[3,4] and directed this momentum to set in place a long-term effort to prepare domestic response for terrorist threats.

The Development of Incident Management Systems

The Incident Command System (ICS) was conceptualized more than 30 years ago, in response to a devastating wildfire in California. The Congress mandated that the U.S. Forest Service design a system that would improve the ability of wildland fire-protection agencies to coordinate interagency action effectively and to allocate suppression resources in dynamic situations. This system became known as the Firefighting Resources of California Organized for Potential Emergencies (FIRESCOPE) ICS. Although FIRESCOPE ICS was originally developed to assist in the response to wildland fires, it was quickly recognized as a system that could help public safety responders provide effective and coordinated incident management for a wide range of situations, including floods, hazardous materials accidents, earthquakes, and aircraft crashes. In 1982 all FIRESCOPE ICS documentation was revised and adopted as the National Interagency Incident Management System (NIIMS). In Homeland Security Presidential Directive 5 (HSPD-5), President Bush called on the Secretary of Homeland Security to develop a national incident management system (NIMS) to provide "a consistent nationwide approach for federal, state, tribal, and local governments to work together to prepare for, prevent, respond to, and recover from domestic incidents," regardless of cause, size, or complexity.[5]

The Development of Disaster Risk-Reduction Strategies

U.S. policy related to terrorism has also developed within a global context of strategies trending over the past two decades toward a more comprehensive approach to disaster risk management that also includes disaster risk-reduction efforts, such as prevention, protection, and mitigation. In 1994, the States Members of the United Nations, having met at the World Conference on Natural Disaster Reduction, in the city of Yokohama, Japan, in partnership with nongovernmental organizations and with the participation of international organizations, the scientific community, business, industry, and the media, affirmed, "Disaster prevention, mitigation, and preparedness are better than disaster response in achieving the goals and objectives of the Decade. *Disaster response alone is not sufficient, as it yields only temporary results at a very high cost*" [emphasis added]. We have followed this limited approach for too long. This has been further demonstrated by the recent focus on response to complex emergencies, which, although compelling, should not divert from pursuing a comprehensive approach. *Prevention contributes to lasting improvement in safety and is essential to integrated disaster management*"[6] [emphasis added]. Although focused on natural disasters, this declaration represented an early recognition of the importance of a more comprehensive approach to managing disasters that also includes pre-event activities of prevention, mitigation, and preparedness.

One decade later, The World Conference on Disaster Reduction was held from January 18 to 22, 2005, in Kobe, Hyogo, Japan, and it adopted the present Framework for Action 2005-2015. The conference provided a unique opportunity to promote a strategic and systematic approach to reducing vulnerabilities and risks to hazards. It underscored the need for, and identified ways of, building the resilience of nations and communities to disasters. The resultant Hyogo declaration concluded, "*an integrated, multi-hazard approach to disaster risk reduction should be factored into policies, planning and programming* (emphasis added) related to sustainable development, relief, rehabilitation, and recovery."[7]

In 2011 the Obama administration released Presidential Policy Directive 8 (PPD-8) that includes "a series of integrated national planning frameworks, covering prevention, protection, mitigation, response, and recovery."[8] The National Prevention Framework describes what the whole community—from community members to senior leaders in government—should do upon the discovery of

intelligence or information regarding an imminent threat to the homeland in order to thwart an initial or follow-on terrorist attack.[9]

Recent Terrorist Events That Have Influenced U.S. Policy

The development of new disaster policy is dependent upon a society's perception of risk. Public perception of risk is known to be higher immediately after the occurrence of a major disaster. Terrorist attacks have a particularly powerful effect on the human psyche and subsequently often result in rapid, sometimes drastic, public policy changes. During such times, there is a notable window of opportunity for change in disaster reduction policy. Table 63-1 is a listing of select major terrorist events that have occurred over the past three decades and their corresponding influence on resultant U.S. policy.

CURRENT PRACTICE AND "LESSONS LEARNED"

PPD-8 was released in March 2011, with the goal of strengthening the security and resilience of the United States through the application of a comprehensive approach for disaster risk management detailed within five National Planning Frameworks: prevention, protection, mitigation, response, and recovery.[9] Risk management is a coordinated activity directed toward assessing, controlling, and monitoring risks. Disaster risk management is a comprehensive all-hazard approach that entails developing and implementing strategies for each phase of the disaster life cycle. The emphasis on a "life-cycle" approach to risk management is important in the case of disasters.[10] All disasters are said to follow a cyclical pattern that includes five stages: prevention, mitigation, preparedness, response, and recovery.[11,12] These phases often overlap each other in time and scope. However, operationally, one can divide the life cycle into *pre-event* disaster risk reduction (prevention, preparedness, and mitigation) and *post-event* disaster risk retention (response and recovery).[13] The underlying drive of disaster management is to reduce risk both to human life and to systems important to livelihood.[14]

Over the past 30 years, U.S. policy has applied lessons learned because of terrorist attacks within a framework based upon the comprehensive approach of disaster risk management. Terrorist attacks have driven U.S. Federal Emergency Management policy toward inclusion of risk-reduction strategies into prevention, protection, preparedness, mitigation, and response efforts. The National Planning Framework has expanded and adopted a National Prevention Framework that includes, "those capabilities necessary to avoid, prevent, or stop a threatened or actual act of terrorism" and a National Mitigation Framework that "establishes a common platform and forum for coordinating and addressing how the Nation manages risk through mitigation capabilities."[9] However, the framework for responding to natural disasters in the United States has not used these pre-event risk-reduction activities to the same extent. Table 63-2 lists key lessons learned from terrorist attacks, as applied to the five phases of disaster risk management: prevention, mitigation, preparedness, response, and recovery. The importance of an all-hazard approach to disaster risk management is also included. Table 63-2 also lists key examples of reports that have identified important lessons, as well as examples of their corresponding effects on U.S. policy.

! PITFALLS

The Public Health and Health Care Sector Is Quite Diverse and Collaboration Has Been Difficult as a Result

Efforts to improve coordination and collaboration efforts have varied among different sectors because of their characteristics and level of maturity. For example, "the public health and health care sector is quite

TABLE 63-1 **Thirty Years of Selected Terrorist Events That Have Influenced U.S. Policy**

DATE	EVENT	DESCRIPTION	CHANGES IN U.S. POLICY
1983	Bombing of Lebanon Marine Barracks	• Truck bomb detonated near U.S. military barracks • Linked to Moslem International Extremists (MIE) • Early asymmetric attack on U.S. military facility by MIE	• National Security Decision Directive 138: Combating Terrorism authorizes "Preemptive Strikes against Terrorists," April 26, 1984
1984	Bahgwan Rajneesh Salmonella Release	• Salmonella bacteria released in restaurants in The Dalles, Oregon • Years later, the outbreak was linked to the Bhagwan Shree Rajneesh religious cult • No deaths, but over 800 were infected • First biological attack in the United States, and with highest morbidity rate	• None; for years, the outbreak went largely unrecognized as an intentional event
1985	Rome and Vienna Airport Attacks	• Abu Nidal terrorists perpetrate nearly simultaneous shooting and bombing terrorist attacks aimed at Israelis in airports in Rome and Vienna • Linked to Libya • The event illustrates the effectiveness of multiple, simultaneous urban attacks using small arms and hand-carried explosives • The terrorist attack is directed at public transportation	• National Security Decision Directive 205: Acting Against Libyan Support of International Terrorism, 1986 • National Security Decision Directive 207: The National Program for Combating Terrorism, 1986
1988	Bombing of Pan Am Flight 103	• A parcel bomb is detonated on a plane en route from London to New York; it explodes over Lockerbie, Scotland • Linked to a Libyan MIE terrorist cell • The event represents state-sponsored (Libyan) terrorism against a primarily U.S. target • The terrorist attack is directed at public transportation	• Executive Order 12686, President's Commission on Aviation Security and Terrorism, 1989 • Public Law 101-604: Aviation Security Improvement Act of 1990 • National Security Directive 47: Counterintelligence and Security Countermeasures, 1990 • Executive Order 12705: Extending the President's Commission on Aviation Security and Terrorism, 1990 • Presidential Decision Directive 2: Organization of the National Security Council, 1993
1993	World Trade Center (WTC) Bombing	• A truck bomb is detonated in the WTC parking garage • Linked to MIE, including multiple Arab nationalities	• Congress enacts the National Defense Authorization Act for Fiscal Year 1995 • It prepares federal response plans and programs for the emergency preparedness of the United States • It sponsor and directs such plans and programs to coordinate with state efforts
1994-1995	Aum Shinrikyo sarin attacks	• In 1994, Japanese religious cult, Aum Shinrikyo, released Sarin nerve agent in a residential area of Matsumoto, Japan, killing seven and injuring hundreds • In 1995, the same group released Sarin in the Tokyo subways, killing 12 and injuring thousands • Evidence of extensively coordinated planning and execution • This was the first time that a nonstate group used a chemical weapon against civilians • Represented the escalation effect of larger attacks • Demonstrated how terrorist groups could recruit scientists, obtain deadly chemicals or biological agents, and put plans into action	• "The Defense Against WMD Act," also known as the "Nunn-Lugar-Domenici Act" • Federal Emergency Management Agency (FEMA) adopts the Terrorist Annex to the Federal Response Plan, 1997 • Executive Order 12938: Proliferation of WMD, 1994 • Executive Order 13094: Proliferation of WMD, 1998
1995	Bombing of the Murrah Federal Building in Oklahoma City	• A truck bomb is detonated near the Alfred P. Murrah Federal Building in Oklahoma City, Oklahoma • The bombing is linked to U.S. right-wing extremists • First instance of large-scale bombing attack by U.S. domestic terrorists • Experts other than foreign policy and security specialists become more involved in terrorist preparedness and response (most notably including disaster medicine) • Increased awareness of occupational health concerns among disaster responders (most notably, including behavioral health)	• First use of the president's authority under the Stafford Act to "self-initiate" an emergency declaration for emergencies with federal involvement • Presidential Decision Directive 39: U.S. Policy on Counterterrorism, 1995 • Public Law 104-132: Antiterrorism and Effective Death Penalty Act of 1996 • Executive Order 13010: Critical Infrastructure Protection, 1996

TABLE 63-1   Thirty Years of Selected Terrorist Events That Have Influenced U.S. Policy—cont'd

DATE	EVENT	DESCRIPTION	CHANGES IN U.S. POLICY
1995	Chechnyan Threat of Using a Radiological Dispersion Device (RDD)	• Chechen separatists direct news reporter to a Moscow park, where a Cesium-137 RDD weapon is found • First credible threat for use of a radiological dispersion device (a.k.a., a "dirty bomb") by a subnational group	• No specific action other than increased awareness and improved threat characterization
1996	Khobar Towers Bombing	• Truck bomb detonated near U.S. military barracks in Dhahran, Saudi Arabia • Linked to MIE • Asymmetric attack on a U.S. military facility by MIE	• No specific action other than increased awareness and improved threat characterization
1996	Crash of TWA Flight	• Explosion of an airliner during takeoff in New York • Initially believed to be result of a terrorist attack using a surface-to-air missile • Later ruled to be accidental • Occurred within days of the start of the 1996 Olympics • Shoulder-fired surface-to-air missiles are later used by MIE to attack aircraft in Kenya, Saudi Arabia, and Iraq during 2003-2004	• In 1997, the White House Commission on Aviation Safety and Security (Gore Commission) considers "aviation security as a national security issue and provide substantial funding for capital improvements": • The Dept. of Homeland Security 2005 budget includes $61 million for research and development of countermeasures to protect commercial aircraft from shoulder-fired and surface-to-air missiles • Airport Security Improvement Act of 2000, Public Law 106-528, November 22, 2000
1996	Bombing of Atlanta Olympic Games	• Pipe bomb explodes at Centennial Olympic Park, in Atlanta, Georgia, during the ninth day of the 1996 Summer Olympics • First incident coordination by federal interagency WMD response teams • First forward staging of a medical stockpile in preparation for WMD casualties during the Atlanta Olympic Games	• Unprecedented State and Federal preparedness activities related to the 1996 Olympic games associated with implementation of Presidential Decision Directive 39: U.S. Policy on Counterterrorism, 1995 • Adoption of Title XIV of the Defense Authorization Act of 1996, "The Defense Against WMD Act," also known as the "Nunn-Lugar-Domenici Act" • Terrorist Annex to the Federal Response Plan adopted by FEMA, 1996
1998	U.S. Embassy Bombings in Kenya and Tanzania	• Truck bombs detonated simultaneously near U.S. embassies in Nairobi and Dar es Salaam • Evidence of extensively coordinated planning and execution • Linked to MIE and the Al Qaeda terrorist network • First large-scale attack on U.S. embassies caused by MIE terrorists	• U.S. responds with cruise missile strikes against Al Qaeda training site in Afghanistan and Khartoum chemical factory, August 1998 • First HHS/CDC public health and medical response to overseas terrorism • Presidential Decision Directive 67: Enduring Constitutional Government and Continuity of Government Operations, 1998
2000	Attack of the U.S.S. *Cole*	• Explosion occurred on the destroyer U.S.S. *Cole*, docked at the harbor in Aden, Yemen • Linked to MIE and the Al Qaeda terrorist network • First asymmetric attack on a U.S. naval warship perpetrated by MIE	• Presidential Decision Directive 75: Counterintelligence for the 21st Century, 2001
2001	WTC and Pentagon Attacks	• Hijacked airliners deliberately flown into the WTC towers and the Pentagon • Linked to MIE and the Al Qaeda terrorist network • Attack has significant and long-term economic and sociopolitical significance for the United States	• U.S. response includes at least 10 pieces of national legislation; 12 Executive Orders; 15 Homeland Security Decision Directives; and one new federal department: the Department of Homeland Security • Major reorganization of U.S. intelligence organizational structure in 2004, consistent with recommendations of the 9/11 Commission report • Public Law 110-53: Implementing Recommendations of the 9/11 Commission Act of 2007 • A series of executive orders provide for a clear order of succession for U.S. cabinet-level officials
2001	Anthrax Letter Attacks	• Letters containing anthrax spores are mailed to news media personnel and Congress • Leads to the first cases of intentional anthrax infection in the United States • Infections follow a 3-year history of over 1500 anthrax-letter hoaxes, many targeting Planned Parenthood clinics • Perpetrators remain unconfirmed	• The Federal Response Plan was never activated • Public Law 107-188: Public Health Security and Bioterrorism Preparedness and Response Act of 2002 • Public Law 108-276: Project BioShield Act of 2004 • Homeland Security Presidential Directive 9: Defense of United States Agriculture and Food, 2004 • Homeland Security Presidential Directive 10: Biodefense for the 21st Century, 2004

(Continued)

TABLE 63-1		**Thirty Years of Selected Terrorist Events That Have Influenced U.S. Policy—cont'd**	
DATE	**EVENT**	**DESCRIPTION**	**CHANGES IN U.S. POLICY**
		• Second largest-scale biological attack in the United States and the highest mortality rate • Reports cite speculation regarding the U.S. domestic origin of the terrorist(s) • Revealed the challenges and shortcomings facing the nation's public health system • The federal Concept of Operations Plan (CONPLAN) for responses to terrorist attacks was not used • The Federal Bureau of Investigations (FBI) did not exercise its crisis-management authority; FEMA did not exercise its consequence-management authority, as called for by PDD 39	• Public Law 109-374: Animal Enterprise Terrorism Act of 2006 • Homeland Security Presidential Directive 18: Medical Countermeasures against WMD, 2007 • Homeland Security Presidential Directive 21: Public Health and Medical Preparedness, 2007 • Presidential Policy Directive 2: National Strategy for Countering Biological Threats, 2009 • Executive Order 13486: Strengthening Laboratory Biosecurity in the United States, 2009 • Executive Order 13527: Establishing Federal Capability for the Timely Provision of Medical Countermeasures Following a Biological Attack, 2009 • Executive Order 13546: Optimizing the Security of Biological Select Agents and Toxins in the United States, 2010
2001	Airliner Shoe Bomb Attempt	• A British man tries to blow up a U.S.-bound airliner with explosives in his shoes but is subdued by passengers and crew • The event illustrates the need for heightened airport security that includes protection against chemical explosives • The event illustrates the value of public awareness in foiling terrorist plots • A terrorist attack directed at public transportation	• Public Law 107-197: Terrorist Bombings Convention Implementation Act of 2002 • Homeland Security Presidential Directive 11: Comprehensive Terrorist-Related Screening Procedures, 2004
2002	LAX Airport Shooting	• Egyptian immigrant shoots and kills two people at the (Israeli) El Al Airlines counter in the Los Angeles (LAX) airport • The event illustrates the need for heightened airport security before security-screening areas • Reminiscent of tactics used during the 1985 Rome and Vienna airport attacks • A terrorist attack directed at public transportation	• No specific action other than increased awareness and improved threat characterization
2002-2004	Bombings and Attacks in Russia, Indonesia, the Philippines, Kenya, Saudi Arabia, Afghanistan, and Iraq	• A series of terrorist bombings and attacks involving numerous nations • Shoulder-fired surface-to-air missiles are used by MIE to attack aircraft in Kenya, Saudi Arabia, and Iraq in 2003-2004 • Most attacks are linked to MIEs, and some to national separatist movements • Events illustrate MIE tactics for attacks against broader pro-Western interests • Events related to national separatist movements reveal a growing level of sophistication in coordination and execution of attacks • Nations other than the United States become frequent targets • Some terrorist attacks are directed at public transportation	• Department of Homeland Security 2005 budget includes $61 million for research and development of countermeasures to protect commercial aircraft from shoulder-fired surface-to-air missiles
2004	Attack on the U.S. Consulate in Jeddah, Saudi Arabia	• A car bomb detonation and subsequent small arms attack of the U.S. Consulate in Jeddah, Saudi Arabia • Linked to MIE, and possibly Al Qaeda	• Recent U.S. activities resulting in hardening and increasing security of U.S. Embassies and Consulates prove valuable in mitigating the effects of the attack
2004	Madrid Train Bombings	• Nearly simultaneous, coordinated bombings against the commuter-train system of Madrid • Linked to an Al Qaeda-inspired cell • Event illustrates the need for heightened security, including modes of public transportation other than airlines • Event illustrates the "lone wolf" phenomenon of U.S. domestic attackers sympathetic with MIE ideals • Nations other than the United States become frequent targets • The terrorist attack is directed at public transportation	• No specific action other than increased awareness and improved threat characterization

TABLE 63-1	Thirty Years of Selected Terrorist Events That Have Influenced U.S. Policy—cont'd		
DATE	EVENT	DESCRIPTION	CHANGES IN U.S. POLICY
2005	London Subway Bombings	• On July 7, nearly simultaneous coordinated bombings of five locations in the London subway system • Two weeks later, four more attacks (unconnected with those on July 7) were attempted but unsuccessful • Both linked to MIE • The events illustrates the need for heightened security, including modes of public transportation other than airlines • Nations other than the United States become frequent targets • Terrorist attacks are directed at public transportation	• Homeland Security Presidential Directive 15 [War on Terrorism], 2006
2008	Mumbai Attacks	• Twelve coordinated shooting and bombing terrorist attacks lasting 4 days across Mumbai, India's largest city • Linked to Pakistani terrorist organization • Event illustrates the effectiveness of multiple, simultaneous urban attacks using small arms and hand-carried explosives • Reminiscent of tactics used during the 1985 Rome and Vienna airport attacks	• No specific action other than increased awareness and improved threat characterization
2009	Shootings at Fort Hood	• Shooting rampage by an Army psychiatrist who killed 13 and wounded 30 more • Perpetrator was a Sunni extremist • Highest number of fatalities for a terrorist attack in the United States since 9/11 • Event illustrates the "lone wolf" phenomenon of U.S. domestic attackers who are sympathetic with MIE ideals • Similar the attacks to military facilities that lead to the creation of the National Joint Terrorism Task Force in 2002	• No specific action other than increased awareness and improved threat characterization
2009	Underwear Bomb Attempt	• A Nigerian man tries to blow up a U.S.-bound airliner with explosives in his underwear but is subdued by passengers and crew • Linked to MIE and the Al Qaeda terrorist network • Event illustrates the need for heightened airport security, including protection against chemical explosives • The event illustrates the value of public awareness in foiling terrorist plots	• No specific action other than increased awareness and improved threat characterization
2010	Times Square Bomb Attempt	• Failed attempt by a Pakistani man to set off a car bomb in Times Square • The event illustrates the "lone wolf" phenomenon of U.S. domestic attackers who are sympathetic with MIE ideals • The event illustrates the value of public awareness in foiling terrorist plots • A terrorist attack on a mass gathering	• No specific action other than increased awareness and improved threat characterization
2010	Parcel Bomb Attempt on Cargo Planes	• Two packages sent by air from Yemen to Chicago, containing bombs placed within printer cartridges • Linked to MIE and the Al Qaeda terrorist network • Event illustrates the ongoing threat posed by Al Qaeda in the Arabian Peninsula • The event illustrates the continued vulnerability of U.S.-bound cargo planes	• Executive Order 13611: Blocking Property of Persons Threatening the Peace, Security, or Stability of Yemen, 2012
2010	Attempted Bombing of a Christmas-Related Mass Gathering	• Failed attempt by a Somali-American to bomb a mass gathering event in Portland, Oregon • The event illustrates the "lone wolf" phenomenon of U.S. domestic attackers who are sympathetic with MIE ideals • Event illustrates the value of public awareness in foiling terrorist plots • Terrorist attack on a mass gathering	• No specific action other than increased awareness and improved threat characterization

(Continued)

TABLE 63-1   Thirty Years of Selected Terrorist Events That Have Influenced U.S. Policy—cont'd

DATE	EVENT	DESCRIPTION	CHANGES IN U.S. POLICY
2011	U.S. Embassy Attack in Benghazi, Libya	• Islamic militants attacked the American diplomatic mission at Benghazi, in Libya, killing a U.S. Ambassador • The third such large-scale attack on U.S. Embassies or Consulates caused by MIE terrorists	• No specific action other than increased awareness and improved threat characterization
2013	Nairobi, Kenya, Shopping Mall Attack	• Mass shooting and bombings by four Islamic militants in an upscale shopping mall • Reminiscent of tactics used during the 1985 Rome and Vienna Airport Attacks and 2008 Mumbai Attack	• No specific action other than increased awareness and improved threat characterization
2013	Boston Marathon Bombing	• Two Chechen-American brothers, working alone, detonate two homemade bombs in a crowd at the Boston Marathon • The event illustrates the "lone wolf" phenomenon of U.S. domestic attackers who are sympathetic with MIE ideals • A terrorist attack on a mass gathering	• No specific action other than increased awareness and improved threat characterization

TABLE 63-2   Disaster Risk-Management "Lessons Learned" as a Result of Terrorist Events

LESSON	REPORTS AND FEDERAL ACTIONS
Need for a Comprehensive and Coordinated Disaster Risk-Management Strategy	**Reports** • Gilmore Report I, December 15, 1999. Identified the "need for national strategy to address domestic response to terrorism" • GAO-01-14: Combating Terrorism: Federal Response Teams Provide Varied Capabilities; Opportunities Remain to Improve Coordination, November 30, 2000 • Gilmore Report II, Restated "The U.S. needs a functional coherent strategy for domestic preparedness against terrorism," December 15, 2000 • U.S. Commission on National Security/21st Century: Seeking a National Strategy—A Concert for Preserving Security; • Promoting Freedom—The Phase II Report on U.S. National Security Strategy for the 21st Century, April 15, 2000 • GAO-01-822: Combating Terrorism: Selected Challenges and Related Recommendations, September 20, 2001 • GAO-01-915: Bioterrorism: Federal Research and Preparedness Activities, September 28, 2001 • Gilmore Report III, recommended clarifying the role of the military for domestic preparedness against terrorism," December 15, 2001 • GAO-02-893 T: Homeland Security: New Department Could Improve Coordination but May Complicate Priority Setting, June 28, 2002 • GAO-02-924 T: Homeland Security: New Department Could Improve Biomedical R&D Coordination but May Disrupt Dual-Purpose Efforts, July 9, 2002 • GAO-02-954 T: Homeland Security—New Department Could Improve Coordination, but Transferring Control of Certain Public Health Programs Raises Concerns, July 16, 2002 • GAO-03-260: Homeland Security: Management Challenges Facing Federal Leadership, December 20, 2002 • GAO-04-100: Homeland Security—Effective Regional Coordination Can Enhance Emergency Preparedness, September 15, 2004 • GAO-07-386 T: Applying Risk Management Principles to Guide Federal Investments, February 7, 2007 • GAO-08-488 T: DHS Improved Its Risk-Based Grant Programs' Allocation and Management Methods, but Measuring Programs' Impact on National Capabilities Remains a Challenge, March 11, 2008 • GAO-08-627SP: Strengthening the Use of Risk Management Principles in Homeland Security, April 15, 2008 • GAO-08-672: National Strategy and Supporting Plans Were Generally Well-Developed and Are Being Implemented (for Maritime Security), June 20, 2008 • GAO-08-852: DHS Risk-Based Grant Methodology Is Reasonable, but Current Version's Measure of Vulnerability Is Limited, June 27, 2008

TABLE 63-2 Disaster Risk-Management "Lessons Learned" as a Result of Terrorist Events—cont'd

LESSON	REPORTS AND FEDERAL ACTIONS
	Federal Actions • National Security Presidential Directive 1: Organization of the National Security Council System, March 2001 • Homeland Security Presidential Directive 1: Organization and Operation of the Homeland Security Council, October 2001 • Homeland Security Presidential Directive 3, Homeland Security Advisory Supplement, March 2002 • National Strategy for Homeland Security, July 2002 • National Security Strategy of the US, Sept 2002 • Public Law 107-296: Homeland Security Act, November 2002 • Homeland Security Presidential Directive 4: National Strategy to Combat WMD, December 2002 • U.S. Department of Health and Human Services Assistant Secretary for Preparedness and Response Strategic Plan (2007–2012), 2006 • National Planning Framework, September 2011
Need for Comprehensive National Analytical Risk Assessment	**Reports** • Gilmore Report I, December 15, 1999 • GAO/NSIAD-98-74: Combating Terrorism—Threat and Risk Assessments Can Help Prioritize and Target Program Investments, April 9, 1998 • GAO/NSIAD-99-163: Combating Terrorism—Need for Comprehensive Threat and Risk Assessments of Chemical and Biological Attacks, September 9, 1999 • GAO-01-822: Combating Terrorism—Selected Challenges and Related Recommendations, September 20, 2001 • GAO-06-91: Further Refinements Needed to Assess Risks and Prioritize Protective Measures at Ports and Other Critical Infrastructure, January 17, 2005 • GAO-07-375: Progress Has Been Made to Address the Vulnerabilities Exposed by 9/11, but Continued Federal Action Is Needed to Further Mitigate Security Risks, January 24, 2007 • GAO-08-373R: DOD's Risk Analysis of Its Critical Infrastructure Omits Highly Sensitive Assets, April 2, 2008 • DHS Allocates Grants Based on Risk, but Its Risk Methodology, Management Controls, and Grant Oversight Can Be Strengthened, July 8, 2009 • GAO-11-873: Quadrennial Homeland Security Review—Enhanced Stakeholder Consultation and Use of Risk Information Could Strengthen Future Reviews, October 5, 2011. • GAO-12-272: Chemical, Biological, Radiological, and Nuclear Risk Assessments—DHS Should Establish More Specific Guidance for Their Use, January 25, 2012 • GAO-13-801 T: DHS Needs to Improve Its Risk Assessments and Outreach for Chemical Facilities, August 1, 2013
	Federal Actions • Homeland Security Act of 2002 creates the Homeland Infrastructure Threat and Risk Analysis Center (HITRAC) • Presidential Policy Directive 8: National Preparedness, 2011 • Strategic National Risk Assessment in Support of PPD #8, December 2011
Importance of Prevention as a Critical Component of Risk Reduction	**Reports** • Report of the White House Commission on Aviation Safety and Security (Gore Commission), February 12, 1997 • Gilmore Report III, December 15, 2001 • Report of the 9/11 Commission, July 25, 2004
	Federal Actions • National Security Decision Directive 138, Preemptive Strikes Against Terrorists, April 26, 1984 • Aviation Security Improvement Act of 1990: P.L. 101-604, November 16, 1990 • Airport Security Improvement Act of 2000: Public Law 106-528, November 22, 2000 • Public Law 107-56: The U.S.A. Patriot Act, October 26, 2001 • Authorization for Use of Military Force Against Iraq Resolution of 2002, October 2002 • Enhanced Border Security and Visa Entry Reform Act: Public Law 107-173, May 14, 2002 • Maritime Transportation Security Act: Public Law 107-295, November 25, 2002 • Homeland Security Act of 2002: Public Law 107-296, November 25, 2002 • CIA Terrorism Threat Integration Center announced in February 2003 • Homeland Security Presidential Directive #10, Biodefense for the 21st Century (initiates U.S. BioShield program), April 28, 2004 • National Prevention Framework, September 2011

(Continued)

TABLE 63-2	Disaster Risk-Management "Lessons Learned" as a Result of Terrorist Events—cont'd
LESSON	**REPORTS AND FEDERAL ACTIONS**
Importance of Mitigation as a Critical Component of Risk Reduction	**Reports** • Critical Foundations: Protecting America's Infrastructure, President's Commission on Critical Infrastructure Protection, 1997 • Gilmore Report III, December 15, 2001 • GAO-01-822; Combating Terrorism: Selected Challenges and Related Recommendations, September 1, 2001 • GAO-030165, Combating Terrorism: Interagency Framework and Agency Programs to Address the Overseas Threat, May 23, 2003 • GAO-04-628 T: Challenges and Efforts to Secure Control Systems, March 2, 2004 **Federal Actions** • Presidential Decision Directive/NSC-63, May 22, 1998 • Executive Order 13130, "National Infrastructure Assurance Council," 3 CFR, 1999 Comp., p. 203, July 14, 1999, • Executive Order 13231 "Critical Infrastructure Protection in the Information Age," October 16, 2001 • National Strategy for Protection of Critical Infrastructure and Key Assets, February 2003 • National Strategy to Secure Cyberspace, April 2003 • Homeland Security Presidential Directive #7: Critical Infrastructure Identification, Prioritization, and Protection, December 2003 • Public Law 109-139: Pre-disaster Mitigation Program Reauthorization Act of 2005 • National Mitigation Framework, 2011
Importance of Preparedness as a Critical Component of Risk Reduction	**Reports** • GAO/HEHS/AIMD-00-36, Combating Terrorism: Chemical and Biological Medical Supplies are Poorly Managed, October 29, 1999 • Gilmore Reports I-IV, December 1999 through December 2002 • GAO-02-141 T, Bioterrorism: Public Health and Medical Preparedness, October 9, 2001 • GAO-02-149 T, Bioterrorism: Review of Public Health Preparedness Programs, October 10, 2001 • GAO-03-373, Bioterrorism: Preparedness Varied across State and Local Jurisdictions, April 7, 2003 • GAO-03-924, Hospital Preparedness: Most Urban Hospitals Have Emergency Plans but Lack Certain Capacities for Bioterrorism Response, August 6, 2003 • GAO-04-152, Bioterrorism: Public Health Response to Anthrax Incidents of 2001, October 15, 2003 • GAO-04-360R, HHS Bioterrorism Preparedness Programs: States Reported Progress but Fell Short of Program Goals for 2002, February 10, 2004 • GAO-04-458 T, Public Health Preparedness: Response Capacity Improving, but Much Remains to Be Accomplished, February 12, 2004 • A National Public Health Strategy for Terrorism Preparedness and Response 2003-2008 Prepared by the Centers for Disease Control and Prevention, the Agency for Toxic Substances and Disease Registry, and the Department of Health and Human Services, March 2004 • GAO-06-559 T: The Status of Strategic Planning in the National Capital Region, March 29, 2006 • GAO-06-1096 T: Assessment of the National Capital Region Strategic Plan, September 29, 2006 • GAO-07-274: Three Entities' Implementation of Capital Planning Principles Is Mixed, March 26, 2007 • GAO-09-369: FEMA Has Made Progress, but Needs to Complete and Integrate Planning, Exercise, and Assessment Efforts, May 29, 2009 • GAO-10-381 T: State Efforts to Plan for Medical Surge Could Benefit from Shared Guidance for Allocating Scarce Medical Resources, January 25, 2010 • GAO-12-276 T: National Capital Region—2010 Strategic Plan Is Generally Consistent with Characteristics of Effective Strategies, December 7, 2011 • GAO-13-116R: Performance Measures and Comprehensive Funding Data Could Enhance Management of National Capital Region Preparedness Resources, January 31, 2013 **Federal Actions** • Homeland Security Presidential Directive 3 (HSPD-3) Homeland Security Advisory System, March 2002 • HRSA National Hospital Bioterrorism Preparedness Cooperative Agreement, 2002-2004 • Homeland Security Presidential Directive 5 (HSPD-5) Management of Domestic Incidents, March 2003 • National Strategy for Integrated Public Warning Policy and Capacity, May 2003 • Homeland Security Presidential Directive #8: National Preparedness, February 2003 • Reorganization of CDC, 2003-2004 • Homeland Security Presidential Directive 9: Defense of United States Agriculture and Food, January 2004 • Homeland Security Presidential Directive 10: Biodefense for the 21st Century, April 2004 • National Preparedness Guidelines, September 2007

TABLE 63-2   Disaster Risk-Management "Lessons Learned" as a Result of Terrorist Events—cont'd

LESSON	REPORTS AND FEDERAL ACTIONS
	• National Capital Region's (NCR) Homeland Security Strategic Plan, September 2010 • Presidential Policy Directive 8: National Preparedness, 2011
Importance of Response and Recovery as a Critical Component of Risk Management	**Reports** • GAO/NSIAD-97-254, Combating Terrorism: Federal Agencies' Efforts to Implement National Policy and Strategy, September 26, 1997 • Gilmore Reports I-IV, December 1999 through December 2002 • GAO-01-822, Combating Terrorism: Selected Challenges and Related Recommendations, September 20, 2001 • GAO-04-904 T: Coordinated Planning and Standards Needed to Better Manage First Responder Grants in the NCR, June 24, 2004 • GAO-05-121: Management of First Responder Grant Programs Has Improved, but Challenges Remain, March 3, 2005 • GAO-06-85: Insurers Appear Prepared to Recover Critical Operations Following Potential Terrorist Attacks, but Some Issues Warrant Further Review, December 20, 2005 • GAO-06-863 T: Challenges in Developing a Public/Private Recovery Plan, July 28, 2006 • GAO-09-996 T: Preliminary Observations on Preparedness to Recover from Possible Attacks Using Radiological or Nuclear Materials, September 19, 2009 • GAO-10-204: Actions Needed to Better Prepare to Recover from Possible Attacks Using Radiological or Nuclear Materials, February 26, 2010 • GAO-12-838: Improved Criteria Needed to Assess a Jurisdiction's Capability to Respond and Recover on Its Own, September 12, 2012 **Federal Actions** • PD 67 of October 21, 1998, "Ensuring Constitutional Government and Continuity of Government Operations" • CDC Public Health Bioterrorism Preparedness Cooperative Agreement, 2002-2004 • Homeland Security Act, November 2002 • Terrorism Risk Insurance Act of 2002 • Homeland Security Presidential Directive 5 (HSPD-5) Management of Domestic Incidents, March 2003 • National Response Plan, December 2004 • National Incident Management System, December 2008 • National Response Framework, July 2013 • National Disaster Recovery Framework, July 2013 • Recovery Policy 9461 1 Disaster Assistance for Child Care, January 2014 • HHS Concept of Operations (CONOPS) for Public Health and Medical Emergencies, March 2014
Importance of an All-Hazard Approach	**Reports** **Chemical Hazards** • GAO-04-410: DOD Needs to Continue to Collect and Provide Information on Tests and on Potentially Exposed Personnel, May 14, 2004 • GAO-04-1068 T: Health Effects in the Aftermath of the WTC Attack, September 8, 2004 • GAO-05-631 T: Federal and Industry Efforts Are Addressing Security Issues at Chemical Facilities, but Additional Action Is Needed, April 27, 2005 • GAO-05-652: DHS' Efforts to Enhance First Responders' All-Hazards Capabilities Continue to Evolve, August 10, 2005 • GAO-07-143: Management Actions Are Needed to Close the Gap between Army Chemical Unit Preparedness and Stated National Priorities, February 20, 2007 **Biological Hazards** • GAO-03-578, Smallpox Vaccination: Implementation of National Program Faces Challenges, April 30, 2003 • GAO-04-239, U.S. Postal Service: Better Guidance Is Needed to Ensure an Appropriate Response to Anthrax Contamination, September 9, 2004 • GAO-04-152, Bioterrorism: Public Health Response to Anthrax Incidents of 2001, October 15, 2003 • GAO-04-788 T: Federal Funds for First Responders, May 13, 2004 **Radiological and Nuclear Hazards** • GAO-06-545R: Investigators Successfully Transported Radioactive Sources Across Our Nation's Borders at Selected Locations, March 28, 2006 • GAO-06-558 T: Challenges Facing U.S. Efforts to Deploy Radiation Detection Equipment in Other Countries and in the United States, March 28, 2006

(Continued)

TABLE 63-2   Disaster Risk-Management "Lessons Learned" as a Result of Terrorist Events—cont'd

LESSON	REPORTS AND FEDERAL ACTIONS
	• GAO-06-1015: Federal Efforts to Respond to Nuclear and Radiological Threats and to Protect Emergency Response Capabilities Could Be Strengthened, September 21, 2006 • GAO-08-72: DOE Has Made Little Progress Consolidating and Disposing of Special Nuclear Material, November 5, 2007 • GAO-08-285 T: Federal Efforts to Respond to Nuclear and Radiological Threats and to Protect Key Emergency Response Facilities Could Be Strengthened, November 15, 2007 **Federal Actions** • Public Law 107-188: Public Health Security and Bioterrorism Preparedness and Response Act of 2002 • Public Law 107-197: Terrorist Bombings Convention Implementation Act of 2002 • Homeland Security Presidential Directive 19: Combating Terrorist Use of Explosives in the United States, 2007 • Homeland Security Presidential Directive 10: Biodefense for the 21st Century, 2004 • Public Law 108-276: Project BioShield Act of 2004 • Homeland Security Presidential Directive 18: Medical Countermeasures against WMD, 2007 • Homeland Security Presidential Directive 21: Public Health and Medical Preparedness, 2007 • Public Law 110-23: Trauma Care Systems Planning and Development Act of 2007 • Presidential Policy Directive 2: National Strategy for Countering Biological Threats, 2009 • Public Law 111-140: Nuclear Forensics and Attribution Act, 2010

diverse and collaboration has been difficult as a result; on the other hand, the nuclear sector is quite homogenous and has a long history of collaboration."[15] Challenges most frequently cited included, "the lack of an effective relationship with DHS," as well as private sector "hesitancy to share information on vulnerabilities with the government or within the sector for fear the information would be released and open to competitors."[15] The federal government's processes for coordination and collaboration continue to evolve in light of the new emphasis on homeland security.

The Process of Developing Coordination among Federal Agencies

Beyond a national strategy, substantial progress has been made in completing operational guidance and related plans to coordinate agencies in their response to acts of terrorism. In 2001 the U.S. Government Accountability Office (GAO) assessed that coordination of federal terrorism research, preparedness, and response programs was fragmented, prompting concerns of whether state and local programs could respond to biological terrorism.[16] Since the terrorist attacks of September 11, 2001, the federal government has invigorated the homeland security missions of many departments and agencies, nearly doubling the amount of federal funds devoted to homeland security. Moreover, the GAO enacted new legislation to create a new department and strengthen transportation security and law enforcement activities, leveraged relationships with state and local governments and the private sector, and began to establish a framework for planning the national strategy and the transition required for implementing the new Department of Homeland Security and other homeland security goals.[17]

Progress also has been made by some individual agencies that have completed or are developing internal plans and guidance.[17] Building on this progress, the federal government continues to develop its practices for managing federal progress and resources to combat terrorism, by working to address and overcome challenges identified by the GAO in 2009. Specifically, the U.S. government found that several inherent challenges remained in managing federal programs and resources to combat terrorism. First, numerous federal agencies have some role in combating terrorism. Second, these federal agencies represent different types of organizations, including those involved in intelligence, law enforcement, military matters, health services, environmental protection, emergency management, and diplomacy.

Occupational Health and Safety Are Critical to Effective Disaster Response

During the anthrax emergency of 2001, nine postal employees associated with two postal facilities that processed tainted letters contracted anthrax and two employees died. The response to anthrax contamination revealed the importance of choosing a course of action that poses the least risk of harm when considering actions to protect people from uncertain and potentially life-threatening health risks.[18] The World Trade Center attack of 2001 also resulted in a very high occupational health risk to workers.[19,20] GAO reports on past disaster responses have identified challenges for occupational health that continue to inform future disaster responses.[21-25]

Interoperability and Robust Methods of Communication Are Difficult to Maintain

The need for common, agreed-upon information and communication standards is widely acknowledged in the health community, and activities to strengthen and increase the use of applicable standards are ongoing. Despite ongoing efforts to address IT standards, many issues remain to be worked out, including coordinating the various standards-setting initiatives and monitoring the implementation of standards for health care delivery and public health. Experts believe that developing and implementing an overall strategy guiding IT development and initiatives could overcome many of the underlying challenges.[26-31]

Disaster Policy and Plans Are Difficult to Integrate

The anthrax incidents of 2001 required an unprecedented public health response. These biological attacks on the nation not only affected our government but also revealed the challenges and shortcomings facing the nation's public health system. It is important to note that during the anthrax emergency, neither the Federal Response Plan nor the federal Concept of Operations Plan (CONPLAN) for responses to terrorist attacks was used. Under the CONPLAN, the FBI and FEMA play major roles as the lead agencies for crisis management and consequence management, respectively. Although the FBI was very heavily involved in the source letter investigations, FEMA did not serve as the federal lead for consequence management because the incident did not meet those Stafford Act criteria necessary for federal declaration of disaster.[3] The U.S. GAO has recognized FEMA's progress and recommended further integration of planning, exercise, and assessment efforts.[32] Expert reports, such as those from the GAO, have highlighted the challenges that response authorities face in integrating community-preparedness programs into their strategic approaches. Progress continues to be made; however, it is an ongoing process.[33,34]

The Ongoing Need to Improve Chemical, Radiological, and Nuclear Capabilities

Even though there have been many accomplishments involving public health and medical countermeasures involving biological terrorism, a significant number of unresolved challenges related to public health and medical response for chemical, radiological, and nuclear terrorism remain.[35,29] "Experts, such as those at the GAO, believe that there are options for overcoming these challenges. Options might include enhancing the security at key emergency-response facilities, improving preparation for radiological and nuclear attacks, and/or establishing specific guidance for chemical, radiological, and nuclear risk assessment and for responding to nuclear or radiological attacks."[30,31,36–40]

Significant Challenges Associated with Protecting Agriculture from a Terrorist Attack

Homeland Security Presidential Directive 9, issued by President Bush on January 30, 2004, establishes a national policy to defend the agriculture and food system against terrorist attacks.[41] In 2006, Congress passed Public Law 109-374, the Animal Enterprise Terrorism Act, as "an act to provide the Department of Justice the necessary authority to apprehend, prosecute, and convict individuals committing animal enterprise terror."[42]

Much is being done to protect agriculture from a terrorist attack, but important challenges remain.[42,43] There are a number of options for addressing these challenges. For example, in 2012 the GAO made recommendations for actions to improve response to potential terrorist attacks affecting food and agriculture.[44,45] Another option for addressing these challenges would be the development of an overall strategy to strengthen disease surveillance in livestock and poultry.[46]

CONCLUSION

The approach to disaster risk management is best viewed as a cycle of continuous capacity building and quality improvement. There have been remarkable accomplishments associated with lessons learned from terrorist attacks to date; however, the threat environment and risk-management tactics are extremely dynamic and constantly changing. Many opportunities remain for improvement of critical national assets and capabilities.

ACKNOWLEDGMENT

A special thank you to my mentor, Kenneth Grey (retired Centers for Disease Control and Prevention [CDC] branch chief and developer of the CDC's first emergency operations unit and center).

REFERENCES

1. Rubin C, Cumming W, Tinmalli R, et al. *Major Terrorism Events and Their U.S. Outcomes (1998-2001)*. Claire Rubin: Arlington, VA; October 2003.

2. Government Accounting Office. *GAO/NSIAD-97-254: Combating Terrorism: Federal Agencies' Efforts to Implement National Policy and Strategy*; Washington, DC; September 26, 1997. Available at: http://www.gao.gov/products/NSIAD-97-254, Accessed 09.06.14.

3. Ember LR. FBI takes lead in developing counter terrorism effort. *Chem Eng News*. 1996;10–16.

4. Sharp TW, Brennan RJ, Keim M, Williams RJ, Eitzen E, Lillibridge S. Medical preparedness for a terrorist incident involving chemical or biological agents during the 1996 Atlanta Olympic Games. *Ann Emerg Med*. 1998;2(32):214–223.

5. White House. *Homeland Security Presidential Directive #5 (HSPD 5) Management of domestic incidents*; February 28, 2003. Available at: http://www.gpo.gov/fdsys/pkg/PPP-2003-book1/pdf/PPP-2003-book1-doc-pg229.pdf, Accessed 09.06.14.

6. United Nations. *Yokohama strategy and plan of action for a safer world: guidelines for natural disaster prevention, preparedness and mitigation*. Japan: World Conference on Natural Disaster Reduction Yokohama; May 23-27, 1994. Available at: http://www.unisdr.org/we/inform/publications/8241, Accessed 09.06.14.

7. United Nations. *Hyogo framework for action 2005-2015: building the resilience of nations and communities to disasters*; 2005. Available at: http://www.unisdr.org/files/1037_hyogoframeworkforactionenglish.pdf, Accessed 09.06.14.

8. White House. *Presidential Policy Directive #8 (PPD-8) presidential policy directive/PPD-8: national preparedness*; March 30, 2011. Available at: http://www.dhs.gov/xlibrary/assets/presidential-policy-directive-8-national-preparedness.pdf, Accessed 14.07.14.

9. Department of Homeland Security. *Overview of the national planning frameworks*; May 2013. Available at: http://www.fema.gov/media-library-data/20130726-1914-25045-2057/final_overview_of_national_planning_frameworks_20130501.pdf, Accessed 14.07.14.

10. King F. The role of risk assessment in life cycle management. In: Martin L, Lafond G, eds. *Risk Assessment and Management: Emergency Planning Perspective*. Waterloo: University of Waterloo Press; 1988:31–38.

11. Hogan D, Burstein J. Basic physics of disasters. In: Hogan D, Burstein J, eds. *Disaster Medicine*. Philadelphia, PA: Lippincott Williams & Wilkins; 2007:5.

12. Ciottone G. Introduction to disaster medicine. In: Ciottone G, ed. *Disaster Medicine*. Philadelphia, PA: Mosby Elsevier; 2006:4.

13. Schipper L, Pelling M. Disaster risk, climate change and international development: scope for, and challenges to, integration. *Disasters*. 2006;30(1):19–38.

14. O'Brien G, O'Keefe P, Rose J, Wisner B. Climate change and disaster management. *Disasters*. 2006;30(1):64–80.

15. Government Accounting Office. *GAO-07-626T: Challenges Remain in Protecting Key Sectors*; 2007. Available at: http://www.gao.gov/products/GAO-07-626T, Accessed 09.07.14.

16. Government Accounting Office. *GAO-01-915: Bioterrorism: Federal Research and Preparedness Activities*; 2001. Available at: http://www.investigativeproject.org/documents/testimony/187.pdf, Accessed 09.07.14.

17. Government Accounting Office. *GAO-03-260: Homeland Security: Management Challenges Facing Federal Leadership*; December 20, 2002. Available at: http://www.gao.gov/products/GAO-03-260, Accessed 09.07.14.

18. Government Accounting Office. *GAO-04-239: U.S. Postal Service: Better Guidance Is Needed to Ensure an Appropriate Response to Anthrax Contamination*;Washington, DC; 09.09.04. Available at: http://www.gao.gov/products/GAO-04-239, Accessed 09.06.14.

19. NY Department of Health, Data Snapshot: Understanding the health impact of 9/11. Available at: http://www.nyc.gov/html/doh/wtc/downloads/pdf/wtc/wtc-report2004-1112.pdf. Accessed 09.06.14.

20. Centers for Disease Control and Prevention. Self-reported increase in asthma severity after the September 11 attacks on the world trade center—Manhattan, New York, 2001. *MMWR Morb Mortal Wkly Rep*. 2002;51(35):781–784.

21. Government Accounting Office. *GAO-04-1068T: Health Effects in the Aftermath of the World Trade Center Attack*; September 8, 2004. Available at: http://www.gao.gov/new.items/d041068t.pdf, Accessed 09.06.14.

22. Government Accounting Office. *GAO-07-1253T: Problems Remain in Planning for and Providing Health Screening and Monitoring Services for Responders*; September 20, 2007. Available at: http://www.gao.gov/products/GAO-07-1253T, Accessed 09.06.14.

23. Government Accounting Office. *GAO-08-429T: Improvements Still Needed in Availability of Health Screening and Monitoring Services for Responders Outside the New York City Area*; January 22, 2008. Available at: http://www.gao.gov/products/GAO-08-429T, Accessed 09.06.14.

24. Government Accounting Office. *GAO-08-610: HHS Needs to Develop a Plan That Incorporates Lessons from the Responder Health Programs*; June 2, 2008. Available at: http://www.gao.gov/products/GAO-08-610, Accessed 09.06.14.

25. Government Accounting Office. *GAO-08-180: First Responders' Ability to Detect and Model Hazardous Releases in Urban Areas Is Significantly Limited*; June 27, 2008. Available at: http://www.gao.gov/products/GAO-08-180, Accessed 09.06.14.

26. Government Accounting Office. *GAO-03-139: Bioterrorism: Information Technology Strategy Could Strengthen Federal Agencies' Abilities to Respond to Public Health Emergencies*; Washington, DC; May 30, 2003. Available at: http://www.gao.gov/products/GAO-03-139, Accessed 09.06.14.

27. Government Accounting Office. *GAO-09-604: Vulnerabilities Remain and Limited Collaboration and Monitoring Hamper Federal Efforts*; June 26, 2009. Available at: http://www.gao.gov/products/GAO-09-604, Accessed 09.06.14.

28. Government Accounting Office. *GAO-10-463R: Establishment of the Emergency Communications Preparedness Center and Related Interagency Coordination Challenges*; March 3, 2010. Available at: http://www.gao.gov/products/GAO-10-463R, Accessed 09.06.14.

29. Government Accounting Office. *GAO-11-940T: Progress Made and Work Remaining in Implementing Homeland Security Missions 10 Years after 9/11*; June 30, 2010. Available at: http://www.gao.gov/products/GAO-11-940T, Accessed 09.06.14.

30. Government Accounting Office. *GAO-04-482T: Federal Action Needed to Address Security Challenges at Chemical Facilities*; February 23, 2004. Available at: http://www.gao.gov/products/GAO-04-482T, Accessed 09.06.14.

31. Government Accounting Office. *GAO-08-285T: Federal Efforts to Respond to Nuclear and Radiological Threats and to Protect Key Emergency Response Facilities Could Be Strengthened*; November 5, 2007. Available at: http://www.gao.gov/products/GAO-08-285T, Accessed 09.06.14.

32. Government Accounting Office. *GAO-09-369: FEMA Has Made Progress, But Needs to Complete and Integrate Planning, Exercise, and Assessment Efforts*; April 30, 2009. Available at: http://www.gao.gov/products/GAO-09-369, Accessed 09.06.14.

33. Government Accounting Office. *GAO-10-193: FEMA Faces Challenges Integrating Community Preparedness Programs into Its Strategic Approach Published*; January 29, 2010. Available at: http://www.gao.gov/products/GAO-10-193, Accessed 09.06.14.

34. Government Accounting Office. *GAO-10-969T: Criteria for Developing and Validating Effective Response Plans*; September 22, 2010. Available at: http://www.gao.gov/products/GAO-10-969T, Accessed 09.06.14.

35. Government Accounting Office. GAO-11-606: DHS and HHS Can Further Strengthen Coordination for Chemical, Biological, Radiological, and Nuclear Risk Assessments. Available at: http://www.gao.gov/products/GAO-11-606, Accessed 09.06.14.

36. Government Accounting Office. *GAO-10-204: Actions Needed to Better Prepare to Recover from Possible Attacks Using Radiological or Nuclear Materials*; February 26, 2010. Available at: http://www.gao.gov/products/GAO-10-204, Accessed 09.06.14.

37. Government Accounting Office. *GAO-12-272: Chemical, Biological, Radiological, and Nuclear Risk Assessments: DHS Should Establish More Specific Guidance for Their Use*; September 8, 2011. Available at: http://www.gao.gov/products/GAO-12-272, Accessed 09.06.14.

38. Government Accounting Office. *GAO-13-801T: DHS Needs to Improve Its Risk Assessments and Outreach for Chemical Facilities*; April 10, 2013. Available at: http://www.gao.gov/products/GAO-13-801T, Accessed 09.06.14.

39. Government Accounting Office. *GAO-13-243: NRC Needs to Better Understand Likely Public Response to Radiological Incidents at Nuclear Power Plants*; January 25, 2012. Available at: http://www.gao.gov/products/GAO-13-243, Accessed 09.06.14.

40. Government Accounting Office. *GAO-13-736: Major Cities Could Benefit from Federal Guidance on Responding to Nuclear and Radiological Attacks*; August 1, 2013. Available at: http://www.gao.gov/products/GAO-13-736, Accessed 09.06.14.

41. White House. Homeland security presidential directive 9: defense of United States Agriculture and Food. Available at: https://www.hsdl.org/?view&did=444013. Accessed 09.06.14.

42. Public Law 109-374: Animal Enterprise Terrorism Act. Available at: https://www.hsdl.org/?view&did=476361. Accessed 09.06.14.

43. Government Accounting Office. *GAO-05-214: Much Is Being Done to Protect Agriculture from a Terrorist Attack, But Important Challenges Remain*; Mar 8, 2005. Available at: http://www.gao.gov/products/GAO-05-214, Accessed 09.06.14.

44. Government Accounting Office. *GAO-11-946T: Challenges for the Food and Agriculture Sector in Responding to Potential Terrorist Attacks and Natural Disasters*; September 13, 2011. Available at: http://www.gao.gov/products/GAO-11-946T, Accessed 09.06.14.

45. Government Accounting Office. *GAO-11-652: Actions Needed to Improve Response to Potential Terrorist Attacks and Natural Disasters Affecting Food and Agriculture*; September 12, 2011. Available at: http://www.gao.gov/products/GAO-11-652, Accessed 09.06.14.

46. Government Accounting Office. *GAO-13-424: An Overall Strategy Is Needed to Strengthen Disease Surveillance in Livestock and Poultry*; May 21, 2013. Available at: http://www.gao.gov/products/GAO-13-424, Accessed 09.06.14.

CHAPTER 64

The Psychology of Terrorism

Robert A. Ciottone

Terrorism is an elusive term to define, one that seems "far too nimble a creature for social science to be able to pin it down in anything like a reliable manner. . . ."[1] Experientially, however, terror has a shared and familiar meaning within everyone's frame of reference. The origins of those feelings may be recent or they may be remote and only dimly recalled under the usual conditions of everyday life. Nevertheless, every individual within a population either is or has been the child who fears monsters lurking in places that cannot be seen clearly. Because of the universality of such experiences, feelings of terror remain potentially resurgent for every person.

Terrorists seek to destabilize population groups by a variety of means. One method is to resurrect through their actions the primitive and enveloping fears associated with the sense that "monsters" may act unpredictably and with impunity. Further, terrorists seek to imbue the destabilizing effects of such events, for both individuals and societal institutions, with sustained, destructive energy. Although terrorist-driven occurrences are temporally circumscribable, the psychological effect of terrorism is more of a process than an event. A host of factors conspire to perpetuate the psychologically destabilizing effect of terrorism, long after a focal event has occurred. These include uncertainty about the potential for, and the possible timing of, renewed attacks, disruption of infrastructure upon which many have relied, fears that health services may become overtaxed and unavailable when they are most needed, and concerns about loved ones in areas presumed to be particularly vulnerable.

Problematic psychological reactions to destructive terrorist-driven occurrences are not restricted to individuals who directly witness the event or are affected by it directly. Indeed, "media coverage of major terrorist events tends to be intense, capturing acute suffering and vulnerability. Unlike fictional stories, it portrays actual events and is sometimes unedited. And it produces the images of death and destruction that instill fear and intimidation in the larger public."[2] At the very least, the psychological effects of disastrous events can severely tax the ability of those affected to function with a level of efficiency that characterized their pre-event baseline.[3] Moreover, erosion of that efficiency may persist for many months and perhaps much longer, particularly with regard to incidence rates of psychiatric dysfunction and/or of stress-related physical illness within an affected population.

HISTORICAL PERSPECTIVE

Terrorism has been defined as violence involving attacks on a small number of victims, to influence a wider audience.[4] Much that has been written about the psychology of terrorism has centered on the emotions, motivations, cognitions, and other aspects of the psychological profile of those who would perpetrate such violence. As Cooper[5] noted, "The true terrorist must steel himself against tender-heartedness through a fierce faith in his credo or by a blessed retreat into a comforting, individual madness." If the presumed gift of a wooden horse that secretly held in its belly attackers who were bent on surprise and violence qualifies by this definition, the roots of terrorism stretch back through antiquity. More recently, in the centuries from the Middle Ages to the Industrial Revolution, warfare was conducted according to an implicit code of rules that sought in its most caricatured instances to render military conflict a "civilized affair." Eventually, international organizations such as the League of Nations, and later the United Nations, came about in part out of a need to hold conflict within some bounds, even if it could not be eliminated entirely. The Geneva Convention sought explicit agreement to rules of conduct on the part of potential adversaries before conflict had even emerged.

The goals underlying such efforts have proved elusive at best. As Crenshaw[6] noted, "significant innovations" in terrorism occurred in 1968, with the onset of relatively routine diplomatic kidnappings and hijackings involving extortion or blackmail. The pattern of increase in terrorist activity since that time has been all too familiar. Silke[1] has strongly argued the importance of researching this phenomenon with all of its implications. However, Silke,[7] like Merrari[8] before him, found that systematic inquiry by psychologists and psychiatrists fell short of what seemed to be needed.

The goal of this chapter is to consider psychological factors related to the effect of terrorism on a population and critical considerations for emergency response personnel. Although some specific guidelines may be derived, the purpose is to develop an awareness of psychologically contextual issues that may productively inform the judgments and decisions of service providers functioning in a terrorist-driven circumstance. First responders and caretakers are clearly among those in the population who can be affected most directly by terrorist events. Not only do they share in the danger of feeling overwhelmed and in the risk for problematic reactions, they also bear the expectations of others to remedy what might seem to be an impossible situation at times. Further, they share with those to whom they provide services, the need that the toll taken by terrorism upon them be monitored and managed. The alternative of implicitly adopting the false notion that first responders and medical practitioners are somehow above or immune to the psychologically harmful effects of terrorism invites multiple problems that have the potential of proliferating because of their effects on the service function. Accordingly, in the context of responding to terrorism, one of the imperatives for emergency medicine personnel must be to attend to the psychological needs of peers and of subordinates. For them, the sustained nature of the problem can exact a toll far exceeding the accustomed demands of providing emergency care.

DEVELOPMENTAL PERSPECTIVES

Although various aspects of the psychological effects of terrorism for both individuals and societal institutions can be considered, an overarching concept would provide coherence to considerations that might otherwise seem scattered. One such conceptually unifying theoretical perspective is the orthogenetic principle, a holistic developmental notion first articulated by Werner[9] and later by Wapner and Werner.[10] Briefly stated, the principle holds that all that occurs through development proceeds from the global and diffuses through increasing states of differentiation and hierarchic integration. In this context, "development" is not temporally defined nor is it tied to chronometry. Instead, the principle applies to any developmental phenomenon ranging, for example, from the microgenesis of thought behind each word spoken to the experience of an overall self-world relationship throughout the life span.

Through the prism of the orthogenetic principle, the developmental continuum from diffuse through integrated is conceived of as a dynamic one, within the context of which is the potential for developmental advance (toward increased integration) and/or dedifferentiation (regression to a more primitive developmental level). Movement forward (developmental advance) and/or movement backward (developmental regression) is not a discrete event but rather an ongoing process. Each advance in the direction of increasing differentiation brings with it the requirement that the parts of experience be hierarchically integrated (i.e., subordination of the differentiated parts to the whole) in a yet more refined fashion. Conversely, dedifferentiation leads to a less integrated experience with a correspondingly less refined sense of part-whole and of means-ends relationships and of the instrumentalities available for transacting with the environment thus construed. Developmental advance along that continuum brings with it an increasing sense of mastery, whereas dedifferentiation or regression to a more developmentally primitive level invites a growing sense of feeling overwhelmed.

Within that frame of reference, terrorism can be seen as an effort to bring about dedifferentiation and correspondingly more developmentally primitive functioning within populations and among the individuals that comprise them. Accordingly, interventions intended to address terrorism and its effects can be characterized as more or less facilitative of developmental advance and, correspondingly, of some increased level of mastery.

Acts of terrorism result psychologically in both direct and indirect destructive consequences of the sort that bring about developmental regression to a relatively less differentiated sense of one's relationship with the surroundings. The direct consequences typically have a powerful immediacy in their effect on the consciousness of affected segments of the population. Those consequences may well prove precipitously dedifferentiating in their assault on the sensibilities of those persons who are affected. Indirect effects, on the other hand, can be less apparent, particularly in the immediate aftermath of the disaster, but their destructive influence on the population and upon its institutions may be equally, if not more, disruptive to the functioning of the society.

The orthogenetic principle provides, in effect, a reference point by which to gauge and monitor the psychological harm done by terrorism, as well as the potential efficacy of efforts intended to mollify the psychological impact of sudden and disastrous terrorist-driven events. Initially, consideration must be given to the psychological vulnerabilities of individuals and/or of groups with regard to the risk of developmental regression. In other words, what has been the effect of trauma and of related fears upon individuals' cognitive, emotional, and valuative perceptions of and transactions with the physical, interpersonal, and sociocultural aspects of their surroundings? Stated differently, what changes have occurred with regard to what those affected by terrorism know with some confidence about the objects and places in their surroundings, how have their feelings about them changed, and what shifts have occurred in their attaching relative importance or unimportance to those objects and places? Likewise, how have knowing, feeling, and valuing shifted with regard to the interpersonal environment and in relation to their perceived environment of customs, responsibilities, and expectations? Second, how might a particular effort foster developmental advance in these areas? In other words, what is the best way to facilitate movement toward an approximation of pre-event psychological baseline?

The direct effects of terrorism are closely linked to the physical realities of the event (explosions, collapse of buildings or other structures, infectious outbreaks, etc.). According to Shalev,[11] however, traumatic events such as acts of terrorism can also be described according to their psychological dimensions. The two are obviously intertwined. Indeed, as Shalev has also noted, "Shortly after exposure, the traumatic event ceases to be a concrete event and starts to become a psychological event."[11] Physical injuries, often of a mangling and grotesque sort, together with the tragic loss of lives, typically become the signature of the event in the popular mind. Those images serve as a reference both for on-site survivors and, as a result of media coverage, for those who learn of the disaster from a distance. Moreover, such images can quickly become an experiential template onto which both proximate and remote observers project their own sense of vulnerability and/or that of their loved ones. In the context of responding to terrorism, therefore, emergency interventions on behalf of victims, as well as the ancillary and administrative procedures established to support them, should emphasize not simply the reactive measures taken, but the proactively oriented steps as well. The goal is to impart the promise of mastery of the circumstance by conveying some sense that those acting as agents for the well-being of the affected remain able to act on their behalf. By the very nature of terrorism, some of those efforts may have to be shaped on an ad hoc basis. Even in that circumstance, however, it is important to establish and maintain an approach that is consistent in both appearance and substance with a relatively differentiated response, rather than one that conveys a global, diffuse, and relatively undifferentiated quality.

The destruction of property and infrastructure, the limits imposed on transportation, and the disruption of communication typically serve to further compound the effects of terrorism on the accustomed behavior patterns of those sectors of society that have been affected directly. Essentially, individuals as well as groups and organizations may be severely limited in the use of accustomed instrumentalities that they have habitually used as a means of transacting with their surroundings. Regression to developmental primitivity is a distinct risk for those persons and institutions thus deprived of the tools by which to manage ongoing experience and to meet needs that have been readily satisfied in the past.

Developmental dedifferentiation in the wake of terrorist-driven events and the resulting increase in stress that may in turn compromise health can also result from sociological factors. In the past, populations could be expected to unite when confronted with a common foe. Attacks or states of siege were typically seen as the work of "outsiders." As a result, those who comprised the population attacked were the "insiders," united at least to that degree and able to take some measure of comfort from the availability and presumed goodwill of neighbors. In a terrorist environment, however, there is the distinct danger that neighbors may seem suspect. "Cells" of terrorists may operate anywhere and, thus, danger may be perceived as potentially stemming even from those who seem to be "insiders" or members of the same targeted population. Therefore the cohesiveness that usually occurs within a population on the heels of an attack may be severely compromised. Further, anyone exhibiting characteristics similar to those associated with the assumed perpetrators of the terrorism may become the object of suspicion, if not attack. Backlash effects can then lead to divisiveness and thereby compound the resulting stress experienced by individuals within the population. Given the demonstrable relationship between stress and health, it is incumbent upon caretakers and service providers to remain mindful of this potential psychosocial complication and to temper their interventions with sensitivity.

These and other direct effects of terrorism can severely tax and compromise the psychological resources and abilities required to cope with the demands of daily living. The resulting dedifferentiation would be further compounded if some semblance of predisaster infrastructure and service capability is not restored relatively soon after the focal event or if no believable estimation is issued as to when such restoration will occur. Accordingly, an important part of an effective emergency response includes providing accurate information regarding system level plans and prospects for returning to a pre-event baseline of service delivery. Although meeting this requirement of comprehensive care might be subsumed under the principle of providing reassurance, it is important from a developmental perspective that it not be trivialized. Further, it is important that information provided not be false or contrived, particularly because subsequent determination of intentionally misleading facts having been provided would probably compound the psychological damage it may have been intended to relieve.[12] Instead, a straightforward acknowledgment that information is not available is much more helpful, particularly when accompanied by an indication that facts will be sought out and shared when they become known.

Offering reassurance without misleading patients is a concern that applies to all aspects of clinical care. Providing services in response to terrorism is no exception. In fact, by virtue of the sense of the potentially overwhelming danger that seems to linger in the wake of terrorist-driven events, that requirement, particularly when viewed from a developmental perspective, becomes a salient one. To err by presenting patients with excessive ambiguity invites the projection of fears that might be much more extreme than the reality, however harsh. Such projections could well prompt developmental regression in the experience of self-world relationships. On the contrary, the other extreme of seeking to reassure patients by straining the limits of believability can not only destroy trust and encourage regression but also render its future restoration difficult at best. Accordingly, patients' psychological well-being and developmental advance are best served by clinicians relating with honesty tempered by empathic consideration for patients' subjective experience.

Observable instances of terrorism differ in terms of the degree and extent of their physical destructiveness. More circumscribed acts of terrorism, such as a bomb being detonated outside a police station or a polling place, would obviously have a correspondingly less-pervasive and/or less-extensive effect on infrastructure and the operation of societal institutions. Developmental regression, however, remains a danger. Those individuals upon whom the event directly impinges by its actual occurrence or by the fear that its having been threatened was intended to cause might well experience a disruption in their perception of "self-world relationships" and their ability to manage themselves productively. Their reaction, in other words, could prove analogous to that which would likely occur on a larger scale in the wake of more extensive incidents. Moreover, even those not directly affected by the event could well come to experience themselves as operating in a context of potentially sudden and unexpected hazard such that their actions might well become more tentative and fearful and less purposefully goal oriented.

Indirect, destructive effects of human-made disasters are often subtle and insidious in their erosive effect on the developmental level of functioning of societal institutions, as well as on that of the individuals within them. The frequent absence of immediate and overt indications of those effects notwithstanding, disruptions in cognitive, emotional, physical, and behavioral functioning in significant segments of the population can be anticipated in the aftermath of a terrorist event.[12] These may be sustained by lingering (if not growing) fear and by feelings of helplessness in the face of an unseen and perhaps unidentified perpetrator who may strike again with no warning. The resulting perception of risk represents a strong challenge to the capacity of individuals and groups to cope with the demands of everyday life with the same level of efficiency that characterized their pre-event behavior. Thus clinicians may well note that lapses will occur in patients' (as well as in peers' and subordinates') previously accustomed patterns of judgment, decisiveness, establishing and maintaining priorities, and other related psychological functions. Organizations, as well as individuals, are likely to experience these changes to varying degrees. Such effects may very well linger for a significant period after the terrorist event. For those in authority to provide supportive oversight of groups assigned various responsibilities therefore takes on an even greater importance than usual.

Indirect effects of a human-made disaster also include a significant increase of pressure upon public health systems for resources and services. Those demands typically occur in two phases. First is an obvious requirement to respond to direct casualties of the disaster. It is necessary, however, to also anticipate a predictable increase in stress-related illness that typically follows such events. In addition to psychiatric reactions, such as depression and posttraumatic stress disorder, rates of physical stress-related illnesses also rise when the psychological resources of a population are taxed by trauma.[13] Psychiatric problems, not restricted in their increased incidence to the immediate aftermath of focal terrorist events, tend to increase within a traumatized population about 3, 6, and 18 months after the event. The increased incidence rates of these and of stress-related physical illnesses in particular may well extend much further.[14] Accordingly, planning for health care within a population exposed to a human-made disaster must adopt a long-term view that takes the continuing effect of trauma on the health of an exposed population into account.

When negligence or incompetence results in death and/or destruction, those who perceive themselves as being at risk from its recurrence are likely to experience emotions ranging from fear and anger to distrust of societal institutions and their stewards. Intentional events of destruction such as acts of terrorism, however, may have even more disruptive immediate and delayed psychosocial effects. Similarly, the devastation wrought by a naturally occurring disaster may be greater in terms of casualties and damage to infrastructure, yet the psychological impact of the terrorist-driven disaster may still prove more extensive. Why is this the case? One reason has to do with perceived intentionality on the part of the potential causal agent of the danger.

A central tenet of most teleologically oriented theoretical perspectives in psychology (including the holistic developmental system of conceptual constructs) is that individuals impose meaning upon their experience and transact with the surroundings thus construed.[15] When the source of a seemingly amorphous but apparently present danger is perceived as intentionally malevolent, the safety of self and others feels particularly at risk. When that potential source of danger is hidden from view and perhaps anonymous as well, feelings of fear and helplessness are further compounded. Moreover, locations usually perceived as safe provide little comfort and do not satisfy the wish to hide in protected places.

It is important to recall that problematic reactions to destructive occurrences are typically not restricted to individuals who directly witness the event. As previously noted, media coverage of events may in some ways leave those who are more distant with an even broader and potentially more destabilizing view than is available to those who are closer to the event but whose view of it is less expansive. In either case, the psychological effects can severely tax the ability of those affected to function with a level of efficiency that characterized their pre-event baseline. Further, persons affected by virtue of their relatedness to victims of a disaster and/or by disruption of their relationship with societal systems affected by the disaster (e.g., supply systems for food, water, and medical services) may be at extreme risk for problematic reactions. Specifically, they may well be left in an ego-dystonic state of perceived inefficacy, vulnerability, and dysphoria.[16] Those effects can be profound. Indeed, those who remain thus affected for 1 year may not recover.[17]

As noted previously, one consequence of the dedifferentiating effect of exposure to critical events upon perception is to reactivate developmentally primitive perceptual tendencies and to vaguely experience a profound and panic triggering sense of helplessness in the face of what seems to be overwhelmingly threatening. Given the continuing availability of that frame of reference, terrorists who are intent on wreaking havoc and who seem to strike without warning may recall the feelings that perhaps long ago were as overwhelming as they might be to the child who was fearful of monsters in the shadows. Just as the child looked to a parent to "put on the light" and check for danger, those affected by a terrorist event look to authorities for reassurance. They seek to put aside their feelings of terror, and, to some degree, to master the ongoing experience. Moreover, just as the child needed reassurance on more than one occasion, populations look to perceived authorities such as service providers, for repeated signals that problems are being addressed.

⚠ PITFALLS

By the nature of their responsibilities, clinicians are obliged to remain alert to the signs that pressures are giving rise to stress that has the power to potentiate physical illness and/or to retard healing. To be sure, "pressure" and "stress" are often used as interchangeable terms, as if they were fully synonymous. To say "I am under stress" carries that implication. In one sense, however, pressure differs from stress in that pressure impinges on people. Stress, contrastingly, can be seen as a quality of the response that is made by individuals trying to manage pressure. The distinction is more than semantic; it is an important one because it implies that some measure of control over stress is possible, independent of the pressures that may operate outside of one's control. The psychological pressures associated with terrorism can obviously be extreme, but an effort needs to be made nonetheless to intervene in ways that, to the extent possible, minimize the extent to which those pressures are translated into stress and thereby into increased vulnerability to related illness.

What might be anticipated when the pressures related to terrorism become pathogenic sources of stress? Among the most frequently occurring, posttraumatic stress disorder (PTSD) represents one very prominent problematic sequela associated with exposure to terrorism.[18] Those who have been directly exposed to traumatic events are at greatest risk for developing PTSD, particularly if they have experienced physical immobility and/or helplessness while trying to escape; or if they have firsthand experience of the sounds, smells, and images; or if their lives have been permanently altered by the death or injury of a loved one.[19] Among those working in concert with emergency medicine providers, even the anticipation of handling of bodies and body parts after violent death can foreshadow PTSD.[20,21]

The signs of PTSD may include excessive excitability and arousal, emotional numbing, repetitive intrusive memories of the trauma,

and a general inability to function with the efficiency that was typical prior to the trauma. From a diagnostic standpoint, PTSD is evident when these and related symptoms persist for at least 1 month, and when significant distress results from them (DSM IV). The persistence of symptoms differentiates PTSD from acute stress disorder (ASD), which involves a clinically significant response to trauma similar to that seen in longer-term stress disorders (i.e., at least 2 days but no longer than 4 weeks).[22] The most recent revision of that diagnostic reference allows for a kind of second-order effect, by including the affected family members of those who suffered the event directly, as well as emergency workers who responded to their needs, as being among those considered potential victims of PTSD.

According to Muldoon,[23] some studies suggest that the distress that foreshadows the development of PTSD in fact may be cumulative in a transgenerational sense. Israeli soldiers for whom one or both parents were holocaust survivors, for example, showed a higher incidence of PTSD.[24] In a potentially related way, children of Vietnam veterans who had experienced particularly high levels of stress in that conflict showed higher levels of behavioral disturbance.[25] Early warning signs of PTSD include memory disturbances that may involve even previously automatized means-ends and part-whole perceptions and behavior sequences. Additional indicators may include flashbacks and traumatic dreams; episodic presentation of a seemingly dissociated or dazed appearance (e.g., the "thousand mile stare"); the emergence of panic attacks, fears, and irritability; and tendencies to "self-medicate" (i.e., substance abuse).

Developmental regression as a function of the effect of terrorism may first emerge as somewhat less specific antecedents to the symptoms associated with PTSD and/or with other problematic sequelae. As outlined by the Critical Incident Stress Foundation,[12] the tendencies that become evident when stress begins to take a toll will most likely include disruptions in cognitive functioning, such as confused thinking, disorientation, indecisiveness, and difficulty establishing priorities. Difficulties with emotional functioning that will most likely become evident may include feeling overwhelmed and unable to manage, extreme anger and/or grief, a pervasively and persistently depressed mood, etc. Physical functioning may well reflect problems that include increased blood pressure, increased heart rate, dizzy spells, rapid breathing, etc. Adverse effects on behavioral functioning may lead to changes in eating and sleep patterns, interpersonal withdrawal, changes in behavior patterns associated with the activities of daily living, etc.

What are the implications of this aspect of a patient's problematic psychological response for clinicians trying to address the consequences of terrorism? How might the lingering perception of continuing risk from recurrent events be managed? How best to mobilize and direct patients' energies to facilitate recovery rather than to allow those energies to be spent in diffuse anger or transformed into feelings of helplessness? In addressing these and related matters, clinicians' efforts should be shaped by an ongoing monitoring of the extent to which developmental dedifferentiation is being averted and developmental advance is instead being fostered.

From the outset, clinicians must adopt a manner, particularly in communication, that conveys a determination to focus on resolving the problem. It is also important to "put on the light," as it were, to offset the potential for resurgence of archaic fears that monsters lurk in the shadows. This can be accomplished in part by providing information that does not compromise honesty but which nevertheless conveys the message that gains are being made. At a systematic level as well (and with particular reference to the needs of peers and subordinates), the efforts made by emergency medicine personnel would be well supported by encouraging that information about perpetrators be made public once some reasonable level of certainty about its accuracy can be assumed. As van der Kork[19] has noted, "After safety is assured, psychological intervention may be needed. People have to learn to put words to the problems they face, to name them and to formulate appropriate solutions."

When ambiguity persists and rumor holds sway, fears can be projected that are so extreme as to invite retraumatization. The importance of dispelling ambiguity notwithstanding, however, identification should not be made in ways that might encourage wariness and distrust because of reliance on categories such as ethnicity, religious affiliation, etc. Such groupings do little or nothing to assuage anxiety and may, in fact, lead to its exacerbation because of their infusing potential alarm into categories that have been otherwise relatively benign within the population affected by terrorism. Instead, citing the allegiance of terrorist groups to shared goals of destabilization and to the use of terrorist methods in the service of a specified cause might be a useful supplement to providing the names of perpetrators if available in the process of identification. By this means, stress is less likely to be compounded by the relatively undifferentiated formlessness of those who would do harm.

To label that which is unknown is to impart some sense of mastery and control. Those who might otherwise be immobilized to some degree by fear can then use the label to perceive an otherwise amorphous threat as one that at least has a name and, thereby, some boundaries and limits to its potential malevolence. Fear then takes on a more circumscribed and seemingly more manageable form. Conversely, in the absence of a name for the potential danger, the sense of jeopardy and the stress-inducing need for sustaining a state of heightened vigilance increases.

Not all victims of terrorist-driven events suffer developmental dedifferentiation resulting in stress-related dysfunction or physical disease. According to van der Kork,[19] however, "almost everyone is perturbed during the aftermath of a trauma, and everyone experiences a degree of intrusiveness and sadness." Many others, however, have a much more difficult time "getting over it." In addition to PTSD, consequences of exposure to such events can include depression and disabling, treatment-resistant symptoms of fear and anxiety, as well as marital crises and other relationship problems.[13] Accordingly, "Understanding the mechanisms of mental traumatization is extremely important when seeking to evaluate and assist the recent survivor."[26]

To rely primarily on the verbal reframing of experience in an effort to provide psychological assistance in the wake of trauma may well prove less than productive, particularly in the early stages of intervention.[27] In fact, studies have shown that high levels of arousal, such as those associated with trauma, result in frontal lobe functions being suppressed,[28,29] as are Broca's area functions, which are needed to put feelings into words.[30] Subcortical centers, however, have been implicated as being more prominent in the neuropsychological mediation of trauma, particularly with regard to the limbic system.[31,32] Accordingly, Shalev[11] has noted that soothing bodily contact with the recently rescued is often helpful, but gender and social boundaries must be respected. Bringing in relatives of victims and others close to them may be especially helpful in this regard, with caregivers serving as coaches. By these means, a relatively more differentiated and integrated sense of the relationship between the self and the physical, interpersonal, and sociocultural aspects of the environment can be fostered and maintained. For this reason, "the first role of a therapist is to assess the strengths and weaknesses of the survivor's immediate supporters"[11] and to provide them with the support needed. Thereafter, interventions derived from the principles of cognitive behavioral therapy have been shown to be of more benefit than supportive counseling alone is during the postacute phase of early syndrome formation.[33]

Having particular relevance to the challenge of precluding developmental regression in the wake of exposure to traumatic events,

approaches referred to as "debriefing" involve semistructured group interventions geared toward alleviating potentially dedifferentiating distress and thereby preventing pathological reactions. Two approaches, one introduced by Mitchell[34] and another by Dyregov,[35] have had relatively extensive application. The first, subsequently advanced through the Critical Incident Stress Foundation, has been presented as a training program for volunteers who might be mobilized for service in the wake of a disaster, whether naturally occurring or terrorist driven. The process involves several phases, beginning with an introduction, during which personal identification takes place, along with a definition of expectations, a setting of limits, and an explanation of confidentiality. There follows a "fact stage," during which each participant is asked to describe the event from his or her own perspective, and a "thought stage," during which each participant is asked to recall first thoughts as the event occurred. In the "reaction phase," each person is asked to identify the worst part of the experience, one that she or he would erase from memory if possible. During the "symptom phase" that follows, each person is invited to explain how he or she is different because of the incident, and to describe how life has been since the event. A "teaching phase" then takes place, during which debriefing team members seek to "normalize" reactions by explaining their predictability as extraordinary characteristics of the circumstance rather than of the experiencing individual. The team also gives suggestions intended to aid recovery (e.g., relaxation and deep breathing exercises). Finally, during a "reentry phase," team members provide a summarization and encourage cognitive reframing of the experience to include some positive outcomes (e.g., lessons learned and insights achieved). Some studies[36-38] have failed to show that debriefing prevents stress disorders. However, those same studies indicate that most participants recall the sessions as helpful and satisfying. Moreover, Shalev et al.[39] found that debriefing significantly reduces concurrent distress and enhances group cohesion.

COMMUNITY PERSPECTIVES

One effect of increased group cohesion is to advance the development of what has been referred to as *community resilience*. As Pfefferbaum[40] and others have noted, resilience of communities implies that individual members are working together in the process of successfully adapting to and recovering from adversity. In that connection, Brown and Kulig[41] have explained that community resilience occurs when individuals engage in cooperative relationships and joint efforts that seek rapid recovery for the whole rather than independently seeking gains. In that manner, the risk of individual community members turning on each other in the wake of a mass trauma, with aggression rooted in panic and couched in an "every man for himself" mentality, can be minimized.

The factors that contribute to resilient and healthy communities have been identified by Gibbon, Labonte, and Lavarack, as well as by others.[42] They include relatedness, connectedness, and commitment to places, groups, organizations, and a shared history and value system. Other factors include participation with a sense of belonging to a community that provides the promise of support, nurturance, and a structure that clarifies roles and responsibilities. The readiness of a community to provide these without concern for the socioeconomic status, ethnicity, educational level, or religion enhances both individual and community resilience. Terrorists target the community in its widest sense. They seek to effect and disrupt not simply a geographic area or even those individuals who comprise the community but, most importantly, their customs, values, alliances, and systems of providing a ready flow of goods and services. Efforts to foster community resilience are, therefore, of paramount importance not only in the wake of an attack but as a pivotal component of preparedness as well.[43]

One barrier to overcome in that effort, however, may be failure on the part of many to recognize the extent to which trauma blurs the arguable but often assumed distinction between mental health and physical health on the part of the populations and even among providers generally. Resulting problems may be compounded by the stigma often associated with mental illness and treatment.[44,45]

As has been argued by Friedman, a perspective-based model of holistic wellness rather than illness is more likely to be effective for both individuals and communities in fostering the resilience needed to manage the effects of traumatic stress. By that means, in both preparedness for terrorism and in response to it, physical and psychological functioning are more likely to be restored and maintained in the wake of terrorism, when community providers make decisions and follow practice patterns informed by awareness of the behavioral and sociological dimensions of the effects of terrorism on health.[46]

Despite resilience within both individuals and communities, the response to adversity and trauma may vary at different times and as a function of the nature of the stressors. Invariably, some adults and children will develop symptoms that approximate the diagnostic criteria for PTSD.[47] Societal health agencies are, therefore, confronted with the question of whether a systematic effort should be made to screen for such problems within the general population in the wake of a terrorist attack.[47] When governmental agencies announced an epidemic of PTSD one week after the 2004 terrorist attack in Spain, under the headline "Marked Forever," it was estimated that between 90,000 and 180,000 persons were likely to manifest the symptoms of PTSD. When such dire symptoms are seen as inevitable in the wake of collective trauma, whether and how an effort should be made to screen for such symptoms can become a focal issue. Several studies, however, caution against overestimation of the probable emergence of clinically significant psychopathology, noting, for example, that high initial emotional responses may be a part of natural recovery, with improvement occurring in a supportive environment without individual professional help.[48,49] There is little doubt that, despite the danger of overestimation of its incidence, significant risk does develop, and large numbers of individuals may well fall victim to PTSD in the wake of a terrorist attack—how then to understand that phenomenon and how best to respond to it?

LEARNING THEORY PERSPECTIVES

One way to conceptualize symptom emergence of that sort is in terms of a Pavlovian classical conditioning paradigm.[50] Viewed from that perspective, the fear-related symptoms of PTSD may be considered the result of the pairing of the experiential events of the trauma, (the unconditioned stimulus) with the unconditioned response of fear and arousal. Cues in the environment at the time of the trauma then become conditioned stimuli that gain the power to elicit a conditioned response of fear and arousal, as persons approximate and recall the unconditioned stimulus. Accordingly, the PTSD symptom of reexperiencing the trauma or reacting to its assumed imminence can be thought of as a persistent conditioned response.[51,52]

Extinction of an acquired fear response of the sort associated with PTSD may sometimes be achieved through systematic desensitization. In that procedure, approximations of the conditioned stimulus are paired incrementally (through imagery and according to a preestablished hierarchy) with an experience of relaxation and calm elicited by a counterconditioning agent such as guided imagery, mindful breathing, or administration of an anxiolytic.

However, as compelling as such conceptual models may seem, a number of studies, nevertheless, suggest that PTSD may often be associated with an impairment in fear inhibition or fear extinction.[53]

Specifically, PTSD patients presented with feared stimuli were found to demonstrate heightened activity in the amygdala but diminished activity in the prefrontal cortex when they were presented with approximations of feared stimuli.[54] Additionally, the hippocampus has been found to be reduced in size in PTSD patients. That finding raises questions about the role of memory in PTSD symptoms and about possible changes in both functional and structural neuroanatomy among those meeting diagnostic criteria for PTSD.[55]

Taken together, studies indicate that no single approach promises consistently broad-ranging efficacy in the clinical response to individuals who develop PTSD. Pharmacologically, the only FDA-approved drugs for the treatment of PTSD are the selective serotonin reuptake inhibitors (SSRI) paroxetine and sertraline. There is some empirical support for other drugs used off label, but they tend to target specific symptoms, such as extremes of mood, anxiety, insomnia, or irritability. Cognitive behavioral therapy or desensitization procedures that are based on a sense of PTSD as the end result of a classical conditioning process may prove helpful, but some symptoms, nevertheless, may persist or recur. The troublesome uncertainty associated with various forms of clinical intervention with individuals presenting with PTSD underscores the overarching importance of developing resilient communities as a context that can enhance the response to treatment among afflicted individuals, as well as coordination among the providers.

In the wake of the April 2014 terrorism in Nigeria, the development of resilience extended to a sense of community that took on global dimensions in its definition and cohesion. "Bring back our girls!" became a rallying cry on social media that was echoed worldwide and that brought with it a potentially formidable counterforce to the efforts of terrorists to divide and destabilize communities. "The Congregation of the People of Tradition for Proselytism and Jihad," is known by its Hausa name, "Boko Haram," which means figuratively "Western education is sin." Like most groups that give rise to terrorism, it attracts those who feel powerless, and it ignites in them a fervor to dominate and/or destroy "out groups," which are, in effect, defined as any other than those who share their mission.[56] As in this instance, it may well prove to be the case in the future that the widespread and rapid dissemination of news of terrorism events, including images of those most directly affected, together with the bourgeoning empowerment of even those distant from the event to unite in their opposition to it, will prove a potent deterrent to terrorists' achieving their goals of destroying the cohesiveness of targeted communities Accordingly, providers serve the community well to facilitate dissemination of verified information by cooperating with well-vetted gatekeepers of far reaching platforms to support the development of community resilience.

CONCLUSION

Terrorists seek to destabilize individuals and societal organizations by undermining the cognitive, affective, and valuative perspectives they have of the physical, interpersonal, and sociocultural aspects of the world. In other words, terrorists seek to reshape the frame of reference by which people know about, have emotional reactions to, and attach relative importance to the world of objects and places, of people and of laws, and of rules, customs, and expectations. To the extent that they succeed, terrorists can compromise the psychological and physical health of individuals and thereby undermine the strength of a society. Accordingly, those in authority, and, in particular, the health service providers within a society, must make decisions and initiate efforts with judgment that is informed by sensitivity to the importance of both avoiding developmental dedifferentiation and fostering developmental advance.

REFERENCES

1. Silke A. Preface. In: Silke A, ed. *Terrorists, Victims and Society.* West Sussex, England: John Wiley and Sons; 2003:xv–xxi.
2. Pfefferbaum B. Victims of terror and the media. In: Silke A, ed. *Terrorists, Victims and Society.* West Sussex, England: John Wiley and Sons; 2003:175–187.
3. Spurrell M, MacFarlane A. Posttraumatic stress disorder and coping after a natural disaster. *Soc Psychol Psych Epidemiol.* 1993;28:194–200.
4. Crenshaw M. How terrorists think: what psychology can contribute to understanding terrorism. In: Howard L, ed. *Terrorism, Roots, Impact, Response.* London: Praeger; 1992.
5. Cooper H. The terrorist and the victim. *Victimology.* 1993;1(2):229–239.
6. Crenshaw M. The logic of terrorism: terrorist behavior as a product of strategic choice. In: Reich W, ed. *Origins of Terrorism.* Washington, DC: The Woodrow Wilson Center Press; 1998.
7. Silke A. The road less travelled: trends in terrorism research 1990–1999. Paper presented at the International Conference on Countering Terrorism through Enhanced International Cooperation, September 22–24, 2000, Courmeyeur, Italy. Cited in Silke A, ed. *Terrorists, Victims and Society.* West Sussex, England: John Wiley and Sons; 2003.
8. Merrari A. Academic research and governmental policy on terrorism. *Terrorism Political Violence.* 2001;3(1):88–102.
9. Werner H. *The Comparative Psychology of Mental Development.* New York: International Universities Press; 1948.
10. Wapner S, Werner H. *Perceptual Development.* Worcester, MA: Clark University Press; 1957.
11. Shalev A. Treating survivors in the acute aftermath of traumatic events. In: Chu J, ed. *Terror in the Nation: The Mental Health Clinician's Role.* April 12, 2002, Publication prepared as part of a conference sponsored by McLean Hospital, Boston, MA.
12. Everly G, Mitchell J. *Critical Incident Stress Management: Advanced Group Crisis Interventions—A Workbook.* 2nd ed. Ellicott City, Md: Critical Incident Stress Foundation; 2000.
13. American Psychological Association. When disaster strikes. In: *Terror in the Nation: The Mental Health Clinician's Role;* April 12, 2002, Publication prepared as part of a conference sponsored by McLean Hospital, Boston, MA.
14. Volkman P. *Presentation of the Basic Critical Incident Stress Management Course and the Advanced Critical Incident Stress Management Course.* Brattleboro, VT: Brattleboro Retreat; Sept. 30-Oct 4, 2002.
15. Wapner S, Kaplan B, Cohen S. An organismic developmental perspective for understanding transactions of man-in-environment. *Environ Behav.* 1973;5:200–289.
16. Everly G. Emergency mental health: an overview. *Int J Emerg Ment Health.* 1999;1:1.
17. Freedman S, Peri T, Brandes D, et al. Predictors of chronic PTSD: a prospective study. *Br J Psych.* 1999;174:353–359.
18. Shalev A, Freedman S, Peri T, et al. Prospective study of posttraumatic stress disorder and depression following trauma. *Am J Psych.* 1998;155 (5):630–637.
19. van der Kork B. The assessment and treatment of complex PTSD. In: Yehuda R, ed. *Psychological Trauma.* New York: Academic Press; 2002.
20. McCarroll J, Ursano R, Wright K, et al. Handling bodies after violent death: Strategies for coping. *Am J Orthopsych.* 1993;63(2):209–213.
21. McCarroll J, Ursano R, Fullerton C. Symptoms of PTSD following recovery of war dead: 13–15 month follow-up. *Am J Psych.* 1995;152:939–941.
22. Sprang G. The psychological impact of isolated acts of terrorism. In: Silke A, ed. *Terrorists, Victims and Society.* West Sussex, England: John Wiley and Sons; 2003.
23. Muldoon O. The psychological impact of protracted campaigns of political violence on societies. In: Silke A, ed. *Terrorists, Victims and Society.* West Sussex, England: John Wiley and Sons; 2003.
24. Solomon Z. Does the war end when the shooting stops? The psychological toll of war. *J Appl Social Psych.* 1990;20/21:1733–1745.
25. Rosenbeck R, Fontana A. Transgenerational effects of abusive violence on the children of Vietnam combat veterans. *J Trauma Stress.* 1998;11(4): 731–742.
26. Shalev A, Ursano R. *Mapping the Multidimensional Pictures of Acute Response to Traumatic Stress.* London: Oxford University Press; 2001.
27. van der Kork B. Beyond the talking cure: somatic experience, subcortical imprints and the treatment of trauma. In: Shapiro S, ed. *EMDR: Toward a Paradigm Shift.* New York: APA Press; 2001.
28. Arnsten A. The biology of being frazzled. *Science.* 1998;280:1711–1712.
29. Birnbaum S, Gobeske K, Aurb LG, et al. A role for norepinephrine in stress-induced cognitive deficits: alpha-1-adrenoceptor mediation in the prefrontal cortex. *Biol Psych.* 1999;46:1266–1274.
30. Rauch S, van der Kork B, Fisher R, et al. A symptom provocation study of posttraumatic stress disorder using positron emission tomography and script-driven imagery. *Arch Gen Psych.* 1996;53:380–387.
31. van der Kork B. The body keeps the score: memory and the evolving psychobiology of posttraumatic stress. *Harv Rev Psych.* 1994;1:253–265.
32. van der Kork B, van der Hart B, Marmar C. Dissociation and information processing in posttraumatic stress disorder. In: van der Kork B, McFarlane A, Weisaeth L, eds. *Traumatic Stress: The Effects of Overwhelming Experience on Mind, Body and Society.* New York: Guilford Press; 1996.
33. Bryant R, Harvey A. Relationship between acute stress disorder and posttraumatic stress disorder following mild traumatic brain injury. *Am J Psych.* 1998;155:625–629.
34. Mitchell J. When disaster strikes. *J Emerg Med Services.* 1983;8:36–39.
35. Dyregov A. Caring for helpers in disaster situations: psychological debriefing. *Disaster Manag.* 1989;2:25–30.
36. Bisson J, Jenkins P, Alexander L, et al. Randomized controlled trial of psychological debriefing for victims of acute burn trauma. *Br J Psych.* 1997;171:78–81.
37. Morbidity and the effectiveness of psychological debriefing. *Br J Psych.* 1994;165:60–65.
38. Shalev A, Freedman T, Peri T, et al. Prospective study of posttraumatic stress disorder and depression following trauma. *Am J Psych.* 1998;155:255–261.
39. Shalev AY, Peri T, Rogel Fuchs Y, et al. Historical group debriefing after combat exposure. *Mil Med.* 1998;163(7):494–498.
40. Pfferbaum B, Pfefferbaum RI, Norris F. Community resilience and wellness for children exposed to Hurricane Katrina. In: Kilmer RP, Gil-Rivas V, Tedeschi RG, Calhoun, eds. *Helping Families and Communities Recover From Disaster: Lessons Learned From Hurricane Katrina and Its Aftermath.* Washington, DC: American Psychological Association; 2010:265–288.
41. Brown DD, Kulig JC. The concept of resiliency: theoretical lessons from community research. *Health Can Soc.* 1996–1997;4(1):29–50.
42. Gibbon M, Labonte R, Laverack G. Evaluating community capacity. *Health Soc Care Community.* 2002;10(6):485–491.
43. Norris FH, Stevens SP, Pfefferbaum B, Wyche KF, Pfefferbaum RI. Community Resilience as a metaphor, theory, set of capacities, and strategy for disaster readiness. *Am J Community Psychol.* 2008;41(1/2):127–150.
44. Pfferbaum B, Flynn BW, Schonfeld D, et al. The integration of mental and behavioral health into disaster preparedness, response and recovery. *Disaster Med Public Health Prep.* 2012;6(1):60–66.
45. Pfferbaum B, Riesman DB, Pfefferbaum RI, Klomp RW. Buiing resistance to mass trauma events. In: Doll LS, Bono SE, Sleer DA, Mercy JA, Haas EN, eds. *Handbook of Injury and Violence Prevention.* New York: Springer; 2007:347–358.
46. Pfferbaum B, Flynn BW, Schonfeld D, et al. The integration of mental and behavioral health into disaster preparedness, response and recovery. *Disaster Med Public Health Prep.* 2012;6(1):60–66.
47. Vazquez C, Perez-Sales P. Planning needs and services after collective trauma: should we look for the symptoms of PTSD? *Intervention.* 2007;5(1):27–40.
48. McNally RJ, Bryant R, Ehlers A. Does early psychological intervention promote recovery from traumatic stress? *Psychol Sci Publ Interest.* 2003;4:45–79.
49. Silver RG, Holman EA, McIntosh DN, Poulin M, Gil-Rivas V. Nationwide longitudinal study of psychological responses to September 11. *JAMA.* 2002;288(10):1235–1244.
50. Norrholm S, Jovanovik T. Translational fear inhibition models of trauma relayed psychopathology. *Currr Psychiatry Rev.* 2011;7.

51. Amstadtler AR, Nugent NR, Koenen KC. Genetics of PTSD: fear conditioning as a model for future research. *Psychiatric Ann.* 2009;39(6):358–3667.

52. Jovanovic T, Resler KJ. How the neurocircuitry and genetics of fear inhibition may inform our understanding of PTSD. *Am J Psychiatry.* 2010;167:648–662.

53. Norrholm S, Jovanovic T. Translational fear inhibition models as indices of trauma related psychopathology. *Curr Psychiatry Rev.* 2011;7.

54. Brenner JD, Vythiligam M, Vermetten E. MRI and PET study of deficits in hippocampal structure and function in women with childhood sexual abuse and PTSD. *Am J Psychiatry.* 2003;160(5):924–932.

55. Felingham K, Kemp A, Williams I, et al. Changes in anterior cingulate and amygdala after cognitive behavior therapy of posttraumatic stress disorder. *Psychol Sci.* 2007;18(2):127–129.

56. Moghaddam, F. The staircase to terrorism: a psychological exploration, *The American Psychologist 60*, 161-169.

SUGGESTED READINGS

1. Wapner S, Kaplan B, Cohen S. An organismic-developmental perspective for understanding transactions of persons-in-environments. *Environ Behav.* 1973;5:255–289.

2. Wapner S, Kaplan B, Ciottone R. Self-world relationships in critical environmental transitions: childhood and beyond. In: Liben L, Patterson A, Newcomb N, eds. *Spatial Representation and Behavior Across the Life Span.* New York: Academic Press; 1981.

3. Wapner S. Transitions of persons-in-environments: some critical transitions. *J Environ Psych.* 1981;1:223–239.

4. Kaplan B, Wapner S, Cohen S. Exploratory applications of the organismic-developmental approach to man-in-environment transactions. In: Wapner S, Cohen S, Kaplan B, eds. *Experiencing the Environment.* New York: Plenum; 1976.

5. Friedman MJ. Every crisis is an opportunity. *CNS Spectr.* 2005;10(2):96–98.

CHAPTER 65

Thinking Outside the Box: Health Service Support Considerations in the Era of Asymmetric Threats

Duane C. Caneva and Pietro D. Marghella

In revising this chapter for the second edition of this text, it is interesting to review our "outside the box" thoughts from nearly 10 years ago. Defining "the box" is a challenge in and of itself. The boundaries of "the box" are further imposed by many, intertwined variables: budgets, policies, personalities, processes, protocols, and unseen interdependencies. Thinking outside "the box" is a lot like "futuring"—identifying drivers, using scenarios, and recognizing emerging themes that direct and refine strategy, development, and execution, and help steer us toward outcomes that are more favorable. These drivers include variables such as knowledge, science, technology, cultural values, geopolitics, environmental changes, and resources, and they factor into a complicated, dynamic, nonlinear system. Throw in innate human factors, and the system becomes complex: the domain of the "wicked problem," where adaptive iteration, that is, repeated consideration and analysis, is required both to refine problem structure and to find the best solution.[1] Some of the drivers have had clear effects on efforts. Goals and objectives have been refined by significant austerity in government spending and grants programs. The windfall of spending in science and technology, homeland security, and related emergency preparedness efforts that occurred after 9/11 is gone. The financial crisis of 2008 further punctuated that decline. In its place are severe cuts to budgets and programs, delays in projected development cycles, and supplies and equipment rapidly becoming outdated. However, the "technology era" offers the worthy goals of integration, innovation, and collaboration as ways for improving preparedness and response cost effectively. Constrained budgets refine priorities and introduce necessity as a driver for invention. Realizing success depends on seeing how things could be, developing a shared vision, aligning efforts, and moving into the right direction.

Our adaptive iterating has gradually added further architecture to our emergency management efforts. The Federal Emergency Management Agency (FEMA) and other government agencies work closely with communities to standardize, customize, and integrate preparedness efforts. Information is readily available to share with individuals, businesses, volunteer organizations, communities, states, and regions on a multitude of disaster preparedness and response activities if senior leadership so desires (see www.fema.gov). The Department of Homeland Security (DHS) works through Sector Coordinating Councils, directly with key members of the private sector in critical infrastructure sectors to coordinate protection, response, and recovery activities.[2] This build out, combining the private sector energy and innovation with the bureaucracy of government, continues to flourish, refining roles, responsibilities, swim lanes, and trust. Unfortunately, progress is still largely captured officially in glossy, paper reports with semantic text. These high-level, "portrait"-oriented documents provide static, snapshot views of ongoing, dynamic, and evolving events occurring in a "landscape" mode, which are of limited value unless operationalized.

Meanwhile, technology continues to advance at a rapid clip. Information management has changed significantly, and, no doubt, will be substantially different 10 years hence. Social networking applications allow for human interaction and establishment of trusted social networks linked around the globe. Search engines put the bulk of current information at our fingertips. Mobile communications allow for near ubiquitous coverage with various modes of talk, data, and streaming video for information retrieval and exchange. The Web is maturing from its early, basic Web 1.0 informational pages to Web 2.0 collaborative wikis, moving on through the semantic Web 3.0 "Internet of Things" (IoT),* where objects in the world are tagged, characterized, and interconnected, to Web 4.0 "Singularity," where computers are capable of independent reasoning, learning, and decision making. In the medical sector, telemedicine, robotics, and point-of-care diagnostics are transforming the way medicine is practiced. Diagnostic algorithms are just around the corner. Genomics is progressing to proteomics, metabolomics, and customized medical approaches geared toward our individual genetic requirements.[3] Electronic health records systems are transforming the way we provide individual and population-based health care. The massive amounts of data now captured in these systems offer enormous potential for innovation, yet also pose incredible security risks.

So what defines the "box" now, and what lies outside of it? In focusing on the need to improve health service support for emerging asymmetric threats, the first steps outside that box must include a leveraging of the benefits to be gained from the confluent areas of information management and technology, opportunities to be gained by embracing network- and coalition-centric hospital and health system architectures, and fully developing public-private partnerships for enhanced preparedness and response collaboration. The goal must be the ability to achieve the change needed to increase "overall resilience," which may be defined as the ability to function as normally as possible in the abnormal environment, across all levels of the operational spectrum.

Information, Integration, Interoperability, and Interdependency

The Wide Area Resiliency and Recovery Program (WARRP), looking at the chemical, biological, radiological, and nuclear defense (CBRN)

---

*The term "Internet of Things" (IoT) refers to uniquely identifiable objects and their virtual representations in an Internet-like structure. The term is used to denote the advanced connectivity of devices, systems, and services that go beyond machine-to-machine (M2M) communications and cover a wide variety of protocols, domains, and applications.

incident scenario set, extended the work done on the Interagency Biodefense Restoration Demonstration (IBRD), using the "whole of community" approach in conforming to FEMA's Disaster Recovery Framework development.[4] IBRD included involvement of the private sector, and it led to some startling revelations for recovery time windows of opportunity that government alone could not have realized. For example, if "big business" corporations cannot regain access and operations within 6 months, they terminate their lease, cut their losses, and abandon the location. Small businesses have about a 3-month window before most are out of business. Both big business and small entrepreneurs are highly incentivized and willing to participate actively in preparedness, response, recovery, and restoration phases; their livelihood in that city depends on it.[5] WARRP uses an engineered approach to further identify key components to Disaster Recovery Frameworks that highlights otherwise nonobvious risk-mitigation actions. Initiatives of this sort raise the thresholds for preparedness and mitigation from disasters, as well as facilitate response and recovery within a given region.

The key lessons from IBRD and WARRP are the importance of public-private partnerships and the creation of mechanisms for efficient data sharing and knowledge management. Orienting the effort through recovery frameworks using a "systems engineering"* approach further leverages the skillsets, tools, and lessons learned within various disciplines, sectors, and stakeholders, often even conforming to or highlighting related best practices across or within those disciplines. Public-private partnering expands the stakeholder pool and promotes broader interoperability efforts that are otherwise missed or ignored. For example, consider building codes in hurricane-prone areas. Insurance analysts, engineering experts, and homebuilders working in partnership with the public sector could determine the right mix of controls, standards, and distribution of homes and buildings able to withstand specific categories of storms. Broad collaboration across government and the private sector is critical. A deliberate planning process then promotes development of common goals and objectives of the partners and stakeholders while still considering the economic impact. These are linked to activities and tasks assigned to specific response plans and requirements. This can be done in real time and modified in crisis planning efforts to adjust to incident specific response requirements.[6] Evolution of the incident management systems permitting further integration and "spread sheet detail" allows for cost/benefit risk analysis, prioritization of objectives, and better decision making. The process established the "new normal." The improved state then provides options for short-term response and longer-term recovery that are better informed and understood, as well as more aspirational. Bringing the private sector into the mix allows for incorporating modernized engineering controls and building codes, dual-use capabilities, and advanced technologies into the next generation of the impacted area. Like the rebuilding of cities in Europe, devastated after World War II, a deliberate planning process propels the "new normal" forward in

modernization, and it confers advantages only seen when the longer view is considered.

The approach for these programs and efforts is sound. Our society is a complex and dynamic system. A systems operations, engineered approach that identifies all potential nodes in the system, where they are, and how they react and interact in crisis, should provide a better understanding of the effects, course, and harm of the disaster. The IoT allows us the potential to identify and monitor any critical node in a system. Many of these monitoring systems are already in place or are being built out. What is more difficult is to capture the cascading, higher-order effects, the interdependencies of these nodes, individually and when acting within a system. Being able to view over 2 million publicly available data layers is in "the box," as can be seen at Collaborate .org (www.collaborate.org). By combining the right combination of these data layers available in the public realm into customized "mash-ups," these data layers that show effective cause and effect, which explain or predict behavior or outcomes, an approach that, currently, is just barely out of the box.

Transform the Public Sector

Governance needs to adopt a network (i.e., "netcentric") or coalition-centric approach to operations with the "pull and smart push" of information.[7] This requires technological platforms that link policy, program management, plans, processes, performance outcomes and metrics, and people—not through paper documents or E-mail, but through integrated, relational data that accounts for the IoT), where machines are linked and functionally integrated. Information needs to be treated as interdependent, constantly updating data elements, with underlying taxonomy and ontology captured in the processes. This information needs to be delivered to the user through an interface that presents more than just a snapshot in time. It needs to capture the context of the information, display any interesting trends, and identify potentially interesting patterns that may indicate a threshold or a warning. The same information systems used on a daily basis should also be used during disaster response. The system should be familiar to the users. The same data and information used in emergency operations centers should be what is used by, and input from, responders on a daily basis and during response, ultimately obviating the need for an operations center at all. Information captured in paper documents no longer reflects the way we work (except when the power goes out). That approach denies us the agility needed for meeting the unique requirements of individual disasters.

Integrated, technology-based planning flows more easily from the common platforms used daily in the workplace, and its use leads to more easily integrated technology-based planning and response. The concept is not new, and it has been demonstrated in practice.[6] Responders are presented the information they need to know for their part of a plan, in a simple, executable format, such as a checklist with specific tasks. These checklists are integrated across the response plan, and responders update the performance of their assigned tasks when completed. A greater amount of background information is easily accessible if it is desired, but it is otherwise treated as "noise" during the response, and is not immediately displayed. The concept of "continual preparedness" builds on this systematic approach, providing the flexibility to modify and update plans, based on real-time response requirements, feedback, or resource availability.[8] Adopting more of a "need-to-share" versus a "need-to-know" approach allows for more effective engagement with the public. Ideally, crowdsourcing ideas and preparedness activities make for preparedness that is more comprehensive, effective, and efficient, although the proper balance between transparency and proliferation of sensitive information must be maintained.

---

*Systems engineering is an interdisciplinary field of engineering that focuses on how to design and manage complex engineering projects over their life cycles. Issues such as reliability, logistics, coordination of different teams (requirements management), evaluation measurements, and other disciplines become more difficult when dealing with large or complex projects. Systems engineering deals with work processes, organizational methods, and risk management tools in such projects. It overlaps technical and human-centered disciplines, such as control engineering, industrial engineering, organizational studies, and project management. Systems engineering ensures that all likely aspects of a project or system are considered and integrated into a whole.

Engaging the Private Sector

Our strength in mustering resources for disaster response lies within our private sector. Large and small businesses have incentive to assist their community's recovery. Business owners and operators represent innovative, engaged citizens, adept at effective problem solving and efficient decision making. Our critical medical sector and infrastructure also largely lies in the private sector, working closely with our public sector emergency services and law enforcement in managing the medical response in disasters. Private sector health care systems and experienced, innovative business leaders need to be actively included in a netcentric operations approach beyond the local emergency planning committee efforts. As WARRP and IBRD demonstrated, the private sector is ready and willing to play in all phases of emergency management. It represents the best way to engage all of the resources in a given community. Private sector partners need to see that investing in community-based preparedness represents an investment in their own continuity of operations, because disruptions to the very environment that they exist in will mean disruptions to the personnel, processes, resources, and infrastructure that support them and, ultimately, directly supports their business strategies and plans.

Engaging the People in Communities

Our communities are comprised of involved, caring, often-altruistic, self-actuating, and self-organizing individuals. These people are important resources. Whether organized through FEMA Community Emergency Response Teams, community organizations, churches, or trusted social networks, they often provide the initial, immediate response to many disasters. Education and training programs continue to evolve with "all get some, some get all" approaches, including advanced degrees and career pathways in emergency management. New focus on the role and effective use of bystanders in initial responses will further improve awareness, resilience, and outcomes. Evolving use of information technology lends itself to near real-time crowdsourcing for situational awareness and emergence of solutions in the chaos of early response activities. Twitter feeds, for example, are now often used to provide insight into incidents as they occur. IT also lends itself to identifying meaningful metrics that allow a community to identify factors contributing to resilience or preparedness for a given incident type. For example, tracking the number, distribution, and accessibility of storm shelters in tornado-prone regions allows a community to measure its risk and prioritization of mitigation activities to drive solutions that are affordable, achievable, and desirable.

Beyond Resilience

Presidential Policy Directive-8 (PPD 8) National Preparedness, introduced the National Preparedness Goal and the National Preparedness System. PPD 8 moved beyond the National Response Framework to a series of linked frameworks.[9,10] As our system increases the level of detail of the interdependencies of items and issues in preparedness, response, and recovery, it necessarily becomes more dependent on a technological environment as the operational platform. It cannot be managed otherwise in any meaningful way. Therefore, smartphone-based telemedicine will soon be used to diagnose ailments based on results from plug-in point-of-care diagnostic tools and actuarial-based medical algorithms gleaned from networked electronic health records; drones will be instructed to deliver customized pharmaceuticals to homes to be administered by personal robots according to the five rights of medication administration (right patient, right drug, right dose, right route, right time); and we will have moved from planning silos to standards-based technological preparedness environments.

CONCLUSION

In the decade since this chapter was first published, it is regrettable to look back and recognize that many of the admonitions contained in the original manuscript for improving the medical and public health readiness posture against large-scale disasters were repeatedly ignored. Each time a new event appeared on our horizon—whether it was the SARS epidemic, Hurricane Katrina, Avian Influenza, the H1N1 Pandemic, the Joplin and Moore tornadoes, or Hurricane Sandy—we found ourselves no better prepared in the critical infrastructure and key resource (CI/KR) sector that we know will always bear the preponderant load in adjudicating the success or failure of our incident management efforts. Moreover, the costs we have borne in both human suffering and loss have been staggering.

It is important to recognize that we are a nation, and a world, that will continue to see only an increase in the frequency, scope, and scale of future disasters. Consider the following:

- It is impossible to ignore what climate change has done to alter the homeostasis of our weather patterns, increasing the diametrically opposite risks of both flooding and drought.
- Significant and steady increases in the human population continue to place increasing demands on the resources necessary to the global population at risk (PAR). These demands only intensify during times of disaster and environmental duress, making competition for scarce resources and their access in "just-in-time" environments all the more difficult.
- The phenomenon of "clustering" in mega-cities intensifies this demand across all defined CI/KR sectors, and places more people in a position of risk when any type of disaster—natural or human made—occurs.
- Right now, more than 50% of the world's population lives within 60 km of the ocean (this is expected to rise to 75% by 2020).[11] Approximately 75% of the world's mega-cities are on the immediate littoral[12] (these same figures hold true for the current United States' population).
- Finally, the British medical historian R.S. Bray points out that "one inexorable truth" exists regarding the spread of disease: it "will always travel along man's lines of transportation."[13] What this truth portends in the era of modern intercontinental air travel has yet to be seen.

The United Nations' Office for Disaster Reduction noted in 2013, "There is no such thing as a natural *disaster*, only natural *hazards*."[14] Disasters occur only at the confluence of where hazards meet vulnerabilities. Said another way, they only occur when we fail to prepare. Their severity is entirely dependent on the choices we make for our lives, property, and environment. Every decision we make can either enhance our posture of preparedness or, conversely, degrade it.

We, therefore, have to stop treating hazards (and the disasters that they can become) as "predictable surprises"[15] and embrace a culture of proactivity that focuses on the gains that may be made in the preparedness and mitigation phases of the disaster management life cycle. Further, we must recognize that the single common denominator to all disasters is human casualties. It follows that the medical and public health infrastructure will bear the preponderant weight of the incident management mission. Embracing this fact must drive our efforts to steel the readiness capacity of the health care capacity of this nation. This chapter focused on gains that may be made by utilizing information management and information technology (IM/IT) systems for enhancing an agile response, the benefits that can be realized when health care organizations and system embrace network-centric and coalition-based architectures to build response capacity and resilience, and the importance of building upon and engaging the public-private partnerships that will increase our ability to withstand the common challenges of duress that future disasters will drive. We must continue to think hyperdimensionally about the interrelatedness of our society and CI/KR sector capacity, as well as how future advances in technology and theory can help to improve our ability to face the challenges yet to come.

REFERENCES

1. US Army TRADOC Pamphlet 525-5-500, Commander's Appreciation and Campaign Design, Jan 2008. Available at: http://www.tradoc.army.mil/tpubs/pams/p525-5-500.pdf.

2. Critical Infrastructure Sector Partnerships. Available at: http://www.dhs.gov/critical-infrastructure-sector-partnerships.

3. Topol E. *The Creative Destruction of Medicine.* Basic Books; 2012. Available at, http://www.medikz.com/Ebook/The%20Creative%20Destruction%20of%20Medicine.pdf.

4. Denver UASI All-hazards Regional Recovery Framework, Oct 31, 2012. Available at: http://www.fema.gov/media-library-data/20130726-1910-25045-8957/51_rrkp_urban_area_recovery_attachment_1_denver_framework___cbr_annexes.pdf.

5. Regional Recovery Framework for a Biological Attack in the Seattle Urban Area, Sep 2010. Available at: http://nwrtc.pnnl.gov/PDFs/RegionalRecoveryBioAttack201009.pdf.

6. Keim ME. An innovative approach to capability-based emergency operations planning. *Disast Health.* 2013;1(1):1–9.

7. Alberts D, Hayes R. "Power to the Edge," Command and Control Research Program, Dept of Defense. Available at: http://www.dodccrp.org/files/Alberts_Power.pdf.

8. Marghella P, Montella A, Josko W. *Dump the 3-Ring Binders: Changing the Planning Paradigm for Enhanced Preparedness and Response.* Available at: http://www.abia.us/articles/index.php?mact=News,cntnt01,print,0&cntnt01articleid=17&cntnt01showtemplate=false&cntnt01returnid=15.

9. Presidential Policy Directive 8, National Preparedness. Mar 2011. Available at: http://www.dhs.gov/presidential-policy-directive-8-national-preparedness.

10. FEMA National Preparedness Goal. Sep 2011. Available at: http://www.fema.gov/media-library-data/20130726-1828-25045-9470/national_preparedness_goal_2011.pdf.

11. UNEP. *Cities and Coastal Areas;* 2013. Retrieved from, www.unep.org/urban_environment/issues/coastal_zone.asp.

12. Laden G. *How Many People Live Near the Ocean?* 2011. Retrieved from, http://scienceblogs.com/gregladen/2011/10/18/how-many-people-live-near-the-/.

13. Bray RS. *Armies of Pestilence: The Impact of Disease Upon History.* New York, NY: Barnes and Noble; 1996, p. 32.

14. UNUSDR. *What Is Disaster Risk Reduction?* 2013. Retrieved from, www.unisdr.org/who-we-are/what-si-drr.

15. Bazerman M, Watkins M. *Predictable Surprises: The Disasters We Should Have Seen Coming.* Cambridge, MA: Harvard Business School Press; 2004.

CHAPTER 66

Integrated Response to Terrorist Attacks

E. Reed Smith, Geoffrey L. Shapiro, and David W. Callaway

The Federal Bureau of Investigation (FBI) defines *terrorism* as "the unlawful use of force or violence against persons or property to intimidate or coerce a government, the civilian population, or any segment thereof, in furtherance of political or social objectives."[1] In total, 2608 terrorist attacks occurred in the United States between 1970 and 2011 (207 from 2001 to 2011). From 2001 to 2011, the most common targets of terrorists in the United States were businesses (62 attacks), private citizens and property (59 attacks), and government entities (43 attacks).[2] Because the focus of this chapter is on operational response, the authors expand on the FBI definition of *terrorism*, and include random acts of mass violence, such as active shooter incidents (ASIs) and active violence incidents (AVIs), as acts of terrorism.

In 2004 Stephen Flynn wrote in Foreign Affairs that "Terrorism is simply too cheap, too available, and too tempting to ever be totally eradicated."[3] The pandemic of global civil strife and irregular warfare, coupled with the expanded Internet capability, is creating a complex and evolving threat matrix. Terrorists are now able to gain "on the job" training in any of a dozen "low-intensity conflicts" ongoing in every time zone. Alternatively, they can simply data-mine the Internet for bomb-making instructions or reviews of prior after-action reports on acts of terrorism.

From 2005 to 2014, the world witnessed a major evolution in the complexity and scope of terrorist attacks (e.g., Mumbai in 2005, the Westgate Mall in Nairobi, Kenya, in 2013, the Boston Marathon Bombing, in 2013, and numerous incidents in Pakistan, Iraq, and Syria). The majority of global terrorist attacks have been designed to destabilize existing political or social paradigms. This is true whether examining Al Qaeda (AQ) and their generational war philosophy, any of the myriad AQ affiliates (e.g., Abu Sayyaf, the Islamic State of Iraq and Syria, and Al Shabaab), domestic extremist groups, or lone-wolf attackers. This evolution emphasizes increasing coordination and sophistication of action; these "complex attacks," by definition, include most or all of the following: diversion, attacks on first responders, use of explosives, use of fire as a weapon, impersonating first responders, and coordination among actors in multiple locations involved. Thus the need for coordination and cooperation among interagency partners in the first-response community has never been clearer.

In his 2001 book, *Fooled by Randomness*, Nicholas Nassim Taleb introduced the concept of "Black Swan" events in terms of financial crises. A *Black Swan* is defined as a major event that is considered in real time to be a surprise, and yet, once examined in hindsight, all of the relevant data reveal that it could have been expected and should have been prepared for. In the first-response community, most if not all of the active violence events since the turn of the century can be considered Black Swan events: they were all major events in their respective communities and were considered a surprise for the community in which they occurred, as well as for first responders, operationally.

Yet, given that these events have occurred at a shockingly high frequency, the possibility of occurrence and the relevant data outlining the risk were never properly accounted for in the emergency-response plans and risk-mitigation programs.[4]

Regardless of jurisdiction or geography, terrorist attacks should no longer be Black Swan events. Our response paradigms must evolve and be proactive rather than reactive, to address this ever-present threat. Successful prevention, response, mitigation, and recovery from terrorist events require a high-level of coordination between all disciplines of public safety, including law enforcement, emergency medical services (EMS), firefighters, and other rescue personnel. Everyone from the first care provider (FCP) through definitive care providers must have a common operating picture that allows for all links in the "violent event chain of survival" to be enacted.[5] Now more than ever, interagency response to acts of domestic terrorism is essential.

This textbook deals extensively with biological, chemical, and radiological response, as well as the federal regulations governing disaster and terrorism response in the United States. This chapter concentrates on U.S. domestic response to terrorist incidents, with a primary focus on the operational aspects of local interagency response to complex terrorist incidents. That said, the chapter draws lessons from international experience with terrorist-incident response and has universally applicable lessons.

HISTORICAL PERSPECTIVE

Federal

Since the 1980s, the terms *consequence* and *crisis management* have been used in differentiating between the roles of rescuers and investigators. The Federal Emergency Management Agency (FEMA) defines *consequence management* as taking action to protect public health and safety, restoring essential government services, and providing relief to governments, businesses, and persons affected by the consequences of terrorism. *Crisis management,* in contrast, is taking measures to identify, acquire, and plan the use of resources to anticipate, prevent, and resolve a threat or act of terrorism.[6]

Consequence management is maintained at the lowest level of government possible. If the consequences of a terrorist incident can be met with resources from the local level, there should be minimal involvement of state or federal resources. If the local government is not able to manage the consequences of the incident adequately, it will turn to the state government for assistance. If the state cannot meet the needs of the incident, it will turn to the federal government. At the federal level, consequence management has been the responsibility of the agency providing civil defense. Since the 1970s, this has been FEMA.[7]

In contrast, crisis management, since its conception, has been considered a function of the federal government. The concept of terrorism as a criminal act evolved from the realm of sabotage and espionage, where an individual, working as an agent of an enemy state, performs an action that is injurious to the government or its people. Acts of terrorism, by extension, are acts committed by transnational or nonstate organizations. Therefore the prosecution of alleged terrorists is conducted in the federal courts under U.S. code. The Department of Justice was appointed the lead federal agency for crisis management in the 1980s, and the FBI assumed lead responsibility for crisis management.[8]

Having the two different response operations to the same incident led to conflicting objectives and incomplete situational awareness for all leaders. Conflict and vertical "stove-piping" of information followed. In an effort to address this challenge, the Stafford Act was passed in 1974, and amended in 1988, to delineate the federal response to a disaster. The Act was not made with a specific reference to terrorism. However, it states that nothing within the Act was to construe an investigatory role for any federal agency other than the FBI.[9] In 1986, in response to the vice president's Task Force on Terrorism, President Reagan issued the first guidance on responding to terrorism, naming the FBI as the lead agency for dealing with acts of terrorism.

The first paradigm-shifting act of terrorism on U.S. territory occurred in 1993. The World Trade Center was the site of an improvised explosive device (IED) detonation that resulted in six deaths and more than 1000 injuries. An area 150-feet wide and five stories deep was destroyed. The incident was initially felt to be a transformer explosion with a resultant fire. Accordingly, the Fire Department of the City of New York (FDNY) performed command and control (C2) of ground operations, drawing on mutual aid for the EMS response. Only later, did the response evolve into a crime scene. The area was then processed initially by four FBI evidence technicians and four Bureau of Alcohol, Tobacco, and Firearms evidence technicians working with a local New York Police Department chemist. After-action reports indicated a minimum number of conflicts between federal and local law enforcement officials. These reports attribute this to an already established joint terrorism task force (JTTF), which had been in existence in New York City since the 1980s.[10-12] Subsequently, JTTFs have been established in 103 metropolitan areas, including all 56 major metropolitan areas that have FBI field offices.[13] Each is made up of FBI special agents, special deputy U.S. marshals, and local law enforcement officers (LEOs). They share in the responsibility of gathering intelligence, investigating, and prosecuting terrorist-related crimes. Funding of the JTTF is largely through the FBI, although the local governments continue to pay the salaries of its officers.[14]

In response to the Oklahoma City Bombing in 1995, President Clinton signed Presidential Decision Directive 39 (PDD-39). However, the response required was greater than the resources available to the local or state governments. Further, the incident was recognized nearly immediately as a criminal action. Although there was immediate involvement of federal agencies, there was little coordination between the consequences and crisis functions. PDD-39 established guidelines for federal C2 in the event of a terrorist incident. Specifically, it designated the Department of Justice as the lead federal agency for operational response and crisis management. The attorney general delegated this role to the FBI. It designated FEMA as the lead federal agency for consequence management. Further, it specified that crisis management would take precedence over consequence management—the FBI would remain in charge of the scene until the attorney general had turned the scene over to FEMA.[15]

Presidential Decision Directive 62 (PDD-62) directed the federal agencies in their preresponse planning to counterterrorism and consequence management. It established a national-level coordinator for security, critical infrastructure protection, and counterterrorism. It provided guidance on the role of the Department of Justice,

Department of Health and Human Services, and Department of Defense in preparing the Metropolitan Medical Strike Teams (now Metropolitan Medical Response System) in the first 120 cities that established them.[16]

The Concept of Operations Plan (CONPLAN) for terrorism, signed in 2000, reaffirmed the role of the Department of Justice as the lead federal agency, a responsibility that is delegated to the FBI, in the response to terrorism. As such, the FBI remained the on-scene commander until the attorney general relinquished control to FEMA. However, there was much to do in terms of transitioning from a focus on crisis management to creating an environment centered on a unified command involving all agencies involved. The FBI would establish a Joint Operations Command (JOC) that would serve as a focus for crisis management in the unified response. It was intended to complement and work with the local agencies' Incident Command System. Further, the National Incident Management System (NIMS) was established to define a common operating language and framework to assure interoperability of local, state, and federal assets.

In 2013 the United States updated the National Response Framework (NRF) to endorse an all-hazards approach to disaster response, which included terrorist incidents. Emergency Support Function #8 (ESF-8) provides a mechanism for the federal government to supplement state, tribal, and local resources in response to public health and medical disasters or potential incidents requiring a coordinated federal response. ESF-8 supports such core functions as rapid needs assessments, health surveillance, medical care personnel, patient evacuation, patient care, blood and blood products, food safety and security, and health, medical, and veterinary supplies. The secretary of Health and Human Services (HHS) leads all federal public health and medical response to public health emergencies and incidents covered in the NRF.

However, the old adage that "all disasters are local" is particularly applicable in the immediate response to a terrorist incident. The move from spectacular attacks to disseminated, "entrepreneurial" attacks (i.e., unaffiliated attackers), "lone-wolf" terrorists, and ASIs and AVIs creates highly dynamic and fluid situations that often do not allow for easy transition between crisis and consequence management. Moreover, areas without JTTF are increasingly at risk. For example, the mass shootings at Virginia Tech (2009) that killed 32 and wounded 17; the Aurora, Colorado, Century 16 shooting (2012) that killed 12 and wounded 70; and the tragic massacre in Newtown, Connecticut (2012), of 26 individuals victims, 20 were children, were all initially managed locally. The migration of terrorist incidents to lower-visibility areas demands immediate, effective, and well-practiced local interagency response to high-threat incidents. Accordingly, it is worth reviewing the evolution of the U.S. Fire Service, EMS, and law enforcement response to acts of terrorism and mass violence.

FIRE SERVICE

Development and History of Response

Organized over a century and a half ago, the U.S. Fire Service initially had the sole task of protecting against property loss from fire. However, in the 1960s and 1970s, as the number of structure fires dwindled—owing to stricter building codes, sprinkler systems, smoke detectors, fire resistant materials, and a push toward more fire prevention and code enforcement—the Fire Service began to evolve to address the operational gaps that were being defined in public safety and response. The concept of an "all-hazards" approach for the U.S. Fire Service was born.

Although commonly labeled as "200 years of tradition unimpeded by progress," the U.S. Fire Service has actually evolved dramatically in the past 40 years. As new risks to public safety were being defined, brave members of the Fire Service often stepped forward to accept the risk associated with mitigation and response. For example, in the 1970s the Fire Service assumed primary lead for management of hazardous material (HazMat) response and developed highly specialized teams of responders trained in recognition of chemical release, decontamination procedures, incident command, and high-threat operations. During the 1980s, the Fire Service identified the need for specially trained personnel to conduct increasingly frequent high-threat rescue operations in urban environments. This gap analysis led to the development of technical rescue, a specialty that includes vehicle extrication, high- and low-angle rope rescue, confined-space rescue, and urban search and rescue (USAR). In the 1990s, the Fire Service took the lead in the development, training, and coordination for integration of prehospital medical personnel into law enforcement specialty tactical teams. As these new response specialties have matured in the Fire Service, regulatory and industry groups have developed guidelines and safety standards to be implemented in an attempt to reduce adverse outcomes and mitigate risk to responders during operations.

Paradigm Change

Given the history of changing the U.S. Fire Service mission to address operational gaps, it is not surprising that the Fire Service sits on the forefront of the need for joint operations with other public safety agencies to mitigate and respond to coordinated terrorism events. Yet, despite the clear operational gaps and the embraced all-hazards response paradigm, resistance remains among the Fire Service to adopting new roles in high-threat operations. This resistance must be addressed and broken down.

The July 7, 2005, coordinated bombings on the London public transportation system provide insight into the consequences of actual, or perceived, coordination gaps in public safety response to a complex attack. The response to the well-planned and well-coordinated bombings involved multiple agencies, including the London Fire Brigade, London Metro Police, City of London Police, London Transit Police, and London Ambulance Service. The official Coroner's Inquest into the bombings revealed the same operational issues seen in almost every major incident: difficult communications, lack of real-time intelligence, equipment issues, and clear operational role tasking.[17] The inquest, as a whole, states that all operational partners performed to the expected standard of their individual disciplines and specialties.

However, the public opinion after the incident was not as supportive. During the initial response to the bombings, citing operational limitations to ensure scene safety, the London Fire Brigade staged outside the train stations while other public safety agencies moved aggressively into the higher threat zone. Newspaper headlines and stories described multiple victims alive after the blast for significant periods, dying in blast wreckage and being tended to only by civilian bystanders or police, while the Fire Brigade staged. The public spokesperson for the victims' families delivered strong critical statements about the Fire Brigade response to the event: "The fact of the matter is that on July 7, 2005, they were operating in the same environment as the other emergency responders and yet did not take or were not willing to take the same calculated risks that were being taken by, for example, British Transport Police at King's Cross.... In our summation the sense has emerged from the inquest that the pendulum may have swung too far in favor of an overly cautious approach."[18] The London Fire Brigade, despite no official criticism, lost the battle in the court of public opinion and lost public confidence.

Public safety entities are a part of the most successful social contract between the government and the people. As such, public safety agencies have been given special status among the citizens; culturally, police,

firefighters, and EMS personnel are heroes who are willing to risk their lives to come to the rescue of the people in their most dire times of need. Public safety agencies are expected to accept mitigated risk in their jobs. Therefore to let citizens die while standing by in the name of safety flies in the face of the social contract upon which these agencies are funded and supported.

In the wake of the event, the London Fire Brigade made rapid and profound operational changes. In preparing for the 2012 London Summer Olympics, their command-level personnel researched international best practices and worked with their public safety partners to develop and implement a new approach to high-threat scenarios (London Fire Brigade, personal communication, 2008). Even though the London Fire Brigade should be applauded for their current approach to high-threat scenario operations, including aggressive police-fire integration for medical rescue and fire suppression, the lasting effects of the loss of public confidence continues to affect the agency even 7 years after the 2005 attacks.

The historical precedent in the U.S. Fire Service is one of ready adoption of new roles once gaps in the public safety response matrix have been identified. The Fire Service of the twenty-first century is one for all hazards, one that researches, studies, and identifies the risks to the public it serves and then builds a response capability to address that risk. This process has started again regarding the gap in response to complex terror attacks on the public. New roles can be accepted and will be integrated into the public safety culture.

EMERGENCY MEDICAL SERVICES

Development and History of Response

The modern EMS system was established in the late 1960s and 1970s, primarily because of a significant number of deaths resulting from motor vehicle collisions on the nation's expanding highway system.[19] The original focus of EMS was to recognize and provide basic care for certain injuries in the field and transport the injured to appropriate care. The role of EMS has evolved over the past 40 years, and it now expands beyond trauma care to include medical emergencies, prevention, education, and specialty services, such as critical care transport, air-medical services, and interfacility medical transports. In addition, EMS organizations are increasingly called upon to provide medical specialists to support technical, tactical, and other rescue activities. Expansion of the levels of certification to include advanced life support (ALS) providers was a pivotal factor in the growth of EMS. In various communities EMS may be provided by the Fire Service, as a stand-alone third service (private or public agency), or, in limited cases, by other public safety entities such as police departments.

In the 1990s, interagency leaders noted the need for specially trained medical personnel to support increasingly high-risk law enforcement special operations and tactical-team missions. These tactical emergency medical support (TEMS) medics, typically cross-trained firefighters or EMS personnel, but in many cases sworn LEOs, provide active medical capability during operations at or near the point of wounding. In many jurisdictions, the TEMS medics have also adopted the role of team occupational health provider, operational medical consultant, and preventative health expert.[20] The role of these specialty providers continues to evolve and expand as their utility is validated across different mission profiles.[21,22]

Paradigm Change

Similar to the Fire Service, EMS must change their paradigm of response and operational risk mitigation. The initiation of TEMS and the expansion of tactical medical support through the 1980s reflected an innovative mind-set to address a changing threat matrix. However, in the past 20 years, TEMS has evolved as a subspecialty of EMS, as opposed to a driving force of change within the specialty. TEMS practitioners have focused on developing support protocols for high-risk SWAT missions and the myriad challenges that accompany planned support in high-threat areas. The EMS community as a whole has remained very risk conscious.

Although scrutiny is generated due to large-scale events such as the 2012 Aurora, Colorado, Century 16 shooting, there has yet to be a sentinel event involving EMS response to drive the needed response paradigm change. Given the evolving terrorist and AVI threat, the national EMS community must embrace expanded, coordinated operations with other first-response disciplines. TEMS specialists have a potentially important leadership role in this transformation, as the designated interagency representatives.

LAW ENFORCEMENT

Development and History

LEOs at all government levels have traditionally held primary responsibility for responding to terrorist attacks and AVIs. LEOs are commonly the initial first responders on scene in any major event, and they are trained early on in risk-mitigation and threat-elimination strategies. Historically, however, most agencies have mitigated risk to the general LEO population by limiting exposure to high-risk scenarios through the utilization of highly trained, specialized tactical teams such as SWAT teams or Violent Criminal Apprehension Teams (VCATs).

The 1966 University of Texas Tower shooting served as the impetus for the creation SWAT teams to address particularly high-risk and dynamic situations. The role of SWAT has expanded and evolved in the past five decades, and they remain an important law enforcement tool. SWAT teams play an important role in planned high-threat operations (e.g., warrant service), static high-threat scenarios (e.g., barricade suspect or bank robbery), and dynamic incidents (e.g., ASI). However, a majority of U.S. SWAT teams are designated "part time," with several members "on call" while filling other roles (e.g., patrol or training). Therefore SWAT takes time to activate and respond. Although SWAT team members have been involved in the response to most domestic terrorism or AVIs since their inception, they have rarely been the first on scene. Even in the 2009 Virginia Tech Massacre, where two local SWAT teams were standing by on campus, the first response was by patrol officers.[23]

Paradigm Change

Columbine was the sentinel event in LEO response to active threats. ASI and active killing events were a well-known public safety risk prior to the 1999 massacre at Columbine High School. However, these incidents were widely considered the responsibility of the highly trained Special Weapons and Tactics teams.

Prior to the Columbine event, the law enforcement response paradigm to ASI and active killing events was based on the concept that the intent of the shooter was not primarily murder and that the operational risk to responders and tactics required to successfully resolve the incident mandated the highly trained tactical teams as the primary responders. As a result, the law-enforcement patrol-officer community response to ASIs was based on the concept of the "five Cs": contain the perpetrator, control the scene, call SWAT, communicate with the perpetrator, and come up with a response plan.

The assault on Columbine High School, which resulted in 12 dead and 24 wounded, forced a change in the LEO ASI response paradigm. The well-planned attack on the school included combined small arms and incendiary devices designed to create a structural collapse and fire that would drive evacuating students into a predesignated "kill zone." The perpetrators planned to shoot these fleeing students as they exited

the building. However, the devices did not explode as intended, so they changed their plan and went in on a shooting spree.[24]

Police responded to Columbine very quickly. In fact, the shooters exchanged fire with LEOs 2 times during their attack: once with the school resource officer and again through the windows of the library, at the police units operating to rescue injured students in the parking lots outside. Tactically, according to the law enforcement paradigm of the day, the law enforcement response went well. As patrol officers responded, an immediate hard perimeter was established. SWAT was requested and was on scene within about 30 to 40 minutes. Plans were rapidly developed to put the SWAT teams into the building. Within an hour of the first shot being fired, SWAT entered the building. However, during the hour prior to LEO entry, as perimeters were established and tactical plans were developed, the shooters had free range of the building. They hunted students, shooting at will with little if any resistance. The two finally committed suicide approximately 46 minutes into the incident, and yet, no significant police entry into the building was initiated for another 15+ minutes.[25]

Even after entry, the response into the school remained slow and methodical. The tactical teams moved slowly through the large and complex school footprint, completing a methodical clearing of the structure. It took almost 4 hours for the building to be declared "safe," thus allowing medical rescue operations inside the building. It is well known that at least one victim died in the interim prior to the police and medical response. Coach David Sanders, during his actions to direct students to safety, was shot in the upper chest and shoulder, suffering damage to several major blood vessels. He was pulled into a room by fellow teachers and students, the door was barricaded, and they waited for rescue. Two hours later, as Coach Sanders's condition became critical, the teachers and students in the barricaded room with him realized that his injuries were grave. In an attempt to communicate the gravity of the situation in the room, they wrote, "1 bleeding to death" on a wipe board, and posted it in the window where it was directly visible to the responding LEOs. Yet, no one came. Coach Sanders died in the classroom after several hours, ironically just minutes before the medical-response assets finally reached him.[26]

The massacre and the perceived lack of action on the part of LEOs horrified the public. Criticism from the Governor's Columbine Commission addressed this directly, "The 46 minute rampage . . . during that period, to the Commission's knowledge, no efforts were made to engage, contain, or capture the perpetrators." Moreover, the conclusions were strongly worded: "Law enforcement policy and training should emphasize that the highest priority of law enforcement officers, after arriving at the scene of a crisis, is to stop any ongoing assault. All law enforcement officers who may be first responders at a crisis, and all school resource officers should be trained in concept and skills of rapid emergency deployment. . . ."[27] Rapidly, the police paradigm of response to ASI and active killing incidents changed.

The new paradigm for law enforcement response became one of rapid deployment into the building or location to aggressively pursue the assailant, and stop the ongoing violence. This new response model was no longer relegated to the highly trained and tactically proficient SWAT teams but the first-arriving officers on scene, most often patrol officers with limited training, limited firepower, and often without high-level ballistic protection. The speed by which this new response paradigm was adopted and implemented by law enforcement agencies was impressive. However, even more impressive was the rapid and absolute acceptance of the burden of immediate response along with the subsequent increased risk by the patrol officer community. This response paradigm represented a completely new role for the patrol officer, and few hesitated at the implications of the job. As a result, the past 14 years have seen a significant shift in the training and culture of the patrol officer as it relates to ASI and active killing event response. Commonplace now across the vast majority of, if not all, law enforcement agencies is training for patrol officers in immediate deployment tactics, single and multiple officer teams, and long weapon training, as well as outfitting with advanced ballistic gear and more firepower.

Study of historical incidents and lessons learned can create a pathway forward to meet the new threat head on. SWAT experts continue to have an important role in the overall response but rarely in the early actions. Instead, the nonspecialized first responder's immediate actions on scene will determine the success of the response. In the United States a majority of AVIs end with LEO and first-responder engagement of the perpetrator.[28] The historical perspective shows that if the attack is not allowed to gain a foothold and develop as planned, there will be less carnage. Addressing this challenge requires a shift in mindset and a change in risk tolerance. It is imperative that first-response agencies shift focus and training to meet this mandate.

CURRENT AND FUTURE BEST PRACTICE: INTEGRATED OPERATIONS

The high-threat scenario is characterized by a multilateral spectrum of potential threats to first responders. These include one or more well-trained and operationally knowledgeable perpetrators often willing to die; well-planned operations using military style tactics with effective communications and external coordination; multicapacity high-velocity weapons; potential for the use of toxic materials and fire to complicate response and increase damage; atypical threats, such as homemade IEDs; and austere conditions created by operational personnel limitations and building and location geography. To address the evolving risk of coordinated terrorism in America, new response paradigms must be accepted among all three public safety disciplines. The traditional single-agency "stove piped" response is ineffective and even dangerous in these unpredictable, chaotic, and fluid events. Success is predicated on a combined Fire-EMS-LEO response, and operational integration among the disciplines must be seamless to prevent the exploitation of the boundaries in the operational picture. The overarching interagency operational priorities must be clear: stop the killing and stop the dying. Supporting priorities such as limitation of physical damage, evidence preservation, and return to routine operations remain important secondary missions. Thus firefighters may be required to fight fire despite an ongoing tactical situation. EMS providers may need to render care in areas that are immediately clear but not entirely secure (e.g., Indirect Threat Zones or "Warm Zones"), and police officers may need to operate in areas of active fire and smoke and assist in rendering medical aid to the wounded.

CHALLENGES TO IMPLEMENTING THE NEW RESPONSE PARADIGM

The challenges to implementing new programs are operational, historical, and political. The major challenge facing first responders is the ability to shift from routine to high-threat operations. These events usually are not clearly defined as such at the onset. The initial dispatch for emergency services may be for what appears to be a routine event such as a "disturbance" at a school, smoke in a subway station, or "trouble unknown" at a mall or hotel. It is imperative for the initial first responders to recognize the event as atypical quickly. In essence, first responders need to have a mental switch in place; for the vast majority of operations, this switch is set to "normal" as routine emergency service is delivered every day. However, when the high-threat incident occurs, these responders must be able to recognize the signs and quickly switch their minds over to a "high-threat operation mode," where all of the operational relationships, rules, and roles are changed.

The second challenge is that the historical model of "stage and wait" for complete scene safety is no longer valid. It is professionally, ethically, and politically unacceptable to allow wounded and dying citizens to lie without care, while those who are tasked with their safety remain in areas of little or no risk. AVIs create a new threat environment for operations that demand rapid deployment into high-threat areas and aggressive risk-mitigation, not risk-avoidance, strategies. Fire and EMS responders must move forward quickly in these scenarios to initiate care and effect rapid rescue of the wounded. This changing requirement does not negate the importance of scene safety, and it mandates aggressive, interagency risk-mitigation procedures. "Scene safety" remains an important concept. However, in the evolving high-threat scenario, leaders and responders must redefine "acceptable" risk and apply safety principles in an incremental fashion based upon the tactical ground reality. This is similar to actions taken on every true fire suppression call, every technical rescue, and every hazardous materials operation where there is a need for immediate life rescue. Fire and EMS operations are rooted in a "culture of safety" that has served to save countless lives over the past several decades. Fire and EMS medical-response and rescue operations in high-threat scenarios are no different, and operations can be developed and delivered within the culture of safety.

Finally, the historical precedence that complex attacks are solely the purview of law enforcement must change. Law enforcement may be the lead agency, but command and operations must be unified across the spectrum of public safety agencies. This level of commitment to unified and integrated operations begins in the offices of the police chief, the fire chief, and the EMS chief. Historically, police and firefighters have viewed their roles as independent. In many jurisdictions interagency rivalry and turf battles—some collegial and healthy, but many malignant and unhealthy—have developed over time, as the different public safety entities have competed for budget, community recognition, and a long legacy of pride. Complex attacks do not allow for rivalries or turf battles. Egos must be put aside among the leadership, and the call for and commitment to integration must be from the top down.

THE MODEL HIGH-THREAT OPERATIONAL PROGRAM

A variety of model high-threat response systems exist. The initial development for an effective well-integrated multidisciplinary high-threat operations program begins at the command level. Agency leaders must conduct a realistic gap analysis and hazard vulnerability assessment (HVA) for the community. This then becomes the road map to set priorities for each individual discipline and their role in high-threat response.

The gap analysis and HVA should articulate a realistic overarching jurisdictional response plan that maximizes individual and combined agency strengths while minimizing the limitations of the organic operational assets. Several work streams must be considered in the development of a high-threat emergency-response plan. These include, but are not limited to, the identification and definition of *complex attacks*, the creation of documents and agency-specific annexes outlining the model response plan, drilling unified and integrated command and control, verifying internal and external communications interoperability, and intelligence gathering, analysis, and sharing, among partners.

The emergency-response plan will lay the foundation for interagency operational coordination. It is critical that this response plan reflects an overarching jurisdictional plan developed jointly by all operational partners with distinct discipline-specific annexes to address the granular operational details of the discipline response. This concept differs from most common current practice of each agency having an individual discipline-specific response plan. The message is then sent to the operational personnel that it is not a "police plan" or "fire plan" but rather a complete coordinated public safety plan. The interagency emergency-response plan improves communication and familiarity while clearly delineating expectations.

In addition to the emergency-response plan, the model public safety high-threat integrated operations program includes six distinct areas of concentration:

1. Intelligence and training
2. Public engagement
3. Fire/EMS Tactical Emergency Casualty Care and Indirect Threat/Warm Zone integrated medical rescue operations
4. Indirect threat or warm zone medical rescue operations
5. Fire as a weapon response
6. Response to mass casualty incidents involving explosives (discussed further in Chapter 71)

Intelligence and Training

Complex attacks are rarely spontaneous. The past defines the future, and perpetrators of complex attacks are professionals; they study historical events, exam response gaps, and "war-game" various attack options. Preparation for violent incident demands close examination of past incidents, critical evaluation of failures (on both the response and perpetrator's side), and a dark creativity to explore the "what ifs." Knowledge is power for operational-response teams. For a high-threat response program to be successful, all members, especially leadership, must understand the true scope of the threat.

Resources such as the First Responder Knowledgebase, created by Mr. Louis Mizell of Mizell & Company International Security, are essential in providing tangible data for analysis by first responders. This knowledgebase consists of more than 48,000 real-life incidents, divided into retrievable topics for easy reference.[29] These incident databases provide institutional memory for crime, terrorism, safety, and security, to preserve the lessons learned and experiences of first responders worldwide. Similar first-responder resources, such as Fire Line, published by FDNY, provide historical and real-time incident analysis that is key in operational planning and training. Considerations, patterns, and details from past incidents, regardless of how long ago they occurred, are not history but rather a blueprint for solid planning.

At least as important as a solid understanding of the past incidents is the need to identify, track, and analyze accidental and unintentional analogous incidents. *Analogous events* are defined as accidental or unintentional events that have profound implications for emergency preparedness. Real-time high-threat incident analysis allows for rapid development of simple and inexpensive training exercises that are easily implemented throughout an agency. For example, the gas line explosion in New York City that destroyed two large residential buildings and killed multiple people in the spring of 2014 was an event that had no nexus of terrorism or intent. However, it had significant effects on the community, as well as requiring multiagency response, posing some degree of dynamic threat, and receiving widespread publicity. Even though the incident was not an act of terrorism, it may have planted the seed or given similar ideas to those intending to do harm to others. As soon as possible after a significant event, the high-threat program's intelligence and training personnel should provide a brief operational synopsis of the event and develop simple discussion points for operational personnel. The general operational details of that incident can then be overlaid onto a similar regional location, and the response can played out through tabletop or guided discussion. These just-in-time exercises can be held at all levels of the operational

response and can be as simple as a 15-minute discussion at role call or around the dinner table at the firehouse. Familiarity with tactics and discussion around response builds a mental thought framework for operational personnel.

Public Engagement

There has been little training or focus on providing basic knowledge of AVI and high-threat events to the civilian populations most at risk: religious facility administration and staff, federal and local government facility staff, large retail facility personnel, and educational facility administrators, faculty, and staff. In any terror or high-threat event, knowledge is power. By training administration and staff in high-risk targets to be familiar with what to expect during these events, as well as giving them a basic framework for personal response, the community itself will be better prepared. The "Run-Hide-Fight" video, produced under a federal grant in 2013, is a strong example of public engagement.[30]

Citizens should be viewed as potential assets rather than liabilities during the response. The goal of public engagement is to turn those uninjured persons affected in these events from bystanders into true FCPs. First responders should not view these citizens as a hindrance to response that needs to be quickly removed from the scene to allow the "professionals" to take over. Instead, these people need to be viewed as force multipliers for the response and should be appropriately incorporated into response by the public agency first responders. Execution first requires a clear, rapid security and screening standard operating procedure (SOP) to mitigate risk of secondary attack, coupled with a well-trained and empowered public. The model for public engagement is the community and citizen preparedness program in Israel. Israelis are given basic public education in organizing response in the first few minutes of an event and providing basic rescue and stabilizing medical techniques for the wounded (Dr. Isaac Ashkenazi, personal communication, 2013).

Patrol Officer Tactical Emergency Casualty Care Training

LEOs operate, often alone, in unsecured and hazardous conditions, interacting with persons who are unstable, unpredictable, and oftentimes potentially deadly. Officers are routinely involved in high-risk operations such as high-speed emergency-response, vehicle pursuits, and traffic stops for violations, where, in addition to being vulnerable from directed violence from the occupants, personnel are minimally protected from continued ongoing vehicular traffic. Traditional prehospital Fire and EMS response may encounter a delay in reaching a downed-officer or injured citizen because of scene safety concerns. This delay in care can cost lives. LEO training must expand to focus on care that must be performed in the first few minutes prior to the arrival of traditional prehospital medical response or additional officers to provide assistance.[31]

Recently, several high-profile mass casualty incidents have demonstrated the benefit of having LEOs trained in and carrying basic medical equipment. First-arriving officers in sufficient numbers, after addressing the immediate tactical threat, may be able to initiate basic lifesaving care for the wounded, in the short time before traditional medical first responders are operational on scene. Prime examples of this theory are the success of the Pima County Sheriff's personnel in providing medical care to the injured during the 2011 Tucson, Arizona, shooting. Further examples are the actions of the Aurora Police Department in the 2012 Century 16 Theater, where over half of the injured were almost immediately transported to trauma centers in the back of patrol cars, and the Boston Police officers who ran immediately into the fray during the 2013 Boston Marathon Bombings. These key examples demonstrate the need for a simple framework and training for LEOs in basic medical stabilization for mass casualty incidents involving ballistics and explosives.

The TECC guidelines represent a set of evidenced-based best practices for the immediate medical management of wounded at or near the point of wounding, for use by all first responders in all prehospital high-risk scenarios.[32] TECC is scalable and can be applied for differing scope of practice and levels of first responders, from the nonmedical layperson to the highly trained physician, nurse, or paramedic. LEOs should be trained in the appropriate concepts of TECC to enable them to assess, identify, and stabilize the immediately preventable life threats in mass casualty incidents, while accounting for the ongoing and dynamic tactical situation in the "first 5 to 10 minutes" prior to the arrival of higher-level medical providers. In addition to the TECC medical training, each LEO should be provided with a standardized individual first aid kit (IFAK). IFAK composition varies, but all LEOs should be equipped with a tourniquet.

Fire-EMS Tactical Emergency Casualty Care and Indirect Threat/Warm Zone Integrated Medical Rescue Operations

All Fire-EMS medical and nonmedical personnel should be trained in tactical emergency casualty care at the appropriate scope of practice and according to local protocols, and should be equipped with the proper TECC medical equipment. TECC is the basis for building a high-threat integrated medical response capability. Public safety officials continue to develop novel ways of responding to, mitigating, and recovering from AVIs. Several models are being fielded in an attempt to provide point-of-wounding care in an expedient manner. These models are designed to deliver lifesaving interventions from easily treated wounds and reduce potentially preventable mortality. "Warm Zone" operations are conducted in areas of indirect threat (i.e., a potential threat to the rescuer exists but is not clearly greater than the life threat from the injuries already sustained). In dynamic high-threat events, zones of care may change suddenly, and rescuers must be able to recognize and react accordingly. Primary response in the indirect threat and warm zone is based on the tenets of TECC. It includes threat mitigation, rapid extremity-hemorrhage control, extraction, and expedited evaluation by higher-level care personnel. There are three primary models for warm zone operations: Escorted Warm Zone care (Rescue Task Force), creation of "warm corridors," and a hybrid model.

Escorted Warm Zone Care

The Rescue Task Force (RTF) model was originally designed in 2007, by the Arlington County Fire Department in Virginia.[33] RTF couples nontactical fire department/EMS providers with patrol officers to enter an indirect threat and warm zone to effect TECC interventions and life rescue. RTF is essentially a Fire/EMS parallel to the existing law-enforcement-response paradigm to AVIs that sends the first-arriving line patrol officers, not specialized tactical assets, into the unsecure environment, to stop the violence by the appropriate use of force. RTF personnel are made up of the first-arriving-line Fire and EMS personnel on scene, not the highly specialized tactical medics deploying with SWAT or other LEO tactical teams.

In the RTF model, the LEO contact teams make immediate entry into the area and attempt to locate, isolate, and stop the violence. Once several of these contact teams have passed through an area without encountering active threats, they declare the area a warm zone and notify incident command of the presence of any casualties. Unified command then decides on the feasibility of deploying an RTF comprised of LEOs and Fire and/or EMS to affect point-of-wounding care and life rescue rapidly.

The combined LEO-Fire-EMS RTF-team personnel have specific functions. LEOs are tasked with movement of the team, monitoring for any immediate threat, and providing force protection to the rescuers; as such, LEOs are specifically instructed not to assist with patient care or movement because it would take their attention away from their primary function. Fire and EMS providers escorted by these LEOs are tasked with the rapid evaluation, TECC stabilization, and coordinated extraction of the wounded. As such, these personnel only carry enough equipment to address the immediately preventable causes of death, such as major hemorrhage, airway and breathing issues, and hypothermia. Depending on the size and geography of the event, an additional command-level Fire or EMS officer may accompany the RTF team to coordinate resources, monitor communications, and provide additional internal command and control.

The initial goal of the first two to three RTF teams is to penetrate as far as possible into the identified warm zone to evaluate and stabilize the nonambulatory wounded. There is essentially little if any triage: patients are treated as they are accessed and, until they are evacuated to areas that are more secure, are considered only to be ambulatory, nonambulatory, or deceased. For these first RTF "treatment teams," no patients are evacuated. Instead, any wounded patient is assessed and stabilized using TECC interventions, positioned appropriately, and left where they lie. Only after all accessible patients have been stabilized will these initial teams begin to evacuate those treated. Depending on the scale of the event, additional RTF teams can be designated "extraction teams" and can be sent in behind the first two to three treatment teams to begin rapid extrication of those treated.

Although several operational variations exist to this model, conceptually, the principles remain consistent throughout all of the jurisdictions and agencies employing the concept. The term *RTF* was chosen to represent this model, the designator of which is NIMS compliant; the model includes multidiscipline entities working together to accomplish a common goal. Certain jurisdictions have used other names for similar types of programs, such as the Philadelphia Fire Department Rapid Assessment Medical Support (RAMS) program.

Indirect Threat and Warm "Island" Care

In this model, Fire and EMS personnel are escorted into tactically secured and hardened areas of the building, such as a cafeteria or library. Once in place, teams of LEOs then function as "rescue teams" to access and extricate the wounded to these secure "islands" in the otherwise unsecure building. This model requires less overall training and interoperability between LEOs, firefighters, and EMS personnel and fewer security personnel for medical operations; however, there can be role confusion for the LEOs. Given the tactical situation, LEOs with the dual role of contact and extrication will have to make a real-time decision on which role to assume when encountering an injured patient in need of extrication in otherwise unsecured, unsearched areas. Additionally, if no actual point-of-wounding care is provided by the LEO rescue teams, there could be significant worsening and delay in care for the wounded during the time required for them to be extricated to care. As such, applications of this model where LEOs do not provide TECC point-of-wounding care prior to moving the patient should be avoided; life-threatening injuries require time-sensitive interventions to prevent death from wounds.

The "Warm Corridor"

The "warm corridor" utilizes LEO contact teams to locate and isolate the potential threat and rapidly do the primary clearing of a wide area. Next, they deploy additional officers for over-watch, who hold tactical domination of a geographic corridor into and out of an otherwise unsecured area. Once this secure corridor is established, firefighters and EMS personnel can then move freely into and out of the area, providing care and extricating the wounded to traditional triage and treatment areas in the outer cold zones. Again, this model requires less direct interoperability between first-responder disciplines, but it takes time and heavy personnel resources to get the corridor in place. Once functioning, tactical dominance of the corridor can be maintained with only a few required security personnel; thus this model allows for redesignation of LEOs in the later stages of the event.

The concepts and execution of Escorted Warm Zone Care continues to evolve. Since 2012, many federal agencies and national organizations, including the Department of Homeland Security, International Association of Firefighters, International Association of Fire Chiefs, and the Urban Fire Forum, have endorsed the operational concepts of point-of-wounding care through Escorted Warm Zone Care response models.

Operational concerns such as personal protective and ballistic equipment, interagency and interdisciplinary communication, and team composition must be considered by each jurisdiction. There is no single solution or answer to these operational concerns, aside from following established best practices, which provides a framework for program development. Ultimately, each jurisdiction must design a response program that considers local resources, operational risk acceptance, and local politics. More importantly, once decided upon, agencies must rehearse all aspects of their operational plans frequently, to assure good outcomes during an event.

Fire as a Weapon

Given the repeated history of the use of fire as a weapon, as well as the magnitude of its effect, the operational paradigm involving fire suppression in high-risk operations must also change. Firefighters must rapidly integrate with law enforcement assets to assess and initiate fire suppression and mitigation activities as needed. This will necessarily include an effective scene size-up, as well as rapid development of a ventilation and fire attack plan in coordination with the law enforcement tactical plan. Depending on conditions and fire load, these fire suppression teams must be capable of performing suppression activities despite an ongoing tactical threat. As with the medical-response paradigm, these personnel should have security provided by LEOs. They require training in basic tactical awareness and movement, appropriate lightweight and innovative suppression equipment, and appropriate personal protective equipment (PPE) to account for both the thermal and ballistic threats.

The required operational paradigm shift for coordination and acceptance of new operational roles is not limited to Fire and EMS. In addition to the current rapid-deployment model, LEO responders must have familiarity with EMS, rescue, and fire suppression operations to be able to assist with escorted medical rescue operations and suppression activities, and they must be able to work in areas of smoke and thermal threats. The role of LEOs in these complex scenarios must be the most flexible, and thus their training must have more breadth. LEO responders should be trained in basic fire awareness and suppression activities, how to move and provide security for firefighters and EMS personnel, and basic medical rescue operations, including being proficient in appropriate scope TECC principles. As with the other disciplines, this will require appropriate equipment and PPE for these responders.

Response to Mass Casualty Events Involving Explosives

The April 15, 2013, Boston Marathon Bombing demonstrates the need for emphasis on preparation and response for operational teams to rapidly deploy into and mitigate the effects of a mass casualty incident involving explosives. To many, this event represented what the emergency preparedness and operational-response community had been bracing for since the attacks on September 11, 2001. The use of explosives against soft targets and mass gatherings has been witnessed for many years. Coordinated attacks against mass transit have been an effective modus operandi of terrorists over the past 10 years, with chilling aftereffects and large fatality counts. The basics of interagency training for response to mass casualty incidents involving explosives (further discussed in Chapter 71) should include the following:

- Basic principles of explosives and blast physics
- Common operational tactics for use of explosives
- Operational use of apparatuses to provide secondary-blast protection for responders and casualty-collection points
- Blast wounding patterns and the effect of immediate geography and structures on injuries
- Common operational risks in the postblast environment
- Rapid point-of-wounding TECC stabilization and extrication
- Israeli principles of postblast triage and evacuation
- Effects on radio transmission and postblast communications
- Evidence preservation and collection

CONCLUSION

In the first part of the twenty-first century, the rapid definition of a new threat matrix for civilian first responders has developed. Incidents and attacks that in the past had been considered problems only for international crisis zones are now the new norm in the United States. The complex attack is the new threat, the new reality, for the entire public safety community. All of the disciplines in the first-response community must develop an integrated, all-hazards approach that can be applied across the threat matrix. Mitigation and response strategies must consider ASI and mass killing events, fire used as a weapon against citizens and responders, IED attacks, and complex attacks that include all of the above.

Normal human behavior is to resist change. Machiavelli, in 1537, said, "There is nothing more difficult to take in hand, more perilous to conduct, more uncertain in its success, than to take the lead in the introduction of a new order of things." The first-response community has a long tradition of growing, evolving, and rising to meet emerging threats. We must draw on this tradition as we modernize our disaster- and terrorism-response strategies. Old response paradigms, politics, risk aversion, and denial are no longer acceptable. Multijurisdictional and interagency response plans that aggressively address dynamic threats while mitigating responder risk are critical—our communities demand it, and our responders deserve it.

⚠ PITFALLS

- Failure to create an interagency plan for response to high-threat, dynamic terrorist incidents
- Failure to address the changing threat matrix and create operational-response programs to mitigate risk in terrorist-incident response
- Overreliance on specialized LEO or technical rescue teams to provide immediate response
- Ignorance of international terrorist attacks and failure to review terrorist tactics, techniques, and procedures, responder after-action reports, and military lessons learned
- Failure to create tiered, interagency response systems that utilize common language and include overlapping tasks for first responders (e.g., provision of basic trauma care, casualty rescue, and communication)

Acknowledgment

We thank Dr. Eric Sergienko for his contributions to the first edition of this chapter; portions of Dr. Sergienko's prior chapter were used in the Historical Perspective section.

REFERENCES

1. National Institutes of Justice. http://www.nij.gov/topics/crime/terrorism/Pages/welcome.aspx. (Accessed June 12, 2014.)
2. Integrated United States Security Database (IUSSD). *Data on the Terrorist Attacks in the United States Homeland, 1970 to 2011 Final Report to Resilient*

Systems Division, DHS Science and Technology Directorate; December 2012. (Accessed December 2013.)

3. Flynn Stephen E. The neglected home front. *Foreign Affairs.* Sept/Oct 2004;83(5):20–33.

4. Callaway DW, Westmoreland TC, Baez AA, McKay SA, Raja AS. Integrated response to the dynamic threat of school violence. *Prehosp Disaster Med.* 2010 Sep-Oct;25(5):464–470.

5. C-TECC Guidelines. www.c-tecc.org. Accessed September 8, 2014.

6. Anonymous. Appendix A: definitions and acronyms. In: *Regional Emergency Coordination Plan.* Washington, DC: Metropolitan Washington Council of Governments; 2002.

7. Clinton W. *Presidential Decision Directive 39: US Policy on Counterterrorism.* Washington, DC, 1995. Available at, www.fas.org/irp/offdocs/pdd39.htm.

8. Carlson J. Critical incident management in the ultimate crisis: counterterrorism. *FBI Law Enforcement Bull.* 1999;68(3):6–8.

9. Sub Chapter IV: B emergency preparedness. In: *The Robert T. Stafford Disaster Assistance and Emergency Relief Act, as amended, 42 USC 5121, et seq*; 1988:36–46. Available at: www.dem.dcc.state.nc.us/mitigation/Library/Stafford.pdf.

10. Fusco A. Overview: chief of department. In: *United States Fire Administration. The World Trade Center Bombing Report and Analysis.* Emmitsburg, Md: Federal Emergency Management Agency; 1993:1–23.

11. Goldfarb Z, Kuhr S. EMS response to the explosion. In: *United States Fire Administration. The World Trade Center Bombing Report and Analysis.* Emmitsburg, Md: Federal Emergency Management Agency; 1993:92–110.

12. Martin RA. The joint terrorism task force: a concept that works-FBI-New York city police department. *FBI Law Enforcement Bulletin.* 1999;68 (3):9–10.

13. http://www.fbi.gov/about-us/investigate/terrorism/terrorism_jttfs (Accessed June 20, 2014).

14. Cumming A, Masse T. *Intelligence Reform Implementation at the Federal Bureau of Investigation: Issues and Options for Congress;* 2005. CRS Report for Congress. Available at: www.fas.org/sgp/crs/intel/RL33033.pdf.

15. The Subcommittee on Economic Development. Public Building and Emergency Management Hearing on Combating Terrorism: Options to Improve the Federal Response. Available at: http://www.house.gov/transportation/pbed/04-24-01/04-24-01memo.html.

16. Anonymous. *White Paper on Presidential Decision Directive 62: Protection Against Unconventional Threats to the Homeland and Americans Overseas.* Washington, DC: 1998. Available at: http://www.fas.org/irp/offdocs/pdd-62.htm.

17. Coroner's Inquest into the London Bombings of 7 July 2005. Presented by Lady Justice Hallett to HM Government on 6 May 2011.

18. Gardham D. *7/7 Inquest: emergency response to bombs "chaotic."* The Telegraph; 2011, May 6. Retrieved from, www.Telegraph.co.uk.

19. Shah MN. The formation of the emergency medical services system. *Am J Public Health.* 2006 Mar;96(3):414–423, Epub 2006 Jan 31. PubMed PMID: 16449600.

20. Jones JS, Reese K, Kenepp G, Krohmer J. Into the fray: integration of emergency medical services and special weapons and tactics (SWAT) teams. *Prehosp Disaster Med.* 1996 Jul-Sep;11(3):202–206.

21. Young JB, Galante JM, Sena MJ. Operator training and TEMS support: a survey of unit leaders in northern and central California. *J Spec Oper Med.* 2013 Fall;13(3):92–97.

22. Young JB, Sena MJ, Galante JM. Physician roles in tactical emergency medical support: the first 20 years. *J Emerg Med.* 2014 Jan;46(1):38–45.

23. Mass Shootings at Virginia Tech. Report of the Review Panel. Presented to Governor Kain, Commonwealth of Virginia. April 16, 2007.

24. Erickson William H. The Report of Governor Bill Owens'. Columbine Review Commission. May 2001. http://www.state.co.us/columbine/Columbine_20_WEBFULL.pdf (Accessed June 22, 2014).

25. Erickson William H. The Report of Governor Bill Owens'. Columbine Review Commission. May 2001. http://www.state.co.us/columbine/Columbine_20_WEBFULL.pdf (Accessed June 22, 2014).

26. Erickson William H. The Report of Governor Bill Owens'. Columbine Review Commission. May 2001. http://www.state.co.us/columbine/Columbine_20_WEBFULL.pdf (Accessed June 22, 2014).

27. Erickson William H. The Report of Governor Bill Owens'. Columbine Review Commission. May 2001. http://www.state.co.us/columbine/Columbine_20_WEBFULL.pdf (Accessed June 22, 2014).

28. Blair JP, Martaindale MH. *United States active shooter events from 2000 to 2010: training and equipment implications*; Oct. 15, 2013. Alerrt.org. Retrieved, from, http://alerrt.org/files/research/ActiveShooterEvents.pdf.

29. Mizell and Associates. (2010). *First Responder Knowledgebase.* Washington, DC: Louis Mizell.

30. Video: Run. Hide. Fight. Surviving an Active Shooter Event. Produced by City of Houston (Tx) Office of Public Safety and Homeland Security. www.FBI.gov, Accessed in September 2014.

31. Robertson J, McCahill P, Riddle A, Callaway D. Another civilian life saved by law enforcement—applied tourniquet. *J Spec Oper Med.* Fall 2014;14 (3):7–10.

32. Callaway DW, Smith ER, Shapiro GL, et al. The Committee for Tactical Emergency Casualty Care (C-TECC): evolution and application of the TCCC guidelines to civilian high threat medicine. *J Spec Oper Med.* 2011;11 (2):95–100.

33. Smith ER, Iselin B, McKay WS. Towards the sound of shooting: the Arlington County Fire Department rescue task force. *JEMS.* December 2009; 48–55.

Multimodality, Layered Attack

Nicholas V. Cagliuso Sr., Jeffrey S. Rabrich, and Thérèse M. Postel

Coordinated simultaneous attacks in multiple geographic locations, both in the United States and abroad, with the intent to kill large numbers of people over minutes, hours, or days have become part of the regular strategy of terrorists. These attacks often employ a combination of conventional and unconventional weaponry and may involve weapons of mass destruction (WMD, including chemical, biological, radiological, nuclear, or explosive [CBRNE] agents and devices). Scenarios of this sort have been effectively carried out since the 1960s, resulting in the deaths of thousands and the psychological impacts that terrorists so eagerly desire. Near-simultaneous or simultaneous attacks utilizing conventional weapons (i.e., small arms and explosives), as witnessed most notably in the Boston Marathon bombings in April 2013, the Oslo attacks and massacre of 2011, the Mumbai attacks in 2008, the Madrid train bombings in March 2004, and the infamous 9/11 attacks, have been used with great success by terrorists.

This chapter discusses emerging tactics, including the coupling of conventional weapons and CBRNE agents in the minutes, hours, or days after the initial attack, in the execution of a "multimodality, layered attack." Rather than targeting locations with a similar threat, those responsible select several types of attack modes. The Iran-Iraq War of the 1980s and the current civil war in Syria provide glaring examples of these tactics, combining conventional and chemical attacks that have significant implications for both the health care system, specifically prehospital and hospital communities, and society as a whole. Given terrorists' motivations to repeatedly highlight their targets' vulnerabilities, and the creative tactics that they use to do so, this chapter meets the urgent need for understanding multimodality, layered attacks and the means to manage their effects.

THE NOTION OF TERRORISM

An agreed-upon definition of terrorism itself must exist in order to understand the concept of multimodal, layered terrorist attacks. Although there is no universally accepted definition of *terrorism*, this chapter uses the U.S. Department of State's definition found in Title 22, Chapter 38, Sec. 2656f, of the United States Code, which states, "the term 'terrorism' means premeditated, politically motivated violence perpetrated against noncombatant targets by subnational groups or clandestine agents."[1-3] Special attention should be paid to the terms *premeditated* and *noncombatant targets,* highlighting that events of this kind are not accidental (see Chapter 36) and are aimed at civilians and off-duty military personnel.

Modes of Attack

Given the diversity of motives for and classifications of terrorism, a review of the two principal modes of terrorist attacks—conventional and unconventional—follows, with particular consideration given to simultaneous deployments within each mode.

Conventional Tactics

Conventional or traditional attack modes include those attacks that do not involve WMD. In conventional attacks, terrorists utilize small arms, explosives, and incendiary devices. Recent terrorist events indicate that these attacks can have a far more considerable impact than those that include WMD.[4] As demonstrated by Faisal Shahzad's attempted Times Square bombing in 2010 and the Boston Marathon bombings of April 2013, intelligence and experience continue to suggest that use of tried-and-true conventional weapons is likely to remain a favored choice of terrorists. This is especially true as the devices employed are inexpensive, are readily available, and require minimal skill to construct. Additional examples of such incidents include the bombings at the World Trade Center in New York City in 1993, the Oslo bombing in 2011, and the bombing of the Alfred P. Murrah Federal Building in Oklahoma City in 1995. One cannot forget the ongoing terrorism and myriad of IED attacks carried out throughout the Middle East.

Unconventional Tactics

Unconventional or WMD attack modes involve the use of CBRNE devices. The Aum Shinrikyo cult attacks utilizing sarin gas in Matsumoto, Japan, in 1994 and again in the Tokyo subway system in 1995, and the recent use of sarin on Syrian civilian populations, are examples of chemical terrorist attacks (see further discussion in Section 11). The sarin attack on the Tokyo subway caused hundreds of people to become ill, resulted in the deaths of 12 persons, and caused psychological harm to many more victims.[5]

The 2001 anthrax attacks in Florida, New York City, New Jersey, Washington DC, and Connecticut represent the most recent large-scale example of a biological agent attack. In the incident, contaminated letters were processed and sent to media outlets and elected officials through the U.S. mail, resulting in several deaths and massive financial consequences. Although the use of biological weapons by terrorists has the potential to harm and kill thousands of people, the extent to which incidents involving weapons of this sort, such as the dissemination of anthrax or smallpox, will occur in the future in the United States or elsewhere is unknown.[6] This is in part because terrorist attacks using biological weapons have been extremely rare, as most terrorist organizations lack both the sophisticated laboratories to develop and the complex delivery systems to disperse such agents.[7] However, the line between chemical weapons and biological weapons is being blurred by rapid developments in biotechnology and the emergence of a new generation of toxins and bioregulators.[8] As a result, the numerous problems in the detection of and response to chemical and biological incidents are now exacerbated by new challenges. Moreover, a follow-up attack that includes the release of an agent such as smallpox could pose threats to large populations because of the potential for person-to-person transmission, enabling spread to other cities and states and exacerbating what would already be a nationwide emergency.[9] The employment of multiple chemical and biological agents is a probable scenario of the future, challenging the medical community to be increasingly proactive in its development of appropriate countermeasures.[10]

Radiological weapons (see Section 10) or "dirty bombs" (see Chapter 77) disperse radioactive materials in a conventional device such as a bomb or other explosive container. To date, the use of nuclear and related weapons has been the sole purview of nation-states.[11] In 1995 Chechen rebels were reported to have buried, but not to have detonated, a 30-lb box of cesium-137 and dynamite near the entrance of a busy Moscow park. More recently, six individuals were arrested after stealing a truck filled with hospital waste cobalt-60 in Mexico, widely considered a potential ingredient for a "dirty bomb." This is only one example of myriad thefts of nuclear material in recent years.[12] The potential use by terrorists of nuclear, radiological, and related weapons expands this threat to new actors with links to the global complex of nuclear weapons and nuclear power facilities.[9]

The use of any or all of these attack modes is not the only issue of concern. The tactics through which they are employed, coordinated with or following a conventional attack, is the key issue at hand. A discussion of the use of multiple modes of attack deployed in a simultaneous or near-simultaneous manner follows.

Categorization of Simultaneous Attacks

Global and domestic affairs dictate that a broad variety of terrorism threats already exist, that others will emerge and develop, and that the United States will be among the targets of such threats for the foreseeable future.[13] The most serious concern about terrorism is that terrorists are seeking to kill and injure more and more people. While this is so, it is also important to note that the desired effects of terrorism transcend physical harm to the victims and the accompanying psychological impacts on the target and the society to which it belongs. The psychosocial impacts of simultaneous attacks (e.g., crippling effects of attacks on energy or information technology infrastructure), even when thwarted, can result in behavioral changes that often affect the economy. These economic effects can have significant impacts, as seen after the 9/11 attacks when many elected officials, including the mayor of New York City, had to make repeated public appeals for people to visit theaters and restaurants and contribute to the local economy again. Unquestionably, mass fatalities that result from simultaneous attacks have an impact, as images and reports of thousands dead or injured are a heinous reality of terrorism, particularly with the proliferation of social media and the ability to instantly provide information and images from incident scenes.

The associated fear and anxiety about one's own safety, concerns about the ability of government to protect its citizens, and the ominous danger brought about by the potential for future acts of terror that are of utmost importance to the terrorist. As a consequence, the terrorist's victims must be carefully selected to ensure the maximum possible psychological impact on the target.[14] While target selection is important (e.g., urban rail hub versus rural elementary school), the timing with which the attacks are carried out—particularly if in a coordinated, simultaneous manner—is also vital to ensuring desired impacts. On 9/11, 2752 people were killed, the most fatalities from any single documented terrorist event in the United States, and the method of attack selected by the terrorists was one that included coordinated, layered attacks across a variety of geographic areas.[15,16]

Although it was a day of utter devastation, one need only think about the effects had the terrorists added follow-up attacks that included a CBRNE event.

A discussion of the two core, but certainly not comprehensive, classifications of simultaneous, layered attacks follows. The first includes "multiple incidents in a single jurisdictional target." Attacks of this sort may commence as a single incident (e.g., a single suicide bus bombing) but can quickly evolve into an attack against multiple targets, including first responders. For example, the March 2004 bombings in Madrid, the deadliest terror strikes in Europe since the bombing of Pan Am Flight 103 over Lockerbie, Scotland, in 1988 killed 270 people, and is the worst terrorist assault in Spanish history. The attacks took place at the height of a weekday rush hour when three separate trains were hit by 10 near-simultaneous explosions. The attacks occurred between 7:39 and 7:54 AM, with multiple explosions at the Santa Eugenia, El Pozo, and Atocha stations. Although three other bombs were found and detonated by police, 192 people were killed and 1800 wounded. In attacks of this kind, multiple weapons or secondary devices are employed with the intention to kill large numbers, drain the resources of the affected jurisdiction by rendering an area insecure, and hamper both rescue efforts and injury control.[17]

In such incidents, first responders become victims as well as they manage the initial event and may be struck by follow-up attacks. According to the National Counter Terrorism Center, "Terrorist groups … may target responders deliberately to enhance the magnitude of their terror attack, creating increased fear and media attention by demonstrating that even would-be rescuers are vulnerable to attack."[18] Given the sophistication of these types of attacks, improved coordination among the perpetrators is required, usually involving multiple people.[19] Include the release of a chemical agent (e.g., tabun, a poison so powerful that even short-term exposure to small concentrations of its vapor results in immediate symptoms and possibly death) in the scenario and the effectiveness of a multimodality, layered attack becomes clear.[20]

The second type of simultaneous attack classification involves "multiple incidents across multiple jurisdictional targets." The incident may begin as one or more concurrent attacks that turns into an attack against multiple targets, again including first responders, in geographically separated areas with multiple weapons or secondary devices. These attacks are aimed at perplexing emergency response systems and draining resources of the local jurisdiction, if not state and federal levels. The coordinated terrorist attacks on Mumbai in 2008 are the most salient example of this tactic. These attacks targeted a train station, a Jewish Center, a theater, and a hospital and lasted over 4 days. The mobile terrorist teams killed over 100 people across multiple "soft targets" including the Cama Hospital and popular tourist destinations across Mumbai.[21]

Although the events of 9/11 illustrate an attack using conventional means, the impact would have been exponentially worse had the perpetrators added the release of a CBRNE agent within the United States later in the day or in the days immediately following the initial attack. The addition of CBRNE agents, even if it added no more casualties, would worsen physical, psychological, and emotional trauma and further complicate and delay response by siphoning resources toward identification of the agent, conduct of an in-depth epidemiologic investigation, and extended incident and resource management.

The use of multiple CBRNE agents or the delivery of chemical and replicating agents or toxins, carefully chosen for their ability to generate specific symptoms and potentiate health effects, further complicates multimodality, layered attacks.[10] Agent detection requires rapid diagnostic methods and procedures (e.g., syndromic surveillance) to identify illnesses that result from multiple agents.[10]

Given the skills necessary to conduct such attacks— timing, organization, and coordination of the perpetrators—and possibly suicide attacks, several persons would be needed to carry out these attacks.

The near-simultaneous bombings of U.S. embassies in Nairobi, Kenya, and Dar es Salaam, Tanzania, which resulted in 224 deaths, are additional examples of multiple-incident, multiple-jurisdiction, layered attacks. The demonstration of an operational capability to coordinate two nearly simultaneous attacks on U.S. embassies in different countries to a large extent has influenced U.S. policy.[22] Many terrorism experts point to the change in targeting and the style of attack as evidence of a possible broadening of the overall strategy from mainly guerilla insurgency against U.S. forces to a coordinated terrorist campaign that includes foreign elements. The evolution of these tactics is difficult to predict.[23] In all cases, the aim of these attacks was to maximize injury and cause complex trauma, thereby elevating the killing ratio.[24] Although the ability to conduct multiple coordinated attacks against several targets is not new for terrorist groups, the manner in which these attacks are being conducted indicates refined capabilities and sophisticated tactics, bringing into focus the reality that future terrorist attacks will likely include even greater use of multimodality, layered attack tactics.[4]

HISTORICAL PERSPECTIVE

Prior to 9/11 approximately one thousand Americans had been killed by terrorist events either in this country or abroad since 1968—the year heralded as the advent of the modern era of international terrorism after the Popular Front for the Liberation of Palestine hijacking of an El Al flight.[25] Simultaneous, large-scale attacks using conventional means such as car bombs are relatively uncommon. For reasons not well understood by scholars or practitioners, terrorists typically have not undertaken such coordinated operations. One thought is that smaller plots are easier to conduct and less likely to be thwarted, thereby improving their chance of completion. Conversely, the historical lack of large-scale, multiple simultaneous attacks may be a reflection of the logistical and other organizational obstacles that most terrorist groups are not able to overcome.[25] In fact, the initial "planes operation" (as it was termed by Al Qaeda operatives) embraced the idea of using suicide operations to blow up planes as a refinement of the original "Manila" air plot. All of the planes hijacked were to be crashed or exploded at or about the same time to maximize the psychological impact of the attacks.[26]

During the 1990s, perhaps only one other terrorist incident evidenced the characteristics of coordination and high lethality: the series of attacks that occurred in Bombay (now Mumbai) in March 1993, where a dozen or so simultaneous car bombings rocked the city, killing nearly 300 persons and wounding more than 700 others.[27] Indeed, apart from the attacks on the same morning in October 1983 of the U.S. Marine barracks in Beirut and a nearby French paratroop headquarters, and the Irish Republican Army's near-simultaneous assassination of Lord Mountbatten and remote-control mine attack on British troops in Warrenpoint, Northern Ireland, in 1979, it is hard to recall many other significant incidents reflecting such operational expertise, coordination, and synchronization.[27]

That is not to say, however, that similar types of operations have not been planned and foiled. Ramzi Ahmed Yousef, the convicted mastermind of the 1993 New York World Trade Center bombing, and 15 other persons reportedly intended to follow that incident in June 1993 with the simultaneous bombings of the Holland and Lincoln tunnels and the George Washington Bridge—vital infrastructure used daily by tens of thousands of commuters between New Jersey and Manhattan.[28] Yousef's plans also included the simultaneous bombings

of 11 U.S. passenger airliners while in flight over the Pacific Ocean in 1995.[29] The importance of simultaneity in attacks is confirmed by these events and, more recently, by the interrogation of Khalid Sheikh Mohammed on August 18, 2003.[16]

In 2010 an Al Qaeda in the Arabian Peninsula (AQAP) plot was disrupted in the latest stages of planning. AQAP placed explosive printer cartridges inside two cargo airplanes, with the intention of detonating these explosives nearly simultaneously while the planes were flying over the continental United States en route to Chicago. The plot was disrupted as a result of intelligence-sharing with Saudi intelligence services. Although few people would have been killed, the impact on world trade would have been tremendous.[30]

Perhaps many people were lulled into believing that mass-casualty, simultaneous attacks in general, and those of such devastating potential as witnessed on 9/11, are beyond the capabilities of most terrorists. Yet, the tragic events of 9/11 demonstrate the profound error of such an assumption.[25] The significance of past successes (e.g., foiling most of bin Laden's terrorist operations between the August 1998 embassy bombings and the November 2000 attack on the U.S.S. *Cole*) and the terrorists' own incompetence and propensity for mistakes (e.g., Ahmad Ressam's attempt to enter the United States from Canada in December 1999) was likely overestimated.[25] The reality demands a robust, comprehensive emergency management strategy that addresses mitigation, preparedness, response, and recovery activities unique to these events to minimize pitfalls.

PREPAREDNESS

Much terrorism preparedness pre-9/11 focused on the comparatively low-end threat posed by car and truck bombs against buildings or the more exotic threats involving biological or chemical weapons or cyber attack. Other preparedness planning continues to (quite possibly erroneously) assume mass-casualty attacks involving biological or chemical agents released at key infrastructures (e.g., air and rail terminals). Mitigating and preparing for myriad attack tactics have been neglected in favor of other, less conventional threats (e.g,. chemical, biological, and radiological) with the possibility of using an aircraft as a suicide weapon almost completely discounted.[25]

Although the so-called WMD were not used in the 9/11 attacks, the destruction was nonetheless "massive."[23] Consequently, the very real prospect of combining modern weapons technology (i.e., CBRNE weapons) with an age-old willingness to die in the act of committing an attack could be unprecedentedly dangerous.[23] Furthermore, with increasing numbers of casualties from multiple suicide attacks occurring globally in places such as Afghanistan, Pakistan, Nigeria, Russia/Chechnya, and Iraq, a discourse on the threat of future suicide attacks is warranted.[23] One need only to examine the Department of State's *Patterns of Global Terrorism* (1983-2001) to see the efficiencies gained by attacks of this sort. Pape found that from 1980 to 2001, suicide attacks represented only 3% of all terrorist attacks but accounted for 48% of total deaths from terrorism.[31,32] Ten years later, in 2011, suicide terrorism had declined to 2.7% of all attacks and 21% of terrorism fatalities.[33]

In retrospect, it was not the 1995 Sarin Nerve Gas Attack on the Tokyo subway and nine attempts to use bioweapons by the Aum Shinrikyo cult that should have had the dominant influence on counterterrorist thinking pre-9/11. Instead, the 1986 hijacking of a Pan Am flight in Karachi and the 1994 hijacking in Algiers of an Air France passenger plane by terrorists belonging to the Armed Islamic Group, reportedly with the intention of crashing the planes into the centers of Tel Aviv and Paris, respectively, should have served as keen indicators of the type, scope, and overall capabilities of those responsible for events to come.[25]

The pendulum has now swung in the other direction. After 9/11, defenses were hardened against conventional threats to the United States. Law enforcement and homeland security focused on "high-probability" incidents and on interdicting these threats. However, a strong argument can be made for continuing to prepare for low-probability, high-impact events. According to Nathan Myhrvold, founder of *Intellectual Ventures*, the attacks of 9/11 pulled our focus away from strategic nation-state threats, such as the Cold War, to tactical terror attacks like that of 9/11. He argues that the defense establishment is overlooking "strategic terrorism." In the past, "strategic terrorism" could only be achieved by state-sponsored actors. However, advances in technology, coupled with the availability of nuclear and chemical material, has undermined the "lethality versus cost curve" and has "democratized" the ability to cause mass deaths. Small groups of people are equipped with an ability to create much greater lethality through their actions than any time in the past.[34] For this reason, it is all the more important to analyze and prepare for multimodal layered terrorist attacks. Not only is it easier for a small group of individuals to wreak havoc; even a single person may have the ability to bring society to a halt with little expertise or money. Myhrvold predicts that this "strategic terrorism" use of chemical, biological, or nuclear weapons can make "9/11 look trivial by comparison."[34]

A commonly held notion is that terrorists are primarily interested in publicity and therefore have neither the need nor interest in annihilating large numbers of people.[25] In 1975 Jenkins noted that "Terrorists want a lot of people watching and a lot of people listening and not a lot of people dead." Just 10 years later, he reiterated, "Simply killing a lot of people has seldom been one terrorist objective. Terrorists operate on the principle of the minimum force necessary. They find it unnecessary to kill many, as long as killing a few suffices for their purposes."[35] The events of 9/11 and far-right, lone-wolf attacks like the Oslo massacre prove such notions now to be wishful thinking, if not dangerously anachronistic.[25]

The primary goals for terrorists today are to instill fear, change patterns of living, and draw attention to their cause. This means maximizing morbidity and mortality. One need not look further than Al Qaeda's first issue of *Inspire* magazine and its article "How to Make a Bomb in the Kitchen of Your Mom." Terrorists today are looking for any attention they can garner—hence the pressure cooker bombs employed by the Boston bombers, built following the instructions in the article."[36] Anders Breivik's acts in Oslo were extremely simple, but caused mass casualties and hysteria. A small explosion in one part of Oslo, followed by a mass shooting spree in a separate jurisdiction, paralyzed law enforcement. The desire to utilize simple tactics to achieve their goals reaches across ideological lines.

CURRENT PRACTICE

Small arms, explosives, and incendiaries are the weapons used in most terrorist acts.[15] Although the use of nonconventional weapons must not be ignored, conventional weapons have had a significant impact in recent terrorist incidents.[4,15,37] Al Qaeda and its affiliates have demonstrated a high level of determination and motivation to conduct high-profile, mass-casualty attacks. Al Qaeda and its franchise terrorist groups are increasingly targeting civilian, noncombatant targets in their attacks. The Bali nightclub bombing (2003), Moscow theater siege (2002), and combined car bombing and surface-to-air missile attacks in Mombasa, Kenya, are indicative of this emerging, increasingly popular tactic.

While Al Qaeda and its affiliates remain a potent threat, far-right extremism represents a burgeoning, and often overlooked, danger. The Oslo terrorist attacks (2011) illustrate the competency of lone-wolf actors to implement multijurisdictional, mass-casualty attacks. Anders Breivik, a far-right neo-Nazi, murdered 77 people by detonating a car bomb in Oslo and then traveled to the island of Utoya, where he shot and killed youths participating in a camp run by the Norwegian Labor Party.[38] By all accounts, those who extol far-right ideology have been "more deadly" than "jihadists" since 9/11.[39]

It must be noted that although damage to a target, or in a multimodality, layered attack, multiple targets, may be relatively small (e.g., a single suicide bomb in a bus or a single aircraft downed), the political and psychological impacts will be significant. To that end, the impact of bombs, and for that matter terrorist acts in general, goes beyond mortality and morbidity.[40] It is the creation of psychological terror, which simultaneous attacks produce so readily, that can cause chaos and panic in both the short and long terms.[41]

Response Strategies

The best response strategy to any emergency is prevention. The omnipresent threat of terrorist acts and their surprise nature demands that key stakeholders craft and implement flexible approaches that they can adjust quickly to respond to these incidents if they do occur. Doing so requires careful coordination of the myriad necessary resources, compatible communication systems, and real-time information feedback to decision makers that permits near-immediate changes in strategy when required.[15] The capacity to respond to a broad technological range of possible adversarial attacks is one of the primary lessons to be learned from all terrorist incidents.

Identifying the threat of terrorism is comparatively new to the United States, and many dimensions of the initial response to this threat have been implemented post-9/11 (e.g., the National Incident Management System and the National Response Framework) but no level of resources will be able to fully prevent the United States from being attacked in the future.[13] Consequently, understanding the full assortment of injuries and disorders, including posttraumatic stress disorder, is critical to responding effectively.[42]

While history does not always repeat itself, it can surely serve as a gauge for what terrorists are capable of and how we should respond. In the case of Al Qaeda, Osama bin Laden has been characterized as a terrorist CEO who organized "spectaculars"—high-visibility, high-casualty operations such as 9/11, the bombing of the U.S.S. *Cole*, and the East Africa embassy bombings.[43] Terrorist activity today does not necessarily follow this, or any, blueprint. From lone wolves to known extremist groups, terrorists always seem to be one step ahead of law enforcement. Attacks on public venues, like the Boston Marathon or a youth camp in Oslo, are an inexpensive yet potent way to gain attention for a cause. As a result, first responders must prepare for simultaneous, geographically distributed attacks. An attack using multiple bombs coordinated to explode in several cities across the country at sites such as stores, schools, hospitals, apartment buildings, and gas stations can no longer be considered an unprecedented or "Black Swan" event. The terrorist attacks we are likely to face will involve not only WMD and weapons of mass disruption, but use of conventional means to attack critical infrastructural targets such as nuclear and chemical plants, agricultural nodes, and the hearts of the American and world economy, with catastrophic human and economic consequences.[32]

Terrorists are also likely to strike at "soft targets" like malls, places of worship, hospitals, and hotels. Al-Shabaab, a terrorist group based in Somalia and affiliated with Al Qaeda, undertook its first "hostage-barricade" attack in September 2013 at Westgate Mall in Nairobi, Kenya. The attack lasted for nearly three days and resulted in over 67 deaths.[44] The attack garnered much media attention for Al-Shabaab and highlighted Shabaab's desire to end Kenya military intervention in Somalia. Soft target attacks like these disrupt the economy, and in a country like Kenya, drain tourism from the country. Soft target attacks, like that on the Westgate Mall, provide a unique challenge for local communities and hospitals not only during the duration of the attack, but throughout the psychological repercussions.

Suicide Attacks

Suicide attacks by terrorist organizations have become more widespread globally, and assessing the threat of these attacks has therefore strategic importance to the United States and its interests at home and abroad.[23] Essentially a punishment strategy, suicide terror has become increasingly prevalent over the past three decades simply because terrorists have learned that attacks of this type work. The success of suicide attacks has two primary consequences. First, it inflicts instant punishment against the target. Second, its success implies a threat for additional punishment in the future and highlights the target's vulnerability. Couched in the act is the message that the attacker(s) could not be deterred and often that the attacker is connected to a broader ideological community. In suicide terrorism, a weaker party, usually a person or small group, acts as the coercer, with the stronger group (e.g., Western society) as the target.

Suicide terrorism represents a small percentage of terrorist attacks (2.7% in 2011) but creates 21% of the fatalities from terrorism.[45] The fact that groups using this tactic are responsible for the majority of high-fatality incidents suggests that they have reached an advanced level of enemy dehumanization and are therefore psychologically closer to perpetrating mass-casualty CBRNE attacks.[46] An innovative use of suicide bombings as a component of multimodality, layered attack methods involves the use of combining self-destructive tactics with CBRNE agents. Suicide tactics could significantly improve the potentiality of a successful CBRNE weapons attack itself. Here, the unimportance of being exposed to extremely dangerous materials permits the attacker to carry out increasingly perilous experiments, thereby expanding the chance of generating and using a potent and effective CBRNE weapon.[46]

Second, notable tactical opportunities arise for terrorists who are indifferent to making contact with a CBRNE agent during delivery. In addition to greater access to the target and enhanced control over the outcome, elimination of shielding measures during the attack, such as personal protective equipment, decreases the risk of early detection and interdiction of the attack. Intelligence agencies have uncovered plots to use the bodies of terrorists as crude delivery systems; the perpetrators are infected with a contagious agent and deployed to crowded areas. Unfortunately, this technique has historic precedent; in 1346 at the Seige of Caffa, bodies infected with the bubonic plague were catapulted over the city walls with a goal of infecting those inside. This form of biological warfare is an ancient tactic that may make a return through terrorism in the future.[47]

MEDICAL MANAGEMENT OF MASS CASUALTY INCIDENTS

In the 17-minute period between 8:46 and 9:03 AM on September 11, 2001, New York City and the Port Authority of New York and New Jersey had mobilized the largest rescue operation in the city's history.[25] In all, over 25,000 people were rescued from the World Trade Center complex on that day, and although the costs in first responders' lives were great, their selfless acts will never be forgotten. During mass-casualty events, terror victims often arrive at hospitals in clusters, whereas during more isolated assaults they arrive either as individuals or a few at a time.[48] The medical management of events of this sort, in which the goal is to save as many lives as possible and to decrease

morbidity, requires that the most senior clinician assume command of the incident and adjust the available resources optimally to the excessive needs.[49]

Hospitals, which exist to serve their communities and care for the sick and injured, can also be soft targets. Relatively easy access to them in the interest of improving the patient experience, the fact that they are already filled with sick and injured, and their roles as cornerstones of communities and as first receivers pose a conundrum for emergency managers and make these facilities particularly attractive terrorist targets. Examples of such realities include the April 2005 incident in the United States involving imposters posing as hospital accreditation surveyors; the November 2005 plot that uncovered a note reading "Hospital = Target" in London; the arrests in 2007 of physicians in Britain for attempting to attack health care facilities; and the thwarted takeover of a Denmark hospital in 2012.

AQAP attacked a military hospital in Yemen, killing 52 people, in December 2103.[50] In June 2014, six people were killed in a foiled attack on another military hospital, days after 15 were killed in simultaneous, coordinated attacks on an airport, a military barracks, and a post office. As noted earlier, a hospital was also targeted during the Mumbai attacks in 2003. If not for quick thinking by nurses and "ward boys" who closed ward doors and ordered mothers to keep their babies quiet as attackers approached, scores of patients would have been killed as terrorists stormed the Cama Hospital for Women and Children, killing security guards.[49] Health care leadership, in conjunction with internal and external emergency management partners, must ensure that staff are cognizant of international trends highlighting hospitals as terror targets and support initiatives for their organizations to minimize the effects of these incidents, if not halt them entirely.

Hospitals and health care organizations will need to continue to develop strategies to detect victims of attacks as well. As terrorists employ varying tactics in a multimodal attack, agents such as biologicals (anthrax, smallpox, plague, etc.) can have insidious onsets and may be difficult to detect, especially the index case. Strategies such as syndromic surveillance to detect disease clusters, as well as radiation portal monitoring, are becoming necessary to help identify biological and radiological agents. Many of the biological agents such as anthrax or plague are rarely seen in naturally occurring states, and the average clinician may not recognize symptoms or make the diagnosis early in an attack. Smallpox, which was eradicated in the 1970s, has never been diagnosed by most practicing physicians. For these reasons it is essential for public health agencies to continuously monitor emergency department activity to detect symptom clusters early on. Failure to detect or understand the causative agent of the symptoms can have serious effects on health care workers, as was the case with the 1995 Tokyo subway sarin attack during which patients were not decontaminated prior to arriving in the emergency department. By the time the agent was identified as sarin, several health care workers had become sick.

Events of this kind require overall medical resource management skills first, rather than clinical capabilities. Here, the aims of saving as many lives as possible and decreasing morbidity dictate skillful prioritization of decisions to restore the balance between needs and available resources. The principles of the medical management of mass-casualty events, where the medical system is overwhelmed and the balance between resources and demands is undermined by terrorist acts, have been fully described elsewhere.[51] Although all terrorist attacks, conventional and unconventional, have the potential to produce significant physical and psychological trauma, simultaneous attacks are far more efficient in overburdening medical systems at the local level, and, if the nature of the simultaneous attacks is on a large scale, on the regional or national level. Consequently, success in the management of large-scale medical events comes from extensive early preparation.[51]

An additional contrast between isolated terrorist events and the multimodal, layered event discussed in this chapter lies in the duration of the events. A short-term event such as the bombing of a single bus can be local in nature, requiring the response of a single jurisdiction's first responders and treatment by a local hospital and, if necessary, specialty centers. Conversely, a multimodal, layered attack may necessitate activation of a national response system in which resources from across the nation are deployed to those areas hardest hit as well as those where intelligence suggests likely follow-up attacks. Dividing the patient load between community hospitals, large urban medical centers, and specialty care centers (e.g., trauma, burns, or hyperbaric centers) will help ensure that no one facility is overwhelmed by the event. Additionally, while many hospital or health care facilities may have the resources to care for victims of a single isolated attack, often they lack the resources and personnel to provide care for a prolonged, sustained, or repetitive attack.

Use of the National Incident Management System and the National Response Framework, each of which provide for the establishment of an Incident Command System/Unified Command, should be engaged at the beginning of the event by the affected local jurisdiction. An interface between prehospital systems and receiving medical centers is paramount. The different modes of terror currently compose a new field of epidemiology that demands ongoing activities at all levels and places increased and unique demands on first responders and in-hospital clinical, management, and support staff.[51]

Mutimodality, layered terrorist acts are capable of producing more victims and higher mortality rates than are seen in natural disasters. Therefore medical personnel must ensure that medical protocols exist for both the daily treatment and transportation of patients as well as for situations that place unexpected demands on the system.[46]

One threat to U.S. citizens comes from the possibility of further attacks orchestrated or inspired by Al Qaeda, either in the United States or abroad.[23] Although those ideologically similar to Al Qaeda remain potent and may continue to grow within Salafi jihadist presence in several failed states throughout the world, rising threats from far-right extremists should be factor into preparedness and counterterrorism, both in the United States and Europe. Contemporary terrorist behavior and tactics seek to destroy those components of our lives that celebrate freedoms. The reality is that we cannot deny terrorists attractive targets. Rather, through effective programs, stakeholders can make attacks more difficult to carry out and less effective.

The events of 9/11 are an egregious reminder of how terrorists can fulfill their aims of death, fear, and intimidation through conventional means. The terrorist of today has the potential to wield conventional and nonconventional WMD—biological, chemical, and nuclear—that damage the body, the mind, and the soul.[48] One needs only to think of the cascading effects a multilayered, simultaneous attack scenario can have on trust in government, the economy, and national security, compared with a single isolated attack. These events demonstrate the ability of even one significant new terrorist incident to instantly reignite worldwide fears and concern.[41]

Israel has long maintained the notion of "mega-terrorism," a concept that embodies the notion of multimodal layered attacks. In "mega-terrorism," not only are the obvious terrorist uses of WMD brought to bear on specific highly symbolic targets, but "soft target attacks" such as attacks on elementary schools or the assassination of political and business leaders are carried out in ways that although not necessarily causing extensive human loss to life in terms of numbers, would nonetheless have profound, far-reaching psychological repercussions on the targeted society.[41] Al Qaeda killed 3000 people with "box cutters and aircraft hijacking" and only five with anthrax spores, to quote Paul Pillar, former National Intelligence Officer.[52] How will terrorists attack next? Strategically, with a large-scale, catastrophic attack? Or tactically, with small attacks that garner media attention? The answer may be murky, but it is generally accepted that if terrorists have the means to attack in a catastrophic way, they will. In the meantime, it is imperative that all those who can be prepared do so for all possibilities.

The fundamental nature and character of terrorism changed with the events of 9/11 and have continued to change and evolve since then. Judging by the simultaneous attacks carried out on that day and the foiled attempts and near misses since, the multiyear planning period of previous Al Qaeda spectaculars suggests that it is premature to write off those who remain inspired by Al Qaeda's ideology.[54] Terrorism is becoming increasingly difficult to characterize as an identifiable phenomenon amenable to categorization or clear distinction. Given the success of the 9/11 attacks, it is difficult to make a case against a similar, more devastating attack using multiple modes of attack that is only now slowly and inexorably unfolding.[54] The masterminds behind the attack proved the impotence of the mightiest military power to protect its citizens against these kinds of devastating blows. From the terrorists' point of view, the attack on America was a perfectly choreographed production aimed at American and international audiences.[20]

THREAT ASSESSMENT

"How do we assess the threat of terrorist events that have not occurred?"[54] Although there is no black-and-white response, today's terrorists are becoming demonstrably more adept in their tradecraft of death and destruction. They are more formidable in their capacity for tactical modification and innovation in their methods of attack (e.g., simultaneous and near-simultaneous deployments), and they have become increasingly competent in operating for sustained periods while avoiding detection, interception, or capture.[53] Moreover, even attacks that are not successful by conventional measures can nonetheless serve as a success for terrorists provided that they are daring enough to garner media and public attention. Given the world's recent hypersensitivity to threats and suspicious incidents, if terrorist action is not completely successful but brings a group publicity, their tenacious pursuit for fresh ways to overcome, circumvent, or defeat governmental security and countermeasures is fueled. Accordingly, attacks at all points along the conflict spectrum—from the crude and primitive to the most sophisticated—must be anticipated and appropriate measures employed to counter them.[53] A limited terrorist attack involving an unconventional chemical, biological, or radiological weapon on a small scale, either isolated or part of a succession of small incidents, may yield disproportionately large consequences, generating fear and serving the terrorists' purpose just as well as a larger weapon or more ambitious attack with massive casualties.[5]

Although many may think of multimodality, layered attacks as restricted to the use of simultaneous suicide attacks, one must examine the use of biological agents, looking specifically at microorganisms that when used in combination have the potential to create a severe disease state.[10] Infection with an agent with a short incubation period that weakens overall resistance may provide an opportunity for infection with a second organism, leading to greater morbidity and mortality.[10] The ability of multiple organisms with different levels of virulence to confuse medical officers looking for a common etiology accentuates the need for sensitive and specific diagnostic tests to be available in the field setting.[10]

Scenarios of the future may be complicated by the possible use of multiple agents or the delivery of chemical and replicating agents or their toxins that have been carefully chosen for stability and ability to generate specific symptoms. From a medical perspective, detection requires the availability of rapid diagnostic methods and procedures to assess illnesses that will be the result of multiple agents.[10] Syndromic surveillance initiatives, which have been in use across the world for decades, track and monitor outbreaks and improve overall situational awareness and resource allocation. The real issue and most likely threat may not be the ruthless terrorist use of some weapon of mass destruction, but the calculated, deliberate, and precisely planned use of some chemical, biological, radiological, or nuclear weapon in conjunction with conventional means in a simultaneous or near-simultaneous time frame to achieve far-reaching psychological effects.[5]

⚠ PITFALLS

- Failure to plan for multimodal attacks that combine conventional and CBRNE weapons.
- Failure to create interagency response plans that address dynamic terrorist attacks. Creation of these plans must be coupled with realistic training that includes law enforcement, emergency medical services, fire personnel, hospital emergency management, and regional and federal resources.
- Planning for the last attack, not the next one. First responders and counterterrorism professionals must continuously "war game" potential threats. A useful adage is to "plan for the most common and the worst-case scenario."

CONCLUSION

Before 9/11, most acts of terrorism resulted in a great deal of publicity in the form of media reporting. Because of the simultaneous, geographically diverse, layered nature of the attacks on that day, the images of commercial airliners crashing as suicide/homicide missiles into symbols of America's economic and military might continue to haunt many people.[20] The attacks could have been scheduled at night, sparing many lives, and still yielded significant publicity, but the bright daylight of that beautiful September morning made certain that the most spectacular of sights and greatest loss of life would occur. In these respects, no previous act of terrorism came close.[20]

Terrorists are well aware how difficult it is to prevent suicide terror. Although the idea that terrorists may obtain and use WMD cannot be ignored, the more immediate concern must be the prospect that geographically diverse and near-simultaneous attacks might well become the most attractive model for terrorism in the near future.[20] The success of follow-up explosions targeting first responders, as seen in Pakistan and Iraq, as well as attacks across multiple jurisdictions such as those in Mumbai and Oslo, may be a harbinger for future attacks in the United States. The ongoing use of such tactics across the globe demands a thoughtfully strategic and boldly operational approach from the disaster medicine perspective. When considering preparedness for and response of hospital systems to such attacks, it is clear that we must continually adjust our efforts and consider the realities of worst-case scenarios. Managing hundreds of casualties, as Boston area hospitals did for 264 victims in the hours after the 2013 Marathon attack, will become exponentially more difficult if the perpetrators introduce a CBRNE agent as well. Therefore the United States must continue to be vigilant when planning for terrorist events and prepare hospital staff to consider their own vulnerabilities. Ultimately, thoughtful emergency management initiatives that make the most efficient use of the health care system's scarce resources is central to local communities' management of future terrorist attacks.

REFERENCES

1. Long D. *The Anatomy of Terrorism.* New York: Free Press; 1990.
2. Parachini J. Comparing motives and outcomes of mass casualty terrorism involving conventional and unconventional weapons. *Stud Conflict Terrorism.* 2001;24:389–406.
3. Legal Information Institute. *U.S. Code Collection, Title 22, Chapter 38: § 2656 f. Annual Country Reports on Terrorism.* September 20, 2004, Available at, http://www4.law.cornell.edu/uscode/22/2656f.html.
4. U.S. Department of Homeland Security. *Statement by the Department of Homeland Security on Continued Al-Qaeda Threats.* November 21, 2003, Available at, http://www.dhs.gov/dhspublic/display?content=3017.
5. Hoffman B. Change and continuity in terrorism. *Stud Conflict Terrorism.* 2001;24:417–428.
6. Kuh S, Hauer J. The threat of biological terrorism in the new millennium. *Am Behav Scientist.* 2001;44(6):1032–1041.
7. Sidel V, Levy B. Biological weapons. In: Levy B, Sidel V, eds. *Terrorism and Public Health: A Balanced Approach to Strengthening Systems and Protecting People.* New York: Oxford University Press; 2003.
8. Spanjaard H, Khabib O. Chemical weapons. In: Levy B, Sidel V, eds. *Terrorism and Public Health: A Balanced Approach to Strengthening Systems and Protecting People.* New York: Oxford University Press; 2003.
9. Lillibridge SR. *Statement on Medical Responses to Terrorist Attacks.* Delivered September 22, 1999, before the House Committee on Government Reform, Subcommittee on National Security, Veterans Affairs, and International Relations. Available at: http://www.hhs.gov/asl/testify/t990922a.html.
10. Takafuji E, Johnson-Winegar A, Zajtchuk R. Medical challenges in chemical and biological defense for the 21st century. In: Zatjchuk R, Bellamy R, eds. *Textbook of Military Medicine.* Washington, DC: Office of the Surgeon General, U.S. Department of the Army; 1996.
11. Sutton P, Gould R. Nuclear, radiological and related weapons. In: Levy B, Sidel V, eds. *Terrorism and Public Health: A Balanced Approach to Strengthening Systems and Protecting People.* New York: Oxford University Press; 2003.
12. Fisher M, Johnson R. IAEA incident and trafficking database and nuclear threat initiative. *The Washington Post.* December 5, 2013.
13. Gillmore Commission. *Forging America's New Normalcy: Securing Our Homeland, Preserving Our Liberty. The Fifth Annual Report to the President and the Congress of the Advisory Panel to Assess Domestic Response Capabilities for Terrorism Involving Weapons of Mass Destruction.* December 15, 2003, Available at, http://www.rand.org/nsrd/terrpanel/.
14. Boshoff H, Botha A, Schonteich M. *Fear in the city: urban terrorism in South Africa, Monograph 63.* Institute for Security Studies. Available at: http://www.iss.co.za/Pubs/Monographs/No63/CONTENT63.HTML.
15. Cukier W, Chapdelaine A. Small arms, explosive and incendiaries. In: Levy B, Sidel V, eds. *Terrorism and Public Health: A Balanced Approach to Strengthening Systems and Protecting People.* New York: Oxford University Press; 2003.
16. McCarthy M. Attacks provide the first major test of USA's national anti-terrorist medical response plans. *Lancet.* 2001;358:941.
17. Christen HT, Walker R. Weapons of mass effect: explosives. In: Maniscalco PM, Christen HT, eds. *Understanding Terrorism and Managing the Consequences.* Upper Saddle River, NJ: Prentice Hall; 2002.
18. NPTC: Worldwide. IED targeting of first response personnel—tactics and indicators; 2012. Available at: https://publicintelligence.net/nctc-first-responder-ieds/.
19. *Weapons of Mass Destruction Incident Management/Unified Command.* Texas Engineering Extension Service; 2003. Available at, http://teexweb.tamu.edu/teex.cfm?pageid=training&area=teex&Division=ESTI&Course=154217&templateid=14&navdiv=ESTI.
20. Nacos BL. The terrorist calculus behind 9-11: a model for future terrorism? *Stud Conflict Terrorism.* 2003;26:1–16.
21. Williams C, Fessenden F, Huang J, Allert M. Mumbai attack sites. *New York Times.* 28 Aug. 2012, Web. 28 June 2014.
22. Lilja GP, Madsen MA, Overton J. Multiple casualty incidents. Available at: In: Kuehl AE, ed. *Prehospital Systems and Medical Oversight.* Dubuque, IA: Kendall/Hunt; 2002:821–827.
23. Kurth Cronin A. *Terrorists and Suicide Attacks. Congressional Research Service.* Report # RL32058, August 28, 2003. Available at, http://www.fas.org/irp/crs/RL32058.pdf.
24. Mintz Y, Shapira SC, Pikarsky AJ, et al. The experience of one institution dealing with terror: the El Aqsa Intifada riots. *Isr Med Assoc J.* 2002;4: 554–556.
25. Hoffman B. Terrorism and counterterrorism after September 11th. *US Foreign Policy Agenda: An Electronic Journal of the US Department of State.* November 2001;6(3).

26. The National Commission on Terrorist Attacks upon the United States. *The 9/11 Commission Report.* Washington, DC: WW Norton; 2004.

27. Dugger C. Victims of '93 Bombay terror wary of U.S. motives. Available at: *New York Times.* September, 24, 2001.

28. Hoffman B. Responding to Terrorism Across the Technological Spectrum. *Strategic Studies Instate Conference Series;* Carlisle Barracks, PA: U.S. Army War College; April 1994.

29. Bone J, Road A. Terror by degree. *Times Magazine (London).* October 18, 1997.

30. Rayner G, Gardham D. Cargo plane bomb plot: ink cartridge bomb "timed to blow up over US." *The Telegraph* Nov, 10, 2010.

31. U.S. Department of State. *Patterns of Global Terrorism, 1983–2001.* 2002.

32. Pape R. *The Strategic Logic of Suicide Terrorism.* Unpublished manuscript; February 18, 2003.

33. National Counterterrorism Center. *Annex of Statistical Information.* U.S. Department of State; 31 July 2012.

34. Myhrvold N. *Strategic Terrorism: A Call to Action.* Lawfare Research Paper No. 2-2013; July 3, 2013.

35. Jenkins B. *The Likelihood of Nuclear Terrorism.* Santa Monica, Calif: The RAND Corporation; 1985 P-7119:6.

36. Anon. Make a bomb in the kitchen of your mom. *Inspire.* 2010;1:13.

37. Mascrop A. Mass hysteria the main threat from bioweapons. *BMJ.* 2001;323:2–5.

38. CBS News. *A Look Back at the Norway Massacre.* CBS Interactive; 18 Feb. 2013.

39. Bergen P. U.S. right wing extremists more deadly than jihadists. *Cable News Network.* 01 Jan. 1970.

40. Meyer M. *The Role of the Metropolitan Planning Organization (MPO) in Preparing for Security Incidents and Transportation System Response.* U.S. Department of Transportation, Federal Highway Administration, Transportation Capacity Building Program. Available at: http://www.planning.dot.gov/Documents/Securitypaper.doc.

41. Stein M, Hershberg A. Medical consequences of terrorism. *Surg Clin North Am.* 1999;79:1537–1552.

42. Abenhaim L, Dab W, Salmi LR. Study of civilian victims of terrorist attacks (France 1982–1987). *J Clin Epidemiol.* 1992;45:103–109.

43. Hoffman B. The leadership secrets of Osama bin Laden: the terrorist as CEO. *Atlantic Monthly.* April 2003; Available at: http://www.theatlantic.com/doc/print/200304/hoffman.

44. START. *Al-Shabaab Attack on Westgate Mall in Kenya. National Consortium for the Study of Terrorism and Responses to Terrorism. Background Report.* Available at: http://www.start.umd.edu/sites/default/files/publications/local_attachments/STARTBackgroundReport_alShabaabKenya_Sept2013.pdf.

45. National Counterterrorism Center. *Annex of Statistical Information.* U.S. Department of State; 31 July 2012, Web. 28 June 2014.

46. Dolnik A. Die and let die: exploring links between suicide terrorism and terrorist use of chemical, biological, radiological and nuclear weapons. *Stud Conflict Terrorism.* 2003;26:17–35.

47. Wheelis M. Biological warfare at the 1346 Siege of Caffa. *Emerg Infect Dis.* 2002;8(9).

48. Shapira S, Mor-Yosef S. Terror politics and medicine: the role of leadership. *Stud Conflict Terrorism.* 2004;27:65–71.

49. Shah J. Nurses presence of mind saved many lives at Cama hospital. *The Indian Express.* 04 Dec. 2008, Web. 28 June 2014.

50. Associated Press. Al-Qaeda branch in Yemen regrets hospital attack. *New York Times.* 22 Dec. 2013, Web. 28 June 2014.

51. Shapira SC, Shemer J. Medical management of terrorist attacks. *Isr Med Assoc J.* 2002;4:489–492.

52. Garwin RL. Nuclear and biological megaterrorism. In: *International Seminar of Planetary Emergencies.* Federation of American Scientists; 2002, 21 Aug. 2002. Web. 28 June 2014.

53. Lesser I, Hoffman B, Arquilla D, et al. *Countering the New Terrorism.* Santa Monica, Calif: The RAND Corporation; 1999.

54. Hoffman B. Al-Qaeda, trends in terrorism, and future potentialities: an assessment. *Stud Conflict Terrorism.* 2003;26:429–442.

68 | CHAPTER

Active-Shooter Response

David W. Callaway and James P. Phillips

The term *active shooter* first entered the medical lexicon after the 1999 Columbine school shootings. A variety of definitions exist for active-shooter events (ASE) and active-shooter and mass-casualty incidents (AS/MCI). An *ASE* is defined as an individual actively engaged in killing or attempting to kill people in a confined and populated area at the time of first responder activation.[1] The term *ASE* is primarily used in the research literature to describe shooting events that may not have resulted in mass casualties, and it excludes gang-related violence. When the ASE injures or kills multiple victims, the scenario becomes an AS/MCI. The distinction between ASE and AS/MCI is relevant in regard to evaluation of the existing literature, but the differences have less operational importance.

The incidence of AS/MCI in the United States varies based upon the definition. The New York Police Department (NYPD) reports 284 ASE from 1996 to 2012.[1] In an FBI-sponsored examination of 110 ASE from 2000 to 2010, Blair noted that ASE occur primarily at businesses (37%), schools (34%), and public outdoor venues (17%). The primary weapons used are pistols (60%), rifles (27%), and shotguns (10%). However, in more than 40% of ASE, the perpetrator used multiple weapons, and in 2% of cases they deployed improvised explosive devices (IEDs).[2]

According to the FBI, the average ASE lasts 12 minutes, and 37% last less than 5 minutes. The study notes average law enforcement (LE) response time was approximately 3 minutes, and a majority of incidents had first LE on scene within 6 minutes. In 20% of the cases, the shooter changes location and in 51% to 57% of the incidents, the violence is ongoing at the time of LE arrival. A majority of ongoing events end within minutes of LE arrival. According to the NYPD, more than 80% of ASE end violently with perpetrator suicide or attempted suicide (40% to 49%) or applied force by LE (17% killed and 34% arrested).[2]

Across ASE in the United States, the median number of victims shot is four, with two being killed (range 0 to 32). Penetrating trauma is obviously the most common cause of injury; however, with the increased use of IEDs and of fire as a weapon, responders must be prepared for high-acuity, complex-trauma patients. These statistics allow planners to assess generalities about AS/MCI. However, most critical is that ASE and AS/MCI are becoming increasingly frequent, complex, and deadly (Fig. 68-1).

HISTORICAL PERSPECTIVE

Columbine represented many of the challenges of AS/MCI: multiple assailants, use of multiple IEDs, potential targeting of first responders, prolonged staging of LE and medical response units, and communication gaps. Columbine resulted in a paradigm shift in LE response to AS incidents. However, emergency medical services (EMS) and fire

department response did not significantly change in the subsequent decade. ASE response is a multiagency process. The increased frequency of high-profile ASE from 2007 to 2014 (e.g., Virginia Tech, Fort Hood Attack, Century Theater, and Sandy Hook) created a heightened sense of urgency and inspired a concerted effort to improve multi-agency ASE response. Throughout this process, it is vital that leaders examine recent international attacks (e.g., Mumbai [2008], Norway [2011], and Nairobi [2013]) when creating response plans. At minimum, plans should address the worst-case scenario (e.g., multiple assailants, multiple jurisdictions involved, and a prolonged dynamic event with multiple weapon systems deployed during a period of high-volume, routine medical requirements) and the most common scenario (e.g., single shooter who remains at a single location and creates an MCI, but dies upon initial police contact).

CURRENT PRACTICE

Pre-Incident Actions
Mitigation

The most effective way to minimize the morbidity and mortality of a mass shooting is to prevent the event from taking place. Prevention is primarily an LE issue, but also a tenet of psychological care. The adage states, "The best defense is a good offense," and it applies to many aspects of crime prevention. We live in a time when firearms are ubiquitous in the United States and many other countries; 2010 National Rifle Association estimates show that approximately 300 million firearms are currently owned in the United States.[3] Firearm ownership is protected by the Constitution of the United States of America, and gun control laws that modify this right have been a cause for debate for decades, and they are beyond the scope of this chapter. Instead, mitigation to reduce casualties must focus on prevention of firearm ownership by potential shooters, aiding LE efforts to find and contain threats before they take action, and to enhance a facility's ability to deter gun violence.

Profiling the Active Shooter

Research into profiling mass-casualty shooters has proven disappointing. Ideally, patterns or precursors could be identified that would serve as a "red flag" that a person is a threat to carry out such an attack. Important academic work has been done in the area of multiple-casualty violence. However, there remains no specific profile of rampage shooters because of the limited number of events to study.[4] Much effort has been put forth to identify such patterns in serial killers, helping to identify sociopaths early to allow attempts at intervention. Meanwhile, the mental health community has identified only vague similarities in the lives of those who go on to become active shooters, including a tendency to be white males with significant life stressors

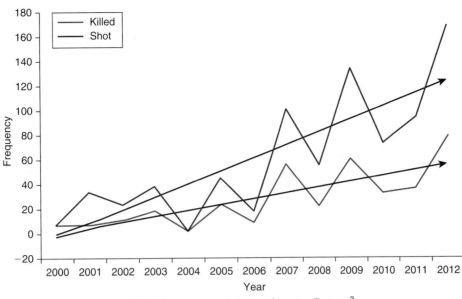

FIG 68-1 Frequency of Active-Shooter Events.[2]

and variable degrees of psychiatric illness.[5] These traits hardly narrow down the American population to a manageable number, and this paucity of unique traits makes profiling the active shooter very difficult. Because of this, families, friends, mental health professionals, and coworkers are likely to be the best source of information to LE regarding potential threats. Verbal threats, social media posts, and accumulation of firearms and ammunition should be taken seriously and reported to authorities for investigation. Lt. Dan Marcou has theorized five phases of ASE in an effort to aid LE intervention.[6] The first four phases, if recognized, could allow police to prevent an attack (Box 68-1).

Target Hardening

The concepts of crime prevention through environmental design (CPTED) and target hardening involve designing structures and spaces and implementing features that make those places less vulnerable to attack or theft.[7] Active shooters in general choose targets that are considered "soft" or easy to attack because of lack of defenses such as secure access points, armed guards, metal detectors, or other means of prevention.[8] Schools such as Virginia Tech University, Columbine High School, and Sandy Hook Elementary School in Connecticut are prime examples. Implementation of hardening features serves as a deterrent to attack and should be considered (Box 68-2).

Hazard Vulnerability Analysis

When planning for disasters and adverse events, performing a hazard vulnerability analysis (HVA) is a valuable tool that allows a planner to determine the most appropriate delegation of limited resources to plan

for hazards with variable levels of probability of occurrence and defensibility. Typically, an HVA is structured to allow the facility to determine which types of events it is most likely to encounter (e.g., earthquakes in San Francisco) and to which it is most vulnerable. Using these calculated likelihoods, agencies can devote appropriate means to protect against certain events. Workplace and school firearm violence should be considered in the HVA for any facility, and the result includes the allocation of funds and time devoted to the mitigation and response to an ASE. Hospitals, and specifically emergency departments, should also include the rapid influx of multiple gunshot wound patients as part of their annual surge capacity training and equipment procurement.

Public Education Drills

The Department of Homeland Security (DHS) and other organizations have developed educational programs designed to educate the public on how to protect themselves during an ASE.[9] The basis for all of these programs is the three options of escape, hide, or fight back. These concepts have been promoted online by an educational video from the city of Houston, Texas, in 2012, titled, Run. Hide. Fight.[10] The essence of the training is to immediately remove oneself from the danger area, as soon as shooting begins. If this is not possible, hide in a secure, protected, locked place in an attempt to deter the shooter. Lastly, and only if confronted with imminent danger, take action against the shooter to subdue him or her. Understanding these concepts is likely to help save lives in future events.

Active-shooter drills are also a critical aspect of preparation. The DHS and others recommend annual workplace violence drills for schools and workplaces.[11–13] ASE are extremely uncommon; there are more people injured by lightning strikes annually than by mass-casualty shooting incidents.[14,15] However, the complexity and frequency of ASE appear to be trending upward (Fig. 68-1). The relatively low-frequency, high-consequence nature of ASE suggests the need for ongoing, integrated all-hazards training for high-threat response. In times of stress, we do not rise to the occasion; we fall to the level of our training.

Schools, workplaces, and public spaces should also develop an active-shooter protocol in the unlikely event that such an incident takes place there. This should include implementation of procedures to keep students and citizens safe. Most commonly this involves immediate notification (public announcement, phone text alerts, auto-calls, etc.), lockdown procedures, evacuation, reaction by on-scene security, notification of LE, and request for prehospital EMS response. In addition, new training programs have been developed for security personnel, including from the DHS and the National Association of School Resource Officers.[11,16] The manner in which police forces respond has undergone sweeping changes, and the adaptation of EMS response into an unsecured tactical environment continues to evolve.[17]

Law Enforcement and Emergency Medical Services Preparation

The massacre at Columbine High School in Colorado in 1999 was the seminal event leading to a paradigm shift in response to ASE. Prior to this attack, police tactics focused on the concept of shooters-as-hostage-takers who are barricaded, not as mass murderers without demands. The traditional response was based on the "Five Cs" of contain, control, communicate, call SWAT, and come up with tentative plan.[18] At Columbine the shooting took place for approximately 45 minutes with no LE entry, despite uniformed officers being on scene very quickly. As SWAT finally entered the building, the shooters killed themselves simultaneously. Following this, training shifted away from containment and negotiation tactics toward immediate response teams of two to four regular service officers making entry with a goal of immediately neutralizing the shooter(s).[6,18]

EMS response has also been identified as a critical area in need of reformatted training to deal with ASE. A tenet of EMS training is the concept of scene safety; standing policy in most jurisdictions is that EMS personnel do not enter scenes that have not been declared secure. Because of the chaos, police must often engage in a systematic search of the attack site before the scene can be declared secure, which may take hours to complete. As seen with the 2013 TSA shooting at Los Angeles International Airport, where a wounded agent hemorrhaged to death for 30 minutes while traditional EMS staged just yards away in the safe zone, the ability to enter and provide medical treatment in an unsecure scene could mean the difference between life and death.[19]

This incident and others like it call for enhanced training of paramedics, in conjunction with LE teams, to provide lifesaving medical treatment within, and evacuation from, unsafe scenes. This requires EMS workers to learn tactics and be properly equipped to enter potentially dangerous sites, under police cover, to render aid to victims. This training includes the use of specialized prehospital medical techniques, adopted from military medic training, for use in the civilian world. Tactical Emergency Casualty Care (TECC) is a training concept adapted for the urban, noncombat environment, derived from the highly effective military program Tactical Combat Casualty Care (TCCC).[17,20]

TCCC, currently taught to military medics, has helped to reduce the preventable-combat-death rate to the lowest of any period of conflict in American history.[21]

To be effective, event drills should include all agencies that would respond in a real-world situation. ASE, hostage situations, and other criminal activities with medical casualties have at their core a need for a combined response from police and EMS. Performing well-planned, multiagency active-shooter drills not only tests the protocols put in place but also allows individuals to interact and become familiar with members of other teams. This undoubtedly leads to better coordination and teamwork. Ideally, the first time these agencies work together should not be during a real event.[22]

Hospital Preparedness

The prehospital preparation for ASE has evolved dramatically over the last two decades. Within the hospital environment, an all-hazards approach to disaster response should be modified to also include a large influx of complex, mixed penetrating-trauma victims. For trauma centers, this is likely not much different than the current surge capacity plans for mass-casualty incidents with heavy surgical needs, such as explosions and multiple vehicle crashes. Nontrauma centers should consider being additionally prepared for simultaneous arrival of multiple unstable gunshot victims brought to the emergency room (ER) for stabilization prior to transfer. Recommendations include mass-casualty drills with victims of projectile injuries, procurement of equipment such as intraosseous access devices and rapid infusers, as well as having readily available tourniquets in the emergency department for application prior to transfer.

Post-Incident Actions

For the purposes of this chapter, the post-incident actions are divided into prehospital and hospital response. In reality, these processes will be executed concurrently.

Prehospital

In active violent incidents such as ASE, responders must rapidly transition from routine to high-threat operations. The initial 5 minutes of response are dynamic and disorganized; however, they are not "chaos." Certain events can be expected (e.g., elevated external threat to life, delayed and conflicting information, high volumes of anxious but non-injured individuals, and highly charged emotions), which require an aggressive yet flexible mission-oriented mind-set that is best developed through extensive interagency training.

The utilization of the Incident Command System (ICS) and Unified Command (UC) is recommended to organize and control the multiagency response.[23] However, given the short time frame in which most of these events develop, agencies must be able to respond dynamically while the UC is being established. LE officers are universally first on scene for ASE. Moreover, even though the initial tactical response is an LE operation, EMS/Fire must be rapidly integrated in order to minimize loss of life. The goals of response are to minimize potentially preventable deaths by mitigating the threat and effectively reducing the distance between casualty and medical provider.

The immediate response can be broken down conceptually into two mission profiles: *stop the killing* and *stop the dying*. Since 2000, LE officers have been trained to rapidly enter the scene and neutralize the shooter(s) in order to stop the killing. Existing data support the rapid entry technique.[1,2,13] With the advent of the TECC guidelines, national efforts are now under way to train LE officers to assist in *stopping the dying* through the application of essential lifesaving interventions such as tourniquet application.[17,22] Appropriate LE application of tourniquets in AS/MCI should be considered standard of care.[17,22,24] The

American College of Surgeons recommends utilization of the acronym THREAT (Threat suppression, Hemorrhage control, Rapid Evacuation to safety, Assessment by medical providers, Transport to definitive care) to reinforce and train the TECC principles.[25]

Historically, EMS/Fire have used the "stage and wait" strategy until LE officers declare the scene secure. This is no longer a tenable operational strategy. As mentioned above, EMS/Fire rescue teams are increasingly expected to assume greater risk and operate in the warm/indirect-threat zone. This expectation should not be taken lightly and proper tactics, techniques, and procedures (TTPs) should be in place to limit unnecessary loss of life. Multiple-risk mitigation strategies exist, and it is incumbent upon leaders to develop a response plan, properly equip their teams, and adequately train the new paradigm.

Traditional models of prehospital trauma care have limited application in high-threat response secondary to several assumptions, including that care begins with patient contact, that patient care is the only operational concern, and that penetrating and blunt trauma are similarly managed. Prehospital care in the high-threat environment such as an ASE requires responders to perform four broad tasks: access, assessment, stabilization, and evacuation of the casualty.

Access is a critical task often overlooked in planning and training. FBI data on ASE suggest that a majority of events end within minutes of LE arrival and contact with the perpetrator. Anecdotally, this is supported by review of events in Platte Canyon (2006), Virginia Tech (2007), and Sandy Hook (2012) (personal communication). The tactical situation determines the barriers to and components of each phase of care. Examples of barriers to access include padlocked doors, ongoing violent attack, IEDs, building layout, fire, and high volume of minimally wounded or noninjured civilians.

Responding teams should immediately perform a rapid risk assessment and initiate an appropriate interagency response. It is critical to note that most AS/MCI end upon initial LE contact, but that the scene is rarely declared secure. "Scene safety" remains an important concept for response. However, traditional practices of "staging and waiting" until LE officers have declared the scene clear are no longer standard of care. Agencies must develop integrated response standard operating procedures (SOPs) for operating in warm or indirect-threat zones (i.e., areas where there exist ongoing, though not imminent, threats to the health and safety of the victim and responder).

A variety of indirect-threat and warm zone operational models exist to shorten the distance between first responders and the victims of AS/MCI. In general, the response paradigms can be classified into *escorted care* or creation of *evacuation corridors*. The prime example of escorted care is the Rescue Task Force (RTF) model, pioneered in Arlington, Virginia. The RTF is composed of specially trained advanced life support (ALS) providers (note: these are not tactical medical personnel) who are provided ballistic PPE and escorted into the warm zone by armed LE officers. Their primary mission is rapid access, assessment, provision of appropriate lifesaving intervention, and rapid extraction of victims.[18] Alternatively, in the Evacuation Corridor model used in other regions, LE officers preliminarily clear immediate threats, creating "warm corridors" and allowing unescorted EMS/Fire to access and extract victims.

Assessment and stabilization should be performed based upon the principles of TECC. The tactical situation and provider qualifications influence the assessment and stabilization phase. In general, rapid control of potentially life-threatening extremity hemorrhage and rapid evacuation are critical. The TECC guidelines are acknowledged as the standard of care principles for response to high-threat events such as AS/MCI.[23,26] The TECC guidelines outline combined medical and operational response principles to reduce potentially preventable causes of death. TECC organizes response into three dynamic threat-based categories: direct-threat, indirect-threat, and evacuation or secure zone. The primary goals during direct- and indirect-threat care are threat mitigation, rapid hemorrhage control, and rapid evacuation.

Despite limited comprehensive data, traumatic hemorrhage is the major cause of death in AS/MCI. Properly applied tourniquets are proven to reduce morbidity and mortality from penetrating extremity trauma.[27–29] TECC guidelines recommend that all first responders, including LE personnel, be trained to use tourniquets aggressively for any potentially life-threatening extremity hemorrhage. Military data suggest that tension pneumothoraces and airway obstructions are the other top-two causes of potentially preventable death in high-threat combat scenarios.[21] There are no corresponding civilian data that confirm similar wounding and mortality patterns. However, given the lack of PPE on most victims of civilian AS/MCI, providers can expect a high volume of penetrating torso trauma.[30]

Triage is a dynamic process that includes an initial sorting of patients, generally during the indirect-threat or evacuation phase of TECC. Regardless of the triage technique (e.g., START, SMART, and SALT), certain universal principles apply in ASE. First, security is paramount. First responders are frequent targets in AS/MCI internationally and increasingly within the United States. Armed LEO should tightly control access to the triage site and triage personnel. All casualties, victims, and bystanders should be searched for weapons or explosive devices prior to being allowed into the triage area. Crowd control is essential and, if absent, can impede proper triage, patient stabilization, and evacuation. Second, conventional MCI-triage tools may initially categorize torso gunshot victims as "green" because they can ambulate. Frequent reassessment is critical, and MCI-triage tools should never trump common-sense clinical decision making. Finally, as triage may occur at several casualty collection points (CCP), communication is paramount for proper patient tracking and resource allocation.

Evacuation is a tiered process in ASE response. Rapid extraction from the direct-threat zone and expeditious transportation to definitive care is critical for casualty survival in AS/MCI. Evacuation includes movement from point of injury to a casualty collection point or evacuation platform (e.g., ambulance or patrol car) and transportation to first-receiving facility. First responders should be trained on proper operational-rescue and casualty-movement techniques. In general, EMS/Fire should initiate damage-control resuscitation (DCR) strategies during transport, which include mechanical hemorrhage control, normotensive or hypotensive resuscitation, hypothermia prevention, and other conventional advanced trauma life support (ATLS) interventions. EMS providers should limit time on scene and, as possible, conduct interventions during transport.

Use of unconventional, nonmedical transport may have a role as an alternate or contingency evacuation platform in AS/MCI. In the initial 30 minutes after the 2012 Century Theater shooting, LE transported 75% (18/24) of the victims to first-receiving facilities with 100% survival.[31] Data from Philadelphia also support selective LE transport with shortened transport times and improved survival for urban gunshot and stabbing victims.[32] Local leaders should determine, via an HVA and gap analysis, whether LE officers and patrol car-based casualty transport will be the primary, alternate, contingency, or emergency (PACE) evacuation platform.

Hospital

Hospitals and health care systems should immediately activate their Hospital Incident Command Center (HICC) on notification of a community AS/MCI. All area hospitals, not just the primary receiving facility, should immediately increase their security posture if there is an AS/MCI in their community. Hospitals are considered a soft target by perpetrators and are known to be a critical component of community response to AS/MCI. Security should initiate controlled-access procedures, assist with searching and clearing of victims, coordinate with local LEO, and provide heightened presence at points of entry to the facility. The public information officer (PIO) should be engaged early in the process and should have experience with handling LE investigations. There will be a huge demand for information. Medical staff should be instructed to follow proper communication procedures, refrain from any use of social medial platforms, and rigorously abide by HIPAA regulations. The PIO should ensure that communication requests do not interfere with providers' ability to care for patients. Communication protocols should plan for loss of cellular phone communication.

AS/MCI events result in a predominance of high-acuity penetrating trauma with overwhelming onsite mortality. Victims may present with orthopedic injuries sustained while fleeing, cardiopulmonary complaints, and severe stress reactions as seen after the 2013 Washington, DC, Navy Yard Shooting (personal communication with hospital and first responders). MCI protocols should be activated, emergency departments cleared, and operating theaters prepped. Note that standard MCI discharge policies may need revision; regardless of complaint, patients may have some reluctance to leave the emergency department (ED) in the aftermath of an ongoing AS/MCI. Research on postbombing events demonstrates a multiple-surge phenomenon where high volumes of low-acuity patients self-present early to local hospitals, overwhelming resources.[33,34] There are no data to support this observation in AS/MCI. More recent information from the terrorist attacks in Aurora and Boston suggest that in AS/MCI, the first-receiving facility should be prepared for a continuous surge of mixed-acuity patients.[35]

Immediate resuscitative care should focus on DCR, mechanical hemorrhage control, balanced blood-product administration for those with hemorrhagic shock, tranexamic acid per protocols, and early operative intervention as needed. Early communication with ancillary services such as the blood bank, patient transportation, and radiology is critical, especially in the setting of restricted access activation. Although infrequent domestically, the concurrent use of IEDs in ASE is increasing globally and should prompt first-receiving facilities to plan for multiple, highly complex-trauma patients.

AS/MCI events frequently occur in small to mid-sized communities and affect people with little exposure to violence. Beyond victims and their families, the psychological toll on first responders, medical providers, and staff can be immense. It is critical that hospitals integrate staff debriefings and early mental health counseling into their response plans.

💡 UNIQUE CONSIDERATIONS

1. AS/MCI events present an active and presumed ongoing threat. Providers should expect ongoing shooting, multiple IEDs, and specific targeting of responders.
2. For first responders, situational awareness is paramount. There may be multiple shooters as was seen in Columbine and the Kenya Westgate Mall attack.[36] Perpetrators may try to escape disguised as victims or choose to take hostages when confronted by LE.
3. ASE are not unique to the United States. Such attacks can occur anywhere firearms are available, as evidenced by the recent high-profile attacks in Kenya, Mumbai, and Norway. In fact, the deadliest mass shooting in history took place on the island of Utøya in 2011, with 69 killed and 110 injured.[36,37]
4. First responders must effectively transition from routine to high-threat operations: traditional EMS "stage and wait" protocols are being replaced by warm or indirect-threat-zone operations.

5. There is an increased requirement for dynamic interagency coordination in the prehospital setting.
6. The shooter(s) may end up as patients in your ambulance or ER, which may cause ethical and security concerns. Plan accordingly.
7. Hospital shootings do occur, but most are targeted, and not random acts of violence; a protocol to address this should be in place for the ER and hospital in general.[38]

⚠ PITFALLS

- General
  - Loss of situational awareness and hyper-focus on initial event leading to vulnerability to ongoing or additional threats
  - Failure to rapidly retriage initially low-priority "greens"
  - Failure to plan, perform, and sustain interagency training for dynamic, high-threat AS/MCI
  - Failure to properly supply first responders with appropriate trauma-response equipment
  - Failure to train LE personnel in AS response including basic trauma management, specifically, hemorrhage control
- Prehospital
  - Failure to aggressively engage the ongoing threat[39]
  - Failure to transition to high-threat medical principles detailed by the TECC guidelines
  - Failure to secure triage points and evacuation routes
  - Failure to perform aggressive early hemorrhage control, including use of tourniquets
  - Failure to rapidly evacuate casualties to appropriate receiving facilities
- Hospital
  - Failure to enact appropriate security measures
  - Failure to train staff in active-shooter response, including patient care
  - Failure to plan for mixed adult and pediatric trauma surge
  - Failure to develop and implement surge plan for blood-product use (e.g., PRBC, FFP, and platelets)
  - Failure to perform regular HVA and to address gaps related to active violent incidents

REFERENCES

1. New York Police Department. *Active shooter: recommendations and analysis for risk mitigation*; Dec. 2012. Retrieved Sept. 24, 2013, from, www.nypdshield.org/public/SiteFiles/documents/Activeshooter.pdf.
2. Blair JP, Martaindale MH. *United States active shooter events from 2000 to 2010: Training and equipment implications*; 2013. Alerrt.org. Retrieved Oct. 15, 2013, from, http://alerrt.org/files/research/ActiveShooterEvents.pdf.
3. Anonymous. national-rifle-association-nra-statistics [Internet]. [cited 2014 Feb 11]. Available from: http://www.statisticbrain.com/national-rifle-association-nra-statistics/. Accessed Feb 9, 2014.
4. Paparazzo J, Eith C, Tocco J. *Strategic Approaches to Preventing Multiple Casualty Violence: Report on the National Summit on Multiple Casualty Shootings.* Washington, DC: U.S. Department of Justice, Office of Community Oriented Policing Services; 2013.
5. Schweit KW. *Addressing the Problem of the Active Shooter.* Available at: *FBI Law Enforcement Bulletin*; 2013. http://www.fbi.gov/stats-services/publications/law-enforcement-bulletin/2013/May/active-shooter [Accessed February 2, 2014].
6. Marcou D. *5 Phases of the Active Shooter Incident*; 2007 Oct 1. Available from: http://www.policeone.com/active-shooter/articles/1672491–5-Phases-of-the-Active-Shooter-Incident/.
7. Atlas RI. *21st Century Security and CPTED.* Boca Raton: CRC Press; 2013, Print.

8. Rivera L. Active shooter's incidents. Retrieved September 12, 2013, from, http://www.endesastres.org/files/Active_Shooter_Incident_FINAL.pdf; 2007.

9. Security UDOH. active_shooter_booklet.pdf [Internet]. 2008 [cited 2013 Sep 15]. Available from: http://www.dhs.gov/xlibrary/assets/active_shooter_booklet.pdf.

10. Run. Hide. Fight. [Internet]. Readyhoustontx.gov. Houston; 2012 [cited 2014 Feb 1]. Available from: http://www.readyhoustontx.gov/trans-runhidefight.html.

11. DHS. active-shooter-preparedness [Internet]. [cited 2014 Feb 11]. Available from: http://www.dhs.gov/active-shooter-preparedness.

12. Badzmierowski WF. *11 Steps to Improve Workplace Violence Prevention Policies [Internet]. campussafetymagazine.com*; 2011. [cited 2014 Feb 13]. Available from, http://www.campussafetymagazine.com/channel/public-safety/articles/2011/04/11-steps-to-better-workplace-violence-prevention-policies.aspx.

13. Columbine Review Commission. The Report of Governor Bill Owens' Columbine Review Commission. May 2001.

14. Davis C, Engeln A, Johnson E, et al. *Wilderness Medical Society Practice Guidelines for the Prevention and Treatment of Lightning Injuries. WEM.* Elsevier Inc; 2012 Sep 1 23(3):260–269.

15. No increase in mass shootings [Internet]. Boston.com. 2012 [cited 2014 Feb 13]. Available from: http://boston.com/community/blogs/crime_punishment/2012/08/no_increase_in_mass_shootings.html.

16. NASRO. SRO Active Shooter Response Training Course [Internet]. nasro.org. [cited 2014 Feb 13]. Available from: http://www.nasro.org/content/sro-active-shooter-response.

17. Callaway DW, Smith ER, Cain J, et al. Tactical Emergency Casualty Care (TECC): Guidelines for the Provision of Prehospital Trauma Care in High Threat Environments. *J Spec Oper Med.* 2011;11(3):104–122.

18. Smith ER. Supporting Paradigm Change in EMS' Operational Medical Response to Active Shooter Events. *JEMS.* 2013 Dec;13.

19. J K. TSA Officer Bled For 33 Minutes in LAX Shooting [Internet]. nbclosangeles.comnewslocal TSA-Officer-Bled-For–Minutes-In-LAX-Shooting-.html. [cited 2014 Jan 2]. Available from: http://www.nbclosangeles.com/news/local/TSA-Officer-Bled-For-33-Minutes-In-LAX-Shooting-232062361.html.

20. Butler FK, Haymann J, Butler EG. Tactical combat casualty care in special operations. *Mil Med.* 1996;161.

21. Butler FK, Blackbourne LH. Battlefield trauma care then and now: a decade of Tactical Combat Casualty Care. *J Trauma Acute Care Surg.* 2012 Dec;73(6 Suppl 5):S395–S402.

22. Jacobs LM, McSwain NE, Rotondo MF, et al. *Improving survival from active shooter events: the Hartford Consensus*; 2013, pp. 1399–1400.

23. Fire/Emergency Medical Services Department Operational Considerations and Guide for Active Shooter and Mass Casualty Incidents. U.S. Fire Administration. September 2013.

24. Doyle GS, Taillac PP. Tourniquets: a review of current use with proposals for expanded prehospital use. *Prehosp Emerg Care.* 2008;12(2):241–256, Apr-Jun.

25. Jacobs LM, McSwain NE Jr, Rotondo MF, et al. Joint Committee to Create a National Policy to Enhance Survivability from Mass Casualty Shooting Events. Improving survival from active shooter events: the Hartford Consensus. *J Trauma Acute Care Surg.* 2013 Jun;74(6):1399–1400.

26. International Association of Fire Fighters Position Statement: Rescue Task Force Training. http://www.iaff.org/Comm/PDFs/IAFF_RTF_Training_Position_Statement.pdf. Accessed January 10, 2014.

27. Kragh JF Jr, Walters TJ, Baer DG, et al. Practical use of emergency tourniquets to stop bleeding in major limb trauma. *J Trauma.* 2008 Feb;64(2 Suppl):S38–S49, discussion S49–S50.

28. Kragh JF Jr, Walters TJ, Baer DG, Fox CJ, Wade CE, Salinas J, et al. Survival with emergency tourniquet use to stop bleeding in major limb trauma. *Ann Surg.* 2009 Jan;249(1):1–7.

29. Beekley AC, Sebesta JA, Blackbourne LH, et al. 31st Combat Support Hospital Research Group. Prehospital tourniquet use in Operation Iraqi Freedom: effect on hemorrhage control and outcomes. *J Trauma.* 2008 Feb;64(2 Suppl):S28–S37, discussion S37.

30. Fierro MF. Mass murder in a university setting: analysis of the medical examiner's response. *Disaster Med Public Health Prep.* 2007 Sep;1(1 Suppl):S25–S30.

31. Aurora Fire Department. (n.d.) Century Theater shooting: Aurora Fire Department preliminary incident analysis. Retrieved Oct. 15, 2013, from www.auroragov.org/cs/groups/public/documents/document/015169.pdf.

32. Band RA, Salhi RA, Holena DN, Powell E, Branas CC, Carr BG. Severity-adjusted mortality in trauma patients transported by police. *Ann Emerg Med.* 2013 Dec 23;13:S0196–S0644, 01582-5.

33. Bloch YH, Leiba A, Veaacnin N, et al. Managing mild casualties in mass-casualty incidents: lessons learned from an aborted terrorist attack. *Prehosp Disaster Med.* 2007 May-Jun;22(3):181–185.

34. Teague DC. Mass casualties in the Oklahoma City bombing. *Clin Orthop Relat Res.* 2004 May;422:77–81, Review.

35. Mass shooting in Colorado: practice drills, disaster preparations key to successful emergency response. *ED Manag.* 2012 Oct;24(10):109–112.

36. Miller Erin. *Al-Shabaab Attack on Westgate Mall in Kenya*; 2013. September, http://www.start.umd.edu/sites/default/files/publications/local_attachments/STARTBackgroundReport_alShabaabKenya_Sept2013.pdf.

37. Sollid SJ, et al. Oslo government district bombing and Utoya island shooting July 22, 2011: the immediate prehospital emergency medical service.

38. Kellen GD, et al. Hospital-based shootings in the United States: 2000 to 2011. *Ann Emerg Med.* 2012 Sep 13;60(6):1–10.

39. Simmons J. *Rapid deployment as a response to an active shooter incident. Scribd.com*; 2003. Retrieved Oct. 15, 2013, from, www.scribd.com/doc/16693309/Rapid-Deployment-as-a-Response-to-an-Active-Incident.

Hostage Taking

Dale M. Molé and Rafael G. Cohen

DESCRIPTION OF EVENT

Since the beginning of recorded history, people have been abducted or held against their will for a variety of reasons. In ancient times, hostages, usually of noble birth, were exchanged to ensure compliance with treaty obligations. Hostage situations in early-American history helped shape both foreign and domestic policy. The plight of American sailors held hostage by Barbar North African states resulted in the Barbary Wars (1801-1805, 1815) and the birth of a permanent U.S. naval force. In 1859 the abolitionist, John Brown, and his followers took 12 hostages in a raid on the Federal Amory at Harper's Ferry. After failed negotiations, federal forces decided to attempt a rescue assault. Colonel Robert E. Lee ordered the Marines in the assault party to unload their rifles and affix bayonets, to lessen the chances of harm to the hostages. Not only were the hostages safely rescued and John Brown captured, but also Lee established the guiding principle for every future on-scene-commander, namely, choose the course of action that is most likely to save the greatest number of lives.[1] Brown's execution barely 2 months later made him a martyr for the antislavery movement, helping foment the American Civil War. From the 1979 Iran Hostage Crisis[2] to the 2002 Dubrovka Theater Crisis to the 2004 Beslan School Crisis, where over 1200 people were held hostage, kidnapping and hostage events continue to occur with increasing audacity.

Some kidnappings/hostage events are politically motivated; others involve simple greed. A few are just the result of being in the wrong place at the wrong time. A Dutch human rights group estimates at least 25,000 people were kidnapped worldwide in 2006. Over 90% of those incidents took place in the top-10 riskiest areas (Box 69-1).[3] According to the U.S. National Counterterrorism Center, in 2011 there were about 2500 kidnappings in Somalia alone.[4] The hijacking of the American-crewed *Maersk Alabama* in 2009, the first United States ship in almost 200 years to be captured by pirates, catapulted modern day piracy into the world news headlines.[5] The rise in kidnappings, hostage taking, and hijackings can be blamed on a combination of factors such as lawlessness, political unrest, and poverty. Kidnapping is an appealing crime for many because the perpetrators are rarely caught, and it is a much easier way to make money compared with drug dealing or robbery. The epidemic of kidnapping/hostage taking is much greater than demonstrated by statistics, because many kidnappings are handled privately and remain unreported.

In about 67% of cases, a ransom is paid, and it usually averages about $2,000,000 in countries where the "business" is well established. If a ransom is not paid, chances of survival for the victim are slim, especially in Latin America. According to insurance industry sources, Americans with kidnapping and ransom insurance are 4 times more likely to survive a kidnapping than are those who have none.

PRE-INCIDENT ACTIONS

Terrorists typically utilize one of three types of hostage scenarios: barricade hostage attacks, kidnapping, or air/land/sea hijackings. In a kidnapping, the location of the hostage(s) is generally not known, strengthening the perpetrator's negotiating position, while avoiding immediate confrontation with a rescue force. A barricade situation, where the location of the hostage(s) and perpetrator(s) is known, provides some advantage to rescue personnel; assuming one of the goals of the hostage takers is to survive. Air/land/sea hijackings are essentially a combination of the two because the terrorists have a mobile platform.[6]

Each year, the U.S. Federal Bureau of Investigation (FBI) is involved in approximately 400 domestic kidnappings, with about one third involving a ransom demand. Branch bank managers and their families appear to be favorite targets.[7] Some kidnapping/hostage taking occurs incidentally to the commission of another crime, with the victim being a target of opportunity for the perpetrator trying to negotiate his way out of a losing situation. Express kidnapping, where a victim is selected at random and held for hours or days and forced to withdraw money from financial accounts, is especially popular in the Third World and Latin America.[8] Because of their relatively short duration, express kidnappings do not require the planning (preattack surveillance, communications for ransom demands, etc.) or infrastructure (such as safe houses or guards) dictated by a traditional kidnapping. These low-budget kidnappings are more dangerous because they are carried out by small-time criminals or inexperienced kidnappers. If something unexpected happens during the abduction, the perpetrators are likely to panic and kill or harm the victim.[9]

With the growing threat of international terrorism and the increasing political value of American hostages, it is the official policy of the U.S. government not to make concessions to individuals or groups holding official or private U.S. citizens hostage. However, the United States will make use of every appropriate resource to ensure the release and safe return of American citizens. The goal is to deny the hostage takers the benefits of ransoms, prisoner releases, policy changes, or other acts of concession, which would increase the risk that other Americans would be taken hostage. The State Department will contact representatives of the captors in an effort to secure release.

Although very dangerous, hostage rescue is sometimes the only viable option. Local, state, and federal law enforcement agencies have specialized teams to rescue hostages or deal with standoff situations. These teams rely on training, speed, coordination, stealth, and overwhelming force to rescue hostages and take control of the situation.[10] The FBI's Hostage Rescue Team (HRT) was established in 1983, and it has been deployed hundreds of times in support of hostage rescue, counterterrorism, stopping violent crime, and other federal law enforcement activities.

POST-INCIDENT ACTIONS

Risk mitigation strategies are critical for individuals and organizations engaged in high-threat activities such as humanitarian aid, disaster response, development work, or security operations.

Individuals

Individuals should undergo basic security and safety training prior to traveling to high-threat regions. This training should cover situational awareness, avoidance of high-risk activities, lodging and travel recommendations, immediate actions, survival strategies, etc. In particular, medical aid workers in conflict or disaster areas should beware of roadblocks. The people controlling the roadblock may desire to extort money or other items of worth. If a person is working with a relief agency, they should ensure proper identification is available, and that they travel in a clearly marked vehicle. Vehicles painted in military colors should be avoided. If a roadblock is encountered, the personnel manning it may be aggressive, undisciplined, untrained, and intoxicated. Travelers should not make any aggressive movements or statements. They should be firm but polite, stating that the authorities have given them permission to travel in the area. If a person is an aid worker, he or she should establish his or her affiliation quickly because it is one of the greatest assets a traveler has.[11]

Survivors who have survived long hostage situations share similar advice. First, the hostage must maintain a positive attitude, a belief that he or she will return to freedom. The ordeal may be long, and seem impossible, but one must maintain faith. The hostage must acquire a sort of daily routine to keep the mind occupied, including a schedule for daily exercise, even if just stretching or moving limbs around. If previously religious, or a newly developed interest because of the situation, prayer may help. In Latin American and Muslim cultures, prayer times or even just the opportunity for prayer is viewed as an individual right that is respected. The hostage-taker may empathize with the hostage's need for prayer, thus establishing rapport. An additional tool to build rapport is casual conversation. That is, when the initial shock of the capture has subsided, the hostage should consider inquiring about the captor's name, his family, his likes and his beliefs.

Two excellent books that illustrate rapport-building in long-term captivities are *Out of Captivity*, by Marc Gonsalves et al., and *News of a Kidnapping*, by Gabriel Garcia Marquez. The first book is a personal recollection of three Americans held captive in Colombia for more than 5 years. The second, by Garcia Marquez, tells the stories of 10 notable Colombians who were kidnapped by Pablo Escobar during the late 1980s.

The two most dangerous times during a hostage situation are at the beginning and at the end, especially if a rescue is attempted. Hostages should help their kidnappers to establish contact with their family or organization as soon as possible. Initially, persons in a hostage situation should make themselves as inconspicuous as possible. They should listen to commands and respond without questioning. "Passive cooperation" should be enacted. Sudden movements or threatening behavior should be avoided, as well as eye contact or any other actions that may single a person out. Hostages should try to remain calm and remember the vast majority of kidnappings end with the hostages released. Death is usually the result of a medical condition, an unsuccessful escape attempt, or perhaps a botched rescue.

Organizations

Risk mitigation is critical. Organizations that operate in high-threat environments should have robust, well-practiced, and well-trained standard operating procedures regarding kidnapping. A majority of nongovernmental organizations (NGOs) have security officers on payroll to accomplish this requirement. The security officer is responsible for permission planning, threat analysis, staff training, site assessments, establishment of contact with local law enforcement/military as needed, and daily operations. For U.S. citizens, organizations should register individuals with the Department of State Smart Traveler Enrollment Program (STEP). In addition, the security officer should conduct safety assessments of lodging, common travel routes, and existing local political or criminal threats. Organizations should seriously investigate kidnapping and ransom (K&R) insurance for operations in semipermissive or high-threat areas. Registering staff with the relevant embassy and having immediate access to important contact information will help reduce the initial chaos that ensues after a kidnapping event.

Responding Agencies

The need for special law enforcement units grew out of the civil unrest in the United States in the 1960s. Tactical emergency medical services (TEMS) emerged as a special interest area within emergency medicine to provide medical services within a civilian law enforcement environment for both law enforcement personnel and suspects. Beyond increasing the chances of successful mission accomplishment, TEMS reduces the morbidity and mortality among innocent persons, suspects, and officers. Medical care in a tactical situation is frequently very different from the care provided by routine civilian emergency medical support (EMS). Richard Carmona and David Rasumoff conducted the first formal TEMS course in Los Angeles for law enforcement special operations units in Los Angeles in 1989.[12] In the 1990s, Frank Butler, a former Navy SEAL and Command Surgeon at the U.S. Special Operations Command, spearheaded a medical research project to improve combat trauma outcomes by optimizing care in the prehospital tactical envrionment.[13] This project gave birth to what is now called Tactical Combat Casualty Care (TCCC) in the military environment or Tactical Emergency Casualty Care (TECC) in the law enforcement environment (Table 69-1). The primary focus of TCCC/TECC is to quickly address the three most common causes of preventable death in a tactical situation: uncontrolled hemorrhage, airway compromise, and untreated tension pneumothorax.[14] A recent article summarizing data from the FBI Uniform Crime Report Law Enforcement Officers Killed and Assaulted for the years 1998-2007 suggests that there may be a larger percentage of preventable deaths from untreated tension pneumothorax than from uncontrolled hemorrhage in the typical law enforcement environment.[15]

Law enforcement agencies manage crisis situations with zones of containment. The inner perimeter is a geographically defined circle around an incident that is controlled by the tactical law enforcement element (i.e., special weapons and tactics teams, special response teams, and the like). The outer perimeter is a larger boundary that excludes the

TABLE 69-1	Focused TECC Training for Rescue Force Operators		
	MEDICAL TRAINING AND QUALIFICATIONS	**LIFESAVING INTERVENTIONS**	**KIT**
All operators	Direct and indirect threat care Recognized preventable causes of death	Tourniquets Hemostatic and pressure dressings Airway adjuncts Chest seals	Individual first aid kit (IFAK)
Operator-medics	All phases of TECC EMT training recommended	All above Needle decompression* Bag-valve-mask ventilation Supraglottic airways	Medical aid bag Soft or semirigid litters
Tactical medic (TEMS Provider)	TECC ALS, others Paramedic or higher	All of the above Advanced airway management IV therapy and fluid resuscitation Pain management Extended care (antibiotic and burn management)	Safety gear similar to operator's (helmets, vests, etc.) Advanced aid bags Modified vehicle equipment, etc.

*Requires approval by medical direction.

public, provides additional safety, and is controlled by patrol or regular uniformed officers.

Similarly, zones of care (i.e., hot, warm, and cold zones) help define appropriate care in a law enforcement or high-threat response environment. The *hot zone* or *inner perimeter* includes those areas where the threat to safety is direct and immediate and the threat for additional injury is high. Examples of hot zones include the area surrounding a sniper's position in a building with a clear field of fire, an area where security forces are actively engaged with an armed threat (e.g., during rescue team entry), and an actively collapsing building, etc. In the hot zones, all operations, especially medical interventions, are extremely hazardous. Hot zone care is defined by the "Direct Threat Care" phase of TECC, with a focus on threat mitigation, extraction, and hemorrhage control. Extraction to a safer area to render medical assistance is critical. Direct Threat Care is provided by tactical team members who are trained in the principals and techniques of TECC. The cold zone or outer perimeter is where limited threat exists and evacuation care can be provided in much the same manner as in any routine civilian situation. The warm zone ("Indirect Threat Care") is an area where the threat is intermediate between these two extremes; this is often the most challenging regarding medical decision making. The benefit of a particular intervention must be considered relative to the risk of additional injury to the patient or the medical tactician. Certain actions considered standard for care in normal situations, such as applying a cervical collar for penetrating neck injuries before moving the patient, make no sense in a tactical environment.[16]

Medical planning is a critical element of the response to a kidnapping/hostage crisis, and it should include plans for point-of-injury care, casualty collection points and casualty movement, movement to civilian EMS, predetermined destinations for injured requiring specialized care, and contingencies that include the evacuation of wounded by assault force/TEMS providers. Medical first-receiving facilities should be ready to care for injured hostages, rescuers, and hostage takers. If possible, a vetted person should be available to provide identification of persons being brought out of the crisis site. There should also be a small contingent of armed personnel providing local security at the casualty collection point.

Having defined the three zones of care, medical training should target those individuals most likely to operate within a particular zone. All members of a rescue force should be trained in TECC and become proficient in providing Direct Threat Care in the hot zone for themselves and their team members. They must recognize and mitigate threats with both marksmanship and medical skills, if required. Additional medical training should be provided to certain members of the tactical team, allowing them to function as Operator-Medics, primarily in the warm zone (Indirect Threat Care). If trained as Emergency Medical Technicians, they would multiply the number of higher-skilled medical providers in the assault force. Not all medical providers supporting the assault force need to be qualified as operators or even be law enforcement agents. TEMS was developed to allow unarmed, nonlaw enforcement medical personnel to be attached to tactical units. The level of expertise of the TEMS provider can vary greatly, but should complement and augment the medical capabilities of the supported unit. A national TEMS curriculum has yet to be implemented, but training should include TECC methodology, remote assessment and surrogate care, rescue and extraction, hemostasis (hemorrhage control), airway management, maintaining adequate ventilation and circulation, medication administration, casualty immobilization, medical planning (threat assessment and medical intelligence), force health protection (including physical fitness), environmental factors, mechanisms and patterns of injury, medicolegal aspects of TEMS, hazardous materials, mass casualties, and tactical familiarization.

Medical intelligence (number of hostages, preexisting medical conditions, current medical status, etc.) is a vital part of the medical planning process; in some cases, it may even be the driving force for the tactical rescue operation. On January 25, 2012, American Jessica Buchanan and Danish citizen Poul Thisted were rescued from Somali pirates by Navy SEALS in a joint U.S. military/FBI operation. In addition to her thyroid problem requiring medication, Jessica had spent 93 days in captivity fully exposed to the harsh environment, had lost 25 pounds from being on a starvation diet, and was suffering from a urinary tract infection. After failed negotiation attempts, recognition of her worsening medical condition prompted the successful rescue operation.[17]

The rescue force must be prepared to deal with the onslaught of the media upon the crisis site. News media will broadcast pictures and video feeds of what the barricade looks like on the outside, directly to the hostage takers located inside. The rehearsal area and the staging area of the force must be obscured from any onlookers. In addition, consider having multiple ambulances and separate egress routes. The medical section should consider the nonmedical general needs of the hostages to include toys for children that can be passed across the barricade; and sunglasses for those hostages who have been held in dark spaces.

MEDICAL TREATMENT OF CASUALTIES

The type and quantity of medical care required depend on the length and conditions of captivity, preexisting illnesses, and whether the hostage was released or had to be rescued. Rescue attempts are inherently very dangerous situations and may result in injury to rescuers, as well as hostages. Special consideration must be given to nontraumatic injuries, including dehydration and malnutrition. In addition consider the possibility of pressure sores on the back, if the hostage has been tied up and not allowed to move or not afforded a chance for personal hygiene.

The difficulty in providing care is greatly affected by the hostage crisis location. Domestic urban settings with robust emergency medical services providing backup support are much less problematic than remote, austere locations where the only medical resources available are those brought by the rescue force. Providing medical care at sea on relatively small vessels in remote parts of the world with impossibly long evacuation routes can prove extremely challenging.[18]

Perhaps most important is the emotional and mental health support required by all hostages, even those not sustaining any physical trauma. The lack of control over one's fate in a highly stressful life-and-death situation will tax the emotional resources of even the most robust person.[19]

UNIQUE CONSIDERATIONS

Being kidnapped or held hostage is perhaps one of the most likely events to cause posttraumatic stress disorder (PTSD). PTSD is characterized by reexperiencing the traumatic event (e.g., vivid nightmares, recurring visual images, and reacting physiologically to stimuli associated with the event), avoidance behavior (i.e., avoiding things associated with the trauma such as activities, places, or people), and hyperarousal symptoms (e.g., insomnia, startle behavior, and attention deficits). PTSD is a normal reaction to an abnormal situation, and it can be prevented or mitigated with timely intervention.

Critical incident stress debriefing (CISD) is an essential component of post-event care. It involves at least one structured meeting with a trained mental health professional, between 24 and 72 hours after release or rescue. The first day after the event is necessary for rest: emotionally and physically. After about 3 days, victims will begin to suppress/repress emotions in an attempt to isolate or compartmentalize the traumatic experience, hence the need to act quickly.

The CISD usually takes several hours and includes an explanation of the purpose of the debriefing, a brief personal history of the people involved in the event, a discussion of what each person saw or experienced and their emotional reactions, a query regarding symptoms associated with PTSD, education regarding PTSD as a normal response to horrific events, and referral of those who require further treatment.

Another unique consideration in a law enforcement environment is the preservation of forensic evidence. A review of 100 patient charts at a Level I trauma center demonstrated poor, improper, or inadequate documentation in 70% of cases; more than a third demonstrated potential evidence was improperly secured, improperly documented, or inadvertently discarded.[20] Proper training of medical personnel in the recognition and handling of evidence, both gross and trace, is essential to avoid the unnecessary destruction of vital evidence.[21]

PITFALLS

Several potential pitfalls exist in response to a hostage-taking event. These include the following:

- Lack of situational awareness in a high-risk environment
- Underestimating the danger or threat posed by female terrorists[22]

- *The Stockholm syndrome:* First described by Professor Nils Bejerot to explain the phenomenon of hostage victims bonding with their captors, following a 6-day ordeal in which two bank robbers held four hostages in Stockholm, Sweden, in 1973 (Symptoms include emotional bonding with captors, seeking approval or favor from the captors, resenting police or other authorities for attempts at rescue, and refusing to seek freedom when the opportunity is available.)
- Lack of properly trained and integrated medical support for specialized law enforcement teams
- Failure to perform a CISD in a timely fashion
- Failure to properly document and preserve forensic evidence

REFERENCES

1. Strentz T. *Hostage/Crisis Negotiations: Lessons Learned from the Bad, the Mad, and the Sad.* Springfield, IL: Charles C Thomas Publisher Ltd; 2013.
2. Farber D. *Taken Hostage.* Princeton: Princeton University Press; 2005.
3. Moor M, Remijnse S. *Kidnapping Is a Booming Business.* IKV Pax Christi: Utrecht, The Netherlands; 2008.
4. National Counterterrorism Center, Kidnapping Trends, Retrieved 10 April 2014 National Counterterrorism Center: http://www.nctc.gov/site/technical/trends.html.
5. Bahadur J. *The Pirates of Somalia.* New York: Pantheon Books; 2011.
6. Dolnik A, Fitzgerald K. *Negotiating Hostage Crises with the New Terrorists.* Westport, CT: Praeger Security International; 2008.
7. Boyle C. In the underworld: kidnapping, hostage-taking, and extortion on the rise. *Insurance J.* July 10, 2000; Available at, http://www.insurancejournal.com/magazines/southcentral/2000/07/10/coverstory/22644.htm.
8. U.S. Department of State, Mexico Travel Warning, Retrieved 10 April 2014. U.S. Department of State: http://travel.state.gov/content/passports/english/alertswarnings/mexico-travel-warning.html.
9. STRATFOR. *How to Live in a Dangerous World.* Austin, TX: STRATFOR Global Intelligence; 2009.
10. Whitcomb C. *Cold Zero: Inside the FBI Hostage Rescue Team.* Boston: Little, Brown and Company; 2001.
11. Green J. Dealing with trouble-the wilder issues. In: Ryan J, Mahoney PF, Greaves I, et al. *Conflict and Catastrophe Medicine: A Practical Guide.* London: Springer; 2002.
12. Schwartz R, McManus J, Swienton R. *Tactical Emergency Medicine.* Philadelphia: Lippincott Williams & Wilkins; 2008.
13. Butler F, Hagman J, Butler E. Tactical combat casualty care in special operations. *Mil Med.* 1996;161(suppl 1):3–16.
14. Butler F, Carmona R. Tactical combat casualty care: from the battlefields of Afghanistan and Iraq to the streets of America. *Tactical Edge.* Winter 2012;86–91.
15. Sztajnkrycer M. Learning from tragedy: preventing officer deaths with medical interventions. *Tactical Edge.* Winter 2010;54–58.
16. Campbell J, Heiskell L, Smith J, Wipfler E. *Tactical Medicine Essentials.* Sudbury, MA: Jones & Bartlett Learning; 2012.
17. Buchanan J, Landemalm E, Flacco A. *Impossible Odds.* New York: Atria Books; 2013.
18. Molé D. Medical support for counter piracy operations. In: *5th International Conference of the Jordanian Royal Medical Services Abstract Book.* Dead Sea, Jordan; 2010:163.
19. Phillips R. *A Captain's Duty: Somali Pirates, Navy SEALs, and Dangerous Days at Sea.* New York: Hyperion; 2010.
20. Carmona R, Prince K. Trauma and forensic medicine. *J Trauma.* 1989; 29(9):1222–1225.
21. Smock W. Penetrating trauma. In: Olshaker J, Jackson M, Smock W, eds. *Forensic Emergency Medicine.* 2nd ed. Philadelphia: Lippincott Williams & Wilkins; 2007.
22. MacDonald E. *Shoot the Women First.* New York: Random House; 1991.

Civil Unrest and Rioting*

Denis J. FitzGerald

Civil unrest, also termed *civil disturbance*, is a spectrum of activities progressively disruptive to public order and tranquility. Civil unrest can occur whenever a group in the community feels, accurately or not, that some aspect of society is antithetic or apathetic to their views, rights, or needs. Examples of civil disturbance include labor strikes, large demonstrations, and riots. As the extreme situation, a *riot* is a violent disruption of the public order that threatens public safety. Proper planning, preparedness, and response strategies can result in significant reductions in violence and injuries, while preserving the fundamental rights of individuals to assemble peacefully. In describing civil unrest, it is valuable to consider first a historical perspective, then to discuss the etiology and evolution of these incidents.

HISTORICAL PERSPECTIVE

Civil unrest has been a part of the fabric of life in the United States since before the country was founded, dating back to the Boston Massacre in 1770.[1] Governed by a set of laws that define mechanisms for expressing constitutional rights and advocating different viewpoints, American society has experienced many instances throughout its history of both peaceful demonstrations and violent riots. Recent notable events include the widespread turbulence of the late 1960s, the civil unrest surrounding the Rodney King incident (1992), the clashes between the police and protesters at World Bank Demonstrations in Washington, DC (2000), and the confrontations surrounding the Occupy Movement (2012). Especially when it turns violent, civil unrest can strain or even shatter the delicate equilibrium between the societal need for public order and the individual's constitutional right to freedom of expression.

Civil unrest arises from the interplay of several factors.[2] It is important to understand that in any large social gathering, all of the factors necessary for violence exist; it is a question of whether these factors will interact with the volatile chemistry necessary to precipitate an actual riot. These factors include confrontational participants, catalyst causes, group dynamics, group leadership, and emotional electricity. To understand the spectrum of civil unrest better, it is important to discuss briefly the role of each causal factor separately and then how they interact together in civil unrest situations.

Across the spectrum of various events, participants in civil unrest span demographic, political, and socioeconomic categories. At baseline, participants are generally connected to the group by a variable degree of investment in a specific cause. Some core persons are highly committed to the issue, whereas others merely become caught up in the frenzied periphery of an event.

Catalyst causes that trigger civil disturbance include any perceived wrongful policy or event felt worthy of active dissent. These issues include special interest topics, perceived law enforcement injustices, and political grievances. Rioting can occur when the group directs its frustration over a given issue toward persons with opposing views or police officers charged with keeping the peace.

As a behavioral dynamic, groups foster an environment in which individual inhibition is lowered because of a collective sense of anonymity, diffusion of personal responsibility, strong social urge toward conformity, and loss of individual decision making. Additionally, during moments of uncertainty or frustration, persons in groups also become more susceptible to suggestion, manipulation, and imitation by strong leaders who are often the first and most assertive agitators. The emotional volatility of a group can also be a powerful unifying force, creating an almost electric connectivity between participants when sparked.

Given the right circumstances and the volatile interplay of these factors, a critical transition can occur in any group that can precipitate violence in civil unrest situations, including large-scale rioting. In any crowd, isolated or progressive violence can occur because of the presence of *agitators*, individuals who incite the crowd by engaging in unlawful disruptive conduct, such as throwing objects. This tactic is increasingly used in international settings, such as Turkey (2013-2014) and Ukraine (2014). The transition from rioting to violence that is widespread hinges on the development of *group cohesion*. Most large groups, such as at demonstrations or sporting events, are considered *crowds*. Crowds are gatherings that lack significant group cohesion. With the evolution of group cohesion, the crowd becomes, in essence, its own autonomous organism with a collective identity, purpose, focus, emotional tone, and coordinated response. At this point, its members are more prone to participate in activities that they would not otherwise do if alone. If the tone of the group shifts toward anger or frustration, a "mob mentality" may take over that converts the crowd into a *mob*; violence can erupt like a contagion, and a riot can ensue. Rooted in group cohesion, this transition from crowd to mob is the central key to the emergence of rioting.

Within this framework, several recognized patterns exist for the development of a riot. First, classically, civil unrest can be a fluid event that escalates along a progressive continuum of disruption. For example, the incident may begin as a planned *demonstration*. A *demonstration* is a group of people (termed *protesters* or *demonstrators*) in a crowd specifically called together for a common purpose, such as to protest a political policy. Under ordinary circumstances in the United States, demonstrations are peaceful expressions of First Amendment rights, and they remain law-abiding entities. However, some demonstrations become increasingly disruptive, with individuals in the group engaging (e.g., agitators) in unlawful activity, such as vandalism or

---

*The content of this chapter exclusively reflects the view of the author and does not represent official policy of the U.S. Department of Health and Human Services or the United States government.

direct violent confrontation with authorities. If violent tactics are adopted, the situation can then degenerate into the anarchy of a riot, and the group becomes a mob. During a tense confrontation, violence can beget violence, requiring law enforcement measures to defuse the situation and to restore order. Second, a crowd may assemble as an unrelated group of people, without common purpose, brought together because of similar circumstances, such as for a sporting event or a court proceeding.[3] A catalyst event, often a verdict in a law enforcement incident or a high-stakes outcome in a sporting event, incites a small ultraviolent group in the crowd to riot in immediate response. Sometimes deep underlying schisms along racial, ethnic, or socioeconomic lines within the community fuel these actions. This core group engages in random acts of violence and looting, subsequently engulfing larger segments of the population. These incidents typically overwhelm the initial public safety resources, requiring an influx of outside support to defuse the situation. Third, and most recently, technology has permitted the formation of *flash mobs*. Coordinated by cellular and Internet technology, flash mobs occur when multiple participants converge abruptly on a given location. These spontaneous gatherings have sometimes focused on demonstrations for specific social issues, but also have resulted in riots characterized by targeted violence and looting.

CURRENT PRACTICE

Pre-Incident Actions

Preplanning saves lives when time counts. It is critical to plan for civil unrest events because time is limited for lifesaving intervention if violence should erupt. Baseline preparation should focus on the development of infrastructure necessary for mitigation of a worst-case scenario, such as widespread rioting. Involving both training and resource coordination, effective medical preplanning for civil unrest involves preparation for the continuum of patient care from the field through initial hospitalization. Important planning aspects include: (1) integration of the field medical response with the law enforcement tactical response; (2) coordination of regional medical resources at all levels; and (3) development of individual hospital response procedures.

Building on this underlying foundation, preparation for specific events (such as announced demonstrations) should involve the completion of a medical threat assessment (MTA). To ensure optimal medical care for all participants on the frontline, it is important that medical support be integrated into the initial law enforcement tactical response. At the flashpoint of a violent incident, the tactical response involves containment and control of the riot through use of a mobile field force (MFF), a special response team for civil disturbance. Successful integration of medical support into the MFF requires the establishment of a working relationship prior to an actual incident. Planning for organic medical support of such tactical operations should focus on many areas, including the following:

- Logistics—deploying, training, and equipping medical personnel for the field
- Preventive strategies—ensuring that needs are met for hydration and adequate protective equipment during deployment of the MFF
- Rehearsal of rescue tactics and techniques—appropriate MFF formations to facilitate extraction of injured individuals from a crowd or mob
- Acute care delivery—coordinating injury treatment and casualty evacuation from the scene
- Decontamination systems—identifying and eliminating contamination thrown by protesters
- Advanced care access issues—connecting MFF field response to the emergency medical system and hospitals

On a regional level, prior planning must ensure that medical resources will be coordinated on all levels of the health care response to function seamlessly within the Incident Command System (ICS). First, the regional disaster plan for large incidents of civil unrest should include a medical annex that focuses on the integration of health care delivery with other public safety functions under such conditions. Resource planning for patient care should address issues related to emergency medical services (e.g., protection of ambulance crews and field rehabilitation logistics),[4] hospital transport (e.g., ensuring safe travel routes), local hospital capabilities (e.g., determining trauma level and diversion status), and mutual aid. Second, the development in advance of a reliable communication system to facilitate information sharing between the lead law enforcement agency, the emergency medical system dispatch, and regional health care facilities is essential. This system may be effectively adapted from preexisting disaster networks to function as well in the limited scope of civil unrest incidents.

Individual hospitals also need to look at planning for civil unrest incidents, particularly in the emergency department setting. In many respects, this preparation may be incorporated into the existing disaster plan, with such provisions as increased staffing and the establishment of an emergency operations center. Unique aspects of preparation for civil unrest include hospital security concerns in the face of violent agitators outside, management of injured disorderly protesters requiring treatment, management of family and friends (nonpatients), contamination issues, the potential for mass casualty situations, and the control of arrested persons.

Regional medical planners should also develop an MTA to address unannounced demonstrations. The MTA is an approach used to prepare for the foreseeable medical issues associated with a particular event by analyzing various health threats, assessing medical vulnerabilities, identifying possible countermeasures, and exploring different resources to optimize health care delivery. Relevant information tied to the anticipated circumstances can be gathered in advance through several methods, such as hospital site surveys, route surveys, open-source material, and information known about the past behavior of the protest group. Specific MTA components may include an analysis of environmental conditions, hospital capabilities, and substances likely to be thrown by demonstrators.

Post-Incident Actions

In the wake of violence associated with widespread civil unrest, the medical community should strive to promote recovery efforts both within its ranks and within the region. In the short term, attention should be paid to responder safety and the emotional effect of the civil disturbance on health care workers. Response efforts should support any persons suffering residual critical incident stress. Hospital personnel should continue to provide care for victims and their families, as well as to release appropriate information to the community as indicated and authorized by the designated public information officer (PIO). Accurate, timely, and strategic communication is critical in the immediate aftermath of dynamic, community disturbances. In the long term, it is valuable for medical professionals to meet with civic representatives to debrief medical aspects of the incident. The focus should be an effort to enhance the medical response to similar situations in the future. By discussing what worked and what did not, lessons learned can be applied to improve patient care delivery in the event of a future civil disturbance.

Medical Treatment of Casualties

Several important factors should be considered with regard to the medical treatment of casualties from civil unrest. For a large-scale incident, the care should be delivered under conditions defined in the disaster plan of the hospital or agency. Important and unique aspects of medical treatment during civil disturbance are the potential for large numbers of patients, the nature of the injuries seen in riots, high likelihood of contamination with crowd control agents such as oleoresin capsicum (e.g., pepper spray), and the use of less-lethal weapons.

The number of casualties from an incident varies widely with the scope of the disturbance. Depending on available resources, medical providers may need to implement mass casualty triage protocols in given situations. The need for this approach may also depend on the timing of the injuries over the course of the incident and the distribution of patients among different hospitals. Particular attention should be paid to scene security and crowd control at the triage and treatment sites.

As exemplified in the civil disturbance surrounding the Rodney King incident,[5] three main patterns of injury have been identified in civil unrest. The first type of injury involves assaults suffered by active participants in rioting or other criminal behavior such as looting. With a mixture of blunt and penetrating trauma, these persons may present with gunshot wounds, stab wounds, or injuries incurred in beatings. A second category of injury that has been noted in civil disturbances involves automobile accidents. Suffering primarily blunt trauma, these patients include struck pedestrians and victims of motor vehicle collisions that result from disruption of traffic patterns, erratic driving, or broken traffic signals. The last group of patients present with an acute decompensation or exacerbation of a chronic medical condition because they were unable to obtain needed care. Included in this group are patients receiving dialysis and persons with diabetes.

Less-lethal weapons are routinely used in the context of modern civil unrest. Less-lethal weapons are devices designed to incapacitate persons or to disperse groups without causing serious harm. As reflected in the term *less lethal*, the potential does exist, however, for serious harm or even death with these devices. There are two general categories of less-lethal agents used in the law enforcement response to civil disturbance. Chemical agents, such as tear gas or pepper spray, cause noxious upper respiratory irritation when deployed. Treatment should focus on removing ongoing contamination, maintaining access to fresh air, and applying cool water. The injury pattern for projectile munitions, such as "bean bag" rounds, ranges from minor lacerations to significant internal injury.[6] It is advisable for health care providers to be familiar with these less-lethal devices and their effects.

Unique Considerations

Medical personnel should remember three unique considerations during a response to civil disturbance. These considerations include awareness of the threat environment, the medical-legal context, and the role of field testing. These three considerations are applicable across the spectrum of medical care settings. The most important consideration for health care providers during civil unrest is to recognize that care is being delivered in a *high-threat environment*. A high-threat environment is a situation in which a person is at risk for harm or injury during the performance of a given task. In civil unrest, there are several personal safety concerns for the provider, such as violent demonstrators, dangerous crowd tactics, contamination from thrown substances (e.g., feces), denial of essential supplies, and the presence of improvised weapons. The provider must provide simultaneous care to different

categories of patients placed in confrontation by the event-arrested demonstrators, injured bystanders, and wounded law enforcement officers. In addition to using appropriate protective equipment, medical providers must continually maintain situational awareness, and practice scene safety in the threat environment posed by civil unrest. During violent demonstrations, protesters may throw a variety of substances at responding police officers. One significant concern with both medical and legal implications is the potential exposure to contaminated blood in this setting. A field blood sampling protocol to assess thrown red liquids can help clarify this issue. This protocol can be developed using screening field assays in conjunction with professional laboratory confirmation.

Providers should also appreciate the medical-legal environment created by civil unrest and the consequent implications for health care delivery. In the care of patients, providers must be careful (to the extent possible) not to destroy evidence such as collected weapons, bullets, or clothing. In the event that court testimony is later required, the medical practitioner should also have a basic understanding of forensics as it applies to recognition of injury patterns.

⚠ PITFALLS

Several potential pitfalls exist in the medical response to an episode of civil unrest. These include the following:

- Failure to understand the dynamics and effects of civil unrest within modern society
- Failure to plan for medical contingencies, communication, and coordination along the continuum of health care delivery before an event occurs
- Failure to understand the nature of medical casualties in civil unrest, including the injury pattern associated with less-lethal weapons
- Failure to promote recovery in the wake of an incident through both short-term and long-term measures
- Failure to consider personal safety while providing care in the threat environment of civil disturbance
- Failure to recognize the unique medico-legal implications of civil unrest

REFERENCES

1. Civil disorder. *Los Angeles County Sheriff Emergency Operations Bureau;* 1997.
2. Civil disturbances. *US Army Field Manual 19-15.* Washington, DC: Headquarters, Department of the Army; 2005.
3. *Law Enforcement Bulletin.* U.S. Federal Bureau of Investigation; March 1994.
4. *Civil Disturbances in Emergency Medical Services: Special Operations Student Manual.* Maryland: Federal Emergency Management Agency. U.S. Fire Administration, National Fire Academy; 2002.
5. Koehler G, Isbell D, Freeman C, et al. *Medical Care for the Injured: The Emergency Medical Response to the April 1992 Los Angeles Civil Disturbance.* State of California Emergency Medical Services Authority; 1993. Available at, http://www.usc.edu/isd/archives/cityinstress/medical/contents.html.
6. Suyama J, Panagos P, Sztajnkrycer M. Injury patterns related to the use of less-lethal weapons during a period of civil unrest. *J Emerg Med.* 2003;25:219–227.

Introduction to Explosions and Blasts

Josh W. Joseph and Leon D. Sanchez

DESCRIPTION OF EVENT

Physics of Blast Injury

Although the exact details of an explosion are rarely available to emergency providers, a basic understanding of explosives and blast-wave physics can help illustrate the underlying pathophysiology of blast injuries and the unique risks facing blast survivors. An explosive blast is an intense exothermic reaction generated by the rapid chemical conversion of a solid or a liquid into a gas. Conventional explosive devices are typically categorized into low- (or "ordinary") and high-order explosives. Low-order explosives include materials such as propellants (e.g., gunpowder), which undergo a process of rapid burning known as *deflagration*, at speeds less than 1000 m/s.[1] If low explosives are ignited in the open, they will often burn rather than result in an explosion. Encasing low explosives in small enclosures such as pipes and pressure cookers significantly increases the speed at which the material is ignited and the amount of pressure generated.[1]

High-order explosives (e.g., trinitrotoluene [TNT]) undergo a process known as *detonation*. In detonation, the ignition of a small amount of the explosive or an igniting agent generates a shock wave, which propagates through the explosive at speeds above 4500 m/s. The remaining explosive ignites within microseconds, releasing tremendous amounts of energy in the form of heat and pressure as the newly formed gas expands, displacing the surrounding air and creating a blast wave.[1,2]

The leading edge of the blast wave, or blast front, consists of a thin layer of compressed air, traveling faster than the speed of sound. When the blast front encounters an object, it causes a virtually instantaneous rise in pressure from ambient pressure to a peak overpressure. This initial wave is followed by a subsonic phase of sustained overpressure, at significantly lesser magnitude than the peak, known as the *positive pressure phase*. Low explosives can generate substantial positive pressure, but will not generate a shock wave. The total duration of overpressure is typically less than 100 ms for conventional explosive devices. This displacement of air generates a "blast wind," which can propel objects and people at speeds in excess of 800 miles per hour (357 m/s). The final portion of the explosion is a negative pressure phase, representing the vacuum created by the gas displaced by the explosion, and a return to atmospheric pressure. Although complex formulae exist for modeling explosions, the Friedlander curve (Fig. 71-1) provides a useful illustration of the phases of a blast.

Several factors govern the destructive effects of an explosion and its potential to cause injury. The most significant is distance from the explosion. The overpressure of the explosion decreases proportionally to the inverse cube of the distance from an explosion; thus a person twice as far away from an explosion experiences approximately an eighth of the overpressure. The medium in which an explosion occurs is also significant. As fluid is incompressible, underwater explosions propagate more quickly, with more energy conserved over distance and time, tripling the lethal radius of an underwater explosion versus an explosion in midair.

Finally, the location of an explosion relative to buildings and other solid surfaces can profoundly increase its lethality. Blast waves may wrap around objects and walls and are often reflected by solid surfaces. Reflected waves can undergo constructive interference, resulting in overpressure amplified far beyond that of the initial blast wave. Victims adjacent to or behind a wall may experience worse injuries than those out in the open. This is particularly acute in enclosed spaces, as the resulting reflections of a blast extend the duration of overpressure leading to very complex wave patterns. If a pressure wave is reflected from a solid object, the pressures generated from the reflecting surfaces may be more than 20 times that of the incident wave. Consequently, a blast wave capable of causing only minor injuries in an open space may be lethal to victims in closed spaces.[1,3,4]

Physiology of Blast Injury

Blast injury is described in terms of primary, secondary, tertiary, and quaternary mechanisms. Blast victims often suffer from multiple mechanisms of injury, and the categories illustrate how the different effects of blasts cause specific patterns of trauma.[2,4] Primary-blast injury (PBI) is a direct result of blast overpressure forces.[4,5] Overpressure forces tend to damage air-containing organs and those with varying internal densities, such as the ear, lungs, intestines, and brain. PBI can be further subdivided into shearing, spalling, and imploding.[1,2,6] Shearing occurs when two adjacent objects of different densities are acted on by the same force. The lighter object accelerates faster than the denser object, creating a shearing stress at their shared boundary. Spalling is the tendency of a dense medium under pressure to displace and fragment into a less-dense medium. The fragments then act as secondary projectiles into the less-dense medium. This occurs frequently in the body when the contents of a fluid-filled organ or vessel are driven into an air-filled or potential space. Implosion occurs when the force of overpressure compresses gas within a tissue. When the period of overpressure ends, the compressed gas expands, disrupting the surrounding tissue.

Secondary blast injury results from projectiles generated by an explosion's overpressure and blast winds. These projectiles have a much greater radius of effect than the explosion itself. An explosion that causes PBI at a radius of tens of meters may launch projectiles hundreds or even thousands of meters away, causing blunt and penetrating trauma. Blast-related debris may include fragments originating from the casing of the charge, intentional shrapnel enclosed with the explosive (e.g., ball bearings and nails), and secondary fragments, such as pieces of glass, wood, stone, and other materials. Even low-order explosives such as pipe bombs can accelerate shrapnel to speeds equivalent to bullets.[7]

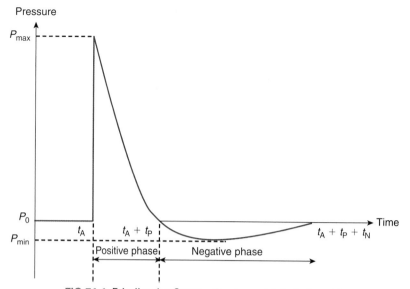

FIG 71-1 Friedlander Curve. (Courtesy of Julia S. Joseph)

Tertiary blast injury results from victims being accelerated by explosions, who are then knocked into hard surfaces or launched into the air. Once a victim's body is in motion, they are also at serious risk of being impaled with stationary objects. Children are at particularly high risk of tertiary injury due to their lower weight. Tertiary injury also encompasses crush injuries from collapsing buildings, and when passengers collide with the inside of a vehicle.[1,4,8]

Quaternary blast injury is a broad category of injury including thermal and chemical burns and inhalational exposure. Heat generated by the initial explosion may cause flash burns. The release of hot gases, secondary fires in the surrounding environment, and contact with hot dust-laden air can also cause conventional burns. Chemical exposures can result from the release of chemicals in the surrounding environment, along with the inhalation of dust, chemically complex smokes, and carbon monoxide.[1,4,9]

HISTORICAL CONTEXT

Increasing Prevalence and Lethality of Explosive Devices

In 1917 the accidental collision of two ships, the *Imo* and the *Mont Blanc*, in Halifax Harbor, Nova Scotia, demonstrated the potential for vast death and destruction from an explosive blast. Their cumulative cargoes included 35 tons of benzene, 2300 tons of picric acid, 10 tons of gun cotton, 200 tons of TNT, and 300 rounds of ammunition. The collision resulted in the largest human-made, nonnuclear explosion in history. Casualties reportedly included over 2000 deaths and 9000 injuries. Parts of the ships were found several miles away; approximately 2.5 km of the city was leveled, and windows were shattered as far as 100 km away.[10]

In the modern era, injuries caused by explosives have become an important issue for civilian health care providers because of the dramatic increase in terrorist bombings worldwide within the past few decades. Throughout the 1990s, terrorist bombings led to approximately 3203 fatalities and 19,329 injuries. In the following decade from 2000 to 2009, there were upwards of 30,992 fatalities and 91,571 injuries resulting from terrorist bombings globally.[11]

Even though the great majority of bombings within the United States have been encased low-explosive devices such as pipe bombs, terrorist bombings against military and civilian targets in Iraq and Afghanistan, as well as in many other recent conflicts, have demonstrated a sharp increase in sophistication and lethality.[7,12] In part, this has stemmed from the wide-scale availability of military-grade munitions in these regions (primarily high explosives). However, observers have also noted that independent terrorist groups worldwide have dramatically increased the rate at which they learn new tactics, techniques, and procedures of improvised explosive devices (IEDs) use. This is attributed to a greater degree of information sharing between terrorist groups, which can result in a rapid sophistication in tactics and technology within months during a bombing campaign.[12]

Prognostic Factors and Critical Mortality Rates

An instructive explosive attack occurred in 1983 in Beirut, Lebanon, where terrorists utilized a truck-borne, ammonium-nitrate-based explosive device equivalent to roughly 6 tons of TNT to bomb the U.S. Marine Corps barracks. The blast resulted in the near complete collapse of a four-story building, and 234 immediate deaths (68% of all victims). Several first responders were killed by sniper fire from waiting terrorists carrying out a "second hit" assault, an asymmetric tactic occurring more frequently in present-day attacks. Most of the survivors had noncritical injuries. However, 19 survivors (17%) suffered critical injuries and 7 of these initial survivors ultimately died. Timing of response is critical for survival. Six of the seven late deaths had been rescued and treated more than 6 hours after the blast. Conversely, only 1 of the 65 initial survivors rescued within 4 hours died. The reported causes of mortality in Marine barrack bombings included the following[1]: head trauma as the leading cause of immediate death (71%) and late death (57%)[2]; chest trauma (29%) (rare among survivors)[3]; and burns (29%).[10]

This event provides important lessons for responding to explosions. Most striking is the effect of early and aggressive resuscitation as a key prognostic factor for long-term survival. Rapid evacuation and treatment must be balanced with operational risks such as terrorist deployment of multiple devices or layered attacks targeting first responders. Building collapse also has a dramatic effect on survival, and the anatomic site and nature of an injury are important prognostic factors. In a review discussing the medical response to terrorist bombings, Frykberg et al. proposed the use of a "critical mortality rate" (the death rate only among those critically injured) as an appropriate measure when calculating vital statistics for a terrorist event. Because the number of noncritical survivors may falsely lower overall mortality rates, the critical mortality rate more accurately describes those victims actually at risk for death.[10]

Triage Efficacy

In 1994 the Argentine Israeli Mutual Association (AMIA) of Buenos Aires, Argentina, was bombed with a large ammonium-nitrate explosive (430 lb TNT-equivalent), leading to the complete collapse of a seven-story building. There were 286 casualties and 82 (29%) immediate deaths.[10,13] In the immediate aftermath of the explosion, the closest hospital emergency department (ED) faced rapid overcrowding by ambulatory survivors and medical personnel offering to help. Of the 204 survivors, 40 were eventually hospitalized, 7% ($n = 14$) in critical condition, among whom 4 later died. These figures represent a 3.4% overall mortality rate and a 29% critical mortality rate.[13]

Among survivors, 58% ($n = 50$) of those who visited the ED suffered minor injuries, 12 of whom were admitted. Moderate injuries were reported among 19% ($n = 16$) of survivors presenting to the ED, with 13 ultimately admitted. Major injuries were reported among 21% ($n = 18$) of presenting patients, 12 of whom were sent directly to the operating room or intensive care unit; 7 later died. A total of five survivors were extricated from rubble, two of whom later died. Only five patients underwent laparotomy, and hepatic lacerations were found in two of these. Three patients were found to have pneumothorax, and two others showed bilateral infiltrates consistent with PBI of the lung.[10,13]

The AMIA bombing demonstrated that hospitals in close proximity to a major explosion suffer rapid and early overcrowding of their EDs with patients who have sustained minor and moderate injuries. Frykberg et al. compared the AMIA bombing with similar events, demonstrating a very strong correlation between the extent to which noncritical patients are overtriaged and mortality.[10] This illustrates the need for disaster management plans that emphasize appropriate and effective triage to be carried out by experienced providers both in the field and at the ED entrance, as well as the need to appropriately manage providers who volunteer to help with the response.

An example of efficient triage can be found in the Boston Marathon Bombing of 2013. During the bombing, two improvised explosive devices, pressure cookers filled with metallic debris and low-order explosives, exploded within 13 seconds of each other near the finish line of the marathon. Three victims were killed immediately. In total, 264 individuals were injured. Although many of the victims suffered traumatic lower-extremity amputations and required critical care and operative management, there were no further fatalities.

The low fatality rate after the Boston bombing was due to several factors. First, the detonations were in close proximity to multiple Level 1 Trauma Centers, allowing for rapid movement to specialized care. Second, emergency medical services (EMS) personnel had established a nearby triage area at the marathon prior to the bombing, and prehospital providers made a concerted effort to distribute critical patients evenly between the area hospitals to avoid overwhelming the services of any one facility. Third, Boston area hospitals and emergency providers had taken significant measures to prepare for a similar disaster, including multiple mass-casualty drills run by the area's hospitals in coordination with emergency medical service providers. Finally, many EMS providers had also received training in the use of tourniquets, which were employed effectively for many of the extremity injuries.[14–16]

Building Collapse

The bombing of the Alfred P. Murrah Federal Building in Oklahoma City, Oklahoma, in 1995 demonstrated the profound effect that structural considerations can play in a bombing. In this incident, an ammonium-nitrate-based bomb exploded with the equivalent of two tons of TNT, causing 759 total casualties with a 21% immediate mortality rate ($n = 162$). Fourteen percent of survivors ($n = 83$) were hospitalized, of which 52 (62%) were critically injured. Five of these later died (representing a 9.6% critical mortality rate). As with the AMIA bombing, the highest mortality and most severe morbidity in Oklahoma City occurred among victims who were located in collapsed portions of buildings at the time of blast.[17]

There were 506 survivors of the bombing. The injury pattern among survivors included 85% who suffered soft-tissue injuries, including lacerations, abrasions, contusions, and puncture wounds. Among survivors, 210 (35%) had musculoskeletal injuries, 60 suffered from fractures or dislocations, and the remainder had sprains or strains. Fewer patients had severe soft-tissue or musculoskeletal injuries. The majority of survivors were injured by flying glass, collapsed ceilings, and other debris.[17]

Open Air Versus Confined Space

Explosions in confined spaces cause markedly different patterns of injury. In a review of open air (OA) versus confined space (CS) terrorist bombings in Israel, Leibovici and colleagues compared 297 victims from two OA bombings and two bus bombings in which similar explosive devices were used. The CS group suffered a significantly greater incidence of PBI, with higher mortality and a greater severity of injury, whereas the OA caused a larger number of less severe injuries. These findings may be due to unique blast wave behavior within the relatively small CSs of buses, and the ability for OA blasts to launch shrapnel in a much wider radius.[3] A study by Golan et al. reviewed 22 terrorist attacks against civilian buses, comparing explosions that occurred adjacent to buses with explosions within them. This study confirmed the earlier group's finding of a higher mortality rate in CS explosions, as well as a higher rate of pulmonary blast injury.[18]

✚ MEDICAL TREATMENT OF CASUALTIES

Most severely injured survivors of blasts have multiple injuries.[1,4] The most common injury patterns seen among explosion survivors are due to secondary and tertiary blast injury. Given the relative similarity of these injury patterns to the patterns of penetrating trauma, blunt trauma, and burns commonly seen in civilian EDs, the following discussion will emphasize PBI. Anatomically, the structures at greatest risk for PBI are the auditory system, thorax, and abdomen.[1,9] PBI may also lead to injuries of the central nervous system (CNS), eyes, and extremities. The greatest potential for avoiding preventable deaths by PBI lies in the appropriate treatment of thoracic PBI. The incidence of PBI varies according to explosive charge, proximity of the victim to the blast, and the environment in which it occurs.[2,9] Survivors of explosions that occur in CSs or underwater may manifest a higher incidence of PBI.[2,3]

Primary Stabilization

The initial response to bombings is a high-risk operation that must address issues of security and casualty care. The principles of Tactical Emergency Casualty Care (TECC), discussed in detail in other sections, offer threat-based principles of prehospital care to address major potentially preventable causes of death in terrorist attacks: specifically, early hemorrhage control, casualty evacuation, and rapid medical assessment. The majority of survivors injured by a blast are likely to have suffered secondary blast injuries from shrapnel. Accordingly, immediate control of potentially life-threatening extremity hemorrhage is critical, and the rapid use of tourniquets has been shown to significantly improve outcomes.[19]

Patients at risk for PBI should not be intubated in the prehospital setting by less-experienced providers, but should receive very limited fluid resuscitation. In the ED, the initial management of blast victims begins with the conventional priorities outlined in the advanced-trauma life-support protocols; however, there are several important exceptions.

Thoracic Injury

The primary organ at risk from PBI to the thorax are the lungs. Blast lung injury (BLI) is a major cause of death in patients who survive initial resuscitation from blast injury. In victims exposed to significant overpressure, blast waves cause an inward displacement of the chest wall that compresses air within the lung parenchyma more slowly than in the hollow respiratory tracts.[1,2] The alveoli implode and reexpand, compromising the alveolar walls, surrounding parenchymal tissue, and capillaries, whereas spalling leads to the extrusion of capillary contents and extravascular fluid into the alveoli. This dramatically decreases lung compliance, and can introduce air emboli into the vascular space.[1,2] The resulting lesions can range from scattered or multifocal petechiae to large confluent hemorrhages involving an entire lung.[1,2] Pleural and subpleural hemorrhages tend to be bilateral, but are usually more extensive on the side facing the source of blast.[4]

Patients with BLI may present with dyspnea, cough, hemoptysis, chest pain, and a clinical picture that resembles pulmonary contusion or acute respiratory distress syndrome (ARDS).[20,21] Clinical signs associated with BLI include tachypnea with rapid, shallow breathing; poor chest wall movement (owing to decreased compliance); dullness to percussion; decreased air movement; hemopneumothorax; subcutaneous emphysema; and retinal artery emboli. Progression of BLI may be due to the cumulative effect of the initial blast injury, inhalation injury, hypovolemic shock, sepsis, aspiration, and aggressive fluid resuscitation.[1] Ultimately, the diagnosis of blast lung is suspected on clinical grounds but confirmed with radiographs. Signs and symptoms usually develop within hours after an explosion, but may be delayed as long as 24 to 48 hours.[2,22,23]

Chest radiography is required for all patients exposed to blast forces to gauge the initial severity of injury and should be obtained in patients with any significant clinical change. Bruising of the intercostal spaces unprotected by ribs often appear on initial chest x-rays as rib markings.[1,2] Diffuse pulmonary opacities may develop within a few hours and will become maximal within 24 to 48 hours. They typically occur in a "butterfly distribution" of bilateral patchy infiltrates. Changes that develop after 48 hours may be due to complications such as ARDS or pneumonia. Other radiological findings may include hemopneumothorax, pneumomediastinum, subdiaphragmatic free air, subcutaneous emphysema, and foreign body impaction.[23] Symptomatic patients without clear radiographic evidence of injury should undergo emergent CT imaging. CT has a higher sensitivity for early parenchymal lesions in patients with nonblast-related pulmonary contusion, and may be useful in predicting which patients will require mechanical ventilation.

The general management of BLI is similar to that of pulmonary contusion and ARDS. However, the relatively higher risk of significant barotrauma (i.e., alveolar rupture, systemic air emboli, and pneumothorax) in patients with BLI is critically important.[1,2,22] Positive pressure ventilation, especially high levels of positive end-expiratory pressure, increases the risk of pulmonary barotrauma and should therefore be avoided when possible. Further, patients with BLI are at increased risk of complications from overly aggressive fluid resuscitation.[1,2]

Several measures have been shown to reduce the risk of complications in BLI. Permissive hypercapnia and lower oxygen saturations coupled with reduced tidal volumes (e.g., 5 to 7 mL/kg) and peak inspiratory pressures have shown good outcomes. High-frequency oscillatory ventilation may benefit refractory cases.[21] Although data are limited, some authors recommend bilateral tube thoracostomy for pulmonary PBI patients requiring aeromedical evacuation.[1,2] The use of dual-lumen endotracheal tubes (i.e., independent lung ventilation) or high-frequency jet ventilation is often recommended for patients diagnosed with bronchopleural fistulae.[4,22]

The treatment of arterial air emboli resulting from BLI also remains controversial. Even though lowered positive end-expiratory pressure (PEEP) should be continued to prevent the entrainment of further emboli, a number of authors recommend the administration of 100% inspired oxygen to aid in the reabsorption of existing emboli.[24] Extracorporeal membrane oxygenation may be indicated in extreme cases.[1,21]

A retrospective study of patients sustaining BLI from explosions on civilian buses in Israel established that the first 24 hours after injury are critical for effective management.[22] The BLI severity score (BLISS), derived from objective signs of hypoxemia, chest radiograph findings, and the presence of bronchopleural fistula, helps to direct treatment and can predict outcome during the initial stabilization phase.[22] Based on the initial BLISS, none of the patients in this study who were classified as mildly injured went on to develop any form of lung injury. Of those classified as moderately injured, 33% went on to develop ARDS. All those classified as severely injured either developed ARDS or later died.[22] This study showed that aggressive and complex interventions, guided by stratification of BLI severity, can lead to dramatic improvements in outcome. Most patients who survive BLI will regain good lung function within 1 year.[1,20]

Cardiovascular Injury

Victims of blast injuries may have hemodynamic instability that is not explained by conventional causes such as hemorrhage. Much of what is known about the PBI of the cardiovascular system has been gleaned from experimental studies in animal models and historical inquiry.[4] A World War II study of 200 casualties assessed immediately after blast exposure showed that more than 25% of them had heart rates of less than 60 bpm and that over 90% had heart rates of less than 80 bpm. This review also found that hypotension was nearly universal, with blood pressures of 80 to 90 mm Hg (systolic) and 40 to 50 mm Hg (diastolic) being common.[25] This bradycardia has been consistently reproduced in animal studies and may be a vagal effect, as experiments have shown the bradycardia can be prevented with bilateral vagotomy.[25,26]

Irwin and colleagues proposed that these vagally mediated cardiovascular changes are initiated by the so-called pulmonary defensive reflex.[26] This reflex acts when acute pulmonary congestion and edema lead to fluid shifts in the lung, stimulating pulmonary C-fibers, and triggering increased cholinergic activity with systemic effects. This mechanism is supported by the clinical observation of brief periods of apnea after blast exposure, followed by rapid shallow respirations.[2] This phenomenon has also been observed in experimental models using artificial stimulation of pulmonary C-fibers.[26] Several studies have reported a greater than 50% decrease in mean arterial pressure in animals immediately after blast exposure, with spontaneous resolution over time.[27]

Various electrocardiographic changes have been observed immediately after blasts and are thought to be due to blunt thoracic trauma and/or coronary air emboli.[26] These may include atrioventricular and bundle branch blocks, nonspecific ventricular ectopy, low-voltage QRS complexes, and T-wave and ST-segment abnormalities. Blast-induced electrocardiographic changes typically revert to normal sinus rhythm within a few minutes, but may deteriorate into sustained dysrhythmias, including lethal ventricular arrhythmias. Ischemic changes may also occur because of complications of air emboli.[26]

Clinically, cardiovascular PBI may be complicated by coexisting hemorrhage. Given the importance of judicious fluid administration (including blood products) in resuscitation, and the potential to exacerbate soft-tissue injury by underresuscitation, invasive monitoring is often necessary to guide therapy.[1,2]

Abdominal Injury

Nonlethal abdominal PBI is almost exclusively found in gas-containing organs and is likely caused by forces including shearing, spalling, and implosion. Solid-organ damage may present as subcapsular hematomas or lacerations of the liver, spleen, and kidney.[2] These injuries are thought to be due to acceleration-deceleration caused by either the initial effects of the blast wave or from secondary and tertiary mechanisms of injury.[4] The incidence of intestinal PBI may be higher in victims of underwater and closed-space explosions.

The classic lesions of intestinal PBI involve small, multifocal intramural hematomas. Initial bleeding in submucosal regions may range from scattered petechiae or large confluent hematomas.[2] Partial- or full-thickness lacerations may occur, as well as separation of individual layers of the intestinal wall, leading to immediate or delayed perforation of the bowel.[4] Shearing may also lead to separation of the intestine from its vascular supply and subsequent ischemia. The cecum and terminal ileum are the most likely areas to contain gas and are the most prone to perforation during blast exposure.[1,28]

Because it is relatively uncommon, intestinal PBI presents a diagnostic challenge. Signs and symptoms of intestinal PBI include abdominal or testicular pain, nausea, vomiting, tenderness, absence of bowel sounds, and other peritoneal signs. Initial evaluation may be complicated by the overall acuity of a multiply injured patient or prior administration of pain-control medication.[1,28] Gastrointestinal injury may be delayed as long as 48 hours after the initial blast exposure. Intestinal hematomas have been reported to rupture up to 2 weeks after the initial injury.[1,28] This may be due to latent injury with delayed perforation as opposed to delayed diagnosis.[29] Currently, no reliable clinical predictors exist to help clinicians determine which patients may progress to delayed perforation.

Ultrasound and abdominal CT are essential for the evaluation of intestinal PBI.[4,22] Although abdominal CT has excellent utility in detecting solid-organ injury and existing perforation, because of the potential for abdominal PBI to result in delayed perforation, a negative abdominal CT should not be used to exclude injury in symptomatic patients.[1,30] Indications for urgent laparotomy are similar to those established for blunt abdominal trauma.[2]

Musculoskeletal/Extremity Injury

Even though most blast injuries involving the musculoskeletal system are due to secondary and tertiary blast injury, many traumatic amputation in blast victims are due to PBI.[31] In traumatic amputations, the initial shock wave may cause diffuse microfractures of bone, whereas sustained positive pressure from the blast wave leads to significant damage to the periosteum, marrow, and surrounding soft tissue. The blast wave also imposes significant shearing stress at the site of the initial microfractures, causing amputation of the limb with a typically oblique pattern. The characteristic blast-related traumatic amputation traverses the proximal third of the tibia, resulting both from the aforementioned forces and the movement allowed by the knee and ankle joints.[31,32] These injuries are associated with very high rates of immediate and delayed mortality and should prompt an extensive search for other injuries.[1] Traumatic amputations should be treated immediately with proximal tourniquets.

Primary blast forces have also been implicated in compartment syndrome. Although the exact mechanism of soft-tissue injury by PBI is unknown, a combination of tissue disruption, the release of inflammatory mediators, and aggressive fluid resuscitation may contribute to the relatively high rate of compartment syndrome in otherwise uninjured limbs exposed to blasts.[1,31,33] Secondary orthopedic blast injury results from materials projected by the blast into tissue and bone. Secondary bony injury commonly results in two patterns of fracture depending on the velocity and size of the object causing the trauma. High-energy objects often cause bones to shatter on impact, leading to comminuted fractures with significant amounts of devascularized fragments, which are frequently contaminated. Lower energy objects have a tendency to result in injuries to a single bony cortex, leading to a characteristic "drill-hole" pattern, which often does not require operative management.[31,34]

When blast fragments pass through soft tissue at high velocity, they tend to create cavities that are much larger than the trajectory of the fragment itself. The passage of the fragment through tissue causes a high-pressure compression wave to travel through the surrounding tissues. The resulting expansion leads to low pressure in the fragment pathway, sucking debris inward through the entry and exit wounds. As the fragments projected by a blast tend to be more irregularly shaped than bullets, they also transfer a much greater amount of energy to the surrounding tissues, further increasing cavity size.[31] In particular, the cavitation associated with gluteal injuries (which are prevalent in ground-level blasts) can extend to involve nearby major vessels.[35]

Tertiary musculoskeletal injuries involve similar forces and mechanisms to blunt trauma in the civilian setting; however, the location and direction of the forces exerted by explosives can lead to patterns of trauma that are less common in civilian blunt trauma. Low-lying explosives can lead to calcaneal fractures and the "umbrella-ing" of the tissue planes of the lower leg (particularly in land mine-related injuries), whereas explosions under vehicles can cause dramatic axial loading of the occupants and significant spinal trauma, including chance and low-lumbar burst fractures, as well as lumbosacral dissociations.[8]

When there is substantial hemorrhage from extremity wounds, tourniquets should be applied immediately. In the prehospital setting, grossly deformed fractures should be reduced if doing so will not significantly delay transport. Open fractures should be externally fixated quickly after irrigation. Fractures of the upper extremities can also be splinted when feasible.[36,37]

Extremity injuries are at high risk of infection. Approximately 15% of patients with extremity injuries will develop osteomyelitis, of which about 17% will develop recurrent infections. Soil contamination of wounds is frequent, and may include multidrug-resistant *Acinetobacter baumannii* and *Pseudomonas aeruginosa*, extended-spectrum β-lactamase-producing *Klebsiella* and *Escherichia coli*, and methicillin-resistant *Staphylococcus aureus*.[38] Current U.S. military and the Infectious Diseases Society of America (IDSA) guidelines derived from casualty data from the conflicts in Iraq and Afghanistan recommend rapid administration of IV or oral antimicrobials as soon as possible. There is considerable evidence that administering antibiotics within 3 hours of injury improves outcomes, and animal models demonstrate improvements with even more rapid administration.[37] As with any soft-tissue injury, updated tetanus prophylaxis should be given to appropriate patients.

Cefazolin remains the initial antibiotic of choice, with clindamycin as an appropriate alternative for patients allergic to β-lactam antibiotics. This is due to the fact that bacteria that initially contaminate wounds are usually gram-positive organisms sensitive to this regimen, and are effectively halted when antibiotics are combined with expedient large-volume low-pressure irrigation and debridement. Most of the bacteria responsible for multidrug-resistant wound and bone infections are actually nosocomial.[37] The current advised regimen consists of 2 g of IV cefazolin every 6 hours for 5 days. If no infection is present on reassessment at day 3, therapy may be halted. Exceptions are made for delayed presentations (after 72 hours) and land mine injuries, for which adding IV metronidazole is recommended.

In the case of suicide bombings, or when the remains of other victims may contaminate wounds, hepatitis B vaccination is prudent for unimmunized individuals. Explosives may be intentionally contaminated with feces or other biological materials.[1] Even though there are no established guidelines for this situation, extensive debridement and irrigation remain appropriate, with the addition of metronidazole to the initial antibiotic regimen.[38] To date, there have been no large-scale accounts of explosives being used to spread specific agents of biological warfare, such as tularemia, smallpox, or anthrax; however, providers should remain aware of this serious possibility.

The conventional military approach to small-fragment wounds has involved treating penetrating wounds in an aggressive fashion with early exploration, debridement, and delayed primary closure. However, recent evidence suggests that a more conservative approach may be appropriate, provided that bacterial colonization is prevented with appropriate antibiotic coverage.[34] This strategy is valid when the following criteria are met[1]: involvement of soft tissue only with no breach of pleura or peritoneum and no major vascular involvement and[2] an entry or exit wound of less than 2 cm in maximum dimension that was[3] not frankly infected[4] and not caused by a mine blast.[39]

Wound closure for blast-related extremity wounds is typically delayed to approximately 5 days from the time of injury to ensure that there is no evidence of infection prior to closure. Exceptions are made for open dural injuries and facial wounds. Studies are currently underway to investigate whether earlier closure may provide lower rates of nosocomial infection, and there are a number of emerging therapies for the treatment of extremity wounds. Early administration of negative pressure wound therapy after debridement has gained widespread acceptance, and antimicrobial-impregnated bead therapy and biofilms are promising technologies currently under investigation.[38]

Central Nervous System Injury

Traumatic brain injury (TBI) is a common result of blasts, and it ranges from minor concussions to fatal intracranial hemorrhage. The primary effects of blast overpressure can lead to neurologic injury; however, the majority of severe TBIs are thought to be due to secondary and tertiary mechanisms. This is due to the fact that the brain (within the skull and cerebrospinal fluid [CSF]) is significantly more tolerant of high pressures than the lungs, and pressures capable of causing fatal pulmonary injuries in a majority of subjects will cause only mild concussive injury to the brain.[40,41]

Mechanisms for isolated PBIs without secondary or tertiary injuries to the brain remain a topic of intense debate. In part, this may stem from the fact that significant PBIs are often associated with other mechanisms of injury. In a study of blast-related TBI survivors by Mac Donald et al., using diffusion tensor imaging to evaluate for axonal injury, all subjects had a mechanism of head injury in addition to PBI.[42] Additionally, more subtle PBIs to the brain may be too small for the resolution of in vivo neuroimaging. Animal models for PBI-induced brain injury suffer from significant differences in the terms of geometry and scale of the human brain versus those of other animals.

Secondary and tertiary mechanisms of TBI can result in penetrating intracranial injury, skull fractures, laceration of major vessels, cerebral contusions (coup and countercoup effects), and acceleration-deceleration injuries as seen in more common causes of TBI. Even though the total contribution of PBI to blast-related TBI remains uncertain, a number of pathological features distinguish blast-related TBI from other causes, such as rapid development of edema, frequent rates of subarachnoid hemorrhage, and a higher tendency toward vasospasm and pseudoaneurysm development.[43-46]

TBIs are classically stratified via the Glasgow Coma Scale (GCS), into severe (below 8), moderate,[9-13] and mild.[14,15,45,47] Severe and moderate TBI patients often have profoundly altered mental status and focal neurologic deficits. The effects of mild TBI are subtle and can be easily missed, as the gross majority of these patients will have no obvious deficits.[48,49] Patients with moderate and severe TBI are at extremely high risk of delayed intracranial hemorrhage and cerebral edema and should be evacuated immediately to a center with neurosurgical capability. Early invasive monitoring and the capability of performing a decompressive craniotomy are vital. Providers should aggressively treat hyperthermia in severe blast-related TBI.[49]

The management of patients with concurrent TBI and hemorrhagic shock is complicated. Even though a degree of permissive hypotension is advocated in the management of uncontrolled hemorrhage in thoracic and abdominal trauma, systolic blood pressures below 90 mm Hg are closely tied to worse outcomes in TBI (pressures at or below 80 mm Hg systolic have also been linked to worse outcomes in blast trauma to the thorax and abdomen).[50] Similarly, both underoxygenation and overoxygenation are problematic in the treatment of TBI. In patients with TBI, oxygen saturation should be kept above 90%, and rapid sequence intubation (RSI) should not be provided in the prehospital setting unless administered by providers with sufficient training in its performance, because of the risk of hypoxia and delayed transport.[51]

Mild blast-related TBI is associated with brief loss of consciousness or awareness and can lead to headache, confusion, amnesia, and anxiety. Although these symptoms often resolve within a few hours or days after the injury, they may lead to long-term changes in personality and intellectual function.[45,48] Patients with mild blast-related TBI may have some minor pathophysiologic and neuropsychiatric differences from those with mild TBI resulting from blunt trauma, although this does not affect immediate management.[52,53] Even though there is an evolving role for neuroimaging in the long-term assessment of blast-related mild TBI, a more promising route for the immediate diagnosis of mild TBI can be found in clinical assessment scales such as the Military Acute Concussion Evaluation (MACE), as well as a number of rapid computer-assisted neuropsychiatric tests under development.[49]

Even though the effects of mild TBI are not by themselves life-threatening, missing a mild TBI can seriously endanger survivors and providers. The deficits caused by mild TBI can significantly impair judgment and concentration, putting victims at risk for repeated head injuries. So-called second impacts dramatically increase the potential morbidity and mortality of even minor head trauma.[54] Accordingly, providers should strongly discourage blast victims at risk for TBI from returning to rescue efforts once they have been evacuated. There is a substantially increased incidence of posttraumatic stress disorder (PTSD) in patients after blast exposure, and the risk is particularly high in patients who have suffered a mild TBI.[55] Providers should refer blast victims to appropriate mental health providers both for general counseling and to help screen for the development of PTSD or "second-victim" syndrome.

Auditory Injury

The ear is the organ most frequently injured by explosions, but auditory PBI is frequently overlooked in the context of more serious coexisting injuries during mass-casualty scenarios.[9] The auditory system is uniquely predisposed to PBI because the tympanic membrane (TM) acts as an efficient means for transmitting pressure waves to the middle and inner ear.[2] Although auditory PBI rarely requires emergent intervention, recognition and appropriate referral can profoundly reduce long-term morbidity.[56] All survivors of a blast should have an otologic assessment and audiometry at some time in their aftercare.[1]

Symptoms of auditory PBI include tinnitus, otalgia, and a feeling of fullness.[56] Perforation of the TM is a hallmark of auditory PBI and is typically seen as multiple "punched out" lesions or radial lacerations. The pars tensa is usually involved.[2,4] Other signs include hearing loss, blood and/or debris in the ear canal, and disruption of the ossicles. The presence of tinnitus and hearing loss may be initially profound; these findings are usually self-limited and tend to improve quickly.[2] Prolonged duration of these symptoms may be seen in survivors of blasts occurring in CSs.[56]

Vertigo is uncommon in auditory PBI, and its presence should prompt evaluation for neurologic injury. The complication of perilymph fistula should be considered in a patient with vertigo and sensorineural hearing loss, particularly if these findings are fluctuating. This is the only component of auditory PBI requiring prompt surgical treatment (i.e., emergent tympanotomy and fistula repair). Cholesteatoma may be a late complication (12 to 48 months) of TM perforation.[2] Eighty percent of TM perforations heal spontaneously, and nonoperative management is appropriate for most cases.[2,56] Large perforations may warrant surgical repair, but elective tympanoplasty can safely be delayed for up to 12 months with good outcomes.[2] Antibiotics are not indicated unless underlying infection is suspected.

Given the relatively low levels of pressure needed to rupture the eardrum relative to the pressure needed to injure other organ systems, a number of authors have suggested using eardrum rupture as a means of triaging patients.[5,9] It is important to note that TM perforation correlates poorly with PBI involving other organ systems and should not be used as a marker of latent PBI elsewhere in the body. This is particularly acute in closed-space explosions, where many survivors may demonstrate pulmonary blast injury without evidence of TM rupture.[5,18] However, in the case of OA blasts, current evidence suggests that patients who present with isolated TM perforation but are otherwise asymptomatic, with a normal chest x-ray, may be safely discharged after 6 hours of observation.[5,9]

⚠ PITFALLS

- *Overtriage is linked to dramatically increased mortality:* Understanding the epidemiology of past explosions can help providers allocate resources appropriately[10,14] (e.g., survivors of closed-space explosions will present with a much higher incidence of PBI than survivors of OA explosions, and will often require a higher proportion of critical care and monitoring, and explosions that cause buildings to collapse will often delay the evacuation of the most critical patients, compared with other survivors).[2,18]
- *Failure to meticulously monitor fluid balance:* Transient hypotension and bradycardia caused by PBI-induced cardiovascular effects can tempt providers into aggressively resuscitating patients, worsening BLI; however, soft-tissue injuries and burns often require intensive fluid resuscitation—therefore invasive monitoring is considered the standard of care in patients with suspected pulmonary PBI who require fluid management.
- *Inappropriate use of oxygen:* Although oxygen is indicated for all patients with signs of respiratory distress or air embolism, providers should remain cognizant of the risks of oxygen toxicity and avoid hyperoxygenating patients with TBIs.
- Failure to aggressively control the airway when patients are in respiratory failure or if their exam suggests a potential airway injury can increase risk to the patient.
- Missed auditory injuries or delayed identification of gastrointestinal injuries: whereas some authors recommend at least 6 to 8 hours of observation, others recommend periods as long as several days in patients with stigmata of blast exposure to the abdomen.[28]
- Providers should guard against failure to address high incidence of psychological stress after an explosion.

REFERENCES

1. Wolf SJ, Bebarta VS, Bonnett CJ, Pons PT, Cantrill SV. Blast injuries. *Lancet.* 2009;374(9687):405–415.
2. Horrocks C. Blast injuries: biophysics, pathophysiology and management principles. *J R Army Med Corps.* 2001;147(1):28–40.
3. Leibovici D, Gofrit ON, Stein M, et al. Blast injuries: bus versus open-air bombings—a comparative study of injuries in survivors of open-air versus confined-space explosions. *J Trauma Acute Care Surg.* 1996;41 (6):1030–1035.
4. Wightman JM, Gladish SL. Explosions and blast injuries. *Ann Emerg Med.* 2001;37(6):664–678.
5. Leibovici D, Gofrit ON, Shapira SC. Eardrum perforation in explosion survivors: is it a marker of pulmonary blast injury? *Ann Emerg Med.* 1999;34 (2):168–172.
6. Cullis I. Blast waves and how they interact with structures. *J R Army Med Corps.* 2001;147(1):16–26.
7. Bors D, Cummins J, Goodpaster J. The anatomy of a pipe bomb explosion: Measuring the mass and velocity distributions of container fragments. *J Forensic Sci.* 2014;59(1):42–51.
8. Kang DG, Lehman RA Jr, Carragee EJ. Wartime spine injuries: understanding the improvised explosive device and biophysics of blast trauma. *Spine J.* 2012;12(9):849–857.
9. DePalma RG, Burris DG, Champion HR, Hodgson MJ. Blast injuries. *N Engl J Med.* 2005;352(13):1335–1342.
10. Frykberg ER. Medical management of disasters and mass casualties from terrorist bombings: how can we cope? *J Trauma Acute Care Surg.* 2002;53 (2):201–212.
11. RAND®-MIPT Terrorism Incident Database [database on the Internet]. RAND® Memorial Institute for the Prevention of Terrorism. [cited (January 12th, 2014)]. Available from: http://www.rand.org/nsrd/projects/terrorism-incidents.html.
12. Barker AD. Improvised explosive devices in Southern Afghanistan and Western Pakistan, 2002–2009. *Studies in Conflict & Terrorism.* 2011;34 (8):600–620.
13. Biancolini CsA, Del Bosco CG, Jorge MA. Argentine Jewish community institution bomb explosion. *J Trauma Acute Care Surg.* 1999;47(4):728.
14. Biddinger PD, Baggish A, Harrington L, et al. Be prepared, the Boston Marathon and mass-casualty events. *N Engl J Med.* 2013;.
15. Kellermann AL. Peleg K. N Engl J Med: Lessons from Boston; 2013.
16. Walls RM, Zinner MJ. The Boston Marathon response: why did it work so well? *JAMA.* 2013;309(23):2441–2442.
17. Mallonee S, Shariat S, Stennies G, Waxweiler R, Hogan D, Jordan F. Physical injuries and fatalities resulting from the Oklahoma City bombing. *JAMA.* 1996;276(5):382–387.
18. Golan R, Soffer D, Givon A, Peleg K. The ins and outs of terrorist bus explosions: injury profiles of on-board explosions versus explosions occurring adjacent to a bus. *Injury.* 2013;.
19. Kragh JF Jr, Littrel ML, Jones JA, et al. Battle casualty survival with emergency tourniquet use to stop limb bleeding. *J Emerg Med.* 2011;41 (6):590–597.
20. Avidan V, Hersch M, Armon Y, et al. Blast lung injury: clinical manifestations, treatment, and outcome. *Am J Surg.* 2005;190(6): 945–950.
21. Mackenzie IM, Tunnicliffe B. Blast injuries to the lung: epidemiology and management. *Philos Trans R Soc Lond B Biol Sci.* 2011;366 (1562):295–299.
22. Pizov R, Oppenheim-Eden A, Matot I, et al. Blast lung injury from an explosion on a civilian bus. *CHEST Journal.* 1999;115(1):165–172.
23. Shaham D, Sella T, Makori A, Appelbaum L, Rivkind AI, Ziv JB. The role of radiology in terror injuries. *IMAJ-RAMAT GAN-.* 2002;4 (7):564–567.
24. Ho AM-H, Ling E. Systemic air embolism after lung trauma. *Anesthesiology.* 1999;90(2):564–575.
25. Barrow DW, Rhoads HT. Blast concussion injury. *JAMA.* 1944;125 (13):900–902.
26. Irwin RJ, Lerner MR, Bealer JF, Mantor PC, Brackett DJ, Tuggle DW. Shock after blast wave injury is caused by a vagally mediated reflex. *J Trauma Acute Care Surg.* 1999;47(1):105–110.

27. Irwin RJ, Lerner MR, Bealer JF, Brackett DJ, Tuggle DW. Cardiopulmonary physiology of primary blast injury. *J Trauma Acute Care Surg.* 1997;43(4):650–655.

28. Owers C, Morgan J, Garner J. Abdominal trauma in primary blast injury. *Br J Surg.* 2011;98(2):168–179.

29. Paran H, Neufeld D, Shwartz I, et al. Perforation of the terminal ileum induced by blast injury: delayed diagnosis or delayed perforation? *J Trauma Acute Care Surg.* 1996;40(3):472–475.

30. Butela ST, Federle MP, Chang PJ, et al. Performance of CT in detection of bowel injury. *Am J Roentgenol.* 2001;176(1):129–135.

31. Ramasamy A, Hughes A, Carter N, Kendrew J. The effects of explosion on the musculoskeletal system. *Trauma.* 2013;15(2):128–139.

32. Hull J, Cooper G. Pattern and mechanism of traumatic amputation by explosive blast. *J Trauma Acute Care Surg.* 1996;40(3S):198S–205S.

33. Ritenour AE, Dorlac WC, Fang R, et al. Complications after fasciotomy revision and delayed compartment release in combat patients. *J Trauma Acute Care Surg.* 2008;64(2):S153–S162.

34. Brown KV, Murray CK, Clasper JC. Infectious complications of combat-related mangled extremity injuries in the British military. *J Trauma Acute Care Surg.* 2010;69(1):S109–S115.

35. Lesperance K, Martin MJ, Beekley AC, Steele SR. The significance of penetrating gluteal injuries: an analysis of the Operation Iraqi Freedom experience. *J Surg Educ.* 2008;65(1):61–66.

36. Caterson E, Carty MJ, Weaver MJ, Holt EF. Boston bombings: a surgical view of lessons learned from combat casualty care and the applicability to Boston's terrorist attack. *J Craniofac Surg.* 2013;24(4):1061–1067.

37. Murray C, Obremskey W, Hsu J, et al. Prevention of infections associated with combat-related extremity injuries. *J Trauma.* 2011;71(2 Suppl 2):S235.

38. Hospenthal DR, Murray CK, Andersen RC, Bell RB, Calhoun JH, Cancio LC, et al. Guidelines for the prevention of infections associated with combat-related injuries: 2011 update: endorsed by the Infectious Diseases Society of America and the Surgical Infection Society. *J Trauma Acute Care Surg.* 2011;71(2):S210–S234.

39. Covey DC. Blast and fragment injuries of the musculoskeletal system. *J Bone Joint Surg Am.* 2002;84(7):1221–1234.

40. Bass CR, Panzer MB, Rafaels KA, Wood G, Shridharani J, Capehart B. Brain injuries from blast. *Ann Biomed Eng.* 2012;40(1):185–202.

41. Moore DF, Jérusalem A, Nyein M, Noels L, Jaffee MS, Radovitzky RA. Computational biology—modeling of primary blast effects on the central nervous system. *Neuroimage.* 2009;47:T10–T20.

42. Mac Donald CL, Johnson AM, Cooper D, et al. Detection of blast-related traumatic brain injury in US military personnel. *N Engl J Med.* 2011;364(22):2091–2100.

43. Bell RS, Vo AH, Roberts R, Wanebo J, Armonda RA. Wartime traumatic aneurysms: acute presentation, diagnosis, and multimodal treatment of 64 craniocervical arterial injuries. *Neurosurgery.* 2010;66(1):66–79.

44. Cernak I, Noble-Haeusslein LJ. Traumatic brain injury: an overview of pathobiology with emphasis on military populations. *J Cereb Blood Flow Metab.* 2009;30(2):255–266.

45. Ling G, Bandak F, Armonda R, Grant G, Ecklund J. Explosive blast neurotrauma. *J Neurotrauma.* 2009;26(6):815–825.

46. Nakagawa A, Manley GT, Gean AD, et al. Mechanisms of primary blast-induced traumatic brain injury: insights from shock-wave research. *J Neurotrauma.* 2011;28(6):1101–1119.

47. Andriessen TM, Horn J, Franschman G, et al. Epidemiology, severity classification, and outcome of moderate and severe traumatic brain injury: a prospective multicenter study. *J Neurotrauma.* 2011;28(10):2019–2031.

48. Elder GA, Cristian A. Blast-related mild traumatic brain injury: mechanisms of injury and impact on clinical care. *Mount Sinai Journal of Medicine: A Journal of Translational and Personalized Medicine.* 2009;76(2):111–118.

49. Rosenfeld JV, McFarlane AC, Bragge P, Armonda RA, Grimes JB, Ling GS. Blast-related traumatic brain injury. *Lancet Neurol.* 2013;12(9):882–893.

50. Garner J, Watts S, Parry C, Bird J, Cooper G, Kirkman E. Prolonged permissive hypotensive resuscitation is associated with poor outcome in primary blast injury with controlled hemorrhage. *Ann Surg.* 2010;251(6):1131–1139.

51. Swadron SP, LeRoux P, Smith WS, Weingart SD. Emergency neurological life support: traumatic brain injury. *Neurocrit Care.* 2012;17(1):112–121.

52. Fischer BL, Parsons M, Durgerian S, et al. Neural activation during response inhibition differentiates blast from mechanical causes of mild to moderate traumatic brain injury. *Journal of Neurotrauma.* 2013.

53. Mendez MF, Owens EM, Jimenez EE, Peppers D, Licht EA. Changes in personality after mild traumatic brain injury from primary blast vs. blunt forces. *Brain Inj.* 2013;27(1):10–18.

54. Blennow K, Hardy J, Zetterberg H. The neuropathology and neurobiology of traumatic brain injury. *Neuron.* 2012;76(5):886–899.

55. Hoge CW, McGurk D, Thomas JL, Cox AL, Engel CC, Castro CA. Mild traumatic brain injury in US soldiers returning from Iraq. *N Engl J Med.* 2008;358(5):453–463.

56. Cohen JT, Ziv G, Bloom J, Zikk D, Rapoport Y, Himmelfarb MZ. Blast injury of the ear in a confined space explosion: auditory and vestibular evaluation. *IMAJ-RAMAT GAN-.* 2002;4(7):559–562.

CHAPTER 72

Suicide Bomber

Evan Avraham Alpert and Shamai A. Grossman

DESCRIPTION OF EVENT

The continued perpetration of suicide bombings by terrorists throughout the world requires that knowledge of the topic be continually updated. Global news services and electronic social networking allow terrorists with fundamentalist ideologies to broadcast their extremist views to an international audience. To achieve their heinous goals of killing and maiming as many civilians as possible, they choose to target high-visibility places where the public is concentrated. Hence, they disproportionately attack urban areas such as buses, malls, and restaurants.

Differences have been noted between bombs prepared by terrorists and those used in traditional warfare. Operating on more limited budgets, terrorists have discovered methods of packing bombs with nails, bolts, and other metal objects so as to inflict maximum injury. These bombs are created to be easily transportable, usually strapped to the terrorist's body. Unfortunately, the ongoing conflicts in places such as Afghanistan, Iraq, and Syria have increased terrorist access to large munitions and resulted in a rapid evolution of suicide bomber tactics, techniques, and procedures (TTPs), such as the use of vehicle-borne improvised explosive devices (VBIEDs) and layered attacks.

PRE-INCIDENT ACTIONS

Suicide bombing attacks present complex planning and response challenges. Pre-incident actions include planning and preparedness activities generally aimed at threat and consequence mitigation. Social policies addressing the roots of terrorism and the psychological profiling of terrorists are critical components to any full-spectrum policy; however, these topics are beyond the scope of this chapter. This section focuses on two main areas: infrastructure hardening and training.

There are multiple strategies to prevent and mitigate the consequences of suicide bombers. Hardening strategies such as security checks and concrete barriers are now common techniques for limiting suicide bomber access to critical facilities such as airports and government institutions. Barriers erected in vehicle approach lanes and around buildings are designed to prevent detonation in close proximity to critical infrastructure. Hardening of structures may work for many pedestrian or vehicle-borne suicide bombings, but not for all bombings; take, for example, the case of the World Trade Center Bombings on September 11, 2001, by which, due to the combination of a large explosive force and building collapse, most of the victims were killed immediately. In addition, terrorists have adapted TTPs, now deploying teams of suicide bombers to attack barriers in waves (e.g., "layered attacks").

Training is essential for improved situational awareness and effective response. Planning activities should include yearly drills so that staffs understand their roles in multicasualty incidents, especially those associated with blast injuries. Command, control, and communication need to be emphasized: the Incident Command System (ICS) should be utilized during response. Training should be interagency, including prehospital staff, law enforcement, emergency management, hospital administrators, and relevant clinical/support departments. Anticipating surge capacity in the emergency department, operating room, and intensive care units is essential. All local hospitals need to be included in contingency plans because the number of severely injured patients may be overwhelming, even for a Level 1 Trauma Center.[1]

POST-INCIDENT ACTIONS

Security is essential at the scene of the event, as well as at the hospital. There have been numerous instances of secondary bombings where an additional intentional device or bomber detonated after prehospital providers entered the scene. This resulted in rescuers then becoming victims. Rescue teams of emergency medical service(s) (EMS) and fire department personnel will naturally assume higher risk than daily operations, but they must work closely with police or security services to ensure appropriate levels of "scene safety" before they enter a scene and begin resuscitation and rescue efforts. Hospitals are vulnerable targets, and staff must remain vigilant after a suicide bombing. Health care facilities are notorious "soft" targets, often lacking armed security and proper blast hardening or mechanisms to effectively limit bomber access.

Blast injury patterns have classically been described based on wartime injuries, with a limited number of survivors requiring medical care.[2-5] In contrast, urban bomb explosions result in many patients arriving alive at the hospital but with devastating injuries. Terrorists know that maximum death and injury can be accomplished by bringing the explosives to closed spaces. There is a direct correlation between the location of the blast and survivability. Open, closed, and sealed spaces result in differential injury patterns based on the standard categories of blast injury.[6,7] Mortality is the highest in ultraconfined spaces such as buses. In general there is a higher injury-severity score for those presenting to the hospital following terrorist attacks than those presenting because of other trauma. Surgical interventions are higher in these patients as well.[6]

The classification of blast injuries is discussed in length in other sections of this text (Box 72-1). Given the suicide bomber TTP of seeking close proximity to victims, there are some issues particularly relevant to suicide bombings. Virtually all patients exposed directly to the blast front will incur primary blast injury. The immediate blast front is dissipated from the center of the explosion based on forces of spalling, acceleration, and implosion mechanisms, as well as pressure differences. Air-containing structures such as the lungs, bowels, and tympanic membranes are often affected. More than 50% of patients

---

BOX 72-1 Types of Blast Injuries

- *Primary:* injury caused by the blast wave
- *Secondary:* injury caused by shrapnel
- *Tertiary:* injury caused by the victim being thrown
- *Quaternary:* injury caused by fire and heat

---

exposed to a blast of greater than 15 to 50 psi will suffer tympanic membrane perforation. This can be a marker of coincident injuries such as a blast lung injury (BLI) that may not be readily apparent (BLI often requires higher pressures of 50 to 100 psi). Primary blast head injury appears to have a higher mortality compared with other conventional head injuries, most probably because of the tremendous force of the initial exposure. Air emboli in the pulmonary and coronary vessels may also be a cause of death.[4-7]

Secondary blast effect results from flying shards of metal, glass, and other explosive objects that inflict injuries similar to those from classic penetrating patterns. Given some limitations in the volume of explosives that suicide bombers can carry, they have historically utilized high volumes of adulterants such as metal bolts, nails, and pellets. As a result, benign appearing skin wounds may signal severe underlying injury. Suicide bombing also significantly increases the risk of biologic foreign body implantation secondary to flying bone fragments from the suicide bomber, other victims, or the patient.[8-11]

Infiltrates on chest x-ray often present a clinical challenge because it may be difficult to differentiate between BLI and lacerated lung caused by secondary blast mechanisms. Both may present as a pneumothorax, but a hemothorax is less common in classic blast injury. Both may also develop significant respiratory difficulties, with persistent air leaks requiring creative ventilator techniques. However, in the early phase of injury, fluid management is different because blast lung requires restrictive management and is nonoperative, whereas lacerated lungs need fluid resuscitation and often surgical repair.[6,7]

Tertiary blast effects, causing the victim's body to be thrown, are accentuated in closed and ultraconfined spaces because the victim's body may be propelled against stationary objects by a supercharged blast front. Immediate amputation or death can occur. Quaternary blast injuries are burns caused by the explosion itself or surrounding flammable area. These may include all types of classical burn injuries, including inhalation, chemical, and contact burns.[6]

Often the patient suffers from a combination of blast injury effects including blunt injury, penetrating trauma, and burns. This is known as the multidimensional injury pattern and is unique to bomb explosions.[6,7] Particularly challenging are visceral blast injuries that may occur from multiple wounding mechanisms. Primary or tertiary blast injury may cause slow dissection along tissue planes, resulting in delayed peritonitis. In contrast, missile trajectory of secondary blast injury may parallel classic penetrating injury resulting from stab or gunshot wounds.[6]

✚ MEDICAL TREATMENT OF CASUALTIES

Prehospital Care

First responders should be versed in Tactical Emergency Casualty Care (TECC). TECC defines threat-based principles of prehospital care, with emphasis on threat mitigation, hemorrhage control, rapid extraction, and rapid evacuation to medical providers for triage and treatment. Triage at the scene is performed based on any number of triage systems, such as the simple triage and rapid transport (START), JumpSTART, SAVE, or Sacco Method.[12] After extensive experience with suicide bombing, Magen David Adom (MDA, Israel's EMS), during the Second

Intifada Palestinian uprising of 2002-2005, successfully adopted the concept of "save and run." The only actions performed at the scene are bandages and tourniquets to stop bleeding and the advanced life support actions of intubation and needle thoracostomy. The most severely injured patients are generally directed to the closest Level 1 Trauma Centers. Other considerations such as the large numbers of casualties or severity of life-threatening injury may result in the patient being taken to the nearest medical centers. A certain percentage of these patients will then undergo secondary transfer to a trauma center.[13] As noted above, with growing concern for multimodal attacks, secondary devices and bombers breaching or detonating at the scene as first responders begin resuscitation, the site should not be approached without a coordinated threat mitigation strategy (e.g., law enforcement/security, EMS, and fire).

Emergency Department Care

Once notification of a suicide bombing occurs, the hospital should begin immediate preparation for incoming casualties. Necessary personnel, from both in-hospital and on-call staff, including doctors, nurses, administrative, and ancillary staff, are recruited through pager or phone. The emergency department is cleared; any patients to be admitted are sent immediately to inpatient units; and those who can be discharged are sent home. Elective surgery, computed tomography (CT), or angiographic cases are delayed.

Space is organized into resuscitation rooms, acute care areas, and observation areas, and room is set aside for expected deceased victims. Staff, including security personnel, should take up designated positions in each of these areas. An emergency physician or senior surgeon is stationed at the entry of the emergency department to triage victims to the appropriate area. One study found that penetrating head and abdominal injuries, as well as injuries to four or more body regions, were associated with a higher rate of BLI or the need for laparotomy. They recommend triage of patients with these criteria, as well as those with hemodynamic instability or respiratory distress, directly to the trauma operating rooms or surgical intensive care units. Patients without those features are sent to either an admitting or observation area.[14]

Emergency care of casualties from a suicide bombing mirrors response to conventional trauma with several nuances. First, even though the Advanced Trauma Life Support (ATLS) principles of ABC (airway, breathing, and circulation) remain critical, the team should consider immediate control of life-threatening extremity hemorrhage with tourniquets within the first 60 seconds of patient arrival. Once an airway has been secured and breathing and circulation established, the primary and secondary physical examination should continue.

Imaging studies such as emergency bedside ultrasound and chest x-ray should be performed. The extended FAST (Focused Assessment with Sonography in Trauma) technique, if positive, can expedite diagnosis of tamponade, pneumothorax, hemothorax, or hemoperitoneum. Prioritization of CT scanning must be established because these tests need to be reserved for immediate, life-threatening, decision-making protocols. Total body fluoroscopy should be used liberally to identify all potential projectiles. A high index of suspicion for life-threatening injury must be maintained when multiple shrapnel pieces are identified on radiograph or fluoroscopy.[6] Routine mapping of such findings is mandatory for documentation and future reference. Radiological studies that are not required for immediate life-saving clinical decisions can be deferred and performed later in the patient's hospital course.

Diagnostic peritoneal lavage (DPL) should also be considered in certain circumstances. It can be rapidly performed at the bedside and performed in the absence of ultrasound. In some cases, injuries are identified after a CT scan with initially negative results. Because of the potential for multiple mechanisms of action, a minimum of 10,000 red blood cells/mL as a lower-level threshold for DPL in blast visceral injury has been suggested.[6]

The multidimensional injury patterns seen in suicide bomb attacks present new dilemmas that demand a reassessment of established techniques to improve patient survival. In evaluating the multidimensional injury pattern with associated abdominal visceral injury, certain patterns have been noted. The injuries in this scenario appear to be more diffuse and necessitate meticulous surgical exploration. This may be particularly difficult in the midst of a multicasualty event involving other injured patients who are waiting to enter the operating room.[15–17] An intensive and persistent search for injury still must be undertaken, with the underlying mechanisms of both blunt and penetrating injuries kept in mind. Clearly, this results in significant surgical burden that is most effectively managed by a system-wide, interdisciplinary approach.

Judicious use of blood products is important. In the violent, traumatic mass casualty incident (MCI), the principles of damage control resuscitation, including hypotensive resuscitation for hemorrhagic shock in the absence of traumatic brain injury, should be encouraged. A retrospective analysis of the transfusion of blood products to suicide bombing victims showed that twice the number of packed red blood cells were ordered than transfused. However, 10% of patients received massive transfusions.[18] Close collaboration between the emergency department, surgery department, and blood bank is critical for creating effective blood product utilization protocols in these complex scenarios.

Tetanus prophylaxis should be given. Because of the potential of infection from human projectile implantation or blood, hepatitis B prophylaxis should be given as well. Counseling for HIV prophylaxis should be considered. If possible, blood from the bomber should be tested for hepatitis B and C, as well as HIV.[8–11]

Because of concern for delayed injury presentation, patients with previously negative examination results require careful reevaluation. Blast injuries may develop exponentially over time, resulting in injuries that are missed initially. For this reason, the tertiary survey has assumed a renewed level of importance in these events. If this examination suggests potential missed injury, further testing with repeat ultrasound or CT is appropriate as soon as the majority of casualties have been admitted and routed through triage.

UNIQUE CONSIDERATIONS

Mechanisms of bomb delivery may be critical in adequately preparing for victims of suicide bombings. Data from Iraq have shown that there is a higher mortality rate in victims of suicide bombers on foot than those in a vehicle.[19] Thus, resources may need to be maximized when caring for these victims in particular.

The subgroup of patients with a multidimensional injury pattern is not predicted adequately by the classic injury-severity score system. Imaging using x-rays, ultrasonography, and CT has been shown to be more frequent in victims of suicide bombing, as compared with other trauma.[20] Parameters such as length of hospital stay, length of stay in the intensive care unit, and mortality appear significantly different from other groups of patients, emphasizing the unique nature of this subgroup.

The management of multidimensional injury can be contrasted with other conventional traumatic injury. Because of the wounding mechanisms, the likelihood that these patients will require some type of surgical intervention is high. Such multiple injuries result in unique challenges in diagnosis, decision making, and treatment. Providing care to a patient with multidimensional injury will often require the careful coordination of multiple surgical teams. This translates into the need for a large operating space to accommodate the teams that must work simultaneously.

Because suicide bombings can be at least as emotionally intense as any other major mass casualty event. Victims frequently suffer from at least short-term posttraumatic stress. Empathetic care must begin from the time the patient arrives in the emergency department and continue throughout the process of their medical care.[21] Multidisciplinary teams should be available for counseling and support of victims, families, community members, and staff.

! PITFALLS

Several potential pitfalls in response to a suicide bomber attack exist. These include the following:
- Failure to aggressively secure first responders and first receiving facilities
- Failure to develop and use protocols to coordinate manpower and medical resources in the post bombing response
- Failure to acknowledge and plan for the complex challenges associated with the combined clinical scenario of head injury, burns, blast lung, and intraabdominal or thoracic injury
- Failure to maintain constant clinical vigilance in the case of combined head and other injuries to time-interventional modalities
- Failure to aggressively monitor and address resuscitation parameters such as acidosis and hypothermia. Aggressive warming mechanisms must be used, and the potential for developing coagulopathy must be recognized[15]
- Overuse of imaging triage such as CT scanning

ACKNOWLEDGMENT

The authors would like to thank Dr. Jeffrey Kashuk for his contribution to the first edition.

REFERENCES

1. Einav S, Feigenberg Z, Weissman C, et al. Evacuation priorities in mass casualty terror-related events: implications for contingency planning. *Ann Surg.* 2004;239(3):304–310.
2. Frykberg ER. Medical management of disasters and mass casualties from terrorist bombings: how can we cope? *J Trauma.* 2002;53:201–212.
3. Frykberg ER. Principles of mass casualty managed following terrorist disasters. *Ann Surg.* 2004;239:319–321.
4. Mellor SG, Cooper GJ. Analysis of 828 servicemen killed or injured by explosion in Northern Ireland 1970–84. The Hostile Action Casualty System. *Br J Surg.* 1989;76:1006.
5. Katz JE, Ofek B, Adler J, Abramowitz HB, Krausz MM. Primary blast injury after a bomb explosion in a civilian bus. *Ann Surg.* 1989;209:484–488.
6. Kluger Y, Kashuk J, Mayo A. Terror bombings: mechanisms, consequences, and implications. *Scand J Surg.* 2004;93:11–14.
7. Kluger Y. Bomb explosions in acts of terrorism—detonation, wound ballistics, triage and medical concerns. *Isr Med Assoc J.* 2003;5(4):235–240.
8. Eshkol Z, Katz K. Injuries from biologic material of suicide bombers. *Injury.* 2005;36(2):271–274.
9. Wong JM, Marsh D, Abu-Sitta G, et al. Biological foreign body implantation in victims of the London July 7th suicide bombings. *J Trauma.* 2006;60(2):402–404.
10. Clint BD. Force protection and infectious risk mitigation from suicide bombers. *Mil Med.* 2009;174(7):709–714.
11. Patel HD, Dryden S, Gupta A, Stewart N. Human body projectiles implantation in victims of suicide bombings and implications for health and emergency care providers: the 7/7 experience. *Ann R Coll Surg Engl.* 2012;94(5):313–317.

12. Jenkins JL, McCarthy ML, Sauer LM, et al. Mass-casualty triage: time for an evidence-based approach. *Prehosp Disaster Med.* 2008;23(1):3.

13. Feigenberg Z. The pre-hospital medical treatment of the victims of multi-casualty incidents caused by explosions of suicide bombers during the Al-Aksa Intifada—April 2001 to December 2004: the activity and experience gained by the teams of Magen David Adom in Israel. *Harefuah.* 2010;149 (7):413–417.

14. Almogy G, Rivkind AI. Surgical lessons learned from suicide bombing attacks. *J Am Coll Surg.* 2006;202(2):313–319.

15. Almogy G, Belzsberg H, Mintz Y, Pikarsky AK, Zamir G, Rivkind AI. Suicide bombing attacks: update and modification to the protocol. *Ann Surg.* 2004;239:319–321.

16. Peleg K. Patterns of injury in hospitalized terrorist victims. *Am J Emerg Med.* 2003;21:258–262.

17. Peleg K, Aharonson-Daniel L, Stein M, et al. Israeli Trauma Group (ITG). Gunshot and explosion injuries: characteristics, outcomes, and implications for care of terror-related injuries in Israel. *Ann Surg.* 2004;239:311–318.

18. Bala M, Kaufman T, Keidar A, et al. Defining the need for blood and blood products transfusion following suicide bombing attacks on a civilian population: a level I single-centre experience. *Injury.* 2014;45(1):5.

19. Hsiao-Rei Hicks M, Dardagan H, Bagnall PM, Spagat M, Sloboda JA. Casualties in civilians and coalition soldiers from suicide bombings in Iraq, 2003–10: a descriptive study. *Lancet.* Sept 3, 2011;378.

20. Aharonson-Daniel L, Klein Y, Peleg K. ITG. Suicide bombers form a new injury profile. *Ann Surg.* 2006;244(6):1018–1023.

21. Dolberg OT, Barkai G, Leor A, Rapoport H, Bloch M, Schreiber S. Injured civilian survivors of suicide bomb attacks: from partial PTSD to recovery or to traumatisation. Where is the turning point? *World J Biol Psych.* 2010;11:344–351.

CHAPTER 73

Improvised Explosive Devices

James P. Phillips and James R. Johnston Jr.

Improvised explosive devices (IEDs) have existed since the first time a person used an explosive material in a different manner than that for which it was originally intended. The term once used primarily by military and law enforcement forces, has now become a part of the civilian lexicon. IEDs have posed serious threats for more than half a century. They have evolved with time and new technologies. However, it is only since they have become a common weapon in the asymmetric warfare tactics used by nonstate combatants in the wars in Iraq and Afghanistan that significant American dollars have been dedicated to studying them. Only the creator's available materials and dark imagination limit the construction of IEDs. Fortunately, the evolution of bomb design through time has also inspired novel countermeasures and disposal techniques.

Experts report various definitions of IEDs. A recent paper by Gill compared 29 different definitions of IED. Nearly all of these had differing and occasionally contradictory inclusion criteria. A new definition, composed of elements from both prior characterizations and novel criteria, was proposed by Gill to provide researchers with uniform criteria for inclusion in future studies:

> An explosive device is considered an IED when any or all of the following—explosive ingredient, initiation, triggering, or detonation mechanism, delivery system—is modified in any respect from its original expressed or intended function. An IED's components may incorporate any or all of military grade munitions, commercial explosives, or homemade explosives. The components and device design may vary in sophistication from simple to complex, and IEDs can be used by a variety of both state and non-state actors. Non-state actors can include (but not be limited to) terrorists, insurgents, drug traffickers, criminals, and nuisance pranksters.[1]

This definition is all encompassing, and it highlights an important point: not all IEDs are used in the military setting. Nonstate combatants and terrorists have used this method of attack for many decades. In recent years, there has been an increase in the incidence of IED attacks globally in the civilian realm. This trend is reminiscent of the period from the 1960s through the 1980s in Northern Ireland known as "The Troubles," a time when bombings became the weapon of choice of the Provisional Irish Republican Army (PIRA). High-profile civilian bombings have become increasingly common: the 1993 World Trade Center Attack, the 1995 Oklahoma City Bombing, the 1996 Atlanta Summer Olympics, the 11-M Train Bombings in Madrid in 2004, the 7/7 Bus Bombings in London 2005, and, most recent to this writing, the 2013 Boston Marathon Bombing.

This chapter will outline the basics of IED construction, and discuss a brief history of improvised explosive devices used in acts of terrorism around the world. Also included are data and lessons learned during U.S. military involvement in the Global War on Terror, including counter-IED advances in training and technology, which are now being adopted domestically. Separate chapters exist in this book detailing blast injuries and vehicle-borne IEDs (VBIEDs), and these should be referenced for highly detailed information on those subjects.

EXPLOSIVES

An explosive is a material that contains a large amount of potential energy stored within its chemical bonds that when released suddenly can cause significant destructive force. During a conventional explosion, the potential energy is released as the chemical bonds are broken, resulting in rapid gas expansion and the production of heat, sound, light, and high-pressure waves. Nuclear explosions share some similarities but have vast differences as well, and they are discussed in other chapters of this textbook.

Explosives are primarily categorized by the speed at which they are consumed during the explosion, differentiating into two broad categories known as high-order and low-order explosives. If the material itself decomposes at a rate faster than the speed of sound, it is considered a high explosive (HE), and the decomposition of the material is referred to as *detonation*. The physics and consequences of HE detonations are significantly different than those that occur as a result of the decomposition of materials at a rate slower than the speed of sound, referred to as low explosives (LEs). The explosion of an LE is not called a detonation, but instead a *deflagration,* or rapid burn. In general, HE explosives are more powerful and more destructive than LE explosives are, thus their use by conventional military forces is common. LE devices still have very important roles in the military as well, but they are primarily used as propellants to launch projectiles, particularly, bullets and shells. Because both types can be used in the creation of IEDs, it is important to have a working understanding of how they are utilized and modified, as well as the effects of their blasts.

ANATOMY OF AN IMPROVISED EXPLOSIVE DEVICE

IEDs can be very simple or very complex. This chapter will focus primarily on the more complex IEDs because these are the types seen most commonly in combat environments and in international terrorism. In general, an IED is composed of four major components (e.g., a power source, trigger, initiator, and explosive material), any of which can be manufactured or improvised for the creation of a bomb. Generally, failure of any of the components will result in failure of the device. A prototypical IED is comprised of a power source, such as a battery, connected by electrical circuit to an initiator, typically embedded within the explosive material itself. One or more "switches" or triggers are integrated into this circuit that act as on/off switches to the device. Closing the circuit allows energy to be transmitted to the initiator, leading to the subsequent detonation or deflagration of the main explosive. A basic understanding of these components is important, especially regarding the different types and physics of explosives themselves.

Power Source

Explosive materials require energy input to begin the decomposition reaction. The amount of energy required to initiate this reaction determines the explosive's *sensitivity*. The sensitivity of a material helps determine its usability. If a material is very sensitive to shock, heat, or friction, it may be too unstable and dangerous for use. Pure nitroglycerin is an example of a highly sensitive explosive. This sensitivity limited its usefulness until a novel production process resulted in a less shock-sensitive state and the creation of dynamite. A few chemicals are so incredibly sensitive that they are unstable in all environments. Nitrogen triiodide, for example, can be detonated by the energy imparted simply from alpha radiation, seemingly spontaneously, rendering it too dangerous for handling or practical use.

Explosives relevant to this chapter are detonated after being supplied with energy, typically in the form of heat, shock, or friction. Energy must be introduced into the system first, and, historically, this energy was supplied from a flame used to light a safety-fuse, such as the type seen in common fireworks. Later, the magneto "dynamite plunger" was invented and later made widely famous by cartoons. Its advanced system generates an electrical current instead of a flame, transmitted to a primary charge, which, in turn, sets off the main charge. This revolutionary design eliminated many of the safety issues associated with gunpowder-based safety fuses. As technology progressed, new circuitry was developed that allowed more options for bomb makers compared with a fuse or a hand-powered generator. Most IEDs now use energy stored within batteries to initiate explosions, allowing the creativity of bomb makers to blossom and develop new types of triggers.

Switch/Trigger

A bomb explosion needs to be "set off" in some way. This event is known as triggering the device. When triggered, energy enters the circuit and is transferred to the explosive. The simplest systems use a fuse, which then directly provides heat to the main charge. More complex devices with electrical power sources function on a closed circuit of electricity, using wires to connect the battery to an initiator, with a switch/trigger placed in the circuit to keep the flow interrupted. In electrical engineering terms, a switch is defined as a device for making, breaking, or changing the connections in an electrical circuit.[2] Activating the switch/trigger, closes the circuit and allows electricity to flow uninterrupted, as happens when a light switch is turned to the on position. The energy from the electrical signal then activates an initiator, such as an electrical filament or a blasting cap, which then leads to the explosion. Many types of triggers exist, and multiple numbers and types can exist within a single device, tailored to the bomb makers desired purposes.

IEDs can also be defined by *how* they are detonated: by command, by time, or initiated through actions by the victim. In command detonation, someone observing the target area triggers the IED by either a wire directly connected to the device or by remote control through wireless devices such as cell phones, pagers, remote car door openers, or garage door openers.[3] An IED can also have a timer built in as a switch, allowing a bomb to be placed well ahead of detonation, and the operator to escape to a safe distance. Finally, a victim-operated IED, also known as a "booby trap," detonates when a person or vehicle triggers the initiator (e.g., trip wire, pressure plate, pressure-release mechanism, or light-sensitive devices such as motions sensors, etc.).[3]

Command switches are the simplest, merely requiring the push of a button. This action can be taken remotely or proximally, as seen in a suicide bomb vest. Increasingly complicated trigger designs exist in multitude. In a "time bomb" the switch is a timer or clock that, when a predetermined time is reached, the circuit closes. Instead of the bell or alarm sounding, the electricity is transmitted to the bomb initiator. The construction of cell phone, remote control, and other remotely detonated bombs uses a similar method of electricity diversion from benign parts to switch components.

Bomb makers may use the cell phone as both the power source and trigger by incorporating the phone vibrator into the circuit. When the phone vibrator is activated via alarm, call, or text, the power flows from the phone battery, through the vibrator, to the initiator. During The Troubles in Northern Ireland during the twentieth century, a period of time when there was much terrorist activity and bomb-making and disposal technologies made rapid advancements, new "antihandling" features were built into the devices to prevent movement or disarming. Mercury "tilt" switches, similar to those seen in thermostats, contain mercury that if tilted in a particular direction will contact two electrodes and complete a circuit between them causing detonation if the IED is moved.

Initiator

The initiator is the component of the bomb that directly transfers the energy (shock, heat, and friction) from the power source directly into the main charge, leading to combustion. The type of initiator required for successful explosion depends on several factors. The primary determinant is the sensitivity of the main charge and how much energy is required of the initiator to begin the explosion. If a sensitive main charge such as gunpowder is used, a simple burning fuse may provide sufficient energy; for example, in IEDs like those used in the Boston Marathon Bombing in 2013, the initiator is the exposed filament of a simple household Christmas tree light. When initiated, electricity causes the filament to glow and give off enough heat to ignite the LE in which the filament is buried.[4]

Some explosives require much more energy to detonate. Therefore, a simple fuse or light filament will not suffice, in which case, a more powerful initiator must be used. The prime example is the commercially available "blasting cap" used in mining and military applications. In this case, the initiator is itself a small explosive device that is embedded into the main charge. When detonated, the cap provides a large amount of energy sufficient to detonate the main charge. Explosives are designed in this way to prevent accidental detonation during transport and handling. In fact, some explosives will only detonate in response to one *type* of energy, such as shock instead of heat. In fact, plastic explosives such as Compound 4 will burn without exploding, as the fire does not impart sufficient heat energy to trigger detonation. This property was useful to soldiers in Vietnam who would allegedly safely burn their C-4 as fuel for warming food when regular fuel supplies became scarce.

Explosive Material

When creating a bomb, first and foremost an explosive material is required. The amount of material used is proportional to the resulting energy released. HEs generate different blast physics than LEs do. The results are different levels of destruction and injury patterns. This is discussed further below and in more detail in other chapters.

As mentioned, sensitivity defines the amount of energy required to initiate the decompensation of the material and subsequent explosion. A *primary* explosive is one that is particularly sensitive to heat and/or shock and is typically used as an initiator, whereas a *secondary* HE is one that requires a much larger amount of energy to begin an explosion.

Primary HEs are less stable, but, in spite of this, they have been used as the main charge in many bombings, most notably a type of very powerful homemade explosive (HME) called triacetone triperoxide (TATP). Secondary HEs, such as TNT, dynamite, and plastic explosives, are designed to be less sensitive to shock and heat so that they are safer for regular use.

Primary explosives, such as lead azide or diazodinitrophenol (DDNP), which are commonly used in blasting cap initiators, can be used as a primer for a larger explosive device utilizing a larger charge of secondary HE. When a small amount of energy is transmitted to the primary explosive (e.g., a blasting cap inserted into plastic explosive) it is exploded, providing the large initiating energy required for the secondary explosive to detonate. This chain reaction is known as the "explosive train."

Some experts include the category of *tertiary* HEs, which require such a substantial amount of energy to detonate that even a typical initiator such as a blasting cap is insufficient. Instead, a "booster" of primary or secondary explosive is needed to detonate the entire device. A very common tertiary explosive used in mining and industry is ANFO (ammonium nitrate, fuel oil mixture). In the 1995 Oklahoma City Bombing, a similar fertilizer mixture using nitromethane and diesel fuel as the main charge was detonated using Tovex booster charges (very similar to dynamite), which were initially triggered by time-delayed nonelectric blasting caps: thus, a three-step explosive train.

Containment

Not all bombs require a container to function effectively. However, the destructive forces may be greatly increased in some cases if a special containment system is created. Containers are much more important in bombs using weaker LE as the main charge. A brick of naked C-4, a powerful HE, will detonate and create a destructive blast pressure wave that can injure people and destroy structures within the blast radius. However, LEs, such as fireworks and gunpowder, do not produce blast pressure waves when they deflagrate. If a naked pile of gunpowder is ignited, it will burn very rapidly, but the destructive force is minimal compared with that of an HE.

However, if that gunpowder is stored inside of a high-strength container, such as a lead pipe or a pressure cooker, the resulting damage is significantly greater. Using such a container can increase the destructive power of LEs in three important ways. First, and most importantly, a sturdy container allows the pressure generated by the rapidly expanding hot gases from a deflagrating LE to build up inside a fixed volume. The pressure will continue to rapidly build for as long as the container can withstand. Once a critical pressure has been reached, the structural integrity of the container will fail, and the pressure will release very quickly in an explosion that is far more powerful than it would be if the same LE were burned "naked." There is still no blast wave generated, as the decomposition is subsonic, but the destructive force is greatly magnified.

In addition to increased explosive force, there are two other important variables that containers allow: *fragments* and *shrapnel.* Simply put, fragmentation is the physical destruction of the container in which the explosive was stored, and these container pieces themselves become ballistic projectiles called *fragments. Shrapnel* are pieces of material added to a bomb for the specific purpose of becoming ballistic projectiles and increasing the deadliness of the bomb. IED makers often use small metallic objects, such as nails, ball bearings, rocks, etc., packed inside the container, to cause maximum damage. This technique was used with devastating results in the Boston and Atlanta bombings.

Importantly, not all IEDs are made completely from scratch. Outside of the United States, IEDs are often created using previously mass-manufactured weapons, such as artillery shells, land mines, and other military ordnance. This ordnance typically uses trinitrotoluene (TNT)

or some derivative of cyclonite (RDX) type of plastic explosive as the main charge, as originally created in the factory. The weapon is simply repurposed in an improvised manner by creating a new type of trigger system or deployment method. A classic example is the use of an unexploded HE artillery shell that is repurposed as a hidden roadside bomb, after attaching an electrical circuit to the intact explosive train, and triggered by cell phone or other remote switch. These types of IEDs were seen almost daily during the earlier years of the Global War on Terrorism (GWOT) in Iraq and Afghanistan.

TYPES OF IEDs

There is debate about the utility of further classification of IEDs beyond the standardized taxonomy for research purposes. Subcategories can be based upon several characteristics of IEDs, including the method of delivery and the mechanism of triggering the explosion. Classification based on delivery method includes the categories of simple IED (roadside bombs), VBIED (vehicle borne), HBIED (house borne), and PBIED (person borne, a.k.a. suicide bombs). An alternative is to categorize them based on how they are triggered, including direct CWIED (command wired), RCIED (radio controlled), timed IED, and VOIED (victim operated).[3]

BLAST INJURIES

IEDs are effective weapons because of their destructive force and large radius of lethality. The damage they cause to living beings, known as blast injuries, can be categorized into five distinct types listed as primary through quinternary. Because no chapter on IEDs would be complete without mentioning blast injuries, a brief summary will be listed here. Chapter 71 is devoted entirely to blast injuries, and it should be referenced for more details.

Primary blast injuries are those caused directly by the supersonic blast wave generated by the detonation of a HE. The profound overpressure created causes compressive and shearing forces to affect the various tissues of the body in different ways, primarily damaging air-filled organs such as the middle ear, lungs, and bowel. Secondary blast injuries are ballistic injuries caused by direct physical contact with shrapnel and fragment missiles. Tertiary injuries occur when a body is thrown by the force of the blast wave and strikes another object, such as a wall or the ground. Additionally, there can be damage caused by structural collapse onto the victim, as well as burns caused by incendiary components, and these are considered quaternary blast injuries. Additionally included in quaternary injuries are those caused by preexisting medical conditions of the victim, such as coronary artery disease that causes a myocardial infarction in a victim, as occurred in a responder during the explosion at the 1996 Atlanta Olympic Games. There is a final category, quinternary injuries, which include effects from dispersed additives such as radioactive material, chemicals, toxins, or biological agents.

HISTORICAL PERSPECTIVE

The term *IED* is a relatively new one that has become widely used during the GWOT.[1] In reality, IEDs existed long before but were simply called by different names. Historical terms include time bombs, booby traps, suicide bombs, and roadside bombs, among others. The change in terminology parallels advancements in manufacturing and sophistication. A look back at some key historical events highlights the evolution of what are now called IEDs.

One of the earliest accounts of improvised explosive use was in the 1927 Bath Consolidated School bombing in Bath, Michigan, still the deadliest school-related mass killing in U.S. history. An employee, upset with the school for several reasons, detonated a large time bomb under the north wing of the elementary school, killing more than 30 children and adults. A second alarm clock–triggered bomb wired to 500 pounds of dynamite and pyrotol had similarly been placed under the south wing of the school but failed to detonate. After murdering his tuberculosis-afflicted wife and firebombing his farm, the bomber drove his dynamite-laden Ford truck to the now-burning school. He had loaded the truck with metal shrapnel then detonated this VBIED as a secondary attack outside the school, killing himself and others. There were a total of 45 deaths and 58 injured.[5]

World War II also saw the use of IEDs. Notably, during what is called Operation Rails War in 1943, hundreds of thousands of miles of German rails were destroyed by improvised explosive charges planted by Belarusian partisans. This resulted in the derailment of thousands of German trains, the destruction of hundreds of bridges, and, ultimately, it helped lead to the Soviet victory in the Battle of Kursk. In addition, an IED was used in a nearly successful assassination attempt of Adolf Hitler in 1944. A plot to kill Hitler using a briefcase bomb filled with plastic explosives was carried out by high-ranking members of the Nazi party who wished to see Hitler overthrown. Hitler managed to survive with only minor injuries.[6]

The 1960s were a decade of political and social unrest in the United States, due in part to the Vietnam War. This conflict was different from previous wars in several ways. Notably, the use of vertical deployment and evacuation by helicopters, the use of primarily guerrilla-type combat in dense jungle environments, and also by the extensive use of booby traps against U.S. soldiers. Booby traps often consisted of rudimentary materials engineered to kill or maim American soldiers such as Punji sticks. However, repurposed mines and IEDs were a hallmark of the Vietnam War and the leading cause of American casualties in some years. These improvised mines were simple to make and were ubiquitous in Viet Cong territories. Some were as simple as hand grenades improvised to have their arming pin pulled out when a soldier stepped through a tripwire. Others, called "toe poppers," consisted of a bullet or shell placed upright in the ground so that when an unsuspecting soldier stepped on it, the primer would press against an improvised firing pin, shooting the bullet upward into the foot. It has been reported by firsthand account that the Viet Cong also created HE IEDs using ammonium nitrate fertilizer and diesel fuel.[7]

During The Troubles (from the late 1960s until 1998) in Northern Ireland, thousands lost their lives due to armed conflict between Catholic Irish nationalist and Protestant loyalist factions that disagreed over how Northern Ireland should be ruled.[8] The Provisional Irish Republican Army (PIRA) was the most notable of the paramilitary groups fighting for independent rule from the United Kingdom. One of the weapons of choice was the IED. Statistics show over 16,000 devices were exploded or neutralized during this period.[9] This conflict saw significant advancements in IED technology, including new triggering devices. In addition to heavy use of victim-triggered vehicle bombs connected to automobile ignition circuits, incorporation of mercury "tilt" switches and micro switches were notable innovations. Radio-controlled IED triggers were seen starting in the 1970s. Based on model airplane controllers, these devices allowed remote detonation from a safer distance than was allowed by the previously used command-wire IEDs. Light-sensitive switches were used in PIRA IEDs; they were placed behind propaganda posters. When British forces would rip down the posters, the light sensitive trigger would detonate the IED.[10]

There have been numerous other high profile IED events targeted at civilians on American soil that warrant mentioning. Ted Kaczynski, a former Berkeley mathematics teacher who became known as the Unabomber, was a well-known serial killer whose method was sending IEDs via the mail to his targets during a 20-year period starting in 1975. He used a combination of rudimentary materials and high technology to further his political agenda. He murdered three people and injured more than twenty others before being captured in 1995.[11]

Several VBIEDs also should be mentioned in this discussion. On foreign soil, there have been several truck bomb attacks on American installations, most notably those against U.S. embassies in Nairobi, Kenya, and Dar es Salaam, Tanzania, by Osama bin Laden in 1998.[12] The most high-profile VBIED used on the mainland was the 1995 Oklahoma City Bombing, where two American citizens detonated a truck bomb adjacent to the Alfred P. Murrah Federal Building in Oklahoma City, killing 168 people. These events led to significant changes in U.S. counterterrorism policy and security. Last, the attacks of September 11, 2001, where terrorists from the group Al Qaeda hijacked four airliners and used them as weapons against the World Trade Center in New York City and the Pentagon in Washington, DC, causing the deaths of thousands of American citizens, can arguably also be classified as IEDs.

CURRENT PRACTICE

The best mitigation to IEDs is to prevent them from going off. Between August 2010 and August 2012, excluding events in Iraq and Afghanistan, there were an average of 527 IEDs found or detonated around the world each month.[13] In the United States, improvised bomb use is second only to arson as the primary weapon of terror.[14] As mentioned above, as IED creators use new technologies and strategies to employ their devices, authorities must parallel these actions by developing new countermeasures. During the later portion of the GWOT, IED explosions caused the majority of American deaths and injuries. Billions of dollars have been budgeted by the government to develop new technologies, disrupt networks, and train against these devices. The U.S. Defense Department has been the home of the new Joint Improvised Explosive Device Defeat Organization (JIEDDO) since its formation in 2006. JIEDDO is a multiagency group tasked with eliminating the IED as a weapon of strategic influence.[15] In addition to the lessons learned in combat, there have also been several recent terrorist attacks against civilians that warrant mention.

Global War on Terror

During the last decade of the wars in Iraq and Afghanistan, the United States encountered significant advancements in the construction and deployment of IEDs used against its forces. In a war with clear asymmetry in troop size, weapons, armor, and experience, guerrilla-style warfare was augmented with roadside bomb use against troops and caravans. The decreased cost of materials and modifications to everyday technologies allowed insurgents to remain at safe distances while still inflicting damage and forcing tactical changes.

IED use against American troops in Iraq were particularly effective in the urban environments of the war, where heavy convoy traffic existed and "presence patrols" were a necessary part of counterinsurgency operations. Initially, IEDs targeted vehicles that lacked armor and earned the moniker "roadside bombs." In the early days of the Iraq War, the bombs were typically constructed as command-wire devices that required someone to remain hidden nearby to push a button to detonate the leftover military ordnance serving as the primary source of explosives for insurgents. They were concealed in rocks, road guardrails, trash, within animal corpses, and buried on the sides of roads. The initial response by the United States was to deploy armored vehicles, reduce route predictability, and develop a strategy of clearing dead spaces on roadways to deny hiding places for IEDs and command-wire triggermen.

To overcome these strategies, insurgents integrated remote detonation technologies, such as garage door openers, car alarm key fobs, walkie-talkies, and other radio frequency (RF) electronic arming and triggering devices, eliminating the need for command-wire triggers. Electronic countermeasures (ECMs) to RF signals were developed to disrupt these remote signals and prevent detonation. These "jammers" emitted electronic interference to disrupt any RF triggering signals and went through numerous iterations under the budget of the JIEDDO, as insurgents were able to adapt and use new frequencies and technologies to remain one step ahead.[16] ECM devices were vehicle based, aircraft based, and some were even developed to be carried by infantrymen. Convoys and infantry developed protocols to clear areas of suspicious objects after stopping, such as the "5-2-5" sweep used by soldiers once they have stopped in an area that may have emplaced IEDs.[17]

Another main goal of the JIEDDO, reminiscent of tactics used by the British during The Troubles, was disruption of bomb-making cells and networks through intelligence, thereby preventing deployment of IEDs. Cells established trends of specialization, such as roadside IEDs, suicide operations, and VBIEDs. Coalition forces could use captured intelligence to improve counter-IED technology and tactics.

Explosively formed penetrators (EFPs), a specialized IED in Iraq, was a particularly effective weapon, based on decades-old technology that was very effective against even tank armor from great distances. An EFP is an IED packed behind a concave platter made from copper or other malleable metal. When detonated the platter deforms into a molten slug that can travel long distances and still penetrate armored vehicles. EFPs could be detonated on command but were increasingly triggered by passive infrared detectors, such as those from security floodlights. Initial countermeasures were improvised by troops, including an ingenious method favorably known as the "rhino," which was an electric heat element attached by a pole to the front of the lead vehicle. The heat from the element would trigger infrared-sensitive EFPs that would then detonate early and miss the target. Insurgents then began offsetting the aiming of the device to project rearward behind the rhino. If resources were plentiful, an additional way they would outsmart this countermeasure was by creating arrays of IEDs or EFPs in series, known as a "daisy chain," detonating multiple devices simultaneously along a road and increasing the likelihood of hitting the target.

Suicide bombings have also been prevalent in the GWOT. Suicide bombings are not limited to this theater; they have been a symbol of terrorism in the Middle East for decades. Also known as person-borne IEDs, they are wearable command-wire bombs typically created as a vest or belt for easier concealment and carry. Further discussion of PBIEDs can be found in Chapter 72.

IEDs in Afghanistan were typically deployed differently than they were in Iraq, owing in part to the terrain. Afghanistan's mountainous landscape lacks the road infrastructure of Iraq. As a result, military tactics included more foot patrols in Afghanistan. U.S. Army Explosives Ordnance Disposal (EOD) technicians saw that one of the most common trigger for these booby traps were variations of "pressure plates," consisting of two slightly separated parallel plates that when stepped on would contact and complete the circuit.

Blast injuries in the GWOT brought the advent of Individual First Aid Kits (IFAKs) issued to all troops on the battlefield. IFAKs increased the amount of medical equipment immediately on hand because each soldier carried dressings and a tourniquet(s). During the Vietnam War, most preventable battlefield deaths were due to extremity hemorrhage. Through the development of Tactical Combat Casualty Care training, many lives are now saved, primarily through the use of battlefield tourniquets on extremity shrapnel injuries and traumatic amputations, which are common in IED strikes. Tourniquets provide an immediate and effective way to manage extremity trauma in patients who require massive hemorrhage control, a lesson that is being learned domestically by emergency medical services (EMS) and police, who are being issued them in increasing numbers.[18]

In addition to the GWOT, there were historically relevant developments on U.S. soil over the most recent decade as well. During the 1990s, methamphetamine use and production escalated rapidly until reaching a peak domestically around 2004, a year in which more than 23,000 meth labs were discovered in the United States.[19] Methamphetamine users and producers have deployed IEDs to booby trap their facilities against intruders and law enforcement. This may be in part due to the extreme paranoia often caused by the use of the drug. Documented methods include tripwires and timed incendiaries.[20,21] First responders are currently being trained to recognize meth labs, in an effort to protect themselves from such devices.

Two unique and highly publicized bombing attempts onboard American commercial jetliners using novel techniques occurred in December 2001 and December 2009, respectively. Al Qaeda affiliates smuggled plastic explosives onboard planes in both attempted bombings. The first was hidden inside a shoe, but the PETN/TATP mixture failed to detonate due to moisture on the fuse. The second device consisted of a 6-inch brick of the same homemade plastic explosive sewn into the underwear of the perpetrator.[22] This device caught fire but did not detonate, and both terrorists were apprehended. Both events led to significant changes in airport screening and security.[23,24]

The addition of incendiary components to IEDs is another technique utilized to cause further injury and property damage through burns and fire. Using flammable liquids in this manner is not a new advancement. In fact, the simplest form of improvised incendiary device, the Molotov cocktail, was first used as an antitank weapon in the 1930s.[25] The concept deserves mention following recent attempts employing such devices against high-profile targets. Most commonly, containers filled with readily available combustible products, such as gasoline or propane, are incorporated into an IED in hopes that the IED explosion will, in turn, ignite the incendiary. In 2010, a rudimentary device with significant destructive potential failed to detonate in Times Square, and, in Oregon in 2013, a terrorist pipe bomb attached to a propane tank detonated but failed to ignite the propane.[26,27]

At the time of this writing, the most-recent significant terrorist act committed in the United States was during the 2013 Boston Marathon. Two brothers created and nearly simultaneously detonated two IEDs in the midst of the crowd of civilian spectators at the race finish line. Three were killed and hundreds injured. Days later, the investigation led to a police chase during which more IEDs were thrown at officers, some of which successfully detonated. One brother was killed and the other was arrested. The devices were comprised of a pressure cooker (container), fireworks (explosive), shrapnel, and an RF trigger taken from a remote control toy car. The surviving brother stated that they were self-trained in bomb making by Jihadist instructions found online, a growing problem, and that they were motivated by their radical Islamist beliefs.[4,28,29]

CONCLUSION

IEDs have grown to become a weapon of choice of insurgent groups around the world. The death and physical destruction they cause are augmented by the psychological toll taken on the general public. Instilling fear with the goals of disrupting normal life and affecting a political outcome is the basis of terrorism, and the nature of the IED makes it perfect for this purpose. The use of IEDs has proliferated in the military arena during the GWOT, and countermeasures developed during this conflict will surely translate to better detection and elimination methods used domestically by law enforcement officers. Continuing education, regular interagency exercises, and incorporation of further technological advances will continue to combat the use of these devices

⚠ PITFALLS

- Avoid tunnel vision after an attack—scene safety is critical to avoid further casualties, and consider limiting access of first responders. IED attacks can occur in phases, to include secondary explosions and/or active shooters intending to target rescuers.[29,30]

- IFAKs and tourniquet training should be considered for police and first responders, particularly those in high-risk occupations, such as SWAT officers, and in rural areas with long hospital transport times.

- Communities and first responders should have regular drills to prepare for IED-type mass casualty incidents to reinforce and critique protocols, improve interdepartmental familiarity, and stay current with evolving terrorist tactics and techniques.

- Responders must consider chemical, biological, and radioactive additives incorporated into IEDs. Numerous bombs in Iraq incorporated chlorine additives to vehicle-borne IEDs, without significant success. Preparation, training, and detection methods of chemical, biological, and radiological additives are essential.

- The future of IEDs used to target airlines and well-protected areas/persons is the "body cavity bomb." There are limitations yet to be overcome, but rectal bombs have been deployed, and surgically implanted bombs will surely follow. Detection methods must continue to adapt.[31] In January 2013, terrorists in India implanted an IED inside the dead body of a murdered police officer, targeting first responders or funeral attendees. It was found by physicians during autopsy and did not detonate.[31]

REFERENCES

1. Gill P, Horgan J, Lovelace J. Improvised explosive device: the problem of definition. *Stud Conflict Terrorism*. 2011;34(9):732–748.
2. Definition of Switch [Internet] [cited 2014 Apr 10]. Available from: http://www.merriam-webster.com/dictionary/switch.
3. Caldwell J. *Understanding the Basics of Improvised Explosive Devices (IED)*. www.cimicweb.org. 2011 Sep 12. Available at: www.cimicweb.org/CounterIE.
4. Make a bomb in the kitchen of your mom. *Inspire, Summer 2010*. 2010;1–67.
5. Peters J. *We Still Look at Ourselves as Survivors*. Crime Blog; Dec. 18, 2012. Available at: http://www.slate.com/blogs/crime/2012/12/18/bath_school_bombing_remembering_the_deadliest_school_massacre_in_american.html Accessed 12.04.14.
6. Jones N. *Countdown to Valkyrie*. Frontline Books; March 2009.
7. Lloyd, P. Viet Cong Booby Traps During the Vietnam War. Retrieved April 13, 2014, from http://peteralanlloyd.com/general-news/viet-cong-booby-traps-during-the-vietnam-war/.
8. Hammer J. In Northern Ireland, getting past the troubles. *Smithsonian*. 2009, March 1. Retrieved April 15, 2014, from http://www.smithsonianmag.com/people-places/in-northern-ireland-getting-past-the-troubles-52862004/?no-ist.
9. Information on "The Troubles." n.d. CAIN: Northern Ireland Conflict, Politics, and Society. Retrieved May 23, 2014, from http://cain.ulster.ac.uk.
10. Dingley J, Allison J. *Combating Terrorism in Northern Ireland*. Taylor & Francis; 2008.
11. Ted Kaczynski Biography. 2014, January 1. *Bio.com*. Retrieved May 2, 2014, from http://www.biography.com/people/ted-kaczynski-578450.
12. Johnson LC. The future of terrorism. *Am Behav Sci*. 2001;44(6):894–913. SAGE Publications.
13. Global IED Monthly Summary, Report. 2012, October 2:1–50.
14. Muhlhausen DB, McNeill JB. *Terror Trends: 40 Years' Data on International and Domestic Terrorism;* 2011 May 19, 1–16.
15. JIEDDO. DoD Directive 2000.19E, February 14, 2006. 1–22.
16. Schachtman N. *The Secret History of Iraq's Invisible War*. Wired.com; 2011, June 12. Retrieved April 23, 2014, from http://www.wired.com/2011/06/iraqs-invisible-war/all/.
17. MNC-1 Counter IED Smart Book. 2008:1–113.
18. CoTCCC. TCCC guidelines and curriculum. *NREMT.org*. 2012. Retrieved May 21 2014, from www.naemt.org/education/TCCC/guidelines_curriculum.aspx.
19. DEA.gov / Methamphetamine Lab Incidents. n.d. *DEA.gov / Methamphetamine Lab Incidents*. Retrieved May 23, 2014, from http://www.justice.gov/dea/resource-center/meth-lab-maps.shtml.
20. No officers injured in booby trapped meth lab explosion. *WBIRcom*. 2014, February 26. Retrieved May 23, 2014, from http://www.wbir.com/story/news/local/kingston-harriman-roane/2014/02/26/no-officers-injured-in-booby-trapped-meth-lab-explosion/5835003/.
21. Reaves S. Police encounter booby traps, weapons stash during meth lab raid. *Wave3.com*. n.d. Retrieved May 23, 2014, from http://www.wave3.com/story/6232338/police-encounter-booby-traps-weapons-stash-during-meth-lab-raid
22. Pelofsky J. Nigerian charged for trying to blow up U.S. airliner. | *World* | *Reuters.com* 2009, December 26. Retrieved April 12, 2014, from http://af.reuters.com/article/worldNews/idAFLDE5BP03M20091226.
23. Gathright A. No small feat, tightening up shoe inspections. *seattlepi.com*. 2003. Retrieved May 6, 2014, from http://www.seattlepi.com/article/No-small-feat-tightening-up-shoe-inspections-1119160.php#src=fb.
24. Schmidt MS. Airplane security debated anew after latest bombing plot. *nytimes.com*. 2012. Retrieved May 6, 2014, from http://www.nytimes.com/2012/05/11/world/americas.
25. Trotter W. The molotov cocktail. *The Molotov Cocktail*. n.d. Retrieved April 14, 2014, from http://www.kevos4.com/molotov_cocktail.htm.
26. Baker A, Rashbaum WK. Police find car bomb in times square. *nytimes.com*. 2010, May 1. Retrieved April 21, 2014, from http://www.nytimes.com/2010/05/02/nyregion/02timessquare.html?pagewanted=all&_r=0.
27. Rollins M. *FBI: Medford Bomb Suspect Confessed After Trying to Cover Plot*. 2013, Nov 23. Retrieved April 20, 2014, from http://www.kgw.com/news/Phone-calls-texts-led-police-suspect-in-DAs-office-bombing-233492181.html.
28. Cooper M, Schmidt M, Schmitt E. Boston suspects are seen as self-taught and fueled by web. *The New York Times*. 2013, April 23. Retrieved May 23, 2014, from http://www.nytimes.com/2013/04/24/us/boston-marathon-bombing-developments.html?pagewanted=all.
29. National Counterterrorism Center. Worldwide Targeting of First Response Personnel—Tactics and Indicators *NCTC Special Analysis Report 2012-34a*. 2012 Aug:1–8.
30. Bhandarwar AH, Bakhshi GD, Tayade MB, Chavan GS, Shenoy SS, Nair AS. Mortality pattern of the 26/11 Mumbai terror attacks. *J Trauma Acute Care Surg*. 2012;72(5):1329–1334.
31. Edwards A. Pathologists find "BOMB sewn into body of Indian soldier killed by Maoist rebels." *Mail Online*. 2013, January 10. Retrieved May 31, 2014, from http://www.dailymail.co.uk/news/article-2260148/Pathologists-BOMB-sewn-body-Indian-soldier-killed-Maoist-rebels.html.

SUGGESTED READINGS

1. Bunker RJ. The projected Al Qaeda use of body cavity suicide bombs against high value targets. *Occas Pap*. March 2011;1–55. GroupIntel.com.

CHAPTER 74

Vehicle-Borne Improvised Explosive Devices

James R. Johnston Jr. and David W. Callaway

Use of vehicle-borne improvised explosive devices (VBIEDs) or "car bombs" have increased in prevalence over the last several decades and most likely will continue to be a significant contributing factor to deaths associated with improvised explosive devices (IEDs). For the purpose of this chapter a VBIED will be limited to ground surface vehicles (e.g., trucks, cars, motorcycles) that have been adapted to deliver a payload of explosives to a target. Vehicles are typically chosen for their ability to carry substantial weights as well as blend into the environment to avoid suspicion. Terrorist bombers can attack any number of targets, including specific buildings of importance or public gatherings. In addition, attackers can use multiple VBIEDs to attack successive gates or barriers of a secured facility in order to allow a final attack proximate to the targeted building.[1] This tactic of tiered attacks gained notoriety in Iraq and Afghanistan.

Components of a VBIED are basically the same as an IED (discussed in detail in Chapter 73). A main charge of explosive with an initiator is triggered by some kind of switch or system using a power source. For instance, the trigger mechanism may be a suicide switch run into the driver's compartment while the explosive payload is in the trunk or bed of a truck. VBIEDs are a versatile and deadly terrorist tool that can be adapted for the mission at hand (e.g., massive civilian casualties, structural compromise, distraction, breaching maneuver). Variations seen during the Global War on Terrorism (GWOT) in Iraq range from motorcycles, police vehicles, ambulances, and taxis, to all different sizes of trucks. At times VBIEDs in Iraq were directly responsible for the upsurge in U.S. casualties.[2] Explosive weights could be as little as one hundred pounds or upward to several thousand pounds. Larger payloads create shrapnel out of the vehicle itself and generate primary blast forces that add destructive force, especially if a building is the target. The VBIED is a very inexpensive and cost-effective terrorist tool.[3] The vehicle can be assembled off site over time while the terrorists maintain a relatively low profile. Further, the main explosive charge is almost always some type of homemade explosive (HME), such as an ammonia nitrate and fuel oil mixture (ANFO) (e.g., used in the Oklahoma City Bombing).

Drivers associated with VBIEDs can play multiple roles. For example, they can drop the vehicle off at a strategic location and disappear into the crowd, allowing for delayed detonation with a timer, as seen in the Wall Street Bombing (1920), the World Trade Center Bombings (1993), and the Oklahoma City Bombing (1995).[4–6] Drivers can also operate as suicide bombers, also known as suicide VBIEDs (or SVBIEDs), for a more precise delivery of an inbound vehicle to a target area, just like a cheaper version of a smart bomb.[7,8] This suicide tactic is primarily the case in VBIED operations in the Middle East but has happened on American soil, as seen in the Bath School disaster in 1927.[9]

The VBIED has been used all over the globe in support of various terrorist and insurgent causes. In all cases, the purpose of this terrorist tactic is destruction, mayhem, and murder. The last decade and a half of the GWOT has brought the VBIED threat to mainstream attention, most notably VBIED use in Iraq. Yet historically many do not realize that VBIEDs have been part of some of America's worst attacks. This chapter will discuss a brief history of some of the pertinent attacks, current first responder operational and clinical practice, and potential pitfalls. This chapter should be read in conjunction with the sections on blast injuries and IEDs for a comprehensive understanding of these types of attacks.

HISTORICAL PERSPECTIVE

The first VBIED attack in the United States was the Wall Street Bombing of 1920 by Italian anarchist Mario Buda. Although not on a motorized vehicle, Buda drove his horse-drawn wagon filled with 100 pounds of dynamite and 500 pounds of cast iron shrapnel into the heart of the financial district in New York City.[3,4] He dismounted the wagon and walked away. The wagon-based VBIED exploded, killing 38 and wounding 143 people.

The first VBIED using a motorized truck was used in what is still America's worst school massacre: the 1927 attack in Bath, Michigan. Andrew Kehoe, angered over a property tax levied to pay for the Bath school, conducted a tiered VBIED/IED attack that set the stage for the future use of improvised explosives in terrorist attacks. In the months preceding the attack, Kehoe staged two 500-pound piles of dynamite and pyrotol in the basement under the north and south wings of the building. He set the devices to explode simultaneously with timers.[9] On May 18, 1927, the timer-detonator triggered an explosion under the north wing. Fortunately, the other charge failed to detonate because of mechanical failure of the second timer. After murdering his wife and firebombing his farm, Kehoe drove to what was left of the Bath Consolidation School in his pickup truck rigged with explosives and extra metal pieces to use as shrapnel. When he arrived, Kehoe called the superintendent over to his vehicle, detonated his VBIED, and killed four more individuals, including another child. In all, this lone wolf killed 38 children and 6 adults, including himself. In addition, he wounded 67 other children and teachers, making this one of the most devastating domestic attacks in U.S. history, excluding the 9/11 attack.

In both these historic bombings, the attackers used a high-order explosive to disperse heavy shrapnel and cause injuries. Kehoe, America's first suicide bomber, also employed the same explosives to cause a building collapse in a multibomb attack. Kehoe's attack portended the modern terrorist deployment of VBIEDs.

Extremists in the Middle East use VBIEDs extensively. Terrorists quickly realized that the capacity and power of the VBIED explosion itself was more destructive than the shrapnel it could create. In Beirut, Lebanon, on April 19, 1983, a bomber drove a truck with 2000 pounds of explosives into the U.S. embassy, killing 63 people.[10] This highly successful attack on the embassy led by the Islamic Jihad Organization encouraged the next attack on the U.S. Marine barracks soon after, on October 23 of that same year.[8] At 6:22 in the morning, a truck disguised to look like a local water delivery truck, but loaded with 12,000 pounds of explosives enhanced with large tanks of butane gas, smashed through a flimsy fence of concertina wire in between two guard posts. The truck smashed into the floor lobby of the Marine barracks.[8,11] Within seconds, the driver detonated the truck-based VBIED, causing seven floors of concrete reinforced with one and three-quarters steel rebar to heave upwards, while the building support columns, measuring 15 feet in diameter, were sheared in half. Due to the building's design and the fact that the vehicle had penetrated so deeply into the structure, a tamping effect of the explosion caused the building to implode onto itself.[11] The collapsed seven stories filled the 8-foot-deep crater measuring 39 feet long by 30 feet wide.

The resulting blast was so powerful that it shattered all the windows of the air traffic control tower of the Beirut International Airport over half a mile away. The Federal Bureau of Investigation (FBI) reported that at that point the blast was the largest nonnuclear explosion seen on earth.[3] Investigation by the FBI revealed large quantities of unburned pentaerythritol tetranitrate (PETN) at the blast site. PETN is not an HME and is produced by a nation-state only for the production of military-grade explosives. Lebanon lacked this capability and Iran was implicated as the main supplier of explosives and training for the bombing of the Marine barracks.[11] This gigantic blast was undoubtedly a win for the Islamic Jihad Organization, who later evolved to operate under the name Hezbollah. The United States withdrew its marines from Lebanon the following February due to the collapse of the supported Lebanese government. Many experts attribute this withdrawal at least partially to the devastating VBIED attacks on U.S. assets and personnel.

The bombing of the Marine barracks served as a template for many extremists in the following years. Attackers took advantage of the lack of sufficient perimeter security and demonstrated, with terrible consequences, the destructive capacity of VBIEDs on community infrastructure. The attack on the Alfred P. Murrah Federal Building in Oklahoma City on April 19, 1995, was the most devastating VBIED attack in America at the time. The attack wounded 680 people and killed 168, including 19 children.[5] Timothy McVeigh parked his 24-foot Ryder moving truck just 16 feet from the building, with approximately four devices composed of 5000 pounds of ANFO. The truck detonated and sheared the concrete support beams. The building suffered a major failure of a girder designed to transfer weight. As a result, successive floors collapsed, creating a complex technical urban search and rescue (USAR) response environment.[12,13] Most of the deaths were due to crush and blunt trauma associated with the collapsed area of the building.[14] The injured and those that were initially extricated from the collapse zone were transferred to receiving facilities via ambulance. During the response, local emergency management services (EMS) had activated "on call" personnel and executed mutual aid agreements with surrounding departments to handle the patient transport load. Many victims with minor injuries were transported via private vehicle and presented to local hospitals in a delayed fashion. This was in part due to the large response from bystanders that swarmed the bombing site to help. Bystander response created a logistic problem for incident command, because the collapse zone was unsecure and unsafe. Bystander presence, in this case, subsequently factored into the 14 additional injuries and 1 fatality suffered during the rescue response.[15]

The Oklahoma City Bombing offers several lessons learned for response to VBIED attacks. First, a majority of the deaths were due to building collapse, causing crush injury, massive head trauma, and torso trauma. In addition, a majority of the survivors suffered from head injuries and orthopedic injuries. Structural collapse is the most lethal aspect of a VBIED attack against a building.[16] There are several ways a structure can collapse, and typically VBIEDs have caused a "pancake" collapse where the floors fall on top of each other. Any collapse scenario is complicated and requires time, special equipment, and highly trained personnel in order to respond effectively. These aspects combined with any security issues associated with a bombing site add to the extended rescue time frame and mortality of trapped victims.[14,16] As a result, VBIED attacks on fixed structures create the potential for complex trauma patients with a mix of penetrating, blunt, and blast pathology, combined with inhalational insults and exacerbation of underlying comorbidities. Second, VBIED attacks can create significant infrastructure damage; in Oklahoma City buildings were damaged up to 16 blocks from the blast site. This devastation can affect response routes (e.g., roads), communication (e.g., loss of cell towers), and coordination. Finally, given the tendency of bystanders to flock to attack sites, the risk of follow-up attack is high.

Ramzi Yousef's February 26, 1993, attack on the World Trade Center (WTC) in New York City demonstrated terrorists' commitment to expanding and evolving their use of VBIEDs. Yousef parked a truck VBIED packed with 1300 pounds of explosives in the basement parking lot of the north tower of the WTC.[6] Yousef and his coconspirators intended to destroy foundation columns of the north tower, causing it to topple into the south tower. This first attack on the WTC resembled techniques used in Beirut, but failed for a variety of technical reasons. The most striking similarity was the use of a gas enhancement of the main charge. In the WTC case, the bombers arranged canisters of hydrogen gas around the main charge of urea nitrate to increase the magnitude of the blast.[17] This use of gas enhancement is commonplace in the military and creates a thermobaric effect that releases an immense amount of energy, heat, and rapidly expanding pressure. The thermobaric effect is especially lethal in confined spaces, such as buildings.

The following investigation and associated arrests in the WTC Bombing also revealed a new aspect to VBIEDs. Along with bomb-making materials, the FBI uncovered a very large amount of sodium cyanide.[6] Yousef denied its use in the WTC bomb but did admit to contemplating its use in the bomb. This new tactic of combining chemical warfare agents and VBIED dramatically complicates first response to VBIED attacks.[18] During Operation Iraqi Freedom (OIF), extremists built upon Yousef's failures, adding chlorine canisters to VBIEDs and attacking both military and civilian targets.

The technique of using multiple or simultaneous VBIEDs in coordinated attacks first gained international notoriety after the bombings of the U.S. embassies in Nairobi, Kenya, and Dar es Salaam, Tanzania. The deadlier of the two attacks was in Kenya. Terrorists equipped with small arms and a VBIED (i.e., Toyota Dyna small haul vehicle) attempted to force their way through the embassy gate and enter the underground parking garage. Their access was blocked and they detonated the VBIED in the rear parking area of the embassy. Despite being outside of the physical structure of the embassy, the area devastation was immense. Although the embassy did not collapse, many of the 44 deaths in the embassy were associated with the secondary blast effects from shattered glass and displaced office furniture. The effects of blasts on surrounding local buildings included major structural damage (or collapse, in the case of the Ufundi building). In addition, the secondary blast effects on pedestrian traffic accounted for another estimated 200 deaths and 4000 wounded. The bomber was not as successful in Dar es Salaam, where the entrance to the embassy happened to be blocked by a water tanker. The bomber detonated his vehicle at the gate entrance, killing 12 and wounding another 85. In both instances the embassy security personnel were ill-prepared for repelling the attack, nor able to physically impede the vehicles by barriers or heavy gates, resulting in an environment for successful attacks.[19] The sequencing of VBIEDs in two different countries continued to follow a trend of larger, far-reaching operations being undertaken by Al Qaeda (AQ) and associated terrorist networks. Both the 1993 WTC Bombing and the dual attacks at American embassies in 1998 seemed to be dress rehearsals for the 9/11 attacks.

Modern terrorists are displaying a tendency to deploy smaller VBIEDs. Passenger car–size bombs employed against targets of opportunity in the general public may be the new path taken by extremists, versus a large-scale target such as a building. On May 1, 2010, Faisal Shahzad, who was a naturalized citizen from Pakistan, left his parked car in a busy area of Times Square in New York City with the engine running and his hazard lights on. He had rigged several different explosive components into his Nissan Pathfinder to include M-80 fireworks, gasoline, three 20-pound propane tanks, and a metal box containing 250 pounds of urea-based fertilizer. Local street vendors noticed popping sounds and smoke coming from within the car. Two local street vendors alerted police, who evacuated and cordoned off the area.[20] Although his device was a failure, it could have been a very devastating attack within any city in America. Similar attacks using incendiary and propane components were seen earlier in London in 2007, creating a noteworthy tactical trend that should be planned for by responders.

Terrorists will continue to have distinct advantages when deploying VBIEDs due to the availability and accessibility of various types of targets. Aggressors actively conduct surveillance on targets and often rehearse undetected beforehand. Active planning, preparation, awareness, and assessment of vulnerabilities for high profile sites are paramount for a good defensive posture. As seen in historical events such as the Beirut and Oklahoma City Bombings, VBIEDs are most effective close to or underneath buildings. In these circumstances, the use of barricades is the most effective countermeasure against a VBIED blast. The casualty-producing potential of a VBIED is equally as high in areas crowded with pedestrians. Unfortunately, these open environments are hard to safeguard. In planned mass gatherings, leaders can limit vehicle access and create tiered, highly regulated entry protocols. However, as seen in the successful Wall Street Bombing and the failed Times Square bombing, an attack can happen on any street in America. Reproduction or variations of any of these attacks will continue to create difficulty for responding municipalities, due to the variability of injuries, blast damage to surrounding infrastructure, and logistical aspects of response.

CURRENT PRACTICE

The first 15 years of the twenty-first century has witnessed an expansion in frequency, sophistication, and severity of VBIED attacks. The highest volume of VBIEDs used in one country occurred in Iraq during the GWOT. However, use by extremists against targets in other countries, such as Syria, Libya, and Somalia, has also increased. In Iraq, as well as Afghanistan, the main charges for large vehicles, such as delivery trucks, are HME. Terrorists use military-grade explosives, such as 105 mm artillery shells, to create more concentrated explosive capacity when deploying smaller VBIEDs. These shells are filled with high-grade explosives and provide a container for tamping of the explosion, as well as fragmentation. The smaller size facilitates concealment and device management. The smaller charges can be "daisy-chained" in series to explode simultaneously or in a coordinated fashion. The main charge in a VBIED itself can vary drastically depending on the group or individual building the device.

Initially, observant soldiers noticed that trucks with low-riding vehicle chassis could signal large VBIEDs weighed down with heavy explosives. However, vehicle modification is now common with more elaborate VBIEDs. Springs of trucks can be stiffened or welded to disguise weight.[21] Also, triggering devices such as fuses or wiring can be passed through tubing from the driver's compartment to the cargo area or truck. As the number of coalition Iraqi police checkpoints increased, some vehicles were extensively modified to smuggle the explosives using such techniques as false floors.

The use of secondary or multiple VBIEDs has become a common technique in attacking fortified checkpoints and buildings. In more than one instance, large trucks laden with explosives have rammed into checkpoints as far as they could go and then detonated, attempting to clear a path for a second VBIED or follow-up ground attack.[1] Fortunately, often the crater from the first truck hinders the second truck's penetration. Regardless, the attacks still prove to be very deadly and destructive. One technique that is effective in hindering deep penetration of VBIEDs into fortified areas is the use of barricades. The lack of barriers and its consequence was a lesson learned in the Beirut bombing. In Iraq, "T-barriers" were typically made of concrete and could stand anywhere from 12 to 20 feet tall. These are enlarged versions of "Jersey barriers" and were erected throughout posts because of VBIED and indirect fire threat, such as mortars. Elaborate S-turns with numerous checkpoints funneled traffic in and out of bases and prevented a VBIED driver from trying to enter the compound at a high rate of speed.

The use of armed personnel to facilitate entry or augment a VBIED attack is also a tactic that has become more common, as seen in multiple cases during the GWOT, Kenya embassy bombing, and the attacks in Riyadh, Saudi Arabia, in 2003.[8,21] Terrorists accompanying an attack can maneuver quickly to targeted areas to engage security forces and disable blockades or countermeasures. Variations of this template include fighters who synchronize shootings or assaults with VBIEDs. These can be deliberate or simply targets of opportunity. A very successful example of an assault with coordinated vehicle bombings was the 2008 Mumbai attacks. Ten highly trained shooters used two timer-detonated bombs in taxis and small arms to wreak havoc at 12 different targets over 4 days, resulting in 166 dead and 308 wounded.[22] Although this incident did not use a preassembled VBIED, attackers did place IEDs into taxis to gain similar effects of a VBIED. Agencies should develop plans for responding to any suspected bombing with adequate preparation for additional bombing, as well as active shooters.

Current (2012-2014) reporting from Syria details the most recent VBIED tactics used by AQ–affiliated extremists. Captured military vehicles, such as Armored Personnel Carriers (APCs), have been turned into VBIEDs. Extremists have also been successful in modifying VBIEDs with remote control steering to deliver the vehicle without a driver. Perpetrators are deliberately attaching makeshift armor (e.g., steel plates attached onto the outside of the vehicles with slits for the driver to navigate).[23] This "Mad Max" style of vehicle armament shows the level of autonomy at which these extremists can operate within unstable countries.

From 2012 to 2014, Al Qaeda in Iraq (AQI) and its affiliated extremist groups (e.g., the Islamic State of Iraq and the Levant [ISIL]) dramatically increased their frequency and variety of VBIED deployment to attack Iraqi security forces, execute prison breaks, assassinate local political leaders, disrupt local political processes, and commit mass atrocities against civilians. The propagation of AQ and ISIL tactics, techniques, and procedures over the Internet and through experiential learning in civil wars across the Middle East and North Africa (e.g., Syria, Iraq, Egypt, Libya, Mali, Somalia) has allowed terrorists to create and effectively deploy VBIED "cells."[24]

The current VBIED threat to responders is higher than it has ever been in history. The U.S. government has urged state and local governments to develop response plans that account for attacks targeting responders.[25] Departments should identify potential high-threat areas and plan for a response using historical and trending tactics as a start point for mitigation tactics. Some examples include use of barriers after an attack, development of combined law enforcement and medical first response protocols, expanded interagency coordination and training, and exercises that test response to multiple simultaneous attacks. Finally, it is critical to plan for and test response techniques for attacks on emergency services, such as hospitals and police departments. All of these aspects of war-gaming should be coupled with ongoing intelligence assessment for indications of a VBIED attacks.

POTENTIAL VBIED INDICATORS[26]

- Vehicles
  - License plates inconsistent with vehicle registration
  - Obviously carrying a heavy load or with a heavy rear end
  - Modification of a truck or van with heavy duty springs to handle heavier loads
  - False papers used for rental of vans
- Community
  - Rental of self-storage space for the purpose of storing chemicals or mixing apparatus
  - Delivery of chemicals directly from the manufacturer to a self-storage facility or unusual deliveries of chemicals to residential or rural addresses
  - Recent theft of explosives, blasting caps, or fuses, or certain chemicals used in the manufacture of explosives
  - Chemical fires, toxic odors, brightly colored stains, or rusted metal fixtures in apartments, hotel or motel rooms, or self-storage units due to chemical activity
  - Small test explosions in rural wooded areas
- Emergency department or urgent care
  - Patients with untreated chemical burns or missing hands or fingers
  - Patients presenting for treatment of chemical burns or missing hands or fingers

⚠ PITFALLS

- Not planning for contingency movements of first responders and casualties. Responders must be prepared to fall back at any time. A VBIED attack is chaotic, and structural collapse, toxic fumes, fire, etc., often compromise scene safety.
- Not planning for additional attacks following a VBIED. A secondary attack targeting responders is a real and prevalent threat, whether via another VBIED, armed shooters, or a combination of attacks. Agencies should have contingencies for security of an attack site, such as rapid barrier emplacement, cordon plans, and rapid incident command setup.
- Lack of tiered response plans. One VBIED can produce hundreds of casualties in a matter of seconds in a crowded environment; casualties will overwhelm communication systems, responders, transportation, and hospitals. Agencies should have primary, alternate, and contingency plans for all aspects of incident command, communication, treatment, and transport to include other surrounding municipalities.
- Failure to prepare for a chemical or biological component of VBIED attacks. Failed attempts in Iraq to build VBIEDs that integrated chlorine tanks highlight the importance of comprehensive preparation, training, and detection methods of chemical, biological, and radiological additives. Even unsuccessful attacks can result in community, bystander, and even first responder panic.

REFERENCES

1. CJTF-7 OIF Smart Card 4. Version 1.A. C3 Training Cell. January 2, 2004.
2. Lewis J. Middle East Security Report 14. Al-Qaeda in Iraq Resurgent. *The Breaking The Walls Campaign, Part I.* Washington, DC: The Institute for the Study of War; 2013 September, pp. 7–20.
3. Davis M. A History of the Car Bomb. *Part 1: The Poor Man's Air Force.* April 13, 2006, Retrieved April 8, 2014, from, http://www.atimes.com.
4. A Fact Sheet from the Worldwide Incidents Team, National Counterterrorism Center. Document No. 20071105-05. November 9, 2007. Retrieved April 5, 2014, from https://www.fbiic.gov.
5. Terror Hits Home: The Oklahoma City Bombing. Retrieved April 8, 2014, from http://www.fbi.gov.
6. FBI 100 First Strike: Global Terror in America. Retrieved April 20, 2014, from http://www.fbi.gov.
7. MNC-1 Counter IED Smart Book. 2008. pp. 1–113.
8. Morgenstern H. Vehicle Born Improvised Explosive Device-VBIED, The Terrorist Weapon of Choice. Retrieved April 2, 2014, from www.nationalhomelandsecurityknowledgebase.com.
9. A Fact Sheet from the Worldwide Incidents Team, National Counterterrorism Center. Document No. 20071008-05. October 8, 2007. Retrieved April 5, 2014, from https://www.fbiic.gov.
10. Flashback: April 18, 1983: U.S. Embassy Attacked in Beirut. Retrieved April 11, 2014, from https://www.cia.gov.
11. Report of the DOD commission on Beirut International Airport Terrorist act October 23, 1983, 20 Dec 1983, pp. 84–119.
12. The Oklahoma Department of Civil Emergency Management After Action Report. 19 April 1995. Retrieved April 20, 2014, from http://www.ok.gov.
13. Terrorist bombing, Murrah Federal Building Oklahoma, 1995. Retrieved April 9, 2014, from http://www.nist.gov.
14. Teague DC. Mass casualties in the Oklahoma City bombing. *Clin Orthop Relat Res.* 2004 May;422:77–81.
15. Maningas P, Robison M, Mallonee S. The EMS response to the Oklahoma City bombing. *Prehosp Disaster Med.* 1997 Apr-Jun;12(2):80–85.
16. Glenshaw MT, Vernick JS, Li G, Sorock GS, Brown S, Mallonee S. Preventing fatalities in building bombings: what can we learn from the Oklahoma City bombing? *Disaster Med Public Health Prep.* 2007 Jul;1(1):27–31.
17. The U.S. Fire Administration/Technical Report Series. Homeland security, USFA-TR-076. *The World Trade Center Bombing Report and Analysis.* February 1993, New York City, NY pp. 30, 87–90.
18. Parachini John V, et al. Tucker Jonathan B, ed. *Toxic Terror: Assessing Terrorist Use of Chemical and Biological Weapons.* Cambridge, MA: MIT Press; 2000:185–206.
19. Report of Accountability Review Boards. Bombings of the U.S. Embassies in Nairobi, Kenya, and Dar es Salaam, Tanzania on August 7, 1998. Retrieved March 26, 2014, from http://1997-2001.state.gov.
20. Esposito J, Carroll T. FDNY Operations at Times Square Car Bomb Scare May 1st 2010. *FDNY Center for Terrorism and Disaster Preparedness.* 2010 May, slides 2-10. Retrieved March 27, 2014, from http://www.iafc.org.
21. Homeland Security Information Bulletin. *Potential Indicators of Threats Involving Vehicle Borne Improvised Explosive Devices (VBIEDs) May 15.* 2003, Retrieved March 31, 2014, from, http://www.sifma.org.
22. Mortality pattern of the 26/11 Mumbai terror attacks. *J Trauma Acute Care Surg.* 2012 May;72(5):1329–1334.
23. Cardash M, Ganor I. Australian Suicide Bomber Initiates Truck SVBIED in Deir ez-Zor, Syria, pp. 2–8. Retrieved April 13, 2014, from http://terrogence.com.
24. Lewis JD. *Al-Qaeda in Iraq Resurgent, Part II. Middle East Security Report 15.* Washington, DC: Institute for the Study of War; October 2013.
25. NCTC. *Special Analysis Report 2012-34a.* Worldwide: IED Targeting of First Response Personnel — Tactics and Indicators; 2012. Retrieved April 16, 2014, from http://info.publicintelligence.net.
26. Morgenstern H: Vehicle-Borne Improvised Explosive Device (VBIED): the terrorist weapon of choice. Security Solutions International. http://www.nationalhomelandsecurityknowledgebase.com/Research/International_Articles/VBIED_Terrorist_Weapon_of_Choice.html. (Accessed June 9, 2014).

CHAPTER 75

Conventional Explosions at Mass Gatherings

Franklin D. Friedman and Erin E. Noste

DESCRIPTION OF THE EVENT

The magnitude and severity of primary injuries from a blast explosion are determined by proximity, the quantity and type of explosive, and whether the explosion is in an open or enclosed space.[1,2] Naturally, when an explosion occurs at a large gathering of people, other factors that strongly affect overall morbidity and mortality include access of rescuers to the injured and the personnel and resources available to care for an overwhelming number of victims in the immediate aftermath.

The increasing prevalence of terrorism and insurgency over the last three decades has increased our understanding of the types of injuries caused by blasts in the civilian environments—injuries once seen only on the battlefield—as well as the predictors of survival and the management techniques for such incidents.[3–5] Primary blast injuries are uncommon by the time blast victims reach the hospital because most primary blast injuries result in immediate death.[6] Because they are so rare, and because a bombing often results in so many casualties converging on a single institution, many physicians and other health care workers with no prior expertise in trauma or disaster management may be pressed into service to care for trauma patients.[7]

Even though many articles in the medical literature describe the effects of blast injuries,[8–11] and others describe medical planning and care for mass gatherings[12–15] (i.e., mass "gatherings of potential patients"[16]), few combine both topics.[17–20] Until recently, most of the literature concerning health care planning for mass gatherings ignored the risk of a major traumatic event such as a bombing, instead focusing on environmental or medical emergencies An incident in which 60,000 spectators are exposed to an exploding bomb demands a different response.

Fortunately, very few incidents of intentional or accidental explosions affecting large gatherings such as sporting or entertainment events (e.g., the Atlanta Olympics in 1996, Bali in 2002, and Boston Marathon in 2013) have occurred. The bombings at the finish line of the 2013 Boston Marathon illustrated just how easily amateurs with readily obtainable supplies can inflict significant damage to a civilian population.[21,22] Many of the terrorist bombings from which we have learned about injury patterns occurred in other settings (i.e., U.S. barracks in Beirut 1983, the Murrah Federal Building 1995, the World Trade Center in New York in 1993, the Madrid train in 2004, and numerous attacks in Israel). By extrapolating from what is known about the nature of explosion injuries, the outcome of explosions that have affected many victims, and the strategies developed to provide medical care at major events, a workable strategy to care for these injuries can be built.

The medical usage rate (MUR; generally reported as numbers of patients per 10,000 in attendance) at a mass gathering is rarely greater than 50 at a spectator event, and it is most often related to weather. By stark contrast, one author documents a mortality of 7.8% for open-air and 49% for closed-space bombings (although these do not refer to mass gatherings with several thousand people in attendance).[23]

In this chapter we present two different case presentations of explosions at mass gatherings that serve to illustrate the differences between low- and high-order explosives.[24,25] One example, the Boston Marathon Bombing in April 2013, is a case where low-order explosives were used. These explosives (e.g., black powder, which is found in fireworks) typically do not detonate but instead burn rapidly. They can still produce a large amount of force. Our second case presentation examines an attack using high-order explosives, the bombing of a nightclub in Bali in 2002, with ammonium nitrate. These explosions do not burn but detonate. They generate high temperature and pressure gases that lead to a shock wave. Please refer to Chapter 71 for more details on the physics of blasts and blast injury patterns.

PRE-INCIDENT ACTIONS

Preparation for conventional explosions at a large gathering is best when it is preventative rather than reactive. The best preparations depend on making conditions unfavorable for the bomber and designing structures that are fire resistant, less likely to collapse, and that offer easy egress in the event of an explosion. Measures can be taken, as in the London Underground, to remove waste receptacles in which an explosive device may be hidden. Similarly, although inconvenient, inspecting the backpacks and the trunks of vehicles of those entering events has become a necessary precaution.

The importance of repeated drilling of all the facets of a hospital and region's disaster plan must not be underestimated. Following the bombing at the 1996 Atlanta Olympics, Atlanta Emergency Medical Services leaders attributed pre-event training and drills practiced during the five years leading to the event as the principal reason why their response went well.[19] All 111 injured patients were evacuated to the area hospitals within just 32 minutes of the explosion.[19] To best prepare for a conventional bombing at a mass gathering, drill a scenario with a large surge of trauma victims, mixing both critically ill and lightly injured victims.

POST-INCIDENT ACTIONS

The potential volume of patients with both critical and noncritical injuries is the greatest risk to successful management of an explosion at a mass gathering. Establishing effective triage, both at the scene and again at the receiving hospitals, will prevent overwhelming limited resources and ensure that the most seriously injured patients are identified rapidly and sent to appropriate medical facilities.

Virtually all civilian bombings constitute a criminal act. Therefore, any material from the explosives found on or inside of victims is evidence that may be useful to investigational authorities to solve the crime. Salvaged clothing may contain identifiable explosive residue. Even corpses may yield important clues; consider performing postmortem x-rays to identify shrapnel. Expect to continue to work with law enforcement after an incident, especially in matters such as evidence collection, and as witnesses as the examining health care providers.

After treatment of casualties is completed, how should outcomes be assessed? Data points of interest include injury severity scores, specific injuries, morbidity, mortality, and location of individuals with respect to the explosive device. By publishing data such as these, as well as lessons learned, it may be possible to improve the response to the next bombing incident.

✚ MEDICAL TREATMENT OF CASUALTIES

When caring for victims of a conventional bombing at a mass gathering, keep in mind the convergence of two types of disasters: injuries unique to conventional explosives and the challenges of caring for the surge of many simultaneously injured patients. Those close to the actual explosion often will die or suffer serious injuries, but the majority of casualties will receive relatively minor injuries, frequently from flying debris.[26] The other traumatic injuries likely seen will be those related to stampede from those trying to escape, or burns from a resulting fire. Despite the variety of serious injuries unique to blast injuries, the most common injuries among blast survivors involve standard penetrating and blunt trauma.

The major medical challenge in caring for the victims of bombs, in addition to the multiple simultaneous casualties, is to identify those who are seriously injured but salvageable, and to realize that they will be mixed in with a large number who are lightly injured or psychologically traumatized.[1] Details concerning the nature, type, and care of injuries common to conventional explosions are available elsewhere in the book.

Case Presentation—Low-Order Explosives: The Boston Marathon Bombing, April 15, 2013

The two bombs that exploded near the finish line of the 2013 Boston Marathon provide an example of the effect of homemade bombs, improvised explosive devices (IEDs), at an urban outdoor mass gathering. The two suspects in this attack brought the devices in backpacks and fashioned the IEDs out of readily available pressure cookers, filled with the powder contained in fireworks purchased in New Hampshire, mixed with metal shrapnel (i.e., nails and ball bearings). The explosions were triggered using the remote controls for toy cars. Instructions for these devices were reportedly found in the online magazine, *Inspire*, an Al Qaeda in the Arabian Peninsula (AQAP) publication.[27,28]

Most of the serious injuries in this open-air attack were severe lower extremity injuries. This is unlike the injuries often seen after a typical high-order bomb explosion, particularly those in confined spaces such as a building or a bus.[29] The bombs were built using low-order explosives (fireworks primarily containing black powder[30]), and were placed on the street, near the facades of buildings, resulting in a high-speed shrapnel blast that was only a few feet from the ground. There were still three fatalities from the explosions.[31]

It is postulated that the low number of fatalities from this event can be attributed to a number of fortuitous circumstances unique to this particular event.[32,33] The explosions took place near the finish line of a well-planned sporting event for which medical tents, medical personnel, and numerous ambulances were already stationed nearby.[34,35] Further, five adult and two pediatric American College of Surgeons verified Level I trauma centers are located in less than a 2.5-mile radius from the incident. The attack took place just before the change of shift

at these hospitals, so in essence they each had double their ordinary staffing. Finally, a number of horrific acts of terrorism had occurred in the past year in the United States, and responders within the Boston hospitals noted that these events had led them to pay special attention to their disaster readiness and training.[36,37]

Case Presentation—High-Order Explosion: The Bali Bombings of October 12, 2002

Shortly before midnight in the town of Kuta on Bali, an electronically triggered bomb exploded in Paddy's Bar, driving the patrons outside, where, moments later, a powerful car bomb (containing ammonium nitrate) exploded in front of the crowded Sari Club. "The place was packed, and it went up within a millisecond" was the description of a visiting Australian football coach[38] (the team was in the club, and half perished). "A huge, massive flame erupted from the floor like a volcano.... Everybody rushed to the back steps, but it was too crowded to get out... everything was on fire."[39] Most of the victims were in their twenties and thirties, and most were foreign visitors (primarily from Australia, although at least 22 countries were represented among the deceased).[40] The death toll was 202, and several hundred more suffered various injuries, including severe burns.

In addition to the actual explosions, the other two principal injury-causing features of this attack were the collapse of the Sari Club (a largely open-sided building), trapping patrons, and the ignition of a huge fire, apparently caused by exploding gas cylinders. Care of the injured was compromised by the limited medical infrastructure in Kuta. (Even though it is one of the best hospitals in Bali, the care offered is still rudimentary.)[41] Many of the foreign nationals were evacuated to Australia and Singapore. Sixty-one patients were transferred to Royal Darwin Hospital in Australia, twenty-eight of whom had major trauma, including "severe burns, missile injuries from shrapnel, limb disruption, and pressure-wave injury to ears, lung, and bowel."[42]

In Bali, beyond the limitations of caring for so many burned and otherwise injured patients, untrained volunteers performed much of the initial mortuary care. Tourists took on the daily responsibility of bringing ice to a makeshift morgue. Unfortunately, they also combined victims' remains in single bags, commingling DNA, making some identification impossible (three unidentified bodies were cremated subsequently).[40]

❓ UNIQUE CONSIDERATIONS

A conventional explosion at a mass gathering presents an emergency medical care situation unlike either that from an explosion with a small number of victims or from a large event with the typical patients presenting (usually medical complaints, minor injuries, or environmental-related problems). A carefully placed explosive device at a major indoor event can result in hundreds, potentially thousands of casualties suffering assorted trauma, including burns. Triage, both at the scene and again at the receiving hospitals is one of the most crucial aspects of the response to care for patients when resources are limited. Keep in mind that unlike a medical emergency at a sporting event, the emergency medical technicians (EMTs) prepositioned in the stadium may be among the victims when a bomb explodes.

Delaying care for those truly in need (i.e., of chest decompression, mechanical ventilation, and operative exploration) while methodically evaluating and bandaging every patient with an abrasion will mean lives lost. The effective disaster response, as for any surge of trauma patients, will rely on a variety of caregivers pressed into service to treat the lesser injuries,[7] while senior, experienced emergency providers perform rapid triage, directing casualties to appropriate sites for care.

⚠ PITFALLS

- Over-triage will rapidly overwhelm hospitals, resulting in needless deaths of those casualties who otherwise might have been saved.
- Failure to consider the possibility of additional explosive devices after the initial detonation can needlessly result in additional casualties.
- Failure to rapidly institute an orderly means to perform triage, both in the field and at hospitals, will result in unnecessary chaos. A military processing station model should be the ideal.

REFERENCES

1. Stein M, Hirshberg A. Medical consequences of terrorism. *Surg Clin North Am.* 1999;79:1537–1552.
2. Leibovici D, Gofrit ON, Stein M, et al. Blast injuries: bus versus open-air bombings—a comparative study of injuries in survivors of open-air versus confined-space explosions. *J Trauma.* 1996;41:1030–1035.
3. Frykberg ER, Tepas JJ 3rd. Terrorist bombings, lessons learned from Belfast to Beirut. *Ann Surg.* 1988;208:569–576.
4. Biancolini CA, Del Bosco CG, Jorge MA. Argentine Jewish community institution bomb explosion. *J Trauma.* 1999;47:728–732.
5. Pahor AL. The ENT, problems following the Birmingham bombings. *J Laryngol Otol.* 1981;95:399–406.
6. Boffard KD, MacFarlane C. Urban bomb blast injuries: Patterns of injury and treatment. *Surg Annu.* 1993;25:29–47.
7. Fisher D, Burrow J. The Bali bombings of 12 October, 2002: lessons in disaster management for physicians. *Int Med J.* 2003;33:125–126.
8. Phillips YY. Primary blast injuries. *Ann Emerg Med.* 1986;15:105–109.
9. Mallonee S, Shariat S, Stennies G. Physical injuries and fatalities resulting from the Oklahoma City bombings. *JAMA.* 1996;276:382–387.
10. Wightman JM, Gladish SL. Explosions and blast injuries. *Ann Emerg Med.* 2001;37:664–678.
11. Gibbons AJ, Farrier JN, Key SJ. The pipe bomb: a modern terrorist weapon. *J R Army Med Corps.* 2003;149:23–26.
12. Milsten AM, Maguire BJ, Bissell RA. Mass-gathering medical care: a review of the literature. *Prehospital Disaster Med.* 2002;17:151–162.
13. Michael JA, Barbera JA. Mass gathering medical care: a twenty-five year review. *Prehospital Disaster Med.* 1997;12:305–312.
14. Arbon P, Bridgewater FHG, Smith C. Mass gathering medicine: a predictive model for patient presentation and transport rates. *Prehospital Disaster Med.* 2001;16:150–158.
15. Nordberg M. EMS and mass gatherings. *Emerg Med Serv.* 1990;19:46–56, 91.
16. Butler WC II, Gesner DE. Crowded venues: avoid an EMS quagmire by preparing for mass gatherings. *JEMS.* 1999;24:62–65.
17. Severance HW. Mass-casualty victim "surge" management: preparing for bombings and blast-related injuries with possibility of hazardous materials exposure. *N C Med J.* 2002;63:242–246.
18. Frykberg ER. Medical management of disasters and mass casualties from terrorist bombings: how can we cope? *J Trauma.* 2002;53:201–212.
19. Feliciano DV, Anderson GV, Rozycki GS, et al. Management of casualties from the bombing at the Centennial Olympics. *Am J Surg.* 1998;176:538–543.
20. Brismar BO, Bergenwald L. The terrorist bomb explosion in Bologna, Italy, 1980: an analysis of the effects and injuries sustained. *J Trauma.* 1982;22:216–220.
21. Arsenault M. 3 killed, 130 hurt by bombs at finish line; area locked down. *The Boston Globe.* 16 April 2013;A1, Print.
22. Eligon J, Cooper M. Blasts at Boston Marathon kill 3 and injure 100. *The New York Times.* 16 March 2013;A1, Print.
23. Leibovici D, Gofrit ON, Stein M. Blast injuries: bus versus open-air bombings—a comparative study of injuries in survivors of open-air versus confined-space explosions. *J Traum.* 1996;41:1030–1035.
24. Wolf SJ, Bebarta VS, Bonnett CJ, Pons PT, Cantrill SV. Blast injuries. *Lancet.* 2009;374(9687):405–415.
25. Horrocks C. Blast injuries: biophysics, pathophysiology and management principles. *J R Army Med Corps.* 2001;147(1):28–40.
26. Kennedy TL, Johnston GW. Civilian bomb injuries. *Br Med J.* 1975;1:382–383.
27. United States of America v. Dzhokhar A. Tsarnaev, 18 U.S.C §232a(a) (2) 2013. http://www.justice.gov/iso/opa/resources/632013627162038513370.pdf; retrieved March 30, 2014.
28. Make a bomb in the kitchen of your mom. *Inspire.* Summer 2010. http://azelin.files.wordpress.com/2010/06/aqap-inspire-magazine-volume-1-uncorrupted.pdf; retrieved March 30, 2014.
29. Victims of the Marathon Bombings. http://www.boston.com/news/local/massachusetts/specials/boston_marathon_bombing_victim_list; retrieved March 31, 2014.
30. Conkling JA. Pyrotechnics. *Sci Am.* July 1990;96–102.
31. The Boston Victims. http://www.nytimes.com/interactive/2013/04/18/us/boston-bombing-victims.html; retrieved March 31, 2014.
32. Gawande A. Why Boston's hospitals were ready. *The New Yorker.* http://www.newyorker.com/online/blogs/newsdesk/2013/04/why-bostons-hospitals-were-ready.html#livefyre; retrieved April 1, 2014.
33. Kellermann AL, Peleg K. Lessons from Boston. *N Engl J Med.* 2013;368:1956–1957.
34. Mitchell EL. Finish line becomes front line at Boston Marathon. *Ann Emerg Med.* 2013;62:543–544.
35. Biddinger PD, Baggish A, Harrington L, et al. Be prepared—the Boston Marathon and mass-casualty events. *N Engl J Med.* 2013;368:1958–1960.
36. Goralnick E, Gates J. We fight like we train. *N Engl J Med.* 2013;368:1960–1961.
37. Walls RM, Zinner MJ. The Boston Marathon response: why did it work so well. *JAMA.* 2013;309:2441–2442.
38. Bonner R. Bombing at resort in Indonesia kills 150 and hurts scores more. *The New York Times on the Web.* 13 Oct 2002; retrieved 29 June 2004, http://travel2.nytimes.com/mem/travel/article-page.html?res=9F06E7DA103AF930A25753C1A9649C8B63.
39. Mydans S. Terror in Bali: the aftermath; survivors of Indonesia blast are left stunned and searching. *The New York Times on the Web.* 14 Oct 2002; retrieved 29 June 2004, http://travel2.nytimes.com/mem/travel/article-page.html?res=9C02E4D9113AF937A25753C1A9649C8B63.
40. 2002 Bali terrorist bombing. *Wikipedia.* Retrieved 29 June 2004. http://en.wikipedia.org/wiki/2002_Bali_terrorist_bombing.
41. Watts J. Bali bombing offers lessons for disaster relief. *Lancet.* 2002;360:1401.
42. Palmer DJ, Stephens D, Fisher DA, et al. The Bali bombing: the Royal Darwin Hospital response. *Med J Aust.* 2003;179:358–361.

Nuclear Disaster Management*

George A. Alexander

The events of September 11, 2001, and the worldwide proliferation of nuclear materials, including theft and smuggling, increase the possibility that a nuclear disaster may occur from the terrorist use of radiation as a weapon. There are two documented incidents of the threatened use of radiation as a terrorist weapon thus far, both of which occurred in Russia.[1] In 1995 Chechen insurgents buried a cesium-137 "dirty bomb" in a Moscow park and alerted the media before it was detonated. In 1998 a container of radioactive materials was found attached to an explosive mine near a railroad line in Chechnya.

The threat of a nuclear terrorist attack with a nuclear device or radioactive materials is not a question of if, but when. Nuclear disasters can have different scenarios. An extreme situation would be the threat of a terrorist attack using a low-yield 10-kiloton nuclear weapon. Many people have become aware of the threat of such an attack because of increased media attention. Successful planning for a nuclear attack or accident is imperative.

This chapter presents important concepts of nuclear disaster management. The aim is to offer a basic understanding of the threat and effect of nuclear disasters, including accidents and terrorist events. This chapter provides a brief historical overview of the development of the nuclear era, the nuclear arms race, and present concerns. It highlights some basic physical and biological principles of radiation injury that are commonly misunderstood by health care professionals. The chapter reviews various nuclear disaster scenarios, summarizes medical management principles, and underscores obstacles to nuclear disaster management.

HISTORICAL PERSPECTIVE

Following the discovery of radioactivity in 1896, the understanding of atomic physics increased rapidly in the early twentieth century.[2] Ernest Rutherford is recognized as the father of nuclear physics. In 1908 he received the Nobel Prize for chemistry for his "investigations into the disintegration of the elements, and the chemistry of radioactive substances."[3] He was directly responsible for training many physicists at Cambridge University in England. In the latter capacity, he was also indirectly responsible for much of the nuclear physics research that was being conducted at many universities by his former students throughout the world and for the development of the nuclear era.

In 1938 Hahn and Strassmann in Berlin described the phenomenon of nuclear fission.[2] They determined that when uranium was bombarded with neutrons, the nucleus split into two parts of comparable

mass with the release of an enormous quantity of energy. This observation would lead to the Manhattan Project and eventually to the production of the atomic bomb (A-bomb).[3] In 1942 Fermi achieved the first controlled self-sustaining nuclear reaction.[3] In August 1945 the first A-bombs (or fission bombs) were detonated over Hiroshima and Nagasaki, Japan.

The development of the A-bomb would lead ultimately to the development of the even more devastating hydrogen bomb (H-bomb). In the 1950s, justification of work on the H-bomb (fusion or thermonuclear bomb) was based on the fact that it produced less radioactive fallout and therefore was considered a "cleaner" nuclear weapon.[4] Enhanced radiation weapons (neutron bombs) were later developed to minimize the effects of blast and heat on buildings and to maximize the effects of the neutrons on living organisms (e.g., to kill tank crews without causing much collateral damage).[4]

During the Cold War era, the nuclear arms race between the United States and the former Soviet Union continued for more than 30 years. By the early 1980s the number of nuclear warheads worldwide was estimated to be in excess of 40,000.[5] The explosive power of these warheads ranged from about 100 tons up to more than 200 million tons equivalent of high explosives. During this same time period the total strength of nuclear arsenals was believed to have been equivalent to about a million Hiroshima bombs or 13,000 million tons of trinitrotoluene (TNT).

With the end of the Cold War in the late 1980s, the threat of Armageddon—a nuclear war between the United States and the former Soviet Union in which 200 million Americans might not survive—was dramatically reduced.[6] However, this apparent relief from the Armageddon syndrome has been short-lived because the twenty-first century now appears to be more dangerous and less predictable. The risk that someone might detonate a nuclear weapon in anger or retribution is probably greater than at any other time since the 1962 Cuban missile crisis.[7] Moreover, nuclear weapons ambitions are spreading not only to states, but also to terrorist groups. Osama bin Laden talked of acquiring nuclear weapons as a "religious duty."[7] By 2000 some 32,000 nuclear weapons were still being deployed and posed new threats from some terrorist groups.[8]

Today, the most likely threat from nuclear weapons is based on a scenario of a terrorist group or rogue nation using a single, low-yield device, such as a suitcase-size tactical nuclear weapon.[9] The second most likely threat is from an improvised nuclear device (IND) used by terrorists and composed of either weapons-grade (enriched) uranium or plutonium-239. The third most likely terrorist nuclear threat is from a radiological dispersal device (RDD), also known as a "dirty bomb." (See Chapter 77 for a more complete discussion of the RDD.) Although the detonation of an RDD does not produce a nuclear yield, RDDs are important because of their potential to cause a nuclear disaster using high explosives to disperse very high levels of

---

*The views expressed in this chapter are those of the author and do not necessarily represent the official policy or position of the National Cancer Institute, the National Institutes of Health, or the Department of Health and Human Services.

radioactivity associated with materials from nuclear reactors, spent fuel storage depots, nuclear fuel reprocessing facilities, high-level nuclear waste sites, or transport vehicles.[9]

The development of human-made radioactive isotopes and nuclear weapons during and after World War II was an important factor in the birth of the nuclear weapons industry in the mid-twentieth century. Most of what we know today about nuclear disasters comes from the A-bomb experience of World War II and from radiation accidents that have occurred over the past 70 years. Information on the effects of nuclear weapons has been obtained from Hiroshima and Nagasaki and from animal experimentation conducted during the atmospheric tests of the 1950s.[8] Data on the consequences of radiation accidents have been obtained from the methodical medical and scientific assessments of radiation accident victims. The existence of national and international registries on accidental radiation injuries has helped to characterize the types and patterns of radiation damage and to provide useful information for optimal medical management of victims.[10] The knowledge gained from these experiences serves as the foundation of nuclear disaster management for the twenty-first century.

CURRENT PRACTICE

Nuclear weapons produce their biological effects through the direct or indirect effects of blast, heat, and radiation.[11-13] The first two effects are fairly simple and the mechanisms of their injury are readily understood. Radiation, on the other hand, is a more complex noxious agent and is generally misunderstood by health professionals. Understanding how radiation interacts with matter provides insights into methods used to detect and measure radiation, reduce the biological hazards, and manage nuclear disasters and their consequences.

Basic Principles
Radiation Physics

After a nuclear weapon detonation, a tremendous amount of energy is quickly released in the form of ionizing radiation. Ionizing radiations are defined as those "types of particulate and electromagnetic radiations that interact with matter and either directly or indirectly form ion pairs."[14] Ionizing radiations can be divided into two categories: directly ionizing and indirectly ionizing. Directly ionizing radiations are charged particles (electrons, protons, beta particles, alpha particles, etc.) that have sufficient kinetic energy to produce ionizations through direct collisions with bound orbital electrons of an atom or molecule. Indirectly ionizing radiations are uncharged particles or photons (neutrons, x-rays, gamma rays, etc.) that can liberate bound orbital electrons, but only indirectly.

Both x-rays and gamma rays are photons, or small quantized packets of pure electromagnetic energy, just like light. However, they have a much higher nonvisible frequency. X-rays and gamma rays differ only in their origin. X-rays are produced in the outer orbital shells of atoms, whereas gamma rays come from within the nucleus of the atoms. X-rays and gamma rays are low linear energy transfer radiations; that is, they deposit relatively low amounts of energy along the track of radiation as they penetrate tissue and deposit energy deep in the body. Many radioactive isotopes decay by emitting several different types of particles. The most common forms of particle radiation are alpha, beta, and neutron.

Alpha particles are massive, charged helium nuclei. Because they deposit all of their energy over a very short distance, alpha particles are classified as high linear energy transfer radiation. Because of their size, alpha particles can easily be stopped using a sheet of paper or light clothing. Beta particles are very lightly charged high-speed electron particles that can penetrate to a depth of a few centimeters. Neutron

radiation is an uncharged particle that is emitted during a nuclear detonation almost exclusively from the fission and fusion processes themselves. Important factors that will prevent or minimize the effects of radiation exposure on humans include the principles of time, distance, and shielding. (See Chapter 105 for a discussion of radiation safety.)

Radiation Biology

Radiation biology is the field of study that describes the many changes that radiation produces in biological material. Charged particles (e.g., electrons, protons, beta particles, alpha particles, fission fragments) are directly ionizing because they can disrupt (ionize) chemical bonds and produce chemical and biological changes.[15] Electromagnetic radiations (e.g., x-rays, gamma rays) are indirectly ionizing because they do not themselves cause any chemical or biological changes. Instead, they deposit kinetic energy into the material through which they pass and produce secondary charged particles (electrons) that can produce subsequent chemical and biological alterations. Radiation can damage a cell by indirectly interacting with water molecules in the body. This leads to the creation of unstable, toxic hyperoxide molecules (i.e., free radicals) that then damage sensitive molecules and subcellular structures. Ionizing radiations transfer energy to biological material by two mechanisms: ionization and excitation.[15]

Alpha radiation is fully absorbed within the first millimeter of exposed skin. It is generally not an external radiation hazard. Alpha radiation poses serious health hazards if it is inhaled, ingested, or deposited in an open wound. If an alpha-emitting radioactive material is internally deposited, all of the radiation energy will be absorbed in a very small volume of tissue immediately surrounding each particle of material. The internal deposition of alpha particles can cause radiation injury over a long period. If a beta-emitting radioactive material is on the surface of the skin, the ensuing beta radiation causes damage to the basal stratum of the skin and produces deep "beta" burns, or lesions similar to superficial thermal burns. If the beta material is incorporated internally into the body, the beta radiation can cause considerable injury. Gamma radiation is highly energetic and penetrating and therefore is both an internal and external radiation hazard. Gamma rays can cause whole-body injury. Neutron radiation is extremely penetrating and can also result in whole-body irradiation. Compared with gamma rays, neutrons can cause 20 times more damage to tissues.[16]

The sensitivity of cells, tissues, and organs to a dose of ionizing radiation depends primarily on two factors: the rapidity of cell division and the radiosensitivity of the cells.[15] Cells are most sensitive to radiation during mitosis, when DNA is being divided. Rapidly dividing cells are more radiosensitive. Tissues and organs that depend on an active stem cell pool will be more radiosensitive than those tissues and organ systems made up of mature cellular pools with little or no stem cell activity.

Radiation Dose and Units

Quantities of radiation can be expressed in several different ways. The term *radiation exposure* applies to air only and is a measure of the amount of ionization produced by x-ray and gamma radiation in air. It is measured in coulombs per kilogram (C/kg) of dry air. The roentgen (R) is an older unit of radiation exposure and applies only to x-rays and gamma rays up to energies of about 3 MeV ($1 \text{ R} = 2.58 \times 10^{-4}$ C/kg).

The *radiation absorbed dose* is the amount of energy deposited in a given mass of absorbing material. The conventional unit for absorbed dose, the *rad*, is equal to the absorption of 100 ergs of energy in 1 g of absorbing medium, typically tissue (1 rad = 100 ergs/g of medium). The International System of Units (SI) unit of absorbed dose, the gray (Gy), is defined as the absorption of 1 J of energy per kilogram of medium (1 Gy = 1 J/kg = 100 rad and 1 rad = 1 cGy).

The term *dose equivalent* is necessary because different radiations produce different amounts of biological damage. It is defined as the product of the absorbed dose and a factor, Q (the quality factor), that characterizes the damage associated with each type of radiation. In the conventional system, the unit of dose equivalent is the *rem*, which is calculated from the absorbed dose (rem = rad × Q). The SI unit of dose equivalent is the sievert (Sv), and Sv = Gy × Q.

Radioactivity is the activity level of a radioactive isotope expressed as the number of atoms that will disintegrate (decay) per second. One becquerel (Bq) is equal to one nuclear transformation per second. The unit in the traditional system is curie (Ci), where 1 Ci = 3.7×10^{10} Bq. The term *dose rate* is the dose of radiation per unit of time.

Nuclear Disaster Scenarios

In light of the terrorist attacks of September 11, 2001, it is important to understand possible nuclear disaster scenarios. September 11 was a "day of unprecedented shock and suffering in the history of the United States. The nation was unprepared."[17] The greatest threat we face in the world today is from nuclear terrorism.[18] The vast stockpiles of nuclear weapons and highly enriched uranium and plutonium in Russia are vulnerable to theft and illicit trafficking. Russia remains the most probable source for a terrorist to obtain a nuclear weapon or materials to construct a weapon, followed by Pakistan and North Korea. North Korea is believed to be the world's most promiscuous nuclear proliferator.[18] The leaking of weapons technologies allows smaller terrorist groups to wreak havoc and cause greater destruction. Globalization has made it easier for terrorists to travel, communicate, and transport weapons. There is a burgeoning and well-organized black market for nuclear technologies and arms. September 11 was a wake-up call to America. Americans fear more terrorist attacks and more Middle East instability.[19] In fact, a poll taken in 2003 found that 4 of every 10 Americans say that they "often worry about the chances of a nuclear attack by terrorists."[20] The threats of terrorist attack will be far more serious, for example, in light of the possibility that North Korea has already developed a nuclear program.

Detonation of Nuclear Weapons

Strategic nuclear weapons. Strategic nuclear weapons are devices constructed by a government or country. This category of arms made up the main strategic arsenal during the height of the Cold War. These weapons generally have a yield (or size) from 170 kilotons to 24 megatons.[5] Interestingly, the Soviets are reported to have had some warheads with yields as high as 100 megatons. Strategic nuclear weapons could be carried to the intended target by various delivery vehicles, including land-based intercontinental ballistic missiles, submarine-launched ballistic missiles, or long-range bombers. The detonation of a strategic nuclear weapon in the United States today is unlikely. However, the risk of such an event would most likely be associated with the accidental launch of a former Soviet Union nuclear weapon resulting from equipment malfunction or warning system failure, or dissidents getting hold of strategic weapons and launching them.

Tactical nuclear weapons. Tactical nuclear weapons are also fabricated by a government or country and have yields from less than 0.1 to more than 100 kilotons.[5] These nuclear systems could be used by a military organization for employment against, for example, military targets in a theater of war. Such weapons are artillery shells, ground-mobile rockets and missiles, and air-launched bombs. Tactical nuclear weapons may be the size of a suitcase or backpack.

Imagine a terrorist scenario in which a 10-kiloton nuclear weapon is stolen from a Russian arsenal and detonated in New York City, San Francisco, Houston, Washington, Chicago, or Los Angeles.[20] If a terrorist group, such as Al Qaeda, rented a van and carried this nuclear weapon into the middle of Times Square in New York and detonated it next to the Morgan Stanley headquarters on Broadway, Times Square would vanish within a second.[20] The resulting fireball and blast wave would destroy instantly the theater district, the New York Times building, Grand Central Station, and every other building within a third of a mile from "ground zero." The resulting firestorm would engulf Rockefeller Center, Carnegie Hall, the Empire State Building, and Madison Square Garden. On a typical workday, more than 500,000 people may crowd into an area within a half-mile radius of Times Square. A noontime detonation could potentially kill all of these people, including hundreds of thousands of others who would die from collapsing buildings, fire, and fallout. The electromagnetic pulse from the blast would destroy phones, radios, and other electronic communications. Emergency medical services and hospitals would be overwhelmed by the injured.

Improvised nuclear device. An IND is fabricated by a nongovernmental organization or terrorist group. It is made up of either highly enriched uranium or plutonium-239. Tens of thousands of potential weapons (softball-size lumps of highly enriched uranium and plutonium) remain today in unsecured storage facilities in Russia, vulnerable to theft by criminals who could sell them to terrorists. Since the collapse of the former Soviet Union, there have been hundreds of confirmed cases of successful theft of nuclear materials. If successful, detonation of an IND could produce a nuclear yield similar to that of Hiroshima, with similar releases of radiation, blast, thermal pulses, and considerable radioactive fallout. Fabrication of such a device would be difficult because of the sophisticated expertise and engineering required. A terrorist organization might be able to produce a partial yield, producing less effect.

Effects of Nuclear Weapons

In this section, the basic characteristics of the effects of nuclear weapons are summarized, with an emphasis on the information of greatest use to nuclear disaster managers. There are numerous other references that treat this subject in much greater detail.[9,16,21,22]

The main physical effects of nuclear weapons are blast, thermal radiation (heat), and nuclear radiation. These effects depend on the yield of the weapon, physical design of the weapon, and method of employment.[22] The altitude at which a weapon is detonated will determine the relative effects of blast, heat, and nuclear radiation. Nuclear detonations are usually classified as airbursts, surface bursts, or high-altitude bursts.

The blast and thermal effects of a detonation produce the greatest number of immediate human casualties.[21] Immediately after detonation the temperature at the center of the fireball reaches 1,000,000 °C, producing a shock wave traveling at supersonic speeds, followed by hurricane-force afterwinds and an intense flash of thermal radiation. A 5-psi blast wave and 160-mph blast winds associated with the blast wave would destroy a two-story brick house, rupture the human eardrum, or hurl a person against stationary structures.[21] A pressure level of 15 psi could produce serious intrathoracic injuries, interstitial hemorrhage, edema, and air emboli as well as serious abdominal injuries, such as hepatic and splenic rupture.

The thermal radiation is associated with burns, including *flash burns* and *flame burns*, and certain eye injuries, including *flash blindness* and *retinal burns*. Flash burns result from the skin's exposure to a large quantity of thermal energy in a very short time, leaving the affected skin with a charred appearance. Flame burns result from the contact with a conventional fire, such as that on clothing. Flash blindness is a temporary condition; however, a retinal burn that results from looking directly at the fireball causes a permanent blind spot.

Detonation of a nuclear weapon produces a variety of nuclear radiations.[21] Initial radiation consists of neutrons and gamma rays produced within the first minute after detonation. The main hazard from initial radiation is acute external whole-body irradiation by neutrons and gamma rays. Residual radiation is generated beyond the first minute after detonation and includes gamma rays, beta particles, and alpha particles. These radiations are produced as highly radioactive fission fragments and activated weapons material. The main hazard from residual radiation is radioactive fallout, which can remain a significant biological hazard long after detonation.

Attacks on Nuclear Reactors

The potential of terrorist attack on a nuclear power plant has been mentioned by the media and is discussed in more detail in Chapters 168 and 194. However, the probability of an attack is low. The low probability is due to the high security surrounding a nuclear reactor and the safety systems incorporated into it. There is extensive shielding around the reactor core and large amounts of explosives would be needed to breach the reactor core. If an accident occurs, reactors are designed to slow down and stop the reaction. A reactor coolant system does contain some radioactivity, which could be released if the coolant system were damaged. Radioactive iodine and noble gases would probably be released. There would be immediate health effects local to the release. The release of large amounts of radioactive iodine could have long-term effects, such as thyroid cancer in children. In fact, this is exactly what happened after the Fukushima nuclear power plant accident, where large amounts of iodine-131, cesium-134, and cesium-137 were released into the environment.[23] It is possible that a jumbo jet could crash into a reactor or adjacent spent fuel storage facilities, but it would be difficult in the latter situation to expose a large population to radiation from spent fuel rods. Recent computer modeling and engineering studies suggest that the construction of most reactors could withstand a direct hit from a commercial aircraft flying into a reactor at less than 300 mph. However, some scientists question these findings and believe that penetration of the containment dome could cause the reactor to melt down. The 1986 Chernobyl and 2011 Fukushima nuclear power plant accidents serve as harsh reminders of scenarios in which terrorists might possibly cause a nuclear disaster by breaching a nuclear reactor and releasing radioactive materials into the environment.

Detonation of a Radiological Dispersal Device

An RDD is a device that combines radioactive materials with conventional explosives. (See Chapter 77 for a more complete discussion of RDDs.) It may be made from traditional dynamite, TNT, ammonium nitrate, or a variety of other explosive materials.[24] When detonated, an RDD kills or injures through the initial blast, which causes damage from the expansion of hot gases, and by dispersing radioactive materials that are highly toxic over a wide geographic area without a nuclear explosion. Some common radioactive sources that have a high probability of being used in an RDD include cobalt-60, strontium-90, cesium-137, iridium-192, radium-226, plutonium-238, americium-241, and californium-252. The dispersal effects of an RDD depend on the amount of explosives, the physical form of the radioactive source, and the atmospheric conditions.[25] RDDs are attractive to terrorists because they are relatively easy to acquire and have the potential of causing casualties, contamination of widespread areas, adverse psychological effects on people, and economic disruption.

Simple Dispersal Device

A simple dispersal device (SDD) contains a high-energy source that irradiates people or spreads radioactive material in a populated area, such as an airport, train station, sports arena, or theater. Use of such a device to cause radiation exposure in unsuspecting people is considered a terrorist act. Common radioactive sources that could be used in an SDD are the same as the sources mentioned previously for RDDs. The threat of radiation exposure from an SDD would have the same psychological effect on people as an RDD: instilling fear.

Radiation Accidents

Information on radiation injuries has been gathered over a period of 70 to 100 years.[26] Important information obtained from previous worldwide radiation accidents is useful in preparing and planning for nuclear terrorism and disasters. Radiation accidents can occur in situations where there are problems with nuclear reactors as well as industrial and medical sources of radiation. From 1946 to 2000, there have been more than 120 documented fatalities resulting from radiation accidents worldwide.[27] Serious radiation accidents in the United States have been rare.[28] From 1944 to June 2000, only 30 persons lost their lives in 13 separate radiation accidents in the United States. There were 233 other, less serious accidents during the same period. In the former Soviet Union 59 deaths occurred from radiation accidents between 1950 and 2000.[29]

There are two categories of radiation accidents.[30] The first category is an *external exposure* accident, that is, external irradiation from a source distant to or in close proximity to the body. Once a person has been removed from the source of radiation or the radiation-producing machine has been turned off, the irradiation stops. This exposed person does not become radioactive and there are no hazards to other people. The second category is a *contamination* accident. A person contaminated with radioactive material will continue to be irradiated until the radioactive material is removed, is eliminated, or decays. Contamination may occur in the form of radioactive gases, liquids, or particles. The contamination can be spread to other parts of the victim's body as well as to others. There is a third category of accident: a combination of the two.

The effects seen in persons who have been exposed in radiation accidents can be categorized as either deterministic or stochastic radiation effects.[31] Direct deterministic effects include the different types of acute and chronic radiation syndromes. The clinical manifestations of radiation injury include the latter as well as characteristic erythema, blistering, and even necrosis caused by local radiation damage. These deterministic effects occur when a specific dose-level threshold has been exceeded. The direct deterministic effects on an individual will depend on the dose of radiation received, the quality or type of radiation, the volume of tissue irradiated, and the time over which the dose is received. The stochastic effects are long term and include, for example, the induction of cancer and potential genetic abnormalities. More in-depth information on the medical management of radiation accident patients can be found in *Medical Management of Radiation Accidents*.[32] In addition, improving health care following a catastrophic radiological or nuclear incident requires more educational training for health responders about ionizing radiation; radiation safety; and managing, diagnosing, and treating radiation-related injuries and illness.[33]

Principles of Medical Management

The optimal medical treatment for injury following detonation of a nuclear weapon can be found in several valuable sources.[8,16,21,22,33–35] Other articles have addressed medical treatment of individuals injured by a terrorist act involving radioactive materials.[25,34,36–41] There is a growing body of evidence that suggests medical personnel in hospitals are unprepared for a large-scale radiological emergency, such as a terrorist event involving nuclear or radioactive materials.[42] Clinicians and medical personnel lack sufficient training on radiological emergency preparedness and have concerns about overloading of clinical systems. The Centers for Disease Control and Prevention have provided a tool kit for use by hospital medical personnel who have to respond to a nuclear or radiological event. The medical response to radiation is the least taught topic in professional schools or civil preparedness organizations.[43] Few medical professionals possess the basic knowledge or skills to identify, diagnose, and treat a radiation victim. Managing radiation injuries requires acute, critical, and long-term care during the course of illness.

Conventional injuries should be treated first, since radiation contamination is not a life-threatening medical emergency. Patients with traumatic blast and radiation injury should be resuscitated and stabilized. Airway, breathing, and circulation always take priority. These patients require more specialized treatment. Decontamination of patients should be carried out according to accepted standards of radiation decontamination. (See Chapter 84 for further discussion.) Specialists in hematology, oncology, radiation, and infectious disease should be consulted. Effective treatment of internally contaminated patients requires knowledge of both the radioactive isotope and its physical form. Treatment should be instituted quickly to ensure effectiveness. However, with a terrorist incidence, initially the radioactive source or sources are not known.[34] Several general approaches may be used to treat internal radiation contamination, including reduction of absorption (Prussian blue), dilution (force fluids), blockage (potassium iodide), displacement by nonradioactive materials (oral phosphate), mobilization as a means of elimination from tissue (ammonium chloride), and chelation (calcium and zinc diethylenetriamine pentaacetate [Ca-DTPA and Zn-DTPA]).[44] Although no drugs have been licensed in the United States to treat acute and long-term radiation injuries in the event of large-scale radiation or nuclear public health emergency, there is a goal to ensure the government stockpiles of medical countermeasures to treat radiation injuries.[44]

Patients who have received a low whole-body radiation dose may develop gastrointestinal (GI) distress within the first 2 days. Antiemetics may be effective in reducing the GI symptoms. Symptoms will usually subside within the first day of treatment. If not, parenteral fluids should be considered. The prognosis for patients who have suffered traumatic blast, burn, and radiation injury is worse than for patients with radiation injury alone.[45] A wound that is contaminated with radioactive materials should be rinsed with saline and treated using conventional aseptic techniques.[25] For example, alpha-emitting radioactive isotopes that contaminate wounds are usually excised. In patients who receive whole-body doses of radiation greater than 100 cGy, the wound should be closed as soon as possible to prevent it from becoming an entry for lethal infection.

In spite of the wide availability of antibiotics, infections from opportunistic pathogens are a major problem among patients exposed to intermediate and high doses of radiation. In these cases the primary determinants of survival are treatment of microbial infections and aggressive resuscitation of the bone marrow.[45]

⚠ PITFALLS

Obstacles to the provision of optimal nuclear disaster management include the following:

- Lack of adequate preparation of nuclear disaster management planning for possible nuclear terrorism and accidents before they occur
- Lack of coordination with local and state emergency response agencies
- Lack of understanding of the physical and biological principles of radiation interaction by medical and public health professionals and nuclear disaster managers
- Lack of involvement of behavior and social health professionals to address the psychological consequences of nuclear terrorism and disasters

- Failure to adequately secure sources of highly enriched uranium and plutonium
- Failure to adequately secure nuclear weapons
- Failure to secure industrial and medical radiation sources and radioactive materials that would prevent any loss of control and consequent misuse

REFERENCES

1. Edwards R. Only a matter of time? *New Sci.* 2004;182(2450):8–9.
2. Wilson W. *A Hundred Years of Physics.* London: Gerald Duckworth & Co; 1950.
3. Weber RL. *Pioneers of Science: Nobel Prize Winners in Physics.* London: The Institute of Physics; 1980.
4. Rotblat J. Digest of nuclear weaponry. In: Cassel C, McCally M, Abraham H, eds. *Nuclear Weapons and Nuclear War: A Source Book for Health Professionals.* New York: Praeger; 1984:76–88.
5. Cassel C, McCally M, Abraham H, eds. Report of the Secretary General. Factual information on present nuclear arsenals. In: *Nuclear Weapons and Nuclear War: A Source Book for Health Professionals.* New York: Praeger; 1984:61–75.
6. Gray CS, Payne K. Victory is possible. In: Cassel C, McCally M, Abraham H, eds. *Nuclear Weapons and Nuclear War: A Source Book for Health Professionals.* New York: Praeger; 1984:48–57.
7. A world wide web of nuclear danger. *Economist.* Feb 28—March 5, 2004;25–27.
8. Holdstock D, Waterston L. Nuclear weapons, a continuing threat to health. *Lancet.* 2000;355:1544–1547.
9. National Council on Radiation Protection and Measurement. *Management of Terrorist Events Involving Radioactive Material.* Report No. 138, Bethesda, MD: National Council on Radiation Protection and Measurement; 2001.
10. Guskova AK. Medical characteristics of different types of radiation accidents. In: Gusev I, Guskova AK, Mettler FA Jr, eds. *Medical Management of Radiation Accidents.* 2nd ed. Boca Raton, FL: CRC Press; 2001:15–22.
11. Glasstone S, Dolan P. Biological effects. In: Cassel C, McCally M, Abraham H, eds. *Nuclear Weapons and Nuclear War: A Source Book for Health Professionals.* New York: Praeger; 1984:91–118.
12. Wald N. Radiation injury. In: Cassel C, McCally M, Abraham H, eds. *Nuclear Weapons and Nuclear War: A Source Book for Health Professionals.* New York: Praeger; 1984:121–138.
13. Beebe GW. Ionizing radiation and health. In: Cassel C, McCally M, Abraham H, eds. *Nuclear Weapons and Nuclear War: A Source Book for Health Professionals.* New York: Praeger; 1984:139–158.
14. Sholtis JA Jr. Ionizing radiations and their interactions with matter. In: Conklin JJ, Walker RI, eds. *Military Radiobiology.* San Diego, CA: Academic Press, Inc; 1987:55–86.
15. Holahan EV Jr. Cellular radiation biology. In: Conklin JJ, Walker RI, eds. *Military Radiobiology.* San Diego, CA: Academic Press; 1987:87–110.
16. Jarrett D, ed. *Medical Management of Radiological Casualties: Handbook.* 1st ed. Bethesda, MD: Armed Forces Radiobiology Research Institute; 1999, AFRRI special publication 99-2.
17. National Commission on Terrorist Attacks Upon the United States. *The 9/11 Commission Report: Final Report of the National Commission on Terrorist Attacks Upon the United States.* New York: W.W. Norton & Company; 2004.
18. Allison G. Nuclear terrorism poses the gravest threat today. *Wall St J Eur.* July 14, 2003;A10.
19. Seib GF. As Bush and Kerry focus elsewhere, atomic threats stew. *Wall St J.* Aug 11, 2004;4.
20. Allison G. *Nuclear Terrorism: The Ultimate Preventable Catastrophe.* 1st ed. New York: Times Books; 2004.
21. Zajtchuk R, Jenkins DP, Bellamy RF, et al, eds. *Medical Consequences of Nuclear Warfare.* vol. 2. Falls Church, VA: TMM Publications, Office of the Surgeon General; 1989.
22. United States Army Center for Health Promotion and Preventive Medicine. *The Medical NBC Battlebook.* USACHPPM Tech Guide 244, 2000.

23. Hachiya M, Tominaga T, Tatsuzaki H, et al. Medical management of the consequences of the Fukushima nuclear power plant incident. *Drug Dev Res.* 2014;75:3–9.

24. King G. *Dirty Bomb: Weapon of Mass Disruption.* New York: Penguin Group; 2004.

25. Mettler FA Jr, Voelz GL. Major radiation exposure—what to expect and how to respond. *N Engl J Med.* 2002;346:1554–1561.

26. Guskova AK. Radiation sickness classification. In: Gusev I, Guskova AK, Mettler FA Jr, eds. *Medical Management of Radiation Accidents.* 2nd ed. Boca Raton, FL: CRC Press; 2001:23–31.

27. Mettler FA Jr, Guskova AK. Treatment of acute radiation sickness. In: Gusev I, Guskova AK, Mettler FA Jr, eds. *Medical Management of Radiation Accidents.* 2nd ed. Boca Raton, FL: CRC Press; 2001:53–67.

28. Ricks RC, Berger ME, Holloway EC, Goans RE. Radiation accidents in the United States. In: Gusev I, Guskova AK, Mettler FA Jr, eds. *Medical Management of Radiation Accidents.* 2nd ed. Boca Raton, FL: CRC Press; 2001:167–172.

29. Soloviev V, Ilyin LA, Baranov AE, et al. Radiation accidents in the former U.S.S.R. In: Gusev I, Guskova AK, Mettler FA Jr, eds. *Medical Management of Radiation Accidents.* 2nd ed. Boca Raton, FL: CRC Press; 2001:157–165.

30. Mettler FA Jr, Kelsey CA. Fundamentals of radiation accidents. In: Gusev I, Guskova AK, Mettler FA Jr, eds. *Medical Management of Radiation Accidents.* 2nd ed. Boca Raton, FL: CRC Press; 2001:1–13.

31. Guskova AK. Medical characteristics of different types of radiation accidents. In: Gusev I, Guskova AK, Mettler FA Jr, eds. *Medical Management of Radiation Accidents.* 2nd ed. Boca Raton, FL: CRC Press; 2001:15–22.

32. Gusev I, Guskova AK, Mettler FA Jr, eds. *Medical Management of Radiation Accidents.* 2nd ed. Boca Raton, FL: CRC Press; 2001.

33. Conklin JJ, Walker RI, eds. *Military Radiobiology.* San Diego, CA: Academic Press; 1987.

34. Leikin JB, McFee RB, Walter FG, et al. A primer for nuclear terrorism. *Dis Mon.* 2003;49:479–516.

35. Fong FH Jr. Nuclear detonations: evaluation and response. In: Hogan DE, Burstein JL, eds. *Disaster Medicine.* Philadelphia: Lippincott Williams & Wilkins; 2002:317–339.

36. Waselenko JK, MacVittie TJ, Blakely WF, et al. Medical management of the acute radiation syndrome: recommendations of the Strategic National Stockpile Radiation Working Group. *Ann Intern Med.* 2004;140:1037–1051.

37. Moulder JE. Post-irradiation approaches to treatment of radiation injuries in the context of radiological terrorism and radiation accidents: a review. *Int J Radiat Biol.* 2004;80:1–8.

38. Turai I, Veress K, Gunalp B, et al. Medical response to radiation incidents and radionuclear threats. *BMJ.* 2004;328:568–572.

39. Dainiak N, Waselenko JK, Armitage JO, et al. The hematologist and radiation casualties. *ASH Education Book.* 2003;1:473–496.

40. Hagby M, Goldberg A, Becker S, et al. Health implications of radiological terrorism: perspectives from Israel. *J Emerg Trauma Shock.* 2009;2:117–123.

41. McCurley MC, Miller CW, Tucker FE, et al. Educating medical staff about responding to a radiological or nuclear emergency. *Health Phys.* 2009;96(5 suppl 2):S50–S54.

42. MeFee R, Leikin JB. Death by polonium-210: lessons learned from the murder of former Soviet spy Alexander Litvinenko. *Semin Diagn Pathol.* 2009;1:61–67.

43. Voelz GL. Assessment and treatment of internal contamination: general principles. In: Gusev I, Guskova AK, Mettler FA Jr, eds. *Medical Management of Radiation Accidents.* 2nd ed. Boca Raton, FL: CRC Press; 2001:319–336.

44. Rios CI, Cassatt DR, Dicarlo AL, et al. Building the strategic national stockpile through the NIAID radiation nuclear countermeasures program. *Drug Dev Res.* 2014;75:23–28.

45. Conklin JJ, Walker RI. Diagnosis, triage, and treatment of casualties. In: Conklin JJ, Walker RI, eds. *Military Radiobiology.* San Diego: Academic Press; 1987:231–240.

Dirty Bomb (Radiological Dispersal Device)*

George A. Alexander

A *dirty bomb* is a device that combines radioactive materials with conventional explosives. Global terrorist organizations are believed to be interested in and capable of constructing dirty bombs and launching attacks with them.[1] There are only two documented cases of terrorist use of dirty bombs in the world today.[2] Both incidents occurred in Russia. In 1995 Chechen insurgents buried a cesium-137 dirty bomb in a park in Moscow and alerted the media before its detonation. In 1998 a container of radioactive materials was found attached to an explosive mine near a railroad line in Chechnya. Dirty bombs are attractive to terrorists because they are relatively easy to acquire and have the potential for causing casualties, contamination of widespread areas, adverse psychological effects, and economic disruption. A dirty bomb threat potentially poses a medical and public health disaster.

A dirty bomb can be made from traditional dynamite, trinitrotoluene (TNT), ammonium nitrate, or a variety of other explosive materials.[3] When detonated it kills or injures by the initial blast, which causes damage from the expansion of hot gases, and by dispersing radioactive materials that are highly toxic over a wide geographic area without a nuclear explosion. The dispersal effects of a dirty bomb depend on the amount of explosives used, the physical form of the radioactive source, and the atmospheric conditions.[4] A dirty bomb is also known technically as a radiological dispersal device (RDD).

Many different radioactive sources can be used to fabricate a dirty bomb. Radioactive sources can be obtained illicitly from hospitals and medical clinics, industrial radiography and gauging devices, food sterilizers, power sources, communication devices, navigator beacons, oil well logging, and scientific research laboratories. Some common radioactive sources that have a high probability of being used as a dirty bomb based on their availability include cobalt-60, strontium-90, cesium-137, iridium-192, radium-226, plutonium-238, americium-241, and californium-252. Alpha-emitting radiation sources pose serious health hazards if they are inhaled, ingested, or deposited in an open wound. Beta-emitting sources can cause deep beta burns on the skin. Gamma rays may penetrate body tissues and cause deep tissue injury.

The most likely dirty bomb scenarios would involve the use of either a few small low-level radioactive sources or a large amount of highly radioactive sources combined with high explosives. The first scenario considers use of a dirty bomb containing a few curies of a gamma-ray source, such as cesium-137,[5] combined with a few kilograms of high explosive. In this case the dirty bomb may be used with the primary intent of causing fear or panic among people and disrupting their community. Because the amount of radioactivity is small, the radiation exposure to individuals would be low and no immediate effects on health would be expected. The probability of long-term health effects would be small.

The second scenario considers use of a dirty bomb containing large sources of penetrating radiation coupled with sophisticated high explosives. The detonation would disperse considerable amounts of radioactive material over a large area. Persons injured by the blast are likely to be contaminated with radioactivity and may receive life-threatening doses of radiation. Such a device is intended to kill tens or hundreds of persons, injure and sicken hundreds or thousands, and cause widespread panic.[6]

Recognizing that a conventional explosive device has been detonated may be simple because of the associated blast. However, it may take considerable time before the radioactive component of the dirty bomb attack is recognized. Therefore it is important that first responders use radiation-detection equipment to identify a radioactive component after any explosion.[7]

Recognition of acute radiation injury is based on the patient's medical history and clinical findings.[8] The extent of radiation injury depends on three factors: depth of penetration of the radiation, dose of radiation absorbed, and volume of tissue irradiated. For localized radiation exposure the initial signs of injury might be a radiation burn, including erythema, blistering, or desquamation. With a low whole-body dose of 0 to 100 cGy from a dirty bomb, a patient would generally have no symptoms. With a moderate whole-body dose of 100 to 200 cGy, the patient may exhibit the prodromal phase (nausea and vomiting) of acute radiation syndrome. At doses exceeding 300 cGy, patients would experience nausea, vomiting, diarrhea, erythema, and fever. A useful method of predicting the clinical severity of radiation injury is the time to onset of vomiting. If the time to vomiting is less than 4 hours, the patient has received a high dose of radiation.

Laboratory data show that early changes in lymphocyte counts are associated with the severity of radiation injury. Absolute lymphocyte counts less than 1000 mm^3 and greater than 500 mm^3 indicate moderate and severe levels of radiation exposure, respectively. Complete blood counts can be repeated every 4 to 6 hours to evaluate lymphocyte depletion kinetics. The appearance of dicentric chromosomes in peripheral blood lymphocytes is also useful in the calculating exposure dose. In patients who have developed acute radiation syndrome, within 2 to 3 weeks bone marrow suppression may occur with associated neutropenia, lymphopenia, and thrombocytopenia.

◀◀ PRE-INCIDENT ACTIONS

One of the most important preemptive actions that emergency medical service agencies, hospital-based emergency departments, and outpatient facilities should do is to determine whether their community is a possible

---

*The views expressed in this chapter are those of the author and do not necessarily represent the official policy or position of the National Cancer Institute, the National Institutes of Health, or the Department of Health and Human Services.

target for a terrorist dirty bomb attack. Coordinating with local and state law enforcement and response agencies should provide a framework in which to assess the dirty bomb threat and develop a medical radiation incident or injury protocol. The protocol should be incorporated into the overall disaster plan. The radiation disaster plan should address decontamination, security, radiation monitoring, and decorporation of radioactive materials. The hospital radiation safety officer should be included in the medical radiation response team. Hospital staff should understand the hazards of radioactive contamination and be trained in radiation-monitoring techniques. Staff would need access to dosimeters, Geiger-Mueller counters, and personal protective equipment. Radiation-detection capabilities are critical to an effective medical response. Hospitals should have a realistic decontamination plan for patients,[9] a lockdown plan to control access, and evacuation plans. A radiation risk communication program is required for the public. As has been shown by the Fukushima Nuclear Plant accident in 2011 the most important task for scientists is to make available to the public scientific knowledge of the level of radiation risk resulting in more understanding of their potential health risks.[10]

POST-INCIDENT ACTIONS

Emergency medical first responders arriving on the scene of a dirty bomb incident should initiate actions to treat or evacuate casualties. All response personnel should be advised of the explosive and radiological hazards that may be present. Health care providers should advise others regarding safety measures to be taken to protect the public and to mitigate the radiation health effects. Patients evacuated from the scene and arriving at hospitals or medical clinics should be routinely monitored for radiation and decontaminated, as needed. Health care providers should control any exposure of hospital personnel to contamination. Moreover effective decontamination procedures are available to reduce the radiation contamination and to avoid an uncontrolled spread of the contamination.[11] Clinicians should seek the assistance and cooperation of state and local authorities and inform them of casualties and possible hazards. Hospital radiation safety staff should periodically monitor the emergency department for radioactive contamination.

MEDICAL TREATMENT OF CASUALTIES

Injuries associated with dirty bombs pose new and significant challenges for clinicians. Because radiation affects many organ systems, it can complicate blast and thermal injuries associated with a dirty bomb. Conventional injuries should be treated first because radiation contamination is not an imminent life-threatening medical emergency. Patients with traumatic blast and radiation injury should be resuscitated and stabilized. The assessment of patient airway, breathing, and circulation always takes priority. Victims of radiation exposure require more specialized treatment, and specialists in hematology, oncology, radiation, and infectious disease should be consulted. Effective treatment of internally contaminated patients requires knowledge of both the relevant radioactive isotope and its physical form. Treatment should be instituted quickly to ensure its effectiveness. However, with a terrorist incident, initially the radioactive source or sources are not known.[12] Several general approaches may be used to treat internal radiation contamination, including reduction of absorption (administer Prussian blue), dilution (force fluids), removal of blockage (use potassium iodide), rectification of displacement by nonradioactive materials (administer oral phosphate), mobilization as a means of elimination from tissue (use ammonium chloride), and chelation (achieve with Ca-DTPA and Zn-DTPA).[13,14]

Patients who have received a low whole-body radiation dose may develop gastrointestinal tract distress within the first 2 days. Antiemetic agents may be effective in reducing the gastrointestinal symptoms, which will usually subside within the first day. If not, the administration of parenteral fluids should be considered. The prognosis for patients who have suffered traumatic blast, burn, and radiation injury is worse than for patients with radiation injury alone.[15] A wound that is contaminated with radioactive materials should be rinsed with saline and treated using conventional aseptic techniques.[4] Wounds contaminated with alpha-emitting radioactive isotopes are usually excised. In patients who receive whole-body doses of radiation greater than 100 cGy, the wound should be closed as soon as possible to prevent it from becoming an entry for lethal infection. The ability for surgical teams to respond to the consequences of combined trauma-radiation blast injury casualties is determined by prior knowledge and training for this type of terrorist event.[16]

In spite of the wide availability of antibiotics, infections from opportunistic pathogens pose a major problem among patients exposed to intermediate and high doses of radiation. In these cases the primary determinants of survival are treatment of microbial infections and aggressive resuscitation of the bone marrow.[15]

UNIQUE CONSIDERATIONS

In contrast to popular belief a dirty bomb is not considered a weapon of mass destruction.[6] Instead it is used as a weapon of mass *disruption*.[3] Because radiation is colorless, odorless, tasteless, silent, and invisible, the uncertainty of not knowing whether one is being or has been exposed to radiation instills fear and panic in most people.[17] The psychological effects of a dirty bomb incident require special consideration. Recognition of the importance of social and psychological issues will be essential in responding to a terrorist dirty bomb attack.[7] Such an incident can cause profound psychosocial effects at every level of society, including individual, family, community, and the nation. A dirty bomb attack has the capability of causing widespread fear, an increased sense of vulnerability, and loss of trust and confidence in societal institutions.[7] The effects can be emotional, physical, cognitive, or interpersonal in nature. Significant numbers of people may suffer chronic distress years after an attack. However, a study of the impact of a long-term (48-hour) shelter-in-place (SIP) simulation on mental health during a dirty bomb detonation provides evidence that SIP is a viable disaster response strategy that does not adversely affect the mental health provided.[18] Although a dirty bomb attack will create unique challenges, basic tenets of disaster mental health should still be followed in treating those affected.

PITFALLS

Obstacles to the provision of optimal medical care include the following:
- Failure to adequately prepare medical response planning for possible terrorist dirty bomb attacks before they occur
- Failure to coordinate with local and state emergency response agencies
- Lack of understanding by medical providers of the basic science of radioactive isotopes
- Failure to consult with specialists who have clinical experience in the medical management of the effects of radiation exposure
- Lack of recognition that anxiety-induced nausea and vomiting may occur after a dirty bomb attack (This phenomenon has been observed after radiation accidents in which people thought they had been exposed to radiation even in the absence of actual exposure.[19])

REFERENCES

1. Meyer J. Al Qaeda feared to have "dirty bombs." *The Los Angeles Times.* February 8, 2003;A1.
2. Edwards R. Only a matter of time? *New Sci.* 2004;182:8–9.
3. King G. *Dirty Bomb: Weapon of Mass Disruption.* New York: Penguin Group; 2004.
4. Mettler FA, Voelz GL. Major radiation exposure—what to expect and how to respond. *N Engl J Med.* 2002;346:1554–1561.
5. Blair JD. Why the dirty bomb is still ticking. *J Healthc Prot Manage.* 2014;30:109–115.
6. Zimmerman PD, Loeb C. *Dirty bombs: the threat revisited. Center for Technology and National Security Policy, National Defense University;* January 2004, Defense Horizons. No. 38.
7. National Council on Radiation Protection and Measurement. *Management of Terrorist Events Involving Radioactive Material.* Bethesda, Md: National Council on Radiation Protection and Measurement; 2001, Report No. 138.
8. Gusev I, Guskova AK, Mettler Jr FA, eds. *Medical Management of Radiation Accidents.* 2nd ed. Boca Raton, Fla: CRC Press; 2001.
9. Levitin HW, Kahn CA. Decontamination. In: Koenig KL, Schultz CH, eds. *Koenig and Schultz's Disaster Medicine: Comprehensive Principles and Practices.* Cambridge: Cambridge University Press; 2010:195–202.
10. Suzuki T. Unconscious exposure to radiation. *Genes and Environment.* 2013;35:63–68.
11. Schneider N. Radiological/nuclear decontamination—reduce the risk. In: Richardt A, Hülseweh B, Niemeyer B, Sabath B, eds. *CBRN Protection: Managing the Threat of Chemical, Biological, Radioactive and Nuclear Weapons.* Weiheim: Wiley-VCH Verlag GmbH & Co KGaA; 2013:411–430.
12. Leikin JB, McFee RB, Walter FG, et al. A primer for nuclear terrorism. *Dis Mon.* 2003;49:485–516.
13. Voelz GL. Assessment and treatment of internal contamination: general principles. In: Gusev I, Guskova AK, Mettler Jr FA, eds. *Medical Management of Radiation Accidents.* 2nd ed. Boca Raton, Fla: CRC Press; 2001:319–336.
14. Yamamoto LG. Risks and management of radiation exposure. *Pediatr Emerg Care.* 2013;29:1016–1026.
15. Conklin JJ, Walker RI. Diagnosis, triage, and treatment of casualties. In: Conklin JJ, Walker RI, eds. *Military Radiobiology.* San Diego, Calif: Academic Press, Inc; 1987:231–240.
16. Williams G, O'Malley M. Surgical considerations in the management of combined radiation blast injury casualties caused by a radiological dirty bomb. *Injury.* 2010;41:943–947.
17. Drukier GA, Rubenstein EP, Solomon PR, et al. Low cost, pervasive detection of radiation threats. 2011 IEEE International Conference on Technologies for Homeland Security, HST 2011; Article number 6107897, pages 365-371.
18. Dailey SF, Kaplan D. Shelter-in-place and mental health: an analogue study of well-being and distress. *Journal of Emergency Management.* 2014;12:121–131.
19. International Atomic Energy Agency. *The Radiological Accident in Goiânia.* Vienna: International Atomic Energy Agency; 1988.

CHAPTER 78

General Approach to Chemical Attack

Duane C. Caneva, Mark A. Kirk, and John B. Delaney Jr.

The risk of chemical attack is no longer confined to the battlefield. The rise of asymmetric terrorist tactics, combined with the dual-use nature of technology and the proliferation of information, makes chemical terrorism a realistic threat for domestic first responders. In addition to conventional chemical warfare agents, the threat now includes the use of toxic industrial chemicals and materials that, as part of an industrial-based economy, are ubiquitous in much of developed society. Prevention, preparation, and response to such an attack requires consideration of a myriad of issues and integration across diverse disciplines to ensure optimal use of limited resources and the development of best practices. Coordination of these efforts into a cogent emergency management program requires various levels of cooperation across communities, jurisdictions, regions, states, agencies, and industries, which will improve our capabilities to respond to all hazard challenges and drive us toward better business practices. This chapter focuses on the basics of preparing for and responding to a chemical attack.

HISTORICAL PERSPECTIVE

Brief History

The history of chemical warfare is both rich and fascinating. An excellent summary of this topic can be found in the *Textbook of Military Medicine*.[1] The modern era" of chemical warfare began during the events leading up to and surrounding World War I. In the United States, the Chemical Warfare Service was established on June 28, 1918, as part of the National Army, with responsibilities for all chemical weapons research, defense, training, medical treatment, and production facilities. The offensive weapons program was officially terminated by signature to the Chemical Weapons Convention (CWC) on January 13, 1993, with Senate approval on April 24, 1997. The existing infrastructure was converted to a strictly passive defense program. Through this infrastructure, the U.S. military has provided valuable input toward preparations for a chemical attack. This, combined with Hazardous Materials (HazMat) response work statutes from the Occupational Safety and Health Administration (OSHA) and the National Fire Protection Administration (NFPA) Guidelines governing fire and emergency services response, have served as the cornerstones of current U.S. doctrine and policy for preparation, training, and response to chemical attacks in noncombat situations.[2,3]

The Chemical Weapons Convention

The United Nations CWC, formally titled the "Convention on the Prohibition of the Development, Production, Stockpiling and Use of Chemical Weapons and on Their Destruction," opened for signature on January 13, 1993, after 20 years of negotiation and entered into force on April 29, 1997. Signed by 182 UN member nations to date, it describes the prohibition of the use of specific chemical warfare agents, production limits for study, measures to ensure compliance, and destruction of stores of chemical stockpiles. The CWC established the Organization for the Prevention of Chemical Weapons (OPCW), located in The Hague, to serve as its operational arm, conducting verification activities, ensuring implementation of convention provisions, and providing a forum for consultation and cooperation.[4]

Chemical Agents

A chemical attack traditionally involves highly toxic chemical warfare agents that are specifically designed to cause morbidity and mortality, are produced in significant amounts, and are coupled with appropriate dispersal technologies. By definition these agents are controlled under the CWC. However, a chemical attack can also involve toxic industrial chemicals that, while not as toxic as chemical warfare agents, are more readily available in larger quantities and are less tightly controlled. Currently, approximately 125,000 chemicals are designated as a toxic industrial chemical. These agents are generally defined as a chemical, excluding chemical warfare agents, that have an LCt50 (lethal concentration for 50% of a population exposed over a given time, *t*) less than 100,000 mg-min/m^3 in any mammalian species and are produced in quantities exceeding 30 tons annually at any one production facility. Of these, approximately 4600 are considered "critical," and almost 400 are "extremely hazardous."[5,6]

Chemical agents can be dispersed in various forms (e.g., vapor, aerosols, smokes, liquids on surfaces, or solids) depending on the characteristics of the agent and the intended exposure route. Most large-scale hazardous chemical incidents (intentional or unintentional) occur through inhalation exposure, but other routes, such as dermal contact or ingestion of contaminated food or water could result in substantial casualties. Individual agents, their characteristics, and treatment are covered later in this section.

Current Practice

Chemical attacks may occur suddenly and unexpectedly, with only local response capabilities available to manage the early phases of the incident. A large-scale intentional chemical attack will require additional resources from the state and federal level. Each community's preparedness efforts should begin with a thorough understanding of all the available resources and methods to rapidly mobilize them if needed. Current tactics, techniques, and procedures (TTP) for emergency management of chemical attack have evolved from a combination of response practices from emergency services, HazMat response, and military chemical warfare defense doctrine.

Various panels have developed consensus "best practices" reports and documents, many compiled and available at the Homeland Defense Information Analysis Center (HDIAC).[7] The National Medical Response Teams (NMRT), part of the National Disaster

Medical System (NDMS), under the Department of Health and Human Services (DHHS), represent civilian teams charged with responding to CBRNE mass casualty incidents (MCI), providing decontamination, medical triage, and treatment. In 1996, the military stood up the U.S. Marine Corps Chemical Biological Incident Response Force (CBIRF) to respond to mass casualty CBRNE attacks.[8] Additionally, the Department of Defense continues to build out its National Guard CBRNE Consequence Management Enterprise, which includes 10 Homeland Response Forces, a Defense CBRNE Response Force (DCRF), 2 command and control consequence management response elements (C2CRE), 57 Weapons of Mass Destruction Civil Support Teams (WMD-CST), and 17 CBRNE-enhanced Response Force Packages (CERFP). Aligned and distributed along Federal Emergency Management Agency (FEMA) regions, the teams are located for timely response to major population centers. These teams represent model constructs for concepts of operations for their particular missions.[8]

DOCTRINE AND POLICY

National Incident Management System

Presidential Policy Directive-8 (PPD-8) for National Preparedness establishes and defines the National Preparedness Goal and National Preparedness System as a network of planning frameworks integrating incident management across critical sectors, jurisdictions, and response organizations. Federal interagency operational plans drive unity of effort through the concept of resilience in further integrating across and through sector and agency channels to state, local, tribal, and territorial governments, nongovernmental organizations, private-sector partners, and the general public.[9] PPD-8 builds on foundations set by Homeland Security Presidential Directive-5 (HSPD-5) defining the National Incident Management System (NIMS) as the comprehensive approach in preventing, preparing for, mitigating, responding to, and recovering from domestic incidents. The Incident Command System (ICS) and Unified Command System (UCS) are used to develop a common operating picture accessible across jurisdictions and functional agencies.[10] The approach is to be used at federal, state, local, and tribal government municipalities.

Emergency Management Programs

HSPD-5 establishes and defines the five phases of emergency management as prevention, preparedness, mitigation, response, and recovery, around which emergency management programs (EMPs) are built. Often called Disaster Response Plans, programs now encompass an "all hazards" approach to disasters. They usually include a comprehensive, overarching plan with specific plans or annexes for various incident types. For incident management response, the Hospital Incident Command System (HICS) has become the standard used by many hospitals, and the HICS organization makes program management materials readily available online.[11] Hospital and health system personnel have significant roles and responsibilities preidentified in preparedness and response activities. Additionally, FEMA has developed standardized training for hospital-based personnel.[12] Health care organizations should further coordinate through their EMP with local and regional partners via local emergency preparedness committees (LEPCs) or other appropriate mechanisms. These programs are further governed by The Joint Commission standards for emergency management oversight.[13]

For chemical attacks, critical actions in pre-incident planning phases include (1) identifying first responders/first receivers for triage, treatment, and decontamination teams; (2) establishing appropriate training, exercise, and evaluation programs; (3) developing respiratory protection and supply programs; (4) identifying key suppliers and

locations for chemical antidotes; and (5) drafting and testing life-cycle management programs, communication plans, operational and evacuation procedures and policies, shelter-in-place procedures, and warning and notification procedures.

The Hazard Vulnerability Analysis (HVA) assists in determining personal protective equipment (PPE) requirements and identifying other specific planning requirements. The HVA is done in conjunction with local municipal efforts. Community planning for hospitals includes coordinating with all other regional hospitals on all aspects of EMPs, including communications, mutual aid agreements, specialized treatments, alternate care facilities, cross credentialing, information management, supplies and logistics, and training exercises.

Finally, the critical step may be networking and information management links that are established during the pre-incident phases; although having a plan is important, having gone through the planning process is the critical step. Such relationships allow for rapid reorganization or self-organization of response systems under catastrophic duress, but they must be established before the incident to be effective. Hospitals should work through their LEPC.

CURRENT STANDARDS AND GUIDELINES

The current operating standards and guidelines applicable in responding to chemical attacks present challenges on several fronts. Statutes established for either the workplace or the battlefield are less than optimal for emergency, life-saving actions in an urban MCI response. The need for multidisciplinary expertise in developing EMPs also requires that various regulatory agencies and professional societies work together in establishing pragmatic statutes and guidelines. Challenges lie in developing standards around so many unknown entities within the response requirements and the limited real-world experience of large-scale incidents. A review of the various agencies with statutory authorities demonstrates the importance of coordination and cooperation, and further details are provided elsewhere in this text.

FEMA now serves as the central integrating agency for incident management at the federal level.[14] It plays a huge role in nearly all aspects of emergency management, including coordinating interagency planning, national training standards, best practices, incident management, grant programs, and lessons learned collection and analysis. It maintains the Lessons Learned Information Sharing (LLIS) portal,[15] which includes the Responder Knowledge Base (RKB) and the Authorized Equipment List (AEL).[16]

The OSHA[17] within the Department of Labor serves as an advocate for worker safety and health by developing standards for workers and workplaces. This includes setting levels for exposure to hazardous chemicals during work cycles, as well as levels for short-term and emergency exposure. OSHA also works with the National Institute of Occupational Safety and Health (NIOSH), other federal agencies, and private industry to develop standards for general emergency planning,[18] Hazardous Waste Operations and Emergency Response Standard (HAZWOPER),[19] and PPE[20] for emergency response personnel. More specific information is available in the OSHA Technical Manual.[21]

The Code of Federal Regulations (CFR) serves as the basis for first responder safety in emergency response to chemical attack. However, OSHA recognizes that statutory code written for emergency first responders at an incident site may be too restrictive for hospital-based "first receivers"[22] or those health care workers who receive contaminated victims at treatment facilities. Accordingly, OSHA promulgated guidelines to provide hospitals with expert consensus regarding safe response practices.[23] In addition, incident commanders (ICs) may use their expertise and experience to make a "risk assessment" that allows responders at hospitals or at an incident site working under their supervision to deviate from standards in order to save lives.[24]

The NFPA[25] develops guides and recommends practices, codes, and standards for the protection of firefighters and emergency medical technicians. Standards are enforced through OSHA promulgation. For example, NFPA defines PPE Levels 1 to 4 (e.g., Level 1 being vapor-protective for hazardous chemical emergencies; Level 2 being liquid splash-protective for hazardous chemical emergencies; Level 3 being liquid splash-protective for nonemergency, nonflammable hazardous chemicals; and Level 4 being standard work clothes).[26] These levels correspond closely to OSHA Levels A-D, respectively. NFPA also has several guidelines regarding competencies for first responders.[27-29] As background, NFPA "owns" their own work as a private, nongovernmental entity developing national firefighter standards that are then adopted by OSHA as federal standards. Meanwhile, OSHA has their own, nonfirefighter regulations. In the hot zone, both levels are used, depending on who you work for (fire and emergency services, HazMat, EPA, etc.). For the most part, manufacturers develop suits that meet both criteria levels.

The NIOSH, a division of the Centers for Disease Control and Prevention (CDC), seeks to prevent work-related illness and injury by ensuring the development, certification, deployment, and use of PPE and fully integrated, intelligent ensembles. Although NIOSH establishes standards, it does not have enforcement authority.[30] The National Personal Protective Technology Laboratory at the NIOSH partners with NFPA, OSHA, the Department of Defense (DoD), the National Institute of Standards and Technology (NIST), and the National Institute of Justice (NIJ) in the development of standards for CBRN respirators and their certification. All respirators used for response in a chemical attack must meet NIOSH certification.[31]

The Office of Law Enforcement Standards (OLES) at NIST, part of the NIJ, works with various agencies and partners to establish objective performance standards and equipment testing programs for critical equipment. CBRNE standards development falls under the "Critical Incident Technologies" program area. Applying technical expertise and "gold standard" laboratory capabilities, OLES works with its partners to identify technical issues, develop standard testing protocols, identify testing labs, and develop standards for such things as communications interfaces for the first responder in protective equipment, tracking first responders, and networking sensors. The standards are then issued out through the appropriate agency with statutory authority, such as NIOSH, the Environmental Protection Agency (EPA), OSHA, FEMA, DoD, or DHS. The OLES also partners with the Interagency Board (IAB, see below). PPE Guidelines are promulgated through the U.S. Department of Justice Law Enforcement and Corrections Standards and Testing Program.[32,33]

The Interagency Board for Standardization of Equipment and Interoperability (IAB), formed in the late 1998 through a partnership with DoD and FBI, ensures standardization and interoperability throughout the response community in preparing for and responding to weapons of mass destruction (WMD) incidents. Although it is not a statutory setting agency, it has an expanded stakeholder list of federal and local partners that includes statutory agencies. Its five subgroups work through a standards coordination committee, in conjunction with a science and technology committee, to develop, maintain, and update a national standardized equipment list (SEL). This SEL is maintained online currently at the IAB's website.[34]

Research, Development, and Support

In addition to many excellent academic research centers, the Technical Support Working Group (TSWG) conducts the U.S. interagency research and development program for combating terrorism, coordinates research and development requirements, disseminates technology information transfer, and influences basic and applied research. The CBRN Countermeasure Subgroup focuses on chemical incident response issues.[35] The TSWG has broad representation from federal agencies and has international participation. Current projects include a comprehensive and novel look at decontamination strategies of medical casualties and development of improved PPE.

Other Departments and Agencies

Specific roles of federal agencies and departments are covered elsewhere in this textbook; however, some specific agencies merit mention here. The DHHS has several entities with relevance for chemical attack. The National Library of Medicine (NLM) provides ready, useful resources for information on chemicals.[36] Their Chemical Hazards Emergency Medical Management (CHEMM) Web portal represents a most useful repository of all pertinent aspects of medical response to chemical incidents.[37] They have leading-edge technology applications, including WISER (Wireless Information System for Emergency Responders), to make information portable and accessible.

The Agency for Toxic Substances and Disease Registry (ATSDR), an agency of the DHHS, serves the public by using the best science, taking responsive public health actions, and providing trusted health information to prevent harmful exposures and disease related to toxic substances. The ATSDR is directed by congressional mandate to perform specific functions concerning the effect on public health of hazardous substances in the environment. These functions include public health assessments of waste sites, health consultations concerning specific hazardous substances, health surveillance and registries, response to emergency releases of hazardous substances, applied research in support of public health assessments, information development and dissemination, and education and training concerning hazardous substances. ATSDR produces toxicological profiles for hazardous substances and includes them on the National Priorities List (NPL), ranked based on frequency of occurrence at the sites, toxicity, and potential for human exposure. The profiles for nearly all of the 275 toxic substances on the NPL are available at the ATSDR website.[38] The DHHS is also home to the Public Health Emergency Medical Countermeasures Enterprise (PHEMCE), which coordinates with federal efforts to enhance preparedness for CBRN threats.[39]

The DoD is covered in more detail in other chapters of this textbook; however, several agencies play significant roles in preparing for and responding to chemical attacks. The Research Development & Engineering Command (RDECOM), formerly known as the Soldier Biological Chemical Command (SBCCOM is the research and development arm of the U.S. Army's Chemical Corps. RDECOM, with the Edgewood Chemical Biological Center (ECBC), applies this R&D effort to develop concepts of operations, training programs, partnering efforts across the chemical-biologic response paradigm, and providing publications addressing significant, challenging issues in chemical incident response.[40] RDECOM also serves as the partnering test facility with NIOSH, to perform official testing of mask/filter combinations against chemical weapons for CBRN certification.

The Army Forces Command 20th Support Command (CBRNE), formerly known as Guardian Brigade, represents an expert team specializing in responding to emergency, nonlifesaving aspects of chemical incidents[41]; although robust, CBRNE response capability now extends to many DoD units around the nation. The U.S. Marine Corps' CBIRF, is a rapid response, antiterrorism unit located in Indian Head, Maryland. The USMC CBRIF serves as a model for CBRNE response teams around the world. CBRIF works closely with partners at the local, state, and federal levels, as well as with private industry, to develop, evaluate, and validate best practice TTPs for "all hazards" emergency management planning, improvement of response equipment, and development of advanced training techniques related to CBRNE.[42] The U.S. Army Medical Research Institute for Chemical Defense (USAMRICD) provides the nation's primary medical laboratories charged with identifying chemical weapons threats and developing medical countermeasures, including antidotes, barrier creams, decontamination solutions, and chemoprophylaxis. The training arm of Institute for Chemical Defense develops and provides the chemical portion of the "gold standard" Medical Management of Chemical/Biological Casualties and the Field Management of Chemical and Biological Casualties Courses.[43]

The Department of Homeland Security also contributes to Chemical Defense through several offices. The Office of Science and Technology coordinates research and development and supports the Chemical Security Analysis Center (CSAC), which among other things, conducts the Chemical Terrorism Risk Assessment.[44] The DHS Office of Health Affairs Chemical Defense Program also works with state, local, and private-sector partners and recently completed National Planning Guidance for Communities for Patient Decontamination in a Mass Chemical Exposure Incident.[45]

THE RESPONSE

A chemical attack will likely occur abruptly and unexpectedly, creating large numbers of casualties. From past incidents it is expected that accurate information about the cause and extent of the event will only become clear over time. Incident command will be forced to make critical decisions about all phases of the response during a period of uncertainty and limited information. The scene perimeter will only be secured after many victims leave the scene potentially contaminated and enter the health care system unannounced. Specialized response teams, mutual aid, and other resources require time to mobilize; therefore, the initial response lies on the shoulders of the local response community. Local resources are likely to become overwhelmed, and additional resources will be necessary to augment the local response capabilities. Even though it is true that many chemicals cause their effects within seconds to minutes after exposure, the efficacy of response actions extends much longer beyond several hours. Ongoing or unpredictable exposures or shifting exposure levels; effects of comorbid medical conditions, partial or improper treatments; or delayed exposures can extend the onset of symptoms. Sublethal doses combined with underlying medical conditions, extremes of age, or coincident trauma or panic can lead to significantly compromised patients. Planning and preparedness assumptions should account for both immediate and ongoing response components.

During the Iran-Iraq War of the 1980s, Iran suffered several chemical warfare mass casualty attacks utilizing nerve agents, mustard agent, or a combination of the two (and sometimes in combination with conventional artillery attacks). The Iranian health system responded to these mass casualties, adjusting strategies and procedures over time by providing medical care closer to the incident site, eventually deploying mobile medical teams to provide care at the scene. Lessons learned from published exploits of response include the need to treat early and far forward in order to confer maximal patient benefit, the need for an integrated system of care, and a rapid response to antidote therapy and recovery for mild, uncomplicated casualties.[46]

Several factors make it difficult to predict response time requirements. Toxicity and lethality data of specific agents are derived from animal models and are not easily translatable to humans. Toxicity curves are likely affected by extremes of age, confounding medical problems, and concomitant trauma, with unknown effects on the course of poisoning and greater potential for effects of sublethal

exposures. Further, the management of large-scale MCI is poorly studied, as well, particularly in a heterogeneous population. The additional site response burden of working in PPE, and having an additional decontamination step in the treatment protocol, adds another dimension of complexity. The critical point is that response time requirements and treatment outcomes are not known; they may be affected by a multitude of factors and they may be extended.

INITIAL ACTIONS

Recognizing an Attack

Execution of a chemical attack may be overt, such as utilization of an explosive device, or more insidious, such as an aerosolized dispersal device. Crude explosive dissemination devices typically use a third of the explosives component as comparable conventional explosive devices, in order to minimize consumption of agent and maximize spread. Consequently, improvised explosive devices (IEDs) that seem to have more smoke than blast or fire might indicate a chemical dispersal device. Vapor clouds, smoke without fires or with color, or more sophisticated spray devices or aerosolizers in unusual places may indicate an attack. Clinically, multiple, unexplained victims with similar symptom patterns (e.g., difficulty breathing, tearing, dimmed vision, muscle weakness, and nausea seen with nerve agent symptoms) may indicate a chemical attack. Seemingly unrelated observations such as multiple dead animals should also raise suspicion of a chemical attack. Critically, any chemical attack is both a HazMat incident and a crime scene. Responders should consider crime scene preservation when practical.

Establishing Scene Safety

Initial actions on scene should include maintaining a high index of suspicion for the presence of a toxic material and additional explosive devices. First on scene and incident command should establish zones of operation. The "cold zone" or low risk area of operations should be established upwind and upgrade from the contaminated "hot zone." A "warm zone" or contamination-reduction corridor defines the area adjacent to the "hot zone" that is initially uncontaminated, but where decontamination will occur. Ambulatory victims can be directed toward safe havens, cold zone locations outside of where the decontamination is and where it is not likely to spread, to await further directions as the response ensues.

RESPONSE CAPABILITIES

Effective response to the chemical attack MCI is best approached by defining the functional capabilities for response requirements at the incident site. These capabilities provide the descriptions of the response resources, the physical first responders with the appropriate training and equipment working in functional squads or units (e.g., decontamination, detection, medical care, or supply). These resources will vary in size and capability, depending on the response requirements driven by the incident, local availability, or as per the IC. The same functional capabilities also define response resources required at remote sites, such as hospitals or alternate treatment sites, where first receivers treat victims who were not evaluated or decontaminated at the incident site. Figure 78-1 demonstrates a typical incident site response scheme.

Command and Control

The Incident Command System or Unified Command System (ICS/UCS) provides a standard framework for responding to a chemical attack. The IC, located at the incident command post, establishes the

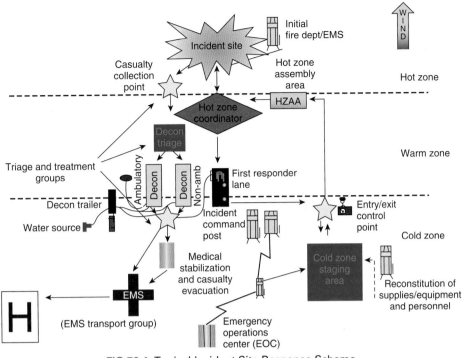

FIG 78-1 Typical Incident Site Response Scheme.

incident action plan following general incident action guides. The NIMS provides guidance on these activities. The IC is responsible for crisis action planning, accountable for the safety and actions of all response personnel, and liable for actions during the response. As per the NIMS, the ICS creates a UCS as the national standard response structure. Under the ICS/UC system, the "best qualified" person initially on scene assumes the role of IC. Transition to a UCS occurs as soon as reasonably achievable. ICS training and Job Aids listing such things as organizational charts, roles, responsibilities, meetings, Response Action Guides, and sample forms are available from various sources and provide excellent guidance for developing response plans to chemical attacks.[37–39] Handheld information technology emergency response tools are also commercially available.[47–49]

As in all incidents, the size and impact of the incident drive the manning of the positions in the ICS, with roles and responsibilities becoming more specific as the size increases. The IC establishes a command post in a safe place near the incident site, analyzes the incident, and incorporates detection and reconnaissance data, plume modeling, and weather effects as available, and then develops and implements the incident action plan and evaluates the progress. Ongoing hazard and risk assessments allow the IC to determine the threats and estimate the potential course and harm in order to develop strategic goals and tactical objectives, as well as to determine the required protective measures and PPE levels and assign team tasking goals and missions to the various response squads, teams, or units. The risk assessment also allows the IC to use experience and expertise to deviate from statutory regulations, if necessary. Leaders are expected to coordinate and integrate their teams into the IC's incident action plan.

Because local resources are likely to become overwhelmed and additional state and federal response capabilities will be necessary to augment the local response capabilities, the community's plan should clearly address how each will be notified/requested, as well as their expected response times and their role in the incident command structure. Every opportunity to build relationships with these response capabilities, such as exercises, will prove invaluable during a real crisis.

Reconnaissance/Hazard Detection and Identification

The reconnaissance teams are responsible for describing the environment of the "Hot Zone" and helping the IC define safe operating parameters for the worksite. "Recon" teams provide critical information, such as oxygen levels, presence of explosive gases, chemical agents, radioactivity, mechanical hazards, and structural integrity of buildings. Further, these teams report on casualty numbers, locations, and conditions, in order to guide IC management of the incident. Typically, the "recon" team works initially in OSHA Level A (NFPA Level 1) or Level B (NFPA Level 2) suites, because the environment is "undefined" and chemical levels are assumed to be an immediate danger to life and health (IDLH).

Various detection/identification technologies are available; however, these are beyond the scope of this chapter. Research is continually being conducted toward making handheld devices capable of detecting and identifying more chemicals faster and more reliably. Technologies range from Drager Tubes to ion mobility spectrometry, flame ionization, surface acoustic wave analysis, and gas chromatography/mass spectrometry (GCMS) in conjunction with solid phase microextraction (SPME) fibers. Information provided by the reconnaissance team allows the IC to determine the appropriate level of PPE for the other elements of the response team. Because quantitative levels of chemicals are difficult to determine rapidly at an incident site utilizing current technology, exposure levels based on concentration are difficult to use, and thus often drive the decision to use higher levels of PPE.

Chemical identification is a critical element to good decision making during a response. Just as important is passing this information to key elements of the response system (e.g., law enforcement, EMS, hospitals, public health, medical examiners, and environmental responders). During the early phases of an emergency response, missing information, misinformation, and the lack of exact chemical identification will challenge the incident command's ability to make critical decisions. The exact chemical name is desirable, but it may not be essential information for decision makers. Early in the response, suspecting a class of agents is better than dealing with an unknown. As the response unfolds over time, the specific chemical identity will be discovered and decision making can be honed. Clinical recognition of toxidromes can complement detector technology, providing more rapid identification of a suspected class of chemical agent. This early information may be sufficient to give medical first responders and first receivers the confidence to administer specific medical countermeasures during a crucial window of opportunity to save lives.

Casualty Extraction

Casualty extraction is likely the most emotionally and physically challenging of the functional elements because it requires the ability to make life-and-death decisions in chaotic environments, while under demanding physical exertion and working in high levels of PPE. Victims who cannot ambulate out of a toxic environment must be carried out to optimize outcome. Current protocols are not evidence based or optimized for survivability. Heat stress and heat exhaustion collapse are significant problems for the extraction teams, particularly on warm or sunny days. The IC should limit work cycles to 30 minutes or less.

Casualty extraction operations should include designated team members as "victim assist teams." The victim assist teams prevent ambulatory victims from wandering outside of established control zones and decontamination corridors to limit cross contamination of clean areas and to mitigate interference with decontamination set up. Such teams then assist with patient flow, transport, care, and crowd control.

Medical Triage, Treatment, and Transport

The medical section of the command post oversees the medical triage, treatment, and transport of patients at the incident site, interfacing with other aspects of the ICS/UCS in carrying out the incident action plan. Depending on the size of the response, there may be branches overseeing triage and treatment or transportation groups, divisions, or task forces.

Most existing chemical response-MCI triage systems lack evidence to support their efficacy. Further, little guidance exists to define crisis standards of care in the chemical attack response environment.[50,51] Recently, evidence-based triage systems employing algorithms that consider medical resources, transport times, and predicted survivability have been proposed to optimize overall survivability.[41] Although correlated to trauma databases, it is not clear whether the same criteria used for triage prioritization would correlate to survivability for a chemical incident.

Although dependent on available resources, triage and treatment teams are best placed at naturally occurring "bottlenecks" in processing victims from the incident site "hot zone" through the contamination-reduction corridor (e.g., "warm zone") to a medical stabilization area in the "cold zone" in preparation for transfer to the emergency medical service(s) (EMS) transportation teams. Depending on distances and specifics of the incident site, a casualty collection point (CCP) might be established at the border between the hot and warm zones, where extractors can transfer victims to initial care in a relatively less-contaminated environment. This provides early access to medical attention for initial triage and treatment, such as administration of antidotes, and it shortens the extraction cycle for the extraction team. Although it may be beneficial to deploy dedicated medical personnel into the hot zone to provide limited triage, medical direction, and antidote administration, there exists little evidence to support this practice as being the best use of limited medical resources. That said, early administration of antidotes by appropriately trained first responders working in the hot zone is likely beneficial.

Medical treatment teams placed on both ends of the decontamination process (in the warm zone and the cold zone) will facilitate better prioritization of patients moving through decontamination, provide medical oversight for patients during the formal decontamination process, and facilitate retriage and treatment in preparation for transfer to emergency medical system transportation units. Naturally occurring bottlenecks in the decontamination process will suggest that a "decon triage" medical treatment area be established on the warm-zone end of the decontamination process for nonambulatory patients. Even though little more than the ABCs (airway, breathing, and circulation management) can be done in the contaminated environment of the warm zone, the results of chemical attacks primarily affect the ABCs, and management of the airway in a contaminated environment should be a primary area of focus for planning and preparation for a chemical attack. Appropriate administration of antidotes is accomplished along the entire medical treatment corridor. Depending on the composition of the medical teams, special protocols requiring specialized training for antidote administration by nonlicensed medical responders may be needed. These should be established during the preparation phase of an emergency management program.

PPE requirements for medical providers in the warm zone are an area of interest to OSHA, although the IC determines the requirement for the level. For response conducted remotely from the incident site, such as at a hospital or alternate care facility, OSHA has promulgated the specific first-receiver guidelines mentioned previously.

Decontamination

Decontamination remains an area of intense research and development. Current best practices rely on physical removal of agents using soap and water. Use of 0.5% bleach solution has fallen out of favor. Several good consensus standards have been promulgated.[52–55] There is evidence, however, to suggest these water-based techniques, if not performed immediately after exposure, may not be effective, and may even cause more harm.[56] Others argue for a more-rational approach that considers high molecular weight solutions optimized for specific agent characteristics including solubilities.[57] A comprehensive review of decontamination guidelines conducted by a joint effort by the DHS Office of Health Affairs and the DHHS PHEMCE provided the "Patient Decontamination in a Mass Chemical Exposure Incident: National Planning Guidance for Communities." This multiyear effort included broad participation of stakeholders in government, the private sector, and the general public, and it should provide national planning guidance for communities on patient decontamination in mass chemical exposure incidents.[58]

Mass casualties requiring decontamination present major challenges to the resources, personnel, and efficiency of a community response. After a chemical attack, potentially contaminated patients may be injured and may remain at the scene, unable to extricate themselves or they may be ambulatory and remain at the scene or they may leave and self-triage to the hospital or leave and go home. Proper decontamination offers the benefit by decreasing exposure dose by diluting or removing chemicals preventing additional absorption and reducing contamination, preventing the spread of contaminants that could jeopardize critical infrastructure such as personnel, ambulances or hospitals. Since decontamination is a first aid procedure, every attempt to accomplish decontamination reduction should start as quickly as possible. A tiered approach provides a method of rapid contamination reduction for a large number of people and may decrease chemical exposure. This approach begins by quickly instructing exposed groups how to perform self-care, followed by rapid gross decontamination and subsequent technical decontamination. Each step along the way requires resource capabilities that are more intense.

For ambulatory patients, most systems essentially represent mass shower sequences through tents for set periods of time, with a range of shower times depending on various factors. Although it is commonly stated that disrobing may provide up to 90% decontamination in and of itself, some care to the process must be applied to prevent cross contamination. Decontamination of nonambulatory patients is time and manpower intensive. Even the most elaborate systems and experienced teams do not provide adequate throughput for true MCI. Roller systems that allow easier, rapid movement of patients through a "car wash"-like system take more than 2 to 5 minutes per patient. Set up times for different teams and systems vary and, if not prepositioned, provide additional challenges because of large footprints and time to set up. In addition, mass casualty decontamination setups require a significant reliable water source, and pose the inability to move easily if necessary.

There are several critical issues in the decontamination process. First, at least three separate lanes for processing people through should be recognized: a lane for ambulatory patients, a lane for nonambulatory patients, and a separate lane for responders. Each group will have different decontamination requirements and priorities and likely use different processes. The responder lane becomes especially critical for responders on supplied air who will usually be near the end of their air supply while processing out. Cutting clothes with "J knives" versus scissors may enhance the throughput capability and avoid hand fatigue. Second, controlling water temperature during the decontamination process can be a challenge given portability, sourcing, and volume requirements. Third, decontamination lanes are typically manned with nonmedical personnel, so medical oversight during the decontamination process needs to be provided with clear protocols for alerting medical providers of any medical issues in patients during the decontamination process. Finally, the environment in decontamination systems can become very hot and humid. The effect on personnel, as well as filter performance, must be considered. Finally, neutralizing solutions such as Reactive Skin Decontaminant Lotion (RSDL) are commercially available and offer significantly more favorable decontamination performance.[59] However, further evaluation needs to be done, including FDA licensing as a medical drug if such solutions are to be used for full-body decontamination

Scene Security/Explosives Ordnance Disposal

Scene security plays several significant roles, including maintaining order and personnel accountability, controlling and maintaining zone boundaries for contaminated areas and scene perimeters, directing traffic flow, and preventing secondary attacks that might jeopardize the initial response. Trained law enforcement personnel should assist with maintaining the integrity of the operational decontamination zones. Explosives Ordnance Disposal (EOD) teams, when available, should provide a sweep for secondary devices such as IEDs that might be targeting responders.

Supplies and Logistics

The role of logistics is to ensure the needed resources (e.g., decontamination supplies, equipment, personnel, or specialized services) get to the proper person or place at the proper time and in the proper amount. Actions range from maintaining and resupplying critical resources, such as PPE suits, boots, filters, and decontamination supplies, to fluids and food to reconstitute the responders. It is crucial that response teams identify and carry items they will need in a given response and not create a logistical burden when they present to an incident. Teams should be able to provide accurate estimates on the duration of their resources, to identify sources to replace consumed supplies, and to identify any critical support requirements that the unit might have. For logistical support of chemical attacks there are several programs worth mentioning in addition to the Strategic National Stockpile (SNS) that can provide critical supplies to a response in a more reasonable time frame.

The Chempack Program, part of the SNS Program, provides forward placement of supplies and equipment specifically needed in the event of a chemical attack, to provide state and local government these critical supplies and improve the response times, spread-loading them across the nation, and place them closer to large population centers where they might be needed. Preplanning with the prehospital, hospital, poison center, and public health communities can activate this resource, ensuring that it will arrive during the crucial window of opportunity to save lives. Chempack Program prepositions medical countermeasures including autoinjectors and multidose vials of antidotes for the treatment of nerve agent and organophosphate insecticide poisonings. Local preparedness activities should include training first responders and first receivers on how to recognize the clinical manifestations of poisoning and provide clearly defined methods to request and mobilize these resources and effective just-in-time training aids and dosing guidance for providers. Poison centers and medical toxicologists are valuable coordination points and subject matter experts for assisting with planning and response to incidents requiring the Chempack.

The Emergency Management Strategic Healthcare Group, under the Veterans Health Administration (VHA) of the Department of Veterans Affairs (VA), addresses emergency management functions for the VHA, including medical support to the DoD, NDMS, and the National Response Plan as needed. VA Medical Centers maintain caches with products to respond to CBRNE incidents for treating veterans, VA staff, and other individuals seeking treatment at a VA facility.

⚠ PITFALLS

Failure of Integration and Coordination: At the federal level, integration for emergency management response and Homeland Security is now the responsibility of the DHS, with the NIMS Integration Center established to oversee the process. It is incumbent on responders and managers at every level in the preparedness and response effort, to ensure understanding of systems architecture, statutes, procedures, roles and responsibilities that affect them, and their integration into their emergency management program as appropriate and needed. Use and integration of information management tools is another area undergoing rapid development, and it should be encouraged with development of standards. Cooperation and compromise are necessary as requirements are identified and capabilities developed.

Failure to participate in a Learning Lessons Learned Process: The Lessons Learned Information Sharing[60] is designed to capture insights from various levels of government response and share the information appropriately with emergency response personnel and Homeland Security officials. Active participation with a lessons learned program should be considered part of the professional responsibilities of emergency response personnel. Lessons learned come not only from actual response experiences but also from standard training, evaluating exercises, and ensuring feedback loops in evolving and improving plans, procedures, protocols, and that the information is shared appropriately.

Emerging Threats

As a parting consideration, it is vital to keep in mind that many of the traditional chemical warfare agents about which we learn and train are over 70 years old. With the further progress of technology and science, it is likely that development of chemical weapons will not necessarily require the resources of a state-sponsored program. Many toxic industrial chemicals are much more readily accessible than traditional chemical warfare agents are, some possessing toxicity profiles with a potential risk of harming large numbers of people. Because of their unique characteristics, these nontraditional chemical weapons may be desirable choices for adversaries. In addition, novel agents may be developed that cause unfamiliar effects and presentations. As part of our preparation, we must foster and maintain our ability for critical reasoning, assessing, adapting, and thinking outside the box.

REFERENCES

1. Joy R. Historical aspects of medical defense against chemical warfare. In: Sidell F, Takafuji E, Franz D, eds. *Medical Aspects of Chemical and Biological Warfare, Textbook of Military Medicine, Part I*. San Antonio, TX: Borden Institute; 1997.
2. 29 CFR 1910 series.
3. National Fire Protection Association: NFPA 471, 472, 473, 1600, 1994.
4. Organization for the Prevention of Chemical Weapons: Available at http://www.opcw.org/html/db/cwc/eng/cwc_frameset.html.
5. National Library of Medicine Hazardous Substances Database. Available at http://toxnet.nlm.nih.gov/cgi-bin/sis/htmlgen?HSDB.
6. Environmental Protection Agency. Alphabetical Order List of Extremely Hazardous Substances (Section 302 of EPCRA). Available at: http://www.ecfr.gov/cgi-bin/text-idx?rgn=div9&node=40:29.0.1.1.11.4.17.3.14.
7. Homeland Defense Information Analysis Center (HDIAC). Available at: www.HDIAC.org.
8. U.S. Marine Corps Chemical Biological Incident Response Force (CBIRF). Available at: http://www.cbirf.usmc.mil.
9. Presidential Policy Directive 8, National Preparedness Goal. Available at: http://www.fema.gov/pdf/prepared/npg.pdf.
10. National Incident Management System, Dept of Homeland Security, 01 Mar 2004. Available at: http://www.fema.gov/nims/.
11. Hospital Incident Command System Available at: http://www.hicscenter.org/.
12. Federal Emergency Management Agency (FEMA) Training IS-100.HCB: Introduction to the Incident Command System (ICS 100) for Healthcare/ Hospitals. Available at: http://training.fema.gov/EMIWeb/IS/courseOverview.aspx?code=is-100.hcb.
13. The Joint Commission, New and Revised Requirements for Emergency Management Oversight. Available at: http://www.jointcommission.org/assets/1/18/JCP0713_Emergency_Mgmt_Oversight.pdf.
14. FEMA. Available at: https://www.fema.gov/.
15. Lessons Learned Information Sharing. Available at: https://www.llis.dhs.gov/.
16. Responder Knowledge Base and Authorized Equipment List, Available at: https://www.llis.dhs.gov/knowledgebase.
17. Occupational Safety and Health Administration (OSHA). Available at: www.OSHA.gov.
18. 29 CFR 1910.38, 29 CFR 1926.35.
19. 29 CFR 1910.120, 29 CFR 1926.65.
20. 29 CFR 1910.132 to 137.
21. Occupational Safety and Health Administration. OSHA Technical Manual, Chapter 1 Section VIII. Available at: https://www.osha.gov/dts/osta/otm/otm_toc.html.
22. Koenig KL. Strip and shower: the duck and cover for the 21st century. *Ann Emerg Med*. 2003;42:391–394.
23. Occupational Safety and Health Administration. *OSHA Guidance for Hospital-Based First Receivers of Victims from Mass Casualty Incidents Involving the Release of Hazardous Substances*. January 2005. Available at: https://www.osha.gov/dts/osta/bestpractices/html/hospital_firstreceivers.html.
24. 29 CFR 1910.120.
25. National Fire Protection Association. Available at: http://www.nfpa.org/index.asp?cookie%5Ftest=1.
26. National Fire Protection Association. NFPA 1990 series.
27. National Fire Protection Association. NFPA 471, Recommended Practice for Responding to Hazardous Materials Incidents. 2002 ed.
28. National Fire Protection Association. NFPA 472, Standards for Professional Competence of Responders to Hazardous Materials Incidents. 2002 ed.
29. National Fire Protection Association: NFPA 473, Standard for Competencies for EMS Personnel Responding to Hazardous Materials Incidents. 2002 ed.
30. National Institute for Occupational Safety and Health. Available at: www.cdc.gov/niosh.
31. CDC, NIOSH Workplace Safety and Health Topics. Available at: http://www.cdc.gov/niosh/topics/respirators/.
32. Office of Law Enforcement Standards Guide for the Selection of Personal Protective Equipment for Emergency Responders, NIF Guide 102–00. Available at: https://www.ncjrs.gov/pdffiles1/nij/191518.pdf.
33. National Institute of Justice. *NIJ Guide 102-00, Guide for Selection for Personal Protective Equipment for Emergency First Responders (Respiratory Protection)*. Nov 2002.
34. Interagency Board. Available at: www.iab.gov.
35. Combating Terrorism Technical Support Office, Technical Support Working Group. Available at: http://www.cttso.gov/?q=cbrne.
36. National Library of Medicine. NLM information on chemicals. Available at: http://sis.nlm.nih.gov/chemical.html.
37. Chemical Hazards Emergency Medical Management. Available at http://chemm.nlm.nih.gov/.
38. Agency for Toxic Substances and Disease Registry. Available at: http://www.atsdr.cdc.gov/about.html.
39. Public Health Emergency Medical Countermeasures Enterprise (PHEMCE). Available at: http://www.phe.gov/preparedness/mcm/phemce/Pages/default.aspx.
40. US Army Research, Development and engineering Command. Available at: http://www.army.mil/info/organization/unitsandcommands/commandstructure/rdecom/.
41. 20th Support Command (CBRNE). Available at: http://www.army.mil/20thcbrne.
42. US Marines CBIRF, Ibid.
43. US Army Medical Research Institute for Chemical Defense (USAMRICD). Available at: http://chemdef.apgea.army.mil/.
44. Chemical Security Analysis Center (CSAC). Available at: https://www.dhs.gov/st-csac.
45. Department of Homeland Scurity Office of Health Affairs Chemical Detection Program. Available at: https://www.dhs.gov/health-threats-resilience-division.
46. Newmark J. The birth of nerve agent warfare. *Neurology*. 2004 May 11;62 (9):1590–1596.
47. FEMA Incident Command System Self-study course. Available at http://www.osha.gov/SLTC/etools/ics/index.html.
48. Occupational Safety and Health Administration. OSHA e-tools: Incident Command System. Available at: http://www.osha.gov/SLTC/etools/ics/index.html.
49. Office of Hazardous Materials Safety. Emergency Response Guidebook. Available at: http://hazmat.dot.gov/pubs/erg/gydebook.html.
50. Institute of Medicine Crisis Standards of Care: A systems Framework for Catastrophic Disaster Response. Available at: http://www.iom.edu/Reports/2012/Crisis-Standards-of-Care-A-Systems-Framework-for-Catastrophic-Disaster-Response.aspx.
51. American College of Emergency Physicians, Guidelines for Crisis Standards of Care During Disasters. June 2013. Available at: http://www.acep.org/uploadedFiles/ACEP/Practice_Resources/disaster_and_EMS/disaster_preparedness/Crisis%20Standards%20of%20Care%200613.pdf.
52. Patient Decontamination Recommendations for Hospitals, Emergency Medical Services Authority, #233, CA, July 2005, Available at: http://www.emsa.ca.gov/aboutemsa/emsa233.pdf.
53. *Best Practices and Guidelines for CBR Mass Personnel Decontamination*. 2nd ed. Technical Support Working Group; Aug 2004. Available at: http://www.tswg.gov/tswg/cbrnc/MPDP Order.html\.
54. NFPA Handbook Supplement 7. Guidelines for Decontamination of Fire Fighters and Their Equipment following Hazardous Materials Incidents, 2002.

55. Guidelines for Cold Weather Mass Decontamination During a Terrorist Chemical Agent Incident, SBCCOM, Jan 2002.

56. Loke W-K, et al. Wet decontamination-induced stratum corneum hydration—Effects on the skin barrier function to diethylmalonate. *J Appl Toxicol.* 1999;19:285–290.

57. Buckley TJ, et al. *A Rational Approach to Skin Decontamination.* Available at http://www.skcinc.com/CLI/A%20Rational%20Approach.pdf.

58. DHS and HHS. *Draft Patient Decontamination in a Mass Chemical Exposure Incident National Planning Guidance for Communities.* Washington, DC; 2014.

59. Clawson RE. *Overview of a Joint US/Canadian Test and Evaluation Program, DECON 2002.* Oct 2002, San Diego, CA.

60. U.S. Department of Homeland Security. Lessons Learned Information Sharing. Available at: https://www.llis.dhs.gov/.

SUGGESTED READINGS

1. Department of Defense Homeland Response Force (HRF) Fact Sheet. Available at: http://www.defense.gov/news/d20100603hrf.pdf.

Biological Attack

Andrew W. Artenstein

Bioterrorism can be broadly defined as the deliberate use of microbial agents or their toxins as weapons. The broad scope and mounting boldness of worldwide terrorism exemplified by the massive attacks on New York City and Washington, DC, on September 11, 2001, coupled with the apparent willingness of terrorist organizations to acquire and deploy biological weapons, constitute ample evidence that the specter of bioterrorism will continue to pose a global threat.

As in other aspects of daily life and the practice of medicine, in particular, the concept of "risk" is germane to considerations regarding an attack using biological agents. *Risk*, broadly defined as the probability that exposure to a hazard will lead to a negative consequence, can be accurately calculated for a variety of conditions of public health importance (Table 79-1). However, the quantification of risk as it pertains to bioterrorism is imprecise because accurate assessment of exposure depends on the whims of terrorists, by nature, an unpredictable variable. Although the probability of exposure to a biological attack is statistically low, it is not zero. Because the negative consequences of an attack are potentially catastrophic, an understanding of biological threat agents and a cogent biodefense strategy are important components of disaster medicine.

HISTORICAL PERSPECTIVE

Biological weapons have been used against both military and civilian targets throughout history, perhaps as early as 600 BC.[1] In the fourteenth century, Tatars attempted to use epidemic disease against the defenders of Kaffa, by catapulting plague-infected corpses into the city. British forces gave Native Americans blankets from a smallpox hospital in an attempt to affect the balance of power in the Ohio River Valley in the eighteenth century.[2] In addition to their well-described use of chemical weapons, Axis forces purportedly infected livestock with anthrax and glanders to weaken Allied supply initiatives during World War I. Perhaps the most egregious example of biological warfare involved the Japanese program in occupied Manchuria from 1932 to 1945. Based on survivor accounts and confessions of Japanese participants, thousands of prisoners were murdered in experiments using a variety of virulent pathogens at Unit 731, the code name for a notorious Japanese biological weapons facility.[3]

The United States maintained an active program for the development and testing of offensive biological weapons from the early 1940s until 1969, when the program was terminated by executive order of then President Nixon. Current efforts continue as countermeasures against biological weapons. The Convention on the Prohibition of the Development, Production, and Stockpiling of Biological and Toxin Weapons and on their Destruction (BWC) was ratified in 1972, formally banning the development or use of biological weapons, and assigning enforcement responsibility to the United Nations.[2] Unfortunately, the BWC has not been effective in its stated goals; multiple signatories have violated the terms and spirit of the agreement. The accidental release of aerosolized anthrax spores from a biological weapons plant in the Soviet Union in 1979, with at least 68 human deaths from inhalational anthrax reported downwind, was proven years later to have occurred in the context of offensive weapons production.

Events within the past 30 years have established bioterrorism as a credible and ubiquitous threat: for example, the 1984 incident in The Dalles, Oregon, involving the intentional contamination of restaurant salad bars with *Salmonella*, by a religious cult attempting to influence a local election.[4] Public fears were additionally heightened by the international events following the Japanese Aum Shinrikyo cult's sarin attack in Tokyo in 1995, especially after investigations revealed that the group had been experimenting with aerosolized anthrax release from rooftops for several months prior. More recently, UN weapons-inspector findings of significant quantities of weaponized biological compounds in Iraq during the Gulf War and the subsequent aftermath has served as sentinel warnings of a shift in terrorism trends. This trend culminated with the October 2001 anthrax attacks in the United States, which elevated bioterrorism to the forefront of international dialogue and heightened public concerns regarding systemic health care preparation against the threat of biological attacks.

CURRENT PRACTICE

Threat Assessment

Biological agents are considered weapons of mass destruction (WMDs) because, as with certain conventional, chemical, and nuclear weapons, their use may result in large-scale morbidity and mortality. A World Health Organization (WHO) model based on the hypothetical effects of the intentional release of 50 kg of aerosolized anthrax spores upwind from a population center of 500,000 (analogous to that of metropolitan Providence, RI) estimated that the agent would disseminate in excess of 20 km downwind and that nearly 200,000 people would be killed or injured by the event.[5] Biological weapons possess unique properties among WMDs. By definition, biological agents are associated with a clinical latency period of days to weeks, in most cases, during which time early detection is quite difficult with currently available technology. Yet, early detection is critical because specific antimicrobial therapy and vaccines are available for the treatment and prevention of illness caused by certain biological weapons. Casualties from other forms of WMDs can generally only be treated by decontamination (with antidotes available for only some types), trauma mitigation, and supportive care. Additionally, the possibility of a biological attack provokes fear and anxiety—"terror"—disproportionate to that seen with other threats, given their often invisible nature.

TABLE 79-1 U.S. Mortality Risk Analysis*

Heart disease	1 in 397
Cancer	1 in 511
Stroke	1 in 1699
Alzheimer's	1 in 5752
Motor vehicle accident	1 in 6745
Homicide	1 in 15,440
Drowning	1 in 64,031
Fire	1 in 82,977
Bicycle accident	1 in 376,165
Lightning strike	1 in 4,478,159
Bioterrorism (anthrax)	1 in 56,424,800

*U.S. Population divided by the number of annual deaths for 2000.
Source: Harvard Center for Risk Analysis, http://www.hcra.harvard.edu ©2004.

TABLE 79-2 Agents of Concern for Use in Bioterrorism

MICROBE OR TOXIN	DISEASE
Highest Priority (Category A)	
Bacillus anthracis	Anthrax
Variola virus	Smallpox
Yersinia pestis	Plague
Clostridium botulinum	Botulism
Francisella tularensis	Tularemia
Filoviruses	Ebola hemorrhagic fevers and Marburg disease
Arenaviruses	Lassa fever and South American hemorrhagic fevers
Bunyaviruses	Rift Valley fever and Congo-Crimean hemorrhagic fevers
Moderately High Priority (Category B)	
Coxiella burnetti	Q fever
Brucella spp.	Brucellosis
Burkholderia mallei	Glanders
Alphaviruses	Viral encephalitis
Ricin	Ricin intoxication
Staphylococcus aures	Staphylococcal toxin illness enterotoxin B
Salmonella spp.	Food- and water-borne gastroenteritis
Shigella dysenteriae	Bacillary dysentery (shigellosis)
Escherichia coli	Gastroenteritis, 0157:H7-induced HUS
Vibrio cholerae	Cholera diarrhea
Cryptosporidium parvum	Cryptosporidiosis
Category C	
Hantavirus	Viral hemorrhagic fevers
Flaviviruses	Yellow fever
Mycobacterium tuberculosis	Multidrug-resistant tuberculosis
Miscellaneous	
Genetically engineered vaccine-and/or antimicrobial-resistant Category A or B agents	
HIV-1	
Adenoviruses	
Influenza	
Rotaviruses	
Hybrid pathogens (e.g., smallpox-plague and smallpox-Ebola)	

Artenstein AW. Bioterrorism and biodefense. In: Cohen J, Powderly WG, eds. *Infectious Diseases.* 2nd ed. London: Mosby; 2003:99-107. Used with permission.

The goals of bioterrorism are those of terrorism in general: morbidity and mortality among civilian populations, disruption of the societal fabric, and exhaustion or diversion of resources. A successful outcome from a terrorist standpoint may be achieved without furthering all of these aims but instead disrupting daily life. The anthrax attacks in the United States in 2001 evoked significant anxiety and diverted resources from other critical public health activities despite the limited number of casualties. In many cases, the surge capacity of our public health system has been inadequate to deal with the emergency needs, resulting in reform and additional planning after the event.

To be used in large-scale bioterrorism, biological agents must undergo complex processes of production, cultivation, chemical modification, and weaponization. For these reasons, state sponsorship or direct support from governments or organizations with significant resources, contacts, and infrastructure would predictably be required in large-scale events. However, revelations have suggested that some agents may be available on the worldwide black market and in other illicit settings, thus obviating the need for the extensive production process.[6] Although traditionally thought to require an efficient delivery mode, recent events, including the 2001 United States anthrax attacks, demonstrated the devastating results that can be achieved with relatively primitive delivery methods (e.g., high-speed mail-sorting equipment and mailed letters).

Numerous attributes contribute to the selection of a pathogen as a biological weapon: availability or ease of large-scale production, ease of dissemination (usually by the aerosol route), stability of the product in storage, cost, and clinical virulence. The last of these refers to the reliability with which the pathogen causes high mortality, morbidity, or social disruption. The Centers for Disease Control and Prevention (CDC) has prioritized biological-agent threats based on the aforementioned characteristics, and this has influenced current preparation strategies (Table 79-2).[7] Category A agents, considered the highest priority, are associated with high mortality and the greatest potential for major effects on the public health. Category B agents are considered "incapacitating" because of their potential for moderate morbidity but relatively low mortality. Most of the category A and B agents have been experimentally weaponized in the past and thus have proven feasibility. Category C agents include emerging threats and pathogens that may be available for development and weaponization.

Another factor that must be addressed in assessing future bioterrorism risk is the historical record of experimentation with specific pathogens, informed by the corroborated claims of various high-level Soviet defectors and data released from the former offensive weapons programs of the United States and United Kingdom.[2,7,8] Information from these sources, combined with the burgeoning fields of molecular biology and genomics, demonstrates that future risk scenarios will likely have to contend with genetically altered and "designer" pathogens intended to bypass current known medical countermeasures or defenses. To this end, a miscellaneous grouping of potential threat agents is added to the extant CDC categories in Table 79-2. The most cautious approach to assessing risk requires public health officials to remain open to additional and novel possibilities in the setting of a suspected bioterrorism event.

BIOTERRORISM RECOGNITION

Bioterrorist attacks are often insidious. Absent of advance warning or specific intelligence information, clinical illness will likely manifest before the circumstances of a release event are known. For this reason, health care providers are likely to be the first responders and reporting agents of this form of terrorism. This is in contrast to the more familiar scenarios in which police, firefighters, paramedics, and other emergency services personnel are deployed to the scene of an attack with conventional weaponry or a natural disaster. Physicians and other health care workers must therefore maintain a high index of suspicion of bioterrorism, and recognize suggestive epidemiologic clues and clinical features to enhance early recognition and guide initial management of casualties. Early recognition and rapid deployment of specific therapy remains the most effective way to minimize the deleterious effects of bioterrorism on both exposed individuals and public health.

Unfortunately, early recognition is hampered for multiple reasons. As previously discussed, it is likely that the circumstances of any event will only be known in retrospect. Therefore responders may be unable to discern the extent of exposure immediately. Also, terrorists have a nearly unlimited number of targets in most open democratic societies, and it is unrealistic to expect any governing body without detailed intelligence of an impending attack to secure an entire population at all times. Certain sites, such as government institutions, historic landmarks, or large public gatherings, may be predictable targets; however, other facilities may fall victim to bioterrorism. In fact, government data support that businesses and other economic concerns were the main targets of global terrorism during the period from 1996 to 2002.[9] Metropolitan areas are traditionally considered especially vulnerable given the dense populations and already existing public gathering areas such as subways and office buildings. Because of the expansion of suburbs and the commuter lifestyle, as well as the clinical latency period between exposure and symptoms, casualties of bioterrorism are likely to present for medical attention in diverse locations and at varying times after a common exposure. An event in New York City on a Wednesday morning may result in clinically ill persons presenting over the ensuing weekend to a variety of emergency departments within a 60-mile radius. Finally, current modes of transportation ensure that there will be affected persons thousands of miles away, at both national and international locations, related to a single common exposure. This adds layers of complexity to an already complicated management strategy and illustrates the critical importance of surveillance and real-time communication in the response to suspected bioterrorism.

Further hindering the early recognition of bioterrorism is that initial symptoms of a biological weapon may be nonspecific and nondiagnostic. In the absence of a known exposure, many symptomatic persons may not seek medical attention early, or if they do, they may be misdiagnosed as having a viral or flu-like illness. If allowed to progress beyond the early stages, many of these illnesses deteriorate quite rapidly, and treatment may be significantly more difficult. Most of the diseases caused by agents of bioterrorism are rarely, if ever, seen in modern first-world clinical practice. Physicians are likely to be inexperienced with their clinical presentation and be less aware of alarming symptomatic constellations. Additionally, these agents by definition will have been manipulated in a laboratory and may not present with the classic clinical features of naturally occurring infection. This was dramatically illustrated by some of the inhalational anthrax cases in the United States in October 2001.[10]

Early recognition of bioterrorism is facilitated by the recognition of epidemiologic and clinical clues. Clustering of patients with common signs and symptoms—especially if regionally unusual or otherwise characteristic of bioterrorism agents—is suggestive of an intentional exposure and should prompt expeditious notification of local public health authorities. This approach will also lead to the recognition of outbreaks of naturally occurring disease or emerging pathogens. The recognition of a single case of a rare or nonendemic infection, in the absence of a travel history or other potential natural exposure, should raise the suspicion of bioterrorism. Finally, unusual patterns of disease, such as concurrent illness in human and animal populations should raise suspicions of bioterrorism or another form of emerging infection. An effective response to bioterrorism requires coordination of the medical system at all levels, from the community physician to the tertiary care center, with rapid activation of public health, emergency management, and law enforcement infrastructures.

THREAT AGENTS

This section provides a broad overview of the biological threat agents thought to be of major current concern—largely, the CDC category A agents. Extensive coverage of specific pathogens can be found in related chapters in this text and in other sources.[11] These agents can possess rapid person-to-person transmission or the potential for rapid dissemination if weaponized, with high-mortality potential, small infective doses, and significant environmental stability.[12,13] Data concerning clinical incubation periods, transmission characteristics, and infection-control procedures for agents of bioterrorism are provided in Table 79-3. Syndromic differential diagnoses for select clinical presentations are detailed in Table 79-4.

Anthrax

Anthrax results from infection with *Bacillus anthracis*, a gram-positive, spore-forming, rod-shaped organism that exists in its host as a vegetative bacillus and in the environment as a spore. Details of the microbiology and pathogenesis of anthrax are found in Chapter 124. In nature, anthrax is a zoonotic disease of herbivores that is prevalent in many geographic regions; sporadic human disease results from environmental or occupational contact with endospore-contaminated animal products.[14] The cutaneous form of anthrax is the most common presentation; gastrointestinal and inhalational forms are exceedingly rare in naturally acquired disease. An additional form, injectional anthrax, represents a potentially lethal, deep soft-tissue infection that has been well described in injection heroin users in several western European countries.[14a] Cutaneous anthrax occurred regularly in the first half of the twentieth century in association with contaminated hides and wools used in the garment industry, but it is uncommonly seen in current-day industrialized countries because of importation restrictions. The last-known fatal case of naturally occurring inhalational anthrax in the United States occurred in 1976, when an individual was exposed to imported wool from Pakistan.[15] Case reports of naturally occurring anthrax do occur within the United States, although they are rare.[16] It has been previously hypothesized that large-scale bioterrorism with anthrax would involve aerosolized endospores with resultant inhalational disease, but the 2001 attacks in the United States illustrate the difficulties in predicting modes and outcomes in bioterrorism. These attacks were on a relatively small scale, and nearly 40% of the confirmed cases were of the cutaneous variety.[17] The serious morbidity and mortality of anthrax is instead related to inhalational disease, as was the case in the Sverdlovsk outbreak in 1979. As a result, planning for larger-scale events with aerosolized agent is warranted given the high-mortality cost of an exposure to this more weaponized form of anthrax.

The clinical presentations and differential diagnoses of cutaneous and inhalational anthrax are described in Table 79-4. The skin lesion

TABLE 79-3 Infection-Control Issues for Selected Agents of Bioterrorism

DISEASE	INCUBATION PERIOD (DAYS)	PERSON-TO-PERSON TRANSMISSION	INFECTION-CONTROL PRACTICES
Inhalational anthrax	2-43*	No	Standard
Botulism	12-72 h	No	Standard
Primary pneumonic	1-6	Yes	Droplet
Smallpox	7-17	Yes	Contact and airborne
Tularemia	1-14	No	Standard
Viral hemorrhagic fevers	2-21	Yes	Contact and airborne
Viral encephalitides	2-14	No	Standard
Q fever	2-14	No	Standard
Brucellosis	5-60	No	Standard
Glanders	10-14	No	Standard

Artenstein AW. Bioterrorism and biodefense. In: Cohen J, Powderly WG, eds. *Infectious Diseases*. 2nd ed. London: Mosby; 2003:99-107. Used with permission.
*Based on limited data from human outbreaks; experimental animal data support clinical latency periods of up to 100 days.

TABLE 79-4 Presentations and Differential Diagnoses of Bioterrorism Agents

CLINICAL PRESENTATION	DISEASE	DIFFERENTIAL DIAGNOSIS
Nonspecific flu-like symptoms with nausea and emesis, without coryza or rhinorrhea, leading to abrupt onset of shock and mental abnormalities (wide mediastinum, infiltrates, pleural effusions)	Inhalational anthrax	Bacterial mediastinitis; tularemia; Q fever; psittacosis; cough with or without chest discomfort; Legionnaires' disease, influenza, *Pneumocystis carinii* pneumonia; viral pneumonia; ruptured aortic respiratory distress with or without aneurysm; superior vena cava syndrome; histoplas-status changes, with chest radiograph mosis; coccidioidomycosis; sarcoidosis
Pruritic, painless papule, leading to vesicle(s), leading to adenopathy	Cutaneous anthrax	Recluse spider bite; plague; staphylococcal lesion; ulcer, leading to edematous black eschar with atypical Lyme disease; orf; glanders; tularemia, without massive local edema and regional rat-bite fever; ecthyma gangrenosum; rickettsialpox; and fever, evolving over 3-7 days; atypical mycobacteria; diptheria
Rapidly progressive respiratory illness with cough, fever, and possible consolidation	Primary pneumonic-plague hemorrhage	Severe community-acquired bacterial or viral rigors, dyspnea, chest pain, hemoptysis, pneumonia, inhalational anthrax, inhalational gastrointestinal symptoms, lung tularemia, pulmonary infarct, and pulmonary infarct without shock
Sepsis, disseminated intravascular coagulation, and purpura	Septicemic plague pneumococcal or staphylococcal	Meningococcemia; Gram-negative, streptococcal, acral gangrene bacteremia with shock; overwhelming postsplenectomy sepsis; acute leukemia; Rocky Mountain spotted fever; hemorrhagic smallpox; hemorrhagic varicella (in immuno-compromised patients)
Fever, malaise, prostration, headache, and myalgias, followed by progressive papular rash on the face, with a hemorrhagic component and system toxicity	Smallpox	Varicella; drug eruption; Stevens-Johnson syndrome; by development of synchronous; measles; secondary syphilis; erythema multiforme, leading to vesicular and then pustular severe acne; meningococcemia; monkeypox; mucous membranes (extremities more than generalized vaccinia; insect bites; Coxsackie virus trunk); the rash may become generalized; infection; vaccine reaction
Nonspecific flu-like illness with pleuropneumonitis; lymphadenopathy	Inhalational tularemia	Inhalational anthrax, pneumonic plague, influenza, bronchiolitis with or without hilar mycoplasma pneumonia, Legionnaire's disease, variable progression to respiratory failure, Q fever, bacterial pneumonia
Acute onset of afebrile, symmetric, descending flaccid pupils; dysarthria; ptosis; dry mucous membranes leading to airway obstruction with respiratory muscle paralysis; clear sensorium and absence of sensory changes	Botulism	Myasthenia gravis, brain stem cerebrovascular paralysis that begins in bulbar muscles; dilated accident; polio; Guillain-Barre syndrome variant; diplopia or blurred vision; dysphagia; tick paralysis; chemical intoxication
Acute-onset fevers, malaise, prostration, myalgias, headache, gastrointestinal symptoms, mucosal hemorrhage, altered vascular permeability, disseminated intravascular coagulation, and hypotension leading to shock with or without hepatitis and neurologic findings	Viral hemorrhagic fever	Malaria, meningococcemia, leptospirosis, rickettsial infection, typhoid fever, borrelioses, fulminant hepatitis, hemorrhagic smallpox, acute leukemia, thrombotic thrombocytopenic purpura, hemolytic uremic syndrome, systemic lupus erythematosus

Artenstein AW. Bioterrorism and biodefense. In: Cohen J, Powderly WG, eds. *Infectious Diseases*. 2nd ed. London: Mosby; 2003:99-107. Used with permission.

of cutaneous anthrax may be similar in appearance to other lesions, including cutaneous forms of other agents of bioterrorism; however, it may be distinguished by epidemiologic, as well as certain clinical, features. Anthrax is traditionally a painless lesion, unless secondarily infected, and is associated with significant local edema. The bite of *Loxosceles reclusa*, the brown recluse spider, shares many of the local and systemic features of anthrax but is typically painful from the outset and lacks such significant edema.[18] Cutaneous anthrax is associated with systemic disease, and it carries an associated mortality in up to 20% of untreated cases, although with appropriate antimicrobial therapy mortality is less than 1%.[14]

Once the inhaled endospores reach the terminal alveoli of the lungs—generally requiring particle sizes of 1 to 5 μm—they are phagocytosed by macrophages and transported to regional lymph nodes. Here the endospores germinate into vegetative bacteria and subsequently disseminate hematogenously.[13] Spores may remain latent for extended periods in the host, up to 100 days in experimental animal exposures.[15] This translates to prolonged clinical incubation periods after respiratory exposure to endospores. Cases of inhalational anthrax occurred up to 43 days after exposure in the Sverdlovsk accident, although the average incubation period is thought to be 2 to 10 days, perhaps influenced by exposure dose.[13,15]

Before the U.S. anthrax attacks in October 2001, most of the clinical data concerning inhalational anthrax derived from Sverdlovsk, the largest outbreak recorded. Although there is much overlap between the clinical manifestations noted previously and those observed during the recent outbreak, data that are more detailed are available from the recent U.S. experience. There were 11 confirmed persons with inhalational anthrax, 5 (45%) of whom died. This contrasts with a case-fatality rate of greater than 85% reported from Sverdlovsk with an estimated 100 deaths. The reliability of reported data from this outbreak is questionable, given Soviet documentation, but a majority of victims were located downwind of the ill-fated weapons plant.[15,18] Patients almost on average present of 3.3 days after symptom onset with fevers, chills, malaise, myalgias, nonproductive cough, chest discomfort, dyspnea, nausea or vomiting, tachycardia, peripheral neutrophilia, and liver enzyme elevations.[11,19,20] Many of these findings are nondiagnostic, and they overlap considerably with those of influenza and other common viral respiratory tract infections. Recently compiled data suggest that shortness of breath, nausea, and vomiting are significantly more common in anthrax, whereas rhinorrhea is uncommonly seen in anthrax but noted in the majority of viral respiratory infections, an important clinical distinction.[21] Other common clinical manifestations of inhalational anthrax include abdominal pain, headache, mental status abnormalities, and hypoxemia. Abnormalities on chest radiography appear to be universally present, although these may only be identified retrospectively in some cases. Pleural effusions are the most common abnormality, although radiographs may demonstrate patchy infiltrates, consolidation, and/or mediastinal adenopathy. The latter is thought to be an early indicator of disease, but computed tomography appears to provide greater sensitivity compared with chest radiographs for this finding.

The clinical manifestations of inhalational anthrax generally evolve to a fulminant presentation with progressive respiratory failure and shock. *B. anthracis* is routinely isolated in blood cultures if obtained before the initiation of antimicrobials. Pleural fluid is typically hemorrhagic; the bacteria can either be isolated in culture or documented by antigen-specific immunohistochemical stains of this material in the majority of patients.[11] In the five fatalities in the U.S. series, the average time from hospitalization until death was 3 days (range, 1 to 5 days), which is consistent with other reports of the clinical virulence of this infection. Autopsy data typically reveal hemorrhagic mediastinal lymphadenitis and disseminated, metastatic infection. Pathology data from the Sverdlovsk outbreak confirm meningeal involvement, typically hemorrhagic meningitis, in 50% of disseminated cases.[22]

The diagnosis of inhalational anthrax should be entertained in the setting of a consistent clinical presentation in the context of a known exposure, a possible exposure, or epidemiologic factors suggesting bioterrorism (e.g., clustered cases of a rapidly progressive illness). The diagnosis should also be considered in a single individual with a clinical illness consistent with anthrax exposure in the absence of another etiology. The early recognition and prompt treatment of inhalational anthrax is likely associated with a survival advantage.[11] Therefore the emergency physician should promptly initiate empiric antimicrobial therapy if infection is clinically suspected. Combination parenteral therapy is appropriate in the ill person for a number of reasons: to cover the possibility of antimicrobial resistance, to target specific bacterial functions (e.g., the theoretical effect of clindamycin on toxin production), to ensure adequate drug penetration into the central nervous system, and perhaps to favorably affect survival.[11] Drainage of pleural effusions is indicated to reduce toxin burden. Detailed therapeutic and post-exposure prophylaxis recommendations have been recently reviewed elsewhere.[22a] A monoclonal antibody targeted at the protective antigen component of anthrax toxin, raxibacumab, is available for the adjunctive treatment of systemic anthrax.[14a] In the future, it is likely that novel therapies such as toxin inhibitors or cell-specific receptor antagonists will be available to treat anthrax post exposure.[23] Detailed therapeutic and postexposure prophylaxis recommendations for adults, children, and special groups have been recently reviewed elsewhere.[15] With regard to postexposure prophylaxis, the Anthrax Vaccine Adsorbed is effective for prevention of cutaneous anthrax in human clinical trials, as well as preventing inhalational disease after aerosol challenge in nonhuman primates.[21] Current studies are investigating the efficacy of this vaccine when paired with antibiotics in the postexposure period. For preexposure prophylaxis, the vaccine is generally very safe, but it requires five doses over 18 months, with the need for annual boosting for ongoing preventative immunity.[24] Preexposure use of the vaccine is currently limited to individuals at high risk for anthrax exposure, such as military personnel and specific laboratory workers. Although not currently available, additional research into second-generation anthrax vaccines is aimed to generate a more easily distributed means of mass prophylaxis following an anthrax exposure.[25]

Smallpox

The last-known naturally acquired case of smallpox occurred in Somalia in 1977. In one of the greatest triumphs of modern medicine, smallpox was officially certified as having been eradicated in 1980, the culmination of a 12-year intensive campaign undertaken by the WHO.[26] However, because of concerns that variola-virus stocks may have either been removed from or sequestered outside of their officially designated repositories, smallpox is considered a potential and certainly dangerous agent of bioterrorism. Multiple features make smallpox an attractive biological weapon and ensure that any reintroduction into human populations would be a global public health catastrophe: it is stable in aerosol form, has a low infective dose, is associated with up to a 30% case-fatality rate, and has a large vulnerable target population because civilian vaccination was terminated in 1972. Smallpox is also especially dangerous because secondary attack rates among unvaccinated close contacts are estimated at 37% to 88% and are only further amplified by the lack of vaccine-induced immunity and a lack of naturally circulating virus to induce low-level booster exposures.[27] Because of the successful eradication, preexposure vaccination is currently limited to specific military and laboratory professionals. There are currently no antiviral therapies of proven effectiveness against this pathogen.

After an incubation period of 7 to 17 days (average 10 to 12 days), patients will develop a prodrome of fever, rigors, headache, and backache that may last 2 to 3 days. This is followed by a centrifugally distributed eruption that generalizes as it evolves through macular, papular, vesicular, and pustular stages in synchronous fashion over approximately 8 days, with umbilication in the latter stages. Enanthem in the oropharynx typically precedes the exanthem by 24 to 48 hours. The rash typically involves the palms and soles early in the course of the disease. The pustules begin crusting during the second week of the eruption; separation of scabs is usually complete by the end of the third week. The differential diagnosis of smallpox is delineated in Table 79-4. Historically, varicella and drug reactions have posed the greatest diagnostic dilemmas; this would likely be further complicated by the absence of this clinical disease and therefore experience in its diagnosis for the past 40 years.[21]

Smallpox is transmitted person to person by respiratory droplet nuclei and (although less commonly) by contact with lesions or contaminated fomites. Airborne transmission by fine-particle aerosols has also been documented under certain conditions.[21] The virus is communicable from the onset of the enanthem until all of the scabs have separated, although patients are thought to be most contagious during the first week of the rash because of high titers of replicating virus in the oropharynx. Household members, other face-to-face contacts, and health care workers have traditionally been at highest risk for secondary transmission, given their proximity to infected individuals during the highly infectious period. As a result, patients with signs and symptoms concerning for smallpox should be placed in negative-pressure rooms with contact and airborne precautions to minimize this risk. Those not requiring hospital-level care should remain isolated at home to avoid infecting others in public places.

The suspicion of a single smallpox case should prompt immediate notification of local public health authorities and the hospital epidemiologist. Containment of smallpox is predicated on the "ring vaccination" strategy, which was successfully deployed in the WHO global eradication campaign. This strategy mandates the identification and immunization of all directly exposed persons, including close contacts, health care workers, and laboratory personnel. Vaccination, if deployed within 4 days of infection during the early incubation period, can significantly attenuate or prevent disease and may favorably affect secondary transmission.[21] Because the occurrence of even a single case of smallpox would be tantamount to bioterrorism, an immediate epidemiologic investigation is necessary to establish a biological perimeter and trace initially exposed individuals for ring vaccination purposes.

Botulism

Botulism is an acute neurologic disease caused by *Clostridium botulinum*, which occurs both sporadically and in focal outbreaks throughout the world related to wound contamination by the bacterium or the ingestion of the foodborne toxin. A detailed discussion of botulism is found in Chapter 154. Aerosolized forms of the toxin are fortunately a rare mode of acquisition in nature, but they have been weaponized for use in bioterrorism.[5] Botulinum toxin is considered the most toxic molecule known; it is lethal to humans in very minute quantities. It is estimated that a single gram of concentrated *Clostridium botulinum* neurotoxin could kill up to 1 million otherwise healthy individuals.[29] The toxin functions by blocking the release of the neurotransmitter acetylcholine from presynaptic vesicles, thereby inhibiting muscle contraction.[30]

Botulism presents as an acute, afebrile, symmetric, descending, and flaccid paralysis. The disease manifests initially in the bulbar musculature and is unassociated with mental status or sensory changes. Fatigue, dizziness, dysphagia, dysarthria, diplopia, dry mouth, dyspnea, ptosis, ophthalmoplegia, tongue weakness, and facial muscle paresis are early findings seen in more than 75% of cases. Progressive muscular involvement leading to respiratory failure ensues. The clinical presentations of foodborne and inhalational botulism are indistinguishable in experimental animals.[24] Fortunately, outside of the toxin itself being utilized for bioterrorism, botulism is not spread directly from person to person. Typically, these patients will recover with supportive care in weeks to months.

The diagnosis of botulism is largely based on epidemiologic and clinical features and the exclusion of other possibilities (Table 79-4). Clinicians should recognize that any single case of botulism could be the result of bioterrorism or could herald a larger-scale "natural" outbreak. A large number of epidemiologically unrelated, multifocal cases should be clues to an intentional release of the agent, either in food sources, water supplies, or as an aerosol.

The mortality from foodborne botulism has declined from 60% to 6% over the last four decades, likely because of improvements in supportive care and mechanical ventilation. Because the need for the latter may be prolonged, limited resources (e.g., mechanical ventilators) would likely be exceeded in the event of a large-scale bioterrorism event. Treatment with an equine antitoxin, available in limited supply from the CDC, may ameliorate disease if given early. There is no currently available vaccine.

Plague

Plague, a disease responsible for multiple epidemics throughout human history, is caused by the gram-negative pathogen *Yersinia pestis*. This pathogen is found in a variety of forms in the natural world. It is extensively covered in Chapter 125. Plague is endemic in parts of Southeast Asia, Africa, and the western United States. Aerosolized preparations of the agent, the expected vehicle in bioterrorism, would be predicted to result in cases of primary pneumonic plague outside of endemic areas. Additional forms of the disease, such as bubonic and septicemic plague, are also concerning from a bioterrorism perspective.

Primary pneumonic plague classically presents as an acute, febrile, pneumonic illness with prominent respiratory and systemic symptoms. Patients will often endorse gastrointestinal symptoms and purulent sputum production, with variable levels of reported hemoptysis.[31] Chest x-rays will typically show patchy, bilateral, multilobar infiltrates or consolidations. Unlike other forms of community-acquired pneumonia, in the absence of appropriate treatment, there may be rapid progression to respiratory failure, vascular collapse, purpuric skin lesions, necrotic digits, and death. The differential diagnosis for these symptoms including rapidly progressive pneumonia is very broad as noted in Table 79-4. Plague is suggested by the characteristic small gram-negative coccobacillary forms found in stained sputum specimens with the bipolar uptake ("safety pin") of Giemsa or Wright stain.[32] Culture confirmation is necessary to establish the diagnosis; the microbiology laboratory should be notified in advance if plague is suspected because special techniques and precautions must be employed. Of note, initial Gram staining of samples can often be negative despite positive culture in *Y. pestis* detection. Serologic testing is also possible if the aforementioned studies are persistently negative.

Treatment recommendations for plague have been reviewed elsewhere.[26] Pneumonic plague can be transmitted from person to person by respiratory droplet nuclei, thus placing close contacts, other patients, and health care workers at risk for secondary infection. Prompt recognition and treatment of this disease, appropriate deployment of postexposure prophylaxis, and early institution of droplet precautions will help to interrupt secondary transmission. Both live and attenuated plague vaccines exist; however, these are not currently approved for commercial use in the United States. High-risk populations, including laboratory and military personnel, may receive a formaldehyde-killed version of the vaccine as prophylaxis in certain situations.[13] Fortunately, new recombinant vaccines are currently in development, although some parts of the world continue to use live versions of the vaccine.[33]

Tularemia

Francisella tularensis, the causative agent of tularemia, is another small gram-negative coccobacillus with potential to cause a primary pneumonic presentation if delivered as an aerosol agent of bioterrorism. This bacterium is commonly found in smaller mammals, most classically hares and rabbits. Humans serve as an accidental host; typically, natural infections occur via insect bites, consuming infected animal products, or direct contact with infected domesticated animals.[34] The causative bacteria can be transmitted between humans by close contact via mucous membrane contact, cutaneous inoculation, and inhalation if patients are exposed to aerosolized forms of the bacteria.[14]

Pulmonary tularemia presents with the abrupt onset of a febrile, systemic illness with prominent upper-respiratory symptoms of a highly variable nature. Patients may exhibit inconsistent development of pneumonia, hilar adenopathy, hemoptysis, pulse-temperature dissociation, malaise, and progression toward respiratory failure and death in excess of 30% of those who do not receive appropriate therapy.[35] The diagnosis is generally based on clinical features after other agents are ruled out, but again it requires a high level of clinical suspicion. Confirmatory serology using various immunologic assays is currently available.[13] Laboratory personnel should be notified in advance if tularemia is suspected because the organism can be very infectious under culture conditions. This agent is discussed in depth in Chapter 126. Moreover, treatment typically consists of antibiotic therapy with streptomycin or gentamicin, with an estimated overall mortality after treatment of only 1%.[13] A live attenuated vaccine against tularemia exists; however, it is not currently available for human use in the United States.[36] Tularemia remains a significant concern, given the lack of current vaccine, especially when coupled with the high infectivity and mortality of pulmonary tularemia.

Viral Hemorrhagic Fevers

The agents of viral hemorrhagic fevers are members of four distinct families of ribonucleic acid viruses that cause clinical syndromes with overlapping features: fever, malaise, headache, myalgias, prostration, mucosal hemorrhage, and other signs of increased vascular permeability with circulatory dysregulation. Unfortunately, they are all capable of leading to shock and multiorgan system failure in advanced cases.[37] Specific agents are also associated with specific target organ effects, although each has a propensity to damage vascular endothelium. These pathogens, discussed in detail in Chapters 142 to 145, include Ebola, Marburg, Lassa fever, Rift Valley fever, and Congo-Crimean hemorrhagic fever.

Hemorrhagic fever viruses have been viewed as being emerging infections because of their sporadic occurrence in focal outbreaks throughout the world; the ongoing epidemic of Ebola hemorrhagic fever in West Africa has resulted in more than 25,000 cases and 10,000 deaths since 2014.[36a] Often in novel outbreak situations, these severe effects of these viruses on humankind are thought to be the results of human intrusion into a viral ecologic niche. They are concerning potential weapons of bioterrorism because they are highly infectious in aerosol form, are transmissible in health care settings,

cause high morbidity and mortality, and are purported to have been successfully weaponized.[9] Blood and other bodily fluids from infected patients are extremely infectious, and person-to-person airborne transmission may occur, as well. As a result, strict contact and airborne precautions should be instituted if viral hemorrhagic fevers are implicated in a terrorism event.[28]

The diagnosis of viral hemorrhagic fevers is complicated, especially in a potential bioterrorist attack, which would lack a known exposure, or following recent travel to Africa. Microbiology studies and immunological testing are difficult to perform routinely, and often require evaluation by CDC laboratories.[38] Treatment is largely supportive, and it includes the early use of vasopressors as needed. Ribavirin is effective against some forms of viral hemorrhagic fevers but not those caused by Ebola and Marburg viruses. For a majority of these diseases, the treatment is largely supportive therapy. Nonetheless, ribavirin should be initiated empirically in patients presenting with a syndrome consistent with viral hemorrhagic fever until the exact etiology is confirmed. Even though there are vaccines available for similar diseases, such as yellow fever and Argentine hemorrhagic fever, there are no current options for preexposure vaccination for viral hemorrhagic fevers. This paired with the highly infectious nature and significant mortality rates make this category of viruses worrisome potential agents of bioterrorism.

MANAGEMENT OF SPECIAL PATIENT POPULATIONS

The approach to the management of diseases of bioterrorism must be broadened to include children, pregnant women, and immunocompromised persons. Specific recommendations for treatment and prophylaxis of these special patient groups for selected bioterrorism agents have been recently reviewed.[14,26,27] A general approach requires an assessment of the risk of certain drugs or products in select populations versus the potential risk of the infection in question, accounting for extent of exposure and the agent involved. The issue extends to immunization because certain vaccines, such as smallpox, pose higher risk to these special groups than to others. This will affect mass vaccination strategies and will likely warrant case-by-case decisions.

Of note, the prevalence of antivaccine sentiments has implications with regard to global biosecurity. A decline in herd immunity against a vaccine-preventable communicable disease could leave even a medically prepared society vulnerable to a terrorist-introduced agent previously well controlled with prophylactic vaccinations. This will be yet another special population to consider in the event of a mass casualty bioterrorist attack.

PSYCHOSOCIAL MORBIDITY

An often overlooked but vitally important issue in bioterrorism is that of psychosocial sequelae. These may take the form of acute anxiety reactions and exacerbations of chronic psychiatric illness during the stress of the event, or posttraumatic stress disorder (PTSD) in its aftermath. Nearly half of the emergency department visits during the Gulf War missile attacks in Israel in 1991 were related to acute psychological illness or exacerbations of underlying problems.[39] Data from recent acts of terrorism in the United States suggest that PTSD may develop in as many as 35% of those affected by the events.[40] In the early period after the 9/11 attacks in New York, PTSD and depression were nearly twice as prevalent as in historical control subjects.[41] Although close proximity to the events and personal loss were directly correlated with PTSD and depression, respectively, there was a substantial burden of morbidity among those indirectly involved. Among individuals working on Capitol Hill following the 2001 anthrax scare, 27% were diagnosed with PTSD, with up to 55% diagnosed with any variety of psychiatric disorder. Moreover, a majority of these patients were not adherent with antibiotics prescribed, perhaps because of a newfound lack of trust in the health care system.[42] Although not always clinically apparent, the psychological effect of a bioterrorism event is certainly a significant and important consideration for ongoing public health management strategies following any biological threat or terrorist attack.

⚠ PITFALLS

The response to bioterrorism is unique among WMDs because it necessitates consequence management that is common to all disasters, as well as the application of basic infectious diseases principles. Disease surveillance, diagnosis, infection control, antimicrobial therapy, post-exposure prophylaxis, and mass preventative vaccinations are all important considerations when managing a bioterrorism event. For these reasons, physicians are likely first responders to bioterrorism and will be expected to be reliable sources of information for their patients, colleagues, and public health authorities.[43]

A remaining number of potential pitfalls regarding disasters involving a biological attack must be identified and managed to optimize the public health response. As alluded to above, the clinical latency period between exposure to an agent and the manifestation of signs and symptoms is approximately days to weeks with most of the CDC category A, B, or C agents. Thus, early diagnoses of the first cases are likely to prove problematic and require heightened clinical vigilance, a difficult task considering a majority of these agents are rarely observed in the developed world.[44] Even after initial victims have been diagnosed, communications among hospitals and other health care institutions on a local, regional, national, and international level will be essential to help define the epidemiology and identify possible exposure sources. Given the extent and ease of rapid individual movement within our globalized world, clinical presentations from a point-source biological attack could occur in widely disparate geographic locations. Additionally it is possible that a terrorist attack would be multifocal in any case, with components of WMDs paired with biological weapons for maximum effect. A fundamental and consistent epidemiologic approach using case definitions, case identification, surveillance, and real-time communications is necessary, whether the event is a malicious attack, emergent from nature, or of unknown etiology.[45]

Other potential bioterrorism management pitfalls reside in the arena of diagnostic techniques, treatment, and prevention of disease related to biological agents. Although an active area of research, the development of field-ready and highly predictive rapid screening tests for many agents of bioterrorism has not yet progressed to the point at which such assays are approved by the U.S. Food and Drug Administration and available in a "point-of-care" format. Treatment and prevention issues such as the absence of effective therapies for many forms of viral hemorrhagic fevers, shortages in the availability of multivalent antitoxin for botulism, projected shortages in the availability of mechanical ventilators to manage a large-scale botulism attack, lack of human data regarding the use of antiviral agents in smallpox, and the unfavorable toxicity profiles of some currently available smallpox vaccines remain unresolved but active areas of research. Emerging molecular biology techniques capable of producing genetically altered pathogens with "designer" phenotypes including antimicrobial or vaccine resistance add additional layers of complexity to an already multifaceted problem. As was vividly illustrated in the 2003 severe acute respiratory syndrome epidemic and previously well recognized when smallpox occurred with regularity, transmission of infection of potential bioterrorism agents within hospitals is common and difficult to control.[46,21] Health care workers, our first line of defense against an attack using biological agents, remain at significant occupational risk.

Research in the field of bioterrorism recognition has demonstrated a perceived weakness among clinicians in recognition of category-A infectious agents.[47] As pathogens of bioterrorism are not frequently encountered in daily practice, they often fall low on the differential without clinician knowledge of an insidious local mass casualty event.[48] Clearly, awareness of a recent local event heightens clinical suspicion, but it is imperative for the front-line clinician to recognize, report, and initiate treatment of affected patients. This will only serve to facilitate the initial containment and facilitate rapid disaster-protocol activation. Early recognition and initiation of a prompt, unified response will remain the primary challenge for all health care providers in the current era of bioterrorism.

REFERENCES

1. Riedel S. Biological warfare and bioterrorism: a historical review. *Proc (Bayl Univ Med Cent)*. 2004;17(4):400–406.
2. Christopher GW, Cieslak TJ, Pavlin JA, Eitzen Jr EM. Biological warfare: a historical perspective. *JAMA*. 1997;278:412–417.
3. Harris SH. *Factories of Death: Japanese Biological Warfare, 1932-45, and the American Cover-Up*. New York, NY: Routledge; 1994.
4. Torok TJ, Tauxe RV, Wise RP, et al. A large community outbreak of Salmonellosis caused by intentional contamination of restaurant salad bars. *JAMA*. 1997;278:389–395.
5. World Health Organization. *Health Aspects of Chemical and Biological Weapons: Report of a WHO Group of Consultants*. Geneva: World Health Organization; 1970. 98–99.
6. Miller J, Engelberg S, Broad W. *Germs: Biological Weapons and America's Secret War*. Simon and Schuster: New York, NY; 2001.
7. CDC. Biological and chemical terrorism: strategic plan for preparedness and response. *MMWR Recomm Rep*. 2000;49(RR-4):1–14.
8. Alibek K. *Biohazard*. New York, NY: Random House; 1999.
9. United States Department of State. *Patterns of Global Terrorism 2001*. Washington, DC: U.S. Department of State; May 2002.
10. Jernigan J, Stephens DS, Ashford DA, et al. Bioterrorism-related inhalational anthrax: the first 10 cases reported in the United States. *Emerg Infect Dis*. 2001;7:933–944.
11. Sidell FR, Takafuji ET, Franz DR, eds. *Medical Aspects of Chemical and Biological Warfare. Textbook of Military Medicine series. Part I, Warfare, Weaponry and the Casualty*. Washington, DC: Office of the Surgeon General, Department of the Army; 1997.
12. Balali-mood M, Moshiri M, Etemad L. Medical aspects of bio-terrorism. *Toxicon*. 2013;69:131–142.
13. Christian MD. Biowarfare and bioterrorism. *Crit Care Clin*. 2013;29 (3):717–756.
14. Dixon TC, Meselson M, Guillemin J, et al. Anthrax. *N Engl J Med*. 1999;341:815–826.
14a. Artenstein AW, Opal SM. Novel approaches to the treatment of systemic anthrax. *Clin Infect Dis*. 2012;54:1148–1161.
15. Inglesby TV, Henderson DA, Bartlett JG, et al. Anthrax as a biological weapon: medical and public health management. *JAMA*. 1999;281:1735–1745.
16. Griffith J, Blaney D, Shadomy S, et al. Investigation of inhalation anthrax case, United States. *Emerg Infect Dis*. 2014;20(2):280–283.
17. Inglesby TV, O'Toole T, Henderson DA, et al. Anthrax as a biological weapon, 2002: updated recommendations for management. *JAMA*. 2002;287:2236–2252.
18. Freedman A, Afonja O, Chang MW, et al. Cutaneous anthrax associated with microangiopathic hemolytic anemia and coagulopathy in a 7-month-old infant. *JAMA*. 2002;287:869–874.
19. Barakat LA, Quentzel HL, Jernigan JA, et al. Fatal inhalational anthrax in a 94-year-old Connecticut woman. *JAMA*. 2002;287:863–868.

20. CDC. Considerations for distinguishing influenza-like illness from inhalational anthrax. *MMWR Morb Mortal Wkly Rep.* 2001;50:984–986.

21. Friedlander AM, Pittman PR, Parker GW. Anthrax vaccine: evidence for safety and efficacy against inhalational anthrax. *JAMA.* 1999;282:2104–2106.

22. Friedlander AM. Tackling anthrax. *Nature.* 2001;414:160–161.

22a. Hendricks KA, Wright ME, Shadomy SV, et al. Centers for Disease Control and Prevention expert panel meetings on prevention and treatment of anthrax in adults. Emerg Infect Dis 2014;20:e130687,doi.org/10.3201/eid2002.130687.

23. Abramova FA, Grinberg LM, Yampolskaya O, Walker DH. Pathology of inhalational anthrax in 42 cases from the Sverdlovsk outbreak of 1979. *Proc Natl Acad Sci U S A.* 1993;90:2291–2294.

24. Wright JG, Quinn CP, Shadomy S, Messonnier N. Use of anthrax vaccine in the United States: recommendations of the Advisory Committee on Immunization Practices (ACIP), 2009. *MMWR Recomm Rep.* 2010;59 (RR-6):1–30.

25. Hopkins RJ, Howard C, Hunter-stitt E, et al. Phase 3 trial evaluating the immunogenicity and safety of a three-dose BioThrax(®) regimen for post-exposure prophylaxis in healthy adults. *Vaccine.* 2014;32(19):2217–2224.

26. Fenner F, Henderson DA, Arita I, et al. *Smallpox and Its Eradication.* Geneva: World Health Organization; 1988.

27. Breman JG, Henderson DA. Diagnosis and management of smallpox. *N Engl J Med.* 2002;346:1300–1308.

28. 2002d. Smallpox response plan and guidelines (version 3.0). Available at: http://www.bt.cdc.gov/agent/smallpox/response-plan/. Accessed April 2, 2014.

29. Dhaked RK, Singh MK, Singh P, Gupta P. Botulinum toxin: bioweapon & magic drug. *Indian J Med Res.* 2010;132:489–503.

30. Arnon SS, Schechter R, Inglesby TV, et al. Botulinum toxin as a biological weapon: medical and public health management. *JAMA.* 2001;285:1059–1070.

31. Artenstein AW, Lucey DR. Occupational plague. In: Couturier AJ, ed. *Occupational and Environmental Infectious Diseases.* Beverly, MA: OEM Press; 2000:329–335.

32. Inglesby TV, Dennis DT, Henderson DA, et al. Plague as a biological weapon: medical and public health management. *JAMA.* 2000;283:2281–2290.

33. Oyston PC, Williamson ED. Prophylaxis and therapy of plague. *Expert Rev Anti Infect Ther.* 2013;11(8):817–829.

34. Cronquist SD. Tularemia: the disease and the weapon. *Dermatol Clin.* 2004;22(3):313–320.

35. Dennis DT, Inglesby TV, Henderson DA, et al. Tularemia as a biological weapon: medical and public health management. *JAMA.* 2001;285: 2763–2773.

36. Skyberg JA. Immunotherapy for tularemia. *Virulence.* 2013;4(8):859–870.

36a. CDC. 2014 Ebola outbreak in West Africa—case counts. http://www.cdc.gov/vhf/ebola/outbreaks/2014-west-africa/case-counts.html, accessed 30 march 2015.

37. Borio L, Inglesby T, Peters CJ, et al. Hemorrhagic fever viruses as biological weapons: medical and public health management. *JAMA.* 2002;287: 2391–2405.

38. Arie S. Polio outbreak leads to calls for a "vaccination ceasefire" in Syria. *BMJ.* 2013;347:f6682.

39. Karsenty E, Shemer J, Alshech I, et al. Medical aspects of the Iraqi missile attacks on Israel. *Isr J Med Sci.* 1991;27:603–607.

40. Yehuda R. Post-traumatic stress disorder. *N Engl J Med.* 2002;346:108–114.

41. Galea S, Ahern J, Resnick H, et al. Psychological sequelae of the September 11 terrorist attacks in New York City. *N Engl J Med.* 2002;346:982–987.

42. North CS, Pfefferbaum B, Vythilingam M, et al. Exposure to bioterrorism and mental health response among staff on Capitol Hill. *Biosecur Bioterror.* 2009;7(4):379–388.

43. Artenstein AW, Neill MA, Opal SM. Bioterrorism and physicians. *Ann Intern Med.* 2002;137:626.

44. Artenstein AW. Bioterrorism and biodefense. In: Cohen J, Powderly WG, eds. *Infectious Diseases.* 2nd ed. London: Mosby; 2003:99–107.

45. Artenstein AW, Neill MA, Opal SM. Bioterrorism and physicians. *Med Health R I.* 2002;85:74–77.

46. Svoboda T, Henry B, Shulman L, et al. Public health measures to control the spread of the severe acute respiratory syndrome during the outbreak in Toronto. *N Engl J Med.* 2004;350:2352–2361.

47. Hartwig KA, Burich D, Cannon C, Massari L, Mueller L, Dembry LM. Critical challenges ahead in bioterrorism preparedness training for clinicians. *Prehosp Disaster Med.* 2009;24(1):47–53.

48. Stephens MB, Marvin B. Recognition of community-acquired anthrax: has anything changed since 2001? *Mil Med.* 2010;175(9):671–675.

CHAPTER 80

Future Biological and Chemical Weapons

Robert G. Darling and Erin E. Noste

HISTORICAL PERSPECTIVE

Biological and chemical weapons have been used throughout history.[1] For millennia, indigenous South American peoples deliberately used plant-derived arrow poisons such as curare and toxins from poison dart frogs, although these preparations were used mainly for hunting. Similar toxins were used in Africa. The ancient Greeks, for whom *toxikon* meant "arrow poison," tipped arrows with winter aconite, and this practice continued into medieval Europe, persisting into the seventeenth century in Spain and Portugal.[2] Soldiers in India used smoke screens, incendiary weapons, and toxic fumes as early as 2000 BCE, and the Sung Dynasty in China employed a wide variety of arsenical smokes and other poisons in battle. The military use of toxins dates from at least the sixth century BCE, when Assyrian soldiers poisoned enemy wells with ergot-contaminated rye. In 423 BCE, during the Peloponnesian War, Thracian allies of Sparta captured the Athenian fort at Delium by using a long tube and bellows to blow poisonous smoke from coals, sulfur, and pitch into the fort. Greek fire (likely composed of rosin, sulfur, pitch, naphtha, lime, and saltpeter) was invented in the seventh century CE and proved to be a very effective naval weapon. Various poisons saw battlefield use during medieval times, and the use of poisons for murder (including assassinations) became widespread. Other examples before the twentieth century include the contamination of water by dumping the corpses of dead humans or animals into wells, the use of snakes and other creatures as poisonous vectors, and occasionally, fomites to transmit infections such as smallpox to unsuspecting victims. This latter technique was used with remarkable success during the French and Indian War (1754-1767), when Sir Jeffrey Amherst was alleged to have given "gifts" (blankets) harboring the pus and scabs from smallpox victims to unsuspecting Native Americans. The Indians possessed no immunity against smallpox and thus experienced very high rates of infection and mortality as smallpox swept through the local tribes.[3]

During the late nineteenth and early twentieth centuries, the science and technology necessary for the development of sophisticated biological and chemical weapons proceeded apace. World War I saw the first large-scale use of "poison gas," including lacrimators, chlorine, phosgene, arsenicals, cyanide, and sulfur mustard. By the end of the war, nearly one in every three rounds was a chemical munition. Dr. Shiro Ishii and other Japanese scientists in the infamous Unit 731 worked on the weaponization of anthrax, plague, smallpox, and tetrodotoxin as well as a variety of chemical agents during World War II. There are even suspicions that the bomb used in the assassination of Reinhard Heydrich in Czechoslovakia in 1942 contained botulinum toxin.[4] After World War II, ricin was used as an injectable assassination weapon, and in the 1970s and 1980s T-2 toxin, a trichothecene mycotoxin, was alleged to have been the toxic component of the "yellow rain" employed against H'Mong refugees from Laos. More recently, Iraq and Iran both

used chemical weapons against each other in the Iran-Iraq War of the 1980s, and Iraq had a weapons program that included the development of sulfur mustard, nerve agents, "Agent 15" (an anticholinergic incapacitating agent), botulinum toxin, epsilon toxin from *Clostridium perfringens*, and aflatoxin.[5] Militia groups in the United States and terrorist groups throughout the world have used ricin for political purposes.

American scientists started developing chemical weapons as a response to the use of chemical warfare in Europe during World War I and conducted both offensive and defensive research on biological and chemical weapons. However, in 1969 the United States unilaterally renounced the first use of chemical agents, halted chemical-agent production, and terminated its offensive biological weapons program.

In 1972 the Biological Weapons and Toxins Convention was created; it was signed by representatives from 104 nations, including the United States (which ratified the Convention in 1975), the Soviet Union, and Iraq, although many signatories did not consider toxins to be biological weapons and did not consider the treaty binding on toxin use. Since that time, at least 140 nations have either signed or ratified this treaty.[6] However, the Soviet Union and Iraq began violating the treaty in short order. In the Soviet Union, weapons scientists stepped up research and development of numerous biological and chemical weapons as part of one of the largest and most comprehensive biological-weapons programs in history. Soviet scientists created large stockpiles of weaponized anthrax, plague, smallpox, tularemia, nerve agent, mustard, and other biological and chemical agents.[5]

In 1979 the world was put on notice of the devastating potential that biological weapons pose to humanity. In that year, a small quantity of weapons-grade anthrax was accidentally released from a manufacturing plant located in the former city of Sverdlovsk (now Yekaterinburg) in Russia, resulting in 77 cases and 66 deaths. Dr. Matthew Meselson, a Harvard scientist, was permitted to study the event many years later and reported the results of his work in a 1979 *Science* article. Meselson determined that the majority of the deaths had occurred among victims living in a narrow, 4-km-wide band downwind from the plant. Animal deaths were confirmed as far as 30 km downwind. Meselson further concluded that less than 1 g of weapons-grade anthrax had been released from the plant.[7] If his calculations are accurate, weaponized anthrax possesses staggering potential as a biological weapon given its stability, its relative ease of production, and its ability to be dispersed in a clandestine manner over great distances.

In March 1995, after having unsuccessfully attempting to deploy biological agents, members of the Aum Shinri Kyo cult executed a coordinated attack with the nerve agent sarin (GB) on the Tokyo subway system. More than 5500 people sought medical treatment, and a dozen died. The Aum Shinri Kyo had used sarin in Matsumoto 9 months earlier in an attack that had exposed more than 300 people and killed 7 in an attempt to assassinate judges unfavorable to their cause.[8,9]

The anthrax attacks in the fall of 2001 involved the use of letters containing weapons-grade anthrax mailed through the U.S. postal system. Five people died, and 17 became ill with either cutaneous or inhalational anthrax. Buildings contaminated with spores included the Hart Senate Office building and the Brentwood postal facilities in Washington, DC. It cost millions of dollars to rehabilitate these buildings. The anthrax used in the attacks was determined to be extremely potent and could have caused far greater numbers of casualties had it been dispersed more widely.[10,11]

The use of chemical weapons also occurred in recent history. In September 2013 the United Nations (UN) released their investigations on the use of chemical weapons in Syria. The UN concluded that sarin gas was used on August 21, 2013, in the Ghouta area of Damascus against "civilians, including children, on a relatively large scale."[12] These findings were based on interviews with survivors and other witnesses, documentation of munitions and their components, collection of environmental samples for subsequent analysis, assessment of symptoms of survivors, and collection of hair, urine, and blood samples.

According to Dr. Ken Alibek, former Deputy Director of Biopreparat, the Soviet Union's nominally civilian medical research institute, Soviet scientists and physicians spent large sums of money and manpower during the 1980s and 1990s developing the most lethal and potent biological weapons known to man. In addition to weaponizing the etiologic agents of anthrax, smallpox, Marburg fever, and others, they created antibiotic-resistant strains of *Yersinia pestis* (plague), *Francisella tularensis*, and other pathogens. Furthermore, by applying genetic engineering techniques, the Soviets are also alleged to have created pathogens with novel characteristics and strains of several organisms capable of defeating certain vaccines.[13]

As we enter the biotechnological revolution of the twenty-first century, our understanding of molecular biology, genetics, and biochemistry is exploding. The human genome has been sequenced, and it is now possible to manipulate genes from disparate organisms to create new and novel pathogens. Scientists are also able to synthesize and weaponize a number of different endogenous biological-response modifiers including cytokines, hormones, neurotransmitters, and plasma proteases. But even nature continues to surprise us. New, naturally occurring infections with the potential to cause large-scale human diseases and death continue to emerge at an ever-increasing rate throughout the world, and it is conceivable that these pathogens could also be weaponized by enterprising scientists.

This chapter briefly reviews the future of chemical and biological weapons as we enter this new era of explosive growth in our understanding of the life sciences. We are presented with an extraordinary opportunity to solve a host of human afflictions or to create new classes of biological and chemical weapons that have the capacity to destroy our civilization as we know it today.

FUTURE BIOLOGICAL WEAPONS

The appearance of a new or reemerging infectious disease has global implications. During the past 20 years, more than 30 new lethal pathogens have been identified.[14] A classic example of this emerging threat is pandemic influenza. In 1918, as World War I was coming to an end, the Spanish flu struck with devastating consequences. In less than 1 year, this virus was able to circumnavigate the globe and kill an estimated 40 million people.[15] More recently, the emergence of severe acute respiratory syndrome (SARS) in Southeast Asia resulted from a coronavirus that jumped species from animals to humans and rapidly spread to 29 countries in less than 90 days. Finally, the 2014 outbreak of Ebola in Western Africa, still raging as of this writing, is an example of

how devastating these agents can be when they emerge in a region previously naïve to them. Novel and dormant infectious agents such as SARS, influenza, and Ebola appear to be emerging or reemerging with increasing frequency and with greater potential for serious consequences. Many factors contribute to the emergence of new diseases: environmental changes, global travel and trade, social upheaval, and genetic changes in infectious agent, host, or vector populations. Once a new disease is introduced into a suitable human population, it often spreads rapidly and has a devastating impact on the medical and public health infrastructure. If the disease is severe, it may lead to social disruption and have a profound economic impact. Outbreaks of emerging or reemerging diseases may be difficult to distinguish from outbreaks resulting from intentional introduction of infectious diseases for nefarious purposes.

As scientists develop more sophisticated laboratory procedures and increase their understanding of molecular biology and the genetic code, the possibility of bioengineering more virulent, antibiotic, and vaccine-resistant pathogens for military or terrorist uses becomes increasingly likely. It is already theoretically possible to synthesize and weaponize certain biological response modifiers (BRMs) as well as to engineer genomic weapons capable of inserting novel DNA into host cells. The potential to cause widespread disease and death with any of these weapons is incalculable and concerning. Scientists and policy makers have begun to address the issue with a robust research agenda to develop medical countermeasures.

Ebola hemorrhagic fever, as of December 4, 2014, had caused 6055 deaths among 17,111 confirmed cases in western Africa. Scientists have debated whether Ebola could be weaponized into a weapon of mass destruction by terrorists. The consensus seems to be that this would be a very difficult undertaking because of the knowledge and laboratory skills that are required. Moreover, the biology of the virus does not lend itself well to weaponization.[16] Of course, nefarious individuals could use Ebola in a number of ways, in much the same way that a suicide bomber straps on a vest laden with explosives. In theory a person could deliberately infect themselves with the virus and then attempt to infect others once they become symptomatic.

Existing Agents and Their Potential for Future Use

Important existing biological agents with the potential for weaponization for military or terrorist use include the following:

1. Biological agents
   a. *Bacillus anthracis* (anthrax; see Chapter 124)
   b. *Yersinia pestis* (plague; see Chapter 125)
   c. *Francisella tularensis* (tularemia[17]; see Chapter 126)
   d. *Brucella* species (brucellosis; see Chapter 127)
   e. *Coxiella burneti* (Q fever; see Chapter 128)
   f. *Rickettsia prowazekii* (typhus fever; see Chapter 129)
   g. *Orientia tsutsugamushi* (scrub typhus; see Chapter 130)
   h. *Rickettsia rickettsii* (Rocky Mountain Spotted Fever; see Chapter 131)
   i. *Vibrio cholerae* (cholera; see Chapter 132)
   j. *Shigella dysenteriae* (shigellosis; see Chapter 133)
   k. *Salmonella* species (salmonellosis; see Chapter 134)
   l. *Salmonella typhi* (typhoid fever; see Chapter 135)
   m. *Burkholderia mallei* (glanders; see Chapter 136)
   n. *Burkholderia pseudomallei* (melioidosis; see Chapter 137)
   o. *Chlamydia psittaci* (psittacosis; see Chapter 138)
   p. *Escherichia coli* O157:H7 (hemorrhagic *E. coli*; see Chapter 139)
2. Viral agents
   a. Viral encephalitides (alphaviruses; see Chapter140)

b. Tick-borne encephalitis virus (see Chapter 141)

c. Viral hemorrhagic fever viruses (arenaviruses, bunyaviruses, filoviruses, flaviviruses; see Chapters 142-145)

d. Chikungunya virus (see Chapter 146)

e. Variola major virus (smallpox; see Chapter 147)

f. Influenza virus (see Chapter 148)

g. Monkeypox (see Chapter 149)

h. Hantavirus pulmonary syndrome (see Chapter 150)

i. Henipavirus (Hendra virus and Nipah virus encephalitis; see Chapter 151)

j. SARS-CoV (see Chapter 152)

3. Toxins

a. Staphylococcal enterotoxin B (see Chapter 153)

b. *Clostridium botulinum* toxin (botulism; see Chapter 154)

c. *Clostridium perfringens* toxin (epsilon toxin; see Chapter 155)

d. Marine toxin (see Chapter 156)

e. T-2 toxin (trichothecene mycotoxins; see Chapter 157)

f. Ricin toxin from *Ricinus communis* (castor beans; see Chapter 158)

g. Aflatoxin (*Aspergillus* species; see Chapter 159)

4. Other biological agents

a. *Coccidioides immitis* (coccidioidomycosis; see Chapter 160)

b. *Histoplasma capsulatum* (histoplasmosis; see Chapter 161)

c. *Cryptosporidium parvum* (cryptosporidiosis; see Chapter 162)

Another way to view the relative importance of the above list of agents and diseases list is to consider The Centers for Disease Control and Prevention (CDC) strategy. The CDC categorizes bioterrorism agents or diseases as category A, B, or C.[17] *Category A* agents pose the highest risk to the public and are characterized as follows:

- Easily disseminated or transmitted from person to person
- Can cause high mortality rates and possess the potential for profound public impact
- Could cause public panic and social disruption
- Require special preparations for adequate public health preparedness Diseases and agents
- Anthrax (*Bacillus anthracis*)
- Botulism (*Clostridium botulinum* toxin)
- Plague (*Yersinia pestis*)
- Smallpox (variola major)
- Tularemia (*Francisella tularensis*)
- Viral hemorrhagic fever: filoviruses (e.g., Ebola and Marburg) and arenaviruses (e.g., Lassa and Machupo)

Category B agents are the next highest priority and are characterized by

- Moderately easy to disseminate
- Cause moderate morbidity and low mortality
- Require specific enhancements of CDC's diagnostic capacity and enhanced disease surveillance Diseases and agents
- Epsilon toxin of *Clostridium perfringens*
- Food safety threats (*Salmonella* species, *Escherichia coli* O157:H7, *Shigella*)
- Glanders (*Burkholderia mallei*)
- Melioidosis (*Burkholderia pseudomallei*)
- Psittacosis (*Chlamydia psittaci*)
- Q fever (*Coxiella burnetii*)
- Ricin toxin (*Ricinus communis*—castor beans)
- Staphylococcal enterotoxin B
- Typhus fever (*Rickettsia prowazekii*)
- Viral encephalitis (alphaviruses: Venezuelan equine encephalitis, eastern equine encephalitis, western equine encephalitis)

- Water safety threats (*Vibrio cholerae, Cryptosporidium parvum*)

Category C agents form the third highest priority and include emerging pathogens that could be engineered for mass dissemination in the future because of the following:

- Availability
- Ease of production and dissemination
- Potential for high morbidity and mortality rates and major health impact Agents
- Emerging and reemerging infectious diseases such as Nipah virus, hantavirus, human influenza, avian influenza, SARS and SARS-associated coronavirus (SARS-CoV), and Middle East respiratory syndrome (MERS)

Selected Emerging and Reemerging Infections with Weaponization Potential

Because emerging diseases are so diverse and endemic to different geographic locations, their complete description is beyond the scope of this chapter. However, some of these infections may become future threats as agents of biological warfare or terrorism. The most worrisome emerging infectious disease may well be the one we do not know about. Recent experience with HIV, Ebola hemorrhagic fever, SARS, monkey pox, West Nile fever, and hundreds of other "new" diseases reveal that we will continue to be surprised.

Avian Influenza

Avian influenza, or highly pathogenic avian influenza, has periodically caused human infections primarily through close contact with avian species, most often through occupational contact at chicken or duck farms in Southeast Asia. A large outbreak of avian influenza involving the H5N1 strain and human cases occurred in 2004 and originated in two countries from this region.[18] No sustained human-to-human transmission was reported, but there is some evidence that isolated episodes did occur, and the potential exists for genetic reassortment between avian and human or animal strains of influenza. A recent report in the journal *Science* linked the influenza virus responsible for the 1918 epidemic to a possible avian origin.[19] If true, avian influenza may pose a much greater danger to human populations than previously reported. The disease presents in humans in a fashion similar to other types of influenza viruses. It usually begins with fever, chills, headaches, and myalgias and often involves the upper and lower respiratory tract with development of cough, dyspnea, and, in severe cases, acute respiratory distress syndrome. Laboratory findings may include pancytopenia, lymphopenia, elevated liver enzymes, hypoxia, a positive reverse transcriptase-polymerase chain reaction (RT-PCR) test for H5N1, and a positive neutralization assay for H5N1 influenza strain. in vitro studies suggest that the neuraminidase (NA)-inhibitor class of drugs may have clinical efficacy in the treatment and prevention of avian influenza infection.[20]

Human Influenza

The threat for pandemic spread of human influenza viruses is substantial. The pathogenicity of human influenza viruses is directly related to their ability to alter their eight viral RNA segments rapidly; the new antigenic variation results in the formation of new hemagglutinin (HA) and NA surface glycoproteins, which may go unrecognized by an immune system primed against heterologous strains.

Two distinct phenomena contribute to a renewed susceptibility to influenza infection among persons who have had influenza illness in the past. Clinically significant variants of influenza A viruses may result from mutations occurring in the HA and NA genes and expressed as minor structural changes in viral surface proteins. As few as four amino acid substitutions in any two antigenic sites can cause such a clinically significant variation. These minor changes result in an altered virus able to circumvent host immunity. Moreover, genetic reassortment between avian and human or avian and porcine influenza viruses may lead to the major changes in HA or NA surface proteins known as antigenic shift. In contrast to the gradual evolution of strains subject to antigenic drift, antigenic shift occurs when an influenza virus with a completely novel HA or NA formation moves into humans from other host species. Global pandemics result from such antigenic shifts.

Influenza causes in excess of 30,000 deaths and more than 100,000 hospitalizations annually in the United States. Pandemic influenza viruses have emerged regularly in 10- to 50-year cycles for the last several centuries. During the last century, influenza pandemics occurred 3 times: in 1918 ("Spanish influenza," an H1N1 virus), in 1957 (Asian influenza, an H2N2 subtype strain), and in 1968 (Hong Kong influenza, an H3N2 variant). The 1957-1958 pandemic caused 66,000 excess deaths, and the 1968 pandemic caused 34,000 excess deaths in the United States. The 1918 influenza pandemic illustrates a worst-case public health scenario; it caused 675,000 deaths in the United States and 20 to 40 million deaths worldwide.[19] Morbidity in most communities was between 25% and 40%, and the case-mortality rate averaged 2.5%. A reemergent 1918-like influenza virus would have tremendous societal effects, even in the event that antiviral medications were effective against this more lethal influenza virus.

SARS and SARS-Associated Coronavirus

SARS-associated coronavirus (SARS-CoV) emerged as the cause of SARS during 2003. That year, SARS was responsible for approximately 900 deaths and more than 8000 infections in people from at least 29 countries worldwide. Before a case definition had been clearly established, Chinese authorities reported to the World Health Organization (WHO) more than 300 cases of an atypical pneumonia with 5 related deaths, all originated from Guangdong province in China during February 2003. The infection quickly spread as infected patients traveled to Hong Kong and from there to Vietnam, Canada, and other locations. Only eight laboratory-confirmed cases occurred in the United States, but there is concern that the U.S. population is vulnerable to a widespread outbreak of SARS such as the one that occurred in China, Hong Kong, Singapore, Toronto, and Taiwan in 2003.[21]

A SARS case definition evolved from this initial report to the WHO by Chinese health authorities in February 2003. A case was initially defined by clinical criteria; a suspected or probable case was defined as an illness that included potential exposure to an existing case and fever with pneumonia or respiratory distress syndrome. In April 2003, a confirmed case was defined as a case from which SARS-CoV was isolated from culture.[22] SARS-CoV infections have an incubation period of 2 to 10 days. Systemic symptoms such as fever and chills followed by a dry cough and shortness of breath begin within 2 to 7 days. Patients may develop pneumonia and lymphopenia by days 7 to 10 of the illness. Most patients with SARS-CoV have a clear history of exposure either to a patient with SARS or to a setting in which SARS-CoV is known to exist. Laboratory tests may be helpful but do not reliably detect infection early during the illness. SARS-CoV should be suspected in patients requiring hospitalization for radiographically confirmed pneumonia or acute respiratory distress syndrome of unknown etiology and one of the following risk factors during the 10 days before the onset of illness: (1) travel to China, Hong Kong, or Taiwan, or close contact with an ill person having a history of such travel; (2) employment in an occupation associated with a risk for SARS-CoV exposure; or (3) inclusion in a cluster of cases of atypical pneumonia without an alternative diagnosis.

A "respiratory hygiene/cough etiquette" strategy should be adopted in all SARS-affected health care facilities. All patients admitted to the hospital with suspected pneumonia should receive the following measures: (1) they should be placed in droplet isolation until it is determined that isolation is no longer indicated (standard precautions are appropriate for most community-acquired pneumonias; droplet precautions for nonavian influenza); (2) they should be screened for risk factors of possible exposure to SARS-CoV; and (3) they should be evaluated with a chest radiograph, pulse oximetry, complete blood count, and additional workup as indicated. If the patient has a risk factor for SARS, droplet precautions should be implemented pending an etiologic diagnosis. When there is a high index of suspicion for SARS-CoV disease, the patient should be treated in terms of SARS isolation precautions immediately (including airborne precautions), and all contacts of the ill patient should be identified, evaluated, and monitored.[22] Although ribavirin, high-dose corticosteroids, and interferons have been used in treatment, it is unclear what effect they have had on clinical outcome. No definitive therapy has been established. Empiric antibiotic treatment for community-acquired pneumonia following the current American Thoracic Society/Infectious Diseases Society of America guidelines is recommended pending etiologic diagnosis. Diagnostic tests for SARS-CoV include antibody testing using an enzyme immunoassay and RT-PCR tests for respiratory, blood, and stool specimens.[23] In the absence of known SARS-CoV transmission, testing is recommended only in consultation with public health authorities. Testing for influenza, respiratory syncytial virus, pneumococcus, chlamydia, mycoplasma, and legionella should be conducted, as the identification of one of these agents excludes SARS by case definition. Clinical samples can be obtained during the first week of illness with a nasopharyngeal swab plus an oropharyngeal swab and a serum or a plasma specimen. After the first week of illness, a nasopharyngeal swab plus an oropharyngeal swab and a stool specimen should be obtained. Serum specimens for SARS-CoV antibody testing should be collected when the diagnosis is first suspected and at later times as indicated. An antibody response can occasionally be detected during the first week of illness, is likely to be detected by the end of the second week of illness, and at times may not be detected until more than 28 days after the onset of symptoms. Respiratory specimens from any of several different sources may be collected for viral and bacterial diagnostics, but the preferred specimens of choice are nasopharyngeal washes or aspirates.[23]

Middle East Respiratory Syndrome (MERS-CoV)

MERS-CoV is a disease caused by a coronavirus and results in severe acute respiratory disease including fever, chills, cough, and dyspnea. Some patients also develop nausea, vomiting, and diarrhea. It has a 30% mortality rate. Most patients who have died had underlying comorbidities and developed pneumonia or renal failure. The illness was first reported in Saudi Arabia in September 2012; most cases appear to be limited to the Arabian Peninsula. The incubation period ranges from 2 to14 days. The illness can spread from person to person but it requires close contact, and no sustained transmission had been reported by late 2014. The virus could evolve and lead to sustained transmission, but this cannot be predicted with certainty. There is no vaccine for MERS-CoV and there is no specific treatment, but there is ongoing research by the National Institutes of Health (NIH) and other entities to fill this gap.[24]

Nipah and Hendra Viruses

The Nipah and Hendra viruses are closely related but distinct paramyxoviruses that compose a new genus within the family Paramyxoviridae. The Nipah virus was discovered in Malaysia in 1999 during an outbreak of a zoonotic infection, now called Nipah virus encephalitis, involving mostly pigs and some human cases.[25] Hendra, the causative agent of Hendra virus disease, was identified in a similar outbreak involving a single infected horse and three human cases in Southern Australia in 1994.[26] It is believed that certain species of fruit bats are the natural hosts for these viruses and remain asymptomatic. Horses and pigs act as amplifying hosts for the Hendra and Nipah viruses, respectively. The mode of transmission from animal to humans appears to require direct contact with tissues or body fluids or with aerosols generated during butchering or culling. Personal protective equipment including gowns, gloves, and respiratory and eye protection is advised for agricultural workers culling infected animal herds. Thus far, human-to-human transmission of these viruses has not been reported.

In symptomatic cases, the onset of disease begins with flu-like symptoms and rapidly progresses to encephalitis with disorientation, delirium, and coma. Fifty percent of those with clinically apparent infections have died from their disease. There is currently no approved treatment for these infections, and, therefore, therapy relies heavily on supportive care. The antiviral drug ribavirin has been used in past infections, but its effectiveness remains unproven in clinically controlled studies.[27] Although no person-to-person transmission is known to have occurred, barrier nursing and droplet precautions are recommended because respiratory secretions and other bodily fluids are known to harbor the virus. The clinical laboratory should be notified before specimens are sent as these may pose a laboratory hazard. Specimens for viral isolation and identification should be forwarded to a reference laboratory. Requests for testing should come through public health departments, which should contact the CDC Emergency Operations Center at 770-488-7100 before sending specimens.

Biological Response Modifiers

BRMs direct the myriad complex interactions of the immune system. BRMs include erythropoietins, interferons, interleukins, colony-stimulating factors, granulocyte and macrophage colony-stimulating factors, stem cell growth factors, monoclonal antibodies, tumor necrosis factor inhibitors, and vaccines.[28] A growing understanding of the structure and function of BRMs is driving the discovery and creation of many novel compounds including synthetic analgesics, antioxidants, and antiviral and antibacterial substances. For example, BRMs are being used to treat debilitating rheumatoid arthritis by targeting cytokines that contribute to the disease process.[29] By neutralizing or eliminating these targeted cytokines, BRMs may reduce symptoms and decrease inflammation. BRMs may also be used as anticarcinogens, with the following goals: (1) to stop, control, or suppress processes that permit cancer growth; (2) to make cancer cells more recognizable, and therefore more susceptible, to destruction by the immune system; (3) to boost the killing power of immune system cells, such as T cells, natural killer cells, and macrophages; (4) to alter growth patterns in cancer cells to promote behavior like that of healthy cells; (5) to block or reverse the processes that change a normal cell or a precancerous cell into a cancerous cell; (6) to enhance the ability of the body to repair or replace normal cells damaged or destroyed by other forms of cancer treatment, such as chemotherapy or radiation; and (7) to prevent cancer cells from spreading to other parts of the body.[30,31]

More of these promising new drugs are currently in development. It can be readily theorized that research to develop various BRMs can be subverted to a malicious end. That is, instead of using BRMs to suppress cancer growth or to decrease disease susceptibility, researchers could develop compounds to cause illness and death. Other drugs could be designed to alter certain metabolic processes or to alter brain chemistry to affect cognition or mood. The opportunity for mischief is limited only by the imagination of the person with ill intent.

Synthetic Biology and Bioengineered Pathogens

The field of synthetic biology had its beginnings near the turn of the millennium with the idea that basic engineering principles could be applied to biological systems at the cellular and genetic levels to create new and improved organisms. Synthetic biology is the "engineering of biology."[32] The goal and end products of the engineering are conventionally to be used for the benefit of humankind. However there has been increasing concern that synthetic biology could be used for nefarious purposes.[33–36]

A precise definition of synthetic biology has not yet been established; however, a consensus is building that synthetic biology is defined as the use of molecular biology tools and techniques to forward the engineering of cellular behavior. There is disagreement among scientists whether the new field of synthetic biology will allow terrorists to create biological agents with more lethal characteristics or create completely novel pathogens with enhanced pathogenicity and weaponization potential in an easier fashion.[37] Some argue that synthetic biology causes "de-skilling" of biological techniques and allows laboratory processes to become easier for less experienced scientists or even laypeople to master.[35] Others maintain that the tacit or unwritten laboratory skills that only a few highly trained scientists possess and which are very difficult to transfer and very difficult for a terrorist to acquire.[38] Social scientists have carefully studied these tacit skills and argue that these techniques are very difficult to pass on from scientist to scientist without considerable effort that is often impossible even under the most ideal circumstances.[38] This difficulty was historically present in both the U.S. and Soviet biological weapons programs each of which were extremely well funded and staffed with competent scientists.

Nevertheless, the rapid advance of synthetic biology has the potential to alter the present and future threat of biological weapons.[9,35,36] Already, complete or partial genomic sequence data for many of the most lethal human pathogens (such as anthrax, plague, and the smallpox virus) have been published and are widely available via the Internet.[39] In addition to the enormous explosion in our knowledge of human pathogens, there is a parallel increased understanding of the complexities of the human immune response to foreign agents and toxins. Such knowledge has led to a deeper understanding of the development of basic immunity to a variety of different human infectious diseases.

With this increase in scientific knowledge has come the power to manipulate the immune system at its most fundamental level. As we prepare for future threats, we must not ignore the potential quantum leap that synthetic biology offers to terrorists for developing new biological-warfare threats. Examples of biological threats that could be produced through the use of synthetic biology include the following: (1) microorganisms resistant to antibiotics, standard vaccines, and therapeutics; (2) innocuous microorganisms genetically altered to produce a toxin, a poisonous substance, or an endogenous bioregulator; (3) microorganisms possessing enhanced aerosol and environmental stability characteristics; (4) immunologically altered microorganisms able to defeat standard threat identification and diagnostic methods; (5) genetic vectors capable of transferring human and foreign genes into human cells for therapeutic purposes[39]; and (6) combinations of these with improved delivery systems.[40–42]

POTENTIAL FUTURE CHEMICAL WEAPONS

Nature of the Problem

The threats associated with the use of chemical weapons as battlefield or terrorist weapons are not easy to assess.[43,44] Risk assessment of use must take into account national laws, international treaties and conventions, and the likelihood of adherence to these legal obligations. Loopholes in existing agreements can be exploited to develop weapons that are technically not prohibited by international law. Goals and objectives may vary depending on whether military use is planned at the strategic, tactical, or operational level and whether the developer is a national government, a breakaway republic, a kidnapped or recruited scientist, or a terrorist cell. Risk of use may also depend on whether the targets are military versus civilian, human versus nonhuman (animals or plants, including livestock and crops), or individual (as in assassinations) versus large groups, and on whether the aim is death versus incapacitation. Risk also depends on agent availability and on the technology available for production, storage, and dissemination; current advances in technology are associated with a higher risk of weaponization. Two examples from the twentieth century and one from the twenty-first can illustrate the fallibility of intelligence:

1. During most of World War II, the Allied perception of risk from possible chemical agent use by Axis powers focused on those agents, primarily pulmonary agents and vesicants, known from World War I. In fact, Germany had developed a new kind of chemical-warfare agent, the compounds later to be called G-series nerve agents. Their existence came as a complete surprise to Western governments when, in the waning days of the European campaign, Allied soldiers advancing into Germany discovered buried nerve-agent munitions and entire nerve-agent factories. Why these agents were never used on the battlefield is a topic of much speculation, but in retrospect they clearly posed the most lethal, yet unrecognized, threat from Germany.[45]

2. Assessment of the chemical threat posed by Saddam Hussein at the time of the Gulf War of 1991 centered on the known Iraqi use of sulfur mustard and nerve agents during the Iran-Iraq War in the 1980s. It was not until 1998 that Reuters News Agency reported the discovery by British intelligence that Iraq had stockpiled large quantities of a "mental incapacitant" (incapacitating agent) known as Agent 15.[18,46]

3. The risk of use of chemical agents by Iraq after 2001 was assessed to be high partly because of the known stockpiles of sulfur mustard and nerve agents (as well as the suspected stockpiles of cyanide and the new revelations about Agent 15) from the time of the 1991 Gulf War. President George W. Bush's summary in October of 2002 of the National Intelligence Estimates (NIE) states, "Baghdad has begun renewed production of mustard, sarin, GF (cyclosarin), and VX. Although information is limited, Saddam probably has stocked at least 100 and possibly as much as 500 metric tons of CW agents." However, in 2006 the Iraq Study Group (ISG) Report was released and reported that "while a small number of old, abandoned chemical munitions have been discovered, ISG judges that Iraq unilaterally destroyed its undeclared chemical weapons stockpile in 1991."[47] Although the initial intelligence proved to be wrong, it does not invalidate the argument that the risk from these agents, if possessed, would be very concerning.

Chemical agents originally used during World War I are sometimes considered obsolete, especially in comparison to the more potent nerve agents and incapacitating agents. However, agent potency is only one part of the story. To deliver the 5 μg that represents an estimated lethal dose for half of an exposed group (LD_{50}) of the nerve agent VX would seem to be easier than delivering the 3 to 7 g that constitute the LD_{50} of sulfur mustard and more difficult than delivering the much smaller lethal doses of toxins such as botulinum toxin.[48] In fact, sulfur mustard is easier to synthesize than is a nerve agent and is easy to disseminate in a clandestine manner to create delayed effects. Thus mustard still lays claim to being the "King of Gases," and it has allegedly been used in a variety of venues since the end of World War II. Most known chemicals

with toxicities equal to or greater than that of ammonia could theoretically be used as chemical warfare or terrorism agents.

Existing Agents and Their Potential for Future Use

Existing chemicals capable of weaponization for military or terrorist use include the following:

1. Battlefield and riot-control agents
   a. Pulmonary agents (see Chapter 114)
   b. Vesicants (see Chapter 113)
   c. Cyanide (see Chapter 115)
   d. Nerve agents (see Chapter 112)
   e. Antimuscarinic agents such as BZ and Agent 15 (see Chapter 116)
   f. Riot-control agents (see Chapter 120)
   g. Defoliants and other herbicides
   h. Novichok
2. New chemicals employed for physicochemical effects
   a. Related compounds
   b. Battlefield incendiary agents, smokes (including standard military white obscurant smoke, or HC smoke), and other combustion products such as oxides of nitrogen and perfluoroisobutylene (PFIB)
   c. Opioids (see Chapter 118) and other anesthetic agents (see Chapter 122)
   d. Cholinergic agents (see Chapter 121)
   e. Psychedelic indoles and other hallucinogens (see Chapter 117)
3. Toxic industrial chemicals or materials (see Chapter 111)
4. Poisons
5. Combination of chemicals
6. Nontraditional agents (see Chapter 119) such as hydrofluoroalkane propellant attack

Existing chemicals remain candidate agents for future use. Some compounds not developed to cause injury or incapacitation nevertheless can be very dangerous; hexachloroethane (HC) smoke, for example, can cause the same type of pulmonary damage induced by phosgene, a chemical weapon used in World War I. The CDC lists nearly 70 separate chemicals, including a variety of toxic industrial chemicals and poisons, as potential agents for terrorism. These include osmium tetroxide, long-acting anticoagulants, heavy metals, toxic alcohols, and white phosphorus.[49] The April 21, 2000, *Morbidity and Mortality Report* included an even longer list of chemical agents that might be used by terrorists.[50] Pyrolysis, the thermochemical change of an organic material in the absence of oxygen by heat, and products from explosions and conflagrations may release large quantities of cyanide and other toxicants that, although different from the original chemicals present, may still cause death. Industrial chemicals are readily available in large quantities as preformed compounds and should be considered high on the list of potential terrorist agents.[51,52] Toxins that are chemicals produced within biological organisms also represent high-threat agents.[53] New chemicals are currently being synthesized on rigid three-dimensional molecular skeletons, the most promising of which are the norbornanes. Norbornane is a bicyclic crystalline hydrocarbon (C7H12).[54] Building on norbornane geometry allows for a modular enhancement of the number of functional sites on a given molecule. Many norbornane derivatives, such as the mixture of chlorobornanes known as the toxaphenes, are persistent and have significant acute and chronic toxicity. These norbornane derivatives have been considered as potential candidates for new agents. Novichok[55-58] (Russian for "newcomer") refers to the alleged Russian development of a highly toxic binary nerve agent or generation of nerve agents (sometimes called "fourth-generation" agents). Only sketchy and unverifiable information is available in the unclassified literature, but the existence of these agents would demonstrate the possibility of creating new chemical compounds toxic enough to be used as chemical warfare or terrorist agents. One of the sources of unclassified information is from a dissident Russian scientist who wrote newspaper articles and published a book about the Novichok program and the types of chemical agents that were produced.[59] So-called GV analogs combining some of the properties of G-series and V-series nerve agents have also been suggested as potential new agents.[38]

The use in 2002 of an incapacitating gas in the siege of a Moscow theater taken over by Chechen rebels was evidence of use of a chemical aerosol.[60,61] The Russian Health Minister at the time, after significant international pressure identified the aerosol as a fentanyl derivative and then stated that use of a fentanyl derivative was not prohibited by the Chemical Weapons Convention. Further investigations of survivors have suggested that carfentanil and remifentanil were possibly used in the siege.[62]

Organofluorines have been investigated because of their reported ability to defeat protective-mask or chemical-filtration systems.[38] Other incapacitating agents under development exert primarily physical rather than chemical effects and include immobilizing agents ("stickums"), antitraction gels ("slickums"), and malodorants.[63,64] An effective incapacitating agent must be highly potent and reversible. It also must have rapid onset, short duration of action, and a high safety margin.[63]

Nontraditional agents (NTAs) are chemicals that do not fall in the traditional chemical weapons category but have been reportedly researched or developed for use as chemical weapons. "NTAs are novel chemical threat agents or toxicants requiring adapted countermeasures," according to Homeland Security Presidential Directive/HSPD-18.[65] Developing defenses against NTAs is a listed priority for the U.S. Department of Defense.[41]

Technological Modifications of Battlefield Chemical Agents and Delivery Systems

Ways in which existing or future battlefield chemical agents and delivery systems could be modified to improve performance must be considered. These modifications include the following:

1. Agent thickening
2. Binarization
3. Micronization: "dusty agents"
4. Developments in delivery systems
   a. Dual-use cyberinsects and biorobots
   b. Nanotechnology

Small quantities of thickening agents, such as acrylates, can be added to chemical agents to increase their viscosity. Thickened agents are more persistent in the environment and in wounds than are nonthickened agents, and they are less easily decontaminated.[66] Although no nation is currently known to stockpile thickened agents, the technology for their production is relatively simple and requires only standard chemical-warfare agents and the right proportion of a thickener.[67] Many industrial chemicals and other poisons could theoretically be rendered more effective as battlefield or terrorist agents by thickening.

In the 1950s, the U.S. Army began to investigate the then-new technology of binarization, although production did not accelerate until the 1960s and deployment was not widespread until the 1980s.[58] A binary chemical weapon did not employ a new kind of agent but rather represented a novel way of producing and storing an already existing type of agent. The idea was to make storage of chemical rounds safer by stopping the production process at the penultimate synthetic step, resulting in two precursor compounds that when mixed would create the desired agent. These two precursors could then be stored separately. Just before use, one component could be inserted into a round, where it would be separated from the other precursor by a thin membrane. The impact and momentum of the launch of the projectile would burst the membrane to allow for mixing of the components and in-flight production of the chemical agent. In practice, this process was often not complete, but the 20% or so of ancillary reaction product was often extremely toxic by itself. Binarization or some similar production-arrest method could theoretically be used by a clandestine terrorist cell to help evade detection and to decrease the risks associated with the production, transportation, and use of chemical agents.

Micronization is a type of particularization involving the production of extremely fine particles onto which a chemical agent can be adsorbed. During World War II, Germany explored particularization of sulfur mustard onto small carrier particles of silica (silicon dioxide), although other powdered silicates (e.g., talc, diatomite, and pumice) and clays (e.g., kaolinite and Fuller's earth) can also be used.[68] The advantages of such "dusty agents" are increased volatility, facilitation of the movement of relatively nonvolatile agents such as sulfur mustard and the persistent nerve agent VX into the alveoli, and increased penetration of clothing and chemical protective equipment.[31] Iraq used a "dusty mustard" composed of 65% sulfur mustard adsorbed onto silica particles ranging in diameter from 0.1 to 10 μm during its war with Iran. Micronization of a variety of chemical, biological, and toxin agents requires a certain degree of technological sophistication that is becoming increasingly easy to acquire.

Agent delivery can potentially be modified in a variety of ways in addition to thickening and micronization. The Jordanian government released a report in 2004 of the discovery of an elaborate plot by Al Qaeda terrorists for a two-stage attack using a massive vehicle-borne improvised explosive device followed by the release of toxic chemicals to include acetones, nitric acid, and sulfuric acid.[69] Similarly, enhanced-fragmentation munitions could be used in combination with chemical agents to drive the agents more effectively into the body.

Innovative new delivery systems taking advantage of advances in robotics include the proposed use of cyberinsects and biorobots to deliver biological agents, chemical agents, or toxins.[70] Engineering on an even smaller scale is the purview of nanotechnology, also called "micromechanical engineering" and "micro-electromechanical systems."[71] Nanotechnology takes advantage of the unique properties of materials on the scale of about a nanometer (10 to 9 m)[72] and deals with the molecule-by-molecule or even atom-by-atom assembly of materials. Nanoparticles behave in unusual and unpredictable ways, are small enough to enter cells easily, and in fact are being developed to provide not only better storage and dispersal of pharmaceutical products but also more efficient transport of both biological organisms (e.g., viruses) and chemical compounds into the body.[71] In some cases they may be surprisingly toxic, partly because of the ease with which they can cross membranes, including the blood-brain barrier, and enter cells.[73] This toxicity could be exploited by governments or terrorist organizations interested not only in small-particle delivery of chemical agents but also in the ancillary and perhaps synergistic effects of the carrier materials themselves.

Nanomaterials can be encapsulation compounds such as fullerenes, or buckyballs, which are hollow 60-carbon geodesic shells; nanoshells (e.g., a gold shell surrounding an inert silica core); a "self-assembled, polyamino acid nanoparticles system" under development in France; or dendrimers, which are onion-like layers of shells surrounding a biologically active core.[72] Any of these materials could be used to deliver existing or new chemical agents. Other nanomaterials include self-assembling liquids composed of cylindrical nanofibers (each 6 to 8 nm in diameter) that solidify upon injection to form structured scaffolds capable of presenting ordered peptide signals to cells. A ferrofluid such as a colloidal suspension of nanoscale ferrous oxide can be coupled with antibodies in a laboratory to detect and concentrate rare human cells in a diagnostic setting, but this technology could easily be adapted to target those cells in vivo.

Quantum dots are nanoscale semiconductor crystals that show promise in the in vitro and in vivo diagnosis of a variety of conditions; although their main use is projected to be in the laboratory, animal experimentation involving injected quantum dots has demonstrated successful targeting of lymph nodes and of prostate-cancer xenografts in mice.

Adverse health effects from any of these kinds of nanoparticles could represent a primary goal for military or terrorist operatives in addition to the toxicity of any other chemicals delivered by the nanoparticles. For example, water-soluble fullerenes (or buckyballs) have caused brain damage in largemouth bass.[74] Also, dendrimers can cause osmotic and membrane damage and can activate the clotting and complement systems. Quantum dots composed of selenium, lead, and cadmium could release those metals into cells, depending on the composition of the surface coating of the dots, and cause damage.[72]

"Designer" Chemicals from Biotechnological Processes

Biotechnology refers to "any technological application that uses biological systems, living organisms, or derivatives thereof, to make or modify products or processes for specific use."[75] Biotechnology includes such time-honored practices as the baking of bread and the brewing of beer, but in the twenty-first century refers in particular to genetic engineering, that is, the artificial transfer of genes from one organism to another and the consequent alteration of the genetic structure of a cell.[76] It is founded on the basic sciences of genomics (the study of the genetic composition of an organism) and proteomics (the study of the expression of the genome by means of protein synthesis). "Designer" chemicals could be produced from biotechnological processes. These processes include the following: (1) combinatorial chemistry and ligand modification; (2) genomics and target identification; (3) microarrays, proteomics, and rational agent design; and (4) toxicogenomics, database mining, and the prediction of toxicity.[77] These developments, if used for chemical warfare agents, would be considered "dual-use technology." This is technology that can be used for both peaceful and military aims.

Combinatorial chemistry is the production of complex sets, or so-called libraries, of related compounds, as in the case of the norbornane derivatives previously described. Automated screening techniques to select for library elements with desired toxic effects on specified target organs can process several hundred thousand compounds a day against several dozen different proteins. This obviously accelerates tremendously the development of new chemical agents.

Genomics has benefited enormously from three modern scientific efforts: the Human Genome Project, the Human Genome Diversity Project, and gene therapy.[78] Identification and cataloging of hundreds of single-nucleotide polymorphisms (individual sequence variations) allow for the selection of genomic sequences to be mass-produced for insertion into cells to create a specific effect. Targeting unusual sequences of high prevalence in certain populations raises the specter of genomic, or ethnic, weapons, as previously described. Less appreciated is the potential for genomics to be used to develop drugs and chemical or toxin agents that can also be targeted to specific variants within a population of humans, animals, or crops. The widespread availability of genome libraries on the Internet makes it nearly impossible to control or restrict access to the already published genomic libraries on over a hundred microbial pathogens.[79]

Proteomics complements genomics by characterizing the protein expression of segments of the genome and by making it easier to develop compounds that target or produce a specific protein. Direct gene insertion, genetic delivery via virus or bacteria, or drug tailoring

to affect a given protein can be used. For example, a scorpion toxin has been successfully engineered into a virus that acts as a pesticide against caterpillars. Protein sequences in toxins are partly responsible for resistance to light, oxygen, moisture, and desiccation; the insertion of genes to create altered proteins or the introduction of chemical agents engineered to cause structural changes in expressed proteins could significantly alter the toxicity of a given compound.[77] Furthermore, the widespread use of DNA microarrays (glass slides or chips imprinted with thousands of specific single-stranded DNA sequences) allows for fast-automated screening of candidate compounds.

Scientists involved in the selection and evaluation of specific chemical agents can now use toxicogenomics (the study of genetic variation of response to toxins) and data mining (the computerized analysis of databases of drug and chemical information via sophisticated neural nets) as tools to eliminate less likely candidates and to algorithmically predict compounds with high toxicity or with other desired characteristics relating to environmental persistence, toxicokinetics (absorption, distribution, biotransformation, and elimination), and toxicodynamics (mechanism of action). Such tools will undoubtedly lead to the development not only of new pharmaceutical agents but also of designer toxins for military or terrorist use.[77]

CONCLUSIONS

If history is any guide, new biological and chemical weapons and novel "mid-spectrum" agents (e.g., toxins, bioregulators, synthetic viruses, and genocidal weapons) will be developed in the future, and new modifications will be found to improve the production, weaponization, storage, delivery, and action of existing agents.[33,80–82] Naturally occurring emerging infectious diseases provide examples of newly identified pathogens with weaponization potential, and midspectrum agents such as toxins and bioregulators will undoubtedly assume more prominence with the accelerating pace of synthetic biology. Agents of any category can theoretically be engineered to target specific genes or proteins with differential population prevalence to produce genomic or ethnic weapons; and advances in proteomics, toxicogenomics, and computerized database mining could be used for the rapid and efficient development of not only new drugs but also new chemical agents for terrorism.[9,17,68] Synthetic biology has now advanced to the point that no special equipment is required beyond that available to any modern molecular-biology laboratory, and the scale of operations is also well within the means of governments and terrorist groups.[78] The threats from future modification of existing agents and from the development of new agents, new agent-development technologies, and innovative delivery systems should not and must not be underestimated.

ACKNOWLEDGMENTS

The authors gratefully acknowledge the previous contributions of James M. Madsen.

REFERENCES

1. Joy RJT. Historical aspects of medical defense against chemical warfare. In: Sidell FR, Takafuji ET, Franz DR, eds. *Medical Aspects of Chemical and Biological Warfare, Part I*. Washington, DC: Borden Institute; 1997:111–128.

2. Mann J. *Murder, Magic, and Medicine. Oxford*. New York, NY: Oxford University Press; 1992.

3. Fenn EA. *Pox Americana: The Great Smallpox Epidemic of 1775-82*. Hill and Wang: New York, NY; 2001.

4. Williams PWD. *Unit 731: Japan's Secret Biological Warfare in World War II*. London: Hodder and Stoughton; 1989.

5. Christopher GW, Cieslak TJ, Pavlin JA, Eitzen EM, Jr. Biological warfare. A historical perspective. *JAMA*. 1997;278(5):412–417.

6. Regis E. *The Biology of Doom: America's Secret Germ Warfare Project*. Henry Holt: New York, NY; 1999.

7. Meselson M, Guillemin J, Hugh-Jones M, et al. The Sverdlovsk anthrax outbreak of 1979. *Science*. 1994;266(5188):1202–1208.

8. Noah DL, Huebner KD, Darling RG, Waeckerle JF. The history and threat of biological warfare and terrorism. *Emerg Med Clin North Am*. May 2002; 20(2):255–271.

9. Tucker JB. *Toxic Terror: Assessing Terrorist Use of Chemical and Biological Weapons*. Cambridge, MA: MIT Press; 2000.

10. CDC. Follow-up of deaths among U.S. Postal Service workers potentially exposed to *Bacillus anthracis*–District of Columbia, 2001-2002. *MMWR Morb Mortal Wkly Rep*. 2003;52(39):937–938.

11. Fennelly KP, Davidow AL, Miller SL, Connell N, Ellner JJ. Airborne infection with *Bacillus anthracis*—from mills to mail. *Emerg Infect Dis*. 2004;10(6):996–1002.

12. UN Secretary General. United Nations Mission to Investigate Allegations of the Use of Chemical Weapons in the Syrian Arab Republic Report on the Alleged Use of Chemical Weapons in the Ghouta Area of Damascus on 21 August 2013. 2013.

13. Alibek KHS. *Biohazard : The Chilling True Story of the Largest Covert Biological Weapons Program in the World, Told from the Inside by the Man Who Ran It*. New York, NY: Random House; 1999.

14. Morens DM, Folkers GK, Fauci AS. The challenge of emerging and re-emerging infectious diseases. *Nature*. 2004;430(6996):242–249.

15. Phillips HKD. *The Spanish Influenza Pandemic of 1918-19: New Perspectives*. London; New York, NY: Routledge; 2003.

16. Hummel S. Ebola: not an effective biological weapon for terrorists. *CTC Sentinel*. 2014;7(9):16–19.

17. Centers for Disease Control and Prevention. *Emergency Preparedness and Response: Bioterrorism Agents/Diseases*. http://emergency.cdc.gov/agent/agentlist-category.asp. Accessed November 23, 2014.

18. Centers for Disease Control and Prevention. *Avian Influenza A Virus Infections of Humans*. 2008. http://www.cdc.gov/flu/avian/gen-info/avian-flu-humans.htm.

19. Stevens J, Corper AL, Basler CF, Taubenberger JK, Palese P, Wilson IA. Structure of the uncleaved human H1 hemagglutinin from the extinct 1918 influenza virus. *Science*. 2004;303(5665):1866–1870.

20. Centers for Disease Control and Prevention. Interim Guidance for Protection of Persons Involved in U.S. Avian Influenza Outbreak Disease Control and Eradication Activities. 2006. Available at: http://www.cdc.gov/flu/avian/professional/protect-guid.htm. Accessed April 11, 2015.

21. Teleman MD, Boudville IC, Heng BH, Zhu D, Leo YS. Factors associated with transmission of severe acute respiratory syndrome among health-care workers in Singapore. *Epidemiol Infect*. 2004;132(5):797–803.

22. CDC. Revised U.S. surveillance case definition for severe acute respiratory syndrome (SARS) and update on SARS cases—United States and worldwide, December 2003. *MMWR Morb Mortal Wkly Rep*. 2003;52 (49):1202–1206.

23. Centers for Disease Control and Prevention. *Severe Acute Respiratory Syndrome: Public Health Guidance for Community-Level Preparedness and Response to SARS*. Version 2. Supplement F: Laboratory guidance. Appendix F8—Guidelines for laboratory diagnosis of SARS-CoV infection. 2005. Available at: http://www.cdc.gov/sars/guidance/. Accessed April 11, 2015.

24. Centers for Disease Control and Prevention. *About MERS*. Available at: http://www.cdc.gov/coronavirus/mers/. Accessed November 23, 2014.

25. Prevention CfDCa. *Hendra Virus Disease & Nipah Virus Encephalitis*. Available at: http://www.cdc.gov/ncidod/dvrd/spb/mnpages/dispages/Fact_Sheets/Hendra_Nipah_Fact_Sheet.pdf. Accessed April 11, 2015.

26. Mackenzie JS. Emerging viral diseases: an Australian perspective. *Emerg Infect Dis*. 1999;5(1):1–8.

27. Snell NJ. Ribavirin therapy for Nipah virus infection. *J Virol*. 2004;78 (18):10211.

28. Kagan E. Bioregulators as instruments of terror. *Clin Lab Med*. Sep 2001;21 (3):607–618.

29. O'Dell JR. Therapeutic strategies for rheumatoid arthritis. *N Engl J Med*. 2004;350(25):2591–2602.

30. Bokan S, Breen JG, Orehovec Z. An evaluation of bioregulators as terrorism and warfare agents. *ASA Newslett*. Available at: http://www.asanltr.com/newsletter/02-3/articles/023c.htm. Accessed April 11, 2015.

31. U.S. Congress, Office of Technology Assessment. *Technologies Underlying Weapons of Mass Destruction*. US GPO: Washington, DC; 1993.

32. Cameron DE, Bashor CJ, Collins JJ. A brief history of synthetic biology. *Nat Rev Microbiol*. 2014;12(5):381–390.

33. Casadevall A. The future of biological warfare. *Microb Biotech*. 2012;5 (5):584–587.

34. Garrett L. Biology's brave new world: the promise and perils of the synbio revolution. *Foreign Affairs* 2013. Available at: http://www.foreignaffairs .com/articles/140156/laurie-garrett/biologys-brave-new-world. Accessed October 29, 2014.

35. Tucker JB. Could terrorists exploit synthetic biology? *New Atlantis*. 2011;31:69–81.

36. Tucker JB, Zilinskas RA. The promise and perils of synthetic biology. *New Atlantis*. 2006;12(1):25–45.

37. Jefferson C, Lentzos F, Marris C. *Synthetic Biology and Biosecurity: How Scared Should We Be*. London: King's College London; 2014.

38. Ouagrham-Gormley SB, Vogel KM. The social context shaping bioweapons (non)proliferation. *Biosecur Bioterr*. 2010;8(1):9–24.

39. Black JL, 3rd. Genome projects and gene therapy: gateways to next generation biological weapons. *Mil Med*. 2003;168(11):864–871.

40. Appel JM. Is all fair in biological warfare? The controversy over genetically engineered biological weapons. *J Med Ethics*. 2009;35(7):429–432.

41. Program DoDCaBD. *2013 Department of Defense Chemical and Biological Defense Annual Report to Congress*; 2013.

42. Roberts MA, Cranenburgh RM, Stevens MP, Oyston PC. Synthetic biology: biology by design. *Microbiol*. 2013;159(Pt 7):1219–1220.

43. Cordesman AH. *Defending America: Iraq and other threats to the US involving weapons of mass destruction*; 2001. Available at: http://csis.org/files/media/csis/pubs/iraq_otherthreatswmd.pdf, Accessed October 15, 2014.

44. U.S. Government Accountability Office. *Combating Terrorism: Need for Comprehensive Threat and Risk Assessments of Chemical and Biological Attacks*. Report to Congressional requesters. Washington, DC. 1999. GAO/NSIAD-99-163.

45. Sidell FR. Nerve agents. In: Sidell FR, Takafuji ET, Franz DR, et al., eds. *Medical Aspects of Chemical and Biological Warfare, Part I*. Washington, DC: Borden Institute; 1997:111–128.

46. Fitzgerald GM, Sole DP. *CBRNE: incapacitating agents, Agent 15*; 2014. Available at: http://emedicine.medscape.com/article/833238-overview, Accessed October 15, 2014.

47. National Intelligence Estimate: Iraq's Continuing Programs for Weapons of Mass Destruction. In: Intelligence DoC, Washington, DC, 2002. Available at: https://www2.gwu.edu/~nsarchiv/NSAEBB/NSAEBB129/nie.pdf; accessed April, 11, 2015.

48. Pitschmann V. Overall view of chemical and biochemical weapons. *Toxins*. 2014;6(6):1761–1784.

49. Centers for Disease Control and Prevention. *Chemical Agents*. 2013. Available at: http://emergency.cdc.gov/agent/agentlistchem.asp. Accessed October 15, 2014.

50. CDC. Biological and chemical terrorism: strategic plan for preparedness and response. Recommendations of the CDC Strategic Planning Workgroup. *MMWR Recomm Rep*. 2000;49(Rr-4):1–14.

51. Burklow TR, Yu CE, Madsen JM. Industrial chemicals: terrorist weapons of opportunity. *Pediatr Ann*. 2003;32(4):230–234.

52. U.S. Department of Health Human Services. Agency for Toxic Substances Disease Registry. Industrial chemicals and terrorism: human health threat analysis, mitigation and prevention. Available at: http://www.mapcruzin .com/scruztri/docs/cep1118992.htm. Accessed April 11, 2015.

53. Madsen JM. Toxins as weapons of mass destruction. A comparison and contrast with biological-warfare and chemical-warfare agents. *Clin Lab Med*. Sep 2001;21(3):593–605.

54. Holderna-Natkaniec K, Natkaniec I, Khavryutchenko V. Neutron spectroscopy of norbornane. *Phase Trans*. 2003;76(3):275–279.

55. Adams JR. Russia's toxic threat. *Wall St J (Midwest Ed)*. 1996;A18.

56. Englund W. Ex-Soviet scientist say Gorbachev's regime created new nerve gas in '91. *Baltimore Sun*. 1992;3A.

57. Sands A, Pate J. CWC compliance issues. In: Tucker JB, ed. *The Chemical Weapons Convention: Implementation Challenges and Solutions.* Washington, DC: Center for Nonproliferation Studies, Monterey Institute of International Studies; 2001:17–22.

58. Smart JK. History of chemical and biological warfare: an American perspective. In: Sidell FR, Takafuji ET, Franz DR, et al., eds. *Medical Aspects of Chemical and Biological Warfare, Part I.* Washington, DC: Borden Institute; 1997:9–86.

59. Mirzayanov V. *State Secrets: An Insider's Chronicle of the Russian Chemical Weapons Program.* Parker, CO: Outskirts Press; 2008.

60. Bismuth C, Borron SW, Baud FJ, Barriot P. Chemical weapons: documented use and compounds on the horizon. *Toxicol Lett.* 2004;149 (1–3):11–18.

61. Coupland RM. Incapacitating chemical weapons: a year after the Moscow theatre siege. *Lancet.* 2003;362(9393):1346.

62. Riches JR, Read RW, Black RM, Cooper NJ, Timperley CM. Analysis of clothing and urine from Moscow theatre siege casualties reveals carfentanil and remifentanil use. *J Anal Toxicol.* 2012;36(9):647–656.

63. Pearson A. Incapacitating biochemical weapons. *Nonproliferation Rev.* 2006;13(2):151–188.

64. Harigel GG. *Introduction to Chemical and Biological Weapons.* Washington, DC: Carnegie Endowment for International Peace; 2001. *http:// carnegieendowment.org/2001/01/18/introduction-to-chemical-and-biological-weapons.* Accessed April 11, 2015.

65. Department of Homeland Security. Homeland Security Presidential Directive/HSPD-18. *Medical Countermeasures Against Weapons of Mass Destruction* January 31, 2007.

66. Hurst CG. Decontamination. In: Sidell FR, Takafuji ET, Franz DR, et al., eds. *Medical Aspects of Chemical and Biological Warfare, Part I.* Washington, DC: Borden Institute; 1997:351–359.

67. Takafuji ET, Kok AB. The chemical warfare threat and the military healthcare provider. In: Sidell FR, Takafuji ET, Franz DR, et al., eds. *Medical Aspects of Chemical and Biological Warfare, Part I.* Washington, DC: Borden Institute; 1997:111–128.

68. Dando MR. *The danger to the Chemical Weapons Convention from incapacitating chemicals. First CWC Review Conference Paper No. 4.*

Strengthening the Chemical Weapons Convention. Bradford, UK: University of Bradford Department of Peace Studies; 2003.

69. Jordan "was chemical bomb target." 2014. Available at: http://news.bbc.co .uk/2/hi/3635381.stm. Accessed April 11, 2015.

70. DaSilva EJ. Biological warfare, bioterrorism, biodefence and the biological and toxin weapons convention. *Electronic J Biotech.* 1999;2(3):9–128.

71. Jane's Chem-Bio Web. News: Nanotechnology: the potential for new WMD. Available at: http://chembio.janes.com [subscription required]. Accessed April 11, 2015.

72. Perkel J. The ups and downs of nanobiotech. *Scientist.* 2004;18(16).

73. Weiss R. Nanotechnology precaution is urged: miniscule particles in cosmetics may pose risk, British scientists say. *Washington Post.* July 30, 2004, A02.

74. Oberdorster E. Manufactured nanomaterials (fullerenes, C60) induce oxidative stress in the brain of juvenile largemouth bass. *Environ Health Perspect.* 2004;112(10):1058–1062.

75. Wikipedia, The Free Encyclopedia. *Biotechnology.* Available at: http://en .wikipedia.org/wiki/Biotechnology. Accessed April 11, 2015.

76. Convention on Biological Diversity, United Nations Environment Program. Governments to advance work on Cartagena Protocol on Biosafety [press release]. Available at: http://www.biodiv.org/doc/meetings/ bs/iccp-03/other/iccp-03-pr-en.pdf. Accessed April 11, 2015.

77. Wheelis M. Biotechnology and biochemical weapons. *Nonproliferation Re.* 2002;9(1):48–53.

78. Barnaby W. *The Plague Makers: The Secret World of Biological Warfare.* 3rd ed. Continuum International: New York, NY; 2000.

79. Russo E. NRC wants genome data unfettered. *Scientist.* 2004. http://www .the-scientist.com/?articles.view/articleNo/23067/title/NRC-wants-genome-data-unfettered/. Accessed October 15, 2014.

80. Aas P. The threat of mid-spectrum chemical warfare agents. *Prehosp Disaster Med.* 2003;18(4):306–312.

81. Caves JP, Carus WS. *The Future of Weapons of Mass Destruction: Their Nature and Role in 2030.* Washington, DC: National Defense University Press; 2014, Occasional Paper 10.

82. Kagan E. Bioregulators as prototypic nontraditional threat agents. *Clin Lab Med.* 2006;26(2):421–443.

CHAPTER 81

Directed-Energy Weapons

M. Kathleen Stewart and Charles Stewart

A directed-energy weapon (DEW) emits energy in an aimed direction without the means of a projectile. A DEW transfers the energy to a target for the desired effect. Most DEWs rely on electromagnetic waves or subatomic particles that impact at or near the speed of light. The energy can be delivered in various forms:

- Electromagnetic radiation (e.g., radio frequency devices, microwave devices, lasers, and masers)
- Particles with mass (e.g., particle beam weapons; theoretical, no known weapons exist)
- Sound (e.g., sonic weapons)

Several of these weapons have already been tested in combat and are now potentially available to terrorists. As new technology becomes available and the military uses become apparent, terrorists will adopt it and often increase its lethality.

Whatever the form of electromagnetic energy used for the DEWs, they all share certain characteristics that make them revolutionary weapons:

- They hit a target at the speed of light.
- They are line-of-sight weapons.
- The price of use is typically a small fraction of what it costs to fire a missile or a large gun. Low- and medium-power lasers can be cheaply obtained.
- They are able to engage many different targets because of their instantaneous effects and the ease of reaiming them.

HISTORICAL PERSPECTIVE

Lasers

Immediately after the development of the first functional laser, the military (and hence terrorist) potential of the laser was apparent. Modern pulsed lasers can reach energy levels of up to millions of watts in a fraction of a second. In many cases, the laser is not intended as a weapon per se, but rather as a targeting device for another weapon, such as a missile or a "smart bomb." The properties of the laser are particularly suited for this purpose. The military in many nations developed lasers for use as range finders and target designators. Laser light has special qualities, including the following:

- The light released is *monochromatic*; it contains one specific wavelength of light (one specific color). The wavelength of light is determined by the amount of energy released when an electron drops to a lower orbit. This wavelength depends on the material of the laser and the method by which it was stimulated to emit light. The frequency of the wave multiplied by its wavelength equals the speed of light.
- The light released is *coherent*. It is "organized"; each photon moves in step with the others (i.e., the waves of the electromagnetic radiation are in phase in both space and time). This means that all of the photons have wave fronts that launch in unison and the beam is parallel.

- The light is *directional*. A laser light has a tight beam and is very strong and concentrated. A light bulb, on the other hand, releases light in many directions, and the light is weak and diffuse.
- The light does not disperse over long distances because of the coherent nature (collimation) of the laser beam.

Military laser devices can easily cause retinal injury, even at a distance of many miles.[1-3] Military planners found that this optical effect can be used as an antipersonnel system to actively disable personnel by blinding or "dazzling" them.[2] By 1985, the British Navy had developed an unclassified weapon that was fitted aboard ships to blind oncoming enemy pilots at ranges up to 3 miles. Deployment of lasers designed specifically to blind is now banned by the Protocol on Blinding Laser Weapons, adopted by the United Nations in 1995.[4,5] Many thousands of target-designation and distance-ranging lasers have been manufactured and sent out with troops of multiple countries.[6] Because of this availability, they may find their way into the hands of terrorists and be used against U.S. civilians.

Civilian lasers can be easily adapted to similar purposes. For example, muggers in England have used simple laser pointers to blind victims before robbing them.[7] There have been many anecdotal reports of eye pain and headaches lasting for several weeks after brief ocular exposures to laser pointer beams.[8] The pathology of this pain is difficult to understand, because lasting pain is not a common consequence of retinal laser treatment for diabetes, when a considerable amount of laser energy is delivered to the retina.[9,10]

Lasers have already been used to blind helicopter pilots and commercial pilots.[11,12] It would be no great stretch for a terrorist to mount a relatively powerful laser on a truck or within a car and attempt to blind pilots who are landing at a commercial civilian airport.[13] Likewise, simple lasers may destroy vision in law enforcement officers responding to a terrorist attack.

Microwave-Radiation Emitters

Long-term exposure to high-intensity microwaves can produce both physical and psychological effects on humans, including sensations of warmth, headaches, generalized fatigue, weakness, and dizziness. The effect depends on the power output of the weapon and the distance between the generator and the person. The U.S. Air Force has fielded a microwave system (Active Denial System, or ADS) that uses the surface heat production of high-power, very high frequency (VHF) microwaves to induce people to leave an area.[14] The military currently has this weapon only mounted on a truck but is working on a more portable version.

The destruction of electronic devices by high-intensity microwave devices is well understood, and multiple weapons have been developed to exploit this vulnerability. These include the Bofors HPM Blackout, a commercially available electromagnetic pulse weapon.[15] Smaller devices using similar technology have been proposed to disable vehicles in police chases.[16]

Sonic Weapons

The Long Range Acoustic Device (LRAD) was designed to "hail, warn, and notify" vehicles and sea vessels at a distance.[17] It uses high-intensity, highly focused acoustic output to communicate beyond the effective range of small arms. LRAD's main function is as a hailing device, being basically a super-bullhorn. But it can also be used in what has been termed a *warning tone*: an extremely loud and unpleasant sound said to resemble a fire alarm. Despite the device's nonviolent purpose, media has termed it a *sound cannon* or *sonic cannon*.[17] Extremely high power sound waves can disrupt or destroy the eardrums of a target and cause severe pain or disorientation. This is usually sufficient to incapacitate a person. According to the National Institute on Deafness and Other Communication Disorders, any sound over 90 dB can damage a person's hearing, so the LRAD can damage hearing.[18] Less powerful sound waves at certain frequencies can cause humans to experience nausea or discomfort. The use of these frequencies to incapacitate persons has occurred both in counterterrorist and crowd-control settings. There is no medical treatment for these effects except removal from the source. Although many popular writings have postulated acoustic weapons with internal effects such as cavitation of tissue, practical application appears to require higher energy than currently available.[19]

Particle Beam Generators

A particle beam is a directed flow of atomic or subatomic particles. These high-energy particles, when concentrated into a beam, can melt or fracture metals and plastics. They also may generate x-rays at the point of impact. These weapons are in development stages only.[20]

CURRENT PRACTICE

There is no foolproof countermeasure for a blinding laser. Each of the available protective efforts will hinder to some degree a person's ability to see and to carry out activities requiring sight.[21,22] Laser radiation does not travel through opaque objects. Any opaque cover will provide protection against all but very high power military lasers. Avoid looking directly at any laser beam or its reflection, if at all possible. Reflections off shiny surfaces may cause damage, despite forward cover. Wearing an eye patch on one eye offers partial protection from blinding lasers; unfortunately, it also deprives the wearer of depth perception and peripheral vision. Patching only prevents blinding in the patched eye.

The present method of protection from the laser threat is quite simple: a pair of protective sunglasses can be fashioned that reflect the laser light but let other wavelengths through so that the wearer can see sufficiently to do tasks. These helmet visors or goggles would prevent laser radiation from damaging the wearer's eyes. This works well if the laser threat has been previously identified and is limited to one or two wavelengths. However, there are multiple frequencies available in lasers; each additional frequency "protected" is a wavelength that is dimmed for vision. The management of casualties from the effects of laser light is discussed later in this chapter. The triage of these casualties can be accomplished by use of the triage algorithm shown in Fig. 81-1. Casualties from consequent events, such as a blinded driver or pilot crashing his or her vehicle, are managed in the customary fashion covered by trauma protocols. There would be no difference in management of these casualties if they had a concomitant eye injury.

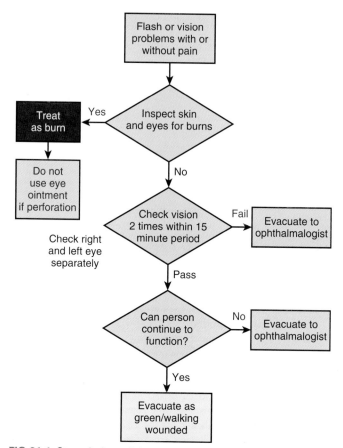

FIG 81-1 Steps in laser injury triage.

KEY MANAGEMENT ISSUES

Laser Eye Injury

The eye is the part of the body most vulnerable to laser hazards. When a person is exposed to laser light, he or she can be temporarily blinded (as a result of dazzling), be blinded for a prolonged period of time (as a result of photolysis), or incur changes in visual function from cataracts, retinal lesions, or hemorrhages. This damage may be either temporary or permanent, depending on the wavelength and power of the laser. Because the eye is more sensitive and the pupil is larger during darkness, laser weapons have a greater effect at night than during the day. Eye damage can occur at much lower power levels than those causing changes to the skin, and ocular injuries are generally far more serious than injuries to the dermis.[23] If the person is using a see-through optical device, such as binoculars, the beam strength is magnified and greater injury to the eye can result. Even modestly powered lasers can temporarily blind an unprotected human looking through a telescope or binoculars.[23] Higher-power lasers can be used to destroy objects in flight or on the ground.

Examination of the eye in part depends on available tools. In the field, examination may be limited to direct vision with magnification supplied by loupes or magnifying glasses. Corneal injuries may be assessed with fluorescein staining and ultraviolet light. In the emergency department, further assessment with a slit lamp is appropriate, and if available, use of a retinal camera may be appropriate. If any abnormalities are found, referral to an ophthalmologist is appropriate.

Retinal Damage

Retinal damage primarily occurs in the 400- to 1400-nm wavelength range (i.e., in the visible and near-infrared [IR-A] region). Laser light between visible and the IR-A region can cause damage to the retina. These wavelengths are also known as the "retinal hazard region." Radiation in these wavelengths is the most hazardous because it is transmitted by the optical components of the eye. The infrared spectrum is often used for military target-designation lasers. IR-A radiation is transmitted by the cornea to the lens of the eye, which narrowly focuses it on the retina, concentrating the radiant exposure of the laser by up to 100,000 times. It is this considerable optical gain of the lens arrangement of the eye that increases the hazard when laser beams enter the eye. In the retina, most of the radiation is absorbed in the retinal pigment epithelium and in the choroid, a dark brown layer with exceptionally large blood vessels and high blood flow rate. Because the tissue structures of the retina are unable to undergo any repair, lesions caused by the focusing of visible or IR-A light on the retina may be permanent. The most critical area of the retina is the central portion, which includes the macula and the fovea.

Damage to the retina or hemorrhaging from retinal damage can cause a complete loss of vision. Persons who see large dark spots at or near the center of their vision, who have a large floating object in their eye, or who have an accumulation of blood in the eye should be promptly evacuated to a hospital with ophthalmological support. There is no currently accepted treatment for laser- or light-induced eye injuries. However, hemorrhage into the eye noted on either direct examination of the eye or with a slit lamp should be treated by positioning the patient in a head-up position to allow the blood to settle into the lower part of the eye. Laser burns to the retina do not require an eye patch. Indeed, an eye patch may reduce the person's remaining vision. A laser eye injury can worsen with time, so anyone with a suspected laser eye injury should be evaluated promptly and again at regular intervals.

Cornea and Lens

Laser light in either the ultraviolet (UV) or far-infrared spectrum can cause damage to the cornea or the lens. Selective, sensitive portions of cells in the cornea absorb UV light (i.e., 180 to 400 nm), resulting in photochemical damage. Many proteins and other molecules (such as DNA and RNA) absorb UV light and are "denatured" by the radiation. Excessive exposure to UV light can cause photophobia, redness of the eye, tearing, discharge, stromal haze, and other effects. These adverse effects are usually delayed for several hours but will occur within 24 hours. The lens principally absorbs UVA (315 to 400 nm). The lens is particularly sensitive to the 300-nm wavelength. XeCl excimer lasers operating at 308 nm can cause cataract with an acute exposure. The cataracts are delayed and may not occur for years.

Far-infrared radiation (IR-B) (i.e., 1400 nm to 1 mm) is produced by CO_2 lasers and is also absorbed primarily by the cornea (Fig. 81-2). Thermal damage is caused by the heating of the tears and tissue water of the cornea by the infrared light. Excessive exposure to infrared radiation results in a loss of transparency of the cornea or surface irregularities. A high-energy laser pulse may severely burn or perforate the cornea. Severe burns or perforations should not be patched, and the eye should be protected to ensure that the vitreous humor does not leak out. Minor laser burns to the cornea may be treated with an eye patch and appropriate eye antibiotics. Some infrared radiation in the IR-A range (700 to 1400 nm) and the IR-B range (1400 to 3000 nm) is absorbed directly by the lens. These effects are delayed and do not occur for many years (e.g., cataracts).

Laser Skin Burns

Dermal injury is more likely, though generally less severe, than ocular laser injuries. With enough power and duration, a laser beam of any wavelength in the optical spectrum can penetrate the skin and cause deep internal injury. The pain from thermal injury to the skin by most

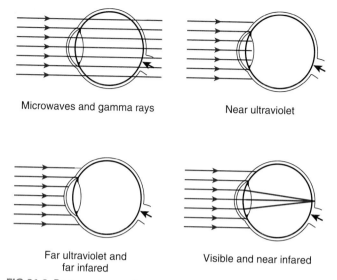

Microwaves and gamma rays

Near ultraviolet

Far ultraviolet and far infrared

Visible and near infared

FIG 81-2 Damage to eye tissue may vary with the wavelength of the laser.

targeting lasers is enough to alert a victim to move out of the beam path. Unfortunately, a number of high-power visible-light and infrared lasers are now used in industry. These are capable of producing significant skin burns in less than a second. These burns are treated as any other thermal burn.

Electromagnetic Beam Weapon Clinical Effects

The ADS microwave system has not yet been deployed in the field, but over 11,000 volunteers have been exposed to effects of the nonionizing radiation from this weapon. According to the Department of Defense, only eight injuries have occurred with this system: six minor injuries and two requiring hospitalization.[24] The system's long-term effects on humans have not been studied, and there is some worry about potential ocular damage.[25–27] The medical treatment of the burns caused by this device would be unchanged from that of usual burn care.

Clearly, devices with directed microwave energy sufficient to disable or destroy vehicle computers would be detrimental to neurostimulators, insulin pumps, and other nonshielded computerized devices. Although pacemakers are shielded from some microwave interference, the high energy of vehicle-disabling microwave devices would have a strong likelihood of causing some pacemaker malfunction.[28] Nonlocalized effects of electromagnetic pulse (EMP) generators are covered elsewhere (see Chapter 198). Treatment of the effects of a disabled medical device would depend on device function and mode of malfunction. For example, the failure mode of an insulin pump may be to overdose the patient with continuously injected insulin or to shut down completely.

⚠ PITFALLS

Knowing the type of laser involved in an injury may be very valuable. Tables 81-1 and 81-2 provide a breakdown of biological effects by laser type. It must be stressed that, to be effective, laser protective goggles or glasses must be donned before exposure to the laser and must have the appropriate wavelength-rejection characteristics for the laser used. This presents a difficult problem for law enforcement and providers of emergency medical services, who may be faced with any wavelength of lasers in a terrorist threat. It is expected that a tunable (frequency/wavelength agile) laser threat will also be developed soon. The technical approach used to protect against fixed-wavelength lasers cannot be applied to

TABLE 81-1   Biological Effects of Laser by Wavelength

The potential location of injury in the eye is directly related to the wavelength of the laser radiation entering the eye

RADIATION TYPE (WAVELENGTH)	BIOLOGICAL EFFECTS
Near ultraviolet UVA (315-400 nm)	Most of the radiation is absorbed in the lens of the eye. The effects are delayed and do not occur for many years (e.g., cataracts).
Far ultraviolet UVB (280-315 nm)	Most of the radiation is absorbed in the cornea. Keratoconjunctivitis (snow blindness/welder's flash) will result if sufficiently high doses are absorbed.
UVC (100-280 nm)	Keratoconjunctivitis (snow blindness/welder's flash) will result if sufficiently high doses are absorbed.
Visible (400-760 nm)	Most of the radiation is transmitted to the retina.*
Near-infrared (IR-A) (760-1400 nm)	Overexposure may cause flash blindness or retinal burns and lesions.
Far-infrared (IR-B) (1400 nm to 1 mm)	Most of the radiation is transmitted to the cornea. Overexposure to these wavelengths will cause corneal burns.

*Radiation in the visible and IR-A (400 nm to 1,400 nm) is the most hazardous and is transmitted by the optical components of the eye Most of the radiation is absorbed in the retinal pigment epithelium and in the choroid plexus.

TABLE 81-2   Biological Effects of Commonly Used Lasers

LASER TYPE	WAVELENGTH (μM)	BIOLOGICAL PROCESS	TISSUE AFFECTED SKIN	CORNEA	LENS	RETINA
CO_2	10.6	Thermal	X	X		
HFl	2.7	Thermal	X	X		
Er-YAG	1.54	Thermal	X	X		
Nd-YAG*	1.33	Thermal	X	X	X	X
Nd-YAG	1.06	Thermal	X			X
Gas (diode)	0.78-0.84	Thermal	†			X
He-Ne	0.633	Thermal	†			X
Ar	0.488-0.514	Thermal or photochemical	X			X‡
XeFl	0.351	Photochemical	X	X		X
XeCl	0.308	Photochemical	X	X		

Ar, argon; *CO₂*, carbon dioxide; *Er*, Erbium; *He-Ne*, helium-neon; *HFl*, hydrogen fluoride; *Nd*, neodymium; *XeCl*, xenon chloride; *XeFl*, xenon fluoride; *YAG*, yttrium aluminum garnet.
*Wavelengths at 1.33 nm or more, common in some Nd-YAG lasers, have demonstrated simultaneous cornea/lens/retina effects in biological studies.
†Power levels not normally sufficient to be considered a significant skin hazard.
‡Photochemical effects dominate for long-term exposures to retina (exposure times more than 10 seconds).

protection from the agile threat or even for protection from a larger number of fixed-wavelengh threats. As more wavelength-rejection filters are built into protective goggles, transmission of light through the lens at other wavelengths decreases also, making it unusable at night and limiting its utility in the daytime.

REFERENCES

1. Sunder KS, Shetty N, Singh VK, Chaudhary VS, Sharma S. Laser range finder can cause retinal injury. *Indian J Ophthalmol*. Jun 2004;52 (2):169–170.
2. Eggertson L. Military claims laser dazzlers have "negligible" risk. *CMAJ: Canadian Medical Association Journal = journal de l'Association medicale canadienne*. May 26 2009;180(11):1099–1100.
3. Johnson TE, Keeler N, Wartick AL. Laser eye injuries among U.S. military personnel, *Proc SPIE*. June 18, 2003;4953, Laser and Noncoherent Light Ocular Effects: Epidemiology, Prevention, and Treatment III, 51. http://dx.doi.org/10.1117/12.477900.
4. Doswald-Beck L. *Blinding weapons: report of the meeting of experts convened by the International Committee of the Red Cross on battlefield laser weapons 1989-1991*. Geneva: ICRC; 1993.
5. Doswald-Beck L. New Protocol on Blinding Laser Weapons. *International Review of the Red Cross*. 30 Jun 1996.
6. Chandra P, Azad RV. Laser rangefinder induced retinal injuries. *Indian J Ophthalmol*. Dec 2004;52(4):349.
7. Killer pens. *Newsweek*. 1997(Nov 24):8.
8. Seeley D. Laser point causes eye injuries? In: *Laser Institute of America: Proceedings of International Laser Safety Conference*. Orlando, FL USA: ILSC; 1999:129–135.
9. Mainster MA, Sliney DH, Marshal J. But is it really light damage? *Ophthalmology*. 1997;104:179–190.
10. Yolton R, Citek K, Schmeisser E, et al. Laser pointers: toys, nuisances, or significant eye hazards? *J Am Optom Assoc*. 1999;70(5):285–289.
11. Daly v Fesco Agencies NA, Inc., C01–0990C (United States District Court, Western District of Washington, 2001).
12. Laser Aviation incidents. 2014; http://www.laserpointersafety.com/news/news/aviation-incidents_files/category-did-not-realize-hazard.php. Accessed 05.02.14.
13. "Russian ship's laser caused eye injury, Navy officer says." http://www.aeronautics.ru/nws002/ap036.htm. Accessed 21.08.03.
14. AFRL's Directed Energy Directorate HPMD, Applications, Branch KAN. Active Denial Technology. http://www.afrlhorizons.com/Briefs/Sept01/DE0101.html. Accessed 03.01.04.
15. Karlsson MU, Olsson F, Aberg D, Jansson M, Bofors HPM. blackout—a versatile and mobile L-band high power microwave system. Paper presented at: Pulsed Power Conference, 2009, PPC '09. IEEE; June 28 2009-July 2 2009.

16. Montecuollo G. Cutting to the Chase: Are ignition-disabling systems the future for stopping pursuits? 2007. http://lib.post.ca.gov/lib-documents/cc/39-Montecuollo.PDF. Accessed 04.02.14.

17. Schrantz J. The Long Range Acoustic Device: Don't Call It a Weapon—Them's Fightin' Words. *The Army Lawyer.* 2010;27:50–447.

18. Noise-Induced Hearing Loss. http://www.nidcd.nih.gov/health/hearing/pages/noise.aspx. Accessed 24.03.14.

19. Jauchem JR, Cook MC. High-intensity acoustics for military nonlethal applications: a lack of useful systems. *Mil Med.* Feb 2007;172(2):182–189.

20. Geis JP. Directed energy weapons on the battlefield: A new vision for 2025. Occasional Paper No. 32: Center for Strategy and Technology. 2003.

21. Nakagawara VB, Wood KJ, Montgomery RW. Laser exposure incidents: pilot ocular health and aviation safety issues. *Optometry.* Sep 2008;79(9):518–524.

22. Whitmer DL, Stuck BE. Directed energy (laser) induced retinal injury: current status of safety, triage, and treatment research. *U.S. Army Medical Department Journal.* Jan-Mar 2009;51–56.

23. Marshall J. Blinding laser weapons; Still available on the battlefield. *BMJ.* 29 November, 1997;315:1392.

24. Active Denial System FAQs. http://jnlwp.defense.gov/About/FrequentlyAskedQuestions/ActiveDenialSystemFAQs.aspx. Accessed 24.03.14.

25. D'Andrea JA, Adair ER, de Lorge JO. Behavioral and cognitive effects of microwave exposure. *Bioelectromagnetics.* 2003;(suppl 6):S39–S62.

26. Dovrat A, Berenson R, Bormusov E, et al. Localized effects of microwave radiation on the intact eye lens in culture conditions. *Bioelectromagnetics.* Jul 2005;26(5):398–405.

27. Chalfin S, D'Andrea JA, Comeau PD, Belt ME, Hatcher DJ. Millimeter wave absorption in the nonhuman primate eye at 35 GHz and 94 GHz. *Health Phys.* Jul 2002;83(1):83–90.

28. Niehaus M, Tebbenjohanns J. Electromagnetic interference in patients with implanted pacemakers or cardioverter-defibrillators. *Heart.* September 1, 2001;86(3):246–248.

82 CHAPTER

Chemical, Biological, Radiological, and Nuclear Quarantine

Jeffrey D. Race, Carey Nichols, and Susan R. Blumenthal

Although the term *quarantine* is familiar to most physicians, nurses, and emergency medical services (EMS) personnel from their core training, it may mean many different things depending on where, to what level, or from which discipline or perspective someone was trained. The meanings of quarantine and isolation are quite often different between first responders and first receivers (i.e., those who work in hospitals). Within each first responder discipline (e.g., emergency medical technician [EMT] and paramedic, firefighter, and police officer), there are different roles to play and connections or responsibilities, as determined by position, training, and/or experience. Confusion often occurs between the terms isolation and quarantine; many people use the term quarantine to mean either isolation or quarantine. Both are public health measures used to control the spread of contagious disease:

- *Isolation* is used to separate and restrict the movement of those who are ill with a communicable disease.
- *Quarantine* is used to separate and restrict the movement of those who are still well but who may have been exposed to a communicable disease.

For the purpose of this chapter we will be using the term quarantine to refer to both isolation and quarantine because we will discuss quarantine in terms of both biological and nonbiological exposures.

The quarantine of any population is a troublesome matter for both the society involved and the government agencies overseeing the containment efforts. At a moment's notice a nation must mobilize significant resources to help triage, treat, and contain any communicable and potentially epidemic diseases or exposures. Making the decision to identify and then contain individuals certainly cannot be taken lightly and will have both political and logistical repercussions. For the purposes of this chapter the idea of quarantine will include the management of those exposed to chemical, biological, radiological, and nuclear (CBRN) disasters. In particular this chapter will examine and discuss processes to help control the spread of societal hazards, giving particular attention to medical triage and containment.

In the event of a terrorist attack or growing natural epidemic, a rapid quarantine effort can certainly help to mitigate the damage. Proper deployment and specific targeting will be of critical importance to successfully reduce the overall number of casualties by preventing secondary cases. Obtaining data by examining and monitoring exposed individuals can help to predict the clinical trajectory of future cases and also help medical providers rapidly identify any new cases. This information could also be of tremendous significance should the exposure be more occult in nature to help epidemiologists determine the origins of a previously undetected initial event.

As with any government-mandated health care policy, quarantines of any variety will certainly raise questions regarding ethics. Although restrictive measures discussed in this chapter may be of significant benefit to the afflicted society as a whole, they may meet resistance and raise ethical dilemmas. This may be alleviated by attempting to induce voluntary compliance by always proposing restrictive measures that are proportional to a given threat and providing transparency at all stages of a restrictive quarantine.[1] In the United States in particular, balancing personal liberties with societal benefit rapidly becomes an ethical dilemma without a clear resolution. The word quarantine often carries a stigma and negative connotation—to restrict movement, isolate, and maintain a safe distance from "contaminated" individuals. This becomes especially problematic when a rapid quarantine is clearly the safest option for the nation as a whole following a significant communicable exposure event.

The purpose of quarantine is clearly to prevent additional spread of contagious disease or environmental toxins within a specific population. Quarantine success demands tailoring preventative measures to specific features of a given exposure. With the overall goal of quarantine being a significant reduction in total casualties, a successful quarantine will look to accomplish the following:

- Identify what and who has been exposed
- Determine which exposed people, animals, and/or goods are likely to be contaminated or infected
- Prevent transmission by managing those who are contaminated or infected
- Prevent subsequent exposures and contaminations

Frequently employed measures to accomplish the above goals include the following:

- Identification of potentially infected or contaminated persons, animals, and goods
- Initiation of protective measures to prevent further transmission of infectious agents
- Initiation of protective measures to prevent exposed persons from becoming infected

CBRN incidents are those due to weaponized or nonweaponized CBRN materials that have the ability to cause significant harm to life, health, or the environment. Traditionally in the United States and Canada, nonweaponized materials are referred to as dangerous goods (DG) or hazardous materials (HazMat) and can also include items such as contaminated food, livestock, and crops. The term *CBRN* includes DG or HazMat plus the same materials weaponized into explosive threats. Typically spills or accidental releases or leakages are considered DG or HazMat, whereas intentional spills, releases, or leakages (whether explosive or not) are considered terrorist incidents.[2] Although the approach to dealing with the consequences of both types of incidents may be similar, the terrorist incident will involve additional agencies as well as concerns for public and national security and safety.

Advances in technology and training, years of planning, and billions of dollars spent on that training and equipping response agencies has advanced domestic preparedness for an incident requiring quarantine. This level of training and preparedness has dramatically changed current strategies and tactics in the management of incidents that may require quarantine. Countless lives could thus be saved.[3]

HISTORICAL PERSPECTIVE

The popular media have shaped lay public perceptions of quarantine. Dramatic portrayals of military personnel in personal protective equipment (PPE) and armored vehicles patrolling city streets create a sense of fear and anxiety. If not managed properly, this anxiety can evolve into panic and chaos.

For thousands of years humankind has recognized the need to isolate from the general population persons, animals, and goods that have been exposed to contagious elements. As early as 583 AD, authorities restricted the association of lepers and healthy people, building on the biblical sources in Leviticus.[1] History reveals that the use of the term quarantine only recently entered the first responder lexicon despite its having been in practice back to biblical times.[4]

In the fourteenth century, Europe endured repeated episodes of the plague, with an estimated loss of one third of the population. The plague spread rapidly throughout Europe, beginning in the south in 1347, and reaching England, Germany, and Russia within 3 years.[5] Fear, combined with the severe impact of the plague, led to the development of intense measures to attempt to control the spread of the disease—measures we would currently call infection control. Some of the more severe measures include the abandonment of the ill in the fields outside Reggio, Italy, in 1374. By order of Viscount Bernabo, patients were left in the fields to recover or die on their own.[6]

Similarly, in the area currently occupied by the modern city of Dubrovnik, Croatia, the chief physician of the city, Jacob of Padua, advocated the establishment of an area outside of the city walls for those needing treatment for the "black death."[7] This separation was motivated by an early theory of contagion; however, the efforts were only modestly effective. It was this lack of effectiveness that prompted the Great Council of the city to develop more aggressive methods to prevent the spread of future epidemics.[6]

In 1377 the Great Council established a four-pillared approach to a trentino, or 30-day isolation period.[6] The four pillars include the following:

1. The exclusion of citizens or visitors from plague-endemic areas from the city of Ragusa until they had been in isolation for 30 days
2. The restriction that no person from Ragusa could go to the isolation area without remaining there for 30 days
3. That any person who was not assigned by the Great Council to care for those in quarantine was not permitted to bring food or other items to someone in isolation without having to remain there for 30 days
4. That anyone who did not follow these regulations would be fined and subjected to isolation for 30 days

Similar laws were introduced in Marseilles, Venice, Pisa, and Genoa during the following 80 years,[8,9] although during this time the period of isolation was extended from 30 to 40 days. This 40-day period was known as a quarantino, which was derived from the Italian quaranta or forty.[3,10] Although the rationale for extending the period to 40 days is not known, it has been suggested that the shorter trentino period of 30 days was found to not be long enough to prevent the spread of the plague.[11] Others have suggested that the change was related to the 40-day period of the Christian observance of Lent[4] or the 40-day period associated with many other significant biblical events (the great flood,

Moses' time on Mount Sinai, or Jesus' time in the desert).[12] Still others have suggested that the foundation for the quarantino came from the Greek doctrine of "critical days," which stated that contagious disease occurs within 40 days of exposure.[5,11] Regardless of the rationale, the duration embodied within quarantino provides the fundamental concept for our present-day quarantine.

The identification of the pathogenic agents of epidemic diseases between the nineteenth and twentieth centuries led to a turning point in the history and development of more modern quarantine. Cholera, plague, and yellow fever began to be thought of as individual pathogenic agents to be considered separately in the development of regulations. International regulations were rewritten in 1903 by the Eleventh Sanitary Conference, at which the convention of 184 articles was signed.[13] Modern planning, identification, and response to individual pathogenic agents of concern comes out of this historical separation. Additionally with the emergence of severe acute respiratory syndrome (SARS) in the twenty-first century, traditional measures were once again utilized because a global public health crisis arose as a result of international travel of people and goods.[14]

CURRENT PRACTICE

First responders now have tools to rapidly and accurately identify the nature of an incident (e.g., chemical, biological, or radiological). As a result, the strategies and tactics (policies and procedures) have dramatically evolved from those of the past. First responders can rapidly test potential exposures and determine preliminary information on the nature of the offending agent. Often these rapid tests are definitive. However, most standard operating procedures call for confirmatory testing and follow-up identification procedures in specialized laboratories in order to increase accuracy and specificity. This strategy allows first responders to rapidly determine whether the incident is of a biological, chemical, or radiological/nuclear etiology and adjust quarantine recommendations accordingly. Although the first responder community continues to educate themselves, broad knowledge of signs and symptomatology has become a baseline for education and identification, even without the use of these technologies as a backup.

Quarantine is technically for those incidents involving biological exposures. However, in modern practice, the term also applies to detention, in holding areas, following exposures and prior to decontamination for chemical and radiological or nuclear events. Modern quarantine may be initiated whenever an individual or group is known or suspected to have contracted, or been exposed to, a highly contagious or dangerous disease or a chemical contamination. Public health authorities must ensure that there are resources available to provide care for those in quarantine and to implement and maintain the quarantine. It is also imperative that authorities provide for the expeditious provision of health care for those in quarantine, including coordination with the local health care delivery system, heightened surveillance and monitoring, expedited diagnosis and treatment, and preventive treatment (vaccination, prophylactic antibiotics, and PPE).[15,16]

Within any potential circumstance in which a modern quarantine might be issued, the primary goal is to reduce disease transmission by increasing the "social distance" between persons (i.e., reducing the number of people each person comes into contact with).[17] To accomplish this there are a wide variety of strategies for disease control that may be implemented individually or in combination with one another. These strategies include shelter-in-place, short-term voluntary home curfew, restrictions on public gatherings and events (including travel and mass transit restrictions), and cordoning off an area with a sanitary barrier.[18] Modern quarantine can be effective in some cases even when it is only partial quarantine (i.e., where many or most, but not all, exposed persons are quarantined).[17] This partial or "leaky" quarantine, particularly when combined with a program of vaccination, has been effective in slowing the rate of the spread of disease, including SARS and smallpox.[19]

Distance and duration of exposure are commonly found to be important predictors of transmission. Accordingly public health authorities employ modern quarantine procedures that involve limited numbers of exposed persons in small areas. These small areas or zones are designed as "rings" or concentric circles drawn around individual disease cases.[20] Only those who fall within the ring of exposure duration or distance would be quarantined along with the individual disease case, with the most intensive disease control activities in the inner ring.

Implementation of modern quarantine also requires the trust and participation of the public. Compliance with quarantine is lowest in areas with little to no experience with quarantine in their recent past. In the United States, obstacles to compliance include difficulties with PPE and preventive measures, issues with compensation for lost income because of missed work, and lack of communication from trusted public officials.[21,22] The public must be informed about the dangers of contagious diseases subject to quarantine before an outbreak or intentional release of biological agents occurs and throughout an actual event.

Authority for Quarantine

Whereas all aspects of the first responder community provide a rapid response to 911 emergencies when called upon, state and federal governments have enormous resources and jurisdictional laws, rules, and regulations that are utilized to protect and respond to incidents throughout the United States. They also respond in support of first responders, as needed. These federal, state, and local jurisdictional laws govern the specifics of incident command and control in response to a biological incident.

Federal Law

The Commerce Clause of the U.S. Constitution provides the authority for utilization of quarantine and isolation by the federal government. The U.S. Secretary of Health and Human Services is also authorized to take measures to prevent the entry and spread of communicable diseases from foreign countries into the United States and between states, as stated in section 361 of the Public Health Service Act (42 U.S. Code § 264).[23] The authority to carry out these functions is delegated to the Centers for Disease Control and Prevention (CDC), including the authority to detain, medically examine, and release persons who are suspected of carrying a communicable disease and are arriving into the United States or traveling between states (42 CFR, parts 70 and 71). Twenty U.S. quarantine stations are located at ports of entry and land border crossings, enabling the CDC to routinely monitor people at these locations for signs or symptoms of communicable disease. When necessary the CDC can institute public health practices to stop or limit the spread of disease through the use of isolation and quarantine.[21]

Although isolation and quarantine are well understood as medical functions, they are less well known as "police power" functions. These police power functions come from the right of the state to take actions affecting individuals for the benefit of society and empower the government to detain or constrain people who may be contagious with a communicable disease.

Federal isolation and quarantine are authorized by executive order of the president and currently exists for the following communicable diseases (this list may be revised by executive order of the president):

- Cholera
- Diphtheria
- Infectious tuberculosis

- Plague
- Yellow fever
- Smallpox
- Viral hemorrhagic fevers (e.g., Ebola)
- SARS
- Pandemic influenza

State, Local, and Tribal Law

Similar to the federal government, individual states have police power functions to protect the health, safety, and welfare of people within their jurisdiction and to enforce the administration of isolation and quarantine.[21] Laws vary between states, and the authority to enforce state law can be at the state or local level, although breaking quarantine is a criminal offense in most states. In the United States, Indian tribes also have police power authority to take actions to establish and enforce their own isolation and quarantine laws within tribal lands.[21]

Who Is in Charge?

In a quarantine situation the federal government has authority over the states and tribal lands and likewise the states have authority over local governments. In addition federal authorities may either assist state and local authorities in infection control operations or request assistance from state and local authorities in enforcing federal isolation and quarantine.

It is possible for federal, state, local, and tribal health authorities to each have legal quarantine power over the same incident at the same time. Whenever this occurs, however, federal law and authority supersede all others.[24]

Federal Enforcement

When a communicable disease that is authorized for quarantine is suspected or identified, the CDC may issue a federal isolation or quarantine order. Enforcement of such a public health order may require assistance from police or other law enforcement. The issuing authorities may request domestic law enforcement assistance at any time in the quarantine process. U.S. Customs and Border Protection and the U.S. Coast Guard are also authorized to assist with the enforcement of federal quarantine orders.[21] Failure to follow a federal quarantine order is punishable by fines and imprisonment, although federal law does allow for conditional release from quarantine when possible if the individuals agree to comply with medical monitoring and surveillance.[21] Although federal authorities have the capability to declare such events, large-scale isolation and quarantine have not been initiated since the influenza ("Spanish Flu") pandemic in 1918-1919.[21]

State and Local Enforcement

State and local authorities respond in a similar manner to federal authorities with regard to the issuance of a quarantine order. Assistance with enforcement may be requested from local law-enforcement agencies and from the federal level, when necessary. Failure to follow quarantine orders can lead to fines and/or detention, depending on the local or state statutes.

First Responders

First responders will be early on the scene and expected to initiate a response. It is critical that as they arrive, first responders have the capability to properly assess the situation and recognize the signs and indications that a potential CBRN incident has occurred. First responders have to rely on the strength of their training to guide them in their next decisions about the incident. Standard operating guidelines and procedures will likely provide the basis for much of these decisions, including a predetermined level of response to suspected or confirmed CBRN incidents, when to initiate a public health response, how to assess the extent of damage and risk, how to determine exposure pathways and the need for mutual aid, and criteria for activating an emergency operations center (EOC) and incident command post (ICP).

Once determinations are made that there is a CBRN incident requiring the activation of an EOC/ICP and involving public health, the local resources will continue to operate using the incident command system (ICS) and remain in control of the scene for rescue and public safety. The incident commander should coordinate with local and state emergency management officials to request additional resources from state or federal assets in the event that quarantine becomes necessary. First responders may be called upon by the incident commander to assist with provision of needed services throughout the duration of the incident and/or quarantine. Scene management for the first responder requires an understanding of quarantine for potentially contaminated or infected persons, establishment of decontamination and triage areas, and isolation of contaminated areas. For each of these items, it is critical that the first responder understands the signs, symptoms, and effects of CBRN substances (weaponized or nonweaponized CBRN materials that can cause significant harm) and is familiar with HazMat management.[1]

Under control of their respective governor, each state possesses assets that may be deployed to assist in the event of an incident. The National Guard Civil Support Teams (CSTs) are one of the most critical components for quarantine responses. A state's Office of Emergency Services coordinates the request for and deployment of the CSTs. When an incident exceeds the states' capabilities, they may request federal assets through their Federal Emergency Management Agency (FEMA) Regional Operations Center.

Training and Response of First Responders: Quarantine

Agencies and organizations, such as the Occupational Safety and Health Administration (OSHA), Environmental Protection Agency (EPA), National Fire Protection Agency (NFPA), and FEMA, have many different levels of training on this topic, ranging from basic awareness courses up through specialist and advanced formal courses. Current guidelines and training emphasize the need to be knowledgeable of all types of Haz-Mat and their management. Recognition is the first line of defense in an incident. Recognition not only protects each individual and other first responders, but also enables first responders to initiate the system-wide responses necessary to manage these incidents. Most training also emphasizes the adherence to established protocols designed to detect hazardous agents on a minute level by the first arriving units. One aspect of these protocols establishes the criteria for involving the highly advanced capabilities of specialized HazMat and weapons of mass destruction (WMD) teams and state and federal resources, if necessary. Recognition that an incident is beyond the management capability of local resources and involves HazMat or WMD would be an initial reason for an incident commander to reach out through an EOC for state or federal resources. This is particularly true when combined with patients exhibiting signs and symptoms of exposure to HazMat or WMD. State resources that may be called upon include agencies such as CSTs. Federal assistance may be requested by the incident commander in coordination with an EOC at the local and state levels through the proper channels. State and federal authorities throughout a state's Office of Emergency Management and Department of Homeland Security (DHS) monitor incidents of significance and of larger magnitudes. This includes fusion centers, which serve as focal points within the state and local environment for the receipt, analysis, gathering, and sharing of threat-related information between the federal government and state, local, tribal, territorial (SLTT), and private sector partners.

Further knowledge of protocols and procedures provides guidance on protection of the scene for the purpose of limitation and/or reduction of further injuries and illness through limiting ongoing or subsequent exposure and contamination. Finally first responders' knowledge of their own agency-specific guidelines and those of other related agencies will assist in the speed of implementation of these protocols. It is this knowledge of protocols and procedures that provides a first responder with the ability to take the initial actions toward isolation and quarantine procedures. These actions must be guided by stated policies and procedures and supported by training guidelines and principles.

When referring to CBRN incidents, there are continual changes in the management of these incidents based on improvements in education, training, experience, and, most significant of all, technology. Best practices have also led to advances in management. However, the United States is a diverse country, and scenarios in different parts of the country have to be managed based on their locale and its related procedures. Many different factors, such as weather, population, location, infrastructure, and nature of the incident, come into play in different locations. However, the basic facts of exposure and contamination remain constant. Below is a short summary of exposures and contaminations that have relevance to quarantine and isolation.

Types of Quarantine

Following an exposure or contamination, the greatest concern for the first responder is to limit the number of people already affected or who could potentially be affected. The nature of the agents and the methods of exposure determine the risk level and the actions necessary to mitigate that risk. Quarantine and isolation are the most extreme actions for risk mitigation. Technically quarantine most closely fits biological exposures due to the method of transmission, incubation, and infection by biological agents. However, quarantine is also used when detaining exposed or contaminated personnel for decontamination following a chemical, radiological, or nuclear exposure (Boxes 82-1 to 82-4).

Biological

There are many biological agents that are pathogenic and can cause harm. Rapid identification of potentially infected persons and the biological agents involved increases the effectiveness of methods to control the spread of disease (isolation, quarantine, barrier methods [gloves, filter masks, and eye protection], and hand washing). When quarantine is

---

BOX 82-1 Examples of Vaccine-Related Quarantine Measures

- Unimmunized children exposed to measles are excluded from school until one full incubation period after the last case. Children who accept immunization with live virus vaccine within 72 hours of exposure or with immune globulin within 6 days of exposure may return to school. Children immunized outside these time frames are excluded from school until a full incubation period from the last exposure of that child has passed.

- Persons exposed to smallpox without fever or exanthemata may be vaccinated and continue normal activity while being monitored until a vaccine "take" is ensured (discharge from quarantine) or until fever and/or skin lesions appear (isolation required).

- Immunized domestic and farm animals exposed to rabies are revaccinated and confined for observation if owners are willing and able to restrict the animal's contact with other animals and humans until an incubation period has expired. Unimmunized pets have to be quarantined in a controlled facility for 10 days, observed for onset of illness, and, if well, vaccinated before being released from quarantine.

BOX 82-2 Examples of Prophylactic Treatment as Quarantine Measures

- Persons with household and face-to-face contact to pneumonic plague and those exposed through a terrorist act should receive prophylactic antibiotics as quickly as possible and be placed under surveillance for 7 days. If unprotected exposure continues, prophylaxis may need to be extended. Those who refuse or cannot receive prophylactic antibiotics must be placed in strict isolation and monitored closely for 7 days.
- Persons with tuberculosis may be required to remain isolated until antibiotics have effectively sterilized the sputum, at which time isolation ceases, but directly observed therapy continues for the full course of treatment.

BOX 82-3 Examples of Travel-Related Quarantine Measures

- A child on a long airplane trip may develop symptoms suspicious of measles. Data must be collected on the immunization status and current health status of all travelers. Data on the seating arrangements and movements within the plane of the child and other occupants are useful. Immunization can be provided to any unimmunized person. If immunization is unavailable or refused, detailed contact information for the next 3 weeks for any susceptible person is collected, as is precautionary information.
- In a more complex scenario, the diagnosis of measles is made after the debarkation and airline manifests must be used to find and notify fellow passengers.
- Travelers with suspected SARS provide recent examples. Temperature screening at embarkation and debarkation of travelers from areas with reported cases provide an opportunity to detect cases before passengers are dispersed to many destinations. The quarantine officers need data to decide whether to detain any passengers if there is a suspected case. Data are collected on the body temperature, current health status, seating arrangements, and movements within the plane of all travelers. Detailed travel plans and contact information for all nonfebrile travelers for the next 10 days are obtained in some instances. Before being released from quarantine, travelers receive "fever watch" instructions and directions to report to medical care if fever develops.

BOX 82-4 Useful Resources

- Selected Federal Legal Authorities Pertinent to Public Health Emergencies. Prepared by the Public Health Law Program, U.S. Department of Health and Human Services. Centers for Disease Control and Prevention. Updated February 2014. http://www.cdc.gov/phlp/docs/ph-emergencies.pdf.
- Centers for Disease Control and Prevention. U.S. Department of Health and Human Services. http://www.cdc.gov.
- Federal Emergency Management Agency. U.S. Department of Homeland Security. http://www.fema.gov.

---

necessary it is critical that there is continuity of provision of care and command and control in order to ensure the best possible outcomes.

Chemical

Following a chemical exposure, first responders often need to detain exposed people in a quarantine area to isolate them from nonexposed people and areas and to provide rapid decontamination and medical treatment. By treating exposed people according to their clinical syndrome, rather than waiting on the identification of the specific chemical involved, first responders can provide the most rapid, aggressive, and clinically relevant care.[25] This alignment of treatment modalities based on syndromic categories is believed to provide for better outcomes and faster release of exposed persons.

Radiological and Nuclear

Radiological and nuclear incidents are often confused with one another. For the purposes of emergency management and disaster medicine, a nuclear incident involves a nuclear detonation, whereas all other radiation incidents are called radiological incidents.[26]

Although the sources may differ between the two, the exposure requiring isolation, quarantine, decontamination, and treatment is the same for both incidents. With radiological and nuclear exposures, first responders will need to detain exposed people in a quarantine area to provide rapid assessment of injuries. Injured people should receive immediate medical treatment and transportation to a hospital facility for additional treatment and appropriate decontamination. The noninjured will be assessed for level of contamination for determination of type of decontamination process (emergency decontamination on site or at hospital or delayed decontamination at home).[27]

Execution of Quarantine
Control of Individual, Animal, and Environmental Movements

The actual conditions and stipulations of any quarantine depend on a variety of factors. In particular the type, natural history, contagious period, environmental spread, and specific routes of transmission will all influence the type and variety of restrictive measures that may be necessary. Typically these decisions will arise from state or federal public health authorities, but only after careful review of the currently available clinical data. A multidisipinary approach will include physicians, nurses, law enforcement officers, and likely military personnel for adequate containment and restriction enforcement. Although the United States has predetermined exposures that do not require additional federal approval to instigate a local quarantine, many jurisdictions require a court order to initiate or enforce movement restrictions or property confiscation.

Implementing a proper quarantine to separate the unexposed from exposed populations, a variety of measures may be useful. Within the quarantine area, unexposed individuals can utilize personal protective measures, including face masks and gloves. Removing individuals from a nuclear quarantine area is obviously ideal; however, preventing additional radiation exposure with both personal and regional decontamination methods can help to limit the number of exposures. Unexposed individuals within a quarantine zone may benefit from immunization or prophylactic therapies. These prophylactic measures do not have to include the entire at-risk population; however, as evidenced by the 2009 U.S. H1N1 and oseltamivir programs, it may be of benefit to prophylactically treat vulnerable populations, including those with high risk of exposure and immunocompromised individuals, depending on the agent of concern.[28] The decision to offer prophylaxis to some members of the population must be done carefully and with clear dissemination of public information to avoid confusion and unnecessary treatments. For example, the public fear of radiation exposure and misguided rush for iodine tablets following the 2011 Fukushima nuclear disaster caused undue stresses and unnecessary treatments even in distant European nations.[29]

Close, at-home observation remains a viable option, as does the performance of serial examinations on those with known exposure to a contagion or environmental toxin. Individuals who develop signs and symptoms may be hesitant to seek care, especially with knowledge that this may lead to isolation. Every effort must be made to ensure that a quarantined population is well informed and understands that treatment and social support are readily available during this stressful time.

Those who develop evidence of infectivity may qualify for additional restrictive measures, including isolation. However, depending on the type of exposure it may be acceptable to enforce at-home isolation with relief of work duties and other activities that would place a known contagious individual in public spaces. Depending on the natural history of the disease, any isolative measures should be lifted as soon as possible once a contagious period has passed to avoid any further public distrust.[1]

Restricting movement in any capacity will likely displace individuals from their homes, as may already be the case in any large-scale disaster associated with nuclear or airborne toxins. Shelter provisions should clearly be provided to those displaced by circumstance, though front-line medical care teams must remain vigilant for signs of communicable exposures. If water sources and other sanity conditions decline, the ease of disease transmission will exponentially increase. As a result disaster response teams should consider ways to quarantine and potentially isolate infectious individuals under even the worst conditions, if at all possible, to help reduce new cases in a refugee shelter situation.

Events involving highly contagious strains of influenza demonstrate the potential impact of movement restrictions. For example, during the 2009 H1N1 outbreak, the United States and Canada instigated voluntary home quarantine of sick individuals and closed public meeting places, including schools and malls, with moderate success. In comparison China enacted a strict quarantine lasting 60 days in many major urban areas, including Beijing, with military enforcement to restrict personal movement until the quarantine period was cleared.[30] Although differences in governmental policies and ability to rapidly restrict travel and public space usage exist, restricting the movement of individuals in and out of a quarantine zone will be critical to help prevent additional spread of the targeted exposure. In particular, careful screening of major air and seaport passengers will likely become necessary, again depending on the type of contagious material and natural history of the disease. Travel restrictions can be especially effective in the early phases of a quarantine to help limit the rapid spread of undetected cases, though sensitive measures are difficult to discern early in a disease process, as evidenced by the questionably ineffective efforts during the 2009 H1N1 outbreak to fever screen airport passengers at airports.[31,32] Restriction of clearly symptomatic individuals from making both local and international travel can be a method to help prevent rapid spread, though as with any restrictive measure this must be carried out in an evidence-based method and tailored to the pathogen at hand.

If an exposure is suspected to involve any animals responsible for producing food or other goods, public health officials must also seek to establish livestock quarantines. Although this may be difficult in the early stages of a previously unknown or undetected pathogen, many novel diseases are ultimately found to be harbored or spread via animal vectors toward humans. For example, given initial suspicions that the SARS pandemic of 2002 and 2003 may have originated in civet cats sold in public markets, China quickly moved to ban the sale or transport of these animals. Civet farms were closed until additional information became available, to prevent any further animal-born spread of SARS cases.[33] In the present-day, globalized economy, this prospect can be especially difficult, making strict port-of-entry precautions, including freight examination, testing, and quarantine, necessary to combat a given zoonotic exposure.[34] These policies will certainly come with economic consequences and the decision to enact mandatory culling, isolation, or trade restrictions on a specific animal or animal product must not be taken lightly, but instead enacted with clear intentions and clear public information regarding necessity.

Regardless of the source, in any unfolding epidemic or mass exposure, controlling the movements of populations is challenging but can be of tremendous benefit for preventing additional spread of the contagion. However, inappropriate quarantine is likely to create civil distrust and unrest. In addition a poorly planned quarantine, which unintentionally exposes healthy individuals or animals with the infected or afflicted, can have disastrous consequences and spark further distrust. Actions intended for the greater good of a society can be easily perceived as inequitable if poorly understood, and every effort must be made to encourage voluntary compliance and reduce panic with equitable means of population control. Trust becomes a vital commodity during times of crisis, and it will become the duty of front-line medical professionals and public health officials to minimize novel cases after an event by providing reasonable yet effective methods of controlling the movements of people and their property following an exposure disaster.

Management and Protection of Community Assets

As with any significant natural disaster or terrorist attack, management of community assets in the immediate post-event period is critical for effective exposure control. When considering a quarantine or isolation, health care officials must take into account any limitations on existing health care and community assets. It is also possible to instigate voluntary and less-invasive means, such as closure of public schools and transportation, to help alleviate the spread of a concerning pathogen. With this in mind, one can best utilize existing infrastructure for triage and treatment of the exposed, while looking to minimize exposure of healthy individuals by best managing public facilities.

Health Care Assets

Following a mass-exposure event, protecting and managing health care assets in a given community is of utmost importance. Decontamination (discussed in Chapters 83 and 84) will certainly be the initial and primary strain placed on hospitals and emergency departments after a mass-casualty event. Once these patients are triaged and decontaminated, proper management and placement within the health care system can help to minimize secondary exposures. In addition to standard hospital policies already in place for infection isolation and environmental decontamination, quarantine measures may include cohorting of patients and health care workers among institutions to reduce the exposure spread to all institutions. Should the number of infected or exposed individuals overwhelm the isolation capacity of regional hospitals, setting up separate temporary facilities to care specifically for disaster victims can be an effective means to simultaneously treat and quarantine populations. This strategy does require significant resources and predetermined disaster management plans.

Measures to protect and maintain the availability of medical care following an exposure are also of utmost importance. Basic means, including hand washing and equipment disinfection, gloves and masks, and spatial separation of suspected or confirmed victims, can assist with intrahospital quarantine. Effective infection isolation within a care facility can maintain the overall function of that clinic or hospital. It is important to remember that more typical emergencies and community health care demands will continue despite a recent exposure event, and all efforts must be made to maintain normal function while also preventing exposure spread. Additional strategies, including measures to avoid patient-to-patient exposures entirely by nonfacility care, can also be effective, and include telephone screening, home visits, and public-place examination clinics. With growing public fears people may seek out unnecessary health care visits, only furthering the risk of contamination. As a result, aggressive public communication and clear reasoning are necessary to help alleviate these fears and prevent unnecessary health care access.

Schools

In any crisis schools become a source of significant anxiety for parents and students. Because of close contact with their peers and family members, school children are a rapid means of spreading infection. An immediate local school closure following an exposure event can be of tremendous benefit to help prevent novel cases and also prevent unnecessary travel and further public exposure to a given pathogen. Schools can also be temporarily repurposed as shelters, outbreak clinics, or government rally points for further management after a major disaster. The decision to close individual or entire systems of schools should be based on the nature of the exposure and the need for facility repurposement. Simulated influenza pandemic models also suggest that school closures can alleviate strain on local health care assets by reducing new cases in both children and adults.[35]

After schools are reopened it is prudent to instruct school officials regarding signs and symptoms of exposure-related illness in order to detect any new cases early and prevent further spread. School events, including sports and social gatherings, should be treated like other mass gatherings after a major disaster with quarantine rules extending to these events as well. Isolation measures within schools could help to facilitate ongoing educational concerns; however, the logistics of effective isolation inside of most schools are likely near impossible. It is likely of greater benefit to reopen schools only once a threatening pathogen or exposure has been adequately controlled and new cases have already started to subside.

Travel

Travel management of exposed or infected patients is critical to any adequate quarantine process. Unfortunately this will also likely become a major point of social contention, given concerns of government oppression of a specific population. The modern, globalized era has made rapid international travel both easy and affordable, a major risk for ongoing infection spread. In the immediate post-event phase, grounding all air travel to and from areas of concern can help to prevent contagion transmission; however, this will likely be met with significant amounts of public fear as unexposed individuals attempt to rapidly leave the area. As discussed previously, effective quarantine requires the close management of population movement. Depending on the variety of disaster exposure, screening methods may be effective to still allow travel while preventing additional spread. The same principles can be applied to roadways, seaports, and other means of public transportation.

Once a quarantine or travel stoppage is ordered, there will be individuals previously traveling through the area or visiting that cannot leave as previously planned. Providing a safe shelter for these travel refugees is not only ethical, but also important to help manage the travel quarantine. If screening methods are effective at ruling out exposure or infection, these individuals can be safely moved back to their home regions. It is also important for neighboring areas to establish their own quarantine and screening practices to help evaluate and manage people leaving from a contaminated area. As mentioned previously, traveler quarantine and isolation has been a recurrent theme throughout human history and is an effective means to prevent introduction of pathogens to a new area. Management of private vehicle movements can certainly be a daunting task, but if an infection or environmental exposure is allowed to enter a new geographic region, the ultimate containment process will become exponentially more difficult. As with all forms of quarantine or isolation, clear explanations and equitable treatment of all impacted by the restrictive measures will help to alleviate any growing public distrust.

Business and Agriculture

Businesses and other places of work that are fundamental level areas of community gathering are capable of expediting the spread of a contagious material. In times of quarantine, many businesses will voluntarily close based on school closures, which can be a helpful means to limit person-to-person interaction. Despite this, some daily business will certainly continue, and every effort should be made to encourage worker safety and special precautions should be made to identify and prevent infected individuals from exposing their coworkers. Business closures and mandatory sick days can be difficult to enforce, especially in open-market settings with many small business owners operating independently. As evidenced by China's actions to ban the sale or transport of civet cats during the SARS pandemic, direct interventions on commerce can help to alleviate further exposure spread during a quarantine.[33]

It is also important to note the impact of quarantine measures on local business and commerce. Areas highly dependent on tourism and international travel can be dramatically impacted by public fears associated with voluntary or mandatory quarantine. Some estimates place Beijing at a U.S. $1.4 billion loss with regards to tourism alone as a result of the SARS outbreak of 2003.[36] Ideally, rapid action and site control can help to minimize the spread of a radiological, nuclear, or biological agent, with hopes to minimize the spread initially and prevent any need for long-term quarantine with significant financial impact. As a quarantine continues, business will suffer from supply shortages and product stagnation—things that must be considered and will certainly account for ongoing financial losses. Imposing mandatory embargos and trade restrictions can help both sides of a trade agreement prevent the introduction of HazMat within their borders. An effective quarantine will also look to utilize existing business resources to better understand and control the movement of goods, animals, and individuals to minimize contagion spread.

Food production and agricultural supply are not only necessary for ongoing exposure dissemination, but also for providing a quarantined population with adequate goods of daily living. Many agents of biological terrorism can compromise food production without directly impacting humans, as can effects of nuclear fallout if water supplies are contaminated. Initial decontamination and rescue efforts will appropriately focus on humans, but the surrounding livestock exposed to hazardous or contagious materials can also spread disease and radioactive material if their products are not removed from circulation. Guidance from public health officials will be critical in the management of agricultural resources, and importing in sufficient supplies during a quarantine is a critical action for effective societal support. Plants and other crops may exhibit long-term, though silent, contamination and ultimately require destruction. Restricting the movement of livestock in and out of a quarantined area should follow that of humans, with special attention in situations where asymptomatic animals may pass disease to their human counterparts.

⚠ PITFALLS

- *Balancing civil liberty with quarantine:* Any quarantine or isolation will fundamentally restrict certain civil liberties. In the health care setting, specific policies regarding patient isolation are at the discretion of the treating facility, but in the public sphere, isolation measures become ethically challenging. As previously emphasized, the principle of utilizing the least restrictive means possible to accomplish public protection must be at the forefront of any quarantine planning. This strategy will ideally optimize voluntary compliance, which in turn will yield an overall higher protection rate than an overly aggressive quarantine with very poor public compliance. As with any public health crisis, every effort should be made to maintain personal privacy, especially regarding infectious status, whenever possible. Throughout history, quarantines and restriction of societal rights have been utilized in ethical atrocities, and this must be guarded against with well-defined checks and balances to prevent any unintended consequences of a public health effort.

- Restricting personal movement and travel capabilities can quickly lead to civil unrest and social stigma. It is important to differentiate and remove any growing blame on infected individuals and redirect focus toward treatment and prevention of further spread. A study of the 2003 SARS outbreak quarantine in Toronto demonstrated that those entering an enforced quarantine were especially concerned with their ability to maintain work wages, obtain groceries, and continue their prior way of life after the quarantine was lifted. All of these concerns are certainly legitimate and are exacerbated by the intentional interruption of daily routine and removal of routine civil rights. Regardless, during times of significant natural disaster, nuclear fallout, or biological terrorism, civil rights may need to be temporarily restricted to help protect the interests of society as a greater whole. The challenge for public officials will be to ensure that this is done in an equitable and reasonable fashion, with allowances and appropriate support for those placed within a quarantine zone, and removal of restricted measures as quickly as the situation permits.

- *Obtaining compliance:* Whenever rights or activities are restricted by a governing body, a significant amount of civil unrest can result. This can be especially problematic following a major disaster when societal fears and media frenzy have reached maximum levels. Utilizing quarantine as a means of greater public defense and disaster response must always take the forefront of any restrictive efforts with careful attention to ensure that it is not being utilized as a punishment or political tool against a specific population. Clear public communication forums to reinforce that the goal of any isolation or restriction is to prevent the spread of disease and minimize the overall impact of a natural or terrorist-driven exposure.

- Unified and consistent statements and stances regarding the best methods for preventing new cases, treating those already exposed, and minimizing civil disruption are critical for the front-line physicians and public health officials. Issues of compensation for lost wages, care for family members, and similar concerns of persons subject to quarantine cannot be ignored. As evidenced by the North American influenza pandemics of 2008 and 2009, education and communication with the public are key components to encourage voluntary cooperation. Public health officials must ensure that restrictive measures are appropriate and proportional for the targeted exposure, implemented uniformly across all socioecomonic statuses, and followed with highly transparent official communications to maintain public engagement.[1] Just as careful planning is required to set up an appropriate and effective quarantine, health policy makers must be equally prudent as they deescalate any restrictive measures. Emphasis on resumption of normal routine and the importance of continued monitoring throughout all levels of the health care system can assist in this transition and help to reduce the chances of post-event turmoil.

- *Attention fatigue:* Constant vigilance is necessary to maintain quarantine, isolation, and infection control measures following a mass-exposure event. Initial disbelief, even if scientifically justified, can lead to a low index of clinical suspicion. This is especially true in the early phase of a major disaster when the exact details and etiology behind a patient's symptoms may be unclear. In the modern era of sophisticated biological weapons and the potential for multiple-modality terrorist events, clinicians cannot allow tunnel vision to prevent them from noticing and differentiating pathology. It is also worth noting that even during a mass-exposure disaster, there will

still be more typical medical problems requiring emergency intervention. As a result, front-line physicians and other health care providers must maintain attention to clinical details and prevent diagnostic momentum from building based on recent local events. That being said, erring on the side of caution is likely prudent given an unexplained clinical picture with undifferentiated terrorist or natural exposures and with an accepted number of false positives receiving treatment or isolation for precautionary measures.

- *Conflicting goals:* Physicians and other medical professionals are already accustomed to placing the needs of their patients first. This becomes especially difficult when a specific diagnosis mandates additional isolative measures. After any anxiety-provoking disaster, there will be a significant number of patients seeking reassurance following the development of suspected symptoms. Making decisions that will require treatment can be compounded by additional ethical dilemmas given a patient's entire socioeconomic sphere, in particular if removing a breadwinner from standard duties. It becomes difficult for the front-line physician to protect an entire population from further exposures while also advocating for their individual patients. Preexisting relationships with patients and community members can also exacerbate a clinician's ethical dilemma, especially when a particular diagnosis holds isolating repercussions.

- This conflict between medical responsibility to individuals and entire populations creates many of the pitfalls surrounding a mass-exposure event. It is especially difficult to maintain professional relationships with patients when trust is questioned following instigation of restrictive measures. Clinicians must communicate clearly and provide effective education to their patients, especially regarding prophylaxis and treatment options. In the initial phase of a mass-exposure event, the front-line provider will be faced with difficult decisions, only further compounded by often conflicted goals of individual and community protection.

- *Communication:* Communication between health care professionals (including first responders) and law enforcement, between the health care professionals and the community, and between governmental authorities and the public require honesty, clarity of message, and frequent updating. Trust, consistency, and credibility are essential. Professional public information officers (PIOs) should manage all communication strategies.

CONCLUSION

There are many options for a CBRN incident response, and quarantine is the most extreme of these options. For this reason the criteria for initiating quarantine is clearly delineated in federal, state, and local laws, regulations, and policies. Although states may differ regarding their laws on quarantine and emergency response and operations, each state has established laws regarding quarantine. Federal laws and regulations outline parameters by which they would supersede state law in support of a local incident. It is incumbent on all disaster medicine providers to know and understand these laws, regulations, and policies, including local and agency-specific procedural guidelines and how they interact with one another.

REFERENCES

1. Smith MJ, Bensimon CM, Perez DF, Sahni SS, Upshur RE. Restrictive measures in an influenza pandemic: a qualitative study of public perspectives. *Can J Public Health.* 2012;103(5):e348–e352.
2. Public Safety Canada. *The Chemical, Biological, Radiological and Nuclear Strategy of the Government of Canada.* http://www.publicsafety.gc.ca/cnt/rsrcs/pblctns/rslnc-strtg-rchvd/index-eng.aspx; Accessed 23.04.14.

3. EMS makes a difference: improved clinical outcomes and downstream healthcare savings. A position statement of the national EMS advisory council. December 2009.

4. Books of Leviticus chapter 13, and Numbers chapter 5, requires expulsion from camp for everyone with a skin disease or bodily discharge. *The Bible New American Standard.* 1977.

5. Kilwein JH. Some historical comments on quarantine: part one. *J Clin Pharm Ther.* 1995;20:185–187.

6. Jewell W. *Historical Sketches of Quarantine.* Philadelphia: TK and PG Collins; 1957.

7. Stuard SM. *A State of Deference: Ragusa/Dubrovnik in the Medieval Centuries.* Philadelphia: University of Pennsylvania Press; 1992.

8. Matovinovic J. A short history of quarantine (Victor C. Vaughan). *Univ Mich Med Cent J.* 1969;35:224–228.

9. Bolduan CF, Bolduan NW. *Public Health and Hygiene: A Student's Manual.* Philadelphia: WB Saunders; 1941.

10. Kilwein JH. Some historical comments on quarantine: part two. *J Clin Pharm Ther.* 1995;20:249–252.

11. Gordis L. *Epidemiology.* Philadelphia: WB Saunders; 1995.

12. *Foundations of Public Health: History and Development.* Baltimore: Johns Hopkins University Bloomberg School of Public Health; 2001.

13. Howard-Jones N. *The Scientific Background of the International Sanitary Conferences, 1851–1938.* Geneva: World Health Organization; 1975. http://whqlibdoc.who.int/publications/1975/14549_eng.pdf.

14. Rothstein MA, Alcalde MG, Elster NR, et al. *Quarantine and Isolation: Lessons Learned from SARS, A Report to the Centers for Disease Control and Prevention.* Louisville (KY): Institute for Bioethics Health Policy and Law, University of Louisville School of Medicine; 2003, 1–160.

15. The Seattle-King County Advanced Practice Center (APC). http://www.kingcounty.gov/healthservices/health/preparedness/apc.aspx.

16. *Understand Quarantine and Isolation: Facts Sheet.* U.S. Department Of Health And Human Services. Centers for Disease Control and Prevention. Emergency Risk Communication Branch (ERCB), Division of Emergency Operations (DEO), Office of Public Health Preparedness and Response (OPHPR); February 10, 2014. http://emergency.cdc.gov/preparedness/quarantine/facts.asp.

17. Cetron M, Maloney S, Koppaka R, et al. Isolation and quarantine: containment strategies for SARS 2003. In: Institute of Medicine (U.S.) Forum on Microbial Threats , Knobler S, Mahmoud A, Lemon S, et al., eds. *Learning from SARS: Preparing for the Next Disease Outbreak: Workshop Summary.* Washington (D.C.): National Academies Press (U.S.); 2004.

18. Cetron M, Maloney S, Koppaka R, et al. Isolation and quarantine: containment strategies for SARS 2003. In: Institute of Medicine (US) Forum on Microbial Threats, Knobler S, Mahmoud A, Lemon S, et al., eds. *Learning from SARS: Preparing for the Next Disease Outbreak: Workshop Summary.* Washington (DC): National Academies Press (US); 2004.

19. *Principles of Modern Quarantine in: Learning from SARS: Preparing for the Next Disease Outbreak—Workshop Summary.* Forum on Microbial Threats, Board on Global Health, Institute of Medicine. National Academies Press; April 26, 2004.

20. Rea E, Laflèche J, Stalker S, et al. *Epidemiol Infect.* 2007;135(6):914–921.

21. Blendon RJ, DesRoches CM, Cetron MS, Benson JM, Meinhardt T, Pollard W. DataWatch: attitudes toward the use of quarantine in a public health emergency in four countries. *Health Aff.* March 2006;25(2). doi:10.1377/hlthaff.25.w15,w15-w25; published ahead of print January 24, 2006.

22. DiGiovanni C, Conley J, Chiu D, Zaborski J. Factors influencing compliance with quarantine in Toronto during the 2003 SARS outbreak. *Biosecur Bioterror.* 2004;2(4):265–272.

23. *Legal Authorities for Isolation and Quarantine. Fact Sheet.* U.S. Department of Health and Human Services. Centers for Disease Control and Prevention. http://www.cdc.gov/quarantine/pdf/legal-authorities-isolation-quarantine.pdf.

24. *National Incident Management System.* U.S. Department of Homeland Security. Federal Emergency Management Agency; December 2008, FEMA Publication P-501.

25. *The Public Health Response to Biological and Chemical Terrorism Interim Planning Guidance for State Public Health Officials.* U.S. Department of Health and Human Services. Centers for Disease Control and Prevention; July 2001. http://emergency.cdc.gov/Documents/Planning/PlanningGuidance.pdf.

26. *Radiation Basics Made Simple. Segment 8: Responding to Radiation Emergencies.* U.S. Department of Health and Human Services. Centers for Disease Control and Prevention. Oak Ridge Associated Universities. http://orau.gov/rsb/radbasics/downloads/transcripts/chapter_8.html.

27. *Emergency Response Plan.* U.S. Department of Homeland Security. Federal Emergency Management Agency. http://www.ready.gov/business/implementation/emergency.

28. Sullivan SJ, Jacobson RM, Dowdle WR, Poland GA. 2009 H1N1 influenza. *Mayo Clin Proc.* 2010;85(1):64–76.

29. Crépey P, Pivette M, Bar-Hen A. Quantitative assessment of preventive behaviors in France during the Fukushima nuclear crisis. *PLoS One.* 2013;8 (3):e58385.

30. Li X, Geng W, Tian H, Lai D. Was mandatory quarantine necessary in China for controlling the 2009 H1N1 pandemic? *Int J Environ Res Public Health.* 2013;10(10):4690–4700.

31. Gunaratnam PJ, Tobin S, Seale H, Marich A, Mcanulty J. Airport arrivals screening during pandemic (H1N1) 2009 influenza in New South Wales, Australia. *Med J Aust.* 2014;200(5):290–292.

32. Hui DS, Lee N, Chan PK. Clinical management of pandemic 2009 influenza A(H1N1) infection. *Chest.* 2010;137(4):916–925.

33. Zhong N. Management and prevention of SARS in China. *Philos Trans R Soc Lond B Biol Sci.* 2004;359(1447):1115–1116.

34. Meslin FX. Surveillance and control of emerging zoonoses. *World Health Stat Q.* 1992;45(2–3):200–207.

35. Jackson C, Mangtani P, Hawker J, Olowokure B, Vynnycky E. The effects of school closures on influenza outbreaks and pandemics: systematic review of simulation studies. *PLoS One.* 2014;9(5):e97297.

36. Beutels P, Jia N, Zhou QY, Smith R, Cao WC, de Vlas SJ. The economic impact of SARS in Beijing, China. *Trop Med Int Health.* 2009;14 (suppl 1):85–91.

CHAPTER 83

Chemical Decontamination

Peter McCahill, Barbara Vogt, and John Sorensen

Decontamination is defined as the reduction or removal of chemical (or biological) agents by physical means or by chemical neutralization (detoxification) so that agents are no longer hazardous.[1] The major objectives of decontamination of victims exposed to a hazardous chemical is the prevention of further harm from the substance and the optimization of the chance for full clinical recovery.[2] An important secondary objective is to avoid spreading contaminated material to others or the health care facility (HCF). Although accidents from the manufacture, storage, or transportation of chemicals account for most instances of patient contamination, HCFs must now anticipate the intentional use of chemicals (including chemical warfare agents) to contaminate potentially large numbers of victims who may enter the facility individually or en masse, with or without prior decontamination. This chapter focuses on the decontamination of patients exposed to chemical warfare agents before entry to an HCF and the issues associated with preventing secondary or cross contamination of health care providers and their facilities. Also discussed are the problems associated with treating contaminated patients while wearing personal protective equipment (PPE).

Chemical agents exist in liquid, solid, or vapor form. Inhalation of vapors is the most likely route of exposure. Depending on the chemical's characteristics, physical properties, and exposure pathway, treatment for chemical warfare agent–contaminated patients is similar to other chemical casualties in the HCF environment. The management of terrorist-related events is more complex. A chemical attack would likely occur without warning, with an unknown substance, and in a location where large numbers of people are present or likely to pass through. These "outrage" factors elevate the perception of risk and safety-related fears, resulting in heightened psychological harm.[3,4] Other factors—a sense of helplessness and fear of unknown consequences from the exposure to oneself and others—may also result in large numbers of the "walking wounded" converging on an HCF without prior decontamination.

Given the covert measures usually employed by terrorists, health care providers should routinely be alert for signs and symptoms of contamination on patients and take immediate steps to protect themselves and their facility from becoming secondary victims. Facility managers, especially emergency department directors, should communicate early with first responders about unusual incidents to ensure prompt notification about any potentially contaminated patients. The same personnel should have the authority to lock down the HCF and reroute response teams and self-presenting victims to appropriate decontamination areas.

Field decontamination is generally the task of first responders (e.g., firefighters and hazardous materials [HazMat] teams) trained to use PPE and to process victims through decontamination units at the site of the chemical release. After an accidental release, the chemical's characteristics (including toxicity, persistence, and health effects) are frequently known through information on material safety data sheets or from managers or employees at the release site. Conversely, in a terrorist event, the chemical substance will likely be unknown, the dose uncertain, and the subsequent health effects undetermined. If the victims include children and infants, input from pediatricians and poison specialists will be needed. All victims will require debriefing (even if the chemical agents remain unknown at the time) after decontamination and treatment.

Field decontamination procedures are carried out in both rural and urban settings by full-time first responders or part-time volunteers with or without special equipment or training. Field decontamination of the potentially exposed often occurs as a precautionary measure, especially when health effects are unclear. Working with the hypothesis that removal of clothing reduces the majority of contaminants, most field decontamination efforts involve clothing removal and showering, either in a special decontamination unit (e.g., trailer on expedient setup) or by hosing off from firefighting hoses.[5] The objective of field decontamination is to transfer a clean victim to an HCF without contaminating the conveying vehicle or exposing others. Given the large uncertainty of field decontamination effectiveness, most victims undergo another round of decontamination at the HCF to ensure the level of cleanliness needed to protect the facility. Patients are often frightened during this process and may question the need for a second round of decontamination. First-receiving facilities should include an aggressive information operation campaign in all of their chemical attack response activities. It is essential that the HCF be able to lock down as soon as the potential for arrival of contaminated victims is detected, to protect critical assets such as health care providers, the HCF, and the existing patient population.

The most important element of treatment after exposure to a chemical warfare agent is to immediately remove the agent through decontamination. Decontamination that is delayed or ineffective can escalate the number of casualties when very toxic substances, such as nerve agents, are involved. If injuries are life threatening, victims are sometimes transported with minimal attention to the decontamination unit before arrival at the HCF. This problem can be exacerbated if communications between the field response units and medical facility fail to describe the event so that the HCF can take advance precautions, such as suiting up personnel in PPE, performing lockdown, and initiating decontamination setup. In a terrorist event, the number of victims transporting themselves to emergency departments could quickly overwhelm resources, as happened in the Tokyo subway incident.[6]

Treating a chemical warfare agent–contaminated patient is similar to handling patients contaminated by other hazardous chemicals, such as organophosphate pesticides, and requires similar precautions. Over

95% of surface contaminants can be eliminated by removing clothing and showering.[7] Although the process is well known and easy to accomplish with ambulatory victims, injured patients require increased numbers of personnel and resources to perform decontamination.[8]

The three primary types of decontamination important to the health care provider are as follows:

- Personal decontamination (i.e., self-decontamination or buddy decontamination when one is exposed)
- Casualty decontamination (i.e., decontamination of casualties)
- Personnel decontamination (generally, decontamination of noncasualties)

Personal decontamination may or may not involve PPE.[9] More often, personal decontamination (i.e., disrobing and bagging clothing, then showering with copious amounts of soap and water) is needed after an unprotected health care provider is exposed while caring for a contaminated patient who presents to an emergency department without alerting the admitting staff. If PPE is worn, all equipment including outer garments, gloves, boots, and respiratory apparatus should be decontaminated after removal. This will avoid the unnecessary cost of replacing expensive and individually fitted PPE. Health care providers should also be instructed in the proper donning and doffing of PPE to prevent exposing themselves or others to contaminated clothing surfaces.

Decontamination of chemical casualties and other exposed personnel requires a substantial outlay of resources and personnel.[10,11] Not all decontamination efforts will involve health care providers directly because HazMat teams are the general providers. However, medically trained personnel should provide overall supervision. The decontamination of each person should be monitored for adequate removal of agents and not left to the subjective evaluation of victims, especially children.[12,13] This process requires sensitivity and tact when handling civilian casualties, especially in the stressed environment of the disaster aftermath.

DECONTAMINATION SOLUTIONS

Many substances have been evaluated for their ability to remove contaminants from the skin. Compared with washing the skin with copious amounts of soap and water and irrigating the eyes with clean water, most have been found lacking. The most common problems are skin irritation, toxicity, ineffectiveness, and high cost. Although the military has used substances (such as special wipes) to determine whether the contaminant is removed, most health care providers must rely on subjective evaluations to assess decontamination effectiveness.

Disposal of contaminated solutions from decontamination of victims should follow the same procedures as disposal of other hazardous materials. If the contaminant is unknown or is suspected as benign at the time of decontamination, precautions such as holding secured drums of solution until a definitive result is obtained from later laboratory analysis can save the considerable expense of sending the wastewater to an HazMat disposal site. The U.S. Environmental Protection Agency (EPA) notes that in special circumstances where the protection of populations is critical, contaminated water can be diverted to storm sewer or sanitary disposal.[14] Although this is likely not an option for persistent biological agents, most chemical agents would likely be dispersed in this way without causing further harm.

It is often assumed that trained HazMat personnel perform normal decontamination procedures outside the emergency department; however, during an emergency, those same providers will likely be involved in search and rescue activities, with decontamination of exposed victims a low priority. Many victims will likely self-evacuate to the nearest medical facility without advising emergency department personnel.

After the Tokyo subway release of sarin, it was estimated that more than 10,000 victims presented to medical facilities on their own without any form of decontamination before arrival.[6]

SECONDARY CONTAMINATION

Because of the potential for secondary contamination, it is essential that medical personnel understand the need for and undergo training in the actual use of PPE. Surgical masks are not sufficient to protect against hazardous vapors from a contaminated patient's fluids or body parts.[15] This is also a problem if the contaminant was purposely ingested and regurgitated in vomitus. Some persistent chemical warfare agents are not immediately symptomatic or visually evident on a patient's skin, hair, or clothing. For example, sulfur mustard is a persistent oily substance producing signs and symptoms that can be delayed for 2 to 24 hours after exposure. It is also important that deceased victims of chemical agent events (even in body bags) be decontaminated prior to release to prevent secondary contamination of unsuspecting forensic or funerary workers.

A serious issue regarding chemical agents is the general absence of criteria to determine the effectiveness of decontamination efforts. Field decontamination performed by HazMat personnel is generally considered gross decontamination and should not be considered adequate for admitting patients to a medical facility. This is a serious problem if the medical facility has not planned for decontamination of patients being admitted and health care providers respond without determining the cleanliness of patients.[16] Reports of emergency departments being closed for several hours after health care providers were sickened by fumes from patients who were only field decontaminated suggest this could be a very real problem in large-scale disasters. Not only would the loss of health care providers create difficulties but also certifying that the HCF was clean enough to reopen could take several hours or, in the worst cases, several days. In a major disaster that disrupts normal infrastructure channels and communications, medical facility deliveries could be delayed for several days.

Chemical agents that might be used in a terror event include a wide variety of substances, ranging from chemical warfare agents such as nerve and sulfur mustard agents to riot control and choking agents. (Some consider toxins such as ricin from the castor bean plant a chemical derivative, but most authorities characterize toxins as biological agents because they are derived from living matter.) The individual chemical's characteristics and mode of release and the victim's own characteristics will determine how decontamination is performed. For example, most victims exposed but not symptomatic can accomplish decontamination on their own. But patients who are injured, wheelchair bound, elderly, or very young will require assistance. Decontaminating victims on litters often requires a team effort to coordinate the lifting required to move the victim from the dirty (hot) to clean (cold) zones.

An issue with most health care providers, especially in emergency departments, is the lack of training on wearing PPE while treating victims. PPE is becoming more available in emergency departments because The Joint Commission requires an emergency response incident management system that is integrated with the community response system. However, periodic training in the actual use of equipment during patient treatment is still lacking. Having enough equipment for each person and providing the necessary training (8 hours for some PPE) are often restricted by budgets and the common misperception that a mass chemical casualty event will not occur in one's hometown. As respirators must be fitted for individual use to prevent leakage around the face to protect the mouth and eyes, use of individual pieces of respiratory equipment by multiple persons is not acceptable.

Each wearer must also be trained in the proper decontamination of the PPE and how to don and doff the equipment effectively. Otherwise the facility, victims, and other health care providers will be placed at risk of secondary contamination.

Communication with patients and with other health care providers is difficult when wearing a full face mask respirator.[17] Handling equipment and providing care are severely hampered when wearing the recommended 7-mm-thick gloves instead of the more common latex ones. Movements are often hindered by cumbersome outerwear, especially if the facility uses a common air line for the supplied air for respirators. Those who do not want to wear PPE and instead rely on common barrier practices should not be allowed into the arena because the threat of secondary contamination from victims is too serious to allow the practice. Appropriate training in PPE can alleviate the feelings of confinement and dread that often affect first-time users. Enacting policies and publicizing them within the facility will help eliminate problems with noncompliant personnel during an actual event.

The Occupational Safety and Health Administration (OSHA) mandates specific stay and rest times while wearing PPE, especially in hot or cold environments. This adds to the total number of health care providers needed during the event. PPE and wear-time requirements dictated by state health authorities or OSHA may be more stringent than federal regulations and should be addressed in training sessions. Jurisdictional disputes over appropriate PPE and the training required should be addressed in reviewing yearly plans and in all Memorandums of Understanding (MOUs) and Memorandums of Agreement (MOAs) with other facility managers.

HISTORICAL PERSPECTIVE

The earliest documented use of gas warfare in the West occurred during the Peloponnesian War in the fifth century BC. Spartan forces besieging an Athenian city burned a mix of wood, pitch, and sulfur, in an effort to incapacitate the inhabitants.[18] World War I (WWI) saw the advent of modern chemical weapon usage. Substances included chlorine, phosgene, and mustard gas. It is estimated that over 124,000 tons of different agents were deployed during the conflict, resulting in 1.3 million casualties. As a result of the threat posed by these weapons, researchers began to look at ways to counteract them and treat patients who were exposed. On the day of the declaration of American involvement in WWI, the National Research Council subcommittee on noxious gases was created. Their mission was not only to develop compounds that could be weaponized but to find treatments and antidotes as well.[19] Due to fear of retaliatory use, chemical weapons were not seen on the battlefield again until the 1980s, during the war between Iran and Iraq. The sarin attacks in 1994 and 1995 in Japan represented the advent of chemical weapons–based terrorism.

CURRENT PRACTICES

To prevent the spread of contamination, knowing when and how to decontaminate patients is critical. Decontamination usually requires multiple teams to fully decontaminate victims. Factors to be considered in planning for a decontamination facility at HCFs include the number of patients to be processed, the number of personnel in PPE needed, the frequency of rotating those personnel, and the availability of PPE for rotating shifts.[20,21] This section discusses current decontamination practices at an HCF. This includes the physical layout of a decontamination area for handling both ambulatory and nonambulatory patients, mass-decontamination techniques, and self-decontamination and buddy decontamination procedures.

Physical Layout

Figure 83-1 shows one example of a casualty-receiving decontamination station. This can be situated in a field setting in an area safely distant from the accident site or at a hospital. The areas used for a station should be identified during the planning phase. A properly sited station will permit drainage from the decontamination process to be directed into a sump or a holding pond or container that can be emptied later during the recovery phase. The hot zone is the area considered to be contaminated. The cold zone is free from contamination. Plan the cold zone to be upwind, uphill, and upstream from the hot zone. Walk-in patients and those who cannot be confirmed as receiving decontamination from a certified HazMat unit in the field go to screening and triage stations in the hot zone before proceeding through the decontamination line. Medical personnel should determine whether those decontaminated in the field should be decontaminated again or whether they can proceed directly to the triage area.

Site location and layout for decontamination should be predetermined and well known to operators. Maintaining secure perimeter control and clean work areas are important. All staff should be aware of the potential problems of cross or secondary contamination and should know how to process patients through decontamination stations. All of this requires planning and practice through live drills. At an HCF, the decontamination station could be temporarily set up in a parking lot outside the emergency department using a portable unit, or a more permanent decontamination facility could be constructed adjacent to the emergency department. Macintyre and colleagues discuss descriptions of permanent facilities.[8] Common features of most stations include separate lines for ambulatory patients and nonambulatory patients. Each is discussed in more detail below.

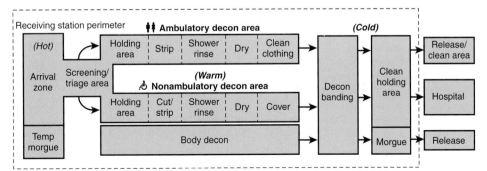

FIG 83-1 Layout of a Decontamination Station Outside a Health Care Facility. (From Federal Emergency Management Agency: Don't be a victim: medical management of patients contaminated with chemical agents [training video], Oak Ridge, Tenn., 2003, Oak Ridge National Laboratory.)

Ambulatory Patient Decontamination

Medical personnel should make the decision about who should proceed through the ambulatory line. The "walking wounded" and others tagged *minimal* can usually be sent to the ambulatory decontamination area, where fewer personnel are needed to supervise the self-decontamination process.

Medical personnel may decide to decontaminate ambulatory victims' wounds and remove bandages before allowing victims to shower. Keep in mind that bandages can readily absorb liquids or aerosols, so passing a victim with bandages across the contamination control line to relatively unprotected personnel could create a secondary hazard. Open wounds should never be decontaminated with a normal soap-and-water solution. First, remove previously applied dressings and foreign bodies from the wound. Then, flush the wound and surrounding areas with water and a tincture of green soap. Carefully decontaminate around the wound by wiping outward, pack the wound, and then seal with occlusive dressing before proceeding to full body decontamination.

Ambulatory patients should be instructed to remove all clothing and to bag personal effects. To avoid contamination of the eyes and mucous membranes, contaminated clothing should not be removed over the head but should instead be cut away and discarded. The patient should then shower with copious amounts of soap and water from the head down, leaning the head back to reduce the chance of residue contacting the eyes, nose, or mouth. Encourage careful cleaning of warm, moist areas such as under the armpits and the groin, followed by a thorough overall rinse with clean water.

Once decontaminated, patients should don clean clothing; Tyvek disposables or scrubs work well. Patients then should receive a standardized wristband indicating that decontamination has been completed and move to the cold zone staging area for screening and medical treatment. The best assurance that a victim is free of contamination is verification that they went through a thorough decontamination process. Most ambulatory patients will be capable of walking through the ambulatory decontamination lines, but some may need assistance. If possible, separate decontamination lines should be set up for males and females. When only two lines are possible, designate the second line for nonambulatory patients, such as people with wheelchairs or walkers, those on stretchers, or anyone else requiring assistance or supervision.

Decontamination is not necessary for patients who were never in the path of a plume or in a contaminated area and who are without signs and symptoms of exposure. However, if some persons are still concerned about possible contamination, they should be instructed to remove their outer layers of clothing and take a quick, 3- to 4-minute shower. Because much of the contamination, whether from liquid or vapor exposure, is removed by discarding clothing, that action followed by a rapid shower will likely eliminate 99% to 100% of the contaminant.

Nonambulatory Patient Decontamination

Nonambulatory patients displaying serious signs and symptoms of chemical exposure will be the first ones decontaminated in the nonambulatory area. Rapid decontamination is initiated, involving removal of clothing and a quick, high-volume shower focusing on exposed areas, such as skin, hair, and wounds. This should take a maximum of 5 to 10 minutes per patient. Health care providers should follow universal precautions when treating these victims, and they may decide to more thoroughly decontaminate a patient if severe signs and symptoms continue. Patients exhibiting moderate signs, or who have a confirmed liquid exposure, will be processed in the normal fashion once the rapid-decontamination patients have completed the process. Those with minimal signs and symptoms will follow those with moderate exposures.

Normal decontamination of nonambulatory patients usually takes two to four staff members and 10 to 20 minutes. The casualty's backboard or stretcher should be elevated to limit the amount of runoff exposure to the patient. Each staff member focuses on a quadrant of the victim's body, perhaps using the waist as a midline. Clothing is cut away or otherwise removed. Starting at the midline, spray or wipe the victim laterally or to the side or back of the victim. The sponge or brush used to decontaminate should be rinsed in the decontamination solution after each wipe. Once the front is finished, roll the victim to the side and proceed to decontaminate the back from the highest to lowest point.

Once the actual wiping process is complete, a liberal amount of solution should be used to rinse the patient, and then the patient is dried. The process requires 35 to 50 gallons per patient, and fresh decontamination solution should be used for each patient. Once the patient is cleaned, roll him or her onto a clean stretcher or backboard and transfer across the hotline into the cold area.

Mass Decontamination

Alternatively, victims may be decontaminated in one or more large groups; this is called *mass decontamination*. Chemical warfare agents can cause large numbers of casualties if dispersed in a vapor or aerosol, as manifested in the Tokyo subway incident. Such a situation could also occur in a high-profile event at a stadium, concert, or airport. The mass-decontamination process requires cordoning off several areas where a decontamination corridor can be set up with fire department aerials and/or deluge guns in close proximity. The nozzles are set at low volume so as not to inflict damage while maximizing the amount of water to which each victim is exposed. Ambulatory victims progress through the deluge so that they may be grossly decontaminated. In conjunction with removal of clothing, this will likely suffice to decontaminate those victims not exhibiting signs or symptoms of chemical agent exposure.

Another mass-decontamination method is to set up a sprinkler head near the exit point of the hot zone as a rudimentary decontamination shower. In this scenario, water delivered at 500 gallons per minute will produce 8 gallons per second. If the victim remains in the shower for 3 seconds on average, this equals 12 gallons—the amount used in a normal shower. In both scenarios, some clothing is left on, which reduces the effectiveness if vapor has penetrated to the skin.

Potentially contaminated runoff from mass-decontamination stations generally must be disposed of in compliance with local or state environmental regulations. The EPA has also published guidelines on this issue when conditions warrant otherwise.[14] The agency concluded that based on the "Good Samaritan" provision in the Comprehensive Environmental Response, Compensation, and Liability Act, Section 107d, first responders should undertake any necessary emergency action to save lives and protect the public and themselves. Section 107d states that no person will be liable for costs or damages resulting from actions taken or not taken rendering care, assistance, or advice under the National Contingency Plan or at the direction of the on-scene coordinator. This does not preclude liability for damages resulting from negligence. The EPA recommends that once imminent threats to human life are addressed, reasonable attempts should be made to contain wastewater and prevent environmental insult.

Self-Decontamination and Buddy Decontamination

If resources cannot be mobilized quickly enough to perform systematic and assisted decontamination, it is crucial to have a plan to instruct potentially exposed members of the public to either perform self-decontamination or assist another to decontaminate ("buddy decontamination"). Instructions should inform people to remove and bag all clothing and personal items, such as watches and jewelry, and thoroughly wash with copious amounts of soap and water followed by a clean water rinse. People should then don clean clothes and follow official instructions. To decontaminate eyeglasses, soak them in household bleach and then rinse with clean water. Although self-decontamination and buddy decontamination will not suffice for entry into an HCF, it will minimize health impacts to the exposed person and help avoid cross contamination.

⚠ PITFALLS

Decontamination of victims of a hazardous chemical release is fraught with problems, many of which can be alleviated with appropriate planning. Appropriate PPE is expensive, and maintaining the appropriate level of trained personnel for 24-hour operations will strain budgets and resource allocations.[22] Mass decontamination of victims of a chemical warfare agent release will likely exhaust even the most well-prepared medical facility, and currently there is inadequate evidence in the literature for making recommendations on the management of these scarce resources during a mass casualty event.[23] If the event is terrorist-instigated, there is also the possibility of the perpetrator(s) initiating a secondary hazard or hiding among the casualties. This increases the stress on health care providers accustomed to dealing only with a patients' medical issues. If the victims include a large number of fatalities, instructions for handling the deceased must be clearly detailed to prevent secondary contamination among medical personnel.

Communications may be difficult between health care providers and HazMat responders when the substance is unknown or widespread. The potential chaos caused by a chemical release makes the prior establishment of relations between HazMat teams and HCFs important. Founded understanding of equipment and practices between the two groups can simplify communication and minimize misunderstanding during an actual event.

Wearing protective respirators complicates communication between patients and health care providers. The situation is exacerbated by the potential conflict in agenda between crisis and consequent management teams. Deciding what takes priority—crime investigation or medical care—can be problematic, especially if the event is labeled an act of terrorism. Victims exposed to high levels of chemical warfare agents particularly need immediate care to offset rapid and potentially fatal effects, a need that may not be readily apparent to crime scene investigators.

An issue not often considered by health care providers is the special decontamination needs of the more vulnerable populations, such as elderly persons, children and young adolescents, or immune-compromised persons. Children may compose a significant portion of casualties in a terrorist attack because of their higher breathing rates, thinner skin, larger surface-to-mass ratio, smaller fluid reserves, and lower circulating blood volumes.[22,24] Such groups may also be more vulnerable to negative psychological effects.[25] Likewise, elderly persons may have underlying health problems, such as asthma, that exacerbate the health effects from a chemical release. Decontamination solutions and areas for disrobing and showering may not be heated. Care should be taken to avoid the necessity of treating victims for exposure (e.g., hypothermia). Having access to personal records of victims may be impossible in mass care situations, and health care providers may need to rely on subjective evaluations of stressed victims.

Lack of victim privacy when media personnel are on the scene has also been a problem.[26] Graphic photographs and videos of victims being decontaminated are sought by media outlets but only increase the stressful situation for victims.[27] Securing external perimeters of

areas for triage and decontamination of victims while the HCF is in lockdown may prevent such intrusion but may delay essential treatment as well. Innovative news correspondents may pose as victims to gain entry and access to victim's stories. Medical facilities that plan to use expedient items such as large trash bags for patient wear after decontamination should be aware that privacy can and will be a major issue for victims already subjected to unfamiliar decontamination procedures.

Preplanning for chemical agent incidents is still not universal.[28] Although planning for and providing resources for responding to a terrorist event have been advocated by The Joint Commission in cooperation with OSHA, studies of health care preparedness have found many facilities not in compliance. The focus of training and perpetrations should be adapted to the local resources and potential threats, while incorporating the knowledge gained from formal disaster research studies.[29]

The casual openness and use of volunteers at many entries to HCFs present significant vulnerabilities for contamination of the HCF, health care providers, and volunteers. A few HCFs provide separate waiting rooms for reasons other than maintaining a space for isolation of contaminated victims. Although this method of receiving patients is not likely to change soon, HCF managers and supervisors should consider reorganizing the environment to more easily adjust to the unexpected influx of contaminated patients after a disaster.

The number of pitfalls that can hinder effective decontamination efforts may seem overwhelming; however, with planning, management support, and appropriate resources and training, such events can be managed with less chaos and confusion. The most important factor is protection of the health care provider and the HCF to optimize the care provided to victims.

REFERENCES

1. Sidell FR, Takfuji ET, Franz DR, eds. Office of the Surgeon General, Department of the Army. In: *Textbook of Military Medicine, Part 1: Medical Aspects of Chemical and Biological Warfare.* Washington, DC: Borden Institute, Walter Reed Army Medical Hospital; 1997:352.
2. National Academy Press. *Chemical and Biological Terrorism: Research and Development to Improve Civilian Medical Response.* Washington, DC: National Academy Press; 1999, 97.
3. Slovic P, Fischhoff B, Lictenstein S. Facts and Fears: Understanding Perceived Risk. In: Schwing RC, Abers WA, eds. *Societal Risk Assessment: How Safe Is Safe Enough?* New York: Plenum; 1980:181–214.
4. Slovic P. *Perception of Risk.* London: Earthscan Pub; 2002, 225–226.
5. Cox RD. Decontamination and management of hazardous materials: exposure victims in emergency departments. *Ann Emerg Med.* 1994;23 (4):761–770.
6. Okamura T, Suzuki K, Fukuda A, et al. The Tokyo subway sarin attack: disaster management, part 2—hospital response. *Acad Emerg Med.* 1998;5 (6):618–624.
7. Keonig K. Strip and shower: the duck and cover for the 21st century. *Ann Emerg Med.* 2003;42(3):391–394.
8. Macintyre AG, Christopher GW, Eitzen E, et al. Weapons of mass destruction events with contaminated casualties: effective planning for health care facilities. *JAMA.* 2000;283(2):242–249.
9. Hick J, Penn P, Hanfling D, et al. Protective equipment for health care facility decontamination personnel: regulations, risks, and recommendations. *Ann Emerg Med.* 2003;42(3):370–380.
10. Burgess JL, Kirk M, Borron SW, et al. Emergency department hazardous materials protocol for contaminated patients. *Ann Emerg Med.* 1999;34 (2):205–212.
11. Hick J, Penn P, Hanfling D, et al. Establishing and training health care facility decontamination teams. *Ann Emerg Med.* 2003;42(3):381–390.
12. Rotenberg J, Burklow T, Selanikio J. Weapons of mass destruction: the decontamination of children. *Pediatr Ann.* 2003;32(4):261–267.

13. Wheeler D, Poss W. Mass casualty management in a changing world: an overview of the special needs of the pediatric population during a mass casualty emergency. *Pediatr Ann.* 2003;32(2):98–105.

14. *Office of Solid Waste and Emergency Response, Environmental Protection Agency. First Responder's Environmental Liability Due to Mass Decontamination Runoff.* Washington, DC: Chemical Emergency Preparedness and Prevention Office; 2000.

15. Burgess JL. Hospital evacuation due to hazardous materials incidents. *Am J Emerg Med.* 1999;17(1):50–52.

16. Brennan RJ, Waeckerle JF, Sharp TW, et al. Chemical warfare agents: emergency medical and emergency public health issues. *Ann Emerg Med.* 1999;34(2):91–204.

17. Moles TM. Emergency medical services systems and HAZMAT major incidents. *Resuscitation.* 1999;42(2):103–116.

18. Mayor A. *Greek Fire, Poison Arrows and Scorpion Bombs: Biological Warfare in the Ancient World.* New York: The Overlook Press; 2003.

19. Fitzgerald G. Chemical Warfare and Medical Response During World War I. *Am J Public Health.* 2008;98(4):611–625.

20. *Agency for Toxic Substances and Disease Registry. Hospital Emergency Departments: A Planning Guide for the Management of Contaminated Patients.* Atlanta: U.S. Department of Health and Human Services, Public Health Service ATSDR; 2000, Managing Hazardous Material Incidents; vol II.

21. Cone DC, Davidson SJ. Hazardous materials preparedness in the emergency department. *Prehosp Emerg Care.* 1997;1(2):85–90.

22. Burklow T, Yu C, Madsen J. Industrial chemicals: terrorist weapons of opportunity. *Pediatr Ann.* 2003;32(4):230–234.

23. Timbie JW, Ringel JS, Fox DS, et al. Systematic review of strategies to manage and allocate scarce resources during mass casualty events. *Ann Emerg Med.* 2013;61(6):677–689.

24. Blaschke G, Palfrey J, Lynch J. Advocating for children during uncertain times. *Pediatr Ann.* 2003;32(4):271–274.

25. Balk SJ, Gitterman BA, Miller MD, et al. Chemical-biological terrorism and its impact on children. *Pediatrics.* 2000;105(3):662–670.

26. Vogt B, Sorensen J. *How Clean Is Safe: Lessons Learned From Decontamination Experiences.* Oak Ridge, Tenn: Oak Ridge National Laboratory; 2002, ORNL/TM-2002/178.

27. DiGiovanni C. Domestic terrorism with chemical or biological agents: psychiatric aspects. *Am J Psychiatry.* 1999;156(10):1500–1505.

28. Treat KN, Williams JM, Furbee PM, et al. Hospital preparedness for weapons of mass destruction incidents: an initial assessment. *Ann Emerg Med.* 2001;35(5):562–565.

29. Der Heide EA. The importance of evidence-based disaster planning. *Ann Emerg Med.* 2006;47(1):34–49.

CHAPTER 84

Radiation Decontamination*

George A. Alexander

Merriam Webster's Collegiate Dictionary, 10th edition, lists 1936 as the year of the earliest known use of the word *decontaminate* in English.[1] *Decontaminate* is defined as follows: "to rid of contamination (as radioactive material)." To better appreciate the meaning of the word, one should first understand the concept of radiation contamination. Contamination occurs when material containing radioactive particles is deposited on skin, clothing, or any surface area of an inanimate object. A person contaminated with radioactive material will continue to be irradiated until the radioactive material (source of radiation) is eliminated or removed. Interestingly, radiation does not spread in a person; instead, it is the radioactive contamination that can spread. *External contamination* of a person may occur if radioactive material is deposited on external body surfaces or clothing. *Internal contamination* occurs if radioactive material is inhaled, ingested, injected into, or absorbed through wounds. The environment can also become contaminated if radioactive materials are uncontained or spread about.

Comprehensive concepts of radiation decontamination are presented in this chapter. The aim is to provide a framework in which to understand the principles of radiation decontamination and their application in controlling exposures to radioactive contamination. The chapter provides a brief historical perspective of radioactivity, summarizes current practices of radiation decontamination, and highlights obstacles to the execution of an optimal radiation decontamination response plan.

HISTORICAL PERSPECTIVE

Radiation injury to human cells was first recognized within months after Roentgen's discovery of x-rays in 1895.[2] In 1896 Becquerel discovered natural radioactivity—the emission of fast electrons from the nuclei of salts of uranium.[3] This mode of radioactive decay was termed *beta decay*. This discovery eventually led to another discovery and isolation of radium by Marie Curie in 1898.[4] In 1899 Rutherford described radioactive decay by the emission of alpha particles (helium nuclei).[5] And in 1900 Villard was the first to describe electromagnetic radiation release during radioactive decay known as gamma radiation.[6] The three major forms of radioactivity are alpha (α), beta (β), and gamma (γ), named for alpha particles, beta particles, and photon energy, respectively.

After their discovery, x-rays and radioactive materials were used with little regard for their biological effects. The consequences of careless handling and use of radiation sources soon became apparent. Many of the early workers who pioneered the medical applications of ionizing radiation experienced firsthand the deleterious effects of radiation. Curie's discovery of radium led her to receive the Nobel Prize for chemistry in 1911 and brought about the introduction of radium use in medicine and industry.[5] Internal contamination from radium caused injury to many workers of the radium watch dial–painting industry in the 1920s.[7]

In the early twentieth century the understanding of atomic physics increased rapidly and culminated in the nuclear era. The development of human-made radioactive isotopes during and after World War II was a factor in the establishment of the nuclear industry that had a workforce of several hundred thousand people. Only 97 cases of clinical radiation injury had occurred in this population by 1969.[7] Knowledge of radiation-monitoring procedures was an integral component of the civil defense programs of the 1960s directed against the threat of nuclear weapons use and thermonuclear war. Most of what is known today about radiation decontamination came about after the atomic bomb explosions of World War II and has evolved from three primary areas: therapeutic radiation exposures, radiation accidents, and military preparedness training directed at nuclear weapons–related injuries. The military experience has provided some of the most comprehensive and useful information on radiation decontamination.[8–10]

CURRENT PRACTICE

Basic techniques of radiation decontamination derived from the military can be applied to nonmilitary settings depending on the situation and resources available. Radiation is given off by radioactive particles, most of which appear as dust or debris as in the case of a detonation of a nuclear weapon or radiological dispersal device (RDD). For decontamination purposes, radiation is generally thought of as a solid. Four categories of decontamination are recognized[8]: (1) personal decontamination is decontamination of one's self; (2) casualty decontamination denotes decontamination of patient casualties; (3) personnel decontamination generally means decontamination of workers who are not patients; and (4) mechanical decontamination includes procedures to physically remove radioactive particulates. Radiation decontamination is not an emergency. Decontamination of casualties is a labor-intensive task. The process demands the dedication of a significant number of personnel and large amounts of time. Appropriate planning and training are a necessity. The demands may require a major contribution of resources.

Monitoring Instruments

A variety of instruments are available for detecting and measuring radiation. Radiation monitoring entails the measurement of radiation fields in the vicinity of a radiation source, measurement of surface

---

*The views expressed in this chapter are those of the author and do not necessarily represent the official policy or position of the National Cancer Institute, the National Institutes of Health, or the U.S. Department of Health and Human Services.

contamination, and measurement of airborne radioactivity. Such monitoring methods are also known as radiation surveys. Radiation survey meters are used to evaluate radiation contamination of patients, equipment, or the environment. Old civil defense instruments, such as the CD V-700 and CD V-715 survey meters, can be used. The CD V-700 meter is used to detect low-intensity gamma and most beta radiation. It can measure only up to 50 mR/h. The CD V-715 meter is used to measure high-intensity gamma radiation. It can measure up to 500 R/h; however, it cannot detect beta or alpha radiation. These instruments are also called Geiger counters or Geiger-Mueller meters.

Newer portable and compact radiation monitor units with digital readouts and alarm systems are commercially available to measure alpha, beta, and/or gamma radiation. Because alpha radiation travels a very short distance in air and is not penetrating, radiation survey instruments cannot detect alpha radiation through even a thin layer of water, blood, dust, paper, or other materials. Most beta emitters can be detected with a survey instrument, such as a CD V-700, provided the metal probe cover is opened. Because gamma radiation or x-rays frequently accompany the emission of alpha and beta radiation from radioactive isotopes, the latter constitute both an external and internal hazard to humans. Gamma radiation is readily detected with survey instruments.

Radiological Assessment

In the period immediately after a detonation of, for example, a nuclear or large RDD, there will be considerable uncertainty about the nature and extent of radioactive contamination. It is imperative that radiation measurements be obtained as soon as possible to implement proper protective actions against potential radiological hazards. On-scene radiological assessments can be easily and rapidly performed using exposure rate measurements. However, assessments of long-term consequences require knowledge of the specific radioactive isotopes and more specialized skills.[11] An RDD that contains nuclear spent fuel as a radiation source will probably release one or a few radioisotopes on detonation. This simple source is easier to measure and characterize than mixed radiation sources potentially released from nuclear reactors or weapons. For nearly a century, epidemiologic studies of various human populations exposed to ionizing radiation have provided significant quantitative information on health risks. Much data are known about radiation and its risks; however, the important unanswered question is what the level of risk is from low dose exposures.[12]

Prehospital Decontamination

Most health care workers, such as emergency first responders, hospital first receivers, and others, lack radiation-related training.[13] These responders have not received sufficient training about ionizing radiation, radiation safety, and managing, diagnosing, or treating radiation-related injuries. The effectiveness of any medical response and recovery effort can be improved by providing a radiation training strategy for the health care delivery team. The detonation of a nuclear or radiological device within a U.S. city would create a national need for health care practitioners to manage radiation casualties. To provide guidance for health care providers about the diagnosis and treatment of radiation injury during nuclear and radiological emergencies the Department of Health and Human Services launched the Radiation Emergency Medical Management (REMM) website in 2007.[14] Since that time REMM content has expanded significantly with a variety of REMM versions having been launched.[15] State radiation safety or health departments should provide field teams to assist in radiation monitoring at the scene of a nuclear or radiological incident. The radiological evaluation of injured patients should be performed by persons with radiation health and safety training under the supervision of on-scene medical personnel.[11] Patient decontamination performed by emergency responders should be brief. The goal should be to remove all gross radioactive dust or debris from body surfaces. If clothing and shoes are contaminated, they should also be removed. These measures may benefit the patient by eliminating sources of radiation exposure and reducing the cumulative absorbed dose the patient would have received. Depending on the severity of injuries and the extent of radiation exposure, these simple decontamination methods may be life-saving while the patient is en route to more definitive care at the nearest hospital emergency department.

Hospital Decontamination

To prevent or minimize the occurrence of radiological contamination of the hospital facility and staff, a decontamination area should be established outside the hospital, preferably downwind from the clean treatment area or hospital entrance. A patient arrival/triage area should be downwind from the decontamination area. Wind direction is vital because resuspension of radioactive dust may occur downwind from the contaminated area. Outdoor patient decontamination is always performed downwind from the patient arrival/triage area.[8] Ideally the decontamination area should be set up to take advantage of the prevailing wind. The setup should be adaptable. Consideration must be given to the security of the decontamination area. An outdoor shower system may also be considered for use of mass decontamination. Portable vacuum units with high-efficiency particulate air filters have reportedly been used to facilitate rapid decontamination outdoors.[16]

An entry control point is necessary to identify and manage movement of clean and contaminated vehicles to the decontamination site. Control of patient and staff movement is critical to ensure that contaminated ambulatory patients and staff do not accidentally contaminate clean areas. A hotline (i.e., division between contaminated and clean zone) should be established and secured. Any people or equipment leaving a contaminated area must undergo radiological monitoring to make sure that radioactive contaminants do not enter clean areas. In addition, a radiation emergency area (a location for indoor decontamination) should be part of the radiation emergency plans in the event that patients contaminate the hospital.[16] Hospitals with nuclear medicine departments have an added resource—a gamma camera. A gamma camera is a perfect device for detecting nuclear fission products from either nuclear detonations or nuclear power plant reactors accidents.

Patient Decontamination

Removal of outer clothing and rapid washing of exposed skin and hair remove 95% of contamination.[8] Standard patient decontamination is normally performed under the supervision of medical personnel.[11] Moist cotton swabs of the nasal mucosa from both sides of the nose should be obtained, labeled, and sealed in separate bags. These swabs can be used as evidence for inhalation of radioactive particles. A 0.5% sodium hypochlorite solution can be used to remove radioactive contamination from intact skin. Radioactive material removed from the patient should be preserved for later analysis to identify the specific radioisotope. Maintain care not to irritate the skin. If skin becomes erythematous, some radioactive isotopes can be absorbed directly through the skin. Surgical irrigating solutions, such as normal saline or lactated Ringer's solution, should be used liberally in wounds, the abdomen, and the chest. These solutions should be removed using suction instead of wiping or sponging. For the eyes, only abundant amounts of water, normal saline, or eye wash solutions are recommended. If feasible, skin wash water should be contained and held for disposal. Contaminated tourniquets are changed with clean ones. Wounds should be covered after adjacent skin is decontaminated to prevent skin contaminants from entering the wound.

Wound Decontamination

During initial decontamination in the receiving/triage area, bandages should be removed and all wounds flushed. If bleeding persists, apply fresh bandages. Highly energetic gamma emitters can present an immediate hazard to contaminated wounds. Particulate matter contaminating a wound should be removed if possible. Alpha and beta emitters left in a wound can cause extensive local injury and may be absorbed into the systemic circulation, where they will be redistributed as internal contaminants; this can cause additional internal organ injury from irradiation. After adequate decontamination of the wound is achieved, it should be copiously irrigated with saline or some other physiological solution. Aggressive surgery, such as amputation, is not necessary and should never be used to manage radioactive contamination of a limb. Partial-thickness burns should be extensively irrigated and cleaned with mild solutions to prevent irritation of burned skin. In full-thickness burns, the presence of radioactive contaminants requires specialized surgical treatment.

Mechanical Decontamination

Radiological contamination may involve one or more radioactive elements. This section addresses the specific decontamination of six common radioactive elements.[9] The decontamination principles discussed here are also applicable to radiological contamination by other elements with chemical properties similar to those discussed below.

Cesium

The most common radioisotope of cesium is cesium-137. It emits beta and gamma radiation, decaying to stable barium-137. Cesium-137 is widely used in gamma sources. It occurs in these sources as cesium chloride pellets. Cesium chloride is a soluble salt. The contamination from a sealed-source leak absorbs water, becomes damp, and creeps. Contamination from a sealed cesium source is best decontaminated by wet procedures unless the contamination is on a porous surface, in which case, vacuuming should precede wet procedures. Cesium is known to adsorb from a solution onto glass surfaces. Decontaminating a liquid cesium–contaminated surface is best accomplished by wetting the surface, absorbing the solution with a rag or other absorbent material, and rinsing the area several times with water. If the contamination persists, use a detergent solution and scrub with a brush.[9]

Cobalt

The most common radioisotope of cobalt is cobalt-60, which is a beta and gamma emitter. Metallic cobalt-60 is commonly used in sealed gamma sources. Particles of cobalt dust adhering to small articles are readily removed by ultrasonic cleaners or by dipping the article in a dilute solution of nitric, hydrochloric, or sulfuric acid. Cobalt dust contamination that exists over a large area is best removed by vacuuming. Sealed cobalt sources may leak as a result of electrolytic action between the cobalt and the container. The result is often a soluble cobalt salt, which creeps and spreads. This is best decontaminated with a detergent or an ethylenediamine tetraacetic acid solution, followed by treatment with mineral acids. Contamination from solutions containing cobalt may be treated with water.[9]

Plutonium

The most common isotope in which plutonium may be present as a contaminant is plutonium-239, which is an alpha emitter. Plutonium contamination may be the result of a nuclear weapons accident, in which case the plutonium will be scattered as a metal or oxide in a dust form. Both forms of plutonium are insoluble. Aging of plutonium-239 contamination is impractical because it has a 24,000-year half-life. Plutonium contamination that covers a small area is best decontaminated by vacuuming. If contamination remains, the area should be washed with a detergent solution. Any contamination that remains can be sealed in a protective coating of paint, varnish, or plastic. Plutonium oxide or metal dust spread over a large area, such as a field, is best decontaminated by removing the top layer of soil and disposing of it as radioactive waste.[9] Because inhalation is generally considered the most likely route of entry of plutonium during a nuclear accident or nuclear terrorist incident there can be considerable harm to humans from plutonium exposure.[17] Personnel should wear respiratory protection when decontaminating or removing the soil.[9]

Strontium

The most common radioisotope of strontium is strontium-90, which is a beta emitter. The daughter particle of strontium-90 is yttrium-90, which is also a beta emitter. Strontium-90-yttrium-90 is commonly used in sealed beta sources. Generally it is present as a chlorine or carbonate. The chlorine is hygroscopic; it absorbs water and creeps out of the container. This contamination is best decontaminated by vacuuming, followed by treatment with water, a complexing agent solution (i.e., substance capable of forming a complex compound with another material in solution), and a mineral acid, in that order. Contamination resulting from a strontium-containing solution is best decontaminated by absorbing the solution with rags or other absorbing materials and washing the area with a detergent solution. If strontium contamination persists, the top layer of the surface should be removed by abrasives or other removal procedures and a sealing coat should be placed over the surface.[9]

Tritium

Tritium is the radioisotope of hydrogen and is a weak beta emitter. If it is released to an area as a gas, the best decontamination method is to flush the area with air. As inhalation tritium can present an internal hazard, personnel entering an area containing tritium gas should wear an appropriate self-contained type of breathing apparatus. Objects in an area exposed to tritium for any great length of time may absorb the gas and should be disposed of, if possible. They may be degassed, under a vacuum, by flushing with helium or hydrogen. A surface that is monitored as clean may become contaminated again in a matter of hours by percolation. There is no practical way of removing tritium oxide (T_2O) from water due to its similarity to natural water.[9]

Uranium

The most probable source of uranium contamination is a nuclear weapon accident in which the fissionable uranium is spread as a metal or oxide dust. The common isotopes of uranium contamination are uranium-235 and uranium-238. This metal or oxide is insoluble and is best removed from a contaminated surface by brushing or vacuuming, followed by a treatment with mineral acids or oxidizing acids, and then the area should be sealed. Large-area uranium contamination is best decontaminated by removing the top layer of the surface or by sealing it.[9]

Equipment and Building Decontamination

In most instances of equipment and building contamination, a mixture of normal household cleaning practices will remove the radioactive material. Vacuum cleaners that can handle wet material and have high-efficiency particulate air filters are suggested.

Personal Protective Equipment

Members of on-scene field radiological decontamination teams and hospital-based teams should have appropriate protective equipment to meet all requirements for radiation decontamination. Emergency medical services and hospital personnel responsible for patient decontamination should also be appropriately equipped to protect themselves from the hazards of radioactive contamination.

Respiratory Protective Devices

There are two types of respiratory protective devices: air-purified respirators, which remove contaminants from breathing air by filtering or chemical absorption, and air-supplied respirators, which provide clean air from an outside source or from a tank. Most air-purified respirators (i.e., protective masks) afford excellent protection from inhalation of radioactive material. Radioisotopes such as radon and tritium gas will pass through these filters. However, short exposures to these gases are not considered medically significant. The device providing the greatest factor of safety for a particular radiation incident should be used.

In nuclear weapons accidents or terrorist incidents, most nuclear weapons will contain high explosives in varying amounts—even as much as hundreds of pounds. Detonation of high explosives in nuclear weapons will cause a major radiological threat—the release of plutonium-239.[18] When associated with a fire, metallic plutonium may burn, producing radioactive plutonium oxide particles and serious inhalation and wound deposition hazards. In these situations use of self-contained breathing apparatuses should be considered.

In RDD incidents in which radioactive contamination is associated with fire and dangerous chemical fumes from burning metals and plastics, use of self-contained breathing apparatuses should be considered. Such devices enable radiation response and decontamination workers to enter a contaminated or oxygen-deficient environment, up to the limits of the respirator. They should be used when it is necessary to enter a highly contaminated environment to rescue persons, for example, from RDD incidents or nuclear power plant accidents.

Protective Clothing

Anticontamination suits are commercially available for use in nuclear and radiological disasters. Chemical-protective clothing provides excellent protection against radioactive contamination while also offering protection from chemical and biological agents or hazards. A wide variety of chemical-protective clothing is available to protect the body, including gloves, boots, coveralls, and total-encapsulation protective suits. Standard hospital barrier clothing that is used in universal precautions is adequate for protection of hospital personnel who provide emergency evaluation and treatment to limited numbers of radiologically contaminated patients. In these instances, hospital personnel should be decontaminated after the patients' emergency treatment and decontamination.

Radiation Dosimeters

There are a variety of detectors used to measure a person's level of radiation exposure.[19] Film badges, thermoluminescent dosimeters (TLDs), pocket dosimeters, or other devices should be used by radiation decontamination personnel, emergency responders, and hospital medical providers who are involved in any nuclear accident or terrorist incident.

Film badges are the most common dosimeter in use. They are worn on the outer clothing and are used to measure gamma, x-ray, and high-energy beta radiation. A badge consists of a small piece of photographic film wrapped in an opaque cover and held in a metal frame. It can be worn as a ring or pinned to clothing. Radiation interacts with the atoms in the film to expose the film. At periodic intervals, the film is removed and is developed to determine the amount of radiation exposure. A film badge provides a permanent record of radiation exposure.

TLDs are used for measuring gamma, x-ray, and beta radiation exposures. They can be worn as rings or body badges. They contain small chips of lithium fluoride, which absorb ionizing radiation energy and displace electrons from their ground state. The electrons then become trapped in a metastable state but can be restored to their original ground state by heating. When heated, the electrons return to their ground state and light is emitted. A TLD readout instrument is used to heat the chips and measure the emitted light. The amount of light emitted is related to the dose of radiation absorbed by the TLD and to the radiation exposure dose of the individual. TLDs are beginning to replace film badges.

A pocket dosimeter is a direct-reading portable unit shaped like a fountain pen with a pocket clip. It is worn on the trunk of the body and is generally used to measure x-ray and gamma radiation. It should be used in conjunction with a TLD rather than in place of TLD use. The pocket dosimeter consists of a quartz fiber, a scale, a lens to observe movement of the fiber across the scale, and an ionization chamber. The quartz fiber is charged electrostatically until it reaches zero on the scale. When the dosimeter is exposed to radiation, some of the atoms of air in the chamber become ionized. This causes the static electricity charge to leak from the quartz fiber in direct response to the amount of radiation present. As the charge is lost, the fiber moves to some new position on the scale that indicates the amount of radiation exposure.

The main advantage of the pocket dosimeter is that it can be read immediately by the wearer, even while working in a radiation-contaminated environment, instead of waiting for processing of a film badge or TLD. However, because pocket dosimeters lose their electrical charge over time, they may give a false indication of radiation exposure. When practicable, use of two dosimeters can prevent false interpretation of a person's exposure. One should assume that the lower reading is the actual exposure.

Basic Radiation Safety

During a nuclear or radiological disaster it is vital that emergency medical responders, decontamination team personnel, and hospital health care providers adhere to the basic principles of radiation safety. These actions will help to prevent or minimize the risk of these persons becoming radiation casualties due to exposure to radioactive contaminants. The three basic principles of radiation protection are time, distance, and shielding.

Time

The longer the exposure to radioactive contaminants, the possibility of radiation injury is greater. There is a direct relationship between the exposure dose received and the duration of exposure. Reducing exposure time in a contaminated area will reduce the radiation exposure. The maximum acceptable exposure time can be calculated based on the exposure dose rate measured using radiation survey meters at a given incident scene and the maximum dose that is needed to accomplish radiation decontamination or other task. In practice the dose received in completing a task may be spread over several workers so that no one person's exposure exceeds guide levels.

Distance

The inverse square law states that the dose from a radiation point source decreases with the square of the distance from the source. For example, doubling the distance from the source of radiation, the exposure would be decreased to $(\frac{1}{2})^2$, or one fourth of the original amount. In nuclear or radiological incidents, the radiation source may not be equivalent to a point source and so the inverse square law can be used as an approximation. In most instances, the approximation should be adequate. Maintaining a safe distance is especially critical. The larger the distance from a radiation source, the lower the dose.

There are certain emergency response operations that cannot be performed without some exposure of workers. In these situations, all unnecessary exposure to radiation should be avoided, even if it means barring workers from entering contaminated areas. These hazardous areas should be barricaded or roped off to form a restricted area that cannot be entered by non–radiation workers or bystanders.

Shielding

Shielding is generally used to safeguard against radiation from radioactive sources. The more mass placed between a source and a person, the less radiation the person will receive. This should be the guiding principle. Proper shielding from a source requires knowledge of the type of radiation hazard.[19] Different types of shielding are required for alpha, beta, and gamma radiation. Light clothing will provide protection and prevent contamination of the body from alpha radiation. Light metals such as aluminum are preferred for shielding from beta emissions. A sheet of aluminum can stop most beta radiation. Plexiglas is another shielding material that is effective against beta particles. Because gamma radiation is more penetrating than alpha and beta particles, higher-density materials such as lead, tungsten, steel, and concrete are ideal for shielding gamma rays. As the thickness of these materials increases, the intensity of the gamma radiation will decrease.

⚠ PITFALLS

Obstacles preventing the delivery of proper radiation decontamination procedures in response to a radiation catastrophe include the following:

- Lack of adequate radiation decontamination planning by emergency medical and hospital responders for possible nuclear or radiological accidents and/or terrorist incidents
- Lack of commitment of resources for radiation decontamination preparedness by emergency and hospital disaster planners
- Lack of consultation and involvement of medical or health physicists in planning radiation decontamination plans and protocols
- Lack of coordination with local and state radiological health and safety agencies
- Lack of understanding by medical providers and assigned decontamination team personnel of the basic science of radioactive isotopes and principles of radiation injury
- Lack of adequate training in radiation decontamination techniques
- Lack of recognition of the importance of radiation safety by emergency medical response personnel
- Lack of proper radiation safety equipment and monitoring devices and instruments

REFERENCES

1. *Merriam-Webster's Collegiate Dictionary*. 10th ed. Springfield, Mass: Merriam-Webster; 1997.
2. Zajtchuk R, Jenkins DP, Bellamy RF, et al, eds. *Medical Consequences of Nuclear Warfare*; Vol 2. Falls Church, Va: TMM Publications, Office of the Surgeon General; 1989.
3. Becquerel H. Sur les radiations émises par phosphorescence. *Compt Rend*. 1896;122:420.
4. Wilson W. *A Hundred Years of Physics*. London: Gerald Duckworth; 1950.
5. Weber RL. *Pioneers of Science: Nobel Prize Winners in Physics*. London: The Institute of Physics; 1980.
6. Villard P. Sur la réfraction des rayons cathodiques et des rayons déviables du radium. *Compt Rend*. 1900;130:1010.
7. Wald N. Radiation injury. In: Cassel C, McCally M, Abraham H, eds. *Nuclear Weapons and Nuclear War: A Source Book for Health Professionals*. New York: Praeger; 1984:121–138.
8. Jarrett D, ed. *Medical Management of Radiological Casualties: Handbook*. Bethesda, Md: Armed Forces Radiobiology Research Institute; 1999, AFRRI special publication 99-2.
9. U.S. Department of the Army and the Commandant, Marine Corps. *NBC Decontamination. Army Field Manual 3-5; Marine Corps Warfighting Publication 3-37.3*; July 28, 2000, Washington, DC.
10. U.S. Army Center for Health Promotion and Preventive Medicine. *The Medical NBC Battlebook. USACHPPM Tech Guide 244*; 2000, Washington, DC.
11. National Council of Radiation Protection and Measurement. *Management of Terrorist Events Involving Radioactive Material: Report No. 138*. Bethesda, Md: National Council on Radiation Protection and Measurement; 2001.
12. Boice JD Jr. Radiation epidemiology: a perspective on Fukushima. *J Radiol Prot*. 2012;32:N33–N40.
13. Blumenthal DJ, Bader JL, Christensen D, et al. A sustainable training strategy for improving health care following a catastrophic radiological or nuclear incident. *Prehosp Disaster Med*. 2014;29:80–86.
14. Bader JL, Nemhauser J, Chang F, et al. Radiation event medical management (REMM): website guidance for health care providers. *Prehosp Emerg Care*. 2008;12:1–11.
15. National Library of Medicine, National Institutes of Health. Radiation Emergency Medical Management (REMM) Website http://www.rem.nlm .gov. Accessed June 24, 2014.
16. Fong FH Jr. Nuclear detonations: evaluation and response. In: Hogan DE, Burstein JL, eds. *Disaster Medicine*. Philadelphia: Lippincott Williams & Wilkins; 2002:317–339.
17. Scott BR, Peterson VL. Risk estimates for deterministic health effects of inhaled weapons grade plutonium. *Health Phys*. 2002;85:280–293.
18. Berger M, Byrd B, West CM, et al. Transport of Radioactive Materials: Q&A About Incident Response. Oak Ridge, Tenn: Oak Ridge Associated Universities; 1992.
19. Martin JE. *Physics for Radiation Protection*. New York: John Wiley & Sons; 2000.

85 CHAPTER

Military Lessons Learned for Disaster Response*

David W. Callaway and Paul M. Robben

Military medicine has often driven advancements in the provision of medical care in austere environments. Military medicine encompasses all aspects of health care required to keep the fighting force healthy and deployed. The result is a diverse requirement, including response to complex polytrauma, management of large numbers of patients in a short period of time, care for patients during prolonged transports, and the prevention, recognition, and management of endemic communicable diseases. These attributes are shared with the characteristics of clinical care for patients following a humanitarian crisis or disaster situation. Though the fields are drawing ever closer together, humanitarian assistance (HA) and disaster response (DR) remain somewhat distinct in practice and scope. This chapter focuses on the U.S. military experience and relevant lessons learned for domestic DR and international HA/DR missions.

HISTORICAL PERSPECTIVE

The U.S. Department of Defense (DoD) has a long history of applying the unique capabilities of the individual armed services to HA and DR efforts following both natural and human-made disasters. In 1882 the U.S. Army Corps of Engineers provided support to the Army Quartermaster Corps' efforts to rescue people and property during flooding of the Mississippi River.[1] In 1899 the U.S. Army Medical Department's role in the response to a severe hurricane in Puerto Rico was guided by the military governor's chief surgeon and involved the disbursement of more than 60 tons of medical supplies.[2] DoD elements executed Operation Damayan in November 2013 as part of a broad multinational response to the devastation wrought upon the Philippines by Typhoon Yolanda or Haiyan.

The U.S. military's medical system has long played a part in response efforts, treating local populations abroad during and after complex emergencies, providing logistical support for governmental and private aid organizations, and ensuring secure operating space for humanitarian actors. Despite this long history of participation in HA/DR to natural disasters and complex emergencies, the role of the DoD and its impact on the practice of HA/DR has been questioned both internally and by civilian agencies.[3] Historically the HA community has argued against military involvement in HA/DR operations, citing the Geneva Convention and International Humanitarian Law (IHL),

which emphasize neutrality, impartiality, and independence. This philosophy has many valid supporting arguments, but practically has resulted in distinct professional approaches to HA/DR. In addition, the increased prevalence of intrastate conflict and the proliferation of nonstate actors utilizing service-restriction tactics (e.g., destroying health care facilities, restricting water and food deliveries, and gender-based violence) have worsened the "dilemma of neutrality" and are challenging the historic concepts fundamental to IHL.[4]

Traditionally the civilian medical intervention in fragile regions was divided into DR, HA, and international development (ID). Each sphere defined their role vis-à-vis crisis response in somewhat narrow terms. DR was largely short-term, high-intensity interventions meant to stabilize populations in the post-event phase. The DR field was dominated by government organizations, such as the Department of Health and Human Service's (DHHS) Disaster Medical Assistance Teams (DMATs), the U.S. Agency for International Development (USAID) Disaster Assistance Response Teams (DARTs), and the Office of the United Nations Disaster Relief Coordinator (UNDRC), now part of the U.N. Office for the Coordination of Humanitarian Affairs (OCHA). Emergency medicine professionals (e.g., physicians, paramedics, and emergency department [ED] nurses) dominated the dynamic DR field. HA developed in response to longer-term "creeping crises," such as droughts, famines, and large-scale population migrations. The U.N. Department of Humanitarian Affairs (DHA) ultimately merged with the UNDRC to form OCHA, which covers HA and DR missions. The HA industry largely defined and developed the principles of IHL and applied these principles across decades of global response. The HA professionals tended to have stronger interests in public health, primary care, and infectious diseases. ID as a generality is comprised of policy experts, public health specialists, and health economists approaching broad issues via activities that will span years and require decades to achieve the desired effects.

Multiple factors are driving the evolution of the military medical system's role in HA and DR. The most significant shaping factor has been the engagement of the United States in the broadly defined Global War on Terrorism (GWOT) since 2001. In addition to large-scale conventional operations in Afghanistan and Iraq, the U.S. military has engaged in counterinsurgency (COIN) engagements and stability operations across the Middle East, Africa, and Southeast Asia. Each mission profile adds unique contributions to the development of medical systems, mission planning, and logistical support for medical operations.

---

*The views expressed in this article are those of the authors and do not necessarily reflect the official policy or position of the U.S. Army, Department of Defense (DoD), or the U.S. government.

Operation Iraqi Freedom began on March 19, 2003, and major combat operations lasted less than 2 months, ending with President George W. Bush's now infamous declaration of "mission accomplished" on May 1, 2003. The initial stage of Operation Enduring Freedom was similar in length. The first Pentagon-acknowledged ground action occurred on October 19, 2001, the Taliban lost Kabul on December 7, 2001, and the birth of the U.N.-authorized International Security Assistance Force and swearing in of Hamid Karzai marked the birth of the new transitional central government before the end of December 2001. The exceedingly short period of time required for domination of the battlefield contrasts starkly with the more than 10 years of irregular warfare, including COIN, counterterrorism, foreign internal defense activities, and the peacekeeping and stability operations that have followed. The persistent, long-term execution of these missions has resulted in changes in practice and procedure through trial-and-error discovery of best practices. Lessons derived from COIN and stability operations, including the establishment of tiered treatment facilities, development of streamlined patient transport systems, utilization of electronic patient tracking, forward deployment of mobile critical care capabilities, emphasis on local capacity-building partnerships, and interagency coordination, often have applicability to HA and DR efforts.

The second factor driving the convergence of military and DR medicine is current U.S. National Security Strategy (NSS). The U.S. NSS outlines the nation's major security concerns and the authoring presidential administration's goals and preferred methods for addressing those challenges. The current NSS is built upon the three pillars of *defense, diplomacy,* and *development.*[5] DR is represented in all three key pillars. After the conclusion of the Cold War, the 1999 NSS authored by President Bill Clinton's administration referenced DR and disaster relief efforts multiple times, placing them in the context of affecting both the important national interests and humanitarian interests of the United States.[6] President George W. Bush's 2002 document focused primarily on response to the September 11, 2001, attacks and gave little mention to DR. However, in President Bush's 2006 update to the NSS, reference is again made to DR, most notably recognizing that coordinated disaster relief efforts have contributed to improvements in regional conflicts in Indonesia and between India and Pakistan.[7] An NSS published by the Obama administration in 2010 references disaster relief efforts several times, but often commenting on the need to focus inward on the domestic preparedness of the United States. In practice, however, the U.S. government (USG) has used DR as a tool of diplomacy and soft-power exertion in multiple high-profile events since 2010, including responses to the Haiti earthquake, Japan earthquake, and 2014 Philippines hurricane.

The current U.S. foreign affairs policy articulates a "whole of government" approach to development and DR, closely aligning subordinate components of the Department of State (DoS), USAID, and DoD. Department of Defense Directive (DoDD) 3000.5 (November 28, 2005) is the guiding directive that articulates the importance of integration of civilian and military efforts to achieve successful stability operations. DoDD 3000.5 also outlines the manner in which the DoD will interact with foreign governments and security forces, global and regional international organizations (IOs), nongovernmental organizations (NGOs), private sector individuals, and for-profit companies. Title 10, US Code, Section 401 governs U.S. military involvement in international HA/DR and articulates the manner in which the DoD may be activated to support operations and the technical assistance that the DoD may lawfully provide during HA/DR missions. This "whole of government" strategy drives funding requirements and therefore programmatic development. The result has been increased DoD engagement in the HA/DR space. According to Dr. Stewart Patrick, the DoD is now the major

provider of official development assistance (ODA). Between 1998 and 2005 the Pentagon's share of total U.S. ODA rose from 4% to 22%, or to $5.5 billion, with the majority spent in Iraq and Afghanistan. This percentage has since declined to 18%.[8]

Third, intrastate conflict has emerged as one of the most significant challenges in modern DR (e.g., conflict as either an initiating factor or consequence of disaster). A brief survey of major humanitarian crisis and disaster zones from 2013 to 2014 includes civil wars and massive population displacements in Syria, the Central African Republic, the Democratic Republic of Congo, South Sudan, and Somalia.[9] In 2013-2014 infectious disease outbreaks, such as cholera in Nigeria, polio in Syria, and measles in the Sahel, can also be directly linked to ongoing violence. With human conflict an impetus for, or a direct consequence of, many modern disasters, the world's militaries are increasingly working side by side with civilian HA/DR and development organizations.

Finally, beyond these geopolitical realities, military medicine and DR share a variety of similar operational challenges and often demand overlapping skill sets. Both combat and DR present multimodal challenges to the delivery of care, including, but not limited to, logistics, security, multiagency coordination, data collection, rapid modification of medical care protocols, and disciplined adherence to the mission at hand. However, perhaps the most unifying challenge is the "tyranny of distance" that affects all aspects of combat and DR.

CURRENT PRACTICE

Domestic Response Systems

Military medicine has had a fundamental role in the development of domestic DR strategies, especially in the United States. The military's influence on civilian disaster management can be broadly categorized into operational systems and clinical care. Key among the systems contributions are the Incident Command System (ICS) and principles of high-reliability organizations (HROs). The ICS is an all-hazards incident management approach for the command, control, and coordination of emergency responses. The ICS is based upon limited span of control and is a fundamental tenet of DR. The ICS concept, initially proposed in 1970 by California fire chiefs as a strategy for coordinated battling of forest fires, was based on the U.S. Navy hierarchical chain of command.[10] In the past 45 years the ICS emerged as the key operational paradigm for prehospital, health care facility, and governmental response to crisis.[11,12] Both in the prehospital environment and in health care facilities (e.g., hospital ICS) the ICS system is used to standardize the management of complex, interagency, or interdepartmental responses. Briefly, the ICS system creates flexibility of action, clear accountability, and clear operational span of control. ICS mirrors the military command system by identifying and empowering an incident command (e.g., commanding officer), operations officer (e.g., staff 3 [S3]), planning officer (e.g., staff 5 [S5]), logistics officer (e.g., staff 4 [S4]), finance and administration officer (e.g., staff 1 [S1]), and information officer (e.g., staff 6 [S6]). The ICS principles are discussed at length in Chapter 38.

During the past 5 years, disaster management practitioners have gained increased awareness of the principles of HROs. The theory of HROs began in the 1970s but gained traction with the study of the aircraft carrier USS Carl Vinson and Capt. Thomas Mercer.[13–15] The study examined the notion that "accidents" in high-risk environments were considered normal. Capt. Mercer and his team faced highly complex operational environments, uncertain threats, frequent turnover of staff, and catastrophic consequences for failure. Their approach embodied the principles of HROs, leading to fewer significant adverse outcomes and improved safety. An in-depth discussion of HROs is beyond the scope of this chapter; however, the five core concepts of HROs include the following[16,17]:

- *Sensitivity to operations:* Constant awareness by leaders, practitioners, and staff about the state of the systems and key processes that affect patient care. Accidents are rarely the result of a single error by a single person, but rather errors "latent in the system."
- *Reluctance to simplify:* Clinical and response operations are inherently complex. Development of simple processes can reduce error, but oversimplification of the root cause of errors is dangerous. Categorizing challenges is unavoidable, but should not constrain skepticism or investigations.
- *Preoccupation with failure:* Constant vigilance about viewing near misses within the system as early signs of failure. This is not a preoccupation with avoiding failure. Rather, this acknowledges that errors will happen and focuses attention on avoiding complacency and limiting adverse outcomes.
- *Deference to expertise:* Willingness of leaders and managers to listen and respond to the expertise of front-line staff. Expertise is not based on position, but rather knowledge, experience, and credibility.
- *Commitment to resilience:* Organizations must maintain function during periods of high demand or system failures and grow from prior episodes.

These HRO principles are applied in intensive care units (ICUs),[18] emergency medical service (EMS) agencies,[19,20] EDs, and DR.[21] They have also become a component of the Agency for Healthcare Research and Quality (AHRQ) standards for achieving clinical quality, safety, and efficiency.[10]

Clinical Care Advances

The practice of military medicine has advanced tremendously in the past decade. The GWOT has provided a generation of military medical providers with expeditionary experience. During this period, the military often looked to civilian HA/DR providers for lessons learned, best practices, and gap analysis. However, where civilian practice is frequently limited by lack of funding, the GWOT provided the unique opportunity to align defense funding and training requirements with these identified gaps, therefore accelerating the advancement of medical care delivery in austere or high threat environments, both military and civilian.

In the prehospital environment the influential example is the creation of the Tactical Combat Casualty Care (TCCC) guidelines. TCCC stems from efforts by U.S. Special Operations units in the 1990s to adapt prehospital care techniques to the battlefield environment where disciplined adherence to tactics often determines mission success versus failure. The TCCC guidelines were the first modern medical guidelines to align medical care and operational constraints—in this case the tactical combat scenario—to address potentially preventable causes of death.[22,23] The tiered application of TCCC guidelines to nonmedical personnel, medics, and physicians resulted in the lowest case fatality rate in modern combat history.[24] Over the past decade the TCCC Guidelines expanded beyond point-of-injury care to address issues related to standardized field surgical care, analgesia, damage control resuscitation, and tiered hemorrhage control. The CoTCCC also drove initiatives, such as the DoD implementation of tourniquets, hypothermia prevention, expanded use of tranexamic acid (TXA), and utilization of intranasal ketamine for analgesia.[25-27]

The military experience has clear and direct application to mass casualty incidents (MCIs), acts of terrorism, and management of complex polytrauma in the civilian setting. The civilian Committee for Tactical Emergency Casualty Care (C-TECC) was established in the United States to serve as a best practice development group for translating combat lessons learned to civilian response to high threat prehospital care. The C-TECC guidelines emphasize an integrated, threat-based

response to prehospital care with emphasis on threat mitigation, early hemorrhage control (e.g., aggressive tourniquet application), rapid extraction, and tiered initiation of damage control resuscitation principles.[28] The TECC guidelines represent a critical paradigm shift in civilian care, especially in regards to aggressive tourniquet use, which had been considered an anathema in trauma care. Multiple studies have demonstrated the efficacy and safety of properly applied tourniquets, leading to more widespread adoption as part of MCI plans.[29,30] Since, organizations such as the American College of Surgeons have looked with increasing frequency to the military to provide lessons learned on management of traumatic MCI events.[31,32] The 2013 Boston Marathon Bombing illustrated the critical importance of proper, aggressive tourniquet application—a key lesson learned from combat experience and articulated in TECC.[33]

One of the other critical military care advancements with direct application in the civilian DR community is the conceptualization and development of damage control resuscitation (DCR) strategies. DCR emerged in the early years of the U.S. conflict in Afghanistan as forward-deployed surgical units began to manage large volumes of complex, polytrauma patients in resource-poor environments. The principles of DCR include early hemorrhage control, permissive hypotension, prevention of acidosis and hypothermia, and early damage control surgery (DCS).[34,35] The apparent reductions in mortality noted by implementation of DCR and DCS principles in combat led to the widespread adoption of these techniques in civilian trauma centers, especially as part of MCI and disaster plans.[36-38] Though DCR principles continue to be fine tuned, they certainly have a role in the provision of high-quality care in austere, resource-challenged, and crisis situations.

Humanitarian Assistance

The U.S. DoD has a long history of conducting and supporting HA missions. The DoD provides much of its routine humanitarian aid through the Overseas Humanitarian, Disaster and Civic Action (OHDACA) account. Outside of overt war zones, these DoD operations are generally conducted in "semi-permissive" environments defined by elevated threat scenarios but not outright combat operations. Academic, operational, and policy stakeholders actively debate the impact, consequences, and implications of the "militarization" of HA missions. However, there are clear lessons learned from military operations that inform modern and future civilian HA missions.

Operations Management and System Design

The DoD is a clear global leader in logistics and mission support. Frequently, components of the U.S. military must work with other branches of the U.S. Armed Forces, USG civilian agencies, foreign governments, nonstate responders, and IOs to achieve mission success. In response, the DoD creates various interagency task forces and provides guidance on roles, responsibilities, and operational span of control. Clear chains of command, effective communication, and cooperation are critical to success. This mission profile mirrors that of the HA community during large-scale response operations. The largely ineffective U.N. cluster system was and is an attempt to provide a similar coordination infrastructure by identifying key stakeholders within each sector and identifying sector "leads." Limitations to the U.N. cluster system include a lack of regulatory and command authority. In Jordan the U.N. High Commissioner for Refugees (UNHCR) has begun to implement, with some success, issue-specific task forces, innovation and problem solving teams (similar to Red Cell teams in the military), and contracted lead agencies with execution authority within specific areas of operation.

The U.S. military is also an expert at the development and deployment of trauma systems in crisis zones. In Iraq and Afghanistan the

U.S. military has created an integrated, tiered trauma system that provides exceptional care from point of wounding through evacuation to the United States. The DoD system combined trauma training for nonmedical personnel, rapid evacuation using various modalities (e.g., trucks, helicopters, and fixed-wing aircraft), far-forward deployment of surgeons and critical care staff, mobile ICUs, modern information management systems, and a properly resourced logistics and support system to reduce combat mortality to the lowest rate in modern combat history.[39] The system design focused around the critical issues of prolonged evacuation time and resource limitation. In particular the ability to provide critical care in austere environments was a major advance in combat, and thus HA medicine. These principles focused on diligent resource management, aggressive infection control, practiced interdisciplinary team care, and leveraging of air-evacuation platforms.[40] In disaster zones from postearthquake Haiti to posttyphoon Philippines these lessons are critical for success and should be closely studied by HA leaders.[41,42]

Innovation and Technology

Plato wrote, "Necessity, the mother of invention." Jonathan Schattke expanded on Plato, writing that "Necessity, it is true, but its father is creativity, and knowledge is the midwife." The September 11, 2001, attacks drew into the military some of the most creative, knowledgeable, and motivated individuals in the United States. The subsequent decade of complex urban operations, counterinsurgency, and mixed national policy goals demanded from leaders at all levels the rapid development of expertise and application of creativity in order to both achieve mission success and to survive.

Reliable energy is critical to effective HA mission execution. Oftentimes HA/DR operations occur in remote regions or areas where the energy infrastructure has been destroyed. The U.S. military faced a similar challenge in Afghanistan, where the logistical system required to provide power to forward-operating bases was expensive, deadly, and unreliable. In 2009 the Pentagon estimated the average cost to provide one gallon of fuel to a vehicle in Afghanistan was $400/gallon.[43] The officials also estimated that one casualty was sustained every 24 missions.[44] So pressing is the issue that the Defense Advanced Research Projects Agency (DARPA) is developing a mobile integrated sustainable energy recovery (MISER) system. The applications in HA missions is direct and obvious. Unfortunately, the cost of large-scale solar projects and antiquated funding mechanisms have prevented the large-scale deployment of renewable energy solutions beyond solar lamps, solar water heaters, and the occasional solar street lamp. For example, during 2014, UNHCR spent an estimated $700,000 USD on electricity for the Za'atari refugee camp in northern Jordan.[45] Jordan has an abundance of solar energy with average annual daily solar irradiance ranges from 5 to 7 kWh/m^2. The scenario is primed for widespread application of clean energy technology, such as solar and wind. The increased interest from the U.S. military is driving research and development, creating a private sector market for mobile renewable energy and providing case studies for application in austere environments.

In HA/DR missions one of the most significant challenges is tracking refugees, casualties, and at-risk populations. In Haiti the Operational Medicine Institute (OMI) identified a critical gap in the interagency/U.N. cluster system capacity to track volunteers, patients, and displaced populations.[46] As a result, the OMI developed an iPhone-based tracking application that gained widespread utilization. However, the issue of accountability repeated itself in the Philippines, South Sudan, and countries responding to the massive Syrian refugee crisis. In 2013 the HA community again looked to the military for a solution. During the conflicts in Iraq and Afghanistan, the U.S. military deployed portable biometric identification devices to identify criminals, track insurgents, and vet potential political allies.[47] Again this drove development and technology transfer to the civilian sector. In Jordan the UNHCR contracted with Iris Guard to provide biometric registration of refugees, allowing greater situational awareness, the efficient deployment of cash and food voucher systems, and the identification of potential security threats from insurgents posing as refugees.[48,49]

CONCLUSIONS

The military's depth of experience providing care in conflict zones and austere environments, coupled with an institutional reliance on systems design and rapid operational improvement on the ground can significantly inform modern and future HA and DR efforts. Civilian HA/DR practitioners should examine best practices for crisis response from the global military community and balance these observations with personal experience and critical evaluation of civilian HA/DR past performance.

! PITFALLS

- Confusion of civilian and military operational space: coordination and sharing of lessons learned are critical; however, consideration must also be given to the various implications of not just what is done, but by whom it is done.
- Unintended consequences of overlapping military, humanitarian, and development goals can lead to wasted money, redundant care, recipient population disillusionment, and conflict.
- Reluctance to share best practices across civil-military operational spheres.

REFERENCES

1. Responding to Natural Disasters. www.usace.army.mil/About/History/BriefHistoryoftheCorps/RespondingtoNaturalDisasters.aspx. Accessed May 9, 2014.
2. The Demands of History: Army Medical Disaster Relief; Foster, Gaines, 1983. http://history.amedd.army.mil/booksdocs/misc/disaster/default.html. Accessed May 31, 2014.
3. The Military Sector's Role in Global Health: Historical Context and Future Directions; Derek Licina, Global Health Governance, Volume VI, Issue 1, Fall 2012.
4. Leaning J. The dilemma of neutrality. *Prehosp Disaster Med.* 2007 Sep-Oct;22(5):418–421.
5. National Security Strategy. 2010. http://www.whitehouse.gov/sites/default/files/rss_viewer/national_security_strategy.pdf. Accessed March 17, 2014.
6. *A National Security Strategy of Engagement and Enlargement. The White House.* 1996, http://www.fas.org/spp/military/docops/national/1996stra.htm. Accessed May 31, 2014.
7. The National Security Strategy. March 2006. http://www.comw.org/qdr/fulltext/nss2006.pdf. Accessed May 31, 2014.
8. Patrick S. Impact of the department of defense initiatives on humanitarian assistance. *Prehosp Disaster Med.* July-August 2009;24(2):S238–S2243.
9. http://reliefweb.int/. Accessed March 17, 2014.
10. Cole, D. The Incident Command System: A 25 year evaluation by California practitioners. http://www.usfa.fema.gov/pdf/efop/efo31023.pdf. Accessed June 2, 2014.
11. National Incident Management System. http://www.fema.gov/incident-command-system. Accessed June 1, 2014.
12. Chertoff, M. National Incident Management System. December 2008. http://www.fema.gov/pdf/emergency/nims/NIMS_core.pdf. Accessed June 2, 2014.

13. Van Stralen D, Mercer T. Why being a high-reliability organization is important in EMS. *JEMS*. Tuesday, June 11, 2013. http://m.jems.com/article/administration-and-leadership/why-being-high-reliability-organization. Accessed June 2, 2014.

14. Desai VM, Roberts KH, Ciavarelli AP. The relationship between safety climate and recent accidents: behavioral learning and cognitive attributions. *Hum Factors*. 2006 Winter;48(4):639–650.

15. Roberts KH. Some characteristics of one type of high reliability organization. *Organ Sci*. 1990;1:160–176.

16. Weick K, Sutcliffe K. *Managing the unexpected: Resilient performance in an age of uncertainty.* San Francisco, CA: Jossey Bass; 2007.

17. Hines S, Luna, K, Lofthus J, et al. Becoming a High Reliability Organization: Operational Advice for Hospital Leaders. (Prepared by the Lewin Group under Contract No. 290-04-0011.) AHRQ Publication No. 08-0022. Rockville, MD.

18. Roberts KH, Madsen P, Desai V, Van Stralen D. A case of the birth and death of a high reliability healthcare organisation. *Qual Saf Health Care*. 2005 Jun;14(3):216–220.

19. Van Stralen D, Mercer TA. EMS & high reliability organizing. Achieving safety & reliability in the dynamic, high-risk environment. *JEMS*. 2013 Jun;38(6):60–63.

20. Heightman AJ. A win for HROs. Employing high-reliability organization characteristics in EMS. *JEMS*. 2013 Jun;38(6):12–13.

21. Morrison JB, Rudolph JW. Learning from accident and error: avoiding the hazards of workload, stress, and routine interruptions in the emergency department. *Acad Emerg Med*. 2011 Dec;18(12):1246–1254.

22. Butler FK Jr., Blackbourne LH. Battlefield trauma care then and now: a decade of Tactical Combat Casualty Care. *J Trauma Acute Care Surg*. 2012 Dec;73(6 Suppl 5):S395–S402.

23. Butler FK Jr., Hagmann J, Butler EG. Tactical combat casualty care in special operations. *Mil Med*. 1996 Aug;161(Suppl):3–16.

24. Kotwal RS, Montgomery HR, Kotwal BM, et al. Eliminating preventable death on the battlefield. *Arch Surg*. 2011 Dec;146(12):1350–1358.

25. Deal VT, McDowell D, Benson P, et al. Tactical combat casualty care February 2010. Direct from the Battlefield: TCCC lessons learned in Iraq and Afghanistan. *J Spec Oper Med*. 2010 Summer;10(3):77–119.

26. Butler FK, Kotwal RS, Buckenmaier CC 3rd, et al. A triple-option analgesia plan for Tactical Combat Casualty Care: TCCC guidelines change 13-04. *J Spec Oper Med*. 2014 Spring;14(1):13–25.

27. Butler FK Jr., Holcomb JB, Giebner SD, McSwain NE, Bagian J. Tactical combat casualty care 2007: evolving concepts and battlefield experience. *Mil Med*. 2007 Nov;172(11 Suppl):1–19.

28. Callaway DW, Smith ER, Cain J, et al. Tactical Emergency Casualty Care (TECC): guidelines for the provision of prehospital trauma care in high threat environments. *J Spec Oper Med*. 2011 Summer;11(3):104–122.

29. Kragh JF Jr, O'Neill ML, Walters TJ, et al. Minor morbidity with emergency tourniquet use to stop bleeding in severe limb trauma: research, history, and reconciling advocates and abolitionists. *Mil Med*. 2011 Jul;176(7):817–823, PubMed PMID: 22128725.

30. Doyle GS, Taillac PP. Tourniquets: a review of current use with proposals for expanded prehospital use. *Prehosp Emerg Care*. 2008 Apr-Jun;12(2):241–256.

31. Elster EA, Butler FK, Rasmussen TE. Implications of combat casualty care for mass casualty events. *JAMA*. 2013;310:475–476.

32. Jacobs L, Burns KJ. The Hartford Consensus to improve survivability in mass casualty events: process to policy. *Am J Disaster Med*. 2014 Winter;9(1):67–71.

33. Caterson EJ, Carty MJ, Weaver MJ, Holt EF. Boston bombings: a surgical view of lessons learned from combat casualty care and the applicability to Boston's terrorist attack. *J Craniofac Surg*. 2013 Jul;24(4):1061–1067.

34. Rappold JF, Pusateri AE. Tranexamic acid in remote damage control resuscitation. *Transfusion*. 2013 Jan;53(Suppl 1):96S–99S.

35. Duchesne JC, Holcomb JB. Damage control resuscitation: addressing trauma-induced coagulopathy. *Br J Hosp Med (Lond)*. 2009 Jan;70(1):22–25.

36. Campion E, Pritts T, Dorlac W, et al. Implementation of a military derived damage control resuscitation strategy in a civilian trauma center decreases acute hypoxia in massively transfused patients. *J Trauma Acute Care Surg*. 2013;75:S221–S227.

37. Jenkins D, Stubbs J, Williams S, et al. Implementation and execution of civilian remote damage control resuscitation programs. *Shock*. 2014 May;41(Suppl 1):84–89.

38. Duke MD, Guidry C, Guice J, et al. Restrictive fluid resuscitation in combination with damage control resuscitation: time for adaptation. *J Trauma Acute Care Surg*. 2012 Sep;73(3):674–678.

39. Bailey JA, Morrison JJ, Rasmussen TE. Military trauma system in Afghanistan: lessons for civil systems? *Curr Opin Crit Care*. 2013 Dec;19(6):569–577.

40. Grathwohl KW, Venticinque SG. Organizational characteristics of the austere intensive care unit: the evolution of military trauma and critical care medicine; applications for civilian medical care systems. *Crit Care Med*. 2008;36(Suppl 7):S275–S283.

41. Jawa RS, Heir JS, Cancelada D, Young DH, Mercer DW. A quick primer for setting up and maintaining surgical intensive care in an austere environment: practical tips from volunteers in a mass disaster. *Am J Disaster Med*. 2012 Summer;7(3):223–229.

42. Venticinque SG, Grathwohl KW. Critical care in the austere environment: providing exceptional care in unusual places. *Crit Care Med*. 2008 Jul;36(7 Suppl):S284–S292.

43. Tiron R. $400 per gallon gas to drive debate over cost of war in Afghanistan. The Hill. October 16, 2009.

44. Goossens E. Exploding Fuel Tankers Driving US Army to Solar Power. Bloomberg October 1, 2013. http://www.bloomberg.com/news/2013-09-30/exploding-fuel-tankers-driving-u-s-army-to-solar-power.html. Accessed June 2, 2014.

45. UNHCR Jordan country team. Personal Communication. May 2014

46. Callaway DW, Peabody CR, Hoffman A, et al. Disaster mobile health technology: lessons from Haiti. *Prehosp Disaster Med*. 2012 Apr;27(2):148–152.

47. Harward RS. *Commander's Guide to Biometrics in Afghanistan*. Center for Army Lessons Learned; April 2011. No. 11-25, https://info.publicintelligence.net/CALL-AfghanBiometrics.pdf, Accessed June 2, 2014.

48. Vrankulj A. UNHCR adopts IrisGuard technology for refugee registration. Biometric Update. http://www.biometricupdate.com/201402/unhcr-adopts-irisguard-technology-for-refugee-registration. Accessed June 2, 2014.

49. Kleinschmidt K. UNHCR Head of Sub Office- Mafraq, Jordan. Personal communication. May 2014.

CHAPTER 86

Integration of Law Enforcement and Military Resources with the Emergency Response to a Terrorist Incident

Cord W. Cunningham, Donald Keen, Chetan U. Kharod, and Neil B. Davids

In a terrorist incident, medical and rescue personnel will respond to locate, extricate, treat, and transport patients. Simultaneously, law enforcement resources will respond to investigate, interview, and collect evidence. Medical operations can interfere with the investigation and successful prosecution of terrorist activity. Movement through the scene can disrupt or destroy evidence. At the same time, by limiting access to the scene, law enforcement can impact the ability of medical responders to effectively treat patients and move them from the scene. Secondary or delayed attacks as part of a terrorism event in particular can create more casualties from the responders themselves, further complicating and delaying treatment to all patients. Yet, rapid response and extrication from the point of injury is critical to treating victims and preventing further injuries.

Integrating the law enforcement response with the medical response requires cooperation at all levels of the operation: tactically, where individual personnel must work side by side; operationally, where a unified command must smoothly coordinate resources at the incident site; and strategically, where resource and response decisions must be made. Emergency medical technicians (EMTs), nurses, and physicians need to be aware of evidence preservation and crime scene management. Mass fatality management must also coincide with evidence processing.

In a large-scale incident, regardless of its type, military resources may also respond to the scene. The military has unique assets that can respond to terrorist incidents, including personnel trained for decontamination, mitigation, and detection of weapons of mass destruction (WMD). They can serve to augment the medical, rescue, and law enforcement capabilities of the civilian community. However, both the military responder and their civilian requester must understand the processes that allow the use of military resources and the rules under which they function.

The potential conflicts between medical responders and law enforcement officials must be addressed prior to the actual incident. The relation between military assets and the civilian government must be established. By recognizing the distinct roles that each agency plays in responding to a terrorist incident, the responder can better address his or her mission and the incident commander can better utilize resources.[1,2]

In the wake of 9/11 and subsequent attacks, there has been ongoing change in the legal and administrative framework that organizes the U.S. federal and state response to terrorist incidents. To better understand these changes, it is helpful to look at the trends in the response to terrorism as a crime and terrorism as a mass casualty event over the last few decades.

HISTORICAL PERSPECTIVE

Law Enforcement

Since the 1980s, the terms *consequence management* and *crisis management* have been used when differentiating between the roles of rescuers and the roles of investigators. The Federal Emergency Management Agency (FEMA) defines consequence management as the actions taken to protect public health and safety, restore essential government services, and provide relief to governments, businesses, and persons affected by the consequences of terrorism. Crisis management, in contrast, is the measures taken to identify, acquire, and plan the use of resources to anticipate, prevent, and resolve a threat or act of terrorism.[3]

Consequence management is maintained at the lowest level of government possible. If the consequences of a terrorist incident can be met with resources from the local level, there should be minimal involvement of state or federal resources. If local government is not able to adequately manage the consequences of the incident, it will turn to the state government for assistance. Similarly, if the state cannot meet the needs of the incident, it will turn to the federal government. At the federal level, consequence management has been the responsibility of the agency providing civil defense; since the 1970s this has been FEMA.[4]

In contrast, crisis management has always been a function of the federal government. The concept of terrorism as a criminal act evolved from the realm of sabotage and espionage where an individual, working as an agent of an enemy state, performs an action that is injurious to the government or its people. Acts of terrorism, by extension, are acts committed by transnational or nonstate organizations and individuals. As a result, these crimes are prosecuted in the federal courts under U.S. Code. The Department of Justice was appointed the lead federal agency for crisis management in the 1980s. The Federal Bureau of Investigation (FBI) was then delegated the responsibility for crisis management.[5]

The difficulty with having two different response operations to the same incident is that each entity, rescue and investigation, has a different set of objectives. Neither feels the other has a complete view of the incident. Conflict in managing the incident is an inevitable consequence of these unshared objectives.

The Stafford Act was passed in 1974 and amended in 1988 to delineate the federal response to a disaster. The act was not made with a specific reference to terrorism. It did, however, state that nothing within the act was to construe an investigatory role for any federal agency other than the FBI.[6]

In 1985 George H.W. Bush, acting in his capacity as vice president, led the Task Force on Combatting Terrorism, which made many recommendations for further actions, including clarification of lead agencies and available resources for various aspects of combating terrorism, both foreign and domestic.[7] The following three decades have displayed an ongoing refinement of government structure in response to terrorism. The first large-scale act of modern terrorism on U.S. territory occurred in 1993, and it is an example of an event during which there was minimal conflict between the crisis and consequence management entities. The World Trade Center was the site of a vehicle-borne improvised explosive device detonation that resulted in six deaths and more than 1000 injuries. An area 150 feet wide and 5 stories deep was destroyed. The cause of the explosion was initially identified as a transformer explosion with a resultant fire. Because of this, command and control was largely initially performed by the fire department of the city of New York (FDNY). Fire ground operations were handled with resources from the FDNY only, with mutual aid being required for the emergency medical services (EMS) response. Only later, after the discovery of a car bomb as the source, did the site evolve into a crime scene. The area was then processed by four FBI evidence technicians and four Bureau of Alcohol, Tobacco, and Firearms evidence technicians working with a local New York Police Department chemist. After-action reports indicated a minimum number of conflicts between federal and local law enforcement officials. These reports attribute this to an already established Joint Terrorism Task Force (JTTF), which had been in existence in New York City since the 1980s.[7-9]

JTTFs have been established in 103 cities, including an office in each of the 56 major metropolitan areas that have FBI field offices. Seventy-one of these offices opened after 9/11. Each is made up of FBI special agents and local law enforcement officers functioning as Special Deputy U.S. Marshals. They share in the responsibility of gathering intelligence, investigating, and prosecuting terrorist-related crimes. Funding of JTTFs is largely through the FBI, although the local governments continue to pay the salaries of their officers.[10]

Two months after the Oklahoma City Bombing in 1995, President Clinton signed Presidential Decision Directive 39 (PDD-39). PDD-39, still mostly a classified document, established guidelines for federal command and control in the event of a terrorist incident. Although local agencies were mainly responsible for search and rescue, FEMA deployed multiple urban search and rescue teams.[11] Furthermore the incident was recognized nearly immediately as a criminal action. Specifically, the directive designates the Department of Justice as the lead federal agency for operational response and crisis management, and the attorney general delegated this role to the FBI. It designates FEMA as the lead federal agency for consequence management. Furthermore, it specifies that crisis management will take precedence over consequence management: the FBI would remain in charge of the scene until the attorney general had turned the scene over to FEMA.[12]

Presidential Decision Directive 62 (PDD-62) directs the federal agencies in their preresponse planning to counterterrorism and consequence management. It established a national level coordinator for security, critical infrastructure protection, and counterterrorism. It provided guidance to the Department of Justice, Department of Health and Human Services, and Department of Defense (DoD) in preparing the Metropolitan Medical Strike Team (now Metropolitan Medical Response System) in the first 120 cities that established them.[13]

The Concept of Operations Plan (CONPLAN) for terrorism, signed in 2000, reaffirmed the role of the Department of Justice as the lead federal agency in the response to terrorism. As such, the FBI remained the on-scene commander until the attorney general relinquished control to FEMA. The FBI would establish a Joint Operations Command (JOC) that would serve as a focus for crisis management in the unified response. It was intended to complement and work with the local agencies' Incident Command System (ICS).[14]

On September 11, 2001, the World Trade Center was attacked for a second time. It was a much larger and clearly more destructive attack; the response was large and difficult to manage. Again, the JTTF was crucial in providing a guiding framework for the crisis management response. There was a coordinated response to evidence processing that seemed to have had minimal effect on the rescue efforts. The most serious concern with the response to 9/11 was not a conflict between law enforcement and rescue, but the lack of coordinated communications that may have led to unnecessary morbidity and mortality. The police commander ordered the evacuation of his personnel from the building after receiving information pointing to the potential for collapse, but this was not relayed to the firefighters, contributing to the loss of 343 firefighters' lives in the eventual collapse.[15] The success of the management of the response to the 9/11 Pentagon attack can largely be attributed to the ability of the first responders, the Arlington Fire Department, to assert themselves as the incident commanders. Until the initial rescue and recovery operations were completed, the command remained with one agency as the lead, while other agencies actively contributed to the management of the incident.[16]

The Initial National Response Plan (INRP) was enacted in September 2003, while a final National Response Plan (NRP) was being developed.[17] After it was signed, the NRP became the guiding document for federal response to terrorism, supplanting the Federal Response Plan, the INRP, and the CONPLAN. It delineated the role of the Department of Homeland Security in the response to terrorism. It also proposed moving toward a unified command, with a designated principal federal official (PFO) as the overall senior federal official at the scene.[18]

The NRP was enacted in 2004; it underwent subsequent revisions in 2006, incorporating lessons from the Hurricane Katrina response. It evolved into the National Response Framework (NRF) in 2008, with its current version released in May 2013. The change from the NRP to the NRF reflected feedback from local emergency management entities that the NRP was not a detailed response plan, nor did it stress the importance of local resources.[19] The NRF stresses an all-hazards approach and provides guidance for local to large-scale terrorist events.

Military

The military has been involved in support to civilian disasters since the inception of the union. The use of the military for non–law enforcement response is legal and well established in both statute and case law. The military has performed ad hoc relief missions to natural disasters both as an immediate response to emergencies in adjacent civilian communities (as in the San Francisco earthquake of 1906) or in sustained efforts as approved by Congress. It was not until the Federal Civil Defense Act of 1950 that Congress codified the military's standing role in civilian disasters. This military role was later expanded in the Stafford Act of 1974, and it has been supported in periodic amendments and revisions.[20]

However, there is often concern about the use of military in support of civilian law enforcement. Originally, the states were concerned about the federal government maintaining a standing army. In the Reconstruction Era after the Civil War, the Union Army was used to maintain order in the Southern states. Southern states' reaction to the continued presence of martial law during this time was to limit the future use of the army in civilian law enforcement. Feeling that the army's enforcement of polling laws led to the party's loss of the presidency, a Democratic Congress passed the Posse Comitatus Act in 1878. A *posse comitatus* (Latin for "power of the county") historically is a collection of able-bodied citizens working under the county sheriff to enforce the laws. Currently, under Title 18, Section 1385 of the U.S. Code, the U.S. Army and U.S. Air Force are prohibited from serving as a posse or other form of law enforcement. By DoD policy, this has been extended to the U.S. Navy and the U.S. Marine Corps.

Since the passing of the Posse Comitatus Act, the military has continued to respond to natural disasters to support civilian communities in non–law enforcement roles. Importantly, the Posse Comitatus Act does not completely eliminate the use of the military as an aid to law enforcement: it does allow for the suppression of riots and controlling of crowds. The last large-scale use of this provision of the U.S. Code, Title 10, Chapter 15, Section 332, was in 1992, when President George H.W. Bush responded to the Los Angeles riots by deploying U.S. Army and Marine troops and "federalized" (used as part of the U.S. Army) California National Guardsmen.[21] Furthermore, it is important to note that the Coast Guard is excluded from the Posse Comitatus Act. The Coast Guard, part of the Department of Homeland Security, is the United States' leading maritime law enforcement agency. Its duties include drug enforcement, immigration control, and port security.[22]

The Stafford Act identifies the DoD as a resource that may be requested by the state governor from the president through a state disaster declaration. In an incident in which a disaster declaration is expected, the president can direct the secretary of defense to provide military resources to the response for a period of up to 10 days. Once a declaration has been made, the resources are available through the established Joint Field Office (JFO). Expenses that the DoD incurs in either of these response modes are reimbursable.

Additionally, under the concept of *immediate response,* a local military commander can use assets available to him or her to provide aid to an adjacent civilian community. Traditionally, the period of time in which an immediate response can be performed is generally considered the first 3 days of a disaster. After that period, it is expected that requests for assistance will come through the channels established for crisis or consequence management (e.g., a state governor will request assistance from the president, then the president tasks the military with providing support). Under the concept of immediate response, the local commander can provide support to law enforcement when there is the possibility of loss of life or wanton property destruction, or to restore the functions of government.[23]

Although the military is a very large entity, they do not automatically take command in the rare instance when they respond to a civilian jurisdiction. The 9/11 Pentagon response is one such example of incident command remaining with a local fire department. The Fort Hood shooting event in 2009, although not legally categorized as an act of terrorism, highlighted the importance of immediate response memorandums of agreement between local EMS and military personnel that allowed transport and distribution of patients to both local hospitals and to the on-base military hospital.

CURRENT PRACTICE

Law Enforcement

In the moments immediately following a domestic terrorist attack, it may not be clear that a terrorist event has taken place. Local law enforcement will likely respond to the scene as they would to any other major crime scene. A command post will be established early in the incident according to the National Incident Management System (NIMS).[24] This command post will be scaled to the size of the incident and be expanded as needed. As part of law enforcement's response, efforts will be made to limit the contamination of evidence by keeping the number of responders entering the scene to a minimum. An internal and external perimeter will be established as soon as practical. Also, it is expected that rescuers will need to enter the scene of a terrorist

attack, and the chaotic movement of patients and rescuers carries an inherent risk of contamination of an active crime scene. To minimize the risk of adulteration of evidence at the scene, multiple courses are available to teach the EMS and firefighter to recognize a criminal or terrorist incident, minimize scene contamination, and to relate crime scene information to law enforcement officials.[25] As the incident develops, additional resources may be mobilized at the local, state, and federal level. Depending on the type of incident, other local law enforcement assets (e.g., Special Weapons and Tactics [SWAT], canine [K-9], Explosive Ordnance Disposal [EOD], and hazardous materials [HazMat] units) may require entry into the scene as well, and this requires coordination if evidence is to be preserved.

At the federal level, the lead authority for the investigation of domestic terrorist events is the FBI. When notified of a possible terrorist incident, the FBI will send agents from its local field office to the scene separately or as part of an existing local JTTF.[26] The Special Agent in Charge (SAC) for the FBI will be the primary investigator to determine if the incident is related to terrorism. Initially, an FBI command post will be established to coordinate efforts with the local first responders' command post. Ideally, this will evolve into a unified command structure supported by the Department of Homeland Security's JFO and by local, state, and regional emergency operations centers.[27] The Department of Homeland Security (DHS) will establish a JFO within 4 to 12 hours of determining that a terrorist incident has occurred. The JFO functions in essence as an area command as established in the ICS, or similar to a regional emergency operations center (Fig. 86-1). It functions as the Unified Coordination Group (UCG) which incorporates a coordination group, operations group, administration and finance group, logistics group, and a planning management group paralleling the ICS used at the local level.

The PFO coordinates the efforts of the command group, which incorporates the senior representative from FEMA as the federal coordinating officer and the SAC from the FBI as senior federal law enforcement officer. There are liaisons from all involved federal agencies, as well as state and local representatives.

The Domestic Emergency Support Team (DEST) is a rapidly deployable interagency support team that brings to the on-scene commander the breadth of expertise available from the federal government. The makeup of the DEST depends greatly upon the specific need of the incident, and usually command remains with the FBI. Typically, the DEST will deploy immediately to an incident that may require federal support. The DEST may then become the nucleus of the JFO.[28,29]

The FBI has had a Hazardous Materials Response Unit (HMRU) since 1996 to collect evidence in a hazardous environment. Deployed from FBI headquarters to any hazardous materials release, the HMRU is capable of operating in a hostile environment to process it as a crime scene. In addition to the HMRU, designated FBI field offices maintain smaller but similarly equipped HazMat response teams to act as an immediate response resource to local incidents. In addition, the FBI response will include an evidence response team, a team of 8 to 50 members from a local field office that will process evidence from a crime scene.[30]

At the tactical level, local SWAT teams have the need for integrated EMS support. Typically, either SWAT officers are trained to the EMT or paramedic level, or an experienced EMS provider is trained to operate in a tactical environment. Training for the medical provider is aimed at providing emergency care in an austere tactical environment. In addition, the EMS provider gives preventive care as well, measuring heat stress and injury potential, and enforcing work/rest cycles. Some agencies have developed a local joint task force to respond to a WMD release. Made up of local fire, EMS, law enforcement, and EOD personnel, this task force trains personnel to provide a unified initial response

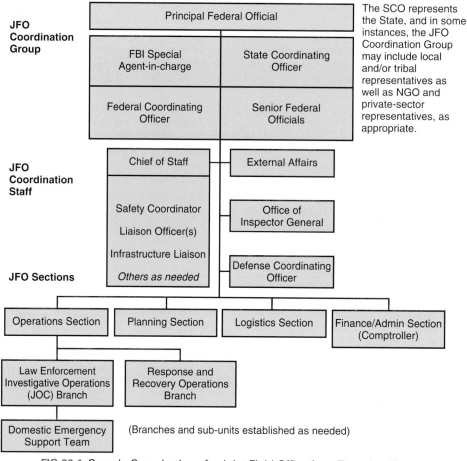

JFO Coordination Group

Principal Federal Official

FBI Special Agent-in-charge

State Coordinating Officer

Federal Coordinating Officer

Senior Federal Officials

The SCO represents the State, and in some instances, the JFO Coordination Group may include local and/or tribal representatives as well as NGO and private-sector representatives, as appropriate.

JFO Coordination Staff

Chief of Staff

External Affairs

Safety Coordinator
Liaison Officer(s)
Infrastructure Liaison
Others as needed

Office of Inspector General

Defense Coordinating Officer

JFO Sections

Operations Section

Planning Section

Logistics Section

Finance/Admin Section (Comptroller)

Law Enforcement Investigative Operations (JOC) Branch

Response and Recovery Operations Branch

Domestic Emergency Support Team

(Branches and sub-units established as needed)

FIG 86-1 Sample Organization of a Joint Field Office for a Terrorism Event.

within the hot zone. It has many of the capabilities of the National Guard's WMD–Civil Support Team (WMD-CST), including agent identification, hazard mapping, and plume modeling.

Military

Civil support is the provision of DoD support to U.S. civil authorities for domestic emergencies and for designated law enforcement and other activities. When its involvement is appropriate, and when a clear end point for its role is defined, the DoD undertakes civil support missions. Defense Support of Civil Authorities (DSCA) as governed by DoD Directive 3025.18 (which supersedes 3025.1 and 3025.25) was previously split into Military Support to Civil Authorities (MSCA) and Military Assistance to Civil Authorities (MACA) and encompasses the following[31,32]:

Military aid to civil disturbance is the use of military force to quell a civil disturbance. The use of federal military assets requires an executive order from the president specifically indicating the location where assets are to be deployed, and is influenced by the Posse Comitatus Act of 1878 (18 U.S.C. § 1385) modified in 1981 to apply specifically to the armed forces of the United States.[33] DSCA planning will consider command and control options that will emphasize unity of effort and authorize direct liaison if authorized by the secretary of defense.[32]

Military support to law enforcement agencies is technical assistance rendered by the military to civilian law enforcement agencies. This can include military resources that are not available to civilians (such as aerial surveillance), technical assistance, and tactical advice. The military can be granted law enforcement powers within the United

States by the president of the United States under Title 10 U.S. Code, Sections 331 to 335, known as the Insurrection Act, and does not specifically require governor consent or request.[34] Of note, the U.S. Army and Air National Guard do not require presidential authority in order to be mobilized for law enforcement. The guard is commanded and mobilized by the state governor, but can be brought under federal control and armed (a National Guardsman is a state employee, but when "federalized" becomes an asset of the regular military forces). A special situation in which the DoD aids law enforcement agencies involves the U.S. Secret Service. The DoD has authority to provide support to the U.S. Secret Service in support of the president of the United States. Types of support may include, but are not limited to, airlift, communications, medical, and EOD.

Improvised nuclear device (IND) response is delineated in DoD Directive 3150.5. It assumes that any IND release is an act of terrorism and establishes the FBI as the overall lead federal response agency in U.S. territories. The U.S. Department of State is the designated lead agency in any situation outside of FBI purview. DoD Directive 3150.5 establishes specific roles for each armed service in the event of IND incidents.

The largest repository of resources for WMD release response resides in the DoD total force (active duty, reserve, and National Guard components), despite growth in the civilian response to WMD. The DoD's initial response depends on the local military commander having available resources to respond. Local governments with adjacent DoD assets should establish memorandums of understanding and mutual aid agreements in advance so that resources used in the immediate response mode can freely flow across territorial boundaries.

Requests for support using this mode are made from local or state governments to the base commander or regional commander.[35]

Other than initial response mode (in which local governments interact directly with local DoD commanders), the primary pathway to request military resources is by request of the state governor to the U.S. president. The president declares a disaster, which triggers involvement of a lead federal agency, which would then request DoD assistance if required. This request will go to the secretary of defense (SecDef), who will then task the director of military support (DOMS). The DOMS oversees an operational staff within the DoD for the coordination of military assets in a civil emergency. Until a JFO is established with a defense coordinating officer (DCO) in place, the DOMS validates all mission requests, identifies available units, and initiates the mission assignment (MA) and deployment orders (Fig. 86-2). The DCO serves as the senior DoD representative within the JFO. Typically, the DCO is a senior military officer who is responsible for coordinating all DoD elements at an incident. He or she is responsible for validating any requests made from the federal coordinating officer (FCO) or PFO. A defense coordinating element comprised of an experienced staff of emergency managers and planners assists the DCO.

The emergency preparedness liaison officer (EPLO) is a senior military officer, typically a reservist, who serves to coordinate federal planning with state and local agencies. Each state and each FEMA region has an associated EPLO. EPLOs participate in federal planning, as well as the development of tabletop and full-scale exercises. In the event of an actual incident, the EPLO would be activated to serve as a full-time liaison between the DoD and the local and state response. If a JFO is established with a DCO in place, the EPLO is attached to continue his or her role within the organized response under that office.[36]

U.S. Northern Command (NORTHCOM) is the command and control structure for organizing DoD assets into an effective homeland security response. Established in October 2002, NORTHCOM has minimal assets under its operational control. Rather, it serves as a clearinghouse for planning and coordinating response by DoD assets. During an incident, NORTHCOM would receive tasks either from DOMS (prior to the establishment of a DCO) or from the DCO after he or she has been activated.

In the event of a chemical, biological, radiological, nuclear, or explosive (CBRNE) incident, the Joint Task Force Civil Support (JTF-CS) is the NORTHCOM subcommand that would provide command and control of DoD assets. It is a standing joint task force located at Fort Monroe, Virginia, commanded by a "federalized" National Guard general. When directed by the commander of NORTHCOM, JTF-CS would deploy to the incident site and establish command and control of DoD forces to provide military assistance to civil authorities. JTF-CS focuses on consequence management and would report to and work closely with the lead federal agency in this response. Typically, the DCO would be attached to the JTF-CS staff as a special assistant. The DCO would continue his or her focus of validating missions and authorizing the use of DoD assets.

The Marine Corps' Chemical Biological Incident Response Force (CBIRF) is a battalion-sized unit able to deploy to a WMD scene. It has a large integrated medical unit with emergency physicians, environmental health specialists, and medical technicians. Currently, CBIRF is based south of Washington, DC, however, it can be staged elsewhere in support of national special security events.[37]

The U.S. Army previously organized its WMD response into a single organization known as the Guardian Brigade. In 2004, the U.S.

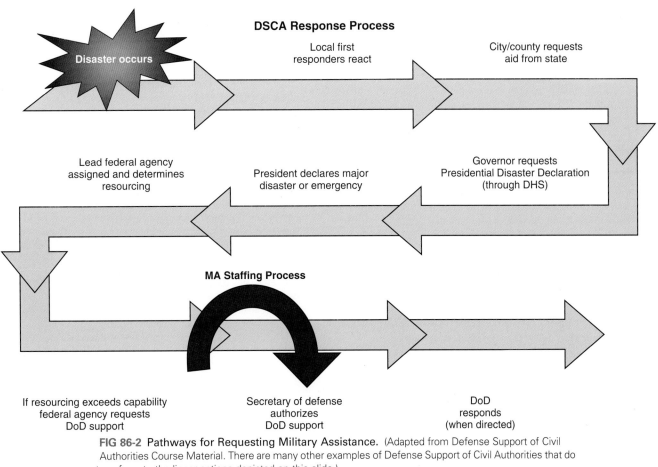

FIG 86-2 Pathways for Requesting Military Assistance. (Adapted from Defense Support of Civil Authorities Course Material. There are many other examples of Defense Support of Civil Authorities that do not conform to the linear actions depicted on this slide.)

Army consolidated all of its CBRNE response elements under one command. The 20th Support Command is comprised of a headquarters element, a Chemical Biological Rapid Response Team (C/B-RRT), the 22nd Chemical Battalion (Technical Escort), and the 52nd Ordnance Group. The army's C/B-RRT is a rapidly deployable asset to provide assessment of a potential chemical or biological incident. The mission of C/B-RRT is to coordinate the activities of all DoD assets responding to a CBRNE incident.[38]

WMD-CSTs are full-time National Guard teams that support the local incident commander "by identifying CBRNE agents/substances, assessing current or projected consequences, advising on response measures, and assisting with appropriate requests for additional follow-on state and federal military forces."[39] They are a state asset and report to the governor via the state's adjutant general (the commander of the state's National Guard). As a team, they can provide identification, threat modeling, mitigation, medical assessments, and recommendations while interfacing with subject matter experts and the incident commander. Once in place, they can act as the initial liaison between the local incident command structure and arriving DoD resources. It is essential to note the WMD-CSTs are not designed to provide mass decontamination, treatment, or care.[39]

The U.S. Air Force's Radiation Assessment Team (AFRAT) is a deployable team from Wright-Patterson Air Force Base (AFB), Ohio. It is designed to respond to incidents involving radiation emergencies. They are activated to respond to scenarios ranging from the accidental or intentional release of radioactive isotopes to large-scale WMD events. The AFRAT can provide a spectrum of capabilities "to deliver radiological risk assessment for contingency planning, consequence management, and site recovery."[40]

In addition to a monumental in-garrison health care mission, the medical commands of the U.S. Army, U.S. Air Force, and the U.S. Navy maintain deployable medical assets. An example is the U.S. Air Force's Expeditionary Medical Support (EMEDS) system. EMEDS is a modular response field hospital that is built around a central resuscitation area, operating room, and intensive care unit module. The basic EMEDS can deploy in hours, is transportable by air in a single C-130 aircraft, and has enough material to do multiple resuscitations and 10 surgeries. Additional beds and ancillary capabilities can be added to increase the health care delivery capacity in a sequential manner.[41]

! PITFALLS

Law Enforcement
Failure to Ascribe to the Incident Command System
There is an increasing but not universal use of unified command or the ICS. Failure to ascribe to the ICS leads to potential confusion of command and lack of standard terminology and structure, all of which can further complicate an already chaotic event.

Jurisdictional Confusion
An overall goal is a fluid response and rapid identification of the lead agency, especially at the first determination of an incident being a terrorist event. This requires a concentrated effort to work closely with law enforcement and other agencies as the incident develops.

Patient Care versus Evidence Preservation
When involved in the response to a terrorist incident, the EMS responder must stop to assess the scene not only from a mass casualty management standpoint, but also from a forensic viewpoint. It is likely that the EMT or firefighter may be the first, and perhaps only, witness to a particular piece of evidence. However, the primary goal of both law enforcement and medical providers is "preserving life or minimizing risk to health."[42]

Military
Presuming the Role of Lead Agency
Although the military is well suited to immediate response, the role of the military is to support local authorities, and they must not undermine that authority.

Inappropriate Immediate Response Authority
The use of the military is a well-described process. For forces that are proximate to an emergency, regardless of whether it involves terrorist activity, the local commander can operate under the auspices of immediate response. These are actions that can be taken to save life or limb or to preserve property, but are limited to 72 hours duration unless a formal disaster declaration ensues. If the event does not fall into either of these categories, the military should not be asked to deploy, nor should they agree to.

Violation of the Posse Comitatus Act
Although it is clear that the Posse Comitatus Act does not apply to the use of military resources in non–law enforcement situations, there will always be a concern expressed that the military is involved in civilian affairs. To minimize these concerns, the military should be used only for validated missions. Furthermore, military assets should not be placed in a potential situation where lethal force may be needed without clear instructions from higher authority under standing rules of force (SRUF).

REFERENCES

1. Anonymous. Preface. In: *National Interagency Management System.* Washington, DC: Federal Emergency Management Agency, Government Printing Office; 2004.
2. *Homeland Security Presidential Directive 5: National Strategy for Homeland Security.* Washington, DC: Office of the White House; 2002.
3. Anonymous. Appendix A: definitions and acronyms. In: *Regional Emergency Coordination Plan.* Washington, DC: Metropolitan Washington Council of Governments; 2002.
4. Clinton W. *Presidential Decision Directive 39: US Policy on Counterterrorism.* Washington, DC, 1995. Available at, www.fas.org/irp/offdocs/pdd39.htm. 22.01.14.
5. Carlson J. Critical incident management in the ultimate crisis: counterterrorism. *FBI Law Enforcement Bull.* 1999;68(3):6–8.
6. Sub Chapter IV: B emergency preparedness. In: *The Robert T. Stafford Disaster Assistance and Emergency Relief Act, as amended, 42 USC 5121, et seq.* 1988:36–46. Available at, www.dem.dcc.state.nc.us/mitigation/Library/Stafford.pdf. accessed 24.01.14.
7. Fusco A. Overview: chief of department. In: United States Fire Administration, ed. *The World Trade Center Bombing Report and Analysis.* Emmitsburg, Md: Federal Emergency Management Agency; 1993:1–23.
8. Goldfarb Z, Kuhr S. EMS response to the explosion. In: United States Fire Administration, ed. *The World Trade Center Bombing Report and Analysis.* Emmitsburg, Md: Federal Emergency Management Agency; 1993:92–110.
9. Martin RA. The joint terrorism task force: a concept that works—FBI–New York City police department. *FBI Law Enforcement Bull.* 1999;68(3):9–10.
10. *Protecting America from Terrorist Attack: Our Joint Terrorism Task Forces.* Available at: http://www.fbi.gov/about-us/investigate/terrorism/terrorism_jttfs; Accessed 22.01.14.
11. FEMA Website. http://www.fema.gov/oklahoma-city-bombing-1995; Accessed 18.06.14.
12. The Subcommittee on Economic Development. *Public Building and Emergency Management Hearing on Combating Terrorism: Options to Improve the Federal Response.* Available at: http://www.house.gov/transportation/pbed/04-24-01/04-24-01 memo.html. 22.01.14.
13. Anonymous. *White Paper on Presidential Decision Directive 62: Protection Against Unconventional Threats to the Homeland and Americans Overseas.* Washington, DC, 1998. Available at, http://www.fas.org/irp/offdocs/pdd-62.htm. 22.01.14.

14. Anonymous. Chapter IV: concept of operations. In: *United States Government Interagency Domestic Terrorism. Concept of Operations Plan (CONPLAN)*; 2001:19–26. Washington, DC. Available at, www.fbi.gov/publications/conplan/conplan.pdf. Accessed 22.01.14.

15. Kean T, Hamilton L, Ben-Veniste R, et al. Chapter 9.2: September 11, 2001. In: *The 9/11 Commission Report*. Washington, DC: Government Printing Office; 2004:285–313.

16. Kean T, Hamilton L, Ben-Veniste R, et al. Chapter 9.3: emergency response at the pentagon. In: *The 9/11 Commission Report*. Washington, DC: Government Printing Office; 2004:311–314.

17. Department of Homeland Security. *Initial National Response Plan*. Washington, DC: Department of Homeland Security; 2003. Available at, https://www.crcpd.org/Homeland_Security/Initial_NRP_100903.pdf. Accessed 16.01.14.

18. Department of Homeland Security. *National Response Plan*. Washington, DC: Department of Homeland Security; 2004. Available at, http://www.dhs.gov/dhspublic/display?content=3611. Accessed 16.01.14.

19. Department of Homeland Security. *National Response Framework*. Washington, DC: Department of Homeland Security; 2008, 2013. Available at, http://www.fema.gov/pdf/emergency/nrf/nrf-core.pdf and http://www.fema.gov/media-library-data/20130726-1914-25045-1246/final_national_response_framework_20130501.pdf. Accessed 16.01.14.

20. Buchalter AR. *Military Support to Civil Authorities: The Role of the Department f Defense in Support of Homeland Defense*, vol. 13. Washington, DC: The Library of Congress; 2007, February.

21. Presson W. *Enhancing Security-Projecting Civil Authority into America's Uncontrolled Spaces*. No. ATZL-SWV-GDP, ARMY COMMAND AND GENERAL STAFF COLL FORT LEAVENWORTH KS; 2012.

22. Brake JD. *Terrorism and the Military's Role in Domestic Crisis Management: Background and Issues for Congress*. Washington, DC: Congressional Research Service; 2003.

23. Anonymous. Immediate response. In: *Department of Defense Emergency Preparedness Course Handbook*. Fort MacPherson, Ga: Department of Defense; 2004.

24. Department of Homeland Security. *National Response Framework*. Washington, DC: Department of Homeland Security; 2013. Available at, http://www.fema.gov/media-library-data/20130726-1914-25045-1246/final_national_response_framework_20130501.pdf. Accessed 16.01.14.

25. Anonymous. *Compendium of Federal Terrorism Training: For State and Local Audiences*; January 2007, Available at, http://develop.oes.ca.gov/WebPage/oeswebsite.nsf/699b301869389a02882573c900817d70/17056e559defd1398825767f00767279/$FILE/compendium.pdf. Accessed 26.01.14.

26. Department of Homeland Security. *National Response Framework*. Washington, DC: Department of Homeland Security; 2013. Available at: http://www.fema.gov/media-library-data/20130726-1914-25045-1246/final_national_response_framework_20130501.pdf. Accessed 16.01.14.

27. Rohen G. WMD response: integrating the joint operating center and the incident command system. *Police Chief Mag*. 2001; Available at, www.iacptechnology.org/Library/WMDResponseIntegratingJointOpsandIncidentCommand.pdf. Accessed 26.01.14.

28. Anonymous. Emergency preparedness and response. In: *The National Strategy for Homeland Security*. Washington, DC: Department of Homeland Security; 2003:41–45.

29. Anonymous. National response plan. In: *Department of Defense Emergency Preparedness Course Handbook*. Fort MacPherson, Ga: Department of Defense; 2004.

30. Fletcher WD, Field VW, Wade C. *FBI Laboratory*. Available at: http://www.fbi.gov/hq/lab/labhome.htm. Accessed 22.01.14.

31. Anderson MR. *Twenty Years of Evolutionary Change in the Department of Defense's Civil Support Mission*. ARMY COMMAND AND GENERAL STAFF COLL FORT LEAVENWORTH KS SCHOOL OF ADVANCED MILITARY STUDIES; 2013.

32. Anonymous. *Defense Support of Civil Authorities (DSCA): Department of Defense Directive 3025.18*. Washington, DC: Department of Defense; 2010 (incorporating Change 1, 2012).

33. The Posse Comitatus Act: setting the record straight on 124 years of mischief and misunderstanding before any more damage is done. *Mil Law Rev*. 2003;175.

34. Elsea JK. *The Use of Federal Troops for Disaster Assistance: Legal Issues*. LIBRARY OF CONGRESS WASHINGTON DC CONGRESSIONAL RESEARCH SERVICE; 2006.

35. Taft WH. *DOD Response to Improvised Nuclear Device (IND) Incidents: Department of Defense Directive 3150.5*. Washington, DC: Department of Defense; 1987 (incorporating review 2004).

36. Anonymous. *Army Emergency Preparedness Liaison Officer (EPLO) Program. FORSCOM Regulation 140-12*. Fort Mac-Pherson, GA: Department of Defense; 2001.

37. Anonymous. *Chemical Biological Incident Response Force*. Website http://www.cbirf.marines.mil/About/History.aspx; Accessed 17.01.14.

38. Anonymous. *20th Support Command (CBRNE)*. Website http://www.cbrne.army.mil/aboutus/history.html; Accessed 17.01.14.

39. Anonymous. *Weapons of Mass Destruction Civil Support Team Factsheet*. http://www.nationalguard.mil/media/factsheets/2013/WMD-CST-March-2013.pdf; Accessed 17.01.14.

40. Anonymous. *Air Force Radiation Assessment Fact Sheet*. http://www.wpafb.af.mil/library/factsheets/factsheet.asp?id=18146; Accessed 17.01.14.

41. Anonymous. *The EMEDS Handbook*. Wright-Patterson AFB, OH: The US Air Force School of Aerospace Medicine; 2003.

42. Anonymous. *Radiological/Nuclear Law Enforcement and Public Health Investigation Handbook—September, 2011*. Washington, DC: Centers for Disease Control; 2011. Available at, http://emergency.cdc.gov/radiation/pdf/radiological%20nuclear%20handbook%2009%2001%2011.pdf. Accessed 17.01.14.

87 | CHAPTER

Tactical Emergency Medical Support

Jason Pickett

Tactical emergency medical support (TEMS) draws its roots from military medics in conflicts in the Napoleonic wars. Later conflicts, such as World Wars I and II, the Korean War, and Vietnam War, saw the role and capability of the combat medic expand. Medical care and evacuation became an essential part of the battle plan. The modern day infantry medic participates in combat alongside other infantrymen as a fully integrated member of the platoon.

The National Tactical Officers Association defines TEMS as "the provision of preventative, urgent, and emergent medical care during high-risk, extended-duration and mission-driven law enforcement special operations."[1] Although models vary from one team to another, the basic premise of TEMS includes medical personnel integrated with tactical units to provide on-site medical care and assist in the planning process.[2] This may include police officers who are cross-trained in medical care, paramedics or physicians who are fully integrated into teams but lack police powers, or medical support that remains outside of the inner perimeter. Each model has advantages and disadvantages that will be discussed later. TEMS medics have tactical training that enables them to enter high threat environments with the team.

The importance of having medical support embedded with the team is most evident when one examines scene safety doctrine among conventional emergency medical services (EMS). EMS are often ill-trained to function in a high-threat setting, such as one where active hostile fire is present, and will therefore wait outside the "hot zone" until their safety can be guaranteed. Without tactical medical support, long delays in care may result as EMS wait for the tactical situation to be resolved before making patient contact. A short distance of 100 yards may still prove deadly to a victim who is actively hemorrhaging in an unsafe area. In the Columbine High School Massacre in 1999 a teacher was wounded inside the school and bled to death as he waited more than 3 hours for medical care to arrive at his side. His family later settled a lawsuit with the Jefferson County Sheriff's Office for the delay in care, receiving a settlement of $1.5 million.[3] In the 2013 Los Angeles International Airport shooting a Transportation Security Administration (TSA) agent was shot by a lone gunman; 30 minutes passed before medical care was rendered due to the concern for additional threats.[4] In the North Hollywood shootout of 1996, one perpetrator bled to death for 30 minutes after being shot at close range by police. Because there were two mobile, heavily armed shooters firing indiscriminately at police and civilians, it was felt that the situation was too volatile for EMS to enter. His family sued, which resulted in a hung jury, and later dropped the suit in exchange for an assurance to provide additional training for officers.[5] Whether any of these victims could have been saved with earlier care is uncertain, but this highlights the difficulty in bringing care to the hostile environment.

HISTORICAL PERSPECTIVE

In the 1960s and 1970s high profile incidents, such as the 1966 Texas Bell Tower Incident, where a lone shooter climbed the clock tower at the University of Texas in Austin, killing 17 people and wounding 31 more with a high-powered rifle,[6] created the impetus to form specialized, highly trained, and versatile police tactical teams to intervene on high-risk incidents. The Los Angeles Police Department and Los Angeles Sheriff's Department organized two of the first tactical law enforcement teams in the United States in the latter part of 1966.[7,8] Hostage rescue, apprehension of violent, armed criminals, special reconnaissance, clandestine drug lab operations, and protection of special assets or high profile persons are among the missions that law enforcement tactical teams may be asked to accomplish. These special weapons and tactics (SWAT) teams are comprised of law enforcement and support personnel under a unified command structure for maximum versatility. With the high likelihood of injury and death posed by these missions, it was not long before embedded medical support was part of the SWAT team profile. Teams drew on the military medical model of line medics who are closely aligned with tactical team members to minimize the distance to competent medical care from the point of injury. To operate in this high threat environment, additional training must be provided so that the medic does not become a liability to the team. The top priority always remains: mission first. The mission is what will prevent more casualties and loss of life. The medic may therefore defer medical care or bypass casualties in order to continue the mission and eliminate the threat.

CURRENT PRACTICE

Delivery Models

The basic premise of medical support on tactical teams remains constant: to reduce death, injury, and illness through care, training, and preventive measures. The composition and training of TEMS units remain diverse at the local level. Not all SWAT teams have organic medical support embedded in their organization. This is sometimes due to funding, lack of available trained personnel, or jurisdictional conflict between the police department and other organizations that may provide support. There are some team commanders who incorrectly believe that providing medical care is inconsistent with the organizational mission and that doing so would invite additional liability. The opposite appears to be true, however, and rapid medical treatment and stabilization will improve liability posture. Table 87-1 illustrates some common delivery models with advantages and disadvantages of each.

TABLE 87-1 TEMS Delivery Models

ADVANTAGES	DISADVANTAGES
Sworn Police Officers Cross-Trained in Emergency Prehospital Medicine	
Role flexibility: can perform enforcement duties and change to TEMS when needed.	Potential role confusion if both duties are required.
Can go where the team goes.	Cross-training dual roles could mean less expertise than their single-role counterparts.
Have statutory authority to arrest and carry weapons where they may otherwise be prohibited.	Training programs for police vary from 120 hours to over 700 hours. EMT requires 140 hours, and paramedics an additional 1000-2000 hours. These courses represent a substantial investment of time that may be prohibitive.
Can provide for their own defense.	
Training standard for weapons is defined in state or federal law.	
Statutory liability protections may exist.	
Nonsworn Medical Personnel (Physicians, Physician Assistants, Paramedics)	
Can go where the team goes.	Poor clarity on legal liabilities, and may have limitations on carrying firearms in all places (government buildings, schools).
Typically have continuous practice in their field.	
No role confusion or arrest powers.	If unarmed, another operator must provide defense.
Conventional EMS Units Staged for Support	
Little to no cost burden for the law enforcement agency.	Inadequate for tactical medical support.
Law enforcement agency can refute liability for medical care.	No tactical training, weapons, or rescue skills.
No role confusion.	Must remain far from the danger area and cannot enter the hot zone, which can delay care.
	No training in team health, operational sustainment, temporizing treatments to maintain mission profile.
	Limited understanding of unique SWAT personality types, and limited trust due to lack of regular training with the team can be detrimental to care.
	Lack of ability to train SWAT officers in tactical medicine for self-care.
	Ambiguity in chain of command, and leadership confusion when a medical emergency occurs.

Training, Preventive Medicine, and Mission Sustainment

A core function of TEMS includes advising the commander and team members of hazards that may compromise mission success and lead to undesirable outcomes. Gathering medical intelligence about the operational area is paramount. Weather, food and water sources, endemic illnesses, and likely patient population to be encountered will factor in to equipment selection and training. The TEMS provider has the responsibility to educate the commander and tactical operators on

medical issues and procedures that will enhance mission effectiveness and prevent injury. All team members should be taught by their TEMS provider how to perform basic bleeding control, application of chest seals, use of basic airway tools, and drags and carries for moving injured casualties. Hydration, prevention of heat and cold injuries, poisonous fauna, and management of simple ailments are other items of interest to the tactical team.

The TEMS provider will have to consider hygiene, toileting, and food and water sources for extended operations. In a disaster setting these may provide significant challenges. Management of minor injuries and illnesses must be considered, particularly if evacuation is onerous or not tactically feasible.

Echelon Staging of Medical Gear

One way the medic can maintain maximum mobility is by determining where in each phase of care certain equipment will be needed. For example, direct threat care items, such as tourniquets, chest seals, and nasal airways, might be located on the medic's primary load carriage or vest. Additional equipment for multiple casualties may be kept in a medical bag that can be dropped and then quickly retrieved at a point of entry into a building, whereas more advanced equipment for extended care may be kept in a kit in a vehicle.

Mission profile will greatly dictate what and how much equipment is carried. A high-risk arrest warrant executed in an urban house is likely to encompass few issues when it comes to casualty evacuation and handoff to civilian EMS. The same warrant on a rural methamphetamine lab may involve significant travel by vehicle and on foot to avoid detection. In some missions tactical teams and their medical support may need to shelter in place to remain hidden until it is time to make contact with the target. Body armor, helmet, water, weapons, ammunition, and other protective gear may weigh upwards of forty pounds. Equipment selection is therefore of utmost importance. TEMS medics will often repackage gear to reduce space and weight. Packing equipment that can be utilized for multiple purposes, sometimes in unusual ways, will help maintain the medic's mobility. Some techniques are listed in Box 87-1.

Many of the principles from military and SWAT team medical support can be applied in any high-threat situation, such as a disaster or civil disturbance. Conventional EMS and local health care facilities may be severely impacted or nonexistent in a disaster. Disaster medical resources may become targets in severe civil unrest or terrorism.[9,10] Modifying care protocols based on the surrounding circumstances is a core principle in disaster care.[11]

There are times when good medicine can be bad tactics—procedures or practices common in EMS may expose the victim or team member to additional hazards. An example of this would be the victim who is lying wounded in an area vulnerable to sniper fire. Whereas traditional EMS doctrine might dictate performing a full assessment and stabilizing treatment prior to moving the victim,[12] in the tactical setting it may be wiser to provide very limited care such as hemorrhage control while rapidly moving the victim to cover. Good tactical field care may sustain a victim for hours or days in an area where EMS cannot be brought in to effect evacuation.

Principles of care in the tactical setting follow a doctrine as put forth by the Committee for Tactical Emergency Casualty Care (C-TECC).[13] These protocols were developed by physicians, physician assistants, medics, and law enforcement for application in the civilian environment and are derived from military protocols for Tactical Combat Casualty Care (TCCC). These treatment recommendations are based on available research and lessons learned from decades of combat.

BOX 87-1 Techniques to Reduce Load Size and Weight

1. Pack gauze with a vacuum food sealer to reduce space and protect from water. Make a small cut in the edge so that it is easy to tear open.
2. Limit the amount of intravenous fluid carried and be cautious about unnecessary over-resuscitation with crystalloids.
3. Hetastarch and freeze-dried plasma colloids are administered in smaller volumes, and therefore may reduce the overall fluid weight carried.
4. Divide the medical load among team members. Increasingly SWAT operators are being issued an individual first aid kit with tourniquet(s), etc., for personal use.
5. If battery-powered tools, such as laryngoscope handles or intraosseous drivers, will be carried, select the smallest, with the smallest batteries.
6. Surgical instrument sets, such as surgical airway kits or wound repair kits, can be broken into small packages and sterilized in small pouches.
7. A Foley catheter can be utilized for hemorrhage control at a noncompressible site, such as the subclavian area.
8. Padded, malleable aluminum splints are highly versatile.
9. Limit the size options of equipment. Half-sizes of items, such as endotracheal tubes, may not be necessary.
10. A carabiner and 550 cord (paracord) make for a compact dragline that can be thrown to a casualty to drag him or her behind cover.
11. Duct tape is one of the most useful things you can carry.
12. A roll of cellophane food wrap has many uses: securing dressings and equipment, making occlusive dressings, and packaging patient medications.

TECC grew out of a need to develop treatment guidelines specific to the civilian environment where regulatory issues (scope of practice of providers, civil liability) and patient population (pediatrics, geriatrics, comorbid disease) differ from the military setting.

As in disasters, equipment, space, and medical resources in the tactical environment may be limited, and these must be factored in when planning and equipping for the mission. Light and noise discipline must be practiced to avoid detection of covert operations, whereas in a disaster, light may not be available due to infrastructure damage or time of day. Time and distance to resupply may be problematic, so the TEMS medic should plan and equip for casualty care with this in mind.

Direct Threat Care

The direct threat zone, or "hot zone," is an area where the victim and medic may be subject to accurate hostile fire or explosive threats. Emphasis here is on expedited treatment of immediate life threats at the point of wounding, such as active hemorrhage, airway obstruction, or tension pneumothorax. Tourniquets, nasal airways, occlusive chest seals, and hemostatic dressings are lightweight items that should be carried by all tactical team members, who regardless of any other medical training, should be trained in their use. Use of these for injuries must be followed by rapid extraction to cover to begin field resuscitation in the indirect threat zone, or "warm zone." Evacuation to definitive care should be undertaken as soon as practical, but may be delayed by the mission.

Indirect Threat Care

Care in the indirect threat zone, or "warm zone," is provided in an area where the victim and medic are protected from direct fire, but mobility is hampered, or where evolution in the tactical situation may expose them to direct fire. This zone may be a point of cover, such as behind a wall or berm, inside an armored vehicle, or inside a building in an otherwise hostile area. Indirect threat care may be brief if local medical resources are available to take the patient to definitive care or may be prolonged if the tactical situation isolates the team from EMS or health care facilities due to location.

Core principles of care in this setting include advanced airway management, pain control, resuscitation, injury stabilization, and antibiotic administration. Self-administration of oral fluids and pain medication can free the medic to concentrate on advanced care of more serious casualties.

Pain management at the point of wounding has been shown to reduce posttraumatic stress disorder in combat casualties. Side effects of narcotics, such as hypotension and respiratory depression, which are somewhat more difficult to manage in the tactical setting, have led to the development of pain control protocols using ketamine. Often used for procedures in the emergency department setting, ketamine is a dissociative anesthetic that does not tend to cause hypotension or respiratory depression in trauma casualties. Transmucosal fentanyl "lollipops" enable a casualty to self-administer pain medication as needed, are very lightweight, and take up very little space in the medical pack. Self-titration of fentanyl frees the medic to perform other tasks as needed.

Intravenous fluids take up significant amounts of weight and space in the medical pack, which may hamper mobility of the medic. Patients with trauma often have worse outcomes when even relatively small amounts of crystalloid fluids (Ringer's lactate, normal saline) are given.[14-16] It may therefore be prudent to limit crystalloid infusion in the trauma patient, despite significant blood loss when the patient is not in severe shock. The concept of "permissive hypotension" has gained ground in recent years in treatment of the trauma patient to limit continued hemorrhage when it cannot be directly controlled. The TEMS medic must balance the capability for large volume fluid resuscitation with limitations of the equipment set. Hypertonic crystalloids (3% saline), hetastarch (Hespan or Hextend), and freeze-dried plasma are some options that may reduce fluid volume but maintain perfusion in the trauma patient.

Early administration of antibiotics may be prudent.[17] The Battle of Mogadishu on October 3-4, 1993 (as seen in the Mark Bowden book and movie, *Blackhawk Down*) saw a 38% wound infection rate, though all casualties received definitive care within 15 hours of the start of the operation.[18] Fluoroquinolones, carbapenems, and third and fourth generation cephalosporins have broad-spectrum coverage of gram-positive and gram-negative bacteria and relatively infrequent dosing (every 24 hours for some).[19]

Casualty Evacuation

Movement of the casualty to definitive surgical care or extended inpatient medical care will be necessary for all but minor injuries and illnesses. The current tactical situation, availability and skill level of local EMS, and distance to a functioning hospital will determine the timing and means of transport. If route security is an issue, travel by air may be necessary. Vehicles of opportunity can serve as impromptu medical evacuation platforms, when needed. The need for en route care must also be weighed, along with the medic's ability to do so in a vehicle not designed for medical care. It may be better in the long run to stabilize in the field as much as possible before transport if en route care will be restricted.

Tactical Rescue

Movement of patients out of the direct threat zone is the most important step in being able to provide advanced medical care to a casualty. Casualties may be able to effect self-rescue, by crawling or running to the nearest point of cover. This can be accomplished without additional team members exposing themselves to fire. If the casualty is unable to move to cover, then a dragline may be thrown to the casualty, who may then be pulled behind cover without exposing the team.

For movement of 10 yards or less, a "hasty drag" of the victim by an extremity or clothing will get them quickly to cover. Most tactical vests have built in handles for just this purpose. The rescuer will not be able to provide for his own defense while dragging the victim, so additional personnel will have to provide security and return fire, if needed. Ideally the victim may provide additional cover fire while being extracted, if physically possible. Rescue team members must remain exposed for as little time as possible. They should move quickly from one point of cover to another and not stop in the open for any reason.

For movements up to 75 yards or so, a flexible litter may be used to move the casualty. A litter is a piece of fabric with handholds for rescuers to lift or drag a nonambulatory casualty. This can be a commercial litter with heavy-duty handles, or an improvised one utilizing a sheet or tarp. This enables multiple rescuers to carry the casualty and prevent fatigue.

For movements over greater distances, a poled litter or vehicle is best. Some techniques for utilizing vehicles of opportunity may allow greater cover for rescuers from direct fire or carry the weight of the casualty to enable the team to move faster out of the threat zone.

Armored vehicles may serve as a shooting platform and can be interposed between the medical team and a potential threat. Armored cars commonly used by banks may be commandeered if a tactical armored vehicle is unavailable. Other, more technical tactical rescue techniques are discussed elsewhere in this textbook.

⚠ PITFALLS

Liability

Arming of nonsworn TEMS providers remains a controversial topic. In military settings noncombatant medical providers are still permitted to be armed and use deadly force to protect themselves and their patients.[20] Any team member who carries a weapon should have training in safe weapons handling, marksmanship, weapon retention, and proper use of deadly force. Laws regarding use of deadly physical force do not differ greatly between police officers and citizens, with a few narrow exceptions, and typically may only be used if there is an imminent threat to life. Any SWAT team member who uses physical force in the course of duties will expose the organization to some degree of liability. A failure to act may also invite liability, so the team commander must balance these factors to decide if arming the nonsworn TEMS provider is prudent. Regardless of whether the tactical medical provider is personally armed, he or she should be trained to properly disarm and store all weapons carried by the SWAT operators, particularly if the injured operator has altered mental status.

SUMMARY

The tactical environment and disaster environments have much in common, and skills that are applicable during tactical operations are useful in any high-threat, limited-resource setting. Focused initial-injury or illness mitigation in direct threat settings, followed by focused care and stabilization in preparation for evacuation, with limited multipurpose equipment and creative application, are critical skills not only for TEMS providers, but also disaster responders.

REFERENCES

1. National Tactical Officers Association. NTOA.org.
2. Heiskell LE, Carmona RH. Tactical emergency medical services: an emerging subspecialty of emergency medicine. *Ann Emerg Med.* 1994;23 (4):778–785.
3. Abbott K, Able C. Sanders settles Columbine suit. *Rocky Mountain News.* Aug 21, 2002.
4. Kandel J. *NBC Los Angeles;* Nov 15, 2013. www.nbclosangeles.com/news/local/TSA-Officer-Bled-For-33-Minutes-In-LAX-Shooting-232062361.html.
5. Rosenzweig D. *Los Angeles Times.* June 20, 2000. http://articles.latimes.com/2000/jun/20/local/me-42801.
6. National Public Radio. npr.org.
7. National Tactical Officers Association. NTOA.org.
8. Ramirez E. *Police Magazine.* Published online May 1, 2003. http://www.policemag.com/channel/swat/articles/2003/05/point-of-law.aspx.
9. Relief workers confront "Urban Warfare" *CNN.* Sept 1, 2005. http://www.cnn.com/2005/WEATHER/09/01/katrina.impact.
10. Stoddard A, Harmer A, DiDomenico V. *Providing Aid in Insecure Environments: 2009 Update. Trends in Violence Against Aid Workers and the Operational Response.* Humanitarian Policy Group, Overseas Development Institute; 2009.
11. *Crisis Standards of Care: A System Framework for Catastrophic Disaster Response.* Institute of Medicine of the National Academies; March 2012.
12. *Emergency Medical Technician National Standard Curriculum.* National Highway Transportation and Safety Administration. NHTSA.gov.
13. Callaway DW, Smith ER, Cain J, et al. Tactical emergency casualty care (TECC): guidelines for the provision of prehospital trauma care in high threat environments. *J Spec Oper Med.* 2011 Summer;11(3):104–122.
14. Morrison CA, Carrick MM, Norman MA, et al. Hypotensive resuscitation strategy reduces transfusion requirements and severe postoperative coagulopathy in trauma patients with hemorrhagic shock: preliminary results of a randomized controlled trial. *J Trauma.* 2011;70(3):652–663. http://dx.doi.org/10.1097/TA.0b013e31820e77ea.
15. Kasotakis G, Sideris A, Yang Y, et al. Inflammation and Host Response to Injury Investigators. Aggressive early crystalloid resuscitation adversely affects outcomes in adult blunt trauma patients: an analysis of the Glue Grant database. *J Trauma Acute Care Surg.* 2013;74(5):1215–1221. http://dx.doi.org/10.1097/TA.0b013e3182826e13. discussion 1221–1222.
16. Ley EJ, Clond MA, Srour MK, et al. Emergency department crystalloid resuscitation of 1.5 L or more is associated with increased mortality in elderly and nonelderly trauma patients. *J Trauma.* 2011;70(2):398–400. http://dx.doi.org/10.1097/TA.0b013e318208f99b.
17. Butler FK, Holcomb JB, Giebner SD, McSwain NE, Baglan J. Tactical combat casualty care 2007: evolving concepts and battlefield experience. *Mil Med.* November 2007;172(suppl).
18. Mabry RL, Holcomb JB, Baker AM, et al. United States Army Rangers in Somalia: an analysis of combat casualties on an urban battlefield. *J Trauma.* 2000;49(3):515–528. discussion 528–529.
19. *Infections. Emergency War Surgery Handbook, 4th United States Revision 2013.* Washington, DC: Borden Institute. Walter Reed Army Medical Center; 2004.
20. FM 4-02.2. *Medical Evacuation.* US Army Publishing Directorate.

88 CHAPTER

Medicine beyond the Barricade

Michael D. Mack and James P. Phillips

A SWAT team is a group of highly trained individuals used by their respective agency to complete missions that are beyond the scope and expertise of the general officer. The origin of SWAT can be traced back to the University of Texas Bell Tower Shooting that took place in 1966. Since that time, SWAT has developed not only new tactics but also specialized roles including proactive mobilization for high-risk warrant serving, reactive deployment against violent offenders, planned staging for show-of-force purposes, and situations in which criminals take hostages or barricade themselves from law enforcement.

In a parallel manner, the development of the current hostage negotiation team (HNT) occurred following the failed attempt to rescue members of the Israeli Olympic Team taken captive by terrorists at the 1972 Munich Games. During this incident, a group of Palestinian terrorists invaded an Olympic dormitory and seized 11 Israeli athletes as hostages. Once the terrorists' political demands had been refused, the Munich police resorted to firepower, resulting in the death of 22 people, including all 11 of the hostages. This event highlighted the distinct lack of protocol or procedure to deal with crises in a controlled way and limit death or injury to hostages.[1]

The purposeful barricading of wounded people from law enforcement and emergency medical service (EMS) and the unique role of the medical provider in such situations is the focus of this chapter. Such medical events have fortunately been rare, but certainly, they do occur. Therefore it is important that physicians involved in Tactical Emergency Medical Support, military operations, EMS direction, and Urban Search and Rescue (US&R) be familiar with the concepts and skills so that they can be best prepared if called upon.

HISTORICAL PERSPECTIVE

"Medicine beyond the barricade" refers to the unique, specialized skills that are required to assess a patient and provide medical care in a situation in which there is no direct contact between the patient and the provider. As stated in the above paragraph, this phrase refers primarily to situations in which a hostage is injured or ill, law enforcement has contained the area, and an armed suspect(s) prevents emergency rescuers access to those in need. The term *barricade* refers to a barrier created to impede the advance of an enemy.[2] In a hostage situation, it is common for hostages to have suffered injuries that require attention. In fact, published data from a retrospective review of crisis and hostage situations by Feldman demonstrated that 88% of such of incidents ended in injury or death to either some or all of the hostages and perpetrator(s).[3] Hostage situations occur not only domestically with police departments but also in military operations overseas. Notably, there is some crossover with US&R missions, as well as modern telemedicine. Concepts taught to prepare for medical assessment and treatment during barricade and hostage situations can be applied to noncriminal

situations. US&R providers train extensively, and part of that training involves the assessment of injured and trapped victims with whom they may not be in visual contact because of situations following accidents, terrorism, and natural disasters.

Medicine beyond the barricade conceptualizes the process of assessing and rendering aid to those who are out of direct physical and visual contact of the provider. Providing emergency medical care to patients in a typical combat environment is challenging for numerous reasons, including the lack of advanced diagnostic tools, limited supplies, the probability of severe injuries, austere environments, and the unique complexities of being under fire.[4] Typically, providers have the opportunity to assess patients using all of their senses; however, when the medic and the patient are separated by a physical barrier there are additional factors to consider that are widely variable depending on the particular situation. Tactical emergency medical support (TEMS) providers must be flexible, with the ability to adapt to unexpected situations and perform a remote medical assessment, which involves assessing a patient without being able to visualize the patient.[5] These scenarios are not typically encountered by physicians or paramedics in routine practice. It is unlikely that a non-TEMS–related provider would ever be called upon to perform in such a way, as successful outcomes in barricade medicine require unique training, and the provider must keep these skills sharp through frequent drilling. To be successful and prevent worsening of a crisis situation, the provider must incorporate competencies from other disciplines that are not taught in standard medical education, including negotiation tactics, interpersonal skills, stress management, and medical care improvisation. In addition, it is highly unlikely that a provider who has not been intimately trained to work with Special Forces law enforcement (SWAT, Hostage Negotiation Team [HNT], and Hostage Rescue Team [HRT]) would be given consent by the incident commander to take part in the crisis process.

Several models of training in the performance of remote medical assessments have been published, and some of the tactical medicine schools in the United States, including Counter Narcotics and Terrorism Operational Medical Support (CONTOMS), incorporate medicine across the barricade as part of their formal curriculum.[5,6] Remote assessment is not a skill unique to US&R or TEMS providers. Remote assessments are performed many times per day by professionals who answer the phones for 911 centers across the country. These emergency medicine dispatchers (EMDs) are trained and certified to perform remote assessments for each call, including those that are primarily medical in nature. Their training includes the concept of Dispatch Life Support, which represents the sum of knowledge, procedures, and skills used by trained EMDs to provide care via prearrival instructions given to callers.[7] Many dispatchers use specialized computer software with protocols in the form of question-prompts based on the chief complaint of the caller, which allows them a step-by-step way to render aid according to a script. EMDs must also maintain a current Healthcare Provider–level CPR certification. There are other professions where medical specialists may encounter the need for remote assessment of patients, as well. Among the more interesting programs are NASA, the International Space Station, the Antarctic Research Station, and those used during in-flight medical emergencies on commercial airliners.

CURRENT PRACTICE

Access to the Patient

The very nature of barricade medicine implies that there is severely limited access to the person or persons requiring medical help, and in most cases, there is no direct or visible contact. In the search and rescue realm, the situation may have different threats and limitations, but the techniques and technology may overlap with a hostage crisis. For the sake of this chapter, the focus will be on situations in which the provider and the injured are completely separated with only voice communication. Access can be accomplished by a variety of means including voice communication, radio, telephone, or Internet communication. US&R personnel sometimes secure access to a patient by creating a small caliber borehole into void spaces where the patient is trapped. The holes can be used for passing food, water, and medical supplies.[8] The teams are trained to deploy hardline phones (also known as "throw phones"), cell phones, radios, and microphones. They can even lower fiber optic cameras through such openings to obtain visual data. These methods are also used by law enforcement agencies during crises as needed, with traditional landlines and cell phones being the primary means used when infrastructure is not disrupted by the disaster or other causes. Additionally, LE agencies may use fiber optic cameras to see inside barricaded structures or use robot-mounted cameras of various types.

Several factors should be considered regarding the use of cell phones during a crisis. For instance, if law enforcement is concerned that an explosive device may be present, cell phone towers may be taken out of service to prevent remote detonation by the perpetrator. Additionally, if the event is ongoing and high profile, the cellular networks may be overwhelmed with local civilian traffic, effectively jamming communication across the barricade. While a cellphone could be very useful if a hostage can use it to provide photos, video, or video conferencing of wounded persons to expedite remote care, their utility may not outweigh the risks of battery depletion, inopportune signal loss, and illegal signal interception. For scene and personal security reasons, it is important to consider the potential danger of outside monitoring of the radio and cellular signals.[2,8] This may seem innocuous, but civilians or media may gain information and subsequently reveal details of an ongoing event or investigation without proper corroboration or clearance.

Many SWAT teams use robots to assist in high-threat environments. Some are simple and consist of little more than a camera attached to a radiocontrolled, wheeled vehicle. Others are significantly more complex, with features such as video and infrared optics, two-way communications, and even weaponry. They may also have special functions, such as using robotic arms to open doors and deliver hardline telephones or radios to gain access and communication without putting an officer in harm's way. These could be used to deliver medicines and medical supplies in a similar way.

Communications

All communications in and out of a crisis should be directly monitored by the Incident Commander (IC) or hostage negotiator. If needed, they will reach out to medical support to provide assistance. It is most likely that in an ongoing, tense hostage situation, a specialized negotiator will be the primary person in contact with any suspects or hostages, by either phone or radio, and any medical involvement will be in the form of advice from tactical EMS to the IC. In the extremely rare event that a TEMS provider would be required to have direct communication with perpetrators or hostages, the provider chosen should have some prior TEMS training and, ideally, familiarity with barricade medicine and remote assessment and treatment.

As part of their EMT-tactical training program, CONTOMS teaches a specific section called Medicine across the Barricade.

Several key points are taught to the provider. First, it is critical, using the EMD model of orderly assessment, that the provider focuses immediate lifesaving interventions. The acronym "XABC" is used among tactical medicine providers to remember the order of care given. It is modified from the typical first aid approach to include control of "eXsanguinating hemorrhage," then airway, breathing, and circulation. The IC should ensure that a medical provider chosen for this stressful task be well versed in emergency care and communication under stress.

Second, it is fundamental to prevent role confusion by the provider. There is ongoing debate outside the TEMS world regarding the ethics and utility of a physician acting as a police officer who is placed in a situation where lethal force may be required of that provider. In that same vein, it is critical that in a barricade medicine situation the physician knows his or her role is to provide medical assistance only, and *not* to attempt any tactical maneuvers, such as making promises, negotiating, or performing overt reconnaissance. Again, all communications should be monitored and controlled by the IC.

Medical Assessment

It can be assumed that the vast majority of crises with medical needs will be because of trauma to hostages or suspects, but it cannot be forgotten that hostages also may have chronic medical conditions and medication needs that must be addressed. The amount of time the crisis lasts may dictate the attention needed for different types of preexisting medical conditions. Insulin and food for diabetics becomes a problem early on. Some hostages may have needs that require several days to manifest, such as ongoing dialysis therapy or alcohol dependence with withdrawal symptoms. These things should be considered at the outset of a crisis, and every attempt should be made to contact relatives of known hostages to get medical information as early as possible.

Once verbal communication is established with the medical provider, that provider must use the information he has been given and that he can obtain over the phone to direct care. The role of the person with whom the physician is communicating will dictate the flow of the situation. The easiest encounter would involve direct verbal interaction with the injured person. A complete history and descriptive exam is clearly best obtained if the patient is conscious and talking on the phone. In a situation like this, the patient can provide care to him- or herself and can easily verbalize information regarding his past medical history and medication needs. However, if the person in need is not responsive or otherwise incapacitated, another person must act as an intermediary to relay historical information and to provide the care directly. The provider must be able to ask questions and give instructions in concise, simple, layperson vernacular, taking special care to avoid complexity. Three competencies are critical. These include the ability to remain calm, to avoid the use of medical jargon, and to complete a head-to-toe assessment using another's eyes, ears, and hands.[2,5] Should the provider have to speak directly with a perpetrator, the situation may be much more complex and volatile, depending on perpetrator's state of mind. This added layer of complexity requires direct supervision of the entire conversation by a trained IC or negotiator, to avoid misspeaking or agitation of the suspect. In such a high-stress situation, even the coolest heads may not perform at their peak. One protocol recommends a team approach to medical assessment and treatment; that is, always work with a partner. The role of the partner is to act as a "coach" to help the speaking provider stay calm and to provide reminders and notes to ensure no details are missed.

They can listen in by speakerphone or headset and can provide silent, written notes to the speaker as needed. If the proxy being spoken to is the perpetrator, the partner can step in and take over the provider role if the relationship between the perpetrator and the first provider turns sour.

There are different approaches to a remote, systematic evaluation of a patient. For the purpose of this chapter, we will assume the patient is unable to provide any information, and the proxy is a hostage. The medic must first introduce him- or herself, his partner, and provide calm reassurance. The medic asks the proxy his or her name or how he or she to be addressed, and if he or she has any prior medical or first aid training.

Next, the medical provider should ask for a quick overview of the state and position of the patient keeping in mind the XABC protocol as above. Some key considerations include whether the patient is injured or ill, presence of significant bleeding, state of breathing, presence of pulse, and level of consciousness. The rescuers must first treat any life-threatening injuries with emergency interventions, such as applying tourniquets, opening the airway, and/or occluding open chest wounds as needed.[8] The ability to improvise materials may save a life. Therefore the provider must get information from the proxy regarding the presence of medical supplies, first aid kits, and other accessible nonmedical equipment that can be used for tourniquets and splints.

After the XABC survey, the proxy must be coached through a rapid head-to-toe assessment, noting as many physical findings as possible. These include, but are not limited to, reactivity of pupils, general appearance of head, eyes, ears, nose, and throat (HEENT), trachea, presence of bulging neck veins, motion of chest during breathing, visual appearance of abdomen, whether the abdomen is soft to the touch, pelvic stability, bony deformities, and the presence of central and distal pulses. Appearance of the skin, including color, temperature, and moisture, may help the provider determine the presence of shock. Armed with a summary of injuries and findings, the provider can now work to give instructions to render aid, knowing that all interventions must be accomplished as dictated by necessity and availability of equipment.[9]

There may be no other situation during which communication is the most vitally important consideration for the outcome of the patient and the overall mission. There should be regular updates to the IC to keep him or her apprised on the patient's condition.[2] Be prepared to supply information in a clear, concise form, remembering that the IC may not have a medical background. The TEMS provider has no role in discussing the case with anyone, including the media, unless specifically put in that position by the IC, and remembering that Health Insurance Portability and Accountability (HIPPA) patient confidentiality rules still apply.

Equipment and Training

Similar to most TEMS missions with SWAT teams, the primary choice for a piece of medical equipment and supplies may be extremely limited or altogether unavailable. Therefore the rescuers must either deliver diagnostic and therapeutic equipment to the involved parties or be able to *describe* how to improvise equipment from items available in the victim's environment. Being able to find creative solutions to complex problems using rudimentary or improvised materials (such as a tourniquet from a cravat and stick, or a cervical collar made of a structural aluminum malleable splint) could be the difference between life and death.[4,10] Even when equipment is available, resupply may be hindered or impossible.

Training is essential to master the medical and communication skills necessary to be successful in these situations.[4,9–12] Drills for these skills should be constructed and performed at least annually by TEMS providers, as most likely, they will be selected by the IC or police to serve as the primary physician or medic on scene. These training scenarios only require low-tech equipment and imagination, and can be as simple as a story and two rooms connected by a telephone. Alternatively, they can be incorporated into a larger, multiagency disaster drill. Important training concepts should include having nonmedical personnel acting as the hostage and perpetrator on the phone and ensuring that there is no visual contact between the TEMS provider and the patient.[5] Also recommended, train with both standard and improvised equipment. In line with this, it is proposed that certain fixed and malleable traits, such as personality, coping style, decision-making style, emotion regulation, and emotional intelligence, may play a role in the ability of individuals to successfully perform and cope with their role.[1]

Documentation

Documentation, even if unable to be written in real-time, should be recorded as soon as possible. This may be helpful for use by emergency physicians after transport from the area and could be used as criminal evidence. Conversations on phones can and should be recorded. The after-action report (AAR) should be as complete and detailed as possible, as these records can also be valuable as training tools. The paperwork should include key points of the history and physical examination by proxy, notes between provider teammates, interventions recommended, and tourniquet times if applicable.

⚠ PITFALLS

Training for this extremely rare occurrence is paramount. Medicine across the barricade constitutes uniquely stressful situations with numerous, fluid variables.[2] Assuming success without training will assure failure.[5] At the other end of the spectrum, attempting to train every possible unique scenario will waste resources without significantly enhancing skills and knowledge. Maintaining these skills will help facilitate a remote medical assessment in most scenarios and give broad-based exposure to varied situations without compromising fidelity.

Becoming upset, excited, or flustered may compromise the situation. It is important to keep calm and collected, and to work with a partner who can provide relief if the communications turn unfavorable.

It is critical that the IC choose the most qualified, experienced, and well-trained provider for the task. A paramedic with street experience may be better qualified than a physician who works only clinically, and ego should have no influence in who is given the phone.

REFERENCES

1. Grubb A. Modern day hostage (crisis) negotiation: the evolution of an art form within the policing arena. *Aggress Viol Behav.* 2010;15(5):341–348.
2. Faure GO. Negotiating with terrorists: the hostage case. *Intl Negot.* 2003;8(3).
3. Feldmann TB. Implications for negotiation strategies and training. *J Police Crisis Negotiat.* 2001;1(1):3–33.
4. Kragh JF, Walters TJ, Baer DG, et al. Survival with emergency tourniquet use to stop bleeding in major limb trauma. *Ann Surg.* 2009;249(1):1–7.
5. Mack MD, Springer B, Eyck Ten R. Medicine Across the Barricade. *MedEdPORTAL Publications;* 2013.
6. Medicine Across the Barricade. In: *Counter Narcotics and Terrorism Operational Medical Support Student Manual;* 2014, CONTOMS EMT-T Provider Course.

7. Clawson JJ, Hauert SA. *Dispatch Life Support: Establishing Standards That Work;* 1990. Available at: www.emergencydispatch.org.

8. Colantoni A. Personal communication. Mack DO ed.

9. Gildea JR, Janssen AR. Tactical emergency medical support: physician involvement and injury patterns in tactical teams. *J Emerg Med.* 2008;35 (4):411–414.

10. Moore FA. Tourniquets: another adjunct in damage control? *Ann Surg.* 2009;249(1):8–9.

11. Mullins J, Harrahill M. Use of a tourniquet after a gunshot wound to the thigh. *J Emerg Nurs.* 2009;35(3):265–267, 271.

12. Ramirez ML, Slovis CM. Resident involvement in civilian tactical emergency medicine. *J Emerg Med.* 2010;39(1):49–56.

Operational Rescue

Jeff Matthews and Sean D. McKay

Operational rescue, or as it is sometimes referred to, *contingency* or *hasty rescue*, is a multidisciplinary approach to rescue while operating within dynamic, often high-threat, and asset-depleted environments. This category often includes Special Operations Forces (SOF) personnel, tactical law enforcement personnel, and/or civilian specialized rescue elements (fire and rescue, disaster response, mountain rescue, USAR, counter-terror response, etc.), which are the first-line response to an unforeseen or outlier event that requires immediate rescue. Often this "immediate rescue" requirement is dictated by heightened threat and environmental variables that increase the risk of morbidity and mortality to not only the casualty but also the rescuer. These variables include but are not limited to enemy threat or gunfire, secondary collapse, toxic atmospheric conditions, weather, fire, and explosive devices.

Observations of training, review of mission After Action Reports (AARs), and ad hoc discussions with state and federal disaster response teams, federal law enforcement officers, and returning military units indicate that there exists a significant gap in terms of how first responders access and extract casualties in the tactical and technical environment. This work suggests that there is a requirement within the disaster and mass casualty response to develop foundational principles of rescue and to build appropriate tactics, techniques, and procedures (TTPs) for the evolving operational environment.[1]

When we examine casualty management within an austere environment as a whole, it can be divided into four distinct categories: *access*, *assess*, *stabilize*, and *extraction and evacuation*. Operational rescue primarily focuses on the access and extraction and evacuation categories, although all are interdependent on one another.

Access issues may include gaining access to a casualty within an elevator shaft or a collapsed structure, or needing to breach into reinforced doors. Access is a real problem in terrorism-related events, both international and domestic. In fact, most active-shooter responses contain some type of access hurdle for responders to overcome. A prime example of this is the campus shooting at Virginia Tech on April 16, 2007. At this event, the shooter, Seung-Hui Cho, used locks and chains to prevent quick access by law enforcement. It should be noted that the Virginia Tech incident was the third in a series of school attacks within a 6-month period. Attacks at Platte Canyon High School and Nickel Mines Amish School occurred in the preceding months to the Virginia Tech incident. Each attack progressively increased in fortification, subsequently lengthening the "time-to-entry" of law enforcement.

Assessment requires a rapid systematic search for potentially preventable causes of death from which the casualty may be suffering. An example would be an uncontrolled arterial hemorrhage from an extremity that is amenable to a tourniquet or hemostatic agent.

Stabilize describes the required and appropriate treatment modalities based on the assessment. The term *stabilize* is dynamic. Stabilization will look different depending on the threat level within the rescue operational space. The goal of this phase will most likely not be to return to homeostasis but rather to keep the casualty alive through evacuation. If the casualty is outside of a direct-threat environment and minimal danger is present for the casualty and rescuer, care that is more thorough can be provided. For the casualty inside a collapsed structure, where a potential for secondary collapse exists, only limited, lifesaving techniques should be applied prior to extraction. What constitutes these "lifesaving techniques" has and will continue to be modified. As medical technology and capabilities increase, additional evidence-based skills may become part of the standard of tactical medical care.

Extrication or Evacuation describes the process of packaging and removing the casualty from the environment to transport or a secured casualty staging area. This could take the form of a high-angle rope rescue, confined-space movement, or removal from various vehicles to include armored wheeled and rotary or fixed winged aircraft.

HISTORICAL PERSPECTIVE

We define three distinct rescue categories. It is important to appreciate the differences between them to understand the rescue environment and how it might affect first-responder response.

RECREATIONAL RESCUE

Examples of recreational environments would be climbing, canyoneering, and mountaineering. By true definition, recreational does not qualify as a rescue category, although safe recreational climbing requires the expert to use safety techniques to mitigate accidents, which can be categorized as "preventative rescue" or "reactive rescue." Rock climbing anchors are an example of equipment used for such a preventative purpose, and the use of these in recreation can easily translate into high-angle rescue techniques during an emergency response. In the recreational context, the climber is not responding to any kind of emergency, he or she is simply making his or her best attempt at preventing an emergency. He or she has time to engage in the analysis of the pathway, to weigh the pros and cons, reevaluate, and rig his or her best option. The climber also has evaluated and often specifically chosen his or her desired route. Some of these routes may also have pre-drilled, permanent fixed anchors available. Owing to the operational parameters listed, the safety-factor capability in this realm (although a rock face is demanding) is a luxury because of available time and lack of many variables that face disaster-response personnel (enemy fire, building collapse, flood, limited organic assets, etc.).

Situational Rescue

Situational rescue refers to a dedicated, organized element with the sole mission to respond to catastrophic events requiring rescue. This would include Fire Department Technical Rescue, Federal Emergency Management Agency (FEMA), Urban Search and Rescue (US&R), hazardous materials, and certain combat search and rescuer (CSAR) responses. These are groups of highly trained individuals with specific skill sets in various disciplines of rescue. Their gear typically has a high specificity and in many instances is prepackaged or cached in response vehicles, tractor trailers, aircraft cargo planes, or helicopters, ready for an immediate response. In many cases, the personnel are able to fill in within close proximity of the emergency or objective, and are not required to "pack-in" their equipment and supplies physically over great distances. In addition, once these personnel are activated, they function solely as a rescue element. This makes their posture reactive and specific to rescue. Their gear, "loadout," and assets are rescue centric and mission specific.

Operational Rescue

This category describes personnel who are first responders to an unforeseen or outlier event that requires immediate action to save a life. Often these rescues would be conducted in extremis. As stated previously, for the rescuers involved, "Specialized Rescue" may not be their primary, secondary, or even tertiary role or responsibility in the mission. Rescuers must consider that a chaotic problem is unfolding in front of them, and they may be part of the problem. In addition, rescuers must recognize that they are rescuing within a complex environment with unknown hazards and constantly changing variables.[2,3]

In the past, both Department of Defense (DoD) and civilian-response capabilities were constructed around the "Situational Rescue" paradigm. The need for operational-rescue techniques is becoming more evident as active-shooter incidents become more commonplace and involve the response of the entire public-safety response system. No discussion on active-shooter response would be complete without mentioning Columbine High School and the events that unfolded on April 20, 1999. This incident changed the way responders, particularly law enforcement, responded to these types of incidents. The theory of confining the perpetrator to the building and trying to negotiate to free hostages was no longer applicable for this type of violence.

Recall the outcry from parents and loved ones of the injured and deceased for answers on why it took so long for law enforcement and medical providers to reach those inside the building. The most notable example involved David Sanders, a teacher killed in the Columbine High School attack. At approximately 11:40 AM, David Sanders was shot while encouraging students to evacuate the cafeteria and directing them through a stairway. Mr. Sanders, along with 50 other students and teachers, took refuge in Science Room 3. While in the science room, students and teachers administered first aid and made contact with 911 emergency-services operators. The first direct outside contact was delivered to David Sanders at 4:00 PM, 3.5 hours after the first 911 calls were made requesting help.

In all, it would be over 45 minutes before the first law enforcement officer would make entry. It would be even longer before the first medical personnel would make patient contact. The delay was so great, the last victim was removed from Columbine High School 4.5 hours after the attack started, and 3 hours after the perpetrators, Klebold and Harris, committed suicide.[4]

Operational-rescue techniques are well suited for the active-shooter environment. First, active-shooter incidents are highly stressful for the responder. Studies have shown that humans do not become smarter when they are confronted with a highly stressful situation.[5]

As Lt. Col. Dave Grossman puts it, "we do not rise to the occasion, we sink to our training." Not only do stress and/or self-preservation not help our intelligence and decision making, hormone-induced tachycardia also decreases our ability to perform fine and complex motor skills. For this reason, operational-rescue techniques are built around very simple equipment and very basic techniques. It is important that no operational-rescue procedure requires extreme dexterity or technical calculations.

Another reason established operational-rescue techniques are desirable in an active-shooter situation is due to the specialized equipment involved. Typical fire-rescue and rope-rescue equipment weighs in at nearly 60 lbs., for a typical equipment bag, and another 40 lbs. for two ropes. Using operational-rescue equipment and techniques, responders are able to decrease the weight of the equipment from roughly 100 lbs. to only 8 to 15 lbs. The hardware in operational rescue is aluminum (versus stainless steel for traditional rescue), and the rope is much thinner (7.5 to 9 mm vs. 12.5 mm). From the perspective of technique, a typical urban-rescue-team rope rescue would include using a two-rope system. One rope would be the mainline supporting the victim, the other rope is considered a safety rope, should the mainline system fail.[6] With regard to operational rescue, only one rope is used to facilitate hasty setup. If a second rope is available during the execution of an operational rescue, it should be used to rescue additional civilians or personnel.

No discussion regarding operational rescue during an active-shooter response would be complete without mentioning the development of the Rescue Task Force (RTF) concept; this concept is born out of the Department of Homeland Security (DHS). In 2008 DHS stated, "The first officers to arrive on scene will not stop to help injured persons. Expect rescue teams comprised of additional officers and emergency medical personnel to follow the initial officers. These rescue teams will treat and remove any injured persons."[7]

In 2009, the Arlington Fire Department, under the direction of Dr. Reed Smith, was perhaps the first organization to develop RTF's into what they are now. The RTF concept is that the initial on-scene officers will go directly to the threat. This direct-threat area is the area where active violence is taking place and/or a location where the threat has unrestricted movement. The direct-threat area could also be where a known hazard, such as improvised explosive devices (IED), could be located.[8]

Once the threat is confined, barricaded, or eliminated, remaining officers will pair with teams of firefighters and emergency medical services (EMS) personnel to create an RTF. The RTF, under the protection of law enforcement, will enter the building, treating and extracting victims as quickly as practical. Treatment of victims should include the use of Tactical Emergency Casualty Care protocols.[9]

In 2013 the U.S. Fire Administration published *Fire/Emergency Medical Services Department Operational Considerations and Guide for Active Shooter and Mass Casualty Incidents*.[10] The purpose of this document was to support planning and preparation for active-shooter and mass casualty incidents. One section of this document titled Maximizing Life references a joint effort between the American College of Surgeons and the Federal Bureau of Investigation to develop a concept to maximize the survivability in a mass-shooting event. The consensus paper (known as the Hartford Consensus) identified the simple act of hemorrhage control as core treatment to improve survival. In an effort to facilitate rapid treatment and extraction, the U.S. Fire Administration (USFA) references the THREAT acronym.

- **T**—threat suppression (law enforcement direct to threat)
- **H**—hemorrhage control (Tactical Emergency Casualty Care [TECC] protocol and tourniquet application)

- **RE**—**r**apid **e**xtrication to safety (through traditional or operational-rescue means)
- **A**—assessment by medical providers (exterior triage and treatment)
- **T**—transport to definitive care

Even though medical treatment is an important part of the RTF response, it is only one piece of the puzzle. The evacuation of the injured is equally important. The traditional methods used to move casualties are not at the core of operational rescue. One would not be able to use traditional patient packaging methods, such as the use of backboards and stretchers, in the direct-threat environment. Standard techniques would require the caregiver to be exposed for too long, and the techniques are too cumbersome for quick extraction. This is especially true when casualties must be removed from multistory buildings, where stairwells would be the most direct routes out of the building. The use of stretchers and backboards would simply be too difficult and too slow. However, operational-rescue techniques would be highly applicable should a gain in extraction time occur, or threats reemerge during the RTF's deployment. Remember, operational-rescue techniques could be deployed when organic assets such as equipment, and personnel resources are at their minimum. In a multistory structure, teams should be prepared to use hasty rope systems to accomplish the emergency evacuation of victims and the RTF itself. This can be accomplished using a rope system and a very basic casualty extraction strap to conduct a basic stairwell evacuation, or as complicated as rigging a full rope-based lowering system. The size and complexity of the event will dictate the rescue system used. Personnel can easily carry a basic, lightweight, and capable rope system in a fanny pack, in addition to the medical equipment appropriate for TECC.

Another environment primed for operational rescue is the structural collapse. Structural collapse can occur through various means, including weather or other environmental emergencies, human-made causes, such as terrorism, fires, and even simple accidents, such as driving a vehicle through a house. When the topic of structural collapse comes up, many emergency personnel think of the FEMA US&R system. However, this great resource only responds when an incident is declared a federal disaster. Many structural collapse responses are staffed only by state and local responders, typically standard fire and EMS professionals, who are unlikely to have specialty training in advanced rescue techniques. Some departments do train specialty operators for search and rescue, but this is likely to be found only in larger metropolitan areas. Should a local jurisdiction have a rescue team, it may be ill-equipped for a structural collapse. Once again, we can look to the operational-rescue approach to make these local responders more effective in their response.

As an example, it may occur that to enter a collapsed building, a rescuer needs to place shoring material to keep collapsed walls, floors, and roofs stabilized. For the FEMA US&R team, this would involve deploying engineers and shoring teams along with thousands of dollars' worth of equipment to make the building safe for entry. However, for the first responder, these resources are likely not readily available. They must rely on a more asymmetric approach, such as using debris from the collapse as shoring material to make an area safe, or using pipe found in the pile along with concrete block as a lever and fulcrum to lift an item off a victim. Known or unknown, this rescuer is using the concept of operational rescue to make a difference.

The most frequent user of operational-rescue techniques is the U.S. military. The Global War on Terror brought with it a battlefield that presented many types of hazards of rescue. This includes, but is not limited to, the following:

- Remote mountainous terrain (including altitude problems)
- Rivers
- Deserts
- Lack of infrastructure (drinking and sanitation wells)
- Threat of improvised explosive devices

Many of the operational-rescue techniques used now were derived from AARs or interviews with military personnel. An example where ad hoc operational-rescue techniques were utilized is during the U.S. Consulate attack in Benghazi, Libya, on September 11, 2012. The attack moved from the U.S. Consulate to the CIA annex, and Americans were wounded and trapped on a rooftop. A small element of operators hastily created a rope-rescue system using "rope they had cut from gym equipment," and they lowered the casualty.[11] This operation was a prime example of operational rescue. The rescue occurred in a highly stressful environment, and was executed with few personnel and limited equipment. In addition, the equipment used was an improvised organic asset, or an asset that was found on the scene, versus carried to it.

CURRENT PRACTICES

After examining examples of operational rescue, it should be evident that key performance parameters for both techniques and equipment dictate nontraditional solutions. Specialized training with a specialized kit becomes the mandate, just as it is within TCCC/TECC. After 4.5 years of research and development of mission-specific techniques for operational-rescue situations, with end-users ranging from DoD SOF to civilian and federal assets, the solution was not only creating new techniques but also the creation of appropriate gear to facilitate the required techniques. Complicating the development of standardized training and equipment is that these organizations respond in every conceivable environment, including remote villages, multistory urban buildings, schools, and high-altitude mountainous regions. Because of this research and development, a few mandatory requirements became evident for training and technique selection. The first requirement is a de-emphasis on the memorization of numerous techniques, which are difficult for the end user to sustain and execute under stress: for example, identify those knots, hitches, and bends with a broad-spectrum use that can be tied incorrectly and still have a large element of safety for application. Second, techniques, equipment, and foundational understanding are simplified to increase sustainability of skill sets. Third, an emphasis is now placed on only the proven evidence-based techniques (i.e., lowering and hauling systems) that are realistic in tactical situations. Fourth, techniques and capabilities based on previous operation AAR's with a minimalist equipment preference, and layering specific techniques based on available resources, ranging from optimal to nonexistent, should be emphasized. Fifth, allow foundational techniques to permeate through various mission profiles with minimal adjustment (e.g., the same 3:1 mechanical advantage can be used for mountain-hauling, confined-space, and maritime operations).

The equipment to be used during a potential rescue is often restricted to only what is carried or staged in close proximity to the objective, requiring it to be lightweight, modular, multiuse, and simple because of the elevated sympathetic nervous system response and the dynamic situation. It is vital for operators in this realm to understand "how to think" through operational-rescue complexities versus a cookbook of "what to think" contained in formatted standard operating procedures (SOPs). Rescue efficacy is directly proportional to the individual's capability to rapidly problem solve under extreme stress and expeditiously utilize organic assets; therefore a thorough knowledge of key rescue principles and practices must be foundational. These principles and practices originate from disciplines such as mountaineering, canyoneering, climbing, technical rescue, fire department rapid-intervention crews, caving, alpine, US&R, vehicle extrication, confined space, structural collapse, and others.

These specialized skills must be used under the most difficult conditions and in extreme environments. Training organizations must take this outcomes-based model and apply it to all training evolutions to make the participants perform complex skills under stress. Most commercial and many military training and education programs exist for encoding a specific response to a specific problem, which effectively teaches the student a very narrow perspective on a very dynamic problem.

Operational-rescue skills can be directly correlated to civilian protocol using the National Fire Protection Standard for Technical Rescuer Professional Qualifications (NFPA 1006). This standard establishes the minimum job-performance requirements necessary for fire service and other emergency response personnel who perform technical rescue. An important feature of NFPA 1006 (and all NFPA professional qualification standards) is the inclusion of job-performance requirements (JPRs). JPRs are simply a task list of skills that the candidate should be capable of completing as part of the certification process. For instance, NFPA 1006 6.1.8 states a technical rope rescuer should be capable of "descending a fixed rope in a high-angle environment, given an anchored fixed-rope system, a specified minimum travel distance for the rescuer, a system to allow descent of a fixed rope. . . ." Note the lack of direction on *how* the skill is to be completed. This is important, as it allows various end-users flexibility in accomplishing the task in their own unique fashion; military personnel may choose to descend using a hitch and a carabineer, whereas a civilian rescuer may choose a piece of hardware designed for descending ropes. Many of the rescue courses offered to our special operations units now are slightly modified civilian-based high-angle, confined-space, climbing, and even rapid-intervention team curriculums. These stand-alone concepts, although effective in certain situations, do not template success in the operational setting.[2,6]

When unrealistic training paradigms are coupled with a static training environment, low stress, and limited knowledge of the problematic nature of current operational deployments, few useful capabilities are transferred to the students. Instruction should focus on encoding principles, require performance under stressful and varied conditions, and result in giving the student operational skills that are the result of being shown how to think in an asset-depleted dynamic environment. The world is dynamic and ever changing, and thus training for the domain of friction and violence involving asymmetric combat actions must incorporate exercises that require participants to think, engage chaos, solve problems rapidly, and perform skills under stress.

Operational rescue is a critical component of trauma-casualty management. Trauma care in the disaster and tactical environment is complex; it requires a unique blend of situational awareness, foresight, medical skill, multitasking, and physical strength. The TECC & TCCC model illustrates the shift of paradigm from civilian-based trauma guidelines to tactical adaptive principles that consider environmental and physiological challenges specific to the operational realm. Although overarching "principles" remain constant, medical standard practices cannot be transposed successfully into all arenas, just as standard rescue practices require improvisation for operational success.

As with the above examples of TECC & TCCC, the principles of rescue remain the same, whereas the practices and application vary depending on operational environment. An example of this can be found in the JPR from NFPA 1006 *Standard for Technical Rescuer Professional Qualifications 2013 Edition,* JPR 5.5.2: Construct a single-point anchor system. This principal should be foundational to all rescuers, but depending on the environmental variables present, it could vary dramatically. The fire department response to a high-angle incident may dictate a single-point anchor constructed of 1-inch flat webbing for the main line and an identical second system rigged for the belay line as the appropriate technique. Conversely, during a hasty or contingency rescue within a tactical environment, the single-point anchor may be a 1-inch tubular webbing, rigged to be releasable for a single-rope technique.

⚠ PITFALLS

The largest problem with operational rescue is the difficulty in preparing for an outlier event. Too often, rescue teams deploy to "bread and butter" operations, only to find the situation is much more complex than anticipated. Revisiting the Benghazi attack as an example, even though intelligence personnel may have foreseen a potential for an armed conflict, they did not foresee the building being set ablaze and the subsequent need to perform rescue within a burning building.[11] Moving forward, it will be critical for all responders to embrace this new response paradigm: operational rescue.

REFERENCES

1. McKay SD, Johnston J, Callaway DW. Redefining technical rescue and casualty care for SOR: part 1. *J Spec Oper Med.* 2012;12:86–93.
2. NFPA. *NFPA 1006: Standard for Technical Rescuer Professional Qualifications.* 2013 ed. National Fire Protection Association: Quincy, MA; 2013.
3. NFPA. *NFPA 1983: Standard on Life Safety Rope and Equipment for Emergency Services.* 2012 ed. Quincy, MA: National Fire Protection Association; 2012.
4. Mell HK, Sztajnkrycer MD. EMS response to Columbine: lessons learned. *Internet J Rescue Disaster Med.* 2005;5.
5. Grossman D, Christensen L. *On Combat: The Psychology and Physiology of Deadly Conflict in War and Peace.* Human Factor Research Group: Milstadt; 2004.
6. Matthews J. *Technical Rescuer: Rope Levels I and II.* Delmar, Cengage Learning: Clifton Park; 2009.
7. Department of Homeland Security. Active shooter: how to respond. http://www.dhs.gov/xlibrary/assets/active_shooter_booklet.pdf; 2008 Accessed June 2014.
8. Smith ER, Iselin B, McKay WS. Toward the sound of shooting: Arlington County, VA., rescue task force represents a new medical response model to active shooter incidents. *JEMS.* 2009;34:48–55.
9. Callaway DW, Smith ER, Cain J, et al. Tactical emergency casualty care (TECC): guidelines for the provision of pre-hospital trauma care in high threat environments. *J Spec Oper Med.* 2011;11:104–122.
10. Fire Administration US. *Fire/emergency medical services department operational considerations and guide for active shooter and mass casualty incidents;* 2013.
11. Murphy W. *Benghazi: The Definitive Report.* Harper Collins: New York, NY; 2013.

Operations Security, Site Security, and Incident Response

Paul M. Maniscalco and Scott D. Weir

In preparing organizations and persons for response to a high-impact emergency incident, two of the most often overlooked requirements are operations security (OPSEC) and site security. Bound inextricably with coordination and integration strategies for response, OPSEC and site security are often compromised in the "heat of the battle." Well-intentioned responders frequently converge on the scene of the disaster, unbidden, and they implement strategies without addressing OPSEC and site-security considerations. The discipline to apply the principles of OPSEC and site security following a preestablished, organized, and well-practiced plan is crucial given the nature of the threat and the variety of conditions that may present themselves. Failing to address these priorities before an event amounts to failing to protect the protectors. It jeopardizes the viability of the response mission itself. Terrorist attacks present the contemporary emergency services manager or chief officer with challenges that are more complex and risks of greater magnitude.

Site security and OPSEC are multifaceted and diverse concepts, ranging from protecting an organization's information concerning activities, intentions, or capabilities to controlling scene access, traffic control, and evidence protection. Because this involves so many different aspects of disaster response, and because it cannot be completely achieved without full integration of each of those aspects, site security is best understood broadly. Robust control of the incident and surrounding areas should be the desired goal. This includes controlling the human and material flow into, out of, and around the site; providing for the security and safety of responding personnel; providing these responders with the ability to perform their jobs; and ensuring personnel accountability and the fulfillment of performance requirements. It is recognized that OPSEC infrastructure and strategies may necessarily develop over the course of the event response. Much like safety, OPSEC is the responsibility of every provider. Both the discipline of the initial responders and adherence to key principles provide the initial security until assessments and mitigation strategies that are more deliberate are implemented.

For an OPSEC program to be effective, personnel must be aware of OPSEC concerns. They must implement OPSEC countermeasures when appropriate and be observant of potential intelligence collection activities directed at their organization. This is only possible if the members understand the range of threats affecting their organization and actively support the OPSEC program.[1]

Under these definitions, the framework that makes for effective and successful deployment of OPSEC and site-security strategies is the Incident Management System/Unified Command (IMS/UC) as articulated in the National Response Framework (NRF) and the National Incident Management System (NIMS). Many OPSEC and site-security issues can be addressed merely by properly applying these disciplined and standard structures, practices, and protocols. For example, interagency integration problems involving the establishment of a chain of command, which produced many of the issues that plagued security at the World Trade Center site in the aftermath of the September 11, 2001, events, could have been significantly ameliorated by the implementation of an effective IMS/UCS early in the event, as well as the requisite immediate establishment of a workable security perimeter. Simply restating the requirement for implementing the IMS/UCS structure, which has already been established with the release of the NRF and the resulting NIMS, is not the purpose here. Moreover, this chapter seeks to address the roles that OPSEC and site security play in the response to a terrorist incident within the framework of the IMS/UCS process.

INCIDENT MANAGEMENT/UNIFIED COMMAND AS THE FOUNDATION

All people who choose to devote their life's work to responding when others are fleeing must resist the urge to "run in" without fully understanding what lies beyond that door, on the other side of that cloud of smoke, or around the next corner. Although difficult in a terrorist event, the success of the response mission and the survival of responders depend on projecting or knowing what threats lie ahead. The organizational protocol established by IMS/UCS is simply the framework by which OPSEC and site security can be established efficiently, effectively, and successfully; in other words, IMS/UCS is required but not sufficient on its own. Although not a panacea, IMS/UCS implementation is crucial for us to remediate the hard lessons learned in the recent past, fixing the problems inherent in past responses and implementing standards for OPSEC and site security.

The adoption and implementation of the NIMS-IMS/UCS framework addresses and corrects a large portion of site-security issues by the incorporation of the talents and services provided via the law enforcement community at the command post; it is important to note, however, most (or many) of these concerns are not limited to terrorism-related events, and the UC concept is appropriate at most emergency scenes.[2,3] Many of the difficulties inherent in the massive response of multiple agencies are just as prevalent in an earthquake as in a dirty bomb attack or other disaster. It is the particular nature of the threat that makes OPSEC and site security so salient, and unique in the context of terrorism is the particular nature of the threat.

The unique challenges posed by acts of terrorism create conditions that are fluid, requiring speed and flexibility of thought and action, as well as thorough planning and preparation. These attributes must be institutionalized in the response doctrine and responding personnel to achieve safe, effective, and sustainable responses to an incident. Moreover, the After Action Reporting (AAR) from the Boston Marathon Bombing further amplifies this requirement when leaders from all disciplines reported that the response performance really emerged from intuitive reactions by their personnel who had been training for years using a variety of evolving scenarios to achieve adaptability of response. Further, it is critical to remain mindful that the targeting of responders and "soft targets," such as health care facilities and schools, makes this an even more complex matter to address and manage to ensure one's own safety and the safety of those responders that are being coordinated at the scene.

HISTORICAL PERSPECTIVE

By analyzing the experience from the major recent terrorist attacks, particularly the 1993 World Trade Center Bombing and those following, numerous areas of concern consistently emerge. By focusing on each of these identified areas of concern and the pitfalls encountered during event response, we can identify opportunities to improve and lessons to be learned, and can develop best practices to shape future responses. As just noted, these concerns fall into two general categories. The first elements to consider are those that are universal to all event types and that can be remedied by the proper implementation of IMS/UCS. These include the following:

- Perimeter establishment and access control.
- Traffic and crowd control.
- Victim rescue in the immediate aftermath of an incident.
- Personnel needs including work-rest cycle, shift duration, feeding, watering, hygiene, adequate personal protective equipment (PPE), as well as the continuation of normal emergency medical services (EMS), law enforcement, and fire services operations over the course of the event.
- Organizational integration and interoperability communication issues.
- Public relations, including interactions with dignitaries, media, charities, and families of the victims and the missing.
- OPSEC and site security.
- Staffing support for other elements.

Second, some considerations are particularly relevant following terrorist events and cannot be addressed simply by the implementation of IMS/UCS; these therefore require further attention and creativity and are listed as follows:

- Search for secondary devices and hostile threats to the scene and responders.
- Perimeter establishment and access control (although relevant in all emergency events, it takes on special significance following terrorist events).
- Traffic and crowd control (although relevant in all emergency events, it takes on special significance following terrorist events).
- Evidence recovery and protection.

CURRENT MEDICINE

Operations Security and Site Security: Challenges of a General Nature

The important role IMS/UCS plays in enabling successful OPSEC and site security cannot be overstated. Perhaps the essential component in OPSEC and site security is communication and coordination among responders, and IMS/UCS, by design, provides a mechanism for exactly that. The following section addresses each aspect of OPSEC and site security that can be helped by the implementation of IMS/UCS, including multiple examples from recent terrorist attacks, where such implementation would have directly resulted in saved lives or property. Suggestions are then made as to how these issues can be dealt with in future events.

Victim Rescue

The first challenge to OPSEC and site security is victim rescue in the immediate aftermath of an incident. This is the initial and most dramatic problem faced by all responders during and immediately after a terrorist attack or large-scale event. A driving characteristic common to most responders is the natural instinct to rush forward, nobly intentioned, to do whatever one can to quickly save as many lives as possible. However, for both the safety of the responders and the victims, as well as the sustained good of the mission, some deliberate restraint and organization must be exercised. Absent this disciplined wisdom, the overall incident management may be negatively affected, and people may die needlessly. Among the lasting images from the events of 9/11 and the Boston Marathon attack are the hundreds of first-responder personnel rushing to the scene to help all who were impacted by these horrible attacks. The counterpoint is the striking example of misguided good intentions observed at the Shanksville, Pennsylvania, United Airlines flight 93 crash site, which on September 11, 2001, became overwhelmed and severely congested because of both on- and off-duty units responding, making their way to the scene either by self-dispatch or by convincing dispatchers to send more help. The resulting chaos clogged the scene, severely complicating command and control, and confusing perimeter maintenance.[4]

This area of OPSEC and site security primarily deals with ensuring an effective response rather than an unorganized, potentially dangerous, and surely less-effective response. Implementation of IMS/UCS could have diminished the reported congestion because it states that off-duty response personnel should not respond to an event unless directed to do so. Although operational doctrine dictates that you "man your post" until otherwise directed, the reality is that such a situation rarely exists.[5]

The instinct to respond is powerful and is complicated by the "touch the plane" phenomenon,[6] in which people feel they have to be at the disaster scene so they can tell anyone who will listen that they were indeed there "when it happened." Therefore it is incumbent on the agency and organizational leaders to stress and practice operational discipline that demands coordination and adherence to strict deployment protocol. Another relevant example is provided by the Bali Bombing of October 2002. As with other examples, the Bali responders rushed in to help victims, with the intention to save as many lives as possible, and, in doing so, rendered OPSEC and site security nonexistent, and it placed many more lives in danger in the event of another coordinated secondary attack. Even though it is difficult to find fault with the selfless actions of such responders, it is, however, crucial that this emotional response be tempered by reason and the knowledge that restraint and discipline are essential. They are necessary for a measured and effective response, in addition to ensuring an effective investigation to bring the perpetrators to justice.

Finally, there is the example of the brave responders to the World Trade Center attacks. In their zeal to charge into the scene and save as many people as possible, the "tunnel vision" they experienced allowed them to neglect properly assessing the danger to their own lives. Based upon this historical experience, responders must consider the full gamut of threats posed by formal secondary attacks or secondary effects of the primary attack mindfully. This includes the possibility that the initial event is actually a precursor to a campaign of attacks, as well as the expanded implications of fire, hazardous materials, and associated infrastructure failures. Any one of these elements presents daunting challenges for a responder, and the collective effects of multiple known and unknown operational variables further complicate the response exponentially. The potential confluence of events compounds the threats to environmental safety, and demands that the responsible emergency-response chief establishes and maintains aggressive safety policies throughout the event.

OPSEC and site security involve understanding the situation as accurately possible, including the possibility that attempting to rescue victims immediately may not be the wisest, safest, or most appropriate course of action. Although it may seem that delaying rescue efforts is tantamount to abandonment of our duty to act and is contrary to the oath many of us swear to, in the end, lives may be saved by taking the time to assess the situation fully, in a coherent fashion, before executing operational response.

Personnel Needs

The security needs of response personnel are a major issue to be addressed when planning a response to a high-impact and high-yield emergency incident. These needs are varied and can be very complex, complicated, and resource intensive, particularly during and after a terrorist event.[7] These demands are further increased given the likelihood of hazardous materials being present, and the intent of the terrorist to hurt or kill as many people as possible, including responders.

One very good example of this occurred during the 1997 Tokyo Sarin attacks in the subway. Japanese medical personnel lacked proper PPE; more than 20% of the staff of St. Luke's International Hospital exhibited detrimental physical effects after treating victims of the attack.[8] Had the hospital planned properly and equipped the facility and personnel, in addition to regularly training all employees, the instances of secondary contamination may have been greatly reduced once a nerve-agent attack was recognized.

Another well-known example of responders lacking proper PPE was the September 11, 2001, attacks. Early in the response, heavy particulate asbestos was found at the site, and later, Freon, cadmium, and other hazardous materials were identified, yet there were many personnel operating without proper protective equipment.[9] This can be attributed to poor planning, poor operational discipline, and/or lack of threat awareness. Logistics-acquisition problems also contributed because there was simply not enough equipment to go around. This suggests that planners failed to conceive or believe that an attack of this scale could possibly occur. Poor logistics further contributed because the equipment that was present was not distributed properly.[8]

Another critical aspect of protecting responders in a traditional sense involves personnel rest and rehabilitation, which are critical to the success and sustainability of an operation. Although rescuers are often willing to work to the point of exhaustion, this is dangerous to the responders, the victims, and the effectiveness of an operation. Fatigue creates more casualties through impaired decision making, increased stress and frustration, and impaired judgment. The medical profession continues to address the effects of sleep deprivation and fatigue, because of errors directly traceable to exhausted health care providers. Several well-publicized studies chronicling the effects of long work hours in life-and-death stressful environments reveal that errors have produced increased morbidity and mortality in the patients being cared for by these well-meaning professionals. Studies conducted over the last several years reveal that moderate sleep deprivation produces impairments in cognitive and motor performance equivalent to legally prescribed levels of alcohol intoxication.[10–13]

To help ensure safe and effective sustained operations, IMS/UCS empowers the Incident Commander to plan for sustained operations by dividing the available workforce across shifts. Work-rest cycles are implemented, and shift durations deliberately established, allowing for the necessary rest and rotation of personnel, even if it must be mandated. The final strategic and operational concern addressed in this chapter is the continuation of public services, including EMS, medical, law enforcement, and fire service, through the end of the incident and into the recovery stage. Sustaining 911-response capacity for an entire community should be a necessary goal that agencies and first responders must accept

and embrace. Just because one is being confronted with a large disaster in one's community does not alleviate the obligation to ensure that "all" emergencies in the community are managed appropriately.

Clearly, and especially in the case of EMS, the fiscal implications of having a sustainable and robust response system that can handle any and all 911 calls at all times is strictly prohibitive. Burden sharing has become accepted widely by way of mutual aid compacts between communities, regions, and now states under the Emergency Management Assistance Compact.[14] The key to successful sustained operation is embracing this concept and employing it, as required, on a regular basis. Further, reviewing scene-safety response protocols for commonality, ensuring interoperability, and having a shared vision of OPSEC and site-security tactics are integral during the duress of a real event.

Hospitals share the same concerns for their facilities and staff. During the planning phase for disaster response, hospital planners must consider a number of issues that previously did not require their attention. Such matters include increased security, physical management of patient flow, PPR, decontamination strategies, and staff training and support. One hospital failure that drew much national media attention occurred in Florida during the hurricane season of 2004. Florida Hospital Ormond Memorial fired and/or suspended more than 20 nurses for not working during Hurricane Frances. The nurses were fired for not calling in, not showing up, or refusing to work, whereas others were suspended for not completing a shift.[15] The hospital stated that hospital policy required critical care employees to work during a disaster. In media accounts, some nurses alleged that they were not trained to deal with these extreme scenarios, and they questioned who would protect their families. Nevertheless, in a crisis, staffing rosters based on the internal disaster plan were not followed, leaving the facility poorly positioned to cover staff vacancies and sustain operations.

Another unfortunate occurrence in the aftermath of disasters is the potential for civil unrest and criminal activity. Police resources are often allocated elsewhere, concentrated at the site of the disaster. Coverage is degraded in the areas where law enforcement officers would normally patrol or deploy, and if the presence is weakened enough, citizens may loot nearby houses, commercial districts, and in some cases emergency-response equipment. Examples of this can be found in the history of countless disasters, including the looting after Hurricane Sandy in 2012, Hurricane Charley's August 2004 landfall in Florida, the events in the aftermath of Hurricane Katrina 2005, as well as the unsubstantiated accusations of looting by the responders themselves following the 9/11 attacks on New York City.[16]

Community planners, responders, and emergency services personnel must also consider the potential for events to have rendered a large-scale area too dangerous even for emergency responders to enter. Such examples might include significant hazardous materials release or large radiological incidents. Responders must ask themselves two questions and answer them honestly: (1) In such a situation, what are the primary responsibilities of responders in getting people out, keeping people from entering, and making sure that the area remains contained? (2) Are the responders prepared to evacuate, relocate, secure, and effectively close a significant portion or an entire city, as was necessary during the Chernobyl disaster?

Proper and effective deployment of law enforcement officers is a key aspect of the incident management, NIMS, and NRF. Successful integration of law enforcement partners firmly within the Unified Command framework promotes effective coordination among responders of different disciplines. It affords greater cohesiveness and security for all personnel operating on site. Moreover, it facilitates integrated operations and the investigative process and provides for sustained reliable evidence collection. Similar concerns exist for fire services in the wake of a disaster, particularly in fire-heavy disasters. The standard fire service response is to rush to the scene of a major working fire and engage to control the threat and resolve the problem rapidly. This traditional response strategy was illustrated in the 2001 World Trade Center response. One can imagine the collateral dangers if concurrent fires were to emerge in other parts of the city, particularly in the event of a secondary terrorist attack. The effectiveness and value of mutual aid are clearly apparent in the responses to any number of large-scale disasters, but this was particularly evident on September 11, 2001. There is also precedent for terrorists using fire as a weapon to drive victims from positions of security or to hamper the emergency response.[17,18]

INTEGRATION

Integration issues are a crucial consideration in any response to an emergency, but they are critical for a large-scale incident. The most obvious example of this is in the immediate aftermath of the 9/11 attacks. Interoperability between fire and police radios was found to be a major problem during the response to the 1993 bombing of the World Trade Center, and, unfortunately, the problems recurred on September 11, 2001. Because of overloaded radio equipment, firefighters in Tower 1 of the World Trade Center were unaware of reports of the imminent collapse of the tower from a New York Police Department (NYPD) helicopter and therefore did not initiate their own evacuation. This lack of communication may have contributed to an increased number of casualties.

The proper implementation of IMS/UCS, which stresses both horizontal and vertical information sharing, would have required interoperable radios, and the NYPD helicopter in the air above the World Trade Center would have been able to relay the information regarding the collapse to the fire department, affording firefighters better situational awareness and the opportunity for earlier evacuation.[19]

The Moscow Theater siege of October 2002 is another tragic example illustrating the consequences of poorly integrated response operations. Chechen terrorists took over the theater, and claimed the patrons as hostages. When Russian law enforcement pumped a toxic gas into the theater that rendered both terrorists and hostages unconscious, it resulted in the deaths of both hostages and hostage takers. The initial refusal by Russian authorities to release information regarding the gas used to subdue and incapacitate the Chechen terrorists hampered efforts to properly diagnose and treat the nearly 650 hostage victims of the gas. Thus 117 perished in the rescue.[20,21] The unfortunate reality is authorities in the Spetsnaz (Russian Special Forces, who carried out the raid) did not involve the medical community. If they had coordinated or included a medical component in their tactical operations, the critical medically relevant communication and coordination would have allowed medical support of tactical operations. Lives could have been saved because medically relevant threat analysis would have identified this predictable result of tactical operations, and medical countermeasures could have been made available and implemented in a coordinated fashion, in support of tactical operations. If medical personnel had been notified that narcotic gas was to be used, the opiate antagonist naloxone could have been available on scene and would have prevented unnecessary deaths.

THE PRESS AND DIGNITARIES

Public relations are an important aspect of OPSEC and site security because outside factors such as the media and the family of victims can seriously complicate a response. One representative example of the lack of OPSEC and site security regarding the media was during the "Beltway Sniper" shootings of October 2002 in the Virginia, Washington, DC, and Maryland area. The sniper pair left notes for the police, with specific instructions not to be relayed to the press. In addition, they allegedly made numerous requests for the media not to be involved in the interaction between the snipers and police.[22] The press obtained this information through the notorious "unnamed source" and went public with information that not only jeopardized the investigation but also put many lives in danger. The resulting lack of trust between the sniper and the police interfered with communication between investigators and the perpetrators and slowed the investigation as authorities shifted focus toward damage control. The Alcohol, Tobacco, and Firearms operation Trojan horse in Waco, Texas, in 1993 similarly was hampered by lack of information security. The Branch Davidians were tipped off regarding the raid, leading to the standoff and subsequent deadly shootout and fire.[23-25]

The media can be a great asset when responding to an incident, provided relations take place in a controlled, efficient manner. An example of the positive and negative roles the media can play in responding to an event occurred during the sarin attacks in Tokyo. Lack of communication complicates many responses, causing frustration and mistakes, and the Tokyo incident was no exception. Personnel at local hospitals had yet to identify the chemical cause of the medical problems they were encountering. The health care personnel became aware of the substance from watching the local television broadcasts; coincidentally, physicians who had experience with sarin and its effects on humans had also been watching and called in. The communication between the physicians viewing the news coverage and the hospitals correctly identified the offending agent. At the time, the media was criticized for filming while people suffered and died, instead of helping them to the hospital.[26]

Media coverage of terrorist events can be a double-edged sword. Planners must ensure that the benefits of having the media present are not outweighed by the disadvantages. This requires having a public information officer (PIO) who is trained prior to an incident on the successful discharge of the PIO duties. The PIO is integrated into the command structure to assist with dissemination of response information and management of the media.

In the event of a major disaster, it is common practice for officials of all levels to visit the site to offer reassurance: for example, President Obama flying to New York and New Jersey to visit the areas devastated by Superstorm Sandy in the Fall of 2012; and President Bush visiting New York City, Shanksville, Pennsylvania, and Arlington, Virginia, after September 11, 2001. It is necessary to have strict OPSEC and site security to maintain the safety of these dignitaries. Efforts must be made to ensure they and their entourages do not disturb the on-scene operations or hinder the investigation. Although such dignitary visits are important to reassure the public, it must not come at the cost of successfully executing the response plan at a local, state, or national level.

Planning must not take place in isolation; plans to deal with the onslaught of media and dignitaries must be a part of the standard disaster planning and drills. Therefore pre-incident introductory and planning meetings should be conducted with all involved stakeholders, including the local media. The primary goal of such meetings is to achieve shared understanding that all participants have a job to do, and planning before the worst-case scenario occurs will allow for the completion of the mission in a safe and cooperative manner.

OPSEC AND SITE-SECURITY DEMANDS FOR OFF-SITE OPERATIONS

Finally, there is the issue of security and staffing support for elements of the response not located directly at the event site, such as joint or regional operation centers, joint or regional information centers, multiagency coordination centers, morgues, and food distribution and donation reception sites. Although these sites may not be physically located inside the incident perimeter, they are no less vulnerable to endemic threats. In the context of terrorism events, they may represent even more attractive and less fortified targets. These critical areas are vulnerable to being compromised or attacked by a variety of means, including but not limited to physical attacks with arms, explosives, criminal acts, and hazardous material dispersal.

Law enforcement officials of some type, whether federal or local police or security forces, must be present to provide force protection to ensure sustained operation of these services. It is vital to the success and continuation of the response that community planners (local, city, and county emergency managers) and all those who will respond (paid and volunteer) meet regularly before a catastrophic emergency occurs. Such forums and open dialogue foster the development of a prudent operational response doctrine, to ensure OPSEC and site security and to test proposed response strategies periodically through comprehensive exercising.

OPSEC AND SITE SECURITY FOR A TERRORIST INCIDENT

It is not enough to simply adopt and implement the NIMS-IMS/UCS framework as the sole means to control and overcome the OPSEC and site-security challenges posed by a terrorist incident. However, it is important to note that the majority of challenges faced by EMS, medical, law enforcement, security, and fire services following terrorism or weapons of mass destruction (WMD) events are common to large-scale nonterrorism events, as well. The adoption of a response plan and/or a response system is only as good as the training provided to familiarize all those who will use the plan and/or system.

It is irresponsible if not impossible to expect that people, agencies, departments, and communities will be able to use plans designed to place everyone on the "same page" without meaningful and frequent training and exercising. The organizational structure afforded by NIMS-IMS/UCS structure provides the means by which proper measures can be successfully implemented. It is a proven operational-management framework to deal with such complex events. The critical priority must be given to OPSEC and site security at all incidents, not just those eventually identified as terrorism or WMD related. This will create a familiarity with OPSEC and site security for all responders, as well as institutionalize these policies. Effective scene management includes perimeter establishment, access and egress control, personnel accountability, evidence protection and chain of custody, and the search for secondary devices and threats. Addressing vulnerabilities in these areas requires not just the existence of an organizational structure but also that it be integrated in a prominent position within the Incident Command structure.

ESTABLISHING A PERIMETER

The effective establishment of a perimeter is often a crucial aspect of gaining control over the scene. Establishing a perimeter has ramifications in all aspects of maintaining OPSEC and site security. Force protection cannot be ensured, evidence cannot be protected, chain of custody cannot be guaranteed, and access to the scene cannot be controlled with a porous or haphazard creation of a perimeter. The overall response to the 1995 terrorist bombing of the Alfred P. Murrah Building in Oklahoma City is an excellent model of what was right and what was wrong. There were three layers of perimeters, quickly established by morning on the day after the bombing: the inner perimeter was designed to provide limited access to only those personnel authorized to participate in the rescue and recovery work and the criminal investigation. Second, a staging area served as a buffer for workers, and, third, a cordon limited traffic access.[27] Unfortunately, an effective perimeter was not established immediately, and the site quickly became overwhelmed with hundreds of well-meaning people who wanted to help in any way they could. Because no control yet existed over the entire area of the dangerous site, one convergent responder, a nurse, was killed by fallen debris. The eventual establishment of an effective perimeter was accomplished by close coordination of disparate agencies, along with the construction of fencing.[17,28]

At the World Trade Center site on 9/11, in admittedly more trying circumstances, "Perimeter security was not adequately established, allowing large numbers of unnecessary personnel to enter," in large part because of a 5-day delay in the creation of an adequate credentialing system and the construction of a fence.[29] It took an extra 4 days at the World Trade Center to establish security, even approaching the perimeter set up at the Murrah Building. The potential repercussions of this sort of inattention are massive. The presence of large numbers of unnecessary personnel hampered effective operations, distracted from other objectives, depleted already taxed resources, and placed the unnecessary personnel themselves at undue risk of exposure and injury.

The 1997 bombing of a women's clinic in suburban Atlanta provides a striking example of the potential consequences of inattention to perimeter security. Eric Rudolph allegedly planted a secondary explosive device timed to detonate on the arrival of personnel responding to the initial explosive event. A CNN camera crew filming an interview with a witness of the initial blast caught the nearby second explosion on film. The media and civilians were endangered because they were allowed access to an area surrounding the scene that should have been secured. The uncontrolled scene increases the potential and likelihood that persons not involved in the initial catastrophic event will be injured in a secondary attack. Failure to control the scene increases the likelihood that hazardous materials (if present) will be spread to a wider area of the city, and that the criminal investigation will be hampered or destroyed. Ground zero of a terrorist attack demands special attention to the formation of perimeters as a necessary requirement to full OPSEC and site security.

The cooperation and discipline required to ensure security and safety does not, and will not, happen overnight or because it is the right thing to do. All aspects of scene control must be carefully planned, practiced, and exercised on an ongoing basis. It is impossible to expect two response disciplines with divergent objectives to come together and cooperate without the right training and education. One large group of people is running in to tear the scene apart to look for victims, survivors, and treat the injured. The other large group requires the meticulous preservation of evidence and maintaining the site just as it was found. There is no question that each group has vital and incredibly important roles and responsibilities, no one more important than another is. Nevertheless, it is naive and irresponsible for any responding person, agency, group, or department to expect these two parallel forces to eventually meet in the middle without long-term focused efforts aimed at settling the differences and ensuring that both jobs are completed efficiently and in a timely manner. This can only be accomplished through regular meetings, educational sessions, and training. It is imperative that this functional integration is achieved well in advance of the event. Failure to address this coordination factor before an event will result in a response that resembles a cacophony rather than the desired symphony.

EVIDENCE PROTECTION

As already stated, ensuring the preservation of evidence is another fundamental aspect of OPSEC and site security following a terrorist or WMD attack. Consider the Oklahoma Department of Civil Emergency Management After Action Report, which outlines the problems encountered when a large number of volunteers were incorporated into rescue operations without being registered or identified. "Since the site was a crime scene, all our volunteers were required to be critically screened before they could work at the bomb site," the report stated.[17] Fortunately, authorities were able to quickly implement this system to rectify the unimpeded access people had previously been afforded; about 30 unauthorized "convergent responder" volunteers were evicted from one floor alone.

This was not handled as well at the site of the 2002 Bali bombings. There, "the crime scene was seemingly ruined and unprotected." In part, this was due to the unavoidable circumstances involved in the response, but it was made worse by "the public's curiosity," which was allowed to hinder the investigation. This occurred despite police efforts to establish a security perimeter around the site.[30] The removal, addition, destruction, or alteration of material could prove to be a major hindrance to the proper conduct of the criminal investigation and identification of those responsible. Whether the adulteration of the scene is intentional, unintentional, or simply the byproduct of an inexperienced volunteer seeking a souvenir is immaterial. Even the most minute and seemingly unimportant pieces of material can prove to be evidence in these situations and their compromise cannot be afforded. To the untrained eye, the aftermath of a terrorist attack is a pile of debris or a chaotic mass of humanity. To the trained criminal investigator, the scene is a road map that tells the complete story of the circumstances. The control of access to the site of an incident through well-guarded perimeters and a secure credentialing system that does not allow for forgeries is the only way to guarantee the integrity of the crime scene.

INFORMATION SECURITY AND TRAFFIC AND CROWD CONTROL

Information security and dispersal interacts with traffic and crowd control to make up an extremely important aspect of OPSEC and site security in the event of a terrorist attack. In this case, OPSEC and site security take on a much broader scope because activity elsewhere affects the flow of people and materials in and out of the site itself. It also affects the flow about the city or general area in which the attack has occurred. The frightening nature of terrorism could and will result in mass hysteria and chaos, especially for cases associated with the use of a WMD, whether confirmed or merely by speculation. In the absence of accurate, timely information from authorities, rumors fill the information vacuum, leading to potentially disastrous public panic. Uncontrolled, large-scale attempts to flee a city in the midst of reports of a chemical or biological outbreak could prevent quarantine and allow further spread of the agent.

Traffic control can also be a statewide or regional issue, particularly with large natural disasters. The following is a description of the evacuation of coastal Florida at the approach of Hurricane Floyd in 1999: "Even many of those not in evacuation zones fled at the sight of satellite images on the news, which depicted a monstrous Floyd larger than the entire state of Florida. The result was a transportation nightmare."[31] Combined with sensationalized speculation of a hurricane engulfing a state or the imminent citywide release of a chemical agent, loss of message control can easily produce wholesale disorder. Traffic and crowd control of the entire surrounding area must be fused with information control to ensure that on-site efforts receive proper support and aid.

Control of pedestrian traffic also has great importance in its localized form. In the rush to leave a scene to avoid injury or seek medical attention, it is very possible that citizens will unintentionally carry biological or chemical hazards with them. Depending on the nature of the agent that has been introduced, the failure to contain contaminated people or other material could lead to secondary injury and illness. The 1995 sarin attack on the Tokyo subway system illustrates the difficulties and effects associated with the uncontrolled vector of contaminated victims. In that incident affecting over 4000 people, some of the contaminated and off-gassing victims showed up seeking medical treatment without official transport.[32] The lesson is clear: in responding to an attack in which biological, chemical, or radiological weapons are suspected, establishing control of the traffic of people both in and out of the area is crucial for the protection of the scene victims and those would-be victims in the surrounding communities.

SECONDARY DEVICES OR THREATS

Perhaps the most pressing and worrying element of concern is that of secondary devices and threats targeting responders and evacuating civilians. Terrorist attacks pose a distinct, dangerous hazard, further complicated by the potential for secondary attacks aimed at first responders. Secondary attacks are growing in number, so the use of such a "follow-up" attack should not be addressed as merely a marginal possibility but as a primary consideration incorporated into training and drills.

The previously mentioned example of Eric Rudolph and his alleged involvement in abortion clinic bombings is relevant here as well. The detonation of a bomb outside of an Atlanta nightclub occurred 1 week after the women's clinic blast, where a secondary attack had targeted responders. Responders astutely suspected a similar threat in Atlanta. Fortunately, the responders remained diligent, and a secondary device was found and disarmed before it could kill or injure responders. Similar terror tactics have been used extensively by several international terrorist organizations, most notably the "Real Irish Republican Army" (RIRA) and the Colombian paramilitary guerilla group known as the Revolutionary Armed Forces of Colombia (FARC). RIRA guerilla forces have operated a two-bomb strategy, hoping secondary devices "catch" security forces rushing to the scene of the first.[33] The adoption of such tactics by the enemies of the United States, given their resourcefulness and excellent access to information, should certainly not be discounted.

Preparation for such a scenario has been found lacking. In the aftermath of the collapse of the World Trade Center towers, the initial rescue phase was followed by a massive recovery effort. Within a day or so after the two towers collapsed, there were already thousands of workers on the scene. Estimates place the number of volunteers and workers at ground zero after the attacks at 30,000 to 40,000.[5] At the same time, however, "risk of secondary attack was not made a priority as the rescue effort was vigorously pursued."[23] The buildings in the immediate vicinity were not searched for 4 days, and then it took months for them to be cleared. There was no standard procedure for obtaining resources such as military aid. Failure to immediately secure a perimeter and control site access left avenues open through which additional strikes could come.

In addition, the majority of the nation's federal response to the disaster was housed in one Manhattan hotel surrounded by response vehicles brightly decorated with a wide variety of responding agency's logos, decals, and identifying placards. The worst-kept secret in

New York City was where all the federal responders were resting, recuperating, and spending their downtime. A well-planned or even a last-minute secondary attack could have been carried out, and it would have produced a very high number of casualties because of the large number of vulnerable personnel in the area. Such an attack would have crippled the New York response, but, more importantly, the secondary attack at that particular time would have crippled the nation's morale. The devastating emotional effects would further extend to those not directly affected by the events in New York and Washington, DC.

CONCLUSION

OPSEC and site security are mission-critical concepts that are best achieved through a deliberate effort to secure vital infrastructure before, during, and after a catastrophic event. To promote awareness and acceptance of OPSEC and site-security concepts, it must be institutionalized into the response culture through training, everyday practice, and exercising.

It is essential that dialogue with all traditional and nontraditional response agencies occurs on an ongoing basis, well in advance of an event. The creation of Memoranda of Understanding that detail the roles, duties, and responsibilities of all agencies and responders will assist in the development of long-term working relationships. Through deliberate and unified effort, our shared objectives of security, safety, and the preservation of life and limb will be achieved.

REFERENCES

1. *Operations security: intelligence threat handbook.* Available at: http://www.fas.org/irp/nsa/ioss/threat96/part01.htm.
2. Maniscalco PM, Christen HT. *Understanding Terrorism and Managing Its Consequences.* Prentice Hall: Upper Saddle River, NJ; 2001.
3. Maniscalco PM, Christen HT. *Homeland Security: Principles and Practices of Terrorism Response.* Sudbury, MA: Jones and Bartlett Publishers; 2011.
4. Federal Emergency Management Agency. Responding to incidents of national consequence: recommendations for America's fire and emergency services based on the events of September 11, 2001, and other similar incidents. FA-282-May 2004:34. Available at: http://www.usfa.fema.gov/downloads/pdf/publications/fa-282.pdf.
5. Cone DC, Weir SD, Bogucki S. Convergent volunteerism. *Ann Emerg Med.* 2003;41:457–462. http://www.smrrc.org/PDF%20files/Convergent%20Volunteerism.pdf.
6. Federal Emergency Management Agency. Responding to incidents of national consequence: recommendations for America's fire and emergency services based on the events of September 11, 2001, and other similar incidents. FA-282-May 2004:34. Available at: http://www.usfa.fema.gov/downloads/pdf/publications/fa-282.pdf.
7. Maniscalco PM, Christen HT. *Homeland Security: Principles and Practices of Terrorism Response.* Sudbury, MA: Jones and Bartlett Publishers; 2011.
8. Ohbu S, Yamashina A, Takasu N, et al. Sarin poisoning on Tokyo subway. *South Med J.* 1997;90:587–593.
9. McKinsey & Company. Improving NYPD emergency preparedness and response. August 19, 2002. Available at: http://911depository.info/PDFs/McKinsey%20Reports/Improving%20NYPD%20Emergency%20Preparedness%20and%20Response.pdf.
10. Williamson AM, Feyer AM. Moderate sleep deprivation produces impairments in cognitive and motor performance equivalent to legally prescribed levels of alcohol intoxication. *Occup Environ Med.* 2000;57(10):649–655.
11. Steele MT, Ma OJ, Watson WA, Thomas Jr HA, Muelleman RL. The occupational risk of motor vehicle collisions for emergency medicine residents. *Acad Emerg Med.* 1999;6(10):1050–1053.
12. Mansukhani MP, Kolla BP, Surani S, Varon J, Ramar K. Sleep deprivation in resident physcians, work hour limitations, and related outcomes: a systematic review of the literature. *Postgrad Med.* 2012;124(4):241–249.
13. NIH, NHLBI—National Center on Sleep Disorders Research and Office of Prevention, Education and Control, Working Group Report on Problem Sleepiness, August 1997.
14. Emergency Management Assistance Compact Web site. Available at: http://www.emacweb.org/.
15. The Associated Press. *Nurses fired or suspended for not working during Hurricane Frances. Sun-Sentinel.* Available at: http://www.hirenursing.com/c/nursing/newsdetailx/nurses-fired-for-not-working-hurricane9417.htm.
16. WCBS-TV NY. *Looting reported at WTC;* September 21, 2001. Available at: http://www.cbsnews.com/news/looting-reported-at-wtc/.
17. Pfeifer JW. *Fire as a weapon in terrorist attacks.* http://www.ctc.usma.edu/posts/fire-as-a-weapon-in-terrorist-attacks.
18. Protecting the Homeland against Mumbai-style Attacks and the Threat from Lashkal-E-Taiba. Hearing before the Subcommittee on Counterterrorism and Intelligence of the Committee on Homeland Security House of Representatives, One Hundred Thirteenth Congress, First Session, June 12, 2013 Serial No. 113-21. Available at: http://www.gpo.gov/fdsys/.
19. Fire Department of the City of New York. *Increasing FDNY's preparedness.* McKinsey & Company; August 19, 2002. 32. Available at: http://www.nyc.gov/html/fdny/html/mck_report/toc.html.
20. *Russia: Gas was fast-acting opiate fentanyl. Associated Press.* October 30, 2002. Available at: http://usatoday30.usatoday.com/news/world/2002-10-30-russia-gas_x.htm.
21. *Hostage drama in Moscow: the toxic agent; U.S. suspects opiate in gas in Russia raid. New York Times.* October 29, 2002. Available at: http://www.nytimes.com/2002/10/29/world/hostage-drama-in-moscow-the-toxic-agent-us-suspects-opiate-in-gas-in-russia-raid.html.
22. Shepard AC. *Terror in October: a look back at the DC Sniper Attacks. Washingtonian,* September 26, 2012. Available at: http://www.washingtonian.com/articles/people/terror-in-october/.
23. Labaton S, Verhovek SH. *Missteps in Waco: A raid re-examined/a special report; US agents say fatal flaws doomed raid on Waco cult.* March 28, 1993. Available at: http://www.nytimes.com/1993/03/28/us/missteps-waco-raid-re-examined-special-report-us-agents-say-fatal-flaws-doomed.html.
24. Thomas P, Schneider H. *ATF agents knew before raid that Koresh may have been tipped off. Washington Post.* 1993;113(17). Available at: http://tech.mit.edu/V113/N17/koresh.17w.html.
25. Bryce R, Ellis J, Moore J. *Killing the messenger; who's really to blame for the botched raid in Waco? Austin Chronicle.* June 23 2000. Available at: http://www.austinchronicle.com/news/2000–06–23/77697/.
26. Japan-101. *Sarin gas attack on the Tokyo subway.* Available at: http://www.japan-101.com/culture/sarin_gas_attack_on_the_tokyo_su.htm.
27. The City of Oklahoma City After Action Report: Alfred P. Murrah Federal Building Bombing, July 1996. Available at: http://www.ok.gov/OEM/documents/Bombing%20After%20Action%20Report.pdf.
28. Maniscalco PM, Christen HT. *Homeland Security: Principles and Practices of Terrorism Response.* Jones and Bartlett: Sudbury, MA; 2011.
29. Fire Department of the City of New York. *Increasing FDNY's Preparedness.* McKinsey & Company; August 19, 2002:32. Available at: http://www.nyc.gov/html/fdny/html/mck_report/toc.html.
30. *Timetile: The Bali bombing, a comprehensive overview. Jakarta Post.* January 3, 2003. Available at: http://www.thejakartapost.com/news/2003/01/03/timetile-the-bali-bombing-a-comprehensive-overview.html.
31. U.S. Department of Transportation, Federal Highway Administration, Officer of Operations; 21st Century Operations Using 21st Century Technologies; 4.2.6.1 Evacuation of Special Needs Evacuees. Available at: http://ops.fhwa.dot.gov/publications/fhwahop08015/lit4_2_6_1.htm.
32. Organization for the Prohibition of Chemical Weapons. *Chemical terrorism in Japan: the Matsumoto and Tokyo incidents.* Available at: http://www.opcw.org/news/article/the-sarin-gas-attack-in-japan-and-the-related-forensic-investigation/.
33. Examiner.com. *Terror tech: the abominable secondary device.* October 12, 2009. Available at: http://www.examiner.com/article/terror-tech-the-abominable-secondary-device.

CHAPTER 91

Medical Intelligence

Gregory R. Ciottone

BACKGROUND

Medical intelligence can be defined as follows:

[. . .]that category of intelligence resulting from collection, evaluation, analysis, and interpretation of foreign medical, bio-scientific, and environmental information which is of interest to strategic planning and to military medical planning and operations for the conservation of the fighting strength of friendly forces and the formation of assessments of foreign medical capabilities in both military and civilian sectors. Also called MEDINT.[1]

Medical intelligence related specifically to the threat of public health emergencies, including terrorism, has obvious applicability to civilian sectors as well. It involves information applied to the identification, characterization, and management of a risk, as applied to both medical and nonmedical countermeasures.

The collection of medical intelligence may include both classified and open sources. Evaluation may involve preexisting publications or ongoing public health surveillance and may also include analysis and/or interpretation of well-established or newly gained data. Characterizations may include situational awareness of current events, as well as descriptions of both foreign and domestic medical and public health capabilities and capacity.[2]

HISTORICAL PERSPECTIVE

The Importance of Medical Intelligence

The greatest threat to military forces is often not enemy weapons, but rather the type of casualty referred to as a "disease and nonbattle injury." The statistics regarding the impact of disease on military operations are remarkable. During the Civil War, there were an estimated 414,152 deaths due to disease, outranking battle deaths by a ratio of over 2:1.[3]

The following statistics reveal that the threat of disease during military operations had not ceased by the twentieth century.[4]

- Influenza killed 43,000 U.S. military personnel in World War I. In the U.S. Army, influenza accounted for 80% of all casualties during the war.
- Of the U.S. marines deployed to Lebanon in 1958, 50% were incapacitated with severe diarrhea.
- Of the U.S. sailors deployed to the Suez in 1975, 80% were stricken with dysentery.
- Of the U.S. soldiers deployed to the Sinai in 1982, 30% became dehydration casualties.

Llewellyn Legters and Craig Llewellyn of the Uniformed Services University of the Health Sciences (USUHS) highlighted the four main objectives of a successful preventive medicine program[4]:

- To determine the nature and magnitude of the disease and injury threats in the planned area of operations before deployment.
- To identify the principal countermeasures that must be emphasized to reduce the threats to acceptable levels.
- To train individuals in the use of these countermeasures.
- To enforce rigorously these countermeasures in the operational area.

These measures correspond nicely with processes of analytical risk management: including risk assessment, countermeasure determination, risk communication, and countermeasure implementation.

CURRENT PRACTICE

Civilian Medical Intelligence

The cause of a disease or even the occurrence of something unusual may be very difficult to determine, especially if the initial cases are few. However, surveillance needs to be more than routine because even relatively small and well-documented outbreaks of disease have the potential to go unrecognized as a bioterrorist attack.[5] This initial investigation does not always have to be time consuming or involve law enforcement. Investigating the facts surrounding the outbreak to determine if anything seems unusual or indicative of bioterrorism will suffice in most cases.[6] Infectious disease criteria for differentiation of bioterrorism from natural outbreaks have been well defined in the literature.[6-11] The most important factors affecting early detection of a bioterrorist event are likely to be the rate of accrual of new cases at the outset of the epidemic, geographic clustering, the selection of syndromic surveillance methods, and the likelihood of making a diagnosis quickly in clinical practice.[10]

National, regional, and local public health departments must be linked in a network of real-time communication with the medical response community, public safety, regional poison control centers, and regional laboratory capacities for integration of information management, passive and active surveillance systems, and epidemiological investigation. In 1998, Keim, Kauffman, and Rodgers were the first to propose the development of such a comprehensive system as part of the U.S. Public Health Service.[12] Over the past decade, a "fusion center" process has been widely implemented in the United States as a method of managing the flow of information and intelligence across levels and sectors of government for integration of intelligence and knowledge management.[13] Moreover, there has been a growing trend toward integration of medical intelligence into multisectoral systems for knowledge management.[14]

Sources of Medical Intelligence

The primary source of civilian medical intelligence in the United States is the Centers for Disease Control and Prevention (CDC) and the Agency for Toxic Substances and Disease Registry (ATSDR). Table 91-1 represents a comprehensive listing of traditional sources of civilian medical intelligence available in the United States.[15-27]

The Origin of Modern Civilian Medical Intelligence in the United States

The role of the U.S. public health system has evolved significantly since 9/11 and the anthrax attacks of fall 2001. The public health threat associated with the release of chemical, biological, and radiological and nuclear agents has drawn the CDC and the entire public health system into a national security role. The safety and health of people across the United States and around the globe demand the best science, immediate public health service, and a sound strategy to prepare and respond to terrorist threats.

In 2000, with the realization that the threat of bioterrorism was increasing, the CDC developed its first strategic plan for preparedness and response to terrorism. The CDC centers, institutes, and offices contribute their expertise toward this effort by improving[28]:

- Detection and investigation
- Prevention programs
- Worker safety
- Laboratory sciences research
- Communication
- Workforce development
- Long-term consequence management

Terrorism-preparedness activities described in the CDC's 2000 strategic plan included the development of a public health communication infrastructure, a multilevel network of diagnostic laboratories, and an integrated disease surveillance system,[28] all consistent with the 1998 recommendations of Keim, Kauffmann, and Rodgers.[12] Surveillance systems now collect and monitor data for disease trends and/or outbreaks so that public health personnel can protect the nation's health. Multiple agencies now maintain effective surveillance tools and systems that can be used to gain medical intelligence for the detection and characterization of outbreaks.

Key Components of Civilian Medical Intelligence

Methods for conducting public health surveillance may often differ considerably by program and disease. Regardless of these differences, all surveillance activities share many common practices in the way data are collected, managed, transmitted, analyzed, accessed, and disseminated. For many nations, the long-term vision is that of complementary electronic information systems, which routinely gather health data from a variety of sources on a real-time basis and facilitate the monitoring of the health of communities, assist in the ongoing analysis of trends and detection of emerging public health problems, and provide information for setting public health policy.

There must be multiple systems in place to support communications for public health labs, the clinical community, and state and local health departments. Each information system has demonstrated the importance of being able to exchange health information. However, it is possible for many of these systems to operate in isolation, not capitalizing on the potential for a cross-fertilization of data exchange between the various systems. There should therefore also be numerous, ongoing efforts among public health agencies to provide an integrated and unifying framework to monitor these data streams better for early detection of public health issues and emergencies. Ensuring the security of this information is critical, as is the ability of the network to work reliably in times of national crisis.

A bioterrorist attack, like other public health threats, is likely to be detected first at the local level.[6] Health departments throughout the nation must therefore be prepared to detect and respond to those threats. Communications, information sharing, distance-learning, and organizational infrastructure established among health organizations are necessary to provide for an adequate and timely public health emergency response, including the possibility of bioterrorism. Federal officials, state and local health departments, poison control centers, and other public health professionals should be capable of accessing and sharing preliminary health surveillance information quickly and securely. Users should also be actively notified of breaking health events as they occur. Veterinarians are also considered as a key part of the disease surveillance system.[29]

In the United States, most bioterrorism agents can be diagnosed at standard hospital clinical laboratories.[30] The CDC Laboratory Response Network (LRN) represents a consortium of laboratories comprised primarily of state, local, and federal public health laboratories, each with different capabilities and levels of expertise.[31] National laboratories, including those operated by the CDC and the U.S. Army Medical Research Institute of Infectious Diseases (USAMRIID), are responsible for specialized strain characterizations, bio-forensics, select agent activity, and handling highly infectious biological agents and toxic chemicals. Reference laboratories are responsible for investigation and/or referral of specimens. They are made up of more than 100 state and local public health, military, international, veterinary, agriculture, food, and water testing laboratories. In addition to laboratories located in the United States, facilities located in Australia and Canada also serve as reference laboratories abroad. Sentinel laboratories are hospital-based, clinical institutions, and commercial diagnostic laboratories. These sentinel laboratories now play a key role in the early detection of biological agents. Sentinel laboratories provide routine diagnostic services, as well as rule-out, and referral steps in the identification process.[28]

To investigate unusual epidemics, information is often required about the ecological and biological characteristics of the pathogen, the natural routes of infection, the pathogenesis, the clinical picture and immunology of certain diseases, the epidemic foci, and the special characteristics of an artificial dissemination of the pathogen. It is also essential that there is an adequate and efficient field analysis of the epidemic, an examination of the clinical picture and the epidemiological situation, and a collection of representative samples and data for statistically sound epidemiological, epizootiological, medical, and laboratory analysis. This necessitates properly trained mobile investigation teams with appropriate technical equipment.[8]

Integration of Medical Intelligence into National-Level Knowledge Management Systems
Fusion Centers

Because of the 2007 National Strategy for Information Sharing, many states and urban areas have established fusion centers.[32] The fusion process is postulated as a method of managing the flow of information and intelligence across levels and sectors of government to integrate information for analysis.[13] Most notably, this process directs the flow of information gathered from state, local, and tribal levels to U.S. federal agencies such as the U.S. Department of Justice, the Federal Bureau of Investigation, the U.S. military, and the Central Intelligence Agency (CIA). The intelligence component of a fusion center focuses on the intelligence process, where information is collected, integrated, evaluated, analyzed, and disseminated. The concept is based upon the assumption that nontraditional collectors of intelligence (such as public health) do in fact possess a form of intelligence that can be fused with

TABLE 91-1 Sources of Medical Intelligence

Centers for Disease Control and Prevention (CDC) and Agency for Toxic Substances and Disease Registry (ATSDR) Resources

Public Health Information Network (PHIN)	The PHIN is a national initiative to increase the capacity of public health agencies to exchange data and information electronically across organizations and jurisdictions (e.g., clinical care to public health, public health to public health, and public health to other federal agencies). It is intended to harmonize the National Notifiable Diseases Surveillance System (NNDSS), and the Public Health Emergency Preparedness (PHEP) Cooperative Agreement for case notifications, as well as the CDC Health Alert Network (HAN).
NNDSS	The NNDSS is a public health surveillance system for infectious conditions operated in all 50 states, New York City, the District of Columbia, and five U.S. territories by the CDC in collaboration with the Council of State and Territorial Epidemiologists (CSTE). It serves as a core, routine surveillance activity that utilizes PHIN standards for electronic transmission of case notification data from reporting jurisdictions to the CDC.
PHEP cooperative agreement	The PHEP provides funding to build and upgrade the preparedness infrastructure of public health departments to improve their ability to respond to the public health emergencies and it supports core surveillance capabilities.
CDC Epidemic Information Exchange (EPI-X)	Epi-X is a secure web-based communications network for public health professionals: CDC officials, state and local health departments, poison control centers, and other public health professionals can access and share preliminary health surveillance information quickly and securely, 24 h, 7 days/wk (24×7). Users can also be actively notified of breaking health events as they occur. Key features of Epi-X include unparalleled scientific and editorial support, controlled user access, digital credentials and authentication, rapid outbreak reporting, and peer-to-peer consultation.
CDC PulseNet	The CDC PulseNet is a U.S. national laboratory network made up of 87 laboratories—at least one in each state. It connects food-borne illness cases together to detect and define outbreaks. PulseNet tracks what is being reported to the CDC on any given day and compares it to what was reported in the past to look for changes through use of its cumulative database representing nearly half a million isolates of bacteria from food, the environment, and human food-borne illness. PulseNet International now spans more than 80 countries, to establish similar networks in Canada, Europe, Latin America, the Caribbean, Asia Pacific, the Middle East, and Africa. These networks collaborate with one another and with PulseNet USA.
BioWatch	BioWatch is a Department of Homeland Security program intended to perform 24×7 environmental surveillance using existing Environmental Protection Agency and Department of Energy (DOE) air quality monitoring systems. Air samples will be tested in cities for the presence of biological pathogens to generate early warnings of possible attacks. The CDC Laboratory Response Network (LRN) labs test filters from these samplers.
CDC Laboratory Response Network (LRN)	The LRN is a consortium of more than 150 laboratories comprised primarily of state, local, and federal public health laboratories, each with different capabilities and levels of expertise. As a network, they provide immediate and sustained laboratory testing and communication in the event of public health emergencies, particularly in response to acts of terrorism. Members belong to different agencies and jurisdictions but are unified by a common system of operations.
CDC Health Alert Network (HAN)	The HAN is a public health alerting system that serves as the primary way of getting validated information to federal, state, territorial, and local public health practitioners; clinicians; public information officers; and public health laboratories about urgent public health incidents that are occurring or have occurred. PHIN Communication and Alerting (PCA) describes the capabilities needed by the CDC and state and local health departments to issue alerts and emergency communications to their own staffs, to other organizations, to people within their jurisdictions that are critical to emergency response, and to other affected public health jurisdictions.
ATSDR National Toxic Substance Incidents Program (NTSIP)	The NTSIP is system for collecting and combining information from many resources to protect people from harm caused by spills and leaks of toxic substances. The NTSIP has three components: National Database, State Partners, and Incident Investigation.
CDC Emergency Communications System (ECS)	The ECS ensures rapid, effective, and consistent CDC/ATSDR communication response to the news media, the public, and key stakeholders in the event of a national public health emergency.
CDC Morbidity and Mortality Weekly Report (MMWR)	The MMWR is a weekly publication containing data on specific diseases as reported by state and territorial health departments and reports on infectious and chronic diseases, environmental hazards, natural or human-generated disasters, occupational diseases and injuries, and intentional and unintentional injuries.

Other Resources

American Association of Poison Control Centers (AAPCC) National Poison Data System (NPDS)	The AAPCC and NPDS form a national near-real-time surveillance system that improves situational awareness for chemical and poison exposures, according to data from U.S. poison centers.
WHO Weekly Epidemiological Record (WER)	The WER is an instrument for the rapid and accurate dissemination of epidemiological information on cases and outbreaks of diseases under the International Health Regulations and on other communicable diseases of public health importance, including newly emerging or reemerging infections.

law enforcement data to provide meaningful information and intelligence about threats and criminal activity.[33]

The focus for sharing of this information is the fusion center, a facility-based center designed to promote information sharing at the federal, state, and local levels of government of the United States. According to the National Fusion Center Association, as of 2014, there are 74 fusions centers operating in the United States.[34]

The role of the public health sector within the fusion center is to gather, analyze, and relay health-related information routinely, including health security risks associated with the detection of suspicious biological or chemical agents within a community, and share this information with other sectors of government.[35] From a national perspective, this collective epidemiological network is intended to contribute to the execution of various national plans to defend against biological attacks.[36]

Medical Intelligence and Risk Management

Risk assessment is a systematic process for quantifying the likelihood of adverse health effects in a population following exposure to a specified hazard. A risk assessment is a decision-making support tool that is used to establish requirements and prioritize program investments. Analytical risk management is the process of selecting and implementing prevention and control measures to achieve an acceptable level of that risk at an acceptable cost (Table 91-2).

It is virtually impossible to avoid all possible risk of terrorism. As compared to risk avoidance, which seeks to counter all possible vulnerabilities, risk management instead weighs the risk of loss against the cost of control measures. Risk management is composed of three main elements: risk assessment, cost-benefit analysis, and risk communication. The components of analytical risk assessment about terrorism include asset and loss effect assessment, threat assessment, and vulnerability analysis.[37]

Well-integrated medical intelligence provides the preexisting public health and intelligence systems with the ability to recognize and characterize a population's risk for terrorism in advance of any subsequent countermeasures in the form of prevention and control. Soundly performed risk assessments help ensure that specific programs and related expenditures are justified and targeted according to the threat and risk of validated terrorist attack scenarios generated and assessed by a multidisciplinary team of experts.[38]

Intelligence and law enforcement threat information is a key input into a risk assessment process that involves criminal or conflict-related activity. Risk assessments are widely recognized as valid decision-support tools to establish and prioritize program investments and are grounded in risk management. Medical intelligence may be applied within the process of analytical risk management in an effort to protect populations as well as private business against the risk of public health emergencies.[39–41]

A threat analysis, the first step in determining risk, identifies and evaluates each threat based on various factors such as its capability and intent to attack an asset and the likelihood and the severity of the consequences of a successful attack. Valid, current, and documented threat information in a risk assessment process is crucial to ensuring that countermeasures or programs are not based solely on worst-case scenarios and are therefore out of balance with the threat. Risk management principles acknowledge that although risk generally cannot be eliminated, it can be reduced by enhancing protection from validated and credible threats. Moreover, even though many threats are possible, some are more likely to be carried out than others are. Risk assessments form a deliberate, analytical approach that results in a prioritized list of risks (i.e., threat-asset-vulnerability combinations) that can be used to select countermeasures to create a certain level of protection or preparedness. Because threats are dynamic and countermeasures may become outdated, it is highly recommended to reassess threat and risk periodically.[39–41]

To perform a realistic risk assessment of terrorist threats, a multidisciplinary team of experts would require several inputs, including written foreign and domestic threat analyses from the intelligence community and law enforcement, as well as civilian public health and medical intelligence.

TABLE 91-2	Elements of Analytical Risk Management	
PROCESS	**ACTIVITIES**
Impact assessment	• Determining critical assets (i.e., a population)
Asset assessment	• Identifying undesirable events and expected loss or damage
Loss assessment	• Prioritizing assets based on consequence of loss
Threat characterization	• Identifying indications, circumstances, or events with the potential to cause the loss of or damage to an asset
Hazard identification	
Adversary intent	• Assessing intent and motivation of each adversary
Adversary capability	• Assessing capabilities of each adversary
Adversary history	• Determining frequency of past events
	• Estimating threat relative to each critical asset
Vulnerability analysis	• Identifying potential weaknesses that may be exploited by an adversary to gain access to an asset
Potential vulnerabilities	• Identifying existing countermeasures and their level of effectiveness which may be used in reducing vulnerability
Existing countermeasures	• Estimating degree of vulnerability to each asset and threat
Countermeasure determination	• Identifying potential actions or physical entities that may be used to eliminate or lessen one or more vulnerabilities
Prevention	
Control	
Cost-benefit analysis	• Identifying countermeasure costs and benefits
	• Conducting cost-benefit and tradeoff analyses
	• Prioritizing options
Risk communication	• Preparing a range of recommendations for decision makers and/or the public

⚠ PITFALLS

Incomplete Integration of Veterinary Medicine into Medical Intelligence Systems

Although recent reports have emphasized the need for improving the ability to detect a biological terrorist attack on human populations, the use of veterinary services in this effort and the potential for the targeting of livestock (e.g., horses, cattle, sheep, goats, swine, and poultry) have been addressed only superficially. Improving surveillance for biological terrorist attacks that target livestock, as well as detection and reporting of livestock, pet, and wild animal morbidity and mortality are important components of preparedness for a covert biological terrorist attack. Although veterinarians have been mentioned as an integral part of biological terrorism-preparedness planning, the importance of improving surveillance among livestock, pet, and wild animal populations has not been emphasized. Any improvement in detection of a covert biological terrorist attack should be a goal of human and veterinary health programs. Even though a system for detecting and reporting nonendemic or foreign animal diseases exists in the United States, the system needs strengthening to increase the likelihood of detecting a covert biological terrorist attack on humans or other mammals. Following a covert bioterrorist attack with an agent targeting livestock or human populations, the front line of practicing human and veterinary health care providers will be essential for detection, reporting, and response.[42]

Inherent Difficulties in the Natural Course of Bioterrorism-Related Illness

Inherent difficulties in the natural course of bioterrorism-related illness might limit the utility of medical intelligence to recognize the clues of a bioterror attack rapidly. In one example, the steep epidemic curve expected in a bioterrorism attack is similar to that seen with other point source exposures, such as foodborne outbreaks.[6]

Even in the presence of known indicators of a bioterror attack, it may not be easy to determine that an attack occurred through nefarious means. For example, in spite of a CDC-led investigation, it took months to determine that an outbreak of salmonellosis in Oregon was caused by intentional contamination of salad bars.[5] Other naturally occurring outbreaks, such as the hantavirus outbreak in the Four Corners area of the United States and the tularemia outbreak in Kosovo, have been mistakenly thought of as possible results of intentional contamination.[8,43]

Lack of Clinical Training among Medical Personnel

Lack of clinical training among medical personnel with respect to illness related to chemical and biological terrorism may limit the timeliness of medical intelligence. Even emergency medicine residency training programs have exhibited a less than optimum capability for training physicians to diagnose and treat rarely seen maladies.[34]

Inherent Difficulties of Syndromic Surveillance

Inherent difficulties of syndromic surveillance may limit the usefulness of early warning in outbreaks related to bioterror attack. Passive disease-reporting systems that are not directly linked to the laboratory could result in delays in the recognition of disease outbreaks. Other difficulties with current surveillance systems include incomplete data capture; inaccurate data; gaps in provider appreciation for the importance and usefulness of surveillance activities, data and information; difficulty in geographic localization of an outbreak and tracking geographic locations of patients; inadequate indicators to serve as triggers for a response; limited surveillance of response personnel; limited feedback to reporting installations; and suboptimal laboratory integration.[44,45]

The signs of a terrorist attack may also appear insidiously, with primary-care providers witnessing the first cases. However, emergency room personnel might not be the first to detect a problem. The first to notice could be a hospital laboratory seeing unusual strains of organisms, a county epidemiologist keeping track of hospital admissions, pharmacists distributing more antibiotics than usual, 911 operators noticing an increase in respiratory distress calls, or funeral directors with increased business.[6]

Despite the small number of patients, the published descriptions of 11 persons with inhalational anthrax in the United States may offer four lessons for detecting a bioterror epidemic.[46] First, a key objective of syndromic surveillance is to detect early stage disease, but fewer than half of these patients sought care in the early stage of illness before hospitalization was necessary. Second, emergency room data are a common source for syndromic surveillance, but detecting an increase in visits coincident with hospital admission may not provide an early warning because the time needed to process surveillance data and investigate suspected cases would be at least as long as the time for admission blood cultures to be positive for *Bacillus anthracis*. Third, the four patients who received early care, and then were discharged to home, were assigned three different diagnoses, suggesting that syndromic surveillance systems must address the potential variability in how patients with the same infection may be diagnosed during the prodrome. Finally, rapid diagnosis after hospitalization was possible only in those patients who had not received antibiotics before cultures were taken.

Challenges Integrating Public Health and National-Level Knowledge Management Systems

According to Lenart et al., "As no standards exist to establish the types of public health and medical information that need to be collected and disseminated, or the qualifications of those collecting the information, the value of information is often questionable."[35] There are several barriers to the development of competency among public health and medical liaisons in the fusion center. One challenge is that it is difficult to acquire the necessary experience because of limited access to training and guidelines. Another barrier for development of public health medical intelligence competencies is their routine lack of security clearance, which is required for admission into the fusion center.[35]

Violation of Civil Liberties and Right to Privacy

In a 2005 survey, the Governors Association Center for Best Practices revealed that states ranked the development of state intelligence fusion centers as one of their highest priorities.[34]

However, significant civil concern with four areas of fusion center aspects has arisen, which is summarized in a 2007 ACLU report on the fusion center process[47]:
- "Ambiguous lines of authority"
- Allowance of authorities "to manipulate differences in federal, state, and local laws to maximize information collection while evading accountability and oversight through the practice of 'policy shopping'"
- Use of private sector and military participation in the surveillance of U.S. citizens through fusion centers
- Likelihood to engage in poorly contained data mining

In 2008, the Department of Homeland Security (DHS) identified a number of risks to privacy presented by the fusion center program[48]:
- Justification for fusion centers
- Ambiguous lines of authority, rules, and oversight
- Participation of the military and the private sector
- Data mining
- Excessive secrecy
- Inaccurate or incomplete information
- Mission creep

By 2012, the U.S. Senate Permanent Subcommittee on Investigations concluded, "the fusion centers often produced irrelevant, useless, or inappropriate intelligence reporting to DHS, and many produced no intelligence reporting whatsoever." The same report presented evidence of three separate occasions where fusion centers may have hindered, not aided, federal counterterrorism efforts.[49] The subcommittees also cited multiple reports of violations of civil liberties and privacy associated with the operation of fusion centers.

ACKNOWLEDGMENT

The author wishes to acknowledge guidance provided by Mark Keim, MD, MBA. Dr. Keim's assistance proved invaluable for the author's development of this chapter.

REFERENCES

1. *Department of Defense Dictionary of Military and Associated Terms, Joint Publication 2-01.* Available at: http://www.dtic.mil/doctrine/dod_dictionary/; March 15, 2014. Accessed 04.05.14.

2. Walden J, Kaplan EH. Estimating the size of bioterror attack. *Emerg Infect Dis.* 2004;10(7):1202–1205.

3. *Casualties in the Civil War.* http://www.civilwarhome.com/casualties.htm. Accessed 04.05.14.

4. Sanftleben K. *The Unofficial Joint Medical Officer's Handbook. Uniformed Services University of the Health Sciences.* 2nd ed. 1997. Available at: http://www.au.af.mil/au/awc/awcgate/usuhs/ujmo_handbook.pdf. Accessed 04.05.14.

5. Torok T, Tauxe R, Wise R, et al. A large community outbreak of salmonellosis caused by intentional contamination of restaurant salad bars. *JAMA.* 1997;278:389–395.

6. Pavlin JA. Epidemiology of bioterrorism. *Emerg Infect Dis.* 1999;5(2):528–533.

7. Noah DL, Sobel AL, Ostroff SM, et al. Biological warfare training: infectious disease outbreak differentiation criteria. *Mil Med.* 1998;163(4):198.

8. Grunow R, Finke EJ. A procedure for differentiation between intentional release of biological warfare agents and natural disease outbreaks of disease: its use in analyzing the tularemia outbreak in Kosovo in 1999 and 2000. *Clin Microbiol Infect.* 2002;8(8):510–521.

9. Treadwell TA, Koo D, Kuker K, Khan AS. Epidemiologic clues to bioterrorism. *Public Health Rep.* 2003;118:92–98.

10. Buehler JW, Berkelman RL, Hartley DM, Peters CJ. Syndromic surveillance and bioterrorism-related epidemics. *Emerg Infect Dis.* 2003;9(10):1197–1204.

11. Walden J, Kaplan EH. Estimating the size of bioterror attack. *Emerg Infect Dis.* 2004;10(7):1202–1205.

12. Keim M, Kaufmann A, Rodgers G. *Recommendations for Office of Emergency Preparedness/CDC Surveillance, Laboratory and Informational Support Initiative.* Atlanta, GA: Centers for Disease Control and Prevention, National Center for Environmental Health; 1998.

13. Carter D, Carter J. The intelligence fusion process for state, local and tribal law enforcement. *Crim Justice Behav.* 2009;36(12):1323–1339.

14. Lenart B, Albanese J, Halstead W, Schlegelmilch J, Paturas J. Integrating public health and medical intelligence gathering into homeland security fusion centers. *J Bus Contin Emer Plan.* 2012 Autumn-2013 Winter;6(2):174–179.

15. Centers for Disease Control and Prevention. *Emergency Preparedness and Response.* Available at: http://www.bt.cdc.gov/. Accessed 04.05.14.

16. Centers for Disease Control and Prevention. *Public Health Information Network.* Available at: http://www.cdc.gov/phin/about/faq2.html. Accessed 04.05.14.

17. Centers for Disease Control and Prevention. *National Notifiable Diseases Surveillance System (NNDSS).* Available at: http://wwwn.cdc.gov/nndss/default.aspx. Accessed 04.05.14.

18. Centers for Disease Control and Prevention. *Epidemic Information Exchange.* Available at: http://www.cdc.gov/epix/. Accessed 05.04.14.

19. Centers for Disease Control and Prevention. *PulseNet.* Available at: http://www.cdc.gov/pulsenet/. Accessed 04.05.14.

20. Centers for Disease Control and Prevention. *Examples of the Laboratory Response Network (LRN) in Action: BioWatch.* Available at: http://emergency.cdc.gov/lrn/examples.asp. Accessed 04.05.14.

21. Centers for Disease Control and Prevention. *The Laboratory Response Network Partners in Preparedness.* Available at: http://emergency.cdc.gov/lrn/. Accessed 04.05.14.

22. Centers for Disease Control and Prevention. *Health Alert Network (HAN).* Available at: http://emergency.cdc.gov/HAN/. Accessed 04.05.14.

23. Agency for Toxic Substances and Disease Registry. *ATSDR National Toxic Substance Incidents Program (NTSIP).* Available at: http://www.atsdr.cdc.gov/ntsip/. Accessed 04.05.14.

24. Centers for Disease Control and Prevention. *CDC Emergency Communication System.* The Risk Communicator. Available at: http://www.bt.cdc.gov/ercn/02/pdf/rcnewsletterissue2.pdf. Accessed 04.05.14.

25. Centers for Disease Control and Prevention. *Morbidity and Mortality Weekly Report (MMWR).* Available at: http://www.cdc.gov/mmwr/. Accessed 04.05.14.

26. American Association of Poison Control Centers (AAPCC). *National Poison Data System (NPDS).* Available at: http://www.aapcc.org/data-system/. Accessed 04.05.14.

27. World Health Organization (WHO). *The Weekly Epidemiological Record (WER).* Available at: http://www.who.int/wer/en/. Accessed 04.05.14.

28. Centers for Disease Control and Prevention. Biological and chemical terrorism: strategic plan for preparedness and response; recommendations of the CDC strategic planning workgroup. *MMWR Recomm Rep.* 2000;49(RR-4):1–14.

29. Noah DL, Noah DL, Crowder HR. Biological terrorism against animals and humans: a brief review and primer for action. *J Am Vet Med Assoc.* 2002;221(1):40–43.

30. Pavlin JA. Bioterrorism and the importance of the public health laboratory. *Mil Med.* 2000;165(7 suppl 2):25–27.

31. Lillibridge SR. *Testimony presented to the Government Reform and Oversight Committee, Subcommittee on National Security;* September 22, 1999, Washington, DC.

32. White House. *National Strategy for Information Sharing.* October 2007, Available at: http://georgewbush-whitehouse.archives.gov/nsc/infosharing/, Accessed 04.05.14.

33. *Fusion Center Guidelines.* US Department of Justice. Available at: http://it.ojp.gov/documents/fusion_center_guidelines_law_enforcement.pdf. Accessed 04.05.14.

34. National Association of Fusion Centers. Available at: https://nfcausa.org/. Accessed 04.05.14.

35. Lenart B, Albanese J, Halstead W, Schlegelmilch J, Paturas J. Integrating public health and medical intelligence gathering into homeland security fusion centers. *J Bus Contin Emer Plan.* 2012 Autumn-2013 Winter;6(2):174–179.

36. Noah DL, Ostroff SM, Cropper TL, Thacker SB. U.S. military officer participation in the Centers for Disease Control and Prevention Epidemic Intelligence Service. *Mil Med.* 2003;168(5):368–372.

37. Keim M. *Intentional Chemical Disasters, Disaster Medicine.* [Hogan D, Burstein J, eds.]. Philadelphia, PA: Lippincott, Williams & Wilkins; 2002.

38. *Combating Terrorism: Need for Comprehensive Threat and Risk Assessments of Chemical and Biological Attacks.* NSIAD-99-163. 28 pp. plus 3 appendices (8 pp), September 7, 1999. Available at: http://www.gao.gov/products/GAO/NSIAD-99-163. Accessed 04.05.14.

39. Yi H, Zheng'an Y, Fan W, et al. Public health preparedness for the world's largest mass gathering: 2010 World Exposition in Shanghai, China. *Prehosp Disaster Med.* 2012;27(6):589–594.

40. Sun X, Keim M, He Y, Mahany M, Yuan Z. Reducing the risk of public health emergencies for the world's largest mass gathering: 2010 World Exposition, Shanghai China. *Disast Health.* 2013;1(1):21–29.

41. Sun X, Keim M, Dong C, Mahany M, Guo X. A dynamic process of health risk assessment for business continuity during the World Exposition Shanghai China 2010. *J Bus Contin Emer Plan.* 2014;7(4):347–364.

42. Ashford DA, Gomez TM, Noah DL, et al. Biological terrorism and veterinary medicine in the United States. *J Am Vet Med Assoc.* 2000;217(5):664–667.

43. Horgan J. Were four corners victims biowar casualties? *Sci Am.* 1993;269:16.

44. Pesik N, Keim M. Do emergency medicine residency training programs provide adequate training for bioterrorism? *Ann Emerg Med.* 1999;34(2):173–176.

45. Kortepeter MG, Pavlin JA, Gaydos JC, et al. Surveillance at US military installations for bioterrorist and emerging infectious disease threats. *Mil Med.* 2000;165:238–239.

46. Buehler JW, Berkelman RL, Hartley DM, Peters CJ. Syndromic surveillance and bioterrorism-related epidemics. *Emerg Infect Dis.* 2003;9(10):1197–1204.

47. American Civil Liberties Union. *What's Wrong With Fusion Centers—Executive Summary.* Available at: https://www.aclu.org/technology-and-liberty/whats-wrong-fusion-centers-executive-summary. Accessed 04.05.14.

48. US Department of Homeland Security. *Department of Homeland Security State, Local, and Regional Fusion Center Initiative;* December 11, 2008, Available at: http://www.dhs.gov/xlibrary/assets/privacy/privacy_pia_ia_slrfci.pdf. Accessed 04.05.14.

49. US Senate Permanent Subcommittee on Investigations. *Federal Support for and Involvement in State and Local Fusion Centers;* October 3, 2012, Available at: http://www.hsgac.senate.gov/download/?id=49139e81-1dd7-4788-a3bb-d6e7d97dde04. Accessed 04.05.14.

CHAPTER 92

Preventive Medicine for Providers in High-Threat Environments

Laura Ebbeling and James P. Phillips

It can be said that the primary role of any tactical emergency medical support (TEMS) provider is to render aid so that others may remain in the fight. Mission success is the ultimate goal, and so much of that depends on the ability of the operators to participate effectively and, if injured, minimize the burden placed on the other team members. This chapter will focus on the area of preventive medicine for those who respond to emergencies in dangerous environments. Preventive tactical medicine (PTM) incorporates ideas from military medicine, international and humanitarian relief, epidemiology, infectious disease, and wilderness medicine. Incorporating these concepts into the regular maintenance and training of a team of operators will ensure that those members selected for a given mission will start at the best baseline health possible and thereby will have the highest probability for operational success.

HISTORICAL PERSPECTIVE

Preventive medicine has long had a role in the military. Periods of advancement in battlefield medicine and trauma surgery have routinely paralleled the involvement of the United States in foreign military actions. It is well described that the field of emergency medical service(s) (EMS) has incorporated lessons and concepts developed during wars to improve domestic medicine, both through medical care as well as means of transport of the sick and injured. In a similar fashion the U.S. military medical community has improved their protocols for preventive medicine during these periods of intense and rapid adaptation to the dangers of enemy forces in hostile environments.

Disease and nonbattle injury (DNBI) is a term used by the U.S. Army to describe what practitioners in the civilian world simply call "illness" and is the primary cause of missed workdays in the military. In this realm there are two major goals: health of the individual patient and success of the unit's mission. A healthy team of operators primed for success is one who begins a mission at baseline health without impairment from medical illness or medicine, mental illness, deconditioning, preexisting injury, high-risk chronic disease, incomplete vaccination status, or lack of clarity regarding local health threats. A solid knowledge of how to prepare a medical threat assessment (MTA) includes understanding the concepts of PTM. And although the TEMS provider typically does not have rank or authority within the team, he does serve as the "medical conscious" to the commander, and medical readiness recommendations on behalf of each soldier should be provided when necessary.

CURRENT PRACTICE

Operator Selection

For a special weapons and tactics (SWAT) or special operations team to remain vigilant, ready to rapidly deploy, and formidable, each member must be healthy and unrestricted by preexisting medical conditions. For the good of the mission, operators chosen for teams should be very healthy at baseline, and exclusion criteria should be clear and obeyed. The maintenance of individual health is the key to team health. The U.S. Army uses specific criteria for the selection of general soldiers, and there are numerous disqualifying medical conditions for enlistment. A subsection of the document discusses the particularly stringent health requirements to be considered for special operations.[1] Many police organizations use similar screening processes to disqualify candidates applying for employment, maintenance of job readiness, and for selection to special operations teams.

At this time there is no national standard of disqualifying medical conditions for the selection of police special operators, although recommendations have been made.[2] Thus it is the responsibility of each department to decide which individuals are medically suited to fulfill particular job requirements. Such guidelines are used to evaluate each candidate to determine suitability before training. Conditions are divided into two types based on the extent to which the condition affects an individual's ability to perform essential functions of the job. The first precludes an individual from performing the essential functions of the job and disqualifies a candidate from the selection process. The second is a medical condition that based on its severity may or may not preclude an individual from performing the essential functions of the job.[3]

The most effective preventive medicine program begins with constructing a team of officers who meet the rigid medical standards and are therefore at low risk of missing workdays or compromising a mission due to a preexisting condition. There are absolute contraindications, such as hearing loss, vision impairment, cardiac conditions, and amputated fingers. Just as those pilots chosen for military duty have specific medical ailments that will preclude them from flying duty,[1] job-specific standards for law enforcement SWAT teams should focus on preventing potential crises. For example, should SWAT officers develop diabetes mellitus, their ability to perform extended missions without refrigeration and regular meals would be severely compromised, and they should be removed from operations secondary to the resulting personal and team risks. This could similarly apply to those afflicted with conditions such as asthma, alcohol dependence, seizure disorders, symptomatic cholelithiasis, and a plethora of other diseases. Selection of team members with nondisqualifying medical conditions, such as essential hypertension, should take place with the caveat that the operator has access to and is able to carry and take necessary medications regularly on sustained operations. Those with environmental allergies (e.g., anaphylaxis to bee stings) should be approved with caution, and consideration should require desensitization therapy as well as availability of antidotes. Even seasonal allergies must be considered particularly because sedating antihistamines should be avoided for all nonemergencies in the tactical environment.

Mental health disorders warrant special discussion here. The Global War on Terrorism has shed new light on the seriousness and incidence of posttraumatic stress disorder (PTSD), which in previous decades has gone by several names: hysteria, soldier's heart, irritable heart, shell shock, combat fatigue, stress response syndrome, Vietnam veterans syndrome, and ultimately PTSD. This disorder is, unfortunately, not uncommon after combat. It is critical for the military and for law enforcement agencies to conduct thorough and exhaustive psychological testing for recruits before selection because we have learned now that the fear and stress caused by combat has the ability to worsen preexisting mental illness and may not only compromise the team and mission but also cause permanent problems for the individual. The U.S. military has strict standards regarding mental illness as exclusionary criteria for enlistment, as noted in the 2011 Standards of Medical Fitness, which defines nearly any preexisting mental health disorder, from attention-deficit disorder (ADD) requiring medication to depression to nocturnal enuresis after age 13, as disqualifying features. Law enforcement agencies should consider similar standards.[1]

Health Maintenance

Following the selection process the key concept in preventive medicine for responders in high-threat environments is general health maintenance. Physical standards should exist to remain on a team, and these should be tested on a regular basis. Each person on the team needs to remain physically fit in order to prevent injury and to ensure the team operates at its peak. Fitness includes not only strength-training and bodybuilding exercises but also regular physical conditioning with stretching and aerobic and anaerobic exercises. Although prevention of deconditioning is paramount, proper nutrition and maintaining a healthy weight with a low total body fat index are also vital.[4,5] In order for a unit to function at maximum capacity the team leader or medical officer should ensure all individuals are taking their home medications, receiving regular physical examinations/treatments, and receiving counseling on smoking cessation and drug and alcohol use.[4] Drug and alcohol dependence, although uncomfortable topics for many, must be addressed within the team and should function as automatic disqualifiers from special operations. All efforts should be made to provide treatment and reinstatement, if possible.

Immunizations

Immunizations are another important aspect of health maintenance for disease prevention and team health. The Department of Defense requires certain immunizations for military personnel and most civilian employees. These include the following, and some are location specific: anthrax, hepatitis A/B, pneumococcus, meningococcus, measles, pertussis, smallpox, diphtheria, typhoid fever, yellow fever, mumps, polio, rabies, rubella, varicella, tetanus, adenovirus types 4 and 7, *Haemophilus influenzae* serotype B, influenza, and Japanese encephalitis.[6] There are certain individuals who are unable to tolerate vaccines, such as those with egg allergies. The CDC provides a concise summary to help guide physicians in this matter and can be referenced on their website at http://www.cdc.gov/vaccines/recs/vac-admin/contraindications-adults.htm. Immunization policies should be in place for all teams functioning in foreign countries.

Medical Threat Assessment

After team selection, immunizations, and health maintenance have been addressed, team leaders must prepare for individual missions. Part of that preparation is performed by the medical team or TEMS provider and is called an MTA. The MTA is an all-hazards approach evaluation tool that provides a standardized mechanism for identifying and risk stratifying potential threats to the health and safety of those involved in the mission. It is a flexible framework for information collection and can be used as a checklist to ensure that preventive medicine measures are completed during the planning phase.[7] An MTA should be performed as far in advance of a mission as possible and should address environmental risks and available assets. Failure to perform a proper MTA could leave the team unprepared for climate extremes, weather, local flora and fauna, local infectious disease risks, and problems with food and water.

Environmental Exposure

Location of missions must be taken into account when considering threats, such as cold and heat extremes, environmental moisture, and sun exposure. Environmental injury can hinder a team's effectiveness and pose severe health threats.[8]

During cold weather missions the primary preventive medicine concerns regard frostbite and hypothermia. It is important for team members to be outfitted with appropriate clothing, gear, water availability, and protection.[8] Hypothermia occurs when the body loses heat faster than it is able to generate it. Core body temperature falls below normal, typically defined as a core temperature below 95 °F. It is critical to understand that freezing environmental temperatures need not be present for hypothermia. It tends to occur during cold, windy weather, rapidly changing weather environments, and in those who are wet, exhausted, and poorly dressed. Prevention includes proper clothing, staying dry, avoiding wind, getting rest, and monitoring your fellow team members.[9] Operators are very likely going to be wearing heavy gear and armor that will lead to perspiration. Sweat will lead to evaporative and conductive heat loss and significantly increase the risk of developing hypothermia. Proper head coverage is essential. The TEMS provider must help team leaders to remember work-rest cycles on sustained operations and has a responsibility to ensure that operators have a place to rewarm periodically. These cycles are particularly important for those with extended exposure roles, most notably snipers, spotters, and countersnipers. Warm drinks should be made available if possible. Critically the prevention of a team philosophy of "toughing it out" will help assure that members in need of help will ask for it.

Frostbite occurs at temperatures below freezing in those who are wet, underprepared, and poorly dressed. Frostbite injuries occur on a spectrum from superficial injury to severe, full thickness skin injuries, which can lead to loss of limb or extremity.[9] For the purposes of tactical medicine, recognizing the early stages, known as frostnip, allows the TEMS provider to perform actions to reverse the condition before development of true frostbite.

Frostnip is a superficial, nonfreezing cold injury associated with intense vasoconstriction on exposed skin, usually cheeks, ears, or nose. By definition, ice crystals do not form in the tissue nor does tissue loss occur in frostnip. The numbness and pallor resolve quickly after covering the skin with appropriate clothing, warming the skin with direct contact, breathing with cupped hands over the nose, or gaining shelter that protects from the elements. No long-term damage occurs. The appearance of frostnip signals conditions favorable for frostbite, and appropriate action should be undertaken immediately to prevent injury.[10]

Frostbite occurs when tissue freezes, forming intracellular ice crystals and leading to variable degrees of tissue damage. Although outside the scope of this chapter, there are well-defined degrees of frostbite that correlate somewhat to the better-known descriptions of the severity of burns.[10] Contributing factors to frostbite include the amount of tissue exposed, ambient temperatures, nutritional status, wind chill, nicotine use, previous cold injury, physical activity, and tight-fitting clothing or boots.[11] Severe frostbite can require evacuation for hospital evaluation and result in loss of a team member.

Immersion injury, such as trench foot, can occur during extended operations as well. This disease process was defined during World War I and is caused by prolonged exposure to dampness and cold temperatures. Improper footwear and hygiene are the primary preventable risk factors. The ambient temperature need not be below freezing. Symptoms of trench foot include a tingling and/or itching sensation, pain, swelling, cold and blotchy skin, numbness, and a prickly or heavy feeling in the foot. The foot may be red, dry, and painful after it becomes warm. Blisters may form, followed by skin and tissue dying and falling off. In severe cases, untreated trench foot can involve the toes, heel, or entire foot.[12,13] Preventative measures, such as waterproof boots, dry socks, massage, and early recognition, are key.

Heat injuries are a serious concern during prolonged operations in warm climates. In hot environments body temperature increases, which places stress on the body's ability to regulate temperature and can lead to failure of compensatory mechanisms in the body.[8] High humidity interferes with sweat evaporation, leaving radiation of heat as the primary method of cooling. The layers of gear and heavy equipment required in tactical operations reduce the ability to radiate heat to the environment and block wind-driven convection heat loss, adding to the cumulative heat stress and thus increasing the risk of heat injury. By overwhelming the body's ability to maintain temperature equilibrium, heat illness can occur. The spectrum of disease includes heat cramps, heat exhaustion, and ultimately heat stroke. It is very important for tactical teams to prevent heat-related illness, starting with the MTA consideration of environmental temperature, humidity, and air movement.[9] Prevention of temperature-related injury involves reducing exposure times, work-rest cycling, heating or cooling areas for operators, moisture-wicking base layer garments, and adequate hydration. It is critical that officers feel comfortable informing their commander if they develop early temperature injury to prevent progression to more severe forms. Lastly, overexposure to ultraviolet (UV) light from the sun can lead to sunburn and also contributes to heat injury. Use of high sun protection factor (SPF) sunscreen before deployment and reapplying often can prevent sunburn. Finding shade when available will also reduce UV burden and lessen the individual's heat stress.

Dehydration

Dehydration occurs when fluid losses exceed intake. Those under high stress and in warm environments lose most of this fluid through sweating but also through insensible means, such as respiration. Heavy gear and hard exertion can lead to fluid losses of 1 L/h. Replacing lost water is necessary in order to maintain an adequate hydration status and avoid heat injury. Any exposed operator is at risk, and command-driven oral hydration should be mandated by the commander and TEMS provider. This is primarily important because unfortunately thirst is not the ideal indicator of hydration status. Headache is a likely first indicator of dehydration and must be addressed as such. Preventive medicine dictates that all team members prehydrate and carry adequate supplies on their person, typically in the form of a backpack bladder. Rehydration with water or 0.5- to 0.25-strength diluted sports drinks will work for minor cases of dehydration, and the dilution will prevent the gastrointestinal (GI) upset sometimes seen with heavy carbohydrate drinks. Although weather conditions and individual variation in sweating may dictate different fluid requirements, a safe recommendation is 1 L/h of work, and the urine color concentration can be used as a rough guide for hydration status.

Infectious Diseases

In the tactical environment the most likely infectious diseases to be encountered are those transmitted by insect vectors. For missions within the United States the greatest risks for mosquito and tick-borne illnesses are West Nile virus and Lyme disease, respectively.[8] However, other tick-borne illnesses, such as babesiosis and rickettsial Rocky Mountain spotted fever, are also important diseases to consider when operating in endemic areas. American trypanosomiasis, also known as Chagas disease, is a protozoal disease caused by transmission from the bite of the "kissing bug" found in the southern United States and Latin America.[9]

Because of the variable incubation periods of vector-borne diseases, acute transmission of these diseases are unlikely to take an operator out of action during a mission. But that does not obviate the TEMS provider of the responsibility of making sure team members undergo proper evaluation for these infections if symptoms develop days or weeks later. All of these diseases can lead to significant impairment, including fevers, encephalitis, myocarditis, neurologic impairment, or sometimes death. The best treatment is prevention. Team members should prepare appropriately with protective clothing, application of high concentration N,N-diethyl-meta-toluamide (DEET) to all exposed skin, and using appropriate pest control with netting and sprays at home base.[8]

Viral infections typically cause self-limited disease; however, more significant infections leading to influenza, measles, hepatitis, and weaponized smallpox could possibly occur. Fortunately vaccination has helped to decrease the risk of infection with hepatitis A, hepatitis B, influenza, measles, poliomyelitis, rabies, smallpox, and mumps when exposed.[6] But, in an era where fringe thinkers are increasingly choosing to ignore science and forgo vaccinating their children, it is imperative that operators stay up to date with immunizations. Adenovirus is very contagious and leads to a spectrum of respiratory illnesses. However, vaccination in some populations and good hygiene in close corridors can prevent the spread of disease. Similarly many viral infections can lead to gastroenteritis, with diarrhea and vomiting, which can ultimately cause dehydration and impair the ability to fight. Good hygiene, including proper toileting away from camp and waste disposal, is a critically important piece of disease prevention.

Bacteria can lead to severe infections and often do not resolve without proper treatment with antibiotics. Since the terrorist attacks in the United States, anthrax has become a true terrorist threat. It is a spore-forming bacterium leading to cutaneous, GI, or inhalational infection. Vaccination in the appropriate population helps to prevent infection when exposed. In addition, caution with human and animal blood and bodily fluids and disinfection of the premises are important aspects in avoiding the spread of disease.[6,9] Bubonic plague, a zoonotic bacterial infection caused by *Yersinia pestis*, is transmitted from rodents via a flea vector and is endemic to parts of the southwest United States. The more deadly pulmonary form, called pneumonic plague, is transmitted person to person by droplet inhalation. Vaccination does not protect against pneumonic plague but can help prevent contraction of the bubonic form from fleas. Other preventative measures include pest control, avoidance of dead animals, and protective gear.[9,6] Tetanus, a neurotoxin-based illness caused by the spore-forming bacterium *Clostridium tetani* found in soil and animal GI tracts, is introduced through contaminated wounds and infection and leads to acute, lethal central nervous system disease. Cleaning wounds and maintaining current immunizations is an important aspect of prevention of tetanus.

For tactical operational teams, such as military special forces or groups deploying for disaster response internationally, additional region-specific illnesses must be considered which can cause significant morbidity and mortality. Malaria is a potentially lethal protozoal infection endemic to tropical and subtropical areas and is caused by species of the *Plasmoidium* genus. It is widespread across developing countries, particularly in Africa, and is transmitted by Anopheles mosquito bites. Symptoms vary but typically include fever, chills, myalgias, abdominal pain, and diarrhea. Prophylactic medications, such as mefloquine, Malarone, and doxycycline, can help prevent infection while in these areas and should be mandatory for all operators before travel and after return.

Dengue fever is a viral infection spread via mosquitos in tropical urban centers. Infectious symptoms include fevers, headaches, myalgias, hemorrhage, and sometimes shock or death. Prevention is similar to avoiding other mosquito-borne illnesses but typically involves the avoidance of outdoor activities while mosquitos are active and using protective clothing, nets, and DEET spray.[9,6]

Yellow fever virus causes a viral hemorrhagic fever and is endemic to tropical jungle environments in Africa and South America. Prevention with immunizations and boosters are important and should be given before travel to any endemic area because the mortality rate for unvaccinated patients is as high as 50%.[14] Another infection, typhoid, is caused by *Salmonella typhi* and is spread from human to human via fecal contamination and shared food. It causes a febrile illness characterized by abdominal pain and sometimes rash. It is encountered both domestically and abroad, typically when exposed to contaminated drinking water in developing countries. Vaccination is available. Otherwise, preventive measures include properly cooking and washing food, drinking appropriate water, and practicing good fecal hygiene.[15]

Parasitic infections are typically contracted through contact with or ingestion of contaminated water. The most common infections include amebiasis, ascariasis, giardiasis, and schistosomiasis, all of which can lead to significant diarrhea, abdominal pain, and in some cases liver failure or death.[9] Prevention with filtering water, boiling water, good hand washing and hygiene, avoidance of fresh water, and safe food preparation is vital. Domestic tactical operations are typically short in duration, close to urban centers, and well within reach of clean water and sanitation. In other operational environments, such as disaster deployment and military missions, these illnesses may be encountered and should be part of the MTA.

Tropical environments lend themselves to more exotic animals and exposure risks. Within the United States the vast majority of poisonous snakebites are caused by pit vipers, such as rattlesnakes, copperheads, and cottonmouth snakes. However, most deaths within the United States are caused by diamondback rattlesnakes. There is a correlation between envenomation dose and rapidity of onset of illness. Symptoms can range from mild swelling of the extremity with localized pain, to diarrhea, confusion, and severe cardiovascular collapse and shock.[9] Prevention includes appropriate leather boots and situational awareness. In the case of envenomation the TEMS provider should arrange medical evacuation to the nearest hospital for supportive care and antivenin, as needed. Venomous spiders, which in the United States are primarily the infamous black widow spider and the brown recluse ("fiddleback") spider, which are the only two endemic species capable of human envenomation, are rarely life or limb threatening. The black widow produces a painful bite and injects a neurotoxin. The brown recluse bite is typically painless, and the necrotoxin injected can cause variable degrees of tissue loss from small ulcers to loss of fingers or toes.

Preventive medicine is a key concept to be understood by all practitioners in the tactical medicine realm. Similar to military and flight medicine, TEMS providers are the medical conscious of the team and for the commander. As such, it is the responsibility of the team's medical expert not only to respond to injured officers, suspects, and civilians but also to engage the team in the important concepts of preventive medicine. In doing so the provider helps to ensure that the operators are in peak fighting condition and are able to participate safely in the mission at hand. Ensuring that each member is screened appropriately before acceptance to the team and before each relevant mission maximizes the probability of mission success and safe return of each participant.

! PITFALLS

Improper selection of team members can lead to mission failure and injury or death. The TEMS provider or team physician must keep abreast of new diagnoses within the team. Should a new medical problem arise that meets exclusionary criteria, the team member should not be allowed to function in a capacity that puts the mission or others at risk. This may be difficult for the team and commanders, but it is vital.

Failure to perform an adequate MTA before the mission is the major error in tactical medicine. Understanding the local medical threats, expected exposures, mission duration, and available infrastructure is critical to preventing mission-based illness and disease. A stepwise checklist will ensure the TEMS provider has considered each aspect of the MTA and preventive medicine, including food, water, rest, sanitation, exposure, and baseline health status of each operator. Team commanders will use this information to help make decisions before each major mission in an effort to maximize the chances of success without injury.

REFERENCES

1. Army HDOT. *Army Regulation 40-501 Standards of Medical Fitness*. Washington, DC: Department of Army; 2011. 1–152.
2. Adamitis, JA. General physical requirements for applicants seeking an occupational career in municipal, county or state law enforcement. Law Enforcement Physical Requirements. N.p., n.d. Web. 14 May 2015. http://www.wright.edu/~jim.adamitis/physical_req/req.
3. Jacobs EB. Physical and Medical Standards for Law Enforcement. Available at: http://www.ebjacobs.com/PrintablePages/standards_le_print.html.
4. Heiskell LE, Olesnicky BT, Welling LE. *Wilderness Medicine*. Philadelphia, PA: Elsevier; 2011. 552–273.
5. Heiskell LE, Carmona RH. Tactical emergency medical services: an emerging subspecialty of emergency medicine. *Ann Emerg Med*. 1994;23(4):778–785.
6. Headquarters Departments of the Army TNTAF, Guard TC. *Army Regulation 40-562 Immunizations and Chemoprophylaxis for the Prevention of Infectious Diseases*. med.navy.mil; 2013. 1–41.
7. Band RA, Callaway DW, Connor BA, Haughton BP, Mechem CC. Dignitary medicine: adapting prehospital, preventive, tactical and travel medicine to new populations. *Am J Emerg Med*. 2012;30(7):1274–1281.
8. Heck JJ. Role of preventative medicine in TEMS. *Top Emerg Med*. 2003;25(4):299–305.
9. US Special Operations Command, ed. *Special Operations Forces Medical Handbook*. 1st ed. CreateSpace Independent Platform, 2001.
10. McIntosh SE, Opacic M, Freer L, et al. Wilderness medical society practice guidelines for the prevention and treatment of frostbite: 2014 update. *Wilderness Environ Med*. 2014;25(4 Suppl):S43–S54.
11. Heiskell L. Hypothermia and frostbite: considerations in cold weather special operations. *Tactical Edge*. 1992;10:26–29.
12. CDC. Trench Foot or Immersion Foot. Available at: http://emergency.cdc.gov/disasters/trenchfoot.asp.
13. Adnot J, Lewis CW. Immersion foot syndromes. *Mil Dermatol*. 1917.
14. Yellow fever. Available at: http://www.who.int/mediacentre/factsheets/fs100/en/.
15. Typhoid Fever. Available at: http://www.cdc.gov/nczved/divisions/dfbmd/diseases/typhoid_fever/.

PART II

Management of Specific Event Types

93 | CHAPTER

Introduction to Natural Disasters

Ali Ardalan and Debra D. Schnelle

This text is designed as a comprehensive study of disaster medicine that also includes ready-made resources for the practitioner of disaster medicine. The goal of this section is to provide a reference for an exhaustive list of the most important natural disaster scenarios. This introductory chapter provides an overview on natural disasters in terms of risk drivers, burden, classification, and international initiatives. It also presents the analytical framework common to all disasters, that is, the disaster management cycle that includes prevention and mitigation, preparedness, response, and recovery. Thus each scenario can be understood within a common frame of reference.

Natural disasters are the major consequences of occurrences of natural hazards. However, all natural hazards do not necessarily cause disasters. In addition to a populations' exposure to hazard, the conditions of vulnerability and insufficient capacity are the factors that determine if a natural hazard leads to a disaster. Natural disasters cause death, injury, or other health impacts; damage to the environment, services, and properties; and social and economic disruption. The well-being of populations and the status of health care systems can be both directly and indirectly impacted by natural disasters.

HISTORICAL PERSPECTIVE

From 1990 to 2013, natural disasters affected approximately 4.8 billion people worldwide. They caused about 1.6 million deaths and 5.3 million injuries and left over 109 million people homeless. During this period, while geophysical disasters were responsible for 52% of total mortality, water- and weather-related disasters accounted for 97% of the people who were in need of immediate assistance; that is, the affected population (Fig. 93-1).[1] Moreover, adverse impacts of climate change are predicted to increase the risks of hydrometerological disasters by increasing the intensity of hurricanes and cycles of droughts and floods.[2]

Natural disasters are a part of the human experience, and as the size of the human population increases, it can be predicted that the impact of natural disasters on society will grow, for the following four reasons[3]:

- Disasters are continuing to increase in frequency and/or intensity
- Disasters are affecting more population centers in the world community
- The economic costs associated with disasters are increasing at an alarming rate

- More people are moving to areas subject to natural hazards such as cyclone- and tsunami-prone coastlines, flood-prone river basins, and earthquake-prone cities

The risks associated with disasters can be intensive or extensive.[4] *Intensive risk* refers to the risk of high-severity, mid- to low-frequency disasters, mainly associated with major hazards. Examples include the 2010 Haiti earthquake, the 2011 Japan earthquake and tsunami, Hurricane Katrina in 2005, and Hurricane Sandy in 2012. *Extensive risk* is used to describe the risk of low-severity, high-frequency disasters, mainly but not exclusively associated with highly localized hazards. While these events have significant cumulative impacts on the societies and health of populations, unfortunately most often they do not receive enough attention by media and community planners. The loss and damage associated with extensive risks are increasing because of poor urbanization, environmental degradation, poverty, inequality, and weak governance.[5] According to the 2009 *Global Assessment Report on Disaster Reduction*, extensive risk events were responsible for about 65% of damages to hospitals.[6] A study on the impacts of natural disasters on primary health centers revealed that extensive risk hazards were responsible for moderate to severe damages in about 26%, 28%, and 59% of structural damages, nonstructural damages, and functional failure, respectively.[7]

CURRENT PRACTICE

Natural disasters obtain their names from the hazards that trigger them. Accordingly, natural hazards can be characterized by their magnitude or intensity, speed of onset (rapid or slow), duration, and area of extent. The Center for Research on the Epidemiology of Disasters (CRED) provides a classification for natural disasters based on the hazard's origin as follows[1]:

1. *Geophysical disasters* are those originating from solid earth events such as earthquakes, tsunamis, and mass movements (dry).
2. *Hydrological disasters* are events caused by deviations in the normal water cycle and/or overflow of water caused by wind. This category includes floods (river flood, flash flood, and storm surge or coastal flood) and mass movements (wet).
3. *Meteorological disasters* are due to short-lived, small- to medium-scale atmospheric processes, that is, from minutes to days. Meteorological disasters include tropical storms, thunderstorms/lightning, snowstorms/blizzards, sand/dust storms, and tornados.

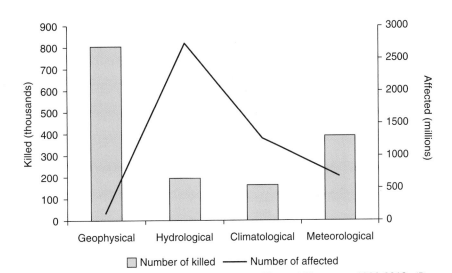

FIG 93-1 Number of People Killed and Affected Due to Natural Disasters, 1990-2013. (Data source: EM-DAT: *The OFDA/CRED International Disaster Database*. Brussels [Belgium]: Université Catholique de Louvain. Available at: http://www.emdat.be.)

4. *Climatological disasters* are those caused by long-lived, medium- to large-scale processes that range from intraseasonal to multi-decade events. This category includes the following hazards: extreme temperature (heat waves and cold waves including frost), extreme winter conditions (snow pressure, icing, freezing, rain debris, and avalanche), drought, and wildfires (forest and land fires).

5. *Biological disasters* are due to the exposure of living organisms to germs and toxic substances. Examples are bacterial or viral epidemics, insect infestations and animal stampedes.

As expected, there are variations in terminology. For instance, the term *hydroclimatological hazards* includes both water- and weather-related hazards. The United Nations International Strategy for Disaster Reduction (UNISDR) defines a hydrometeorological hazard as a process or phenomenon of atmospheric, hydrological, or oceanographic nature.[4] Moreover, biological disasters such as epidemics most often are not included in natural disaster reports.

In some cases, one hazard may result in another, as the case of a tsunami created by an earthquake, a flood caused by a hurricane, or a landslide following an earthquake or a hydrological event. Rockfall, landslides, avalanches, and subsidence can be classified both as geophysical and hydrological hazards depending on the original physical forces.[1] The term *socio-natural hazard* refers to human activities that increase the probability and/or intensity of a natural hazard.[4] Examples include increased flood occurrence following deforestation and increased intensity of cyclones following global warming induced by emission of greenhouse gases. Natural disasters can also trigger the occurrence of technological disasters. The 2011 Japan earthquake and tsunami damaged the power and cooling systems of nuclear power plants and caused an International Nuclear Event Scale (INES) Level 7 accident. About 20% of nuclear reactors worldwide are operating in high seismic zones.[8]

Natural disasters are among the most serious global challenges. The international community has taken initiatives to reduce risk of disasters at the country and local levels and those that cross state boundaries. The second Wednesday of October has been designated as the International Day for Natural Disaster Reduction. The Yokohama Strategy for a Safer World, adopted in 1994, was among the first consolidated international initiatives aimed toward disaster risk reduction. The lessons learned from implementation of the Yokohama Strategy led to development of the Hyogo Framework for Action (HFA) during the World Conference on Disaster Reduction was held in January 2005 in Kobe, Hyogo, Japan. The HFA is an agreed upon international framework for the period of 2005 to 2015.[9] Since 2005, many countries have made some progress in terms of enhancement of capacities in early warning, disaster preparedness, and response that accordingly has contributed to a decreasing trend in mortality risk. Despite these advances, the risk of disasters is still high, causing people to suffer from the associated economic loss and damages, both in developed and less developed nations.[5]

To follow up with the HFA, based on a conference that was held in March 2015 in Sendai, Japan, the United Nations developed the Sendai Framework for Disaster Risk Reduction for the 2015–2030 period.[10] This new framework aims to achieve the following outcome: "the substantial reduction of disaster risk and losses in lives, livelihoods, and health and in the economic, physical, social, cultural, and environmental assets of persons, businesses, communities, and countries." According to the framework, to attain this outcome, the following goal must be pursued: "Prevent new and reduce existing disaster risk through the implementation of integrated and inclusive economic, structural, legal, social, health, cultural, educational, environmental, technological, political, and institutional measures that prevent and reduce hazard exposure and vulnerability to disaster, increase preparedness for response and recovery, and thus strengthen resilience."[10] Because of a proactive contribution by health experts in development of the Sendai Framework, led by the World Health Organization, the health-related subjects have been well highlighted in this global initiative.

Management of natural disasters follows the same tenets of the disaster management cycle described in Chapter 1 of this textbook. The four phases of this cycle include prevention/mitigation, preparedness, response, and recovery.

! PITFALLS

Health systems can play a significant role in disaster risk reduction, particularly for natural disasters. This can be done not only through public health response to disasters and risk reduction of health facilities, but also via assessment and monitoring of community vulnerability and public awareness campaigns. Health systems also need to ensure that risk reduction related to natural disasters is considered by public policies and enforced by law. Unfortunately, to date, health systems have predominantly focused more on response to natural disasters and less on reducing the risks, especially to the general population. Furthermore, despite international efforts toward preparedness of health facilities for natural disasters, less-developed countries still suffer from a lack of high-quality health care infrastructure.[11] The other main challenge is that national health information systems often lack disaster risk management indicators. This fact makes health systems unable to monitor and evaluate the effectiveness of their interventions and resilience of their health facilities and populations to natural disasters. Fortunately, there are some new initiatives in this regard such as a metrics system for disaster risk management that has been developed by health system of Iran and has been integrated to the national health information system.[12]

While natural disasters share common characteristics that require standard response and risk reduction measures, they may also have unique characteristics or consequences that require a specific set of actions. Each of the following chapters in this section focuses on a particular type of natural disaster and presents the associated practical considerations for pre-incident and post-incident actions.

REFERENCES

1. EM-DAT. *The OFDA/CRED International Disaster Database.* Brussels (Belgium): Université Catholique de Louvain. Available at: http://www.emdat.be.
2. National Aeronautics and Space Administration (NASA). The impact of climate change on natural disasters. Available at: http://earthobservatory.nasa.gov/Features/RisingCost/rising_cost5.php.
3. Task Force on Quality Control of Disaster Management, the World Association for Disaster Emergency Medicine, the Nordic Society for Disaster Medicine. Health Disaster Management: Guidelines for Evaluation and Research in the Utstein Style. Volume I. Conceptual Framework of Disasters. *Prehospital Disaster Med.* 2003;17(Suppl 3):1–177.
4. United Nations International Strategy for Disaster Reduction (UNISDR). *Terminology on Disaster Risk Reduction.* Geneva, Switzerland: UNISDR; 2009.
5. United Nations International Strategy for Disaster Reduction (UNISDR). *Global Assessment Report on Disaster Reduction.* Geneva, Switzerland: UNISDR; 2013.
6. United Nations International Strategy for Disaster Reduction (UNISDR). *Global Assessment Report on Disaster Reduction.* Geneva, Switzerland: UNISDR; 2009.
7. Ardalan A, Mowafi H, Yousefi Khoshsabeghe H. Impacts of natural hazards on primary health care facilities of Iran: A 10-year retrospective survey. *PLoS Curr.* 2013;5. http://dx.doi.org/10.1371/currents.dis.ccdbd870f5d1697e4edee5eda12c5ae6.
8. World Nuclear Association (WNA). Nuclear power plants and earthquakes. Available at: http://www.world-nuclear.org/info/Safety-and-Security/Safety-of-Plants/Nuclear-Power-Plants-and-Earthquakes.
9. United Nations International Strategy for Disaster Reduction (UNISDR). Hyogo framework for action 2005-2015: building the resilience of nations and communities to disasters. Available at: http://www.preventionweb.net/files/1037_hyogoframeworkforactionenglish.pdf.
10. United Nations International Strategy for Disaster Reduction (UNISDR). Sendai Framework for Disaster Risk Reduction 2015–2030. Available at: http://www.wcdrr.org/uploads/Sendai_Framework_for_Disaster_Risk_Reduction_2015-2030.pdf.
11. Ardalan A, Kandi M, Talebian MT, et al. Hospitals' safety from disasters in I.R. Iran: the results from assessment of 224 hospitals. PLoS Curr. 2014;6. http://dx.doi.org/10.1371/currents.dis.8297b528bd45975bc6291804747ee5db.
12. Ardalan A. Evidence-based integration of disaster risk management to primary health care, the case of I.R.Iran. UNISDR Scientific and Technical Advisory Group, Case Studies, 2014. Available at: http://www.preventionweb.net/files/workspace/7935_ardalanirancasestudy.pdf.

CHAPTER 94

Hurricanes, Cyclones, and Typhoons

Mark E. Gebhart

DESCRIPTION OF EVENT

Hurricanes, cyclones, and typhoons are all tropical weather systems formed by overly warm water in tropical oceans. Each, characteristically, exhibits rotary circulation and can be described as a low-pressure system. In the northern hemisphere, rotation is counterclockwise. Tropical weather systems can be immense in size, with the average storm reaching 600 km in diameter. These weather systems also exhibit characteristically high wind speeds, reaching a sustained velocity of up to 350 km/h. Research has also shown an average low pressure of 950 mb, with a range of 870 to 990 mb at the storm's center. Hurricanes are classified by the strength of their sustained winds. The Saffir-Simpson scale rates hurricanes on a scale from 1 to 5 (Table 94-1).

The structure of a tropical weather system is primarily defined around the eye and the eye wall of the storm. The eye is the storm's center, and it may be up to 30 km in diameter. It is characterized as the area of lowest pressure, as well as by warmth, lack of precipitation, and air compression. The eye wall is an area extending, on average, 10 to 20 km from the center of the eye; there are thick clouds and heavy rain in the eye wall, and wind speeds are the highest there.

Hurricanes can be described as originating from a large number of thunderstorms. These storms arrange in a pinwheel formation, leading to heavy convection and precipitation, separated by areas of weaker uplift and less precipitation. As a hurricane continues to strengthen, temperature increases toward the center of the storm. The center of the storm is kept warm by the release of latent heat. In the center, mostly clear skies predominate with divergence and sinking air. Near the eye wall, the air rises, cools, and releases latent heat. This latent heat is the primary source of energy for further development. Latent heat requires warm water oceans, generally >27 °C.

PRE-INCIDENT ACTIONS

Planning for a tropical storm involves preparations for all of the threats associated with the storm: high winds, flooding, landslides, thunderstorms, and storm surge.

Preparations for tropical weather should be an ongoing activity, occurring throughout the entire year. Specific preparations may be made at the start of the season, whereas others may be implemented when storm activity is anticipated. Typical hospital emergency management plans are organized based on a time line that starts at the beginning of the storm season and continues through the arrival of storm-force winds and to the poststorm recovery efforts.

Facility infrastructure considerations are essential during construction or remodeling efforts. Hospitals in areas where storms occur should be constructed to withstand high winds and flooding. Storm shutters should be used to protect all exterior openings. Alternate power sources should be an essential component of the facilities infrastructure. Redundant communications systems with civil defense and emergency medical services are essential because multiple system failures can occur.

Another consideration for medical facilities, regardless of size, is the evacuation of patients and staff further inland and away from the predicted storm track. Therefore the facility's evacuation annex should include relocation of patients to a distant facility.

At the start of the storm season, sandbags should be available to barricade low-lying doors susceptible to flooding. Damage control equipment should be available. Plywood sheeting for blown-out windows, two-by-fours for reinforcing doors and other structures that may be stressed by prolonged winds, and vacuums that can handle water (wet/dry vacuum) are essential. Facility engineers and damage control parties must be designated as essential personnel, and they must receive training on mitigation of storm damage. Generators should be fully fueled and maintained.

Before a storm, employees should be alerted to bring in personal items that may be required for a prolonged stay in the medical treatment facility. This should include food, bedding, and medications. Employees who are in the facility during the storm should ensure that their families and residences are prepared before the storm.

Enough durable and expendable medical equipment and pharmaceuticals should be stocked to allow for unsupported operations for up to 72 hours. Disposable equipment (e.g., suture sets) should be considered if sterilization systems should fail. Alternative means of cleaning, such as alcohol-based hand sanitizers, should be obtained. Food and water must be stocked to feed and hydrate staff, patients, and family members of patients. The fuel tanks of vehicles, both personal and hospital-associated, should be filled. Waste systems may be damaged, so alternative means of disposing of liquid and solid waste, including biohazard material, must be considered.

Traditionally, pregnant women, who are either at least 36 weeks' gestation or are in the third trimester and expecting complications with delivery, have been advised to report to the hospital before the storm's arrival. Precipitous labor may occur due to decreased barometric pressure, although this has never been validated.

During the Storm

Generally, damage control predominates during the passage of a tropical cyclone over a medical facility. In an intense storm, there will be minimal movement outdoors, so new patients will not be arriving in large numbers.

Local officials will determine the most effective and safest response method during tropical weather events. Conditions may become so severe that rescue and emergency medical services operations may cease for a period of time. Communications will deteriorate during

TABLE 94-1   Saffir-Simpson Hurricane Scale

CATEGORY	SUSTAINED WINDS	DAMAGE	DESCRIPTION	EXAMPLE
Tropical storm	39-73 miles/h 64-118 km/h			
1	74-95 miles/h 119-153 km/h	Minimal	No real damage to buildings; damage to unanchored mobile homes	Allison, 1995
2	96-110 miles/h 154-177 km/h	Moderate	Damage to building roofs, doors, and windows; considerable damage to mobile homes; flooding damage; trees down	Bonnie, 1998
3	111-130 miles/h 178-209 km/h	Extensive	Some damage to small residences and buildings; mobile homes destroyed; coastal flooding causing destruction to smaller buildings; damage to larger buildings; flooding inland	Opal, 1995
4	131-155 miles/h 210-249 km/h	Extreme	Complete roof failure on small buildings; major erosion; flooding well inland	Hugo, 1989
5	156+ miles/h 250+ km/h	Catastrophic	Roof failure on residences and industrial buildings; building failures possible; flooding on shoreline structures	Andrew, 1992

Adapted from National Weather Service National Hurricane Center. The Saffir-Simpson Hurricane Scale Available at: www.nhc.noaa.gov/aboutsshs.shtml.

the storm. Cellular systems will go down as repeater cells are destroyed. The same is true for handheld radios beyond the line of sight as their repeaters are damaged. Amateur radio operators may serve as a valuable source of redundant communication.

Deaths during the storm will occur due to multiple causes. The largest cause of death in flat areas is flooding. Oftentimes, these deaths involve the drowning of persons trapped in vehicles. In areas with hills, landslides may be the most prominent cause of death. Drownings from swimming, boating, or surfing in storm waters do occur, despite warnings to the contrary. Deaths that can occur poststorm may be indirectly due to power outages because people are electrocuted when power lines are reenergized, and, from the use of candles, which can lead to house fires. Equally frustrating are deaths related to carbon monoxide, resulting from the use of generators or charcoal stoves/grills without proper ventilation.[1,2]

POST-INCIDENT ACTIONS

A rapid needs assessment for the hospital and the community should be performed. Repairs required for maintaining hospital operations should be done. Durable and expendable medical equipment destroyed or damaged during the storm should be noted, and replacement equipment should be ordered. Typically, power will be out, so consideration should be made for patients with medications that require refrigeration. Poststorm morbidity in the community is associated with disruption in the infrastructure and attempts to restore normal function. Those with chronic medical problems or patients who require regular routine medical procedures such as dialysis may experience an exacerbation due to the stresses of the uncontrolled environment and/or loss of medications and durable medical equipment. Injuries occur during cleanup of storm damage and may include lacerations, concussions, and plantar puncture wounds. Illnesses are associated with lack of safe water sources or proper food handling and the inability to dispose of waste. In developing countries, cholera and other diarrheal diseases often occur. Finally, anxiety and posttraumatic stress can occur among survivors.[3,4]

MEDICAL TREATMENT OF CASUALTIES

There may be a greater likelihood to admit patients who are unable to take care of themselves at home until the community's infrastructure has been reestablished. Additional resources such as sheltering may be present to alleviate nonmedical hospital admissions.

There also is a tendency to use antibiotic wound prophylaxis and to administer early updates of tetanus poststorm because of the increased concern over wound contamination and the inability to properly clean the wound. It may be more appropriate to use delayed primary closure.[5]

It may be difficult to obtain ancillary or laboratory studies in a hospital that is stressed by a surge in patients or damaged radiology or laboratory spaces. Consideration for prioritizing studies may be necessary in these situations.

Foodborne and waterborne diseases are possible, even in developed countries. Most of these are spread through fecal-oral contamination. Public health actions may prevent an outbreak. Notices to boil or chlorinate water should be posted. Both depression and posttraumatic stress disorder (PTSD) are common after large storms. Mental health effects after a disaster such as a major hurricane may vary across the exposed population.[6] In one survey after Hurricane Andrew, the incidences of depression and PTSD among survivors were 36% and 30%, respectively. Although there is significant debate over which methods are most effective in minimizing the psychological sequelae of a disaster, cognitive therapy and supportive psychotherapy may be useful, along with short-term use of antianxiety and sleep medications. Recognition that health care providers could be part of the disaster and may need intervention is also important in maintaining a functional disaster response.[6-8]

UNIQUE CONSIDERATIONS

Medical facilities of any sort in at-risk areas need to take preparedness actions before being impacted by tropical weather systems. Pre-Event activities range from staff education to facility infrastructure preparations. A well-prepared and rehearsed disaster plan is essential for medical facilities. This plan should include specific guidelines regarding operations before, during, and after the storm.

PITFALLS

- *Failure to perform preplanning:* Many communities and governmental agencies fail to adequately prepare for hurricanes. Leadership, both governmental and private sector, must appreciate the substantial impact that a tropical weather system may have. Planning for excessive demands upon many systems is essential. Education of citizens at an early age is essential.

- *Failure to evacuate:* This can lead to significant loss of life. Additionally, excessive demands will be placed upon first responders and first receivers. Medical facilities that fail to develop and implement evacuation plans place patients at undue risk.
- *Failure to plan for the delivery of basic needs:* Many planners concentrate efforts on search, rescue, and response. Basic human needs will place excessive demand on systems, such as public health and medical and emergency management. The provision and delivery of basic needs, such as safe shelter, nutritious food, clean water, and effective sanitation, are essential. Establishing long-term shelters for people moved great distances from their homes must be part of the planning process.[9]
- *Failure to plan for long-term effects:* Large tropical weather systems often have long-term effects on communities. Critical infrastructure can be heavily impacted. Critical infrastructure includes and is not limited to medical and public health resources. Specific areas within a medical system requiring significant preplanning efforts that include the provision of primary care across the spectrum of ages, emergency medical care, trauma care, and specialty medical services. These specialty services can include the provision of renal dialysis services, oxygen delivery, home-based care services, and hospice services.

REFERENCES

1. George-McDowell N, Landron F, Glenn J, et al. Deaths associated with Hurricanes Marilyn and Opal—United States, September-October 1995. *MMWR Morb Mortal Wkly Rep.* 1996;45(2):32–34.
2. Carmichael C, Neasman A, Rivera L, et al. Morbidity and mortality associated with Hurricane Floyd—North Carolina, September-October 1999. *MMWR Morb Mortal Wkly Rep.* 2000;49(17):369–372.
3. Hopkins RS. Comprehensive assessment of health needs 2 months after Hurricane Andrew—Dade County. *MMWR Morb Mortal Wkly Rep.* 1993;42(22):434–435.
4. Waring SC, desVignes-Kendrick M, Arafat RR, et al. Tropical Storm Allison rapid needs assessment—Houston, Texas, June 2001. *MMWR Morb Mortal Wkly Rep.* 2002;51(17):366–369.
5. Capellan O, Hollander JE. Management of lacerations in the emergency department. *Emerg Med Clin North Am.* 2003;21(1):205–231.
6. Nates JL. Combined external and internal hospital disaster: impact and response in a Houston trauma intensive care unit. *Crit Care Med.* 2004;32(3):686–690.
7. Garakani A. General disaster psychiatry. *Psychiatr Clin North Am.* 2004;27(3):391.
8. Raphael B. Debriefing: its evolution and current status. *Psychiatr Clin North Am.* 2004;27(3):407.
9. Redlener E, Reilly M. Lessons from Sandy—Preparing Health Systems for Future Disasters. *N Engl J Med.* 2012;367:2269–2271.

Earthquake

Khaldoon H. AlKhaldi

DESCRIPTION OF EVENT

Earthquakes are among the most devastating natural disasters. In many regions of the United States imperceptible earthquakes occur frequently. Historically, massive earthquakes have led to some of the most devastating loss of life, limb, and physical infrastructure and have had an overwhelming economic impact on affected communities. When earthquakes occur in oceans or seas they have the potential to cause a large displacement of water, which may trigger a series of giant waves known as a *tsunami*. Every year there are approximately 500,000 earthquakes worldwide, of which only approximately 20% are perceptible.[1] The potential for disaster exists when an earthquake or subsequent tsunami occurs in a heavily populated area. Although earthquake magnitude plays an important role in the resulting damage, it is not the only factor. The 2010 Haiti Earthquake measured 7.0 on the Richter scale and caused more than 200,000 deaths and thousands of injuries. The 2011 Japan Earthquake measured 9.0 on the Richter scale and caused a tsunami which together caused more than 12,000 deaths and displaced tens of thousands more.

There are critical factors at play other than just magnitude, such as earthquake depth, proximity of the epicenter to population centers, and construction and building codes.[2] The exact mechanism of an earthquake is still largely unknown, but there is the "elastic-rebound theory," which describes the process that creates the energy release of the earthquake. According to this theory, the tectonic plates of the Earth's crust are in constant motion and slip along each other tangentially. At the boundary between plates, called *faults*, friction causes the plates to adhere to each other, while the natural movement of the plates creates strain on this interlocked area. The plates then suddenly and violently move laterally with respect to each other, releasing the potential energy stored at the interface, known as an *earthquake hypocenter*. This is the place from which the seismic waves are generated that radiate out in all directions. The epicenter of the earthquake is the location on the Earth's surface directly above the underground hypocenter.

There are two commonly used scales to describe the strength of an earthquake: the Richter scale and the moment magnitude scale (MMS). Both scales range from 0 to 10 and are logarithmic.[1] Earthquakes with magnitudes 6.0 or greater are generally considered significant events and have the potential to cause widespread damage. Geographically the Asian Pacific Rim (from Japan to Indonesia), also known as the Ring of Fire, is the most seismically active area in the world.

PRE-INCIDENT ACTIONS

Pre-incident actions in earthquake-prone regions fall into two categories. The first focuses on structural preparations and engineering and design issues intended to strengthen and improve buildings to decrease the likelihood of massive destruction in the face of an earthquake event.

These engineering decisions may also focus on the positioning, strengthening, and layout of utility pipes, roadways, and power plants and the relative proximity of potentially dangerous structures, such as factories producing or storing toxic materials and fuel storage facilities, to fault lines and potential earthquake epicenters.

The second set of pre-incident actions for a country with populous regions and cities in the area of large earthquake faults is the development and implementation of a disaster response plan that should include training medical providers and stockpiling equipment to facilitate rapid action in the event of an earthquake.

Most earthquakes strike with little or no warning, and they can occur at any time. Despite constant monitoring of seismic and geologic activity, the ability to predict or detect a significant earthquake in time to mitigate its effects on the community is limited. Improvements in our ability to predict the timing and location of earthquakes, thereby mitigating their impact and preventing loss of life, are continuing and will hopefully play a bigger role in future preparedness. At this moment, however, educating the community, updating building codes, and improving land-use legislation remains the most viable way to mitigate the impact of earthquakes.

POST-INCIDENT ACTIONS

One of the most important concepts in disaster response today is that of command and control. There must be a central authority that oversees the disaster response and controls the overall operations, communications, logistics, requests for and distribution of resources, distribution of information, and allocation of search and rescue teams. Temporary health care facilities may need to be constructed and medical and surgical equipment, primary care and subspecialty health care physicians, and other health care workers allocated. This central authority is also responsible for the control, preparation, and distribution of other vital public health elements of the relief efforts, including sanitation, water, shelter, food, clothing, and psychosocial support. Large-scale international disaster responses are well intentioned and somewhat successful in providing lifesaving interventions; nevertheless, they are often inefficient, disorganized, and resource intensive. One problem that responders sometimes encounter is that many of the teams from different countries do not share a common language or system in their approach to the response. They may have different equipment and drugs that cannot be shared across systems and are often unknown to health care practitioners in the host country. This lack of coordination can lead to extensive duplication of some services and the lack of other services completely. Disaster responders from different countries are sometimes reluctant to submit to a central command and control or Incident Command System that is being directed by administrative personnel from a country other than their own. Following the response period a new stage called the *resilience period* has been recognized, which builds the capacity of a system to absorb future events and maintain civil functions and minimize loss of life and property. This stage takes a long time between onset of the disaster and something close to full recovery.

✚ MEDICAL TREATMENT OF CASUALTIES

Demand for health care is greatest in the period immediately after the earthquake, with studies showing peaks between 12 hours and 3 days after the event. There are two studies from Japan and Taiwan suggesting that serious injuries are most common among the very young and elderly.[3,4] Those studies also suggest that people with preexisting disabilities are at high risk for injury, due to their inability to quickly flee the collapsing structures or to free themselves effectively. Another study following the Taiwan earthquake indicates that casualties are higher in areas close to the earthquake epicenter with fewer physicians and hospitals.[3] If local hospitals are still operational after an earthquake, emergency departments are likely to have a surge of patients within the first 24 to 48 hours after the event. Data from the 1999 Marmara, Turkey, Earthquake found that 645 patients were seen at area hospitals for earthquake-related trauma in the 50 days following the disaster, and a total of 271 (42%) were seen in the first 24 hours.[5]

Care for casualties in the immediate aftermath of an earthquake is typically focused on orthopedic and soft tissue trauma, including management of fractures. Due to the prevalence of head injuries requiring surgical procedures, surgeons and anesthesiologists are important components of the early medical response. In addition, deep sedation and pain management with narcotic medication are important in treating earthquake injuries.

In the Armenian Earthquake of 1988 the acute injuries, as clearly witnessed in the cities of northern Armenia, were caused by collapsing buildings, falling rubble, fire, and dust inhalation. Most people caught in collapsing buildings due to earthquakes, especially structures greater than two stories, are killed instantly or trapped in pockets. Some of those trapped have body parts pinned under extremely heavy loads, timbers, or stone. Even when rescued, they will often have crush syndrome and acute renal failure. Others are caught up in the flash fires that accompany the rupture of natural gas pipes and suffer extensive body burns or smoke inhalation, leading to severe morbidity and mortality. A third group of patients suffers acute and chronic respiratory disease from the inhalation of the large amount of particulate matter that is aerosolized by the collapse of concrete and stone buildings and mixed with smoke from the generalized fires throughout a region. Depending on climatic conditions, hypothermia can also be a consideration.

The cities affected by the earthquake in Armenia were located in a mountainous, snowy region; the earthquake occurred in winter. Five hundred thousand people were homeless, and of those, many had minor to moderate orthopedic and soft tissue injuries. One of the unique acute medical problems associated with earthquakes is crush syndrome. In some ways the timing of the Armenian earthquake was quite fortuitous, considering the large incidence of crush syndrome and secondary renal failure. The American Society of Nephrology was having its annual meeting December 11, 1988. The official Soviet request for dialysis was made to the nephrologists at that meeting, and the international nephrology community responded.[6] Hospitals in Yerevan had 10 antiquated dialysis machines. The system was overwhelmed by the almost 400 patients with acute renal failure from crush syndrome who were extricated from the rubble of the earthquake. Approximately 150 of these patients were flown to Moscow for dialysis treatment. Many others were treated by machinery sent by the international nephrology community rendering humanitarian assistance in response to the earthquake.[7] This acute response also had positive

long-term outcomes for Armenia, in that an extensive sustainable dialysis program was set up in the postearthquake days that continues to exist today.[8,9]

Subacute injuries and medical illnesses after the impact of an earthquake often include those that patients sustain while attempting to rescue other victims trapped in the rubble. These injuries are quite common because many of the buildings in a zone devastated by an earthquake are rendered structurally unstable and are subject to further collapse if people attempt to enter them to perform hand excavation and rescue; aftershocks are common. There are also many new hazards created by the collapse of building structures and the rupture of underground utility pipes and underground or aboveground electric wires. These secondary injuries are less severe than those sustained during the earthquake; nevertheless, they require appropriate intervention if patients are to heal properly without infection and long-term disability. Illness in the subacute phase includes exacerbation of chronic medical problems no longer being treated with appropriate medications or equipment destroyed during the disaster. These illnesses may include diabetes, hypertension, coronary artery disease, and pulmonary disease. Asthma and chronic obstructive pulmonary disease often flare in response to deteriorating air quality and the rapid spread of acute respiratory illness through a population weakened by compromised nutrition, sleep deprivation, lack of clothing, housing, and food, and stress. Smoke from fires caused directly by the disaster as well as smoke from open fires used for cooking and keeping warm exacerbate these problems. Other infectious disease entities of concern include gastroenteritis from the consumption of spoiled food when refrigeration is not available and contaminated water from ruptured water mains and surface water contaminated by toxins and fecal run-off.

Chronic medical problems are seen in the weeks and months of the postimpact phase of an earthquake and include the ramifications of chronic disease entities untreated or partially treated during that time and the infectious complications of a population displaced into temporary and congested housing lacking proper food, clothing, and shelter. In addition, disruption of the social milieu may lead to psychiatric illness, including posttraumatic stress disorder (PTSD) and depression. PTSD and depression may persist for months to years after the impact.[9,10] In fact treatment for these problems both in children and adults has been ongoing for years after the Armenian earthquake.[11,12]

❓ UNIQUE CONSIDERATIONS

There are several considerations that are unique to the disaster medical response to an earthquake.

1. A small but salvageable number of persons are often trapped by falling building debris in an earthquake. Rapid deployment of appropriately trained search and rescue teams with dogs and high-tech listening devices is necessary to locate and save these people. Search and rescue equipment was very limited initially in response to the Armenian earthquake. It was on scene after considerable delay during the rescue effort. Consequently most people trapped in the rubble in Gyumri and Spitak died.

2. The most common injuries in an earthquake are traumatic injuries to the head and body, including closed head injury and orthopedic injuries. Disaster medical response teams must be prepared to handle these neurosurgical, orthopedic, and soft tissue injuries to provide appropriate medical treatment to casualties. Crush syndrome is more common in earthquakes than in any other disaster. The response team should have appropriate intravenous solutions and the equipment and skills to evaluate tissue compartment syndromes, perform fasciectomies, and treat crush syndrome. Laboratory capacity is necessary to monitor renal function and provide dialysis, if necessary.

3. Other injuries commonly seen in earthquakes, especially in urban areas, are burns, inhalation injuries from smoke, and exacerbation of chronic or subacute respiratory illness, including asthma from the inhalation of dust, smoke, and debris. Disaster medical response teams must be prepared to treat patients with these problems.

4. Earthquakes massively destroy infrastructure, rendering hospitals and medical clinics inoperable and unusable. Basic utilities are also usually devastated, including gas lines, water mains, sewage facilities, and electrical power plants. The disaster response team must be prepared to provide these basic services, including water, shelter, and energy as well as temporary equipped medical facilities. Even if hospitals and clinics remain standing after an earthquake, they may be structurally unusable and extremely dangerous to enter.

5. The earthquake site is quite dangerous for rescue workers. Building debris, loose wires, and leaking gas, water, and sewage are common. Rescue workers entering buildings to perform search and rescue operations or to unearth buried casualties are often putting themselves at risk if the buildings are structurally unstable. Aftershocks are common after the initial impact of an earthquake and can trigger the collapse of structures that remain standing.

6. The sheltering system also has an effect on the health outcome of the affected population. People who are living in temporary shelters were almost 1.7 times as likely to seek care as those living in permanent shelters.[13] The Haiti Earthquake in 2010 serves as yet another illustration of the need for more permanent sheltering options.[14] Living in temporary shelter and separation from family members prolong full recovery. These data emphasize the need for psychological first aid and other mental health interventions as part of effective earthquake response.[14,15]

⚠ PITFALLS

- Not implementing search and rescue operations early. Search and rescue personnel with heavy earth-moving equipment can be very effective if mobilized in a timely fashion and are available proximate to the impact of the earthquake. These operations have discovered and unearthed survivors trapped in the rubble; however, this part of the disaster response is very cost-intensive, and generally the number of victims saved is small relative to the total number of casualties that requires intensive short- and long-term medical care.[16]

- Identification and treatment of crush syndrome. Crush syndrome is common in patients pinned under small or large amounts of debris and trapped for extensive periods, leading to necrosis of the pinned extremities. Rescue workers should be fully educated and carry protocols on how to respond properly to patients who potentially have crush syndrome and incipient renal failure. The response team needs to have access to dialysis and nephrology consultation.

- Even though major orthopedic injuries, crush syndrome, hemodialysis, and other major medical subspecialty interventions are interesting and often grab media attention, the most important part of the medical response to earthquakes is couched within public health and primary health care. The major issue facing most survivors of an earthquake is the restoration of infrastructure, including water, shelter, food, sanitation, and basic medical facilities with primary health care services. Any relief effort that ignores these issues will only have a short and expensive impact for a small number of patients without any sustained impact on the short-, medium-, or long-term health of the affected population.[17,18]

- Early attention to anxiety and psychological stress imposed by the disaster can ameliorate the long-term disability and impaired functional capacity associated with PTSD, chronic anxiety, and depression on the population. Disaster medical response teams must engage psychologists and psychiatrists to participate actively from the very beginning of the response.[19]

- Although human nature calls for an immediate active *intervention*, the best disaster medical response to an earthquake demands a rapid and immediate *assessment* with communication of information back to planning entities removed from the disaster site so that appropriate allocations of equipment, medicines, medical personnel, search and rescue teams, and other resources can be made.

- Disaster systems concepts, such as an Incident Command System and Command and Control, must be imposed on any disaster response to avoid ineffective and inefficient interventions resulting in duplication, waste, miscommunication, and unnecessary further loss of life.

REFERENCES

1. US geological Survey (USGS). Earthquake Facts. Available at: http://earthquake.usgs.gov/learn/facts.php.
2. Rosenberg M. Haiti death toll could reach 300,000: Preval. *Reuters.* February 22, 2010.
3. Liang N-J, Shih Y-T, Shih F-Y, et al. Disaster epidemiology and medical response in Chi-Chi earthquake in Taiwan. *Ann Emerg Med.* 2001;38:549–555.
4. Osaki Y, Minowa M. Factors associated with earthquake deaths in the great Hanshin-Awaji Earthquake. *Am J Epidemiol.* 1995;153:153–156.
5. Bulut M. Medical experience of a university hospital in Turkey after the 1999 Marmara Earthquake. *Emerg Med J.* 2005;22:494–498.
6. Eknoyan G. The Armenian earthquake of 1988: a milestone in the evolution of nephrology advances in renal replacement and therapy. *Adv Ren Replace Ther.* 2003;10(2):87–92.
7. Tattersall JE, Richards NT, McCann M, Mathias T, Samson A, Johnson A. Acute hemodialysis during the Armenian earthquake disaster. *Injury.* 1990;21(1):25–28.
8. Eknoyan G. Acute renal failure in the Armenian earthquake. *Ren Fail.* 1992;14(3):241–244.
9. Irvine J, Buttimore A, Eastwood D, Kendrick-Jones J. The Christchurch earthquake: dialysis experience and emergency planning. *Nephrology (Carlton).* 2014;19(5):296–303.
10. Kako M, Arbon P, Mitani S. Disaster health after the 2011 great East Japan earthquake. *Prehosp Disaster Med.* 2014;29(1):54–59.
11. Haga N, Hata J, Yabe M, et al. The Great East Japan Earthquake affected the laboratory findings of hemodialysis patients in Fukushima. *BMC Nephrol.* 2013;14:239.
12. Goenjian AK, Karayan I, Pynoos RS, et al. Outcome of psychotherapy among early adolescents after trauma. *Am J Psychiatry.* 1997;154 (4):536–542.
13. Goenjian AK, Yehuda R, Steinberg AM, et al. Basal cortisol, dexamethasone, suppression of cortisol, and MHPG in adolescents after the 1988 earthquake. *Am J Psychiatry.* 1996;153(7):929–934.
14. Goenjian AK, Pynoos RS, Steinberg AM, et al. Psychiatric co-morbidities in children after the 1988 earthquake in Armenia. *J Am Acad Child Adolesc Psychiatry.* 1995;34(9):1174–1184.
15. Goenjian AK, Najarian LM, Pynoos RS, et al. Post-traumatic stress reactions after single and double trauma. *Acta Psychiatr Scand.* 1994;90(3):214–221.
16. Guha-Sapir D, van Panhuis WG, Lagoutte J. Short communication: patterns of chronic and acute diseases after natural disasters—a study from the International Committee of the Red Cross field hospital in Banda Aceh after the 2004 Indian tsunami. *Trop Med Int Health.* 2007;12:1338–1341.
17. Broach J, McNamara M, Harrison K. Ambulatory care by disaster responders in the tent camps of Port-au-Prince Haiti, January 2010. *Disaster Med Public Health Prep.* 2010;4:16–121.
18. Autier P, Ferir MC, Hairapetien A, et al. Drug supply in the aftermath of the 1988 Armenian earthquake. *Lancet.* 1998;335(8702):1388–1390.
19. Goenjian AK. A mental health relief programme in Armenia after the 1988 earthquake: implementation and clinical observations. *Br J Psychiatry.* 1993;163:230–239.

CHAPTER 96

Tornado

Charles Stewart, M. Kathleen Stewart, Michael D. Jones, and James Pfaff

DESCRIPTION OF EVENT

The American Meteorological Society defines a tornado as "a violently rotating column of air, in contact with the ground, either pendant from a cumuliform cloud or underneath a cumuliform cloud, and often (but not always) visible as a funnel cloud."[1] A tornado is not necessarily visible, but the intense low pressure caused by the high wind speeds and rapid rotation will usually cause the water vapor in the air to condense into a visible funnel-shaped cloud.

The damage from a tornado is a result of both the high wind velocity and wind-blown debris. Tornados can touch the ground with winds greater than 300 miles per hour (mph).[2] Even though winds from the strongest tornados far exceed that from the strongest hurricanes, the latter typically cause much more damage individually and over a season and over far bigger areas. Hurricanes tend to cause much more overall destruction than tornados because of their much larger size, longer duration, and their greater variety of ways to damage property. The destructive core in hurricanes can be tens of miles across, last many hours, and damage structures through storm surge- and rainfall-caused flooding, as well as from wind. Tornados, in contrast, tend to be a few hundred yards in diameter, last for minutes to hours, and primarily cause damage from their extreme winds.[3,4]

The United States averages approximately 1000 tornados per year. "A distant second is Canada, with around 100 per year. Other locations that experience frequent tornado occurrences include northern Europe, western Asia, Bangladesh, South Africa, far eastern Asia and Japan, Argentina, Paraguay and Southern Brazil, Australia and New Zealand. In fact, the United Kingdom has the most tornadoes per land area with an average of about 30 per year. Fortunately, most U.K. tornadoes are relatively weak."[5]

Tornado damage was previously measured on the Fujita Scale or Fujita-Pearson Tornado Scale (F-Scale) until the National Weather Service (NWS) adopted the use of the Enhanced Fujita Scale (EF-Scale) on February 1, 2007.[3] The F-Scale is named after the most noted researcher of tornados, Dr. Fujita of the University of Chicago. The scale ranges from F0 (very weak) to F12 (at wind speed of Mach 1, an unimaginable force). The strongest tornados observed to date have been F5 (261 to 318 mph).[6] An update to the original F-Scale by a team of meteorologists and engineers was implemented in the United States on February 1, 2007.[3] The EF-Scale is based on 28 damage indicators and is considered more replicable and accurate than the F-Scale. Because no storms greater than F-5 have been recorded, the enhanced F-Scale stops at EF-5.[7] The F-Scale and EF-Scale are shown in Table 96-1.

Conditions favorable for tornado development often occur over the central U.S. Plains during spring and summer. As the season goes on, tornados are likely farther and farther north on the Plains and in the Midwest, but in April and May tornados are common in both the South and on the Plains and in the Midwest.[8] Often a large storm system can create tornado conditions for several days in a row.[9]

Tornados are most common in spring and least common in winter.[8] Because autumn and spring are transitional periods from warm to cool and vice versa, there are abundant chances of cooler air meeting warmer moist air, creating thunderstorms and increased risk of tornados.[8,9]

In the United States and Canada, warning of a tornado is given in two phases[3]:

A Tornado Watch is a message that indicates that the conditions are favorable for formation of a tornado. Because tornados are spawned from severe thunderstorms a tornado watch therefore implies that it is also a Severe Thunderstorm Watch.[3] The watch boxes (or weather watches, WWs) are usually issued in the format of *x* miles north and south, or east and west, or either side of a line from *y* miles *direction* of *city, state,* to *z* miles *another direction* of *another city, state.* For example, "THE TORNADO WATCH AREA IS APPROXIMATELY ALONG AND 110 STATUTE MILES NORTH AND SOUTH OF A LINE FROM 45 MILES NORTHWEST OF BARTLESVILLE OKLAHOMA TO 50 MILES NORTHEAST OF HARRISON ARKANSAS."[10] ("Either side" means perpendicular to the center line.) In addition, a list of all counties included in its area of responsibility is now issued by each NWS forecast office for each watch (Fig. 96-1).[11,12]

When severe hail (at least 0.75-inch diameter) or damaging winds (at least 50 knots or 58 mph) appear imminent, local NWS offices will issue a Severe Thunderstorm Warning. The warning is rapidly disseminated over National Oceanographic and Atmospheric Administration (NOAA) weather radio, commercial radio, and television (TV) stations and news wires, so that people in the warning area can find safe shelter to take cover from the storm.[12]

If SKYWARN watchers sight a tornado or the Doppler radar picture shows the characteristic "hook" of a tornado (threshold strong with a tight rotation signature), then a Tornado Warning is issued. A tornado warning means there is immediate danger for the warned and the immediately surrounding area (because the path may not be completely predictable), if not from the relatively narrow tornado itself, then from the severe thunderstorm. All in the path of such a storm are urged to take cover immediately because it is a life-threatening situation. A tornado warning will also be issued if a tropical cyclone is making landfall with winds in excess of 115 mph (185 kph). When a tropical cyclone makes landfall both the extreme wind and the likelihood of accompanying tornados can cause damage.[12]

In the event that the conditions that lead to a tornado watch are likely to form a major outbreak of tornados along with the thunderstorm's destructive winds and hail, the tornado or thunderstorm watch may be enhanced with the words "particularly dangerous situation" (PDS) added to the watch.[12]

TABLE 96-1   Enhanced Fujita Scale for Tornado Damage*,†

| F NUMBER | FUJITA SCALE | | COMMENTS | DERIVED ENHANCED FUJITA SCALE | | OPERATIONAL ENHANCED FUJITA SCALE | |
	FASTEST 0.25-MILE KPH (MPH)	3-SECOND GUST (MPH)		EF NUMBER	3-SECOND GUST (MPH)	EF NUMBER	3-SECOND GUST (MPH)
0 Weak	65-118 (40-73)	45-78	Damage is light. Chimneys on houses may be damaged; trees have broken branches; shallow-rooted trees pushed over; some windows broken; damage to sign boards.	0	65-85	0	65-85
1 Weak	119-181 (74-112)	79-117	Shingles on roofs blown off; mobile homes pushed off foundations or overturned; moving cars pushed off roads.	1	86-109	1	86-110
2 Strong	182-253 (113-157)	118-161	Considerable damage. Roofs torn off houses; mobile homes destroyed; train boxcars pushed over; large trees snapped or uprooted; light objects thrown like missiles.	2	110-137	2	111-135
3 Strong	254-332 (158-206)	162-209	Damage is severe. Roofs and walls torn off better constructed homes, businesses, and schools; trains overturned; most trees uprooted; heavy cars lifted off ground and thrown some distance.	3	138-167	3	136-165
4 Violent	333-419 (207-260)	210-261	Better constructed homes completely leveled; structures with weak foundation blown off some distance.	4	168-199	4	166-200
5 Violent	420-513 (261-318)	262-317	Better constructed homes lifted off foundations and carried considerable distances where they disintegrate; trees debarked; cars thrown in excess of 100 meters.	5	200-234	5	>200
6 Unimaginably Violent	Although F6 and above are theoretically possible in the Enhanced Fujita Scale, they are not used.			N/A—The Enhanced Fujita Scale does not provide for greater than F5		N/A	

*An update to the original F-Scale by a team of meteorologists and wind engineers was implemented in the United States on February 1, 2007.
†**Important note about Enhanced Fujita Scale winds**: The Enhanced Fujita Scale still is a set of wind estimates (not measurements) based on damage. It uses 3-second gusts estimated at the point of damage based on a judgment of eight levels of damage to the 28 indicators listed below. These estimates vary with height and exposure. **Important**: The 3-second gust is not the same wind as in standard surface observations. Standard measurements are taken by weather stations in open exposures, using a directly measured, "1 minute mile" speed.

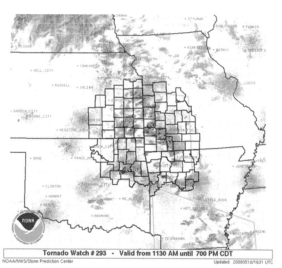

Tornado Watch # 293 · Valid from 1130 AM until 700 PM CDT
NOAA/NWS/Storm Prediction Center   Updated: 20080510/1631 UTC

FIG 96-1 Map of Tornado Watch #293 for May 10, 2008.[10]

PRE-INCIDENT ACTIONS

The issuing of appropriate warnings and the need for the population to take appropriate action on the basis of those warnings are the most important factors in preventing tornado-related death and injury.[13-19] In the United States the NWS has acquired sophisticated instrumentation, such as Doppler radar, which permits them to identify conditions conducive to the formation of a tornado and to issue warnings.[3] A tornado watch means that conditions are conducive to tornado formation in a given area, and a tornado warning means that a tornado has been sighted in a given area and those residing in that area should take appropriate shelter, which entails going to the basement if one exists, going to an inside room or closet, or if outside going to a ditch or gully.[12] See Box 96-1 for detailed shelter advice.

Communication
Command and Control

Designate a clear command and control structure involving police, fire, emergency medical service (EMS), and local hospital emergency rooms with capability for these entities to communicate on radio devices that do not depend on the local power grid for functionality. Remember that the winds of the tornado and associated thunderstorm can also destroy

BOX 96-1 Sheltering Guidelines in Case of Tornado Warning

In General
- Stay away from windows.
- When a warning is issued, move to the safest area immediately.
- If you have access to a motorcycle, bicycle, or climbing helmet, in all cases, put it on. Get under a sturdy piece of furniture and cover yourself with a blanket, pillows, or mattress.

IF YOU ARE	YOU SHOULD
Outside	Get inside a building. If stuck outside, stay away from cars and trees. Lie down in a ditch or culvert and cover your head and neck with your hands. If you have a motorcycle, bicycle, or climbing helmet, wear it.
In a mobile home	Leave the mobile home. Go to a community home shelter. If no shelter is available, see "Outside" above.
In a car	Move the car off the road. Leave the vehicle. Do not seek shelter under an overpass. If stuck outside, see above.
At work or school	Go to the designated interior room or hallway away from windows, and get under a sturdy piece of furniture.
In a house	Go to the basement. If there is no basement, go to an interior room or hallway away from windows, get under a sturdy piece of furniture, and cover yourself with a blanket. Get into an interior bathroom, and get in the tub as an appropriate alternative.

cell towers and antennae for emergency services. Communications in the local area may require supplemental, portable base stations and repeaters to be rapidly emplaced to replace those destroyed by the tornado.

Warning Systems

Ensure that all emergency services have real-time access to Internet data for weather updates and warnings of the actual path taken by the storm. Moving EMS, police, and fire vehicles out of base stations and out of the projected and actual path of the storm is significantly more fruitful than relying on mutual aid, Memorandums of Understanding (MOUs), and insurance to cover for damaged or destroyed vehicles. It is not uncommon for multiple tornados to touch down in a region over a period of several hours. The emergency response teams and emergency departments should have access to Internet-capable computers with uninteruptable power supplies and should constantly monitor the storm. Heavy flooding and/or hail, road damage, and debris on highways may alter the emergency response as well.

Make certain all public buildings, trailer home parks, nursing homes, and all hospitals also have 24-hour/7-days-a-week access to local weather reports and a method for receiving the same severe weather-warning information. Active warning systems (weather alert sirens, weather alert radios, and loudspeakers) appear to be more effective than passive warning systems (conventional radio and TV).[20]

Injury Prevention
Focused Education

Public health education regarding tornado warning systems and safe sheltering during tornados should be provided to the populations most at risk. These include the following:

1. People in mobile homes
2. The elderly, very young, and physically or mentally impaired
3. People who may not understand the warnings because of a language barrier[21]

Sheltering Guidelines

The Federal Emergency Management Agency (FEMA), Centers for Disease Control and Prevention (CDC), and NWS have published guidelines detailing the safest sheltering actions to take in case of a tornado warning. These are summarized in Box 96-1.

Health Care Provider Training

One of the most important things that responsible administration can do in a tornado-prone area is to ensure that the health care providers know, understand, and have been trained on how to protect themselves and their patients during the onslaught of these violent storms. Rapid action drills should be conducted routinely at day, evening, and night shifts. The staff should be provided with tools and equipment to rapidly evacuate patients from high-rise hospitals with the assumption that the power has been destroyed and backup system is inoperable. The staff must practice this difficult task so that all know their duties during the storm and after the storm has passed. The devastating, nearly 1-mile-wide, category EF-5 tornado that struck Joplin, Missouri, in 2011 resulted in exactly this scenario when it struck the St. John's Regional Medical Center, resulting in loss of all power and near-total destruction of the hospital.[22,23]

Emergency Medical Response

As seen in the Joplin EF-5 event, medical facilities are not immune from tornado damage.[22,23] Hospitals should have plans for evacuation and sheltering of patients. Discharge of patients may not be an option if the patient would be discharged to a destroyed or damaged home or during the active storm.

An organized trauma system with a centralized communication system has been shown to be highly effective and efficient in ensuring that the sickest patients go to the most appropriate facilities following a tornado disaster.[18] Even with such a system in place a significant minority of patients will require transfer from community hospitals to higher-level trauma centers. Hospitals must be ready to assimilate patients from damaged areas and possibly transfers from nearby damaged hospitals. Agreements for such transfers should be worked out before a mass casualty incident occurs.

Traffic Control at Hospitals

Traffic control has consistently been reported as a problem in and around emergency departments following a tornado disaster. Disaster plans should include directions for hospital security or local police to secure the access and egress routes from local hospitals. These agencies should understand where to direct the walking wounded, privately owned vehicles, and EMS vehicles for appropriate triage and evaluation.[24,25] Ensure contingency plans have been developed for damage to and/or around the hospital and surrounding community.

POST-INCIDENT ACTIONS
Search and Rescue

Reports of tornado disasters—including the 1970 tornado in Lubbock, Texas, and the 1996 tornado in Topeka, Kansas—support the intuitive idea that the most severely injured victims and the majority of those killed will be found in the core area of the tornado strike.[26] Flying debris from tornados causes most deaths and injuries.[27] Severely injured victims are likely to be thrown by the tornado, struck by flying debris, or found in buildings with the greatest structural damage. These victims may be found in the open or buried under rubble. Impact-related injury or death is defined as an injury or death that is caused by the direct mechanical effects of the tornado. Most mortalities and injuries occur during the impact phase of tornado, but some will happen during cleanup and remediation.[27]

Tornados may shear buildings from foundations with rupture of power lines and natural gas piping. Electrical connections may or may not remain energized. The combination of wet areas, leaking natural gas, and potential electric spark is exceedingly dangerous. Containers of toxic substances can be ruptured and spread across wide areas. Search-and-rescue teams and first responders should protect themselves from hazards, such as downed power lines, gas leaks, and potentially unstable building structures. Sharp debris is quite common and can lacerate feet, hands, and other exposed body parts.

Emergency Medical Service Triage

EMS units should be deployed carefully along the area of the tornado strike. Early responding units will likely become overwhelmed with casualties and must be supported by other units or aeromedical transport systems that can move the severely injured patients to the area hospitals and resupply the units in the field. Frequently EMS units will need to set up triage and collection points, with subsequent arriving units bringing supplies and taking patients to hospitals.

Casualty collection points should be set up using mobile EMS vehicles or public buildings, such as schools or churches. If possible these collection points should be selected to avoid radio blackout zones so that the medical command and control personnel can stay in close contact with the providers in the field to coordinate evacuation resources and resupply of essential equipment and medical materials. Extensive use of improvised patient transport from collection points to major hospitals has been common in large tornados.

Aeromedical transport is often relatively ineffective due to weather (particularly early and when multiple storms are present), inability to land close to the incident, and quite limited capacity to carry multiple patients. If aeromedical transport is to be used, personnel must be trained in selecting and marking safe landing zones for the helicopters. Assessment of foreign object debris (FOD) on the ground is essential. FOD is quite common following a tornado and could easily damage the helicopter's engine with subsequent crash and injury to both crew and patients. An aerial survey using fire, EMS, or police helicopters can greatly assist rescue efforts by defining the regions of greatest damage and guiding search teams to locations where the most injured patients are likely to be found. Such surveys may be hindered by severe weather still lingering in the region. Aeromedical helicopters can also aid ground EMS units with location of damage and assessing possible routes into an area cluttered with debris.

Hospital Triage

As in any mass casualty situation, it is imperative that open and precise communication channels are in place to allow triage personnel, emergency department physicians, and operating room personnel and surgeons to communicate as casualties arrive. Casualties following a tornado usually arrive in a bimodal fashion, with the least severely injured arriving first, usually within 5 to 30 minutes after the disaster. The severely wounded will arrive by EMS transport and by privately owned vehicles usually 1 to 4 hours after the tornado strike.[24,25] Plans should be designed to allocate appropriate resources to the least injured without overwhelming personnel and space that will be needed by critically injured patients.

Even if the hospital has been damaged, patients will continue to come to the hospital until word of the damage has been widely spread.

This may include ambulances from units responding to the disaster and unaware of damage to the hospital. The hospital must be prepared to accommodate these casualties.

Secondary Response

As noted earlier, tornados damage power lines and natural gas piping. Electrical connections may or may not remain energized and may be reenergized at any time. The combination of wet areas, leaking natural gas, and potential electric spark is exceedingly dangerous.

Likewise much debris has been strewn by high-speed winds over driveways, roadways, and access routes. This debris presents hazards to pedestrians and motor vehicles alike. Unsafe structures due to wind damage are quite common in the periphery of the tornado's path. Post-impact injuries are injuries or deaths that occur within 48 hours of the tornado that would not have occurred in the absence of the tornado. Examples include injuries sustained by walking through debris, during cleanup, or as a result of loss of electrical power.[28]

In addition to these hazards, cleanup activities can involve the usual risks of working with power tools, sharp debris, and potential toxic spills.[29] Cleanup workers should have appropriate familiarity with their tools, appropriate protective equipment, and sufficient crew rest and hydration to minimize worker injuries.

✚ MEDICAL TREATMENT OF CASUALTIES

Types of injuries that commonly occur due to a tornado[25,27,29,30]:
- Trauma to head, extremities, and thorax
- Fractures of long bones
- Severe lacerations and abrasions[29]
- Puncture wounds from high-speed projectiles

The leading cause of death is craniocerebral trauma, followed by crushing wounds of the head and trunk.[25,30] Crush injuries are common with building collapse. It is often impossible to determine if lethal injuries are due to high-velocity projectiles propelled by the wind or by collapse of the structures. Fractures are a frequent form of nonfatal injury.[25,30]

Wounds should be considered as highly contaminated, and prudence may dictate delayed primary closure. Wound infections caused by gram-negative bacteria, such as *Escherichia coli*, *Klebsiella*, *Serratia*, *Proteus*, and *Pseudomonas*, are common in wounds sustained during tornados.[31–34] Management of puncture wounds should include imaging or exploration (or both) to ensure that foreign bodies are removed.

❓ UNIQUE CONSIDERATIONS

Because a tornado is part of a severe thunderstorm and thunderstorms occur all over the Earth, tornados are not limited to any specific geographic location. In fact tornados have been documented in every state in the United States and on every continent, with the exception of Antarctica (even there, a tornado occurrence is not impossible). Wherever the atmospheric conditions are right the occurrence of a tornadic thunderstorm is possible. Then if other conditions are right, the thunderstorm could spin out one or more tornados.[5]

⚠ PITFALLS

- Road debris may prevent rapid deployment, response, and resupply.
  - Roads will be clogged with downed trees, power lines, light poles, and debris from destroyed buildings.
  - Tire punctures in EMS vehicles are common.
- Rescuers must have appropriate protective gear.
  - Helmets, gloves, and boots are mandatory for search and rescue.

- Power lines may automatically "reenergize" and should be considered as live till utility company has shut down regional power feed.
- Training is not optional.
  - Train for protection of patients.
  - Train for evacuation of patients.
  - Train for safety in the posttornado environment.
- Movement of response vehicles out of the storm's path can save these vehicles for actual responses.
  - This requires timely, continuous monitoring of the storm's path and a plan for movement at short notice.
- Soft tissue wounds from tornados should be considered highly contaminated, and
  - Delayed primary closure may be a prudent approach to wound management.
- Consider that puncture wounds still have a foreign body in place.
  - Debris may be propelled at over 200 mph.
  - X-ray or computed tomography (CT) is appropriate evaluation for these wounds.

REFERENCES

1. Glickman TS. *AMS Glossary of Meteorology*. 2nd ed. Allen Press, Boston, MA: AMS; 2000.
2. Wurman J. *DOW Measurements of Extreme Winds in Tornadoes and Hurricanes and Comparison with Damage*. University of Oklahoma, National Severe Storms Laboratory, and Pennsylvania State University; 2003.
3. Edwards R. *The Online Tornado FAQ*. NOAA; 2009.
4. Brooks HE, Doswell III CA. Normalized damage from major tornadoes in the United States: 1890-1999. *Weather Forecast*. 2001;16:168–176.
5. NOAA. *U.S. Tornado Climatology*; 2008. Available at: Accessed 30.09.09. http://www.ncdc.noaa.gov/oa/climate/severeweather/tornadoes.html.
6. Doswell III CA. *A Guide to F-Scale Damage Assessment*. US Department of Commerce, NWS: Silver Spring, MD; 2003.
7. NOAA. *The Enhanced Fujita Scale (EF Scale)*; 2009. Available at: Accessed 11.11.09. http://www.spc.noaa.gov/efscale/.
8. Concannon PR, Brooks HE, Doswell III CA. Climatological risk of strong and violent tornadoes in the United States. In: *Second Conference on Environmental Applications*; Long Beach, California: American Meteorological Society; 2000. 8-12 January 2000, Paper 9.4. found online at: http://www.nssl.noaa.gov/users/brooks/public_html/concannon/.
9. Hamill TM, Schneider RS, Brooks HE, et al. The May 2003 extended tornado outbreak. *Am Meteorol Soc BAMS*. April 2005;2005:531–542.
10. NWS. *Tornado watch number 293*. National Weather Service; 2008.
11. NOAA. *National weather service public & fire weather products*. National Weather Service; 2001.
12. NOAA. *National weather service glossary*; 2009.
13. Merrell D, Simmons KM, Sutter D. Taking shelter: estimating the benefits of tornado safe rooms. *Am Meteorol Soc*. 2001;619–625.
14. Brenner S, Noji E. *Risk Factors for Death and Injury in Tornadoes: An Epidemiologic Approach*. Washington, DC: American Geophysical Union; 1993.
15. Brenner S, Noji E. Tornado injuries related to housing in the Plainfield tornado. *Int J Epidemiol*. 1995;24:144–149.
16. Brenner SA, Noji E. Risk factors for death or injury in tornadoes: an epidemiological approach. In: Church C, Burgess D, Doswell C, Davies-Jone R, eds. *The Tornado; Its Structure, Dynamics, Prediction, and Hazards*. Washington, DC, American Geophysical Union: Wiley; 1993:543–544. Also available online at http://onlinelibrary.wiley.com/book/10.1029/GM079.
17. Duclos PJ, Ing RT. Injuries and risk factors for injuries from the 29 May 1982 tornado, Marion, Illinois. *Int J Epidemiol*. 1989;18(1):213–219.
18. May AK, McGwin GJ, Lancaster LJ, et al. The April 8, 1998 tornado: assessment of the trauma system response and the resulting injuries. *J Trauma*. 2000;48(4):666–672.
19. May OW, Bigham AB. After the storm: personal experiences following an EF4 tornado. *J Pediatr Nurs*. 2012;27(4):390–393.
20. Liu S, Quenemoen LE, Malilay J, Noji E, Sinks T, Mendlein J. Assessment of a severe-weather warning system and disaster preparedness, Calhoun County, Alabama, 1994. *Am J Public Health*. 1996;86(1):87–89.
21. Ahlborn L, Franc JM. Tornado hazard communication disparities among Spanish-speaking individuals in an English-speaking community. *Prehosp Disaster Med*. 2012;27(1):98–102.
22. Kikta KJ. 45 seconds: memoirs of an ER physician. When the deadly EF-5 tornado struck Joplin, May 22, 2011. *Mo Med*. 2011;108(3):150–154.
23. National Weather Service. *Joplin Tornado Survey*; 2011. Available at: Accessed 23.08.11. http://www.crh.noaa.gov/sgf/?n=event_2011may22_survey.
24. Hogan DE. Tornadoes. In: Hogan DE, Burstein JL, eds. *Disaster Medicine*. 2nd ed. Philadelphia, PA: Lippincott Williams & Wilkins; 2007:194–204.
25. Mandelbaum I, Nahrwold D, Boyer DW. Management of tornado casualties. *J Trauma*. 1966;6(3):353–361.
26. Bohonos JJ, Hogan DE. The medical impact of tornadoes in North America. *J Emerg Med*. 1999;17(1):67–73.
27. Brown SP, Archer P, Kruger E, Malonee S. Tornado-related deaths and injuries in Oklahoma due to the 3 May 1999 tornadoes. *Weather Forecast*. 2002;17(3):343–353.
28. CDC. Tornado disaster—Illinois. *MMWR Morb Mortal Wkly Rep*. 1991;40(2):33–36.
29. Kikta K, Lohmeir M. EP's on the ground in Joplin. *Emergency Physicians Monthly*; 2011. Available at: Accessed 13.07.11. http://www.epmonthly.com/features/current-features/eps-on-the-ground-in-joplin.
30. Hight D, Blodgett JT, Croce EJ, Horne EO, McKoan Jr JW, Whelan CS. Medical aspects of the Worcester tornado disaster. *N Engl J Med*. 1956;254(6):267–271.
31. Austin CL, Finley PJ, Mikkelson DR, Tibbs B. Mucormycosis: a rare fungal infection in Tornado victims. *J Burn Care Res*. 2014;35(3):e164–e171.
32. Brenner SA, Noji EK. Wound infections after tornadoes. *J Trauma*. 1992;33(4):643.
33. Gilbert DN, Sanford JP, Kutscher E, Sanders Jr CV, Luby JP, Barnett JA. Microbiologic study of wound infections in tornado casualties. *Arch Environ Health*. 1973;26(3):125–130.
34. Ivy JH. Infections encountered in tornado and automobile accident victims. *J Indiana State Med Assoc*. 1968;61(12):1657–1661.

97 CHAPTER

Flood

Ritu R. Sarin and Sylvia H. Kim

DESCRIPTION OF EVENT

Floods are the most common natural disasters. They cause greater mortality than any other natural disaster.[1] Worldwide, floods account for approximately 40% of natural disasters. In the United States, approximately 146 deaths are caused by floods each year, the majority associated with flash floods.[2] The National Oceanic and Atmospheric Administration (NOAA) estimates an average $8.2 billion in damages per year in the United States because of floods, not including damages from the storm surges of hurricanes.[3]

Floods continue to be the number one natural disaster in the United States in terms of lives lost and property damage. In 1889 more than 2200 deaths were due to flash flooding from a dam break in Johnstown, Pennsylvania. In 1976 a 19-foot wall of water near the Big Thompson River near Denver, Colorado, killed 140 people camping nearby.[4] More recently, in 2005, Hurricane Katrina resulted in 1833 deaths, with an associated $148 billion in total damages and costs. Current estimates of the effects of the 2012 "Superstorm" Sandy in the United States are 159 deaths and $65 billion in damages.[5] The 2010 monsoon floods in Pakistan resulted in 1985 deaths, with estimates of $9.5 billion in economic effects.[6]

Floods may be caused by an abundance of rainfall, melting snow, or the expanding development of wetlands, which reduces absorption of rainfall. Flash floods occur within 6 hours of a rain event, after a dam or levee fails, or after the sudden release of water from an ice or debris jam. Flash floods are the leading cause of natural disaster-related death.[7] Most communities in the United States can experience flooding. In fact, flash floods occur in all 50 states.[8] Communities at greatest risk are those in low-lying areas, near water, and located downstream from a dam.[4] In June 2008 the floods in Eastern Iowa resulted in 18 deaths and 106 injuries. The flooding occurred in known flood plains, resulting in the emergent evacuation of a hospital in Cedar Rapids, Iowa.[9]

PRE-INCIDENT ACTIONS

Hospitals should determine whether they are located in a flood-prone area. The National Weather Service issues flood watches and warnings, organized by state, and publishes these listings at www.nws.noaa.gov. These projections are based on precipitation and lake and river levels.[10] Flood watches are posted 12 to 36 hours before possible flooding events. Flood watches indicate that a hazardous event is occurring or will occur within 30 minutes.[7] A flood watch should be used for early evacuation planning.

Evacuation routes should be planned and practiced. For planning purposes, flood hazard maps are available from the Federal Emergency Management Agency at http://www.fema.gov/national-flood-insurance-program-flood-hazard-mapping. The usual routes of access to and from the hospital may be flooded; therefore alternative routes

should be planned. During intense flooding lasting multiple months in southern Africa in 2008, flooded roadways and downed bridges isolated patients from access to health care in Zambia, leaving them without access to acute and chronic care for months.[11] As with any natural disaster, transport times will likely increase, and hospital personnel should expect ambulance arrival without prior dispatch. There will be greater reliance on alternative means of transport, including aeromedical and marine units.[10]

An emergency communications system should be available. Communication lines among hospitals, prehospital staff, and patients may be affected by floods. Telephone lines, 911 dispatch lines, and emergency medical service communication with hospitals may be impaired. Create a plan for redundant communications capabilities, including two-way radios and dedicated channels, cell phones, and Internet connectivity.[12] An emergency communications system plan should be in place to request further staffing, services, or evacuation assistance. Awareness of social media resources should also be incorporated in community and hospital communications plans. Use of sources such as Twitter and Facebook has been utilized to support both information sharing from health agencies and reporting of health and rescue needs by victims during various disasters, including the Haiti Earthquake in 2010 and the 2009 flu pandemic in the United States. Reliable information on affected areas may be shared by local and state emergency management agencies as well as other health care partners and first responders.[13]

Floods are long-term events that may last days to weeks, or longer.[8] Therefore at least 72 hours of disaster supplies, including nonperishable food and water, should be available. Emergency kits should also include a portable battery-operated radio, flashlights, batteries, first aid kits, personal sanitation items, local maps, and a cell phone with charger or spare batteries, among other items. Further recommendations may be found online at www.ready.gov/kit.[4]

POST-INCIDENT ACTIONS

During a flood, battery-operated radios or televisions should be used. The NOAA Weather Radio broadcasts warnings from the National Weather Service 24 hours a day. Hospitals not equipped with the special radio receiver to pick up the signal can obtain timely information at http://www.nws.noaa.gov/view/nationalwarnings.php or from television and radio news services.

Hospital staff and patients should immediately be evacuated according to a preestablished disaster plan. If no plan is in place, seek shelter at higher ground. Avoid walking or driving through floodwater. The force from 6 inches of floodwater can cause a person to fall. Cars can easily be swept away by just 2 feet of floodwater.[4] Research from the Georgia flood in 1994 showed that 71% of flood deaths were associated with submersion in vehicles.[2]

MEDICAL TREATMENT OF CASUALTIES

Approximately 0.2% to 2% of flood survivors will require urgent medical care.[1] The main cause of death during floods is drowning, with victims typically found some time after the flood recedes. Because it is often difficult to reach victims during the acute phase of a flood, it is relatively uncommon for near-drowning victims to present to emergency departments.[14] Fast-flowing floodwaters carry cars, trees, and other large debris that can result in trauma, including orthopedic injuries and lacerations.[1,14] In addition, there have been reports of floodwaters displacing snakes and other animals, resulting in increased animal bites.[15,16] Moreover, the preponderance of water during the event and still water post-event results in an increase in insect bites and vector-borne illnesses. Floodwaters also may contaminate the local water supply and sewage system.[1,16]

The Centers for Disease Control and Prevention analyzed data from emergency departments in 20 hospitals during Hurricane Floyd in North Carolina during September and October 1999. The medical examiner found that 52 deaths were directly related to the storm. Four causes of injury or illness accounted for 63% of all emergency room visits during this period: orthopedic and soft tissue injury (28%), respiratory illness (15%), gastrointestinal illness (11%), and cardiovascular disease (9%). The majority (24 of 52, or 67%) of deaths were due to drowning, primarily associated with vehicles. There were 19 cases of hypothermia, and 10 cases of carbon monoxide poisoning. There was also an increase in suicide attempts, violence, dog bites, and arthropod bites, compared with the same period the prior year. Finally, five deaths occurred among prehospital personnel.[16]

Unsurprisingly, drowning is the primary cause of death during floods. Patients who are submerged in cold water for 40 minutes have been successfully resuscitated to attain complete neurologic recovery secondary to the neuroprotective effects of hypothermia.[1] Therefore, cardiopulmonary resuscitation should be performed as soon as possible after securing the scene. Cervical spine injuries should be suspected, and immobilization should be maintained.[17] The patient should be rewarmed using external and internal rewarming techniques, as indicated. Resuscitation efforts should be continued until the patient's temperature is 32 °C to 35 °C (90 °F to 95 °F); at that point, decisions regarding the utility of continuing resuscitation are made.[18]

Floodwaters carry a large amount of debris, such as cars and tree limbs, and result in traumatic injuries. Orthopedic injuries should be reduced, splinted, and managed accordingly. Most injuries during floods that require urgent medical attention include lacerations, rashes, and ulcers. These wounds are contaminated and should be conservatively managed by irrigation and healing by secondary intention. Among those lacerations that are closed primarily, the majority require reopening secondary to infection.[1]

Floods cause water contamination and an increase in vector-borne illnesses. Water contamination often results from damage to the water purification and sewage systems. Contaminated water sources result in waterborne disease transmission, including *Escherichia coli*, *Shigella*, *Salmonella*, and hepatitis A virus. The large areas of stagnant water that typically remain days or weeks after the initial flood event create a breeding medium for vector-borne illnesses.[19]

Floodwaters may also result in the spread of chemicals stored above ground. In addition, temporary shelters to house those displaced by flooding may result in crowded and unsanitary living conditions, increasing the incidence of gastrointestinal illness, among other infectious illnesses.[1]

The force from floodwaters may also down power lines, flood electrical circuits, and submerge electrical equipment, increasing the risk of fires and electrical hazards.[4,10]

Finally, victims of floods, as well as other natural disasters, are at an increased risk of mental illness and substance abuse.[20] Analysis after the 2007 flood season in the United Kingdom indicated the prevalence of all mental health symptoms was up to five times higher among those with flooding in their homes. Those with negative financial consequences were also more likely to report psychological complications.[21]

UNIQUE CONSIDERATIONS

Floods are the most common natural disasters, and they affect all countries in the world. Floodwaters can remain for days, weeks, or longer. As a result, flood-related injuries and illnesses may continue to present over a long period. Drowning is the number one cause of death and is often related to persons attempting to cross floodwaters in vehicles. Deaths also occur among health care providers, but increased natural disaster training may decrease this occurrence. In addition to drowning, flood victims are at an increased risk for hypothermia, contaminated wounds, and waterborne infections. Water and sewage treatment facilities may be damaged by floodwaters and result in water contamination.

Most communities in the world can experience flooding. Flash floods occur in all 50 states in the United States and most countries globally. Areas at greatest risk are low-lying, near water, and located downstream from a dam.[4] For planning purposes, flood hazard maps should be obtained in advance, and evacuation routes planned accordingly. In the event of flood warnings, evacuate as early possible because a vehicle can be swept away with the force from as little as 2 feet of water.

PITFALLS

- Failure to plan flood evacuation routes before a flood event
- Delayed evacuation by those in a flood-watch area
- Failure to know who is in command of disaster operations in the local area
- Closing contaminated lacerations
- Failure to continue resuscitation of a patient who is hypothermic
- Failure to notify the unified command or management structure and obtain directions
- Not listening to a radio or television or following social media sources for local flood information
- Not preparing an emergency kit and emergency communication (including a battery-operated radio)
- Failure to plan and communicate with other medical facilities to determine who has the capacity to accept evacuated patients

REFERENCES

1. Noji E. Natural disaster management. In: Auerbach P, ed. *Wilderness medicine: Management of wilderness and environmental emergencies.* 3rd ed. St Louis, MO: Mosby; 1995:644–663.
2. Centers for Disease Control and Prevention. Flood-related mortality-Georgia, July 4-14, 1994. *MMWR Morb Mortal Wkly Rep.* 1994;43 (29):526–530.
3. National Oceanic and Atmospheric Administration. Hydrologic Information Center—Flood Loss Data. April 28, 2014. http://www.nws.noaa.gov/hic/. Accessed April 17, 2014.
4. Ready.gov. Fact Sheet: Floods. Available at: http://www.ready.gov/floods. Accessed April 17, 2014.
5. NOAA National Climatic Data Center. Billion-Dollar Weather/Climate Disasters. http://www.ncdc.noaa.gov/billions/events. Accessed April 17, 2014.
6. Shabir O. A summary case report on the health impacts and response to the Pakistan floods of 2010. *PLoS Curr.* 2013;5.

7. National Disaster Education Coalition. Flood and Flash Flood. Available at: http://www.disastercenter.com/guide/flood.html. Accessed April 17, 2014.

8. U.S. Department of Commerce, National Oceanic and Atmospheric Administration, National Weather Service. Floods: The Awesome Power. Available at: http://www.nws.noaa.gov/om/brochures/Floodsbrochure_9_04_low.pdf. Accessed April 17, 2014.

9. Quinlisk P, Jones M, Bostick N, et al. Results of rapid needs assessments in rural and urban Iowa following large-scale flooding events in 2008. *Disaster Med Public Health Prep.* 2011;5:287–292.

10. Floyd K. Floods. In: Hogan D, Burstein J, eds. *Disaster Medicine.* Philadelphia, PA: Lippincott Williams & Wilkins; 2002:187–193.

11. Schatz JJ. Floods hamper health-care delivery in southern Africa. *Lancet.* 2008;371(9615):799–800.

12. Joint Commission on Accreditation of Healthcare Organizations. Health Care at the Crossroads: Strategies for Creating and Sustaining Community-wide Emergency Preparedness Systems. Available at: http://www.jointcommission.org/assets/1/18/emergency_preparedness.pdf. Accessed February 25, 2015.

13. Merchant R, Elmer S, Lurie N. Integrating social media into emergency-preparedness efforts. *N Engl J Med.* 2011;365:289–291.

14. Pan American Health Organization. *Emergency Health Management after Natural Disaster. Scientific Publication 407.* Washington, DC: Pan American Health Organization; 1981.

15. Ussher J. Philippine flood disaster. *J R Nav Med Serv.* 1973;59(2):81.

16. Centers for Disease Control and Prevention. Morbidity and mortality associated with Hurricane Floyd—North Carolina, September-October 1999. *MMWR Morb Mortal Wkly Rep.* 2000;49(23):518.

17. Braun R, Kristel S. Environmental emergencies. *Emerg Med Clin North Am.* 1997;15:451.

18. Jolly B, Ghezzi K. Accidental hypothermia. *Emerg Med Clin North Am.* 1992;10:311.

19. Alderman K, Turner L, Tong S. Floods and human health: a systematic review. *Environ Int.* 2012;47:37–47.

20. Du W, FitzGerald GJ, Clark M, Hou XY. Health impacts of floods. *Prehosp Disaster Med.* 2010;25(3):265–272.

21. Paranjothy S, Gallacher J, Amlôt R, et al. Psychosocial impact of the summer 2007 floods in England. *BMC Public Health.* 2011;11:145.

CHAPTER 98

Tsunami

Prasit Wuthisuthimethawee

DESCRIPTION OF EVENT

A tsunami is one of the most devastating disasters worldwide. It has huge human, physical, economic, and social impacts.[1] This event usually follows a high-magnitude earthquake of greater than 7.0 on the Richter scale, accompanied by landslides and volcanic eruptions. There are two types of tsunami waves: near-field and far-field. The near-field tsunami is caused by a nearby earthquake that significantly shakes the population. Its wave usually arrives at the shore within 5 to 20 minutes. The far-field tsunami is caused by a faraway earthquake without any significant shaking effects noticed on the shore. This wave usually arrives within 40 to 60 minutes.[2] A powerful harbor wave can exceed 490 miles per hour depending on the water depth, and its height can reach 38 m, resulting in massive destruction.[2]

During the years 1700 to 2000, tsunamis killed more than 420,000 people with thousands more injured or missing.[3] The earthquake near Sumatra Island in Indonesia in 2004, with a magnitude of 9.3 on the Richter scale, was one of the most devastating tsunamis in history (Fig. 98-1). More than 200,000 people died or went missing, more than 400,000 people became homeless, and more than 1.2 million people were displaced.[3] This enormous disaster required response from a diverse group of humanitarian organizations and military troops[3-6] and made some scientists believe that tsunami science and engineering were crucial to saving coastal societies, industries, and environment.[2] The complexity of the large earthquake and the tsunami that caused serious damage to the nuclear power plant in Japan on March 11, 2011, made the disaster relief operation more difficult, shocking the people of Japan and the world.[7-9] It is important to understand the course of this natural catastrophic event. Even though we cannot prevent the disaster from happening, we can prevent its adverse consequences.[10]

PRE-INCIDENT ACTIONS

Tsunami Mitigation and Planning

A tsunami disaster cannot be prevented, but planning and preparedness can mitigate its effects. Well thought-out risk and emergency management, planning, and preparedness can enable the community at risk to be ready to respond to a disaster in an effective manner.[2] The strategies include a detailed hazard vulnerability analysis (HVA), evaluation of risks in the area (risk assessment), learning from previous experience and available data, and coordination with all of the community's stakeholders. The significance of socioeconomic factors in making people vulnerable to a disaster should be recognized and included in action plans. The magnitudes of future tsunamis should be predicted during the planning and preparedness process, which is a combination of three components: defense structure, tsunami-resistant town development, and evacuation based on advanced warning.

Earthquake-resistant and shock-absorbing buildings, with their own electric power supply in tsunami-prone areas, is one strategy to prevent building collapse and mitigate the number of casualties.[9] Concrete seawalls with tsunami-absorbing areas and the relocation of population centers to higher ground areas are other strategies to reduce the effects of a tsunami. Accurate warning systems combined with individual, family, and community preparedness will help a population evacuate to designated routes and shelters more effectively.

Community surge capacity information is necessary for planning and preparedness. A method to gather accurate information on damage, logistics of the evacuation, and supplies should be implemented.[7] Two-dimensional (2D) and 3D technology can be used for run-up simulation to estimate the destruction and make a damage assessment (e.g., destruction of structures and the impact of drifting lumber, cars, or boats).[2] Then tsunami hazard maps can be created to provide information for planning, response, and public education.[2] Community and individual awareness and preparedness are very important in tsunami mitigation,[2] and community readiness is a cornerstone for an effective response.[11] An investment in community disaster education and training needs to be made, along with planning for exercises and drills. It has been proven that preparedness and periodic drills have helped people evacuate more smoothly and safely.[9]

Communication is one of the most important components for a more effective response when a tsunami strikes. The chaotic environment in a tsunami disaster makes communication more complex with greater possibilities for failure. Redundancy in communication backup systems (e.g., amateur radio communication, satellite communication systems, and walkie-talkies) is necessary in a plan for disaster response.[12]

In a large-scale disaster with a multiple number of agencies responding, good strategic planning to coordinate all of the responders can facilitate a more effective response.[7] When expanding the preparedness to regional, national, and international levels, a well-organized effort depends on effective command and control. The incident command system (ICS) is the cornerstone for disaster-response readiness. The command and coordination protocols should be prepared before a tsunami strikes, or set up immediately in the aftermath using prior liaisons with external organizations to mobilize their resources for the stricken community.

Financing is one of the challenging issues in a disaster. Public health planning has to ensure that victims can seek medical care without health insurance cards and with co-pays waived.[7]

Community hospitals should prepare and create graded mass casualty or disaster plans to operate the hospitals at full capacity for at least 48 to 72 hours without any external resource requirements. Regular training and mass casualty exercises and drills will help hospitals be ready to respond to any disaster.

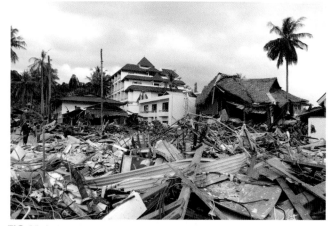

FIG 98-1 Area Destroyed by Tsunami in Thailand.

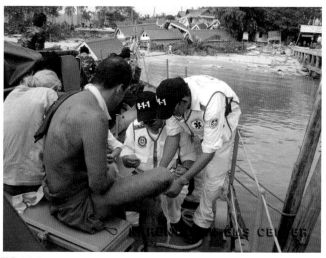

FIG 98-2 Basic Health Care Provided to Victims.

POST-INCIDENT ACTIONS

In the immediate aftermath of a tsunami, the local government should be the first to respond and set up an emergency operation center, apply the ICS, secure the affected area, establish the search and rescue procedure, commit resources to assess the damage, evacuate residents to designated shelters, provide first aid and relief to victims,[7] and establish the standard internal and external community communication systems. The incident commander needs to mobilize all of the available necessary resources to the affected area.[2] In a complex tsunami with damage to the infrastructure, the initial rescue and response will be less effective because of destruction of transportation systems and the lack of gasoline and supplies. Local health care facilities should be prepared with flexible surge capacity plans to respond to a disaster for at least 48 to 72 hours before external agencies or a disaster medical assistance team (DMAT) can reach the affected area. In the early stages of a disaster, local health care facilities need to prepare for a maximum influx of patients within the first 24 to 48 hours.[12] Enabling health care facilities to treat and support victims while also providing for basic needs (shelter, food, clean drinking water, and sanitation) is crucial for injured and uninjured survivors.

The emergency phase is usually followed by the reconstruction and rehabilitation phase. The large-scale influx of aid workers often comes later, and this foreign aid will have an impact on all levels of society during the recovery process.[1] Disasters by nature are intermittent, happen unexpectedly, and require massive recovery efforts,[13] especially in the developing world, which does not have the same capacity and ability to recover from disasters as more developed countries.[1] Recovery activities include restoring the infrastructure, reestablishing communication systems, and rebuilding socioeconomic systems with the main purpose of returning the affected community to its pre-incident state.

Immediately after the response to a tsunami or any other disaster, an after action review (AAR) should be performed to identify good practices and windows of opportunity for improvement. Combining this review with a community risk assessment for pre-incident action will create a more effective response in future tsunami disasters.

Currently, only a small number of research papers with good methodology are available. Conducting basic and advanced research in a tsunami disaster will provide valuable knowledge and information for the future.

MEDICAL TREATMENT OF CASUALTIES

Providing medical relief and understanding the medical needs for an affected area in a timely manner is not easy. The roles of governmental health agency in a disaster include securing medical and nursing care,

providing public health services with maximal safety protocols, ensuring the safety of food and water supplies,[7] and conducting surveillance of endemic diseases. All health institutions in disaster-prone areas should be equipped with emergency care facilities able to provide care when needed (Fig. 98-2).[14] The triage system normally establishes patient priorities by the severity and number of victims versus response assets available in the event of a large influx of patients in the immediate aftermath of a tsunami. On scene or in-hospital initial treatment and stabilization procedures are required. Patient transportation to other hospitals may be necessary for some victims. In the first few days after a tsunami, the immediate health care requirement is treating life-threatening and emergency conditions (e.g., aspiration, blunt and penetrating trauma, and wounds), while in the following weeks, medical assistance usually requires taking care of acute exacerbations of chronic diseases with minor injuries,[7] endemic disease prevention, and psychological support. The deployment of DMATs from the external community or central government is necessary to provide emergency medical assistance at the local hospitals and support for transporting patients in an affected area.

Wound Management

The powerful waves cause many people to be injured.[15] Victims usually suffer from aspiration, drowning and near drowning, blunt and penetrating trauma, and musculoskeletal injuries that include both fractures and dislocations.[16] Most wounds are severely contaminated with foreign bodies, mud, dirt, sand, debris, seawater, seaweed, feces, and saliva.[3,15,17] Contaminated wounds are prone to infection by the *Clostridium tetani* organism. The incidence of tetanus infection significantly increases in: wounds more than 1 cm long, wounds that are left without management at least 6 hours, wounds of the avulsion type, cases involving massive devitalized tissue, and wounds that are grossly contaminated.[18,19]

The disaster response team from Songklanagarind Hospital working at the Krabi Provincial Hospital (one of the most affected areas from the 2004 tsunami in Thailand) found that at least 67% of the contaminated wounds were infected as early as within 24 hours;[15,17,19-21] the most common procedure done was aggressive wound debridement. The infection rate remained high even though some victims initially received antibiotics.[15,17] Mixed organisms were the most common pathogens causing wound infection, with a high rate of antibiotic resistance.[3,17,19-24] The most effective antibiotics for these organisms were third- or fourth-generation cephalosporins, aminoglycoside, and

TABLE 98-1	**Summary of Wound Infection Information for Tsunami Disasters**			
AUTHORS (YEAR)	**POPULATION**	**INFECTION RATE**	**ORGANISM**	**ANTIBIOTIC-SUSCEPTIBLE**
Hiransuthikul[15]	777 patients	66.3%	Polymicrobial Aeromonas	Aminoglycoside Quinolone
Kespechara et al.[21]	391 patients	89%	*Klebsiella pneumoniae, Proteus* species, *Escherichia coli, Aeromonas*	Aminoglycoside Quinolone 3rd, 4th generation cephalosporin
Johnson[20]	777 patients	66%	*Aeromonas*	Aminoglycoside Quinolone 3rd, 4th generation cephalosporin
Katnimit[25]	59 patients	100%	N/A	N/A
Llewellyn[3]	17 patients	100%	*Acinetobacter E. coli*	Ceftazidime, carbapenem
Edsander-Nord[19]	75 patients	Most (esp. primary closure)	Unusual organism, *Mycobacteria, Acinetobacter, Aeromonas,* fungus	N/A
Prasartritha[24]	2311 patients	70%	Polymicrobial *Aeromonas* *Vibrio* *Klebsiella*	Gentamicin, ciprofloxacin
Doung-Ngern[17]	523 patients (1013 wounds)	66.5%	45% polymicrobial	Aminoglycoside Quinolone
Janda[22]	305 patients	N/A	*Aeromonas*	Aminoglycoside Quinolone

quinolone (Table 98-1).[15,17,22,23] Many victims developed wound infections associated with complications and needed aggressive wound management (i.e., surgical wound debridement, limb amputation, and intensive care).[17]

Recommendations for initial wound management in this setting are (1) initial cleaning of the wound with clean water (boiled, drinking, or sterile water or normal saline),[17,19,23,26–27] (2) removal of devitalized tissue and foreign bodies,[15,19,27] (3) leaving the wound open,[3,19,27] (4) dressing the wound with soaked saline or clean water,[15,27] (5) splinting fractures or dislocations,[24,27] (6) giving broad-spectrum antibiotics either orally or intravenously,[15,17,23,27] (7) tetanus vaccination,[18,27] (8) frequent wound evaluation,[17,27] (9) daily wound cleaning,[25,27] and (10) health education for wound care.[17,27]

Other Health Problems
Acute Illnesses and Exacerbation of Chronic Illnesses

Cough, stomachache, headache, general aches and pains, and feeling generally unwell are common symptoms that usually occur in people living in a transitional camp. Displaced people living in transitional camps are a vulnerable population, and specific interventions need to be targeted at this population to address the health inequalities.[28]

In the days and weeks following a devastating natural disaster, the threat of an infectious disease outbreak is high. An outbreak of influenza after a severe natural disaster presents unique challenges and needs prompt implementation of a systemic approach with a bundle of control measures in evacuation settings and hospital settings.[29] The spread of malaria in Indonesia after the 2004 tsunami was due to the increased salinity of inland water. The incidence was high in late infant and early childhood patients. Mass radical therapy is effective for acute control in this setting.[30]

Medical teams providing relief after acute tsunami disasters should be prepared not only to treat acute injury or diseases but also to provide health care for chronic diseases. A delay in the presentation of many acute conditions has implications for the long-term health consequences suffered by victims of disasters.[13] The International Committee of the Red Cross field hospital in Aceh, Indonesia, reported that in 2005, the ratio of chronic versus acute diseases being treated increased by 16.4% per day from January 15 to 23 and then decreased.[11] In people with underlying diabetes, emergency food supplies that usually contain high levels of glucose may exacerbate complications, especially diabetic retinopathy.[8]

Mortuary Operations

The immediate hit by a tsunami wave causes many sudden and subsequent deaths. For example, in Aceh, Indonesia, the highest mortality rate was in the younger and older populations: 0 to 9 years and more than 70 years old. Risk factors for heightened mortality were geographic (close to the shoreline), extreme in age, and female gender.[4] The use of geographic information system (GIS) models, with environmental variables coupled with predisaster population estimates, can create a map of spatial distribution of a population at risk and expected mortality in a tsunami. Mortality estimates from the displaced population are more accurate than estimates based on the size of the population at risk. Such a GIS model covered 97.5% of the reported mortalities in Aceh.[31]

Management of the dead bodies in this situation is also a challenge due to many corpses, lack of containers or temporary areas with high security, lack of transportation, and difficulty in identification of the victims.

Psychosocial Problems

A tsunami disaster causes significant destruction to the community and has significant psychosocial consequences. Along with the loss of property, the disaster causes medical and psychological problems in trauma victims and impacts relatives and health care personnel.[1,14] A tsunami can exacerbate any underlying socioeconomic or psychological problems, as well as create new psychiatric problems. Regardless of their initial socioeconomic status, the impact of the tsunami was interpreted by most of the affected people as *total damage,* which signifies the extent of the consequences on their lives and serves as a metaphor for the losses suffered in terms of human, social, financial, political, and natural capital.[1] This issue should not be underestimated, and it is recommended that the victims be aided in their efforts to cope with the situation.[1]

Psychological symptoms in tsunami victims vary from sleep disturbance, mood disorders, anxiety, and depression, to posttraumatic stress disorder (PTSD).[32,33] It is critical not only to examine for symptoms of trauma in children but also to collect sleep duration and disaster damage condition data following natural disasters.[34] The prevalence of clinically significant PTSD, depression, and anxiety in the survivors from the 2004 tsunami disaster was 21%, 16%, and 30%, respectively.[32] Significant risk factors for developing PTSD in the aftermath of a tsunami include poor socioeconomic status associated with poor baseline mental health, living in an urban area, the magnitude of property or community destruction, being female or a child, death of relatives, and injury to self or family members.[14,33] The protective parameters that prevent development of PTSD are absence of fear of the recurrence of a tsunami, counseling received more than 3 times, and satisfaction with services provided.[14]

Mental health care for this population is a major challenge for health care providers in a disaster.[33] Mental health aspects of relief and rehabilitation are increasingly recognized as an integral part of a disaster response[13] that are necessary in order to develop rational surveillance and interventions.[32] The World Health Organization recommends training and strengthening of the infrastructure for psychosocial capacity building as a fundamental part of public health relief and reconstruction programs for survivors of human-made or natural disasters in developed and developing countries.[13] Psychological support facilities and interventions should be planned for the areas that are prone to natural disasters. A plan for psychological assistance of survivors from a disaster includes community participation as well as a plan for systematic management of the people in the affected areas.[35]

A disaster mental health response team has roles that have evolved from identifying and treating psychiatric cases to focusing on women, children, and the low-socioeconomic-status population.[13,14,32] Family is considered to be a coping unit in this stressful situation.[14] A person's own strength, family and friends, a Western-style hospital, and religious practices are considered to be the most helpful coping aids.[32] A community-based self-help group trained by local community health care providers is crucial to strengthen the coping abilities of survivors and provide individual treatment to prevent psychiatric morbidity.[13] Key factors for promoting mental health services include having nurses be responsible for providing mental health services in the affected areas, having strong community networking and health volunteers, and learning management strategies from other areas.[35]

Therapeutic components of psychosocial care include venting of emotions, normalization of emotional responses, and cognitive processing of the event within a supportive group environment.[13] Psychosocial care in disasters involves (1) community self-help groups for emotional support and reestablishment of social connections, (2) relaxation exercises for controlling and mastering physiological and psychological stress reactions including hypervigilance and avoidance, and (3) cultural metaphors and spiritual beliefs to facilitate cognitive processing and coming to terms with an overwhelming experience.[13] Kid Narrative Exposure Therapy (KIDNET), a brief trauma-focused approach, has proven to be effective in refugee camps and in preventing PTSD in children.[33]

UNIQUE CONSIDERATIONS

The occurrence of a large-scale tsunami is estimated to be every 800 to 1000 years.[9] Tsunami archeology has succeeded in excavating geologically recorded tsunamis during the past 5500 years in eastern Hokkaido. This technique is being applied in countries where tsunami occurrences are rare and no historical documents are available.[2]

The Council on Earthquake Disaster Prevention (CEDP) in Japan proposed a total system of tsunami disaster mitigation including 10 countermeasures as follows:[2]

1. *Relocation of dwellings to high ground:* This is the best measure against a tsunami
2. *Coastal dikes:* Dikes may become too large and financially impractical, but they are effective in reducing the power of a wave
3. *Tsunami control forests:* This method is for tsunami power damping
4. *Seawall:* This is only effective for smaller tsunamis
5. *Tsunami-resistant area:* The construction of concrete buildings at the front line of the area is similar to the use of tsunami control forests
6. *Buffer zone:* Rivers and lowlands designed as buffer zones for the force and water drainage when a tsunami attacks
7. *Evacuation signs and routes* (Fig. 98-3)
8. *Tsunami watch*
9. *Tsunami evacuation:* Vulnerable groups are evacuated to safe areas as a first priority
10. *Memorial events:* Keep events alive in people's minds

PITFALLS

- No previous experience or shared information in some affected areas, leading to less awareness and more loss
- Weaknesses in all levels of preparedness that include individual, community, regional, and national levels and poorly organized response and recovery responses that become exacerbated when a tsunami strikes

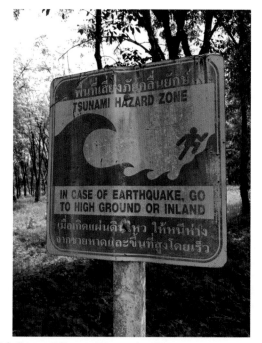

FIG 98-3 Tsunami Sign and Evacuation Route.

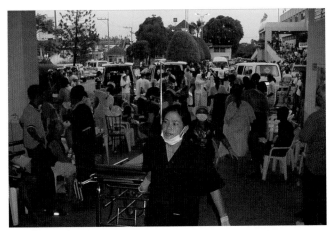

FIG 98-4 Crowded Provincial Hospital with Victims and Relatives.

- Complexity of the event causing infrastructure damage (e.g., communication, transportation, and massive basic sanitation damage).
- Difficulty in multiorganization coordination due to a variety of organizations, agency structures, and protocols.
- Ability to handle patient surge in hospitals; one hospital documented a threefold to fourfold increase of services from its baseline capacity (Fig. 98-4)
- Overwhelming response of volunteers and donations
- Lack of psychosocial support in the immediate aftermath and long term
- Information for public relations that is not totally accurate and probably confusing
- Difficulty in victim identification and management of dead bodies

SUMMARY

A tsunami is one of the most devastating natural disasters, and one which cannot be prevented. A systematic approach using science and emergency management knowledge will mitigate its effects on the population, resulting in lower morbidity and mortality. Public education, training, drills, and exercises are processes to develop community readiness in response to a disaster. A holistic response from safety and search and rescue teams during the response and recovery processes is the cornerstone for the most effective results.

ACKNOWLEDGMENTS

The author thanks Kingkarn Waiyanak for the literature search and retrieval, Glenn K. Shingledecker for his help in editing the manuscript, and the staff personnel at Krabi Hospital, Krabi, and Wachira Phuket Hospital, Phuket, Thailand, for providing valuable pictures.

REFERENCES

1. Fauci AJ, Bonciani M, Guerra R. Quality of life, vulnerability and resilience: a qualitative study of the tsunami impact on the affected population of Sri Lanka. *Ann Ist Super Sanita.* 2012;48:177–188.
2. Shuto N, Fujima K. A short history of tsunami research and countermeasures in Japan. *Proc Jpn Acad Ser B Phys Biol Sci.* 2009;85:267–275.
3. Llewellyn M. Floods and tsunamis. *Surg Clin North Am.* 2006;86:557–578.
4. Doocy S, Rofi A, Moodie C, Spring E, Bradley S, Burnham G, et al. Tsunami mortality in Aceh Province, Indonesia. *Bull World Health Organ.* 2007;85: 273–278.
5. Hawkes AD, Bird M, Cowieb S, Grundy-Warrc C, Hortona BP, Hwaid ATS, et al. Sediments deposited by the 2004 Indian Ocean Tsunami along the Malaysia-Thailand Peninsula. *Mar Geol.* 2007;242:169–190.
6. Kumar MS, Murhekar MV, Hutin Y, Subramanian T, Ramachandran V, Gupte MD. Prevalence of posttraumatic stress disorder in a coastal fishing village in Tamil Nadu, India, after the December 2004 tsunami. *Am J Public Health.* 2007;97:99–101.
7. Saito T, Kunimitsu A. Public health response to the combined Great East Japan Earthquake, tsunami and nuclear power plant accident: perspective from the Ministry of Health, Labour and Welfare of Japan. *Western Pac Surveill Response J.* 2011;2:7–9.
8. Oshima CR, Yuki K, Uchida A, Dogru M, Koto T, Ozawa Y, et al. The Vision Van, a mobile eye clinic, aids relief efforts in tsunami-stricken areas. *Keio J Med.* 2012;61:10–14.
9. Shibahara S. Revisiting the March 11, 2011 earthquake and tsunami: resilience and restoration. *Tohoku J Exp Med.* 2012;226:1–2.
10. Hafstad GS, Haavind H, Jensen TK. Parenting after a natural disaster: A qualitative study of Norwegian families surviving the 2004 tsunami in Southeast Asia. *J Child Fam Stud.* 2012;21:293–302.
11. Guha-Sapir D, van Panhuis WG, Lagoutte J. Short communication: patterns of chronic and acute diseases after natural disasters—a study from the International Committee of the Red Cross field hospital in Banda Aceh after the 2004 Indian Ocean tsunami. *Trop Med Int Health.* 2007;12:1338–1341.
12. Wattanawaitunechai C, Peacock SJ, Jitpratoom P. Tsunami in Thailand-disaster management in a district hospital. *N Engl J Med.* 2005;352:962–964.
13. Becker SM. Psychosocial care for women survivors of the tsunami disaster in India. *Am J Public Health.* 2009;99:654–658.
14. Pyari TT, Kutty RV, Sarma PS. Risk factors of post-traumatic stress disorder in tsunami survivors of Kanyakumari District, Tamil Nadu, India. *Indian J Psych.* 2012;54:48–53.
15. Hiransuthikul N, Tantisiriwat W, Lertutsahakul K, Vibhagool A, Boonma P. Skin and soft-tissue infections among tsunami survivors in southern Thailand. *Clin Infect Dis.* 2005;41:e93–e96.
16. Johnson LJ, Travis AR. Trimodal death and the injuries of survivors in Krabi Province, Thailand, post-tsunami. *ANZ J Surg.* 2006;76:288–289.
17. Doung-ngern P, Vatanaprasan T, Chungpaibulpatana J, Sitamanoch W, Netwong T, Sukhumkumpee S, et al. Infections and treatment of wounds in survivors of the 2004 Tsunami in Thailand. *Int Wound J.* 2009;6:347–354.
18. Afshar M, Raju M, Ansell D, Bleck TP. Narrative review: tetanus—a health threat after natural disaster in developing countries. *Ann Intern Med.* 2011;154:329–335.
19. Edsander-Nord A. Wound complications from the tsunami disaster: a reminder of indications for delayed closure. *Eur J Trauma Emerg Surg.* 2008;34:457–464.
20. Johnson LJ, Travis AR. In the wake: tsunami pathology—then and now, Krabi province, southern Thailand. *Int J Disast Med.* 2005;3:61–65.
21. Kespechara K, Koysombat T, Pakamol S, Phoungchit P, Panyaphul W. Infecting organisms in victims from the tsunami disaster: experiences from Bangkok Phuket Hospital, Thailand. *Int J Disast Med.* 2005;3:66–70.
22. Janda JM, Abbott SL. The genus *Aeromonas*: taxonomy, pathogenicity, and infection. *Clin Microbiol Rev.* 2010;23:35–73.
23. Okumura J, Kai T, Hayati Z, Karmil F, Kimura K, Yamamoto Y. Antimicrobial therapy for water-associated wound infections in a disaster setting: gram-negative bacilli in an aquatic environment and lessons from Banda Aceh. *Prehosp Disaster Med.* 2009;24:189–196.
24. Prasartritha T, Tungsiripat R, Warachit P. The revisit of 2004 tsunami in Thailand: characteristics of wounds. *Int Wound J.* 2008;5:8–19.
25. Katnimit C, Nualsrithong P, Teabput S. The management of wounds caused by the 2004 tsunami. *WCET J.* 2006;26:38–41.
26. Fernandez RS, Griffiths R, Ussia C. Water for wound cleansing. *Int J Evid Based Healthc.* 2007;5:305–323.
27. Wuthisuthimethawee P, Lindquist SJ, Sandler N, Clavisi O, Korin S, Watters D, et al. Wound management in disaster settings. *World J Surg.* 2015;39:842–853.
28. Turner A, Pathirana S, Daley A, Gill PS. Sri Lankan tsunami refugees: a cross sectional study of the relationships between housing conditions and self-reported health. *BMC Int Health Hum Right.* 2009;9:16.
29. Hatta M, Endo S, Tokuda K, Kunishima H, Arai K, Yano H, et al. Post-tsunami outbreaks of influenza in evacuation centers in Miyagi Prefecture, Japan. *Clin Infect Dis.* 2012;54:e5–e7.

30. Manimunda SP, Sugunan AP, Sha WA, Singh SS, Shriram AN, Vijayachari P. Tsunami, post-tsunami malaria situation in Nancowry group of islands, Nicobar district, Andaman and Nicobar Islands. *Indian J Med Res.* 2011;133:76–82.

31. Doocy S, Gorokhovich Y, Burnham G, Balk D, Robinson C. Tsunami mortality estimates and vulnerability mapping in Aceh, Indonesia. *Am J Public Health.* 2007;97(Suppl 1):S146–S151.

32. Hollifield M1, Hewage C, Gunawardena CN, Kodituwakku P, Bopagoda K, Weerarathnege K. Symptoms and coping in Sri Lanka 20-21 months after the 2004 tsunami. *Br J Psychiatry.* 2008;192:39–44.

33. Catani Cl, Kohiladevy M, Ruf M, Schauer E, Elbert T, Neuner F. Treating children traumatized by war and Tsunami: a comparison between exposure therapy and meditation-relaxation in North-East Sri Lanka. *BMC Psychiatry.* 2009;9:22.

34. Usami M, Iwadare Y, Kodaira M, Watanabe K, Aoki M, Katsumi C, et al. Sleep duration among children 8 months after the 2011 Japan earthquake and tsunami. *PLoS One.* 2013;8:e65398.

35. Seeherunwong A, Yuttatri P, Wattanapailin A, Pornchaikate A. Thai Nurses' experiences in providing mental health services to survivors of the 2004 tsunami six months post-disaster. *J Nurs Sci.* 2012;30:16–27.

CHAPTER 99

Heat Wave

Terrance T. Lee

DESCRIPTION OF EVENT

A *heat wave* is defined in meteorological terms as a prolonged period of unusually hot weather. The duration and intensity of the heat play an important role in how people are affected. Illness tends to occur within 2 days of excessive heat. However, there are certain populations who are at increased risk and who may exhibit symptoms earlier. The elderly, children, infants under 1 year of age, persons with preexisting diseases, those taking various drugs and medications, and urban dwellers are more susceptible to heat-related illness. Prolonged exposure to heat can exacerbate preexisting chronic conditions, including various respiratory, cerebral, and cardiovascular diseases. Heat waves have a greater observable effect on respiratory mortality than on cardiovascular mortality, but the underling mechanisms remain unclear. Risk factors for serious heat-related injury are outlined in Box 99-1.[1,2]

Each year, an average of about 700 people die from heat-related illnesses in the United States, with greater mortality during heat wave events. The Centers for Disease Control and Prevention estimated that from 1999 to 2009 there were about 7000 U.S. deaths attributable to extreme heat.[3] There were 600 deaths during the Chicago Heat Wave of July 1995. The next summer, during the 1996 Summer Olympics in Atlanta, Georgia, 1059 people were treated for heat-related illness.[4] During summer 2003, Europe experienced one of the worst heat waves in history, with an estimated mortality between 25,000 and 70,000 deaths in Western Europe.[5] A 2010 heat wave in Moscow, Russia, which lasted 44 days, became a public health crisis when it caused major wildfires and resulted in 11,000 deaths.[6,7]

The human body is able to dissipate heat by four mechanisms. *Radiation* is the passive transfer of heat by electromagnetic waves. This accounts for 65% of heat transfer. *Evaporation* is the transition of liquid into gas. This only occurs when the outside temperature reaches 95 °F, and it accounts for 30% of heat transfer. *Convection* is heat loss to air and water vapor molecules surrounding the body, and it accounts for 10% of heat transfer. Finally, *conduction* is heat transfer via direct physical contact. It is only responsible for 2% of heat transfer.[8]

Heat waves are among the most common emergencies and are the leading environmental cause of death in the United States, followed by cold-related deaths during winter months. Within the twenty-first century, exposure to heat is expected to increase as the average global temperature rises at least 3 °F. Moreover, climate change is expected to increase the frequency and severity of heat waves.[9] Given the projected increase in global prevalence of chronic respiratory and cardiovascular disease and the aging of the U.S. population, an increased proportion of the population will be susceptible to heat-related morbidity.[10] Heat wave mortality risk is ultimately influenced by multiple factors, including intensity and duration of heat, physical acclimatization of various communities, community preparation such as heat wave warning systems, and public willingness to take protective measures.[11]

PRE-INCIDENT ACTIONS

The most important action in preventing illness during a heat wave is proper preparation and public education before the heat wave begins. Proactive heat wave response plans are crucial in reducing heat-related morbidity, and many states have developed their own effective interventions to heat wave events. One should identify vulnerable populations (e.g., the elderly, socially isolated, chronically ill, mentally ill, or homeless) and target interventions to those most at risk. Interventions should include staying cool, hydrated, and informed about heat alerts in the area, as well as remaining cognizant of symptoms of heat illness. Some states have launched campaigns encouraging residents to check on their at-risk neighbors, whereas other efforts have included enlisting local students or the National Guard to participate in home visits. Utility companies should be represented in emergency operations centers to work with states in prioritizing power restoration to vulnerable populations. Multiple media formats, including press releases, social media, calls, and web updates, should be used to disseminate up-to-date information about resources.[3]

Educating the public allows people to protect themselves from excessive heat exposure. People should reduce strenuous activity or reschedule outdoor activities until the coolest time of day. They should wear lightweight clothing and light colors, and avoid restrictive hats that will block sweating and evaporation of heat. They should drink large amounts of water or other nonalcoholic beverages while avoiding alcohol intake. They should know the forecasted temperature and continuously monitor their dwelling's indoor temperature in case cooling systems fail. Finally, people should spend as much time as possible in air-conditioning and avoid direct sun exposure.[12]

Hospitals and emergency departments should be prepared for an influx of patients presenting with heat-related illnesses. Administrators should consider activating their emergency operations center, and should ensure that staffing and resources are adequate. Heat waves are associated with higher levels of emergency medical services (EMS) activity and may require a coordinated regional disaster response.[13] Emergency medicine providers are engaged at a regional and national level, through Disaster Medical Assistance Team (DMAT) deployments, and in triage and care for evacuated patients.[14]

POST-INCIDENT ACTIONS

In the prehospital setting, remove the patient from the heat. Disrobe the patient and apply ice packs to the neck, axilla, and groin. If a prehospital medical tent is immediately available, a patient should be cooled to

---

> **BOX 99-1** **Risk Factors for Serious Heat-Related Injury**
>
> - Dehydration
> - Obesity
> - Heavy clothing
> - Poor physical fitness
> - Cardiovascular disease
> - Skin diseases (burns, eczema, scleroderma, and psoriasis)
> - Febrile illnesses
> - Hyperthyroidism
> - Alcoholism
> - Drug use (cocaine, amphetamines, opiates, LSD, and PCP)
> - Poor socioeconomic conditions
> - Medications (antipsychotics, anticholinergics, calcium-channel blockers, beta-blockers, diuretics, alpha agonists, and sympathomimetics)

> **BOX 99-2** **Methods of Cooling**
>
> **External**
> *Evaporative or Convective Cooling*
> Fanning the undressed patient at room temperature
> Spraying mist or applying a fine, wet sheet on patient while continuously fanning
>
> *Conductive Cooling*
> Application of cold packs to body
> Cooling blankets
> Cold-water immersion
>
> **Internal**
> Iced gastric lavage
> Iced peritoneal lavage

under 104 °F (40 °C) before transport, as every minute of hyperthermia increases morbidity. Otherwise, transfer to an emergency department should be made rapidly. Intravenous (IV) fluid should be started, and blood sugar should be measured.

Always assess vital functions and obtain an accurate core temperature with a rectal probe. Temperature, neurologic status, and vital signs should be monitored continuously. Laboratory evaluation should include a complete blood count, electrolyte and lactate levels, and a urinalysis. Hyponatremia or hypernatremia can occur depending on the patient's salt and water balance. Acute renal failure and myoglobinuria may be present with rhabdomyolysis. If heat stroke is suspected, liver function tests and coagulation studies are needed to assess for hepatic necrosis or disseminated intravascular coagulation.[15]

Further diagnostic tests should include an electrocardiogram, computed tomography of the head for patients with undifferentiated altered mental status, and a chest x-ray in cases of respiratory distress.[16]

✚ MEDICAL TREATMENT OF CASUALTIES

The spectrum of heat-related illnesses ranges from heat cramps, rash, or syncope to heat exhaustion and heat stroke. Heat cramps are painful spasms of heavily used muscle groups with normal serum sodium levels. The victim has often been sweating heavily with insufficient fluid repletion for several days. Treatment is oral or IV fluids and salt replacement. Rhabdomyolysis and electrolyte abnormalities should be excluded.

Heat rash is an intensely pruritic, red, papular dermatitis that, if extensive, increases the risk of heat exhaustion or heat stroke as a result of sweat gland malfunction. Patients should keep their skin cool and dry, and antihistamines can be used for pruritus. Secondary infections should be treated with antibiotics. Heat syncope is a transient loss of postural tone often preceded by dehydration. It is treated with rest, fluids, salt, and gradual return to activity. Heat syncope often occurs early during exposure to high heat.

Heat exhaustion is generally caused by both water and salt depletion. Symptoms include thirst, weakness, anxiety, muscular incoordination, headache, vomiting, diarrhea, and muscle cramps. Treatment centers on replacement of fluid and electrolyte losses with isotonic saline. Severe hyponatremia may require hypertonic saline.

Heat stroke usually develops over several days, although exertional heat stroke can occur in a younger person after a few hours of severe heat stress. It is defined clinically as a core body temperature above 104 °F (40 °C), along with hot, dry skin and central nervous system abnormalities such as delirium, convulsions, or coma. However, assume heat stroke in any patient with changes in mental status during heat stress, even if his or her core temperature is <40 °C. Vital sign abnormalities can include tachycardia, tachypnea, and hypotension. Every organ system can be affected. Other signs and symptoms include liver failure, coagulopathy, hypoglycemia, renal failure from rhabdomyolysis, lactic acidosis, disseminated intravascular coagulation, or respiratory distress syndrome.[17]

The most important part of the treatment of heat stroke is rapid cooling. Every minute counts, as when core temperature is very high, body and brain cells begin to die. The ultimate goal is to get the body temperature under 104 °F (40 °C) within 30 minutes of collapse (or faster if possible). Covering the patient's body in ice is not recommended because vasoconstriction and shivering could increase core temperature. Antipyretics and dantrolene are also ineffective in heat stroke. Instead, ice water immersion should be used in severe cases. In mild cases, cooling should include spraying the disrobed patient with cool mist; fanning mist with bedside fans; and applying ice packs to the neck, axilla, and groin. Iced peritoneal lavage and cardiopulmonary bypass should be considered in refractory cases. A patient can be cooled from 108 to 110 °F (42.2 to 43.3 °C) to 102 °F (38.9 °C) in 15 to 30 minutes. The average length of cooling for a heat stroke victim is about 1 °F every 3 minutes or about 1 °C every 5 minutes. The key to maximizing cooling rate during cold-water-immersion therapy is constant and aggressive stirring of the water, and to stay cognizant that the patient's head stays above water. Cooling is continued only until the temperature drops to 102.2 °F (39 °C) to avoid overshooting to hypothermia. Thus continuous rectal temperature monitoring is recommended. Box 99-2 describes different approaches to cooling a patient suffering from a heat-related illness.

While active cooling is taking place, patients often need sedation and large amounts of IV normal saline. Pediatric patients should receive 20-mL/kg boluses. A central venous pressure line and Foley catheter may be necessary to monitor fluid therapy. Medications to consider include analgesics for muscle cramps; chlorpromazine, benzodiazepines, or thiopental for shivering; benzodiazepines for seizures; and glucose, thiamine, and naloxone for altered mental status.

Patients with minor heat-related problems can be discharged. Patients with heat exhaustion, persistently abnormal vital signs or laboratory abnormalities, or significant comorbid conditions should be admitted to a floor bed. Patients with evidence of heat stroke should be admitted to an intensive care unit.[15–17]

❓ UNIQUE CONSIDERATIONS

Patients at extremes of age are at increased risk of heat-related illnesses. Children have an increased body surface area to mass ratio, which increases their risk. Hydration of pediatric patients consists of 20-mL/kg boluses of IV fluid. If hypoglycemia is present, give 2 mL/kg of D25W over 1 minute, intravenously.

Elderly patients are at increased risk secondary to underlying medical conditions and medications that worsen heat illness. Taking a thorough history and a physical examination will help guide therapy.

Climate-sensitive diseases also include respiratory diseases, such as asthma and chronic obstructive pulmonary disease (COPD), and gastroenteritis from spoiled food. Health care providers may expect a rise in the incidence of these diseases during times of extreme heat.[15,16]

⚠ PITFALLS

Consider other causes of hyperthermia in patients with altered mental status. The differential diagnosis includes alcohol withdrawal, neuroleptic malignant syndrome, malignant hyperthermia, toxicities (anticholinergics, salicylates, PCP, cocaine, and amphetamine), infectious sources (tetanus, sepsis, encephalitis, meningitis, brain abscess, typhoid fever, and malaria), endocrine abnormalities (thyroid storm and diabetic ketoacidosis), status epilepticus, and cerebral hemorrhage.

For patients with hyperthermia, do not forget to consider an acute cardiac event or a severe electrolyte abnormality.

Consider other causes of altered mental status, including hypoglycemia, thiamine deficiency, or opiate overdose.[15]

REFERENCES

1. Michelozzi P, Accetta G, De Sario M, et al. High temperature and hospitalizations for cardiovascular and respiratory causes in 12 European cities. *Am J Respir Crit Care Med.* 2009;179(5):383–389.
2. Anderson GB, Dominici F, Wang Y, McCormack MC, Bell ML, Peng RD. Heat-related emergency hospitalizations for respiratory diseases in the Medicare population. *Am J Respir Crit Care Med.* 2013;187 (10):1098–1103.
3. Centers for Disease Control and Prevention (CDC). Heat-related deaths after an extreme heat event-four states, 2012, and United States, 1999-2009. *MMWR Morb Mortal Wkly Rep.* 2013;62(22):433–436.
4. Wetterhall SF, Coulombier DM, Herndon JM, et al. Medical care delivery at the 1996 Summer Games. *JAMA.* 1998;279:1463–1468.
5. D'Ippoliti D, Michelozzi P, Marino C, et al. The impact of heat waves on mortality in 9 European cities: results from the EuroHEAT project. *Environ Health.* 2010;9:37.
6. Moran DS, Gaffin SL. Clinical management of heat-related illnesses. In: Aurebach PS, ed. *Wilderness Medicine.* 4th ed. St Louis: Mosby; 2001:290–317.
7. Shaposhnikov Dmitry, Bellander T, et al. Mortality related to air pollution with the Moscow heat wave and wildfire of 2010. *Epidemiology.* 2014;25 (3):359–364.
8. Osborn A. Moscow smog and nationwide heat wave claim thousands of lives. *BMJ.* 2010;341:c4360.
9. Interagency Working Group on Climate Change and Health (US). A human health perspective on climate change: a report outlining the research needs on the human health effects of climate change. *Environ Health Perspect.* 2010.
10. Vincent GK, Velkoff VA. *The next four decades: the older population in the United States: 2010 to 2050 (No. 1138).* US Department of Commerce, Economics and Statistics Administration, US Census Bureau; 2010.
11. Anderson GB, Bell ML. Heat waves in the United States: mortality risk during heat waves and effect modification by heat wave characteristics in 43 US communities. *Environ Health Perspect.* 2011;119(2):210.
12. Bittner MI, Matthies EF, Dalbokova D, Menne B. Are European countries prepared for the next big heat-wave? *Eur J Public Health.* doi:10.1093/eurpub/ckt121 [Epub Oct 4, 2013].
13. Dolney TJ, Sheridan SC. The relationship between extreme heat and ambulance response calls for the city of Toronto, Ontario. Canada. *Environ Res.* 2006;101(1):94–103.
14. Hess JJ, Heilpern KL, Davis TE, Frumkin H. Climate change and emergency medicine: impacts and opportunities. *Acad Emerg Med.* 2009;16 (8):782–794.
15. Schmidt EW, Nichols CG. Heat-related illness. In: Wolfson AB, Hendey GW, Ling LJ, eds. *Harwood-Nuss' Clinical Practice of Emergency Medicine.* Philadelphia: Lippincott Williams & Wilkins; 2012.
16. Waters TA, Al-Salamah MA. Heat emergencies. In: Cydulka RK, Meckler GD, eds. *Tintinalli's Emergency Medicine: A Comprehensive Study Guide.* 7th ed. New York, NY: McGraw-Hill; 2011 [chapter 204].
17. Bouchama A, Knochel JP. Heat stroke. *New Engl J Med.* 2002;346 (25):1978–1988.

Winter Storm

Srihari Cattamanchi and Alison Sisitsky Curcio

DESCRIPTION OF EVENT

Winter weather varies across the globe. All people living on high mountains close to seas and oceans or anywhere in the mid to upper latitudes of the earth are likely to experience winter storms at least once in their lives. They usually occur during the winter climatological season between October 15th and April 15th. Winter storms range from moderate snow to blizzards with blinding, wind-driven snow sometimes over a few hours to several days. Winter storms may also occur along with very low temperatures, icing, very strong winds, sleet, and freezing rain.[1]

For winter storms to form, three components are required: moisture, cold air, and lift. First, moisture is produced from the evaporation of water, primarily from the seas and oceans. The moisture forms clouds that are capable of producing precipitation. Second, the temperatures must be below freezing both at the ground level and in the clouds to produce snow or ice. The wet air mass cooled by the freezing temperatures in the clouds and the water vapor turn into snow. It can and does snow over deserts but never reaches the ground due to high temperatures on the surface. Finally, lift is necessary for a winter storm. Moist air is lifted from the clouds and causes precipitation. An example of lift is air flowing up a mountain.[2] One assumes Antarctica receives heavy snowfall every year. On the contrary, it receives very little snowfall because it has a huge mass of ice with most of its mass far away from seas and oceans, and the air is dry. Mid to upper latitudes of North America, Europe, China, and Russia/Siberia receive most of the snowfall globally. Table 100-1 lists different types of snow storms.[3,4]

The Northeast Snowfall Impact Scale (NESIS) and the Regional Snowfall Index (RSI) provide an estimate of the upcoming impact of winter storms in relation to the previous historical storms affecting the region, severity, and population affected by them (Table 100-2).[5,6] These scales provide meteorologists, emergency managers, city administrators, transportation officials, financiers, planners, and journalists the resources to inform and alert the general public and businesses about the severity of the storm and ways to mitigate its impact.[5,6]

Using a newer guide, the Sperry-Piltz Ice Accumulation Index (SPIA Index), one can accurately predict and clearly communicate the impairment that different amounts of ice accumulation can cause in a particular area (Fig. 100-1). The SPIA Index is as accurate an index for predicting severity of ice storms as the Saffir-Simpson Scale is for hurricanes, and the Enhanced Fujita Scale is for tornados.[7] The SPIA Index is a powerful tool to quantify the damage likely due to snow or ice storms long before their impact. This index gives the public, utility companies, and emergency managers a good idea about potential duration of power outages and tree damage.

The incidence of winter storms is approximately 105 per year in the continental United States. The winter storms are referred to as the "deceptive killers" by the National Weather Service[1] because most deaths are related indirectly to the winter storm, such as deaths due to road traffic accidents on icy roads, hypothermia after prolonged exposure to below freezing temperatures, and overexertion while clearing the snow.[8] Of these deaths 70% occur in automobiles, and 25% occur out in the storm.[9] Before a winter storm strikes it is crucial to be prepared for it.

PRE-INCIDENT ACTION

Before a winter storm occurs the public is educated on when to expect it, how to know if a storm is approaching, and how to handle the potential dangers associated with it. The National Weather Service (NWS) issues alerts within 24 hours of a possible storm through local radio news channels and the National Oceanic and Atmospheric Administration (NOAA) weather radio.[10] The alerts are graded from watch to advisory to warning. They warn the public if bad weather is predicted by issuing a watch and, if a hazardous winter storm is predicted, by issuing an advisory. When the weather is very dangerous and potentially life-threatening, the public is alerted by the issuance of a warning.[10]

Every family prepares an emergency plan and a communication plan for use during disasters. Stockpiles of daily medications should be assembled and kept in a safe place. When a disaster strikes, families may not be together; for example, parents might be at work and children at school or play. It is essential for family members to prepare how they will contact each other, where they will gather, and what they will do in case of an emergency.[1] It is prudent to make winter emergency kits and store them at home and in vehicles.

If the plans are to shelter in place, winterize the house to keep it warm (Box 100-1).[11] Stay indoors during a winter storm. If it is essential to go outside, walk carefully on snowy or icy walkways and dress for the winter. Instead of a single-layered, thick jacket, several layers of lightweight, loose-fitting, warm clothing should be worn along with a pair of mittens, warm hat, scarf, and outer waterproof, tightly woven jacket. A pair of mittens keep the hands and fingers warmer than gloves; a warm hat prevents body heat loss, and a scarf covering the mouth protects the lungs.[1]

Overexertion while shoveling snow can bring on a heart attack, which is a major cause of death in the winter.[11] It is crucial to avoid overexertion while shoveling snow. Wet clothing transmits heat rapidly and loses all of its insulating value.[11] Changing wet clothing frequently will keep the body dry and prevent body heat loss. Frostbite appears as numbness and white or pale appearance of distal body areas, such as earlobes, tip of the nose, toes, and fingers.[12] Be alert for signs of frostbite. Also watch for signs of hypothermia, such as uncontrollable shivering, memory loss, disorientation, drowsiness, slurred speech, incoherence, and exhaustion.[13-15] If hypothermia is detected the victim

TABLE 100-1   Nine Types of Snow Storms[3,4]

S. NO	TYPE OF SNOW STORM	DESCRIPTION
1.	Snow flurries	Light snow falling for a short duration, with little to no accumulation.
2.	Snow showers	Snow falls for a brief period with varying intensities. Snow shower accumulation is possible but not always guaranteed.
3.	Snow squall	Occurs when a mass of cold air moves over warmer water, creating an unstable atmospheric temperature. Over the lake, this unstable atmospheric temperature builds clouds that eventually move downward and form snow showers and squalls. Snow squalls are also known as lake effect storms. During the winter on the base of a passing cold front, the freezing Arctic air commonly produces lake effect storms.
4.	Blowing snow	The snow falling through the atmosphere is blown by high-speed winds into almost horizontal bands, and the lighter snows on the ground are picked up by the wind and redistributed, causing a reduction in visibility.
5.	Nor'easters	When continuously strong northeasterly winds blow in from the ocean over the coastal areas, they create strong areas of low pressure. Nor'easters are among winter's most ferocious winter storms for creating heavy rain, snow, and oversized waves that crash onto the beaches, eroding the beaches and damaging nearby infrastructure. The intensity of the wind gusts associated with Nor'easters can exceed a hurricane's force and can occur any time of the year.
6.	Blizzards	Caused by a powerful storm system made from the jet stream dipping far to the south, which allows the warm air current from the south to crash against the cold air current from the north. Blizzards are characterized with wind speeds of 35 mph or higher, temperatures below 20 °F, and heavy falling and/or blowing snow, reducing visibility to 0.25 miles or less. A severe blizzard is characterized with winds exceeding 45 mph, temperatures below 10 °F, and snow reducing visibility to near zero.
7.	Ice storms	Created with accumulation of freezing rain to at least 0.25 inch and accompanied by any other winter precipitation. In many regions of the world, ice storms are often blamed for multiple deaths due to associated losses of power. It is another dangerous winter storm condition.
8.	Sleet	Raindrops freeze into ice pellets before reaching the ground and, on hitting the surface, bounce back and do not stick to any object. Sleet accumulation makes road conditions hazardous.
9.	Freezing rain	Raindrops are made from melting of snowflakes as the snow falls through an above freezing, warm layer in the atmosphere. Right near the surface of the earth, the raindrop passes through a thin layer of below freezing air, and contact with trees, cars, roads, the ground, or other objects allows the raindrop to freeze and form a coating or glaze of ice. This makes a significant hazard due to slippery conditions and weight of solid ice on trees and power lines.

TABLE 100-2   Comparison of NESIS[3] and RSI[4]

CATEGORY	DESCRIPTION	NESIS VALUE	RSI VALUE
1	Notable	1-2.499	1-3
2	Significant	2.5-3.99	3-6
3	Major	4-5.99	6-10
4	Crippling	6-9.99	10-18
5	Extreme	$\geq$10.0	$\geq$18.0

NESIS, Northeast Snowfall Impact Scale; RSI, Regional Snowfall Index. Courtesy: NOAA National Climatic Data Center Website. Adapted from: (a) Kocin, Paul J, Uccellini LW: A snowfall impact scale derived from northeast storm snowfall distributions. *Bull Am Meteorolog Soc.* 2004;85:177-194, Table 5. (b) Squires MF, et al. Regional Snowfall Impact Scale. *NOAA National Climatic Data Center.* v3a, January 25, 2011, Table 3 [Online pdf]. Available at: http://www1.ncdc.noaa.gov/pub/data/cmb/snow-and-ice/rsi/regional-snowfall-impact-scale-27th-iips-v3a.pdf.

is first moved to a warm and safe location. All wet clothing is removed; the victim is dried, warmed from the midpoint of the body to the extremities, and if conscious a warm, nonalcoholic drink is given to the victim. If symptoms of frostbite or hypothermia are identified, medical care should be sought immediately.

During a winter storm driving should be minimized, and in case of travel a disaster "go bag" kit should be prepared and readily available in the car. Winterize the vehicle (Box 100-1).[1] If it is important to go out, drive with a companion and try to travel during the day, keeping others informed of the details of your travel schedule; stay on main roads, avoiding shortcuts. Let someone know the final destination, the exact itinerary, and the expected arrival time at the final destination. In the case of a car breakdown and being stuck in a storm, help can be sent along the predetermined route.[11]

If stranded in the vehicle during a blizzard, try to pull off the road to the side to be safe from traffic, given the decreased visibility. A distress flag should be tied to the antenna or the window, and the hazard lights turned on to caution any oncoming vehicle. It is good to remain inside the car where rescuers are most likely to search. It is important not to go out walking on foot during a winter storm, unless a building is visible close by where shelter can be taken. Beware of distances because blowing snow distorts distances of objects.

Every 10 minutes the engine and heater should be run to keep warm inside the car. When the engine is on, the exhaust pipe should regularly be cleaned to avoid being clogged with snow. The downwind window is best opened slightly for proper ventilation to protect from possible carbon monoxide poisoning inside the car.[1] Exercise to keep up body heat, but do not overexert while stranded in the car. During extreme cold, seat covers, car floor mats, and road maps can be used for insulation and keeping the vehicle warm. The passengers can huddle together and use coats as a blanket to keep them warm. Taking turns sleeping, with at least one person being awake and looking for rescue crews, is a good idea. Drink plenty of fluids to prevent dehydration (avoid alcohol and caffeine) and eat regularly. The car battery power is conserved by balancing energy needs versus supply when utilizing lights, heat, and radio in the vehicle. The lights inside the vehicle are always kept on at night for rescue workers to visualize the victims. If stranded in a remote area, large block letters are to be stomped in the snow in open areas spelling "SOS" or "HELP." To attract rescue personnel surveying by air the "SOS" or "HELP" area is lined with available surrounding material.[11]

The Sperry-Piltz Ice Accumulation Index, or "SPIA Index"–Copyright, February, 2009

ICE DAMAGE INDEX	DAMAGE AND IMPACT DESCRIPTIONS
0	Minimal risk of damage to exposed utility systems; no alerts or advisories needed for crews; few outages.
1	Some isolated or localized utility interruptions are possible, typically lasting only a few hours. Roads and bridges may become slick and hazardous.
2	Scattered utility interruptions expected, typically lasting 12 to 24 hours. Roads and travel conditions may be extremely hazardous due to ice accumulation.
3	Numerous utility interruptions with some damage to main feeder lines and equipment expected. Tree limb damage is excessive. Outages lasting 1 to 5 days.
4	Prolonged and widespread utility interruptions with extensive damage to main distribution feeder lines and some high voltage transmission lines/structures. Outages lasting 5 to 10 days.
5	Catastrophic damage to entire exposed utility systems, including both distribution and transmission networks. Outages could last several weeks in some areas. Shelters needed.

(Categories of damage are based upon combinations of precipitation totals, temperatures, and wind speeds/directions.)

FIG 100-1 The Sperry-Piltz Ice Accumulation (SPIA) Index. Categories of damage are based upon combinations of precipitation totals, temperatures, and wind speeds and directions. (Copyright 2009, Sidney K. Sperry, SPIDI Technologies, LLC.)

⏩ POST-INCIDENT ACTION

It is tempting to go outside immediately when a winter storm clears, especially if stuck inside the house for multiple days. After the storm, the sidewalks, roads, and other hard surfaces are dangerous for days, with frigid temperatures often lingering.[16,17] Weather conditions are carefully monitored. The ill or injured patient should be removed from the cold environment as quickly as possible first. All wet and cold clothes are removed to prevent further heat loss.[15] Food and water are conserved until it is safe to travel and replenish the food supplies. If the area's emergency management authorities issue a "boil water before drinking" alert, this should be continued until advised safe.

Be cautious, and avoid walking outside on hilly or slippery surfaces until all the ice has melted. It may take considerable time for the frozen precipitation on the ground to melt even if there is no snow, sleet, or freezing rain falling.[17] Before setting out on foot, if stranded in a vehicle due to the winter storm, wait for the storm to pass completely. After the storm, snow and ice may melt during the day and refreeze after sunset. It is important to keep roads clear of snow and ice as soon as possible and to be extremely careful when driving after a storm. Use battery-powered flashlights instead of open flames, such as candles, as a light source during a power failure to avoid fire.[16] Many injuries and deaths during winter storms result from accidental fires caused by candles and other types of incendiaries. If suspicious of frozen pipes or a pipe is frozen or burst, the home's water valve should be immediately shut off and a plumber called.

➕ MEDICAL TREATMENT OF CASUALTIES

Medical conditions to consider in a patient caught in a winter storm are hypothermia (mild, moderate, and severe), frostbite, carbon monoxide poisoning, and overexertion injuries.[15] Driveways and sidewalks around the hospital also must be clear to keep patients safe upon arrival.

Assess vital functions, and determine core body temperature. Blood should be evaluated for possible complications, including lactic acidosis, rhabdomyolysis, bleeding diatheses, and toxicology screening. Obtain an electrocardiogram to evaluate for dysrhythmias,[15] prolongation of the intervals, and elevation of the J point (Osborne wave) (Fig. 100-2).

BOX 100-1   Pre-incident Preparations

Winterize the Home

1. Insulate the walls and attic.
2. Install storm windows, and caulk and weather-strip doors and windows to increase the life of fuel supply.
3. Check the roof's structural ability to bear heavy weight due to snow accumulation.
4. Clean the rain gutters; repair roof leaks and cut tree branches that could fall on a house or other structure before a winter storm.
5. Maintain the heating equipment and the chimneys by inspecting and cleaning them yearly.
6. Vent all the fuel-burning equipment, such as kerosene heaters, outside the home to keep the room clear from the smoke and to avoid buildup of toxic fumes.
7. Keep the home cooler than average room temperature and shut off the heat temporarily to some rooms to save fuel.
8. Keep fire extinguishers on hand, and have every person well trained to use it.
9. Insulate the pipes with insulation, plastic, or newspapers, and prevent freezing of pipes by allowing faucets to drip a little during cold weather.
10. Even a trickle of running water prevents freezing of pipes.
11. If pipes freeze, remove insulation and layers of papers and wrap the pipes in rags. Open all taps completely, and pour hot water over the pipes, beginning from where the pipes are most exposed to cold weather.
12. If pipe bursts, water valves must be shut off.

Winterize the Vehicle

1. Check the vehicle for antifreeze levels, ensuring they are sufficient to avoid freezing.
2. Clean the battery and ignition system and keep it in good condition.
3. Check the brakes for fluid level and wear.
4. Check the exhaust system for crimped pipes and any leaks. Carbon monoxide poisoning is deadly; be cautious because it gives no warning.
5. Maintain a full gas tank, replace air filter, and add additives to keep the system free of water.
6. Check the level and weight of oil because at lower temperatures heavier oils congeal more and do not lubricate as well.
7. Check the heater and defroster, and ensure they work properly.
8. Check the lights and flashing hazard lights in the car.
9. Ensure the thermostat works properly.
10. Repair the windshield wiper equipment if required and maintain proper washer fluid level.
11. Equip the vehicle with all-weather radials or snow tires encased with chains or studs.

Winter Emergency Kit

1. Stock an emergency kit with the appropriate quantity of food, snacks, and water, additional matches, and a pocket knife.
2. Have ample warm clothing and blankets to keep warm. Pack an extra pair of mittens and socks, a warm hat, a fully stocked first-aid kit with necessary medications, and enough blanket(s).
3. Have adequate heating fuel, such as a good supply of seasoned dry wood for wood-burning stove or fireplace.
4. A windshield scraper, shovel, small broom, battery-powered NOAA radio, flashlight, and enough extra batteries should be packed.
5. Prepare a winter emergency kit with a sufficient amount of rock salt to prevent ice formation and to melt ice on the walkways.
6. Similarly, a sufficient quantity of sand is stored to improve traction on the driveway, along with the need for snow shovels and other snow removal equipment.
7. Keep a tow chain or rope, booster cables, adequate road salt and sand, a fluorescent distress flag, and a couple of emergency flares in a vehicle's emergency kit.

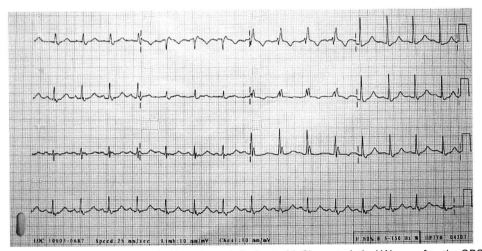

FIG 100-2 Electrocardiogram of a Hypothermic Patient with Characteristic J Waves after the QRS Complexes.

Mild hypothermia is defined as core temperature between 32 and 35 °C. Patients with mild hypothermia may experience tachypnea, tachycardia, shivering, or mild altered mental status. Passive external rewarming should be started after removing wet clothing. Blankets or any other insulation should be enough to assist endogenous thermogenesis.

Moderate hypothermia occurs when the core temperature is between 28 and 32 °C. These patients may have reduced heart rate and cardiac output and generalized central nervous system depression. They are at risk for renal failure, atrial fibrillation, and bradycardia. Immediate passive and active external rewarming should be started. Warm blankets, heating pads, and warm air should be applied to the patient to reduce further heat loss. The heat should be applied to the patient's torso to prevent core temperature from dropping. The goal is to prevent extensive peripheral vasodilation that occurs naturally after the patient is removed from the cold and is rewarmed.

By propelling the cold blood to the heart, contractility is decreased, causing hypotension, decreased cardiac perfusion, and with dropping core temperatures a high risk of ventricular fibrillation.[13,14]

Severe hypothermia is defined as core body temperatures below 28 °C. Patients with severe hypothermia are at risk for hypotension, bradycardia, ventricular fibrillation, pulmonary edema, and coma. Move these patients carefully to avoid inducing ventricular fibrillation. Active internal rewarming is needed for these patients and can be made in addition to the external techniques previously described. Humidified oxygen and warm intravenous fluids are minimally invasive methods to warm the severely hypothermic patient. The peritoneal cavity, pleural spaces, and bladder can be irrigated with 45 °C fluid. Pleural irrigation should be reserved for those without a cardiac rhythm to avoid inducing ventricular fibrillation with chest tube placement. Blood warming by hemodialysis and cardiopulmonary bypass are acceptable means to raise the core body temperature. Protocols for aggressive and invasive rewarming procedures should be developed in cooperation with other departments in the hospital involved in these processes before an incident requiring such measures.[13,14]

Arrhythmias associated with hypothermia were formerly treated with bretylium, but this medication is no longer available. Arrhythmias should be treated according to advanced cardiac life support (ACLS) guidelines and may be refractory until the patient is normothermic.[13]

Cold-induced tissue injuries are common during winter storms. Risk factors include altered mental status, advanced age, malnutrition, and peripheral vascular disease. Tissue injuries range from mild (frostnip) to severe (frostbite). Frostbite is local injury from contact with temperatures below 2 °C. The first phase of frostbite is the initial freeze injury when cell damage occurs. The second phase is the reperfusion injury that occurs while rewarming. The injury severity may not be apparent on first presentation. Do not rub or manipulate the frozen part. Treatment should consist of rapid rewarming in a water bath maintained between 40 and 42 °C. The affected extremity should be immersed for 15 to 30 minutes. Blisters should be left intact, and a sterile dressing with antibiotic ointment should cover any that have burst. Other remedies include aloe vera and ibuprofen. Tetanus status needs to be updated. Patients should be advised to avoid smoking.[12,15,18]

Carbon monoxide poisoning should be considered in patients with headache, dizziness, nausea, vomiting, confusion, seizures, or coma. Apply 100% oxygen, and consider hyperbaric oxygen treatment if the patient's condition is stable and a chamber is easily accessible. Arterial blood gas, base excess, and carboxyhemoglobin levels will help guide treatment.[19] Multiple patients with carbon monoxide toxicity may be encountered when heat and electricity are cut off for prolonged periods due to storms. The indoor use of heat generation utilizing fossil fuels contributes to the high incidence of carbon monoxide poising, as was seen in upstate New York during the 1999 ice storms.

UNIQUE CONSIDERATIONS

Extremes of age are risk factors for cold-induced illnesses. As one ages, the shivering mechanism may not be enough, and therefore there is an increased risk of hypothermia. Infants lose heat quickly because they have a large body surface to mass ratio. The elderly and children may be unable to carry out actions to warm themselves.

Medications, such as barbiturates, benzodiazepines, chlorpromazine, and tricyclic antidepressants, can increase the risk of hypothermia.

PITFALLS

- Always evaluate the entire patient, looking for evidence of frostbite, hypothermia, underlying illness, or trauma.
- Accurate assessment of core temperature in the field is very challenging. Assume that unresponsive patients who are not shivering are severely hypothermic.
- Remember that no prognostic neurologic scale, including the Glasgow Coma Scale, is valid during hypothermia because many patients have recovered completely after prolonged resuscitation.
- Think of other causes of altered mental status and consider giving naloxone, thiamine, and glucose.
- Peripheral pulses are difficult to palpate in profoundly bradycardic vasoconstricted patients. Check the monitor for at least 1 minute before starting compressions because iatrogenic ventricular fibrillation is a real hazard.
- Computer software usually misdiagnoses J waves as injury current on 12-lead electrocardiograms (Fig. 100-2). Prehospital thrombolytic therapy in hypothermia could exacerbate coagulopathies and be fatal.
- Cold hearts fibrillate easily. Avoid rough handling, such as rolling gurneys quickly or rapid transport over rough terrain. Consider aeromedical evacuation in rough terrain.
- Premature termination of thawing is a common error in the treatment of frostbite. Avoid prehospital thawing if there is a possibility of refreezing. Refreezing after thawing leads to increased injury. Rubbing frostbitten tissue increases damage through mechanical injury.

REFERENCES

1. Winter storms & extreme cold. Available at: http://www.ready.gov/winter-weather. Updated 2014. Accessed 18.01.14.
2. Oblack R. The 3 ingredients of snow storms—what is the real cause of severe winter weather? Available at: http://weather.about.com/od/winterweather/p/3winterelements.htm. Updated 2014. Accessed 02.02.14.
3. Oblack R. Types of snow storms. Available at: http://weather.about.com/od/winterweather/p/stormtypes.htm. Accessed 02.02.14.
4. Types of storms. Available at: http://www.weather.com/encyclopedia/winter/types.html#ice. Accessed 03.02.14.
5. Kocin JP, Uccellini WL. A snowfall impact scale derived from northeast storm snowfall distributions. *Bull Am Meteorol Soc.* 2004;85:177–194.
6. Squires FM, Lawrimore HJ, Heim Jr RR, Robinson AD, Gerbush RM, Estilow WT. The regional snowfall index. *Bull Am Meteorol Soc.* April 17, 2014.
7. What is the Sperry-Piltz Ice Accumulation Index? Available at: http://www.spia-index.com/. Accessed 16.01.14.
8. Spitalnic JS, Jagminas L, Cox J. An association between snowfall and ED presentation of cardiac arrest. *Am J Emerg Med.* 1996;14:572–573.
9. Oblack R. The causes of winter storm deaths. Available at: http://weather.about.com/od/winterweather/p/winterdeaths.htm. Updated 2014. Accessed 06.02.14.
10. Winter weather tip sheet. Available at: http://www.nws.noaa.gov/om/winter/winter1.shtml. Updated 2014. Accessed 12.03.14.
11. During winter storm & extreme cold. Available at: http://m.fema.gov/during-winter-storms-extreme-cold. Accessed 02.02.14.
12. Arnold P. Frostbite. In: Schaider JJ, Hayden RS, Wolfe ER, Barkin MR, Rosen P, eds. *Rosen and Barkin's 5-Minute Emergency Medicine Consult.* 2nd ed. Philadelphia, PA: Lippincott Williams & Wilkins; 2003:436–437.
13. Currier JJ. Hypothermia. In: Harwood-Nuss A, Wolfson BA, Linden HC, eds. *The Clinical Practice of Emergency Medicine.* 3rd ed. Philadelphia, PA: Lippincott Williams & Wilkins; 2001:1664–1667.
14. Danzl FD. Accidental hypothermia. In: Auerbach SP, ed. *Wilderness Medicine.* 4th ed. St Louis: Mosby; 2001:135–177.

15. Schaider JJ. Hypothermia. In: Schaider JJ, Hayden RS, Wolfe ER, Barkin MR, Rosen P, eds. *Rosen and Barkin's 5-Minute Emergency Medicine Consult.* 2nd ed. Philadelphia, PA: Lippincott Williams & Wilkins; 2003:584–585.

16. Winter storms: after the storm. Available at: http://www.weather.com/life/safety/winter/article/winter-after-the-storm_2011-10-04. Updated 2011. Accessed 28.01.14.

17. Dolce C. Ice storms: Why they're so dangerous and how to stay safe. Available at: http://www.weather.com/news/weather-winter/ice-storm-damage-impacts-20121123. Updated 2012. Accessed 14.02.14.

18. Gonzalez F, Leong K. Cold-induced tissue injury. In: Harwood-Nuss A, Wolfson BA, Linden HC, eds. *The Clinical Practice of Emergency Medicine.* 3rd ed. Philadelphia, PA: Lippincott Williams & Wilkins; 2001:1661–1664.

19. Chang SA, Hamilton JR. Direct relationship between unintentional workplace carbon monoxide deaths and average U.S. mean monthly temperature. *Acad Emerg Med.* 2002;9:531.

Volcanic Eruption

Gregory Jay, Kevin King, and Srihari Cattamanchi

DESCRIPTION OF EVENT

Volcanic eruptions have the potential to produce significant loss of life and far-reaching medical and socioeconomic disruption. More than 270,000 volcano-related fatalities have been recorded since 1700, with the number of fatal eruptions averaging two to four events per year.[1-3] Eighty percent of the world's active volcanoes are located around the Pacific Basin where continental and seafloor plate subduction occurs.[1,4] In 1990 approximately 10% of the world's population lived within 100 km of an active volcano. This continued growth in world population and urbanization will increase the risk of injury and death from volcanic eruptions over time.

The energy of a volcanic eruption determines the characteristic of injuries produced. Volcanic eruption encompasses the ejection of gases and solid material from a vent or hole in the earth's surface. Outgassing, or release of volatile gas dissolved in magma, provides the motive force for an eruption. While magma rises to the earth's surface, the decreasing pressure around molten rock allows volatile gases in the melt to be released.[5] The higher the silica content of the melt, the more viscous and polymerized it remains, stabilizing volatile melt.[1] When pressure is suddenly released on magma with a high dissolved gas concentration, rapid and explosive outgassing may occur. This produces the typical violent or explosive eruption during which lava bombs and plumes of ash are ejected. When magma has a low silica content, outgassing occurs more gradually, and a more gentle, or effusive, eruption ensues.[6] The volcanoes located along plate subduction zones tend to produce more violent eruptions because of the high silica and dissolved gas concentration in their magma.[1]

A variety of physical and chemical hazards are associated with volcanic eruptions. Lava is responsible for very few fatalities. The flow is often slow and can be easily avoided. Pyroclastic flows are responsible for most deaths.[2] A pyroclastic flow is a mass of hot volcanic ash, lava fragments, and gases that erupts from a volcano and moves rapidly down its slope at speeds of up to a few hundred miles per hour (Figure 101-1).[6-8] Rocks and debris within the flow may be hurled at great speed, causing severe secondary blast injury. Pyroclastic flows are extremely destructive and fatal to nearly all life in the area through which they travel. The temperatures in a pyroclastic flow may be as high as 600° to 900°C, causing severe, if not fatal, burns.[6]

Pyroclastic flows may extend a great distance from the site of an eruption. Flows commonly travel up to 15 km from a vent; during the Mount St. Helens eruption in 1980, flows reached 17 miles.[7] Pyroclastic flows often occur multiple times during an eruption and have also been reported in the absence of violent eruption.[9,10]

Another common cause of volcanic eruption-related fatalities is tephra. Tephra includes all of the solid fragments of magma and volcanic rock ejected from a volcano during an eruption.[6,8] Ejecta can cause severe head injury, burns, and blunt trauma.[11] Tephra fragments less than 2 mm in size are termed *ash*, 2- to 64-mm fragments are called *lapilli*, and fragments larger than 64 mm are often called *lava bombs* or *blocks*. Lava blocks and bombs generally follow a more ballistic trajectory after ejection, landing a few meters to several kilometers away from the site of eruption. The path and final point of impact is dependent on the initial "muzzle velocity" of the fragment.[6] Ballistic fragments are a serious hazard near a vent but become a more minor hazard as distance increases from the site of eruption. Air resistance also prevents ballistic fragments less than a few centimeters in diameter from being hurled more than a few hundred meters from a vent.[6]

Ash clouds pose a potential health hazard. Small particles of tephra rise on convection currents within a hot eruption cloud and may drift for hundreds of kilometers downwind from the active volcano.[6] Tephra deposits tend to become finer grained farther downwind because the coarser particles of ash and lapilli fall nearer the volcano.[6] In enormous eruptions, tephra accumulations may reach several meters in depth, and the associated lapilli and ash fall may be thick enough to induce darkness at midday.[6] Although the mean diameter of tephra grains decreases with distance from a vent, the percentage of respirable ash, particles less than 10 μm in diameter, does not necessarily increase.[6]

Currently, very little research is available regarding the respiratory effects of volcanic ash. There was concern about the development of acute silicosis from exposure to ash with high silica and cristobalite content.[12,13] However, no cases of acute silicoses were reported in studies of eruptions at Soufriere Volcano in Montserrat and of the Mount St. Helens eruption in 1980, where high concentrations of cristobalite and silica were recorded in ash samples.[12,13] These studies did note a slight increase in bronchial reactivity and wheeze in children during the Montserrat eruptions and a doubling of asthma- and bronchitis-related emergency department (ED) visits, compared with the previous year, during the Mount St. Helens eruption.[13,14] There were no cases of acute silicosis reported because people were not exposed to high enough concentrations of silica-laden ash for a long enough duration to develop the condition.[13] The risk of silicosis from prolonged ash exposure may be more substantial, but it is difficult to quantify.[13]

During ashfalls, the amount of total suspended particles (TSP) in the air is a useful predictor of ED visits for some respiratory conditions. The number of ED visits for respiratory complaints during the Mount St. Helens eruption was highest when the TSP concentrations was greater than 30,000 μg/m^3.[14] The number of ED visits did decline with decreasing TSP levels, but it did not return to normal levels until 3 weeks after peak TSP levels were recorded.[14] The increase in ED visits during high TSP levels was greatest for asthmatics.[14] (An important factor to remember is that rain significantly reduces TSP levels.[14])

Volcanic gases also have severe health effects. To determine the hazards from volcanic gas, the composition of the volcanic gas emissions

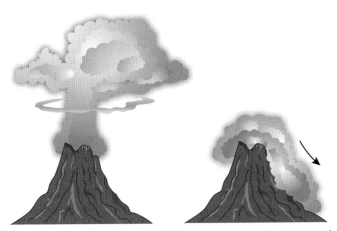

FIG 101-1 Pyroclastic flow ensues when the ash column created by an eruption collapses upon the flanks of the volcano. This "reversal" of flow occurs without warning. The cloud of ash, particulates, and gases is superheated and moves with great speed.

and the prevailing weather conditions should be assessed.[6,15,16] Water vapor is the most plentiful volcanic gas released, followed by carbon dioxide and sulfur dioxide.[5,6] Volcanic emissions may also include smaller amounts of carbon monoxide, helium, hydrogen, hydrogen chloride, hydrogen fluoride, hydrogen sulphide, and trace amounts of other gases.[5]

Hydrogen fluoride also induces an irritant response in the upper and lower respiratory tracts, but it is of greatest risk to livestock secondary to ingestion. Ash becomes impregnated with hydrogen fluoride, and upon ingestion, the fluoride produces fluorosis and death of the animal.[5] Fluorosis is a theoretical risk to a human population posteruption, but it can be avoided by cleaning ash off of food before ingestion and checking the fluoride levels of local drinking water.

Carbon dioxide is the second most common gas released during volcanic activity. Carbon dioxide is odorless, colorless, and heavier than air; thus it will collect in low-lying areas. Breathing air with a carbon dioxide concentration greater than 20% to 30% can rapidly induce unconsciousness and death through asphyxiation.[5] If a substantial release of carbon dioxide has occurred or is suspected, venturing into depressions or cellars in the affected area should be avoided. The carbon dioxide and air boundary can be sharply demarcated, with one step placing a person within a lethal concentration of carbon dioxide.[5]

The other gases tend to be released in much smaller quantities during an eruption. An important consideration is hydrogen sulfide. It is a highly toxic gas that is relatively dense and may collect in depressions and low-lying areas.[6] Hydrogen sulfide gives off a "rotten egg" odor and can cause eye and upper respiratory tract irritation, pulmonary edema with prolonged exposure, and death through cellular asphyxiation.[5,17] By contrast, sulfur dioxide may not have a lasting effect in reactive airway diseases.[18] It is important to determine the emissions spectrum of a volcano to ensure that larger concentrations of dangerous trace gases are not present.

Volcanic debris flows, termed *lahars,* and mudslides can be very destructive. Loose fragments of rock mixed with water from rainfall, melted snow peaks, or another source forms a thick slurry that travels down the mountainside or valley at speeds that may be higher than 50 km per hour.[6,19] The high sediment concentration of the flow destroys buildings, bridges, and other structures, which would usually survive a flood. People caught in the flows almost universally perish.[6]

Lahars can also occur when a volcano is quiescent. A combination of heavy rainfall and the disruption of volcanic debris and sediment by earthquakes have produced lahars and mudslides.[20,21] Lahars may also be formed by lake breakouts. This happens weeks to months after an eruption when a river blocked by a mudslide or other volcanic deposit overflows the newly formed dam.[22] Erosion of the blockage and the walls of the river channel downstream from the initial surge of water allows tremendous volumes of sediment to be incorporated into the flow. This is termed a *cold lahar;* in comparison, the lahars formed by hot volcanic debris may remain hot far downstream.[6]

Volcanoes pose a unique threat in regard to gas release in the absence of visible eruption. In 1984 at Lake Monoun in Cameroon 73 people were killed by carbon dioxide released by lake water turnover.[23] A similar event occurred in 1986 at Lake Nyos in Cameroon, a crater lake. Approximately 1700 people in low-lying areas were killed by a massive release of carbon dioxide.[23] Carbon dioxide is believed to have gradually collected in the deep waters of the lake. Rain or a landslide may have been responsible for the lake water turnover and gas release at Lake Nyos.

Other risks associated with volcanic eruptions are lightning, tsunamis, and earthquakes. Lightning discharges and strikes from ash clouds occur during eruptions and have caused electrocution injuries.[24] Please see the chapters on tsunamis and earthquakes for further information about these forms of disaster. Tsunamis are mostly caused by fault displacements on the sea floor, but underwater volcanic eruptions have caused many. The eruption of Krakatau in 1883 generated a massive pyroclastic flow, which displaced the ocean and initiated tsunamis, which killed 36,000 people.

As the Richter Magnitude Scale is for earthquakes, the Volcanic Explosivity Index (VEI)[25] indicates the severity and explosivity of volcanoes. It is a simple, increasing explosivity index from 0 to 8 with each interval representing an increase of approximately a factor of 10 (Figure 101-2).[25] The VEI combines total volume of eruptive cloud height, explosive products, descriptive terms, and other measures. There is some intentional overlap in criteria for VEI assignments and a combination of data used wherever possible.

VEI 0-1 eruptions produce eruptions that cover an area of only approximately 10,000 m^3, whereas the VEI 7-8 eruptions produce massive eruptions that cover an area of 1,000,000,000,000 m^3 (Figure 101-3). A VEI 7-8 eruption is 10 million times more productive than a VEI 0-1. However, only six eruptions in the past 10,000 years make it into the VEI 7-8 category, whereas there have been at least 2215 VEI 0-1 eruptions.

In the preceding 200 years, there have been over 200,000 deaths in volcanic eruptions (Table 101-1). Ninety-one percent of the fatalities resulted from the following four causes: famine and epidemic disease (30%), pyroclastic flows (27%), lahars (17%), and tsunamis (17%). High-risk regions for volcanoes are Latin America and the Caribbean. Seventy-six percent of the deaths caused worldwide in the twentieth century by volcanic eruptions were in this region. Half of the strongest volcanic eruptions in the world in the past 10 years occurred in Latin America and the Caribbean.

PRE-INCIDENT ACTIONS

Each volcano presents its distinct risks, and each hazard can have a different consequence. Opportunely, most volcanoes are carefully observed, and scientists can usually provide some warning before a serious event. A little knowledge and preparation can reduce injury and mortality.[26] It is an enormous challenge to plan for a volcanic crisis,

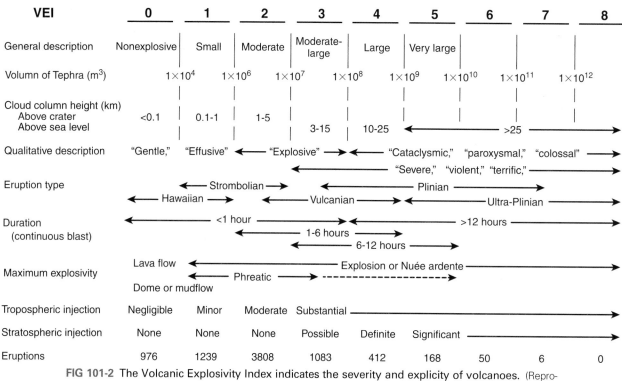

FIG 101-2 The Volcanic Explosivity Index indicates the severity and explicity of volcanoes. (Reproduced with permission from Newhall CG, Self S. The volcanic Explosivity Index (VEI): an estimate of explosive magnitude for historical volcanism. *J. Geophys Res (Oceans Atmos)*. 1982;87:1231-1238. John Wiley & Sons, Inc.)

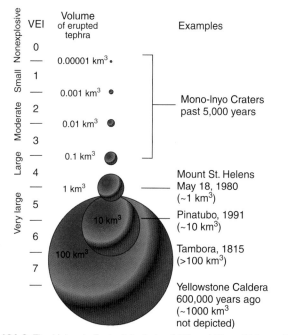

FIG 101-3 The Volcanic Explosivity Index (VEI) and Ejecta Volume Correlation. (With kind permission from USGS.)

but it is critical to be finished before the event and take adequate measures to prevent or minimize its consequences.[27]

Pyroclastic flows and mudflows cause 99% of fatalities due to a volcanic eruption. However, medical attention is often diverted to other risks, such as ash and acid rain. Although they are of concern to the public depending on their proximity to the volcano, they are not as serious a threat to public health.[27]

The best approach to prevent mass casualties and enormous losses from volcanic eruptions is by making sure populations are far away from volcanic areas.[27] It can be accomplished by working with the planning officials and the local government to pass laws and make policies not to allow people settling or communities and health care facilities to be built near volcanic areas. These laws and policies not only will save the governments millions in later costs but also will prevent injuries and deaths due to volcanic eruptions.[27]

In preparing for volcanic emergencies the health sector plays an important role and has enormous responsibilities.[27] Gathering vital information about the volcanic areas surrounding the health facility is the first step in planning for such an emergency. A health sector emergency plan must be created for all areas with risk of volcanic eruptions. The health sector emergency plans are to be designed by the first responders and the stakeholders responding to a volcanic crisis. This includes medical treatment plans, financial arrangements, and creation of temporary evacuation sites.[27] Plans for mass evacuation of people from communities already established in the volcanic area are to be incorporated in to the emergency plan. An effective way of promoting the evacuation of populations is through the exchange of good public information. The accurate, objective information of the volcanic hazard facing the community along with steps taken to help them are presented through community meeting and mass media.[27]

Identifying populations at highest risk is crucial when preparing a disaster plan.[28] Moreover, to identify these high-risk populations, it is imperative to identify potential trouble spots. The local emergency committee and civil defense members along with volcanologists are consulted to understand the history of eruptions, current status, and potential activity of nearby volcanoes. Available hazard maps for a particular area, which help in identifying whether settlements are built in the path of former mudflows or pyroclastic flows, should be incorporated in the emergency plan.[28] If a medical center requires evacuation during an eruption, an evacuation plan is to be prepared and

RANK	DEATH TOLL	VEI*	EVENT	LOCATION	DATE
1	92,000	7	Mount Tambora	Indonesia	April 10, 1815
2	36,000	6	Krakatoa	Indonesia	August 26-27, 1883
3	33,000	5	Mount Vesuvius	Pompeii and Herculaneum, Italy	August 24, 79 AD
4	29,000	4	Mount Pelée	Martinique	May 7 or 8, 1902
5	23,000	3	Nevado del Ruiz	Colombia	November 13, 1985
6	15,000	2	Mount Unzen	Japan	1792
7	12,000	4	Mayon Volcano	Philippines	1814
8	10,000	4	Mount Kelud	Indonesia	1586
9	9,350 (killed approximately 25% of the population)	6	Laki (killed approx. 25% of population)	Iceland	June 8, 1783
10	6,000	6	Santa Maria	Guatemala	1902

TABLE 101-1 **Top 10 Deadliest Volcanic Eruptions in the Past 200 Years**

*VEI, Volcanic Explosivity Index.

coordinated with the appropriate nearest health centers outside of the potential fallout zone.[27]

The emergency plans are prepared with the cooperation of volcanologists, local leaders, first responders, and disaster professionals.[27] Monitoring of CO_2 and SO_2 gas emissions can be useful in predicting whether an eruption is imminent. The preeruptive degassing of CO_2 by rising magmas increases the CO_2/SO_2 ratio which is both measureable and predictive of eruption. Thus volcanologists play a critical role in both planning and activating emergency plans.[28]

The preparedness plan should take into account the ash fall lasting for a prolonged period, blocking roads and reducing visibility for days or weeks until rainfall clears the atmosphere. The plans should look into the possibility of disruption in essential utilities (such as water and electricity), telecommunications and radio blackouts, and satellite communications. The contingency plans should anticipate and plan for shortage of supplies and personnel because most supplies will not be available at the required time. Flexibility to overcome aspects of the plan that may fail is crucial in a successful plan because many things go wrong even with excellent plans.[27]

Ongoing training should be incorporated in contingency plans for every personnel involved in first response, mass casualty management, incident command systems, psychosocial management, public health, and local government.[27] Continuous training of personnel helps build muscle memory that is very much needed to keep everyone safe and calm during a disaster. The emergency plans should be tested and drilled upon with the medical staff and first responders to make them comfortable and prepared and also to develop this muscle memory. The emergency plans are regularly updated based on the after action report developed after a drill and also on the hazard vulnerability assessment of the area. The contingency plans should help create adequate internal resources in the facility for a continued operation for a minimum of 96 hours if isolated due to disruption of local infrastructure.[27]

Water and air quality are to be monitored continually, keeping the people well informed about safety issues.[27] Ash and toxic gases can cause severe air pollution, for which many people seek medical help. The emergency plan should take into account environmental health issues, such as clean air, water supply, healthy food, proper sewage and solid waste disposal, vector control, and proper disposal of the dead.[27]

In the aftermath of a volcanic eruption, people living in the affected area and the workers will need particular protective gear and information to protect themselves.[28] People suffering from respiratory problems are directed to stay indoors and wear lightweight masks protecting them from inhaling fine particles. Emergency first responders and those working to remove ash and debris from the streets and roofs are to be provided with personal protective equipment, such as masks, protective eyewear, hard gloves, hard hats, and boots. If heavy ash fall is observed in the area, high-efficiency lightweight masks are distributed to everyone in the affected area.[27]

Health care facilities should be equipped with sensors and detectors to monitor for carbon dioxide, carbon monoxide, hydrogen sulfide, and sulfur dioxide in case of hazardous gas release from the volcanoes.[16] Particulate masks do not provide adequate protection. Special masks may be needed for protection from the toxic gases and dust. The New York Committee for Occupational Safety and Health based on the 9/11 World Trade Center disaster experience recommended the use of National Institute for Occupational Safety and Health (NIOSH)-approved air-purifying respirators of N-100 or N-95 grade.[29] Other useful protective equipment would include hard hats or helmets and heat-resistant clothing.[11]

Health needs assessment and epidemiological surveillance are essential for health administrators.[27] It is also crucial to determine among the affected population the types of injuries and illnesses by keeping track of reports from health centers, EDs, hospitals, and shelters. It gives the first responders an opportunity to target key services and resources where they are needed the most. The affected population and evacuees are likely to suffer from depression and other mental disorders. It is critical to include mental health issues in the emergency plan. Medical personnel and disaster first responders will also need access to these support services.[27]

Providing medical attention is an essential part of the health sector emergency plans. The health sector emergency plan includes urban search and rescue plans, triage instructions, and mass casualty management plans. The emergency plan takes into account the need for emergency field stations and mass fatality management (temporary morgues), and plans for transporting the critically ill or injured patients to hospitals and emergency clinics.[27] Preparation is crucial, considering that the majority of the deaths during an eruption occur within the first 24 hours.[2]

Managing information about the situation is accomplished by maintaining transparency.[27] Public health effects of any actions being deliberated is shared with the emergency officials and mass media. The information shared to the emergency officials and mass media alleviate fears, dispel myths, and educate the people about the dangers they are facing.[28]

⟫ POST-INCIDENT ACTIONS

1. Activate the disaster plan with appropriate allocation of resources.
2. Distribute and use appropriate personal protective equipment.
3. Be aware of the surroundings and protect from pyroclastic materials. Avoid low-lying areas where lahars or pyroclastic flows have occurred because of the risk of repeat episodes. It is essential to keep a watch, and take precautions to shield from pyroclastic materials while getting to higher ground. It is safe during an eruption to remain under the ridgelines on the hillside opposite to the volcano. Protect the head with arms, a backpack, or anything else one can find, and duck down on the ground facing away if caught in a hail of smaller pyroclastic materials.[26]
4. Be alert for repeat eruptions. The volcano may erupt multiple times.
5. Unless it is prudent to evacuate, the safest place is to be inside a sturdy structure with all the doors and windows closed to protect from ash and burning cinders. Ash and tephra accumulation on buildings are monitored because they cause most injuries through building collapse. If ash clearing is undertaken, make sure that appropriate personal protective equipment is worn and that the conditions are safe enough to allow removal of the ash. If there is any concern about the risk of building collapse, consider evacuating the facility or building.
6. Volcanoes release a number of hazardous gases, and avoiding these gases is of paramount importance. Breathe through a mask, respirator, or moist piece of cloth[30] that protects the lungs from clouds of ash. Most of these hazardous gases are heavier than air and accumulate close to the ground.[30] Avoid staying near to the ground or basements or depressions where toxic gases may have accumulated unless air quality has been tested. Monitor air and water quality and provide appropriate public health warnings. People at risk of asthma exacerbation and chronic obstructive pulmonary disease may benefit from staying indoors if it is harmless to do so when TSP concentrations are high.
7. Once safe from a volcano, waste no time to get prompt medical examination and treatment for gas or ash inhalation, injuries, and burns. Keep in mind, however, that waiting time will be long because there will be many people with more serious injuries requiring urgent care.[26]

✚ MEDICAL TREATMENT OF CASUALTIES

Casualties during a volcanic eruption can be complex and require sophisticated and intensive multisystem trauma care. Detailing all of the medical treatments potentially required is beyond the scope of this chapter. The important factor to consider is the mechanism of volcanic–related injury in anticipating patient care needs. The broad categories of injuries seen are burns, crush injuries, head trauma, inhalation injuries, toxic exposures to gases, blunt force trauma, and amputations. For further information and recommendations please refer to the basics of disaster management of this book (Part 1) and the chapters on the Accidental Disaster, Accidental versus Intentional Events, Building Collapse, Bridge Collapse, Landslide, and Structure Fires.

❓ UNIQUE CONSIDERATIONS

1. Gas release from lake water turnover in the absence of visible volcanic activity.
2. Dormant or suspected dormant volcano reactivation.
3. Significant numbers of deaths throughout history are linked to volcanic activities, such as pyroclastic flow, landslides, tsunamis, and debris flows.[33]

4. Acute respiratory distress/illness results from exposure to volcanic ash, especially in those with preexisting respiratory disease; however, the long-term effects are uncertain and differ from one volcano to another.[33]
5. Health issues in places far from volcanoes occur due to the discharge of toxic aerosols and gases that are dispersed hundreds of miles away.[33]
6. In large volcanic eruptions the gases and particles are discharged into the upper atmosphere, causing global climatic changes.[33]
7. In order to improve management of health risks and hazards due to volcanoes, there has been an increase in multidisciplinary research.[33]

⚠ PITFALLS

1. Failure to assess whether the community and the medical facility is at risk from volcanic eruption and failure to incorporate this eventuality into the disaster plan.
2. Failure to deliberate on a volcano's past eruptive pattern when preparing a disaster plan.
3. Failure of the community and the medical facility to procure adequate and appropriate supplies to deal with a volcanic eruption. Personal protective equipment should include heat-resistant coveralls, hard hats, and NIOSH-recommended respirators.
4. Failure to appreciate the risk for volcano-related injuries in the absence of visible volcanic activity. Examples include mudslides, lahars, and volcanic gas release. A person can be in danger even hundreds of miles away from the volcano.[31,32] Failure to incorporate these details in the disaster plans.
5. Failure to consider the need to evacuate a hospital post–volcanic eruption and to determine whether the receiving facility is in a safe zone that will not be endangered by future or repeated eruptions.
6. Failure to clean the roof of ash intermittently because several feet of ash can fall within a couple of hours, causing the roof to collapse. Look out for the hazard of roof collapse if heavy ash amasses.[31,32]
7. Failure to watch out for signs of fire if sheltering indoors. A red-hot pyroclastic rock can ignite a roof very quickly.

REFERENCE

1. Small C, Naumann T. The global distribution of human population and recent volcanism. *Environmental Hazards*. 2001;3:93–109.
2. Simkin T, Siebert L, Blong R. Disasters: volcanic fatalities – lessons from the historical record. *Science*. 2001;5502:255.
3. US Geological Survey. Types and Effects of Volcanic Hazards. Available at: http://volcanoes.usgs.gov/hazards/what/hazards.html.
4. Bernstein RS, Baxter PJ, Buist AS. Introduction to the epidemiological aspects of explosive volcanism. *Am J Public Health*. 1986;76(3 Suppl):3–9.
5. US Geological Survey. Volcanic Gases and Their Effects. Available at: http://volcanoes.usgs.gov/hazards/what/volgas/volgas.html.
6. Newhall CG, Fruchter JS. Volcanic activity: a review for health professionals. *Am J Public Health*. 1986;76(3 Suppl):10–24.
7. US Geological Survey. Effects of Pyroclastic Surge at Mount St Helens, Washington, May 18, 1980. Available at: http://volcanoes.usgs.gov/hazards/effects/MSHsurge_effects.html.
8. Decker RW, Decker BB. *Mountains of Fire: The Nature of Volcanoes*. New York: Cambridge University Press; 1991:1–40.
9. US Geological Survey. Dome Collapses Generate Pyroclastic Flows at Unzen volcano, Japan. Available at: http://volcanoes.usgs.gov/hazards/what/pf/PFUzn.html.
10. US Geological Survey. Effects of Pyroclastic Flows and Surges at Soufriere Hills Volcano, Montserrat. Available at: http://volcanoes.usgs.gov/hazards/effects/SoufriereHills_PFeffects.html.
11. Baxter PJ, Gresham A. Deaths and injuries in eruption of Galeras Volcano, Colombia, 14 January 1993. *J Volcanology Geothermal Research*. 1997;77:325–338.

12. Martin TR, Covert D, Butler J. Inhaling volcanic ash. *Chest.* 1981; 80(1 Suppl):85–88.

13. Searl A, Nicholl A, Baxter PJ. Assessment of the exposure of islanders to ash from the Soufriere Hills volcano, Montserrat, British West Indies. *Occup Environ Med.* 2002;59:523–531.

14. Baxter PJ, Ing R, Falk H, Plikaytis B. Mount St. Helens eruptions: the acute respiratory effects of volcanic ash in a North American community. *Arch Environ Health.* 1983;38(3):138–143.

15. Baxter PJ, Berstein MD, Buist AS. Preventative health measures in volcanic eruptions. *Am J Public Health.* 1986;76(3 Suppl):84–90.

16. US Geological Survey. Long-lasting Eruption of Kilauea Volcano, Hawai`I Leads to Volcanic-Air Pollution. Available at: http://volcanoes.usgs.gov/hazards/what/VolGas/Volgaspollution.html.

17. Olson KR, et al. *Poisoning and drug overdose.* 3rd ed. Stamford, Conn: Appleton & Lange; 1999:181–188.

18. Mannino DM, Ruben S, et al. Emergency department visits and hospitalizations for respiratory disease on the island of Hawaii, 1981 to 1991. *Hawaii Med J.* 1996;55:48–54.

19. US Geological Survey. "What's That Cloud Upriver?" An Eyewitness Account of a Lahar by USGS Geologist Jeff Marso. Available at: http://volcanoes.usgs.gov/hazards/what/lahars/santiaguito_89.html.

20. US Geological Survey. *Intense Rainfall During Hurricane Mitch Triggers Deadly Landslide and Lahar at Casita Volcano,* Nicaragua, October 30, 1998. Available at: http://volcanoes.usgs.gov/hazards/what/lahars/casitalahar.html.

21. US Geological Survey. Earthquake on June 6, 1994, Triggers Landslides and Catastrophic Lahar Near Nevado del Huila Volcano, Colombia. Available at: http://volcanoes.usgs.gov/hazards/what/lahars/huilalahar.html.

22. US Geological Survey. Lahars Caused by Lake Breakouts. Available at: http://volcanoes.usgs.gov/Hazards/What/Lahars/LakeLahar.html.

23. Baxter PJ, Kapila M, Mfonfu D. Lake Nyos disaster, Cameroon, 1986: the medical effects of large scale emission of carbon dioxide? *BMJ.* 1989;298:1437–1441.

24. Dent AW, Davies G, Barrett P, de Saint Ours PJ. The 1994 eruption of the Rabaul volcano, Papua New Guinea: injuries sustained and medical response. *Med J Aust.* 1995;163:536–539.

25. Newhall CG, Self S. The Volcanic Explosivity Index (VEI): an estimate of explosive magnitude for historical volcanism. *J Geophys Res (Oceans & Atmospheres).* 1982;87:1231–1238.

26. How to survive a volcanic eruption. Available at: http://www.survivethat.com/how-to-survive-a-volcanic-eruption/. Accessed 03/14, 2014.

27. Pan American Health Organization. Volcanoes: Protecting the Public's Health. Available at: http://www.mona.uwi.edu/cardin/virtual_library/docs/1258/1258.pdf. Accessed 03/14, 2014.

28. Aiuppa A, Moretti R, Federico C, Giudice G, Gurrieri S, Liuzzo M, Papale P, Shinohara H, Valenza M. Forecasting Etna eruptions by real-time observation of volcanic gas composition. *Geology.* 2007; 35(12):1115–1118.

29. New York Committee for Occupational Safety and Health. NYCOSH WTC Factsheet 4: Cleaning Up Indoor Dust and Debris in the World Trade Center Area. Available at: http://www.nycosh.org/environment_wtc/wtc-dust-factsheet.html.

30. Geography of Volcanoes. Volcanoes - Blogspot.com. Available at: http://www.geographyofvolcanoes.blogspot.com/. Accessed 03/14, 2014.

31. Extreme Survive. Volcano Survival - Croatian Outdoor Survival School. Available at: https://sites.google.com/a/extremesurvive.com/extreme-survive/not-usual-tips/volcano-survival. Accessed 03/14, 2014.

32. Clyde. How to Survive a Volcano. Available at: http://www.doomsdayprepperforums.com/index.php?threads/how-to-survive-a-volcanic-eruption.78/. Accessed 03/14, 2014.

33. Hansell AL, Horwell CJ, Oppenheimer C. The health hazards of volcanoes and geothermal areas. *Occup Environ Med.* 2006;63(2):149–156, 125.

102 | CHAPTER

Famine

Laura Macnow and Hilarie Cranmer

DESCRIPTION OF EVENT

Famine is the most extreme form of food insecurity (i.e., lack of access to enough food). It is often the result of natural or human-made disasters. Famine has been defined as "a condition of populations in which a substantial increase in deaths is associated with inadequate food consumption."[1] Natural disasters such as droughts and floods, crop infestations, and livestock diseases that limit a population's food production are often considered as events that precipitate a famine. However, insufficient access to food is now more commonly seen as the result of war, civil strife, and economic collapse. A famine is usually caused by an exacerbation of the preexisting conditions of poverty, debt, underemployment, and high malnutrition in a population; so when additional burdens arise, widespread starvation can occur rapidly.[2]

Famine is a complex emergency often involving massive population displacements between and within countries, and, as such, a famine complicates the ability of agencies to coordinate relief efforts and provide ongoing surveillance of the emergency. While famine is understood as an extreme manifestation of the food insecurity of a population, the term "famine" has been controversial. Ambiguities in the definition and usage of the term have resulted in far-reaching and sometimes tragic implications for timely response and accountability of relief agencies in a number of recent food crises.[3] The development of a common standard by which the intensity and magnitude of food insecurity can be measured has been of great consequence in mobilizing relief during periods of such severe food crises, and these measurements are now tied to the livelihoods of the population as well as the medical outcome of lack of food.

The usual medical consequences of mass starvation during a famine are increased malnutrition and mortality.[4] The manifestations of starvation depend on the individual's previous nutritional status, age, and the severity of food deprivation.[5] The objective physical or laboratory findings of physical deterioration as the result of inadequate nutrient intake are referred to as malnutrition, which encompasses a range of conditions, including severe acute malnutrition (characterized by wasting), chronic malnutrition (characterized by stunting or nutritional edema), and micronutrient deficiencies.[6]

To assess the prevalence of moderate to severe malnutrition in a population, it is a commonly accepted practice to carry out anthropometric surveys in a random sample of children younger than 5 years using the weight-for-height (WFH) index.[2,6] These data are a reliable indicator of malnutrition in the wider population. Because weight is more sensitive to sudden changes in food availability,[2] the WFH index is used instead of height-for-age (which measures stunting). The mean upper arm circumference (MUAC) can also be measured to screen for acute malnutrition. This parameter has been endorsed by the World Health Organization (WHO) as an independent criterion for admission in therapeutic feeding programs (TFPs).[7] Measurement of MUAC is simple and can be easily taught to community-based workers, making early screening and treatment possible in resource-poor areas.[8] The presence of nutritional edema (*kwashiorkor*), however, may confound these indices, and clinical judgment must be used in their evaluation. Additionally, anthropometric data may be skewed by concurrent mortality rates. Anthropometric data are commonly interpreted using z-scores (or standard deviation [SD] scores) where

$$z\text{-score (or SD score)} = \frac{\text{Observed measured value} - \text{Average value in reference population}}{\text{SD value of reference population}}$$

The WHO Global Database on Child Growth and Malnutrition[9] uses a z-score cut-off point of less than −2 SD to classify low weight-for-age, low height-for-age, and low WFH as moderate and severe undernutrition, and less than −3 SD to define severe acute malnutrition.[9] If more than 8% of the children samples have a z-score of less than −2, a nutritional emergency exists. An excess of even 1% of children with z-scores of less than −3 indicates a need for immediate action.[2] When using MUAC, a measurement of <115 mm in children 6 months to 5 years of age is a reliable indicator of severe acute malnutrition that reflects high mortality risk and requires immediate therapeutic intervention including food and antibiotics.[8]

Famines are often assessed and reported in terms of cases, rates, or degrees of malnutrition, or the number of deaths from malnutrition and its complications. The Integrated Food Security Phase Classification (IPC) categorizes an "emergency" as a condition in which severe acute malnutrition is seen in 15% to 30% of the population, and the crude mortality rate (CMR) is 1 to 2 deaths per 10,000 population per day or children under 5 mortality rate (U5MR) is 2 to 4 deaths per 10,000 population per day; "famine" has severe acute malnutrition seen in >30% of the population, with a CMR of >2 deaths per 10,000 population per day or U5MR of >4 deaths per 10,000 population per day.[10]

Although the most direct and obvious results of famine are severe malnutrition and death, the immediate cause of death in affected individuals is usually a communicable disease, most commonly measles, diarrheal illness, acute respiratory infections (ARIs), and malaria. Displaced populations almost always experience higher CMRs compared with nondisplaced populations, and this is likely due to the increased risk of communicable disease associated with crowded and often unsanitary camps, interruption in vaccination programming, and lack of access to basic health care and treatment strategies. Malnutrition predisposes individuals to certain micronutrient deficiencies, notably vitamin A deficiency; communicable diseases such as measles and diarrhea further deplete vitamin A stores and can cause worsening immune compromise and xerophthalmia, corneal xerosis, and ulceration and scarring, and can eventually lead to blindness.[2] Other important micronutrient deficiencies include vitamin C, niacin, iron, iodine, and thiamine deficiency. Updated guidelines include treating children with human immunodeficiency virus (HIV) and infants under 6 months.

PRE-INCIDENT ACTIONS

- Advance detection and monitoring of economic, social, and environmental factors that influence the development of food shortages and famine.
- Early warning systems may rely on community involvement. Local people can collect data on what they see as the signs of growing food insecurity. For example, an increase in the number of animals sold in local markets may indicate that families need cash to buy food because their crops have failed.[11] The Famine Early Warning Systems Network (FEWS NET) has been a provider of early warning analysis on acute food security issues by collecting data from local reporters and a variety of sources, including national ministries of trade and agriculture, international organizations, nongovernmental organizations (NGOs), and U.S. science agencies such as National Aeronautics and Space Administration (NASA), National Oceanic and Atmospheric Administration (NOAA), and U.S. Geological Survey (USGS), to create specialized reports on weather and climate changes, regional market and trade data, and agricultural production information. FEWS NET utilizes IPC standards to track likely crises and create maps and reports that detail current and projected food insecurities. Level 5 is considered to be the most severe. IPC uses both livelihood measures (or means of self-support) and measurements of mortality and child malnutrition to categorize a situation as food secure, food insecure, food crisis, famine, severe famine, and extreme famine. The number of deaths determines the magnitude designation, with under 1000 fatalities defining a "minor famine" and a "catastrophic famine" resulting in over 1,000,000 deaths.[12]
- Support of socially responsible community development, including education about preserving the huge local ranges of hardy crop types and encouraging food production of a wide variety of crops that are bred to be hardy and which are grown together in a robust mixed-crop pattern.
- These pre-incident actions will help communities recover quickly in the event of natural disasters.[11] Monocropping can increase vulnerability in times of natural or economic disasters, as can deforestation, desertification, and poor agricultural practices.[2]
- Coordination of relief agencies
- Development of standard case management protocols
- Establishment of reserves of essential supplies (medical and nutritional)
- Development of environmental management plans

POST-INCIDENT ACTIONS

- Media and worldwide notification
- Perform field assessment: determine total displaced population, age-sex breakdown, and average family-household size; identify at-risk groups (children <5 years old including infants under 6 months, pregnant and lactating women, the elderly, disabled or wounded persons, and those with HIV). This information is needed to estimate quantities of relief supplies and for effective surveillance of mortality and morbidity rates.
- Initiate health and nutrition surveillance systems

- Assess prior health and nutritional status, and determine prevalence of severe acute malnutrition and micronutrient deficiencies in children and infants younger than 5 years old (this serves as a proxy for malnutrition in the general population)
- Calculate crude, age-, sex-, and cause-specific mortality and morbidity rates of diseases
- Assess local community resources, and determine important health beliefs and traditions
- Evaluate livelihood measures and means of self-support in the community
- Evaluate environmental conditions, such as water sources, sanitation arrangements, local disease vectors and epidemiology, and availability of materials for shelter and fuel
- Evaluate resources such as food supplies and distribution systems, and assess logistics for food transport and storage
- Ensure ongoing surveillance of communities' health and nutritional status and evaluate the effectiveness of the intervention and quality of care delivered[2]

MEDICAL TREATMENT OF CASUALTIES

Medical treatment of victims of famine must include preventive as well as curative measures. Regardless of immunization status, all children up to age 16 should be immunized against measles. If vaccine supplies are limited, higher-risk children (up to age 5) should be immunized preferentially. One should never withhold immunization because of fever, ARI, diarrhea, HIV, or malnutrition. Vitamin A treatment should be instituted concomitantly. All children with clinical measles should receive 200,000 International Units of oral vitamin A (half-dose for children <12 months); children with complicated measles should receive a second dose on day 2. Individuals with eye symptoms of vitamin A deficiency should receive 200,000 International Units of oral vitamin A on day 1, day 2, and then again 1 to 4 weeks later (half-dose for children <12 months).

Diarrheal illness in malnourished populations is generally caused by the same pathogens that cause diarrhea in developing countries: *Escherichia coli*, *Shigella*, and *Salmonella*. Oral rehydration therapy (ORT) is a mainstay in the treatment of diarrhea, and chemotherapy should not be used for routine treatment of uncomplicated, watery diarrhea unless cholera, *Shigella*, *Giardia*, or amoebic dysentery is suspected. Preventive measures are extremely important in control of diarrheal illness. These measures include providing adequate quantities of clean water, good sanitation, personal hygiene education, and promotion of breast-feeding of infants.[2,6]

Nutritional interventions can be categorized as general ration distribution to the affected population, blanket supplementary feeding to all members of an identified risk group, targeted dry (take-home) supplementary feeding centers for the moderately malnourished, and therapeutic feeding centers for the severely malnourished. General rations must supply at least 2100 kcal per person per day, of which 17% of calories are in the form of fats and 12% of calories are derived from protein.[6]

Food should ideally be distributed in a community setting so as to avoid the risk of communicable disease associated with mass feeding centers, and adequate fuel and cooking utensils should be made available. Supplemental feeding programs should be provided to acutely undernourished children younger than 5 years old, pregnant and lactating women, elderly individuals, and chronically ill individuals. The disadvantage of dry (take-home) supplemental feedings is that sharing of the rations among family members is likely. TFPs are reserved for children with severe acute malnutrition (z-score of less than −3, clinical edema); feedings and antibiotics are provided on-site, rather than at resource-intensive centers. These children should receive 150 kcal and 3 g of protein for each kilogram of body weight in four to six feedings per day.[2] Nasogastric feedings may be needed. Close monitoring is essential, and weight gain should be targeted to 10 g per 1 kg of body weight per day.

There has been a movement toward treating severely malnourished individuals without complications in a community setting. Children with severe acute malnutrition with complications are defined as having any of the following conditions:

1. Severe generalized pitting edema
2. Marasmic kwashiorkor (i.e., both MUAC <115 mm and mild to moderate edema)
3. MUAC <115 mm or mild to moderate edema with one of the following: anorexia, lower respiratory infection, anemia, fever, severe dehydration, or lethargy[8]

TFPs have serious limitations, and there have been suggestions that community-based therapeutic care is likely to be more successful. TFPs are resource intensive and require skilled staff and imported therapeutic products. International standards require one care provider for every 10 patients, with a maximum of 100 patients per center.[13] Criticisms of TFPs include that they take months to become operational, have low coverage, are extremely expensive, undermine local health infrastructure, disempower communities, and promote the congregation of people around them, increasing the risk of communicable diseases.[13] Admitted children usually depend on the presence of their mothers to care for them around the clock, taking the mothers away from their community and decreasing their ability to look after their other children. Community-based therapeutic care, on the other hand, may be as successful overall as TFPs in decreasing overall mortality, while being more cost effective and less disruptive for communities and families. A ready-to-use therapeutic food (RUTF) made from peanuts, dried skimmed milk, sugar, and a specially formulated mineral and vitamin mix can be distributed in the form of a paste, which prevents it from spoiling for several months, and is equally nutritious as TFP feedings. Proponents of community-based therapeutic care suggest that, when used to complement TFPs, overall death rates from starvation can be reduced while providing socioeconomic and educational benefits for the families of the malnourished.[13]

UNIQUE CONSIDERATIONS

The demographic groups that are most at risk during famine are young children and women, and it is important that the establishment of maternal and child health (MCH) care be given high priority to provide care for pregnant and lactating women and children younger than 2 years of age. Services should include health education as well as routine monitoring, immunization, nutritional rehabilitation, micronutrient supplementation, and curative care. Breast-feeding should be encouraged for children, minimally up to the age of 6 months, and preferably up to 2 years of age regardless of the HIV status. Local female health workers should be trained to provide culturally appropriate education and care. Ideally, one MCH clinic per 5000 population should be set up.[2]

! PITFALLS

- Failure to recognize early warning signs of famine including the consideration of livelihoods and childhood indicators of severe acute malnutrition and mortality
- Failure to mobilize resources and coordinate relief agencies
- Neglect of preventive programs (e.g., immunizations, ORT, and hygiene education), and failure to prevent communicable diseases
- Failure to preferentially target vulnerable populations
- Lack of variety in basic relief rations (risk of micronutrient deficiencies)
- Underutilization of community-based therapeutic care
- Failure to recognize the importance of cultural practices, beliefs, and taboos, and failure to involve the displaced community and its leaders in relief work

REFERENCES

1. Toole MJ, Foster S. Famines. In: Gregg MB, ed. *The Public Health Consequences Disasters*. Atlanta: US Department of Health and Human Services, Public Health Service, Centers for Disease Control and Prevention; 1989:79–89.
2. Centers for Disease Control and Prevention. Famine-affected, refugee, and displaced populations: recommendations for public health issues. *MMWR Recomm Rep*. 1992;41(RR-13):1–76.
3. Howe P, Devereux S. Famine intensity and magnitude scales: a proposal for an instrumental definition of famine. *Disasters*. 2004;28:353–372.
4. Noji EK. *The Public Health Consequences of Disaster*. New York: Oxford University Press; 1997.
5. Graham G. Starvation in the modern world. *N Engl J Med*. 1993;328:1058–1061.
6. The Sphere Project. Minimum standards in food security, nutrition and food aid. In Sphere Handbook, 2011 Revised Edition. Available at: http://www.sphereproject.org/handbook/.
7. Mogeni P, Twahir H, Bandika V, et al. Diagnostic performance of visible severe wasting for identifying severe acute malnutrition in children admitted to hospital in Kenya. *Bull World Health Organ*. 2011;89:900–906.
8. Collins S, Dent N, Binns P, et al. Management of severe acute malnutrition in children. *Lancet*. 2006;368:1992–2000.
9. World Health Organization. WHO Global Database on Child Growth and Malnutrition. Available at: http://www.who.int/nutgrowthdb.
10. IPC Global Partners. *Integrated Food Security Phase Classification: Technical Manual Version 2.0*. Available at: http://www.ipcinfo.org/fileadmin/user_upload/ipcinfo/docs/IPC-Manual-2-Interactive.pdf. Accessed July 20, 2014.
11. International Federation of Red Cross and Red Crescent Societies. *World disasters report: focus on reducing risk*. Geneva: International Federation of Red Cross; 2002.
12. Famine Early Warning Systems Network. Available at: http://www.fews.net/our-work. Accessed August 10, 2014.
13. Collins S. Changing the way we address severe malnutrition during famine. *Lancet*. 2001;358:498–501.

CHAPTER 103

Landslides*

Mark E. Keim

DESCRIPTION OF EVENT

Type of Events

The term *landslide* includes a wide range of ground movements. This chapter uses the landslide terminology presented by Varnes[1] and Cruden and Varnes[2] to include all types of gravity-induced mass movements, ranging from rock falls through slides and slumps, avalanches, and flows. The term includes both subaerial and submarine mass movements triggered mainly by precipitation (including snowmelt), seismic activity, and volcanic eruptions. These mass movements may be further categorized as wet and dry. Dry mass movements are gravity-induced slope failures, rock falls, slides, and slumps that are not associated with precipitation or surface water. Wet mass movements (also known as "debris flows") include mudflows, debris torrents, and lahars (volcanic debris flows). Debris flows are fast-moving landslides that occur in a wide range of environments. A debris flow contains water and material that is mainly sand, gravel, and cobbles, but typically also includes trees, cars, small buildings, and other anthropogenic material. A debris flow typically has the consistency of wet concrete and moves at speeds in excess of 16 meters per second (35 miles per hour).[3]

Although the primary reason for a landslide is gravity acting on an oversteepened slope, there are other contributing factors[4]:

- Erosion by rivers, glaciers, or ocean waves creates oversteepened slopes.
- Rock and soil slopes are weakened through saturation by snowmelt or heavy rains.
- Earthquakes create stresses that make weak slopes fail.
- Earthquakes of magnitude 4.0 and greater have been known to trigger landslides.
- Volcanic eruptions produce loose ash deposits, heavy rain, and debris flows.
- Excess weight from accumulation of rain or snow, stockpiling of rock or ore, waste piles, or human-made structures may stress weak slopes to the point of failure.

Historical Events

The world's largest landslides are prehistoric. Their remains are displayed as significant morphological features on the earth's surface. Most very large landslides were triggered by earthquakes or volcanic eruptions.[5]

The world's largest historic landslide is the 1980 Mount St. Helens rock slide-/debris avalanche in the Cascade Range of southwestern Washington State in the United States, which was triggered by a catastrophic volcanic eruption.[6] This 24-km long, 2.8 km³ landslide buried about 60 km² of the North Fork Toutle River valley under hummocky, poorly sorted debris ranging from clay to blocks of volcanic rocks with individual volumes as large as several thousand cubic meters.[1]

SCOPE OF IMPACT

Landslides occur annually in every state and U.S. territory. The Appalachian and Rocky mountains, the Pacific coastal ranges, and some parts of Alaska and Hawaii have severe landslide problems. Landslides cost an estimated $1 billion to $3 billion per year in the U.S. alone. From 1990 to 1999, landslides were second only to hurricanes as the leading cause of death due to environmental disasters in the hazard-prone Pacific basin (four times more than earthquakes and thirty times more than volcanoes).[7]

Landslides and debris flows triggered by earthquakes accounted for most of the fatalities and serious injuries in several major earthquakes of the twentieth century, including those in Peru (1970), Tajikistan (1989), the Philippines (1990), and Colombia (1994).[8]

Wet mass movements have a much greater human impact than dry mass movements. Between 1900 and 2014, the world's 10 largest wet mass movements affected 11.6 million people, killing 26,348; during the same time period, the ten largest dry mass movements affected a total of 26,570 people and killed 3553.[9] During one recent decade (2002-2011), 197 mass movements were reported worldwide. One quarter of these events occurred in nations categorized as having very high or high human development according to the United Nation Development Program Human Development Index.[10] Slightly over half of these 197 mass movements occurred in medium human development countries and the remainder occurred in countries with low human development indices. All but seven of these events were wet mass movements that affected 3.9 million people and caused 9552 deaths. The remaining seven were dry mass movements that affected 4000 and caused 271 deaths.[11]

Landslides may also produce flash floods as a result of debris striking surface water or causing dam failures.[12] In 1985, a lahar from the Nevada del Ruiz volcano traveled over 30 miles and killed at least 23,000 people.[13] In 1999, rainstorms induced thousands of landslides along the coast of northern Venezuela and resulted in a death toll estimated at 19,000 to 30,000 people and total damage estimated at $1.9 billion (Fig. 103-1).[3,14]

Common Health Impacts

Landslides impact public health by causing injuries and severe property destruction. Landslide mortality is largely related to trauma and asphyxiation. Landslide morbidity is largely associated with traumatic

---

*The material in this chapter reflects solely the views of the author. It does not necessarily reflect the policies or recommendations of the Centers for Disease Control and Prevention or the U.S. Department of Health and Human Services.

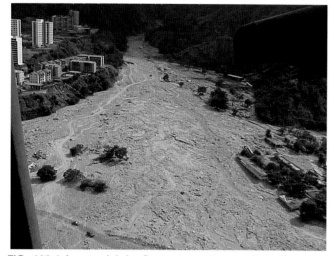

FIG 103-1 Large debris flow channel caused during 1999 Venezuela landslides. (Photo courtesy of Mark Keim, MD 2000.)

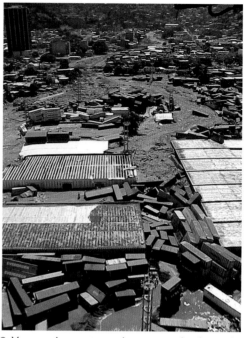

FIG 103-3 Venezuelan port warehouses storing hazardous materials were inundated by debris flow in 1999. (Photo courtesy of Mark Keim, MD 2000.)

injuries and a disruption of water, sanitation, shelter, and the locally grown food supply for the affected population.[15] There have also been case reports of crush syndrome associated with landslides.[16]

Besides direct injury, landslides also have a direct impact on the public health of the affected population by way of displacement. In 2010 multiple landslides in eastern Uganda displaced a total of over 5000 people. The majority of these people sought shelter in impromptu camps with limited access to safe water and poor conditions for sanitation and hygiene.[17]

Survivors of landslides that occurred in Taiwan in 2010 had an increased incidence of mental illness, including posttraumatic stress disorder and major depressive disorder, as well as a higher risk for suicide. Female gender and lack of family support were identified as key risk factors (Fig. 103-2).[18]

Unusual Health Impacts

Landslides triggered during the 1994 Northridge earthquake resulted in an outbreak of 203 cases of coccidiodomycosis when arthrospores were spread in dust clouds.[19] The levels of cultivable *Vibrio cholera* counts in suspended particulate matter and their distribution in the Karnaphuli

estuary, Bangladesh, were compared before and after a strong cyclone in mid-May 2007 and again after a monsoon-triggered landslide a month later. The cyclone did not significantly change previous fecal coliform abundance; however, there was a tenfold increase in cultivable *V. cholera* counts (CVC) after the landslide.[20] While this event was not associated with a notable cholera outbreak, these findings illustrate the potential for spread of waterborne pathogens as a result of landslides, specifically in low human development nations.

Debris flows associated with massive floods in northern Venezuela on December 16 and 17, 1999, destroyed part of the port facilities in La Guaira. The port facilities contained customs warehouses known to store hazardous materials including corrosives, organic solvents, oxidants, compressed gases, heavy metals, and explosives. These chemicals were inundated by the debris flow and came dangerously close to causing an explosion and toxic exposure, with the potential to affect 80,000 nearby residents, as well as close that nation's largest airport and second largest seaport (Fig. 103-3).[21,22]

◀◀ PRE-INCIDENT ACTIONS

Landslides usually strike without warning. Pre-incident actions toward prevention, preparedness, and mitigation are therefore by far the most effective means of protecting life and property.

Although the physical cause of many landslides cannot be removed, geological investigations, good engineering practices, and effective enforcement of land use management regulations can reduce landslide hazards.[4]

Two mitigation strategies can be implemented to protect property: (1) large structural flood control measures and (2) avoidance of the affected area. Land use regulations can reduce hazards by limiting the type or amount of development in high risk areas. Landslide risk analysis offers a quantitative procedure for zoning that can also be used as a preventive tool, through its application to strategic environmental impact analysis (SEIA) of land use plans.[23] In high-risk zones where development and reconstruction are inevitable, steps such as orienting

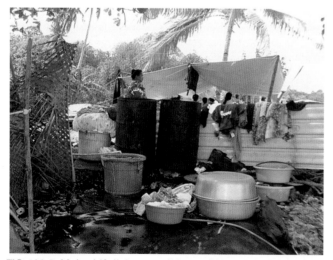

FIG 103-2 Makeshift living conditions of homeless family after 2002 landslides in Chuuk, Micronesia. (Photo courtesy of Mark Keim, MD 2002.)

buildings and streets parallel to the downslope direction of debris flows will minimize the width of the building exposed and allow streets to serve as overflow channels.[3]

Monitoring, warning, and evacuation are nonstructural approaches to hazard mitigation that can reduce potential loss of life. Early warning systems based on weather forecasts and rainfall information can substantially improve emergency managers' ability to warn and evacuate threatened communities. Many cities, including Hong Kong, San Francisco, and Denver, use warning systems such as sirens and radio bulletins to alert residents of potentially threatening conditions.[3] The public, first responders, emergency managers, and decision makers should be educated regarding potential hazards as well as emergency preparedness, mitigation, and response measures.[24]

Box 103-1 provides a list of areas that are generally more prone to landslide hazards.[3,25] Box 103-2 provides a list of things homeowners should do if they suspect that their home is at risk from a potential landslide.[25] Box 103-3 is a list of landslide warning signs.[25]

BOX 103-1   Areas Generally More Prone to Landslide Hazards[4,25]

- On existing old landslides
- On existing alluvial fans
- On or at the base of slopes
- In or at the base of minor drainage hollows
- At the base or top of an old fill slope
- At the base or top of a steep cut slope
- Developed hillsides where leach field septic systems are used

---

BOX 103-2   What to Do if You Suspect That Your Home Is at Risk for Landslide Danger[25]

- Learn to recognize warning signs of a landslide (Box 103-3).
- Purchase flood insurance policies from the National Flood Insurance Program.
- Do not build near steep slopes, close to mountain edges, near drainage ways, or in natural erosion valleys.
- Contact local officials, state geological surveys or departments of natural resources, and university departments of geology. Ask for information on landslides in your area and areas vulnerable to landslides. Request a professional referral for a detailed site analysis of your property with corrective measures you can take if necessary.
- Watch the patterns of stormwater drainage near your home. Note the places where runoff water converges and increases flow in channels. These are areas to avoid during a storm.
- Learn about the emergency response and evacuation plans for your area. Develop your own emergency plan for your family or business. Develop an emergency communication plan in case family members get separated.
- Minimize home hazards.
  - Plant groundcover on slopes and build retaining walls.
  - In mudflow areas, build channels or deflection walls to direct the flow around buildings.
    - If you build walls to divert debris flow and the flow lands on a neighbor's property, you may be liable for damages.
  - Have flexible pipe fittings installed to avoid gas or water leaks, as flexible fittings are more resistant to breakage. Only the gas company or professionals should install gas fittings.

BOX 103-3   Landslide Warning Signs[4,25]

- Springs, seeps, or saturated ground in areas that have not typically been wet before
- New cracks or unusual bulges in the ground, street pavements, or sidewalks, especially at the base of a slope
- Soil moving away from foundations
- Ancillary structures such as decks and patios tilting or moving relative to the main house
- Tilting or cracking of concrete floors, tile, brick, or foundations
- Broken water lines or other underground utilities
- Leaning telephone poles, trees, retaining walls, or fences
- Offset fence lines
- Sunken or dropped roadbeds
- Rapid increase in creek water levels
- Sudden decrease in creek water levels though rain is still falling or just recently stopped
- Sticking doors and windows and visible open spaces indicating jambs and frames out of plumb for the first time
- A rumbling sound that increases in volume as the landslide nears

---

POST-INCIDENT ACTIONS

Landslides in populated areas are associated with high rates of traumatic injury and mortality. If there is an imminent risk of landslides, individuals should stay alert and awake. Many debris-flow fatalities occur when people are sleeping. Those who live within the United States can listen to a National Oceanographic and Atmospheric Administration (NOAA) Weather Radio or a portable, battery-powered radio or television for warnings of intense rainfall. They should be especially alert when driving. Embankments along roadsides are particularly susceptible to landslides.[25] During a landslide, persons at risk should take immediate steps to get out of the downslope path of the flow or, if unable to evacuate, to protect themselves inside of a building. If escape is not possible, individuals should attempt to curl up into a ball and protect their heads.[25] Box 103-4 contains a list of recommendations for actions to be considered after a landslide has occurred.[25]

Whenever possible, search and rescue operations should be performed by properly trained and adequately equipped professional rescuers. Incident commanders need to establish safety zones immediately. Soil engineers should be called and an emergency warning system, such as a siren blowing steadily for 30 seconds, immediately implemented. In the safety briefing on the Incident Action Plan, the incident commander should stress that evacuation and "all-clear" signals must be obeyed immediately.

The literature on landslide rescues is scanty. The following general guidelines for safety zones are recommended[24]:

1. *Cold zone:*
   a. 100 feet from the outside edge of each side of the debris flow in situations involving stream order 1 situations ("stream order" is the geological classification of drainages, the number increasing as the size and number of drainages increase)
   b. 1000 feet from the sides and base of debris flows that are occurring on slopes that are 26 degrees or greater and involve areas with stream orders 2 to 4
   c. 500 feet from the sides and base of flows in stream order 5 and above that occur at the mouth of large canyons and have largely ceased flowing

All of these recommendations are based on weather reports of diminishing or ceasing rainfall. If it continues to rain, all distances should be

---

BOX 103-4 Actions to Be Considered After a Landslide Has Occurred[25]

- Avoid the landslide area as much as possible. There may be a danger of additional slides.
- Check for injured or trapped persons near the slide area. Survival is more likely near the slide periphery.
- Provide first aid to injured persons and activate emergency medical services if necessary.
- Report the event to your local fire, police, or public works department.
- Inform and assist affected neighbors, especially those that may require special assistance such as infants, the elderly, or persons with disabilities.
- Listen to a battery-operated radio or television for the latest emergency information.
- Watch for flooding, which may occur after a landslide or debris flow.
- Look for and report broken utility lines to appropriate authorities.
- Check the building foundation, chimney, and surrounding land for damage.
- Replant damaged ground as soon as possible because erosion caused by loss of groundcover can lead to flash flooding.
- Seek the advice of a geotechnical expert for evaluating landslide hazards or designing corrective techniques to reduce landslide risk in future.
- Support your local government in efforts to develop and enforce land use and building ordinances that regulate construction in areas susceptible to landslides and debris flows.

---

increased. The margin of safety is dependent upon variables at the specific site including soil, topography, precipitation, and vegetation.

2. *Warm zone:* Inside the distances above, up to the edge of the flow. Safety gear should be worn by all personnel in that zone.
3. *Hot zone:* On the debris field. All personnel on the field should have complete safety gear. All personnel should be logged in and out of warm and hot zones.

With respect to personal safety equipment for rescuers: some sort of foot and leg protection is mandatory. Personal flotation devices should be worn if there is danger of further flows. Helmets and harnesses should be worn on steep slopes. A harness—at a minimum, a tubular webbing "hasty" harness—should be worn, even on reasonably flat terrain, in case the rescuer becomes entrapped. Additional equipment might include work gloves, a small backpack or load-bearing rig for water bottles or a "camelback" irrigation system, small folding shovels, face masks, and goggles. All rescuers should be tethered from dry ground if possible.

Small inflatable rafts can assist rescuers crossing soft mud, as can a stable work platform. An air-filled hose can be laced back and forth through a roof ladder and then filled with air to make a field-expedient raft, or simply pulled out onto the mud as a handhold. Technical and urban search and rescue (USAR)-type gear that can be used includes ropes, A-frames and confined-space tripods, plywood and shoring materials, and rescue hardware such as carabiners and pulleys.

Chances of survival in a debris flow or mudslide are best on the edges and decrease toward the center. Most survivors are found in a zone that makes up about a quarter of the flow width, immediately along its edges. As a result, most rescues can be conducted using simple techniques from dry ground.

If a victim is mired more than waist deep, shore-based thrown lines are not likely to work as there is too much suction on the victim. Thus rescuers need to go out to the victim. Extrication techniques rely on breaking the suction. The two best techniques use water or air. The water technique requires a 1-inch-diameter fire hose with a metal "root wand" affixed to the end. This is shoved into the debris along the edge of the victim's body. When the water is turned on, it creates a "slurry" next to the victim and releases the suction. The air technique involves use of a self-contained breathing apparatus (SCBA) bottle and a rigid hose that can be shoved down into the mud. Air charged into the mud creates large air bubbles that help break the suction. It may become necessary to build an "island" around the victim so a vertical pull can be attempted, using either a ladder A-frame or a tripod. A combination of air and water techniques may free victims trapped all the way to their necks. Rescuers should also remain vigilant of the possibility of exposure to hazardous materials and should plan appropriately for HazMat response and facilities for gross decontamination of rescuers at the scene.

✚ MEDICAL TREATMENT OF CASUALTIES

The treatment of landslide casualties is the same as that for other causes of traumatic injury. In the case of mass casualties, an incident management system should be established and a system for triage of casualty care should be in place. After extended entrapments, extricated victims may have medical complications including hypothermia, impaired airway, crush syndrome, and compartment syndrome.

❓ UNIQUE CONSIDERATIONS AND PITFALLS

The single most important issue to keep in mind regarding landslides is the priority of pre-incident prevention and mitigation efforts. Landslide morbidity and mortality can be high, yet many of these deaths and injuries are preventable with an appropriate level of pre-incident intervention. In most cases, emergency response is often too little and too late to have a significant impact. The major pitfall of emergency management related to landslides is an over-reliance upon response instead of the much more cost-effective method of prevention and mitigation. This challenge is exacerbated by an unrealistically low perception of risk frequently found in populations that live in significant danger from landslide disasters.[26,27]

Global climate change will increase the probability of extreme weather events and thus landslides associated with high precipitation events.[28,29] Such events create significant public health needs that can exceed the local capacity to respond, resulting in excess morbidity or mortality and in the declaration of disasters. Because adaptation must occur at the community level, local public health agencies are uniquely placed to build human resilience to climate-related disasters, including landslides.[30]

Another pitfall is underestimating the public health needs of those populations displaced by the disaster.[15] In addition to an obvious lack of food, security, shelter, and adequate sanitation, these populations are prone to additional injuries, disease, and lingering mental illness (Fig. 103-2). Identification of landslide fatalities can be quite difficult, complicated by the fact that recovered remains can be fragmented or severely degraded with few morphological features present. DNA typing of remains and relatives may be a necessary component of fatality management and must be considered when planning disaster mortuary response.[31]

ACKNOWLEDGEMENT

A special thank you to Ritu Sarin, MD, for her assistance involving with the literature search for this chapter.

REFERENCES

1. Varnes DJ. Slope movement types and processes. In: Schuster RL, Krizek RJ, eds. *Landslides: Analysis and Control. Transportation Research Board Special, Report 176.* Washington, DC: National Research Council; 1978:11–33.

2. Cruden DM, Varnes DJ. Landslide types and processes. In: Turner AK, RL Schuster RL, eds. *Landslides: Investigation and Mitigation. Transportation Research Board Special, Report 247.* Washington DC: National Research Council; 1996:36–75.

3. Larsen M, Wieczorek G, Eaton L, et al. *Natural Hazards on Alluvial Fans: The Venezuela Debris Flow and Flash Flood Disaster.* U.S. Department of the Interior; US Geological Survey Fact Sheet 103-01. http://pubs.usgs .gov/fs/fs-0103-01/fs-0103-01.pdf; Accessed 07.07.04.

4. US Geological Survey. *Landslide Hazard Fact Sheet.* http://pubs.usgs.gov/fs/ fs-0071-00/fs-0071-00.pdf; Accessed 30.01.14.

5. Schuster RL. Engineering geologic effects of the 1980 eruptions of Mount St. Helens. In: Galster R, ed. *Engineering Geology in Washington*; 1989:1203–1228. Wash Div Geol Earth Res Bull; vol. 78(2).

6. Voight RB, Janda RJ, Glicken H, Douglass PM. Nature and mechanisms of the Mount St. Helens rock-slide avalanche of 18 May 1980. *Geotechnique.* 1983;33(3):243–273.

7. Red Cross. *World Disasters Report 2000.* Geneva: International Federation of Red Cross and Red Crescent Societies; 2000.

8. Noji E. Earthquakes. In: Noji E, ed. *Public Health Consequences of Disasters.* Oxford: Oxford University Press; 1997.

9. Center for Research on the Epidemiology of Disasters. *EM-DAT Database.* http://www.emdat.be/disaster-profiles; Accessed 30.01.14.

10. United Nations Development Program. *Human Development Index.* http:// hdr.undp.org/en; Accessed 30.01.14.

11. Red Cross. *World Disaster Report 2012.* Geneva: International Federation of Red Cross and Red Crescent Societies; 262–269.

12. Guzzetti F, Stark C, Salvati P. Evaluation of flood and landslide risk to the population of Italy. *Environ Manag.* 2005;36(1):15–36.

13. Voight B. The 1985 Nevada del Ruiz volcano catastrophe: anatomy and retrospection. *J Volcanol Geotherm Res.* 1990;44:349–386.

14. Sancio R. Disaster in Venezuela: the floods and landslides of December 1999. *Nat Hazards Obs.* 2002;24(4).

15. OCHA. *Tropical storm Chata'an, Federated States of Micronesia.* UN Office for the Coordination of Humanitarian Affairs Situation Report No. 2, July 16, 2004. http://archive.is/zfwe; Accessed January 30, 2014.

16. Donato V, Noto A, Lacquaniti A, et al. Levels of neutrophil gelatinase-associated lipocalin in 2 patients with crush syndrome after a mudslide. *Am J Crit Care.* 2011;20:405–409.

17. Atuyambe L, Ediau M, Orach C, et al. Land slide disaster in eastern Uganda: rapid assessment of water, sanitation and hygiene situation in Bulucheck camp, Bududa district. *Environ Health.* 2011;10:38.

18. Tze-Chun T, Cheng-Fang Y, Chung-Ping C. Suicide risk and its correlation in adolescents who experienced typhoon-induced mudslides: a structural model. *Depress Anxiety.* 2010;27:1143–1148.

19. CDC. Coccidioidomycosis following the Northridge earthquake—California, 1994. *MMWR.* 1994;43:194–195.

20. Lara R, Neogi S, Islam M, et al. Influence of catastrophic climatic events and human waste on Vibrio distribution in the Karnaphuli estuary, Bangladesh. *EcoHealth.* 2009;6:279–286.

21. Keim M, Humphrey A, Dreyfus A, et al. Situation assessment report involving the hazardous material disaster site at LaGuaira Port, Venezuela. *CDC Report to Office of Foreign Disaster Assistance, US Agency for International Development.* January 10, 2000.

22. Anonymous. Venezuela seeks contractors for hazardous cleanup. *Hazardous Substances Spill Report.* 2000;3(2).

23. Bonachea J, Remondo J, Díaz de Teran JR, et al. Landslide risk models for decision making. *Risk Anal.* 2009;29(11):1629–1643.

24. Segerstrom J. A dirty job: rescuers face the growing problem of debris flows, mudslides and estuary rescues. *Adv Rescue Technol.* Feb./Mar. 2004;41–47.

25. Anonymous. *Landslide Preparedness. US Geological Survey.* http:// landslides.usgs.gov/learn/prepare.php; Accessed 30.01.14.

26. Boholm M. Risk and causality in newspaper reporting. *Risk Anal.* 2009;29 (11):1566–1577.

27. Fabien N. Risk perception, risk management and vulnerability to landslides in the hill slopes in the city of La Paz, Bolivia. *Disasters.* 2008;32 (3):337–357.

28. Parry ML, Canziani OF, Palutikof JP, van der Linden PJ, Hanson CE, eds. *Climate Change 2007: Impacts, Adaptation and Vulnerability. Contribution of Working Group II to the Fourth Assessment Report of the Intergovernmental Panel on Climate Change.* Cambridge UK: Cambridge University Press; 2007. www.ipcc.ch/ipccreports/ar4-wg2.htm.

29. Yumul G, Cruz N, Servando N, et al. Extreme weather events and related disasters in the Philippines, a sign of what climate change will mean? *Disasters.* 2011;35(2):362.

30. Keim M. Building human resilience: the role of public health preparedness and response as an adaptation to climate change. *Am J Prev Med.* 2008;35(5):508–516.

31. Chun-Yen L, Tsun-Ying H, Hsuan-Cheng S, et al. The strategies to DVI challenges in Typhoon Morakot. *Int J Legal Med.* 2011;125:637–641.

Avalanche

Ali A. Hosin and Jason A. Tracy

DESCRIPTION OF EVENT

Avalanches are rapid flows of large amounts of snow down a sloping surface. They are most commonly triggered when forces on a body of snow exceed its strength. They are primarily composed of flowing snow and air, but in some cases they may also collect trees, rocks, and ice as they progress down a mountain.

Avalanches are responsible for approximately 150 deaths per year in North America and Europe alone[1]; this figure is on the rise as more recreationalists are undertaking "extreme" outdoor sporting activities. Climbers, backcountry skiers, out-of-bounds skiers, and snowmobilers comprise a majority of these fatalities.[2] As many as 80% of these casualties are due to asphyxiation after snow burial[3–5]; time to extrication is the critical factor to survival. The International Commission for Mountain Emergency Medicine (ICAR MEDCOM) has established evidenced-based guidelines for resuscitation of avalanche victims.[2] There is a 92% chance of survival in open areas if victims are found within 15 minutes; however, this decreases to 30% after 35 minutes.[4,6]

This statistic differs dramatically for building-confined avalanche victims, for whom there is only a 31% chance of survival if extricated within 190 minutes.[6] Although rare, avalanches triggered by topographic or meteorologic conditions can be devastating to ill-prepared building inhabitants or to those traveling on exposed roadways.[7] Professional rescue teams, as opposed to recreationalists, can improve survival of these victims, since time to extrication can be dramatically improved to within the "golden 15 minutes." Depth of burial is also a critical survival factor; approximately 50% of individuals who are completely buried (head and chest under the snow) will likely die, whereas only 4% of those who are partially buried will succumb to death.[5] No avalanche victim buried to depths greater than 7 feet has ever survived in the United States.[5]

Asphyxiation from burial or from sudden burial-site airway obstruction causes the majority of avalanche deaths. However, it is clear from autopsy studies that blunt trauma also plays a significant role, not only as a cause of death, but also as a critical consideration during rescue efforts.[5,8] Injuries most commonly sustained by avalanche victims include craniofacial trauma with a high likelihood of closed head injuries,[8] as well as chest and abdominal trauma.[9] Trauma is reportedly the cause of death in up to 13% of all avalanche disaster cases.[10]

Creating an air space in the entombment site has been postulated as the reason that 7% of all victims survive for as long as 130 minutes post-burial.[6] As long as icing of the air space ("ice lensing") does not occur, carbon dioxide diffusion can commence and delay asphyxiation.[5,11] Appropriate survival training and readily available rescue equipment can reduce the time to rescue and prolong the oxygen supply.

Although hypothermia may prevent hypoxic damage,[7] it can also cause vascular instability and death when core body temperatures fall below the 32 °C hypothermic threshold.[12] In hypothermia-inducing conditions, body temperatures will fall predictably by approximately 3 °C/h. Complete burial limits the time up to which hypothermia avoidance is possible (90 minutes). Beyond the 90-minute cutoff, significant hypothermia in these conditions will occur.[7]

PRE-INCIDENT ACTIONS

Avalanche avoidance through appropriate training is the mainstay of prevention. Local weather conditions should be verified before any backcountry traveling. Training for at-risk individuals includes condition analysis, as well as proper safety and rescue equipment usage. Individuals in an avalanche area should carry a snow shovel, which is used not only for rescue purposes but also for building "snow pits" to analyze conditions. Long probes (10 to 12 feet in length when extended) and/or personal avalanche beacons, both of which are useful to teams searching for buried victims, are also requisite recreationalist trekking gear. Personal avalanche beacons have become the most widely used personal rescue devices worldwide. When buried, these devices emit a signal that can be received by active rescuers.[13] Newer survival equipment includes the artificial air pocket device (AvaLung), the ABS-Avalanche Airbag System, and the Avalanche Ball. Each of these devices provides a unique way of preventing death.[5] As previously discussed, professional rescue teams improve avalanche victim survival through their ability to rapidly locate and extricate a buried victim. Regardless of the extrication team's training, it is critical that potential burial-site air pockets be preserved during extrication because any loss of this space will lead to rapid death.

POST-INCIDENT ACTIONS

Rapid location and extrication of buried victims are the keys to survival. The last known location of a victim should be marked before launching the search and rescue effort. Subsequent topological scanning for body parts or debris and probing or rescue-beacon searching should immediately ensue. If a limited number of rescuers are in an isolated location, all immediate efforts should be focused on victim location. If rescuers have a phone or if there is rescuer surplus, then a makeshift contact team can be organized and sent quickly to notify a professional rescue team. Once victims are extricated, medical treatment should occur immediately.[13]

MEDICAL TREATMENT OF CASUALTIES

Initial management of all avalanche victims should focus on the ABCs (airway, breathing, and circulation) of resuscitation followed by spinal stabilization. Immediate entrapment-site airway protection is critical;

airway obstruction or respiratory arrest must be managed immediately using standard advanced cardiac life support (ACLS) guidelines. Due to potential cardiac instability, gentle handling of all hypothermic patients is mandatory.[14] Core temperature and electrocardiogram monitoring should commence as soon as qualified personnel are available. Core temperature monitoring is best achieved via esophageal or rectal measurement, although the less-reliable epitympanic method is an acceptable alternative.[14,15]

Prehospital assessment and treatment of hypothermia will likely be required for victims with prolonged burial (greater than 35 minutes). Assessment of hypothermia using the Swiss Society of Mountain Medicine guidelines can be performed by those with limited medical training and is based on the patient's mental status and presence or absence of shivering. In a patient who is alert and shivering, the core temperature is presumably 32 to 35 °C. Drowsiness and the absence of shivering are causes for concern, since this combination is symptomatic of a very low core body temperature (potentially as low as 28 °C). If the temperature is less than this, the patient is likely to be unconscious and/or not breathing.[7,15,16]

Rapid triage of multiple victims is determined on-scene, with cessation of resuscitative efforts applied to appropriate patients. Death determination on-scene limits futile use of resources and the risk to rescue teams during patient extrication. Burial time, the presence or absence of a burial-site air pocket, and core body temperature are all used as death determination factors. The duration of snow burial and/or the patient's core body temperature are the principal determinants of the rescue strategy. All patients with a burial time of less than 35 minutes and/or a core body temperature greater than 32 °C should undergo ACLS treatment with rapid hospital transfer. Death pronouncement can occur in asystolic patients with no evidence of an air pocket or the presence of obvious airway obstruction, with a burial time greater than 35 minutes, and/or with a body temperature of less than 32 °C. If there is any evidence of an air pocket, hospital transport should occur regardless of burial time. The receiving facility should have extracorporeal membrane oxygenation (ECMO) or cardiopulmonary bypass (CPB) capabilities, since these methods of active internal rewarming have had the best success[7,15,16]; ECMO is associated with a higher survival rate compared to CPB in hypothermic cardiac arrest patients.[17]

Treatment of hypothermia should commence as soon as extrication occurs; the type of treatment will depend on the available equipment and training level of on-site rescuers. Passive rewarming occurs through the removal of wet clothes; shielding from the wind; and application of blankets, aluminum foils, or bivouac bags. Initial warming procedures should be performed on all hypothermic patients and is commonly the only treatment required for patients who can shiver.[14] Active external rewarming occurs with forced air or with heat packs applied to the trunk. Warm, sugar-containing drinks should be provided to those who are conscious.[7,15,16] ACLS recommendations limit active external warming applications to the trunk area only, for fear of "afterdrop" hypothermia. Afterdrop hypothermia, caused by warming of the extremities, can lead to recirculation of cold peripheral blood to the central circulation system, culminating in a substantial decline in core body temperature.[13] Active internal rewarming in the field is best achieved through the use of warm, humidified oxygen. This can be achieved through either application of a mask or through endotracheal intubation.[6,15,16] Hospital treatment of severe hypothermia victims (less than 30 °C by ACLS guidelines) should be more aggressive and includes warm intravenous fluids and warm lavage of the peritoneum, pleural cavity, and gastric mucosa, with cardiopulmonary bypass being the ultimate goal. Internal rewarming should continue until the core temperature reaches 35 °C or there is return of spontaneous circulation.[14]

Severely hypothermic patients with confirmed ventricular fibrillation should not receive any intravenous medications but should receive a maximum of three attempts at defibrillation. Intravenous medications and defibrillation are ineffective at this temperature. Once the core temperature reaches 30 °C, normal ACLS protocols should be followed.[14] Serum potassium levels should be carefully monitored after avalanche burial because hyperkalemia is expected and is predictive of survival for hypothermic cardiac arrest victims.[14] All resuscitation efforts should cease for patients with both substantially prolonged burial times (greater than 35 minutes) and high serum potassium levels (greater than 12 mmol/L).

Although hypoxia and hypothermia usually prevail as initial treatment priorities, attention to other life threats should not be overlooked. Traumatic injuries should be assessed as previously discussed. In victims with obvious traumatic injuries, transport to a trauma center should occur per local protocols. In-hospital evaluation of these patients includes complete trauma and medical requirement assessments in accordance to the Advanced Trauma Life Support (ATLS) algorithm.

UNIQUE CONSIDERATIONS

Hypothermic patients with prolonged burial in an oxygen-available tomb are potentially salvageable with active internal rewarming. Otherwise, resuscitative efforts among severely hypothermic patients or among patients with airway obstructions and burial times of greater than 35 minutes should cease.

PITFALLS

- Inadequate avalanche training of backcountry explorers
- Improper rescue techniques
- Failure to preserve a victim's air pocket
- Inappropriate triage of avalanche victims
- Inappropriate treatment of hypothermic patients

REFERENCES

1. Etter HJ. *Report of the Avalanche Subcommission at the General Meeting of the International Commission for Alpine Rescue;* 2010.
2. Page CE, Atkins D, Shockley LW, Yaron M. Avalanche deaths in the United States: a 45-year analysis. *Wilderness Environ Med.* 1999;10(3):146–151.
3. Ammann WJ. Epidemiological trends in avalanche accidents. *Wilderness Environ Med.* 2001;12(2):139 [Abstract].
4. Falk M, Brugger H, Adler-Kastner L. Avalanche survival chances. *Nature.* 1994;368(6466):21.
5. Radwin MI, Grissom CK. Technological advances in avalanche survival. *Wilderness Environ Med.* 2002;13(2):143–152.
6. Falk M, Brugger H, Adler-Kastner L. Calculation of survival as a function of avalanche burial. *Wilderness Environ Med.* 2001;12(2):140–141 [Abstract].
7. Brugger H, Durrer B, Adler-Kastner L, Falk M, Tschirky F. Field management of avalanche victims. *Resuscitation.* 2001;51(1):7–15.
8. Grossman MD, Saffle JR, Thomas F, Tremper B. Avalanche trauma. *J Trauma.* 1989;29(12):1705–1709.
9. Johnson SM, Johnson AC, Barton RG. Avalanche trauma and closed head injury: adding insult to injury. *Wilderness Environ Med.* 2001;12(4):244–247.
10. Stalsberg H, Albretsen C, Gilbert M, et al. Mechanism of death in avalanche victims. *Virchows Arch A Pathol Anat Histopathol.* 1989;414(5):415–422.
11. Radwin MI, Grissom CK, Scholand MB, Harmston CH. Normal oxygenation and ventilation during snow burial by the exclusion of exhaled carbon dioxide. *Wilderness Environ Med.* 2001;12(4):256–262.
12. Danzl DF, Pozos RS. Accidental hypothermia. *N Engl J Med.* 1994;331(26):1756–1760.

13. Williams K, Armstrong BR, Armstrong BL. Avalanches. In: Auerbach PS, ed. *Disaster Medicine.* 4th ed. St Louis: Mosby; 2001:44–73.

14. American Heart Association. Part 8: advanced challenges in resuscitation. Section 3: special challenges in ECC 3A: hypothermia. *Resuscitation.* 2000;46(1-3):267–271.

15. Brugger H, Durrer B. International Commission for Mountain Emergency Medicine. On-site treatment of avalanche victims ICAR-MEDCOM-recommendation. *High Alt Med Biol.* 2002;3(4):421–425.

16. Brugger H, Durrer B, Adler-Kastner L. On-site triage of avalanche victims with asystole by the emergency doctor. *Resuscitation.* 1996;31(1):11–16.

17. Ruttmann E, Weissenbacher A, Ulmer H, et al. Prolonged extracorporeal membrane oxygenation-assisted support provides improved survival in hypothermic patients with cardiocirculatory arrest. *J Thorac Cardiovasc Surg.* 2007;134:594–600.

SUGGESTED READINGS

1. Brugger H, Durrer B, Elsensohn F, et al. Resuscitation of avalanche victims: evidence-based guidelines of the international commission for mountain emergency medicine (ICAR MEDCOM): Intended for physicians and other advanced life support personnel. *Resuscitation.* 2013;84:539–546.

2. Dohrmann G. A deadly avalanche. *SI Adventure.* February 17, 2003.

CHAPTER 105

Introduction to Nuclear and Radiological Disasters

Dale M. Molé

In March 2011, three of six nuclear reactors at the Fukushima Daiichi Nuclear Power Plant suffered a meltdown and began releasing substantial amounts of radioactive material. Although the largest nuclear event since Chernobyl in 1986, this disaster released only 10% to 30% of the radiation of the previous incident, thanks to the concrete containment vessels surrounding the Japanese reactors.[1] For weeks, this triple disaster of earthquake, tsunami, and nuclear reactor meltdown captivated the world's attention. Despite this tragedy raising concerns regarding engineering safety within the nuclear power industry, the global appetite for energy remains unabated, and nuclear energy is needed to help fulfill the demand. In addition to the rapidly increasing number of nuclear power reactors under construction, the once unthinkable use of nuclear or radiological devices against innocent noncombatants by terrorist groups or rogue nations becomes more likely with each passing day.[2] Underscoring this concern is the disturbing trend of increased geopolitical instability in this new millennium, the rampant proliferation of nuclear weapons technology within the Third World,[3] the likelihood of stolen or black market tactical nuclear weapons from the former Soviet Union,[4] and the diversion of ubiquitous industrial and medical radioactive sources for nefarious uses.[5] For these reasons, a familiarity with the medical aspects of nuclear or radiological incidents is essential for any clinician in the twenty-first century.

In an age of global terrorism, few things generate as much fear in the public as radiation and its potential to produce painful death, malignant disease, or genetic mutations. The 2006 assassination of Russian dissident Alexander Litvinenko with tea laced with polonium-210 (at 200 times the median lethal dose) served to reinforce the public perception of a slow, gruesome death by radiation.[6] Because radiation is undetectable by our normal senses, when used, its psychological effectiveness to achieve sinister goals is enhanced. Public perceptions, or in most cases misperceptions, regarding the risk of even low-dose radiation exposure makes the use of radioactive materials a very effective terror weapon.

Few in the public realize that we live in a world surrounded by natural radiation sources. Cosmic rays from outer space, radioactive minerals on Earth, and some radioactivity in food, water, and air provide the majority of radiation exposure we receive. Additional exposure may be the result of medical procedures (e.g., radiographs and nuclear medicine studies). Even the human body contains small amounts of natural radioactive materials, such as carbon-14, potassium-40, and polonium-210.[7] With the exception of radon—found in excessive amounts in poorly ventilated dwellings in some parts of the United States—no adverse clinical effects of this low level of radiation have been demonstrated.

RADIATION PHYSICS

Radiation consists of either particles or electromagnetic waves, both of which deposit energy when interacting with matter. Radiation of sufficient energy to displace electrons from atoms, creating an ion and a free electron, is called *ionizing radiation*. *Particulate ionizing radiation* is made up of any atomic or subatomic particles, but the ones of clinical interest are alpha particles, beta particles, and neutrons. X-rays and gamma rays are types of *electromagnetic radiation* energetic enough to produce ionization. Forms of electromagnetic radiation that are less energetic (radiant heat, light, lasers, radio, and microwaves) expend energy mainly in the form of heat when interacting with matter, but they do not produce ions; hence, these are classified as *nonionizing radiation*.

Matter consists of atoms. All atoms have a small central nucleus composed of protons (positive charge) and neutrons (no charge) that are surrounded by orbiting clouds of electrons (negative charge). The atomic number, unique for each element and descriptive of its particular physical and chemical characteristics, is equivalent to the number of protons in the nucleus (e.g., hydrogen has one proton and its atomic number is 1). The atomic mass is essentially equivalent to the number of protons plus the number of neutrons (e.g., ordinary carbon has six protons [atomic number 6], but it has an atomic mass number of 12 [six protons plus six neutrons]). Because ordinary carbon-12 is electrically neutral, it has six orbital electrons. Atoms of the same element (the same number of protons) having different atomic mass (different numbers of neutrons) are called isotopes. The isotopes of hydrogen include hydrogen-2, or deuterium, with one proton and one neutron and hydrogen-3, or tritium, with one proton and two neutrons.

The forces between various components of the nucleus determine the stability of an atom. Neutrons appear to play an important role in binding protons together, with the ratio of protons to neutrons determining the stability of an atom. Too many or too few neutrons in the nucleus cause the atom to be unstable, which then decays or emits particles and/or energy to become more stable.

Alpha radiation consists of a helium nucleus (two protons and two neutrons). This relatively massive particle is only able to travel a short distance in air (1 to 2 cm), and it is stopped by a sheet of paper or the top layer of skin. However, if inhaled or ingested, it can produce large exposures to internal organs.

Beta radiation is an electron emitted from an unstable nucleus. Beta particles penetrate deeper into tissue than alpha particles do, but usually not beyond the few top layers of skin. They are completely absorbed by thin layers of glass, plastic, cloth, or metal foils. Beta particles of high energy can cause skin burns ("beta burns") and are hazardous if ingested or inhaled.

Neutron radiation is produced when a neutron is emitted from the unstable nucleus of an atom, usually during nuclear fission in an atomic bomb or nuclear reactor. Being electrically neutral, neutrons are very penetrating and cause secondary beta and gamma radiation to be emitted when interacting with matter.

Gamma rays and *x-rays* are ionizing forms of electromagnetic radiation. Both are very penetrating and capable of delivering significant radiation doses to internal organs without ingestion or inhalation. Identical except for place of origin, gamma rays are emitted from an unstable nucleus, whereas x-rays originate from the outer electron shells of the atom.

The amount of ionizing radiation deposited in tissue or matter is called the *absorbed dose*, conventionally expressed in units of *radiation-absorbed dose* (rad). The International System of Units for absorbed radiation is the gray (Gy). One Gy is equal to 1 J/kg and is equivalent to 100 rads.

The biological effect produced by each type of ionizing radiation depends on the mass, electrical charge, and energy of the radiation. Hence, the same absorbed dose of one type of ionizing radiation can result in more or less biological damage than the same absorbed dose of another type. This is because the *linear energy transfer* (LET), the amount of energy deposited in a unit of track length, is different for different types of radiation. One Gy of alpha radiation will result in more damage to cells than 1 Gy of beta radiation. To standardize the tissue damage produced by the different types of radiation, we use a measure of equivalent biological effects produced or equivalent dose. The absorbed dose multiplied by a quality factor produces an equivalent dose. The quality factor for most x-rays, gamma rays, and beta particles is 1, so the absorbed dose and equivalent dose are essentially equal. Alpha particles have a quality factor of 20, and neutrons have quality factors between 5 and 20, depending on their individual energies. Expressed in conventional units, rads multiplied by the quality factor for that particular type of radiation equals *radiation equivalent man* (rem). The international unit is the sievert (Sv). Because gamma radiation has a quality factor of 1, 1 Gy (100 rad) of gamma radiation equals 1 Sv (100 rem).

Important factors in reducing radiation exposure are time, distance, and shielding. The absorbed dose is directly proportional to the length of time an individual is exposed and inversely proportional to the square of the distance from the radioactive source. Doubling the distance decreases the absorbed dose by a factor of 4. The use of lead, concrete, or other shielding material significantly reduces or eliminates exposure.

Radioactivity decreases or decays with time. The *half-life* of a particular radioisotope is the length of time required for one-half of the radioactive material to decay. Some radioisotopes have half-lives of hours or days; others have half-lives of years or centuries. The decay rate can have an important effect on medical management decisions regarding decontamination and/or treatment.

Biological Effects

Ionizing radiation interacts with living cells by producing charged water molecules (i.e., free hydroxyl radicals) or by direct ionization of deoxyribonucleic acid. Clinical symptoms (acute radiation syndrome) occur if enough cells are damaged and die, or if the cells killed are essential for human survival. Rapidly dividing cells, such as bone marrow cells or the intestinal mucosa, are the most sensitive to radiation, whereas slowly dividing cells (e.g., central nervous system) are the most radio-resistant. Nonlethal radiation doses may cause some cells to undergo malignant transformation, leading to radiation-induced cancers years or decades after exposure.[8]

Nuclear or Radiological Scenarios

History is replete with accidents involving radioactive materials. Fortunately, most involved exposure to only a few people. An exception was the Chernobyl incident in 1986, when reactor unit number 4 exploded, exposing the reactor core and dispersing radioactive material over a wide area. One hundred thirty-four people developed acute radiation syndrome, with 28 deaths directly related to radiation exposure. A dramatic increase in thyroid cancers among those who were either very young or in utero at the time of exposure has been noted.[9] Follow-up studies demonstrated decreased life expectancy from 65 years to 58 years among those in the area around Chernobyl; not as a result of radiation exposure, but rather the psychological consequences of the event resulting in more depression, alcoholism, and suicide. In contrast, the Fukushima Daiichi disaster produced no short-term radiation fatalities. The World Health Organization estimates radiation related health effects in the 300,000 people evacuated will likely be below detectable levels because most were exposed to very little radiation.[10]

Occasionally, individuals without criminal intent can create radiological hazards for themselves and the community. Such was the case of David Hahn, the "radioactive Boy Scout," who attempted to build a breeder reactor in his backyard shed and ended up causing an expensive Environmental Protection Agency cleanup, as well as terrifying his neighbors.[11]

Terrorist groups such as Aum Shinri Kyo and Al-Qaeda, as well as state sponsors of terrorism, have tried to acquire radiological or nuclear material and technology. The father of the Pakistani atomic bomb, A. Q. Khan, peddled nuclear weapon expertise to many rogue nations and terror organizations.[12]

In addition to Third World countries or terror groups trying to develop a nuclear weapons program beginning with uranium ore,[13] an expensive and technologically intensive undertaking, there are other more likely nuclear or radiological scenarios:

- Using highly radioactive materials to fabricate a radiation emission device (RED)
- The detonation of a radiological dispersion device or "dirty bomb" (RDD)[14]
- Sabotage of nuclear facilities (e.g., nuclear power plants) with the subsequent release of large amounts of radioactivity[15]
- The detonation of an improvised nuclear device made from fissile material acquired by theft or purchased[16]
- The detonation of an intact nuclear weapon acquired by theft or on the black market[17]

An RED irradiates passersby with high levels of radiation. Such a device is highly radioactive and poses a significant threat to those who place it. It therefore requires some degree of sophistication to safely construct and deploy. A device using "induced criticality" could expose those nearby to lethal doses of neutron radiation and gamma rays in just moments.[18]

RDDs are often referred to as weapons of mass *disruption* because their psychological and economic effects far outweigh the physical damage to life or property.[19] The so-called dirty bomb, or RDD, consists of radioactive material surrounding or mixed in a conventional explosive. Those injured by blast effects from the explosion are contaminated by the radioactive material, as are the rescue workers.

The accidental contamination of the village of Goiânia, Brazil, in 1987 from an orphaned cancer radiotherapy source provides an insight to the consequences of an RDD. Junkyard workers broke open the lead shielding surrounding a medical radioactive source and exposed the 20-g cesium-137 chloride capsule. Soon afterward, 13 people became ill and sought medical care. Four people died. By the time authorities discovered what had happened, 249 people were affected by radiation, and thousands more rushed to emergency departments fearing contamination. Economic damage because of clean up ran into the millions of dollars: 6000 tons of clothing, furniture, soil, and other materials had to be packed into steel drums and buried in an abandoned quarry.[20]

A nuclear reactor accident (e.g., Chernobyl or Fukushima Daiichi) or sabotage remains an ongoing concern. In August 2003, 19 individuals were arrested for plotting to destroy a nuclear power plant on the shore of Lake Ontario, Canada. The method of attack used on September 11, 2001, raised concerns that terrorists could use a commercial airliner as a guided missile against a nuclear power plant. A study produced for the Nuclear Energy Institute using the Boeing 767-400 as the attacking aircraft suggests that the reactor containment building, as well as irradiated fuel storage facilities, would survive a direct impact.[21] However, other reports are not as reassuring. A Congressional Research Service report[22] outlines three primary areas of vulnerability: (1) controls on the nuclear chain reaction, (2) cooling systems that prevent hot nuclear fuel from melting even after the chain reaction has stopped, and (3) storage facilities for highly radioactive spent nuclear fuel. Although a successful assault on a nuclear power plant would be difficult, a well-executed physical or cyberattack might still achieve its goal.

A nuclear weapon detonation is the ultimate terrorist nightmare. The destructive effects from a nuclear explosion include visual problems from flash blindness (depletion of photopigments in the retinal receptors) and retinal burns, physical trauma from blast effects, burns from the initial flash and burning debris, and ionizing radiation from the fission process initially, followed by radioactive fallout. Estimates indicate a 10-metric ton weapon detonated at Grand Central Station in Manhattan would kill 500,000 people immediately, injure hundreds of thousands more, force the evacuation of all of Manhattan, and result in direct economic damage of well over $1 trillion.

Terrorists may achieve a nuclear detonation by obtaining highly enriched uranium (HEU) and constructing a crude atomic bomb (improvised nuclear device [IND]). Many experts believe a technologically sophisticated terrorist group could construct a nuclear weapon from HEU without state support. A plutonium bomb is much more difficult to construct and probably exceeds the abilities of substate organizations. Given the cost and complexity of a nuclear materials enrichment program, making a bomb from uranium ore is not currently feasible for a substate organization. Of concern, however, is the 130 research nuclear reactors around the world using HEU in the reactor core, many with minimal security and vulnerable to theft. The International Atomic Energy Agency reports 1340 confirmed incidents of illicit trafficking in nuclear materials between 1993 and 2007, including a few involving kilogram quantities of weapons-usable HEU or plutonium.[23]

Nuclear fission is the process underlying the explosive power of an atomic bomb; pound for pound, it is about 10-million times more powerful than a chemical explosion. When atoms of a fissile material (e.g., uranium-235 [U-235] or plutonium-239 [Pu-239]) absorb a neutron, they split or fission into two atoms of roughly equal mass, producing enormous amounts of energy, as well as additional neutrons that cause other atoms to fission. If enough fissile material is present (i.e., *critical mass*), a *chain reaction* will progress at a geometric rate, resulting in the liberation of tremendous quantities of energy in the form of heat, light, and radiation. The critical mass required for a self-sustaining chain reaction is a function of the shape, density, and type of fissile material.

By surrounding the bomb core with a neutron reflector or tamper, the amount of material required to reach critical mass is significantly reduced. The critical mass for a bare sphere of U-235 is 56 kg, but with a thick tamper, this is reduced to about 15 kg. For Pu-239, critical mass is 11 and 5 kg, respectively.

Because the critical mass of a particular fissile material decreases as the density increases by an inverse square relationship, an implosion device requires much less material compared with one using a gun assembly method.

Fission weapons require the "assembly" of a supercritical mass from a subcritical mass to occur in a very short period; otherwise, the weapon is blown apart before significant amounts of material have undergone fission, significantly lowering the yield. There are two classical assembly methods: gun and implosion. Gun assembly is useful only for U-235, and it involves firing a subcritical projectile of U-235 into a subcritical target of U-235 to create a supercritical mass. This is the easiest type of atomic bomb to make. It did not even require testing before operational use over Hiroshima, Japan.[24]

An implosion device uses high explosives to create an inwardly directed shock wave that compresses a sphere of fissile material, increasing density to supercritical levels. Although very efficient, it requires technology that is much more sophisticated because the explosive "lenses" must detonate at exactly the same instant to produce a nuclear explosion. In addition, a neutron generator emits a burst of neutrons to initiate the chain reaction at the point of maximum compression.[25]

For response planning purposes, it is assumed an IND would have an explosive power ranging from a fraction of a kiloton of TNT to as much as 10 kilotons. A ground detonation is the least effective method, but it is the easiest to achieve for a nonstate-sponsored attack. The IND would most likely be transported and detonated in a vehicle or vessel. The nuclear fireball from a 10-metric ton device has a temperature in the millions of degrees and a diameter of about 500 m. In an urban area, the buildings surrounding the explosion would provide some shielding from the flash, blast, and prompt radiation effects. Residual radiation or fallout would consist of mostly of fine sand-sized grains deposited within about 20 miles of ground zero. Survivors of the initial blast would have about 10 minutes to seek cover from the highly radioactive fallout, either somewhere below ground or in the center of a structure. Radiation decreases rapidly with time, hence the 7 to 10 rule; for every sevenfold increase in time, there is a tenfold decrease in radiation. After the first 7 hours, the level of radioactivity is only one tenth of the original amount. The electromagnetic pulse (EMP) effects, which can disable electronics and communication infrastructure, are attenuated with a ground detonation.

Russia has many tactical nuclear weapons that are more widely dispersed and not as well guarded as strategic weapons. With the dissolution of the Soviet Union, there is uncertainty regarding the whereabouts of every weapon. It is not known whether any were sold on the black market, and, if so, whether they remain fully functional. Detonating a "procured" nuclear weapon would likely prove challenging. Most nuclear powers design the devices with electronic locks (permissive action links or PALs) to prevent unauthorized use. A code or password is required to operate the device, and too many incorrect entries or attempts to tamper with the lock will permanently disable the firing circuit.

HISTORICAL PERSPECTIVE

X-rays were first discovered in 1895 by Wilhelm Roentgen while experimenting with cathode-ray tubes and were used in medical diagnosis only a few months later. The following year, Henri Becquerel, while conducting some experiments with uranium salts, discovered radioactivity.[26] The danger of this mysterious new force was not fully appreciated. Initially, radiation was viewed as healthy, perhaps because of the small amounts of radium and radon detected in waters in the health spas of Europe. Despite some evidence of the harmful effects of excessive radiation, such as the deep skin burns to those scientific pioneers who handled unsealed radioactive sources, radioactive material was added to everything from toothpaste to drinking water in an effort to provide a healthful, stimulating effect. Shoe salespersons used portable x-ray machines to check shoe fit. Radium was painted on tonsils and adenoids to reduce the size of lymphoid tissue. Radium was also used together with surgery to provide the "Curie therapy" for cancer patients before the development of effective chemotherapy.

With the discovery of nuclear fission by Otto Hahn, Lise Meitner, and O. R. Frisch in 1939 came the realization that this process could be used to make a bomb.[27] On December 2, 1942, Enrico Fermi succeeded in creating the world's first self-sustaining nuclear chain reaction under the squash courts at the University of Chicago. During World War II, both Germany[28] and Japan[29] pursued atomic bomb development. The world changed forever on July 16, 1945, with the detonation of the atomic bomb in the New Mexico desert.[30]

The following month, World War II ended with the use of atomic weapons on Hiroshima and Nagasaki, Japan. The pictures of the devastation in Japan helped shape public perception regarding the dangers of radiation. This was further enhanced by decades of science fiction movies and antinuclear literature. Movie images, from giant ants and humans to reactor cores melting through the Earth or melting flesh from bones, convinced many in the public that any amount of radiation is an immediate threat to life.

CURRENT PRACTICE

External irradiation is the exposure of the entire body or just a part of it to an external source of penetrating radiation. Unless exposed to high-intensity neutron radiation, a patient is not radioactive from external irradiation and no special protective measures are required of medical personnel.

Acute radiation syndrome (ARS) is the primary threat to life after exposure to major doses of radiation.[31] The diagnosis of ARS is based on a history of exposure and clinical findings (Box 105-1). ARS occurs when the entire body is exposed to a large dose of penetrating external radiation over a short period. There are three classic ARSs.

Bone marrow or *hematopoietic syndrome* usually occurs with doses higher than 2 Sv (200 rem), depending on the premorbid state of health. Destruction or depression of the bone marrow produces a pancytopenia, resulting in increased susceptibility to infection and clotting abnormalities. As long as the bone marrow is not destroyed completely, granulocyte-stimulating factors may enhance regeneration.

The Radiation Injury Treatment Network (RITN) was formed in 2006 to leverage the expertise of hematologists, oncologists, and stem cell transplant practitioners in preparing for and responding to a mass casualty radiological or nuclear event.[32] These specialists are accustomed to providing the intensive supportive care required by patients with suppressed bone marrow function.

Gastrointestinal syndrome occurs with doses greater than 6 Sv (600 rem). Cell death and sloughing of the intestinal mucosa result initially in nausea, vomiting, and diarrhea. Because gastrointestinal symptoms coincide with hematologic abnormalities, dehydration, electrolyte imbalances, and sepsis are part of the natural disease course. Severe bloody diarrhea is an ominous sign.

Cardiovascular (CV)/central nervous system (CNS) syndrome occurs with doses exceeding 20 Sv (2000 rem). The almost immediate nausea, vomiting, ataxia, and convulsions are the result of diffuse microvascular leaks in the CNS, causing edema and increased intracranial pressure. Cardiovascular collapse from a transient postirradiation vasodilation has been observed.[33]

ARS progresses through the following four clinical phases:

- *The prodromal phase* occurs within hours of exposure and may last for up to 2 days. Symptoms are a function of the total rad dose and include anorexia, nausea, vomiting, diarrhea, fatigue, fever, respiratory distress, and agitation. Treatment should be symptomatic.
- *The latent phase* is a transitional period in which the patient is asymptomatic. This may last as long as 3 weeks, but is much shorter with higher radiation exposures.
- *The illness phase* produces overt clinical manifestations, including infection because of leukopenia, bleeding from thrombocytopenia, diarrhea, electrolyte imbalances, altered mental status, and shock.
- *The death or recovery phase* often occurs over weeks or months.

The clinical phases of ARS are related to cell reproduction, with the fastest-dividing cells affected earliest. The time of onset after exposure of general signs and symptoms related to the hematopoietic and gastrointestinal systems are good markers for prognosis. After exposure, a shorter time until symptom onset is associated with a poorer prognosis. One should remain aware that anxiety and pain might also produce nausea and vomiting.

Biodosimetry is a method of determining radiation exposure that is more objective. Although cytogenetic chromosome aberration assay remains the gold standard, current technology does not provide the throughput capacity required for a mass casualty situation. Determining the absolute lymphocyte count (ALC) initially, then every 6 hours for 2 to 3 days, then every 12 hours for 4 days is a useful approach.[34] A 50% drop in lymphocytes at 24 hours postexposure is indicative of significant radiation injury.[35] At 48 hours postexposure, if the ALC is greater than 1200, the patient likely received a nonlethal dose. An ALC between 300 and 1200 indicates significant exposure and the need for hospitalization. If the ALC is less than 300, the patient is critically ill and should be considered for colony-stimulating factors. The ALC may be an unreliable indicator in a patient with combined injuries.

The Armed Forces Radiobiology Research Institute developed a Biodosimetry Assessment Tool (BAT)—available for download at their website—that provides for the recording of peripheral blood lymphocyte counts and then converts them into radiation dose predictions using lymphocyte depletion kinetic models (Box 105-2).

BOX 105-1 Initial Assessment for Radiation Injuries

- Address immediate life threats
- Monitor and measure exposed individuals for radionuclide contamination
- Observe and document prodromal signs and symptoms
- Obtain a complete blood count with differential
- Where appropriate, sample blood for chromosome aberration cytogenetic biodosimetry
- If internal contamination is suspected, conduct bioassay sampling

---

BOX 105-2 Resources

Armed Forces Radiobiology Research Institute (AFRRI). Available at: http://www.usuhs.edu/afrri

Centers for Disease Control and Prevention. Available at: http://www.bt.cdc.gov/radiation/

Radiation Emergency Assistance Center/Training Site (REAC/TS). Available at: https://orise.orau.gov/reacts/

Radiation Event Medical Management. Available at: http://www.remm.nlm.gov

Radiation Injury Treatment Network. Available at: http://www.ritn.net

Cutaneous radiation syndrome (CRS) is the constellation of symptoms resulting from acute exposure to beta radiation or x-rays. This can occur when radioactive isotopes contaminate the patient's clothes or skin. Although similar in appearance to thermal burns, radiation burns may take several days to appear. Dermal changes can help estimate the dose of radiation received, so it is important to observe for signs of erythema, pain, blister formation, and necrosis. Sequelae from CRS include vascular insufficiency developing months or years after exposure and causing necrosis or ulceration of previously healed tissue, and sometimes requiring hyperbaric oxygen therapy, plastic surgery, or amputation. Because of radiation's effect on dividing cells, if a radiation patient requires emergency surgery, it should be done within the first 24 to 48 hours after the radiation injury; otherwise, the surgery should be delayed for 3 months.

Radioactive contamination occurs if radioactive materials are deposited internally, externally, or both. Patients can be radioactive and require decontamination when radioisotopes are inhaled, ingested, or deposited in wounds. *Incorporation* occurs if radioactive materials are taken up by cells and incorporated into tissues or organs.

Effective treatment of internal contamination requires knowledge of the type and chemical form of the radioisotope. The goal is to hasten elimination and prevent incorporation. This is accomplished by reducing absorption (with Prussian blue in the case of cesium), by using dilution techniques (forcing fluids with tritium), chelation (plutonium), or blocking agents (potassium iodide for radioactive iodine). The use of potassium iodide as a blocking agent is especially important for nuclear reactor accidents because of the amount of iodine-131 discharged, the tendency for biological uptake via inhalation or ingestion of contaminated food or water, and its rapid accumulation in the thyroid gland resulting in significant irradiation.[36]

External contamination is not usually a medical emergency. Simply removing clothing will eliminate 90% of the contamination. Water and detergent effectively remove skin contamination. Uncontaminated wounds should be covered before decontamination. Contaminated wounds should be treated conventionally with pressurized normal saline irrigation. Residual radioactivity often comes off with dressing changes, in exudates, or with the eschar. If the wound remains contaminated with long-lived radioisotopes, wound excision should be considered. All contaminated clothing and materials should be placed in labeled plastic bags for proper disposal.

Successfully treating radioactive-contaminated injured people requires teamwork and practice. In addition to the usual emergency medicine personnel, the hospital health physicist or radiation safety officer is essential, both for assistance in conducting surveys of the patient with radiation detection equipment and in providing additional advice regarding decontamination. Emergency department patient decontamination and treatment exercises should occur at least annually to ensure proper decontamination technique, reinforce appropriate treatment priorities, and provide familiarity with radiation detection equipment and personal dosimeters.

It is likely that patients will present with mixed injuries (i.e., trauma or burns combined with significant radiation exposure or contamination). Evaluate, resuscitate, and stabilize the patient before completing decontamination.

Triage decisions based on radiation exposure can be difficult when there are large numbers of casualties because the individual exposure is unknown. Early onset of ARS symptoms portends a poor outcome. Patients with mixed injuries have a much poorer prognosis than do those sustaining an isolated trauma, burn, or radiation insult. Triage assistance tools can be found at the resource websites listed below.

Surgeons operating on irradiated patients should consider them immunocompromised. Impaired wound healing, as well as fluid balance, electrolyte, and clotting abnormalities, should be expected. The earlier the patient is operated on after exposure, the better. If operations are performed early, surgical wounds should be in the healing phase when the immune system is at its nadir. Because of the high potential for sepsis, wound debridement must be meticulous.[37] Prophylactic antibiotics should be considered for any patient with combined injuries of radiation exposure, burns, and classical trauma, and should be continued until the absolute neutrophil count rises above 500 and the patient is afebrile for at least 24 hours. The use of hematopoietic growth factors shortens the duration of neutropenia, and it should be started as soon as significant radiation exposure is identified.

Over the last several years, the Office of the Assistant Secretary for Preparedness and Response, Department of Health and Human Services has done a masterful job developing an integrated medical response plan to a radiological or nuclear event. In collaboration with other government and nongovernment partners, they developed a comprehensive planning framework and online "just-in-time" medical response guidance called Radiation Event Medical Management. The five-part response plan includes (1) basic radiation biology, (2) tailored medical responses, (3) delivery of medical countermeasures for postevent mitigation and treatment, (4) referral to expert centers for acute treatment, and (5) long-term follow-up.[38]

⚠ PITFALLS

- Failure to treat life-threatening injuries or stabilize a patient because of concern regarding radioactive contamination on clothing or skin
- Failure to plan, train, and exercise the emergency management of radiological events
- Lack of personal dosimetry equipment for medical workers
- Poor decontamination skills
- Failure to set and monitor radiation boundaries to prevent the spread of contamination throughout the hospital
- Failure to provide timely and appropriate risk communication regarding the hazards of radiation exposure
- Failure to seek shelter from fallout immediately after a nuclear detonation if within 20 miles from ground zero
- Attempting to evacuate from a nuclear disaster site too early or without official direction

REFERENCES

1. Fukushima Daiichi Nuclear Disaster. Available at: http://en.wikipedia.org/wiki/Fukushima_Daiichi_nuclear_disaster#CITEREFWHO2013.
2. Richelson J. *Defusing Armageddon: Inside America's Secret Nuclear Bomb Squad.* New York, NY: W.W. Norton; 2009.
3. Albright D. *Peddling Peril.* New York, NY: Free Press; 2010.
4. Sokov N, Potter W. *"Suitcase Nukes": A Reassessment.* Monterey, CA: Monterey Center for Nonproliferation Studies; 2004.
5. Wald M. *Uranium reactors on campus raise security concerns.* New York Times; August 15, 2004. Available at: http://ucnuclearfree.org/articles/2004/08/15_wald_uranium-reactors-campus.htm.
6. Cowell A. *The Terminal Spy: A True Story of Espionage, Betrayal, and Murder.* New York, NY: Broadway Books; 2009.
7. Ford J. *Radiation, People and the Environment.* Vienna: International Atomic Energy Agency; 2004.
8. Mettler F, Upton A. *Medical Effects of Ionizing Radiation.* Philadelphia, PA: Saunders; 1995.
9. Gusev I, Guskova A, Mettler F. *Medical Management of Radiation Accidents.* Boca Raton, FL: CRC Press; 2001.
10. WHO. *Health Risk Assessment From The Nuclear Accident After The 2011 Great East Japan Earthquake and Tsunami.* Geneva: World Health Organization; 2013.

11. Silverstein K. *The Radioactive Boy Scout.* New York, NY: Random House; 2004.

12. Ferguson C, Potter W. *The Four Faces of Nuclear Terrorism.* Monterey, CA: Monterey Center for Nonproliferation Studies; 2004.

13. Bhatia S, McGrory D. *Brighter Than the Baghdad Sun.* Washington, DC: Regnery Publishing; 2000.

14. Edwards R. Risk of radioactive "dirty bomb" growing. *New Scientist.* June 2004; Available at: http://www.newscientist.com/article.ns?id=dn5061.

15. Brown D. Canada arrests 19 as security threats. *Washington Post.* August 23, 2003; page A20.

16. Mark JC, Taylor T, Eyster E, Maraman W, Wechsler J. Can terrorists build nuclear weapons? In: Leventhal P, Alexander Y, eds. *Preventing Nuclear Terrorism.* Lexington, MA: Lexington Books; 1987.

17. Alexander B, Millar A. *Tactical Nuclear Weapons.* Washington: Brassey's; 2003.

18. Mettler F, Voelz G, et al. Criticality accidents. In: Gusev I, Guskova A, Mettler FA, eds. *Medical Management of Radiation Accidents.* Boca Raton, FL: CRC Press; 2001.

19. Levi M, Kelly H. Weapons of mass disruption. *Sci Am.* November 2002;77–81. Available at: http://www.fas.org/resource/03212005140554.pdf.

20. O'Neill K. *The Nuclear Terrorist Threat.* Washington, DC: Institute for Science and International Security; 1997.

21. Hardy G, Arros J, Merz K. *Aircraft Crash Impact Analyses Demonstrate Nuclear Power Plant's Structural Strength.* San Diego, CA: ABS Consulting/ANATECH; 2002.

22. Holt M, Andrews A. *Nuclear Power Plant Security and Vulnerabilities.* Washington, DC: Congressional Research Service; January 3, 2014, Report RL 34331.

23. IAEA. *Illicit Trafficking Database.* Geneva: International Atomic Energy Agency; 2007.

24. Henriksen P, Westfall C. Critical assemblies and nuclear physics. In: Hoddeson L, Henriksen PW, Meade RA, Westfall CL, eds. *Critical Assembly: A Technical History of Los Alamos During the Oppenheimer Years, 1943-1945.* New York, NY: Cambridge University Press; 1993.

25. Serber V. *The Los Alamos Primer: The First Lectures on How to Build an Atom Bomb.* Berkeley, CA: University of California Press; 1992.

26. Sacks O. *Uncle Tungsten.* New York, NY: Alfred A. Knopf; 2001.

27. Hahn O. From the natural transmutations of uranium to its artificial fission. *Nobel Lecture.* December 13, 1946; Stockholm. Available at: http://nobelprize.org/chemistry/laureates/1944/hahn-lecture.pdf.

28. Irving D. *The German Atomic Bomb.* New York, NY: Da Capo Press; 1967.

29. Wilcox R. *Japan's Secret War.* New York, NY: William Morrow & Company; 1985.

30. Rhodes R. *The Making of the Atomic Bomb.* New York: Simon & Schuster; 1986.

31. Mettler F, Voelz G. Major radiation exposure—what to expect and how to respond. *N Engl J Med.* 2002;346(20):1554–1561.

32. Ross J, Case C, Confer D, et al. Radiation Injury Treatment Network. *Int J Radiat Biol.* 2011;1–6, Early Online.

33. Hawkins R, Cockerham L. Postirradiation cardiovascular dysfunction. In: Conklin J, Walker R, eds. *Military Radiobiology.* San Diego, CA: Academic Press; 1987.

34. Mickelson A. *Medical Consequences of Radiological and Nuclear Weapons.* Fort Detrick, MD: The Borden Institute; 2012.

35. Jarrett D. *Medical Management of Radiological Casualties.* Bethesda, MD: Armed Forces Radiobiology Research Institute; 1999.

36. Christodouleas J, Forrest R, Ainsley C, et al. Short-term and long-term health risks of nuclear power plant accidents. *N Engl J Med.* 2011;364: 2334–2341.

37. Eiseman B, Bond V. Surgical care of nuclear casualties. *Surg Gynecol Obstet.* 1978;146:877–883.

38. Coleman C, Hrdina C, Bader J, et al. Medical response to a radiologic/nuclear event: integrated plan from the Office of the Assistant Secretary for Preparedness and Response, Department of Health and Human Services. *Ann Emerg Med.* 2009;53(2):213–222.

CHAPTER 106

Nuclear Detonation

Yasser A. Alaska, Abdulaziz D. Aldawas, and William E. Dickerson

DESCRIPTION OF EVENT

The detonation of a nuclear device is, perhaps, the most ominous of potential terrorist scenarios that could result from the most destructive of human-made weapons. As President Obama stated at the Nuclear Security Summit in April 2010, "Two decades after the end of the Cold War, we face a cruel irony of history: the risk of a nuclear confrontation between nations has gone down, but the risk of nuclear attack has gone up."[1] If a terrorist organization were to detonate a nuclear device equivalent to 10 kton of trinitrotoluene (TNT) in a truck parked in a large city, there would be a predictable—and horrific—series of consequences. The blast, heat, and radiation would cause immediate casualties and near-complete destruction within a half-mile radius. Moderate infrastructure damage would occur within approximately one mile, and light damage could occur for 3 miles or more.[2] Because the terrorist use of a nuclear weapon would most likely be a surface burst, radioactive fallout would also be produced, which would travel for 10 to 20 miles or more, depending on the size of the particles and weather conditions.[3] The Hiroshima nuclear detonation in August 1945 was equivalent to approximately 15 kton of TNT and was an air burst that produced minimal fallout. Approximately 100,000 people died within 4 months in a city with a population of about 310,000.

PRE-INCIDENT ACTIONS

Given the potential consequences of a nuclear detonation, planning for such a scenario is extremely challenging. Nonetheless, the U.S. government postulates that "local and state community preparedness to respond to a nuclear detonation could result in life-saving on the order of tens of thousands of lives."[4] In the unlikely event that there is a forewarning of a detonation, the at-risk population must quickly be instructed to find appropriate shelter, or possibly evacuate, depending on the population's location and anticipated travel conditions. Technological systems that can rapidly deliver messages with specific instructions to very large segments of the population quickly would be of great value to help achieve this goal, as would preplanned and well-marked urban evacuation routes. Given the practical limitations on a rapid mass evacuation of an urban population, it is generally recommended that initial public warnings advocate sheltering as the first recommended public action. Emergency and health managers should attempt to educate the public on how best to seek shelter in a disaster situation, how to evaluate what is an adequate shelter, and how to get additional emergency instructions when needed.

Local and state emergency planners are advised to assume that, in the event of a nuclear detonation, federal resources may not be available for at least 24 hours, and full federal resources may not be available for days. Therefore local communities and states should anticipate the need to rely on their own resources and plans. It is expected that citizen responders will be required to play an important relief role during nuclear events, due to the shortage of trained responders and possible restrictions on access to the contaminated zone. Hence, pre-event public education and training regarding mass casualty preparedness and basic first aid training may enhance the community's resiliency in such an event.[1] An example of radiation protection guidance that could be distributed to community groups, citizens, and first responders can be found in Box 106-1.

From a health and medical perspective, hospitals' planning efforts for radiation events, blast injuries, and mass casualties can all support their preparation for a nuclear detonation. Hospital plans should include provisions for how patients with radiation exposure and contamination are identified, decontaminated, and managed while limiting exposure and contamination of the facility. Selected medical staff should be educated on radiation injuries, as well as blast injuries, and all staff should be familiar with the institution's mass casualty plan. As with all aspects of emergency planning, subsequent training and exercises are necessary after plans are constructed. Hospitals should have access to a medical or health physicist and subject matter experts who can guide the treatment of radiation casualties.

POST-INCIDENT ACTIONS

After a nuclear disaster, local responders and facilities will undoubtedly be overwhelmed. Civil infrastructure is highly likely to be damaged, and chaos would be expected. As in many disasters, the majority of patients may self-present to hospitals that may quickly become overcrowded. Emergency operations may be limited or nearly nonexistent around the highly radioactive zones. Some severely injured victims will probably not receive timely life-saving medical care. A federal emergency would be declared, and the National Response Plan and/or Federal Radiation Emergency Response Plan would be activated.

When available, satellite surveillance will identify the "double bubble" signature of a nuclear detonation. Seismology will also show specific patterns unique to kton-size explosions. The nominal distribution of energy from a nuclear detonation is approximately 50% blast, 35% thermal radiation, 4% initial ionizing radiation (first minute), 10% residual nuclear radiation (fallout), and 1% electromagnetic pulse (EMP).[5]

In the immediate area, there will be an extensive zone of complete destruction stretching at least a 1-km radius from ground zero; however, blast winds will be felt many kilometers away from ground zero. The probable appearance of a mushroom cloud will indicate to others farther away that there has been a nuclear detonation. Nuclear weapons with a yield of 10 kton or less have a higher percentage of radiation casualties than do nuclear weapons with a yield of more than 10 kton.

BOX 106-1   Radiation Protection Guidance

1. Time, distance, and shielding.
   - *Time:* Limit the time exposed to radioactive material.
   - *Distance:* The radiation dose received from a source decreases as the inverse square of the distance from the source increases.
   - *Shielding:* The more material (especially earth, water, concrete, or dense metal) between a radiation source and a victim, the less dose to a victim. Therefore one of the best places to take shelter from initial radiation and fallout is in an underground basement away from any windows.
2. Do not look at a nuclear fireball, even from a distance: Flash-blindness and retinal burns may occur up to 20 km from the source during the daytime and up to 50 km at night.
3. The 7/10 rule: For every sevenfold increase in time after a nuclear detonation, the dose rate of early fallout decreases by a factor of approximately 10.[11] For example, if the radiation dose 1 hour after a detonation is taken as a reference, then the radiation dose at 7 hours would be 0.1 of the dose rate at 1 hour. The radiation dose at 49 hours would be $0.1 \cdot 0.1 = 0.01$, and the radiation dose rate at 343 hours ($7 \cdot 7 \cdot 7$, or about 14 days after a detonation) would be $0.1 \cdot 0.1 \cdot 0.1$ or 1/1000 of the radiation level at 1 hour. Therefore maintaining shelter for 14 days would significantly reduce the radiation exposure from fallout.
4. Take shelter or evacuate: Due to radioactive fallout, the government may initially advise people to take shelter if they are within a specific radial distance, such as 30 miles, from the hypocenter. Later, after radiation plume data are available, the government may direct some population areas to take shelter and others to evacuate based on the predicted downwind path of the plume. There is no agreement on the decision of evacuation versus shelter after nuclear detonation. In contrast to informed evacuation, advising everyone to shelter seems to be the most reasonable response due to expected traffic congestions and inadequate citizen compliance. In addition, a recent response model to nuclear detonation has shown that sheltering in place and medical care can be synergistic mitigation schemes and medical care is more likely to save lives when people shelter in place.[12]
5. Should potassium iodide be taken to block the uptake of radioactive iodine? In general, the answer is no. The fission products that make up fallout include more than 300 different isotopes of 36 elements. Radioactive iodine is no more of a problem than other radioactive isotopes unless the radioactive iodine is inhaled or ingested. In this case, it will concentrate in the thyroid gland.[11] The best measure to take is to avoid inhaling radioactive fallout or ingesting crops or milk contaminated with radioactive iodine. The food supply should be monitored for radioactive contamination. In a situation such as a nuclear reactor accident where large amounts of radioactive iodine might be released, potassium iodide would more likely be beneficial for those persons close enough to the source of radioiodine to inhale significant amounts (see Chapter 109).

Thermal radiation is the primary cause of injury from weapons larger than 10 kton because the thermal envelope extends well beyond the radiation contours.[5] Any combination of blast, burn, and radiation injury will cause synergistic effects worse than if there were to be only one type of injury.

First responders will need to evaluate the areas near victims and assess for high levels of radioactivity. A common recommendation for first responders is to use a radiation dose of 0.1 sieverts (Sv) per hour as a "turn-around" (i.e., do not enter) dose. However, for life-saving purposes, a dose of 0.5 Sv or more may be received if the situation warrants and the responder is aware of the potential health effects.[6]

In an effort to help planning response priorities and guide operational actions based on anticipated health and survival implications, an interagency committee in the United States has proposed a description of predicted structural damage zones following a model 10 kton ground nuclear detonation.[4]

Light damage (LD) zone: Damage in the LD zone is mainly caused by the forceful shock waves produced by the explosion. As a result of overpressures of 0.5-2 psi, which corresponds to a distance of around 3 miles (4.8 km), windows and doors will be blown in, and lightly constructed buildings will have significant damage. Injuries in this zone will mostly be related to flying glass and wooden fragments. As one moves closer toward ground zero, debris and rubble, car crashes, and building collapse will increase, and emergency vehicles passage will become more difficult, indicating transition to the moderate damage zone.

Moderate damage (MD) zone: MD zone damage may correspond to a distance of about 1 mile (1.6 km) from ground zero. Blast overpressures in the MD zone are 2 to 5 psi, and only reinforced concrete buildings will be standing; other residential buildings will sustain severe damage and will be structurally unstable. Blown-out buildings' interiors and utility lines, crashed and overturned automobiles, fires, and decreased visibility will be observed. This zone will have elevated radiation levels, but most casualties who survive will benefit from urgent medical care in comparison to other zones. Evacuation and passage of rescue vehicles will be difficult, and roads might require clearing.

Severe damage (SD) zone: The SD zone may have a radius of around 0.5 miles (0.8 km) and will have the greatest blast overpressure (5 to 8 psi and greater). Most buildings will be collapsed in the SD zone, and streets will be blocked with deep, impassable rubble, making timely response unfeasible. Chances of survival in the SD zone are very low, and survivors, if any, are at increased risk due to high fallout radiation levels and their prompt dose exposure. Responders should enter this zone only with extreme caution to rescue confirmed survivors.

✚ MEDICAL TREATMENT OF CASUALTIES

Following a nuclear detonation, medical facilities closest to ground zero may not be functional or may be severely damaged, and the local medical facilities that are functional can be expected to be overloaded. All medical facilities should expect to see large numbers of victims well in excess of their planned surge capacity. Victims may present with a combination of blast, burn, and radiation injuries. The victims with blast and thermal injuries may initially outnumber victims with radiation injury due to the latent nature of manifest radiation injury.

Blast Injury

Important differences exist between the blast effects from a nuclear weapon and the effects from a conventional high-explosive bomb, although many of the basic principles of blast management are still valid. With a nuclear weapon, the combination of high peak overpressure, high wind (or dynamic) pressure, and longer duration of the positive (compression) phase of the blast wave results in "mass distortion" of buildings similar to that produced by earthquakes and hurricanes. By contrast, an ordinary explosion will usually damage only part of a large structure, but the blast from a nuclear weapon can surround and destroy whole buildings.[5] While victims of a nuclear detonation may be more likely to have severe traumatic injuries more associated with earthquakes, it is important for clinicians to look for and treat the pulmonary and other complications of overpressure and blast injury (see Chapter 163).

Burn Injury

Thermal (burn) injury may be difficult to differentiate from skin injury due to radiation, although one important difference is that thermal injury occurs early, and radiation skin injury may not appear for several days. Conventional flame burns may occur due to fires ignited by the explosion. The combination of thermal burns and radiation burns significantly increases mortality.[7] Thermal injury from the infrared pulse may also cause significant eye injury. Two types of eye injuries are well known: temporary blindness, which occurs if a person indirectly sees the flash of a nuclear fireball, and permanent blindness, which occurs from looking directly at a fireball and results in retinal damage[8] (see Chapter 173).

Acute Radiation Injury

The degree of radiation injury depends on the total radiation dose, dose rate, radiation quality, and irradiated fraction of the body.[2] Radiation injury may occur alone or in combination with blast and/or thermal burn injuries. Combined injuries result in a significantly worse prognosis than radiation injury alone. For the diagnosis and treatment of acute radiation injury, the following principles should be used (see Chapter 105):

- Treat life-threatening injuries (e.g., airway, breathing, circulation) first.
- Decontaminate. The removal of clothes may remove up to 90% of external contamination.
- Anticipate combined injuries (e.g., radiation plus blast and/or thermal).
- Close open wounds within 48 hours of the event for best results.
- Base early dose estimates on symptoms and changes in lymphocyte counts. The Biodosimetry Assessment Tool (BAT) is a computer program that assists with dose estimates and is available free at the Armed Forces Radiobiology Research Institute (AFRRI) website (www.afrri.usuhs.mil).[9]

Acute Radiation Syndrome

Patients with acute radiation syndrome (ARS) classically go through four clinical phases: prodrome, latency, manifest illness, and either recovery or death. During the prodromal phase, they usually present with nausea, vomiting, fatigue, and even loss of consciousness at higher doses. Organ systems that are mostly affected by radiation injury are the hematologic, gastrointestinal, and central nervous systems (CNS) and cardiovascular systems (CVS). Even with low radiation levels, peripheral blood cytopenias can occur. Lymphocytes are the most sensitive among blood cells, and lymphocyte count can be used to measure the degree of radiation exposure. The dose at which only 50% of adult humans will survive for at least 60 days without any supportive care (LD50/60) is around 3.5 Gy.[2] ARS may require early use of hematopoietic colony-stimulating factors such as filgrastim. ARS may occur miles from an incident due to radioactive fallout (Figure 106-1). There will probably be no major role for the use of potassium iodide, Prussian blue, or diethylenetriamine pentaacetic acid (DTPA) after a nuclear detonation. (See Chapters 83 and 84 for a more thorough discussion of ARS.)

Delayed Radiation Effects (2 to 4 Weeks after Event)

Due to the delayed onset of the hematopoietic subsyndrome of ARS, some patients may do well for 2 to 4 weeks before developing symptoms of bone marrow suppression and even failure, with neutropenia and infections. These patients should be identified as soon as possible so that they may be transferred to appropriate facilities for treatment of their illness. The Radiation Injury Treatment Network (RITN) is a national organization that coordinates specially prepared bone marrow transplant programs to respond to such an emergency.

Risk of Malignancy

Following a nuclear detonation, persons exposed to radiation will have concerns about their potential risk for developing malignancy. While

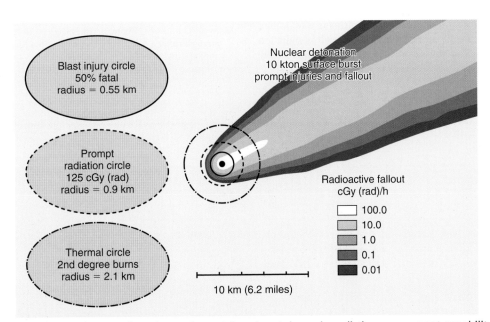

FIG 106-1 A 10 kton nuclear detonation, surface burst, hazard prediction assessment capability (HPAC) plot[10] with wind 10 mph from the southeast. The plot shows both prompt effects and fallout 4 hours after detonation. Prompt effects include blast injury fatal in 50% of victims out to a radius of 0.55 km, radiation injury of 125 cGy (rad) out to a 0.9 km radius, and second-degree burns out to a 2.1 km radius. Fallout shows a 100 cGy/h area out to about 5 km downwind and much longer distances for 10 cGy/h and less.[10]

there is indeed an increased risk of malignancy, it is generally less than commonly thought by the public. It will be important for medical, public health, and emergency management leaders to establish a registry of victims to track their health status, as well as to provide ongoing medical information and monitoring. Creation and administration of the registry will likely require very significant resources, and federal agencies such as the Centers for Disease Control (CDC) and the Agency for Toxic Substances and Disease Registry (ATSDR) may be needed to provide assistance in establishing, coordinating, and maintaining the registry.

Psychological Injury

Long-term follow-up care will be necessary to identify late effects from radiation injury and trauma and to assist with posttraumatic stress symptoms (see Chapter 10).

UNIQUE CONSIDERATIONS

The following should be considered when treating patients as a result of a nuclear detonation event:

- Hospital surge capacity for all services will be exceeded, and many hospitals may have severe damage.
- Hospitals will need to use a combination of their mass casualty, radiation, burn, and blast plans to respond to a nuclear detonation.
- Patients with life-threatening injuries should have assessment and management of their airway, breathing, and circulation performed before radiation decontamination. Medical personnel should wear appropriate personal protective equipment (PPE) and dosimeters for their own safety and monitoring.
- Triage should be performed outside the medical facility, if possible, to avoid contaminating the facility. Decontamination of all but the immediately life-threatening injuries should also occur outside the clinical areas of the facility if possible.
- Mass deaths will exceed immediate storage and burial capacity.

PITFALLS

In the event of a nuclear detonation, there will be damage to the community infrastructure, with limited communications and limited services. Failure to secure the medical center may result in radiation contamination throughout the facility. Health professionals may fail to anticipate the manifest illness phase of isolated radiation casualties.

REFERENCES

1. Subbarao I, James JJ. Nuclear preparedness. *Disaster Med Public Health Prep.* 2011;5(S1):S8–S10.
2. DiCarlo AL, Maher C, Hick JL, et al. Radiation injury after a nuclear detonation: medical consequences and the need for scarce resources allocation. *Disaster Med Public Health Prep.* 2011;5(S1):S32–S44.
3. Radiation Effects Research Foundation. Frequently Asked Questions about the Atomic-bomb Survivor Research Program. Available at: http://www.rerf.or.jp/general/qa_e/index.html.
4. *Planning Guidance for Response to a Nuclear Detonation: National Security Staff Interagency Policy Coordination Subcommittee for Preparedness & Response to Radiological and Nuclear Threats.* 2nd ed. June 2010:40-49. Available at: http://www.remm.nlm.gov/PlanningGuidanceNuclearDetonation.pdf.
5. *The Medical NBC Battlebook. Tech Guide 244.* Aberdeen Proving Ground, MD: U.S. Army Center for Health Promotion and Preventive Medicine; 2002, 2-23.
6. *Management of Terrorist Events Involving Radioactive Material. NCRP Report No. 138.* Bethesda, MD: National Council on Radiation Protection and Measurements; 2001, 23:95-98.
7. Armed Forces Radiobiology Research Institute. *Medical Management of Radiological Casualties Handbook.* 2nd ed. Bethesda, MD: Armed Forces Radiobiology Research Institute; 2003. 39. Available at: http://www.afrri.usuhs.mil.
8. Walker RI, Cerveny TJ, eds. *Textbook of Military Medicine: Medical Consequences of Nuclear Warfare.* Falls Church, VA: TMM Publications, Office of the Surgeon General, Department of the Army; 1989 6, 7. Available at: http://www.afrri.usuhs.mil.
9. Armed Forces Radiobiology Research Institute. Biodosimetry Assessment Tool (BAT). Available at: http://www.afrri.usuhs.mil.
10. Specialized Radiological Monitoring and Hazard Assessment Capabilities. Office of the Assistant Secretary of Defense for Nuclear, Chemical, and Biological Defense Programs/Nuclear Matters. http://www.acq.osd.mil/ncbdp/narp/Radiation_Data/Specialized_Radiological.htm.
11. Glasstone S, Dolan PJ. *The Effects of Nuclear Weapons.* 3rd ed. Washington, DC: U.S. Department of Defense and U.S. Energy Research and Development Administration; 1977.
12. Wein LM, Choi Y, Denuit S. Analyzing evacuation versus shelter in place strategies after a terrorist nuclear detonation. *Risk Anal.* 2010;30(9):1315–1327.

CHAPTER 107

Radiation Accident—Isolated Exposure

Jeanette A. Linder and Lawrence S. Linder

DESCRIPTION OF EVENT

Ionizing radiation is capable of creating ions. These ions then cause cell damage to varying degrees, depending on the total dose, the portion and proportion of body exposed, the duration of exposure, and comorbidities. Isolated radiation exposure is defined as a single event in which a person is externally exposed to ionizing radiation without having any radioactive material deposited on or in the body (i.e., there is no contamination). Dispersed exposure occurs when a patient is exposed and either externally or internally contaminated with radioactive material; this is discussed in Chapter 108.

Intentional radiation exposure of non-humans is an integral part of industrial monitoring, calibration, signage, nuclear reactors, sterilization of agricultural products, and x-ray screening of luggage and cargo. Intentional radiation exposure of humans is also a common and essential element of current medical care, but all intentional radiation exposure must be done in controlled settings and be carefully monitored. Sealed radioactive sources and radiation generators (diagnostic and therapeutic x-ray machines) can cause external radiation without contamination. X-ray machines do not deposit lasting radioactivity in a person. Radioactive sources, on the other hand, are sometimes implanted into patients, permanently or temporarily. High-activity sources are also used in industry for imaging. Sources can be sealed within metal or unsealed in liquid or powder form. Unsealed or damaged sources can transfer radioactivity (i.e., contaminate) and are discussed in Chapter 108.

Accidental exposure from radioactive sources and x-ray–producing machines, however, can easily occur with minor variations in practice, loss of custody of radioactive sources, or equipment malfunction. Although such accidents are infrequent, rapid recognition of an exposure and intervention can prevent potentially significant, and sometimes fatal, possible outcomes.

The most commonly encountered forms of radiation are the following:
- *A*lpha: Topical, absorbed or shielded by clothing or paper
- Beta: *B*arely penetrate only a few millimeters
- *G*amma: *G*o all the way through, deeply penetrate
- Neutrons: *N*astiest and *n*uclear, deeply penetrate and cause more damage than gamma

Sealed sources containing iridium-192, cesium-137, and cobalt-60 are commonly used in industry and medicine. These beta and gamma emitters are the primary cause of isolated exposure without contamination.[1] Alpha and neutron emissions usually occur in nuclear reactions, such as nuclear detonations and nuclear power plant accidents, and are discussed in Chapters 106 and 109.

PRE-INCIDENT ACTIONS

Preparation for a rare event, such as isolated radiation exposure, involves ensuring rapid access by frontline responders to an early warning system for incident recognition and to infrequently used references for access to specialty information. Any facility using radioactive materials or x-ray equipment must have a detailed plan to minimize all exposures and to respond to unintentional exposure. Exposure limits are defined by Occupational Safety and Health Administration (OSHA) guidelines and vary for the general public, radiation workers, and disaster recovery workers.[2,3] Incorporating the radiation safety plans of nearby industrial facilities, including mines, nuclear facilities, municipal landfills, metal works, and radiation therapy accelerators, may help emergency responders, hospitals, and other medical providers prepare for the most likely accidents and incidents.

Basic precautions, such as shielding from radioactive sources, minimal handling of radioactive sources, and maintaining exposure at a maximal distance and minimal time, must be taken to provide primary prevention of radiation accidents. This is best achieved in a controlled environment where the radioactive source is known to be located and is appropriately in the custody of trained and authorized staff. An orphan source is defined as a radioactive source not under the custody of an authorized radiation safety officer (RSO). To help prevent orphan sources, all radioactive sources, both sealed and unsealed, should be registered, clearly labeled, inventoried, and stored in a locked facility that is clearly marked as radioactive storage with access limited to authorized personnel. Orphan sources are further addressed in Chapter 108.

Hospitals should post radiation detectors at strategic locations around diagnostic and therapeutic radiation use areas.[2] These detectors must clearly signal the removal of a source or failure to turn off a radiation generator. Hospitals may also consider placing detectors at hospital entrances or at other strategic locations. Alarm levels are suggested in the National Council on Radiation Protection and Measurements (NCRP) *Report No. 138—Management of Terrorist Events Involving Radioactive Material*.[3] The benefits and consequences of detection alarms, and the possible disproportionate emotional reactions to them, should be considered when choosing a threshold for alarms or whether to post monitors at all. Hospitals should discuss the alarm positions and alarm levels with their RSO, as well as the desired method of rapidly communicating the alarm (audible vs. electronic message to a remote authority, on-site or off-site).

Hospitals must also have a communication plan for recognizing, alerting, and communicating information about radiation that includes their RSO and an appropriate radiation specialist. If a hospital does not have specialists who can recommend treatment for radiation injury, there are several national resources available, including the Radiation Emergency Assistance Center/Training Site (REAC/TS) in Oak Ridge, Tennessee (865-576-1005), or the Medical Radiobiology Advisory Team (MRAT) (301-295-0316 daytime; 301-295-0530 after hours) at the Armed Forces Radiobiology Research Institute (AFRRI) for advice. Local and federal authorities may also need to be notified. If there is a significant patient exposure, either in terms of a large dose or if there are multiple victims, REAC/TS (for civilian incidents) or MRAT (for military incidents) should be notified. Simple forms are available online and in multiple texts for documentation of signs, symptoms, and details of exposure (i.e., isotope or beam generator, direct contact or exposure to a beam, time of exposure, distance, whole versus partial body, single incident, intermittent exposure, or ongoing exposure with contamination).[4,5]

As with all other essential elements of emergency preparedness, preparedness plans for radiation exposure should be reviewed and tested periodically, and necessary supplies should be inventoried.

There are numerous high-quality references on the basic care of radiation accidents that are available in both hard copy and electronic formats. Some of the most commonly accessed references include:

- U.S. Centers for Disease Control and Prevention (CDC): www.bt.cdc.gov/radiation.
- U.S. Food and Drug Administration (FDA): http://www.fda.gov/Drugs/EmergencyPreparedness/BioterrorismandDrugPreparedness/ucm063807.htm.
- The Biodosimetry Assessment Tool (BAT) is detailed later in this chapter and is an extremely useful resource.
- AFRRI: www.usuhs.edu/afrri/. A pdf file of the *Medical Management of Radiological Casualties: Handbook*, 2nd ed., can be downloaded from: www.usuhs.edu/afrri/outreach/pdf/4edmmrchandbook.pdf.
- REAC/TS: www.orise.orau.gov/reacts/.
- American College of Radiology (ACR) *Disaster Preparedness Primer* can be downloaded from: http://www.acr.org/~/media/ACR/Documents/PDF/Membership/Legal%20Business/Disaster%20Preparedness/Primer.

Basic medical fact sheets for providers and patient handouts regarding isolated radiation exposure are available on the CDC website. The available patient education materials address:

1. Short- and long-term health risks of radiation exposure: physical and psychological
2. Signs and symptoms requiring medical intervention, especially subacute to chronic
3. References to websites and other literature for further support
4. Ways to prevent further exposure
5. Referral to a radiation specialist

▷▷ POST-INCIDENT ACTIONS

The most common accidental single exposures occur with previously identified sources and beam generators.[1,6] Most medical and nuclear reactor facilities can immediately identify the radioactive source(s) (usually iridium-192, cobalt-60, or cesium-137) or a generated beam and an approximate dose. Questions regarding the details about the isotope and form of exposure (topical, inhaled, ingested, or absorbed through skin) will focus medical care on the critical organ for that particular isotope and exposed body site. Irradiation by a completely removed isotope, such as a sealed source or a machine-generated beam over a finite period is much simpler than ongoing exposure with contamination and is the focus of this chapter.

Recognition of a radiation accident may be exceedingly difficult. Unrecognized exposure to radiation is uncommon, but can be deduced from signs and symptoms over time.[6] The signs and symptoms of radiation sickness are similar to many common syndromes, including thermal burns, gastroenteritis, vague malaise, nausea, and vomiting.[1] Burns without previous thermal or solar exposure, nausea, vomiting, epilation, and/or bone marrow suppression, especially in clusters of patients, may be due to unidentified radiation exposure. The history and physical should address therapeutic, diagnostic, and occupational sources of radiation, particularly in close proximity to nuclear reactors, scientific laboratories, particle accelerators, or other facilities with high radiation exposure.

Whole-body radiation exposure causes predictable and proportional declines in blood counts, increasing constitutional symptoms, and other factors, as noted below.[7] Once a radiation accident has been confirmed, hospitals and emergency responders should follow their prespecified communication protocol and notify at least the RSO, a radiation specialist, and possibly REAC/TS (civilian) or MRAT (military).

✚ MEDICAL TREATMENT OF CASUALTIES

Initial emergency care is the same for both the nonradiation and the radiation casualty. Airway, breathing, and circulation are always the first priority.[3] Radiological exposure does not cause immediate loss of consciousness; responders should assess for other toxic exposures or trauma if presented with an immediately unconscious patient. As the patient's condition is stabilized, the next most important distinction for initial medical management will be to distinguish whether the patient was only irradiated (i.e., exposed but not contaminated), versus exposed and contaminated. Again, irradiated patients have no detectable radioactivity and pose no risk to providers.[6]

The history and accompanying documentation are usually quickly able to help identify the source, machine or isotope, the form of isotope (sealed or unsealed), the body distance and position from the source, and the approximate dose. One must determine whether the exposure was whole-body, local, or both. Small portions of the body can tolerate much larger radiation exposures than can the whole body. Sequelae of whole-body irradiation can quickly escalate, whereas partial-body exposures can often be observed and treated days to weeks after the exposure when local symptoms occur, if necessary.[1,8,9]

Localized Exposure

Acute treatment of uncontaminated local exposures is similar to the treatment of thermal burns or other local trauma.[9,10] Further physical trauma of the irradiated area must be avoided. The development of erythema, epilation (hair loss), desquamation, and blistering typically requires days to weeks. These signs usually result in predictable cutaneous changes, which vary depending on the dose and distribution of exposure. Consequences of exposure and the time delay until those consequences become clinically apparent will vary with the volume of tissue exposed and the dose absorbed.[8] Epilation occurs in 2 to 3 weeks at doses greater than approximately 3 Gy (gray, a measurement of absorbed dose of radiation in International Units).[9] The threshold for erythema visible on day 1 is 10 Gy; this erythema rapidly dissipates at relatively low doses, then recurs days to weeks later. Local irradiation of 20 Gy causes moist desquamation and possibly ulceration in about 2 weeks. Delayed or lack of healing of ulceration is caused by 25 Gy and greater. Higher doses shorten the time in which these changes develop. Local radiation tissue injury can be treated in a manner similar to thermal burns, but manipulation of erythematous tissue should only be undertaken with severe trepidation. Ulcerated areas will gradually expand to include surrounding erythematous regions as the tissue injury is expressed over time. Follow-up care should be transferred to a radiation specialist.[8,10,11]

Patients with signs of local exposure may also have lesser degrees of whole-body exposure. Other injuries will hinder recovery from whole-body exposure. All patients should be monitored for acute radiation sickness or some other phase of radiation exposure, as noted below. In patients with concomitant total body exposure, closure of wounds should be done either within 36 to 48 hours before bone marrow suppression occurs, or several weeks to months later once the marrow has recovered.[10–12]

Whole-Body or Large Partial-Body Exposure

Radiation exposure of ~1 Gy or more to large portions of the body causes predictable syndromes. The time to first vomiting after exposure (time or emesis [TE]), lymphocyte depletion kinetics, and chromosome aberrations are dose-dependent over time.[7,9,11] A sophisticated but user-friendly software program, BAT, is a free download from the AFRRI website (www.afrri.usuhs.mil) and is based on these indicators.[11,13] Signs and symptoms and validated data can be systematically recorded in the program at varying intervals. The program will provide a calculation of estimated doses based on input data and physical parameters.

Initial symptoms of acute radiation sickness can occur within minutes to days after whole-body exposure. Affected systems increase with increasing dose in the following order: hematopoietic, gastrointestinal, cardiovascular, central nervous system.[7,9,10] Each syndrome has four phases: (1) prodromal, (2) latent, (3) manifest illness, and (4) recovery or death. The prodromal phase is predictive of the severity of subsequent phases. Prodromal symptoms include nausea, vomiting, diarrhea, fatigue, weakness, headache, parotid pain, and erythema. The time between exposure and TE often correlates with general ranges of total body dose. A TE of less than 4 hours may indicate a significant whole-body dose of 3.5 Gy or more. Without appropriate medical treatment, a whole-body dose of approximately 3.5 Gy is generally considered lethal to 50% of patients within 60 days ($LD_{50/60}$). The $LD_{50/60}$ may nearly double to 6 to 7 Gy with aggressive intervention.[10,11] Without medical care, this 6- to 7-Gy dose would allow few survivors. A TE of less than 1 hour possibly indicates a lethal exposure even with intensive medical care; palliative care is recommended if the supralethal dosage is confirmed by clinical evaluation. Healthy adults with a TE of more than 4 hours, which implies a whole-body dose of less than 1 to 2 Gy, will probably survive without medical care, unless additional medical factors complicate the issue. If there are mass casualties, patients without concomitant injuries who have a TE of more than 4 hours can be triaged to delayed evaluation in 24 to 72 hours, but reevaluation is mandatory.[14]

The speed at which lymphocyte counts decrease is directly proportional to the whole-body dose. An absolute lymphocyte count (ALC) decline of 50% or more within 24 hours indicates at least a moderate whole-body dose. If the victim has other injuries, then ALC is a less reliable predictor.[7,10,13]

Physical Examination

Initial physical examination should focus on vital signs (fever, hypotension, orthostasis), skin manifestations (erythema, blistering, onycholysis, edema, desquamation, petechiae), central nervous system deficits (motor, sensory, ataxia, mental status, cognition), and abdominal signs (pain or tenderness).[10]

Laboratory Studies

A complete blood count with differential and platelet count should be drawn immediately and at least three times per day for several days in anyone with prodromal symptoms. Blood samples for cytogenetic studies should be drawn around 24 hours after exposure. The proper tube in which tube to collect blood (e.g., 40 mL in tubes containing lithium-heparin), as well as the proper labeling and storage temperature should be verfied with the institution's RSO or external expert.[11]

Treatment

Treatment is stratified by the estimated total body dose in addition to treatment of known injuries or infections. Estimated dose, probability of survival, and treatment are based on signs, symptoms, and approximate blood counts as outlined in Table 107-1 or by the results of serial data input into the BAT program.[1,13,15]

The Strategic National Stockpile Radiation Working Group (SNS-RWG) has consolidated the seminal literature on radiation injury. It recommends treatment of neutropenic or anticipated neutropenic patients with: (1) broad-spectrum prophylaxis using a fluoroquinolone with streptococcal coverage or augmented with penicillin or amoxicillin; (2) acyclovir; and (3) fluconazole. Known sites of infection should be managed according to established guidelines. Underlying foci of current or new infection are likely to be due to loss of integrity of the integument or gastrointestinal tract. Anaerobic coverage should be added when there is known bowel injury.[10]

The SNS recommends supportive care with cytokines (G-CSF, Peg-G-CSF, GM-CSF), prophylactic and therapeutic antibiotics, leukoreduced and irradiated transfusions, antiemetics, antidiarrheals, opiates, parenteral fluids, and nutrition.[10] In patients with concomitant total-body exposure, closure of wounds should be done either within 36 to 48 hours before bone marrow suppression occurs or months later when the marrow has recovered.[10–12] Treatment should be transferred to a radiation specialist or should continue under the guidance of REAC/TS, MRAT, or other response teams. Long-term care should be transferred to a specialist center in radiation injury. Many such centers participate in the Radiation Injury Treatment Network (RITN). When chronic, nonhealing wounds present as late effects of exposure to radiation, consideration of hyperbaric oxygen therapy should be made before and after attempts at flaps or skin grafts, and consultation from a specialist in hyperbaric medicine should be sought as part of a multispecialty approach to wound healing.[16,17]

❓ UNIQUE CONSIDERATIONS

All radiation accident victims carry some increased risk of an induced malignancy.[3] This risk is usually far less than anticipated and only slightly greater than the pre-incident risk, because radiation is a relatively weak carcinogen.[3] Risk is related to quality and dose of radiation, affected organs, age at the time of exposure, and other risk factors.[3] Education about the typically small increase in risk may diminish stress significantly. General educational materials can initially allay fears, and subsequent consultation with a radiation specialist can better define risks and proper surveillance.

Loss of fertility is common with irradiation of the gonads. This may be temporary or permanent, depending on dose, depth of penetration, age, and maturation of the patient.[3] Doses to the testes of 0.15 Gy are likely to cause temporary sterility, but 3.5 Gy or more will cause permanent sterility. Ovarian doses for permanent sterility range from 2.5 to 6 Gy.[3] There has been some recovery of fertility even in major radiation accidents, as was seen in Chernobyl recovery workers.[18]

Fetal doses should be estimated separately from whole-body and local doses to a pregnant woman. In some cases, the fetus receives a lower whole-body dose than the mother due to natural shielding of the baby by surrounding structures. Very low doses of only 0.1 to 1 Gy can be very harmful to the fetus, depending on the stage of gestation. Exposure to ionizing radiation before implantation usually results in undetectable death of the fetus or failure to implant. Exposure during organogenesis (weeks ~3 to 7) may cause malformations. Later exposure during weeks

TABLE 107-1   **Response Categories**

RESPONSE CATEGORY	WBE	PROBABILITY OF SURVIVAL*	CLINICAL SIGNS[†]	ALC[‡]	ANC[§]	TREATMENT
1	~0.4-1.4 Sv	~100% without treatment	None or minimal	0.5-2	>2	Follow-up as outpatient
2	~1.3-5.5 Sv	>60 days with treatment	Mild N, V, D, F	0.3-0.8	Initial↑ days 10-20, ↓25-30	Antibiotics; transfuse platelets (prn); follow-up for infections; antiemetics
3	~4.4-8.0 Sv	Survival with intense treatment	N, V, F, Er, D, Ep	0.2-0.5	Initial ↑, then↓ days 15-25	Reverse isolation; replacement/transfusions; growth factors; fluids; gut bacterial decontamination; antiemetics
4	~9-11 Sv	10-15 days 100% mortality without transplant	N, V, D, early Er and edema, CNS	0-0.1 in 3 days	Early ↑, then↓ in 6 days	Reverse isolation; gnotobiotic tx; fluids and electrolytes stem cell transplants; antibiotics, antifungals, antivirals; transfusions; cytokines; antiemetics
5	>11 Sv	<7-12 days	CNS, shock, edema, N/V	0-0.1 within hours	Initial↑, then↓ by day 5	Palliative only

WBE, Whole-body exposure in sieverts (Sv), which include a radiobiological quality factor (equivalent to Gy for most radiation exposure); ↓, nadir. Nausea and vomiting can be quite severe after large doses to the abdomen or moderate whole body doses.[12] The most effective antiemetics are 5HT-3 antagonists.[15]

*Survival may be reduced with concomitant injuries and comorbidities.

[†]Clinical signs are N, nausea; V, vomiting; D, diarrhea; F, fatigue; Er, erythema; Ep, epilation; CNS, central nervous system perturbations.

[‡]*ALC,* Absolute lymphocyte count in units of 10^9/L.

[§]*ANC,* Absolute neutrophil count in units of 10^9/L.

Data from Turai I, Veress K. Radiation accidents: occurrence, types, consequences, medical management, and the lessons to be learned. *Central Eur J Occup Environ Med.* 2001;7:3-14; Blakely W, Prasanna P, Miller A. Update on current and new developments in biological dose-assessment techniques. In: Ricks R, Berger M, O'Hara F, eds. *The Medical Basis for Radiation-Accident Preparedness: The Clinical Care of Victims.* Proceedings of the Fourth International REAC/TS Conference on the Medical Basis for Radiation-Accident Preparedness. New York: Parthenon Publishing Group; 2002:23-32; and Mettler F, Guskova A. Treatment of acute radiation sickness. In: Gusev I, Guskova A, Mettler F, eds. *Medical Management of Radiation Accidents.* 2nd ed. Boca Raton, FL: CRC Press; 2001:53-67.

8 to 25 causes decreasing IQ with increasing dose. There is a small increased risk of childhood cancers and leukemias.[3]

Patients, family members, co-workers, recovery workers, and even health care providers often require some psychological intervention. The emotional trauma and possible stigma of radiation exposure can be intense and outlast the physical manifestations. Acute stress reactions of insomnia, impaired concentration, and social withdrawal should be anticipated. If the radiation accident is associated with an act of terrorism, then psychological effects will increase. Patients should be followed over the long term for signs of posttraumatic stress disorder. Groups at particularly high risk are children, mothers of young children, pregnant women, emergency personnel, recovery and cleanup workers, and those with a history of mental illness. Education and early intervention can prevent much of this psychological stress.[9,19]

⚠ PITFALLS

- Failure to prepare a radiation response plan or to learn basic radiation medicine
- Failure to recognize an accidental or intentional radiation incident
- Failure to access the multiple educational resources and emergency expertise available when needed, and/or to use a sample emergency plan from the websites listed in this chapter[20]

REFERENCES

1. Turai I, Veress K. Radiation accidents: occurrence, types, consequences, medical management, and the lessons to be learned. *Central Eur J Occup Environ Med.* 2001;7:3–14.

2. United States Department of Labor, Occupational Safety & Health Administration. *Ionizing Radiation.* Available at: https://www.osha.gov/SLTC/radiationionizing/.

3. National Council on Radiation Protection and Measurements. *Report No. 138—Management of Terrorist Events Involving Radioactive Material.* Bethesda, MD: National Council on Radiation Protection and Measurements; 2001.

4. National Council on Radiation Protection and Measurements. *Report No. 65—Management of Persons Accidentally Contaminated with Radionuclides.* Bethesda, MD: National Council on Radiation Protection and Measurements; 1980.

5. Centers for Disease Control and Prevention. *Radiation Emergencies.* Available at: http://www.bt.cdc.gov/radiation.

6. Mettler F, Kelsey C. Fundamentals of radiation accidents. In: Gusev I, Guskova A, Mettler F, eds. *Medical Management of Radiation Accidents.* 2nd ed. Boca Raton, FL: CRC Press; 2001:1–13.

7. Guskova A, Baranov A, Gusev I. Acute radiation sickness: underlying principles and assessment. In: Gusev I, Guskova A, Mettler F, eds. *Medical Management of Radiation Accidents.* 2nd ed. Boca Raton, FL: CRC Press; 2001:33–51.

8. Guskova A. Radiation sickness classification. In: Gusev I, Guskova A, Mettler F, eds. *Medical Management of Radiation Accidents.* 2nd ed. Boca Raton, FL: CRC Press; 2001:15–22.

9. Mettler F, Voelz G. Major radiation exposure—what to expect and how to respond. *N Engl J Med.* 2002;346:1554–1561.

10. Waselenko J, MacVittie T, Blakely W, et al. Medical management of the acute radiation syndrome: recommendations of the Strategic National Stockpile Radiation Working Group. *Ann Intern Med.* 2004;140:1037–1051.

11. Jarrett D, ed. *Medical Management of Radiological Casualties: Handbook.* 4th ed. 2013. Bethesda, MD: AFRRI Special Publication. Armed Forces Radiobiology Research Institute; 2013. Available at: http://www.afrri.usuhs.mil.

12. Barabanova A. Local radiation injury. In: Gusev I, Guskova A, Mettler F, eds. *Medical Management of Radiation Accidents.* 2nd ed. Boca Raton, FL: CRC Press; 2001:223–240.

13. Blakely W, Prasanna P, Miller A. Update on current and new developments in biological dose-assessment techniques. In: Ricks R, Berger M, O'Hara F, eds. *The Medical Basis for Radiation-accident Preparedness: The Clinical Care of Victims. Proceedings of the Fourth International REAC/TS Conference on The Medical Basis for Radiation-Accident Preparedness*, New York: Parthenon; 2002:23–32.

14. Department of Homeland Security Working Group on Radiological Dispersal Device (RDD) Preparedness. *Medical Preparedness and Response Sub-Group.* Available at: http://www.acr.org/~/media/ACR/Documents/PDF/Membership/Legal%20Business/Disaster%20Preparedness/Counter%20Measures.

15. Mettler F, Guskova A. Treatment of acute radiation sickness. In: Gusev I, Guskova A, Mettler F, eds. *Medical Management of Radiation Accidents.* 2nd ed. Boca Raton, FL: CRC Press; 2001:53–67.

16. Marx RA. Radiation injury to tissue. In: Kindwall EP, Whelan HT, eds. *Hyperbaric Medicine Practice.* 2nd ed. Flagstaff, AZ: Best; 1999:665–723.

17. Feldmeier JJ, Matos LA. Delayed radiation injuries (soft tissue and bony necrosis). In: Feldmeier JJ, ed. *Hyperbaric Oxygen 2003—Indications and Results: The Hyperbaric Oxygen Therapy Committee Report.* Kensington, MD: Undersea and Hyperbaric Medical Society; 2003:87–100.

18. Guskova A, Gusev I. Medical aspects of the accident at Chernobyl. In: Gusev I, Guskova A, Mettler F, eds. *Medical Management of Radiation Accidents.* 2nd ed. Boca Raton, FL: CRC Press; 2001:195–210.

19. Berger M, Sadoff R. Psychological support of radiation accident patients, families, and staff. In: Gusev I, Guskova A, Mettler F, eds. *Medical Management of Radiation Accidents.* 2nd ed. Boca Raton, FL: CRC Press; 2001:191–200.

20. Appendix 1. sample radiation emergency plan for a medical facility. In: Gusev I, Guskova A, Mettler F, eds. *Medical Management of Radiation Accidents.* 2nd ed. Boca Raton, FL: CRC Press; 2001:557–570.

Radiation Accident—Dispersed Exposure

Jeanette A. Linder and Lawrence S. Linder

DESCRIPTION OF EVENT

Dispersed exposure to radiation occurs when a patient is exposed to ionizing radiation and contaminated either externally or internally with radioactive material. As discussed in Chapter 107, *isolated exposure* is a single event in which a person is externally irradiated without any contamination. Dispersed ionizing radiation accidents are caused by either unsealed or damaged radiation sources. Contamination can be external (on the skin and hair) or internal (i.e., occurring by injection, ingestion, inhalation, or absorption through intact skin or wounds). The most common dispersed exposures have been in medical and industrial accidents.[1] Less commonly, orphan sources, defined as those radiation sources no longer in the custody of a radiation safety officer (RSO), have also been the cause of dispersed exposures, whether knowingly or unwittingly transported and/or altered by unauthorized persons. Coupling an orphan source with a conventional explosive will create a dirty bomb. Fortunately, the small amounts of radioactivity that would be dispersed by a dirty bomb or from spraying radioactive powders or liquid are unlikely to cause significant illness beyond the psychological terror caused by the event.[2] Radiation dispersal devices and other intentional dispersion events are addressed in this chapter. The most lethal and fear-causing form of radiation exposure would be caused by a nuclear explosion, which is addressed in Chapter 106.

Medical or industrial sources are the types of sources most likely to be dispersed, either accidentally or intentionally, in a dirty bomb.[1] At baseline in medical or industrial use, these sources are usually sealed in metal. Beta, gamma, and minimal neutron exposures are the most prevalent exposures in industry and medicine, whereas alpha and neutron emitters usually occur in nuclear reactions, such as those in nuclear power plants or nuclear detonations. Accidents with medical or industrial sources can involve, in decreasing order of frequency, iridium-192, cobalt-60, and cesium-137, which emit penetrating gamma and minimal beta radiation.[1] Iodine-125 and palladium-103 seeds are weak gamma and beta emitters. These sources are commonly used in radiation oncology for permanent implantation of the prostate gland and other organs and usually pose little to no risk. Many unsealed sources are used in scientific laboratories and nuclear medicine testing and treatment, including tritium-3, iodine-131, iodine-125, strontium-90, and technetium-99 m. The chemical and radiation characteristics of each isotope will determine which organs are affected and what the resulting illness may be. The effective time of exposure without intervention depends on the body's incorporation and/or excretion of that substance or the vehicle on which the isotope is carried. Incorporation of an isotope into tissues may be temporary or permanent, and it depends on the chemical nature, size of the particles, phase state (liquid versus solid), and route of entry. As examples, radium can be permanently incorporated into bone matrix, whereas iodine is taken up into the thyroid. Others may eventually be excreted in the urine or feces without intervention. Table 108-1 provides basic facts for the most commonly encountered isotopes in accidents.[3-6] The RSO and agencies such as the Radiation Emergency Assistance Center/Training Site (REAC/TS) in Oak Ridge, Tennessee (865-576-1005), will provide detailed information on detection, dose estimation, decontamination, and consequence prevention and management.

PRE-INCIDENT ACTIONS

As discussed in Chapter 107, preparation for a rare event, such as isolated radiation exposure, involves ensuring rapid access by frontline responders to an early warning system for incident recognition and to infrequently used references for access to specialty information. In the case of an event causing contamination with dispersed radioactive materials, patients may know that they were contaminated, especially during medical or industrial accidents. In the rare case of accidental or intentional contamination that goes initially unidentified, mounted radiation monitors at strategic entrances to the hospital may detect undeclared or unrecognized radioactivity. Alarm levels for such detectors are suggested in the National Council on Radiation Protection and Measurements (NCRP) report number 138.[7] However, both the likelihood of and potential for immediate radiation detection and the possible consequences of false alarms and anxiety that might result should be considered when deciding to place such an alarm system. Placing portal radiation monitors requires choosing a threshold for alarm alerts, a well-thought-out architectural plan, and detailed plans for handling alarms, response, and notification of appropriate authorities, including the local RSO and radiation specialists. Sample emergency plans are available on various websites and in radiation texts.[8] Hospital and clinic emergency preparedness exercises should periodically include a radiation-exposed patient or scenario to ensure familiarity with and provide practice of the radiation response, containment, and treatment procedures by the emergency department and other hospital staff members.

First responders to any detonation should always survey for radioactivity on arrival.[7] First responders at the accident site may receive significant doses if they are unaware of the presence of radiation. However, with proper real-time monitoring, limited on-scene time, and maximal distance, exposures can be acceptable. When following simple procedures, providers can receive very little exposure even while caring for large numbers of contaminated victims. It is reassuring that no U.S. health care worker who has adhered to simple barrier precautions has become contaminated from handling a contaminated patient.[9] Habitual use of gowns, double gloves, masks, and hair and shoe covers by all responders, and remaining within the contaminated zone until cleared for exit by the RSO will keep exposures well within

TABLE 108-1 Decontamination of Common Elements in Industrial and Medical Accidents*

ELEMENT	EMISSIONS	CRITICAL ORGAN	EFFECTIVE $t_{1/2}$[†]	DECONTAMINATION
Cesium-137	Beta, gamma	Total body	70 days	Prussian blue (Radiogardase) 3 g po 3 times/day (adults and adolescents); 1 g po 3 times/day (2-12 yr old); consider lavage and purgatives
Cobalt-60	Beta, gamma	Total body	10 days	Lavage, purgatives, penicillamine
Iodine-125, iodine-131	Beta, gamma	Thyroid	Iodine-125, 42 days; iodine-131, 8 days	Potassium iodide: 0-1 mo, 16 mg/day; >1 mo to 3 yr, 32 mg/day; >3 mo to 3 yr, 32 mg/day; >3 to 12 yr and <70 kg, 65 mg/day; adults or ≥70 kg, 130 mg/day; consider lavage
Iridium-192	Beta, gamma	Lung	74 days	Lavage for large quantities
Technetium-99 m	Gamma	Total body	5 hours	Potassium perchlorate to reduce thyroid dose
Tritium-3	Beta	Total body	12 days	Forced fluids
Uranium-235, uranium-238	Alpha	Kidney,[‡] bone, liver, lung	Can be permanent if in bone	Bicarbonate to alkalinize the urine

po, Per os; *qd,* once per day.

*See Chapter 107 for a description of possible elements and types of radioactivity.

[†]Effective $t_{1/2}$ combines radioactive and chemical properties and rates of elimination without decontamination efforts.

[‡]The kidney is most vulnerable to large amounts of uranium because of the chemical properties of this heavy metal. Uranium can ultimately be deposited in bone.

Data from U.S. Food and Drug Administration. Prussian blue, Radiogardase, package insert. Available at: http://www.fda.gov/cder/drug/infopage/prussian_blue/default.htm; U.S. Food and Drug Administration. Guidance: Potassium iodide as a thyroid blocking agent in radiation emergencies. Available at: http://www.fda.gov/cder/guidance/4825fnl.htm; *Management of Persons Accidentally Contaminated with Radionuclides.* NCRP Report No. 65. Bethesda, MD: National Council on Radiation Protection and Measurements; 1980; and Jarrett D, ed. *Medical Management of Radiation Casualties: Handbook.* 2nd ed. AFRRI Special Publication 03-1. Bethesda, MD: Armed Forces Radiobiology Research Institute; 2003. Available at: http://www.afrri.usuhs.mil.

limits in nearly all scenarios.[10] After a radiation contamination incident, if the patient is alive, then the quantity of radioactive contamination is generally thought to be too low to injure a provider who follows standard barrier protocol.[6] The definition of the incident scene may be much larger than it initially appears, and any site the patient has visited before decontamination must be considered radioactive and therefore a hot zone. An adjacent transitional or warm zone should be designated for step-off as protective clothing and gear are removed. Radioactive materials deposited on clothing and skin can be quickly decontaminated largely by simply removing clothing and washing the skin gently with soap and water. Contaminated clothing should be individually bagged and stored separately away from all traffic. Personnel should then be monitored to ensure minimal to no residual radioactivity exists before they step into the cold zone.[5,6]

The hospital floor plan and anticipated personnel and patient flow should be detailed in an accident-preparedness plan. Only essential equipment, personnel, and other necessary items should be in the hot zone. A defined pathway from the entry point or ambulance reception area to the treatment area should be covered in plastic and roped off with radioactive warning signs. Traffic through the emergency department must be tightly monitored to minimize the possibility of spread of contamination. A detailed security plan restricting admittance to authorized personnel and patients should be clearly defined before any incident occurs.[11] If the radioactive contaminant is in a form that may be airborne, air handlers and ventilation should be isolated, if possible.

Background radiation levels for various hospital locations should be documented well in advance of an accident, because knowing when measured radiation levels are above background level will be important for guiding the response.[12] Plans must map the locations and use of beta-gamma detectors and alpha detectors. Plans should also include provisions for use of personal dosimeters of varying types (defined by the RSO), a large supply of sealable plastic containers, various sizes of plastic bags, radiation warning signs, ropes, plastic for covering the

floor, gowns, gloves, tape, and current references on management of contaminated patients.[7,11] The websites, agencies, and literature mentioned in Chapter 107 are often very helpful.

Protective clothing and gear against radiation hazards in the hospital setting is nearly the same as that used for universal precautions. The biggest exception is often double gloving. Detailed instructions on donning and removing protective clothing and gear are available from the Centers for Disease Control and Prevention (CDC).[13] Lead aprons are not recommended. The weight of the aprons may cause overheating, accelerate fatigue, and slow down providers, and generally aprons provide little to no benefit.

Details of whom to notify, education of providers and patients, and other details of the disaster plan are summarized in Chapter 107 and detailed in multiple other references.[5-9,11]

▶ POST-INCIDENT ACTIONS

The initial emergency medical care is the same for both nonradiation and radiation casualties. Airway, breathing, and circulation are always the first priorities. In other words, in radiation incidents, as long as medical personnel are wearing appropriate personal protective equipment, patients with life-threatening conditions are treated first and decontaminated second. Stable patients can be decontaminated first.[6] Radiological exposure generally does not cause immediate loss of consciousness, and therefore responders should assess for other toxic exposures or trauma when encountering the immediately unconscious patient. One exception is that there may be transient incapacitation after extremely high doses to the head or whole body.[14] Once the patient is stabilized, the most important distinction for initial medical management is to determine whether there is contamination (radioactive material present on or within the body) versus simply a history of irradiation (previous exposure without any radioactive material deposited on or within the body).

Usually, the incident history and accompanying documentation from the scene can be used to identify quickly the source, machine, or isotope; form of isotope (sealed or unsealed); body distance and position from the source; and approximate dose. One must determine whether the exposure was whole body or local. Sequelae of whole-body irradiation can quickly escalate without immediate intervention, whereas partial-body exposures can often be observed and treated days to weeks later, when or if signs and symptoms develop.[1,11,15]

First responders should complete an identification tag specifying the usual triage information plus any radiation-specific details that may be available. Information regarding internal contamination should include the radionuclide, route of contamination, nasal counts, wound counts, whole-body counts, bioassay samples already collected, and treatment initiated. Data for external exposure to penetrating radiation should include the location and position of the patient with respect to the source, exact time, and duration of exposure; whether a dosimeter was used and where it was located; who has the dosimeter and its current location; type of symptoms; time to onset of symptoms; and treatment at the accident, assessment, and facility site.[5]

Stable ambulatory patients should be decontaminated, if possible, before transport to the hospital, especially if they are present at a facility with its own decontamination process. A radiation dispersal device may potentially contaminate 1000 victims or more,[2] most of whom will be ambulatory. The few who are not ambulatory will be most likely to have significant blast injuries. Ambulatory patients should remove clothing in a manner that minimizes further contamination, taking care not to contact undergarments, skin, and/or hair with the external surfaces of the garments being removed. Removing clothing and washing gently with soap and water will remove significant amounts of surface contamination. Splashing into eyes, mouth, nose, and open wounds must be avoided to minimize internal contamination. All wounds should be covered to prevent further contamination. Decontamination should generally be repeated until the radioactivity is less than twice that of the background activity, until it is unwise to continue due to medical conditions or impending skin abrasion, or until further measures fail to decrease activity significantly. Wastewater and any shiny or metallic particles should be retained and identified as radioactive contaminant. Abrasions and shaving should be avoided. Hair can be clipped, if necessary. All clothing articles and hair should be individually sealed in a labeled bag for assessment by the RSO.[5,6] When decontamination efforts fail to reduce any radioactivity, suspect internal contamination with a gamma-emitting isotope.[5]

Patients requiring transport by stretcher, if stable, should have their clothing cut off in a manner designed to limit the further spread of contamination as described above.[6] The patient should then be wrapped in cloth sheets, not plastic, to minimize the spread of radioactive material and minimize hyperthermia.[6,13] First responders should notify the hospital before arrival that a contaminated patient is on the way. They should also provide additional medical information including the following:

1. Other injuries and medical conditions besides radioactive exposure or contamination
2. Whether toxic or corrosive chemicals are involved in addition to the radionuclides
3. Whether the compounds are soluble or insoluble, as well as the size of the particles
4. Measurements from the site of the accident that will help determine dose
5. What decontamination efforts have already been attempted, and whether they were successful
6. Verification that clothing removed at the site has been saved to allow identification of isotope and dose estimation

7. Which excreta, swipes, and samples have been collected, time of collection, current location, when analyses will be completed and by whom
8. Any previous radiation therapy or accidental exposure[5-7,9]

Comorbidities may affect the clearance, absorption, or tolerance of decontamination measures (e.g., renal disease may affect the tolerance of chelators).[5] Once the patient is stable, either first responders or hospital providers should swab nasal cavities and collect multiple samples of excreta and blood, as documented below. All metal fragments should be removed with forceps and measured for radioactivity. If these are contaminated debris or particles from a damaged source, your RSO will direct you to seal high-activity sources in lead containers or at least 6 feet from personnel.[2]

✚ MEDICAL TREATMENT OF CASUALTIES

As stated above, the initial emergency medical care is the same for both the nonradiation and the radiation casualty. Once airway, breathing, and circulation are stable, radiation surveys and decontamination can be considered. First, one must identify and/or confirm that a radiation accident has occurred. Occupational and therapeutic exposures may be easily identified after a brief history is taken or a discussion with supervisors or treating physicians is undertaken. More elusive to diagnosis are accidental exposures to unsealed or damaged orphan sources in the community at landfills or construction sites or in malfunctioning equipment. One should include radiation exposure in the differential diagnosis of unexplained bone marrow suppression; skin burns or desquamation with no history of thermal injury; and clusters of people with unexplained nausea, vomiting, and decreasing blood counts currently or several days to weeks earlier.[1] Radiation detectors mounted at hospital entrances may possibly identify persons with significant contamination.

The determination as to whether there is external or internal contamination will determine the subsequent interventions needed. It is important to note that there may also be a combination of external penetrating radiation with concomitant contamination. Prodromal symptoms and serial peripheral blood counts generally correlate with the overall total body dose received, including external components not necessarily identified at the time of presentation.

Once the patient is stable, surface surveys and nasal swabs with a moist cotton-tipped applicator or filter paper swab can be obtained by gently rotating the swabs over accessible surfaces. This should not be done by the patients, who might contaminate the swab with material already on their hands and clothing.[5] Nasal swab counts represent approximately 5% of lung activity.[2]

Medical intervention should be orderly and should include the following:

1. Triage and medical stabilization
2. External decontamination—remove clothing, wash skin, irrigate wounds (collect bandages and attempt to collect drainage), and clip and collect hair if stubborn to shampooing
3. Documentation of signs and symptoms of local exposure (erythema and dry and moist desquamation)
4. Initial complete blood count with differential and platelet count immediately and every 4 to 6 hours for at least 24 to 48 hours
5. Collection of all excreta for at least 48 hours
6. Nasal swabs
7. Internal decontamination (Table 108-1)
8. Documentation of prodromal symptoms or whole-body exposure—nausea, time to emesis, diarrhea, transient incapacitation, hypotension (the presence of all indicates a very high dose), parotid pain, and erythema
9. Collection of blood at 24 hours for cytogenetics

Localized External Contamination

Removing clothing and gently washing with soap and water will remove significant amounts of external contamination. When the skin is unbroken and levels fall below twice background levels, decontamination can stop. Even with broken skin and other injuries, there are generally no immediate consequences of localized exposure.

Patients with localized external contamination may have also had significant external radiation and may manifest acute radiation syndrome (ARS). Only those casualties who were in intimate contact with the source before its dissemination are likely to exhibit this level of injury. Evaluation and treatment of ARS are the same as described in Chapter 107. Radiation specialists and agencies (REAC/TS for civilian events and/or the Medical Radiobiology Advisory Team, MRAT, for military events) should be contacted upon confirmation of a dispersed exposure.

Internal Contamination

The initial evaluation and treatment are the same as that for the externally irradiated patient with respect to ARS. Once a patient's condition is stabilized, measures to reduce internal contamination and incorporation (binding radioactive material into tissues or bone) can proceed. The route of entry and particular isotope will determine decontamination methods. Currently recommended interventions and drugs for each isotope can be found on numerous websites, such as those maintained by the CDC and the U.S. Food and Drug Administration (FDA). The four main mechanisms of internal decontamination are as follows: (1) reducing uptake, (2) isotopic dilution or use of blocking agents, (3) mobilizing agents, and (4) chelation.[5] See Table 108-1 for specific interventions.

Reducing Uptake

Nasopharyngeal, bronchoalveolar, and gastric lavage (within 1 to 2 hours of ingestion); emetics; purgatives; and enemas may significantly reduce contamination.[2,5-7] Prussian blue, approved by the FDA as Radiogardase®, prevents absorption of cesium-134 and cesium-137 and promotes excretion in stool.[3]

Blocking Agents

Blocking uptake of the radioactive material, also called *isotopic dilution*, can decrease uptake into stable metabolic pools, such as bone, where uptake becomes permanent. For instance, potassium iodide will block radioactive iodine if given before or within 4 to 6 hours of exposure. Potassium iodide will not block any other isotopes, although patients and families may request it.[4,5,16] It has no medical value except for the emergency treatment of radioiodine exposure. See Table 108-1 for doses of potassium iodide.

Mobilizing Agents

Mobilizing agents accelerate excretion in feces or urine. Forced fluids will reduce uptake and increase the excretion of tritium-3 in the urine. Alkalinizing the urine with bicarbonate can increase excretion of uranium.[5,7]

Chelation

Americium-241, plutonium-238-239, and curium can be chelated with pentetate calcium trisodium and pentetate zinc trisodium. Care must be exerted because these agents also bind endogenous metals in the body, (i.e., zinc, magnesium, and manganese), and plasma levels should be monitored. Depletion of these trace metals can interfere with necessary cellular mitotic processes. Mineral and vitamin supplements may be indicated. In animal studies, chelates with uranium and neptunium were less stable than chelates of americium, plutonium, and curium, in vivo, resulting in deposition of uranium and neptunium in tissues including bone, and thus they are *not* expected to be effective for uranium or neptunium.[17-21] Ethylenediaminetetraacetic acid can also be used, on the recommendation of REAC/TS or a radiation specialist. Chelated salts are then excreted by glomerular filtration in the urine.[5,7]

Providers should collect blood, urine, feces, wound exudates, and dressings at least 3 times per day for at least 48 hours for patients with significant exposures. Initial excreta may underestimate exposure before transit through the intestines. Any initial orifices with activity above background should be swiped periodically. Care providers must be careful not to cause abrasions, which could cause further internal contamination. At approximately 24 hours after exposure, it is recommended to collect blood for cytogenetics. Decisions about which patients require blood and other body fluid sampling can be made in conjunction with the institutional RSO and radiation specialists that will also help identify those patients who require subsequent surveys. Patients who are not hospitalized but have internal contamination must be given containers and be instructed to collect all excreta. Each sample must be labeled with the time and date for proper dosimetry assessment. All contaminated instruments, specimens, clothing, and equipment should be saved in separate containers and labeled with patient name, time, and date. These samples will contribute to identifying isotopes and approximate dose. Radioactive tissue should NOT be removed as a means of decontamination unless under the guidance of a trained radiological physician. Extreme measures, such as amputation, are rarely indicated except for embedded highly radioactive particulate contamination with long-lived sources that cannot be removed otherwise. Destructive surgeries should only be performed after complete evaluation by and on recommendation of a radiation medicine specialist.[5,7] Clinicians may wish to consider installing the Internal Contamination Clinical Reference (ICCR) application on their smart phone or tablets for quick reference. This reference quickly and simply estimates reference concentrations of radionuclides in the urine.[22] The program is free, and it can be found on the CDC website.

💡 UNIQUE CONSIDERATIONS

The number of casualties involved in a radiation accident may range from one patient to thousands who have been potentially contaminated by a dirty bomb. The number of patients with significant exposure will usually be quite small, however. The only people exposed to very high-activity contamination from a dirty bomb are usually those who were involved in its production or delivery (i.e., the terrorists themselves). Triage may differ depending on the number of casualties and total whole-body doses. The Strategic National Stockpile Radiation Working Group (SNS-RWG) has published guidelines for triage of fewer than or more than 100 casualties.[9]

Accidents involving pregnant women or young children are unique. Internal contamination of the pregnant woman can increase or decrease the relative fetal dose, depending on the element, route of exposure, and age of gestation. Internal contamination with elements excreted in the urine may increase the fetal dose because of the proximity to the bladder. Developing organs in the fetus or young child may have greatly increased uptake of particular elements, especially iodine. The threshold dose for giving potassium iodide is much lower for them (=0.05 Gy expected dose) compared with adults 18 to 40 years old (=0.1 Gy expected dose) and adults older than 40 years (5 Gy).[4]

All radiation accident victims carry some increased lifetime risk of an induced malignancy.[7] This is usually far less than anticipated and only slightly above the pre-incident risk because radiation is a relatively weak carcinogen.[7] Risk is related to quality and dose of radiation, affected organs, age at the time of exposure, and other risk factors.[7]

Education about the usual small increase in risk may diminish the patient's stress significantly. General educational materials can initially allay fears, and subsequent consultation with a radiation specialist can better define risks and proper surveillance.

Mortuary procedures and burial of contaminated corpses must be coordinated with an RSO. The NCRP and the Disaster Mortuary Operational Response Team provide guidelines (see http://www.phe.gov/Preparedness/responders/ndms/teams/Pages/dmort.aspx) for handling deceased patients with radioactivity significantly above background levels.[2,7] Most decedents can be decontaminated for conventional burial; however, cremation may be restricted. All corpses must be stored in the hot zone until decontaminated and released by an RSO.[7]

Finally, psychological stress can be intense and long-lasting in victims, relatives, co-workers, first responders, and providers.[7,16] Counseling and educational handouts can allay many fears. The stigma of radiation exposure and posttraumatic stress disorder may require long-term psychological follow-up.[5,16] Preparation of general and specific educational handouts in advance can provide quick reassurance. The CDC website has excellent resources for the public and professionals. Local electronic storage is appropriate, as authoritative Internet sites will likely be overloaded during an incident. Your facility may find it helpful to prepare specific instructions in advance, relative to the known industrial and medical radiological hazards in your region.

! PITFALLS

- Rapid assessment and limited contamination will only be possible by providers who recognize radiation accidents promptly and institute a predetermined response plan appropriately.
- Failure to have detection equipment available and accessible can lead to delays in initial clinical and decontamination interventions.
- Failure to consider radiation scenarios in disaster exercises can lead to inadequate responses in the event of a true radiological emergency.

REFERENCES

1. Turai I, Veress K. Radiation accidents: occurrence, types, consequences, medical management, and the lessons to be learned. *CEJOEM.* 2001;7:3–14.
2. Department of Homeland Security Working Group on Radiological Dispersal Device (RDD) Preparedness, Medical Preparedness and Response Sub-Group. Available at: http://www.acr.org/~/media/ACR/Documents/PDF/Membership/Legal%20Business/Disaster%20Preparedness/Counter%20Measures.
3. U.S. Food and Drug Administration. Prussian blue, Radiogardase, package insert. Available at: http://www.accessdata.fda.gov/drugsatfda_docs/label/2008/021626s007lbl.pdf.
4. U.S. Food and Drug Administration. Guidance: Potassium iodide as a thyroid blocking agent in radiation emergencies. Available at: http://www.fda.gov/downloads/Drugs/GuidanceComplianceRegulatoryInformation/Guidances/UCM080542.pdf.
5. NCRP. *Management of Persons Accidentally Contaminated with Radionuclides.* Bethesda, MD: National Council on Radiation Protection and Measurements; 1980, NCRP Report No. 65.
6. AFRRI. *Medical Management of Radiological Casualties: Handbook.* AFRRI Special Publication. 4th ed. 2013. Bethesda, MD: Armed Forces Radiobiology Research Institute; 2013. Available at: http://www.afrri.usuhs.mil.
7. NCRP. *Management of Terrorist Events Involving Radioactive Material.* Bethesda, MD: National Council on Radiation Protection and Measurements; 2001, NCRP Report No. 138.
8. Appendix 1: Sample radiation emergency plan for a medical facility. Gusev I, Guskova A, Mettler F, eds. *Medical Management of Radiation Accidents.* 2nd ed. Boca Raton, FL: CRC Press; 2001:557–570.
9. Waselenko J, MacVittie T, Blakely W, et al. Medical management of the acute radiation syndrome: recommendations of the Strategic National Stockpile Radiation Working Group. *Ann Intern Med.* 2004;140:1037–1051.
10. Mettler F, Kelsey C. Fundamentals of radiation accidents. In: Gusev I, Guskova A, Mettler F, eds. *Medical Management of Radiation Accidents.* 2nd ed. Boca Raton, FL: CRC Press; 2001:1–13.
11. Mettler F, Voelz G. Major radiation exposure—what to expect and how to respond. *N Engl J Med.* 2002;346:1554–1561.
12. United States Department of Labor, Occupational Safety & Health Administration. Available at: https://www.osha.gov/SLTC/radiationionizing/.
13. Centers for Disease Control and Prevention. Emergency preparedness and response: radiation emergencies. Available at: http://www.bt.cdc.gov/radiation.
14. Guskova A, Baranov A, Gusev I. Acute radiation sickness: underlying principles and assessment. In: Gusev I, Guskova A, Mettler F, eds. *Medical Management of Radiation Accidents.* 2nd ed. Boca Raton, FL: CRC Press; 2001:33–51.
15. Guskova A. Radiation sickness classification. In: Gusev I, Guskova A, Mettler F, eds. *Medical Management of Radiation Accidents.* 2nd ed. Boca Raton, FL: CRC Press; 2001:15–22.
16. Berger M, Sadoff R. Psychological support of radiation accident patients, families, and staff. In: Gusev I, Guskova A, Mettler F, eds. *Medical Management of Radiation Accidents.* 2nd ed. Boca Raton, FL: CRC Press; 2001:191–200.
17. Package insert: pentetate calcium trisodium injection. Hameln, Germany: Hameln Pharmaceuticals GmbH. Available at: http://dailymed.nlm.nih.gov/dailymed/lookup.cfm?setid=6052c707-a8a3-43a7-80c2-7ad1ad9391a4.
18. Package insert: pentetate zinc trisodium injection. Hameln, Germany: Hameln Pharmaceuticals GmbH. Available at: http://www.fda.gov/downloads/Drugs/EmergencyPreparedness/BioterrorismandDrug Preparedness/UCM131639.pdf.
19. Centers for Disease Control and Prevention. CDC fact sheet on DTPA. Available at: http://www.bt.cdc.gov/radiation/dtpa.asp.
20. Fasano A. Pathophysiology and management of radiation injury of the gastrointestinal tract. In: Ricks R, Berger M, OHara F, eds. *The Medical Basis for Radiation-Accident Preparedness: The Clinical Care of Victims.* New York: Parthenon; 2002:149–160, Proceedings of the Fourth International REAC/TS Conference on the Medical Basis for Radiation-Accident Preparedness.
21. Voelz G. Assessment and treatment of internal contamination: general principles. In: Gusev I, Guskova A, Mettler F, eds. *Medical Management of Radiation Accidents.* 2nd ed. Boca Raton, FL: CRC Press; 2001:319–336.
22. Centers for Disease Control and Prevention, Internal Contamination Clinical Reference (ICCR) Application. Available at: http://emergency.cdc.gov/radiation/iccr.asp.

CHAPTER 109

Nuclear Power Plant Meltdown

William Porcaro

📄 DESCRIPTION OF EVENT

Nuclear power plants provide energy to many areas of the globe. Whereas only about 20% of U.S. power is nuclear generated, the French create about 75% of their energy by the nuclear route. Nuclear power plants provided about 11 percent of the world's electricity production in 2012, down from about 14% in 2009.[1,1a] Nuclear power plants have the unlikely, but real, potential to cause massive disasters, both through accidents and terrorist events. A catastrophic meltdown would pose many threats, ranging from various kinds of radiation escaping into the atmosphere to more conventional dangers, such as steam and fire. Commercial U.S. nuclear reactors have been cited numerous times in the media as potential targets for terrorist attacks.

The risk for radiation leak and exposure exists at many points. Figure 109-1 shows a schematic of a typical nuclear power plant. In the most dangerous situation, a fire, coolant failure, control rod failure, or sabotage could allow a reactor to overheat and melt. If the reactor self-destructs, radioactive solids and gases could be released into the environment. Volatile radioactive isotopes may also be released from the core, including those of iodine and the noble gases. The most dangerous and longest-lasting isotopes are of iodine, strontium, and cesium, which possess half-lives of 8 days, 29 years, and 30 years, respectively.

Over the past 50 years, there have been several instances of nuclear power plant disasters and near disasters. In 1952, the Chalk River nuclear reactor near Ottawa, Ontario, sustained a partial meltdown of the uranium fuel core after four control rods were accidentally removed. Millions of gallons of radioactive water accumulated inside the reactor, but no injuries occurred. In 1957, fire in a graphite-cooled reactor north of Liverpool, England, spewed radiation over the countryside. In 1976, near Greifswald, East Germany, the radioactive core of a reactor nearly melted down due to the failure of safety systems during a fire. At Three Mile Island, near Harrisburg, Pennsylvania, coolant loss allowed overheating and partial meltdown of the uranium core in one of two reactors, and some radioactive water and gases were released.

On April 26, 1986, the worst nuclear accident in history occurred at the Chernobyl power plant near Kiev, U.S.S.R. (now Ukraine). During a shutdown for routine maintenance, a test was performed to see whether enough energy could be maintained to operate emergency equipment and cooling pumps. As workers tried to compensate, they accidentally caused a power surge estimated at 100 times nominal power output. This surge caused part of the fuel rods to rupture and react with water, creating a steam and hydrogen gas explosion and a subsequent graphite fire that destroyed the core. The lack of a containment facility and thermal loft resulted in the release of tremendous amounts of radioactive material into the atmosphere. The failure of officials to acknowledge the incident to the general public resulted in the ingestion of contaminated foodstuffs during the days immediately after the meltdown. The estimated death toll was 31, but the total number of casualties is unknown. Over 100 radioactive elements were sent into the atmosphere during the core fire caused by exploding gases in the number 4 reactor at Chernobyl. The vast majority of these isotopes decayed quite quickly; however, some of the longest-lasting isotopes of iodine, strontium, and cesium remain in the environment and will pose a risk for many years.[2]

A more recent nuclear crisis occurred at the Fukushima Daiichi nuclear complex in Japan. A natural disaster led to several core meltdowns. On March 11, 2011, a magnitude 9.0 earthquake occurred off the east coast of the island of Honshu. Shortly after the quake a series of massive tsunami waves flooded the island and nuclear facility. While several of the operating reactors automatically shut down as programmed when the earthquake occurred, the subsequent tsunamis flooded the complex's backup power diesel generators that maintained cooling systems. Several reactor cores suffered fuel rod meltdown, triggering production of hydrogen gas and leading to structural damage to the plant. Radioactive iodine and cesium leaked from the damaged reactors and in some cases deliberate discharge of radioactive water and steam was allowed to protect the reactors from further deterioration. Of note, a number of plant workers received significant radiation doses, and large zones of evacuation around the facility were required due to the spread of radioactivity into the environment.[3,4]

In addition to nuclear power plants, many TRIGA (Training Research Isotopes, General Atomics, a brand name) nuclear reactors used for research exist primarily in universities throughout the world. They are often located in densely populated urban areas with relatively minimal security. TRIGA reactors are considered "inherently safe." Their safety profile is based on the construction of their fuel rods, which force overheating fuel to limit the fission process and stop the nuclear reaction. Even when all of the control rods are simultaneously removed by accident or deliberate intent, the reactor cannot generate enough heat to cause a problem; it simply shuts down.[5]

◀ PRE-INCIDENT ACTIONS

Hospitals that may receive victims after a nuclear power plant incident should have the capability to detect radioactivity, primarily through the use of Geiger counters. Large institutions should have a radiological emergency response team that can be activated when needed to assist with detection of radiological contamination and with decontamination. This group may be composed of emergency department providers, security personnel, radiation safety officers, maintenance personnel, and laboratory support. Staff should be fitted with appropriate

THE PRESSURIZED-WATER REACTOR (PWR)

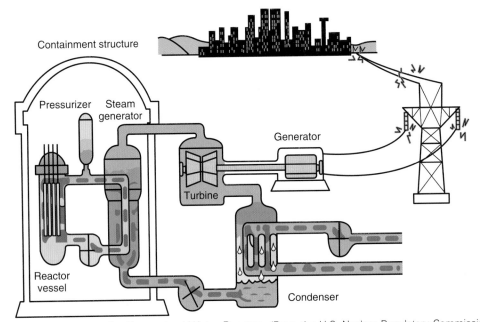

FIG 109-1 Anatomy of a Pressurized Water Reactor. (From the U.S. Nuclear Regulatory Commission website. Available at: http://www.nrc.gov/reading-rm/basic-ref/students/reactors.html.)

anticontamination clothing, including double gloving so that the outer pair can be removed when contaminated. Personnel should also be issued dosimeters to track their exposure. A radiation decontamination area should be prepared with plastic lining and plastic waste containers to limit the further spread of contamination. Flooring should be covered and cordoned off. Special ventilation to isolate the area is desirable but not necessary because there is very low likelihood that radioactive material will become aerosolized.[6]

Community evacuation plans are paramount when preparing for a nuclear power plant meltdown. All Nuclear Regulatory Commission (NRC)–regulated power plants have community contingency plans as a requirement for licensure. In addition to local and state authorities, the Federal Emergency Management Agency (FEMA) also plays a role in orchestrating these strategies. One of the special concerns surrounding nuclear power plant meltdowns involves exposure of the thyroid gland to radioactive iodine. Appropriate plans must be in place for the prophylaxis or treatment of persons who live in close proximity to nuclear power plants to decrease their risk of thyroid cancer if a release occurs, by providing prompt potassium iodide to compete with released radioactive iodine for binding sites in the thyroid. Preparedness should be practiced through exercises involving power plants and area hospitals.

In the United States, the NRC requires that emergency planning zones (EPZs) be established for nuclear reactors. EPZs are defined as the area surrounding a nuclear power plant for which plans required by the NRC have been made in advance to ensure that prompt and effective actions are taken to protect the health and safety of the public in case of an incident. More specifically, the NRC categorizes EPZs.[7] The Plume Exposure Pathway EPZ encompasses a 10-mile radius around the reactor, and the Ingestion Exposure Pathway EPZ extends to a 50-mile radius around the plant. Depending on the type and extent of the incident, various orders for the zones may be issued, such as complete evacuation, shelter-in-place (limiting ventilation, sealing windows, etc.), food restrictions, or medical countermeasures.[8]

POST-INCIDENT ACTIONS

In addition to the health hazards posed by radioactive materials, nuclear power plants harbor many other potential hazards to responders and to the community. The steam and high pressures that exist in the reactor coolant systems and heat exchangers in pressurized water reactors may cause severe thermal burns because either simple steam or radioactive steam may be produced. After a nuclear power plant incident has occurred, containment of radioactive contaminants in and around the facility should continue to be a priority. The Chernobyl Exclusion Zone served as an evacuation area and continues to use natural and human-made boundaries to prevent migration of radionuclides and to control the illegal harvesting of contaminated foodstuffs. Evacuation of the at-risk population will lead to the need for shelter and medical care for large numbers of evacuees and screening for necessary prophylaxis.

Numerous other details must be considered after a meltdown, including radioactive and hazardous waste removal, economic sustainability in the surrounding areas, and food supply and agriculture. Contaminated soil will lead to contamination of plants and animals and their products, such as milk and beef.[9]

MEDICAL TREATMENT OF CASUALTIES

Victims from a nuclear power plant meltdown or potentially exposed persons from the surrounding area must be evaluated for possible contamination. Internalized strontium may lead to leukemia. Cesium may cause liver and spleen pathology.[7] Experience from previous nuclear incidents and nuclear medicine accidents has proved the long-term health implications of a significant release, most notably the increase in childhood thyroid cancer attributed to radioactive iodine.[2] However, immediate medical attention must be paid to serious or life-threatening problems. At triage, a brief radiological survey should be performed to determine exposure. Medical personnel wearing appropriate personal protective equipment and dosimeters generally may safely provide immediate life-saving care to victims who require it, even when external contamination is present. Nonacutely ill victims should have clothing removed and sealed in plastic bags by staff wearing proper protective equipment. Wounds that may be contaminated should be cleansed, after thorough draping to avoid the spread of radioactive material. Cleansing of intact skin must be performed in a manner that limits mechanical or chemical irritation to avoid deeper spread of the radioactive material. Contaminated orifices may require special attention; for example, decontaminating the mouth may require aggressive brushing with toothpaste or gargling with 3% hydrogen peroxide.[6] Irrigation solutions used to clean open contaminated wounds must be carefully retained and surveyed, so they can be disposed of properly.

Victims who are believed to have suffered radioactive exposure and/or contamination should have several basic laboratory studies. All specimens must be sealed in plastic and sent in properly labeled containers that specify a name, the date, the time of sampling, the area of samples, and the size of sample areas. A complete blood count with stat differentials must be obtained to follow absolute lymphocyte counts, and this should be repeated approximately every 6 hours for 2 days to monitor for bone marrow suppression in any patient suspected to have suffered whole-body irradiation. Serum and urine assays should also be performed on all victims of radiological injury to ensure proper renal function, which is necessary to clear possible internal contamination. Externally contaminated patients should have swabs from wounds and all body orifices sent to be monitored for radioactivity. In cases where internal contamination is suspected (i.e., inhalation, ingestion, or absorption), 4 days of 24-hour urine and feces may be sampled for detection of radionuclides excreted from the body.

Acute radiation syndrome may be seen in victims who were in close proximity to the reactor meltdown, such as plant workers, first-responder firefighters, and law enforcement officers, or EMS officials who were unable to use appropriate precautions. Signs and symptoms may arise secondary to cellular deficiencies and the reactions of various cells, tissues, and organ systems to ionizing radiation.

In addition to radiological injuries, traditional injuries may also result from a nuclear power plant incident. Steam is a real and present danger in all power plants. From a nuclear standpoint, radioactive steam may serve as a medium to rapidly spread nuclear fallout and allow it to penetrate the body through burns and inspiration. However, the dangers of injuries inflicted by nonradioactive steam should not be underestimated. Severe thermal skin burns, as well as inhalational burns to the distal airway causing stridor and respiratory distress and failure, should be anticipated. In August 2004, nonradioactive steam leaked from a nuclear power plant in Mihama, Japan, killing four workers and severely burning seven others.

As discussed below, patients from areas of radioactive iodine fallout should be treated with potassium iodide, ideally within 4 hours of exposure.

UNIQUE CONSIDERATIONS

In the event of a significant nuclear incident with a core meltdown, there is likely to be some lead time after the disaster begins before there is a biologically dangerous leak of radioactive material from the containment structures. This window of opportunity allows for meaningful activation of evacuation plans and staging of an emergency medical response.[8]

As with all nuclear or radiological events, the factors of time, distance, and shielding are crucial to determining human exposure and ultimately disease and the outcome of a nuclear power plant meltdown. Simple actions such as rapid and orderly evacuation from contaminated areas, rapid and effective decontamination, and containment

of hazardous waste can greatly reduce risk. As alluded to above, any time there is a leak of radioactive material into the environment, concerns about soil and plant and animal food sources come into play. Therefore, an adequate, noncontaminated food and water supply must be ensured.

An increased risk of thyroid cancer in children must be anticipated. Strong consideration must be given to the treatment of children and infants with potassium iodide when there is risk for inhalation of contaminated air or ingestion of contaminated food. Administered before or within 4 hours after the intake of radioactive iodine, potassium iodide can block or reduce the accumulation of radioactive iodine in the thyroid, thereby reducing the risk of cancer.[10] In the event of a nuclear power plant meltdown, children would also be at risk for greater internal exposure to radioactive gases given their higher minute ventilation. Attention must also be paid to the psychological needs of children and parents during a nuclear incident as they are at higher risk of developing enduring psychological injury.[11]

If a true nuclear power plant meltdown has occurred, the public will be understandably most eager to obtain as much information as possible regarding the incident. When instructions are given, they must be clear and repeated, and the rationale for the warnings and instructions must be provided. They must also be appropriate for the community in terms of format, language, and mechanisms of communication.[12]

⚠ PITFALLS

Well-crafted and rehearsed strategies are the key to success during a nuclear plant incident. Studies suggest that proper planning of evacuation time estimates is crucial for optimal emergency response. Evacuation time estimates must consider many factors, ranging from traffic management to uncontrollable events such as weather, when projecting for an event.[12] "Shelter in place" should also always be considered. Additionally, a community's or hospital's failure to appropriately set up decontamination areas or inadequate decontamination procedures may lead to dispersing contaminated patients throughout the hospital, further exposing these patients as well as contaminating the staff and personnel caring for them.

Although treatment or prophylaxis with potassium iodide is relatively safe for children, there are some risks, including gastrointestinal effects or even hypersensitivity reactions. Additionally, thyroidal adverse effects may result from stable iodine administration, especially in iodine-deficient patients or in connection with thyroid disorders, such as autoimmune thyroiditis or Graves' disease.[10]

REFERENCES

1. Brain M. How nuclear power works. Available at: http://science.howstuffworks.com/nuclear-power.htm.
1a. Nucelar Energy Institute – http://www.nei.org/Knowledge-Center/Nuclear-Statistics/World-Statistics.
2. Mettler FA Jr., Voelz GL. Major radiation exposure: what to expect and how to respond. N Engl J Med. 2002;346(20):1554–1561.
3. Nuclear Energy Agency (NEA). Timeline for the Fukushima Dai-ichi nuclear power plant accident. Available at: http://www.oecd-nea.org/press/2011/NEWS-04.html.
4. Fisher J. Another Earthquake Shakes Japan, Fukushima Evacuated: A Timeline of Key Events. Christian Science Monitor; March 15, 2011. Available at: http://www.csmonitor.com/World/Asia-Pacific/2011/0315/Japan-s-nuclear-crisis-A-timeline-of-key-events.
5. TRIGA nuclear reactors, General Atomics Cooperation website. Available at: http://triga.ga.com.

6. Oak Ridge Institute for Science and Education. Radiation Emergency Assistance Center/Training Site (REAC/TS). Available at: http://www.orau.gov/reacts.

7. International Atomic Energy Agency. *Chernobyl 15, Frequently asked questions.* Available at: http://www.iaea.org/NewsCenter/Features/Chernobyl-15/index.shtml.

8. Radiation Emergency Medical Management, U.S. Department of Health and Human Services. Nuclear Power Plant/Nuclear Reactor Incidents. Available at: http://www.remm.nlm.gov/nuclearaccident.htm.

9. International Conference, 15 Years After the Chernobyl Accident. *Lessons Learned: Executive Summary.* Kyiv, Ukraine: April 18-20, 2001. Available at: http://www.iaea.org/NewsCenter/Features/Chernobyl-15/execsum_eng.pdf.

10. World Health Organization. *Guidelines for Iodine Prophylaxis Following Nuclear Accidents, Update 1999.* Geneva: World Health Organization; 1999.

11. Balk SJ, Best D, Johnson CL, et al. Radiation disasters and children. *Pediatrics.* 2003;111:1455–1466.

12. Mileti DS, Peek L. The social psychology of public response to warnings of a nuclear power plant accident. *J Hazard Mater.* 2000;75:181–194.

SUGGESTED READINGS

1. CNN Timeline: How Japan's nuclear crisis unfolded. Available at: http://www.cnn.com/2011/WORLD/asiapcf/03/15/japan.nuclear.disaster.timeline/index.html.

2. Initial Medical Response to the Fukushima Nuclear Accident at Fukushima Medical University Hospital. Presentation by Arifumi Hasegawa, MD, PhD. Available at: http://www.fmu.ac.jp/radiationhealth/conference/index.html.

3. IAEA—Japan's Nuclear Regulation Authority Reports on Conditions at TEPCO's Fukushima Daiichi Nuclear Power Station. Available at: http://www.iaea.org/newscenter/news/2013/japan-basic-policy-full.html.

4. Catlett CL, Rogers J. Radiation injuries. In: Tintinalli JE, Stapczynski J, Ma O, et al. *Tintinalli's Emergency Medicine: A Comprehensive Study Guide.* 7th ed. New York, NY: McGraw-Hill; 2011, Chapter 11.

5. International Atomic Energy Agency. Promoting safety in nuclear installations. Available at: http://www.iaea.org/Publications/Factsheets/English/safetynuclinstall.pdf.

6. International Atomic Energy Agency. The International Nuclear Event Scale for prompt communication of safety significance. Available at: http://www.iaea.org/Publications/Factsheets/English/ines-e.pdf.

7. Nuclear Energy Institute: Source Book: Soviet-Designed Nuclear Power Plants, 5th Edition, 1997 - http://www.nei.org/corporatesite/media/filefolder/soviet_plant_source_book.pdf.

8. Family Education Network. Nuclear and Chemical Accident. Boston, MA: Family Education Network; 2005. Available at: http://www.infoplease.com/ipa/A0001457.html.

9. Urbanik T. Evacuation time estimates for nuclear power plants. *J Hazardous Mater.* 2000;75:165–180.

10. US Government Information for Nuclear Power Plant Emergencies - http://www.ready.gov/nuclear-power-plants.

Introduction to Chemical Disasters*

Katherine Farmer, Lawrence Proano, James M. Madsen, and Robert Partridge

This chapter provides a historical perspective to chemical disasters and offers a broad overview of the management of persons exposed to toxic chemicals in a mass casualty incident. These disasters occur both unintentionally, through industrial or environmental accidents, and also intentionally through terrorist strikes or attacks related to war. Whereas the specific chemicals and mode of dispersal vary widely, the overall clinical approach remains fairly uniform.

Historically, the majority of large-scale chemical release events have come from industrial accidents. However, there is now wide acceptance that there is an ongoing and increasing threat of chemical terrorist acts or chemical warfare in the United States and abroad.[1] This is evidenced by the recent deliberate use of chemical weapons in other regions of the world.[2,3]

In a potential disaster scenario, the variety of chemical agents harmful to humans is enormous, but a common general approach is taken to these exposures. An appropriate response to any large-scale chemical release relies on the coordination of many different groups of people, including emergency medical service(s) (EMS) providers, law enforcement, firefighters, HazMat (hazardous material) teams, public health professionals, and in-hospital providers. These various teams must come together quickly and work in hectic and often frightening situations. The providers must rapidly establish scene safety and crowd control, begin field triage assessments, set up large-scale sites for decontamination, extricate victims from the scene, and provide definitive medical care to a large number of victims, many of whom require simultaneous care. During this process, these providers must adhere to specific guidelines to ensure the safety of both prehospital and hospital providers, protect the environment, and avoid disruption of a potential crime scene.

Preparation for a chemical disaster involves pre-event planning, frequent drills, and post-event debriefing. Adequate preparation can help improve a coordinated disaster response, allowing for more rapid identification and triage of victims, timely decontamination, faster access to care, and appropriate medical management. The ultimate goal is for any geographic area and any hospital to be prepared to handle the surge of patients that may potentially be seen in either a minor or more significant chemical release event, regardless of the cause.

---

*The views expressed in this chapter are those of the author(s) and do not reflect the official policy of the Department of Army, Department of Defense, or the U.S. Government.

HISTORICAL PERSPECTIVE

Historically, the majority of chemical releases have resulted from industrial accidents, many of which led to a large number of casualties. For instance, in 2005 a train derailed in the middle of the night near a textile mill in Graniteville, South Carolina. Nearly 60 tons of chlorine gas, classified as a pulmonary agent, was released near the town center, causing several hundred victims to fall ill with respiratory symptoms. State and federal environmental officials responded with the Centers for Disease Control and Prevention (CDC) to quickly conduct an assessment of those who had fallen ill, determine the sequelae of the event, and assess the needs of the community. In contrast, a leak of methyl-isocyanate gas from a pesticide plant in Bhopal, India, in 1984 killed over 5000 people, sickened 14,000 people, and decimated the medical and social infrastructure.[4]

The continuous production, transportation, and use of hazardous chemicals in the industrial sector represent an ongoing public health concern. Annual data on these events are collected through the U.S. Department of Transportation Pipeline and Hazardous Materials Safety Administration (PHMSA). In the United States in 2013, a total of 16,004 chemical events were reported that caused 12 fatalities and 165 injuries. The total cost of the HazMat events during 2013 alone was over $78.2 million. Over the past 10 years, there has been a total of 129 fatalities, 2772 injuries, and over $739 million in damages resulting from chemical exposures. The Agency for Toxic Substances and Disease Registry (ATSDR), an agency of the U.S. Department of Health and Human Services, also collects data for the National Toxic Substance Incidents Program (NTSIP) through collaboration with seven state governments (Louisiana, New York, North Carolina, Oregon, Tennessee, Utah, and Wisconsin). In 2011, 3128 events occurred at fixed facilities and during transportation, resulting in 1177 injuries and 62 fatalities. Nearly 70% of the events occurred at fixed facilities and accounted for about 90% of all injuries. Approximately 60% of incidents occurred as the result of exposure to the 20 most frequently used chemicals, with natural gas, carbon monoxide, chemicals involved in the production of illicit methamphetamine, and ammonia at the top of the list. In addition, approximately half of all injuries occurred among the general public. Among transportation-related incidents, most occurred from alkaline hydroxides, including sodium hydroxide and potassium hydroxide; other common incidents included the release of hydrochloric acid, sulfuric acid, and hydrogen peroxide. These data

BOX 110-1 Brief History of Chemical Warfare

- 1000 BC: Use of arsenic smoke by the Chinese.
- 600 BC: Hellebore roots used to poison offensive in First Sacred War in Greece.
- 1847: First international attempt to control chemical arms with the drafting of the International Declaration Concerning Laws and Customs of War.
- 1915: First large-scale use of chemical weapons near Yves, Belgium, during WWI, when chlorine gas was used in an attack by Germany. Both sides later used phosgene and then sulfur mustard among other agents.
- 1918: Chemical Warfare Service (CWS) formed in United States under the National Army.
- 1925: Development of the Geneva Protocol, preventing the use of chemical weapons, but does not prohibit producing and stockpiling them. The treaty was not ratified by the United States at this time.
- 1936: Synthesis and development of first nerve agent, tabun, by Gerhard Schrader in Germany.
- 1943: Attack on the U.S.S. *John Harvey* in Bari Harbor, Italy, releasing large quantities of sulfur mustard.
- 1939-1945: Widespread use of hydrogen cyanide and other asphyxiant agents in the Holocaust.
- 1974: Geneva Protocol ratified by United States.
- 1984: International ban on chemical weapons called for by President Ronald Reagan.
- 1988: The nerve-agent sarin used in the Kurdish city of Halabja in the Iran-Iraq War, killing thousands.
- 1993: Geneva Protocol wording is changed, prohibiting production and stockpiling of chemical weapons.
- 1995: Release of Sarin into Tokyo subway system by the Aum Shinri Kyo cult, killing 12 and injuring thousands.
- 2013: Use of sarin in Damascus during the Syrian civil war.

suggest that whereas overall morbidity and mortality are low from chemical releases, the high number of incidents continues to be a persistent issue.[5,6]

The overall low morbidity and mortality of industrial accidents lie in stark contrast to those incurred through intentional chemical releases, the goals of which are injury and loss of life. In addition, psychological trauma from such events for both victims and communities can be long-standing. To date, there has not been a large-scale mass casualty incident from an intentional chemical release on U.S. soil, but chemical warfare has been employed countless times throughout history.

Chemical warfare dates back as early as 1000 BC in China, with the release of smoke containing arsenic, and 600 BC, when hellebore roots were used to poison water during the First Sacred War in Greece (Box 110-1).[7] Following this, many small-scale attacks using a variety of chemicals have been recorded. The first international movement to control chemical and biological weapons occurred as early as 1874, with the signing of the "International Declaration Concerning the Laws and Customs of War," which banned wartime use of poison or poisoned armaments.

Despite this ban and subsequent resolutions, World War I marked the beginning of the use of chemical weapons in war on an unprecedented scale. On April 22, 1915, near Ypres, Belgium, German troops released a total of 168 tons of chlorine gas over the Allied lines, resulting in hundreds of deaths. Germany soon escalated the use of chemical weapons to include phosgene, another pulmonary agent capable of causing severe and often fatal pulmonary

edema. Later in the war, sulfur mustard was used. This agent exists as a solid and a liquid at ambient temperatures and can remain in the environment for weeks, thus inhibiting troop movements. In 1918, soon after entering the war, the United States formed the Chemical Warfare Service (CWS), responsible for the development and deployment of toxic chemicals during the war. With the formation of this agency, the United States was able to employ chemical weapons, develop detectors and alarms for these agents, and improve protective gear for troops. Even with the formation of the CWS, by the time the armistice of November 1918 ended World War I, there had been over 272,000 U.S. casualties, 72,000 of which are thought to be caused by chemical-warfare agents.[7]

In 1925, in the interim between World Wars I and II, the Geneva Protocol was drafted. An update to the Hague Convention, it prohibited the use of "asphyxiating, poisonous or other gasses. . ." but was not ratified by the United States at that time. During this same time period, in 1936 a German scientist named Gerhard Schrader developed the first organophosphorus nerve agent, an anticholinesterase named tabun, while attempting to refine an insecticide. Since this initial discovery, nerve agents have been refined and strengthened and now comprise the nonpersistent G-series agents such as sarin and the environmentally persistent V agents such as VX. To date, nerve agents remain the most potent traditional chemical-warfare agents.

During World War II, chemical weapons were not used extensively on the battlefield, but both Germany and the Allies stockpiled large quantities of these agents. It is estimated that Germany amassed 78,000 tons of chemical weapons, including tabun, sarin, and nitrogen mustards. The United States collected nearly 146,000 tons of phosgene, sulfur mustard, and Lewisite. During the war, the United States followed a "no first-use rule" designated by President Franklin D. Roosevelt that no chemical weapons were to be used unless they were used first by the enemy. However, preparations for possible use resulted in several near-miss incidents and one major disaster during the transport and storage of these agents. In December of 1943, the U.S.S. *John Harvey* was loaded with 2000 mustard agent bombs and positioned in Bari Harbor, Italy. After a direct air-raid strike by Germany, the ship sank and the agent was released, causing an unknown number, probably hundreds, of military and civilian deaths. The most alarming use of chemicals during World War II, however, was the use of gas chambers by Nazi Germany as a means of systematically murdering probably at least 3 million Jewish civilians (up to 6000 a day at Auschwitz alone) in the Holocaust. These chambers, full of people, were sealed and Zyklon B pellets were introduced, releasing hydrogen cyanide. This resulted in asphyxiation within minutes.

In 1974, following the Vietnam War, the United States ratified the Geneva Protocol, which banned the use of poisonous substances in war. Initially, the United States reserved the right to retaliate if attacked, but in 1991, President George H.W. Bush renounced any use of chemical weapons by the United States even in retaliation. Since this time, under the auspices of the Organization for the Prohibition of Chemical Weapons (OPCW), there have been ongoing efforts to dismantle worldwide supplies of chemical weapons, and this effort continues today under President Barack Obama.[8]

In spite of worldwide treaties to prohibit the development, stockpiling, and use of chemical weapons as well as efforts to dismantle existing stockpiles, these weapons continue to be used by terrorist groups and in recent wars. The use of nerve agents alone has been seen in multiple instances since World War II. Near the end of the Iran-Iraq War in 1988, between 3000 and 5000 people perished when sarin was used in an act of genocide on the Kurdish city of Halabja by the regime of Saddam Hussein. In 1995 members of the Aum Shinri Kyo cult of Japan released sarin into the Tokyo subway system during rush hour, killing 12 and flooding the Tokyo medical system with more than 5000 casualties. Much was learned from this attack regarding pre-event planning, victim decontamination, and appropriate triage, as nearly 80% of victims presented for care outside of the EMS system and an estimated 20% of health care workers at local facilities near the attack presented for medical treatment.[9,10] Most recently, in August of 2013 during the Syrian civil war, a large-scale attack took place during the Syrian civil war in the city of Damascus. The Syrian regime is suspected of using sarin in this chemical attack on rebel-controlled and contested areas of the city. It is estimated that between 300 and 1700 people died, and more than 3500 were treated for symptoms consistent with nerve-agent poisoning.[3] It remains clear that whereas worldwide efforts continue in attempts to dismantle stockpiles of chemical weapons, these agents remain a persistent threat.

CURRENT PRACTICE

Chemical disasters present unique challenges that can change the dynamic of scene response in a mass casualty incident. Chemical agents, whether inhaled or absorbed through the skin, can cause both immediate and delayed effects. Whereas biological and radiological exposures are more frequently characterized by delayed effects, such that definitive care can often await arrival at a hospital, many chemical exposures require lifesaving interventions at or near the scene of the event. This difference has significant implications for the pre-event planning and management of chemical disasters. In all mass casualty events, different teams of people need to organize quickly to provide effective care for patients while keeping health care workers safe. After a large mass casualty incident, it has been estimated that within the first hour of the event between 50% and 80% of acute casualties will arrive at the closest medical facility.[11] Outlying hospitals are unlikely to receive a significant number of casualties; for this reason, significant pre-event planning and frequent training drills are important.[12]

Triage of victims in any disaster is based on the severity of injury. Classically, victims are triaged or "tagged" in one of four colors: *black* if they are not expected to live even if definitive care is achieved within a short time frame, *red* if immediate medical treatment is required for survival, *yellow* if a serious condition is suspected but the victim is not expected to deteriorate within the next several hours, and *green* for less severe conditions in medically stable patients. SALT (sort, assess, lifesaving interventions, treatment or transport) is a mass-casualty triage system recommended by the U.S. government.[13] In the initial sorting, those who are motionless or have an obvious life-threatening condition are assessed first, followed by those who can wave and have purposeful movement; lastly, those who can walk are evaluated. Subsequently, individual assessments are made to determine severity of injury, and formal triage decisions are made to prioritize transport to hospitals. SALT and other triage systems were developed primarily to sort trauma casualties and may benefit from modifications for chemical disasters.

The initial triage, management, transport, and definitive care of victims exposed to toxic chemicals is limited by the risk of contamination of health care workers and other persons. Protection of and, if necessary, decontamination of health care providers are crucial. Hot, warm, and cold zones should be established immediately outside hospitals and at the scene of the event. Anyone entering the hot or warm zones where decontamination takes place must don personal protective equipment (PPE). However, these formal decontamination facilities do take time to erect; in an estimated 20% of cases, they can take up to 10 hours to finalize.[14] Because many chemical agents begin penetrating skin and causing tissue damage within minutes, decontamination should take place at the scene of the event or at least be started by EMS. With chemical casualties, immediate spot decontamination of suspicious areas on the body becomes a priority equal to those of airway, breathing, and circulation. Along with timely administration of drugs or antidotes, the ABCDDs (Airway, Breathing, Circulation, immediate Decontamination, and Drugs) become the initial critical actions in caring for victims in a chemical disaster. Any clothing and shoes should be removed from victims to prevent ongoing contamination and absorption of the chemical. Any visible liquid should be blotted off, and then skin should be cleansed with soap and water. Commercial decontamination solutions such as Reactive Skin Decontamination Lotion (RSDL) do exist and are effective against many agents. In other circumstances, dilute bleach solutions, generally 1 part household bleach to 9 parts water, can be effective. However, because bleach has the potential to cause more tissue damage, as a general rule physical or mechanical decontamination should be emphasized over chemical decontamination. Showers with soap and water may be useful when large numbers of casualties arrive.

In addition, any hospital that may receive victims must limit entrance and egress to reduce the risk of wider contamination. Those with noncritical injuries and symptoms may attempt to leave the scene of the event quickly, and many will present for care outside of the EMS system. This complicates the triage system, as these patients will often arrive at hospitals before the most seriously injured and can delay care of the seriously ill. They also have the potential to contaminate unsecured areas of the hospital grounds. Ensuring that all victims must first pass through the decontamination center is essential.

A problem with all mass casualty incidents is that they result in a large simultaneous surge of patients into the medical system, disrupting the flow of patients in need of medical care for other reasons as well as those related to the disaster. Protocols for prehospital teams and the receiving facility should be in place before any event. Alternative sites of care should be identified, and prehospital diversion by EMS should be employed when possible. Plans should be in place at any hospital to manage a large influx of low-acuity patients and the "worried well" so that they can be seen and released expediently or reassessed at appropriate intervals. Although these events are rare, education, drills, and training exercises are essential because they can increase confidence in caring for victims exposed to toxic chemicals.

Physical properties of chemicals contribute to their effects. These include physical state at ambient temperature, volatility, environmental persistence, flammability, and other properties that help define the hazards associated with a particular chemical. Other important features of a chemical disaster include mode of dispersal, concentration of agent dispersed, amount disseminated, length of exposure, and the environment into which the agent was released. The CDC has divided toxic chemical agents into 13 main categories (Box 110-2).[15] These groups are based on two primary factors: the physical properties of the chemical and the

---

BOX 110-2 Categories of Chemical Agents[13]

- Biotoxins
- Blister agents/vesicants
- Blood agents
- Caustics (acids)
- Choking/lung/pulmonary agents
- Incapacitating agents
- Long-acting anticoagulants
- Metals
- Nerve agents
- Organic solvents
- Riot control agents/tear gas
- Toxic alcohols
- Vomiting agents

physiological effects induced in humans. Agents often have characteristic scents, physical properties in the environment, or specific recognizable physiological effects. Many produce very nonspecific symptoms including nausea, vomiting, shortness of breath, coughing, or dizziness; a more limited number of compounds or classes of compounds can result in characteristic constellations of signs and symptoms, or toxidromes. Some types of chemical exposures may require specific critical actions or specific antidotes, such as atropine and pralidoxime (2-PAM) for a nerve-agent exposure. It is essential that prehospital providers be able to recognize important toxidromes and report them to the receiving facility to allow clinicians to prepare the appropriate antidote if possible. The U. S. Department of Health & Human Services Chemical Hazards Emergency Medical Management (CHEMM) group is developing an online algorithm (CHEMM-IST) for use by EMS and first responders to help identify specific chemical toxidromes. By asking about specific clinical features unique to a toxidrome, such as level of consciousness, presence of seizure activity, pinpoint pupils, diaphoresis, wheezing, and other elements, CHEMM-IST aids in the potential recognition of a defined toxidrome.[16] This algorithm, in prototype testing as of this writing, highlights the importance of early recognition of specific groups of signs and symptoms by first responders.

It is also incumbent on the physicians treating victims of these events to recognize common toxidromes, to understand the appropriate medical management, and include this treatment as part of the ABCDDs. In addition, it is essential for clinicians to have an understanding of the various toxicologic properties of the chemicals involved, including toxicokinetics, toxicodynamics (mechanisms of action), differences in physiological effect depending on routes of exposure (e.g., cutaneous versus inhalation), and immediate versus possible latent clinical effects. In the event of an industrial exposure, a material safety data sheet (MSDS) with information about the specific chemical involved may be available. Consultation with a medical toxicologist or the local poison control center is advised.[17] Acronyms such as ASBESTOS, TOXICANT, and POISON can assist in a systematic assessment of chemical casualties and can help guide assessment and ensure that important toxicologic principles are not overlooked

(Box 110-3). These acronyms may be printed and displayed in emergency departments.

Following triage, decontamination, transport, and treatment of victims in a chemical attack, many other issues will remain, including the future environmental effects (leaching of chemicals into soil, water table, nearby structures, etc.) and potential for future contamination of victims. In some circumstances, the location of the chemical release should be treated as a crime scene. Although this should not affect treatment of casualties, clothing and other items from the scene could potentially be important legal evidence. Lastly, all victims and providers involved in a chemical disaster should undergo a stress debriefing. The long-standing psychological effects of these events are often dramatic. The role of mental health providers and their ability to provide emotional support should not be underestimated.

After any mass casualty incident, the various providers involved in managing victims should debrief and plan for a future event. Whether the event was intentional or accidental, small or large, each event should be treated as a learning experience, with close examination of the pre-event planning process, as well as the decontamination and management of victims. The treatment of victims in a chemical release requires a highly coordinated effort and is dependent on the ability of first responders and first receivers, including hospital staff, to recognize the possibility of a chemical release and to implement the procedures necessary for an effective response. Through planning, appropriate training, and regular drills, both prehospital and hospital providers can be prepared and confident in caring for victims involved in the accidental or intentional release of toxic chemicals in a mass casualty incident.[18]

⚠ PITFALLS

- Failure to quickly recognize a potential chemical disaster when multiple patients begin to experience similar symptoms
- Failure to begin immediate decontamination of victims involved in chemical disasters both at the scene of the release and in formal decontamination centers

---

BOX 110-3 Acronyms to Assist in Assessment of Casualties from Chemical Agents or Toxins

ASBESTOS

• Agent(s):	Type: Is a toxidrome present? Estimated dose?
• State(s):	Solid? Liquid? Gas? Vapor? Aerosol? Combinations?
• Body site(s):	Route(s) of entry? [exposure and absorption]
• Effects:	Local? Systemic? Both? [distribution]
• Severity:	Of effects? Of exposure?
• Time course:	Past (onset, latent period)
	Present (getting better or worse? Stable?)
	Future (expected prognosis)
• Other diagnoses?	Instead of? [differential diagnosis] In addition to? [coexisting diagnoses]
• Synergism:	Combined effects of multiple exposures?

TOXICANT

• Toxicant:	Type: Is a toxidrome present? Estimated dose?
• Outside the body:	Solid? Liquid? Gas? Vapor? Aerosol? Combinations?
• Xing into the body:	Route(s) of entry? [exposure and absorption]
• Into/inside the body:	Local? Systemic? Both? [distribution]

• Chronology:	Past (onset, latent period)
	Present (getting better or worse? Stable?)
	Future (expected prognosis)
• Additional diagnosis?	Instead of? [differential diagnosis] In addition to? [coexisting diagnoses]
• Net effects:	Combined effects of multiple exposures?
• Triage:	How long can the casualty afford to wait?

POISON

• Poison(s):	Type: Is a toxidrome present? Estimated dose?
• Outside the body:	Solid? Liquid? Gas? Vapor? Aerosol?
• Into/inside the body:	Route(s) of entry? [exposure and absorption]
	Local/systemic effects? Both? [distribution]
• Sequence of events:	Past (onset, latent period)
	Present (getting better or worse? Stable?)
	Future (expected prognosis)
• Severity:	Of effects? Of exposure?
• Other diagnoses?	Instead of? [differential diagnosis] In addition to? [coexisting diagnoses]
• Net effects:	Combined effects of multiple exposures?

- Failure to provide for urgent medical treatment (ABCDDs) of unstable casualties before thorough patient decontamination
- Failure to secure hospital grounds and entrances to prevent inadvertent contamination of health care workers and unaffected patients
- Failure to recognize specific toxidromes that require expedient treatment with specific antidotes
- Failure to understand that chemical exposures may cause immediate and delayed symptoms, and that initially asymptomatic patients may later develop life-threatening symptoms
- Failure to contact a medical toxicologist or poison control center regarding specific expected short-term and long-term effects of exposure to a specific chemical
- Failure to coordinate pre-event and post-event planning, education, drills, and training exercises for potential accidental and intentional chemical disasters
- Failure to provide training for prehospital and hospital providers in the medical management of chemical casualties

REFERENCES

1. Statement by Director of Central Intelligence, George J. Tenet, Before the Senate Foreign Relations Committee on The Worldwide Threat in 2000: Global Realities of Our National Security "as prepared for delivery"; March 21, 2000. Available at: http://www.cia.gov/cia/public_affairs/speeches/2000/dci_speech_032100.html.
2. Human Rights Watch. *Rain of Fire: Israel's Unlawful Use of White Phosphorus in Gaza.* New York: Human Rights Watch; 2009. Available at: http://www.hrw.org/sites/default/files/reports/iopt0309webwcover.pdf.
3. Dolgin E. Syrian gas attack reinforces need for better anti-sarin drugs. *Nat Med.* 2013;19:1194–1195.
4. Svendsen E, Runkle J, Dhara V, et al. Epidemiologic methods lessons learned from environmental public health disasters: Chernobyl, the World Trade Center, Bhopal, and Graniteville, South Carolina. *Int J Environ Res Public Health.* 2012;9(8):2894–2909.
5. U.S. Department of Transportation—Pipeline and Hazardous Materials Safety Administration—Incident Statistics. Data as of May 2, 2014. Available at: http://phmsa.dot.gov/hazmat/library/data-stats/incidents.
6. U.S. Department of Health and Human Services. National Toxic Substance Incidents Program (NTSIP)-Annual, Report 2011.
7. Smart, J. *History of Chemical and Biological Warfare: An American Perspective.* Available through the Borden Institute, Office of the Surgeon General, U.S. Army Medical Department (AMEDD) Center and School, http://www.cs.amedd.army.mil/borden/Portlet.aspx?ID=bddf382f-3ca0-44ba-bd67-fdc48bfa03de.
8. Organisation for the Prohibition of Chemical Weapons (OPCW): www.opcw.org.
9. Yangiasawa N, Morita H, Najajima T. Sarin experience in Japan: acute toxicity and long-term effects. *J Neurol Sci.* 2006;249(1):76–85.
10. Ohbu S, Yamashina A, Takasu N, et al. Sarin poisoning on Tokyo subway. *South Med J.* 1997;90(6):587–593.
11. U.S. Centers for Disease Control and Prevention. *Mass Casualties Predictor.* Available at: http://www.bt.cdc.gov/masscasualties/predictor.asp.
12. *U.S. Centers for Disease Control and Prevention Emergency Response Guide.* Available at: http://www.cdc.gov/nceh/ehs/Docs/EH_Emergency_Response_Guide.pdf.
13. U.S. Department of Health and Human Services. *Chemical Hazards Emergency Medical Management.* Available at: http://chemm.nlm.nih.gov/index.html.
14. Chilcott R. Managing mass casualties and decontamination. 2014; *Environ Int.* Epub ahead print. http://dx.doi.org/10.1016/j.envint.2014.02.006.
15. U.S. Centers for Disease Control and Prevention. *Emergency Preparedness and Response Guide.* Available at: http://www.bt.cdc.gov.
16. U.S. Department of Health and Human Services. *Chemical Hazards Emergency Medical Management* (CHEMM). Available at: http://chemm.nlm.nih.gov. And the *CHEMM Intelligent Syndromes Tool* (CHEMM-IST) available at: http://chemm.nlm.nih.gov/chemmist.htm.
17. World Health Organization (WHO). *Interim Guidance Document: Initial Clinical Management of Chemically-Contaminated Patients.* Available at: http://www.who.int/environmental_health_emergencies/deliberate_events/Initial_Management_of_Contaminated_Patients.pdf?ua=1.
18. Madsen JM, Greenberg MI. Preparedness for the evaluation and management of mass casualty incidents involving anticholinesterase compounds: a survey of the emergency department directors in the 12 largest cities in the United States. *Am J Disaster Med.* 2010;5:333–351.

Industrial-Chemical Disasters*

Mark E. Keim

DESCRIPTION OF EVENT

Definitions

Industrial-Chemical Disasters

An industrial-chemical disaster is defined as the release or spill of a toxic chemical that results in an abrupt and serious disruption of the functioning of a society, causing widespread human, material, or environmental losses that exceed the ability of the affected society to cope using only its own resources.

Industrial-chemical disasters may occur as the result of fire, explosion,[1] and chemical releases or spills.[2] The chemical release itself may be acute or chronic in duration. It can be overt or insidious in its onset. Although less dramatic than an explosion, environmental contamination from the toxic residue of industrialization has resulted in health and environmental problems of immense proportions.[3]

Hybrid Disasters

The naturalistic perspective of disasters categorizes disasters in three main types: natural, industrial-technological, and conflict disasters.[4] However, it soon becomes clear upon deeper examination that no disaster exists in strictly one element. This becomes especially evident as disaster risk is increasingly considered to originate from a combination of dysfunctional developmental policies and environmental processes.[5,6] There is now increasing concern about HazMat releases resulting from natural disasters, as well as increases in the population density in disaster-prone areas and technological and industrial expansion.[7,8] Unintentional HazMat releases that result from technological emergencies created by natural disasters have been referred to as natural-technological or hybrid events.[9–14]

There are numerous examples of hybrid disasters triggered by natural (meteorological or seismic) hazards. In one example, in December 1999, several days of torrential rain in Venezuela triggered landslide debris flows of mud, boulders, water, and trees that killed 30,000 people.[15]

In addition to destroying large spans of residential areas, a debris flow descended from nearby mountains into La Guaira, the nation's second largest port near Caracas. The landslide crushed and buried shipping containers known to contain a large amounts of hazardous chemicals.[16] The government of Venezuela requested technical assistance from the United States to perform a site characterization, a preliminary risk assessment, and to advise the Venezuelan government.[17]

Subsequent modeling of the potential for explosion predicted a potential blast radius 5-km wide and a resultant toxic plume emanating from the fire that could kill up to 80,000 people (over double the number of fatalities already caused by the landslide disaster) and engulf Venezuela's largest international airport, as well as all of La Guaira seaport).[17] The incident was successfully resolved without incident, through careful planning and multinational collaboration of emergency response and site rehabilitation measures.

Scope of the problem. The Deepwater Horizon oil spill and the Japanese earthquake/tsunami radiation disaster have increased public concerns regarding the effects of industrial disasters on public health. Industrial-chemical disasters are known to impose a unique set of challenges for public health emergency responders. There are critical gaps in scientific knowledge regarding assessment and control of public health disasters related to industrial releases of hazardous materials. There is also a fundamental lack of familiarity regarding industrial disasters among the public health and medical communities, in general.

Incidents involving either slow or explosive releases of chemicals are common and on the increase.[18] Prior to World War II, these occurrences mainly affected people engaged in specific occupations (e.g., miners). The technological sophistication and industrialization of both developed and developing countries have grown, and with it the potential for industrial disasters.[19] The manufacturing storage, transportation, and use of large amounts and varying types of flammable, explosive, or toxic chemicals has increased. Many of these chemicals are either new or the result of chemical syntheses involving highly reactive and toxic intermediates. There has been a trend toward the centralization of industries and the quantities of chemical stored. Growing population densities in areas where chemicals are manufactured and transported have increased the numbers of persons potentially exposed.[20]

Nonpetroleum Releases

In 1990, the U.S. government Agency for Toxic Substances and Disease Registry (ATSDR), established the Hazardous Substances Emergency Events Surveillance (HSEES) system to collect and analyze information about hazardous material releases in the United States.[21] An HSEES event is any release or threatened release that results in a public health action, such as an evacuation (excluding releases involving only petroleum products). Fifteen state health departments participate in HSEES. Between 1993 and 2008, the HSEES system information reported that:

- Approximately 9000 hazardous substances releases occur annually in the 15 states reporting.
- More than 90% of events involve the release or threatened release of only one hazardous substance.

---

*The material in this chapter reflects solely the views of the author. It does not necessarily reflect the policies or recommendations of the Centers for Disease Control and Prevention or the U.S. Department of Health and Human Services.

- The substance was most frequently a volatile hydrocarbon compound.
- Releases of hazardous substances most often injure employees, followed by the general public and, less frequently, first responders and schoolchildren.
- Approximately 50% of people who reported developing symptoms or injuries from an HSEES event are treated at a hospital and released.[21]

Between 2003 and 2008, the HSEES also reported that the number of fatalities caused by hazardous-substance events increased, with the highest number of fatalities, 69 deaths, occurring in each of the years 2005, 2006, and 2007. In addition, the number of events with victims increased over time. During 2008, the number of events with victims was the highest in the history of the HSEES (948). During 2007, the number of victims was the highest it had been in the preceding 6 years.[21]

The HSEES program concluded in 2009. The National Toxic Substances Incidents Program (NTSIP), which began in 2010, is modeled partially on the HSEES, with additions suggested by stakeholders to have a more complete program. During 2010 and 2011 (the last years for which data are currently available), 6109 NTSIP incidents occurred in fixed facilities or during transportation, resulting in 2366 injured persons, of which 110 (4.6%) were fatalities.[22,23] More than half (50.9%) of all injuries were among the general public. During both years, more incidents, injuries, and fatalities occurred in fixed facilities than during transportation.

In 2010, a total of 722 (24%) incidents were caused by four chemicals: ammonia ($n = 133$), carbon monoxide ($n = 125$), chlorine ($n = 99$), and petroleum ($n = 365$).[22] Most notably this changed in 2011, when the top-four chemicals were carbon monoxide ($n = 256$), illicit methamphetamine-production chemicals ($n = 78$), paints and dyes ($n = 61$), and petroleum ($n = 205$).[23]

Petroleum-Based Releases

An oil spill is a release of a liquid petroleum hydrocarbon into the marine or terrestrial environment due to human activity. Oil spills include releases of crude oil from tankers, offshore platforms, drilling rigs, and wells, as well as spills of refined petroleum products and their byproducts.[24]

Oil spills happen all around the world. Spills of at least 10,000 gallons (34 tons) have occurred in the waters of 112 nations since 1960.[25] Oil spills happen more frequently in certain parts of the world:

1. The Gulf of Mexico (267 spills)
2. The Northeastern United States (140 spills)
3. The Mediterranean Sea (127 spills)
4. The Persian Gulf (108 spills)
5. The North Sea (75 spills)
6. Japan (60 spills)
7. The Baltic Sea (52 spills)
8. The United Kingdom and the English Channel (49 spills)
9. Malaysia and Singapore (39 spills)
10. The west coast of France and north and west coasts of Spain (33 spills)
11. Korea (32 spills)

The incidence of large spills is relatively low, and detailed statistical analysis is rarely possible. Consequently, emphasis is placed on identifying trends. However, it does appear that the number of medium (7 to 700 metric tons) and large (>700 metric tons) spills from oil tankers, combined carriers, and barges has decreased significantly in the last 41 years during which records have been kept.[26]

During the past decade (since 2004), 71 oil spills (with a volume ranging from 2 to 820,000 metric tons) have been reported worldwide. Of these spills, 33 (46%) occurred in the United States (15 since the 2010 Deepwater Horizon spill).[27–31] Of these spills over the past decade, 13 (18%) occurred as hybrid disasters associated with U.S.

hurricanes: 3 were caused by Hurricane Ivan; 9 by Hurricane Katrina; and 1 from Hurricane Sandy.

The largest oil spill in U.S. history occurred in 1910, as an out-of-control oil well in California released more than 378 million gallons of oil. This event was over twice the size of the Deepwater Horizon disaster.[32]

Situational Factors

Timing, site location, and local weather conditions are natural factors that have a significant effect on the severity and occurrence of chemical disasters. Most releases in the United States occur on weekdays between 6 AM and 6 PM. Releases tend to increase in spring and summer, when more shipments of pesticides and fertilizers for agricultural activities occur.[21] Thermal inversion or wind may serve to concentrate or disseminate atmospheric chemical releases, respectively.

Between 1993 and 2008, facilities accounted for 70% to 75%, and transportation-associated releases account for 25% to 30% of reported HSEES events.[21] Causal factors differed by location: for fixed-facility events, the leading factor was equipment failure; for transportation-related events, the leading factor was human error.[21] During the same time frame, the manufacturing industry (consisting of wood, paper, printing, petroleum and coal, chemical, plastic and rubber, and nonmetallic mineral manufacturing) accounted for the largest proportion of the events.[21]

Socioeconomic Factors

In many rapidly industrializing countries, less elaborate measures for the protection of the environment, human health, and safety have been important items in economic negotiations; these have often led to unfair international division of risks.[1,33,34] This "comparative powerlessness of certain societies to control risk" has been described as sociopolitical amplification of risk.[33]

Between 1945 and 1991, India, Brazil, Mexico, and China led the world in the number of chemical releases resulting in greater than five fatalities.[34] The largest industrial-chemical disaster in world history occurred in Bhopal, India, in 1984. The Bhopal disaster killed more than 2500 persons and affected an additional 200,000 to 300,000.[35]

In general, poverty is the single most important risk factor for vulnerability to disasters.[36] In one study of over 15,000 industrial facilities located in some 2333 counties in the United States between 1994 and 2000, higher-risk facilities were more likely to be found in counties with sizeable poor and/or minority populations that disproportionately bear the collateral environmental, property, and health risks.[37]

◀ PRE-INCIDENT ACTIONS

Risk Management Strategies

In recent years the overall approach to emergencies and disasters has shifted from ad hoc postimpact activities to a more systematic and comprehensive process of risk management that also emphasizes the importance of preimpact activities, including prevention, mitigation, and preparedness.[36] Risk management is the process of selecting and implementing prevention and control measures to achieve an acceptable level of that risk at an acceptable cost. In general, risk management is composed of four main elements: risk assessment, countermeasure determination, cost-benefit analysis, and risk communication.

Emergency Preparedness

Elements of emergency preparedness typically include emergency planning, training and education; warning systems; specialized communication systems; surveillance activities; information databases, and resource management systems; resource stocks; emergency exercises; population protection measures; and incident management systems.

Emergency Planning

During an emergency, time constraints place a premium on available plans, data, and record-keeping systems. Planning and preparedness are essential, and carefully crafted procedures and checklists can help; at the same time, prior training in how to respond during emergency situations will aid in handling the difficult circumstances involved.[38] Disaster plans should also be developed for all special facilities, such as schools, hospitals, and nursing homes, which may be at risk for industrial-chemical disasters.[38–40]

Information Databases and Resource Management Systems

There are several available software and Internet-based tools that have been used widely to rapidly access information regarding hazardous materials.

Table 111-1 includes a list of other information resources that planners and responders may use in the event of industrial-chemical disasters.

Specialized Communication Systems

Coordination of the activities of an on-site facility with those located off-site is essential in an emergency.[41] National, regional, and local public health departments must be linked in a network of real-time communication with the medical response community, public safety, regional poison control centers, and regional laboratory capacities for integration of information management, passive and active surveillance systems, and epidemiological investigation.[42–45]

Resource Stocks

A lack of hospital preparedness for chemical casualty care has been well documented in regions throughout the United States.[46–51] In 1999, Congress charged the Department of Health and Human Services (HHS) and the Centers for Disease Control and Prevention (CDC) with establishing the National Pharmaceutical Stockpile (NPS). In March 2003, the NPS became the Strategic National Stockpile (SNS), managed jointly by the Department of Homeland Security (DHS) and HHS.

Training and Education

Caregivers should be familiar with basic principles of toxicology, trauma, burn care, mass casualty management, occupational safety and health, and hazardous materials (HazMat) decontamination, as well as incident management systems. Public health officials should also be aware of population protection measures, information resources, environmental health, environmental law, public warning systems, and risk communication.

Warning Systems

In order to mount a safe and timely evacuation in the event of an industrial-chemical disaster, there must first be an effective system in place for warning the population at risk.[1,38,39,44] The system must

TABLE 111-1   **Resources for Information Related to Industrial Chemical Releases**

INFORMATION RESOURCE	APPLICATION
Major Hazardous Incident Data Service (MHIDAS)	A database of incidents involving hazardous materials that had an off-site effect or had the potential to have an off-site effect.
Environmental Protection Agency (EPA) Toxic Release Inventory (TRI)	A publicly available EPA database that contains information on toxic chemical releases and other waste management activities reported annually by certain covered industry groups and federal facilities.
The National Toxic Substance Incidents Program (NTSIP)	Collects and combines information from many resources to protect people from harm caused by spills and leaks of toxic substances.
CHEMTREC	Provides its preregistered customers with a 24-hour emergency telephone number for shipments of hazardous materials or dangerous goods assistance in identifying the hazardous substance and precautionary measures. There is an annual fee for this service.
The National Library of Medicine	Offers many electronic databases such as MEDLINE and TOXLINE, which provide literature references; and CHEMLINE and TOXLIT, which provide information from books and journals, as well as information on other hazardous-materials databases.
The NIOSH Pocket Guide to Chemical Hazards	Intended as a source of general industrial hygiene information on several hundred chemicals/classes for workers, employers, and occupational health professionals.
U.S. Department of Transportation (DOT) Emergency Response Guidebook 2008 (ERG2008)	Provides guidance to first responders on how to identify the types of hazardous materials that may be involved in an incident and how to respond to the threats those materials might pose to emergency crews and the public.
The National Response Center (NRC)	The sole federal point of contact for reporting all hazardous substances releases and oil spills. The NRC receives all reports of releases involving hazardous substances and oil that trigger federal notification requirements under several laws.
Agency for Toxic Substances and Disease Registry (ATSDR)	Provides 24-hour assistance to emergency responders who require assistance in managing hazardous-materials emergencies. Such assistance includes information on treatment protocols, laboratory support, and emergency consultation related to assessment and decontamination.
National Pesticide Information Center (NPIC)	NPIC provides objective, science-based information about pesticides and pesticide-related topics to enable people to make informed decisions about pesticides and their use. NPIC is a cooperative agreement between Oregon State University and the U.S. Environmental Protection Agency.
Centers for Disease Control and Prevention (CDC)	The National Report on Human Exposure to Environmental Chemicals provides an ongoing assessment of the exposure of the U.S. population to environmental chemicals using bio-monitoring.
National Poison Data System (NPDS)	A comprehensive poisoning surveillance database compiled by the American Association of Poison Control Centers (AAPCC). AAPCC owns and manages a large database holding information from all informational and human-poison-exposure case phone calls into all poison centers across the country.

use redundant methods of communication, including direct contact. It must also address the needs of special populations, such as persons with disabilities and extremes of age, as well as those with language differences.

Exercises

Exercises are a common way of monitoring and evaluating parts of emergency preparedness programs. The purpose of an exercise and the aspect of emergency preparedness to be tested must be carefully decided and fairly specific. Adequate predrill instruction and training are vital for success. Special attention should be given to the training of personnel on the use and wearing of personal protective equipment at the decontamination and initial triage sites.[40]

►► POST-INCIDENT ACTIONS

Detection and Management of the Consequences of Industrial-Chemical Disasters

The primary functions that must be performed at any toxic release remain fairly consistent. Box 111-1 contains a listing of these actions.[38,41,52]

Activities of a rapid assessment should focus on information objectives that can be undertaken consecutively and/or concurrently. Box 111-2 lists examples of such objectives.[1,38,53–56]

Table 111-2 describes several commonly used modeling tools.

Once modeling has been completed for potential areas at risk, the decision can then be made regarding the need for evacuation or shelter-in-place contingencies.[39]

Population protection measures may include population evacuation, sheltering in place, and individual protection measures. Sheltering in place may be necessary when sufficient time for evacuation is not available. Generally, providing individual protection measures in the way of protective gear is impractical and potentially dangerous to the general population.[59]

The effectiveness of shelter-in-place strategies is time dependent and is not always applicable. Indoor shelters may initially provide protection from atmospheric releases as compared to the outdoor

environment immediately after a chemical release. However, 30 to 60 minutes after the plume dispersion has ceased, chemical levels indoors may actually then exceed outdoor concentrations. Recommendations for population protection measures should, therefore, be based on an accurate exposure modeling system and should not remain static over time. Box 111-3 is a list of recommendations for implementing effective population evacuations.[3,56]

Risk Communication

The public will have obvious concerns about their exposure to fire, smoke, and hazardous materials.[60] Public health and medical personnel should anticipate this need for information and develop public advisories and risk communication strategies for early implementation during such an event. A well-executed risk-communication-response effort will increase an organization's credibility.[61]

✚ MEDICAL TREATMENT OF CASUALTIES

In spite of the enormous challenges presented in the identification of chemical hazards, there are certain generalizations that may be made to simplify disaster medical response. Toxic chemicals may be categorized by their known health effects. For ease of case and incident management, a broad variety of hazardous chemicals may be divided into 13 basic categories (Box 111-4).

Outside of an extremely limited number of antidote therapies, medical management of nearly all toxic chemical exposures would involve mostly supportive therapy.[44] Even if there may be an antidote available for a specific exposure, many times the clinician may not be able to identify the offending agent in enough time to guide effective therapy.

Thus the acute health effects of a very broad variety of hazardous chemicals, as categorized in Box 111-4, may actually be expected to invoke demands for medical resources that address a very narrow range of medical conditions. Table 111-3 represents four main basic medical conditions that may be expected to occur as major short-term sequelae following severe exposures to any of these chemical hazards. It then also identifies a mere eight categories of emergency medical therapeutics that would become necessary to treat these four syndrome complexes.[44]

BOX 111-1 The Primary Functions That Must Be Performed at Any Toxic Release

- Rapid assessment
- Scene control and establishment of a perimeter
- Product identification and information gathering
- Preentry examination and characterization of site
- Selection and donning of appropriate personal protective clothing and equipment
- Establishment of a decontamination area
- Entry planning and preparation of equipment and supplies
- Victim rescue from release area
- Containment of spill

- Neutralization of spill/release
- Decontamination of victims and responders
- Triage of injured
- Consultation with toxicologist/Emergency Department (ED)/Poison Control Center
- Medical care, including antidotes
- Transport of patients
- Postentry evaluation of rescuers and equipment
- Delegation of final cleanup to responsible party
- Record keeping and after-action reporting

BOX 111-2 Information Objectives for Rapid Assessment Following Chemical Disasters

- Determine the types, size, and distribution of the release
- Identify the specific type(s) of chemicals and their byproducts
- Characterize the hazardous release site
- Identify human exposure pathways
- Define the populations at risk
- Conduct a toxicological evaluation and assessment
- Describe morbidity and mortality

- Identify appropriate treatment regimens
- Evaluate emergency medical care and health service capabilities
- Ensure provision of appropriate medical care
- Identify and evaluate environmental control strategies
- Evaluate evacuation and mass care strategies
- Develop criteria for defining comprehensive databases

TABLE 111-2   Software Applications Commonly Used for Chemical Emergency Preparedness and Response

APPLICATION	DESCRIPTION
Computer-aided management of emergency operations (CAMEO)[57]	The CAMEO system integrates a chemical database and a method to manage the data, as well as an air dispersion model and a mapping capability. This suite includes 4 components: CAMEOfm, a database and information management tool; CAMEO Chemicals, an extensive chemical database with critical response information; ALOHA; and MARPLOT (see below).
Areal Locations of Hazardous Atmospheres (ALOHA)[57]	ALOHA is an atmospheric dispersion model used for evaluating releases of hazardous chemical vapors.
Mapping Applications for Response, Planning, and Local Operational Tasks (MARPLOT)[57]	MARPLOT is a mapping application that allows users to view their data (e.g., roads, facilities, schools, and response assets), display this information on computer maps, and print the information on area maps.
Consequence Assessment Tools Set (CATS)[58]	CATS is a tool for assessing the consequences of technological disasters on population, resources, and infrastructure. It analyzes the damage to the environment and the risk to the well-being of the exposed population, and it provides real-time resource allocation information to mitigate the consequences.
The Incident Command Tool for Drinking Water Protection (ICWater)[58]	ICWater is a GIS-based software tool for tracking and identifying the source of water contaminants using hydraulic modeling to assess the movement and dispersion of contaminants in streams and rivers in real time.

BOX 111-3   Recommendations for Implementing Effective Evacuations

- Make populations aware of existing emergency operations plans well in advance of any potential industrial disaster
- Ensure that evacuation warning messages include the following:
  - Emphasis that the authorities will prevent looting
  - Emphasis of the dangers of staying home
  - Indication of a place to go and how to get there
- Facilitate the departure of families, even if all members are not present
- Provide public transportation that is suitable for children, the elderly, and handicapped persons
- Consider potential problems of pets and livestock and provide services for taking care of pets during evacuations
- Facilitate access to medical care for evacuees
- Strictly enforce limitations on access to the restricted area after evacuation
- Implement social support services

BOX 111-4   Toxic Materials Categorized According to General Health Effects

- Metals and metallic compounds
- Incendiaries
- Irritant gases
- Asphyxiant gases
- Metabolic asphyxiants
- Radiologicals
- Teratogens
- Corrosives
- Explosives
- Oxidizers
- Pharmaceuticals
- Carcinogens
- Pesticides

TABLE 111-3   Emergency Medical Conditions and Needs Associated with Chemical Exposures

SYNDROME AND CAUSATIVE AGENTS	MEDICAL THERAPEUTIC NEEDS
Burns & Trauma	
Corrosives, vesicants, explosives, oxidants, incendiaries, and radiologicals	Intravenous fluid and supplies Pain medications Pulmonary products Splints and bandages
Respiratory Failure	
Corrosives, military agents, explosives, oxidants, incendiaries, asphyxiants, irritants, pharmaceuticals, and metals	Pulmonary products Ventilators and supplies Antidotes (when available) Tranquilizing medications
Cardiovascular Shock	
Pesticides, asphyxiants, and pharmaceuticals	Intravenous fluids and supplies Cardiovascular products Antidotes (when available)
Neurologic Toxicity	
Pesticides, pharmaceuticals, and radiologicals	Antidotes (when available)

UNIQUE CONSIDERATIONS

Industrial-chemical disasters are also unique in the degree of complexity that the event entails. Decision making becomes less centralized and more interdependent, and it may be influenced by local and distant theaters of operation. Responders are forced to act in a collective and integrated fashion within an unconventional network of personnel also unfamiliar with this catastrophic breakdown phenomenon.[44,62]

In addition, the public tends to judge all technological hazards more harshly than they do natural hazards of a similar magnitude and to attach to them much more of a public concern and perception of risk.[56,18,62–64] In the public eye, these categories of technological catastrophes no longer represent localized emergencies but rather "trends which unravel the very fabric of existing organized systems."[62] There are also special problems with respect to exactly how to handle the overwhelming numbers of mass media representatives.[18] For this reason, risk communication and public information become even more critical and labor-intensive components of the response to these incidents.

Industrial disasters may be unintentional (due to mechanical failure or worker error) or they may be intentional in nature. In effect, the main difference between industrial disasters and those of sabotage, warfare, and terrorism may be a distinction only of malicious intent.[9]

Finally, industrial-chemical disasters are unique among environmental disasters in general, in their potential to affect the long-term environmental viability of a large area. These sites may have lingering toxic effects for many years to come.[1]

⚠ PITFALLS

Lack of Knowledge

One major pitfall involving industrial-chemical disasters is the relative lack of knowledge regarding the adverse health effects of many of the chemicals that are currently on the market. More than 600 new chemical substances enter the marketplace each month.[65] Researchers estimate that only 7% of all known chemical substances have been fully investigated.[35] Measuring human exposure to chemical substances through laboratory sampling also has its limitations.[2] In some cases, consequences can be revealed only by means of formal, sometimes complex, and often long-lasting investigations.[56]

Lack of Familiarity

Another pitfall of industrial-chemical disasters is a fundamental lack of familiarity among the medical community (including emergency care providers). Baxter observes that health professionals are more used to planning for trauma than for mass chemical exposure.[66] The direct effects of the disaster can be compounded by ineffective management or leadership, legal difficulties, economic or political limitations, and psychological stress.[38]

Lack of Community Preparedness

There is also a fundamental and endemic lack of preparedness among communities at risk for industrial-chemical disasters.[2,46–51] An additional impediment to local planning efforts is the fact that the most relevant resources rest in the hands of extra-community groups (i.e., state and federal assets) rather than with the community organizations that invariably are confronted with the immediate post-incident response.[18]

High Occupational Health Risk Posed to Responders

Workers and first responders are often the most frequently injured populations in the case of industrial-chemical-release events.[2,60,67–69] Most injuries of this group of emergency personnel occur in the first few minutes of responding, with firefighters and police being the most frequent victims.[69] Injuries from hazardous-substances-emergency events are also becoming increasingly more common among hospital personnel as a result of secondary contamination.[70]

REFERENCES

1. Hull D, Grindlinger G, Hirsch E. The clinical consequences of an industrial plant explosion. *J Trauma*. 1985;25(4):303–307.
2. Duclos P, Sanderson L, Thompson F, et al. Community evacuation following a chlorine release, Mississippi. *Disasters*. 1987;11(4):286–289.
3. Lillibridge S. Industrial disasters. In: Noji ER, ed. *The Public Health Consequences of Disasters*. New York: Oxford; 1997:354–369.
4. Hogan D, Burstein J. General concepts. In: Hogan D, Burstein J, eds. *Disaster Medicine*. 2nd ed. Philadelphia, PA: Lippincott, Williams & Wilkins; 2007:8.
5. Schipper L, Pelling M. Disaster risk, climate change and international development: scope for, and challenges to, integration. *Disasters*. 2006;30 (1):19–38.
6. World Bank. *Natural Hazards, Un-Natural Disasters*. Washington, DC: World Bank; 2010. Available at: http://www.gfdrr.org/gfdrr/nhud-home, Last Accessed 27.04.14.
7. International Federation of Red Cross and Red Crescent Societies (IFRC). *World Disasters Report 2001*. Geneva, Switzerland: IFRC; 2001.
8. Wijkman A, Timberlake L. *Natural Disasters: Acts of God or Acts of Man*. New York: Earthscan Paperback; 1984.
9. Keim M. Intentional chemical disasters. In: Hogan D, Burstein J, eds. *Disaster Medicine*. Philadelphia: Lippincott, Williams & Wilkins; 2002:340–348.
10. Brown H, Himelberger J, White A. Development of environment interactions in the export of hazardous technologies. *Technol Forecast Soc Change*. 1993;43:125–155.
11. Berren M, Beigel A, Ghertner S. Typology for the classification of disasters. *Community Health J*. 1980;16:103–111.
12. Showalter PS, Myers MF. Natural disasters in the United States as release agents of oil, chemicals, or radiological materials between 1980–1989: analysis and recommendations. *Risk Anal*. 1994;14:169–182.
13. Velimirovic B. Non-natural disasters—an epidemiological review. *Disasters*. 1980;4:237–246.
14. Young S, Balluz L, Malilay J. Natural and technological hazardous material releases during and after natural disasters. *Sci Total Environ*. 2004;322:3–20.
15. Sancio R. Disaster in Venezuela: the floods and landslides of December 1999. *Nat Hazards Obs*. 2002;24(4).
16. Larsen M, Wieczorek G, Eaton L, et al. *Natural Hazards on Alluvial Fans: The Venezuela Debris Flow and Flash Flood Disaster*. US Department of the Interior; US Geological Survey Fact Sheet 103-01. http://pubs.usgs.gov/fs/fs-0103-01/fs-0103-01.pdf. Last Accessed 27.04.14.
17. Keim M, Humphrey A, Dreyfus A, et al. *Situation assessment report involving the hazardous material disaster site at LaGuaira Port, Venezuela*. CDC Report to Office of Foreign Disaster Assistance, US Agency for International Development; January 10, 2000.
18. Quarantelli E, Gray J. Research findings on community and organizational preparations for and responses to acute chemical emergencies. *Publ Manag*. 1986;68:11–13.
19. National Environmental Law Center and the US Public Research Interest Group. *Chemical Releases Statistics*. Washington, DC: Associated Press International; 1994.
20. Sanderson L. Toxicologic disasters: natural and technologic. In: Sullivan JB, Krieger GR, eds. *Hazardous Materials Toxicology: Clinical Principles of Environmental Health*. Baltimore: Agency for Toxic Substances and Disease Registry; 1992:326–331.
21. Agency for Toxic Substances and Disease Registry. *HSEES Annual Report. Hazardous Substances Emergency Events Surveillance (HSEES)*. Atlanta: U.S Department of Health and Human Services; 2007–2008. Available at: http://www.atsdr.cdc.gov/hs/hsees/annual2008.html. Last Accessed 27.04.14.
22. ATSDR (Agency for Toxic Substances and Disease Registry). *National Toxic Substances Incidents Program (NTISP) Annual Report 2010*. Atlanta, GA: US Department of Health and Human Services Available at: http://www.atsdr.cdc.gov/ntsip/docs/ATSDR_Annual%20Report_031413_FINAL.pdf. Last Accessed 27.04.14.
23. ATSDR (Agency for Toxic Substances and Disease Registry). *National Toxic Substances Incidents Program (NTISP) Annual Report 2011*. Atlanta, GA: US Department of Health and Human Services available at: http://www.atsdr.cdc.gov/ntsip/docs/ATSDR_Annual%20Report_121013_508%20compliant.pdf. Last Accessed 27.04.14.
24. NOAA Office of Response and Restoration. *Oil and Chemical Spills*. Available at: http://archive.orr.noaa.gov/topic_subtopic_entry.php?RECORD_KEY%28entry_subtopic_topic%29=entry_id,subtopic_id,topic_id&entry_id(entry_subtopic_topic)=358&subtopic_id(entry_subtopic_topic)=8&topic_id(entry_subtopic_topic)=1. Last Accessed 27.04.14.
25. Etkin DS. *Oil Spills from Vessels (1960–1995): An International Historical Perspective*. Cambridge, MA: Cutter Information Corporation; 1997, p. 72.
26. International Tanker Owners Pollution Federation, Limited. *Statistics*. Available at: http://www.itopf.com/information-services/data-and-statistics/statistics/index.html. Last Accessed 27.04.14.

27. NOAA Office of Response and Restoration. *Oil and Chemical Spills.* Available at: http://archive.orr.noaa.gov/faq_topic.php?faq_topic_id=1#2. Last Accessed 27.04.14.

28. Etkin DS. *Oil Spills from Vessels (1960–1995): An International Historical Perspective.* Cambridge, MA: Cutter Information Corporation; 1997, 72.

29. US Coast Guard. *Oil Pollution Control Act.* Available at: http://www.uscg.mil/d13/dep/news/oil_pollution_act_of_1990.htm. Last Accessed 27.04.14.

30. International Tanker Owners Pollution Federation, Limited. *Statistics.* Available at: http://www.itopf.com/information-services/data-and-statistics/statistics/index.html. Last Accessed 27.04.14.

31. Mariner Group. *Oil Spill History.* Available at: http://www.marinergroup.com/oil-spill-history.htm. Last Accessed 27.04.14.

32. San Joaquin Geological Society. 23 September 2002. Available at: http://web.archive.org/web/20061019100520/http://www.sjgs.com/lakeview.html. Last Accessed 27.04.14.

33. Firpo de Souza Porto M, Machado de Freitas C. Major chemical accidents and industrializing countries: the socio-political amplification of risk. *Risk Anal.* 1996;16(1):19–29.

34. Glickman T, Golding D, Terry K. *Fatal Hazardous Materials Accidents in Industry: Domestic and Foreign Experience from 1945 to 1991.* Washington, DC: Center for Risk Management; 1993.

35. Mehta PS, Mehta AS, Mehta SJ, et al. Bhopal tragedy's health effects. *JAMA.* 1990;264(21):2781–2787.

36. Clack Z, Keim M, MacIntyre A, Yeskey K. Emergency health and risk management in sub-Saharan Africa: a lesson from the embassy bombings in Tanzania and Kenya. *Prehosp Disast Med.* 2002;17(2):59–66.

37. Elliott M, Wang Y, Lowe R, et al. Environmental justice: frequency and severity of US chemical industry accidents and the socio-economic status of surrounding communities. *J Epidemiol Community Health.* 2004;58:24–30.

38. Falk H. Industrial/chemical disasters: medical care, public health and epidemiology in the acute phase. In: Bourdeau P, Green G, eds. *Methods for Assessing and Reducing Injury from Chemical Accidents.* New York, NY: John Wiley and Sons Ltd; 1989:105–114.

39. Rogers G, Sorensen J, Long J, et al. Emergency planning for chemical agent releases. *Environ Prof.* 1989;11:396–408.

40. Tur-Kaspa I, Lev E, Hendler I, et al. Preparing hospitals for toxicological mass casualty events. *Crit Care Med.* 1999;27(5):1004–1008.

41. McCunney R. Emergency response to environmental toxic incidents: the role of the occupational physician. *Occ Med.* 1996;46(5):397–401.

42. Keim M, Kaufmann A, Rodgers G. *Recommendations for Office of Emergency Preparedness/CDC Surveillance, Laboratory and Informational Support Initiative.* Atlanta, GA: Centers for Disease Control and Prevention, National Center for Environmental Health; 1998.

43. Brennan RJ, Waeckerle JL, Sharp TW, Lillibridge SR. Chemical warfare agents: emergency medical and emergency public health issues. *Ann Emerg Med.* 1999;34(2):191–204.

44. Keim M. Intentional chemical disasters. In: Hoganand D, Burstein J, eds. *Disaster Medicine.* Philadelphia, PA: Lippincott, Williams & Wilkins; 2002:340–348.

45. Delgado R, Gonzalez P, Alvarez T, et al. Preparation for response to an industrial disaster in Spain. *Public Health.* 2003;117:260–261.

46. Ghilarducci DP, Pirrallo RG, Hegmann KT. Hazardous materials readiness of United States level 1 trauma centers. *J Occ Env Med.* 2000;42(7):683–692.

47. Wetter DC, Daniell WE, Treser CD. Hospital preparedness for victims of chemical or biological terrorism. *Am J Publ Health.* 2001;91:710–716.

48. Chyka PA, Conner HG. Availability of antidotes in rural and urban hospitals in Tennessee. *Am J Hosp Pharm.* 1994;51:1346–1348.

49. Dart RC, Stark Y, Fulton B. Insufficient stocking of poisoning antidotes in hospital pharmacies. *JAMA.* 1996;276:1508–1510.

50. Woolf AD, Chrisanthus K. On-site availability of selected antidotes: results of a survey of Massachusetts hospitals. *Am J Emerg Med.* 1997;15:62–66.

51. Keim M, Pesik N, Twum-Danso N. Lack of hospital preparedness for chemical terrorism in a major US city: 1996–2000. *Prehosp Disast Med.* 2003;18(3):193–199.

52. Staten C. *Emergency Response to Chemical/Biological Terrorist Incidents.* Emergency Response & Research Institute; 1997. Available at: *http://wearcam.org/decon/no_contaminated_person_allowed_to_leave.htm.* Last Accessed 27.04.14.

53. Sanderson L. Toxicologic disasters: natural and technologic. In: Sullivan JB, Krieger GR, eds. *Hazardous Materials Toxicology: Clinical Principles of Environmental Health.* Baltimore: Williams & Wilkins; 1992.

54. Levitin H, Siegelson H, Dickinson S, et al. Decontamination of mass casualties—evaluating existing dogma. *Prehosp Disast Med.* 2003;18(3):200–207.

55. Curreri P, Morris M, Pruitt B. The treatment of chemical burns: specialized diagnostic, therapeutic, and prognostic considerations. *J Trauma.* 1970;10:634–642.

56. Bertazzi P. Industrial disasters and epidemiology. *Scan J Work Environ Health.* 1989;15:85–100.

57. Environmental Protection Agency. *Computer Aided Management of Emergency Operations (CAMEO)* homepage. Available at: http://www2.epa.gov/cameo. Last Accessed 27.04.14.

58. Leidos. *Consequence Assessment Tool (CATS).* Available at: https://www.leidos.com/products/security/cats. Last Accessed 27.04.14.

59. Golan E, Shemer J, Arad M, et al. Medical limitations of gas masks for civilian populations: the 1991 experience. *Mil Med.* 1992;157:444–446.

60. Hsu E, Grabowski J, Chotani R, et al. Effects on local emergency departments of large scale urban chemical fire with hazardous material spill. *Prehosp Disast Med.* 2002;17(4):196–201.

61. Fernandez L, Merzer M. *Janes Crisis Communications Handbook.* Surrey, UK: Janes Information Group; 2003.

62. Lagadec P. *Accidents, Crises, Breakdowns.* Paper presented at the Society of Chemical Industry, London. January 9, 1998.

63. Slovic P. Perception of risk. *Science.* 1987;236:280–285.

64. Glickman TS, Golding D, Silverman ED. *Acts of God and Acts of Man: Major Trends in Natural Disasters and Major Industrial Accidents.* Discussion paper, Washington, DC: Center for Risk Management, Resources for the Future; 1991.

65. Doyle C, Upfal M, Little N. Disaster management of possible toxic exposure. In: Haddad L, ed. *Clinical Management of Poisoning and Drug Overdose.* Philadelphia, PA: WB Saunders Co; 1990:483–500.

66. Baxter P. Major chemical disasters: Britain's health services are poorly prepared. *Br Med J.* 1991;302:61–62.

67. Doyle C, Upfal M, Little N. Disaster management of possible toxic exposure. In: Haddad L, ed. *Clinical Management of Poisoning and Drug Overdose.* Philadelphia, PA: WB Saunders Co; 1990:483–500.

68. Baxter P. 1991 Major chemical disasters: Britain's health services are poorly prepared. *Brit Med J.* 1991;302:61–62.

69. Zeitz P, Berkowitz Z, Orr M, et al. Frequency and type of injuries in responders of hazardous substances emergency events, 1996 to 1998. *J Occup Environ Med.* 2000;42:1115–1120.

70. Cox R. Decontamination and management of hazardous materials exposure victims in the emergency department. *Ann Emerg Med.* 1994;23:761–770.

CHAPTER 112

Nerve-Agent Mass Casualty Incidents

Brian C. Geyer

DESCRIPTION OF EVENT

Nerve agents have been used numerous times against civilian populations, with catastrophic outcomes.[1,2] Although these are relatively rare events, the willingness of totalitarian regimes and terrorist organizations to deploy these weapons as an act of desperation seems limited only by their access to nerve-agent stockpiles or precursors. As recently as August 2013, an estimated 1400 people were killed in a nerve-agent attack in Syria.[3] In addition to these more high-profile events, there remains the more likely possibility of an industrial accident releasing acetylcholine-modulating agents onto an unsuspecting populace.[4] The history of these agents is rooted in the development of increasingly sophisticated pesticides for agricultural use in the early twentieth century, with subsequent weaponization during World War II. When planning for the possibility of a nerve-agent mass casualty incident, it is important to consider both intentional and unintentional scenarios.

The toxicity of nerve agents arises from their inhibition of acetylcholinesterase (AChE) at the neuromuscular junction. AChE is the primary negative regulator of the cholinergic system. It functions by degrading acetylcholine (ACh). Physiological neuronal stimulation ejects stored ACh into synapses and neuromuscular and neuroglandular junctions, and the released ACh fits into postsynaptic and postjunctional nicotinic and muscarinic ACh receptors (nAChR and mAChR, respectively). This receptor binding stimulates skeletal muscle (nAChR), smooth muscle, and exocrine glands (mAChR), as well as neurons in the central nervous system (CNS; mAChR and nAChR) and sympathetic ganglia (nAChR). AChE normally hydrolyzes ACh to acetate and choline. Nerve agents inhibit AChE by a variety of mechanisms, effectively destroying its catalytic function. ACh accumulates, and its effects are potentiated in an unregulated manner.[5] The physiological manifestation of this toxicity on the nAChR in skeletal muscle is unregulated skeletal-muscle contraction with subsequent muscle fatigue and failure. Even more importantly, fatigue and failure of neurons in the respiratory center of the medulla lead to central apnea. Effects of unregulated muscarinic toxicity include bronchospasm and bronchorrhea, which compound the deleterious effects of the nAChR stimulation on oxygenation and ventilation.

There are three broad classes of nerve agents: carbamates, ammonium alcohols, and organophosphorous esters, commonly called organophosphates. The organophosphates have particularly significant human toxicity and the ability to cause a large mass casualty incident under commonly imagined scenarios. Carbamates and ammonium alcohols are significantly less toxic, in comparison, because of their very brief molecular interactions and inability to cross the blood-brain barrier, respectively.[6-8] The organophosphates include pesticides such as diazinon, malathion, parathion, dichlorvos, and chlorpyrifos, as well as the G- and V-series nerve agents used as chemical-warfare agents. The common structural element in these agents is a phosphoric-acid backbone. When bound to AChE, organophosphates form a very stable complex that is not susceptible to hydrolysis. This is in direct contrast to the carbamates, which may undergo hydrolysis. Further, this AChE-organophosphate bond may then undergo a process called "aging," which creates irreversible inactivation of the phosphorylated AChE.[9] Aging occurs particularly quickly with the nerve agent soman (GD) but takes much longer for the other nerve agents and for organophosphate pesticides.

Organophosphates are variably lipophilic liquids that may smell like garlic or petroleum (OP pesticides) or faintly like fruit (G agents) or rotten fish (VX). These agents can cause toxicity through inhalation, injection, transmucosal (gastrointestinal [GI] and genitourinary [GU]), and transdermal (percutaneous) exposures. Inhalation occurs through direct absorption of nerve-agent vapor or aerosolized droplets into the pulmonary tree. In particular, the classically described G-agent nerve "gases" sarin (GB), GD, and tabun (GA) possess sufficiently high vapor pressures and volatilities to produce lethal vapor concentrations at room temperature.[9,10] Another organophosphate nerve agent, VX, is the most potent chemical warfare agent; a single droplet of VX on the skin can be fatal. VX is a liquid with a low vapor pressure and volatility, and spontaneous evaporation is minimal.[11] However, all organophosphates may be aerosolized with mechanical sprayers, for example, during crop dusting or from the combustion of an explosive device. As these agents persist in the environment, secondary vaporization, so-called off gassing, may occur.[12]

PRE-INCIDENT CONSIDERATIONS

There are two main aspects of preparation for nerve-agent exposure incidents, recognition of the presence of nerve agent in a disaster, and implementation of a plan to treat patients while protecting civilians and health care workers. Recognition may come in many forms, ideally as advance notice from civil or military authorities once an exposure is suspected or verified. The more challenging scenario is identifying the index patient in a crowded first-aid tent or emergency department. Decreased serum cholinesterase activity is highly specific for nerve-agent poisoning, but these tests are not sensitive. They do not correlate with clinical severity and are rarely available in the acute period. Early diagnosis of nerve-agent exposure is clinical, but because of the rarity of the event, very few people have any level of clinical experience. Even though it has not been rigorously evaluated, the nuclear, biological, and chemical (NBC) Indicator Matrix, available in paper and electronic formats, can assist first responders and triage workers in distinguishing between types of NBC agents. In addition, the Chemical Hazards Emergency Medical Management (CHEMM) Intelligent Syndromes Tool

(CHEMM-IST) can provide interactive assistance in the differential diagnosis of clinical presentations in suspected chemical exposures, including nerve-agent poisoning. However, they both presume an initial high index of suspicion for NBC use.[13] In the absence of clear strategies to identify early and atypical presentations of nerve-agent poisoning, organizational and institutional leaders should prioritize continuous retraining of all levels of team members with emphasis on the distinguishing characteristics of the cholinergic toxidrome. This is particularly important for the health care providers triaging the patients and determining the need for immediate isolation.

Once an exposure has been identified, members of the health care team should work quickly to implement a plan to isolate, decontaminate, and treat patients. It is helpful to presume that the first patients encountered are the "walking wounded" and that more critically ill patients will be arriving shortly thereafter. This will often affect decisions to move other patients out of the treatment area quickly, while saving resuscitation bays and equipment for patients needing that level of care. However, it is also important to recognize that liquid nerve agents take time to be absorbed through the skin and that initially asymptomatic individuals may present and even be decontaminated only to collapse and exhibit a full-blown cholinergic crisis later. Large-scale drills can be helpful to reinforce constantly changing protocols that are rarely implemented under normal conditions. Drills can also be a particularly effective way to highlight potential challenges in hospital response, such as the difficulty of providing care for patients because of the decreased visibility, increased weight, and heat stress conferred by the personal protective equipment (PPE) required. Preparation should include reviewing the supply of antidotes, ventilators, PPE, and decontamination facilities (including temporary decontamination tents that may be erected close to but outside of the facility).[14] A more comprehensive outline of decontamination tactics can be found in Chapter 83.

There are several caveats when preparing protocols to handle nerve-agent disasters.[15] Nerve agents are easily absorbed across the epithelium, causing delayed systemic intoxication. Early and aggressive patient decontamination is therefore a high priority, but an agent that has already formed a temporary depot in the stratum corneum may not be removed by all decontaminants, and patients who have been decontaminated and whose skin surfaces demonstrate no residual agent during monitoring may still be at risk for subsequent deterioration. Decontamination proceeds through three ever more aggressive stages of decontamination: Gross, secondary, and definitive decontamination.[14] Gross decontamination involves removing the patient's clothing and performing a 1-minute head-to-toe rinse. Secondary decontamination consists of a full-body wash and rinse. Definitive decontamination is a continuous scrub and rinse until "clean." Irrigation of exposed skin and hair may be performed with saline or soapy water, although in mass casualty situations, water will be the most well-tolerated, abundant, and readily available decontaminating solution. Full-strength sodium hypochlorite (i.e., household bleach) is no longer recommended as a dermal cleansing solution, but is still the solution of choice for decontaminating equipment because it effectively neutralizes organophosphates. Eyes and open wounds should be irrigated with water only. Reactive Skin Decontamination Lotion (RSDL) is a particularly effective decontaminant for organophosphates and is now the standard military chemical-warfare–agent decontaminant. It is also available for civilian use, although it is not yet approved by the U.S. Food and Drug Administration (FDA) for use in the eyes or in wounds. Respiratory exposure prior to decontamination can be minimized either by masking (or intubating) the victim and by removing the victim from the incident site.

The importance of appropriate protective equipment and thorough decontamination should not be underemphasized. There are four levels of PPE in the NIOSH/OSHA/EPA classification system; the highest level, level A, includes full skin protection and full respiratory isolation with self-contained breathing apparatus (SCBA).[14] The lowest level, level D, consists of traditional hospital attire with gloves and eye and face protection, but with vulnerable areas of skin and no respiratory protection. Level A attire is recommended at the release site (the "hot zone"), level C, which includes a full-face or half-mask air-purifying respirator, is needed in the hospital decontamination corridor (the "warm zone"), and level D with standard precautions should suffice once decontaminated patients have crossed a liquid-exposure line ("hot line") to enter the emergency department. However, it should always be kept in mind that apparently decontaminated patients may in fact still be contaminated and that contaminated patients may bypass a decontamination lane to enter the hospital without realizing that they pose a risk to health care providers. Butyl or nitrile rubber gloves, boots, suits, and masks provide protection from nerve-agent absorption; conventional latex and vinyl gloves do not.[16] The U.S. Occupational Safety and Health Administration (OSHA) has published guidelines for choosing appropriate PPE for hospital-based first receivers of chemical casualties.[17]

Several military policies and procedures could have relevance in the civilian world. One is to don PPE immediately after suspecting an exposure.[14] If the probability of attack with the nerve agent GD is high, soldiers may be pretreated with pyridostigmine bromide. Pyridostigmine is a carbamate that when administered before exposure to GD will functionally "protect" some of the AChE by reversibly binding to it. Subsequent spontaneous hydrolysis of the carbamate releases the enzyme for return to normal activity.[18,19] Pyridostigmine is well tolerated with few side effects. It is dispensed in a blister pack containing 30-mg tablets; one tablet is taken every 8 hours for a usual maximum of 14 days. However, pyridostigmine is not useful after exposure, and in an unexpected terrorist release of GD, health care providers will do better to rely upon casualty decontamination and PPE. Provider courses given at the U.S. Army Medical Research Institute of Chemical Defense (USAMRICD) are offered to civilians, as well as to military service members. The courses emphasize attention to the ABCDDs (airway, breathing, circulation, immediate decontamination, and drugs [specific antidotes and antiseizure medications]). The U.S. military issues a combination auto-injector syringe, the Antidote Treatment Nerve Agent Autoinjector (ATNAA). Each autoinjector contains a chamber with 2.1 mg of atropine sulfate and a chamber with 600 mg of 2-pralidoxime chloride. Civilian versions of the ATNAA are available. Benzodiazepine autoinjectors (Convulsant Antidote for Nerve Agent [CANA]) contain diazepam, although midazolam is absorbed more rapidly from intramuscular sites, and a midazolam autoinjector is awaiting FDA approval. In a mass casualty incident, autoinjectors will be the fastest way to administer antidotes in a field setting; however, intravenous administration should be substituted as soon as IV access can be established. Hospital supplies of antidotes must be sufficient for anticipated prehospital and hospital use in the event of a nerve-agent exposure.

▶▶ POST-INCIDENT CONSIDERATIONS

The key action in responding to a nerve-agent attack is to recognize the poisoned patient. Treatment is very time dependent, and delay represents risk for increased morbidity and mortality for both currently exposed individuals and those not yet exposed. Patients can present with signs and symptoms of both nicotinic and muscarinic hyperstimulation. The muscarinic effects are represented with the acronym *DUMBBELLS*: diaphoresis, urinary incontinence, miosis, bronchorrhea, bronchospasm, emesis, lacrimation, loose stools, and salivation.[9,20] Nicotinic effects include weakness, hypertension, hyperglycemia, local or generalized muscle fasciculations, tachycardia, and mydriasis, although with nerve agents, mydriasis is almost inevitably overridden by miosis induced by hyperstimulation of muscarinic receptors. Bradycardia is also a muscarinic effect, but, in humans, it is often overridden by tachycardia from nicotinic stimulation in sympathetic ganglia.

The route of exposure and dose determine the symptom severity and timing. Inhalation immediately leads to bronchorrhea and respiratory difficulty, whereas skin exposure may manifest as local muscle fasciculations and diaphoresis before the onset of systemic symptoms. However, collapse with apnea and convulsions may occur after high doses from either inhalation or percutaneous exposure; the difference is that, for a fatal dose, effects from skin exposure will be delayed for 20 to 30 minutes because of the passage of the agent through the epidermis to the dermal vasculature. The mechanism of death from nerve-agent exposure is primarily respiratory in nature, from progressive bronchorrhea, bronchospasm, direct paralysis of the diaphragm, and especially central apnea. Confusion, seizures, apnea, and coma are ominous CNS symptoms indicative of severe intoxication.[10] Those patients with severe or chronic exposures to organophosphate pesticides may develop a delayed-onset polyneuropathy or chronic organophosphorus-induced delayed neurotoxicity with a stocking and glove distribution. This neuropathy may be permanent but appears to occur seldom if ever with nerve agents.[10,11]

The diagnosis of nerve-agent poisoning is clinical, as laboratory values are of little utility in the immediate management of nerve-agent poisonings. Poison control centers may serve as both a surveillance network to recognize exposures and as a resource for treatment advice. After recognition of the cholinergic toxidrome, postexposure triage can aid in managing mass casualties and in directing initial medical treatment. Exposed victims should be triaged as mild, moderate, or severe, based on their clinical presentation, which will depend in part on the type and route of exposure and the dose of agent (Table 112-1).

Emphasis should be on recognizing the syndrome and broadly grouping casualties to facilitate rapid medical treatment. Initial treatment will be based on triaging casualties into one of these categories.[10,20,21]

MEDICAL MANAGEMENT OF CASUALTIES

After immediate decontamination (the first D of the ABCDDs), medical management of organophosphate exposure is directed at blocking cholinergic-receptor stimulation and reactivating AChE. Management of known quaternary ammonium or carbamate intoxication does not usually require specific medical therapy but rather general supportive measures, although atropine by itself has been used in cases of carbamate poisonings.[22,23] Supportive care should always include the ABCs (airway, breathing, and circulation) and appropriate advanced life-support protocols. Aggressive airway management is often needed. Usually supplemental oxygen and suctioning of airway secretions is sufficient in cases of organophosphate-pesticide poisoning, although high doses of nerve agents will likely require endotracheal intubation and ventilatory support. Bronchospasm may be so severe that efforts to inflate the lungs may be unsuccessful until sufficient atropine is given. Paralytic agents are rarely needed, but if necessary, a short-acting competitive neuromuscular blocker such as vecuronium or rocuronium should be used. Avoid use of succinylcholine, which may have prolonged effects because of concomitant inhibition of serum butyrylcholinesterase (BuChE).[5,9,10]

In cases of ingestion of organophosphate pesticides, early GI decontamination upon arrival at a health care facility will likely be beneficial. When available and indicated, activated charcoal (1 g/kg) should be administered via orogastric and/or nasogastric tube.[24] Oral administration of activated charcoal is not recommended because of the potential for these patients to decompensate, lose their protective airway reflexes, and aspirate the activated charcoal, causing a pneumonitis.

Atropine is a competitive cholinergic blocking agent. When administered, it will aid in alleviating muscarinic symptoms,[9,23] but will not control nicotinic symptoms, such as muscle fasciculations, weakness, or flaccid paralysis. Initial dosing is based on symptoms and triaged categories of victims (Table 112-2). Atropine has a short half-life, and it can be given every 5 to 10 minutes at a dose of 2 mg in adults and 0.05 to 0.1 mg/kg in children. Atropine should be administered until respiratory secretions have dried and airway resistance is minimized.

TABLE 112-1 Nerve-Agent Signs and Symptoms Based on Severity and Route of Exposure*

SYMPTOM SEVERITY AND TRIAGE LEVELS	TYPE OF EXPOSURE	
	LIQUID	VAPOR
Mild	Localized fasciculations and diaphoresis; no miosis	Miosis; dim vision; rhinorrhea
Moderate	Mild symptoms and gastrointestinal symptoms; lacrimation; wheezing; dyspnea; bronchorrhea; and/or bronchoconstriction	Mild symptoms and salivation and cramping; nausea and vomiting; generalized weakness and/or fasciculations
Severe	Mild to moderate symptoms and apnea; convulsions and seizures; confusion, and/or coma; flaccid paralysis	Mild to moderate symptoms and apnea; convulsions and seizures; coma; flaccid paralysis; bowel and bladder incontinence

*Note: The signs and symptoms of severe exposure may occur after progression through mild and moderate effects or may occur suddenly, depending on the dose. Effects from inhalation will be immediate; a latent period of 20 min to 18 h is seen after liquid exposure; the length of this latent period is inversely correlated with dose.

TABLE 112-2 Age-Specific Initial Dosing of Antidotes*

	0-2 YR	2-10 YR	>10 YR, ADULT
Mild to moderate symptoms	Atropine, 0.05 mg/kg every 5 min; pralidoxime, 25 mg/kg	Atropine, 1 mg every 5 min; pralidoxime, 25 mg/kg	Atropine, 2 mg every 5 min; pralidoxime, 25 mg/kg
Severe symptoms	Atropine, 0.1 mg/kg every 5 min; pralidoxime, 25 mg/kg; diazepam, 0.1-0.3 mg/kg	Atropine, 2 mg every 5 min; pralidoxime, 25 mg/kg; diazepam, 0.1-0.3 mg/kg	Atropine, 4 mg every 5 min; pralidoxime, 25 mg/kg; diazepam, 5-10 mg

*Atropine and diazepam may be given intramuscularly (IM) or intravenously (IV). Pralidoxime may be given IM as a single dose or infused IV over 30 min. A second dose of pralidoxime may be given 1 h later if muscle weakness has not improved, then at every 12 h intervals.[9,10]

Organophosphate-pesticide overdose may require as much as 1 to 2 g of atropine, with nerve-agent poisonings expected to require much less, so long as oximes are administered concurrently. Should bolus dosing prove inadequate, continuous atropine infusion can be provided at 0.02 to 0.08 mg/kg/h, titrated to control of hypersecretion.[24] Discontinue atropine 24 hours after control of secretions is achieved. Intravenous beta-blockers or calcium channel blockers may be used for cardioprotection if atropine-induced tachycardia results in cardiac strain, as evidenced by electrocardiogram (ECG) manifestations or positive cardiac biomarkers.

Benzodiazepines are the treatment of choice for organophosphate-induced seizures. Prophylactic administration of benzodiazepines is recommended in all cases of severe organophosphate exposure, to minimize the risk of subsequent seizures. Although benzodiazepines do control convulsions, increased neuronal activity still consumes a significant amount of oxygen, and adequate oxygenation is imperative to preserve CNS function in severely exposed patients. Most experience is with diazepam, but other benzodiazepines, including midazolam, would also be appropriate, and midazolam is preferable to diazepam for intramuscular administration. See Table 112-2 for recommended dosing. Other medical therapies include inhaled nebulized ipratropium bromide, a synthetic analog of atropine. Ipratropium will be helpful in relieving bronchoconstriction and reducing airway secretions. There have been a few case reports of hemodialysis followed by hemoperfusion for direct removal of organophosphate compounds.[9,17]

Fresh frozen plasma (FFP) contains BuChE, also known as pseudocholinesterase, which has chemical affinity for the organophosphate nerve agents. Administration of FFP has decreased mortality for victims of organophosphate poisoning in small preliminary studies.[25] However, this therapy has several significant limitations. First, the quantity of BuChE in FFP is relatively low, and it may result in unfavorable stoichiometry (as a 1:1 ratio of enzyme to agent is required) in doses that do not result in volume overload. Second, BuChE does not cross the blood-brain barrier (BBB), meaning that it may only act on agents that have not yet moved out of the systemic circulation; however, this may be beneficial when there is a large GI or cutaneous exposure. Finally, critically ill patients with organophosphate poisoning often have tenuous respiratory status and may not be able to tolerate a large-volume FFP parenteral infusion.

With organophosphate intoxication, definitive treatment is aimed at reactivating AChE. Reactivation is achieved through the administration of an oxime-containing compound. Oximes reactivate AChE by displacing the phosphorous moiety from the enzyme. However, reactivation is not possible after aging. Although nerve agents begin aging almost immediately, the half-lives of aging are hours to days for most of the agents. The exception is GD, which has an aging half-life of approximately 2 minutes. Thus, the effectiveness of oxime administration in a GD-poisoned patient after five half-lives (about 10 minutes) may be markedly diminished.[20,21] Currently, pralidoxime chloride (2-PAM chloride) is the only oxime approved by the FDA for use in the United States. Again, initial dosing is based on symptom severity. However, because of potential adverse effects (hypertension, laryngeal edema, and muscle spasms) from overdosage, repeat intramuscular administration of oximes after the initial 1800- to 2000-mg dose given to severely intoxicated adults should be delayed for an additional hour. For agents with longer aging times, or delayed absorption secondary to GI exposure, 1 g of pralidoxime may be given every 6 hours.[24] For military exposures, soldiers will have to administer the ATNAA autoinjectors to themselves or to severely exposed colleagues. Those with mild exposures receive one autoinjector; moderate exposures two autoinjectors; and severe exposures (recognized by the presence of significant respiratory distress or of signs or symptoms from systemic distribution)

three autoinjectors, as well as 10 mg of diazepam.[12] Benzodiazepines are synergistic with atropine and pralidoxime, even in the absence of seizure, and they should be given whenever the condition of a casualty requires the addition of three autoinjectors in quick succession. Similar guidelines apply to civilian-use autoinjectors.

A variety of experimental therapies for the prevention and treatment of nerve-agent poisoning are currently being developed. Researchers are testing the Alzheimer's medication galantamine, a competitive AChE antagonist that can cross the BBB, as an alternative to pyridostigmine, which cannot cross the BBB.[3] The expectation is that this approach will be able to protect AChE that is located in the CNS and address the primary neurological manifestations of nerve-agent poisoning. Scopolamine crosses the BBB at much lower doses than atropine does, and it has been shown that even low doses of scopolamine added to the standard antidotal treatment of nerve-agent-exposed animals increases survival and reduces the total dose of atropine needed. A similar antimuscarinic agent, caramiphen, is another promising potential antidote. Another area where a great deal of resources is being invested is in the production of anticholinesterase bioscavengers. The U.S. military has invested a large amount of funding in the manufacture and testing of cholinesterases and the related paraoxonases, with the goal of providing a "molecular sponge" of protection in the circulation that would sequester nerve agents before they can reach the CNS or neuromuscular synapse. Bioscavengers are awaiting FDA approval, a process that will likely take several additional years.

🔍 UNIQUE CONSIDERATIONS

Over the last 40 years, a diverse cadre of individuals, organizations, and foreign governments has demonstrated a willingness to use nerve agents against civilian targets. Unfortunately, in contrast to the well-documented lethality of these agents, there is very little high-quality scientific literature about how to treat patients in a large-scale exposure scenario. Much of the literature involves animal models and case reports or is extrapolated from patients who have ingested large quantities of organophosphates, often intentionally. Many open questions remain, including how coexisting injuries and comorbidities will affect treatment and outcomes of those persons exposed to nerve agents, particularly the synergism that is known to occur between nerve agents and other agents, specifically other chemical, biological, radioactive, and conventional weapons.

Children possess several distinct physiological characteristics that make them particularly susceptible to nerve-agent poisoning. They have lower basal levels of AChE, more permeable skin, and higher minute ventilation compared with adults.[26,27]

With regard to pregnancy, several studies and case reports have shown atropine to be safe during pregnancy. Currently, there is no evidence of atropine having increased teratogenic potential.[28] Atropine is an FDA pregnancy category-C drug.[29] Experience with the oximes is much more limited. Only case reports on the use of pralidoxime during pregnancy exist. Thus far, there have been no reported instances of increased or unexpected teratogenesis related to pralidoxime use. Pralidoxime is also an FDA pregnancy category-C drug.[29] Benzodiazepines have been studied more extensively and have been shown to increase the risk of teratogenesis.[28,29] Consequently, benzodiazepines are FDA pregnancy category-D drugs.[29]

The potential benefits to the patient must always be weighed against the potential risks to the fetus. If a pregnant patient is known to have exposure to a carbamate, atropine may be the only pharmacological therapy needed, and it will be safe. However, in the case of severe organophosphate exposure, none of the previously mentioned therapeutic interventions should be withheld. In mild to moderate organophosphate exposure, benzodiazepines are not indicated, although atropine and pralidoxime should still be used.

! PITFALLS

Several potential pitfalls in response to a nerve-agent attack exist. These include the following:

- Failure to consider nerve agents as a possible etiology for respiratory distress or generalized weakness in the case of exposure to an unknown chemical agent.
- Failure to notify local, state, and federal authorities immediately, including the Federal Bureau of Investigation (FBI) and the Centers for Disease Control and Prevention (CDC), in the event of a suspected nerve-agent attack.
- Failure to wear appropriate protective gear while treating patients with suspected or confirmed nerve-agent poisoning.
- Failure to initiate decontamination immediately—do not delay spot decontamination in favor of later full-body decontamination. Physical or mechanical removal of the agent takes priority over the use of chemical decontaminants such as bleach. If soap is not immediately available, begin irrigation with copious amounts of water.
- Failure to use appropriate clinical ends for atropine administration—administration of atropine should continue until respiratory secretions are clear and airway compromise has resolved. Inappropriate ends for atropine administration include miosis (which may persist for up to 2 months), heart rate, and nicotinic effects, such as twitching or weakness.

REFERENCES

1. Okumura T, Takasu N, Ishimatsu S, et al. Report on 640 victims of the Tokyo subway Sarin attack. *Ann Emerg Med*. 1996;28:129–135.
2. Blanc P. The legacy of war gas. *Am J Med*. 1999;106(6):689–690.
3. Dolgin E. Syrian gas attack reinforces need for better anti-sarin drugs. *Nat Med*. 2013;19(10):1194–1195.
4. Watson WA, Litovitz TL, Rodgers GC Jr, et al. 2002 annual report of the American Association of Poison Control Centers Toxic Exposure Surveillance System. *Am J Emerg Med*. 2003;21:353–421.
5. Miller R. Drugs and the autonomic nervous system. In: *Anesthesia*. 5th ed. Philadelphia, PA: Churchill Livingstone; 2000:550–566.
6. Tafuri J, Roberts J. Organophosphate poisoning. *Ann Emerg Med*. 1987;16:193.
7. Saadeh AM. Metabolic complications of organophosphate and carbamate poisoning. *Trop Doct*. 2001;31:149–152.
8. Mycek M, Harvey RA, Champe PC. Cholinergic agonist and cholinergic antagonist. In: *Pharmacology*. Philadelphia, PA: Lippincott; 2000:40–47. 2nd ed. Lippincott's Illustrated Reviews.
9. Leiken JB, Thomas RG, Walter FG, Klein R, Meislin HW. A review of nerve agent exposure for the critical care physician. *Crit Care Med*. 2002;30:2346–2354.
10. Takala J, de Jong R. Nerve gas terrorism: a grim challenge to anesthesiologists. *Anesth Analg*. 2003;96:819–825.
11. Marrs TC, Maynard RL, Sidell FR. Organophosphate nerve agents. In: *Chemical Warfare Agents: Toxicology and Treatment*. New York, NY: Wiley; 1999:83–100.
12. McKee CB, Collins L. *The Medical NBC Battlebook: USACHPPM Tech Guide 244*. U.S. Army Center for Health and Preventive Medicine (USACHPPM); 2000.
13. U.S. Department of Health & Human Services: Chemical Hazards Emergency Medical Management. http://chemm.nlm.nih.gov. Accessed 24.12.14.
14. Institute of Medicine, National Research Councils. *Chemical and Biological Terrorism: Research and Development to Improve Civilian Medical Response*. Washington, DC: National Academy Press; 1999.
15. Jones J, Terndrup T, Franz D, Eitzen E. Future challenges in preparing for and responding to bioterrorism events. *Emerg Med Clin North Am*. 2002;20:501–524.
16. King JM, Frelin AJ. Impact of the chemical protective ensemble on the performance of basic medical tasks. *Mil Med*. 1984;149:496–501.
17. United States Department of Labor. *OSHA Best Practices for Hospital-Based First Receivers of Victims from Mass Casualty Incidents Involving the Release of Hazardous Substances*. https://www.osha.gov/dts/osta/bestpractices/html/hospital_firstreceivers.html. Accessed 24.12.14.
18. Keller JR, Hurst CG, Dunn MA. Pyridostigmine used as nerve agent pretreatment under wartime conditions. *JAMA*. 1994;266:693–695.
19. Lallement G, Foquin A, Dorandeu F, Baubichon D, Aubriot S, Carpentier P. Subchronic administration of various pretreatments of nerve agent poisoning: I. Protection of blood and central cholinesterase's innocuousness towards blood-brain barrier permeability. *Drug Chem Toxicol*. 2001;24:151–164.
20. Abraham R. Practical guidelines for acute care of victims of bioterrorism: conventional injuries and concomitant nerve agent intoxication. *Anesthesiology*. 2002;97:989–1004.
21. U.S. Army Medical Research Institute of Chemical Defense (USAMRICD). *Medical Management of Chemical Casualties Handbook*. 3rd ed. U.S. Army; 1999.
22. Simpson JR, William M. Recognition and management of acute pesticide poisoning. *Am Fam Physician*. 2002;65:1599–1604.
23. Mokhlesi B, Corbridge T. Toxicology in the critically ill patient. *Clin Chest Med*. 2003;24:689–711.
24. Sungur M, Guven M. Intensive care management of organophosphate insecticide poisoning. *Crit Care*. 2001;5(4):211–215.
25. Guven M, Sungur M, Eser B, Sari I, Altuntaş F. The effects of fresh frozen plasma on cholinesterase levels and outcomes in patients with organophosphate poisoning. *J Toxicol Clin Toxicol*. 2004;42(5):617–623.
26. Henretig F, Cielsak T, et al. Environmental emergencies, bioterrorism and pediatric emergencies. *Clin Pediatr Emerg Med*. 2001;2:211–221.
27. Reigart J, Roberts J. Pesticides in children. *Pediatr Clin North Am*. 2001;48:1185–1198.
28. Bailey B. Are there teratogenic risks associated with antidotes used in the acute management of poisoned pregnant women? *Birth Defects Res A Clin Mol Teratol*. 2003;67:122–140.
29. Hick J. Protective equipment for health care facility decontamination personnel: regulations, risks, and recommendations. *Ann Emerg Med*. 2003;42:370–380.

113 CHAPTER

Vesicant Agent Attack

Charles Stewart, M. Kathleen Stewart, and Lara K. Kulchycki

DESCRIPTION OF EVENT

Vesicants are chemicals that cause skin blisters, or *vesicles*. These chemicals produce severe damage to the eyes, lungs, and skin through direct contact or inhalation of vapor.[1] Vesicant agents include sulfur mustard, nitrogen mustard, arsenical agents (e.g., Lewisite [L]), and halogenated oximes (e.g., phosgene oxime [CX]). The properties and effects of the halogenated oximes are very different from those of the mustard agents.

The mustard agents are a family of sulfur-, nitrogen-, and oxygen-based compounds with similar chemical and biological effects. The prototypical vesicant is mustard agent, of which two types exist: the nitrogen mustards (HN-1, HN-2, and HN-3), which are known for their medicinal uses as chemotherapy drugs, and the sulfur mustards (H, HD, and HT), which are known only for their combat applications. The most dangerous chemical warfare agent of World War I (WWI) was sulfur mustard. Multiple nations maintain stores of these and similar agents because they are simple to manufacture and deploy and can affect large numbers of people with a single deployment. Nitrogen mustard has not been used in chemical warfare, so there is not a large body of literature on the effects of this group of agents from intentional exposure. Because only the sulfur mustard compounds have been used as warfare agents, discussion of *mustard* in this chapter refers to the sulfur compounds. However, there is no reason to believe that a terrorist would not find nitrogen mustard just as attractive as sulfur mustard because they share many properties and there is not as much experience with the management of casualties caused by nitrogen mustard. Other variants of these agents are tabulated elsewhere.[2]

Mustard agent is a yellowish-brown, oily liquid with an odor comparable to that of mustard, garlic, or onion. The English called the chemical mustard after the smell and the yellow-brown color. A more recent casualty described the odor as that of asphalt.[3] It boils at 217 °C (423 °F) and thus is not mustard "gas," but it freezes at 14 °C (58 °F); mustard-Lewisite mixtures remain liquid at lower temperatures. Mustard vaporizes slowly in temperate climates and may be aerosolized by spraying or explosive blasts. The vapor is heavier than air and settles slowly into trenches and other low-lying areas. Because of this low volatility, mustard is considered a persistent agent and may linger for a week or more after dispersal. Mustard agents can be delivered by bomb, artillery shells, mortar rounds, or by release from canisters. It is possible to disseminate mustards that have been adsorbed to small particles ("dusty" mustard). Mustard vapor injury and dispersal is markedly enhanced by high humidity and a hot environment.

Sulfur and nitrogen mustard compounds are bifunctional alkylating agents that bind to DNA. Three different levels of biological activity have been noted following exposure to mustard agents: cytostatic, cytotoxic, and mutagenic effects. Actively proliferating cells are affected most by mustard interactions with DNA, leading many authors to designate these effects as radiomimetic. Basal epidermal cells, hematopoietic cells, and the mucosal lining of the intestine are particularly vulnerable. Mustard causes ocular, respiratory, and dermatological effects in this manner.

Mustard was widely used in WWI by many countries on both sides of the conflict and was outlawed by the Geneva Gas Protocols of 1925.[4] The United States was not a signatory to that agreement. Rumors of possible use of mustard by the German and Italian armies in World War II (WWII) led to the secret production of mustard bombs by the United States to be used only if the Axis forces used them first. Ironically the greatest number of casualties due to chemical agents in WWII occurred when the Nazis bombed the S.S. *John Harvey*, a U.S. Liberty ship loaded with a secret cargo of more than 100 tons of mustard bombs, in the Italian port of Bari in 1943.[5] Over 600 Allied soldiers and sailors and an unknown number of civilians became casualties from mustard released during this attack.[6]

Iraqi forces used sulfur mustard and nerve agents against Iranian forces beginning in 1984 and continuing through the Iran–Iraq War, also known as the First Persian Gulf War.[7,8] Most Iranian chemical casualties were caused by mustard.[9] One source estimates that there were 45,000 casualties from mustard.[10] Some Iranian casualties were cared for in western European medical centers, resulting in many clinical reports. A novel feature of Iraq's use of mustard against Iran was the use of dusty mustard. This was mustard adsorbed onto fine (0.1 to 10 µm) silica particles in a mixture of 65% mustard and 35% silica. This combination produced more serious respiratory injuries than other forms of mustard and a different form of skin injury, with symptoms beginning in 15 minutes to 1 hour (as opposed to 4 to 8 hours).

After WWII large quantities of mustard agents were disposed of by dumping the munitions into the Atlantic Ocean and the Baltic Sea by Allied Forces. Corrosion has weakened the containers, and the resultant leaks have continued to cause numerous casualties among fishermen.[11]

There is a characteristic latent period that lasts from 4 to 12 hours after exposure to mustard before the onset of symptoms. The length of the latent period is inversely correlated to the dose of agent absorbed.[12] Higher concentrations and longer duration exposures cause symptoms that develop more rapidly. The toxic effect of inhaled mustard vapor depends both on the concentration of the mustard in the air inhaled (C) and also on the duration of exposure (t). Early recognition of vesicant agent exposure becomes difficult because the initial effects may be limited to irritation of the mucous membranes similar to the irritation caused by tear gases.[12]

Eye

The eye is the most commonly damaged organ in a mustard attack.[8,13] Eye effects range from tearing and conjunctival irritation to ocular pain, photophobia, corneal ulceration, and blindness. The first complaint of

TABLE 113-1	Incidence Data on Mustard Gas Exposure	
OCULAR FINDING	RECOVERY	INCIDENCE*
Mild conjunctivitis	1-2 weeks	75% of cases
Severe conjunctivitis	2-5 weeks	15% of cases
Mild corneal involvement	2-3 months	10% of cases
Severe corneal involvement	Several months Relapse common	0.1% of cases
Temporary blindness may occur, but permanent blindness is rare.		

From Requena L, Requena C, Sanchez M, et al. Chemical warfare. Cutaneous lesions from mustard gas. *Journal of the American Academy of Dermatology.* Sep 1988;19(3):529-536.
*Data from World War I military statistics.

Iranian troops exposed to mustard gas was usually ocular: photophobia, foreign body sensation, and conjunctivitis (Table 113-1).[9,14]

Respiratory

Mustard respiratory signs and symptoms include rhinorrhea, dysphonia, productive cough, hemoptysis, and dyspnea. The respiratory injuries that develop after the inhalation of mustard vapor (and presumably dusty mustard) primarily affect the laryngeal and tracheobronchial mucosa. After a delay of several hours the victims suffer tracheobronchitis with chest pressure, hacking cough, sore throat, and hoarseness. The severe cough responds poorly to bronchodilators, cough suppressants, or even corticosteroids. There is little effect at low to moderate doses on the lung parenchyma, although large doses may lead to pulmonary edema and to clinical acute lung injury (ALI).

Dermal

The medical provider should clearly understand that the hallmark of mustard exposure is a latent period with development of symptoms hours after the exposure. The duration of the latent period and the severity of the resultant lesions are dependent on the mode of exposure, concentration of the agent, environmental temperature, and to some extent the individual. High temperature and wet skin are associated with more severe lesions and shorter latent periods.

Mustard skin burns are more likely to appear on warm, moist areas of the body, such as the neck, axillae, hand and foot web spaces, and groin. Patients first notice skin erythema, burning pain, and intense pruritus (2 to 48 hours after exposure), followed several hours later by vesiculation. The face, scrotum, and perianal areas are frequently involved, but the thicker skin on the hands may be spared. Nearly half of U.S. survivors of WWI mustard attacks had scrotal and perianal injuries.[9] Full-thickness skin loss is particularly likely to occur on the penis and scrotum. There are no available data about vulvar and perianal involvement in females, but these injuries would be expected to parallel those of males. A "string of pearls" pattern of vesicles surrounding a seemingly normal patch of skin (in actuality so damaged that blisters cannot form) is often seen. Extensive, slowly healing skin lesions place a heavy burden on medical services. The damaged tissues may slough and are extremely susceptible to infection. Regeneration of these tissues is very slow, and healing may take weeks to months—much longer than healing times for comparable thermal or caustic skin burns. Interestingly fluid loss from mustard burns is less than that from thermal burns of the same size.

Bone Marrow Suppression

Because mustards are alkylating agents that interfere with nucleic acid synthesis, high-dose exposures can produce bone marrow suppression, followed by leukopenia 3 to 5 days after exposure. The leukopenia may develop precipitously. This clearly increases the risk for sepsis in the patient with high exposure and widespread skin lesions.

Systemic Effects

Other systemic mustard effects may include nausea, vomiting, tremor, ataxia, and convulsions. Absorption of high doses may result in central nervous system (CNS) excitation leading to convulsions, followed by CNS depression. Cardiac irregularities may also occur.

Death occurs in 1% to 3% of mustard gas victims and usually occurs days after exposure. The lethal dose for 50% (LD$_{50}$) of victims of sulfur mustard is approximately 7 g (about a teaspoon) for a 70-kg adult. The cause of death may be burns, respiratory tract damage, bone marrow suppression, infection, or a combination of these. This statistic underscores that vesicants are maiming agents, intended primarily to disable rather than kill and to generate large numbers of casualties requiring extended medical care.

From a military standpoint (and to a lesser extent applicable to both firefighters and emergency medical services [EMS]), vesicant agents degrade combat effectiveness both by causing direct casualties and also by forcing troops to wear a full protective ensemble. The protective ensemble limits vision and limits exertional and load-bearing capacities. In hot environments the protective ensemble can cause additional casualties because of heat stress and dehydration.

Lewisite was discovered near the end of WWI by a team of Americans headed by Capt. W. Lee Lewis but did not have the chance to be used in WWI before the cessation of hostilities. It is an arsenical vesicant that is a colorless, oily liquid when pure; when impure, it is amber and smells like geraniums. It is less volatile and more persistent than mustard and thus more tactically useful in cold climates; for this reason it was often combined with mustard (HL). However, Lewisite degrades rapidly in wet environments. The HL combination was extensively stocked by former Warsaw Pact countries and causes both rapid and delayed casualties. Significant skin exposure to Lewisite can induce vomiting, making the use of protective masks less reliable. Lewisite can rapidly penetrate the skin and then, like mustard, spread throughout the whole body. After absorption it can act as an arsenical systemic poison. Like mustard, the complete mechanism of action on the body's cells is incompletely known.

Lewisite causes symptoms very similar to those of mustard but is distinguished from mustard by its rapid onset of discomfort—within seconds to a minute or two. The pain on contact has been reported to decrease in severity after blisters form.[15]

Lewisite causes damage to skin, eyes, mucous membranes, and airways with direct contact toxicity. Respiratory injuries may be less likely than with mustard because of the intense immediate irritation caused by Lewisite but when they occur are more likely to progress to acute lung injury with concomitant hypotension ("Lewisite shock"). Mild conjunctivitis due to arsenical vesicants heals in a few days without specific treatment. Lewisite and other arsenicals produce a rapid grayish scarring of the cornea like an acid burn at the point of contact. Severe exposure may cause permanent injury or blindness.

Erythema is like that caused by mustard but is accompanied with more pain. The "string of pearls" distribution of some mustard burns is seldom seen with Lewisite. There is deeper injury to connective tissue and muscle, greater vascular damage, and more severe inflammatory reaction than with mustard. Large deep burns may have considerable necrosis of tissue, gangrene, and sloughing.

As previously mentioned, Lewisite can cause Lewisite shock, probably from arsenic-related increases in capillary permeability and subsequent extensive interstitial fluid losses. Large exposures are notable for causing renal failure, hemolysis with hemolytic anemia, and hepatic necrosis. Lewisite does not suppress bone marrow or immune function, but burns large enough to cause systemic poisoning should be presumed to be life-threatening and to confer a guarded prognosis.

Phosgene oxime is not a true vesicant because it does not cause the blistering seen with mustard and Lewisite. It is more precisely classified as an *urticariant,* or nettle agent, and causes wheals and blanching comparable to nettle stings. It is not to be confused with phosgene (CG), a pulmonary irritant that smells like hay. Phosgene oxime is a colorless solid or yellowish-brown liquid with immediate corrosive effects. Patients experience instantaneous skin blanching and burning, eye pain, and respiratory distress. Phosgene oxime is notable for causing pulmonary edema and pulmonary-vessel thromboses.[16] The German scientists who first developed phosgene oxime as a chemical-warfare agent in the 1920s felt that its respiratory toxicity was more dangerous than its skin effects.[17]

There are no documented battlefield uses of this chemical, and consequently few data exist on the clinical course and optimal treatment regimens. It can be mixed with other agents, such as nerve agents, so that the skin damage caused by phosgene oxime will more readily allow the other agents to penetrate the skin. Phosgene oxime penetrates rubber and garments more quickly than many other agents do.

⏪ PRE-INCIDENT ACTIONS

Every community and each hospital should have a documented disaster plan for mass casualty incidents and release of toxic chemicals. Emergency personnel should be provided with and trained in the use of personal protective equipment and the implementation of the disaster response protocol.

⏩ POST-INCIDENT ACTIONS

Protection

Medical personnel coordinating a disaster response must notify appropriate local and regional health care providers and law enforcement and public health officials. If possible a hotline should be established to disseminate information to the public.

First responders at the scene of a suspected chemical attack will need to create rapid scene control to prevent the spread of contamination and minimize the number of injuries. Any rescuer working in the hot zone will require personal protective equipment to protect against skin exposure as well as a pressure-demand, self-contained breathing apparatus (SCBA) to guard against exposure to liquid and vaporized agents.

Decontamination

Vesicant absorption is both rapid and irreversible. Decontamination occurring within 1 to 2 minutes after exposure is the only known effective means of preventing or decreasing tissue damage from mustard. Decontamination of mustard agents is difficult because mustard is not very water soluble. This means that water alone, and even water with soap, may spread mustard to other parts of the body or other bodies. Decontamination occurring after the first few minutes of exposure may be too late to prevent the eventual development of skin lesions but may prevent systemic absorption of a lethal dose from liquid still in contact with the skin. Late decontamination can also prevent the incapacitation of EMS or fire responders and medical providers by liquid agent or off-gassing vapor from chemical attack victims and may minimize continued absorption of mustard still present on casualties.

Chemical casualties should be removed from the scene and brought to the designated decontamination zone. All contaminated clothing must be removed and double-bagged to prevent off-gassing of mustard vapor.

Mucous membranes

Patients' eyes should be flushed with water for 5 to 10 minutes. No ocular patches or occlusive dressings should be applied. If available, isotonic sodium bicarbonate (1.26%) or normal saline may be used for eye irrigation. The substances used for skin decontamination are usually too irritating for use on mucous membranes and in the eyes.

Skin

The skin should be washed with either soap and water or dilute 0.5% sodium hypochlorite solution (bleach). Water alone, or even soap and water, may not be effective, as noted above. Absorbent materials, such as flour or fuller's earth, can be applied to soak up liquid agent on the skin; these substances should then be washed off after several seconds of contact.[18] Prompt decontamination with Reactive Skin Decontaminant Lotion (RSDL) is very effective for skin decontamination of sulfur mustard; if RSDL is not available, household bleach (Chlorox is 5.25% sodium hypoclorite) is also effective.[19-21] After decontamination, patients can be transferred to the designated medical treatment facility, where they can be retriaged. Contaminated equipment can also be cleaned with dilute sodium hypochlorite.

➕ MEDICAL TREATMENT OF CASUALTIES

Initial medical treatment and stabilization may need to occur in the hot zone, especially for patients with other significant injuries, large chemical exposures, or preexisting airway disease. As always, rapid assessment of the ABCs (airway, breathing, and circulation) is crucial. For sulfur mustard, addition of a D for immediate decontamination is just as crucial.

Constructing a time line of symptom onset can be crucial in determining the agent used in a chemical attack.[22] Immediate onset of lacrimation, blepharospasm, and burning skin pain argues for exposure to Lewisite or phosgene oxime. A latent period of 2 to 12 hours is more consistent with the use of mustard. Despite active investigation, there are currently no sensitive, specific, and readily available laboratory tests to confirm exposure to a particular vesicant,[23] although urinary analysis for thiodiglycol (a metabolite of sulfur mustard) and DNA adducts to mustard is available at military reference-laboratory facilities. Providers must keep in mind that the deployed weapon may have contained multiple chemicals, including nerve agents, each of which may require a different treatment algorithm.

Specific medical management guidelines for exposure to vesicant agents have been compiled by the Agency for Toxic Substances and Disease Registry (ATSDR), a division of the U.S. Department of Health and Human Services designated to assist with emergency medical responses to release of toxic substances. Links to these clinical guidelines can be found on the website for the Centers for Disease Control and Prevention (CDC).[16,24,25]

Eye

Eye injuries require ophthalmic antibiotic ointments to prevent lid adhesion and infection. Corticosteroid ointments are sometimes recommended to decrease inflammation, but these should be administered only after consultation with an ophthalmologist. Short-term visual incapacitation is common after vesicant eye injury, but most patients recover full function.[13] Therefore reassurance for all but the most severely injured is both appropriate and humane.

Use of local analgesics may increase corneal damage and is not recommended. Systemic analgesics should be used as required for pain control. Secondary infection is a serious complication and increases the amount of corneal scarring. Atropine or similar mydriatic agent may be useful in corneal erosions, iritis, cyclitis, or marked photophobia. Occlusive dressings or pressure on the globe should be avoided.

If the agent is known or strongly suspected to be Lewisite, dimercaprol eye ointment may be useful if applied within 2 minutes of exposure. Its value is questionable if applied later.

Respiratory

Respiratory injuries are treated with supportive measures including oxygen, bronchodilators, and ventilatory support, as needed. Pulse oximetry and chest radiographs can aid in clinical assessment. Patients with preexisting reactive airway disease may have more severe reactions to inhalation injury and require careful monitoring. Antibiotics are best withheld until sputum cultures or other clinical evidence confirms infection with a specific organism. Productive cough is a common symptom of chemical bronchitis and by itself does not warrant the use of antibiotics. In severe respiratory injury the airway can become plugged with necrotic debris and urgent bronchoscopy with deep suctioning may be needed.

Skin

Treatment of chemical burns is similar to that required for thermal injuries, including wound care, debridement, topical antibiotics, intravenous fluid replacement, and systemic analgesics. Vesicant skin burns are usually only partial thickness but take nearly twice the time to heal as comparable thermal injuries.[26,27] Maintenance of strict wound hygiene and avoidance of secondary infection is crucial in patients incurring injury from mustard because leukopenia is a delayed effect of exposure to higher doses. The use of systemic antibiotics should be avoided unless there is specific evidence of infection. Involvement of burn specialists would be appropriate for ongoing management of such patients.

Calamine lotion, corticosteroids in solution, or even water can decrease the pain of the skin lesions. Lesions around the genitalia may be quite painful and may macerate and weep. Treatment with exposure to air is desirable and care must be taken to decrease contamination of the area and subsequent secondary infection of these tissues. Analgesics should be given as required. In reviews of the casualties of the Iraq-Iran war, final outcome appeared to be more dependent on the severity of the initial lesions rather than the treatments used.

Data from the Iraq-Iran war suggest that fluid losses occurring in conjunction with vesicant burns are less extreme than those encountered in the case of thermal burns of equivalent body surface area. These data do not include use of mustard/Lewisite combination vesicants. Care providers must be cautious because overzealous fluid replacement can lead to pulmonary edema, further compromising respiratory function in patients with vesicant airway injury.[1,28]

In case of vesicant ingestion, care providers should neither induce emesis nor attempt decontamination with activated charcoal. Symptoms of nausea and vomiting can be treated with standard antiemetic agents.

A set of routine laboratory tests, including a complete blood count (CBC), serum electrolytes, and kidney and liver function tests, is warranted for patients who will be admitted. The CBC is a baseline by which to measure the subsequent leukopenia of patients with mustard injury or the hemolytic anemia of Lewisite-exposed patients. Kidney and liver function tests are particularly important in Lewisite exposure because it is known to cause multiorgan failure.

Of the vesicants, only Lewisite has a specific antidote. The chelating agent British antilewisite (BAL), also known as dimercaprol, enhances urinary excretion of arsenic and improves clinical outcome in exposed patients.[29] BAL chelates unbound Lewisite and reactivates metabolically critical enzymes that have been inactivated by Lewisite

BOX 113-1 Indications for Systemic Treatment in Lewisite Exposure

- Cough with dyspnea and frothy sputum (pulmonary edema)
- Skin burn >1% (palm-sized burn or larger caused by liquid) not decontaminated within 15 minutes (Lewisite is rapidly absorbed)
- Skin contamination of 5% or more total body surface area with immediate skin damage (dead or gray-white blanching of skin) or with erythema occurring within 30 minutes (Lewisite is rapidly absorbed)

(Box 113-1). Similar compounds have been developed but have not been made available for civilian use. The Lewisite protocol suggests a dose of 2.5 to 5 mg/kg delivered intramuscularly (IM) every 4 hours for four doses. Dose frequency can be increased to every 2 hours in cases of severe poisoning. The drug is dissolved in peanut oil and is thus contraindicated in patients with peanut allergy. Water-soluble BAL analogs exist but are still experimental; they are unlikely to be readily available in the instance of a chemical disaster.[30] Side effects of IM administration are both common and dose-related, leading many experts to recommend that BAL be given only to patients with shock or significant pulmonary injury. Side effects include injection site reactions, hypertension, tachycardia, headache, nausea, vomiting, perioral and extremity paresthesias, anxiety, chest pain, and fever.[31] BAL should be used with great caution in patients with renal failure or insufficiency.

Patients with mild symptoms should be observed for 24 hours. If symptoms have not progressed, the patients can be discharged with instructions to return if new manifestations appear. Burns severe enough to cause shock and systemic poisoning are life-threatening. Even if the patient survives the acute effects, the prognosis may be guarded for several weeks.

UNIQUE CONSIDERATIONS

Patients may not show any initial signs of chemical injury. A variable delay in symptom onset can occur with different agents, variations in the amount and route of exposure, and various weather conditions. This latent period can cloud initial clinical evaluation and delay the onset of decontamination procedures. Even if first responders are vigilant and well trained, contaminated patients or equipment may gain entrance to hospitals and cause additional casualties. For sulfur mustard, knowledge of the latent period is useful in estimating absorbed dose because the length of the latent period is inversely correlated with dose. For example, the appearance of respiratory signs and symptoms within 4 hours of inhalational exposure portends a poor outcome.

Proper management of a vesicant attack will require significant medical and financial resources, including facilities equipped for the prolonged hospitalization of casualties and consultation services with specialists in toxicology, burn surgery, ophthalmology, and pulmonary medicine. In addition the psychological burdens to patients, families, and caregivers cannot be ignored. Crisis counseling for victims and debriefing for staff are key components of the disaster response. Chronic medical sequelae, although beyond the scope of this chapter, will add to the toll of a chemical attack.

PITFALLS

Several potential pitfalls in response to a vesicant agent attack exist. These include the following:
- Failure to suspect chemical injury and initiate prompt decontamination because casualties do not yet exhibit the symptoms of vesicant injury. Symptoms should NOT guide decontamination

efforts. Mustard on the skin causes no immediate symptoms, and symptoms may not be present for several hours after exposure. EVERY patient (including EMS, fire, and law enforcement responders) should be checked for mustard and decontaminated if it is found or if detectors are not available.

- Failure to consider that protection of the medical staff is a prime priority[32]
- Failure to consider that mustard is relatively water insoluble. Other decontamination solutions than water have been recommended. Remember that mustard is relatively water insoluble so decontamination must be prolonged.[33] Prolonged washing with water was effective in an Iranian study but in other studies tends to smear the agent. RSDL is the best decontaminant for mustard exposure to the skin, but 0.5% hypochlorite solutions are also effective.[19–21]
- Failure to notify appropriate public health, local government, and law enforcement officials as soon as a chemical attack is suspected
- Failure to treat urgent injuries and respiratory compromise during decontamination
- Failure to maintain a strict hot zone
- Failure to recognize and treat concomitant exposures to other chemical weapons, such as nerve agents. Remember that the terrorist is not constrained to only ONE type of chemical weapon.
- Failure to appreciate the severity of vesicant burns on initial presentation. Rapid onset of dermal symptoms implies a very large exposure to the agent.
- Failure to prevent overhydration in patients with chemical burns
- Failure to involve the appropriate specialty consultants, including toxicologists, burn surgeons, ophthalmologists, and pulmonologists
- Failure to provide counseling and emotional support to victims and medical personnel in the event of a chemical attack[34]

REFERENCES

1. Zajtchuk R, Bellamy RF. *Textbook of Military Medicine.* Washington, DC: Office of the Surgeon General; 1997.
2. Noort D, Benschop HP, Black RM. Biomonitoring of exposure to chemical warfare agents: a review. *Toxicol Appl Pharmacol.* 2002;184:116–126.
3. Le H, Knudsen SJ. Exposure to a First World War blistering agent. *Emerg Med J.* 2006;23(4):296–299.
4. Smith KJ, Skelton H. Chemical warfare agents: their past and continuing threat and evolving therapies. Part II of II. *Skinmed.* 2003;2(5):297–303.
5. Alexander SF. Medical report of the Bari Harbor mustard casualties. *Mil Surg.* 1947;101:1–17.
6. Centers for Disease Control. *Sulfur Mustard Medical Management Guidelines.* Atlanta, GA: CDC.
7. *Report of the Specialists Appointed by the Secretary General to Investigate Allegations by the Islamic Republic of Iran Concerning the Use of Chemical Weapons.* New York: Security Council of the United Nations; Document S/16433 1986.
8. Eisenmenger W, Drasch G, von Clarmann M, Kretschmer E, Roider G. Clinical and morphological findings on mustard gas [bis(2-chloroethyl) sulfide] poisoning. *J Forensic Sci.* 1991;36(6):1688–1698.
9. Requena L, Requena C, Sanchez M, et al. Chemical warfare. Cutaneous lesions from mustard gas. *J Am Acad Dermatol.* 1988;19(3):529–536.
10. Carus WS. *Chemical Weapons in the Middle East.* Washington, DC: The Washington Institute for Near East Policy; 1988 Research Memorandum 9.
11. Centers for Disease Control and Prevention. Notes from the field: exposures to discarded sulfur mustard munitions—mid-Atlantic and New England states 2004–2012. *MMWR Morb Mortal Wkly Rep.* 2013;62(16):315–316.
12. Shakarjian MP, Heck DE, Gray JP, et al. Mechanisms mediating the vesicant actions of sulfur mustard after cutaneous exposure. *Toxicol Sci.* Mar 2010;114(1):5–19.
13. Momeni A-Z, Enshaeih S, Meghdadi M, et al. Skin manifestation of mustard gas: a clinical study of 535 patients exposed to mustard gas. *Arch Dermatol.* 1992;128:775–781.
14. Pierard GE, Dowlati A, Dowlati Y, Pierard-Franchimont C, Hermanns-Le T, Letot B. Chemical warfare casualties and yperite-induced xerodermoid. *Am J Dermatopathol.* 1990;12(6):565–570.
15. Hurst CG, Smith WJ. Health effects of exposure to vesicant agents. In: Romano J. Jr., Lukey BJ, Salem H, eds. *Chemical Warfare Agents: Chemistry, Pharmacology, Toxicology, and Therapeutics.* 2nd ed. New York, NY: CRC Press; 2008:307.
16. Centers for Disease Control and Prevention—Agency for Toxic Substances and Disease Registry. *Phosgene Oxime Medical Management Guidelines.* Atlanta, GA: CDC.
17. Stewart CE. Chemical and biological warfare: improvisational agents. *Emerg Med Serv.* 2002;31(5):88–90.
18. Taysse L, Dorandeu F, Daulon S, et al. Cutaneous challenge with chemical warfare agents in the SKH-1 hairless mouse (II): effects of some currently used skin decontaminants (RSDL and Fuller's earth) against liquid sulphur mustard and VX exposure. *Hum Exp Toxicol.* 2011; 30(6):491–498.
19. Braue EH, Smith KH, Doxzon BF, Lumpkin HL, Clarkson ED. Efficacy studies of Reactive Skin Decontamination Lotion, M291 Skin Decontamination Kit, 0.5% bleach, 1% soapy water, and Skin Exposure Reduction Paste Against Chemical Warfare Agents, Part 1: guinea pigs challenged with VX. *Cutan Ocul Toxicol.* 2011;30(1):15–28.
20. Braue EH, Smith KH, Doxzon BF, Lumpkin HL, Clarkson ED. Efficacy studies of Reactive Skin Decontamination Lotion, M291 Skin Decontamination Kit, 0.5% bleach, 1% soapy water, and Skin Exposure Reduction Paste Against Chemical Warfare Agents, Part 2: guinea pigs challenged with soman. *Cutan Ocul Toxicol.* 2011; 30(1):29–37.
21. Misik J, Jost P, Pavlikova R, Vodakova E, Cabal J, Kuca K. A comparison of decontamination effects of commercially available detergents in rats pre-exposed to topical sulphur mustard. *Cutan Ocul Toxicol.* 2013; 32(2):135–139.
22. Sabelnikov A, Zhukov V, Kempf CR. Airborne exposure limits for chemical and biological warfare agents: is everything set and clear? *Int J Environ Health Res.* 2006;16(4):241–253.
23. Centers for Disease Control. *Lewisite Medical Management Guidelines.* Atlanta, GA: CDC.
24. Mellor S, Rice P, Cooper G. Vesicant burns. *Br J Plast Surg.* 1991;44:434–437.
25. Safarinejad M, Moosavi S, Montazeri B. Ocular injuries caused by mustard gas: diagnosis, treatment, and medical defense. *Mil Med.* 2001;166:67–70.
26. Vilensky J, Redman K. British anti-Lewisite (dimercaprol): an amazing history. *Ann Emerg Med.* 2003;41:378–383.
27. Willems J. Clinical management of mustard gas casualties. *Ann Med Militaris (Belgicae).* 1989;(3 suppl):1–60.
28. Munro N, Watson A, Ambrose KR, et al. Treating exposure to chemical warfare agents: implications for health care providers and community emergency planning. *Environ Health Perspect.* 1990;89:205–215.
29. *Goldfrank's Toxicologic Emergencies.* Stamford, CT: Appleton & Lange.
30. Reminick G. *Nightmare in Bari: The World War II Liberty Ship Poison Gas Disaster and Cover-up.* Palo Alto, CA: Glencannon Press; 2001.
31. Ellison D. *Handbook of Chemical and Biological Warfare Agents.* Boca Raton, FL: CRC Press; 2000.
32. Huelly F, Gruninger M. Collective intoxication caused by the explosion of a mustard gas shell. (Translation US Army). *Ann Med Leg Criminol Police Sci Toxicol.* 1956;36:195–204.
33. Yang Y, Baker JA, Ward JR. Decontamination of chemical warfare agents. *Chem Rev.* 1992;92:1729–1743.
34. Romano J. Jr., King J. *Psychological Factors in Chemical Warfare and Terrorism [Chapter 13].* Boca Raton, FL: CRC Press; 2001.

CHAPTER 114

Respiratory-Agent Mass Casualty Incident (Toxic Inhalational Injury)

Adam J. Janicki and Jason B. Hack

DESCRIPTION OF EVENT

Toxic inhalants are agents that are gases under environmental conditions and that specifically target the lungs. These agents cause dose-related syndromes, ranging from upper-respiratory symptoms of mild cough to acute lung injury (ALI) and acute respiratory distress syndrome (ARDS).[1] This chapter discusses the major pulmonary toxic agents: phosgene (military chemical weapon designation, CG), diphosgene (DP), and chlorine (no military chemical weapon designation).

Phosgene, also known as carbonyl chloride ($COCl_2$), is formed by combining carbon monoxide with chlorine gas, utilizing a carbon catalyst or via the decomposition of DP upon heating. DP ($ClCO_2CCl_3$) is closely related to phosgene; it causes similar symptoms via a similar mechanism but is more easily handled because it is a liquid at normal conditions. Symptoms of exposure include upper-airway symptoms such as cough and bronchoconstriction and lower-airway (respiratory bronchioles, alveolar ducts, alveolar sacs, and alveoli) symptoms such as respiratory failure. Both phosgene and DP are low–water-solubility inhalants that are capable of diffusing deeply into the lungs before reacting; therefore (1) there are often few upper-respiratory symptoms and (2) there may be a significant time delay between exposure and the onset of symptoms. Because phosgene has only subtle irritating warning signs, victims are often left unaware of their exposure.

The mechanism of toxicity of phosgene is incompletely understood; it is postulated to cause injury by two different mechanisms, hydrolysis and acylation.[2] When phosgene contacts water in the respiratory tract, it hydrolyses into hydrochloric acid and carbon monoxide. Hydrochloric acid causes epithelial damage and necrosis in bronchi, small bronchioles, and capillaries, leading to increased permeability of the alveolar and capillary basement membranes with resultant pulmonary edema.[3] The second mechanism occurs through acylation. Phosgene reacts with hydroxyl, thiol, amine, and sulfhydryl groups on proteins, carbohydrates, and lipids, causing significant oxidative damage and quickly depleting glutathione stores to worsen free-radical damage. This initiates a cascade of inflammatory cytokines and other mediators, leading to an increase in vascular permeability, alveolar leakage, and development of pulmonary edema.[2,4] In pulmonary edema, fluid leaks from pulmonary capillaries first into the alveolar-capillary septa and then into the alveoli. From the alveoli, fluid can fill the small and even the large airways. Clinically, this is ALI, which can lead to the ARDS. After a latent period usually of several hours, the first clinical indication of ALI is chest tightness or shortness of breath, typically in the absence of coughing or rhonchi (wheezing).

Chlorine gas is an intermediate-solubility pulmonary irritant. Because it has a slightly higher solubility than phosgene, it often causes upper-airway symptoms including lacrimation, cough, and bronchoconstriction, especially in patients with reactive airway disease or other underlying lung pathology. Further, additional exposure can lead to lower-airway complications of ALI.[1] Chlorine gas, the first chemical respiratory attack agent used in World War I, killed and incapacitated large numbers of soldiers on both sides of the conflict. Although sulfur mustard was used more extensively later in the war and caused more casualties, the case-fatality rate of the pulmonary agents was greater than that from mustard.

Chlorine gas is formed in industry by the electrolysis of sodium chloride dissolved in water; however, this reaction requires membrane cells or diaphragm cells that are not widely available.[5] Chlorine gas can also be generated from household cleaners via the reaction of sodium hypochlorite (bleach) with hydrochloric acid (found in many household products); a similar reaction between bleach and bases creates chloramines, which have similar clinical effects to chlorine. Chlorine gas reacts with upper-airway and alveolar water, generating hydrochloric acid, hypochlorous acid, and oxygen free radicals. The acidic compounds damage the respiratory epithelium of the large airways, leading to sloughing of epithelium, partial airway obstruction, and the clinical signs of coughing, hoarseness, inspiratory stridor, wheezing, and sometimes irritative laryngospasm. The free radicals initiate the release of proinflammatory cytokines and other molecules, causing an increase in alveolar permeability and subsequent pulmonary edema of the lower airways.[6] World War I soldiers exposed to chlorine gas exhibited an almost equal distribution of large-airway and small-airway damage.

Phosgene and chlorine have multiple industrial uses. Since its establishment in 1997, the Organisation for the Prohibition of Chemical Weapons (OPCW) has considered phosgene a Schedule 3 product. Thus, production of more than 30 metric tons per year must be declared to the OPCW, facilities can be inspected, and product export is restricted.[7] Chlorine has no such designation or restriction. Because chlorine gas is easily produced via the mixture of common household products, it has the potential to be an inexpensive chemical weapon for causing casualties and inflicting terror, as demonstrated by its use in World War I, the Iraq War, and the Syrian Civil War.[8-10] These gases could easily be diverted for a large-scale terrorist attack.[11]

A respiratory-agent attack could occur in almost any setting. Closed-ventilation areas, such as public and government buildings, theaters, and shopping malls, are particularly vulnerable. These gases can also be deployed in open areas, as demonstrated during World War I. Because these gases are denser than environmental air, they stay relatively confined to their location of discharge rather than dissipating into the atmosphere.

A respiratory-agent exposure should be suspected when patients with a common point source begin to experience unexpected pulmonary symptoms. In most exposures, tissue damage from these agents begins almost immediately. Initial symptoms in the large airways usually develop within minutes, although the full spectrum of effects can be delayed for several hours, depending upon exposure dose. The coughing, sneezing, voice changes, sore throat, inspiratory stridor, and wheezing from upper-airway damage usually present quickly; in contrast, the dyspnea that heralds emerging pulmonary edema is usually delayed, often for hours. The length of this latent period is inversely related to the dose, and the onset of chest tightness or shortness of breath within 4 hours of exposure indicates a very high dose and predicts a poor outcome.[2]

Characterization of the odor or appearance may help identify the causative agent. Phosgene is colorless but may smell like freshly mown hay; chlorine gas is yellow-green and pungent and has the characteristic odor of bleach or a swimming pool.[12] The toxic effects of phosgene can occur at environmental levels of 1.5 to 2 parts per million (ppm), whereas the odor is detectable at 2 to 3 ppm; hence, toxicity can occur without subject awareness.[13]

◀◀ PRE-INCIDENT ACTIONS

Preparation for a chemical-agent attack includes training of first responders, including emergency medical services (EMS) personnel and staff. Paramedics and emergency medical technicians (EMTs) should be trained how to identify victims, to protect themselves from exposures in the field with personal protection equipment (PPE), and to recognize environmental characteristics, such as odor and color, that may aid in the identification of the agent. However, the perception of odor is very subjective, and its absence should never lead to the assumption that a chemical is not present. This is particularly true of phosgene. Every hospital in the United States should have a disaster plan in place to treat victims of a chemical-agent attack. Such a plan should include a means to identify victims, a procedure to triage them to appropriate areas and control any crowd formation, and a decontamination plan, as well as a treatment and disposition strategy. A hospital pulmonary-care team with respiratory therapists may assist in the monitoring of a surge of patients with respiratory complaints, especially because patients may require ventilatory support. Further, a diversion plan should be established in the event that a hospital is unable to care for the number of victims.

There are no specific antidotes for phosgene or chlorine exposures, and treatment is mainly supportive. Early intubation and ventilatory support may be needed, and access to ventilators is thus essential. ALI, as heralded by delayed-onset chest tightness or shortness of breath, should prompt early evacuation of casualties, who may deteriorate rapidly and who may require specialized management (including intubation, central-line placement, and careful fluid management) in an intensive care unit. Pending evacuation, such casualties need to be kept at rest, since exertion worsens the progress in ALI. Oxygen may be given if available, and positive-pressure ventilation (via a conscious patient or postexpiratory end pressure [PEEP] in a ventilated patient) may help to force fluid from air spaces back into the circulation. N-acetylcysteine (NAC) may improve outcomes in phosgene exposure, and a supply should therefore be ensured. Bronchodilators, normally a treatment for upper-airway effects, may also be effective, by separate mechanisms, for ALI. There are theoretical indications for the use of nebulized sodium bicarbonate and corticosteroids, but their use has not been demonstrated to improve outcomes in patients with large-airway damage. See the section on medical treatment for further details.

▶▶ POST-INCIDENT ACTIONS

Notification of local, state, and federal authorities should occur immediately when a respiratory-agent attack is suspected. Law enforcement, firefighters, and EMS officials will coordinate scene control, triage, evacuation, and containment—crucial steps in the management of any

chemical attack. The Federal Bureau of Investigation or other law enforcement officials will control evidence gathering and the chain of evidence.[14]

The hospital disaster plan should be activated if a significant influx of victims is expected. Crowd control should be initiated, and patients should be triaged to appropriate areas so that decontamination can begin immediately. A medical toxicologist or the regional poison control center (PCC) should also be contacted as soon as possible. PCCs provide early syndromic surveillance that may represent a potential option in monitoring for and responding to chemical-terrorism threats. They are also a vital resource for questions regarding diagnosis and management. In the United States, callers can be automatically connected to the closest regional PCC by dialing 1-800-222-1222.[15]

✚ MEDICAL TREATMENT OF CASUALTIES

The treatment of victims of a respiratory-agent mass casualty incident must begin with their removal from the offending agent to prevent additional exposure. First responders must take caution to avoid exposure as well. These attacks may occur concurrently with detonation of explosive material and may instill panic, causing additional casualties; therefore treatment of any traumatic injuries must occur simultaneously. Treatment continues with standard Advanced Cardiac Life Support and Advanced Trauma Life Support algorithms of assessing and securing the patient's airway, breathing, and circulation.

Airway

A victim with a massive exposure may present in obvious respiratory failure and need immediate intubation. All patients should be monitored for decompensation throughout treatment because progressive deterioration in a patient who was initially stable may necessitate intubation. Sudden dyspnea or stridor should raise concern for acute laryngospasm, and emergent airway management may be necessary.

Breathing

All patients should be placed on high-flow oxygen; this may be weaned or discontinued if the oxygen saturation is found to be normal by transcutaneous pulse oximetry or arterial blood-gas analysis. Wheezing may be present even in the absence of known reactive airway disease and should be treated empirically with beta$_2$-selective agonists such as albuterol. ALI and the ARDS may occur after a respiratory-agent attack and should be managed with lung protective strategies of low (6 mL/kg) tidal volumes.[16]

Circulation

Intravenous (IV) access (18 gauge or larger) should be established and volume resuscitation should occur as necessary in the setting of coexisting trauma. Caution should be taken to avoid iatrogenic volume overload, which may worsen pulmonary edema. Once the airway, breathing, and circulation are secured, other agent-specific treatment strategies may be considered.

Phosgenes

Decontamination and supportive therapy is standard treatment. Nonsteroidal anti-inflammatory drugs (NSAIDs) have been shown to be beneficial in animal studies, albeit at far higher doses than normally given.[2,17] Dosing of ibuprofen 400 mg by mouth (PO) every 6 hours or ketorolac 30 mg given IV every 6 hours is reasonable. Although animal studies have shown inconsistent clinical benefit, corticosteroids are a relatively benign intervention that has been recommended in the treatment of phosgene exposure.[2,18] Early administration is recommended with dosing of prednisolone 1g IV daily until pulmonary toxicity improves, followed by an appropriate taper.[18] NAC has not been shown to affect mortality, but animal studies and human case reports demonstrate decrease in direct toxicity to pulmonary paranchyma.[2,19,20] NAC functions to restore glutathione stores, thereby preventing oxidative damage. Nebulized or IV formulations have been proposed. Dosing of the nebulized solution is 1 to 10 mL of the 20% solution or 2 to 20 mL of the 10% solution every 2 to 6 hours.[17] IV dosing would be similar to treatment of an acetaminophen overdose, with a total dose 300 mg/kg over 21 hours, starting with a 150 mg/kg loading dose, followed by a 50 mg/kg infusion over 4 hours and then a 100 mg/kg infusion over the remaining 16 hours. The use of beta agonists, such as albuterol, isoprenaline, and terbutaline, as well as phosphodiesterase inhibitors, such as aminophylline, have been shown to decrease inflammatory markers but not to affect mortality. These treatments carry significant side-effect profiles and should be used with caution.[2]

Chlorine Gas

Nebulized albuterol, humidified oxygen, and decontamination remain the mainstays of treatment for chlorine gas poisoning. Nebulized sodium bicarbonate, advocated as a means to neutralize the acidic species generated in the alveoli, has been shown to improve pulmonary markers such as oxygenation and forced expiratory volume (FEV_1), but it has no effect on mortality. Patients receiving this treatment must be monitored despite clinical improvement.[6] Reasonable dosing is 4 mL of a 3.75% to 4.2% solution. The efficacy of corticosteroids for ALI caused by chlorine exposure is inconclusive, given the lack of controlled studies and the unclear indications for administration. Animal models have demonstrated improved outcomes with IV or inhaled corticosteroid treatment.[21]

🔅 UNIQUE CONSIDERATIONS

Phosgene and chlorine are true gases and thus require no dispersal mechanism. Although rapid dispersal can be achieved via explosives, these agents require only that the gas container be opened to the atmosphere or that the compounds be synthesized in an open-air reaction. DP can be disseminated as a liquid, which will then evaporate to form vapor that can be inhaled.

Phosgene, DP, and chlorine are also unique in that their toxicity is primarily pulmonary, although chlorine gas may also cause significant ocular and mucous membrane irritation. Other chemical agents may have pulmonary toxicity, but often as a secondary effect. Further, the onset of lower-airway symptoms from respiratory agents is usually delayed significantly after exposure. One must maintain a high index of suspicion and constant vigilance despite a well-appearing patient.

⚠️ PITFALLS

Pitfalls in response to a respiratory-agent attack include the following:
- Failing to consider phosgene and chlorine as potential agents of attack
- Failing to obtain important historical information, such as the presence of an odor of freshly mown hay (phosgene) or bleach (chlorine) or the presence of a yellow-green colored gas (chlorine)
- Assuming that respiratory complaints in patients from a mass casualty incident are secondary to smoke inhalation or panic
- Failing to notify local, state, and federal authorities, as well as PCCs, when a respiratory-agent attack is suspected
- Failing to observe victims of respiratory-agent attack closely in order to monitor for deterioration
- Failing to recognize that patients without signs, symptoms, or laboratory and radiographic evidence of pulmonary injury may have been exposed to a pulmonary agent such as phosgene or chlorine. Patients should be observed (ideally for at least 8 hours) for the

development of shortness of breath and pulmonary edema, even after they show signs of clinical improvement, as when treated with nebulized sodium bicarbonate
- Failure to prepare for a respiratory-agent attack (including failure to train first responders, hospital personnel, and other providers)
- Failure to stock the necessary equipment, including respiratory ventilators, to treat a rapid influx of patients with respiratory-agent exposures

REFERENCES

1. Nelson LS, Lewin NA, Howland MA, Hoffman RS, Goldfrank LR, Flomenbaum NE. *Goldfrank's Toxicologic Emergencies.* 9th ed. New York, NY: McGraw-Hill Professional; 2010.
2. Hardison L, Wright E, Pizon A. Phosgene exposure: a case of accidental industrial exposure. *J Med Toxicol.* 2014;10:51–56.
3. Lewis RJ. *Sax's Dangerous Properties of Industrial Materials.* 9th ed. New York, NY: Van Nostrand Reinhold; 1996:2684.
4. Vaish A, Consul S, Agrawal A, et al. Accidental phosgene gas exposure: a review with background study of 10 cases. *J Emerg Trauma Shock.* 2013; 6(4):271–275.
5. Greenwood NN, Earnshaw A. *Chemistry of the Elements.* 2nd ed. Oxford: Butterworth-Heinemann; 1997.
6. Vajner J, Lung D. Case files of the University of California San Francisco medical toxicology fellowship: acute chlorine gas inhalation and the utility of nebulized sodium bicarbonate. *J Med Toxicol.* 2013;9:259–265.
7. *Guidelines for Schedules of Chemicals. Organisation for the Prohibition of Chemical Weapons.* http://www.opcw.org/chemical-weapons-convention/annex-on-chemicals/a-guidelines-for schedules-of-chemicals/#, Accessed 20.04.14.
8. Rubin A. Chlorine gas attack by truck bomber kills up to 30 in Iraq. *New York Times.* April 7, 2007; http://www.nytimes.com/2007/04/07/world/middleeast/07iraq.html. Accessed 20.04.14.
9. Black I. Chlorine bomb blamed for up to 45 deaths in Iraqi Shia town. *Guardian.* May 16, 2007; http://www.guardian.co.uk/world/2007/may/17/iraq.iraqtimeline. Accessed 20.04.14.
10. Cumming-Bruce N. Syria misses new deadline as it works to purge arms. *New York Times.* April 27, 2014; http://www.nytimes.com/2014/04/28/world/middleeast/syria.html. Accessed 28.04.14.
11. Burklow TR, Yu CE, Madsen JM. Industrial chemicals: terrorist weapons of opportunity. *Pediatr Ann.* 2003;32(4):230–234.
12. *Facts About Chlorine. Emergency Preparedness and Response.* United States Centers for Disease Control and Prevention. http://emergency.cdc.gov/agent/chlorine/basics/facts.asp. Accessed 20.04.14.
13. American Industrial Hygiene Association. *Odor Thresholds for Chemicals with Established Occupational Health Standards.* Akron, OH: AIHA; 1989.
14. DHS (Department of Homeland Security). *National Planning Scenarios.* Raleigh, NC: North Carolina Emergency Management Homeland Security Branch; 2006. https://secure.nccrimecontrol.org/hsb/planning/Planning%20Documents/National%20Planning%20Scenarios%202006.pdf, Accessed 22.04.14.
15. Darracq MA, Clark RF, Jacoby I, Vilke GM, DeMers G, Cantrell FL. Disaster preparedness of poison control centers in the USA: a 15-year follow-up study. *J Med Toxicol.* 2014;10:19–25.
16. Ware LB, Matthay MA. The acute respiratory distress syndrome. *N Engl J Med.* 2000;342(18):1334–1349.
17. Kennedy TP, Rao NV, Noah W, et al. Ibuprofen prevents oxidant lung injury and in vitro lipid peroxidation by chelating iron. *J Clin Invest.* 1990;86:1565–1573.
18. Borak J, Diller W. Phosgene exposure: mechanisms of injury and treatment strategies. *J Occup Environ Med.* 2001;43:110–119.
19. Gutch M, Jain N, Agrawal A, Consul S. Acute accidental phosgene poisoning. *BMJ Case Rep.* 2012; http://dx.doi.org/10.1136/bcr. 11.2011.5233.
20. Sciuto AM, Strickland PT, Kennedy TP, Gurtner GH. Protective effects of N-acetylcysteine treatment after phosgene exposure in rabbits. *Am J Respir Crit Care Med.* 1995;151:768–772.
21. Wang J, Winskog C, Edston E, Walther SM. Inhaled and intravenous corticosteroids both attenuate chlorine gas-induced lung injury in pigs. *Acta Anaesthesiol Scand.* 49:183–190.

Cyanide Attack*

Mark E. Keim

DESCRIPTION OF EVENT

Cyanide—much of it in the form of salts, such as sodium, potassium, and calcium cyanide—is widely used in industry. Hundreds of thousands of tons of cyanide are manufactured annually in the United States alone. The cyanides of military (and possibly terrorist) interest are the volatile liquids hydrogen cyanide (North Atlantic Treaty Organization designation, AC) and cyanogen chloride (CK).[1]

A covert cyanide attack involving food or water contamination with ingestion as a route of exposure would likely initially present in a manner similar to that of a covert biological attack. In this sense the first indications of attack may be an unusual cluster of cases or a more diffuse increase in the number of patients presenting with an initially unknown illness. In this covert scenario forensic and epidemiologic investigation may be necessary to confirm the cause of the event. Obviously an abruptly high incidence, close temporal relationship, or more focal cluster of cases will increase the suspicion of a common causative agent.

Cyanide released as a liquid or an aerosol can pose a liquid hazard via penetration through even intact skin, but the greater risk in a terrorist attack is the inhalation of aerosol, vapor, or gas. A cyanide attack involving inhalational exposure is more likely to present in a manner similar to that of other hazardous materials (HazMat) release events, with a well-localized incident scene and an associated cluster of attack victims. In this scenario an accurate and timely history of the event will be important in guiding response decision making and clinical diagnosis. Lethal concentrations of cyanide vapor or gas typically kill rapidly, dissipate quickly, and leave no toxic residue. It must not be forgotten that smoke-inhalation casualties from any terrorist scenario, even one using only conventional weapons, may also exhibit cyanide toxicity.[2,3]

PRE-INCIDENT ACTIONS

The Importance of Local Preparedness

Preparation for the 1996 Olympic Games in Atlanta demonstrated an ability to stockpile and mobilize resources (including chemical antidotes) given sufficient advance notice.[4] Since then the development of specialized chemical and biological incident-response teams within the National Disaster Medical System as well as the pharmaceutical reserve and delivery systems of the Strategic National Stockpile have augmented regional and national capacity.

---

*The material in this chapter reflects solely the views of the author. It does not necessarily reflect the policies or recommendations of the Centers for Disease Control and Prevention or the U.S. Department of Health and Human Services.

However, with chemical releases (and especially cyanide), lethal effects can occur within minutes after exposure. The characteristically rapid onset of cyanide toxicity offers only a very narrow window of opportunity for clinical intervention, thus limiting the potential effectiveness of resources other than those that are immediately available at the community first-responder level. However, because of their reputed inherent toxicity and narrow therapeutic indices, cyanide antidotes are usually not included in prehospital formularies in the United States.[5] Hospital preparedness for many chemical emergencies and disasters is also reportedly inadequate.[6–10]

The character of HazMat risk has also changed in the wake of recent acts of terror. Emergency responders, including both law enforcement and emergency medical services (EMS) care providers, are not only potential victims but also potential targets.[11,12] Several publications have recently agreed that, "At the community level, planning for chemical-biological catastrophes begins with development of local health resources."[13–15] Boxes 115-1 and 115-2 list recommendations for pre-incident actions that can be undertaken to mitigate the potential impact of a terrorist attack involving cyanide.

POST-INCIDENT ACTIONS

Scene Safety

The first step in the response to any HazMat release incident is to limit any further exposure to the victim and others, including first responders. Despite an increased awareness of chemical terrorism among first responders, in one simulated chemical weapons release in New York City, first responders entered the site without adequate personal protective gear.[21] Despite an extensive prestaging of national assets in preparation for potential terrorist use of mass casualty weapons at the 1996 Atlanta Olympics, many medical and investigational responders entered Olympic Centennial Park immediately after the bomb explosion and before any chemical hazard characterization. A thorough assessment of scene safety is paramount to any subsequent rescue activities. Rescuers should also keep in mind the possibility of secondary devices meant to injure the first responders.[22]

Termination of Exposure and Decontamination

Once the scene has been declared safe for entry or the proper personal protective equipment is employed, the next step is to remove the victims from the area of any potential further exposure. No decontamination is necessary if it is known that the cyanide exposure was in the form of vapor or gas. The health risk from vapor released from clothing contaminated by cyanide gas, vapor, or fine aerosol is not significant. Simple removal of outer clothing will provide an added precaution against any such potential for exposure but should not delay the initiation of emergency medical therapy.

In the case of direct dermal exposures to liquid or dry cyanide compounds, contaminated clothing should be removed immediately and the skin should be decontaminated using copious amounts of water or soap and water. There may also be instances when cyanide contamination is combined with conventional wound injuries. In these cases bandages should be removed in the decontamination area and the wounds flushed. Dressings and tourniquets should be replaced with new ones. Splints should be thoroughly decontaminated (but removed only by a physician).[1] The new dressings should be removed in the operating room and submerged in 5% sodium hypochlorite or placed into a plastic bag and sealed. Cyanide is quite volatile, so although liquid cyanide in a wound may be quickly absorbed and systemically distributed, it is extremely unlikely that cyanide will remain in the wound long enough to be susceptible to decontamination. The risk from vapor off-gassing from chemically contaminated fragments and cloth in wounds is very low and not significant. A chemical protective mask is not required for surgical personnel.[1] The 1978 mass suicide in Jonestown, Guyana, dramatically illustrates the potential for mass casualties from cyanide ingestion. In the case of cyanide ingestion, gastrointestinal decontamination should include gastric lavage, cathartics, and activated charcoal. Although cyanide is not well adsorbed onto charcoal, the toxicity of cyanide means that removal of even a small fraction of the ingested amount may change the internal dose from a fatal one to a survival one. Responders should also take personal protective precautions to avoid dermal exposures to cyanide-contaminated emesis or gastric contents and to avoid mouth-to-mouth resuscitation of suspected cyanide casualties (see "Supportive Care" under "Medical Treatment of Casualties," *infra*).

✚ MEDICAL TREATMENT OF CASUALTIES

Mechanism of Toxicity

The cyanide ion can rapidly bind with certain metallic complexes, particularly those containing cobalt and trivalent (ferric) iron. Cyanide can combine with the ferric iron in the cytochrome-oxidase complex in mitochondria, thus preventing intracellular use of oxygen. The cell must then switch to anaerobic metabolism, creating lactic acid and a high anion gap metabolic acidosis and leading to progressive tissue hypoxia to the point of cell death. The organs most sensitive to this hypoxia are the central nervous system and the heart.

Therapy

The international medical community lacks consensus about the antidote or antidotes with the best risk-benefit ratio. Each of the antidotes shows evidence of efficacy in animal studies and clinical experience. The data available to date do not suggest obvious differences in efficacy among antidotes, with the exception of a slower onset of action of sodium thiosulfate (administered alone) than of the other antidotes.[23,24]

The potential for serious toxicity limits or prevents the use of dicobalt edetate and 4-dimethylaminophenol in prehospital empirical treatment of suspected cyanide poisoning and has led to controversy regarding the prehospital use of the cyanide antidote kit (CAK).[23] Hydroxocobalamin differs from these antidotes in that it has so far not been associated with clinically significant toxicity in antidotal doses. Hydroxocobalamin is an antidote that seems to have many of the characteristics of the ideal cyanide antidote: rapid onset of action, the ability to neutralize cyanide without interfering with cellular oxygen use, tolerability and safety profiles conducive to prehospital use, safety for use with smoke-inhalation victims (although as mentioned later in this chapter concerns about possible harm from the nitrite components of the CAK may have been overstated), lack of demonstrable harm when administered to nonpoisoned patients, and relative ease of administration (although intravenous [IV] access must first be obtained).[23]

Cyanide Antidote Kits

The primary goal of therapy is to remove cyanide from the cytochrome-oxidase complex. Methemoglobin has a high affinity for cyanide, and cyanide will preferentially, although only temporarily, bind to methemoglobin instead of to cytochrome oxidase. Amyl nitrite and sodium nitrite have traditionally been used to induce methemoglobinemia,[24] although their therapeutic effects occur before detectable rises in plasma methemoglobin; in fact, induction of methemoglobinemia is not the only or even possibly the primary mechanism of action of nitrites. Because methemoglobinemia can result in serious side effects, especially in children,[25] methemoglobin levels should be monitored and not allowed to exceed 35% to 40%.[26]

A secondary goal is to bind cyanide irreversibly so that it cannot reenter mitochondria. This detoxification is produced by administration of sodium thiosulfate, which binds to cyanide irreversibly in a one-way reaction that is catalyzed by the enzyme rhodanese and that produces thiocyanate and sulfites, which are rapidly excreted by the kidneys.

Amyl nitrite, sodium nitrite, and sodium thiosulfate are commercially available in the form of a CAK. The CAK itself is not without its own inherent toxicity and adverse effects. Sodium nitrite can cause severe hypotension.[27] High thiocyanate levels (>10 mg/dL) have been associated with vomiting, psychosis, arthralgias, and myalgia. Anaphylaxis is a rare event. The most serious potential adverse effect from the use of a CAK is the production of toxic levels of methemoglobin, although concentrations greater than 40% are identifiable by the appearance of cyanosis and can be treated by the administration of methylene blue. The methemoglobin-induced decrease in the oxygen-carrying capacity of the blood has led to recommendations of caution when the CAK is used to treat smoke-inhalation victims,[28] but risks of nitrite use in this situation may be overstated.[29] Moreover, waiting for laboratory confirmation of cyanide exposure before beginning to administer the CAK may represent a potentially fatal delay in life saving intervention. Nevertheless, fatal methemoglobinemia from an iatrogenic overdose of sodium nitrite has claimed the life of at least one child who consumed a sublethal dose of cyanide.[25] On the positive side, the CAK has a proven track record of efficacy, and amyl nitrite is the only currently available cyanide antidote that can be administered by inhalation (including via an Ambu bag in an apneic patient). Because IV access may be difficult to obtain in a convulsing and hypotensive cyanide casualty, this advantage is not a trivial one.

Hydroxocobalamin

Hydroxocobalamin has been recognized as an antidote for cyanide toxicity for more than 50 years.[30-33] It is in active use in France as an antidote for cyanide intoxication, and excellent data about its efficacy, safety, and adverse reactions are available. Hydroxocobalamin reacts stoichiometrically with cyanide to form cyanocobalamin (vitamin B_{12}). Hydroxocobalamin was initially rarely used in the United States as a cyanide antidote,[33] but after the publication of articles advocating its use for cyanide disasters[5] and after approval of a new formulation by the Food and Drug Administration in 2006, one major pharmaceutical company released a formulation for such use in the United States. Hydroxocobalamin predictably raises blood pressure, but because most cyanide casualties are hypotensive, this could be seen as a therapeutic effect rather than an adverse effect in these casualties.

Anticonvulsants

Cyanide inhibits brain glutamate decarboxylase, which contributes to convulsions by causing a decrease in the inhibitory neurotransmitter gamma-aminobutyric acid (GABA). Therefore anticonvulsant drugs, such as benzodiazepines and barbiturates, which act at the GABA receptor complex, can help control seizures.[34]

Supportive Care

Supportive care for cyanide toxicity is also an important goal during the resuscitative phase of therapy and usually involves ventilation, oxygenation, and possibly sodium bicarbonate for correction of the metabolic acidosis.[35] Ventilation of apneic patients in the field is obviously critical; however, secondary poisoning from cyanide released in the breath of victims has occurred in those attempting to administer mouth-to-mouth resuscitation to cyanide casualties, and ventilation in a prehospital setting should be via bag-valve mask.

Unlike carbon monoxide, inhibition of cytochrome oxidase by cyanide is thought to be noncompetitive. Therefore oxygen has antidotal efficacy in human cyanide poisoning, possibly through altering the affinity of cyanide for cytochrome oxidase.

Patients should be treated with at least 100% oxygen. Humidified oxygen may be beneficial to victims of CK inhalation who are experiencing airway irritation or those with significant signs of cyanide toxicity. In addition, inhaled beta$_2$-agonists may be used to treat bronchospasm resulting from the irritant effects of CK on the respiratory tract.[34]

Potentially Promising Therapies

Hyperbaric oxygen (HBO) has been shown to induce a delayed increase in whole-blood cyanide concentrations and to prevent respiratory distress and restore blood pressure during cyanide intoxication. Animal studies indicate that a combined administration of HBO and hydroxocobalamin has a beneficial and persistent effect on the cerebral metabolism during cyanide intoxication.[36] HBO use may be considered for patients with cyanide toxicity that is refractory to other antidotes, especially in the setting of concomitant carbon-monoxide poisoning. However, because no human studies have been performed to date, its use in pure cyanide poisoning remains controversial.[34] Animal studies involving two new cyanide antidotes (cobinamide, a vitamin B_{12} analog, and sulfanegen, a 3-mercaptopyruvate prodrug) show promise as a new approach to treat cyanide poisoning. Both drugs can be given by intramuscular administration and therefore could be used to treat a large number of people quickly. The effects of the two drugs appear to be additive when used together in both the nonlethal and lethal models. Drug doses that yielded 40% survival with either drug alone resulted in 80% and 100% survival in injection and inhalational models, respectively.[37] The discovery of the highly water-soluble sulfanegen triethanolamine is also a promising lead for development as an intramuscular-injectable cyanide antidote.[38] In another study both hydroxocobalamin and cobinamide rescued severely cyanide-poisoned swine from apnea in the absence of assisted ventilation. The dose of cobinamide was one fifth that of hydroxocobalamin. Time to return of spontaneous breathing after antidote was similar between hydroxocobalamin and cobinamide. Blood cyanide concentrations became undetectable at the end of the study in both antidote-treated groups.[39] Riboflavin has also been found to normalize many of the cyanide-induced neurological and metabolic perturbations in early animal studies.[40] Table 115-1 provides a list of recommendations for detection, decontamination, and therapy for cyanide toxicity.

Triage of Cyanide Mass Casualties

Mass casualty events may necessitate the triage of casualties. In most cases, given the rapidity of the effect of cyanide, by the time the

TABLE 115-1 Overview of Recommendations for Detection, Decontamination, and Therapy of Cyanide Exposures

Likely method of dissemination	1. Liquid, aerosol, vapor, or gas 2. In water or food
Odor	Bitter almonds (although description is variable and the characteristic odor is not universally detectable)
Vapor heavier than air	AC: no CK: yes
Persistency in soil >24 hours	Nonpersistent
Detection equipment	*Military:* AC vapor or gas—M256A2 kit, Individual Chemical Agent Detector (ICAD) CK vapor or gas—M256A2 kit *Commercial:* Draeger Civil Defense Simultest (CDS) kit
Skin decontamination solution[41]	Wet decontamination is usually not necessary for vapor exposure. *For liquid or solids:* water with or without soap (preferred); 0.5% sodium or calcium hypochlorite solution (usually not necessary; do not use full-strength bleach on skin)
Onset of symptoms	Immediate after inhalation; slightly longer after ingestion
Mild effects	Dizziness, nausea, feeling of weakness
Severe effects	Gasping, syncope, seizures, trismus, opisthotonus, apnea, asystole
Adult therapy[34]	*Hydroxocobalamin:* 70 mg/kg (usually 5 g) IV infusion over 15 minutes; additional 5 g IV may be given. Not to exceed a cumulative dose of 10 g *Amyl nitrite:* 1 amp (0.3 mL) for 30 to 60 seconds along with 100% oxygen until IV access is obtained *Sodium nitrite:* 300 mg (10 mL 3% sol) IV over 5 to 20 minutes; slow infusion if patient develops hypotension *Sodium thiosulfate:* 12.5 g (50 mL) slow infusion delivered over 10 minutes immediately following sodium nitrite; slow infusion if patient develops hypotension; repeat at half initial dose in 1 hour if symptoms persist *Lorazepam (other benzodiazepines may also be effective):* 4 mg slow IV at 2 mg/min. If seizure persists after 10-15 minutes, administer 4 mg again
Pediatric therapy[34]	*Hydroxocobalamin:* Pediatric safety and efficacy not established; in non-U.S. marketing experience, a dose of 70 mg/kg IV over 15 minutes has been used *Amyl nitrite:* Pediatric dose not established *Sodium nitrite:* 6 mg/kg (i.e., 0.2 mL/kg of 3% solution) IV infused at rate of 2.5-5 mL/minute; not to exceed 10 mL (300 mg) *Sodium thiosulfate:* 250 mg/kg (i.e., 1 mL/kg of 25% solution) slow IV infusion (over 10 minutes) immediately following sodium nitrite; adjust infusion rate according to blood pressure; repeat in 1 hour at half initial dose if symptoms persist *Lorazepam (other benzodiazepines may also be effective):* Infants and children: 0.05-0.1 mg/kg slow IV over 2-5 minutes; not to exceed 4 mg/dose; may repeat every 10-15 minutes, as needed Adolescents: 4 mg slow IV; if seizure persists after 10-15 minutes, administer 4 mg IV again
Supportive therapy	Assisted ventilation with 100% oxygen

TABLE 115-2 Triage Recommendations for Cyanide Mass Casualties[35]

TRIAGE CATEGORY	CLINICAL SIGNS	RECOMMENDED INTERVENTION
Minimal	Conscious and breathing	No antidotes, no oxygen
Immediate	Convulsions and apnea	Antidotes and oxygen
Delayed	Unconscious but breathing	Antidotes and oxygen
Expectant	No cardiac activity	No care unless resources are available for resuscitation

responder arrives on the scene of an aerosol or vapor release, the casualties will be asymptomatic, exhibiting acute effects, recovering from acute effects, or dead. Table 115-2 lists a triage scheme that may be applied to these four categories.[35]

Case Presentation

A highly charged political meeting was held in a town hall. The meeting was attended by 60 men, women, and children. Everyone was seated in the middle of the hall. During the meeting most of those present began to experience dizziness, lightheadedness, nausea, and weakness. Within minutes a 54-year-old man seated near the back of the hall lost consciousness and fell off his chair. An ambulance was called. Within the next few minutes, many others in the hall also became unconscious, starting with those seated immediately surrounding the 54-year-old casualty. On entering the hall, one emergency medical technician (EMT) complained of feeling dizzy and stumbled to the ground. His partner saw several of the casualties from outside the hall and immediately called for backup before entering to rescue his fallen co-worker.

Thereafter a fleet of ambulances was dispatched to the scene. After they had arrived, police and ambulance services established that a large number of people, including both of the previously dispatched EMTs, were affected. A major incident was declared, and the local HazMat response team was dispatched while police established and maintained a perimeter around the scene.

A HazMat response team arrived, entered the building, and found 62 patients. Twelve patients, including one of the EMTs, were conscious and breathing but weak. Twenty-eight patients, including one EMT, were apneic and convulsing, although all still had a pulse. Ten patients were unconscious but breathing. Twelve patients were apneic and asystolic. The HazMat response team opened all doors and windows to the room and immediately removed everyone but the 12 asystolic patients.

Fifty patients were transferred to a warm zone for removal of outer clothing before evacuation. Thirty-eight patients were triaged for immediate transport to the hospital. While en route, oxygen therapy was initiated for all 38 patients, several of whom also required assisted ventilation. At the hospital 28 patients were found to be dead on arrival, eight patients remained unconscious but breathing, and two had regained consciousness. The hospital had enough CAKs on hand to care for one patient. Antidotal therapy was initiated for one patient, and the rest were treated with 100% high-flow oxygen. All eight recovered.

❓ UNIQUE CONSIDERATIONS

During World War I, both AC and CK were used as chemical warfare agents. Neither form of cyanide was highly successful as a weapon partly because of the incomplete filling of projectiles and partly because of the use of bursting charges that set most of the hydrogen cyanide on fire.

AC is formed when a cyanide salt is mixed with an acid. Hydrogen cyanide is a liquid that boils at 25.6 °C (78.1 °F) but evaporates rapidly at usual temperatures. The vapor and gas are lighter than air and persist for only a few minutes in the open atmosphere. These factors made AC difficult to disperse in a lethal concentration using relatively small payloads on the open battlefield.

CK is similarly released when a saturated solution of potassium-cyanide salt is mixed with chlorine. Cyanogen chloride boils at 13.8 °C (56.8 °F), and its vapor and gas are heavier and less volatile than AC. The toxicity of CK is similar to that of AC, but CK has the additional mucosal irritant and pulmonary effects of its chlorine component.

During World War II the Nazis used AC adsorbed onto Zyklon B, a dispersible pharmaceutical base, as a means for mass murder of prisoners within the confined space of death-camp gas chambers. During the 1980s Iraq is reported to have used cyanide-like agents in incidents involving Syria,[42] Iraqi Kurds,[43] and possibly Iran.[44] (The largest industrial chemical disaster in world history occurred in Bhopal, India, in 1984. The Bhopal disaster killed more than 2500 persons and affected an additional 200,000 to 300,000.[45] Although methyl isocyanate contains a cyanide moiety, methyl isocyanate itself is primarily a pulmonary agent that causes pulmonary edema at moderate doses and has additional irritative effects on larger [central] airways at higher doses.)[45,46]

AC is still used in present-day gas chambers for capital punishment in a process involving the generation of hydrogen cyanide from the reaction of cyanide salts with acid. Precursors of AC were also found in several Tokyo subway restrooms in the weeks after the 1995 sarin nerve agent attack in that city.[1] Cyanide has been implicated in the covert poisoning of commercial foodstuffs[1] and drug products,[47] and terrorists are reported to have expressed an ongoing interest in the use of cyanide compounds—including chemicals from industrial sources—as weapons.[48]

Inhalation and ingestion are the most likely routes of exposure in mass casualties during a terrorist event. Dermal toxicity can occur with cyanide but is less likely to affect large numbers compared with inhalation or ingestion. Dispersing a respirable aerosol in the open atmosphere requires a system that generates high energy to produce the small particle size, appropriate weather conditions to ensure that the aerosol cloud stays near the ground (cyanide is lighter than air), and adequate concentrations of the agent to produce the toxic effect.[1] The release of cyanide vapor or gas within an enclosed public space or building would likely maximize its potential toxicity and minimize the difficulty of its deployment for inhalational exposure. However, a large amount of liquid is required to produce vapor sufficient to cause mass casualties.[1]

Introduction of cyanide, probably as cyanide salts, into the food and water supply may be another feasible scenario that could seek to exploit the physical and toxicological characteristics of cyanide. Inhalational exposure to lethal concentrations of cyanide gas usually kills within minutes. Odor thresholds for AC are highly variable, and 40% to 60% of adults lack the gene that confers the ability to detect its characteristic smell of bitter almonds.[49,50] CK may be more readily detectable by the victim because of its chlorine-like irritation of the eyes, lungs, and mucous membranes. After exposure to lower concentrations, or after exposure to lethal amounts via ingestion, the effects are slower to develop. Ingestion of a lethal dose of cyanide may allow for a 15- to 60-minute window of survival time during which antidotes may be administered, although loss of consciousness has been reported in as little as one minute following ingestion of a high dose of liquid cyanide or cyanide in solution.

⚠ PITFALLS

Pitfalls in Diagnosis

There are several factors that may complicate a timely and accurate diagnosis in the event of a cyanide attack. These include the following:

- Cyanide toxicity is not a common patient presentation and clinicians may have little or no experience in diagnosis. Sublethal symptoms are often nonspecific, and lethal exposures may present as nonspecific cardiorespiratory arrest.
- Measurements of blood cyanide levels are almost never available during the treatment phase, although laboratory determination of a decreased arteriovenous oxygen gradient can usually be performed relatively quickly and can serve as a valuable indicator of exposure.
- Cyanide levels tend to fall in stored samples because of the short half-life of the compound.

Signs and symptoms of cyanide toxicity are often relatively nonspecific and may offer little indication of causation in the absence of other historical data. Early signs and symptoms may include transient hyperpnea, headache, diaphoresis, flushing, weakness, vertigo, dyspnea, and findings of central nervous system excitement progressing to seizures. With high inhalational doses, gasping may be nearly immediate and may progress to collapse, apnea, and convulsions within 30 to 60 seconds, with death ensuing within six to eight minutes. In the case of CK exposure, victims may also complain of irritation of the eyes and mucous membranes. Cyanide casualties are classically described as having flushed skin rather than cyanosis, but many patients are nevertheless cyanotic.[49] The telltale odor of bitter almonds may not always be appreciated because 40% to 60% of the population lacks the gene that enables detection of this odor.[50,51] Late-appearing indications of central nervous system depression, such as coma and dilated pupils, are prominent but nonspecific signs of cyanide intoxication.

Animal studies have indicated the potential diagnostic use of inosine to serve as a biomarker of cyanide exposure.[40] Because the onset of cyanide toxicity is fast, a rapid, sensitive, and accurate method for the diagnosis of cyanide exposure is necessary. A field sensor for the diagnosis of cyanide exposure has been developed based on the reaction of naphthalene dialdehyde, taurine, and cyanide, yielding a fluorescent beta-isoindole. In 2014 the sensor was found to be 100% accurate in diagnosing cyanide poisoning for acutely exposed rabbits.[52]

Pitfalls in Antidote Availability

Unfortunately hospital preparedness for many chemical emergencies and disasters is also reportedly inadequate.[6-10] There is often little incentive to stock antidote for this rare poisoning event. One particular study noted a decrease in hospital-based availability of cyanide antidotes in a major U.S. city between 1996 and 2000.[10] Another study performed in 2013 revealed that only 16% of 238 hospitals surveyed were found to have sufficient stocking of cyanide antidotes (defined as at least four antidote kits).[53]

One investigation of perceived and actual availability of antidotes recommended for stocking in emergency departments (EDs) in England revealed that knowledge of common antidote locations was variable, and stocking of antidotes did not universally meet the College of Emergency Medicine recommendations.[54]

Pitfalls in Treatment

The international medical community lacks consensus about the antidote or antidotes with the best risk-benefit ratio. Critical assessment of cyanide antidotes is needed to aid in therapeutic and administrative decisions that will improve care for victims of cyanide poisoning (particularly poisoning from enclosed-space, fire-smoke inhalation) and enhance readiness for cyanide toxic terrorism and other mass casualty incidents.[23]

The potential for serious toxicity limits or prevents the use of dicobalt edetate and 4-dimethylaminophenol in prehospital empiric treatment of suspected cyanide poisoning and has generated controversy over the appropriate use of the CAK.[5,23] One retrospective review of cases more than 7 years as reported to 61 poison centers in the United States revealed that antidotes were not used, particularly in critically ill patients and especially in the prehospital setting. Out of 1741 exposures, only 13% of all cases and 26% of cases arriving at a health care facility received an antidote. In 35% of cases of cardiac arrest or hypotension and in 74% of intentional ingestions, antidotes were not given. Research is needed to improve outcomes of cyanide-induced hypotension and cardiac arrest and to reduce barriers to antidote use.[55] This is particularly challenging because cyanide toxicity often requires rapid administration of antidote for survival. Hydroxocobalamin has not been associated with clinically significant toxicity when used in antidotal doses for cyanide casualties but is expensive and must be given IV. Amyl nitrite is currently the only cyanide antidote that can be given inhalationally, before an IV line is placed. Thus amyl nitrite can buy time in settings in which rapid administration of antidotes is paramount but IV access is difficult. Unsafe plasma levels of methemoglobin from nitrites can be recognized by cooximetry or clinically by the appearance of cyanosis (not a classic finding from cyanide alone). Concerns about the possibility of undue depression of oxygen-carrying capacity from concomitant inhalation of carbon monoxide by smoke-inhalation victims may be overstated, although it is always wise to use caution in this setting. Although hydroxocobalamin and the CAK are both very effective in cyanide poisoning, antidotes are often not available in a prehospital setting, and even in hospitals there may be insufficient antidotes to treat large numbers of cyanide casualties. It is important for the clinician to understand that with careful attention to supportive care, including management of the airway, breathing, circulation, and seizures, some patients may survive even without antidotes.

REFERENCES

1. Baskin SI, Brewer TG. Cyanide poisoning. In: Zajtchuk R, Bellamy R, eds. *Textbook of Military Medicine*. Washington, DC: Office of the Surgeon General, Department of the Army; 1997:Sidell FR, Takafuji ET, Franz DR, eds. Medical Aspects of Chemical and Biological Warfare; vol. 1.
2. Koschel MJ. Where there's smoke, there may be cyanide. *Am J Nurs*. 2002;102:39–42.
3. Alcorta R. Smoke inhalation and acute cyanide poisoning: hydrogen cyanide poisoning proves increasingly common in smoke-inhalation victims. *JEMS*. 2004;29(8 suppl):6–15, quiz suppl 16–17.
4. Sharp TW, Brennan RJ, Keim M, et al. Medical preparedness for a terrorist event involving biological or chemical agents during the 1996 Atlanta Olympic games. *Ann Emerg Med*. 1998;32:214–223.
5. Sauer SW, Keim ME. Hydroxocobalamin: improved public health readiness for cyanide disasters. *Ann Emerg Med*. 2001;37:631–641.
6. Cone DC, Davidson SJ. Hazardous materials preparedness in the emergency department. *Prehospital Emerg Care*. 1997;1:85–90.
7. Burgess JL, Blackmun GM, Bodkin CA. Hospital preparedness for hazardous materials incidents and treatment of contaminated patients. *West J Med*. 1997;167:387–391.
8. Ghilarducci DP, Pirrallo RG, Hegmann KT. Hazardous materials readiness of United States level 1 trauma centers. *J Occup Environ Med*. 2000;42:683–692.
9. Wetter DC, Daniell WE, Treser CD. Hospital preparedness for victims of chemical or biological terrorism. *Am J Public Health*. 2001;91:710–716.
10. Keim ME, Pesik N, Twum-Danso N. Lack of hospital preparedness for chemical terrorism in a major US city 1996-2000. *Prehospital Disaster Med*. 2003;18(3):193–199.
11. Eckstein M. The medical response to modern terrorism: why the "rules of engagement" have changed. *Ann Emerg Med*. 1999;34(2):219–221.
12. Nakajima T, Sato S, Morita H, et al. Sarin poisoning of a rescue team in the Matsumoto sarin incident in Japan. *Occup Environ Med*. 1997;54:697–701.
13. Nozaki H, Hori S, Shinosawa Y, et al. Secondary exposure of medical staff to sarin vapor in the emergency room. *Intensive Care Med*. 1995;21:1032–1035.
14. American Academy of Pediatrics. Chemical-biological terrorism and its impact on children: a subject review. *Pediatrics*. 2000;3:662–670.
15. Brennan RJ, Waeckerle JF, Sharp TW, et al. Chemical warfare agents: emergency medical and emergency public health issues. *Ann Emerg Med*. 1999;34(2):191–204.
16. Keim ME, Kaufmann AF. Principles of emergency response to bioterrorism. *Ann Emerg Med*. 1999;34:177–182.
17. Keim ME, Kaufmann AF, Rodgers GC. *Recommendations for OEP/CDC Surveillance, Laboratory and Informational Support Initiative*. Atlanta: U.S. Centers for Disease Control and Prevention, National Center for Environmental Health; 1998.
18. Joint Commission on Accreditation of Healthcare Organizations. *2000 Comprehensive Accreditation Manual for Hospitals*. Oakbrook Terrace, Ill: JCAHO; 2000.
19. Anonymous. *29 Code of Federal Regulations Part 1910.120. Occupational Safety and Health Standards*. Washington, DC: U.S. Government Printing Office; 1995.
20. Adler J. The protection and sheltering policy in hospitals. *Prehospital Disaster Med*. 1990;5:265–267.
21. American Hospital Association. *Hospital Preparedness for Mass Casualties: Summary of an Invitational Forum, Final Report*. Washington, DC: American Hospital Association; 2000.
22. Tucker JB. National Health and Medical Services response to incidents of chemical and biological terrorism. *JAMA*. 1997;278:396–398.
23. Hall A, Saiers J, Baud F. Which cyanide antidote? *Crit Rev Toxicol*. 2009;39(7):541–552.
24. Reade M, Davies S, Morley P. Review article: management of cyanide poisoning. *Emerg Med Australas*. 2012;24(3):225–238.
25. Berlin Jr. CM. The treatment of cyanide poisoning in children. *Pediatrics*. 1970;46:793–796.
26. Bunn HF. Disorders of hemoglobin. In: Braunwald E, Wilson JD, Martin JB, et al. *Harrison's Principles of Internal Medicine*. 11th ed. New York: McGraw-Hill; 1987:1518–1527.
27. Bowden CA, Krenzelok EP. Clinical applications of commonly used contemporary antidotes: a US perspective. *Drug Saf*. 1997;16:9–47.
28. Hall AH, Kulig KW, Rumack BH. Suspected cyanide poisoning in smoke inhalation: complications of sodium nitrite therapy. *J Toxicol Clin Exp*. 1989;9:3–9.
29. Kirk MA, Gerace R, Kulig KW. Cyanide and methemoglobin kinetics in smoke inhalation victims treated with the cyanide antidote kit. *Ann Emerg Med*. 1993;22:1413–1418.
30. Mushett C, Kelley KL, Boxer GE, et al. Antidotal efficacy of vitamin B12a (hydroxo-cobalamin) in experimental cyanide poisoning. *Proc Soc Exp Biol Med*. 1952;81:234–237.
31. Lovatt E. Cobalt compounds as antidote for hydrocyanic acid. *Br J Pharmacol*. 1964;23:455–475.
32. Yacoub M, Faure J, Morena H, et al. Acute hydrocyanic acid intoxication: current data on the metabolism of cyanide and treatment by hydroxocobalamin [French]. *Eur J Toxicol Environ Hyg*. 1974;7:22–29.
33. Litovitz TL, Klein-Schwartz W, Caravati EM, et al. 1998 annual report of the American Association of Poison Control Centers Toxic Exposure Surveillance System. *Am J Emerg Med*. 1999;17:435–487.
34. Murphy-Lavoie H. *Cyanogen Chloride Poisoning*. Medscape 2013. Available at: http://emedicine.medscape.com/article/832939-medication; Last Accessed 27.04.14.
35. Anonymous. Cyanide. In: Sidell FR, Patrick WC, Dashiell TR, eds. *Janes Chem-Bio Handbook*. Alexandria, Va: Janes Information Group; 1998:122–123.
36. Hansen M, Olsen N, Hyldegaard O. Combined administration of hyperbaric oxygen and hydroxocobalamin improves cerebral metabolism after acute cyanide poisoning in rats. *J Appl Physiol*. 2013;115(9):1254–1261, 1985.

37. Chan A, Crankshaw D, Monteil A. The combination of cobinamide and sulfanegen is highly effective in mouse models of cyanide poisoning. *Clin Toxicol (Phila)*. 2011;49(5):366–373.

38. Patterson S, Monteil A, Cohen J. Cyanide antidotes for mass casualties: water-soluble salts of the dithiane (sulfanegen) from 3-mercaptopyruvate for intramuscular administration. *J Med Chem*. 2013;56(3):1346–1349.

39. Bebarta V, Tanen D, Boudreau S. Intravenous cobinamide versus hydroxocobalamin for acute treatment of severe cyanide poisoning in a swine (Sus scrofa) model. *Ann Emerg Med*. 2014 Apr 15; http://dx.doi.org/10.1016/j.annemergmed.2014.02.009, pii: S0196-0644(14)00119-X. [Epub ahead of print].

40. Nath A, Roberts L, Liu Y. Chemical and metabolic screens identify novel biomarkers and antidotes for cyanide exposure. *FASEB J*. 2013; 27(5):1928–1938.

41. Anonymous. Cyanide. In: *Medical Management of Chemical Casualties*. Aberdeen Proving Ground, Md: Chemical Casualty Care Office, U.S. Army Medical Research Institute of Chemical Defense; 1995:15.

42. Lang JS, Mullin D, Fenyvesi C, et al. Is "the protector of lions" losing his touch? *US News and World Report*. November 1986;10:29.

43. Heylin M, ed. US decries apparent chemical arms attack. In: *Chem Eng News*. 1988;66:23.

44. Anonymous. Medical expert reports the use of chemical weapons in Iran-Iraq War. *UN Chronicle*. 1985;22:24–26.

45. Mehta PS, Mehta AS, Mehta SJ, et al. Bhopal tragedy's health effects. *JAMA*. 1990;264:2781–2787.

46. Anderson N. Disaster epidemiology: lessons from Bhopal. In: Murray V, ed. *Major Chemical Disasters: Medical Aspects of Management*. London: Royal Society of Medicine Services Limited; 1990:183–195.

47. Wolnick KA, Fricke FL, Bonnin E, et al. The Tylenol tampering incident: tracing the source. *Anal Chem*. 1984;56:466A–470A, 474A.

48. Averted New Year's attack included use of poison gas bombs. *Newsweek*. February 7, 2000; Available at: http://www.prnewswire.com/news-releases/newsweek–bin-laden-procurement-agent-in-us-arrested-by-jordan-role-was-to-get-computers-satellite-phones-surveillance-equipment-72284777.html. Last Accessed 27.04.14.

49. van Heijst AN, Douze JM, van Kesteren RG, et al. Therapeutic problems in cyanide poisoning. *J Toxicol Clin Toxicol*. 1987;25:383–398.

50. Gonzalez ER. Cyanide evades some noses, overpowers others [letter]. *JAMA*. 1982;248:2211.

51. Dhames MS. Acute cyanide poisoning [letter]. *Anaesthesia*. 1983;38:168.

52. Jackson R, Oda R, Bhandari R. Development of a fluorescence-based sensor for rapid diagnosis of cyanide exposure. *Anal Chem*. 2014;86(3): 1845–1852.

53. Gasco L, Rosbolt MB, Bebarta V. Insufficient stocking of cyanide antidotes in US hospitals that provide emergency care. *J Pharmacol Pharmacother*. 2013;4(2):95–102.

54. Mitchell L, Higginson I, Smith J, et al. *Emerg Med J*. 2013;30(1):43–48.

55. Bebarta V, Pitotti R, Borys D. Seven years of cyanide ingestions in the USA: critically ill patients are common, but antidote use is not. *Emerg Med J*. 2011;28(2):155–158.

CHAPTER 116

Antimuscarinic Agent Attack

Fermin Barrueto Jr. and Lewis S. Nelson

DESCRIPTION OF EVENT

Five recognized muscarinic receptor subtypes (M1 through M5) are located primarily within the parasympathetic nervous system and the brain: peripherally, postsynaptically on secretory organs and glands and within the central nervous system (CNS), concentrated in various areas, such as the striatum, cerebral cortex, and hippocampus. Muscarinic antagonists, such as atropine, scopolamine, hyoscyamine, and 3-quinuclidinyl benzilate, cause a constellation of signs and symptoms known as the *antimuscarinic*, or *anticholinergic*, toxidrome. Because cholinergic activation of end organs is partially blocked (these agents do not usually affect nicotinic receptors significantly, *anticholinergic* is technically too broad a term; nevertheless, it is more commonly encountered than *antimuscarinic* is in reference to this toxidrome). The clinical presentation is generally the opposite of that seen in the muscarinic aspects of the cholinergic crisis induced by nerve agents. The peripheral antimuscarinic effects are well described. They include mydriasis, loss of visual accommodation leading to blurred vision, drying of mucous membranes, urinary retention, anhidrosis, hyperthermia, tachycardia, and hypertension. The central antimuscarinic effects include confusion, delirium, memory loss, paresthesias, speech difficulty, characteristic hallucinations (e.g., concrete, describable, and Lilliputian, i.e., decreasing in size over time), as well as disrobing, picking, and plucking (so-called phantom behaviors, or "woolgathering") and, with very high doses, seizures.[1]

Antimuscarinic chemical warfare agents were developed precisely because of these central effects. The anticholinergic toxidrome is sometimes summarized as being exemplified by patients who are "blind as a bat" (from mydriasis and paralysis of accommodation), "dry as a bone," "hot as hades," "red as a beet," and "mad as a hatter"—the first four representing peripheral effects, and the later description referring to effects in the CNS. (Bladder distension and tachycardia have given rise in some circles to the additional appellations "full as a flask" and "tacky as a leisure suit," respectively.) These agents are classified as *incapacitating* (i.e., they are neurotoxic, but were not designed to cause death or serious injury; however, because under certain circumstances, including high doses, death can occur, these compounds should not be described as *nonlethal* agents). The intent of dispersing these agents is to prevent a military force from performing its duties efficiently or to disrupt a military or civilian infrastructure. A similar syndrome seen after the ingestion of jimson weed is caused by natural scopolamine-like agents found in the seeds; this plant could theoretically be used as a source for antimuscarinic agents.

Although atropine is the prototypical antimuscarinic agent, 3-quinuclidinyl benzilate (QNB) (North Atlantic Treaty Organization [NATO] code, BZ) is the prototype for use as an incapacitating agent because of its physicochemical properties (which allow it to be dispersed easily and make it resistant to heat and persistent in the environment for weeks), its potency, and its high safety ratio.[1] BZ was produced in the United States in the early 1960s. It purportedly received its NATO code either because it was a benzilate or because of the "buzz" associated with its use (it was also known as "Agent Buzz").[1,2] Destruction of U.S. stockpiles of BZ began in the 1980s when it was realized that this agent was unpredictable and had little practical utility.[2] BZ is now primarily used as a research marker for single photon emission computed tomography (SPECT) nuclear imaging in Alzheimer's and Parkinson's diseases.[3,4]

BZ is an odorless crystalline solid that can be absorbed by many routes (e.g., intramuscular, intravenous, inhalation, oral, and transdermal, especially if BZ is mixed with a solvent such as dimethylsulfoxide [DMSO]), but a chemical attack would likely involve inhalation of aerosol or ingestion of contaminated food or water.[2] This agent is a more-potent competitive antagonist of muscarinic acetylcholine receptors compared with atropine. The onset of peripheral antimuscarinic signs and symptoms after inhalation of an aerosol is usually between 20 minutes and 4 hours after exposure, but it can be delayed if delivery occurs by other routes.[2] Hallucinations appear approximately 6 hours after exposure and may persist for up to 3 to 4 days. BZ is very potent, but it has a wide safety profile, with an ICt_{50} (the concentration-time product at which half of an exposed group will become incapacitated) of only 112 mg/min/m^3, but an LCt_{50} (the concentration-time product at which 50% of those exposed will die) of 200,000 mg/min/m^3—a safety factor of nearly 2000.[2] Moreover, its intraperitoneal LD_{50} (the dose at which 50% of those exposed will die) in mice is 18 to 25 mg/kg.[5]

It has been alleged that Bosnian Serbs used BZ in July 1995 against 15,000 Bosniak civilians fleeing from Srebrenica to Tuzla.[6] Even though survivors experienced hallucinations and believed that they were victims of a chemical attack, others believe that stress, starvation, and exhaustion were more likely causes.[6]

PRE-INCIDENT ACTIONS

The temporally related presentation of a group of patients with the combination of peripheral and CNS signs and symptoms of the antimuscarinic toxidrome should raise the suspicion of a chemical attack with an antimuscarinic agent. Such an event should prompt notification of local and state health departments. The local hospital disaster plan should be implemented immediately so that proper measures can be taken for decontamination, prevention of secondary exposures, and efficient management of a mass casualty event. The availability of the antidote, physostigmine, should be checked, and the number of patients who could be treated in the event of a mass exposure should be ascertained.

POST-INCIDENT ACTIONS

Physical examination, history, and epidemiology are the primary tools to assist with diagnosis. Hospital-based laboratory confirmation of BZ is not readily available, and no standard laboratory tests will assist with the diagnosis. A gas chromatography and mass spectrometry confirmatory urine test is available through health authorities,[7] although the results will not be available in a clinically relevant fashion. Clinical response to the administration of physostigmine can be a practical diagnostic aid.

MEDICAL TREATMENT OF CASUALTIES

Initial treatment involves removing patients from the exposure, along with external decontamination. The removal of clothes and the decontamination of skin with water or with soap and water are indicated if the exposure occurred through ambient aerosol exposure or from transdermal exposure but not if contaminated food was the source. Standard precautions with the addition of eye protection and neoprene or butyl rubber gloves should be used by health care providers to prevent secondary exposure.[2] Assessment of the patient's hemodynamic status and airway are necessary; however, the most challenging issue may be controlling the patient's agitated delirium. Behavioral control should be easily accomplished by titrating a benzodiazepine, such as diazepam, lorazepam, or midazolam, to sedation, along with judicious use of soft physical restraints. It should be remembered that use of physical restraints could exacerbate body heat retention from excess muscular activity, if a patient is attempting to resist restraint, and it may contribute to hyperthermia. Benzodiazepines should be in plentiful supply for most hospitals, and can be as practically efficacious as the antidotal use of physostigmine.[8] Physostigmine requires both cardiac and respiratory monitoring and may be in short supply. Given the limited clinician familiarity with administration of physostigmine, benzodiazepines are a more practical medication to use in a mass casualty event. However, in a patient with an known exposure to BZ or a related antimuscarinic agent, intravenous administration of physostigmine, 1 to 2 mg over 5 minutes, while assessing for cholinergic effects (see the case below) may reduce the need for additional evaluation and treatment. Antipsychotic sedatives such as haloperidol are probably best avoided because of the potentiation of the antimuscarinic effects, or used only in combination with benzodiazepines. Patients can die from too high a dose of BZ, from self-injury related to hallucinations or illusions, or from heat stress caused by anhidrosis. Careful attention to body temperature should always be a component of supportive care of patients who have been exposed to BZ.

The antidote to poisoning by an antimuscarinic agent is physostigmine, an acetylcholinesterase inhibitor. Physostigmine, a nonpolar tertiary-amine carbamate, crosses the blood-brain barrier, reversibly binds with tissue acetylcholinesterase in postsynaptic membranes, and temporarily increases the concentration of acetylcholine in the synapse. This extra acetylcholine competes with BZ for occupancy of postsynaptic muscarinic receptors and helps to overcome the cholinergic blockade induced by BZ.[8] Although physostigmine is clinically beneficial, its reversible binding mandates multiple repeat intramuscular dosing every 30 to 60 minutes (or careful calibration of an intravenous drip), and it makes its use labor-intensive and practical only with a few patients at a time. For example, a patient given 6.4 mg of BZ intramuscularly required 200 mg of physostigmine over 72 hours to maintain normal functional competence.[9] Although safe when used in small titrated amounts and with frequent clinical reassessment, physostigmine can cause cholinergic effects such as dyspnea, apnea, bradycardia, and seizures if administered too rapidly. In a mass casualty incident, physostigmine and the personnel to administer it and to monitor its use would be in short supply. In these situations, benzodiazepines would be a better option for safe, rapid, and effective management.

Vomiting should not be induced, even if the agent has been ingested. The use of orally activated charcoal in this situation, although likely safe in an alert patient, has not been evaluated and is not generally recommended. Clinical laboratory investigation, including cerebrospinal fluid analysis, should be performed as indicated, at least until the diagnosis is clear. This will allow the clinician to exclude other diagnoses, including infectious etiologies, because BZ-exposed patients will often present with temperature elevation (from psychomotor agitation and anhidrosis) and an altered mental status.

UNIQUE CONSIDERATIONS

Complications resulting from exposure to BZ include acute-angle closure glaucoma secondary to the mydriasis, rhabdomyolysis from psychomotor agitation, ileus, urinary retention requiring Foley catheterization, pneumonia or hypoxia because of prolonged stupor or aspiration, and hyperthermia secondary to anhidrosis.

A bicyclic ester, 3-quinuclidinyl benzilate will hydrolyze in an alkaline solution of pH > 11 to benzylic acid and 3-quinuclidinol within minutes; both of these hydrolysis products are much less toxic than the parent compound (Figure 116-1),[5,10] which may be relevant in the decontamination of surfaces and medical equipment.

PITFALLS

Several potential pitfalls in response to a nerve agent attack exist. These include the following:

- Disorganization of hospital and local emergency medical services, should they become overwhelmed by many patients with agitated delirium.
- Failure to recognize that numerous patients requiring attention (including restraint in many cases) will mandate efficient allocation of hospital resources and personnel to avoid resource depletion and staff exhaustion.

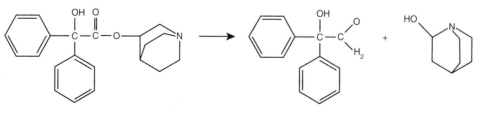

3-Quinuclidinyl benzilate   Benzilic acid   3-Quinuclidinol

FIG 116-1 Hydrolysis of 3-Quinuclidinyl Benzilate (BZ) will Occur at pH > 11.

- Inadequate decontamination of patients exposed externally, resulting in secondary exposure to health care workers, particularly rescue workers and paramedics.
- Failure to be diligent in identifying other injuries when confronted with multiple patients.
- Failure to suspect the diagnosis of an antimuscarinic agent, resulting in the administration of medications with antimuscarinic effects (e.g., haloperidol) that may worsen the patient's condition.
- Failure to restrain potentially disruptive patients who have been exposed to BZ.
- Failure to recognize the potential for heat stress in anhidrotic patients who have been exposed to BZ.

REFERENCES

1. Ketchum JS. *The Human Assessment of BZ*. Edgewood Arsenal, Md: Chemical Research and Development Laboratory; 1963. Technical Memorandum 20–29. Cited in: Ketchum JS, Sidell FR. Incapacitating agents. In: Sidell FR, Takafuji TE, Franz DR, eds. *Textbook of Military Medicine: Medical Aspects of Chemical and Biological Warfare*. Falls Church, VA: Office of the Surgeon General, U.S. Army; 1997:287–305.

2. *U.S. Army Center for Health Promotion and Preventive Medicine: Psychedelic Agent 3: Quinuclidinyl Benzilate (BZ)*. The Deputy for Technical Services, Publication: Detailed Chemical Facts Sheets; 1998. Available at: http://chppm-www.apgea.army.mil/dts/dtchemfs.htm.

3. Norbury R, Travis MJ, Erlandsson K, et al. SPET imaging of central muscarinic receptors with (R, R)[123I]-I-QNB: methodological considerations. *Nucl Med Biol*. 2004;31(5):583–590.

4. Colloby SJ, Pakrasi S, Firbank MJ, et al. In vivo SPECT imaging of muscarinic acetylcholine receptors using (R, R) 123I-QNB in dementia with Lewy bodies and Parkinson's disease dementia. *Neuroimage*. 2006;33 (2):423–429, Epub Sep 7, 2006.

5. Guidelines for 3-quinuclidinyl benzilate. In: *Guidelines for Chemical Warfare Agents in Military Field Drinking Water*. Subcommittee on Guidelines for Military Field Drinking-Water Quality, Committee on Toxicology, Board on Environmental Studies and Toxicology, National Research Council. Wahington, DC: The National Academies Press; 1995:15–18.

6. Hay A. Surviving the impossible: the long march from Srebrenica. An investigation of the possible use of chemical warfare agents. *Med Confl Surviv*. 1998;14:120–155.

7. Byrd GD, Paule RC, Sander LC, et al. Determination of 3-quinuclidinyl benzilate (QNB) and its major metabolites in urine by isotope dilution gas chromatography/mass spectrometry. *J Anal Toxicol*. 1992;16:182–187.

8. Burns MJ, Linden CH, Graudins A, et al. A comparison of physostigmine and benzodiazepines for the treatment of anticholinergic poisoning. *Ann Emerg Med*. 2000;35:374–381.

9. Ketchum JS. *The Human Assessment of BZ*. Technical Memorandum 20–29, Edgewood Arsenal, MD: Chemical Research and Development Laboratory; 1963.

10. Hull LA, Rosenblatt DH, Epstein J. 3-Quinuclidinyl benzilate hydrolysis in dilute aqueous solution. *J Pharm Sci*. 1979;68:856–859.

Mass Casualty Incidents from LSD, Other Indoles, and Phenylethylamine Derivatives

Patrick J. Maher and Fiona E. Gallahue

DESCRIPTION OF EVENT

d-Lysergic acid diethylamide (LSD), an indole alkylamine, also known as LSD-25, was discovered by Albert Hofmann in 1938 while he was working for the Sandoz Company. In 1943 Hofmann became intoxicated by LSD through accidental exposure, and 3 days later he intentionally took LSD. His experience with LSD paved the way for neuropsychiatric studies using LSD and later, in 1951, for U.S. Central Intelligence Agency (CIA) experimentation with human subjects using LSD and similar mind-altering drugs. Declassified CIA documents from these programs describe how the American government experimented with the use of LSD as a psychotropic weapon for use in espionage and interrogation. Psilocin and psilocybin, indole alkylamines derived from hallucinogenic mushrooms, as well as mescaline, a phenylethylamine derived from the peyote cactus, were also reportedly selected for testing on human subjects. Because these agents have somewhat similar (although not identical) effects, and because they were once considered by the American government as potential chemical weapons, we will narrow our focus to these hallucinogens rather than including the entire spectrum of phenylethylamine derivatives (e.g., 3,4-methylenedioxy-*N*-methylamphetamine [MDMA] and related amphetamines) or the other indole alkylamines (e.g., bufotenine, ibogaine).[1-3]

LSD, mescaline, peyote, psilocin, and psilocybin have all been classified as Schedule I drugs since the passage in 1970 of the Controlled Substance Act. These agents differ widely in potency: 1000 µg of mescaline is equivalent to 100 µg of psilocybin and to 1.0 µg of LSD.[4,5] LSD, the most potent of these drugs, produces psychedelic effects at doses between 1 and 1.5 µg/kg, with a typical dose taken of approximately 25 to 100 µg.

LSD is odorless and tasteless and is usually ingested orally, although it can be smoked, snorted, or injected. It has a plasma half-life of 2 to 4 hours and is metabolized in the liver, with urinary excretion of metabolites.[6] Although LSD has a therapeutic index (dose that produces toxicity in 50% of the population divided by the effective dose in 50% of the population) approaching 1000, it is not considered a safe drug.[6,7] It may induce episodes of anxiety, panic disorder, major depression, or psychosis in susceptible individuals.[6] Trauma resulting from accidents or self-destructive behavior, suicide, or homicide can occur; morbidity from LSD is more likely from these effects than from the direct toxicity of the compound.[2,8] Standard toxicological detection methods with gas chromatography and mass spectrometry (GC/MS) are sensitive even for small doses of LSD, and extremely sensitive detection of LSD via radioimmunoassay (RIA) or enzyme-linked immunosorbent assay (ELISA) may be performed on samples for forensic confirmation.[9]

The clinical effects of LSD begin within 30 to 60 minutes and peak at 2 to 4 hours; the majority of the symptoms resolve within 8 to 12 hours.[6,8] Studies conducted in simulated military settings demonstrated that even well-trained units become totally disorganized after ingesting total oral doses of less than 200 µg.[10] Affected persons usually cannot carry out a series of instructions or concentrate on a complex task, but they might be capable of isolated impulsive actions. Their behavior is said to be "well-coordinated" but unpredictable.[10]

LSD resembles serotonin chemically and acts on serotonin and dopamine receptors. Sympathomimetic effects commonly seen with LSD intoxication include dilated pupils, tachycardia, hypertension, and hyperreflexia.[6] The mind-altering properties of LSD can cause euphoria, anxiety, and paranoia with intense visual and auditory hallucinations that tend to be abstract, colorful, and expansive. Geometric patterns as well as distortion, blurring, or "melting" of physical objects are commonly described. Synesthesia (sensory crossover) is frequently present, although tactile hallucinations are uncommon. Severe manifestations of toxicity include hyperthermia, seizures, and rhabdomyolysis.[6,8] Abnormalities of serotonin-induced platelet aggregation may result in abnormal clotting and poor clot retraction. Although cardiovascular complications are infrequent, reports exist of supraventricular tachycardia and myocardial infarction.[11]

Mescaline is a hallucinogenic alkaloid that is derived from the North American peyote cactus (*Lophophora williamsii*) and that also occurs in several species of the genus *Trichocereus* of South American cacti. Mescaline, or 3,4,5-trimethoxyphenylamine, can be taken directly from the peyote cactus or derived synthetically. The ritual use of mescaline-containing cacti is documented from the sixteenth century, and peyote cactus is still used in ritual fashion by members of Native American churches in the southwest United States. Mescaline itself was first isolated from peyote in 1896 and was first synthesized in 1918. Peyote is commonly ingested in the form of brown discoid "mescal buttons," which are the sun-dried crowns of the cactus. Each button may contain 45 to 50 mg of mescaline. The hallucinogenic dose is 5 mg/kg. Taken orally, mescaline has an unpleasantly bitter taste and is rapidly absorbed from the gastrointestinal tract. It can also be taken intravenously with similar effects and with a similar duration of effects.[6,8]

The effects of mescaline begin within 30 minutes of ingestion and peak at about 2 to 4 hours, with a total duration of 8 to 14 hours. Like LSD, mescaline is metabolized in the liver, but it is also excreted unchanged in the urine. Clinically, the effects are similar to those of LSD but with the additional initial symptoms of nausea, vomiting, sweating, generalized discomfort, dizziness, and headache, all of which generally occur during the first hour after ingestion and shortly before the onset of hallucinogenic effects. Large doses can produce hypotension, bradycardia, and respiratory depression.[8,9]

Psilocybin (4-phosphoryloxy-*N*,*N*-dimethyltryptamine), as well as its active metabolite psilocin (4-hydroxyl-*N*,*N*-dimethyltryptamine) to which it is rapidly converted after ingestion, is a member of the indole alkylamine hallucinogens derived from tryptophan. These drugs were first isolated in 1958 from hallucinogenic mushrooms used by Mexican Indians for centuries. Their popular use was encouraged by Dr. Timothy Leary during the psychedelic movement of the 1960s. Psilocybin is more resistant to oxidation than psilocin and retains its activity in dried mushrooms. Psilocin is approximately 1.5 times as potent as psilocybin, but otherwise these two drugs are pharmacologically similar. A 100-μg dose of psilocybin is equivalent to 1 μg of LSD and 1000 μg of mescaline. The lethal dose (LD_{50}) of intravenous psilocybin has been reported to be 280 mg/kg.[4]

Peyote mushrooms can be ingested raw, dried, as a brew, or stewed. The dose to produce hallucinogenic effects in nontolerant adults is approximately 6 to 12 mg. Little correlation has been found between clinical effects and the number of mushrooms ingested. Approximately 50% of the hallucinogenic compounds are absorbed via the gastrointestinal tract, and distribution occurs to most tissues, including the brain; most excretion is renal. Signs and symptoms develop within 30 to 60 minutes, with the psychedelic effects peaking between 30 minutes and 2 hours and lasting from 4 to 12 hours.[4,6,7] Both compounds primarily affect serotonergic neurotransmission. Sympathomimetic clinical effects are more prominent than with LSD and include pupillary dilation, piloerection, tachycardia, and hyperreflexia. The hallucinations are usually visual but may be auditory or tactile. Both dysphoria and euphoria are commonly reported mood alterations. Nausea, cramping, abdominal pain, and a sensation of swelling of parts of the body are potential adverse responses. Deaths from psilocin and psilocybin are rare, with one death reported from neurologic sequelae in a patient with high serum psilocin concentration and one other in a patient who had previously undergone a heart transplant.[12]

All of these drugs have cross-tolerance to each other; the tolerance develops rapidly (within days) without the development of physical dependence and also regresses rapidly, within 3 to 4 days of withdrawal.

LSD, psilocybin, and psilocin all chemically resemble serotonin and interact with the 5-hydroxytryptamine, or 5-HT, receptor. As might be expected, some cross-reactivity exists between LSD and various antidepressants for this reason.[13] Notably, patients taking selective serotonin reuptake inhibitors (SSRI agents) and monoamine oxidase inhibitors have reported decreased responses to LSD, whereas those taking tricyclic antidepressants and lithium may show increased responses. Administration of antidepressants as therapy in response to LSD reactions has not been attempted in humans.

Flashbacks, or recurrences of hallucinogenic imagery days to years after the initial experience, have been described often with LSD but also with mescaline. Known formally as Hallucinogen Persisting Perception Disorder (HPPD), their etiology remains unknown. Flashbacks can be precipitated by triggers such as stress, exercise, and illness. They decrease in intensity with time and can be treated adequately with benzodiazepines in significantly affected patients. Risperidone and the SSRIs have been noted to exacerbate this condition.[6]

LSD is the most potent of the typical hallucinogenic agents, the most difficult to detect (being odorless and tasteless), and the compound that was reportedly most tested by governmental agencies in the 1960s. Thus this agent may be the most likely of the indoles and phenylethylamine derivatives to be used in an attack.[1] However, difficulties in covert and effective distribution of LSD limit its utility as a chemical weapon. The compound could be released into water, but impossibly high quantities would be needed to contaminate a large water source such as a reservoir. Moreover, chlorine in concentrations found in water-treatment plants can deactivate LSD by oxidation. Delivery distal to such treatment facilities is possible but also impractical (because of dilution) even for someone intent on targeting a single building.[2,14] LSD could also be delivered in an aerial drop so that a bomb filled with LSD would explode at ground level or several feet above the ground. The local population would become intoxicated through inhalation.[2] LSD could potentially be aerosolized, but it would have to be dispersed relatively close to the intended targets, a mode of delivery that might be acceptable to some but perhaps not all terrorists, depending on the situation. If an immediate effect in a particular location is desired, the fact that LSD has a latent period of 30 minutes or longer might be a disadvantage, because exposed victims might well have moved to different areas by the time that they begin hallucinating. However, this delay in action might be advantageous in a covert release of agent. With a particle size of approximately 5 μm, the dose that incapacitates 50% of the exposed population) was estimated to be 5.6 μg/kg, approximately twice the ID_{50} of the parenteral route.[10]

PRE-INCIDENT ACTIONS

Hospitals and emergency personnel should be well trained for response to a potential attack by psychedelic indoles and related compounds. Protocols for these events should include removal of the victims from the contaminating source and the use of protective equipment to avoid inhalation, ingestion, or transdermal exposure to the toxicant. Although person-to-person transmission of LSD from a terrorist attack would not be expected, aerosolized LSD could theoretically remain on skin, clothing, or environmental surfaces; whether secondary aerosolization would be significant for this compound would depend on a multitude of as-yet-uninvestigated variables. If settling of aerosolized product on skin or clothing is of concern, washing of the skin with water (with or without soap) and washing of clothes would likely suffice. If LSD detection equipment is not readily available, the detection of small amounts covertly released into the environment could be difficult.

POST-INCIDENT ACTIONS

LSD and similar hallucinogenic agents in a mass casualty event should be relatively easy for most clinicians to detect clinically, given the onset of action of approximately 30 to 60 minutes, the sympathomimetic effects, and the types of hallucinations induced. LSD intoxication would be difficult to distinguish from poisoning by the other psychedelic indoles and by phenylethylamine derivatives, but management of all these types of cases is similar. The differential diagnosis also includes acute panic reactions, schizophrenia, and exposure to phencyclidine (PCP), amphetamines, and anticholinergic compounds. The nature of the hallucinations can help distinguish between hallucinations from psychedelic indole and phenylethylamine compounds and anticholinergic hallucinations; the latter are typically concrete, easily describable, often Lilliputian (decreasing in size over time), socially contagious (sharing of illusions and hallucinations is common), and accompanied by picking or plucking movements (phantom behaviors, "woolgathering"). Evidence of hypotension, seizure, coma, or significant respiratory depression in patients should prompt consideration of alternate or additional agents.[6] The appropriate authorities should be contacted to identify and eliminate the contaminating source.

MEDICAL TREATMENT OF CASUALTIES

Treatment is usually supportive, and patients can often be managed adequately without medications if they can be reassured and treated in a calm, quiet area.[13] Some patients with more severe agitation may require medication. In this situation, a moderately long-acting benzodiazepine such as lorazepam or diazepam administered intravenously is the treatment of choice.[6] Although haloperidol and other antipsychotic medications can also be used effectively for LSD-induced agitation not responding adequately to benzodiazepines, they should not be used routinely for drug-induced hallucinations. Haloperidol and the phenothiazines are contraindicated in patients with anticholinergic poisoning, which could be mistaken for LSD psychosis without a careful examination.

UNIQUE CONSIDERATIONS

Because LSD can be oxidized by large amounts of chlorine, contaminated water sources could potentially be appropriately treated and used safely.

Because LSD, mescaline, and psilocybin are rapidly metabolized and are excreted primarily in the urine, these drugs are most easily detected in the urine through gas GC/MS or via ELISA or RIA for forensic confirmation.[9]

Prolonged adverse effects to exposure with these agents are uncommon. Negative or anxiety-provoking hallucinations ("bad trips") may be treated by movement to a quiet area and by reassurance with statements that convey a sense of security and calm.[6,13]

Use of a related form of synthetic cathinones, sometimes marketed as "bath salts," has more recently been reported with increasing frequency, particularly among young people. Constituting a range of designer substances with clinical effects similar to amphetamines, these drugs have benefited from increased media attention and a variable legal status, which has led to a perception of availability as a "legal high." Although clinical data on these drugs are relatively lacking, their ease of acquisition and potential for abuse have raised concern. The Synthetic Drug Abuse Prevention Act placed 26 synthetic cathinones and related compounds into Schedule I status.[15] Potential for attacks using these substances remains unknown. Treatment is the same as the indole alkylamines and is primarily supportive, with benzodiazepines recommended for agitation.

PITFALLS

Several potential pitfalls exist in responding to an attack. These include the following:

- Failure to notify the appropriate agencies to find the source of the contaminating drug
- Failure to use proper protective equipment in removal of patients, causing additional victims
- Failure to remove hallucinating patients to a quiet, controlled area
- Failure to consider amphetamines, anticholinergic agents, schizophrenia, and acute panic reactions in the differential diagnosis
- Use of haloperidol for hallucinations without being certain of the cause

REFERENCES

1. Marks J. *The Search for the "Manchurian Candidate."* New York, NY: Norton; 1991, 1979.
2. Buckman J. Brainwashing, LSD, CIA. Historical and ethical perspective. *Int J Soc Psychiatry.* 1977 Spring;23(1):8–19.
3. Lee MA, Shlain B. *Acid Dreams: The Complete Social History of LSD, the CIA, the Sixties and Beyond.* London: Pan; 2001, 1985.
4. Passie T, Seifert J, Schneider U, Emrich HM. The pharmacology of psilocybin. *Addict Biol.* 2002;7(4):357–364.
5. Schlicht J, Mitcheson M, Henry M. Medical aspects of large outdoor festivals. *Lancet.* 1972;1(7757):948–952.
6. Shannon MW, Borron SW, Burns MJ. Hallucinogens. In: Haddad LM, Winchester JF, eds. *Clinical Management of Poisoning and Drug Overdose.* 2nd ed. Philadelphia, PA: Saunders; 1990:793–802.
7. Binh TL, Clark RF, Williams SR. Hallucinogens. In: Marx JA, Hockberger RS, Walls RM, Adams J, Rosen P, eds. *Rosen's Emergency Medicine.* 7th ed. Philadelphia, PA: Mosby/Elsevier; 2010:2010–2018.
8. Williams LC, Keyes C. Psychoactive drugs. In: Ford MD, ed. *Clinical Toxicology.* Philadelphia, PA: Saunders; 2001:640–649.
9. Passie T, Halpern JH, Stichtenoth DO, Emrich HM, Hintzen A. The pharmacology of lysergic acid diethylamide: a review. *CNS Neurosci Ther.* 2008 Winter;14(4):295–314.
10. Ketchum JS, Sidell FR. Incapacitating agents. In: Zajtchuk R, ed. *Textbook of Military Medicine, Part I: Warfare, Weaponry, and the Casualty: Medical Aspects of Chemical and Biological Warfare.* Washington, DC: Office of the Surgeon General, U.S. Army: TMM Publications, Border Institute; 1997:293.
11. Ghuran A, Nolan J. Recreational drug misuse: issues for the cardiologist. *Heart.* 2000;83(6):627–633.
12. Lim TH, Wasywich CA, Ruygrok PN. A fatal case of "magic mushroom" ingestion in a heart transplant recipient *Intern Med J.* 2012;42 (11):1268–1269.
13. Johnson M, Richards W, Griffiths R. Human hallucinogen research: guidelines for safety. *J Psychopharmacol.* 2008;22(6):603–620.
14. LSD and water supply. *J Am Water Works Assoc.* 1967;59(1):120–1222.
15. Musselman ME, Hampton JP. "Not for human consumption": a review of emerging designer drugs. *Pharmacotherapy.* 2014;34:745–757.

CHAPTER 118

Opioid Agent Attack

Debra Lee and Rick G. Kulkarni

DESCRIPTION OF EVENT

Opium is a mixture of alkaloids extracted from the sap of unripened seedpods of *Papaver somniferous* (the Asian, or opium, poppy). Natural derivatives of these alkaloids, such as morphine, codeine, and heroin, are referred to as opiates. The term opioid was originally reserved for synthetic derivatives such as oxycodone, meperidine, and fentanyl, but the term is increasingly applied to natural as well as synthetic narcotics.[1]

Opioid receptors are widely distributed throughout the central nervous system (CNS) and gastrointestinal (GI) tract. Postsynaptic binding of opioids to receptors leads to hyperpolarization of neuronal cell membranes, inhibition of neurotransmission, and, depending on the affected cell population, depression or excitation of end organs. The effects of opioids are mediated through three opioid receptors: μ (mu), κ (kappa), and Δ (delta) (Table 118-1).[1] Most of the characteristic clinical effects—analgesia, sedation, euphoria, respiratory depression, and reduced GI motility—are largely mediated through the μ receptor; stimulation of κ receptors is chiefly responsible for opioid-induced miosis. The opioid antagonists (e.g., naloxone, nalmefene, naltrexone) have greater affinity for the μ receptors and are all effective in reversing the respiratory depression and sedation associated with acute opioid overdoses.[1,2] Opioid toxicity characteristically presents with a depressed level of consciousness and should be suspected when the clinical triad of CNS depression, respiratory depression, and miosis are present. Respiratory impairment presents with bradypnea or hypopnea and can progress to complete respiratory arrest. Because the initial respiratory response may be a depression of tidal volume in the presence of a normal respiratory rate, assessment of respiratory depth as well as rate is important. CNS depression can be profound and result in airway compromise.[3,4] Although miosis is classically seen in opioid intoxication, the clinical picture may be obscured with exposure to atypical opioids (e.g., meperidine, propoxyphene, pentazocine, and tramadol), after exposure to multiple agents such as an opioid and an anticholinergic, or from concomitant trauma or hypoxia. Less common effects of opioid administration include chest-wall rigidity and seizure activity, both of which can contribute to further respiratory compromise while complicating the clinical picture.[1] It may be helpful to remember the opioid toxidrome by remembering "depression." Opioids cause depression of (1) vital signs (temperature, pulse, blood pressure, respiratory depth, respiratory rate); (2) mental status; (3) pupil size; (4) peristalsis (hypoperistalsis, with constipation and decreased or absent bowel sounds); and (5) reflexes.

Opioid agents have not been used in a large-scale terrorist attack, but the potential of these agents to create mass casualties is illustrated by their use in October 2002 by special forces of the Russian Federal Security Service (FSB) against Chechen separatists who had entered the Moscow Dubrovka Theater Center and taken over 900 hostages.

Approximately 50 Chechen terrorists, half of whom were strapped with suicide bombs serving as triggers for centralized heavy bombs, were strategically positioned throughout the theater. After a 3-day siege, Russian forces introduced a "knockout gas" through the theater's ventilation system, effectively incapacitating the hostages and terrorists. Troops were then able to enter the theater, killing the terrorists and preventing detonation. Russian troops escaped injury and the hostages were freed. The mission was initially heralded as a success but in the end, 125 hostages died from opioid-induced respiratory depression associated with suboptimal attention to airway maintenance, problems with evacuation and transport, and initial clinical misdiagnosis.[5–8]

Although the composition of the compound or compounds used remains unknown, there was early speculation that an opioid agonist was involved; and 4 days after the rescue mission the Russian Health Minister announced that "a fentanyl based substance was used to neutralize the terrorists."[9,10] A subsequently published case review used analyses of clothing, blood, and urine samples from three of the survivors to identify traces of the fentanyl derivatives, carfentanil, a potent opioid currently used in veterinarian medicine to sedate large animals through intramuscular injection, and remifentanil, an ultra–short-acting intravenous agent typically used as an anesthetic for short procedures.[11]

A separate analysis of samples taken from two survivors suggested that the aerosol used likely contained halothane or another anesthetic agent mixed with a powerful fentanyl derivative.[12] Although a number of other pharmacological agents such as anesthetics and sedative-hypnotics have been studied for their potential uses as incapacitating weapons,[13–15] the scope of this chapter will be limited to opioid agonists. The emergency responder should be aware of the possibility of a mixed toxidrome secondary to the use of agents in multiple classifications; some of these agents will be discussed later in this text (Chapter 122).

The use of fentanyl derivatives has been a longstanding area of interest in the development of incapacitating agents because of their rapid onsets of action, short durations of effect, wide therapeutic indices, and varied distribution methods (Table 118-2).[5,12,13,15] Fentanyl has been administered via intravenous, intramuscular, intranasal, buccal, transdermal, and nebulized aerosol preparations. Aerosolized preparations of fentanyl specifically have been found to exhibit significant variations in plasma concentrations, an effect that complicates dosing on a mass scale.[16,17] This effect is largely due to high lipid solubility and a large volume of distribution. The therapeutic index (the ratio of the lethal dose to the effective dose) of fentanyl should theoretically allow for estimation of the margin of safety, but the outcome of the Dubrovka Theater assault suggests otherwise. While these drugs are safe in monitored settings, aspects of their pharmacokinetics and the inability to provide uniform dosing to individuals when administered on a large scale would result in a range of clinical effects among mass casualties.[5]

TABLE 118-1   Clinical Effects of Opioid Receptors

OPIOID RECEPTOR	CLINICAL EFFECT
μ (mu)	Analgesia, euphoria, sedation, respiratory depression, nausea, reduced GI motility, and miosis
κ (kappa)	Modest analgesia, dysphoria, and mild respiratory depression
Δ (delta)	Anxiolysis and central pain relief

TABLE 118-2   Characteristics of Opioids, Including Fentanyl Derivatives Compared with Morphine

	OPIOID POTENCY	THERAPEUTIC AGENT INDEX*
Morphine	1	70
Fentanyl	300	300
Remifentanil	220	33,000
Carfentanil	10,000	10,600

*Therapeutic index = median lethal dose (LD_{50})/lowest median effective dose (ED_{50}).

Casualty management was a contributing factor to many of the deaths in the Dubrovka incident. Preparatory measures were taken to increase surge capacity at area hospitals, and a few prehospital providers were staged at the scene, but activation of hundreds of first responders was delayed until well after the assault was under way.[8] While there are reports that some of the first responders knew that a gas or aerosol had been deployed and that some were equipped with an opioid reversal agent, still more were not. The effort to deploy the opioid antagonist was inconsistent, with some victims receiving multiple injections and others none. The identification of the incapacitating agent as "nonlethal" agent may also have affected the ways in which casualties were viewed. The knockout agent was correctly viewed as incapacitating in the sense of not being intended to kill or cause serious effects, but as circumstances demonstrated, it was certainly not "nonlethal." Opioids and anesthetic agents are known to be lethal in higher doses, an effect which is typically mitigated by close monitoring of a patient's respiratory status. Post-event analysis indicates that a number of deaths could have been prevented with a coordinated rescue effort where a specific action plan tailored to an opioid agent attack was utilized.[8]

Many casualties appear to have been removed from the theater and placed into positions either on the ground or in buses, in which their airways were left unsecured and the patients were unmonitored. Multiple sources indicate that the use of an opioid derivative was not reliably conveyed to staff at receiving hospitals; and some clinicians may have misinterpreted the apnea, convulsions, and pinpoint pupils as signs of nerve-agent exposure and administered nerve-agent antidotes.[5-8]

PRE-INCIDENT ACTIONS

Preparedness is the single most important action that can be taken to prevent mass casualties from an opioid attack. Preparedness begins with the development, implementation, and activation of an all-hazards emergency management plan that includes an action plan specific to opioid attacks in communities considered at high risk for such attacks.

(The risk of a terrorist attack is in many ways difficult to predict, but large cities or those with politically or economically significant institutions or landmarks can be considered high-risk communities.) Opioid intoxication is commonly encountered in clinical practice and must be recognized in an unlikely scenario. The potential for a large-scale opioid attack and the presentation, differential diagnosis, and treatment of persons exposed to such an agent should be reviewed with first responders. Confronted with large numbers of unconscious patients with respiratory depression and miosis, nerve agents may be the first consideration given their relatively high profile as a chemical weapon. The absence of salivation, lacrimation, diaphoresis, diarrhea, and seizures classically seen prior to the flaccid paralysis and apnea in organophosphate poisonings may be noted, although those who suddenly collapse from high doses of a nerve agent may not have time to exhibit increased secretions. Failure to respond to antidotes for nonopioid agents can help providers widen their differential, and reversal of CNS and respiratory depression in response to naloxone would be diagnostic as well as therapeutic. Critical factors in minimizing the number of casualties include (1) reaching casualties as soon as possible to prevent permanent effects of hypoxia, (2) securing the airway, (3) implementing assisted ventilation, and (4) instituting prompt treatment with an opioid antagonist. High-risk communities should maintain adequate staffing and supplies to provide ventilatory support either invasively or noninvasively and should maintain sufficient stockpiles of naloxone. Because naloxone will be needed early in casualty management, its availability in prehospital settings is particularly important, and plans to use pre-incident mutual aid agreements or the Strategic National Stockpile should focus on resupply of preplaced naloxone.

POST-INCIDENT ACTIONS

Once an attack is identified, a preformulated emergency management plan must be activated. Information about the offending agent will likely come from the field and should be widely disseminated to rescue personnel and receiving hospitals, although initial reports from the site and from news media often misidentify the agent used. First responders must wear appropriate personal protective equipment including supplied air respirators in cases of an inhaled agent. An attack with an opioid agent will likely take place in an enclosed space, and prevention of further exposure to the offending agent may require ventilation or evacuation. Patients who can extricate themselves should be advised to retreat to a specified, unaffected area for later evaluation. Rescue personnel should implement rapid control measures even before the arrival of medical personnel. Affected patients should be removed from confined spaces and positioned in the left lateral decubitus position to help prevent aspiration of gastric contents and airway obstruction. Naloxone is becoming increasingly available for administration by the layperson, and nonmedical rescue personnel should be equipped to administer it when necessary. Additional supplies of naloxone should be requested from adjoining communities, facilitated by prearranged mutual aid agreements. Appropriate local, state and federal public health and law enforcement authorities should be notified.

MEDICAL TREATMENT OF CASUALTIES

Treatment should be tailored to the clinical presentation of victims. Those who are awake and oriented may need only to be escorted into an open area outside the zone of contamination. Those who are sleepy or lethargic but easily arousable should also be escorted to an open area and kept under observation, including monitoring of respiratory depth as well as respiratory rate, for progression of symptoms. Patients who are unconscious and with respiratory depression (manifested by shallow breathing or by a rate of 12 or fewer breaths per minute) should receive naloxone via either the intranasal or the intramuscular route in 2.0-mg increments until the respiratory depression resolves.[2,18] The onset of antidotal effects after naloxone administration is typically 1 to 3 minutes, with maximal effect usually observed within 5 minutes. Repeat doses are indicated for partial responses. The clinical efficacy of naloxone can be limited to as little as 45 minutes; therefore patients should be monitored and re-dosed as needed.[3] Patients who are unconscious with significantly depressed respirations or who are apneic should immediately receive assisted ventilations. They should then be given naloxone until they breathing spontaneously; complete arousal is not the primary objective. Patients exhibiting signs of severe opioid intoxication, those with an initial presentation of CNS and respiratory depression, or those who require repeated doses of naloxone should be triaged and transported to local hospitals for continued administration of naloxone and monitoring as needed. All patients should be assessed for secondary injuries (e.g., blunt trauma resulting from opioid-induced unconsciousness) and for complications due to prolonged hypoxia and should be treated appropriately.

❓ UNIQUE CONSIDERATIONS

Opioid agonists as incapacitating agents are compelling tools for counterterrorism and police applications. Their inherent lethality has been demonstrated, and the potential use in a terrorist attack must be considered. Although there has been only a single known episode of large numbers of victims from opioid inhalational exposure, providers in mass casualty incidents must maintain a heightened level of awareness for a commonly seen toxidrome in an unusual setting.

In an attack, an opioid agent is likely to be aerosolized in an enclosed space with hundreds of people who will exhibit varied responses to the agent based on their individual exposures, preexisting conditions, and agent pharmacokinetics. Because respiratory depression is the usual mechanism of death from opioid intoxication, rapid access to casualties, with maintenance of airway and ventilation during and after evacuation from the scene, is crucial. Modification of triage protocols to include limited rescue breaths and a pulse check should be considered in action plans for specific events. Naloxone should be administered as soon as is practical, but its administration is secondary to securing and maintaining an open airway and ensuring adequate ventilation.

❗ PITFALLS

- Failure to create and implement an emergency management plan
- Failure to recognize or report an attack from an opioid agent
- Failure to consider the differential diagnosis of miosis in mass casualties
- Failure to recognize the clinical presentation of opioid toxicity and to institute assisted ventilations and specific antidotal treatment
- Delay in reaching casualties with respiratory depression or apnea
- Failure to position victims properly and to attend to airway and ventilatory compromise

REFERENCES

1. Freye E. *Opioids in Medicine. Mechanism of Action of Opioids and Clinical Effects.* Dusseldorf: Springe; 2008, 90–172.
2. Schumacher MA, Basbaum AL, Way WL. Opioid analgesics & antagonists. In: Katzung BG, Masters SB, Travor AJ, eds. *Basic & Clinical Pharmacology.* 12th ed. New York, NY: McGraw-Hill; 2012:543–564.
3. Holstege CP, Borek HA. Toxidromes. *Crit Care Clin.* 2012;28:479–498.
4. Barry JD, Wills BK. Neurotoxic emergencies. *Neurol Clin.* 2011;29:539–563.
5. Wax PM, Becker CE, Curry SC. Unexpected "gas" casualties in Moscow: a medical toxicology perspective. *Ann Emerg Med.* 2003;41:700–705.
6. Krechetnikov A. Moscow theatre siege: questions remain unanswered. *BBC News Europe.* October 24, 2012. Available at: http://www.bbc.com/news/world-europe-20067384 February 26, 2014.
7. Leung R. Terror in Moscow. *CBS News.* October 24, 2003. Available at: http://www.cbsnews.com/news/terror-in-moscow/ February 26, 2014.
8. Finogenov and Others v. Russia. *European Court of Human Rights.* April 06, 2012. Available at: http://hudoc.echr.coe.int/sites/eng/pages/search.aspx?i=001-108231 April 27, 2014.
9. Miller J, Broad W. Hostage drama in Moscow: the toxic agent; US suspects opiate in gas in Russia raid. *New York Times.* October 10, 2009.
10. Russia names Moscow siege gas. *BBC News World Edition.* October 31, 2002. Available at: http://news.bbc.co.uk/2/hi/europe/2377563.stm February 26, 2014.
11. Riches TR, Read RW, Black RM, et al. Analysis of clothing and urine from Moscow theatre siege casualties reveals carfentanil and remifentanil use. *J Anal Toxicol.* 2012;36(9):647–656.
12. Enserink M, Stone R. Questions swirl over knockout gas used in hostage crisis. *Science.* 2002;298(5596):1150–1151.
13. Committee for an Assessment of Non-Lethal Weapons Science and Technology, National Research Council. *An Assessment of Non-Lethal Weapons Science and Technology.* Washington, DC: National Academies Press; 2003.
14. Lakoski J, Murray J, Bosseau W, et al. *The Advantages and Limitations of Calmatives for Use as a Non-Lethal Technique.* Penn State College of Medicine Applied Research Laboratory; 2000.
15. Wheelis M. "Nonlethal" chemical weapons: a Faustian bargain. *Iss Sci Technol.* 2003;74–78.
16. Higgins MJ, Asbury AJ, Brodie MJ. Inhaled nebulized fentanyl for postoperative analgesia. *Anaesthesia.* 1991;46:973–976.
17. Worsley MH, Macleod AD, Brodie MJ, Asbury AJ, Clark C. Inhaled fentanyl as a method of analgesia. *Anesthesia.* 1990;45:449–451.
18. Merlin MA, Saybolt MT, Kapitanyan R, et al. Intranasal naloxone delivery is an alternative to intravenous naloxone for opioid overdoses. *Am J Emerg Med.* 2010;28:296–303.

119 CHAPTER

Hydrofluoric Acid Mass Casualty Incident

Paul P. Rega

DESCRIPTION OF EVENT

On October 30, 1987, in Texas City, Texas, part of a hydrofluoric alkylation heater was accidentally dropped from a crane. This resulted in the shearing of two relief valves of a storage tank and the ultimate release of 40,000 to 53,000 pounds of anhydrous hydrogen fluoride (HF) and a couple of hundred barrels (approximately 6000 pounds) of isobutane. A toxic cloud spread across certain residential areas of the community.[1,2]

Within 20 minutes local citizens living within a radius of 0.8 km of the plant were forced to evacuate. Eventually the evacuation zone was expanded to a five-square-mile area. Ultimately 41,000 residents living in an area encompassing 200 city blocks were forced to evacuate for approximately 2 days.[3]

A study of the victims of the incident revealed that nearly 1000 people (845 nonhospitalized and 94 hospitalized) sought care at one of two local hospitals. As one might expect from a hazardous materials (Haz-Mat) airborne release of an acidic compound the predominant topical manifestations were, in order of decreasing frequency, ocular irritation, pharyngeal burning, headache, dyspnea (17% of all cases were hypoxemic), chest pain, cough, nausea and vomiting, dizziness, skin burning, and rash. In addition, 16.3% of the patients were mildly hypocalcemic (7.5 to 8.4 mg/dL); antidotes consisting of calcium gluconate and calcium chloride were administered.[2]

The additional complication of hypocalcemia demonstrates that exposure to HF or hydrofluoric acid is not a typical toxic chemical exposure. Its management goes beyond decontamination and supportive therapy into the realm of the efficacious utilization of antidotal therapy in all its iterations. This is particularly imperative if the exposure involved a liquid spill or an intentional attack with a high risk of dermal contact, inhalation, or both. Delay in definitive therapy could lead to more prolonged pain, chronic morbidity, or an early demise.

HF and hydrofluoric acid are unique corrosives in terms of their mechanism of action and degree of toxicity. First prepared in 1809, HF actually is a weak acid that typically can be found in both anhydrous and aqueous forms. Although not flammable, it can be explosive within a wide range of concentrations.[4] Because of the ease with which "hydrofluoric acid" and "hydrochloric acid" can be confused, the current convention is to use HF to refer to HF or to hydrofluoric acid.

HF is ubiquitous. Its inherent properties are useful to a wide assortment of industries and products, including glass etching and polishing, sand removal, environmental cleaning, fabric rust removal, stone and marble cleaning, electropolishing, ceramic manufacture, semiconductors, dyes, plastics, tanning, fireproofing, microelectronics, pesticide production, and the production of high-octane fuel.[4,5] Much of our current knowledge is based on occupational exposures to the compound in the United States and internationally.[6–8] Pure HF is a liquid with a boiling point of 19.5 °C (67.1 °F); solutions usually contain 3% to 40% HF.

Upon contact of the skin, mucous membranes, airway,[8,9] or GI tract,[4,10,11] HF, unlike other acids, does not cause initial damage via coagulation necrosis[12]; rather, it penetrates deeply like an alkali and induces liquefactive necrosis. Because it is a weak acid it has a chance to penetrate deeply into the skin before fully dissociating into hydrogen and fluoride ions; the penetration of the intact HF molecule facilitates entry of the fluoride anion into fascia, muscle, bone, and the general circulation. Thus HF exhibits not only local but also regional and systemic effects:

$$HF \leftrightarrow H^+ + F^-$$
$$2F + Ca^2 \leftrightarrow CaF_2$$
$$2F + Mg^2 \leftrightarrow MgF_2$$

After HF dissociates, the fluoride anion chelates available calcium and magnesium cations as well as manganese cations. The resultant depletion of these ions within the cell along with the rise in intracellular fluoride from diffusion from extracellular fluid disrupts cellular enzymatic activity and can also cause local pain from neuroexcitation; this pain can be exacerbated by regional ischemia secondary to calcium depletion. As hydrogen ions enter the cells potassium anions exit. Hypocalcemia, hypomagnesemia, and hyperkalemia can systemically lead to life-threatening dysrhythmias. Specifically hypocalcemia can induce tetany, seizures, myocardial dysfunction, ventricular tachycardia, and ventricular fibrillation.[4,5,8,11–16]

Morbidity and mortality from HF are dependent upon three factors:
- The concentration of the hydrofluoric solution[13,17]
- The total body surface area (TBSA) in dermal exposures
- The duration of exposure

Although unusual, even minimal exposure to a relatively low concentration of HF can have disastrous results. One worker suffered a first-degree burn of 3% of his TBSA when he was splashed on the right thigh with 20% HF. Despite receiving immediate irrigation and topical calcium gluconate gel, he developed hypocalcemia, hypomagnesemia, and hypokalemia. Following a period of bradycardia, he became asystolic 16 hours after exposure. Timely administration of calcium, magnesium, and potassium led to a successful resuscitation.[18]

HF exposure results in specific pathophysiology. H^+ causes superficial necrosis, which allows F^- to penetrate and chelate with Ca^{2+}:CaF_2. The F^- anion is rapidly absorbed into cells via nonionic diffusion. It interferes with the function of many cellular enzymes, leading to cellular hypoxia (e.g., direct cardiotoxicity), and it binds to the divalent cations: Ca and Mg.

Clinically, local pain from HF may be immediate with high HF concentrations but may be delayed for several hours after exposure to more dilute solutions. The pain is typically felt as deep, burning, severe, and unremitting. Local and regional blanching is often apparent. Local irritation of eyes, nose, mouth, and throat along with large-airway signs of coughing, hoarseness, inspiratory stridor, and wheezing occur after inhalation of HF. Irritative laryngospasm may occur. Even with burns <2.5% TBSA, hypocalcemia can develop within 1 to 2 hours.

Historically the majority of toxic exposures have involved dilute HF and only small body surface areas. Those precedents can easily promote a cloud of complacency leading to lack of preparedness should a community be faced with an accidental mass casualty incident or a deliberate attack involving high concentrations of HF. Both unintentional releases and deliberate attacks can result in dermal exposure to HF liquid and to inhalation of HF vapor or gas.

Treatment goals include the following:

- Prevention of further absorption of HF on and through body surfaces
  - Standard decontamination procedures: mechanical and dilutional
  - Copious irrigation of the affected areas (15–30)[4,5,12]
- Chemical sequestration of the fluoride ion by forming an insoluble salt in order to prevent major tissue destruction and deadly electrolyte imbalances
  - Antidotal therapy[4,12]
  - Fluid and electrolyte management

◀◀ PRE-INCIDENT ACTIONS

1. Hazard vulnerability analysis
2. Risk assessment

The first two processes may suggest that a community is at risk for an accidental or intentional HF release by reason of, for example, nearby industrial plants using HF. The threat of terrorist use of HF is largely informed by community size and the presence of important political or economic institutions or landmarks that might offer attractive targets for terrorism.

3. Mitigation
   a. Identify sources and caches of local HF suppliers.
   b. Ensure that the storage facilities are secure and meet federal, state, and local safety requirements.
4. Preparedness
   a. Determine personal protective equipment (PPE) requirements for all responders and receivers.
   b. Identify sources and amounts of calcium gluconate and chloride potentially available for use in a mass casualty incident. (Supplies of magnesium sulfate should also be considered.)
   c. Determine how quickly it would take to prepare and deliver various forms of antidotes (pharmacological consultations).
      i. Topical
      ii. Aerosol nebulizer
      iii. Parenteral
   d. Develop triage guidelines, especially in the event of antidote shortages.
   e. Using sort, assess, lifesaving interventions, treatment and/or transport (SALT) triage as a precedent, consider developing guidelines to administer HF antidotes during the initial triage process, possibly within the hot zone, and at the very minimum during the decontamination process.
   f. Develop educational content to address the unique properties of HF, its pathophysiology and clinical effects, recommended antidotes, and the various modes of antidotal administration.
      i. Within the hospital, include emergency medicine, nephrology, orthopedics, radiology, and medical-toxicology services.

g. Once training is completed develop a tabletop exercise for both prehospital and hospital personnel to test the guidelines and modify as warranted.
h. After the tabletop exercise, proceed to a functional exercise.

▶▶ POST-INCIDENT ACTIONS

1. Establish and maintain scene safety.
   a. Consider potential evacuation.
2. Identify hot, warm, and cold zones.
3. Don appropriate PPE.
4. Determine triage methodology.
   a. Simple triage and rapid treatment (START)
   b. SALT
   c. Other
5. Establish prehospital triage categories for nontraumatic HF casualties.
   a. *Red:* Victims in severe pain
      i. Antidote (parenteral, aerosol) indicated
   b. *Yellow:* Victims in moderate pain or with limited areas of TBSA contamination
      i. Antidote (parenteral, aerosol) indicated
   c. *Green:* Victims with little to no pain
      i. Antidote (topical) indicated
   d. *Black:* Absence of vital signs
      i. No antidote indicated

✚ MEDICAL TREATMENT OF CASUALTIES

Whether the incident involves a few victims or hundreds, emergency management can be disastrous unless the basic principles are taught and retained. These guidelines can be modified depending on the number of victims and the amount of resources. Therefore some basic guidelines are presented followed by treatment considerations.

1. Manifestations (summary)[5]
   a. Inhalational exposure:
      i. Ocular, nasopharyngeal, and pulmonary irritation
      ii. Tearing, coughing, stridor, and wheezing (bronchospasm)
   b. Dermal exposure:
      i. Immediate pain: Concentrations usually greater than 50%
      ii. Delayed pain:
         (1) 1 to 12 hours after exposure
         (2) Redness, swelling, blanching
         (3) Pain
   c. Ingestion:
      i. Unlikely in a mass casualty incident

As always, the ABCs (i.e., airway, breathing, and circulation) take precedence once medical personnel have taken appropriate personal safety measures.[5] In tandem with that, cardiac and electrolyte monitoring is crucial.[5]

1. Consider hypocalcemia, hypomagnesemia, and hyperkalemia in the following HF exposures and initiate appropriate monitoring:
   a. >1% TBSA with >50% [HF]
   b. >5% TBSA with any [HF]
   c. Vapor inhalation with >60% [HF]
   d. In all instances of inhalation, ingestion, or in burns >25 square inches of skin
   Note: Ventricular fibrillation has been reported with dermal exposure of between 2.5% and 22% TBSA.[12]

2. Pain may be the best guide in determining triage priorities and allocation of antidotal resources. If the pain (which is described as

"incredibly intense") is immediate, assume an exposure to an HF concentration of at least 50%.[4,12] Should pain develop within minutes to hours of exposure, assume the HF concentration to have been between 20% and 50%. If pain develops between 12 and 24 hours after exposure, assume an HF concentration of <20%.[12] Therefore an awake and alert mass casualty incident victim with no pain may be triaged and decontaminated, but the immediate administration of antidotes may be considered premature and wasteful.

3. Specific therapies
  a. Topical[17,19,20]
    i. Calcium gluconate powder: 3.5 g in 150 mL of sterile water-soluble lubricant[4,12]
    ii. Calcium gluconate 10% solution: 25 mL in 75 mL of sterile water-soluble lubricant[4,12]
      (1) Notes:
        (a) Calcium chloride, calcium hypochlorite, and benzalkonium chloride are alternative topical treatments if calcium gluconate is unavailable.[4,12]
          (i) Dressings soaked in a solution of effervescent tablets of 20 g calcium in 2 L of water have been suggested if nothing else is available.
        (b) The gel will not penetrate intact skin well or be absorbed through a nail.
          (i) Dimethyl sulfoxide (DMSO) has been used anecdotally to mitigate this problem, but there are no controlled studies[5,21,22] and there are concerns about its toxicity.[4]
        (c) Topical hexafluorine is used in Europe, but it is neither well studied in the United States nor approved for use.[4]
        (d) Pain should be relieved within 30 minutes of an intense period (approximately 10 to 15 minutes) of massage. If there is no relief or if the pain recurs the application may be repeated or more aggressive therapy may be instituted.
        (e) Ocular exposure:
          (i) Normal saline: Copious irrigation for 30 minutes
          (ii) Use 1% calcium gluconate irrigation solution (50 mL of 10% calcium gluconate in 500 mL of normal saline)
            [1] Irrigation should continue for at least 30 minutes[4]
            [2] Efficacy is not fully established[5]
          (iii) Short-term care: 1% calcium gluconate drops every 2 to 3 hours for several days
          (iv) Ophthalmological consult[5]
  b. Subcutaneous or intradermal: Usually reserved for large (>160 cm²) areas, more severe exposures, or refractory pain[20]
    i. Using a 30 gauge needle, inject a 5% calcium gluconate solution (10% standard concentration diluted 1:1 with normal saline) in and around the burned area[4,12]
      (1) Use 0.5 to 1.0 mL of the solution per square centimeter of skin and no more than 0.5 mL per digit
      (2) Notes:
        (a) Diminution of pain indicates successful therapy
        (b) The limit on the injection amount is to avoid pain and vascular compromise.
        (c) Calcium chloride should not be used[5]
        (d) With fingertip injuries the nail may need to be removed in order to inject the nailbed[20,23]

        (e) Iontophoresis has been shown to be efficacious experimentally and may even be more effective than topical or parenteral delivery systems[24]
  c. Regional (indicated for extensive extremity burns, especially those of the hands or feet)
    i. Intraarterial[12,23,25–27]
      (1) Consult with interventional radiology
        (a) Consider possible digital subtraction arteriography
      (2) Infuse 10 mL of 10% calcium gluconate in 40 mL of normal saline over 2 to 4 hours.
        (a) Avoid calcium chloride
          (i) Calcium solutions may induce serious skin necrosis should extravasation occur[5,12]
      (3) Regional intravenous with Bier block[4,12,22,28]
      (4) Consider orthopedic consultation
      (5) Infuse 10 mL of calcium gluconate 10% in 30 to 40 mL of normal saline over 2 to 4 hours
        (a) Calcium chloride is not recommended[5]
    ii. Nebulization: Inhalational exposure[4,5,9,19]
      (1) Use 1.5 mL (10% calcium gluconate) in 4.5 mL of normal saline.
      (2) Use 2.5% nebulized solution
      (3) Use of 5% nebulized solution is also recommended
    iii. Steroids may be beneficial for inhalational exposure
    iv. Hemodialysis[29–33]
    v. Early consultation with nephrology
      (1) High concentrations of HF, significant TBSA affected, or a severe clinical deterioration
    vi. Use fluorine-free water if possible

💡 UNIQUE CONSIDERATIONS

An HF exposure secondary to an industrial or transportation mishap or due to an intentional release should be considered *prima facie* evidence that the HF concentration will be high. This assumption will be supported by conscious victims who are crying out in pain or by atraumatic victims with no obvious signs of life. Scientific studies on human tissue explants have indicated that the explants are completely penetrated by HF within only 5 minutes of contact.[13] In addition, ventricular fibrillation and death with dermal exposures as limited as 2.5% of TBSA have been reported. Death has also been reported within 30 minutes of inhalation of 70% HF.

In a mass casualty incident it may be reasonable and possibly lifesaving to mitigate the development of symptomatic hypocalcemia before and at hospital arrival by empirically administering prophylactic calcium gluconate 10% (0.2 to 0.4 mL/kg) or calcium chloride 10% (0.1 to 0.2 mL/kg) intravenously[5,14] or even by nebulizer as mentioned above (nebulizers achieve good systemic absorption).[4,5,9,19] These may be the safest prophylactic routes when a low serum calcium level is suspected but not proven. However, when the signs of hypocalcemia are present, the intraosseous route may also be utilized (intramuscular administration of calcium is too damaging to soft tissue). Bear in mind that 10 mL of calcium gluconate contains 90 mg elemental calcium and that the equivalent amount of calcium chloride contains 272 mg elemental calcium.

Reliance on detection of a prolonged QT interval from low serum ionized calcium or of peaked T waves from hyperkalemia may be difficult in a prehospital setting, but cardiac monitoring should be instituted on arrival at the hospital.

Establishing intravenous access when feasible or at least administering a calcium gluconate aerosol may buy time for multiple patients while blood is being drawn and ECG leads are being applied.

Meanwhile in the hospital, patients can be individually evaluated for pain, location of burns, and additional antidotal therapy by one or more routes. In addition, each person must undergo continuous cardiac monitoring to look for QT prolongation or peaked T waves. Each patient should also have hourly determinations of serum calcium, potassium, and magnesium until symptoms have peaked. Other recommended laboratory studies include tests of liver and renal function and coagulation studies.[4]

⚠ PITFALLS

Pitfalls specific to HF include but are not limited to the following:

- Underrecognition in the hospital vulnerability analysis (HVA) and in prehospital and hospital planning of potential risks from HF in the nearby community
- Lack of development and review of specific HF guidelines[4]
- Failure to educate, train, and drill prehospital and hospital staff on the unique aspects of HF
- Confusion of HF with hydrochloric acid
- Failure to recognize the possible delayed onset of HF signs and symptoms
- Underappreciation of the potential systemic effects of HF
- Not setting up a decontamination area early
- Not establishing continuous cardiac monitoring and frequent monitoring of electrolytes[4]
- Failure to retrieve and replenish sufficient caches of antidote for rapid administration
- Delay in notifying the local poison control center, medical toxicology, nephrology, respiratory care, pathology (lab), cardiology, and pharmacy
- Failure to consider alternative medications, such as magnesium sulfate, as an alternative to calcium when calcium stockpiles are insufficient[34]
- Delay in administering antidote in order to await laboratory confirmation of electrolyte imbalances

REFERENCES

1. Dayal HH, Brodwick M, Morris R, et al. A community-based epidemiologic study of health sequelae of exposure to hydrofluoric acid. *Ann Epidemiol.* 1992;2(3):213–230.
2. Wing JS, Brender JD, Sanderson LM, Perrotta DM, Beauchamp RA. Acute health effects in a community after a release of hydrofluoric acid. *Arch Environ Health.* 1991;46(3):155–160.
3. Dayal HH, Baranowski T, Li YH, Morris R. Hazardous chemicals: psychological dimensions of the health sequelae of a community exposure in Texas. *J Epidemiol Community Health.* 1994;48(6):560–568.
4. Harchelroad FP Jr, Rottinghaus DM. Chemical burns. In: Tintinalli JE, Stapczynski J, Ma O, Cline DM, Cydulka RK, Meckler GD, eds. *Tintinalli's Emergency Medicine: A Comprehensive Study Guide.* 7th ed. New York, NY: McGraw-Hill; 2011. Chapter 211, http://0-accessmedicine.mhmedical.com.carlson.utoledo.edu/content.aspx?bookid=348&Sectionid=40381693. Accessed January 23, 2014.
5. Ly BT. Hydrogen fluoride and hydrofluoric acid. In: Olson KR, ed. *Poisoning & Drug Overdose.* 6th ed. New York: McGraw-Hill; 2012. Chapter 81, http://0-accessmedicine.mhmedical.com.carlson.utoledo.edu/content.aspx?bookid=391&Sectionid=42069895. Accessed January 23, 2014.
6. Blodgett DW, Suruda AJ, Crouch BI. Case report: fatal unintentional occupational poisonings by hydrofluoric acid in the U.S. *Am J Ind Med.* 2001;40:215–220.
7. Wu ML, Yang CC, Ger J, Tsai WJ, Deng JF. Acute hydrofluoric acid exposure reported to Taiwan Poison Control Center, 1991-2010. *Hum Exp Toxicol.* 2013 Jul 25, Epub ahead of print.
8. Dote T, Kono K, Usuda K, et al. Lethal inhalation exposure during maintenance operation of a hydrogen fluoride liquefying tank. *Toxicol Ind Health.* 2003;19(2–6):51–54.
9. Tsonis L, Hantsch-Bardsley C, Gamelli RL. Hydrofluoric acid inhalation injury. *J Burn Care Res.* 2008;29(5):852–855. http://dx.doi.org/10.1097/BCR.0b013e3181848b7a.
10. Kao WF, Dart RC, Kuffner E, Bogdan G. Ingestion of low-concentration hydrofluoric acid: an insidious and potentially fatal poisoning. *Ann Emerg Med.* 1999;34(1):35–41.
11. Stremski ES, Grande GA, Ling LJ. Survival following hydrofluoric acid ingestion. *Ann Emerg Med.* 1992;21(11):1396–1399.
12. Bouchard NC, Carter WA. Caustics. In: Tintinalli JE, Stapczynski J, Ma O, Cline DM, Cydulka RK, Meckler GD, eds. *Tintinalli's Emergency Medicine: A Comprehensive Study Guide.* 7th ed. New York: McGraw-Hill; 2011. Chapter 194, http://0accessmedicine.mhmedical.com.carlson.utoledo.edu/content.aspx?bookid=348&Sectionid=40381675. Accessed January 23, 2014.
13. Burgher F, Mathieu L, Elian Lati E, et al. Experimental 70% hydrofluoric acid burns: histological observations in an established human skin explants *ex vivo* model. *Cutan Ocul Toxicol.* 2011;30(2):100–107.
14. Sanz-Gallén P, Nogué S, Munné P, Faraldo A. Hypocalcaemia and hypomagnesaemia due to hydrofluoric acid. *Occup Med (Lond).* 2001;51(4):294–295.
15. Caravati EM. Acute hydrofluoric acid exposure. *Am J Emerg Med.* 1988;6:143–150.
16. Dünser MW, Öhlbauer M, Rieder J, et al. Critical care management of major hydrofluoric acid burns: a case report, review of literature, and recommendations for therapy. *Burns.* 2004;30:391–398.
17. Dalamaga M, Karmaniolas K, Nikolaidou A, Papadavid E. Hypocalcemia, hypomagnesemia, and hypokalemia following hydrofluoric acid chemical injury. *J Burn Care Res.* 2008;29(3):541–543.
18. Wu ML, Deng JF, Fan JS. Survival after hypocalcemia, hypomagnesemia, hypokalemia and cardiac arrest following mild hydrofluoric acid burn. *Clin Toxicol (Phila).* 2010;48(9):953–955.
19. Kono K, Watanabe T, Dote T, et al. Successful treatments of lung injury and skin burn due to hydrofluoric acid exposure. *Int Arch Occup Environ Health.* 2000;73(Suppl):S93–S97.
20. Ohata U, Hara H, Suzuki H. 7 cases of hydrofluoric acid burn in which calcium gluconate was effective for relief of severe pain. *Contact Dermatitis.* 2005;52(3):133–137.
21. Hatzifotis M, Williams A, Muller M, Sotoude H, Mirfazaelian H. Hydrofluoric acid burns. *Burns.* 2004;30(2):156–159.
22. Zhang Y, Wang X, Ye C, et al. The clinical effectiveness of the intravenous infusion of calcium gluconate for treatment of hydrofluoric acid burn of distal limbs. *Burns.* 2014;40:e26–e30. http://dx.doi.org/10.1016/j.burns.2013.12.003.
23. Vance MV, Curry SC, Kunkel DB, Ryan PJ, Ruggeri SB. Digital hydrofluoric acid burns: treatment with intraarterial calcium infusion. *Ann Emerg Med.* 1986;15(8):890–896.
24. Yamashita M, Yamashita M, Suzuki M, Hirai H, Kajigaya H. Iontophoretic delivery of calcium for experimental hydrofluoric acid burns. *Crit Care Med.* 2001;29(8):1575–1578.
25. Capitani EM, Hirano ES, Zuim Ide S, et al. Finger burns caused by concentrated hydrofluoric acid, treated with intra-arterial calcium gluconate infusion: case report. *Sao Paulo Med J.* 2009;127(6):379–381.
26. Zhang Y, Ni L, Wang X, et al. Clinical arterial infusion of calcium gluconate: the preferred method for treating hydrofluoric acid burns of distal human limbs. *Int J Occup Med Environ Health.* 2014 Jan 24, Epub ahead of print.
27. Lin TM, Tsai CC, Lin SD, Lai CS. Continuous intra-arterial infusion therapy in hydrofluoric acid burns. *J Occup Environ Med.* 2000;42(9):892–897.
28. Graudins A, Burns MJ, Aaron CK. Regional intravenous infusion of calcium gluconate for hydrofluoric acid burns of the upper extremity. *Ann Emerg Med.* 1997;30(5):604–607.
29. Björnhagen V, Höjer J, Karlson-Stiber C, Seldén AI, Sundbom M. Hydrofluoric acid-induced burns and life-threatening systemic poisoning—favorable outcome after hemodialysis: case report. *J Toxicol Clin Toxicol.* 2003;41(6):855–860.

30. Antar-Shultz M, Rifkin SI, McFarren C. Use of hemodialysis after ingestion of a mixture of acids containing hydrofluoric acid. *Int J Clin Pharmacol.* 2011;11:695–699.

31. Berman L, Taves D, Mitra S, Newmark K. Inorganic fluoride poisoning: treatment by hemodialysis. *N Engl J Med.* 1973;289(17):922.

32. Yolken R, Konecny P, McCarthy P. Acute fluoride poisoning. *Pediatrics.* 1976;58:90–93.

33. Usuda K, Kono K, Watanabe T, et al. Hemodialyzability of ionizable fluoride in hemodialysis session. *Sci Total Environ.* 2002;297:183–191.

34. Williams JM, Hammad A, Cottington EC, Harchelroad FC. Intravenous magnesium in the treatment of hydrofluoric acid burns in rats. *Ann Emerg Med.* 1994;23(3):464–469.

CHAPTER 120

Mass Casualties from Riot-Control Agents

Sam Shen and Stephen P. Wood

DESCRIPTION OF EVENT

Riot-control agents are commonly known as "tear gas," irritants, harassing agents, and lacrimators. These agents are used by the military for training purposes and by law enforcement officers for riot control. The North Atlantic Treaty Organization (NATO) has assigned these compounds two-letter codes. The agents include 1-chloroacetophenone (NATO code, CN), *o*-chlorobenzylidene malononitrile (CS), bromobenzylcyanide (CA), and dibenz (b,f)-1:4-oxazepine (CR). Oleoresin capsicum (OC), an oily extract of the capsaicin found in pepper plants, is also used by law enforcement officers. It is often mixed with CN in products for personal protection. Because of their long chemical names, the agents are generally referred to by their NATO codes, except for OC, which is often called pepper spray. These compounds are similar in the following respects[1]:

- Production of sensory irritation causing severe discomfort
- Quick onset of action
- Short duration of effects after exposure
- High safety profile (ratio of lethal to effective dose)

Diphenylaminearsine, or Adamsite (DM), an agent used for riot control, differs in several aspects from CA, CS, and CR[1]:

- Its onset of action is delayed for several minutes after exposure.
- It produces nausea, vomiting, diarrhea, abdominal cramping, and other systemic effects (including headache and depression), in addition to the mucosal irritation characteristic of the other riot-control agents.
- It produces effects on the skin that are less severe compared with those caused by the other agents.

Although not considered riot-control agents by definition, there are recent reports of the use of the opiates carfentanil and remifentanil in an aerosolized form. They were believed to have been used in one rescue operation to free hostages taken in a kidnapping. However, suboptimal prehospital medical care contributed to the deaths of many of the hostages extracted from the release site.[2] There have been no other documented uses of opioids in either crowd or riot control in other events.

When properly used, conventional riot agents can cause extreme discomfort and temporarily disable the victim.[3] Because of their high safety profile, riot-control agents constitute an attractive option for incapacitation by military and law enforcement personnel. They are sometimes called nonlethal or less-lethal agents because the intent behind their use is to incapacitate rather than to produce serious injury or death and because of their high safety ratios; however, sufficiently high doses can prove fatal.

The first agent to be used widely was CN, which was developed in 1871. In about 1912, ethyl bromoacetate was used to control riots in Paris.[1] As Mace, CN was also subsequently marketed for personal protection. Subsequent agents were developed that produced similar results but possessed better safety profiles, higher potencies, or both.[4] CS is potent but of low toxicity.[4] Introduced for common civil use in 1967, it is now the agent most commonly used.[5,6] CA was developed toward the end of World War I, but it is rarely used now. CR, the newest compound in this class, is also the most potent, but it has a high safety profile and such low volatility that its effects deep in the lungs are minimal.[1] Even though DM is primarily a vomiting agent, it will be discussed further as a riot-control agent because of its similar effects and management steps.

Riot-control agents are solids ("tear gas" is a misnomer), and they can be dispersed as fine droplets or particles or in solution. They may be combined with an explosive substance in grenades or released as a smoke of particles from handheld devices; solutions may also be sprayed.[7,8] Effects are from direct contact with the skin, eyes, or mucous membranes and from inhalation.

EFFECTS OF RIOT-CONTROL AGENTS

Riot-control agents are nonlethal when used properly. Reports of death are infrequent and are usually secondary to toxic pulmonary damage leading to pulmonary edema and acute respiratory distress syndrome (ARDS), including acute lung injury (ALI).[3] Symptoms usually occur within a minute of exposure and last approximately 30 minutes.[7] These agents usually have minimal long-term effects.[6] The predominant systems affected are the eyes, nose, lungs, and skin.[4]

Eyes

The eyes are extremely sensitive to irritants. Exposure to an agent will produce an intense burning sensation leading to tearing, blepharospasm, photophobia, periorbital edema, and conjunctival injection.[7,9,10] The victim will subsequently close his or her eyes reflexively. Although the vision of the victim will be near normal, the blepharospasm will hinder the ability of the victim to see. Most of these effects disappear in 20 minutes, although conjunctivitis may persist for 24 hours.[4] In addition to the sensory effects, the ejection of the agent particles can cause blunt trauma to the cornea, and small particles can be embedded in the tissue of the eye.

Nose

If riot-control agents make contact with the mucous membranes of the nose, they will produce rhinorrhea, sneezing, and burning.[4,9]

Lungs

One of the more serious effects of riot-control agents involves the airways. In addition to a burning sensation, irritation of the bronchial lining can produce bronchoconstriction, coughing, and dyspnea. Effects from higher doses include chemical pneumonitis and, in particularly high doses, pulmonary edema, manifesting as ALI.[3] The agents can also worsen underlying lung disease such as asthma or chronic obstructive pulmonary disease.[3]

Because of reported deaths in custody patients who had been exposed to OC, many of whom had been restrained, pulmonary function testing was studied in normal subjects given OC or placebo to inhale. OC does not result in abnormal spirometry, hypoxemia, or hypoventilation in the sitting or the prone-maximal restraint position.[11]

Skin

If riot-control agents make contact with the skin, they will produce erythema and a burning or tingling sensation.[3] Prolonged exposure can produce vesicles and burns similar to thermal burns. These symptoms are exacerbated in hot or humid weather, as well as when the agent on the skin is not removed by brushing, rinsing, or washing.[3]

Metabolic System

Some studies have suggested that CS can be metabolized to cyanide in peripheral tissues.[3,12] However, the risk of cyanide toxicity from inhalational exposure to CS appears to be minimal.[1]

Gastrointestinal System

Exposure can produce nausea, vomiting, and diarrhea.[3] DM is the riot-control agent responsible for predominantly gastrointestinal symptoms, in addition to mucosal irritation.

Pregnancy

One animal study showed no significant effects from CS on pregnancy.[3,9]

LABORATORY INVESTIGATION

There is typically no indication for laboratory testing or for any imaging. Evaluation of the eye with fluorescein may be indicated if there is concern for subsequent corneal abrasions or foreign bodies. Chromatography has been utilized to detect the metabolites of CS, but the utility of this is limited to forensic applications.[13]

PRE-INCIDENT ACTION

The effects of riot-control agents are usually self-limiting. Therefore, victims often will not seek medical care initially. Victims may seek assistance if symptoms persist or if complications develop. Emergency-medicine physicians should wear impermeable gloves and goggles to avoid exposure to the agents before treating casualties.[4,7] Facilities should be prepared for the disrobing and showering of patients before they enter the emergency department.[9]

It is important that providers potentially on the scene of riot-control-agent use are knowledgeable about the effects of various agents and the initial care of exposed victims, as well as the use of personal protective equipment including respirators ("gas masks" in military parlance).[14] Providers should know how to properly don and use respirators to protect themselves against these agents. Many agencies are now providing personal respirators to emergency medical technicians (EMTs) and paramedics for this purpose. Ongoing training including practical application is important to maintain this skill set.

POST-INCIDENT ACTION

Because the agents are released into the air, evacuation is important to eliminate further exposure. Therefore, victims must be advised to do the following[15]:

- Immediately leave the scene where riot-control agents were released.
- Move upwind if possible, to an area where fresh air is available.
- Move to higher ground because riot-control agents can linger as dense, low-lying clouds.

MEDICAL TREATMENT OF CASUALTIES

There is no antidote for riot-control agents. Their effects are self-limiting and usually last no more than 15 to 30 minutes; however, erythema of the skin may persist longer.[1] Medical management consists primarily of supportive care for each affected system. Initially, it is important to decrease any possible further contact with the agents through the following decontamination methods[15]:

- Remove clothing that may have agent particles on it. Do not pull clothing over the victim's head. Instead, clothing should be cut off to minimize potential further contact.
- The victim should be washed with copious amounts of soap and water, even though wetting of the skin may temporarily increase the severity of the burning sensation from CS and OC.

The specific management steps are directed to each system affected.

Eyes

Empirical data suggest that the first step should involve blowing dry air into the eyes with a fan to help the dissolved agents to vaporize.[7,16] This should be followed by irrigation of the eyes with cold water or saline. If irrigation is performed before drying the eyes, it can prolong the burning sensation in the eyes. A Morgan Lens can be used effectively to deliver irrigation to both eyes simultaneously. Although 5% sodium bisulfite was once recommended for treatment of exposure, its use is no longer advised.[17] A careful slit-lamp examination should be performed to evaluate for corneal impaction injuries secondary to the blast of the agent particles. If a corneal injury is present, any visible foreign bodies should be removed, and topical antibiotics should be prescribed.

Airway

There is at least one case report of a victim of CS experiencing significant laryngeal and vocal-cord edema resulting in airway obstruction. This case described edema of the vocal folds and distal bronchial structures, and these effects were prolonged, lasting upward of 21 days.[18] There is also one case study of an anesthesiologist who experienced symptoms after extubating a patient exposed to CS. The patient also exhibited significant laryngeal spasm and edema that necessitated reintubation.[19]

Lungs

The most serious complications occur in the lungs. Initially, humidified oxygen can provide relief. Inhaled beta-2 agonists may be given for dyspnea and bronchospasm.[7] Because the clinical onset of pulmonary edema can be delayed, patients should be admitted for observation. Victims should also be admitted if they have respiratory complaints or underlying lung disease.[3]

Skin

Any solid powder or smoke particles should be gently brushed from the skin. After copious irrigation with soap and water (a measure that may be briefly painful), burns should be treated the same as any other types of burns. If dermatitis or erythema persists, topical steroids or antipruritic agents may be applied.[3,7]

UNIQUE CONSIDERATIONS

Riot-control agents are fast-acting compounds that cause significant discomfort but are nonlethal when used properly. Whereas other chemical agents may cause worsening of symptoms over time, symptoms of riot-control agents often recede with time. Death is rare, and, when it occurs, it usually ensues from pulmonary complications. Typically, symptoms will improve over time without long-term sequelae; thus supportive care is the main treatment.

PITFALLS

Several potential pitfalls exist in treating injuries involving riot-control agents. These include the following:
- Failure to evacuate victims from the area of exposure.
- Failure to remove clothing or any materials that may have been exposed to the agents from the victims.
- Failure to blow dry eyes before irrigating them with water or saline after exposure.
- Failure to brush affected skin before washing with soap and water to eliminate further exposure.
- Use of bleach for skin decontamination.[20]
- Failure to admit patients with respiratory symptoms or underlying lung disease.
- Failure to decontaminate any patient with riot-control agent contamination before loading the patient onto a medical helicopter; the spread of such agents around the cockpit during flight could affect the pilot and endanger the lives of the patient and crew.

REFERENCES

1. Sidell F. *Riot Control Agents. Medical Aspects of Chemical and Biological Warfare.* Borden Institute, Walter Reed Army Medical Center Office of the Surgeon General, U.S. Army U.S. Army Medical Dept. Center and School, U.S. Army Medical Research and Material Command Uniformed Services University of the Health Sciences; 1997, 307-324.
2. Riches JR, Read RW, Black RM, Cooper NJ, Timperley CM. Analysis of clothing and urine from Moscow theatre siege casualties reveals carfentanil and remifentanil use. *J Anal Toxicol.* 2012;36(9):647–656. http://dx.doi.org/10.1093/jat/bks078, Epub Sep 20, 2012.
3. Hu H, Fine J, Epstein P, Kelsey K, Reynolds P, Walker B. Tear gas: harassing agent or toxic chemical weapon? *JAMA.* 1989;262:660–663.
4. Beswick FW. Chemical agents used in riot control and warfare. *Hum Toxicol.* 1983;2:247–256.
5. Kalman SM. Riot control agents. Introduction. *Fed Proc.* 1971;30(1):84–85.
6. Karagama YG, Newton JR, Newbegin CJ. Short-term and long-term physical effects of exposure to CS spray. *J R Soc Med.* 2003;96:172–174.
7. Yih J-P. CS gas injury to the eye. *BMJ.* 1995;311:276.
8. Smith J. The use of chemical incapacitant sprays: a review. *J Trauma.* 2002;52:595–600.
9. Sanford JP. Medical aspects of riot control (harassing) agents. *Ann Rev Med.* 1976;27:421–429.
10. Schep L, Slaughter R, McBride D. Riot control agents: the tear gases CN, CS and OC—a medical review. *J R Army Med Corps.* 2013. http://dx.doi.org/10.1136/jramc-2013-000165, Epub ahead of print.
11. Cucunell SA, Swentzel KC, Biskup R, et al. Biochemical interactions and metabolic fate of riot control agents. *Fed Proc.* 1971;30:86–91.
12. U.S. Army Medical Research Institute of Chemical Defense. *Riot control agents. Medical Management of Chemical Casualties Handbook.* 2nd ed Aberdeen Proving Ground, MD: Medical Research Institute of Chemical Defense; 1995.
13. Riches JR, Read RW, Black RM, et al. The development of an analytical method for urinary metabolites of the riot control agent 2-chlorobenzylidene malononitrile (CS). *J Chromatogr B Analyt Technol Biomed Life Sci.* 2013;928:125–130. http://dx.doi.org/10.1016/j.jchromb.2013.03.029, Epub Mar 30, 2013.
14. Hout JJ, Kluchinsky T, LaPuma PT, White DW. Evaluation of CS (o-chlorobenzylidene malononitrile) concentrations during U.S. Army mask confidence training. *J Environ Health.* 2011;74(3):18–21.
15. Lee BH, Knopp R, Richardson ML. Treatment of exposure to chemical personal protection agents. *Ann Emerg Med.* 1984;13:487–488.
16. Svinos H. Towards evidence-based emergency medicine: best BETs from the Manchester Royal Infirmary. BET 1: the best treatment for eye irritation caused by CS spray. *Emerg Med J.* 2011;28(10):898. http://dx.doi.org/10.1136/emermed-2011-200635.
17. Harrison JM, Inch TD. A novel rearrangement of the adduct from CS-epoxide and dioxin-2-hydroperoxide. *Tetrahedron Lett.* 1981;22:679–682.
18. Karaman E, Erturan S, Duman C, Yaman M, Duman GU. Acute laryngeal and bronchial obstruction after CS (o-chlorobenzylidenemalononitrile) gas inhalation. *Eur Arch Otorhinolaryngol.* 2009;266(2):301–304. http://dx.doi.org/10.1007/s00405-008-0653-5, Epub Mar 26, 2008.
19. Davey A, Moppett IK. Postoperative complications after CS spray exposure. *Anaesthesia.* 2004;59(12):1219–1220.
20. Chan TC, Vilke GM, Clausen J, et al. The effect of oleoresin capsicum "pepper spray" inhalation on respiratory function. *J Forensic Sci.* 2002;47:299–304.

Cholinergic Agent Attack (Nicotine, Epibatidine, and Anatoxin-a)

Sage W. Wiener and Lewis S. Nelson

DESCRIPTION OF EVENT

Nicotine has long been recognized as a toxin acting as a direct agonist at the nicotinic family of acetylcholine receptors (a family in fact defined by the affinity for nicotine). These receptors are present at the neuromuscular junction (NMJ), in both sympathetic and parasympathetic ganglia, and in the central nervous system (CNS).[1]

More recently recognized nicotinic acetylcholine receptor agonists include epibatidine and anatoxin-a.[1-3] Epibatidine is derived from the skin of the *Epibatobades* frog (a species of "poison dart" frogs) and has been studied as an analgesic that acts through incompletely understood central nicotinic cholinergic pathways.[4] Anatoxin-a is found in species from several genera of cyanobacteria (formerly known as blue-green algae).[3] It should not be confused with *amatoxin*, a cyclopeptide RNA polymerase inhibitor found in several hepatotoxic mushrooms, or with *anatoxin-a(s)*, a cyanobacterial toxin that acts purely as a cholinesterase inhibitor with prominent muscarinic effects (the *s* refers to the *salivation* caused from excess acetylcholine at muscarinic receptors).

Anatoxin-a and epibatidine differ from nicotine primarily in potency. The LD_{50} (the dose required to kill 50% of those exposed) of anatoxin-a is 200 to 250 µg/kg body weight (mouse, intraperitoneally),[3] and the LD_{50} of epibatidine (rat, intravenously) is less than 125 nmol/kg.[5] By comparison a lethal dose of nicotine has traditionally been estimated to be between 0.5 and 1.0 mg/kg in humans.[6] However, the true lethal dose may be as much as 10-fold higher.[7] Epibatidine is also more specific than nicotine at the ganglionic and CNS subtypes of nicotinic receptor and does not act directly at the NMJ, although neuromuscular paralysis can be seen clinically.[1] Another difference between these agents is that in vitro, epibatidine appears to have some agonist action at muscarinic acetylcholine receptors as well.[8] It is unclear, however, whether muscarinic effects would be seen clinically after human exposure. In animals epibatidine also causes a pronounced antinociceptive effect not blocked by naloxone and at only slightly higher doses hypertension, apnea, seizures, and death ensue.

Although nicotine may never have been developed as a chemical weapon by any government, it has a long history of use in human poisoning and has been weaponized more than once by domestic and international criminals. The earliest known malicious use of nicotine was the murder of Gustave Fougnies in 1850, a case notable at that time because no one had yet been able to detect plant alkaloids in blood or human tissues.[9] In 1997 Thomas Leahy was found to possess ricin and botulinum toxins as well as a spray bottle filled with nicotine sulfate dissolved in dimethyl sulfoxide (DMSO, an organic solvent). Because his intent with the other agents was difficult to prove, he was initially charged and convicted only for the weaponization of the nicotine sulfate, although he subsequently pled guilty to the other charges.[10] In 2003 a disgruntled former meat cutter poisoned ground beef with Black Leaf 40, a widely available pesticide containing 40% nicotine. The meat tested contained 300 mg/kg of nicotine, making approximately one-third pound a potentially lethal dose. Ninety-two people were ultimately determined to have been poisoned by the beef.[6] In 2011 Anders Behring Breivik, a Norwegian right-wing extremist and mass murderer, claimed to have obtained 99% pure liquid nicotine from a Chinese online supplier; he discussed in his manifesto his intent to inject several drops of the liquid nicotine into hollow-point rifle bullets to turn them into lethal chemical weapons.[11] Neither epibatidine nor anatoxin-a is known to have been developed for state, terrorist-group, or individual use.

The potential for the use of nicotine in a chemical attack is highlighted by its many possible means of delivery and routes of absorption. Nicotine freebase is an oily liquid but is relatively unstable in air. Nicotine salts, however, are solids that are readily dissolved in water or organic solvents. Therefore these salts could potentially be dispersed as an aerosol of liquid or powder. Nicotine can be absorbed transdermally, as evidenced by "green tobacco sickness." In this illness acute nicotine toxicity occurs in those who harvest wet tobacco without protection for their skin.[12] Nicotine patches for smoking cessation take advantage of this route. Clearly if nicotine were suspended in a solvent with good dermal penetration (DMSO, for example) and then aerosolized, the potential for systemic toxicity from dermal exposure would be great. The nicotine liquid used in e-cigarettes is an example of such a solution, and it is widely available in concentrations up to about 10%.[13] The solvent in these solutions is typically glycerin or propylene glycol. Nicotine is also stable to pyrolysis and may be absorbed through inhalation, as occurs with tobacco smoking. Nicotine is absorbed transmucosally (e.g., chewing tobacco) and is orally bioavailable if swallowed, and numerous case series exist of children with nicotine toxicity from oral exposure to tobacco products.[14-22] Much less is known about the absorption and bioavailability of epibatidine and anatoxin-a through different routes. Epibatidine is available as an off-white powder and is soluble in organic solvents including alcohol. Anatoxin-a is a light brown solid that is soluble in water. Anatoxin-a appears to be capable of causing illness through ingestion in animal models.[23] Few data exist regarding the oral bioavailability of epibatidine or the inhalational absorption of either toxin. One feature of anatoxin-a that might make it ill-suited to chemical terrorism is that it is susceptible to photolysis, rapidly breaking down in the presence of sunlight.[24] Thus, although an incident involving contamination of food is possible, an incident involving outdoor dispersion of an aerosol seems extremely unlikely.

The clinical effects of nicotinic poisoning depend in part on the route of absorption. Most data have been gathered in the context of exposure through ingestion, in which significant nausea and vomiting are early features. In one review of 143 children with symptoms after ingestion of cigarettes or cigarette butts 99% (138 children) vomited; 74% (104 children) did so within 20 minutes.[14] Data suggest that ingestion of liquid nicotine preparations for e-cigarettes is increasingly common and will likely soon surpass cases of cigarette ingestion. Calls to poison centers involving e-cigarettes are more likely to be associated with adverse health effects than calls about cigarettes.[25] A 10-year-old child who ingested "a small amount" of a combination preparation of nicotine and methylsalicylate developed vomiting, tachycardia, grunting respirations, and truncal ataxia.[26] Clinical features of toxicity associated with ingestion also occur from dermal absorption but may not be the first sign of exposure. Other early findings include dizziness and dyspnea. In one reported case of dermal exposure dizziness, dyspnea, "unsteadiness," and nausea occurred within 30 minutes.[27] Flushing and pallor of the skin have both been reported after nicotine exposure, and diaphoresis may be present as well.[15,16,18] Cardiac effects include both hypertension and hypotension as well as palpitations and dysrhythmias ranging from sinus bradycardia and tachycardia to sino-atrial block, atrial fibrillation, and asystole.[14,16-18,20,21] These seemingly contradictory effects are better understood when one considers that the effects of nicotine on the autonomic nervous system are mediated through its action at both sympathetic and also parasympathetic ganglia. Which effects predominate in any individual patient can be difficult to predict. Nicotine also acts as a depolarizing neuromuscular blocker at the NMJ.[1] Thus early muscle spasms and fasciculations may occur, followed by weakness, hypotonia, and even flaccid paralysis.[14,16,17] Nicotinic cholinergic agonism in the CNS leads to seizures and altered mental status. In children both lethargy and irritability have been reported after tobacco ingestion.[14-18,20] Patients with less severe poisoning may present with headache or dizziness.[14,15,19] Seizures are uncommon in typical cases of cigarette ingestion and when present suggest a more severe exposure.[14] Severe exposures can lead to permanent neurological devastation.[28] Although the lethal dose has traditionally been reported as 50 to 60 mg for an adult (LD_{50} of 0.8 mg/kg), it has recently become clear that this number is somewhat arbitrary and based on few data. The true lethal dose may be as much as 10 times higher, although substantial morbidity may occur with much lower doses.[7]

Little is known about clinical findings in humans after poisoning with epibatidine because there are no reported cases. One 17-year-old boy is thought to have died of anatoxin-a poisoning and another boy was sickened, but the cases were reported only in the lay press, so details of their presentations are limited; the boy who died "went into shock and had a seizure before his heart failed," and the surviving boy had severe diarrhea and abdominal pain.[29] Because of the greater potency of epibatidine and anatoxin-a, patients with a significant exposure would presumably clinically resemble those with severe nicotine toxicity. If epibatidine were used it is possible that muscarinic findings would be present as well, which would make the distinction from nerve-agent poisoning even more challenging. However, sudden collapse from epibatidine or anatoxin-a may occur before either muscarinic or nicotinic signs can manifest themselves.

⏪ PRE-INCIDENT ACTIONS

Disaster planning and education are the most important pre-incident actions that can be taken in preparation for an attack involving cholinergic agents. Coordination between the U.S. Department of Agriculture, the Food and Drug Administration, and law enforcement and counterterrorism agencies is likely to facilitate early detection of incidents involving food and water contamination. Syndromic surveillance of emergency department triage complaints may also play a role because food and water contamination may initially appear as gastrointestinal (GI) illness. Although atropine is already stockpiled in many

hospitals because of preparations for nerve agent attack this measure is unlikely to be helpful because muscarinic effects will be inconsequential in most patients. Other than basic preparedness for chemical terrorism, such as personal protective equipment and decontamination facilities, no specific physical infrastructure or supplies are required in the hospital for preparation for a nicotinic agonist attack.

Technology originally developed for workplace monitoring exists for detection of small amounts of nicotine in the air.[30] It is also possible to test water supplies for cyanobacteria,[3] and anatoxin-a can be detected by gas chromatography with an electron-capture detector.[31] In the future it may be possible to deploy chemical detectors in strategic sampling locations to provide early warning of a chemical attack.

⏩ POST-INCIDENT ACTIONS

The most important actions after a nicotinic agent attack (besides rescue and care of exposed patients) are prompt notification of the appropriate authorities and decontamination of affected areas. This differs little from the response to other types of chemical attacks. If anatoxin is known to have been the agent involved, maximizing exposure of the involved area to sunlight will help to rapidly destroy the toxin; anatoxin-a spontaneously degrades in direct sunlight, with a half-life of approximately 1 hour.[24]

✚ MEDICAL TREATMENT OF CASUALTIES

Although nicotinic cholinergic antagonists exist, there are no clinical data on their use in human poisoning with nicotinic agents. In addition, of the ganglionic blockers, hexamethonium and trimethaphan are not available for clinical use, and mecamylamine is available in tablet form only, making it unsuitable for use in an emergency. Furthermore nicotinic cholinergic antagonists at the NMJ are not useful to treat paralysis because they are themselves paralytic agents. There is thus no useful antidote to nicotine or nicotinic agonist exposure, and supportive care is the mainstay of therapy.

As in most chemical-attack scenarios, rapid removal of at least visibly affected clothing and of agent visible on the skin (local, or "spot," decontamination) is crucial to prevent continued absorption and should be accomplished in concert with attention to airway, breathing, and circulation. Patients without a secure airway or who need ventilatory support need these interventions at approximately the same time that local decontamination is being done and before full-body disrobing and decontamination. Mouth-to-mouth ventilation should never be performed because it can pose risks to the rescuer, particularly after a GI exposure.[32] For full-body decontamination, removal of the patient's clothes, shoes, belt, watch, and jewelry should be followed by irrigation of the skin with copious amounts of water with or without soap (soap may be useful for oily substances, such as nicotine freebase or any of these agents dissolved in an organic solvent). Reactive Skin Decontamination Lotion is stocked by some hospitals as a decontaminant for spot decontamination of nerve-agent casualties and is superior to most other decontaminants for that purpose, but it has not been evaluated for efficacy against nicotinic compounds.

Hemodynamic support should include intravenous fluid boluses followed by vasoconstrictors, such as norepinephrine, as needed to treat hypotension. Therapy for hypertension should be approached with caution because hemodynamic collapse may be precipitous.[33] In the absence of end-organ effects of severe hypertension, pharmacological intervention should probably be avoided. Dysrhythmias should be managed according to the usual practice. Seizures should be treated with benzodiazepines or barbiturates. Other anticonvulsants are unlikely to be helpful and are not indicated. Vomiting should be managed with antiemetics, and oral activated charcoal should be administered, particularly after GI exposures.[34] Because nicotine exhibits a certain degree of enteroenteric circulation, oral activated charcoal, even after dermal or inhalational exposure, may be beneficial.[33]

Suspected cases should be reported to the regional poison control center. Poison control centers can recognize developing epidemics, assist with patient management, and help contact other health and law enforcement authorities in the event of an attack. Because symptoms occur early after exposure, minimal observation is required for patients who present with no clinical abnormalities.

Poisoning by a nicotinic agonist may be difficult to distinguish from nerve-agent poisoning, and it is possible that patients exposed to these agents might conceivably be treated in the field with autoinjectors containing atropine and pralidoxime. Antidote Treatment Nerve Agent Autoinjector (ATNAA) is such an autoinjector available for military use, and DuoDote is the civilian counterpart. If possible, autoinjectors that combine different antidotes in a fixed ratio, such as atropine and pralidoxime, should be used cautiously, particularly after the initial phase of therapy. Although there may be some role for atropine in patients with bradydysrhythmias, bronchorrhea, or other severe muscarinic symptoms, there is no role for pralidoxime, an oxime cholinesterase reactivator. In fact aggressive oxime therapy may do more harm than good because pralidoxime is itself a weak cholinesterase inhibitor with the potential to cause cholinergic excess. Similarly in patients with nerve agent exposure, in which muscarinic effects are likely to be limited, overdosing with atropine while attempting to administer sufficient pralidoxime may lead to anticholinergic toxicity.

❓ UNIQUE CONSIDERATIONS

The most notable feature of nicotinic agonist poisoning is its similarity to poisoning by cholinesterase inhibitors, such as organophosphate pesticides and nerve agents. Enhanced parasympathetic outflow (with resulting muscarinic effects) due to ganglionic stimulation may further confuse the clinical findings and mimic organophosphate poisoning. Without identification of the product at the scene it is unlikely that this distinction will be possible in the event of a chemical attack. Failure to respond to atropine and oximes (or worsening of symptoms with oxime therapy) may be the only clue. Because there is no specific therapy for nicotinic agonist poisoning, chemical attacks with these agents are otherwise managed as are any generic chemical exposure; good decontamination and supportive care is the only therapy needed.

⚠ PITFALLS

Several potential pitfalls exist in responding to a cholinergic agent attack. These include the following:

- During disaster planning and provider education, failure to consider the possibility of nicotinic agonists as mass casualty chemical agents
- Failure to consider a chemical attack with a nicotinic agonist after an epidemic of a GI illness
- Misdiagnosis of nicotinic agonist poisoning as poisoning by organophosphate pesticides or nerve agents
- Administration of atropine therapy to patients with nicotinic agonist poisoning and with no significant muscarinic signs or symptoms
- Administration of oxime therapy to patients with nicotinic agonist poisoning
- Failure to involve public health and law enforcement authorities when a chemical attack is suspected
- Failure to call the regional poison control center to report cases and to get assistance with management

REFERENCES

1. Hoffman BB, Taylor P. Neurotransmission. In: Hardman JG, Limbird LE, Gilman AG, eds. *Goodman & Gilman's The Pharmacological Basis of Therapeutics.* 10th ed. New York, NY: McGraw-Hill Medical Publishing Division; 2001:115–153.
2. Rupniak NM, Patel S, Marwood R, et al. Antinociceptive and toxic effects of (+) epibatidine oxalate attributable to nicotinic agonist activity. *Br J Pharmacol.* 1994;113:1487–1493.
3. Hitzfeld BC, Höger SJ, Dietrich DR. Cyanobacterial toxins: removal during drinking water treatment, and human risk assessment. *Environ Health Perspect.* 2000;108:113–122.
4. Dukat M, Glennon RA. Epibatidine: impact on nicotinic receptor research. *Cell Mol Neurobiol.* 2003;23:365–378.
5. Kassiou M, Bottlaender M, Loc'h C, et al. Pharmacological evaluation of a Br-76 analog of epibatidine: a potent ligand for studying brain nicotinic acetylcholine receptors. *Synapse.* 2002;45:95–104.
6. Boulton M, Stanbury M, Wade D, et al. Nicotine poisoning after ingestion of contaminated ground beef. *MMWR Morb Mortal Wkly Rep.* 2003;52:413–416.
7. Mayer B. How much nicotine kills a human? Tracing back the generally accepted lethal dose to dubious self-experiments in the nineteenth century. *Arch Toxicol.* 2014;88:5–7.
8. Kommalage M, Hoglund AU. (+/−) Epibatidine increases acetylcholine release partly through an action on muscarinic receptors. *Pharmacol Toxicol.* 2004;94:238–244.
9. Blum D. Nicotine and the chemistry of murder. Wired Science Blogs/Elemental 5/25/2012. Available at: http://www.wired.com/2012/05/nicotine-and-the-chemistry-of-murder/. Accessed 23.04.14.
10. Threat of Bioterrorism in America. *Statement for the Record of Robert M. Burnham, Chief, Domestic Terrorism Section before the United States House of Representatives Subcommittee on Oversight and Investigations.* May 20, 1999, Available at: http://www.fas.org/irp/congress/1999_hr/990520-bioleg3.htm.
11. Msnbc.com news services. "Did Norway shooter inject bullets with poison? NBC News. Available at: http://www.nbcnews.com/id/43902300/ns/world_news-europe/t/did-norway-shooter-inject-bullets-poison/#.U2-gwC-Gc5g. Accessed 12.05.14.
12. Ballard T, Ehlers J, Freund E, Auslander M, Brandt V, Halperin W. Green tobacco sickness: occupational nicotine poisoning in tobacco workers. *Arch Environ Health.* 1995;50:384–389.
13. Richtel M. E-cigarettes spawn poison sold by barrel. *New York Times.* Available at: www.nytimes.com/2014/03/24/business/selling-a-poison-by-the-barrel-liquid-nicotine-for-ecigarettes.html. Accessed 23.03.14.
14. McGee D, Brabson T, McCarthy J, Picciotti M. Four-year review of cigarette ingestions in children. *Pediatr Emerg Care.* 1995;11:13–16.
15. Lewander W, Wine H, Carnevale R, et al. Ingestion of cigarettes and cigarette butts by children—Rhode Island, January 1994-July 1996. *MMWR Morb Mortal Wkly Rep.* 1997;46:125–128.
16. Smolinske SC, Spoerke DG, Spiller SK, Wruk KM, Kulig K, Rumack BH. Cigarette and nicotine chewing gum toxicity in children. *Human Toxicol.* 1988;7:27–31.
17. Oberst BB, McIntyre RA. Acute nicotine poisoning. *Pediatrics.* 1953;11:338–340.
18. Mensch AR, Holden M. Nicotine overdose after a single piece of nicotine gum. *Chest.* 1984;86:801–802.
19. Haruda F. "Hip-pocket" sign in the diagnosis of nicotine poisoning. *Pediatrics.* 1989;84:196.
20. Malizia E, Andreucci G, Alfani F, Smeriglio M, Nicholai P. Acute intoxication with nicotine alkaloids and cannabinoids in children from ingestion of cigarettes. *Human Toxicol.* 1983;2:315–316.
21. Petridou E, Polychronopoulou A, Kouri N, Karpathios T, Trichopoulos D. Childhood poisoning from ingestion of cigarettes. *Lancet.* 1995;346:1296–1297.
22. Sisselman SG, Mofenson HC, Caraccio TR. Childhood poisoning from ingestion of cigarettes. *Lancet.* 1996;347:200–201.
23. Stevens DK, Krieger RI. Effect of route of exposure and repeated doses on the acute toxicity in mice of the cyanobacterial nicotinic alkaloid anatoxin-a. *Toxicon.* 1991;29:134–138.

24. Stevens DK, Krieger RI. Stability studies on the cyanobacterial nicotinic alkaloid anatoxin-a. *Toxicon.* 1991;29:134–138.

25. Chatham-Stevens K, Law R, Taylor E, et al. Notes from the field: calls to poison centers for exposures to electronic cigarettes—United States, September 2010-February 2014. *MMWR Morb Mortal Wkly Rep.* 2014;63:292–293.

26. Bassett RA, Osterhoudt K, Brabazon T. Nicotine poisoning in an infant. *N Engl J Med.* May 7, 2014. EPub ahead of print Available at: http://www.nejm.org/doi/full/10.1056/NEJMc1403843.

27. Davies P, Levy S, Pahari A, Martinez D. Acute nicotine poisoning associated with a traditional remedy for eczema. *Arch Dis Childhood.* 2001;85:500–502.

28. Rogers AJ, Denk LD, Wax PM. Catastrophic brain injury after nicotine insecticide ingestion. *J Emerg Med.* 2004;26:169–172.

29. Behm D. Coroner cites algae in teen's death. *Milwaukee Journal Sentinel.* September 6, 2003. Available at: Accessed 23.04.14. http://www.whoi.edu/science/B/redtide/notedevents/bluegreen/bluegreen_9-5-03.html

30. Pendergrass SM, Krake AM, Jaycox LB. Development of a versatile method for the detection of nicotine in air. *AIHAJ.* 2000;61:469–472.

31. Stevens DK, Krieger RI. Analysis of anatoxin-a by GC/ECD. *J Anal Toxicol.* 1988;12:126–131.

32. Koksal N, Buyukbese MA, Guven A, Cetinkaya A, Hasanoglu HC. Organophosphate intoxication as a consequence of mouth-to-mouth breathing from an affected case. *Chest.* 2002;122:740–741.

33. Soghoian S. Nicotine. In: Nelson LS, Lewin NA, Howland MA, et al. *Goldfrank's Toxicologic Emergencies.* 9th ed. New York, NY: McGraw-Hill Medical Publishing Division; 2010:1185–1190.

34. Geller RJ, Singleton KL, Tarantino ML, Drenzek CL, Toomey KE. Nosocomial poisoning associated with emergency department treatment of organophosphate toxicity—Georgia, 2000. *J Toxicol Clin Toxicol.* 2001;39:109–111.

Anesthetic-Agent Mass Casualty Incident

Kinjal N. Sethuraman, Jerrilyn Jones, and K. Sophia Dyer

DESCRIPTION OF EVENT

The 1830s saw the first use of Ether, the earliest anesthetic agent, for sedation and pain control in the United States.[1] Today, ether and various other anesthetics such as chloroform and cyclopropane are no longer in use because of the danger of explosion and the potential for fatal consequences. Initially, they were replaced by nonflammable agents such as halothane and nitrous oxide; however, halothane itself, because of its hepatotoxicity and cardiotoxicity, has now been largely superseded by halogenated ethers such as isoflurane, enflurane, desflurane, and sevoflurane. These drugs are typically delivered via inhalation after intravenous sedation. A major advantage of inhaled anesthetics for anesthesiologists is that the level of sedation can be rapidly modified to remain within the therapeutic window and to achieve desired analgesia, amnesia, muscle relaxation, and paralysis.[2]

Anesthetic agents are not known to have been used on the battlefield or by terrorists; however, the Nord-Ost siege in Russia in October 2002 brought the topic of anesthetic agents as potential mass casualty weapons into sharp focus.[3–5] A "knockout gas," bluish-gray in color and with a sweet taste, was used by the Russian army to incapacitate Chechnyan hostage-takers while elite Spetsnaz forces attempted to rescue 800 hostages in a Moscow theater.[6] While the exact composition of the gas or aerosol remains a state secret, it has been speculated that the gas contained halothane or another anesthetic agent mixed with an opioid compound (see Chapter 118).[7,8] Analysis of clothing and urine samples from casualties of the event revealed the use of carfentanil and remifentanil, which are both synthetic opiates.[9] A total of 127 hostages, including several children, died from the agent or agents, which were reportedly released for more than 20 minutes at an unknown concentration. The pre-incident health of some of the victims may have led to the high mortality rate, but some hostages had virtually no response to the agents.[7] Hospitals that received victims of the attack were allegedly not informed of the compounds used and thus had to experiment with reversal agents.[8,10] As television footage shows, many affected hostages removed from the theater were placed onto the ground or onto buses in positions that risked airway compromise, which underscores the necessity of attention to airway and breathing in these casualties quite apart from considerations of specific antidotal treatment.[7] It is still unclear whether or to what extent a volatile anesthetic gas was used in the formulation employed by the Spetsnaz unit.

Although newer anesthetic gases are relatively safe, older agents have several properties that could make them appealing for criminal purposes:
- Ease of availability
- Portability
- Volatility
- Ease of mass dissemination
- Rapid onset of action
- Ineffective warning properties
- Potential to incapacitate or kill
- Possible use of a remote trigger
- Novelty to first responders

In this chapter, we will focus on some of the more common agents. If a terrorist attack occurs with any agent, first responders need to be well prepared. The response team must act quickly to triage, evacuate, and attend to airway and breathing in affected casualties and to determine which agent or agents were used, the method of distribution, and the approximate dose received. The odor, taste, color, signs, and symptoms will vary by agent. Therefore interviewing victims can be helpful in identifying the gas or gases used. As these agents share significant inhalational hazards with a quick onset of action, they could pose a hazard both to original victims and to first responders.

CHARACTERISTIC PROPERTIES OF POTENTIAL TERROR AGENTS

The physicochemical properties and effects of the agents to be discussed in this chapter illustrate the diversity of the many compounds that have been used as inhalational anesthetics. Clinicians should always be aware of potential interactions from combinations of agents, as may have occurred in the Moscow theater incident. Attention to presenting symptoms, descriptions by victims, and information from hazardous materials specialists can aid in clarification of the chemical used.

Victims of inhaled anesthetic agents will experience confusion, relaxation, dizziness, drowsiness, and various respiratory symptoms that can include choking, a burning sensation in the mouth or nose, and respiratory distress. Agents that are less soluble in water, such as nitrous oxide, will stealthily cause delayed effects in the smaller, peripheral airways but less pronounced skin, mucous membrane, or central airway damage.[11]

The mean alveolar concentration (MAC) is used as a measure of the strength of an anesthetic. It represents the *minimal* concentration necessary to cause unresponsiveness in 50% of the general population.[12] Simply put, the higher the MAC, the less potent the gas. The MAC is influenced by many factors including age, comorbidities and metabolism, preexposure vital signs, and the use of the agent in combination with another anesthetic or analgesic agent.[2] The solubility of an anesthetic in blood is described by the blood-gas partition coefficient (BGPC), a unitless ratio of the concentration of the agent in blood to the concentration in gas in contact with that blood when the partial pressure in both compartments is equal. The lower the BGPC, the faster the onset of an anesthetic and the faster it will wear off.

Diethyl Ether

Diethyl ether ($C_4H_{10}O$) is a flammable, volatile, and colorless liquid with a sweet taste and characteristic odor.[13] It is soluble in alcohol, acetone, benzene, and chloroform. Its boiling point is 94 °F (34.5 °C). When exposed to fire or heat, ether releases carbon monoxide (CO); exposure to light causes ether to break down into flammable peroxides.[13] Ether, with a BGPC of 12, is more soluble in blood than either halothane or nitrous oxide. The MAC of ether is 2.0%. Because of the explosive nature of ether, the National Fire Protection Association has given it a flammability rating of 4, corresponding to an extreme fire hazard.[14] Although ether works well as an anesthetic, its propensity to explode prompted anesthetists to find alternative inhaled agents such as chloroform, cyclopropane, and halothane.

Anesthesia induction occurs at a concentration of 100,000 to 150,000 ppm and is maintained with 50,000 ppm.[14] Very small doses to eyes or skin can cause corneal injury and burns.[15] Toxic exposures to ethers (as with other anesthetics) can occur through inhalation, eye or skin contact, and ingestion. The effect of ether is dose-dependent. Symptoms consist of skin, eye, and mucosal irritation leading to an increase in bronchial secretions. Dizziness, drowsiness, bradycardia, hypothermia, or acute excitement may also occur. Laryngospasm, loss of consciousness, and death may result. The aftereffects of emergence from ether-induced anesthesia include nausea, vomiting, and headache.[16]

Newer ethers are halogenated and include enflurane, desflurane, and sevoflurane. They are not flammable, have fewer side effects, are efficient as anesthetic agents, and cause less end-organ damage.[1] They may be potentially used by terrorists as incapacitating agents.

Nitrous Oxide

Nitrous oxide (N_2O)[17] is a weak anesthetic (MAC of 105%) often combined with other agents to produce adequate analgesia and anesthesia. Induction and maintenance of anesthesia with nitrous oxide alone require very high concentrations of this anesthetic, and hypoxia may result if high concentrations of oxygen are not coadministered. During minor procedures, lower concentrations are used for sedation. Nitrous oxide is commonly provided in aerosol sprays, and its abuse potential is accordingly high. Prolonged use can cause peripheral nerve damage, psychosis, perceptual impairment, and hyperpyrexia.[18]

Nitrous oxide administered in high doses has been found to cause arrhythmias, malignant hyperthermia, seizures, pneumomediastinum, and subcutaneous emphysema. Nausea and vomiting are early signs of nitrous-oxide toxicity.[19]

Chloroform

Chloroform ($CHCl_3$)[19] is a colorless, volatile chlorinated hydrocarbon that is often mixed with ethanol. It has a sweet, burning taste and a pungent odor. As a byproduct of chlorination, chloroform is present in low concentrations in chlorinated water,[20] but exposure to these low concentrations is insufficient to cause anesthesia. It is also produced from the reduction of carbon tetrachloride (CCl_4) with moist iron.

Although no longer used as an anesthetic,[1] chloroform is still used as an intermediate in chemical syntheses. It is currently used as a component of polyfluorotetraethylene (PTFE, Teflon) and as a component of Freon refrigerants. Moreover, chloroform, with its relatively low MAC of 0.5%, has been widely popularized as a knockout agent to induce unconsciousness when poured onto a handkerchief or other cloth and held over the mouth and nose. Its well-known use for this purpose may make it a likely choice for terrorists for either small-scale or mass casualty use.

The toxic dose of chloroform is 7 to 25 mg/dL (0.59 to 2.1 mmol/L).[21] At inhaled concentrations of less than 1500 ppm, physical effects of dizziness, tiredness, and headache are reported; anesthesia occurs at a range of 1500 to 30,000 ppm. Chloroform causes irritation to the respiratory tract. It will cause dry mouth, sedation, confusion, and loss of consciousness within 5 to 10 minutes, and unconsciousness may last up to 30 minutes after removal from exposure. Fatalities occur after 5 to 10 minutes at doses of 25,000 ppm or greater by inhalation.[21] Often, death is sudden ("sudden sniffing death") from ventricular dysrhythmias thought to be induced by sensitization of the myocardium to catecholamines.

Death can occur from cardiac arrest and hepatic toxicity with peak elevation of hepatic enzymes 3 to 4 days after exposure and a subsequent return of liver-function tests to normal in survivors.[21] Pulmonary toxicity from intravenous injection of chloroform peaks after 3 days. Renal and hepatic toxicity may also occur from phosgene ($COCl_2$), a product of the exposure of chloroform to sunlight and air (see Chapter 114).[22] Other byproducts include hydrochloric acid (HCl), CO, inorganic chloride, and formaldehyde.[23] Pulmonary exposure to HCl and phosgene can result in bronchial pneumonia and pulmonary edema, respectively, and subsequent lung abscesses.

Victims exposed to chloroform need supportive care, including cardiac and pulmonary monitoring in an intensive care unit as clinically indicated. While there is no antidote for chloroform, liver toxicity in animals has been prevented by using N-acetylcysteine (NAC) after exposure, since chloroform and its byproducts deplete glutathione stores.[21,23] However, no studies have evaluated the use of NAC for this purpose in humans.[24]

Cyclopropane

Cyclopropane (C_3H_6) is a hydrocarbon ring that was discovered in 1882; it began to be used as an anesthetic in 1933.[1] It is extremely flammable and is thus no longer used clinically. A gas at room temperature, it is caustic to the eyes but not to the skin. At concentrations greater than 40%, cyclopropane irritates the eyes and the large airways. Its density is greater than air; if released into the environment, it will hug the ground.[15] At higher concentrations it causes nausea, disorientation, dizziness, and incoordination. If released in a closed area, cyclopropane, like all hydrocarbons, can displace oxygen and cause asphyxiation.[25]

Autopsies following accidental death after cyclopropane ingestion have showed hemorrhagic edema of the lungs.[15] Cardiac output, stroke volume, and heart rate are all affected by high concentrations of cyclopropane, but these parameters return to normal a few minutes after the agent is removed.[26] Cyclopropane causes decreases in renal blood flow and glomerular filtration rate.[27] Malignant hyperthermia from cyclopropane has been reported; it is managed with cooling and if necessary by the administration of dantrolene.[28] Cyclopropane has also been shown to alter cognitive function, especially the ability to learn, for up to a week after exposure.[29]

Halothane

Halothane ($C_2HBrClF_3$), a colorless, volatile, nonflammable liquid unique for its sweet taste and odor, continues to be used occasionally as an anesthetic, analgesic, and amnesic. With an MAC of 0.77%, it is the most potent of the currently used inhaled anesthetics.[2] The MAC is commonly reduced even further by administering an additional agent. The MAC for patients who are older, hypothermic, hypotensive, or hypoxic will be lower than that for young, healthy adults.[30] Halothane is highly soluble in both blood and fat; this behavior accounts for prolonged emergence from anesthesia with this agent.[2] When exposed to light, heat, flames, or acids, halothane will decompose into toxic substances (e.g., bromide, chlorine, and fluorine). The dose used for anesthesia ranges from 5000 to 30,000 ppm,[31] or 0.5% to 3% concentration in oxygen.[32,33]

Even if victims are exposed to less than 5000 ppm, they will show impaired manual dexterity and word-finding difficulties.

Acute exposure to this agent causes severe irritation to all exposed areas. Hypotension, dizziness, somnolence, lethargy, and changes in mental status are all possible symptoms. Exposure to halothane may lead to mild and self-limited hepatic dysfunction, to rare but life-threatening hepatic failure, to cardiac arrhythmias, and to malignant hyperthermia.[32,34,35] Liver failure from other halogenated anesthetics is less common. Long-term, chronic exposure to halothane can increase the risk of some cancers and can increase rates of spontaneous abortions and congenital abnormalities in newborns of exposed mothers.[36]

Diagnosis of halothane toxicity is based mainly on history, physical examination, and basic laboratory analyses. Attributing hepatic failure to halothane is difficult, as the clinical presentation is identical to other causes of hepatitis. An assay for halothane-related antibodies is available for experimental use but is not practical in emergency or disaster settings. Halothane metabolites can be detected in the urine up to 1 week after exposure.[32]

PRE-INCIDENT ACTIONS

Because terrorist attacks are for the most part unpredictable, emergency medical services, law-enforcement resources, and local, state, and national agencies must be prepared for any type of attack at any given time. For attacks using anesthetic agents, the focus should be on rapid access to casualties, prompt evacuation, careful attention to airway and ventilation (especially during transport and positioning), general supportive care, the identification of the agent, and, in the case of opioids, an ample supply of reversal agents (see Chapter 118). In Moscow, although the Russian military had an "antidote" (probably naloxone) to the agents used, claims were made that there were not enough medical personnel to administer the drug.[7] There are no antidotes to ether, chloroform, cyclopropane, or halothane; again, the importance of attention to airway, breathing, and circulation cannot be overemphasized.

The first military gas masks were developed as a response to the use of inhaled gases in Belgium during World War I.[3] In any given situation, appropriate respiratory protection should be worn by emergency medical services personnel, health care workers, and law enforcement personnel until the area in question has been cleared of inhalation risk. Many first responders may not have available detection equipment to identify the exact type of anesthetic gas used or even the general class of anesthetic gases used, thus making it even more important to use proper protective equipment. The typical canister respirator either with a full face piece or partial face piece will not offer protection in an atmosphere of depleted oxygen. If oxygen displacement has occurred, a supplied-air respirator (either through a tank or airline) is the only appropriate respiratory protection. Many portable sensors are available for measuring ambient oxygen concentrations, either as individual items or components in other detection equipment. Most medical first responders will not enter the actual site of release to extract casualties—that task is primarily the responsibility of HazMat response teams—and therefore would not be subject to an oxygen-deficient environment, but it is possible that some first responders might.

Several companies market canister respirators for application in event of the use of weapons of mass destruction. In general, these products are not specifically tested against many of the anesthetic agents discussed in this chapter at the time of this writing. An organic-vapor canister might trap some of these agents, with the obvious exception of the inorganic nitrous oxide. However, the effectiveness of such a canister will depend on concentration values within the acceptable range. In addition, the canister testing information should be evaluated to see whether it has been tested against the known agent. Given that such an

evaluation might be difficult to accomplish in a critical time period, a self-contained breathing apparatus offers the best protection for an unknown environment.

POST-INCIDENT ACTIONS

As with any potential exposure to an inhalational toxicant, protection of the victims from further exposure and guarding against exposure in responders is vital. If in doubt as to the type of chemical, the highest level of respiratory protection is recommended—in many cases, this is a supplied-air respirator. Because some of these products are volatile, precautions against direct flame and any equipment that could potentially generate a spark are prudent. The most important immediate actions to take are to reach victims (who may already be apneic) as soon as possible, to ensure a patent and protected airway, to support ventilation, to decrease exposure, and to provide oxygen to victims.

MEDICAL TREATMENT OF CASUALTIES

It is important to interview survivors and gather as much data as possible to determine the agent used. The volatility of anesthetic agents may decrease the utility of air samples, but such samples can help to identify other agents that may have been used in combination with the agents. It is important to consider the potential of a mixture of agents even after the identification of a specific agent. Once victims are at a hospital, laboratory studies that can be obtained relatively quickly can be helpful in the management of exposed patients. These studies include arterial blood-gas and carboxyhemoglobin determinations, liver function tests, a complete blood count, and a comprehensive metabolic panel. A chest radiograph is also useful in the setting of suspected chemical pneumonitis or pulmonary edema, although delayed-onset shortness of breath or chest tightness is usually the first indicator of incipient pulmonary edema.

PITFALLS

Several potential pitfalls exist in response to an anesthetic opioid-agent release. These include the following:

- Failure to recognize that a release has taken place
- Failure to reach potentially apneic patients as soon as possible
- Failure to attend adequately to airway, breathing, and circulation in casualties before, during, and after transport to medical treatment facilities
- Failure to notify proper local, state, national, and international agencies
- Failure to follow up on the identification of a specific nonanesthetic chemical agent by consideration of the possibility of simultaneous use of an anesthetic agent
- Failure to identify the agent or agents used
- Failure to remove igniting factors or flammable objects from scene
- Failure to use gloves and appropriate respiratory protection
- Failure to evacuate or ventilate the area
- Failure to notify hospitals
- Failure to have enough personnel available

REFERENCES

1. Vandam L. History of anesthetic practice. In: Miller RD, ed. *Anesthesia.* vol. V. Philadelphia, PA: Churchill Livingston; 2000.
2. Schwinn DA, Shafer SL. Basic principles of pharmacology related to anesthesia. In: Miller RD, ed. *Anesthesia.* vol. V. Philadelphia, PA: Churchill Livingston; 2000.

3. Gas killed hostages in raid. *CNN Website*. October 27, 2002. http://www.cnn.com/2004/WORLD/europe/02/06/russia.timeline/.
4. Moscow doctor: gas killed 116 hostages. *CBS News Website*. October 27, 2002. http://www.cbsnews.com/stories/2002/10/28/world/main527107.shtml.
5. Bismuth C, Borron S, Baud FJ, Barriot P. Chemical weapons: documented use and compounds on the horizon. *Toxicol Lett*. 2004;149:11–18.
6. Reed D. *Terror in Moscow*. HBO Documentaries; June 2004.
7. Wax PM, Becker CE, Curry SC. Unexpected "gas" casualties in Moscow: a medical toxicology perspective. *Ann Emerg Med*. 2003;41:700–705.
8. Lethal Moscow gas an opiate? *CBS News Website*. October 29, 2002. http://www.cbsnews.com/stories/2002/10/29/world/main527298.shtml.
9. Riches JR, Read RW, Black RW, Cooper NJ, Timperley CM. Analysis of clothing and urine from Moscow theatre siege casualites reveals carfentanil and remifentanil use. *J Anal Toxicol*. 2012;36:647–656.
10. Anger grows over gas tactics. *CNN Website*. October 28, 2002. http://edition.cnn.com/2002/WORLD/europe/10/28/moscow.gas/index.html.
11. Greenfield RA, Brown BR, Hutchins JB, et al. Microbiological, biological, and chemical weapons of warfare and terrorism. *Am J Med Sci*. 2002;323:326–340.
12. Marshall BE, Longenecker DE. General anesthetics. In: Hardman JG, Limbird LE, Molinoff PB, et al., eds. *Goodman and Gilman's the Pharmacological Basis of Therapeutics*. vol. IX. New York, NY: McGraw-Hill; 1996.
13. Occupational Safety and Health Administration, US Department of Labor. *Ethyl Ether: Material Data Safety Sheet*. April 27, 1999. http://www.osha.gov/SLTC/healthguidelines/ethylether/.
14. Hathaway GJ, Proctor NH, Hughes JP, et al. *Proctor and Hughes' Chemical Hazards of the Workplace*. vol. III. New York, NY: Van Nostrand Reinhold; 1991.
15. Grant WM. *Toxicology of the Eye*. Springfield, IL: Charles C Thomas; 1962.
16. Clayton G, Clayton F. *Patty's Industrial Hygiene and Toxicology*. 3rd ed. New York, NY: Wiley; 1981.
17. OSHA Health Guidelines. *Occupational Safety and Health Guideline for Nitrous Oxide*. http://www.osha.gov/SLTC/healthguidelines/nitrousoxide/recognition.html.
18. Murray MJ, Murray WJ. Nitrous oxide availability. *J Clin Pharmacol*. 1980;20:202–205.
19. Haddad K, Pearson C. Chlorinated hydrocarbons. In: Ellenhorn MJ, Barceloux DG, eds. *Medical Toxicology: Diagnosis and Treatment of Human Poisonings*. Philadelphia, PA: Saunders; 1998.
20. Rook JJ. Formation of haloforms during chlorination of natural waters. *Water Treat Exam*. 1974;23:234–243.
21. Maynard SM. Appendix D: drugs and toxins: therapeutic and toxic levels. In: Ford MD, ed. *Clinical Toxicology*. vol. 1. Philadelphia, PA: Saunders; 2001.
22. Van Dyke RA. On the fate of chloroform. *Anesthesiology*. 1969;30:264–272.
23. el-Shenawy NS, Abdel-Rahman MS. The mechanism of chloroform toxicity in isolated rat hepatocytes. *Toxicol Lett*. 1993;69:77–85.
24. Flanagan RJ, Meredith TJ. Use of N-acetylcysteine in clinical toxicology. *Am J Med*. 1991;91:131S–139S.
25. Barasch ST, Booth S, Modell JH. Hypercapnia during cyclopropane anesthesia: a case report. *Anesth Analg*. 1976;55:439–441.
26. Cullen DJ, Eger EI, Gregory GA. The cardiovascular effects of cyclopropane in man. *Anesthesiology*. 1969;31:398–406.
27. Deutsch S, Pierce EC, Vandam LD. Cyclopropane effects on renal function in man. *Anesthesiology*. 1967;28:547–558.
28. Lips FJ, Newland M, Dutton G. Malignant hyperthermia triggered by cyclopropane during cesarean section. *Anesthesiology*. 1928;56:144–146.
29. James FM. The effect of cyclopropane anesthesia without surgical operation on mental function of normal man. *Anesthesiology*. 1969;30:264–272.
30. Dale O, Brown BR. Clinical pharmacokinetics of the inhalational anesthetics. *Clin Pharmacokinet*. 1987:145–167.
31. OSHA Health Guidelines. *Occupational Safety and Health Guidelines for Halothane*. http://www.osha.gov/SLTC/healthguidelines/halothane/recognition.html.
32. *Halothane: Drugdex Drug Evaluations*. DRUGDEX® System. Greenwood Village, Colo: Thomson MICROMEDEX.
33. *Product Information: Fluothane®, Halothane (liquid for vaporization)*. Philadelphia, PA: Wyeth-Ayerst Laboratories; 1998.
34. Viitanen H, Baer G, Koivu H, Annila P. The hemodynamic and Holter-electrocardiogram changes during halothane and sevoflurane anesthesia for adenoidectomy in children aged one to three years. *Anesth Analg*. 1999;87:1423–1425.
35. Humphrey DM. *Technical Info Fluothane®, Halothane*. Philadelphia: Wyeth-Ayerst Laboratories; 2002.
36. *Material Safety Data Sheet 2-Bromo-2-Chloro-1,1,1-Trifluoroethanes*. Milwaukee, WI: Aldrich Chemical; May 1992.

123 CHAPTER

Introduction to Biological Agents and Pandemics

Alexis Kearney and Catherine Pettit

HISTORICAL PERSPECTIVE

Biological agents have been used as weapons since antiquity. In 600 BC Solon of Athens poisoned the wells of his adversaries with hellebore—a purgative herb—during the siege of Krissa. Similarly the Assyrians contaminated the wells of their enemies with rye ergot.[1-3] In the fourteenth century corpses of plague victims were hurled over walls to infect enemies, and in the seventeenth and eighteenth centuries smallpox-laden blankets were used to target Native Americans. Biological agents played a role in military offenses into the twentieth century and have been used in terrorist actions around the world.

In 1969 President Richard Nixon halted offensive biological and toxin research and production in the United States. Stockpiles of various biological agents and toxins, including *Bacillus anthracis*, botulinum toxin, and *Francisella tularensis*, were subsequently destroyed. In 1972 the United States, the United Kingdom, the USSR, and more than 100 other nations ratified the Biological Weapons Convention (BWC). The BWC prohibits the development, production, and stockpiling of weapons of mass destruction.[1,3] Despite this, during the last 40 years, multiple signatory nations have violated the pact set forth by the BWC. Additionally, there has been a rise in the use of biological agents in terrorist attacks, including the anthrax attacks in 2001, which resulted in few deaths but widespread fear.[2]

The U.S. Centers for Disease Control and Prevention have organized biological weapons into three categories (Table 123-1). Category A, or high-priority agents, include organisms that can be easily disseminated, result in high mortality, and have the potential to cause significant public panic. Anthrax, botulism, smallpox, tularemia, and the viral hemorrhagic fevers are included in category A. Category B agents, including food and water safety threats, are moderately easy to disseminate. Although mortality rates due to these agents are lower they may result in significant morbidity. Finally, category C agents are considered emerging pathogens. These agents may be adapted in the future to take full advantage of their pathogenicity, availability, and lethality.

In general, biological weapons are characterized by low visibility, high potency, and relative ease of delivery and dissemination.[4] The agents must also be easily obtained, cultured, or reproduced and be relatively stable in the environment.

SURVEILLANCE

A good surveillance system is essential to any public health effort and is recognized as the single most important factor in identifying events of global concern.[5] Historically, surveillance systems relied on manual reporting of notifiable diseases or suspicious cases from clinicians, hospitals, and laboratories. There has been a shift to focus more on automated surveillance of readily available data to improve the timeliness, sensitivity, and specificity of the system.[6] The exponential increase in social media use and availability of web-based applications has added another potential surveillance domain, which is being utilized for research and communication.

Syndromic Surveillance

In an effort to better identify and track potential outbreaks related to infectious diseases, both naturally occurring and those related to biowarfare and terrorism, public health practitioners developed surveillance systems designed to analyze routinely collected health information. Syndromic surveillance, as it has come to be known, includes a wide range of surveillance activities, from monitoring over-the-counter medication purchases to tracking discharge diagnoses from emergency departments and analyzing Internet search queries.[1,7] True syndromic surveillance monitors syndromes—or constellations of symptoms—that may represent the prodromes of biological agents or emerging epidemics.[7] It relies on the automated analysis of routinely collected data to detect aberrancies in expected trends in near real-time. This process has been streamlined with the increased availability of electronically collected and exchanged data. It is frequently used in conjunction with alternative surveillance methods and verification techniques to improve outbreak detection.

The goal of syndromic surveillance systems is to enable more timely detection of outbreaks by identifying trends before these patterns are recognized clinically and a formal diagnosis is made.[7] This allows a more rapid response, ultimately decreasing morbidity and mortality.[8] Once an outbreak is suspected public health responders must proceed with a thorough epidemiological investigation to further describe the outbreak and implement control measures.[1]

Although syndromic surveillance complements the more time-consuming and burdensome conventional surveillance systems that rely on physician and laboratory reporting, there are significant limitations, including frequent false alarms.[9] If the system is sensitive enough to detect small outbreaks, it may result in false alarms, which consume resources and make it difficult to separate true outbreaks from daily variation.[6,7,9] Additionally, the ability of a surveillance system to detect an outbreak depends on a variety of factors, including the size of the outbreak, pattern of population dispersion following exposure to the

TABLE 123-1 Bioterrorism Agents, as Categorized by the Centers for Disease Control and Prevention

CATEGORY	DEFINITION	AGENTS/DISEASES
Category A	High-priority agents include organisms that pose a risk to national security because they can be easily disseminated or transmitted from person to person, result in high mortality rates and have the potential for major public health impact, might cause public panic and social disruption, and require special action for public health preparedness.	Anthrax (*Bacillus anthracis*) Botulism (*Clostridium botulinum* toxin) Plague (*Yersinia pestis*) Smallpox (variola major) Tularemia (*Francisella tularensis*) Viral hemorrhagic fevers (e.g., Ebola, Marburg, Lassa, Machupo)
Category B	Second highest priority agents include those that are moderately easy to disseminate, result in moderate morbidity rates and low mortality rates, and require specific enhancements of the CDC's diagnostic capacity and enhanced disease surveillance.	Brucellosis (*Brucella* species) Epsilon toxin of *Clostridium perfringens* Food safety threats (e.g., *Salmonella* species, *Escherichia coli* O157:H7, *Shigella*) Glanders (*Burkholderia mallei*) Melioidosis (*Burkholderia pseudomallei*) Psittacosis (*Chlamydia psittaci*) Q fever (*Coxiella burnetii*) Ricin toxin from *Ricinus communis* (castor beans) Staphylococcal enterotoxin B Typhus fever (*Rickettsia prowazekii*) Viral encephalitis (e.g., Venezuelan equine encephalitis, eastern equine encephalitis, western equine encephalitis) Water safety threats (e.g., *Vibrio cholerae*, *Cryptosporidium parvum*)
Category C	Third highest priority agents include emerging pathogens that could be engineered for mass dissemination in the future because of availability, ease of production and dissemination, and potential for high morbidity and mortality rates and major health impact.	Emerging infectious diseases, such as Nipah virus and hantavirus

agent, and data sources and syndrome definitions used in the analysis.[8] Methods have been developed to analyze data using time and time-space relationships to take into account baseline variability; however, these methods have not been standardized across surveillance systems.[6–8] Each community utilizing syndromic surveillance must ultimately set its own threshold level for activation. These thresholds should be set using historical data, hazard vulnerability analysis, and risk-benefit calculations for each syndrome.

Environmental Surveillance

Environmental surveillance systems rely on the remote detection of aerosol clouds or point detection systems to collect and analyze data. Remote detection systems identify and analyze the components of clouds, subsequently transmitting that information to public health personnel on the ground. Point detection systems sample an environmental area using high speed particle concentration methods and rapid diagnostic modalities to detect and identify potential agents.

In 2003 the Department of Homeland Security launched BioWatch, an environmental air sampling program currently under way in more than 30 U.S. cities, with the goal of facilitating detection of specific agents that could be aerosolized and used in a biological attack.[10] Bio-Watch is intended to complement current surveillance activities at the state and local levels. However, in its current design, it is unlikely that the BioWatch system will result in more timely detection of biological agents unless there is a large-scale aerosol attack in a location monitored by BioWatch using biological agents detectable by the system.

The U.S. postal service also instituted point detection systems in high volume mail distribution hubs after the 2001 anthrax incident.

PREPAREDNESS

Since the turn of the century we have faced numerous outbreaks—both naturally occurring and intentional—that have changed the landscape of public health surveillance and preparedness. In 2001 *B. anthracis* spores were sent to various locations around the United States, resulting in 22 cases and 5 deaths.[11] This was followed by the epidemic of severe acute respiratory syndrome (SARS) in 2002, an outbreak of novel influenza A H1N1 in 2009, and in 2012 Middle East respiratory syndrome (MERS-CoV), which continues to spread. Since the anthrax attacks, a significant amount of money and resources has been poured into improving public health infrastructure. However, despite this focus, it is unclear if improvements have actually been achieved. In part this stems from conflicting goals, shifting priorities, and the lack of a clear definition of what it means to be prepared.[12,13] Ultimately reactionary response programs have less impact than hardening all hazards public health infrastructure, which has been neglected for decades.

In 2007 a diverse expert panel convened by the RAND Corporation developed the following definition of public health emergency preparedness (PHEP) in order to strengthen accountability and streamline preparedness efforts. They define PHEP as

the capability of the public health and health care systems, communities, and individuals, to prevent, protect against, quickly respond to, and recover from health emergencies, particularly those whose scale, timing, or unpredictability threatens to over-whelm routine capabilities. Preparedness involves a coordinated and continuous process of planning and implementation that relies on measuring performance and taking corrective action.[12]

The panel further argued that PHEP must cover a full range of activities, including prevention, mitigation, response, and recovery. Additionally, it must take into account not only capacity (i.e., infrastructure, trained personnel), but also capability—the ability to implement preparedness plans in real time.[12]

Large-scale public health emergencies occur infrequently; as a result, it is difficult to execute, assess, and refine preparedness plans based on experience. Furthermore there is no universally agreed upon standard of preparedness. Federal, state, and local organizations have all established their own conflicting requirements, and there are few data to support one set of standards over another.

Written assessments and exercises have frequently been used to assess preparedness. Although written assessments are easily administered to large groups of people and the data obtained are generally easier to analyze, they frequently focus on the capacity as opposed to the capabilities of a system. Although important, these factors do not ensure an effective emergency response. Exercises, in contrast, may be discussion based or operations based and generally provide a more realistic view of an organization's capability to mobilize resources and infrastructure. However, real-time exercises are rarely evaluated with standard metrics to identify and address performance gaps.[13]

Moving forward it is essential to incorporate evaluations into routine public health functions.[14] In 2009 public health practitioners in both Los Angeles and New York City embedded assessments into influenza A H1N1 vaccination campaigns.[15] As a result, invaluable information was gained about the optimal placement of points of dispensing influenza vaccines within a community and the potential for scaling up electronic immunization information systems to better track immunization progress and manage supply and distribution of vaccines in a pandemic.[16,17] Although it may be difficult to identify questions and develop research protocols in the midst of an emergency, the time between events can serve as an opportunity to engage leaders, develop template protocols, and prioritize areas for investigation.[14]

SUMMARY

Ultimately, leaders must make decisions regarding public health responses with imperfect, limited data. The information provided by surveillance systems, used in conjunction with clinical data, will ultimately help public health practitioners identify an etiologic agent. As preparedness strategies become more standardized and evidence based, our ability to respond to public health emergencies, including biological attacks, will improve. Each chapter in Section 12 will cover a specific biological agent. The authors will outline what is known about the agent currently and, from this, attempt to extrapolate how this agent might be used in a bioterrorism attack.

REFERENCES

1. Dembek ZF, Alves DA, Cieslak TJ, eds. *Medical Management of Biological Casualties Handbook*. Fort Detrick, Frederick, MD: US Army Medical Research Institute of Infectious Diseases; 2011.
2. Riedel S. Biological warfare and bioterrorism: a historical review. *BUMC Proceedings*. 2004;17:400–406.
3. Christopher GW, Ciestak TJ, Pavlin JA, Eitzen E. Biologic warfare: a historical perspective. *JAMA*. 1997;278(5):412–417.
4. Joseph B, Brown CV, Diven C, Bui E, Aziz H, Rhee P. Current concepts in the management of biologic and chemical warfare casualties. *J Trauma Acute Care Surg*. 2013;75(4):582–589.
5. Kman NE, Bachmann DJ. Biosurveillance: a review and update. *Adv Prev Med*. 2012. http://dx.doi.org/10.1155/2012/301408, Epub Jan 2, 2012.
6. Bravata DM, McDonald KM, Smith WM, et al. Systematic review: surveillance systems for early detection of bioterrorism-related diseases. *Ann Intern Med*. 2004;140(1):910–922.
7. Buehler JW, Berkelman RL, Hartley DM, Peters CJ. Syndromic surveillance and bioterrorism-related epidemics. *Emerg Infect Dis*. 2003;9(10):1197–1204.
8. Henning KJ. What is syndromic surveillance? *MMWR Morb Mortal Wkly Rep*. 2004;53(Suppl):5–11.
9. Chretien JP, Tomich NE, Gaydos JC, Kelley PW. Real-time public health surveillance for emergency preparedness. *Am J Public Health*. 2009;99 (8):1360-1363.
10. Institute of Medicine and National Research Council. *BioWatch and Public Health Surveillance: Evaluating Systems for the Early Detection of Biological Threats*. Washington, DC: The National Academies Press; 2011. Abbreviated version.
11. Kman NE, Nelson RN. Infectious agents of bioterrorism: a review for emergency physicians. *Emerg Med Clin North Am*. 2008;26:517–547.
12. Nelson C, Lurie N, Wasserman J, Zakowski S. Conceptualizing and defining public health preparedness. *Am J Public Health*. 2007;97(Suppl 1):S9–S11.
13. Nelson C, Lurie N, Wasserman J. Assessing public health emergency preparedness: concepts, tools, and challenges. *Annu Rev Public Health*. 2007;28:1–18.
14. Lurie N, Manolio T, Patterson A. Research as a part of public health emergency response. *N Engl J Med*. 2013;368(13):1251–1255.
15. Shumabukuro TT, Redd SC. Incorporating research and evaluation into pandemic influenza vaccination preparedness and response. *Emerg Infect Dis*. 2014;20(4):713–714.
16. Saha S, Dean B, Teutsch S, et al. Efficiency of points of dispensing for influenza A(H1N1)pdm09 vaccination, Los Angeles County, California, USA, 2009. *Emerg Infect Dis*. 2014;20:590–595.
17. Marcello RK, Papadouka V, Misener M, Wake E, Mandell R, Zucker JD. Distribution of pandemic influenza vaccine and reporting of doses administered, New York City, New York, USA. *Emerg Infect Dis*. 2014;20:525–531.

CHAPTER 124

Bacillus anthracis (Anthrax) Attack

Selwyn E. Mahon

DESCRIPTION OF EVENT

Bacillus anthracis is a category A bioterrorism agent that causes anthrax and tops the list of potential threat agents. In 2001, 1 week after the September 11 terrorist attacks, it was used against U.S. citizens. Powdered spores were placed in envelopes and sent through the U.S. mail to several news media offices in New York City and Florida. Three weeks later, anthrax-laced letters were sent to two Democratic U.S. senators. The letters sent to the media contained a coarse brown material, while the letters sent to the senators contained a fine powder.[1,2] Anthrax spores found in the media letters were less concentrated, but the anthrax spores in the senators' letters were very pure, sophisticated, and smaller. Tests indicated the presence of additives that reduced static electricity and made the spores lighter, more likely to hang in the air, and more easily absorbed into the lungs; in other words, weaponized-grade anthrax.

The American anthrax attacks, nicknamed "Amerithrax," resulted in infection of 22 people, including mail handlers, and five deaths from inhalation of anthrax. Dozens of buildings were contaminated with anthrax as a result of the mailings. The incident closed down mail delivery hubs and office buildings, disrupting normal activities until those areas were freed of anthrax spores. The U.S. Environmental Protection Agency spent $41.7 million to clean up government buildings in Washington, DC. One Federal Bureau of Investigation (FBI) document estimated that the total costs of the attacks exceeded $1 billion.[3] In the aftermath of this attack, the clinical and public health approach to epidemics caused by anthrax and bioterrorism in general was rewritten. Significant increases in U.S. government funding for biological warfare research and preparedness occurred. Biowarfare-related funding at the National Institute of Allergy and Infectious Diseases (NIAID) increased by $1.5 billion in 2003. In 2004 Congress passed the Project Bioshield Act, which provides $5.6 billion over a period of 10 years for the purchase of new vaccines and drugs.[4]

The United States was not the only country terrorized by anthrax letters; internationally, powdered lace letters caused panic. In October 2001 in Berlin, German Chancellor Gerhard Schröder's office was sealed off after a white powder leaked from a letter in the mailroom. In Paris, similar discoveries led to 55 people being taken to hospitals. In the United Kingdom, the Canterbury Cathedral was evacuated; in Canada, the main Parliament building was evacuated; and in Vienna, the international airport terminal was closed after questionable letters or packages were found. The Netherlands, Israel, Mexico, and Brazil also reported anthrax scares; in November 2001, a letter that tested positive for anthrax was mailed to a pediatrician in Chile.[5]

The discovery of envelopes or packages containing a "powder" creates chaos and fear, often paralyzing public health departments, hospitals, and communities with a significant potential to disrupt the economy, the national infrastructure, public confidence, or public health and safety. While the differential diagnosis of the "powder" includes ricin and other malevolent materials, few powders evoke the fear of anthrax.

Anthrax is a zoonotic disease caused by *B. anthracis*, an aerobic, nonmotile, spore-forming, gram-positive bacillus that is ubiquitous in soil. Anthrax is primarily a disease of herbivores, including sheep, cattle, goats, horses, and, less commonly, pigs. Humans usually become infected through contact with infected animals or contaminated animal products and hides. Anthrax features prominently throughout history. The first known description of anthrax (approximately 1400 BC) is in the Old Testament where it represented the fifth plague in Egypt, the killing of the Egyptian cattle. One of history's most serious anthrax outbreaks was the "Black Bane," a terrible epidemic that swept Europe in the 1600s. The "Black Bane" outbreak (named after the black eschars caused by cutaneous anthrax) killed 60,000 people and many more animals.

Anthrax was the first disease in history proven to be caused by a microbe. French bacteriologist Casimir-Joseph Davaine first observed the presence of anthrax bacilli in infected sheep's blood in 1863. In 1876 Robert Koch proved empirically that the anthrax bacillus was the etiological agent of anthrax. Around 1877, John Bell first described inhalational or pulmonary anthrax in England. "Woolsorter's disease," as it became commonly known, was one of the first recognized occupational hazards caused by a microorganism. In 1881 Louis Pasteur successfully produced a vaccine to protect livestock against anthrax, the first effective live bacterial vaccine to be developed.

Anthrax still occurs naturally and is most common in agricultural regions of Central and South America, Sub-Saharan Africa, Central and Southwestern Asia, Southern and Eastern Europe, and the Caribbean. There are 2000 to 5000 cases of anthrax worldwide, but less than five cases a year in the United States. The world's largest recorded anthrax epidemic in humans occurred during the civil war in Zimbabwe (1979-1980). More than 9400 cases (most of them cutaneous), resulting in 182 fatalities, were reported in a 2-year period. Anthrax is endemic in Zimbabwe (formerly called Rhodesia), but less than 500 cases had been reported in the 50 years before the war.[6] The dramatic increase in the number of anthrax cases in 1978 has been partly attributed to the effects of war in the country, including lack of food, which forced people to handle and eat diseased animals. Other sporadic outbreaks of anthrax occur worldwide. Human infections often result directly from contact with infected livestock or contaminated animal materials. Although several countries with endemic anthrax have implemented successful control strategies, anthrax remains a reemerging threat to public health in areas with weak health systems. Sick and dying animals are often slaughtered and brought to market quickly to mitigate economic losses, resulting in increased anthrax exposure risk while limiting livestock reporting. Contaminated meat is brought into urban areas and sold at informal meat markets that because of fiscal constraints have little to no regulation. Reemergence of anthrax infections is postulated to result from decreased public health funding and agricultural reform resulting in a shift to private ownership from collectivization.[7] These factors, coupled with limited veterinary control and the cessation of compulsory livestock vaccination, have played plausible roles in the continued incidence of human anthrax infections.

B. anthracis tops the list of potential biological warfare and bioterrorism agents. Weaponization of anthrax requires milling the spores into particles small enough to ensure that they remain suspended in the air for long periods of time. Anthrax makes an almost perfect biological weapon and has been used in that context. The microscopic spores are so small, with a spore size of approximately 1 to 2 μm, that humans are usually unable to see, smell, or taste them.

Anthrax is readily available. B. anthracis was relatively easy to obtain from commercial, academic, and government laboratories until recently, but now it is mostly obtained from natural sources since it is still endemic in many parts of the world. Anthrax is also easy to disseminate. It can be put into powders, food, or water and can be aerosolized and released quietly, without anyone knowing. Anthrax has a high mortality rate and the spores are highly resistant to drying, heat, gamma radiation, ultraviolet light, and many disinfectants. Additionally, the spores can remain dormant in the environment for up to 40 years.

Several countries have developed weaponized anthrax. Its first modern military use occurred when Scandinavian rebels supplied by Germany used anthrax with unknown results against the Imperial Russian Army in Finland in 1916.[8] During World War II, anthrax (designated at the time as Agent N) was used by the Japanese in Manchuria. In the 1940s several allied forces investigated the military application of anthrax. In 1942 British bioweapons trials severely contaminated Gruinard Island in Scotland with anthrax spores, making it a quarantine area until it was decontaminated in 1990. Weaponized anthrax was part of the U.S. stockpile before it was destroyed per presidential order in 1969. In 1978-1979 the Rhodesian government used anthrax against cattle and humans during its campaign against black rebels.

Concern about the use of anthrax spores as a biological weapon was heightened dramatically in 1979. Despite the Soviets signing the 1972 agreement to end bioweapon production, on April 2, 1979, some of the inhabitants of Sverdlovsk (now called Yekaterinburg), about 850 miles east of Moscow, were exposed to an accidental release of anthrax from a biological weapons complex located nearby. Sverdlovsk has a population of more than 1 million people; 68 people died. The first victim died 4 days after the release, and the last death occurred 6 weeks later. Extensive cleanup, vaccinations, and medical interventions managed to save about 30 of the infected victims.[9]

Subsequent evaluation of this catastrophe provided significant insight into the use of anthrax as a bioweapon. Scientists have developed models of what an anthrax attack might look like. Anthrax sprayed from a plane or truck onto a city is one likely scenario. An attack that used 2 kg of anthrax, about the size of a 5-pound bag of sugar, could infect 100,000 people or more. It is estimated that the release of 100 kg of anthrax spores in a major city could cause up to 3 million deaths, making anthrax potentially as lethal as a hydrogen bomb. The Soviet Union was known to have created and stored 100 to 200 tons of anthrax. It is estimated that Iraq had 8500 L of concentrated B. anthracis in 1991, all of which was subsequently destroyed.

Anthrax continues to be used as a weapon and to create psychological unrest. In 2012 the New York Times reported that the Pakistani Prime Minister received a postal package confirmed to contain anthrax. Currently soldiers in Afghanistan face the threat of anthrax, as Taliban commanders have claimed that homemade bombs are being loaded with anthrax. Several suspected biological weapons laboratories have been found in Afghanistan, and anthrax is endemic to the area.

Anthrax continues to invoke fear worldwide. It has been the named agent in many threats and hoaxes. It has been mentioned as the lethal agent in sophisticated weaponized delivery systems and in crude systems, for example, improvised explosive devices (IEDs) attached to anthrax-infected carcasses.

Transmission

Anthrax infection occurs by four methods: contact with broken skin, inhalation of spores, ingestion, and injection. Naturally occurring infections are due mainly to contact with infected animals or animal products, such as hides or poorly cooked meats. Historically, the number of inhaled spores required to cause infection in 50% of individuals was thought to be approximately 10,000. More recent data suggest that as few as 1 to 3 spores may be sufficient to cause disease, depending on particle size. This estimate is tempered somewhat by the observation that many hide and wool workers are exposed to high concentrations of aerosolized spores on an ongoing basis with subsequent infection occurring only in a minority of individuals. There is no person-to-person transmission of anthrax, with the exception of the cutaneous form, which can be spread by skin contact.

Virulence

The virulence of anthrax is dependent on its ability to produce three distinct proteins: lethal factor (LF), protective antigen (PA), and edema factor (EF). Edema toxin, formed when EF and PA bind, interferes with water homeostasis, causing the severe, localized edema seen in cutaneous anthrax. Edema toxin also inhibits neutrophil function, impairing the host's ability to defend itself against infection. Lethal toxin is also formed by the binding of two subunits: LF and PA. Lethal toxin is responsible for, among other things, the release of tumor necrosis factor (TNF)-alpha and interleukin B-1, which are responsible for the systemic reaction leading rapidly to death. One area of investigation has been the search for an inhibitor that can block the binding of PA with LF and EF, thus preventing the formation of lethal toxin and edema toxin.

Inhaled Anthrax

Inhaled anthrax is the most serious form of infection likely to occur after a bioterrorism event and one of the deadliest. Without treatment, only about 10% to 15% of patients with inhalation anthrax survive. Inhalational anthrax victims typically present 1 to 5 days after exposure, with a median incubation time of 4 days,[10] but cases have occurred up to 2 months after exposure to anthrax spores (thus the suggestion for prolonged prophylaxis). Inhaled anthrax does not cause a true pneumonia. Rather, the lungs act only as a portal for infection. After the inhalation of anthrax spores into the alveoli, the spores are picked up by macrophages that transport them to the mediastinal and peribronchial lymph nodes. Activated spores divide rapidly, causing hemorrhagic mediastinitis and subsequent dissemination to the rest of the body via the blood, causing toxemia and sepsis.[11] Presenting complaints are that of a nonspecific flulike illness, often including occasional nonproductive cough, fevers, chills, sweats, malaise, myalgia, and chest discomfort. Rhinorrhea is notably absent. If untreated, this prodrome can last for 48 to 72 hours, after which the patient's condition may improve before a severe and precipitous decline. Within 24 to 48 hours of the onset of respiratory disease, patients develop bacteremia, with disease progression to hemorrhagic mediastinitis, pleural effusions, and septic shock. Patients often become dyspneic and cyanotic, with increasing chest and/or abdominal pain and diaphoresis. Stridor may also be present because of obstruction of the trachea by enlarged lymph nodes. Up to 50% of patients with pulmonary anthrax develop meningitis with associated subarachnoid hemorrhages.

The detection of hemorrhagic cerebrospinal fluid with gram-positive bacilli and polymorphonuclear pleocytosis can aid in making the diagnosis.[12] Chest radiographs characteristically show a widened mediastinum with pleural effusions and relative sparing of the lung parenchyma. Computed tomography (CT) of the chest should be considered if inhalation anthrax is suspected and the diagnosis is in doubt. CT scan is more sensitive and specific for detecting mediastinal lymphadenopathy, in which there is a normal white cell count or a mild leukocytosis with a left shift.[13] The differential diagnosis of inhalational anthrax is wide and includes mycoplasma, influenza, legionella, tularemia, and psittacosis. Characteristics that differentiate anthrax from influenza and other influenza-like illnesses include the following: wide mediastinum on radiograph (70%), pleural effusion (80%), absence of rhinorrhea (only 10% of patients with anthrax infection will have rhinorrhea), absence of sore throat (found in only 20%), dyspnea (80%), and nausea and/or vomiting (80%). Before September 2001, inhalation anthrax was estimated to have a mortality rate of up to 95%. With modern antibiotics and aggressive supportive care, the mortality rate has been reduced to 55%. This reduction in mortality is attributed to prompt recognition of the disease, aggressive concomitant antimicrobial therapy, and improvements in supportive care techniques. However, in the face of a major attack, medical services will likely be overwhelmed and it will not be possible to provide intensive care for all cases. Thus, the mortality of cases will likely be higher than 55%.

Cutaneous Anthrax

Cutaneous anthrax represents 95% of background cases of anthrax in the United States. Cutaneous anthrax presents as a painless pruritic papule generally appearing the first week, but not later than 12 days after exposure, in an area of compromised skin integrity. Within 48 hours, vesicles containing a serosanguineous fluid surround the papule, with extensive associated edema. The vesicles rupture, necrose, and enlarge, forming the characteristic painless, black (hence "anthrax" from the Greek "anthracis," or coal), ulcerated lesion. Debridement of such lesions should be avoided because this may facilitate bacteremia. However, with concurrent administration of antibiotics, this prohibition does not extend to diagnostic skin biopsies, which are part of the recommended evaluation for cutaneous anthrax.[14] The eschar dries and falls off in 1 to 2 weeks, leaving little or no scar. Lymphangitis and painful lymphadenopathy associated with systemic symptoms occur in some patients. Mortality is due to systemic invasion and may be as high as 20% in those with untreated cutaneous anthrax. Even though antibiotics do not affect the course of the local eschar, they can prevent systemic infection. The differential diagnosis of cutaneous anthrax includes ecthyma gangrenosum, brown recluse spider bite, orf (parapox virus disease), and glanders. The presence of purulence suggests an etiology other than anthrax unless there is a secondary infection.

Gastrointestinal Anthrax

Gastrointestinal anthrax occurs 2 to 5 days after ingestion of poorly cooked, contaminated meat or poisoned food sources. Patients generally develop ulcers in the mouth, esophagus, terminal ileum, or cecum. Symptoms initially include nausea, vomiting, fever, and abdominal discomfort that progresses rapidly to bloody diarrhea and signs suggestive of peritonitis. Gastric ulcers with associated hematemesis, hemorrhagic mesenteric lymphadenitis, and massive ascites may also occur.[15] Gastrointestinal anthrax can mimic an acute abdomen, ascites with peritonitis, and a perforated viscus. The mortality rate of gastrointestinal

anthrax approaches 100%. It has been suggested that early aggressive therapy may reduce the mortality rate. However, the diagnosis is often overlooked until the patient's condition is already terminal.

Injectional Anthrax

Injectional (blood) is a new type of anthrax caused when contaminated heroin is injected, usually under the skin. During 2009-2010, a total of 119 (47 laboratory confirmed) drug abuse–related cases of anthrax were reported in the United Kingdom and Germany. Of the 47 patients with confirmed cases of injectional anthrax acquired during this outbreak, 19 died from the disease. In June 2012, after a 20-month gap, two new cases of injectional anthrax in heroin consumers were reported in Bavaria. Additional cases have been reported since then from Germany, Denmark, the United Kingdom, and France, leading to 26 deaths as of August 2013.[16] Between 2009 and 2010, more than 30 cases of injectional anthrax, leading to 11 deaths, were confirmed among heroin users in the United Kingdom. Severe infections of the skin and blood have been reported. Patients with injectional anthrax show severe symptoms, and death rates are high. Treatment is more effective when infections are diagnosed before they spread to the bloodstream. Investigators believe that injectional anthrax isolates likely came from the same source. The heroin that arrived in Europe was contaminated with anthrax spores at some unknown point during transport of the drug from Afghanistan, where anthrax occurs naturally.[16]

Specimen Collection and Organism Identification

Anthrax can be seen on a Gram's stain of blood. Cultures of blood, pleural fluid, and cerebrospinal fluid may be used to identify the organism in suspected cases. Surveillance cultures in exposed individuals (e.g., nasal swabs) are used as an epidemiological tool and should not be routinely obtained. If possible, cultures should be obtained prior to the initiation of antibiotic therapy, since blood can be sterilized after only one or two doses of antibiotics. The organism can be easily cultured on 5% sheep blood agar or MacConkey's agar; growth can be expected in 6 to 24 hours. Treatment, however, should be initiated on clinical grounds. Withholding treatment while waiting for culture results will lead to increased mortality.

Although initial identification of the organism can be done in a local laboratory, specialized testing must be done in certified laboratories. Environmental identification of anthrax spores at the site of an attack is improving but problematic. Many handheld identification devices are not sensitive, requiring 10,000 or more spores for detection; also, their results may be affected because of cross-reactivity between anthrax and other bacillus species. But since 2001, several rapid identification techniques have been developed, including a nucleic acid-based test that can identify as few as 10 spores within 4 hours. Autonomous detection systems (ADS) for anthrax have also been developed to help minimize anthrax exposure via mail and are being deployed in many high-speed mail-handling facilities. The system collects air surrounding mail-handling equipment and uses polymerase chain reaction (PCR) analysis to look for anthrax DNA. The system can return a result on sampled air in as little as 30 minutes, and each batch of mail is held until it is found to be anthrax-free. A positive result would cause the system to stop mail processing and isolate the potentially contaminated batch of mail.

Isolation

There are no data suggesting that person-to-person transmission of inhalational anthrax occurs; hence, patients with suspected anthrax may be hospitalized in a standard hospital room with standard universal precautions. Contact precautions should be used with patients who have cutaneous lesions because direct exposure to vesicle secretions of such lesions may result in secondary cutaneous infection.[17]

✚ MEDICAL TREATMENT OF ANTHRAX

Prior to 2001, mortality rates for patients with inhalation anthrax approached 90%. Since then, patients with inhalation anthrax have had significantly better survival due to earlier diagnosis, treatment with a combination of antimicrobials to eradicate the bacteria and inhibit toxin production, and aggressive pleural effusion management. Guidelines for therapy are subject to change and may vary at the time of an anthrax attack. This is because weaponized *B. anthracis* may be engineered to be resistant to multiple antibiotics. For specific treatment guidelines clinicians should consult their health department or the Centers for Disease Control and Prevention (CDC) website.

The approach to prevention and treatment of anthrax differs from that for other bacterial infections. The production of toxin, potential for antimicrobial drug resistance, frequent occurrence of meningitis, and presence of latent spores are all factors when selecting postexposure prophylaxis (PEP) or treatment of anthrax. In patients with inhalation anthrax, antimicrobial drug combination therapy is more likely to be curative. Patients hospitalized for anthrax should be immediately treated with a combination of broad-spectrum intravenous antimicrobial drugs pending confirmatory test results because any delay may prove fatal. Treatment should include at least three antimicrobial drugs with activity against *B. anthracis*. All should have good central nervous system penetration, at least one drug should have bactericidal activity, and at least one should be a protein synthesis inhibitor. Intravenous combination treatment should continue for at least 2 to 3 weeks (Table 124-1).

Doxycycline does not penetrate the central nervous system; therefore ciprofloxacin should be the drug of choice for central nervous system anthrax. This recommendation may be extended to all patients with inhalational anthrax, given the high rate of associated meningitis. Penicillin, cephalosporins, and trimethoprim-sulfamethoxazole should not be used for treatment because of significant drug resistance. The presence of a spore form of *B. anthracis* requires prolonged antimicrobial drug prophylaxis. Persons exposed to aerosolized *B. anthracis* are at risk for inhalation anthrax from ungerminated spores retained in their lungs after the initial exposure, hence the need to continue antimicrobial drug therapy for 60 days to clear germinating organisms. Surgical (chest tube) drainage of the recurrent, often hemorrhagic, pleural effusions has been shown to lead to quite dramatic clinical improvement and should be strongly considered.

Exposure to anthrax can also lead to cutaneous anthrax. A single oral dose of fluoroquinolone may successfully treat uncomplicated cutaneous anthrax. Ciprofloxacin, levofloxacin, moxifloxacin, and doxycycline are equivalent first-line agents.[18]

Pregnant, postpartum, and lactating women require special consideration with respect to the prevention and treatment of infectious diseases. However, given the severity of anthrax, even this unique population of women should receive the same PEP and treatment as other adults. Ciprofloxacin is preferred over doxycycline for first-line anthrax PEP for pregnant, postpartum, and lactating women. Antimicrobial drug treatment for any of these women with a clinical or laboratory diagnosis of anthrax would be the same as for other adults. Other critical care measures and procedures include hemodynamic support, mechanical ventilation, and antitoxin treatment.[19]

Similar to adults, all children believed to be exposed to aerosolized *B. anthracis* spores should receive ciprofloxacin or doxycycline (or, if pathogens are documented to be susceptible to penicillin, oral amoxicillin or phenoxymethyl penicillin may be used). A limited supply of oral suspension formulations of recommended PEP antimicrobial agents will be available, and distribution strategies will be determined by public health authorities. If oral suspensions are not readily available, directions will be given by the Food and Drug Administration (FDA) or similar

health authority on how tablets can be crushed and added to a food or liquid for those who are unable to swallow a tablet. Tetracycline-based antimicrobial agents, including doxycycline, may cause permanent tooth discoloration in children younger than 8 years if used for repeated treatment courses. Doxycycline binds less readily to calcium compared with older tetracyclines, and in some studies, doxycycline was not associated with visible teeth staining in younger children. A single 10- to 14-day course of doxycycline is not routinely associated with tooth staining. However, the benefits of preventing life-threatening anthrax infection outweigh the potential risks of injury to teeth. Similarly, although no prospective data exist on the risks of cartilage toxicity with ciprofloxacin, particularly for a 60-day course, the benefits of an extended course for prophylaxis in children outweigh the concerns for potential cartilage toxicity.[20]

Special considerations: Some experts believe that if the incidence of adverse events is equal between doxycycline and ciprofloxacin, the potential for tooth staining is less serious than the potential for long-term cartilage injury.[20] Also, liquid amoxicillin is widely more available than liquid forms of doxycycline and ciprofloxacin, so urgent susceptibility studies should be done before choosing among ciprofloxacin, doxycycline, or amoxicillin.

TABLE 124-1 Intravenous Treatment for Systemic Anthrax with Possible/Confirmed Meningitis*,†,‡		
BACTERICIDAL AGENT (E.G., FLUOROQUINOLONE)	**BACTERICIDAL AGENT (E.G., β-LACTAM)§**	**PROTEIN SYNTHESIS INHIBITOR**
Ciprofloxacin, 400 mg every 8 h	**Meropenem, 2 g every 8 h**	**Linezolid, 600 mg every 12 h**
OR	or	or
Levofloxacin, 750 mg every 24 h	Imipenem, 1 g every 6 h†	Clindamycin, 900 mg every 8 h
OR	or	or
Moxifloxacin, 400 mg every 24 h	Doripenem, 500 mg every 8 h	Rifampin, 600 mg every 12 h§
		or
		Chloramphenicol, 1 g every 6-8 h
	Alternatives for penicillin-susceptible strains	
	Penicillin G, 4 million units every 4 h	
	or	
	Ampicillin, 3 g every 6 h	

*Duration of treatment: ≥2 to 3 wk until clinical criteria for stability are met.
†Patients exposed to aerosolized spores will require prophylaxis to complete an antimicrobial drug course of 60 days from onset of illness. Systemic anthrax includes anthrax meningitis; inhalation, injection, and gastrointestinal anthrax; and cutaneous anthrax with systemic involvement, extensive edema, or lesions of the head or neck.
‡Preferred drugs are indicated in **boldface**. Alternative drugs are listed in order of preference for treatment for patients who cannot take first-line treatment or if first-line treatment is unavailable.
§For all strains, regardless of penicillin susceptibility or if susceptibility is unknown
Data from Centers for Disease Control and Prevention Expert Panel Meetings on Prevention and Treatment of Anthrax in Adults.

Vaccination

While there is a vaccine licensed to prevent anthrax, it is not typically available for the general public. Anthrax Vaccine Adsorbed (AVA) protects against cutaneous and inhalation anthrax, according to limited but well-researched evidence. The vaccine is approved for at-risk adults before exposure to anthrax. The vaccine does not contain any anthrax bacteria and cannot cause anthrax infections. Even though in some countries the vaccine is not approved for use after exposure, in an anthrax emergency, people who are exposed might be given anthrax vaccine to help prevent disease. Current recommendations for exposed individuals are three doses of anthrax vaccine over a period of 4 weeks. The vaccine should be administered subcutaneously initially (day 0), then at 2 and 4 weeks.

The Advisory Committee on Immunization Practices reviewed all safety data and concluded that AVA is safe to administer to anthrax-exposed women during pregnancy. However, in the pre–anthrax event setting, during which the risk for anthrax exposure is low, vaccination of pregnant women is not recommended. In the setting of an anthrax event that poses a high risk for exposure to aerosolized *B. anthracis* spores, pregnancy is neither a precaution nor a contraindication to vaccination. Pregnant women at risk for inhalation anthrax should receive AVA therapy regardless of pregnancy trimester. Furthermore, there is no biological reason to suggest that breast-feeding women or breast-fed infants have an increased risk for adverse events after vaccination with AVA. Therefore, breast-feeding is neither a precaution nor a contraindication to vaccination in the post–anthrax event setting.[19]

AVA is not recommended for children younger than 6 weeks. It is recommended that children older than 6 weeks get the three-dose AVA series postexposure. For children younger than 6 weeks of age, the vaccine series should be delayed until the child reaches 6 weeks of age.

Special considerations: During an emergency, the only people who should not get the vaccine after exposure are those who have had a serious allergic reaction to a previous dose of anthrax vaccine and children under the age of 6 weeks.

Antitoxin

Anthrax antitoxins are effective when given without and with antimicrobial drugs. Although anthrax antitoxin has a role in treatment for systemic anthrax, data on the optimal time to initiate it are lacking, and the opinions of expert panelists were mixed on this issue. Given that systemic anthrax has a high case-fatality rate and the risk for antitoxin treatment appears to be low, the potential benefit achieved by adding antitoxin to combination antimicrobial drug treatment outweighs the potential risk. An antitoxin should be added to combination antimicrobial drug treatment for any patient for whom there is a high level of clinical suspicion for systemic anthrax. At this time there are no major medical, operational, or logistical considerations that clearly favor the use of a specific antitoxin over another for systemic anthrax.

Treatment of Exposed Individuals

Treatment is not advocated for asymptomatic persons unless public, health, or law-enforcement authorities have ascertained that there is a risk of exposure. Ciprofloxacin 500 mg orally twice daily for 60 days and AVA vaccination are recommended. AVA boosters should be given at 6, 12, and 18 months and yearly thereafter if needed. Compliance with treatment during anthrax attacks has been found to be problematic. The majority of patients who receive prophylaxis cannot tolerate the therapy. At 30 days, as few as 40% of individuals continued their prophylactic medications (70% of high-risk exposures). Common side effects at 14 days include "severe" gastrointestinal symptoms (13% to 19%); fainting, dizziness, and lightheadedness (7% to13%); and heartburn and gastroesophageal reflux disease (8%).[21,22]

PRE-INCIDENT ACTIONS

Personal protective equipment should be available. Stockpiling of antibiotics in local or national stores and rapid distribution systems can prevent delays in PEP. Prophylactic vaccination is indicated only in individuals who will be repeatedly exposed to anthrax spores, such as those in Bioterrorism Level B laboratories; those working with animals, animal products, imported rawhides, and wool (for example wool cleaning crews and some veterinarians); and finally, some military members.

POST-INCIDENT ACTIONS

Anthrax exposures may occur with or without warning. Doctors, emergency room staff, and other frontline medical professionals may be the first to encounter a bioterrorist victim. For people known to have been exposed to anthrax but have no signs of systemic anthrax, PEP should start as soon as possible after exposure. Ciprofloxacin, levofloxacin, and doxycycline are recommended for the antimicrobial drug portion of PEP for inhalation anthrax in adults. A three-dose series of anthrax vaccine is also recommended for long-term protection following exposure to anthrax.

Clinicians should now routinely consider whether patients have been the victims of an attack by biological agents. In the 2001 anthrax attacks, several people died primarily because those treating them, quite understandably, never considered anthrax infection as a possible diagnosis. In today's bioterrorism treatment paradigm, clinicians should screen every patient and identify patients who may have been exposed to dangerous pathogens, order infection control precautions that will prevent spread to others, collect clinical information and laboratory specimens, immediately notify public health authorities, and arrange appropriate treatment and follow-up care. It is the responsibility of the treating physician to report all suspected or confirmed cases of anthrax to the local and state public health departments and laboratories as well as the local police department.

For decontamination, sporicidal solutions, such as commercially available bleach or 0.5% hypochlorite solution (a 1:10 dilution of household bleach), should be used. These substances may be corrosive to some surfaces. Dressings used for cutaneous lesions are considered a biohazard. Re-aerosolization of *B. anthracis* spores is uncommon. Cleansing of the skin, potentially contaminated clothing, and the environment may reduce the risk of acquiring cutaneous and gastrointestinal forms of disease.[23]

ANTHRAX PREVENTION

Well-timed and effective PEP can potentially save thousands of lives (Table 124-2). PEP of asymptomatic persons should ideally start as soon as possible after exposure because its effectiveness decreases with delay in implementation. To ensure adequate and continued protection, everyone exposed to aerosolized *B. anthracis* spores should receive a full 60 days of PEP antimicrobial drugs, whether they are unvaccinated, partially vaccinated, or fully vaccinated.

UNIQUE CONSIDERATIONS

Isolation of the source of infection may be valuable for public health and law enforcement officials. If, for example, an envelope is the source of infection, the source should be placed in a plastic bag. If a plastic bag is not available, the source should be covered with a sheet or other barrier. All windows in the infected building should be closed, the ventilation system should be turned off, and exposed individuals should be

TABLE 124-2 Oral Postexposure Prophylaxis for Infection with *Bacillus anthracis

ADULTS[†]	CHILDREN 1 MO OF AGE AND OLDER[†]	TERM NEWBORN INFANT (BIRTH TO 4 WK)[‡]
Ciprofloxacin, 500 mg every 12 h OR **Doxycycline, 100 mg every 12 h** OR Levofloxacin, 750 mg every 24 h OR Moxifloxacin, 400 mg every 24 h OR Clindamycin, 600 mg every 8 h	**Ciprofloxacin, 30 mg/kg/ day every 12 h (not to exceed 500 mg/dose)** OR **Doxycycline, <45 kg: 4.4 mg/kg/day every 12 h (not to exceed 100 mg/ dose) >45 kg: 100 mg/ dose every 12 h** OR Clindamycin, 30 mg/kg/day every 8 h (not to exceed 900 mg/dose) OR Levofloxacin, <50 kg: 16 mg/ kg/day every 12 h (not to exceed 250 mg/dose) >50 kg: 500 mg every 24 h	**Ciprofloxacin, 30 mg/ kg/day every 12 h** Doxycycline, 4.4 mg/kg/ day every 12 h Clindamycin, 0-1 wk of age, 15 mg/kg/day every 8 h Clindamycin, 1-4 wk of age, 20 mg/kg/day every 6 h
Alternatives for penicillin-susceptible strains Amoxicillin, 1 g every 8 h OR Penicillin VK, 500 mg every 6 h	For penicillin-susceptible strains **Amoxicillin, 75 mg/kg/day every 8 h (not to exceed 1 g/dose)** OR Penicillin VK, 50-75 mg/kg/day every 6-8 h	For penicillin-susceptible strains **Amoxicillin, 75 mg/kg/ day every 8 h Penicillin VK, 0-1 wk of age, 75 mg/kg/day every 8 h** Penicillin VK, 1-4 wk of age, 75 mg/kg/day every 6-8 h

*Preferred drugs are indicated in **boldface**. Alternative drugs are listed in order of preference for treatment for patients who cannot take first-line treatment or if first-line treatment is unavailable.
[†]Data from Centers for Disease Control and Prevention. Expert Panel Meetings on Prevention and Treatment of Anthrax in Adults.
[‡]Data from J. Bradley, G Peacock, S Krug, et al. AAP Committee on Infectious Diseases and Disaster Preparedness Advisory Council. Pediatric Anthrax Clinical Management. Pediatrics 2014;133;e1411.

instructed to remove possibly contaminated clothing and shower before presenting to the emergency department.

⚠ PITFALLS

- Failure to remain vigilant
- Failure to treat for an adequate length of time and with multidrug regimens
- Failure to consider inhalation anthrax as the cause of flulike symptoms
- Failure to notify appropriate authorities in suspected or confirmed cases of anthrax

REFERENCES

1. Letters carried fresh anthrax. *Baltimore Sun.* June 23, 2002, http://articles.baltimoresun.com/2002-06-23/news/0206230062_1_anthrax-spores-powder-leahy. Retrieved 27 September 2012.
2. Massive cross-contamination feared. *New York Daily News.* October 26, 2001, http://www.nydailynews.com/archives/news/nbc-anthrax-case-news-aide-opened-tainted-brokaw-letter-article-1.932811. Retrieved September 27, 2012.
3. Lengel A. Little progress in FBI probe of anthrax attacks. *Washington Post,* http://www.washingtonpost.com/wp-dyn/content/article/2005/09/15/AR2005091502456_pf.html. Accessed 08.04.08.
4. President Bush signs Project Bioshield Act of 2004. www.whitehouse.gov. Accessed 07.04.08.
5. Erlanger S. The powder: from Berlin to Brazil, the 'anthrax' letters. *New York Times.* October 16 2001.
6. Davies JCA. A major epidemic of anthrax in Zimbabwe. *Cent Afr J Med.* 1982;28:291–298.
7. Kracalik I, Malania L, Tsertsvadze N, et al. Human cutaneous anthrax, Georgia 2010-2012. *Emerg Infect Dis.* 2014;20(2):261–264.
8. Bisher J. During World War I, terrorists schemed to use anthrax in the cause of Finnish independence. *Mil Hist.* 2003;20:17–22.
9. Guillemin J. Anthrax: the investigation of a deadly outbreak. *N Engl J Med.* 2000;342:1373.
10. Dixon TC, Meselson M, Guillemin J, Hanna PC. Anthrax. *N Engl J Med.* 1999;341:815.
11. Inglesby TV, Henderson DA, Bartlett JG, et al. Anthrax as a biological weapon: medical and public health management. [Erratum appears in *JAMA.* 2000;283:1963]. *JAMA.* 1999;281:1735–1745.
12. Friedlander AM. Anthrax: clinical features, pathogenesis, and potential biological warfare threat. In: Remington JS, Swartz MN, eds. *Current Clinical Topics in Infectious Disease*; vol. 20:Malden, MA: Blackwell Science; 2000:335–349.
13. Jernigan DB, Raghunathan PL, Bell BP, et al. Investigation of bioterrorism-related anthrax, United States, 2001: epidemiologic findings. *Emerg Infect Dis.* 2002;8:1019–1028.
14. CDC. Update: investigation of bioterrorism-related anthrax and interim guidelines for clinical evaluation of persons with possible anthrax. *MMWR Morb Mortal Wkly Rep.* 2001;50:941–948.
15. Swartz MN. Recognition and management of anthrax—an update. *N Engl J Med.* 2001;345:1621–1626.
16. Berger T, Kassirer M, Aran AA. Injectional anthrax—new presentation of an old disease. *Euro Surveill.* 2014;19(32):pii, 20877.
17. CDC. Bioterrorism alleging use of anthrax and interim guidelines for management—United States, 1998. *MMWR Morb Mortal Wkly Rep.* 1999;48:69–74.
18. Hendricks KA, Wright ME, Shadomy SV, et al. Centers for Disease Control and Prevention expert panel meetings on prevention and treatment of anthrax in adults. *Emerg Infect Dis.* 2014;20(2), http://dx.doi.org/10.3201/eid2002.130687.
19. Meaney-Delman D, Zotti M, Creanga A, et al. Special considerations for prophylaxis for and treatment of anthrax in pregnant and postpartum women. *Emerg Infect Dis.* 2014;20(2):e130611.
20. Bradley J, Peacock G, Krug S, et al. and AAP Committee on Infectious Diseases and Disaster Preparedness Advisory Council. Pediatric anthrax clinical management. *Pediatrics.* 2014;133:e1411.
21. Bell DM, Kosarsky PE, Stephens DS. Conference summary: clinical issues in the prophylaxis, diagnosis and treatment of anthrax. *Emerg Infect Dis.* 2002;8:222–225.
22. CDC. Use of anthrax vaccine in response to terrorism: supplemental recommendations of the Advisory Committee on Immunization Practices. *MMWR Morb Mortal Wkly Rep.* 2002;51(45):1024–1026.
23. APIC Bioterrorism Task Force, CDC Hospital Infections Program Bioterrorism Working Group. Bioterrorism readiness plan: a template for health care facilities. http://www.cdc.gov/ncidod/hip/Bio/13apr99APICCDCBioterrorism.PDF.

CHAPTER 125

Yersinia pestis (Plague) Attack

Kimberly A. Stanford and Jonathan Harris Valente

DESCRIPTION OF EVENT

A bioterrorism event leading to multiple cases of the plague would likely result from airborne dispersal of a weaponized form of *Yersinia pestis* and would cause a pulmonary variant of the plague called *pneumonic plague*.[1] Outbreaks of pneumonic plague have also been reported following natural disasters, such as after the 1994 earthquake in Maharashtra, India, and in war-torn regions, such as the Congo, as recently as the first decade of the twenty-first century.[2] During World War II, in two separate incidents, the Japanese dropped clay pots filled with *Y. pestis*-contaminated rice and fleas over the Chinese cities of Shusien, in Chekiang province, and Changteh, in Hunan province. This tactic led to outbreaks of bubonic plague.[3,4] However, it would not be the optimal way for terrorists to spread the plague because bubonic plague requires a bite from a flea. In addition, bubonic plague is not spread directly from person to person as is the pneumonic form.

Pneumonic plague may occur as a secondary pneumonia due to hematogenous spread from bubonic plague. This is the most common form of naturally occurring pneumonic plague. Primary pneumonic plague occurs after inhalation of aerosolized *Y. pestis* bacilli, either from person-to-person transmission or via an intentional attack. Pneumonic plague is rapidly progressive, and it can spread from person to person via aerosolized droplets. The incubation period for pneumonic plague (1 to 6 days) is shorter than that of the bubonic form (2 to 8 days).[5,6] Control of the disease would be complex because affected people without knowledge of the exposure could spread disease by travel to other regions.[7–9]

Pneumonic plague presents clinically as a rapidly progressive respiratory syndrome that is often associated with fever, cough, shortness of breath, chest pain, hemoptysis, malaise, myalgia, nausea and vomiting, sputum or blood cultures with gram-negative rods, and radiographic findings of pneumonia. Chest roentgenograms of patients with pneumonic plague usually show patchy bronchopneumonic infiltrates as well as segmental or lobar consolidation with or without confluence. They may show cavitary lesions or bilateral diffuse infiltrates characteristic of acute respiratory distress syndrome.[10] Time from onset of symptoms to fulminant disease is generally less than 24 hours, rapidly progressing to disseminated intravascular coagulation (DIC), circulatory collapse, and respiratory failure.[11]

It has been estimated that if 50 kg of weaponized *Y. pestis* were released as an aerosol over a city of 5 million people, pneumonic plague could occur in as many as 150,000 persons, 36,000 of whom would be expected to die.[12]

PRE-INCIDENT ACTIONS

An intentional plague outbreak should be considered one of the most likely bioterrorism scenarios for which emergency providers need to prepare. Pneumonic plague would most likely occur naturally as a complication of bubonic plague in the setting of a major bubonic plague outbreak.[13] Warning the public to avoid contact with dead animals, especially rodents such as marmots, is an important preventive measure following a natural disaster such as a large earthquake.[14] *Y. pestis* is not stable in the environment, and it is readily destroyed by drying and sunlight exposure. If *Y. pestis* were released into the air in a bioterrorism attack, it would likely survive for less than an hour. Because of these factors, preparation for environmental decontamination is less important than it would be in other similar attacks, such as with anthrax.[8,9,12]

No vaccine is currently available. The U.S. manufactured vaccine, a killed whole-cell vaccine (Greer), was discontinued in 1999 because of significant adverse effects and because it was not protective for the pneumonic form of the plague. Subunit vaccines based on rF_1V and LcrV antigens are currently undergoing clinical trials, and these are the most promising prospects, but efficacy against pneumonic plague, specifically, is unclear. Live attenuated vaccine is likely the best option in this regard, but it carries the risk of reversion to virulence, limiting its utility.[15]

There are no early-warning systems for the detection of *Y. pestis* if an aerosolized form were dispersed. A real-time PCR has been developed with the potential for identification of *Y. pestis* in less than 5 hours, from blood or sputum, including identification of specific strains such as ciprofloxacin-resistant.[16–18] However, newly engineered strains for use as bioterrorist agents might not be detected by this assay, and thus culture and biochemical identification must still be used for confirmation.

POST-INCIDENT ACTIONS

All cases of pneumonic plague should be considered terrorism-related until proven otherwise. Hospital infection control officers and local and state, national health, and law enforcement officials should be notified immediately of any suspected cases of the plague.

The risk for reaerosolization of *Y. pestis* from the contaminated clothing of exposed persons is low. Under ideal conditions, *Y. pestis* can survive in the environment for about 1 hour, and since patients will present with symptoms after 24 hours, there is no need for routine decontamination. In situations where there may have been recent, gross exposure to *Y. pestis*, decontamination of skin and potentially contaminated fomites (e.g., clothing or environmental surfaces) may be considered to reduce the risk of cutaneous or bubonic forms of the disease.

The plan for decontaminating patients may include several steps. Patients should be instructed to remove contaminated clothing. Clothing should be stored in labeled, plastic bags and gently handled to avoid dispersal of *Y. pestis*. Patients should be instructed to shower thoroughly with soap and water. Environmental surface decontamination may be performed using an Environmental

Protection Agency-registered, facility-approved sporicidal/germicidal agent or a 0.5% hypochlorite solution (one part household bleach added to nine parts water).[1,19,20] In addition to standard decontamination procedures, chlorine dioxide gas has been shown to rapidly deactivate almost 100% of *Y. pestis* in a hospital environment, but further studies are needed regarding safe usage.[21]

In its natural form, pneumonic plague is transmitted person to person via large droplets (not via fine-particle aerosol), and it requires close personal contact (2 m or less) for effective transmission.[5,22,23] Patients with symptoms suggestive of pneumonic plague should be isolated using droplet precautions in addition to standard precautions. Patients with suspected pneumonic plague should be placed in a private room when possible. It is appropriate to cohort symptomatic patients with similar symptoms and the same presumptive diagnosis (i.e., pneumonic plague) when private rooms are not available. Maintain spatial separation of at least 3 feet between infected patients and others when cohorting is not possible. Avoid placement of patients requiring droplet precautions in the same room with an immunocompromised patient. Special air handling is not necessary, and doors may remain open. Patient transport should be limited to essential medical purposes. When transport is necessary, minimize dispersal of droplets by placing a surgical-type mask on the patient. Isolation precautions should be continued for 2 days after initiation of antibiotics and until some clinical improvement occurs in patients with pneumonic plague.[9]

✚ MEDICAL TREATMENT OF CASUALTIES

Specific antibiotic treatment must be initiated within 24 hours after symptom onset, otherwise pneumonic plague is nearly uniformly

TABLE 125-1   Recommendations for Antimicrobial Treatment of Pneumonic Plague*

PATIENT CATEGORY	RECOMMENDED THERAPY
Contained Casualty Setting	
Adults	Preferred choices
	Streptomycin, 1 g IM twice daily
	Gentamicin, 5 mg/kg IM or IV once daily or 2 mg/kg
Loading dose followed	By 1.7 mg/kg IM or IV 3 times daily[†]
	Alternative choices (first choice for postexposure prophylaxis)
	Doxycycline, 100 mg IV twice daily or 200 mg IV once daily
	Ciprofloxacin, 400 mg IV twice daily[‡]
	Chloramphenicol, 25 mg/kg IV 4 times daily[§]
Children[‖]	Preferred choices
	Streptomycin, 15 mg/kg IM twice daily (maximum daily dose, 2 g)
	Gentamicin, 2.5 mg/kg IM or IV 3 times daily[†]
	Alternative choices
	Doxycycline
	If > 45 kg, give adult dosage
	If < 45 kg, give 2.2 mg/kg IV twice daily (maximum, 200 mg/d)
	Ciprofloxacin, 15 mg/kg IV twice daily[‡]
	Chloramphenicol, 25 mg/kg IV 4 times daily[§]
Pregnant women[¶]	Preferred choice
	Gentamicin, 5 mg/kg IM or IV once daily or 2 mg/kg
Loading dose followed	By 1.7 mg/kg IM or IV 3 times daily[†]
	Alternative choices
	Doxycycline, 100 mg IV twice daily or 200 mg IV once daily
	Ciprofloxacin, 400 mg IV twice daily[‡]
Mass Casualty Setting and Postexposure Prophylaxis[#]	
Adults	Preferred choices
	Doxycycline, 100 mg orally twice daily[††]
	Ciprofloxacin, 500 mg orally twice daily[‡]
	Alternative choice
	Chloramphenicol, 25 mg/kg orally 4 times daily[§,**]

TABLE 125-1   Recommendations for Antimicrobial Treatment of Pneumonic Plague—cont'd

PATIENT CATEGORY	RECOMMENDED THERAPY
Children[‖]	Preferred choice
	Doxycycline[††]
	If <45 kg, give adult dosage
	If >45 kg, then give 2.2 mg/kg orally twice daily
	Ciprofloxacin, 20 mg/kg orally twice daily
	Alternative choices
	Chloramphenicol, 25 mg/kg orally 4 times daily[§,**]
Pregnant women[¶]	Preferred choices
	Doxycycline, 100 mg orally twice daily[††]
	Ciprofloxacin, 500 mg orally twice daily
	Alternative choices
	Chloramphenicol, 25 mg/kg orally 4 times daily[§,**]

*These are consensus recommendations of the Working Group on Civilian Biodefense and are not necessarily approved by the Food and Drug Administration. One antimicrobial agent should be selected. Therapy should be continued for 10 days. Oral therapy should be substituted when patient's condition improves. IM indicates intramuscularly; IV, intravenously.
[†]Aminoglycosides must be adjusted according to renal function. Evidence suggests that gentamicin, 5 mg/kg IM or IV once daily, would be efficacious in children, although this is not yet widely accepted in clinical practice. Neonates up to 1 week of age and premature infants should receive gentamicin, 2.5 mg/kg IV twice daily.
[‡]Other fluoroquinolones can be substituted at doses appropriate for age. Ciprofloxacin dosage should not exceed 1 g/d in children.
[§]Concentration should be maintained between 5 and 20 µg/mL. Concentrations greater than 25 µg/mL can cause reversible bone marrow suppression.[24,25]
[‖]Refer to "Management of Special Groups" for details. In children, ciprofloxacin dose should not exceed 1 g/d, chloramphenicol should not exceed 4 g/d. Children younger than 2 years should not receive chloramphenicol.
[¶]In neonates, gentamicin loading dose of 4 mg/kg should be given initially.[26]
[#]Duration of treatment of plague in mass casualty setting is 10 days. Duration of postexposure prophylaxis to prevent plague infection is 7 days.
[**]Children younger than 2 years should not receive chloramphenicol. Oral formulation available only outside the United States.
[††]Tetracycline could be substituted for doxycycline.
(From Inglesby TV, et al. Consensus Statement: Plague as a Biological Weapon: Medical & Public Health Management. *JAMA.* 2000;283[17]: 2281-90.)

fatal.[7,9] Table 125-1 shows the Working Group on Civilian Biodefense's antibiotic recommendations for pneumonic plague.[9] These consensus-based recommendations cover contained exposures, mass casualty exposures, and postexposure prophylaxis. They are based on the best available evidence. However, it should be noted that there is a lack of published trials in treating plague in humans, and a limited number of studies in animals. A number of possible therapeutic regimens for treating plague have not been prospectively studied or approved by the Food and Drug Administration.

In a contained casualty setting, parenteral antibiotics are recommended for all symptomatic patients. In a mass casualty incident, local resources must be evaluated, and, if sufficient supplies of parenteral antibiotics are not available, oral antibiotics may be used. Oral antibiotics should also be given for 7 days as postexposure prophylaxis. Individuals refusing postexposure antibiotics should be observed for fever or cough for 1 week, although isolation is not recommended.[7,9] Several antibiotics that should not be used for pneumonic plague include rifampin, aztreonam, ceftazidime, cefotetan, and cefazolin.[27]

Laboratory testing is needed to confirm pneumonic plague. A sputum Gram's stain should be used emergently because it may reveal bipolar staining gram-negative bacilli or coccobacilli. *Y. pestis* is described as having a bipolar (also termed *safety pin*) staining best seen with Giemsa or Wayson stains.[28] The only gram-negative bacilli to cause rapidly progressing pulmonary symptoms are *Y. pestis* and *Bacillus anthracis*. Blood or sputum cultures should demonstrate growth within 24 to 48 hours, although some laboratory systems may misidentify *Y. pestis*.[29] Laboratory personnel should be notified when *Y. pestis* is suspected, to decrease the chance of laboratory exposure and to increase the diagnostic yield. Biosafety Level 2 conditions are acceptable for routine laboratory procedures.[9] Rapid PCR, if available, can expedite diagnosis.[15-17] Serologic tests are useful for bubonic plague, but, because patients do not seroconvert until between 5 and 20 days postexposure, they would be of little use in a pneumonic plague outbreak.[5]

Because of the severity of pneumonic plague, patients may require advanced supportive measures, including mechanical ventilation, pressors, and invasive monitoring. During the first few hours after initiation of antibiotics, patients must be monitored closely for shock due to bacteriolysis and endotoxin release.[11,30] However, continued clinical deterioration despite appropriate antimicrobial treatment should raise the possibility of an antimicrobial-resistant strain of *Y. pestis*. Multidrug resistant strains have increasingly been reported to occur naturally, as well as via genetic engineering by former Soviet scientists.[31] Because of increasing antibiotic resistance, several alternative therapies continue to be investigated, including antibody, phage and bacteriocin therapy, antiinflammatory therapies to mediate the cytokine storm leading to septic shock and death, and compounds that prevent adhesion to the alveolar epithelium or other key cell membranes.[11]

UNIQUE CONSIDERATIONS

Y. pestis must be considered one of the most likely bacteria to be used as a bioterrorism agent. *Y. pestis* has been used as a biowarfare agent throughout history; it is readily available worldwide in nature and biologic laboratories, and mass production is relatively simple. Although aerosolized *Y. pestis* is not known to have ever been used, it has been successfully weaponized by the former Soviet Union, and it could be effectively dispersed as an aerosol.[9,31] Under proper conditions, such a release could lead to widespread epidemic pneumonic plague with continued human-to-human transmission. Cases would not present for at least 24 hours after exposure. Pneumonic plague is highly contagious and virulent, and antimicrobial treatment must be initiated

within 24 hours to improve survival. Without appropriate antibiotic treatment and supportive care, numerous casualties would result.

⚠ PITFALLS

- Failure to notify appropriate public health and law enforcement agencies when an outbreak of pneumonic plague is suspected or confirmed
- Failure to consider pneumonic plague as the etiologic agent in major pneumonia endemics or pandemics
- Failure to use droplet precautions and standard precautions in potential cases of pneumonic plague
- Failure to initiate specific antibiotic therapy within 24 hours of symptom onset
- Failure to provide postexposure antibiotic prophylaxis

REFERENCES

1. APIC Bioterrorism Task Force, CDC Hospital Infections Program Bioterrorism Working Group. *Bioterrorism Readiness Plan: A Template for Healthcare Facilities.* Available at: http://emergency.cdc.gov/bioterrorism/pdf/13apr99APIC-CDCBioterrorism.pdf.
2. Butler T. Plague gives surprises in the first decade of the 21st century in the United States and Worldwide. *Am J Trop Med Hyg.* 2013. Sept;89(4):788–793.
3. Noah DL, Huebner KD, Darling RG, et al. The history and threat of biological warfare and terrorism. *Emerg Med Clin North Am.* 2002;20(2):255–271.
4. Williams P, Wallace D. *Unit 731: Japan's Secret Biological Warfare in World War II.* New York: The Free Press; 1989.
5. Dennis DT, Gage KL, Gratz N, et al. *Plague Manual: Epidemiology, Distribution, Surveillance and Control.* Available at: http://www.who.int/csr/resources/publications/plague/whocdscsredc992a.pdf.
6. Gani R, Leach S. Epidemiologic determinants for modeling pneumonic plague outbreaks. *Emerg Infect Dis.* 2004;10(4):608–614.
7. Miller JM. Agents of bioterrorism: preparing for bioterrorism at the community health care level. *Infect Dis Clin North Am.* 2001;15(4):1127–1156.
8. US Centers for Disease Control and Prevention. *Frequently asked questions (FAQ) about Plague.* Available at: http://www.bt.cdc.gov/agent/plague/faq.asp.
9. Inglesby TV, Dennis DT, Henderson DA, et al. Plague as a biological weapon: medical and public health management. *JAMA.* 2000;283(17):2281–2290.
10. Mettler FA, Mann JM. Radiographic manifestations of plague in New Mexico, 1975-1980. A review of 42 proved cases. *Radiology.* 1981;139:561–565.
11. Anisimov A, Amoako K. Treatment of plague: promising alternatives to antibiotics. *J Med Microbiol.* 2006;55:1461–1475.
12. *Health Aspects of Chemical and Biological Weapons.* Geneva, Switzerland: World Health Organization; 1970: 98–109.
13. Cunha BA. Anthrax, tularemia, plague, ebola, or smallpox as agents of bioterrorism: recognition in the emergency room. *Clin Microbiol Infect.* 2002;8:489–503.
14. Lohmus M, et al. Rodents as potential couriers for bioterrorism agents. *Biosecur Bioterr.* 2013;1(1):S247–S257.
15. Sun W, Roland K, Curtiss R. Developing live vaccines against *Yersinia pestis. J Infect Dev Ctries.* 2011;5(9):614–627.
16. Tomaso H, Reisinger E, et al. Rapid detection of *Yersinia pestis* with multiplex real-time PCR assays using fluorescent hybridisation probes. *FEMS Immunol Med Microbiol.* 2003. Sept;38(2):117–126.
17. Lindler LE, Fan W, Jahan N. Detection of ciprofloxacin-resistant *Yersinia pestis* by fluorogenic PCR using the LightCycler. *J Clin Microbiol.* 2001;39:3649–3655.
18. Loiez C, Herwegh S, et al. Detection of *Yersinia pestis* in sputum by real-time PCR. *J Clin Microbiol.* 2003. Oct;41(10):4873–4875.

19. US Centers for Disease Control and Prevention, the Hospital Infection Control Practices Advisory Committee (HICPAC). Recommendations for isolation precautions in hospitals. *Am J Infect Control.* 1996;24:24–52.

20. American Public Health Association. *Control of Communicable Diseases in Man.* Washington, DC: American Public Health Association; 1995.

21. Lowe J, Gibbs S, Iwen P, Smith P, Hewlett A. Decontamination of a hospital room using gaseous chlorine dioxide: *Bacillus anthracis, Francisella tularensis,* and *yersinia pestis. J Occup Environ Hyg.* 2013;10(10): 533–539.

22. Meyer K. Pneumonic plague. *Bacteriol Rev.* 1961;25:249–261.

23. Doll JM, Zeitz PS, Ettestad P, Bucholtz AL, Davis T, Gage K. Cat-transmitted fatal pneumonic plague in a person who traveled from Colorado to Arizona. *Am J Trop Med Hyg.* 1994;51:109–114.

24. American Hospital Formulary Service. *AHFS Drug Information.* Bethesda, Md: American Society of Health System Pharmacists; 2000.

25. Scott JL, Finegold SM, Belkin GA, et al. A controlled double blind study of the hematologic toxicity of chloramphenicol. *N Engl J Med.* 1965;272: 113–142.

26. Watterberg KL, Kelly HW, Angelus P, Backstrom C. The need for a loading dose of gentamicin in neonates. *Ther Drug Monit.* 1989;11:16–20.

27. Byrne WR, Welkos SL, Pitt ML, et al. Antibiotic treatment of experimental pneumonic plague in mice. *Antimicrob Agents Chemother.* 1998;42:675–681.

28. McGovern TW, Friedlander AM. Plague. In: Sidell FR, Takafuji ET, Franz DR, eds. *Medical Aspects of Chemical and Biological Warfare.* Washington, DC: Office of The Surgeon General; 1997:479–502. Available at: https://ke.army.mil/bordeninstitute/published_volumes/chemBio/Ch23.pdf.

29. Wilmoth BA, Chu MC, Quan TC. Identification of *Yersinia pestis* by BBL Crystal Enteric/Nonfermenter Identification System. *J Clin Microbiol.* 1996;34:2829–2830.

30. Jacobs RF, Sowell MK, Moss MM, Fiser DH. Septic shock in children: bacterial etiologies and temporal relationships. *Pediatr Infect Dis J.* 1990;9:196–200.

31. Alibek K, Handelman S. *Biohazard.* New York: Random House; 1999.

CHAPTER 126

Francisella tularensis (Tularemia) Attack

Irving "Jake" Jacoby

DESCRIPTION OF EVENT

Tularemia, known also as rabbit fever, hare fever, deerfly fever, or lemming fever, is a zoonotic bacterial illness caused by a small, gram-negative coccobacillus, *Francisella tularensis*. It infects more than 150 animal species, can be transmitted to humans, and is associated with a wide variety of clinical presentations. It received its name following a plague-like illness of ground squirrels in Tulare County, California, in 1911. Reservoirs for this disease include terrestrial and aquatic mammals, such as rabbits, hares, ground squirrels, voles, muskrats, skunks, and water and other rats. Most recently, it has been identified in prairie dogs.[1] Additionally, *F. tularensis* survives in amoebae, which may explain the association of this bacterium with swamps and waterways.[2] The primary vectors are ticks, mosquitoes, and biting flies, such as the deerfly.

Four subspecies are currently recognized by microbiologists, with somewhat different geographic distributions. *F. tularensis* subspecies *tularensis*, also known as Type A, is found almost exclusively in North America and is considered a more virulent strain in humans, whereas the *F. tularensis* subspecies *holarctica* (Type B) is found throughout the northern hemisphere, predominantly in Europe, and is associated with a milder disease state. *F. tularensis* subspecies *novicida* is also found in North America, and subspecies *mediasiatica* is found in Kazakhstan and Uzbekistan. Transmission to humans occurs in a number of ways, including the handling of infected animal tissues or fluids; bites from infected arthropods, particularly ticks and mosquitoes that have fed on infected animals; direct contact or ingestion of contaminated water or food; and via the inhalation of infective aerosols. Examining an open culture plate has resulted in human infection in laboratory workers, and Biosafety Level 3 facilities must be used for work with the organism. Historic origins related to human infection have been presented elsewhere.[3] No human-to-human transmission has ever been documented; therefore, isolation is not required. Most naturally occurring cases in the United States are seen from May to September, although infection can occur at any time.

During the decade from 2001 to 2010, a total of 1208 cases of naturally occurring tularemia were reported to the Centers for Disease Control and Prevention (CDC) via the National Notifiable Diseases Surveillance System (NNDSS). Cases were reported from 47 states, with the six Midwestern states of Missouri (19%), Arkansas (13%), Oklahoma (9%), South Dakota (5%), and Kansas (5%) accounting for over 50% of all cases.[4]

Tularemia is high on the list of dangerous weaponizable biologic agents due to its extreme infectivity once aerosolized, the ease of dissemination, and its substantial capacity to cause morbidity and mortality. One of the most infectious pathogens known, as few as 10 to 50 inhaled organisms have been shown to be capable of producing disease.[5,6] Tularemia has historically been a part of biologic weapons programs in the last century. It was one of the agents studied at Japanese germ warfare research units operating in Manchuria between 1932 and 1945. Ken Alibek suggests that the tularemia outbreak that infected thousands of Soviet and German soldiers before the Battle of Stalingrad in 1942 was related to weaponized tularemia developed by the Soviets, which spread out of control by wind changes,[7] although this claim remains controversial.[8] *F. tularensis* weapons were produced and stockpiled in the biologic warfare production facility of the U.S. Army at the Pine Bluff Arsenal, Arkansas, from 1954 to 1955, but were destroyed by 1973.[9] Vaccine-immune and antibiotic-resistant strains of tularemia were prepared by Biopreparat, the covert Soviet biologic weapons effort, in the 1980s.[10]

Clinical manifestations of disease in humans are varied and often depend on the mode of transmission, site of infection, and the virulence and dose of the infecting organism. Presenting syndromes are glandular, ulceroglandular, oculoglandular, oropharyngeal, pneumonic, typhoidal, and septic.

The most common forms of naturally acquired disease are ulceroglandular and glandular. A cutaneous papule forms at the site of the bite or cutaneous inoculation from an infected animal hide or carcass, and involvement of regional lymph nodes occurs. The pustule suppurates and ulcerates within a few days. Lymph nodes can swell to a large size and resemble the buboes of bubonic plague or the adenopathy of cat scratch disease. An eschar may form and resemble anthrax. Symptoms include fever, chills, headache, and myalgia. Glandular tularemia is present when there is adenopathy without ulceration. Mortality rates for ulceroglandular and glandular forms of the disease were 4.4% and 4.3%, respectively, in the preantibiotic era.[11] In treated cases, the mortality rate was 1.6% in Oklahoma.[12]

Oculoglandular disease occurs when inoculation takes place directly into the eye, often by a finger that has viable organisms on it, and ulceration of the conjunctiva may be seen. Pronounced chemosis and preauricular node enlargement are prominent.

Oropharyngeal tularemia occurs after ingestion of contaminated water or food. Stomatitis, exudative tonsillitis, or pharyngitis may occur with or without ulceration. Lymphadenopathy of cervical or retropharyngeal nodes can be marked.

Tularemia pneumonia follows either inhalation of contaminated aerosols or is secondary to bacterial spread from a local site and is a much more serious form of tularemia. Mortality rates of 30% are reported for this form. The pneumonia is accompanied by hilar adenopathy, dry cough, shortness of breath, and chest pain, either substernal or pleuritic. The term *lawnmower tularemia* was first used when two cases of pneumonic tularemia were reported to have occurred in adolescent males who mowed over a dead rabbit with presumptive aerosolization and inhalation of contaminated fomites.[13] Both were treated with streptomycin and both recovered. A larger outbreak was reported with patients who had mowed lawns and cut brush on Martha's Vineyard in 2001.[14] Adult respiratory distress syndrome has been reported in association with tularemic pneumonia.[15]

Typhoidal tularemia refers to illness characterized by systemic infectious manifestations of fever and chills, but without cutaneous, ocular, lymphatic, or pulmonary findings. Diarrhea and abdominal pain may predominate.

Tularemic sepsis is severe and often fatal. The patient is toxic-appearing, confused, and may become comatose. Systemic inflammatory response syndrome (SIRS) may occur with shock and disseminated intravascular coagulation.[15]

Standard blood, wound, and body fluid cultures should be sent for detection of *F. tularensis*. Because the organism may grow on conventional culture media, it is important to notify laboratory personnel of your suspicion for this organism because growth on a plate represents a significant contagion risk to the laboratory worker.[16] Notification in advance may also increase the likelihood of detecting the organism because use of special media can enhance growth and recovery. If organisms suggestive of *Francisella* are grown by a standard hospital laboratory, further steps in identification may need to be halted, with referral of the isolate to a state laboratory or to the CDC reference or national laboratory for definitive identification and sensitivity testing. Such laboratories would be part of the CDC's Laboratory Response Network (LRN), where standardized, unpublished protocols are followed when dealing with such suspected agents of bioterrorism.

Other clinical tests for general use can be ordered, such as commercially available serologic tests for *F. tularensis* antibody, antigen capture enzyme-linked immunosorbent assay (cELISA), and polymerase chain reaction/TaqMan assays, for detecting antigen in inactivated clinical samples. If present, pleural fluid should be tapped and sent for staining, culture, and direct fluorescent antibody (DFA) testing. Acute and convalescent titers are often necessary to confirm diagnosis.

F. tularensis is one of the organisms screened for in the BioWatch program, an ongoing program in multiple cities in the United States designed to filter air to detect releases of bioterrorism organisms.[17] The first incident of a positive BioWatch result was reported on October 9, 2003, in Houston, Texas. The Houston Department of Health and Human Services reported detecting low levels of the bacterium that causes tularemia. According to a press release, positive results were detected on 3 consecutive days, with negative results on subsequent days. This was felt to be a nonterrorism event, and no clinical cases were found to have developed.[18]

◀◀ PRE-INCIDENT ACTIONS

Tularemia is typically a rural disease, and, although urban[19] and suburban exposures may occur, occurrence in the latter situations may signal the possibility of a terrorist attack, even when a link to an animal vector can be made, because known contaminated hides or fomites could be circulated as a terrorist act. Animal reservoirs may be identified even in urban areas.[20] Given the greater severity of Type A disease and the inhalational route, as well as the known weaponization of *F. tularensis*, a terrorist attack is most likely to be perpetrated via the aerosolized route. However, identification of an index case is key in defending against a tularemic terrorist attack. An index case may represent autoinoculation by the perpetrator. Detecting an uncommon disease can be enhanced by ongoing public health communications of isolated occurrences or outbreaks in a real-time continuum.[21] The similarity of many of the clinical manifestations of tularemia to other more common syndromic presentations would make it difficult to come up with tularemia as an immediate diagnosis because it is unlikely to be a leading cause

of community-acquired pneumonia or conjunctivitis. The careful history of live or dead animal exposures would be an important source of clues to suggest the need for a diagnostic workup for tularemia. Familiarization with the different syndromic presentations of tularemia remains the most important tool in the physician's armamentarium.

Vaccination before exposure would be an ideal way of preparing for an attack. The Soviet Union used a live-attenuated vaccine strain for decades, starting in the 1930s, to immunize millions of people living in endemic areas. One of these strains was transferred to the United States in the 1950s, further attenuated, and called live vaccine strain (LVS). A retrospective study of laboratory workers working with *F. tularensis* at a U.S. Army research facility found a decrease in risk of infection from 5.70 cases of typhoidal tularemia per 1000 person-years of risk with a killed vaccine to 0.27 cases per 1000 person-years of risk after introduction of the LVS vaccine.[22] However, the incidence of ulceroglandular tularemia was unchanged, albeit cases were moderated. This vaccine is not licensed and is not produced in the United States. Improved vaccines are needed since the earlier LVS vaccine required scarification, was cumbersome, and was difficult to standardize. Current vaccine efforts continue due to the risk of the organism being used as a weapon.[23,24] Recent progress with multiple new live vaccines, and in understanding the immunological characteristics and requirements for protection, is encouraging.[25,26]

In areas endemic for tularemia, protection against tick bites remains one of the key interventions to prevent infection, particularly those at greatest risk for exposure (e.g., campers, hikers, and hunters). Data from Missouri, from 2000 to 2007, found 72% of cases with known exposure source were from tick bites.[27]

▶▶ POST-INCIDENT ACTIONS

The local or state health department should be alerted if tularemia is highly suspected, particularly if multiple patients present with a compatible illness.

If prompt recognition of an attack with a tularemia bioweapon occurs during the early incubation period, exposed persons should be treated prophylactically, with either doxycycline 100 mg po twice daily or ciprofloxacin 500 mg by mouth (po) twice a day (bid) for 14 days. Use of penicillin or ceftriaxone should not be attempted due to known production of beta-lactamases and clinical failures in the past.

If an attack has been identified only after cases are occurring, it has been recommended by the Working Group on Civilian Biodefense that persons potentially exposed should begin a fever watch. Persons who develop an otherwise unexplained fever or flu-like illness within 14 days should begin treatment as noted later in the chapter.[28]

If a laboratory worker has had a potentially high-risk infective exposure to *F. tularensis*, such as via a spill, centrifuge accident, needlestick exposure, or exposure to an open culture plate, oral postexposure prophylaxis should be given.

Laboratory spills of infectious *F. tularensis* broth or suspension should be decontaminated with a 10% bleach solution; after 10 minutes, it is recommended that 70% solution of alcohol be used to further clean the area and reduce the corrosive effects of the bleach.[25]

Isolation is not recommended for infected patients, given lack of human-to-human transmission. Close contacts of patients with diagnosed disease thus do not require prophylaxis.

✚ MEDICAL TREATMENT OF CASUALTIES

Treatment of tularemia is antibiotic-based. The preferred first-line choice of antibiotics for adults is streptomycin 1 g given intramuscularly (IM) twice daily or gentamicin 5 mg/kg given IM or intravenously

(IV) once daily for 10 days.[29] In the rare instances of meningitis, since aminoglycoside levels are poor in the CSF, a fluoroquinolone or chloramphenicol should be used.

For patients allergic to aminoglycosides, alternatives are doxycycline 100 mg given intravenously twice daily for 14 to 21 days; chloramphenicol 15 mg/kg given intravenously four times daily for 14 to 21 days. Ciprofloxacin 400 mg given intravenously twice daily for 10 days; other fluoroquinolones have also been used.[30]

In pregnant women, preferred choices are gentamicin or streptomycin; alternative choices are ciprofloxacin or doxycycline.

For pediatric patients <45 kg, doxycycline 2.2 mg/kg IV twice a day for 14 to 21 days (maximum 200 mg daily); gentamicin 2.5 mg/kg IM or IV thrice a day for 10 days; or ciprofloxacin 15 mg/kg IV twice a day for 10 days; up to a maximum daily dose of 1 g should be given.

Bioterrorist attacks using resistant strains are a possibility. Culturing available specimens (scrapings, swabs or aspirates of ulcers, lymph nodes, or other available tissue; sputum, pleural fluid, bronchial washings for respiratory syndromes; corneal scrapings from ocular disease) to obtain isolates for sensitivity testing is essential. Check with the state lab to confirm the method in use at the time, for transporting specimens. Sending blood for titers is also important in making the diagnosis, as absolute titers over 1:160 are considered diagnostic, as are fourfold changes in titers after 2 to 4 weeks; titers peak at 4 to 5 weeks.

Supportive care is critical for fluid management and the detection and treatment of the complications of sepsis, including shock, acute respiratory distress syndrome, disseminated intravascular coagulation, rhabdomyolysis, and organ failure.

UNIQUE CONSIDERATIONS

It would be expected that tularemia would have a slower progression of illness and a lower case fatality rate than that of inhalational anthrax or pneumonic plague. Presumptive laboratory diagnosis of anthrax or plague would likely be made more rapidly than of tularemia, due to the need for referral to reference laboratories.

Outbreaks of tularemia in patients from an urban setting should trigger suspicion of a bioterrorist attack. A World Health Organization expert committee in 1970 gave an estimate that aerosol dispersal of 50 kg of virulent *F. tularensis* over a metropolitan area with 5 million inhabitants would result in 250,000 incapacitating casualties, including 19,000 deaths.[31]

Painful preauricular lymphadenopathy is a hallmark of oculoglandular tularemia, and it distinguishes tularemia from cat scratch disease, tuberculosis, sporotrichosis, and syphilis.

Epidemiologic workup may be needed to determine the reservoir in a given outbreak. The occurrence of an outbreak of tularemia in a war-torn area, although suggestive of possible bioterrorism, can be related to factors such as environmental disruption, as occurred in Kosovo.[32]

Organisms growing in the lab are a distinct risk to laboratory workers, who must be notified when the organism is suspected, and receive prophylaxis for significant exposures.

PITFALLS

Although intuitively one might think that only pneumonic tularemia would occur from an airborne attack with viable organisms, airborne transmission can result in an initial clinical illness without prominent respiratory symptoms.

Mild inhalational disease in a rural setting can be indistinguishable from Q fever.

Because of the many varied presentations of classical tularemia, the differential diagnosis is very broad. Add to that the unusual manifestations of tularemia, including pericarditis, lymphocytic meningitis, hepatitis, endocarditis, osteomyelitis, rhabdomyolysis, and sepsis with septic shock, it is apparent that tularemia could be missed easily in the urban setting, until laboratory confirmation is made.

Relapses are more common with the bacteriostatic agents doxycycline and chloramphenicol than they are with aminoglycosides.

In the event of a mass exposure and large numbers of cases, and the inability to provide IV therapy to all patients, oral antibiotics may be used, in which case, treatment should be continued for 14 days.

Because caseous necrosis can be seen in pathologic specimens from patients with tularemic cervical lymphadenitis, tularemia should be excluded before the diagnosis of tuberculosis is made.[33]

REFERENCES

1. Avashia SB, Petersen JM, Lindley CM, et al. First reported prairie dog-to-human tularemia transmission, Texas, 2002. *Emerg Infect Dis.* 2004;10:483–486.
2. Titball RW, Sjöstedt A. *Francisella tularensis*: an overview. *Am Soc Microbiol (ASM) News.* 2003;69(11):558–563.
3. Weinberg AN. Commentary: Wherry WB, Lamb BH. Infection of man with *Bacterium tularense. J Infect Dis.* 2004;189:1317–1331.
4. Nelson C, Kugeler K, Petersen J, et al. Tularemia—United States 2001–2010. *Morb Mortal Wkly Rep.* 2013;62(47):963–966.
5. Saslaw S, Eigelsbach HT, Prior JA, et al. Tularemia vaccine study. II. Respiratory challenge. *Arch Int Med.* 1961;107:702–714.
6. McCrumb FR. Aerosol infection of man with *Pasteurella tularensis. Bacteriol Rev.* 1961;25:262–267.
7. Alibek K. *Biohazard.* New York: Dell Publishing; 1999, 15–28.
8. Croddy E, Krcalova S. Editorial: tularemia, biological warfare and the battle for Stalingrad (1942–43). *Milit Med.* 2001;166(10):837–838.
9. Franz DR, Parrott CD, Takafuji ET. The U.S. biological warfare and biological defense programs. In: Sidell FR, Takafuji ET, Franz DR, eds. *Textbook of Military Medicine, Part I: Warfare, Weaponry and the Casualty: Medical Aspects of Chemical and Biological Warfare.* Washington, DC: Office of the Surgeon General, Department of the Army; 1997:425–436.
10. Alibek K. *Biohazard.* New York: Dell Publishing; 1999, 29–38.
11. Pullen RL, Stuart BM. Tularemia: analysis of 225 cases. *JAMA.* 1945;129(7):495–500.
12. Rohrbach BW, Westerman E, Istre GR. Epidemiology and clinical characteristics of tularemia in Oklahoma, 1979 to 1985. *South Med J.* 1991;84(9):1091–1096[Abstract].
13. McCarthy VP, Murphy MD. Lawnmower tularemia. *Pediatr Infect Dis J.* 1990;9:298–299.
14. Feldman KA, Enscore RE, Lathrop SL, et al. An outbreak of primary pneumonic tularemia on Martha's Vineyard. *N Engl J Med.* 2001;345:1601–1606.
15. Sunderrajan EV, Hutton J, Marienfeld D. Adult respiratory distress syndrome secondary to tularemia pneumonia. *Arch Int Med.* 1985;145:1435–1437.
16. Shapiro DS, Schwartz DR. Exposure of laboratory workers to *Francisella tularensis* despite a bioterrorism procedure. *J Clin Microbiol.* 2002;40(6):2778–2781.
17. Kman NE, Bachmann DJ. Biosurveillance: a review and update. *Adv Prev Med.* 2012;9. http://dx.doi.org/10.1155/2012/301408, Article ID 301408.
18. *The BioWatch Program: Detection of Bioterrorism.* Congressional Research Service Report No. RL 32152, November 19, 2003. Viewed online 4/20/14 at http://www.fas.org/sgp/crs/terror/RL32152.html#_1_3.
19. Raimondi A, Koll B, Casau N, et al. Tularemia in New York City: when do we need to suspect bioterrorism? *Am J Infect Control.* 2005;33(5): e44–e45.
20. Sinclair JR, Newton A, Hinshaw K, et al. Tularemia in a park, Philadelphia, PA. *Emerging Inf Dis.* 2008;14(9):1482–1483.
21. Dembeck ZF, Buckman RL, Fowler SK, et al. Missed sentinel case of naturally occurring pneumonic tularemia outbreak: lessons for detection of bioterrorism. *J Am Board Fam Pract.* 2003;16:339–342.

22. Burke DS. Immunization against tularemia: analysis of the effectiveness of live *Francisella tularensis* vaccine in prevention of laboratory-acquired tularemia. *J Infect Dis.* 1977;135:55–60.

23. Nierengarten MB, Lutwick LI. Biowarfare vaccines: developing new tularemia vaccines. *Medscape Infectious Diseases.* 2004; Available at, http://www.medscape.com/viewarticle/431539.

24. Ellis J, Oyston PC, Green M, et al. Tularemia. *Clin Microbiol Rev.* 2002;15(4):631–646.

25. Mahawar M, Rabadi SM, Banik S, et al. Identification of a live attenuated vaccine candidate for tularemia prophylaxis. *PLoS One.* 2013;8(4):e61539. http://dx.doi.org/10.1371/journal.pone.0061539.

26. Marohn ME, Barry EM. Live attenuated tularemia vaccines: recent developments and future goals. *Vaccine.* 2013;31:3485–3491.

27. Turabelidze G, Patrick S, Mead PS, et al. Tularemia—Missouri 2000–2007. *MMWR.* 2009;58(27):744–748.

28. Dennis DT, Inglesby TV, Henderson DA, et al. Tularemia as a biological weapon: medical and public health management. *JAMA.* 2001;285(21):2763–2773.

29. Enderlin G, Morales L, Jacobs RF, et al. Streptomycin and alternative agents for the treatment of tularemia: review of the literature. *Clin Infect Dis.* 1994;19(1):42–47.

30. Johansson A, Berglund L, Gothefors L, et al. Ciprofloxacin for treatment of tularemia in children. *Pediatr Infect Dis.* 2000;19(5):449–453.

31. *Health Aspects of Chemical and Biological Weapons.* Geneva, Switzerland: World Health Organization; 1970, 105–107.

32. Reintjes R, Dedushaj I, Gjini A, et al. Tularemia outbreak investigation in Kosovo: case control and environmental studies. *Emerg Infect Dis.* 2002;8(1):1–8.

33. Yildirim S, Turhan V, Karadenizli A, et al. Tuberculosis or tularemia? A molecular study in cervical lymphadenitis. *Int J Infect Dis.* 2014;18:47–51.

CHAPTER 127

Brucella Species (Brucellosis) Attack

Edward W. Cetaruk and Teriggi J. Ciccone

DESCRIPTION OF EVENT

Brucellosis, also known as Mediterranean fever, undulant fever, and Malta fever, is a zoonotic bacterial infection caused by a number of species within the genus *Brucella*. *Brucellae* are small, gram-negative aerobic, nonsporulating coccobacilli. They are facultative, intracellular organisms that have the ability to survive and multiply within the phagocytic cells of the host. Brucellosis is transmitted to humans by consumption of infected, unpasteurized animal milk or through direct contact with infected animals, their secretions, or aborted fetuses or by inhalational of infectious aerosols. Although there are seven named species of *Brucella*, each typically is (although not strictly) associated with infection of certain animal species. Human brucellosis has been associated with *Brucella suis*, *Brucella melitensis*, *Brucella abortus*, and *Brucella canis*. Clinical cases of brucellosis are rare in North America (there are approximately 110 cases per year in the United States), occurring almost exclusively as an occupational zoonotic illness in workers exposed to livestock. It has a seasonal variation, occurring more frequently during the summer months, and is more common in the southern states and along the border with Mexico.[1] Brucellosis is endemic throughout the world, although it is more common in areas with poor food and sanitation standards, such as in the Middle East, India, Central Asia, and Latin America. Domesticated animals such as cattle, swine, sheep, and dogs comprise *Brucellae*'s natural reservoir. *Brucella* is classified as a category B bioterrorism agent (moderately easy to disseminate, with a low mortality rate) by the Centers for Disease Control and Prevention (CDC).[2]

One of the first biological agents to be weaponized by the United States in 1942, *Brucella* was maintained in the American arsenal until the United States ended its offensive biological weapons program in 1969.[3,4] Although several characteristics of *Brucellae* make them ideal candidates for a biological weapon (e.g., easy to grow in sufficient quantities, stable in culture), their ease of transmisson as an aerosol made them most attractive. It is also important to note that *Brucella* is also considered a likely agent for agroterrorism. A large outbreak of brucellosis in a nation's cattle, sheep, or swine population would result in the loss of many millions of dollars by the agricultural economic sector and would also likely cause human cases as well.

Generally speaking, an effective biological weapon requires a highly infectious biological agent (e.g., bacteria or a virus) that is accessible to the bioterrorist, can be grown in substantial quantity, and can be weaponized and disseminated to attack a target population. The agent may cause a highly lethal infection (e.g., anthrax) or an infection that typically is not lethal (often called an incapacitating agent) such as *Brucella*. Also, the agent may be contagious (e.g., *Yersinia pestis*, the causative agent for plague), which will allow the attack to perpetuate itself by causing additional cases after the initial attack. Once a

biological agent has been obtained and grown in quantities sufficient for an attack, the agent must still be weaponized into a form that a bioterrorist can deliver to the intended target. Weaponization can be either simple (e.g., a liquid preparation containing a high concentration of an infectious agent such as *Salmonella* that can be sprayed directly on food) or sophisticated (e.g., an aerosolizable dry powder that is resistant to environmental stressors and that can be used for a large-scale, open-air attack). An ideal biological weapon intended for an aerosol release would be weaponized into dry particles 1 to 5 μm in diameter and may include various coatings to overcome electrostatic charges that cause clumping or to protect the organism from environmental stressors such as sunlight or desiccation. Particle size is critical, as particles within the 1 to 5 μm size range will travel to the distal airways of the lungs when inhaled, markedly increasing the potential to cause infection. However, even if a terrorist lacks the technical knowledge or access to highly lethal agents to make an "ideal" biological weapon, he can still launch a successful biological weapon attack causing hundreds of casualties or deaths using less effective alternatives. Such an attack can have a significant impact on a medical system and cause a substantial psychological impact on the larger population. A case in point: the anthrax attacks of 2001 caused only 22 cases and five deaths but effectively terrorized a nation of 300 million people, leading to permanent changes in security, disaster planning, etc.

Brucellae can be manipulated in the laboratory and manufactured into particles measuring 1 to 5 μm in diameter. Such weaponized particles are highly virulent, with only 10 to 100 organisms required to cause infection.[5] *Brucellae* species are very hardy organisms and can survive for prolonged periods in storage (e.g., munitions) and under harsh environmental conditions. In soil or water, these organisms may survive for up to 10 weeks.[6] However, unlike the CDC category A agents (*Bacillus anthracis*, *Francisella tularensis*, etc.), *Brucellae* have very low mortality among immunocompetent hosts, with only about a 2% mortality rate.[7,8]

Due to the low mortality and prolonged incubation period, medical and public health officials may not recognize a *Brucella* attack for quite some time. A likely scenario would involve a large number of otherwise healthy individuals presenting over weeks to months with a febrile illness with vague, multisystem complaints (see below). An attack could occur in an urban area where an airborne release could spread over a heavily populated area, causing many primary human infections. In a hypothetical biological attack scenario, it was estimated that a line source release of aerosolized *Brucella* (under optimal conditions) upwind from an urban center would cause 82,500 cases of brucellosis and 413 fatalities, presenting over a period of 16 weeks.[9] Once a significant number of cases of brucellosis are confirmed among persons without exposure to livestock, the possibility of a biological weapon attack should be highly considered.

After respiratory, gastrointestinal, dermal (via cuts or abrasions), or mucous membrane inoculation, the bacteria spread hematogenously to all organ systems, with a predilection for the reticuloendothelial system. Depending upon the size of the inoculum and route of infection, clinical manifestations develop weeks to months later. Patients experience intermittent and irregular fevers (hence the name "undulant fever") over weeks and possibly months. Fever is present in >90% of cases and can be spiking and accompanied by rigors, or it may be relapsing, mild, and/or protracted. Malodorous perspiration is almost pathognomonic. Other constitutional symptoms, such as chills, fatigue, malaise, sweats, and headache, may occur. Pulmonary manifestations are generally rare, even after inhalation exposure.[8] Interstitial pneumonitis, hilar lymphadenopathy, pleural effusions, and empyema may be seen on chest x-ray. Gastrointestinal manifestations are more common and involve nausea, vomiting, anorexia, diarrhea, and abdominal pain.[8,10]

Osteoarticular disease is universally the most common complication of brucellosis, and three distinct forms exist: peripheral arthritis (most often seen in the larger joints), sacroiliitis, and spondylitis (most frequently seen in the lumbar spine).[8] Although uncommon (5% to 7% of cases) neurobrucellosis occurs rarely and may range from depression to meningitis, meningoencephalitis, and brain abscesses and has a poor prognosis.[8,11] Acute orchitis and epididymitis have been reported.[12] Brucellosis in pregnancy poses a significant risk of spontaneous abortion. Although rare, endocarditis most often involves the aortic valve and is the most common cause of death from *Brucellae* infections.[13] Physical examination is generally nonspecific, although lymphadenopathy, hepatomegaly, or splenomegaly is often present.[8]

Laboratory data are generally low yield and nonspecific. White blood cell count is typically characterized by mild leukopenia and relative lymphocytosis, along with mild anemia and thrombocytopenia. Elevated liver transaminases may occur in cases of hepatic involvement. *Brucellae* species grow quite slow in culture media, and cultures should be maintained for 4 to 6 weeks if the diagnosis is suspected. Although bone marrow cultures have been shown to be the best source of *Brucellae* for culture, this method is limited by its difficulty, pain, etc.[8] Therefore, serologic studies are the most commonly used means of diagnosis. Some methodologies (e.g., Brucellacapt) provide rapid results (24 hours).

PRE-INCIDENT ACTIONS

Hospital, emergency department, and outpatient facilities should all have general disaster plans in place in the event of a bioterrorist attack. Mass casualty events require coordination of local, state, and federal public safety resources. Both emergency medical service and hospital-based triage systems may need to be altered in the event of a large number of patients seeking medical care within a brief time period. Isolation procedures should be in place in the event of an attack with known person-to-person transmission. However, transmission of *Brucellae* species between individuals is not believed to occur, and no specific isolation precautions are needed in patients suspected of having brucellosis. The possibility of contracting brucellosis by inhalation of particles in culture among laboratory workers is significant, and negative-pressure isolation measures and Biosafety Level 3 procedures should be used within laboratories. Health care providers should practice universal precautions.

Since a true mass casualty scenario after a *Brucella* attack is unlikely, physicians and other health care providers must remain vigilant in identifying local epidemiological trends that may indicate an outbreak of brucellosis. These trends may only be noted over days to weeks, with an increasing volume of otherwise healthy patients with fever and multiple systemic complaints that came on insidiously and have persisted for prolonged time periods.

POST-INCIDENT ACTIONS

Clinicians with a high level of suspicion of a possible *Brucella* attack or confirmatory data of a case of brucellosis should notify the appropriate local, state, and federal public health and law enforcement authorities. Materials and surfaces possibly contaminated by brucellosis patients should be disinfected with 0.5% hypochlorite solution.[3]

MEDICAL TREATMENT OF CASUALTIES

Antibiotic treatment for brucellosis requires multiple agents (monotherapy is not recommended). Prolonged antibiotic therapy is required to prevent relapse of disease. Most cases can be successfully treated with doxycycline 100 mg twice daily plus rifampin 600 to 900 mg daily for 6 weeks. Streptomycin is often recommended but is difficult to obtain; other aminoglycosides can be considered. Triple antibiotic regimens are recommended for neurobrucellosis. Spondylitis and neurobrucellosis require prolonged treatment (months). In children, substituting doxycycline with trimethoprim-sulfamethoxazole has been used; however, relapse rates are high when compared with the doxycycline-rifampin regimen.[14] Although no formal recommendations exist for postexposure prophylaxis, high-risk patients after a *Brucella* attack may be considered to receive a 3-week course of doxycycline and rifampin. Currently, no vaccine is available for brucellosis.

UNIQUE CONSIDERATIONS

Brucellae species are small, gram-negative bacteria that cause a wide spectrum of clinical symptoms and signs in infected humans. Even though they are considered a potential bioweapon due to their high virulence when inhaled, *Brucellae* species have a disadvantage when compared with other inhaled bacteria due to their low mortality and prolonged incubation period. This makes the identification of a possible *Brucella* attack extremely difficult. In the event of a *Brucella* attack, the only clue may be the presentation of a large number of healthy individuals over days to weeks with prolonged fevers and a myriad of multisystem complaints. Providers should also be aware that treatment for brucellosis requires multiple antibiotic agents and a prolonged treatment regimen to prevent relapse.

PITFALLS

- Failure to prepare adequate systems to respond to possible terrorist attacks before the attacks occur
- Failure to consider brucellosis as the etiologic factor for persistent fever in patients
- Failure to consider a *Brucella* attack in the setting of a large number of otherwise healthy people who present over days to weeks with a wide range of vague complaints
- Failure to treat cases of brucellosis with multiple agents over a prolonged time period to prevent relapse
- Failure to notify appropriate public health and law enforcement agencies when an outbreak of brucellosis is suspected or confirmed among persons with no exposure to domesticated animals

REFERENCES

1. Centers for Disease Control. Morbidity and Mortality Weekly Report summary of notifiable diseases—United States, 2012 (Brucellosis). *MMWR Morb Mortal Wkly Rep.* 2014;61(53):104.
2. Khan AS, Sage MJ. Biological and chemical terrorism: strategic planning, preparedness, and response. *MMWR Morb Mortal Wkly Rep.* 2000;49:1–14.

3. Greenfield RA, Drevets DA, Machado LJ, et al. Bacterial pathogens as biological weapons and agents of bioterrorism. *Am J Med Sci.* 2002;232:299–315.

4. Brucellosis. Dembek ZF, lead ed, Alves DA, Cieslak TJ, Culpepper RC, et al. *USAMRIID's Medical Management of Biological Casualties Handbook.* 7th ed. Fort Detrick, MD: U.S. Army Medical Research Institute of Infectious Disease; 2011:35–43.

5. Bellamy RJ, Freedman AR. Bioterrorism. *QJM.* 2001;94:227–234.

6. Franz DR, Jahrling PB, Friedlander AM, et al. Clinical recognition and management of patients exposed to biological warfare agents. *JAMA.* 1997;278:399–411.

7. Chin J, Asner MS, eds. *Control of Communicable Disease Manual.* 17th ed. Washington, DC: American Public Health Association; 2000.

8. Pappas G, Akritidis K, Bosilkovski M, et al. Brucellosis. *N Engl J Med.* 2005;352:2325–2336.

9. Kaufmann AF, Meltzer MI, Schmid GP. The economic impact of a bioterrorist attack: are prevention and postattack intervention programs justifiable? *Emerg Infect Dis.* 1997;3:83–94.

10. Purcell BK, Hoover DL, Friedlander AM. Brucellosis. In: Lenhart MK, Lounsbury DE, Martin JW, Dembek ZF, eds. *Textbook of Military Medicine: Medical Aspects of Biological Warfare.* Washington, DC: Borden Institute; 2007:185–198. Available at: http://www.cs.amedd.army.mil/borden/Portlet .aspx?ID=66cffe45-c1b8-4453-91e0-9275007fd157.

11. Young EJ. *Brucella* species. In: Mandell GL, Bennett JE, Dolin R, eds. *Principles and Practice of Infectious Disease.* 6th ed. Philadelphia, PA: Churchill Livingstone; 2005:2669–2674.

12. Khan MS, Humayoon MS, Al Manee MS. Epididymo-orchitis and brucellosis. *Br J Urol.* 1989;63:87–89.

13. Al-Harthi SS. The morbidity and mortality pattern of *Brucella* endocarditis. *Int J Cardiol.* 1989;25:321–324.

14. Lubani MM, Dudin KI, Sharda DC, et al. A multicenter therapeutic study of 1100 children with brucellosis. *Pediatr Infect Dis J.* 1989;8:75–78.

SUGGESTED READINGS

1. Ariza J, Gudiol F, Pallares R, et al. Treatment of human brucellosis with doxycycline plus rifampin or doxycycline plus streptomycin. *Ann Intern Med.* 1992;117:25–30.

Coxiella burnetii (Q Fever) Attack

Edward W. Cetaruk and Teriggi J. Ciccone

DESCRIPTION OF EVENT

The name Q fever derives from "Query fever," the original name given to the febrile illness first noted among slaughterhouse workers in Australia in 1933.[1,2] Q fever is caused by the gram-negative, obligate intracellular bacteria Coxiella burnetii. C. burnetii is maintained in a large natural reservoir within mammals, birds, and arthropods. Natural human infection occurs primarily as a zoonotic occupational infection in persons exposed to livestock including sheep, goats, and cattle. The organism is shed in urine, feces, milk, and in especially high concentrations in placentas and birth fluids from infected livestock. Placental tissue contains especially high concentrations of infectious particles, and persons exposed to parturient livestock are at particularly high risk.[3] The largest known Q fever outbreak involved approximately 4000 human cases and occurred during 2007-2010 in the Netherlands. The outbreak was linked to dairy goat farms near densely populated areas and presumably involved human exposure via a windborne route.[3] Infection can also occur via ingestion of unpasteurized milk from infected animals, and, rarely, through an arthropod vector, particularly ticks.[1] Person-to-person transmission has been reported, but is believed to be extremely rare.[4] On average, there are about 125 cases of Q fever in the United States per year, typically occurring as isolated cases.[5] A significant outbreak without a clear association to livestock should raise concern for the use of C. burnetii as a biological weapon.

Generally speaking, an effective biological weapon requires a highly infectious biological agent (e.g., bacteria or virus) that is accessible to the bioterrorist, can be grown in substantial quantity, and can be weaponized and disseminated to attack a target population. The agent may cause a highly lethal infection (e.g., anthrax) or an infection that typically is not lethal (often called incapacitating an agent), such as Q fever. In addition, the agent may be contagious (e.g., Y. pestis, the causative agent for plague), which will allow the attack to perpetuate itself by causing additional cases after the initial attack. Once a biological agent has been obtained and grown in quantities sufficient for an attack, the agent must still be weaponized into a form that a bioterrorist can deliver to the intended target. Weaponization can be either simple (e.g., a liquid preparation containing a high concentration of an infectious agent, such as salmonella, that can be sprayed directly on food) or sophisticated (e.g., an aerosolizable dry powder that is resistant to environmental stressors that can be used for a large-scale open-air attack). An ideal biological weapon intended for an aerosol release would be weaponized into dry particles 1 to 5 μm in diameter that may include various coatings to overcome electrostatic charges that cause clumping or to protect the organism from environmental stressors such as sunlight or desiccation. Particle size is critical because particles within the 1- to 5-μm size range will travel to the distal airways of the lungs when inhaled, markedly increasing the potential to cause infection. However, even if a terrorist lacks the technical knowledge or access to highly lethal agents to make an "ideal" biological weapon, he can still launch a successful biological weapon attack causing hundreds of casualties or deaths using less effective alternatives. Such an attack can have significant effect on a medical system and cause substantial psychological effect on the larger population. Case in point, the anthrax attacks of 2001 caused only 22 cases and five deaths but effectively terrorized a nation of 300 million people, leading to permanent changes in security.

C. burnetii is classified as a category B bioterrorism agent (moderately easy to disseminate with a low mortality rate) by the Centers for Disease Control and Prevention (CDC).[6] Although its use in warfare has never been documented, military personnel have become infected with C. burnetii in endemic areas during warfare.[2] The U.S. military stockpiled C. burnetii in its biological arsenal until 1971, when these agents were destroyed.[2,7] Multiple factors contribute to C. burnetii's appeal as a biological weapon. This agent is highly virulent, with the highest attack rate of any weaponized agent. Inhalation of a single particle is sufficient to cause disease in some patients.[2,7] The spore-like form of C. burnetii is also resistant to heat and desiccation. It can survive in the natural environment for weeks to months and spread over large distances while airborne.[2,5,7-9] The release of infectious particles within or over a major population center could potentially result in tens of thousands of infections.[3,9] However, C. burnetii infection carries a relatively low case fatality rate. In a large case series, Raoult and colleagues reported 13 deaths among 1383 cases of Q fever over a period of 14 years, most frequently from myocarditis.[10]

Identification of a biological attack using aerosolized C. burnetii would be difficult because of lack of a specific clinical syndrome and a variable incubation period. A likely scenario for a C. burnetii biological attack could involve a cluster of previously healthy persons presenting with a nonspecific febrile illness over days to weeks as described above. Once C. burnetii infection is confirmed in the absence of significant risk factors (e.g., exposure to livestock), the possibility of a biological weapon attack must be considered.

Infection with C. burnetii can result in a wide spectrum of human disease. After an incubation period of 2 to 3 weeks, the most common clinical presentation is a nonspecific febrile illness with chills, malaise, fatigue, anorexia, and headache that might occur in conjunction with pneumonia or hepatitis.[2,3,5,7,10] The most frequently reported symptoms include fever, fatigue, chills, and myalgias. The initial picture would be difficult to differentiate clinically from a naturally occurring outbreak of influenza or other causes of atypical pneumonia, such as mycoplasma or viral pneumonia. Acute symptomatic infection occurs in 50% to 77% of victims, with asymptomatic seroconversion occurring in nearly all other victims.[10-12] Disease severity is inversely proportional to the amount of inoculum to which the victim is exposed.[2,7]

Presumably, a biological attack with aerosolized *C. burnetii* would expose victims to a relatively high level of inoculum, and thus result in a greater number of patients with acute disease. Patients frequently recover from this syndrome without treatment.

Q fever pneumonia occurs in 17% to 50% of cases and can range from mild to severe.[7,10] Patients may complain of cough and pleuritic chest pain. Chest radiographs findings are nonspecific; most often consistent with an atypical pneumonia (although consolidation and pleural effusion may be found) and are indistinguishable from other etiologies of community-acquired pneumonia.[13] Frequently, patients will have positive chest radiographic findings without pulmonary symptoms.[14] Moreover 30% to 40% of victims will develop hepatitis[7,10] with abdominal pain and tenderness, hepatomegaly, and elevated serum transaminases. Sonographic liver imaging or liver biopsy may reveal a granulomatous hepatitis. Jaundice is a rare finding.[15]

Endocarditis, myocarditis, meningoencephalitis, and osteomyelitis occur in less than 1% of acute cases of Q fever.[10] Fatalities from acute Q fever are most often the result of myocarditis. Infection in pregnant women is associated with spontaneous abortion.[5,10,16]

Chronic Q fever is uncommon and affects less than 5% to 23% of patients with *C. burnetii* infection.[4,5,10] The most prominent clinical manifestation is endocarditis, affecting 60% to 73% of patients with chronic infection.[10,15] Patients with preexisting valvular disease and prosthetic valves are at the highest risk. Other chronic syndromes include arterial aneurysms, osteomyelitis, chronic hepatitis, and chronic fatigue syndrome.[4,14]

Laboratory data are often nonspecific in acute Q fever. Although up to 25% of patients with acute Q fever have an increased leukocyte count, most patients have normal white blood cell counts. Mild thrombocytopenia occurs in approximately one third of patients and may be followed by thrombocytosis.[4] Increased erythrocyte sedimentation rate, hyponatremia, hematuria, increased creatine kinase, and increased C-reactive protein levels have been reported. The most common laboratory abnormalities are increased liver enzyme levels, which are seen in up to 85% of cases.[5] Elevations in erythrocyte sedimentation rate, smooth muscle antibodies, and antiphospholipase antibodies may be found.[15] Children with Q fever generally have a milder acute illness than adults have and are more likely to have a rash than adults are. Rash has been reported in up to 50% of children with acute Q fever.[5]

Diagnosis of *C. burnetii* infection is confirmed by serologic testing, most commonly by indirect fluorescent antibody assays. Other laboratory methods include complement fixation, enzyme-linked immunosorbent assays (ELISA), and macroagglutination and microagglutination.[5] ELISA is regarded as the most sensitive serologic test, with sensitivities greater than 90%.[15] Culture of *C. burnetii*, technically difficult and potentially hazardous to laboratory personnel, is rarely performed.

PRE-INCIDENT ACTIONS

Preparations for a biological weapon attack require that hospitals, emergency departments, public health systems, prehospital emergency medical services, and law enforcement officials develop and coordinate disaster plans before an attack occurs. Plans for responding to biological mass casualty incidents should be broad enough to respond to all biological agents (or naturally occurring outbreaks such as SARS), including contagious agents, highly lethal agents, and less lethal agents, such as Q fever. More importantly, plan development should include input from all stakeholders and be tested using realistic mass casualty scenarios (e.g., tabletop and field exercises) on an ongoing basis to identify weaknesses and needs in the system. As most biological weapons attacks will present days to weeks after the attack occurred, response plans should include a passive surveillance system to detect

an increased incidence of febrile illnesses that can be changed to an active system that can identify new cases as they present. This is especially critical when the agent is unidentified or potentially contagious.

A clear chain of command should be established in the event of a disaster, to coordinate the actions of these various groups. In contrast to an acute event, such as a chemical attack or bomb blast, infectious disease mass casualty incidents develop over time, and caseloads may increase exponentially days or weeks after the attack, overwhelming local health care resources. Isolation and decontamination procedures should be in place to prevent person-to-person transmission of the infectious agent. Local and regional supplies (or chains of supply) of critical material (e.g., consumable medical equipment and antibiotics) should be established.

Because person-to-person transmission of *C. burnetii* is thought to be extremely rare, no specific isolation precautions are required. However, health care workers should practice universal precautions at all times. Because of its highly infectious nature, all laboratory workers handling clinical specimens with *C. burnetii* should work under Biosafety Level 2 precautions. These include limiting laboratory access to trained personnel, working in safety hoods when contact with potentially aerosolized materials is suspected, and following strict protocols for disposal and autoclaving of all potentially infectious materials.

POST-INCIDENT ACTIONS

Confirmation of *C. burnetii* infection is a "notifiable illness" and should lead to notification of the local health department and CDC involvement. Cases without an exposure to domesticated animals or other "traditional" sources should alert the clinician, and all other agencies involved, to the possibility of a biological attack. Material and surfaces contaminated with *C. burnetii* should be disinfected with a 0.05% hypochlorite solution (household bleach).[17]

MEDICAL TREATMENT OF CASUALTIES

Although most cases of Q fever resolve spontaneously without treatment, antibiotic treatment should be started in confirmed or suspected cases to shorten the course of illness and to reduce the number of complications. Doxycycline is considered the drug of choice for acute Q fever.[2,7] A standard regimen with 100 mg twice daily for 14 to 21 days provides adequate coverage for most adults.[5,12,15] Macrolides, quinolones, trimethoprim/sulfamethoxazole, and rifampin have also been shown to have effect against *C. burnetii*.[2,5,8] Patients with preexisting valvular heart disease or prosthetic heart valves require a prolonged course of treatment to prevent endocarditis. Chronic Q fever should be treated with a combination of doxycycline plus hydroxychloroquine (200 mg 3 times per day) for 1 year.[5,17] Treatment of known Q fever endocarditis requires at least 18 months of treatment with doxycycline and hydroxychloroquine.[5] In pregnant women with Q fever, treatment with co-trimoxazole during the first two trimesters has been shown to reduce the incidence of spontaneous abortion,[18] and treatment with macrolides in the third trimester would be appropriate to avoid kernicterus. In children older than 8 years, doxycycline at 2.2 mg/kg is given twice daily. For low-risk children younger than 8 years trimethoprim/sulfamethoxazole at a dosage of 4 to 20 mg/kg every 12 hours is recommended. Alternative regimens include chloramphenicol 25 mg/kg/day divided every 6 hours, or erythromycin 50 mg/kg/day divided every 6 hours.

A formalin-killed vaccine to *C. burnetii* is available for high-risk persons, such as slaughterhouse workers, veterinarians, and laboratory workers.[2,7] A single vaccination is 95% effective against aerosolized *C. burnetii*, and it offers protection for up to 5 years.[7]

UNIQUE CONSIDERATIONS

Acute infection with *C. burnetii* causes a nonspecific febrile illness. The time of onset after exposure and the severity of disease are proportional to the amount of inoculum. The ability of *C. burnetii* to cause infection with as few as one infective particle, in addition to the spore-like form's ability to be spread as an aerosol over large distances, make this agent a potential biological weapon. The release of *C. burnetii* particles over a large population center would result in a high number of casualties over days to weeks. As the clinical syndrome caused by *C. burnetii* infection is relatively nonspecific, health care, public health, and law enforcement officials should maintain a high index of suspicion for Q fever when a large number of previously healthy persons without exposure to livestock or other domesticated animals become ill with a febrile illness over a brief period. Once cases of Q fever are confirmed in otherwise low-risk persons, the possibility of biological attack should be considered.

PITFALLS

Several potential pitfalls in response to an attack exist. These include the following:

- Failure to establish a coordinated disaster plan (involving input from local health care, public health, and law enforcement systems) for a possible biological attack
- Failure to test the plan with regular and realistic scenarios
- Failure to consider Q fever when a large number of persons present over a brief period with nonspecific febrile illnesses
- Failure to consider Q fever in patients with fever, pneumonia, and hepatitis
- Failure to begin appropriate antibiotic treatment in cases of acute Q fever to prevent chronic forms of disease that are more severe, such as endocarditis
- Failure to notify appropriate infection control, public health, and law enforcement officials when cases of Q fever are diagnosed or suspected

REFERENCES

1. Derrick EH. "Q" fever, new fever entity: clinical features, diagnosis, and laboratory investigation. *Med J Aust.* 1937;2:281–299.
2. Waag DM. Q fever. In: Lenhart MK, Lounsbury DE, Martin JW, Dembek ZF, eds. *Textbook of Military Medicine: Medical Aspects of Biological Warfare.* Washington, DC: Borden Institute; 2007:199–213.
3. Schimmer B, Dijkstra F, Vellema P, et al. Sustained intensive transmission of Q fever in the Netherlands, 2009. *Eurosurveillance.* 2009;14(19):19210.
4. Anderson A and the CDC Q Fever Working Group. Diagnosis and management of Q fever—United States, 2013.
5. Centers for Disease Control. Morbidity and Mortality Weekly Report Summary of notifiable diseases—United States, 2012. *MMWR Morb Mortal Wkly Rep.* 2014;61(53):26.
6. Khan AS, Sage MJ, Groseclose SL, et al. Biological and chemical terrorism: strategic plan for preparedness and response. *MMWR Morb Mortal Wkly Rep.* 2000;49(RR04):1–14.
7. Q fever. Dembek ZF, Alves DA, Cieslak TJ, et al. *USAMRIID's Medical Management of Biological Casualties Handbook.* 7th ed. Fort Detrick, MD: US Army Medical Research Institute of Infectious Disease; 2011:65–73.
8. Franz DR, Jahrling PB, Friedlander AM, et al. Clinical recognition and management of patients exposed to biological warfare agents. *JAMA.* 1997;278(5):399–411.
9. World Health Organization. *Health Aspects of Chemical and Biological Weapons: Report of a WHO Group of Consultants.* Geneva: WHO; 1970.
10. Raoult D, Tissot-Dupont H, Foucault C, et al. Q fever 1985-1998: clinical and epidemiologic features of 1383 infections. *Medicine.* 2000;79 (2):109–123.
11. Dupuis G, Petite J, Péter O, Vouilloz M. An important outbreak of human Q fever in a Swiss alpine valley. *Int J Epidemiol.* 1987;16(2):282–287.
12. Centers for Disease Control and Prevention. Q fever—California, Georgia, Pennsylvania, and Tennessee, 2000-2001. *MMWR Morb Mortal Wkly Rep.* 2002;51:924–927.
13. Franz DR, Jahrling PB, Friedlander AM, et al. Clinical recognition and management of patients exposed to biological warfare agents. *JAMA.* 1997;278(5):399–411.
14. Marrie TJ, Roult D. *Coxiella burnetii* (Q fever). In: Mandel GL, Bennett JE, Dolin R, eds. *Principles and Practice of Infectious Diseases.* 6th ed Philadelphia, PA: Churchill Livingstone; 2005:186, 2296-2303.
15. Raoult D, Marrie T. Q fever. *Clin Infect Dis.* 1995;20:489–495.
16. Raoult D, Stein A. Q fever during pregnancy, a risk to women, fetuses, and obstetricians. *N Engl J Med.* 1994;330:371.
17. Greenfield RA, Drevets DA, Machado LJ, Voskuhl GW, Cornea P, Bronze MS. Bacterial pathogens as biological weapons and agents of bioterrorism. *Am J Med Sci.* 2002;232:299–315.
18. Raoult D, Fenollar F, Stein A. Q fever during pregnancy: diagnosis, treatment, and follow-up. *Arch Intern Med.* 2002;162:701–704.

CHAPTER 129

Rickettsia prowazekii Attack (Typhus Fever)

Devin M. Smith, Lawrence Proano, and Robert Partridge

DESCRIPTION OF EVENT

Typhus fever (TF), otherwise known as epidemic typhus, red louse fever, jail fever, or sylvatic typhus, is caused by the obligate intracellular, gram-negative coccobacillus *Rickettsia prowazekii*.[1] Like other *Rickettsia* spp., *R. prowazekii* is passed to humans from arthropod ectoparasites; the primary vector in the case of TF is the human body louse (*Pediculus humanus corporis*).

The disease is not spread by the bite of an infected louse as may be expected. Rather, the louse defecates shortly after taking a blood meal at the same site. The human host, inclined to scratch the site because of a local inflammatory reaction from the bite, autoinoculates himself with the organism from the fecal matter.[2] Alternatively, crushing an infected louse into a wound or subsequently touching mucous membranes may also result in the transfer of the bacteria to the human host.[3] In the United States, there have been rare cases of TF transmitted after encountering flying squirrels. These are the only known nonhuman reservoir of TF found to date. The mechanism of transmission between human and squirrel has not been determined but likely is related to contact with parasites carried by the flying squirrels.[4]

Those who come into physical contact with or share quarters or clothes with infected victims can acquire the pests and the disease. Incidents causing humans to be in close contact or in less-than-ideal sanitary conditions can lead to an increase in infection rates.[5] TF has been critically important in human history in such situations. The disease has affected the outcomes of wars and has led to epidemics in prison populations and in those who have survived natural disasters. TF tends to have a higher prevalence in colder months, as those without adequate shelter or heating often crowd together for warmth.

Incidents of TF transmission have been reported when aerosols of louse fecal dust are inhaled by physicians and laboratory personnel. *R. prowazekii* has been found to remain infective in louse fecal matter beyond 100 days.[6] The inhalational transmission capability in conjunction with the prolonged active phase makes it functional as an agent of bioterrorism. The National Institute of Allergy and Infectious Diseases (NIAID) has classified TF as a Category B Biodefense Priority Agent because of its moderate ease of distribution, as well as its moderate casualty rates.[7] The mortality rate in untreated patients ranges from 20% to 40%, depending on the severity of the epidemic.[8] Based on the low infective dose required to cause overt disease, the World Health Organization (WHO) estimates that using 50 kg of aerosolized powder containing TF could cause approximately 125,000 casualties (including 8000 deaths) in a well-developed, highly populated urban environment.[9] These figures and estimates are large enough to warrant concern and development of a disaster plan to prepare for and respond to a bioterrorism event with intentional release of TF.

Clinical manifestations of TF can be nonspecific, causing a delay in diagnosis and subsequent increase in morbidity and mortality. There is an approximate 2-week incubation period before overt symptoms develop.[10] The earliest symptoms typically are severe headache and fever. The classic maculopapular, blanching rash that originates around the axilla and trunk within the first week of symptoms is actually present in as few as 25% of cases.[11] This classical rash tends to spread to the entire body, with the exception of the face, palms, and soles. It also may become more confluent and petechial or purpuric in nature if not treated.[3] TF was named from the Greek word for smoke because of the neurologic side effects often seen, including mental dullness, delirium, coma, and seizures.[3,5,11] A mild conjunctivitis and a brown furry tongue have also been described.[10] In severe cases, vasculitis may lead to vascular collapse and multiorgan damage (e.g., cerebral ischemia or necrosis of the digits).[3] The appearance of these symptoms is variable, thus clouding the diagnosis. Outcomes are significantly better if diagnosed early and treated appropriately.

PRE-INCIDENT ACTIONS

In the United States, a surveillance system for TF has not been created.[4] This is primarily owing to the general lack of commercially available accurate tests. As of now, state officials only become aware of TF outbreaks when special testing is requested from state health departments or the Centers for Disease Control and Prevention (CDC). Because category B status is given to TF by the NIAID, the attainment and trafficking of the causative agent are restricted, which offers a level of protection to the public.[8]

Clinical suspicion for TF can be confirmed by means of polymerase chain reaction (PCR), enzyme-linked immunosorbent assay (ELISA) for IgG and IgM antibodies, or culture.[3,12] Historically, Weil-Felix agglutination testing has been used; however, there is significant cross reactivity with other *Rickettsia* spp., rendering it less specific for TF. Western blot testing has been shown to help distinguish *R. prowazekii*.

POST-INCIDENT ACTIONS

Lines of communication between local health facilities and state agencies should be developed early and maintained if there is a suspicion of a multiple or mass casualty event from intentional attack or a natural outbreak of TF. Suspicion of an intentional release should be high if numerous cases of TF present in a nonendemic region.[8] Hospitals and emergency departments should rely on their site-specific triage protocols to maximize treatment and minimize further exposure. Because of the potential of victims harboring infectious louse fecal dust, it is critical that health care workers employ contact and airborne precautions when interacting with patients suspected of exposure to TF.

In a suspected epidemic, people who have likely been exposed to infected lice or their fecal matter should be considered as a source of infection. These individuals should be isolated and decontaminated. Decreased casualty rates have been seen by using 0.5% permethrin powder on contaminated individuals in conjunction with other sanitation techniques.[13] Clothes and linens of the infected should be collected and destroyed to prevent further spread. Using insecticides to clean infested premises in a safe manner has been shown to be effective at reducing louse burden during outbreaks among prisoners in Burundi.

➕ MEDICAL TREATMENT OF CASUALTIES

Correct antibiotic selection is essential in cases of epidemic typhus. Early antibiotic therapy is estimated to reduce the need for hospitalization by 50% and mortality by 70% in developed settings.[9] Doxycycline is considered the treatment of choice for adults and children.[14] The suggested dose is 100 mg twice a day for 5 to 7 days until 48 hours after symptoms resolve.[15,16] For children over 8 years old, dosing is 2.2 mg/kg every 12 hours (max dose 200 mg/day). Additionally, a single dose of 200 mg of doxycycline has been shown to be effective in epidemic conditions.[17] In cases where doxycycline cannot be used, chloramphenicol is the second-line agent.[3] The suggested dose for chloramphenicol is 60 to 75 mg/kg divided into four doses per day for the same duration of treatment as doxycycline.[15] Pediatric dosing is lower and varies considerably, based on the child's age and weight. Chloramphenicol has been found to be less effective than doxycycline, and it can lead to an increased duration of illness.[14] Currently, in the United States, only the intravenous (IV) formulation of chloramphenicol is available.

Administering treatment to those exposed to infected individuals has been part of successful intervention in past events[13] Preventative vaccines for TF have been studied and have been used intermittently for almost a century.[3] A vaccine developed using killed *R. prowazekii* was used successfully in protecting soldiers in World War II. This did not entirely prevent the disease, but it did reduce the illness to a milder form.[18] In addition, during the mid-twentieth century, a live attenuated vaccine was utilized with promising results in South America and Burundi. Unfortunately, approximately 14% of those treated developed symptoms of TF because of the recurrence of the virulent pathway of the pathogen. Research efforts to develop better interventional methods to prevent and treat TF are ongoing. In the event of mass attacks, state agencies would be responsible for determining how to treat low-risk individuals within the public sphere.

❓ UNIQUE CONSIDERATIONS

A certain unidentified population retains a subclinical infection of *R. prowazekii* after treatment. In this group, it is possible to develop a recurrent form of TF known as Brill-Zinnser disease.[3] These individuals serve as a primer for a new epidemic in the absence of initial louse infection. The course and severity of this form of the disease is considered milder, and it is treated in the same manner as the louse borne disease.

❗ PITFALLS

- Failure to consider TF in a patient with fever and headache without the "classical rash"
- Failure to start empiric doxycycline early in clinically suspected cases of TF
- Failure to isolate, decontaminate, and dispose of linens/clothing of infected individuals
- Failure to utilize contact and airborne precautions when treating the infected
- Failure to contact the appropriate state agencies when an attack or outbreak is suspected
- Delaying initiation of treatment while awaiting confirmatory testing

REFERENCES

1. Brooks GF, Carroll KC, Butel JS, Morse SA, Mietzner TA. *Rickettsia* and related genera. In: Brooks GF, Carroll KC, Butel JS, Morse SA, Mietzner TA, eds. *Jawetz, Melnick, & Adelberg's Medical Microbiology.* 26th ed. New York, NY: McGraw-Hill; 2013. http://accessmedicine.mhmedical.com/content.aspx?bookid=504&Sectionid=40999947.
2. World Health Organization. International Travel and Health: Typhus Fever (Epidemic Louse-Borne Typhus). Available from: http://www.who.int/ith/diseases/typhusfever/en/.
3. Bechah Y, Capo C, Mege J-L, Raoult D. Epidemic typhus. *Lancet Infect Dis.* 2008 Jul;8(7):417–426.
4. Reynolds MG, Krebs JW, Comer JA, et al. Flying squirrel-associated typhus, United States. *Emerg Infect Dis.* 2003 Oct; [serial online]. Available from: http://wwwnc.cdc.gov/eid/article/9/10/03-0278.htm.
5. Conlon JM. The historical impact of epidemic typhus. *Insects, Disease, and History.* Available from: http://entomology.montana.edu/historybug/TYPHUS-Conlon.pdf.
6. Raoult D, Roux V. The body louse as a vector of reemerging human diseases. *Clin Infect Dis.* 1999;29(4):888–911.
7. U.S. Department of health and human services, National Institutes of Health, National Institute of Allergy and Infectious Diseases. *NIAID Biodefense Research Agenda for Category B and C Priority Pathogens* (NIH Publication No. 03-5315). 2003.
8. Azad AF. Pathogenic rickettsiae as bioterrorism agents. *Clin Infect Dis.* 2007;45(suppl 1):S52–S55.
9. World Health Organization. Annex 3: Bases of Quantitative Estimates. In: *Health Aspects of Chemical and Biological Weapons.* November 1969.
10. Walker DH, Dumler J, Marrie T. Rickettsial diseases. In: Longo DL, Fauci AS, Kasper DL, Hauser SL, Jameson J, Loscalzo J, eds. *Harrison's Principles of Internal Medicine.* 18th ed. New York, NY: McGraw-Hill; 2012. http://accessmedicine.mhmedical.com/content.aspx?bookid=331&Sectionid=40726928.
11. Raoult D, Ndihokubwayo JB, Tissot-Dupont H, et al. Outbreak of epidemic typhus associated with trench fever in Burundi. *Lancet.* 1998;352(9125):353–358.
12. La Scola B, Raoult D. Laboratory diagnosis of rickettsioses: current approaches to diagnosis of old and new rickettsial diseases. *J Clin Microbiol.* 1997;35(11):2715–2727.
13. Bise G, Coninx R. Epidemic typhus in a prison in Burundi. *Trans R Soc Trop Med Hyg.* 1997;91(2):133–134.
14. Botelho-Nevers E, Raoult D. Host, pathogen and treatment-related prognostic factors in rickettsioses. *Eur J Clin Microbiol Infect Dis.* 2011;30 (10):1139–1150.
15. VanRooyen MJ, Venugopal R. World travelers. In: Tintinalli JE, Stapczynski J, Ma O, Cline DM, Cydulka RK, Meckler GD T, eds. *Tintinalli's Emergency Medicine: A Comprehensive Study Guide.* 7th ed. New York, NY: McGraw-Hill; 2011. http://accessmedicine.mhmedical.com/content.aspx?bookid=348&Sectionid=40381633.
16. Baxter J. The typhus group. *Clin Dermatol.* 1996;14:271–278.
17. Perine PL, Krause DW, Awoke S, McDade JE. Single-dose doxycycline treatment of lous-borne relapsing fever and epidemic typhus. *Lancet.* 1974;2(7883):742–744.
18. Walker D. The realities of biodefense vaccines against *Rickettsia.* *Vaccine.* 2009;27(suppl 4):D52–D55.

CHAPTER 130

Orientia tsutsugamushi (Scrub Typhus) Attack

Selwyn E. Mahon and Peter B. Smulowitz

DESCRIPTION OF EVENT

Scrub typhus is an acute, febrile, infectious illness caused by *Orientia* (formerly *Rickettsia*) *tsutsugamushi*, an obligate intracellular gram-negative coccobacillus. It was first described in China in 313 AD, and first isolated in Japan in 1930. Although scrub typhus was originally recognized as one of the tropical rickettsial diseases, *O. tsutsugamushi* differs from the rickettsiae with respect to cell-wall structure and genetic composition. Scrub typhus, tropical typhus, and tsutsugamushi disease are all names for the same disease. The colorful name "tsutsugamushi" means small and dangerous creature in Japanese. This tiny parasite is transmitted via the bite of larval stage mites of the genus *Leptotrombidium* (also known as chiggers—the "small and dangerous creature"). Scrub typhus derives its name from the scrub vegetation (i.e., terrain between woods and clearings) where traditionally the disease occurs. But this term is not entirely accurate, as scrub typhus can also exist in sandy beaches, mountain deserts, and equatorial rain forests. The disease is endemic in a broad area known as the "tsutsugamushi triangle," which extends from northern Japan and eastern Russia in the north to northern Australia in the south and to Pakistan and Afghanistan in the west.

Currently, it is estimated that approximately one million cases of scrub typhus occur annually and that as many as one billion people living in endemic areas may have been infected by *O. tsutsugamushi* at some time.[1] Focal pockets of infection known as "mite islands" or "typhus islands" are created in endemic areas secondary to the chiggers' general ability to feed only once[2] and the mites' preference for certain habitats (e.g., scrub vegetation, forest clearings, riverbanks, grassy regions).[3] Although rodents are the main host for the mites, humans who enter these "mite islands" are at high risk of disease transmission. There may be no risk to humans in nearby areas because chiggers typically stay within several meters of where they hatch.[2] Once the chiggers attach to a passing host, they prefer to feed where the skin is thin, tender, or wrinkled and clothing is tight. When feeding, chiggers do not usually pierce the skin. They prefer to insert their mouthparts down hair follicles or pores. They then inject a liquid that dissolves the tissue around the feeding site. The chiggers then suck up the liquefied tissue as food. Large numbers of *O. tsutsugamushi* organisms are found in the salivary glands of the chigger and are injected into its host when it feeds. After feeding, the engorged chigger will drop off its host and burrow into the ground to continue its transformation into a nymph.[4]

Scrub typhus is often acquired either through occupational or travel exposure. Occupational or agricultural exposures occur because active rice fields are an important reservoir for transmission.[5] Most travel-acquired cases of scrub typhus occur during visits to rural areas in endemic countries for activities such as camping, hiking, or rafting, but urban cases have also been described. Clinical cases of scrub typhus are exceedingly rare in the United States, limited to travelers returning from endemic areas.

According to the Centers for Disease Control and Prevention (CDC), travelers and health care providers are generally not at risk of becoming infected via exposure to an ill person. Rickettsial species in general are usually not transmissible directly from person to person, although transmission has been documented to occur via blood transfusion.[6] Rickettsial organisms have caused infection via inhalation of laboratory-derived aerosols, suggesting the potential threat of the organisms as an aerosolized bioweapon.[7] The Soviet Union successfully developed *Rickettsia prowazekii* as a biological weapon during the 1930s and investigated a naturally occurring dormant, stable form that is infectious for long periods of time. During the 1930s and 1940s, the Japanese experimented with both *R. prowazekii* and typhus.[7,8] To date, *O. tsutsugamushi* is not known to have been developed as a biological weapon. Theoretically, the organism could be spread by aerosol if it were manipulated to enhance its ability to survive in the environment. It may also be spread via the rodent host or the chigger vector. Despite the propensity of the chigger to feed only once, dissemination into a crowded population could result in numerous infections.

Scrub typhus often presents as a febrile illness that can be clinically indistinguishable from co-endemic diseases such as typhoid, leptospirosis, and dengue. Affected persons typically develop clinical symptoms between 6 and 18 days after inoculation by an infected chigger. Before the development of systemic symptoms, patients may develop a red papule at the site of the bite, which later forms a vesicle or ulcerates and forms a black eschar. The eschar has been reported to occur in 36% to 88% of cases.[3] The lesion may be associated with regional lymphadenopathy initially and generalized lymphadenopathy in the next 4 to 5 days. The finding of an eschar in a traveler should raise the possibility of scrub typhus. However, finding this lesion in a domestic patient should raise the possibility of cutaneous anthrax.

The onset of systemic symptoms in scrub typhus is usually sudden, with the most common findings being fever, myalgia, severe headache, and rash. Fever, in early stages up to 104 to 105 °F, is the most common symptom. The rash typically occurs after about 5 days of illness. A macular and papular or occasionally vesicular rash begins on the trunk and spreads to the extremities. Other symptoms occasionally encountered include nausea, vomiting, diarrhea, tremors, delirium, nervousness, slurred speech, deafness, and nuchal rigidity.[2] The disease has even been reported to present as an acute abdominal process.[9]

Serious complications occurring with untreated scrub typhus are predominantly pulmonary. Interstitial pneumonia and pulmonary edema may occur. Up to 22% of patients develop serious pneumonitis.[10] Cardiac involvement is less common, but patients may develop myocarditis or congestive heart failure. Other serious complications include meningitis, encephalitis, disseminated intravascular coagulation (DIC), shock, acute respiratory distress syndrome, and acute renal failure.

No laboratory test is diagnostic for scrub typhus. Most patients have a normal white blood cell count, although both leukopenia and leukocytosis may occur. Patients with severe disease often develop thrombocytopenia. In one series of 47 patients from Taiwan, 77% of patients demonstrated abnormalities of hepatic enzymes, with 6 patients presenting with a picture similar to acute viral hepatitis.[11] Lumbar puncture is also nondiagnostic, usually revealing a lymphocytic pleocytosis; in one series of 27 patients, the white blood cell count ranged from 0 to 110/mm^3, with about half lymphocytes.[2]

Diagnosis of scrub typhus is made via serologic studies. The oldest test in current use is the Weil-Felix OX-K agglutination reaction, based on cross-reactivity between antirickettsial antibodies and *Proteus* antigens. The test is inexpensive and easy to perform, and results are available overnight; however, it lacks specificity and sensitivity[12] and is not recommended. The indirect fluorescent antibody (IFA) test, which detects antibodies to specific antigens of the bacteria, is used most often due to its simplicity, rapidity, and a specificity approaching 99%.[13] Results are available in a couple of hours; however, the test is expensive and requires considerable training. IFA uses fluorescent antihuman antibody to detect specific antibodies from patient serum bound to a smear of scrub-typhus antigen and is currently the reference standard.[14] Indirect immunoperoxidase (IIP) testing is becoming more widely used. It eliminates the expense of a fluorescent microscope by substituting peroxidase for fluorescein, and results are also available in 2 hours. All currently available serologic tests for scrub typhus have limitations of which clinicians need to be aware, despite their widespread use. Diagnosis is made when there is a $\geq$4-fold increase in antibody titer between two consecutive samples, but such a diagnosis is retrospective and cannot guide initial treatment.[15] Diagnosis, therefore, depends on clinical suspicion, prompting the clinician to request an appropriate laboratory investigation. Failure to consider or diagnose scrub typhus often results in treatment with ineffective β-lactam–based regimens and poor outcomes.

◀◀ PRE-INCIDENT ACTIONS

Scrub typhus was once a feared disease in the preantibiotic era with case fatality rates reaching 50%. It is also an important military disease. Along with dengue and malaria, scrub typhus exacted a significant toll during World War II. In the Pacific Theater, it was second in importance only to malaria, yet was more dreaded by the troops.[16] It caused almost as many deaths as malaria and was the most important rickettsial disease among American troops. In the Southeast Asia Theater, scrub typhus was the leading cause of death from any communicable disease. Some American troops during the epidemic were convinced that scrub typhus was a biological weapon of the Japanese. Rumors were rampant, but there is no evidence to support the claim.[16]

The magnitude of a bioattack using *O. tsutsugamushi* depends on the mode of dissemination: aerosol versus the chigger vector. Populations of patients may present with the eschar or systemic symptoms described. At the phase of illness at which an eschar is present, cutaneous anthrax must be considered. Isolation may be initially required for patients with other symptoms of scrub typhus, which may be similar to the symptoms of bacterial meningitis. Other differential diagnoses to consider include malaria, dengue, leptospirosis, other rickettsial diseases, typhoid fever, endocarditis, tularemia, hemorrhagic fevers, meningococcemia, measles, secondary syphilis, infectious mononucleosis, and rubella.

Transmission of *O. tsutsugamushi* between persons is not believed to occur and poses little risk to health care workers. Preventive measures in endemic areas include the use of protective clothing and insect repellents. Short-term vector reduction using environmental insecticides and vegetation control should be instituted.

▶▶ POST-INCIDENT ACTIONS

Clinicians entertaining a high level of suspicion for a possible scrub typhus attack or who have confirmatory data of a case of scrub typhus should notify the appropriate local, state, and federal public health and law enforcement authorities. Control of the disease depends on control of the trombiculid mites. Focal areas can be treated with chlorinated hydrocarbons such as lindane, dieldrin, or chlordane, although these may cause secondary environmental problems. Insect repellants and miticides such as *N,N*-diethyl-*m*-toluamide (DEET), dusting sulphur, dimethyl phthalate, or benzyl benzoate are effective when applied to both clothing and skin, whereas permethrin and benzyl benzoate are effective when applied to clothing and bedding.[3,4]

✚ MEDICAL TREATMENT OF CASUALTIES

The current treatment for scrub typhus is administration of a tetracycline.[17] Chloramphenicol is also effective, and macrolides have been used as well. Intravenous (IV) antibiotics may be administered to patients who are seriously ill and unable to swallow pills. Azithromycin has been suggested as an alternative therapy in pregnant women and children. Doxycycline is the most commonly used treatment for scrub typhus. The regimen consists of 100 mg given orally or IV twice daily for 7 days. Some studies have advocated short-course therapy, consisting of anywhere from 1 to 3 days of treatment, although the 5- to 7-day course is still recommended to prevent relapse of the disease. Relapse may occur despite proper antibiotic therapy. Likely reasons for relapse include the following: antibiotics are not taken for a long enough period, treatment limited to the first 5 days of the disease, and the emergence of strains of *O. tsutsugamushi* with reduced susceptibility to antibiotics.[18] In resistant strains, limited data have demonstrated the utility of adding rifampin to doxycycline.[20,21] Rifampin and azithromycin have also been used successfully in areas where scrub typhus is resistant to conventional therapy.[18] Due to the serotypic heterogeneity of *O. tsutsugamushi*, no effective vaccine has been developed.

If an attack with the organism is highly suspected, chemoprophylaxis in potentially exposed persons might be successful. Chemoprophylaxis regimens include the following:

- A single dose of doxycycline given weekly, started before exposure and continued for 6 weeks after exposure[19]
- A single oral dose of chloramphenicol or tetracycline given every 5 days for a total of 35 days, with 5-day nontreatment intervals

❓ UNIQUE CONSIDERATIONS

Mass bioattack with the bacteria causing scrub typhus is difficult because the bacteria require the mite vector for dissemination. The larval mites rarely travel far from the place where they hatch, and they usually bite only once. However, focal islands of infection may be created in areas suitable to the mites, and cases have been reported in urban areas of Asia. In 1976 letters containing ticks were found in various U.S. cities. The letter that accompanied the ticks warned of a "dangerous disease" that the ticks carried. It is possible that the mites that carry scrub typhus could be used in similar bioattacks. Scrub typhus should be considered in patients presenting with an eschar or with fever and a rash because early treatment can prevent many of the serious complications of the disease.

! PITFALLS

Several potential pitfalls in response to an outbreak of scrub typhus exist. These include the following:

- Failure to consider scrub typhus in a patient with a cutaneous eschar
- Failure to realize that relapse of the disease can occur if treated early in the course or if doxycycline fails (or is not used) to treat resistant strains
- Failure to consider scrub typhus in the setting of high fever and a rash developing in patients within a focal geographic location
- Failure to avoid serious complications of the disease by delaying necessary antibiotic therapy
- Failure to report suspected cases of scrub typhus to the appropriate health and law enforcement agencies

REFERENCES

1. Raoult D. Scrub typhus. In: Mandell GL, Bennett JE, Dolin R, eds. 6th ed. *Mandell, Douglas and Bennett's Principles and Practice of Infectious Diseases*; vol. 2: Philadelphia, PA: Elsevier Churchill Livingstone; 2005:2309–2310.
2. Saah AJ. *Orientia tsutsugamushi* (scrub typhus). In: Mandell GL, Bennett JE, Dolin R, eds. *Principles and Practice of Infectious Diseases*. 5th ed. Philadelphia, PA: Churchill Livingstone; 2000:2056–2058.
3. Sexton DJ. Scrub typhus: clinical features and diagnosis. *UpToDate online.* 2003. http://www.uptodateonline.com/application/topic.asp?file=tickflea/6173&type=A&selectedTitle=1~7.
4. Devine J. A review of scrub typhus management in 2000–2001 and implications for soldiers. *J Rural Remote Environ Health.* 2003;2:14–20.
5. Watt G, Walker DH. Scrub typhus. In: Guerrant RL, Walker DH, Weller PF, eds. *Tropical Infectious Diseases: Principles, Pathogens and Practice*; 2nd ed. vol. 1. Philadelphia, PA: Elsevier Churchill Livingstone; 2006.
6. CDC Health Information for International Travel Chapter 3: Infectious Diseases Related To Travel. Available at: http://wwwnc.cdc.gov/travel/yellowbook/2014/chapter-3-infectious-diseases-related-to-travel/rickettsial-spotted-and-typhus-fevers-and-related-infections-anaplasmosis-and-ehrlichiosis August 2013.
7. Walker DH. Principles of the malicious use of infectious agents to create terror: reasons for concern for organisms of the genus *Rickettsia. Ann N Y Acad Sci.* 2003;990:739–742.
8. Azad AF, Radulovic S. Pathogenic rickettsiae as bioterrorism agents. *Ann N Y Acad Sci.* 2003;990:734–738.
9. Yang CH, Young TG, Peng MY, Hsu GJ. Unusual presentation of acute abdomen in scrub typhus: a report of two cases. *Zhonghua Yi Xue Za Zhi (Taipei).* 1995;55:401–404.
10. Watt G, Parola P. Scrub typhus and tropical rickettsioses. *Curr Opin Infect Dis.* 2003;16:429–436.
11. Yang CH, Hsu GJ, Peng MY, Young TG. Hepatic dysfunction in scrub typhus. *J Formos Med Assoc.* 1995;94:101–105.
12. Kelly DJ, Wong PW, Gan E, Lewis GE. Comparative evaluation of the indirect immunoperoxidase test for the serodiagnosis of rickettsial disease. *Am J Trop Med Hyg.* 1988;38:400–406 [PubMed: 3128129].
13. Weddle JR, Chan TC, Thompson K, et al. Effectiveness of a dot-blot immunoassay of anti-*Rickettsia tsutsugamushi* antibodies for serologic analysis or scrub typhus. *Am J Trop Med Hyg.* 1995;53:43–46.
14. Blacksell SD, Bryant NJ, Paris DH, Doust JA, Sakoda Y, Day NP. Scrub typhus serologic testing with the indirect immunofluorescence method as a diagnostic gold standard: a lack of consensus leads to a lot of confusion. *Clin Infect Dis.* 2007;44:391–401 [PubMed: 17205447].
15. Koh GCKW, Maude RJ, Paris DH, Newton PN, Blacksell SD. Diagnosis of scrub typhus. *Am J Trop Med Hyg.* 2010;82(3):368–370.
16. Philip CB. Tsutsugamushi disease (scrub typhus) in World War II. *J Parasitol.* 1948;34:169–191.
17. Gupta N, Mittal V, Gurung B, Sherpa U. Pediatric scrub typhus in South Sikkim. *Indian Pediatr.* 2012;49(4):322–324.
18. Cennimo DJ. Scrub typhus treatment & management. *Medscape.* July 2013. http://emedicine.medscape.com/article/971797.
19. Olson JG, Bourgeois AL, Fang RC, Coolbaugh JC, Dennis DT. Prevention of scrub typhus. Prophylactic administration of doxycycline in a randomized double blind trial. *Am J Trop Med Hyg.* 1980;29(5):989–997.
20. Panpanich R. Antibiotics for treating scrub typhus. *Cochrane Database Syst Rev.* 2002;3, CD002150.
21. Watt G, Kantipong P, Jongsakul K, et al. Doxycycline and rifampicin for mild scrub-typhus infections in northern Thailand: a randomized trial. *Lancet.* 2000;356:1057–1061.

Rickettsia rickettsii (Rocky Mountain Spotted Fever) Attack

Mohammad Alotaibi and Siraj Amanullah

DESCRIPTION OF EVENT

Rocky Mountain spotted fever (RMSF), once known as "black measles" and "black fever" for its associated hemorrhagic rash, has been recognized as the most lethal tick-borne illness in the United States. It was first documented in the United States in 1896 after outbreaks in Idaho and Montana and resulted in numerous deaths at the time.[1,2] In 1919 the etiologic infectious agent was named *Rickettsia rickettsii*, an obligate gram-negative intracellular coccobacillus. There are 20 other known species of *Rickettsia* bacteria resulting in illness similar to RMSF throughout the world.[3,4] RMSF is the most significant rickettsiosis in the United States with several hundred cases reported annually to the Centers for Disease Control and Prevention (CDC).[5,6] There has been an overall increase in reported cases over the years that could be attributed to either better identification or a more broad definition of cases required to be reported (required reporting of suspected cases and not just those that are confirmed).[3,7] Case fatality rate has declined from 60% in the preantibiotic age to now less than 0.5% in 2010 (CDC estimates).[8] Mortality rises in untreated cases, if antibiotics are started late in the course of illness, in patients who present in "out of tick season" or without a rash (possibly due to delayed diagnosis and initiation of appropriate treatment), in immunocompromised hosts, and in pediatric patients less than 10 years of age.[9]

R. rickettsii exists naturally in a complex life cycle involving certain ixodid hard tick species and their warm-blooded hosts. Ticks act as both hosts and vectors by passing the organisms to their progeny transovarially. Wild mammals and rodents may become transiently infected when bitten, thus representing another host reservoir for the bacteria. Humans appear to be accidental hosts when bitten by infected ticks with the majority of reported cases in the spring and summer months (more outdoor activities); however, humans may become infected throughout the year. Ticks responsible for transmission of RMSF are primarily dog ticks, including *Dermacentor variabilis*, *Dermacentor andersoni*, and *Rhipicephalus sanguineus*. Humans become infected by coming in contact with these ticks via dogs. Adult ticks can transmit the infection after 6 to 10 hours of feeding.[10] Other reported modes of transmission are direct exposure to the agent from a crushed tick and via human blood transfusions or exposure.[3]

Vascular endothelium is primarily infected by this organism after it is inoculated through the skin and enters the bloodstream via lymphatics. The resultant vasculitis results in vascular leakage, microhemorrhages, and thrombin formation. Clinically it is evident as hypovolemia, edema (e.g., pulmonary edema, increase in intracranial pressure), tissue infarcts (e.g., myocarditis, skin rash), hyponatremia, and thrombocytopenia. However, multiorgan failure is seen only in very sick patients and disseminated intravascular coagulation is rare despite the procoagulation phenomenon due to vascular injury. The first sign of infection after an incubation period of 5 to 14 days is fever, and the presentation is usually abrupt. The classic triad of headache, fever, and rash after tick exposure has been reported in approximately 60% of cases at various points of illness. Other symptoms include anorexia, abdominal pain, nausea, vomiting, diarrhea, myalgias, conjunctivitis, hepatosplenomegaly, and lymphadenopathy. The characteristic rash, which is present in up to 85% of cases, appears early in most pediatric patients, usually in 48 to 72 hours, and around the third to sixth day of illness in adults. It is composed of pink macules on the wrists and ankles and is due to focal skin infection. This may progress to papules and eventually petechiae, which may involve the palms and soles. The petechiae appear late (usually by the sixth day of illness) and is a sign of severe illness. The face is usually not involved and involvement of the palms and soles (not pathognomonic) is reported in up to 50% of cases.[10] Patients with the most severe form of illness have petechiae, hypovolemia, myocarditis, cardiac arrhythmias, pulmonary edema, pneumonitis, acute tubular necrosis and renal failure, seizure, encephalitis, and coma.[11–13]

The diagnosis is usually made clinically, and it is recommended that treatment be started before confirmatory results are obtained, due to severe morbidity associated with the illness. A tick bite is recalled only in approximately half of the patients, and confirmatory diagnosis is based on fourfold or greater elevation of antibody titers between acute and convalescent sera. Laboratory findings are variable and nondiagnostic but may include leukocytosis, thrombocytopenia, anemia, hyponatremia, low albumin, elevation of hepatic enzymes, and cerebrospinal fluid findings of pleocytosis (mononuclear cells), elevated protein, and normal glucose. Skin biopsy (with polymerase chain reaction [PCR] or immunohistochemical stains) and indirect immunofluorescent antibody assay remain the mainstay of diagnosis but are not considered essential for initiation of treatment.[3] Both IgM and IgG antibodies can be cross reactive to other *Rickettsia* infections, and can take about 2 weeks to be detectable.[14] Therefore an early negative test does not rule out RMSF. Also it is essential to perform both IgM and IgG titers because IgM can be false positive.

PRE-INCIDENT ACTIONS

It is unknown whether RMSF has ever been used as a bioweapon. Considering the nature of the causative organism and its dependence on strict host environment (either ticks or mammals), it may be extremely unlikely to convert this agent into a bioweapon. However, just like any other biological agent with the potential of significant morbidity and mortality, a high index of suspicion is required to identify such an attack when there are unusual clusters, increased numbers, or unseasonal presentations of infectious illness consistent with RMSF. *R. rickettsii* is not known to be transmitted by aerosol route. This is in comparison to *R. prowazekii* (causative agent of epidemic typhus) which is considered to be a type B bioterrorism agent due to its ability to be transmitted via aerosol route. As discussed, exposure to infected ticks is the only known risk factor for *R. rickettsii* and human-to-human transmission is only reported by blood exposure.[3]

POST-INCIDENT ACTIONS

As in any other bioterrorism event, there is a need for post-event preparedness involving establishment of communication channels, resource activation, assembly of teams and leadership structure, and initiation of proper triage, decontamination areas, and management planning at hospitals and emergency department levels. RMSF is not considered to be contagious and therefore would not potentially require decontamination unless somehow changed into an aerosolized agent. RMSF has an inexpensive effective treatment. There are no vaccines for rickettsial infections, and the CDC does not recommend any chemoprophylaxis. The diagnosis remains clinical, and treatment should be instituted early based on the clinician's index of suspicion.

MEDICAL TREATMENT OF CASUALTIES

The treatment of choice for RMSF is doxycycline 2.2 mg/kg body weight twice daily for children less than 45 kg (100 lb). For adults the dosage is 100 mg every 12 hours for 7 to 10 days (or until 3 days after the patient is afebrile). RMSF treatment in pediatric patients by doxycycline has not found to result in the dental and bone side effects associated with tetracycline treatment. Hence doxycycline is the first line treatment in pediatric patients. This is also due to the severe morbidity risk of RMSF and studies showing a reduction in mortality only with doxycycline. For pregnant patients or those with tetracycline allergy the alternative drug of choice is chloramphenicol at 50 to 75 mg/kg/day in four divided doses. Chloramphenicol has been found to have lower efficacy than doxycycline for RMSF especially when mortality is compared. Chloramphenicol is also associated with the potential idiosyncratic side effect of aplastic anemia and does not have available oral formulation in the United States. No other antibiotic has been found to be effective against RMSF. Treatment remains supportive for various clinical complications seen in severe cases of RMSF including ventilation, dialysis, and volume resuscitation.[15,16]

UNIQUE CONSIDERATIONS

RMSF agent due to its natural course and need for existence in a living host makes it an unlikely candidate for bioterrorism. It is the agent of the most lethal form of tick-borne illness and therefore should be on the clinical radar when unusual clusters of infections are identified. It is also not known if it could be converted to an aerosol form and if so whether it can be transmitted from human to human.

PITFALLS

Potential pitfalls in response to an *R. rickettsii* attack include the following:

- Failure to consider RMSF as a potential cause of acute, febrile illness with or without rash
- Failure to initiate treatment on clinical suspicion while waiting for laboratory test results

- Failure to report suspected cases to the state department of public health or CDC
- Failure to alert local and state agencies to a suspected biological attack when presented with an usual cluster or unseasonal presentation of RMSF-like acute febrile illness
- Using geographic or seasonal exclusion criteria for the diagnosis as it can present year-wide and from any geographic area
- Failure to use doxycycline in adults and children unless absolutely contraindicated
- Failure to recognize that human transmission has been reported after blood transfusion, needlestick injuries, or laboratory accidents[17,18]

REFERENCES

1. CDC Viral and Rickettsial Zoonoses Branch Web site. Available at: http://www.cdc.gov/ncidod/dvrd/rmsf. Accessed on April 29, 2014.
2. Masters EJ, Olson GS, Weiner SJ, et al. Rocky Mountain spotted fever: a clinician's dilemma. *Arch Intern Med.* 2003;163:769–774.
3. Woods CR. Rocky Mountain Spotted Fever in Children. *Pediatr Clin North Am.* 2013;60:455–470.
4. Walker DH. *Rickettsia rickettsii* and other spotted fever group rickettsia (Rockey Mountain Spotted Fever and other spotted fevers). *Mandell: Mandell, Douglas, and Bennett's Principles and Practice of Infectious Diseases*; 7th ed; Churchill Livingstone; 2009. Accessed MD Consult on May 1, 2014.
5. Paddock CD, Holman RC, Krebs JW, et al. Assessing the magnitude of fatal Rocky Mountain spotted fever in the United States: comparison of two national data sources. *Am J Trop Med Hyg.* 2002;67:349–354.
6. Dalton MJ, Clarke MJ, Holman RC, et al. National surveillance for Rocky Mountain spotted fever, 1981-1992: epidemiologic summary and evaluation of risk factors for fatal outcome. *Am J Trop Med Hyg.* 1995;52:405–413.
7. Centers for Disease Control and Prevention. Summary of notifiable diseases—United States, 2010. *MMWR Morb Mortal Wkly Rep.* 2012;59(53):1–116.
8. http://www.cdc.gov/rmsf/stats. Accessed on April 24, 2014.
9. Kirkland KB, Wilkinson WE, Sexton DJ. Therapeutic delay and mortality in cases of Rocky Mountain spotted fever. *Clin Infect Dis.* 1995;20:1118–1121.
10. Lin L, Decker CF. Rocky mountain spotted fever. *Dis Mon.* 2012;58(6):361–369.
11. Fauci AS, Braunwald E, Isselbacher KJ, et al. *Harrison's Principles of Internal Medicine.* 14th ed. New York: McGraw-Hill; 1998:1045–1047.
12. Helmick CG, Bernard KW, D'Angelo LJ. Rocky Mountain spotted fever: clinical, laboratory, and epidemiological features of 262 cases. *J Infect Dis.* 1984;150:480.
13. Buckingham SC, Marshall GS, Schutze GE, et al. Clinical and laboratory features, hospital course, and outcome of Rocky Mountain Spotted Fever in children. *J Pediatr.* 2007;150(2):180–184.
14. Raoult D, Paddock CD. *Rickettsia parkeri* infection and other spotted fevers in the United States. *N Engl J Med.* 2005;353(6):626–627.
15. Minninear TD, Buckingham SC. Managing Rocky Mountain spotted fever. *Expert Rev Anti Infect Ther.* 2009;7(9):1131–1137.
16. American Academy of Pediatrics. Rocky mountain spotted fever. In: Pickering LK, ed. *Red book: 2012 Report of the Committee on Infectious Diseases.* 29th ed. Elk Grove Village, IL: American Academy of Pediatrics; 2012:623–625.
17. Wells GM, Woodward TE, Fiset P, et al. Rocky mountain spotted fever caused by blood transfusion. *JAMA.* 1978;239(26):2763–2765.
18. Tamrakar SB, Haas CN. Dose-response model of Rocky Mountain spotted fever (RMSF) for Human. *Risk Anal.* 2011;31(10):1610–1621.

Vibrio cholerae (Cholera) Attack

Nishanth S. Hiremath, Srihari Cattamanchi, Vidyalakshmi PR, and Milana Trounce

DESCRIPTION OF EVENT

Cholera is an acute diarrheal illness caused by the bacterium *Vibrio cholerae*. If cholera is left untreated, it leads to dehydration and death. *V. cholerae* is a Centers for Disease Control and Prevention (CDC) category B bioterrorism agent. It is a motile, curved, gram-negative rod that exists in nature independent of a mammalian host and is a normal inhabitant of surface water. More than 99.9% of naturally occurring, waterborne *V. cholerae* organisms are associated with tiny crustaceans: zooplankton called copepods. The cholera bacteria attach themselves to copepods and travel with their hosts as they follow their algae and plankton food source. Attempts to limit cholera transmission have used this fact and led to the active filtering of water through low-tech filters (e.g., eight layers of "sari" cloth in Bangladesh).

Although cholera is virtually nonexistent in North America (0 to 5 cases per year), it is endemic in agrarian areas with poor sanitation, crowding, famine, and war.[1] Areas of occurrence include Sub-Saharan Africa, the Middle East, South Asia, Southeast Asia, and South America.[2] Figure 132-1 displays all countries that reported cholera outbreaks from 2010 to 2013.[3]

Approximately 3 to 5 million cases of cholera occur each year worldwide, with more than 100,000 attributable deaths.[4] During the nineteenth century, the disease spread from the Ganges Delta region in India, the original reservoir of the disease, across the world.[4] Cholera first spread as a pandemic in 1817; subsequently, six pandemics occurred that killed millions of people across all continents.[2] During the seventh pandemic that began in 1961, the El Tor biotype of *V. cholerae* Serotype O1 originated in Sulawesi, Indonesia, and rapidly spread to other countries in Asia, Europe, and Africa, reaching Latin America in 1991.[4] *V. cholerae* O139 Bengal, a new strain identified in India and Bangladesh, caused an outbreak in 1992, which is still confined to Asian countries.[2] The recent Haiti cholera outbreak in October 2010 due to a strain found in South Asia has produced by the date of this writing more than 6631 attributable deaths and 470,000 cases of cholera.[5] The CDC has declared the ongoing Haiti cholera outbreak as the worst outbreak in recent history; it is also the best-documented outbreak in modern public health.[5]

Transmission of cholera occurs via the fecal-oral route. Ingestion of the typical environmental reservoir of *V. cholerae*, undercooked food, especially shellfish, and "burial ceremonies requiring the handling of intestinal contents" have also been implicated in the transmission.[6] Cholera can survive for 24 hours in sewage, about 6 weeks in water containing organic matter, and 16 days in soil. *V. cholerae* can withstand freezing for 3 to 4 days but is readily killed by dry heat at 242.6 °F (117 °C) or by boiling.[7] Of the 18 cholera investigations undertaken by the CDC between 1988 and 1998, four occurred in the United States and involved various factors including patients at nursing homes, raw fish, food imported from other countries, and contaminated food on an international flight.[8] In addition to sporadic cases, epidemics sometimes occur, including several during the 1990s in South and Central America.[8]

Only two serotypes of *V. cholerae* cause epidemic disease: the O1 serotype (divided into two groups, El Tor and "classical") and the O139 serotype. Other serotypes cause sporadic cases of gastroenteritis. Recently, the O139 serotype has spread from India and Asia to the Middle East.[9] At this time, there is no weaponized form of the disease. A bioattack using *V. cholerae* would most likely occur via contaminated water or food source.

Infection can occur after the ingestion of as few as 1000 organisms. Infection is more likely in patients who are receiving acid suppression therapy because gastric acid at a pH of less than 2.5 will effectively kill *V. cholerae* organisms. After ingestion, the incubation period is 4 hours to 5 days, with most patients presenting within 2 to 3 days.[7,10,11] Most *V. cholerae* infections are asymptomatic or present with only mild disease. Depending on the serotype, up to 75% of infected individuals will remain asymptomatic. Of the other 25%, the majority have a mild diarrheal illness not requiring medical attention, 5% require hospitalization, and 2% develop classic cholera (also known as *cholera gravis*) with voluminous "rice water" stools. The symptoms of cholera gravis include a gradual to sudden onset of vomiting, malaise, headache, and intestinal cramping with mild or no fever, trailed by painless and voluminous diarrhea that looks likes rice water. Fluid losses surpass 5 to 10 L/day and up to 1 L/h of diarrhea is not uncommon. Patients with blood type O are more likely to develop severe disease. The mortality rate in the 2% with cholera gravis is 50% to 75%, giving an overall mortality in infected persons of 1% to 1.5%. Patients can die within 2 to 3 hours of the initial signs of infection, but death in the untreated individual usually occurs after several days.[12] The mortality risk is increased in children (10 times greater than in adults), the elderly, and pregnant women. There is also an amplified risk of fetal death.[13]

Definitive testing for *V. cholerae* is performed relatively easily in the laboratory. Stool cultures should be sent and plated on thiosulfate-citrate-bile salts-sucrose (TCBS) agar or tellurite, taurocholate, and gelatin agar (TTGA). Gram stains of stool may show sheets of curved gram-negative rods. Other rapid diagnostic methods primarily used in epidemiological studies include the detection of *V. cholerae* organisms in stool specimens by polymerase chain reaction and monoclonal antibody-based stool tests.[14]

The most likely scenario for an outbreak would involve a large number of otherwise healthy persons presenting over a period of several days with severe diarrhea or gastroenteritis symptoms and dehydration. Once a few cases of cholera are confirmed, the possibility of biological terrorism should be considered.

Cholera should be included in the differential diagnosis of all cases of severe watery diarrhea and vomiting, especially those producing

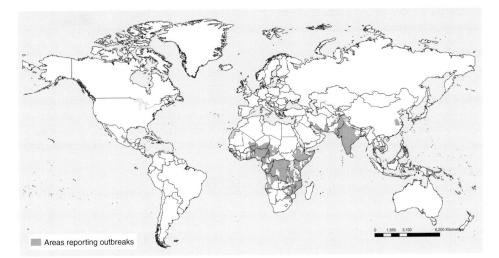

FIG 132-1 Countries Reporting Cholera Outbreaks from 2010 to 2013. (Data from World Health Organization Map Production: Health Statistics and Information Systems [HSI], Copyright World Health Organization.)

severe and rapid dehydration. The possibility of one or more cholera epidemics is a powerful motivation to the development of needed infrastructure for safer water handling, sanitation, and public health capability for surveillance and response to epidemics.

PRE-INCIDENT ACTIONS

A multidisciplinary approach centered on prevention, preparedness, and response laterally with an effectual surveillance structure is crucial for controlling and mitigating cholera outbreaks in endemic areas and reducing deaths.[4] Transmission of cholera-causing species between persons is rare, and no additional precautions beyond universal precautions are required in patients suspected of having cholera. The possibility of contracting cholera by inhalation is extremely unlikely, and personal protective equipment is not essential.

POST-INCIDENT ACTIONS

In some countries individuals with cholera can be legally quarantined, for example in Australia under the Commonwealth Quarantine Act of 1908.[15] If cholera is diagnosed either clinically or by laboratory testing, notify the appropriate local, state, federal, or government public health and law enforcement authorities. Steps ought to be taken to recognize the source of the contamination and to prevent further spread of disease, particularly if there is no history of travel to an endemic region.

From the date of last exposure, contacts are to be observed for 5 days. Contacts include all fellow travelers of the index case. Even if asymptomatic, stool culture of all contacts should be undertaken. It is not indicated to immunize the contacts. Using standard precautions, isolate severely ill patients in the hospital. All articles and linen used by the patients should be disinfected. In the absence of preliminary disinfection, feces and vomitus can be disposed of into toilets linked to a sewage system.[15]

Simple soap-and-water bathing or skin-washing will remove nearly all *V. cholerae* from the skin surface; washing should be performed immediately and often. Chlorine and other antibacterial solutions provide adequate decontamination of surfaces of potentially contaminated objects.

Urgent investigation of potentially contaminated food and water supply should be carried out if there is no history of overseas travel.[15] Cholera is almost unknown where water supplies are properly disinfected (~100 ppm of chlorine). However, it is tolerant to residual

(<2 ppm) chlorine. Water should be boiled if an event warrants necessity of this precaution (e.g., in the event of a water purification infrastructure failure), and all food should be well cooked. Reverse osmosis of water, iodine, chlorine (e.g., chlorine bleach added to drinking water: two drops household bleach [5.25%] per liter), or micropore filters can also be used. Simple filtering procedures (e.g., sari cloth) will not be effective in the event of an epidemic caused by purposefully contaminated water. While simple filtering techniques may limit transmissions associated with copepods in purposefully contaminated water, *V. cholerae* may be transmitted independently.

An outbreak of cholera is a single case of cholera in a person with no history of overseas travel. An investigation is initiated immediately to find the circumstances and vehicle of disease transmission and accordingly plan for control measures. The populations at risk should be educated on precautions to be taken and the need to seek appropriate medical treatment immediately. In order to ensure a safe water supply, emergency measures are taken, and food and drink preparations are to be carefully supervised.[15]

MEDICAL TREATMENT OF CASUALTIES

The degree of dehydration determines the course of treatment. Oral rehydration solutions (ORS) have decreased the mortality rate associated with cholera from more than 50% to less than 1%.[9] ORS take advantage of the fact that adsorption of water, along with sodium, in the small intestine is expedited by glucose and occurs even in the presence of cholera toxin. The World Health Organization (WHO) endorses a solution that contains 1.5 g of potassium chloride, 2.5 g of sodium bicarbonate or 2.9 g of trisodium citrate, 3.5 g of sodium chloride, and 20 g of glucose or 40 g of sucrose per liter of water.[16] A number of studies have investigated alternatives to this WHO ORS and found that ORS containing rice or cereal as the carbohydrate source may be even more effective than glucose-based solutions in shortening the duration of diarrhea and reducing stool volume.[12,16]

Patients who have lost more than 10% of their body weight due to dehydration or who are not able to drink because of vomiting or mental status changes should be started on intravenous rehydration. The ideal solution is lactated Ringer's solution. Normal saline can be used with the realization that bicarbonate and potassium losses are not being replaced. Use of 5% dextrose in water is also suboptimal because it does not replace sodium, bicarbonate, or potassium losses.

Antimicrobial therapy can also be used in the treatment of cholera but should be viewed as an adjunct to appropriate hydration. Antibiotics reduce the volume of diarrhea by 50% and the duration of *V. cholerae* excretion by about 1 day. Thus antibiotics are cost-effective and recommended for severely ill patients (i.e., those with cholera gravis). Antibiotics are given orally when vomiting stops and when initial rehydration is accomplished. Antibiotic susceptibility patterns should guide treatment. Tetracycline and doxycycline are the most commonly prescribed antibiotics. Ciprofloxacin has also been used with equal or greater effectiveness than doxycycline. Risks and benefits need to be weighed when determining treatment in pregnant women and children. Options in children and pregnant women include erythromycin or azithromycin. It is of note that many strains are tetracycline-resistant. It is also likely that any organism used as a weapon may be multidrug-resistant.

Vaccination is also another therapy used in the treatment of cholera. A parenteral killed whole-cell vaccine is available in the United States, but provides less than 50% protection for only 3 to 6 months and is not effective for all types of cholera (such as O139).[17] A number of new vaccines are under investigation. In 1999 WHO recommended that the oral cholera vaccine, that is the whole-cell/recombinant B subunit (WC/rBS) vaccine, should be considered for use in preventing cholera in residents at risk for an epidemic within 6 months but not experiencing a current epidemic.[18] Vaccine use during an epidemic is not recommended.

Although antibiotic prophylaxis seems intuitive for populations at risk in cholera epidemics, it has been shown to be ineffectual and should not be used. Because direct person-to-person transmission does not occur, treating family members is unnecessary. However, if the family is using the same contaminated water source (e.g., in third world countries or with a breakdown of water treatment in the United States), consider prophylactic use of antibiotics if more than one family member becomes infected.

UNIQUE CONSIDERATIONS

The core issues in the treatment of cholera are (1) ensuring an adequate supply of intravenous fluids if a large population of persons becomes symptomatic and (2) adequately measuring stool output in order to calculate replacement. The initial problem can be addressed by using oral rehydration solution in the least sick patients and in all patients who can keep up with fluid output orally. The second problem has been solved in third world countries using "cholera beds." Cholera beds are stretchers with a hole in them through which the patient passes stools. The stool is collected in a bucket so that fluid loss can be measured. Cholera beds can be improvised by cutting holes in simple canvas or nylon stretchers or military cots without too much difficulty. Repulsive as it may seem, this setup is practical and reduces staff time substantially (e.g., time spent getting patients to the commode). Evidently, these would only be used during an epidemic when hospital resources are stretched thin.

PITFALLS

Several potential pitfalls in response to a cholera epidemic exist. These include the following:
- Failure to implement adequate systems (e.g., hospital beds, personnel, local, state, and federal or government resources) to respond to possible bioattacks before they occur

- Failure to have adequate supplies of oral and intravenous rehydration solutions and supplies
- Failure to adequately rehydrate patients, instead relying on antibiotic treatment
- Failure to notify appropriate public health and law enforcement agencies when an outbreak of cholera is suspected or confirmed
- Failure to treat patients with ORS instead of intravenous hydration, when possible (an excessive amount of intravenously treated patients will unnecessarily tie up resources needed by sicker patients in the event of a mass casualty event related to cholera attack)

REFERENCES

1. Cholera: Causes, Symptoms, Treatment and Prevention. Available at: http://www.webmd.com/a-to-z-guides/cholera-faq.
2. Mandal A. Cholera epidemiology. Available at: http://www.news-medical.net/health/Cholera-Epidemiology.aspx.
3. World Health Organization—Global Health Observatory Map Gallery. World: areas reporting cholra outbreaks, 2010-2013. Available at: http://gamapserver.who.int/mapLibrary/Files/Maps/Global_Cholera_outbreaks.png.
4. World Health Organization. Cholera. Available at: http://www.who.int/mediacentre/factsheets/fs107/en/.
5. Centers for Disease Control and Prevention (CDC)—Global Health. Cholera in Haiti: One year later. Available at: http://www.cdc.gov/haiticholera/haiti_cholera.htm.
6. Butterton JR. Pathogenesis of *Vibrio cholerae*. In: Rose BD, ed. *UpToDate*. 2004 Wellesley, MA, Available at: http://www.uptodate.com/contents/pathogenesis-of-vibrio-cholerae-infection.
7. USAMIIRD. *Medical Management of Biological Casualties Handbook*. 7th ed. 2001. Available at: http://www.usamriid.army.mil/education/bluebookpdf/USAMRIID%20BlueBook%207th%20Edition%20-%20Sep%202011.pdf.
8. Tauxe RV, Blake PA. Epidemic cholera in Latin America. *JAMA*. 1992;267:1388.
9. World Health Organization. *Cholera: WHO Report on Global Surveillance of Epidemic-Prone Infectious Diseases*. 2000, Report No.: WHO/CDS/CSR/ISR/2000/1. Geneva, Available at: http://www.who.int/csr/resources/publications/surveillance/en/cholera.pdf?ua=1.
10. Goma Epidemiology Group. Public Health Impact of the Rwandan refugee crisis: what happened in Goma, Zaire, in July 1994? *Lancet*. 1995;345, 359.
11. Lindenbaum J, Greenough WB III, Islam MR. Antibiotic therapy of cholera. *Bull World Health Org Suppl*. 1967;36:871.
12. Molla AM, Ahmed SM, Greenough WBI. Rice-based oral rehydration solution decreases the stool volume in acute diarrhea. *Bull World Health Org Suppl*. 1985;63:751.
13. Hirschhorn N, Chaudhury AKMA, Lendenbaum J. Cholera in pregnant women. *Lancet*. 1969;1:1230.
14. Albert MJ, Islam D, Nahar S, Falklind S, Weintraub A. Rapid detection of *Vibrio cholerae* O139 Bengal from stool specimens by PCR. *J Clin Microbiol*. 1997;35:1633.
15. Department of Health, Victoria, Australia. *Cholera*. Available at: http://ideas.health.vic.gov.au/bluebook/cholera.asp.
16. Ramakrishna BS, Venkataraman S, Srinivasan P, Dash P, Young GP, Binder HJ. Amylase-resistant starch plus oral rehydration solution for cholera. *N Engl J Med*. 2000;342:308.
17. Centers for Disease Control and Prevention. *Health Information for International Travel 1996-97*. Atlanta, Ga: U.S. Department of Health and Human Services; 1997. Available at: http://wonder.cdc.gov/wonder/prevguid/p0000475/p0000475.asp.
18. World Health Organization. *Potential Use of Oral Cholera Vaccines in Emergency Situations: Report of a WHO Meeting*. Geneva: WHO; May 12-13, 1999. Report No. WHO/CDS/CSR/EDC/99.4. Available at: http://whqlibdoc.who.int/hq/1999/WHO_CDS_CSR_EDC_99.4.pdf?ua=1.

CHAPTER 133

Shigella dysenteriae (Shigellosis) Attack

Suzanne M. Shepherd, Steven O. Cunnion, and William H. Shoff

DESCRIPTION OF EVENT

Recognized since ancient times, shigellosis encompasses a broad spectrum of acute bacterial infectious diseases of the intestinal tract, caused by species of the genus *Shigella*. *Shigellae* are nonmotile, rod-shaped gram-negative bacteria. Four groups of *Shigella* are recognized based on serologic and biochemical differentiation: group A (*Shigella dysenteriae*), group B (*Shigella flexneri*), group C (*Shigella boydii*), and group D (*Shigella sonnei*). Groups A, B, and C possess multiple serotypes and subtypes. *S. dysenteriae*, type I, also known as the Shiga bacillus, produces Shiga toxin and causes the most severe clinical illness, including hemolytic uremic syndrome and toxic megacolon. It can harbor R-factor plasmids, conferring resistance to multiple antibiotics and produce pandemics with severe clinical illness and a high case fatality rate in all age groups.

Shigella is endemic throughout the world and hyperendemic in developing countries. *S. sonnei* is the predominant serotype isolated in industrialized nations, whereas *S. dysenteriae* and *S. flexneri* are most commonly isolated in developing countries. The annual worldwide incidence of shigellosis is 200 million cases, most commonly found in children 2 to 3 years of age, with an approximate mortality of 650,000.[1] *S. sonnei* causes approximately 14,000 cases of gastrointestinal infection in the United States yearly, with peak incidence in daycare centers and custodial centers for the mentally ill and physically challenged.[2] *Shigella* is the third-most-common enteric bacterial infection in the United States. Except for captive primates, humans serve as the only natural host and reservoir for *Shigellas*. Disease incidence is seasonal, peaking in summer. *Shigella* is transmitted via fecal-hand-oral spread under conditions of poor sanitation, crowding, and limited personal hygiene. Less frequently, *Shigella* is transmitted via contaminated food and water, including swimming areas and wading pools, and seasonally via houseflies.[3] *Shigella* transmission, primarily *S. flexneri*, is increasingly reported via direct or indirect anal-oral contact in men having sex with men (MSM).[4,5]

Both its virulence and short incubation period make *Shigella* a good candidate for use as a bioweapon. Foodborne diseases remain a major public health problem globally. In the United States, foodborne illness has a yearly incidence between 60 and 80 million, and 500 to 9000 deaths.[6–8] Consequently, identifying an outbreak of shigellosis as an incident of bioterrorism may initially escape local public health and medical community awareness and surveillance modalities because of the large baseline noise produced by the relatively common occurrence of food- and water-borne illness and the larger, often multistate, nature of current outbreaks of foodborne disease. Factors that have been shown to contribute to this include the increasing globalization of the food supply and centralization of food production, processing, and distribution, and increasing consumer consumption of fresh produce, as well as foods not prepared in the home.

Shigellas are an interesting bioweapon candidate because of their low infectious dose; as few as ten *Shigellas* have been shown to produce overt clinical illness in volunteers. This finding supports the clinical observations of the ease at which shigellosis can be transmitted among people via the fecal, hand, or oral route during epidemics, particularly in the midst of conditions of crowding and poor sanitation and when poor personal hygiene is practiced among infected victims. Outbreaks caused by these factors have been reported in daycare centers, prolonged care facilities, and refugee and military camps.[9,10] The low infectious dose coupled with the short incubation period (1 to 4 days; 1 to 8 days for *S. dysenteriae* type 1) sets the stage for a widespread outbreak in a short period, when conditions are appropriate. This also allows for potential widespread dispersion of infected individuals before their symptoms are manifested. Additionally, since many individuals with shigellosis are only mildly ill, they remain in contact with others and can further readily transmit the infection.[10] *Shigella* can infect both immunocompetent and immunosuppressed individuals. Finally, *Shigellas* are hardy organisms that may survive for weeks to months in untreated water.[11]

Shigellas are more acid resistant than other bacterial enteropathogens and therefore have higher survival during passage through the stomach, which explains in part their relatively low infectious dose. After a 1- to 4-day incubation period, the spectrum of illness includes asymptomatic infection; mild, watery diarrheal illness similar to that caused by many other bacterial, viral, and protozoal organisms; and classic, severe dysentery, with frequent, small bloody, mucus-containing stools, tenesmus, significant abdominal cramping, vomiting, high fevers, rigors, and toxemia. Typically, illness progresses through several distinct phases. Initial toxemia, malaise, and high fever, and, less commonly, seizure activity in children are followed by several hours of watery diarrhea and then dysentery. The terminal ileum and colon serve as the most significant sites of pathology, demonstrating *Shigellas'* key ability to invade, and reproduce within, intestinal epithelial cells, ultimately leading to cell death, with resultant ileal, colonic and rectal edema and ulceration, hemorrhages, microabscess formation, and a significant inflammatory infiltrate in the lamina propria. Bacteremia is not common, except in patients with AIDS and in malnourished children infected with *S. dysenteriae* type 1. Although all serotypes can cause any type of illness, *S. flexneri and S. dysenteriae* serotypes tend to be associated with more severe illness, and *S. sonnei* with more mild illness. *Shigellosis* may be complicated by severe dehydration in infants and young children. Other complications include the hemolytic uremic syndrome; severe hypoproteinemia in infants and small children, producing an acute kwashiorkor syndrome with edematous extremities[11]; leukemoid reactions (polymorphonuclear leukocyte counts may reach more than 100,000/mm^3); toxic megacolon and rectal prolapse in infants and young children; and, rarely, Reiter syndrome.

Two enterotoxins (ShET 1 and 2) are responsible for the increased small bowel secretions and watery diarrhea prominent in early shigellosis. *Shigellas* possess both chromosomal genes and a large enteroinvasiveness plasmid that encodes the expression of several outer membrane proteins required for cell entrance, intracellular movement, and access to adjacent cells. Shiga toxin possesses several important activities: it is cytoxic in nanogram quantities, possessing a structural similarity to ricin and abrin and inhibiting protein synthesis by cleaving an adenine residue from ribosomal RNA molecules[12,13]; it acts as a neurotoxin, producing hind-limb paralysis, upon injection into mice or rabbits; and it acts as an enterotoxin, inducing intestinal secretions. The exact role of Shiga toxin is unclear. *S. dysenteriae* type-1 mutants that retain invasive potential but lack Shiga-toxin production cause illness with diarrhea and dysentery almost identical to those strains producing Shiga toxin, except with less blood in the stool. Associated hemolytic uremic syndrome is attributed to Shiga toxin.[12]

No characteristic features delineate shigellosis on clinical examination. Laboratory data are also nonspecific. The white blood cell count is often elevated, with a left shift on the differential. Stool microscopy for fecal leukocytes, done appropriately in areas that contain mucus, usually yields positive results. Patients may develop complications including the hemolytic uremic syndrome with significant proteinuria and Reiter syndrome. A specific diagnosis can usually be made within 48 hours by culture of two fresh stool samples on selective and differential media. Rectal swabs can also be transported in buffered glycerol saline and cultured. Of note, *S. dysenteriae* type 1 can be very difficult to culture. In an outbreak investigation, serodiagnosis of serum antibodies to O antigen of the specific *Shigella* serotype can be performed by enzyme-linked immunosorbent assay (ELISA) or passive hemagglutination.

PRE-INCIDENT ACTIONS

Pre-incident actions focus on public health preparedness, health care provider education, and medical surveillance. The Centers for Disease Control and Prevention (CDC) maintain passive national laboratory-based surveillance for *Shigella* and other food- and waterborne pathogens, using electronic public health reporting. Rapid statistical analysis of this electronically transmitted information can detect unusual disease clusters by geographic area or time. A passive, physician-based reporting system also provides data to monitor trends. These systems are, however, prone to significant under-reporting and lack of timeliness.[7] Realizing this, the CDC designed the Foodborne Diseases Active Surveillance Network (FoodNet) to more precisely determine the incidence of foodborne illness in the United States and to provide a network to identify and respond to new and emerging foodborne diseases and to provide a network to identify and respond to the source of specific foodborne illnesses.[15] Health care providers should remain vigilant in identifying case trends suggestive of a *Shigella* outbreak. Ongoing CDC and World Health Organization (WHO) funding has focused on the development of a vaccine that is well tolerated, has a broad spectrum, and possesses long-lived immunity.[14]

Emergency department, hospital, and outpatient facilities should all have general disaster plans in place that address bioterrorist attack and major infectious disease outbreaks, and these plans should be tested regularly. The importance of staff implementing universal precautions and hand washing procedures should be stressed. Measures should be delineated in these plans for changes in triage guidelines to accommodate a rapid increase in patient census, patient isolation, and procedures to obtain increased antibiotic supplies. These plans should be developed in coordination with those of local, state, and federal emergency medical services and public health and government agencies, carefully specifying leadership and decision-making roles.[15]

Ongoing measures to reduce the availability of *Shigella* for malicious purposes are being developed and implemented. Congress enacted the

Public Health Security and Bioterrorism Preparedness and Response Act of 2002. It requires the Food and Drug Administration (FDA) to develop regulations regarding registration of food manufacturing, processing, packing, or holding companies; prior notification of the FDA for imported food; and individuals involved in all areas of food provision to keep records regarding food sources and recipients. In addition, it outlines procedures by the FDA to detain food deemed a threat.[16] National type collections, hospitals, and research laboratories have developed guidelines for the control of access to areas where these microbiological agents are stored.[17]

POST-INCIDENT ACTIONS

Health care providers with a high level of suspicion that a possible *Shigella* outbreak is the result of a deliberate action should notify their hospital infection control personnel and administration, their local public health officer, and law enforcement authorities. Prepositioning of drug and medical equipment stockpiles may prove critical in responding during very large outbreaks. Appropriate infection control procedures should be strictly enforced. Depending on the nature of the purported attack, materials and surfaces possibly contaminated by *Shigella* should be decontaminated with an appropriate disinfectant solution. During naturally occurring outbreaks of shigellosis, mass antibiotic therapy has not been found to be useful.[11]

MEDICAL TREATMENT OF CASUALTIES

The treatment of patients with shigellosis should be initially focused on emergency management of life-threatening complications, supportive measures, and provision of specific antimicrobial therapy. Rapid intravenous access and infusion of crystalloid should be instituted in patients exhibiting signs and symptoms of shock and acidosis. In less critically ill individuals, oral rehydration with oral glucose-electrolyte solutions is preferred. Seizure activity in children necessitates monitoring for airway compromise, head and neck trauma, and aspiration. Intravenous benzodiazepine administration can be used for initial seizure control. Accompanying fever can be controlled with acetaminophen and cool sponge baths, if needed. Agents that suppress intestinal motility should be avoided, as they may prolong the duration and shedding of *Shigellas*. They should only be used in conjunction with antibiotic therapy.

Appropriate antibiotics significantly decrease the duration of diarrheal illness, fever, and *Shigella* excretion. Only a few antibiotics have been proven clinically useful, and widespread use of these agents has led to the emergence of resistance. *Shigellas* have developed resistance to the sulfonamides, tetracycline, and ampicillin. Current treatment options include the use of parenteral ceftriaxone in severely ill children and oral quinolones or azithromycin. Sporadic ciprofloxacin resistance has been reported since 2002, most recently in an outbreak of shigellosis in men who have sex with men.[18,19] Azithromycin resistance has also been noted.[20-22] Several states require two consecutive negative stool cultures at least 24 hours apart for individuals to return to day care or as staff in child and adult care facilities, food handling, or health care. This requires substantial health care resources. At least one small study suggests that a single culture may be appropriate[23] No formal recommendations exist for postexposure prophylaxis. Currently no vaccine is available for shigellosis.

UNIQUE CONSIDERATIONS

Shigella species have an advantage over other potential enteropathogenic bioweapons because of their low infective dose, short incubation period, and variety of potential disease presentations. Health care providers should be aware of the ability of *Shigellas*, especially those organisms producing Shiga toxin, to develop resistance to commonly employed antibiotics. Further, as relatively common causes of intestinal illness worldwide, the only clue to their use as a bioweapon may be the presentation of a large number of individuals with an unusual strain at an unusual time of year or in an uncommon setting.

⚠ PITFALLS

Several potential pitfalls in response to an attack exist. These include the following:

- Failure to develop, implement, and test emergency response plans that include plans to respond to acts of bioterrorism
- Failure to notify appropriate public health agencies when an outbreak of diarrheal illness is suspected
- Failure to consider *Shigella* as a bioweapon
- Failure to consider *Shigella* in the setting of nondysentery illness
- Failure to monitor *Shigella* for antibiotic resistance
- Failure to instruct patients adequately on appropriate infection control precautions

REFERENCES

1. Institute of Medicine. Prospects for Immunizing Against *Shigella* Spp. Washington, DC: National Academic Press; 1986:329–337. New Vaccine Development: Establishing Priorities; Diseases of Importance in Developing Countries; Vol 2.
2. Centers for Disease Control and Prevention. *Shigella Surveillance: Annual Tabulation Summary, 1999*. Atlanta, GA: U.S. Department of Health and Human Services, CDC; 2000.
3. Cohen D, Green M, Block C, et al. Reduction of transmission of shigellosis by control of houseflies (*Musca domestica*). *Lancet*. 1991;337:993–997.
4. Bader M, Pederson AHB, Williams R, Spearman J, Anderson H. Venereal transmission of shigellosis in Seattle—King County. *Sex Transm Dis*. 1977;4:89–91.
5. Centers for Disease Control and Prevention. *Shigella sonnei* outbreak among men who have sex with men-San Francisco, California, 2000-2001. *JAMA*. 2002;287(1):37–38.
6. Bennett JV, Holmberg SD, Rogers MF, et al. Infectious and parasitic diseases. In: Amler RW, Dull HB, eds. *Closing the Gap: The Burden of Unnecessary Illness*. New York, NY: Oxford University Press; 1997:102–114.
7. Swerdlow DL, Altekruse SF. Food-Borne Diseases in the Global Village: What's on the Plate for the 21st Century. In: Scheld WM, Craig WA, Hughes JM, eds. *Emerging Infections 2*. Washington, DC: ASM Press; 1998:273–290.
8. Jones TF, Pavlin BI, LaFleur BJ, Ingram LA, Schaffner W. Restaurant inspection scores and foodborne disease. *Emerg Infect Dis*. 2004;10 (4):688–692.
9. Green MS, Cohen D, Block C, Rouach Z, Dycian R. A prospective epidemiologic study of shigellosis: implications for the new *Shigella* vaccines. *Isr J Med Sci*. 1987;23:811–815.
10. Mohle-Boetani JC, Stapleton M, Finger R, et al. Communitywide shigellosis: control of an outbreak and risk factors in child day-care centers. *Am J Public Health*. 1995;85(6):812–816.
11. Levine MM. Shigellosis. In: Strickland GT, ed. *Hunter's Tropical Medicine and Emerging Infectious Diseases*. 8th ed. Philadelphia, PA: Saunders; 2000:319–323.
12. Heyworth MF. Pathogenesis of bacterial colitis. *Gut*. 1995;36(1):154–155.
13. Jackson MP. Structure-function analyses of Shiga toxin and the Shiga-like toxins. *Microb Patho*. 1990;8:235–242.
14. Angulo F, Voetsch A, Vugia D, et al. Determining the burden of human illness from foodborne diseases: CDC's emerging infections program Foodborne Diseases Active Surveillance Network (FoodNet). *Vet Clin North Am*. 1998;14:165–172.
15. Inglesby TV, Grossman R, O'Toole T. A plague on your city: observations from TOPOFF. *Clin Infect Dis*. 2001;32:436–445.
16. Acheson DWK, Fiore AE. Preventing foodborne disease—what clinicians can do. *N Engl J Med*. 2004;350:437–440.
17. Kolavic SA, Kimura A, Simons SL, Slutsker L, Barth S, Haley CE. An outbreak of *Shigella dysenteriae* type 2 among laboratory workers due to intentional food contamination. *JAMA*. 1997;278(5):396–398.
18. Gandreau C, Raynayake R, Pilon PA, Gagnon S, Roger M, Lévesque S. Ciprofloxacin-resistant *Shigella sonnei* among men who have sex with men, Canada, 2010. *Cent Disease Control Disp*. 2011;17(9):2034–2041.
19. Pazhani GP, Niyogi SK, Singh AK, et al. Molecular characterization of multi-drug resistant *Shigella* species isolated from epidemic and endemic cases of shigellosis in India. *J Med Microbiol*. 2008;57:856–863.
20. Karlsson MS, Bowen A, Reporter R, et al. Outbreak of infections caused by *Shigella sonnei* with reduced susceptibility to azithromycin in the United States. *Antimicrob Agents Chemother*. 2013;57(3):1559–1560.
21. Özment EN, Ince OT, Örün T, Yalçın S, Yurdakök K, Gür D. Clinical characteristics and antibiotic resistance of *Shigella* gastroenteritis in Ankara, Turkey between 2003 and 2009, and comparison with previous reports. *Int J Infect Dis*. 2011;15:e849–e853.
22. Ud-Din AI, Wahid SU, Latif HA, et al. Changing trends in the prevalence of *Shigella* species: Emergence of multi-drug resistant *Shigella sonnei* biotype G in Bangladesh. *PLoS One*. 2013;8(12):e82601.
23. Turabelidze G, Bowen A, Lin M, Tucker A, Butler C, Fick F. Convalescent cultures for control of shigellosis outbreaks. *Pediatr Infect Dis J*. 2010;29 (8):728–730.

SUGGESTED READINGS

1. Mitscherlich E, Marth EH. *Microbial Survival in the Environment: Bacteria and Rickettsiae Important in Human and Animal Health*. Berlin: Springer; 1984:124–130.
2. Cohen D, Ashkenazi S, Green MS, et al. Double-blind vaccine-controlled randomized efficacy trial of an investigational *Shigella sonnei* conjugate vaccine in young adults. *Lancet*. 1997;349:155–159.

134 | CHAPTER

Salmonella Species (Salmonellosis) Attack

Saleh Ali Alesa

DESCRIPTION OF EVENT

Salmonella organisms are gram-negative, nonspore-forming, facultatively anaerobic bacilli of the family Enterobacteriaceae. In humans, nontyphoidal *Salmonella* (NTS) infections are most often associated with food products and are the most frequently identified agent of foodborne disease outbreaks. Food of animal origin, including meat, poultry, eggs, and dairy products, can become contaminated with *Salmonella*. Eating uncooked or inadequately cooked foods cross-contaminated with these products may lead to human infection. In the developed world, nontyphoidal salmonellosis is most often associated with consumption of poultry and eggs, but many food vehicles have been implicated in transmission to humans. Although foodborne outbreaks predominate, waterborne outbreaks of salmonellosis have also been reported. Salmonellosis associated with exotic pets is a resurgent public health problem, with an estimated 3% to 5% of all cases of salmonellosis in humans associated with exposure to exotic pets, especially reptiles.[1] Transmission between humans is less frequent but can occur. Infection has also resulted from the ingestion of contaminated medications, through the administration of intravenous platelet transfusions, and via direct transmission through inadequately sterilized fiber-optic instruments that have been used on patients undergoing upper gastrointestinal endoscopy.[2] Direct fecal to oral spread can also occur, particularly in children.

Salmonella species are classified as category B biological threat agents according to the Centers for Disease Control and Prevention (CDC). Criteria for this category include moderate ease of dissemination and a lower mortality rate than category A agents such as anthrax, and they require enhancement of the CDC's diagnostic capacity as well as enhanced disease surveillance. Several category B agents pose a threat to the food supply. *Salmonella*'s potential as a bioterrorism weapon is well established. The most prominent example of the use of *Salmonella* as a bioterrorism agent occurred in 1984 in The Dalles, Oregon, when followers of the cult leader Bhagwan Shree Rajneesh attempted to influence a local election by contaminating salad bars in several local restaurants with *Salmonella* cultures. No deaths resulted, but 751 people were sickened.[3]

In many countries, the incidence of human *Salmonella* infections has increased markedly, although accurate population-based surveillance data are mostly lacking, especially from sub-Saharan Africa. In the United States, the incidence rate of NTS infection has not changed in the last 15 years but remains high. NTS species cause an estimated 1.2 million cases of foodborne illness each year in the United States, second only to noroviruses, and are associated with an estimated hospitalization rate of 27% and death rate of 0.5%. The incidence of NTS infection is highest during the rainy season in tropical climates and during the warmer months in temperate climates, coinciding with the peak in foodborne outbreaks.[2]

The development of disease after ingestion of *Salmonella* is influenced by the number and virulence of the organisms ingested, as well as individual host factors. In most cases, a large number of bacteria, in the range of 1 million to 1 billion, must be ingested to cause symptomatic infection.[4] In the case of unusually virulent strains or in a patient with reduced resistance, symptomatic ingestion my result from smaller inocula. Factors that predispose persons to infection include underlying immunocompromising diseases, inflammatory bowel disease, malignancy, or use of antacids or histamine-2 blockers. After ingestion of a sufficient number of bacteria, one or more of several clinical syndromes may manifest individually or concurrently. These clinical syndromes include enterocolitis (gastroenteritis), enteric (typhoid) fever, bacteremia, extraintestinal infection, and the chronic enteric or urinary carrier state.

Acute enterocolitis is the most common clinical manifestation of *Salmonella* infection. Nausea and vomiting are the earliest symptoms and develop 6 to 48 hours after ingestion of contaminated food, milk, or water. These are followed by diarrhea, which can range in severity from a few loose stools to fulminant, bloody diarrhea. Diarrhea usually persists less than 7 days, but rare cases may continue for several weeks. Fever, when present, usually lasts less than 2 days. Prolonged fever combined with diarrhea should suggest a complication or another diagnosis. Electrolyte and water depletion may be severe, leading to hypovolemic shock in some cases.

Enteric fever produced by *Salmonella* serotypes other than *S. typhi* is called paratyphoid fever. The clinical features of paratyphoid fever are essentially the same as typhoid fever, but with milder symptoms. Signs and symptoms of enteric fever develop after an incubation period of 1 to 2 weeks and include fever, bradycardia out of proportion to the fever, myalgias, arthralgias, headache, hepatosplenomegaly, and rose spots, typically on the anterior chest wall. If the patient is not treated, altered mental status may develop.[2]

Salmonella infection can produce an illness characterized by fever and sustained bacteremia without manifestations of enterocolitis or enteric fever. The clinical syndrome of *Salmonella* bacteremia is characterized by a febrile course lasting for days or weeks. In bacteremia, the organism is isolated from the blood, but stool cultures often have negative results. Bacteremia has also been shown to occur in 1% to 5% of patients overall and more frequently in infants and malnourished children.[5] The median duration of persistence of *Salmonella* in stool is 7 weeks for patients younger than 5 years and 3 to 4 weeks for older children and adults.

Extraintestinal manifestations of *Salmonella* infection include meningitis, pleuropulmonary disease, endocarditis, pericarditis, arteritis, osteomyelitis, arthritis, hepatosplenic abscess, urogenital tract infections, and soft-tissue abscesses. Chronic carriers (i.e., persons who continue to excrete the organism for more than a year after infection) are asymptomatic and unusual in nontyphoidal salmonellosis. The frequency of chronic carriage is higher in women and in persons with biliary abnormalities, gallstones, or concurrent bladder infection with *Schistosoma haematobium.*[2]

PRE-INCIDENT ACTIONS

Foodborne diseases present a major challenge to public health authorities. Surveillance for acts of terrorism involving the intentional contamination of food or water with a biological agent is dependent on close cooperation between community clinicians, public health officials, and law enforcement agencies. Clinicians must be able to recognize the unusual disease or disease pattern, order the appropriate laboratory tests and cultures, and report their suspicions or positive culture results to public health officials. The public health officials must then perform an appropriate epidemiological investigation to identify the source. If a bioterrorist incident is suspected or confirmed, the appropriate law enforcement agencies must be notified. Methods to enhance surveillance include promoting awareness of bioterrorism among the medical community and general public, performing appropriate microbiological testing in suspected cases, developing a clearly defined reporting system that facilitates early recognition of outbreaks, and promoting interagency cooperation and communication on local, regional, and national levels.[6]

POST-INCIDENT ACTIONS

Bioterrorism will often resemble a point-source outbreak, with all cases clustering around a single time period. An unusually high incidence may suggest deliberate infection, particularly if several point-source outbreaks occur simultaneously. Several features may suggest that a *Salmonella* outbreak is the result of an act of bioterrorism. These include the following: (1) large numbers of patients seeking care for similar signs and symptoms; (2) unusually high morbidity or mortality, or failure of the infection to respond to standard therapy; (3) multiple clusters of cases of *Salmonellae* in areas that are not geographically contiguous; (4) simultaneous disease outbreaks in human and animal or bird populations; and (5) unusual temporal or geographic clustering of illness (e.g., patients who attend the same public event, live in the same part of town).[6,7] If an act of bioterrorism is suspected, the proper authorities should be notified immediately. Information on salmonellosis should also be disseminated to the general public to prevent further transmission of disease, to identify and treat those affected, and to initiate a disease prevention program.

MEDICAL TREATMENT OF CASUALTIES

The type of syndrome produced by *Salmonella* species influences the selection and duration of antimicrobial therapy. Antimicrobial therapy of uncomplicated gastroenteritis is not indicated in patients without underlying diseases, because this condition is generally self-limiting and there is no evidence of clinical benefit. Furthermore, treatment with antibiotics may increase adverse effects and tend to prolong the carrier state.[8] The most important therapeutic consideration in enterocolitis is fluid and electrolyte replacement. However, therapy should be considered in patients with invasive disease risk, such as neonates, adults older than 50 years, immunosuppressed patients, and patients with vascular abnormalities or prosthetic valves, grafts, or joints. In these cases fluoroquinolone is the first line therapy, and azithromycin, cephalosporins, trimethoprim-sulfamethoxazole, or ampicillin are alternatives. In bacteremia, a third-generation cephalosporin or intravenous fluoroquinolone are recommended for 7 to 14 days. Localized infections require surgical debridement and endovascular infections surgical resection.[2] Treatment concerns are rising globally with the increasing number of multidrug-resistant strains.[9] Feeding of stock animals with food containing antibiotics plays a significant role in the development of multidrug-resistant *Salmonella.* In 1997, the first recognized outbreak of fluoroquinolone-resistant *Salmonella* infection occurred in the United States.[10] The increased number of multidrug-resistant *Salmonella* strains raises significant concerns because infections secondary to these strains may be difficult to treat with conventional antibiotics and as a consequence lead to higher mortality.

UNIQUE CONSIDERATIONS

Salmonellosis is in most cases a disease of morbidity, with an overall mortality rate of 0.4%. However, its appeal as a potential bioterrorism weapon derives from the ability to produce a large number of victims whose care would overwhelm local medical resources. In addition, *Salmonella* is a common pathogen that clinicians encounter routinely, with an estimated 1.2 million cases annually in the United States; of these, approximately 42,000 are laboratory-confirmed cases reported to CDC.[11] Therefore, an outbreak of salmonellosis would be less likely to raise concern over an act of bioterrorism than would a rare pathogen such as anthrax. As a consequence, the recognition of a deliberate release of *Salmonella* organisms would most likely be delayed, increasing the number of victims and decreasing the likelihood that the perpetrators would be apprehended.

PITFALLS

Several potential pitfalls in response to an outbreak exist. These include the following:

- Failure to educate health care providers and the general public on the signs and symptoms of salmonellosis
- Failure of health care providers to maintain a high index of suspicion for intentional salmonellosis infection
- Failure to order appropriate laboratory tests, delaying diagnosis
- Failure to treat with appropriate antibiotics and follow up on stool cultures to verify antimicrobial sensitivity
- Administration of antibiotics when they are not indicated, a practice that can lead to the development of antibiotic-resistant strains
- Failure to notify the proper authorities when an outbreak of salmonellosis is suspected or confirmed

REFERENCES

1. Guerrant RL, Walker DH, Weller PF, eds. Nontyphoidal salmonellosis. In: Moore CC, Baunra P, Pegues DA, et al. *Tropical Infectious Diseases: Principles, Pathogens and Practice.* 3rd ed. Edinburgh: Elsevier Saunders; 2011:128–136.
2. Bennett JE, Dolin R, Blaser MJ, eds. Salmonella species. In: Pegues DA, Miller SI. *Mandell, Douglas and Bennett's Principle and Practice of Infectious Disease,* Volume 1. 8th ed. Cambridge, UK: Saunders; 2015:2559–2568.
3. Torok TJ, Tauxe RV, Wise RP, et al. A large community outbreak of salmonellosis caused by intentional contamination of restaurant salad bars. *JAMA.* 1997;278:389–395.
4. Hook EW. Salmonellosis: certain factors influencing the interaction of salmonella and the human host. *Bull NY Acad Med.* 1961;37:499.
5. Haeusler GM, Curtis N. *Salmonella* species. In: Long SS, ed. Pickering L, Prober C, associate eds. *Principles and Practice of Pediatric Infectious Diseases.* 4th ed. Edinburg; New York: Elsevier Churchill Livingstone; 2012;146, 814–819.
6. Keene WE. Lessons from investigations of foodborne disease outbreaks. *JAMA.* 1999;281:1845–1847.

7. Franz DR, Zajtchuk R. Biological terrorism: understanding the threat, preparation, and medical response. *Dis Mon.* 2002;48(8):493–564.

8. Onwuezobe IA, Oshun PO, Odigwe CC. Antimicrobials for treating symptomatic non-typhoidal *Salmonella* infection. *Cochrane Database Syst Rev.* 2012;11, CD001167.

9. Centers for Disease Control and Prevention. National Antimicrobial Resistance Monitoring System: Enteric Bacteria 2010 Annual Report. http://www.cdc.gov/salmonella/.

10. Olsen SJ, DeBess EE, McGivern TE, et al. A nosocomial outbreak of fluoroquinolone-resistant *Salmonella* infection. *N Engl J Med.* 2001;344:1572–1579. www.cdc.gov/salmonella/.

11. Centers for Disease Control and Prevention. *Salmonella* home page; 2014. http://www.cdc.gov/salmonella/.

CHAPTER 135

Salmonella typhi (Typhoid Fever) Attack

Lawrence Proano

DESCRIPTION OF EVENT

Typhoid fever is a clinical syndrome caused by the bacterium *Salmonella typhi*. These anaerobic, gram-negative, flagellated bacilli possess an antigenic structure consisting of a lipopolysaccharide somatic surface antigen (O) and a flagellar antigen (H). *S. typhi* organisms usually possess a polysaccharide surface antigen (Vi) that coats the O antigen, protecting it from antibody attack.

Salmonella are classified as category B agents by the Centers for Disease Control and Prevention (CDC).[1] This category includes viruses, bacteria, fungi, and toxins that are relatively easy to disseminate, which cause moderate morbidity and in most cases low mortality, and require specific enhancement of diagnostic and surveillance capacities for the laboratory to respond effectively during an outbreak. However, unlike the CDC category A agents, typhoid fever has a relatively low mortality rate among immunocompetent hosts, about a 10% mortality rate if untreated.[1]

The disease is an unattractive weapon from a bioterrorism standpoint because is difficult to spread efficiently on a wide-scale compared with other organisms, which can be transmitted via the aerosol route. Nevertheless, the possibility of an intentionally caused large outbreak of disease spread by the foodborne route of infection or that typhoid might be considered for use as a bioterrorist option must not be ignored. For example, in 1972, a group of college students, influenced by ecoterrorist ideology planned a large-scale attack using typhoid fever, diphtheria, and other agents, targeting many world cities. They later narrowed their plan to five cities near Chicago. Although their plan was ultimately aborted, it demonstrates that typhoid is an agent in the universe of potential consideration for terrorists.[2] Counterterrorism authorities have long been concerned that Al Qaeda is much more likely to attempt to carry out a mass casualty attack using biological agents rather than lethal chemicals or radiological or nuclear weapons[3]

The potential results of such an attack on the food supply can be inferred from some historic examples of unintentional foodborne disease outbreaks. In 1994, an estimated 224,000 people in the United States were infected during an outbreak of *Salmonella enteritidis*, caused by contamination of pasteurized liquid ice cream that was transported nationally in tanker trucks, resulting in one of the largest foodborne disease outbreaks in U.S. history.[4] In 1985, contamination of pasteurized milk from a dairy plant in northern Illinois resulted in more than 170,000 people being infected with an outbreak of *Salmonella typhimurium* that was multidrug resistant.[5]

Because of the lower incidence in the United States, medical and public health officials may not recognize a foodborne attack such as typhoid fever for some time. The incidence of typhoid fever declined steadily in the United States from 1900 to 1960 and has since remained low. From 1975 to 1984, the average number of cases of typhoid fever reported annually in the United States was 464. In that period, 57% of cases were in patients aged 20 years or older, and 67% of cases were acquired while traveling internationally.[6] Several recently reported typhoid cases, along with cases of hepatitis A, cyclospora, *Salmonella* gastroenteritis, and listeria, also highlight the vulnerability of the global food supply chain to contamination with serious pathogens.[7]

The most likely foodborne attack scenario would involve a large number of otherwise healthy persons presenting over days to weeks with vague, multisystem complaints, with some of the cases progressing to syndromes that are more toxic.

The incubation period of typhoid fever varies from several days to longer than 3 weeks, averaging around 14 days. During the first week, there are often nonspecific symptoms such as malaise, anorexia, gradually worsening fever, occasional chills, headache, upper respiratory symptoms, cough, and hearing loss. Patients are often constipated during the first week.

In the second week, fever continues, often accompanied by a relative bradycardia, diarrhea, vomiting, and an appearance of the patient that is more toxic. Rose spots, 2- to 4-mm pink papules visible on the torso of fair-skinned persons, are seen in about 50% of patients. Abdominal pain and distension with hepatosplenomegaly may be present.

During the third week, the patient becomes increasingly toxic, with high fever, delirium, or coma: the so-called typhoid state. Diarrhea may have a "pea-soup" appearance. Multiplication of *S. typhi* in Peyer's patches of the small bowel may result in small bowel hemorrhage or perforation and peritonitis. Sepsis, anemia, leukopenia, pneumonia, and myocarditis may also occur. Death may occur in untreated patients in the third week of illness, usually from gastrointestinal perforation, anemia, toxemia, or, occasionally, meningitis. If the patient survives through the fourth week of illness and gastrointestinal complications do not occur, fever, toxemia, and abdominal symptoms abate over a few days.

Complications of typhoid fever are numerous and can occur at any time during the illness, even after a seemingly benign course.[1] Complications may be the presenting symptom or sign rather than the picture of typhoid fever. Complications include small bowel perforation, gastrointestinal hemorrhage, hemolytic anemia (common in patients with G6PD deficiency), typhoidal pneumonia, meningitis, glomerulonephritis, acute renal failure, nephrotic syndrome, arthritis, osteomyelitis, orchitis, hepatitis, acute cholecystitis, and parotitis. Abscesses may occur virtually anywhere in the body as a late complication, most commonly in the liver, spleen, brain, breast, and bone. Deep venous thrombosis and Guillain-Barre syndrome have been reported in association with typhoid fever.

◀◀ PRE-INCIDENT ACTIONS

Adequate preparation for and response to bioterrorism events require coordination of local, state, and federal public safety resources in the United States. Several agencies are involved in detection and epidemiological investigation of foodborne disease outbreaks, whether intentional or unintentional. These include local and state health epidemiology departments, public health laboratories at the local and state levels, the Council of State and Territorial Epidemiologists, the Association of Public Health Laboratories, and the CDC. The U.S. Food and Drug Administration and the U.S. Department of Agriculture have the primary regulatory authority over food safety, in coordination with state departments of agriculture.[8]

A mass casualty event resulting from an outbreak of typhoid, or most other foodborne illnesses, is less likely to occur compared with what would be expected from the intentional dissemination of a Category-A bioterrorism agent. However, smaller-scale attacks are well within the realm of possibility. Therefore, physicians, health care workers, and health agency personnel must remain vigilant in identifying trends that may correspond with an outbreak of typhoid or any foodborne or waterborne illness, whether terrorist related or not. With some diseases, including typhoid fever, these trends may take days or even weeks to develop, and they may involve somewhat nonspecific systemic complaints that evolve over time.

Numerous unintentional foodborne outbreaks are reported every year. Epidemiological clues to a deliberate, covert act of contamination include the following:

1. The presence of a large epidemic with unexplained morbidity and mortality
2. More severe disease than is usually expected for a specific pathogen or failure to respond to specific therapy
3. Multiple simultaneous or serial epidemics
4. A disease that is unusual for a particular age group
5. Unusual strains or variants of organisms or antimicrobial resistance patterns different from those circulating in the population
6. A similar genetic type among agents isolated from distinct sources at different times or locations

Features that would be suggestive of deliberate contamination might also arise in unintentional outbreaks as well. Confusing matters further, these epidemiological clues might not necessarily be evident in an outbreak due to deliberate contamination.[1]

▶▶ POST-INCIDENT ACTIONS

Clinicians who are suspicious that an outbreak may represent typhoid fever, even before bioterrorism is suspected, should notify the appropriate local, state, and federal public health and law enforcement authorities. This is the proper course of action, even from a public health perspective, because occasional outbreaks of typhoid fever can occur.

Both state and federal regulatory agencies participate in food-specific aspects of outbreak investigation, especially those related to the tracking of suspected foods and their recall. A trace-back investigation locates the origin of the food vehicle to establish the source of contamination, often by review of the records of vendors, shippers, producers, and processors, and by inspection of their facilities.

Integration of data from the epidemiological and trace-back investigations is crucial to identify properly the contaminated food and the mode of contamination, underscoring the need for the closest collaboration between epidemiologists, microbiologists, and food-safety officials.[5]

✚ MEDICAL TREATMENT OF CASUALTIES

Successful treatment of typhoid fever requires rapid diagnosis, antibiotic administration, and supportive care. With prompt treatment, mortality rates have been reduced from between 10% and 15% to between 1% and 4%.[1]

Chloramphenicol is the antibiotic most widely used worldwide for treating typhoid fever. Tetracyclines and aminoglycosides are not effective against *S. typhi,* although they may demonstrate in vitro activity. Ampicillin, amoxicillin, and trimethoprim-sulfamethoxazole have been successfully used to treat this entity. However, in the past decade, fluoroquinolones and third-generation cephalosporins have been shown to be as effective as chloramphenicol is, and, in the developed world, have largely become the antibiotics of choice. Thus fluoroquinolones would be the recommended agent to treat victims diagnosed with typhoid fever.

Aside from antibiotic administration, general supportive care, hydration, and electrolyte management are important in treating this disease. This is especially important because patients with severe typhoid fever have a limited ability to maintain their nutritional and fluid status.

In addition to antibiotic therapy, studies have clearly demonstrated that corticosteroid administration reduces mortality in patients with severe typhoid fever. It does not appear to increase the incidence of complications, relapse rate, or induction of a carrier state among those treated.

❓ UNIQUE CONSIDERATIONS

The features of typhoid fever tend to be nonspecific, and a number of other causes must be considered when encountering febrile illnesses. Malaria would be the most likely consideration in the tropics but would be far less likely in developed countries such as the United States. Tuberculosis and brucellosis can also mimic typhoid fever. Other illnesses to consider in the differential diagnosis of typhoid fever include dengue fever, endocarditis, typhus, and lymphoproliferative disorders. The tests for typhoid fever do not have a high degree of sensitivity or specificity, and because of the relatively low prevalence of this disease in the United States, it would not likely be an early consideration in the minds of most clinicians.

Nonspecific hematologic and biochemical findings can lend support for the diagnosis of typhoid fever. Leukopenia is common. There is often a modest degree of hyponatremia, as well as a mild transaminitis.

❗ PITFALLS

Several potential pitfalls in response to an outbreak of typhoid fever exist. These include the following:

- Failure to prepare adequate state or local systems to respond to possible terrorist attacks before the attacks occur
- Failure to consider typhoid fever as the etiology for patients who present without diarrheal illness (Early typhoid fever often presents initially with constipation, not diarrhea!)
- Failure to consider typhoid fever as a bioterrorism attack in the setting of a large number of people who present over days to weeks with symptoms consistent with this or any foodborne illness
- Failure to notify appropriate public health and law enforcement agencies when an outbreak of foodborne illness is suspected or confirmed

REFERENCES

1. Le TP, Hoffman SL. Typhoid fever. In: Guerrant R, Walker D, Weller P, eds. *Essentials of Tropical Infectious Diseases*. Philadelphia, PA: Churchill Livingston; 2001, Chapter 15.
2. Southern Illinois University School of Medicine, Division of Infectious Diseases, "Overview of Potential Agents of Biological Terrorism. Available at: http://www.siumed.edu/medicine/id/bioterrorism.htm.
3. Available at: http://www.hstoday.us/blogs/the-kimery-report/blog/the-threat-of-bioterrorism-and-the-ability-to-detect-it/bea57df4219d59980fcbd46429f7a918.html. Accessed April 9, 2015.
4. Hennesy TW, Hedberg CW, Slutsker L, et al. A national outbreak of *Salmonella enteritidis* infections from ice cream. *N Engl J Med*. 1996;334:1281–1286.
5. Ryan CA, Nickels MK, Hargrett-Bean NT, et al. Massive outbreak of antimicrobial-resistant salmonellosis traced to pasteurized milk. *JAMA*. 1987;258:3269–3274.
6. Corales R, Schmitt SK. *Typhoid fever;* August 11, 2004. Available at: http://www.emedicine.com/MED/topic2331.htm. Accessed April 9, 2015.
7. Available at: http://emedicine.medscape.com/article/231135-overview. Accessed April 9, 2015.
8. Sobel J, Khan AS, Swerdlow DL. Threat of a biological terrorist attack on the US food supply: the CDC perspective. *Lancet*. 2002;359:874–880.

Burkholderia mallei (Glanders) Attack

John W. Hardin

DESCRIPTION OF EVENT

Burkholderia mallei is a nonmotile, aerobic, encapsulated, gram-negative intracellular bacterium and is the causative agent for the disease known as Glanders.[1,2] Due to a lack of prophylactic vaccine, significant potential morbidity and mortality, and significant virulence as an aerosol, it has been listed as a category B bioterrorism agent by the Centers for Disease Control and Prevention.[3]

B. mallei has been classified and reclassified multiple times since its initial discovery, including *Bacillus, Corynebacterium, Mycobacterium, Loefflerella, Pfeifferella, Malleomyces, Actinobacillus,* and *Pseudomonas,*[4] given its microscopic appearance, which has obviously led to confusion in nomenclature. In 1992 Yabuuchi and co-workers applied the genus of *Burkholderia* based on rRNA genotyping.[5]

B. mallei cultures easily on standard nutrient growth media, and it is often described as having a "safety-pin" appearance on methylene blue or Wright's stain on standard microscopy. Although clinical testing involving chemistry and hematology can be performed safely under biosafety level 2 (BSL-2) conditions, cultures must be handled in BSL-3 containment due to the highly infectious nature of *B. mallei* aerosols.[6]

In addition to nomenclature confusion, there had been some initial debate as to whether *B. mallei* has an external polysaccharide capsule, but this has since been confirmed with additional testing and electron microscopy. Not only is *B. mallei* encapsulated, but this capsule also acts a major virulence factor.[7]

B. mallei is unique in the *Burkholderia* family because it does not survive in soil, instead needing an animal host to survive.[2] Therefore the primary natural reservoir for *B. mallei* is horses because they are highly susceptible to infection. It is from this equine population that the name Glanders originated, stemming from the lymphangitis and lymphadenopathy (glands) that are typically involved, even though the cutaneous manifestations in this group is called Farcy.[8] Although less susceptible, other equines, such as mules and donkeys, may serve as hosts for the bacteria.

The disease of Glanders also has its own distinct historical background both from a laboratory perspective and in warfare. First described in 1882 in the liver and spleen of an infected horse the history and pathogenesis of *B. mallei* have been best described in that area.[8] The use of *B. mallei* as a biological warfare agent has been seen as early as the American Civil War. In World War I it was used with particularly devastating effect on troop and artillery movement on the eastern front. During World War II civilians and prisoners of war in China were purposefully infected with Glanders by the Japanese. Finally, *B. mallei* was used by the former Soviet Union on a limited basis in Afghanistan in the 1980s.[8,9]

The disease was eradicated from equine hosts in the United States by 1942 and in the United Kingdom by 1928 due to strict testing and surveillance. Subsequently the last naturally occurring case of human Glanders in these countries was noted in 1934, but it is still endemic in Asia, Africa, Central and South America, and the Middle East.[2,8] Given the success in eradicating the disease in many first-world countries, it would be prudent to treat any reemergence as a possible bioweapon release.

Human acquisition of disease is essentially limited to those who have close contact with infected animals, such as veterinarians or farmers, or those who are working with isolates in the laboratory setting.[9] Human to human transmission has been reported but very rarely.[8] Even with close contact with infected animals, transmission rates are low, given that 30% of tested horses in China in World War II were positive for *B. mallei* yet human disease was seldom reported.[8]

Given the low human transmissibility rate even when exposed to an endemic equine population, the most logical and effective use of *B. mallei* as a bioweapon agent would be dispersal as an aerosolized agent, which would markedly increase the infectious ability of the bacterium. This would imply, as better described below, that respiratory symptoms would predominate as a presenting complaint. If this were to occur in the middle of another respiratory outbreak (i.e., influenza), it would provide significant confounding and likely delay awareness that an attack has occurred.

With growing percentages of the world population becoming diabetic or otherwise immunocompromised there is escalating interest in these diseases as a public health issue because both *B. mallei* and its close relative *B. pseudomallei* (see Chapter 137) can cause opportunistic infections in these patient populations.[1]

Generally the route of inoculation determines the disease course with skin contact leading to a localized cutaneous infection, and the inhalation of aerosolized *B. mallei* leading to lung infections, followed by overwhelming sepsis. The course in equines is closely mirrored in humans, although the equine form has several names based on presentation. In equines and humans *B. mallei* infection can present as either nasal-pulmonary infections (Glanders) or cutaneous infections (Farcy), and the disease may develop either acutely or chronically.[2]

It is critical to note that regardless of inoculation location, all forms possess the potential to cause overwhelming sepsis. Once systemic infection occurs, there is approximately a 95% fatality rate in untreated cases and upward of 50% in antibiotic-treated individuals.[10]

The clinical course of the disease typically manifests within 1 to 14 days but can be up to 4 weeks, depending on the route of inoculation, with localized and cutaneous forms being on the lower end of the spectrum, pulmonary in the middle, and systemic infection at the longer range.[11] It is exceedingly rare to see isolated cutaneous forms because even those can progress rapidly into lymphangitic and systemic involvement. Clinically the disease manifests as ulcerations progressing to lymphangitis and lymphadenopathy in the cutaneous form. In the inhalational form, expected pulmonary symptoms, such as dyspnea and cough, predominate but can also result in cavitary lung lesions on imaging. Once systemic infection occurs, multisystem involvement, abscess formation, and sepsis are followed by death within 7 to 30 days without adequate treatment. Even with appropriate treatment, prognosis remains quite poor. *B. mallei* is also concerning because in treated and clinically resolved cases there can be chronic infection, which can recrudesce at nearly any time in the future, even with prolonged and appropriate antimicrobial therapy. These patients can then still progress to overwhelming systemic infection and death.[8]

PRE-INCIDENT ACTIONS

There are no specific pre-incident steps to take because ongoing surveillance of the disease already exists. Continued surveillance, especially with the aid of veterinarians may be helpful because equines are the primary reservoir for this disease. The emergence of Glanders in an area where it has been previously eradicated should also alert authorities to the possibility of a bioweapon release. There is no vaccine available, and although there has been some study on the benefit of prophylactic treatment of murine models with trimethoprim-sulfamethoxazole (TMP-SMX), this has not yet been studied in humans.[12]

POST-INCIDENT ACTIONS

Because equines have proven to be a robust reservoir, post-incident containment steps should be aimed at identifying infected members of this group via mallein-purified protein derivative testing (which is widely accepted) and subsequent extermination.[13] Additional actions should focus on persistent surveillance of those geographic areas and the equines therein.

MEDICAL TREATMENT OF CASUALTIES

Initial medical treatment weighs heavily on the assumption that the correct diagnosis is made. If classic symptoms are noted in an area found to have equines positive for *B. mallei*, it would be appropriate to initiate approved treatment empirically given the significant morbidity of untreated disease as definitive diagnosis lags significantly behind symptom onset.

Blood cultures for *B. mallei* are rarely positive, and agglutination testing may take up to 3 weeks to become positive and even then tend to be unreliable. Polymerase chain reaction (PCR) assays are the most reliable but are difficult to obtain.[2]

Antibiotics are the mainstay of treatment and are directed at gram-negative coverage. Favored antibiotics to which *Burkholderia* is sensitive include TMP-SMX, doxycycline, imipenem, ceftazidime, ciprofloxacin, and anti-pseudomonal penicillins, such as piperacillin/tazobactam.[14] Interestingly *B. mallei* appears to be susceptible to aminoglycosides, in contrast to its relative *B. pseudomallei*. This is due to the lack of an efflux pump that confers aminoglycoside resistance. Thus *B. mallei* may be susceptible to antibiotics, such as gentamicin and tobramycin.[15] Given some potential ambiguity in differentiating *B. mallei* from *B. pseudomallei*, it would be prudent to initially avoid aminoglycosides in favor of the antibiotics listed previously.

Although no official Food and Drug Administration (FDA)-approved therapy exists, current recommendations are for an initial intensive parenteral therapy. The current recommendation for therapy is initially a 10 to 14 day intensive phase with intravenous ceftazidime (120 mg/kg/day divided 3 times a day [TID]) or a carbapenem (imipenem: 60 mg/kg/day divided 4 times a day [QID] *or* meropenem: 75 mg/kg/day divided TID) with a switch to oral agents only when there are clear signs of clinical improvement. TMP-SMX at the high end of the dosing regimen (8 mg/kg/day divided 2 times a day [BID]) is often

added as well given the apparent ineffectiveness of single drug therapy and even then must be continued for up to 2 to 6 months, with lifelong follow-up being important.[9] This is followed by eradication therapy with oral doxycycline (100 mg BID) and TMP-SMX (4 mg/kg/day divided BID) for 20 weeks.[6]

UNIQUE CONSIDERATIONS

Specific to Glanders it would be important to consider and monitor the reservoir for illness, long-term follow-up of the human infected, and long courses of antimicrobial therapy with a heightened awareness for recurrence of disease.

PITFALLS

- False identification of the causative organism
- Failure of surveillance of equine reservoir
- Inability to provide BSL-3 conditions for culture
- Failure to provide multiple appropriate antibiotic agents
- Failure to continue the appropriate agents for appropriate duration (20 weeks)
- Failure to adequately follow up with patients in the long-term

REFERENCES

1. Estes DM, Dow SW, Schweizer HP, Torres AG. Present and future therapeutic strategies for melioidosis and glanders. *Expert Rev Anti Infect Ther.* 2010;8(3):325–338.
2. Whitlock GC, Estes DM, Torres AG. Glanders: off to the races with *Burkholderia mallei. FEMS Microbiol Lett.* 2007;277(2):115–122.
3. "Bioterrorism Agents/Diseases." CDC. Web. January 1, 2014. http://www.bt.cdc.gov/agent/agentlist-category.asp.
4. Graves MG, Harrington KS. Glanders and melioidosis. In: Beran GW, ed. *Handbook of Zoonoses.* 2nd ed. Boca Raton, FL: CRC Press; 1994.
5. Yabuuchi E, Kosako Y, Oyaizu H, et al. Proposal of *Burkholderia* gen. nov. and transfer of seven species of the genus *Pseudomonas* homology group II to the new genus, with the type species *Burkholderia cepacia* (Palleroni and Holmes, 1981) comb. nov. *Microbiol Immunol.* 1992;36:1251–1275.
6. (U.S.) AM, Dembek ZF. Glanders/Melioidosis. In: *Medical Management of Biological Casualties Handbook.* Department of the Army; 2012.
7. Deshazer D, Waag DM, Fritz DL, Woods DE. Identification of a *Burkholderia mallei* polysaccharide gene cluster by subtractive hybridization and demonstration that the encoded capsule is an essential virulence determinant. *Microb Pathog.* 2001;30(5):253–269.
8. Gregory BC, Waag DM. Glanders. In: Dembek ZF, ed. *Medical Aspects of Biological Warfare.* Washington, DC: U.S. Government Printing Office; 2007.
9. Srinivasan A, Kraus CN, DeShazer D, et al. Glanders in a military research microbiologist. *N Engl J Med.* 2001;345:256–258.
10. Mandell GL, Bennett JE, Dolin R. *Pseudomonas Species (Including Melioidosis and Glanders).* New York, NY: Churchill Livingstone; 1995.
11. Batts-Osborne D, Rega PP, Hall AH, McGovern TW. CBRNE—Glanders and melioidosis. *Emedicine J.* 2013.
12. Barnes KB, Steward J, Thwaite JE, et al. Trimethoprim/sulfamethoxazole (co-trimoxazole) prophylaxis is effective against acute murine inhalational melioidosis and glanders. *Int J Antimicrob Agents.* 2013;41(6):552–557.
13. De Carvalho Filho MB, Ramos RM, Fonseca AA, et al. Development and validation of a method for purification of mallein for the diagnosis of glanders in equines. *BMC Vet Res.* 2012;8:154.
14. Heine HS, England MJ, Waag DM, Byrne WR. In vitro antibiotic susceptibilities of *Burkholderia mallei* (causative agent of glanders) determined by broth microdilution and E-test. *Antimicrob Agents Chemother.* 2001;45(7):2119–2121.
15. Nierman WC, Deshazer D, Kim HS, et al. Structural flexibility in the *Burkholderia mallei* genome. *Proc Natl Acad Sci U S A.* 2004;101(39):14246–14251.

Burkholderia pseudomallei (Melioidosis) Attack

John W. Hardin

DESCRIPTION OF EVENT

Burkholderia pseudomallei is a saprophytic motile, aerobic, non–spore-forming, gram-negative bacillus and the causative bacterium of the human disease melioidosis. Similar to its close relative *Burkholderia mallei* (see Chapter 136), because of a lack of vaccine, high mortality rate, highly pathogenic nature as an aerosol, and significant antibiotic resistance, it is currently listed as a category B bioweapon agent by the Centers for Disease Control (CDC).[1,2]

Melioidosis was initially described in 1911 in Burma by Captain Alfred Whitmore, who was the namesake for the alternative name "Whitmore's disease," as a Glanders-like illness and was microscopically identified and named *Bacillus pseudomallei*.[3] It was also subsequently named *Pseudomonas pseudomallei* because of the very similar microscopic appearance shared with that genus. This similarity can cause diagnostic confusion even now. When under the microscope, the bacterium is typically described as having bipolar staining or safety-pin resemblance, although the morphology tends to be extremely variable. It was not until 1992 that the bacterium was incorporated into its current genus of *Burkholderia*.[4]

As contributory evidence to its listing as a potential bioweapon, it is known that the United States did study these agents as possible biological warfare agents in 1943-1944 but did not weaponize them. The former Soviet Union is believed to have been interested in Glanders as a potential biological weapon as well, but not specifically melioidosis. During World War I, Glanders was allegedly used to infect horses and mules destined for delivery to France by German agents.[5] The Japanese are believed to have infected civilians, prisoners of war, and horses during World War II.

B. pseudomallei is particularly robust in the environment and able to survive in triple distilled water for years, but is truly deft in its evasion and subversion of immune defenses. It is resistant to complement, lysosomal defensins, and cationic peptides. It produces proteases, lipase, lecithinase, catalase, peroxidase, superoxide dismutase, hemolysins, a cytotoxic exolipid, and at least one siderophore.[6] The quorum-sensing system influencing the behavior of the whole bacterial population is an area of active research and adds to the virulence of *B. pseudomallei*.[7]

Conventional techniques, including Gram's stain and culture, remain the mainstay of laboratory diagnosis for melioidosis, aided by its biological profile that can be demonstrated by an oxidase positive glucose user or using a kit-based system, typically on either Ashdown's media or *Burkholderia cepacia* selective media.[8] Testing can be done on blood, or as a large Thai study determined, a throat swab; if *B. pseudomallei* is isolated a throat swab can approximate 100% sensitivity for clinical melioidosis.[9] Care must be taken when culturing *B. pseudomallei* because of its significant aerosol risk; the current USAMRID recommendation is that it be cultured in a BSL-3 laboratory.[2]

Fortunately, alternatives to culture do exist. In Thailand, an immunofluorescent stain, which can be performed on fresh specimens such as sputum or urine in minutes, was shown to be both sensitive and useful when more advanced laboratory equipment and culture media do not exist.[10] Polymerase chain reaction (PCR) is also extremely useful, sensitive, and specific in diagnosis, but time delay and unavailability of equipment generally preclude its routine use.[11]

B. pseudomallei is endemic in soil and water in tropical regions, primarily in east Asia and northern Australia. In northeast Thailand, for instance, the bacterium is easily cultured in 50% of rice paddies and peaks with the rainy season.[12] Melioidosis poses a significant public health threat in these areas, representing the third most frequent cause of death from infectious disease in northeast Thailand and the most common cause of community-acquired bacterial pneumonia in certain parts of northern Australia.[13,14]

When tested with indirect hemagglutination (IHA), up to 60% to 70% of Thai children are found to be positive for antibodies to *B. pseudomallei*. Thus exposure does not necessarily confer active or even latent disease.[15] In fact, those who are at greatest risk are the functionally immunosuppressed, particularly those with diabetes, chronic renal disease, chronic lung disease (specifically cystic fibrosis), and alcoholism. Interestingly, those who are HIV-positive do not seem to share this predisposition.[16]

The listed characteristics, particularly the ease of obtaining and culturing samples, robust nature and resilience, and the complicated treatment resistance pattern (discussed in further detail below), makes *B. pseudomallei* an excellent choice as a bioweapon agent. Because of the variable presentations of melioidosis, the unpredictable incubation period, and the possibility that many carriers will remain asymptomatic, the medical and public health community may not recognize a bioterrorist attack involving *B. pseudomallei* until the organism is cultured from acutely septic patients. The attack would likely involve aerosolizing media containing *B. pseudomallei* and distributing it over a heavily populated, urban area. Over a period of days to weeks, infected people would visit health care facilities with a diverse symptom set (see below), making initial detection quite difficult.

Inoculation through broken skin and inhalation are the major routes of acquiring *B. pseudomallei*. As demonstrated by the prevalence of antibody-seropositive children the majority of people exposed are asymptomatic.[17] In cases of a specific inoculation event, the mean incubation period was 9 days with a range of 1 to 21 days; clinical presentation early after exposure is the general rule, although the disease can remain latent for years and then reactivate as well.[18,16] The disease recurs with a frequency of 6% in the first year and 13% in following 10 years. Approximately 75% of these cases are relapse of the same infection, while 25% are actually re-infection with a different strain.[19]

Following inoculation, melioidosis can present with a wide spectrum of symptoms. Local abscess or ulceration does occur after cutaneous inoculation, but with less frequency than in Glanders, and there is seldom an infected wound or evidence of trauma. Abscess formation is very common, arising essentially anywhere in the body with a preference for the liver, spleen, kidney, and prostate.[20] The latter two sites demonstrate the utility of urine immunofluorescence in diagnosis. Splenic abscesses provide a good means to differentiate melioidosis from *Entamoeba histolytica* infection, which is endemic in the same areas but seldom creates abscesses outside of the liver.[19]

More common, however, is pneumonia which accounts for 51% of initial disease presentations.[15] Melioidosis pneumonia is diverse on its own accord and can present from purulent cough with localized infiltrates to acute fulminant sepsis with multifocal infiltrates and even chronic infection.[19] This confounding clinical picture in chronic infection can include hallmark tuberculosis symptoms such as fever, night sweats, weight loss, and hemoptysis as well as radiographic findings that lead it to be initially (and easily) misdiagnosed as tuberculosis.[21,22]

Even though patients with secondary pneumonia tend to have higher rates of bacteremia and multilobar involvement, they are less likely to develop septic shock or die; therefore treatment focus is on early aggressive therapy for active disease.[15] Another aspect of the diversity of melioidosis presentation is a unique syndrome of acute suppurative parotitis, which was found to be the initial disease presentation in one third of infected symptomatic children in Thailand.[23]

PRE-INCIDENT ACTIONS

There are no specific pre-incident steps to take other than having a low threshold of suspicion for the disease in the event of a rapidly progressing sepsis from pneumonia-type symptoms in endemic areas, and the education of laboratory workers there. There is no vaccine available; although there has been some study on the benefit of prophylactic treatment of murine models with trimethoprim-sulfamethoxazole (TMP-SMX) for both *B. mallei* and *B. pseudomallei*, this has not yet been studied in humans.[24]

POST-INCIDENT ACTIONS

The recommended post-exposure prophylaxis for those in contact with cultures of *B. pseudomallei* or concern for exposure in those at risk entails the following[25]: TMP-SMX: 2 × 160-800 mg (960 mg) if >60 kg, 3 × 80-400 mg (480 mg) if 40 to 60 kg, and 1 × 160-800 mg (960 mg) or 2 × 80-400 mg (480 mg) tablets if adult <40 kg every 12 hour *or* amoxicillin-clavulanate 20/5 mg/kg/dose. This equates to: 3 × 500/125 tabs if >60 kg every 8 hours and 2 × 500/125 tabs if ≤60 kg every 8 hours.

Early access to critical care and appropriate isolation (BSL-3) of cultures are important.

MEDICAL TREATMENT OF CASUALTIES

There is no Food and Drug Administration (FDA)-approved therapy for melioidosis, but current recommendations are based on current understanding of antibiotic resistance and current susceptibilities and have essentially remained constant since early trials demonstrated the superiority of ceftazidime against the previous regimen of co-trimoxazole–doxycycline–chloramphenicol. Since that time, no antibiotic regimens have been shown to have a mortality benefit.[26]

Thus the current recommendation for therapy is initially a 10 to 14 day intensive phase of IV ceftazidime (120 mg/kg/day divided tid) or a carbapenem (imipenem 60 mg/kg/day divided qid *or* meropenem 75 mg/kg/day divided tid) with a switch to oral agents only when there are clear signs of clinical improvement.[2] The natural course of the disease allows for enlargement of abscesses or appearance of new abscesses, especially in skeletal muscle during the first week of treatment, which is not necessarily a sign of treatment failure. Surveillance blood cultures should be negative by the end of the first week of oral treatment (3 weeks post-initiation of therapy), whereas sputum or draining abscesses can remain culture-positive for 1 month in infections that are actually responding to therapy.[19] Although sporadic cases of ceftazidime resistance have been reported, it remains the recommended first-line therapy. There have been no reported cases of carbapenem resistance, so carbapenem should be considered for cases not responding to ceftazidime.[27]

This intensive parenteral phase is immediately followed by a long eradication phase of least 12 and up to 20 weeks of oral therapy. Dosing for TMP-SMX in the eradication phase is 4 mg/kg/day divided bid. Newer recommendations of single-agent eradication therapy with TMP-SMX have supplanted previous regimens of dual therapy with TMP-SMX and doxycycline.[25,28,29]

New therapies have been explored, including granulocyte colony-stimulating factor at a dose of 300 g IV daily for 10 days, which was associated with a significant mortality benefit when compared with a historical control group. This makes sense given the higher incidence of melioidosis in patients with functional neutrophil defects such as diabetes mellitus and renal disease.[30]

Regardless of therapy, severe melioidosis carries a high mortality rate, up to 50% in northern Thailand and 20% in Australia, and tend to be recalcitrant to antibiotic therapy. The difference in mortality between the above two geographic areas seems to be due to the greater availability in Australia of early intensive care to treat sepsis.[10]

UNIQUE CONSIDERATIONS

It is important to be aware of which areas are endemic for this bacteria. Providing long-term follow-up of the infected person in addition to long courses of antimicrobial therapy must be accompanied by a heightened awareness for recurrence of disease.

PITFALLS

- False identification of the causative organism
- Inability to provide BSL-3 conditions for culture
- Failure to provide multiple appropriate antibiotic agents
- Failure to continue the appropriate agents for the appropriate duration (12 to 20 weeks)
- Failure to adequately follow up patients in the long term

REFERENCES

1. CDC. Bioterrorism Agents/Diseases. Available at: http://www.bt.cdc.gov/agent/agentlist-category.asp.
2. USAMRIID. Glanders/melioidosis. In: Dembek ZF, ed. *Medical Management of Biological Casualties Handbook*. Fort Derick, MD: Department of the Army; 2012.
3. Whitmore A, Krishnaswami CS. An account of the discovery of a hitherto undescribed infective disease occurring among the population of Rangoon. *Indian Med Gaz*. 1912;47:262–267.
4. Yabuuchi E, Kosako Y, Oyaizu H, et al. Proposal of *Burkholderia* gen. nov. and transfer of seven species of the genus *Pseudomonas* homology group II to the new genus, with the type species *Burkholderia cepacia* (Palleroni and Holmes 1981) comb. nov. *Microbiol Immunol*. 1992;36(12):1251–1275.
5. Horn J. Bacterial agents used for bioterrorism. *Surg Infect (Larchmt)*. 2003;4:281–287.
6. Woods DE, DeShazer D, Moore RA, et al. Current studies on the pathogenesis of melioidosis. *Microbes Infect*. 1999;1:157–162.

7. Wiersinga WJ, Currie BJ, Peacock SJ. Melioidosis. *N Engl J Med.* 2012;367 (11):1035–1044.

8. Walsh AL, Wuthiekanun V. The laboratory diagnosis of melioidosis. *Br J Biomed Sci.* 1996;53:249–253.

9. Wuthiekanun V, Suputtamongkol Y, Simpson AJ, Kanaphun P, White NJ. Value of throat swab in diagnosis of melioidosis. *J Clin Microbiol.* 2001;39:3801–3802.

10. Wuthiekanun V, Desakorn V, Wongsuvan G, et al. Rapid immunofluorescence microscopy for diagnosis of melioidosis. *Clin Diagn Lab Immunol.* 2005;12:555–556.

11. Peacock SJ. Melioidosis. *Curr Opin Infect Dis.* 2006;19(5):421–428.

12. Wuthiekanun V, Smith MD, Dance DA, White NJ. Isolation of *Pseudomonas pseudomallei* from soil in north-eastern Thailand. *Trans R Soc Trop Med Hyg.* 1995;89(1):41–43.

13. Limmathurotsakul D, Wongratanacheewin S, Teerawattanasook N, et al. Increasing incidence of human melioidosis in Northeast Thailand. *Am J Trop Med Hyg.* 2010;82(6):1113–1117.

14. Cheng AC, Currie BJ. Melioidosis: epidemiology, pathophysiology, and management. *Clin Microbiol Rev.* 2005;18(2):383–416.

15. Wuthiekanun V, Chierakul W, Langa S, et al. Development of antibodies to *Burkholderia pseudomallei* during childhood in melioidosis-endemic Northeast Thailand. *Am J Trop Med Hyg.* 2006;74(6):1074–1075.

16. Meumann EM, Cheng AC, Ward L, Currie BJ. Clinical features and epidemiology of melioidosis pneumonia: results from a 21-year study and review of the literature. *Clin Infect Dis.* 2012;54(3):362–369.

17. Currie BJ, Fisher DA, Anstey NM, Jacups SP. Melioidosis: acute and chronic disease, relapse and re-activation. *Trans R Soc Trop Med Hyg.* 2000;94 (3):301–304.

18. Currie BJ, Fisher DA, Howard DM, et al. The epidemiology of melioidosis in Australia and Papua New Guinea. *Acta Trop.* 2000;74:121–127.

19. Maharjan B, Chantratita N, Vesaratchavest M, et al. Recurrent melioidosis in patients in northeast Thailand is frequently due to reinfection rather than relapse. *J Clin Microbiol.* 2005;43:6032–6034.

20. White NJ. Melioidosis. *Lancet.* 2003;361(9370):1715–1722.

21. Currie BJ, Dance DA, Cheng AC. The global distribution of *Burkholderia pseudomallei* and melioidosis: an update. *Trans R Soc Trop Med Hyg.* 2008;102:S1–S4.

22. Vidyalakshmi K, Chakrapani M, Shrikala B, Damodar S, Lipika S, Vishal S. Tuberculosis mimicked by melioidosis. *Int J Tuberc Lung Dis.* 2008;12:1209–1215.

23. Dance DAB, Davis TME, Wattanagoon Y, et al. Acute suppurative parotitis caused by *Pseudomonas pseudomallei* in children. *J Infect Dis.* 1989;159:654–660.

24. Barnes KB, Steward J, Thwaite JE, et al. Trimethoprim/ sulfamethoxazole (co-trimoxazole) prophylaxis is effective against acute murine inhalational melioidosis and glanders. *Int J Antimicrob Agents.* 2013;41(6):552–557.

25. Chaowagul W, Chierakul W, Simpson AJ, et al. Open-label randomized trial of oral trimethoprim—sulfamethoxazole, doxycycline, and chloramphenicol compared with trimethoprim-sulfamethoxazole and doxycycline for maintenance therapy of melioidosis. *Antimicrob Agents Chemother.* 2005;49:4020–4025.

26. White NJ, Dance DA, Chaowagul W, Wattanagoon Y, Wuthiekanun V, Pitakwatchara N. Halving of mortality of severe melioidosis by ceftazidime. *Lancet.* 1989;2:697–701.

27. Schweizer HP. Mechanisms of antibiotic resistance in *Burkholderia pseudomallei*: implications for treatment of melioidosis. *Future Microbiol.* 2012;7(12):1389–1399.

28. Peacock SJ, Schweizer HP, Dance DA, et al. Management of accidental laboratory exposure to *Burkholderia pseudomallei* and *B. mallei. Emerg Infect Dis.* 2008;14:e2. http://dx.doi.org/10.3201/eid1407.071501.

29. Chetchotisakd P, Chierakul W, Chowagul V, et al. Trimethoprim-sulfamethoxazole alone or with doxycycline for eradication phase treatment of melioidosis (MERTH-study group). Presented at the VI World Melioidosis Congress, Townsville; 2010.

30. Cheng AC, Stephens DP, Anstey NM, Currie BJ. Adjunctive granulocyte colony-stimulating factor for treatment of septic shock due to melioidosis. *Clin Infect Dis.* 2004;38:32–37.

CHAPTER 138

Chlamydophila psittaci (Psittacosis) Attack

Hans R. House and Olivia E. Bailey

DESCRIPTION OF EVENT

Psittacosis, also known as parrot fever, is caused by *Chlamydophila psittaci*, an obligate intracellular bacterium. Clinical cases of psittacosis are sporadic and have a worldwide distribution. Fewer than 20 cases are reported each year to the Centers for Disease Control and Prevention (CDC).[1] The true incidence, however, is likely higher. Because psittacosis carries a nonspecific presentation and is difficult to culture, many cases go unnoticed or are simply attributed to "atypical pneumonia."

The association of bird ownership or bird exposure with psittacosis is well known. Parrots, parakeets, cockatiels, and canaries are the species most commonly associated with *C. psittaci* infection. More than 130 avian species have been documented as hosts of *C. psittaci*, including pigeons, sparrows, ducks, egrets, chickens, and turkeys.[2] Not all cases of human psittacosis derive from avians; case reports describe transmission from infected sheep, cattle, cats, and dogs as well.[3,4] Human-to-human transmission has been described, but it is rare.[5]

C. psittaci is categorized as a CDC class B biological warfare agent for its potential to spread via aerosol and infect victims with a relatively low mortality rate.[6] The United States, former Soviet Union, and Egypt have all conducted research into its use as a weapon, but none is known to have deployed it. To date, no known incidents of intentional infection by *C. psittaci* have occurred.[7]

The few incidents of large-scale outbreaks of psittacosis involved the distribution or industrial processing of birds. The largest outbreak, from 1929 to 1930, involved 750 to 800 cases and was linked to the importation of exotic birds from Argentina to Europe and the United States. Epidemiological data from the 1970s and 1980s in the United Kingdom, United States, and Sweden show a direct relationship between increased importation of exotic birds and rising numbers of cases of psittacosis.[8,9] Outbreaks have occurred in workers at a duck farm, at turkey processing facilities, and in attendees of a bird fair.[10-14]

C. psittaci is usually acquired by inhalation or direct contact with the infectious discharges from infected animals. Infected birds may transmit the disease while asymptomatic, but the greatest number of organisms are expressed during periods of obvious illness (shivering, emaciation, anorexia, dyspnea, and diarrhea). Because the feces, urine, and discharge from beaks and eyes are all infectious, feathers and dust in and around the birds' cages become infectious.[15] Aerosolization of infectious material, such as bird excreta, is one possible route of infection that might be attempted in a biological attack. In the case of a psittacosis outbreak at a bird fair, closed windows and a lack of ventilation were factors that contributed to the large number of cases.[13] It is possible, however, unlikely, that a weaponized agent could also be used. According to Bill Patrick, who headed a component of the U.S. biological weapons program at Fort Detrick, Maryland, in the 1950s and 1960s, *C. psittaci* was high on the list to be produced and stockpiled as a biological weapon

just before President Richard Nixon terminated the program in 1969 (Bill Patrick, personal communication, July 30, 2004). The organism, measuring 300 nm in its infectious form (or elementary body), is resistant to drying and may be viable for up to 1 week at room temperature.[16]

After inhalation of *C. psittaci* and establishment of an infection in the epithelial cells of the lower respiratory tract, psittacosis may follow one of two routes of pathogenesis. Direct local invasion of the pulmonary parenchyma results in a disease with a relatively short incubation period (1 to 3 days). More commonly a primary bacteremia leads to infection of the reticuloendothelial cells of the liver and spleen. This results in an incubation period of 1 week to 15 days.

Based on this bimodal pathogenesis, it can be presumed that a biological attack on a large population would lead to an epidemic with two spikes in cases. The first, smaller peak would occur only days after the attack, and a second, larger peak may be seen 1 to 2 weeks after the release of the agent.

Cases would probably go unnoticed initially. Although there may be clues on history and physical examination, psittacosis does not have a distinctive presentation; the history of avian exposure remains an essential element in suspecting the disease.[17] It usually presents as an atypical pneumonia with varying degrees of severity—from an unapparent mild disease to a severe, life-threatening systemic illness and respiratory failure. When untreated, up to 20% of cases may be fatal. With proper treatment, however, the mortality rate is approximately 1%.

The most common symptoms of psittacosis are cough, fever, headache, and vomiting. Most patients (approximately two thirds) describe a dry cough with scant sputum. Malaise, anorexia, and diarrhea are also common symptoms. Many other symptoms have been associated with cases of *C. psittaci* infection, including photophobia, tinnitus, ataxia, deafness, sore throat, hemoptysis, epistaxis, and rash.

Typical findings on physical examination include fever, rales, consolidation, and tachypnea.[18,19] Two unusual findings that may alert the examiner to the possibility of psittacosis are splenomegaly and relative bradycardia (a normal heart rate in the presence of a high fever). Many other signs have also been described in reviews of psittacosis cases. These include somnolence, confusion, pleural rub, adenopathy, palatal petechiae, herpes labialis, and Horder's spots. Horder's spots are pink, blanching maculopapular eruptions similar to the rose spots seen in typhoid fever. As the disease progresses, multiple systemic complications may develop (see Post-Incident Actions).

The most important laboratory finding involves the chest x-ray, which usually demonstrates a variable degree of consolidation. Most often, this consolidation exceeds the clinical severity of the patient. The white blood cell count is usually normal, but often demonstrates a left shift. More than half of patients have moderately elevated transaminase levels, and many demonstrate mild hyponatremia.

Although isolation of the organism from the blood in cell culture is possible, it can be difficult and is dangerous for laboratory personnel.

The preferred method of diagnosis has been by serology; antibodies are measured by complement-fixation (CF) or microimmunofluorescence (MIF) during the acute illness and after recovery. A single convalescent titer of 1:32 in a patient with a compatible clinical picture is considered by the CDC to be a presumptive case. A fourfold rise in titer between acute and convalescent specimens in a consistent clinical setting is defined as a confirmed case. The presence of immunoglobulin M (IgM) antibody to *C. psittaci* in either specimen is also considered to be a confirmed case.[20] The disadvantage to these techniques, particularly in an outbreak or biological attack, is that results are not immediately available. Real-time polymerase chain reaction (PCR) has been used for a more rapid diagnosis.[21]

PRE-INCIDENT ACTIONS

A biological attack with psittacosis does not necessarily call for unique preparations. As with any potential incident, the emergency department, hospital, and local emergency services should have an integrated disaster response plan. This plan should provide for security and isolation of the treating facility, the triage of potential patients, a mechanism for liberating hospital beds and other treatment space, and the rapid recruitment of local police, fire, and health care personnel. Above all, the plan should provide for redundancy in communication methods—the element most commonly deficient in disaster scenarios. This plan should be reviewed and practiced annually.

Person-to-person transmission of psittacosis has been documented, but no specific isolation beyond universal precautions is indicated. The treating hospital should have a sufficient supply of antibiotics (tetracycline or doxycycline; see the Medical Treatment of Casualties section) available to initiate therapy in suspected cases. The disaster plan should then include a mechanism for recruiting more doses from local and state suppliers within 1 day. After 48 to 72 hours the federal stockpiles should be mobilized to the affected area.

The most significant challenge in addressing a *C. psittaci* attack is recognizing the event at all. Natural outbreaks are preceded by a large number of bird deaths. This is followed by patients presenting with a nonspecific, febrile, respiratory illness during 1 to 2 weeks.[22] Such a scenario would probably be interpreted as an influenza outbreak. Establishing a local or statewide syndromic surveillance system might assist in identifying psittacosis and other subtle biological attacks using nonspecific diseases. A syndromic surveillance system that depends on observed rates of certain symptoms, such as cough, fever, or shortness of breath, would more rapidly detect a psittacosis attack than the conventional public health reporting system. A surveillance system that monitors pharmaceutical sales (such as the National Retail Data Monitor) may also be helpful. It may detect a spike in sales of antipyretics and analgesics or antitussives.

The hospital laboratory should not be expected to culture *C. psittaci*. The CF, MIF, or PCR test for *C. psittaci* should be readily available. If the local facility cannot provide these tests, it must provide for rapid referral of specimens to the next level in the Laboratory Response Network (LRN). The LRN laboratories are a defined hierarchy of increasingly specialized and sophisticated testing institutions available for the confirmation of suspicious agents.[23] The earlier the outbreak is identified, the sooner specific treatment can be initiated. Early therapy of psittacosis is important to minimize mortality, prevent secondary and recurrent cases, and reduce the rates of systemic complications.

POST-INCIDENT ACTIONS

If a case of psittacosis has been confirmed, the appropriate local public health authority should be notified (psittacosis is considered a reportable disease). In the event that multiple cases from different households are diagnosed, the possibility of a biological attack must be considered. Alerting the disaster chain of command up to the federal level would be indicated.

Isolation of patients is not necessary, but decontamination of the affected area may help to prevent additional cases. Patients' clothing should be discarded in a safe manner. Any surface possibly contaminated by infectious particles should be disinfected with 70% isopropyl alcohol or a 1:100 dilution of household bleach. Note that *C. psittaci* is susceptible to heat and most detergents, but it is resistant to acid and alkali. Avoid using a vacuum cleaner because it can aerosolize particles; sweep or wet mop the floor after spraying it with a disinfectant. The use of an N95 respirator and disposable protective clothing (gown, gloves, and mask) is advisable for those cleaning infectious dust.

If the outbreak is associated with a known bird population, isolate or cull the birds. Infected avians can be successfully treated with medicated water or feed or can be administered antibiotics. Wash and disinfect all cages or other containment areas.

After the initial acute cases have presented, the affected population can expect sporadic complications of systemic *C. psittaci* infection. In addition to the expected respiratory illness, psittacosis has been known to cause pericarditis, myocarditis, and "culture-negative" endocarditis. Unless the diagnosis is specifically sought, a patient with *C. psittaci* endocarditis might be subjected to repeatedly negative evaluations, delaying definitive therapy and risking valve destruction.

Psittacosis has also been associated with hepatitis and jaundice, glomerulonephritis, hemolytic anemia, pancytopenia, and disseminated intravascular coagulation. A reactive, polyarticular arthritis is seen 1 to 4 weeks after the initial illness. Neurologic complications are common and diverse. Cranial nerve palsies, cerebellar dysfunction, transverse myelitis, confusion, meningitis, encephalitis, and seizures have all been described. A lumbar puncture is usually normal, but protein levels may be greatly elevated.

MEDICAL TREATMENT OF CASUALTIES

Tetracyclines are the treatment of choice for psittacosis. Satisfactory response is seen with oral therapy: doxycycline 100 mg twice per day or tetracycline 500 mg 4 times per day. Azithromycin has been demonstrated to be effective in animal models.[24] Intravenous treatment can be initiated in the severely ill with doxycycline 2.2 mg/kg (up to 100 mg) twice per day. Defervescence is expected after 24 to 48 hours of therapy. Treatment should continue for 10 to 14 days after the fever resolves. Relapses can occur, so adequate duration of therapy is essential. Although in vivo data are lacking, erythromycin is presumed to be the best alternative agent for patients with a contraindication to tetracyclines, such as children and pregnant women. Antibiotic prophylaxis is not specifically addressed by psittacosis infection control guidelines, but preventative therapy for exposed persons (doxycycline 100 mg by mouth once per day) was demonstrated to be effective in at least one outbreak.[25] There is no vaccine for psittacosis in either humans or animals.

UNIQUE CONSIDERATIONS

Psittacosis is an unusual disease that is rarely seen. Every medical student recognizes it as the "pneumonia caused by living with a parrot." But would this disease be considered in a large number of patients who lack a history of exposure to birds? Very little has been written about the use of *C. psittaci* as a biological weapon, so most would probably consider other agents before testing for psittacosis. Clinical clues to the possibility of psittacosis include a respiratory illness with unusual systemic symptoms and signs. Severe headache, neurologic abnormalities or complications, splenomegaly, or elevated transaminase levels in a patient with x-ray findings consistent with atypical pneumonia should suggest psittacosis as a possible diagnosis.

⚠ PITFALLS

Several potential pitfalls may occur in response to an outbreak of psittacosis. These include the following:

- Failure to identify that a biological attack has occurred; dismissing a spike in respiratory illnesses as a routine influenza outbreak
- Failure to consider psittacosis as a possible diagnosis in a patient who does not have contact with birds
- Failure to directly test for *C. psittaci* by serology in a patient with a history of bird contact or in a group of patients with similar, unexplained cases of "atypical pneumonia"
- Failure to design, practice, and implement a disaster plan to cope with the increase in patient load seen during a biological attack
- Failure to stock adequate supplies of antibiotics or to request early mobilization of state and federal stockpiles
- Failure to treat infected patients with a sufficient duration of therapy to prevent relapses

REFERENCES

1. Centers for Disease Control and Prevention. Notifiable Diseases and Mortality Tables. Available at: http://www.cdc.gov/mmwr/mmwr_nd/index.html.
2. Macfarlane JT, Macrae AD. Psittacosis. *Br Med Bull.* 1983;39:163–187.
3. Schlossberg D. *Chlamydia psittaci* (psittacosis). In: Mandell GL, Bennet JE, Dolin R, eds. *Principles and Practice of Infectious Diseases.* 4th ed. New York, NY: Churchill Livingstone; 1995:1693–1696.
4. Gresham AC, Dixon CE, Bevan BJ. Domiciliary outbreak of psittacosis in dogs; potential for zoonotic infection. *Vet Rec.* 1996;138:622–623.
5. Ito I, Ishida T, Mishima M, et al. Familial cases of psittacosis: possible person-to-person transmission. *Intern Med.* 2002;41:580–583.
6. U.S. Centers for Disease Control and Prevention. Emergency Preparedness & Response. Available at: http://www.bt.cdc.gov.
7. Davis JA. The looming biological warfare storm. *Air Space Power J.* 2003;17:57–68.
8. Wreghitt TG, Taylor CED. Incidence of respiratory tract chlamydial infections and importation of psittacine birds. *Lancet.* 1988;8585:582.
9. Reeve RVA, Carter LA, Taylor N. Respiratory tract infections and importation of exotic birds. *Lancet.* 1988;8589:829–830.
10. Hinton DG, Shipley A, Galcin JW, Harkin JT, Brunton RA. Chlamydiosis in workers at a duck farm and processing plant. *Aust Vet J.* 1993;70:174–176.
11. Hedberg K, White KE, Forfang JC, et al. An outbreak of psittacosis in Minnesota turkey industry workers: implications for modes of transmission and control. *Am J Epidemiol.* 1989;130:569–577.
12. U.S. Centers for Disease Control and Prevention. Psittacosis at a turkey processing plant—North Carolina, 1989. *MMWR Morb Mortal Wkly Rep.* 1990;39:460–461.
13. Belchior E, Barataud D, Ollivier R, et al. Psittacosis outbreak after participation in a bird fair, Western France, December 2008. *Epidemiol Infect.* 2001;139:1637–1641.
14. Koene R, Hautvast J, Zuchner L, et al. Local cluster of psittacosis after bird show in the Netherlands, November 2007. *Euro Surveill.* 2007;12, E071213.1.
15. Grimes JE. Zoonoses acquired from pet birds. *Vet Clin North Am.* 1987;17:209–218.
16. U.S. Centers for Disease Control and Prevention. *Psittacosis Surveillance, 1975-1984.* Atlanta: Centers for Disease Control and Prevention; 1987.
17. Senn L, Greub G. Local newspaper as a diagnostic aid for psittacosis: a case report. *Clin Infect Dis.* 2008;46:1931–1932.
18. Yung AP, Grayson ML. Psittacosis—a review of 135 cases. *Med J Aust.* 1988;148:228–233.
19. Crosse BA. Psittacosis: a clinical review. *J Infect.* 1990;21:251–259.
20. U.S. Centers for Disease Control and Prevention. Compendium of measures to control *Chlamydia psittaci* infection among humans (psittacosis) and pet birds (avian chlamydiosis), 2000. *MMWR Recomm Rep.* 2000;49 (RR-8):3–17.
21. van der Bruggen T, Kaan JA, Heddema ER, van Hannen EJ, de Jongh BM. Rapid diagnosis of psittacosis using a recently developed real-time PCR technique. *Ned Tijdschr Geneeskd.* 2008;152:1886–1888.
22. Telfer BL, Moberley SA, Hort KP, et al. Probable psittacosis outbreak linked to wild birds. *Emerg Infect Dis.* 2005;11:391–397.
23. Pavlin JA, Gilchrist MJR, Osweiler GD, Woollen NE. Diagnostic analyses of biological agent-caused syndromes: laboratory and technical assistance. *Emerg Med Clin North Am.* 2002;20:331–350.
24. Guzman DS, Diaz-Figueroa O, Tully T, et al. Evaluating 21-day doxycycline and azithromycin treatments for experimental *Chlamydophila psittaci* infection in cockatiels. *J Avian Med Surg.* 2010;24:35–45.
25. Broholm KA, Bottiger M, Jernelius H, Johansson M, Grandien M, Sölver K. Ornithosis as a nosocomial infection. *Scand J Infect Dis.* 1977;9:263–267.

Escherichia coli O157:H7 (Enterohemorrhagic E. coli)

Roy Karl Werner

DESCRIPTION OF EVENT

Escherichia coli is a ubiquitous, gram-negative, rod-shaped bacterium that can be located throughout the environment, including water and soil. It is most commonly found as normal flora of the intestinal tract of most mammals, including humans, where it lives to suppress growth of more harmful bacteria. In addition to the enterohemorrhagic *E. coli* (EHEC), which is of concern as potential biological weapons, there are four other types of *E. coli* that cause gastrointestinal disease.[1] Although a detailed discussion of these other types is beyond the scope of this chapter, their characteristics are summarized in Table 139-1.

E. coli O157:H7, the prototypical enterohemorrhagic strain, would be considered a category B threat by the Centers for Disease Control and Prevention (CDC)[2] because it is easily spread via the fecal-oral route[2,3] and has moderate morbidity but low mortality. The O157:H7 serotype produces a Shiga-like toxin that can cause a significant inflammatory response within the intestines without direct invasion of cells. The toxin is bacteriophage-encoded and can be readily transferred from one bacterium to another.[1] This bacterium is quite facile in its ability to obtain new genetic information and incorporate it into its arsenal for defense and infectivity in its hosts. *E. coli* O157:H7 can persist for significant lengths of time in hostile environments and may even require a slightly acidic environment to grow.[4–6] Most *E. coli* O157:H7 outbreaks are linked to fecal-oral transmission caused by poor hand washing techniques and unhygienic food handling. Sources of human infection have included, among others: poorly cooked meat (especially hamburger), apple juice, water (including water parks), vegetables and fruit from salad bars, and milk products such as yogurt and unpasteurized milk.[7–11] There are reported cases of the aerosolized spread of *E. coli*, usually in sewage, but only under very specific circumstances and conditions.

E. coli O157:H7 can infect anyone, but more severe symptoms are found among patients at the extremes of age or in immunocompromised individuals.[12] The endotheliocidal properties of *E. coli* O157:H7 affect the intestinal endothelium, as well as the renal and vascular endothelium, leading to the development of hemolytic uremic syndrome (HUS) and thrombotic thrombocytopenic purpura (TTP).[1,2,7,12–14] It is noteworthy that other EHEC exist with different serotypes. Thus a bioterrorism attack need not use the O157:H7 serotype. For purposes of this chapter, the term *E. coli* O157:H7 will be used because it is the most common serotype, but the reader should understand that the clinical syndrome could be caused by other enterohemorrhagic serotypes, as well.

Symptomatic *E. coli* O157:H7 infection affects approximately 75,000 individuals in the United States yearly. It was first identified as a human pathogen in 1982, when it was isolated in the stool of individuals who had eaten raw or undercooked meat. In 1993 there was an outbreak from hamburgers served at a regional fast food chain, causing HUS and several deaths.[8,15,16]

The incubation period of *E. coli* O157:H7 is between 3 and 9 days.[6,14] Patients initially complain of symptoms similar to viral gastroenteritis: abdominal cramping with significant abdominal pain and tenderness, flatulence, elevated temperatures, and voluminous, watery diarrhea. The diarrhea eventually becomes bloody: 91% of patients report bloody stools at some time during the course of the disease. This likely overestimates the prevalence of bloody diarrhea because patients with less severe disease likely do not present to physicians. Approximately 30% of symptomatic patients require hospitalization, and the mortality rate is approximately 1%. *Shigella*, *Vibrio parahaemolyticus*, *Campylobacter*, and *Salmonella* species; cancerous lesions; ulcerative colitis; incomplete obstruction; gastrointestinal bleeding; and recent antibiotic usage (e.g., for *Clostridium difficile*)[13] should all be included in the differential diagnosis of hemorrhagic diarrhea.

Treatment for *E. coli* O157:H7 infection is limited to supportive measures to prevent dehydration and other complications. The use of antibiotics is contraindicated and has been associated with increased incidence of hemolytic complications.[2,7,13,14,17,18] Antimotility medications are appropriate in afebrile patients without bloody diarrhea. Early refeeding of patients with a lactose-free diet can reduce the duration of diarrhea. The disease is generally self-limited and resolves approximately 1 week after the onset of symptoms.

The most feared sequela of EHEC is HUS, a triad of acute renal failure, thrombocytopenia, and microangiopathic hemolytic anemia. This is more common in infants and children, and some studies have linked antibiotics to many of these cases. Patients with the additional findings of fluctuating neurologic symptoms and fever are classified as having TTP. This may be more common in geriatric or infirmed populations.[19] Blood urea nitrogen (BUN) should be monitored because an increase may signal extraintestinal endothelial involvement and potential progression to TTP or HUS. Urine should also be monitored for hematuria and/or proteinuria, again suggesting progression to TTP or HUS. Discussion of the treatment of TTP and HUS is beyond the scope of this chapter.

All *E. coli* are easily cultured on Sorbitol MacConkey agar. Laboratory analysis will seldom identify the causative organism unless *E. coli* O157:H7 is specifically sought. However, the CDC recommends that all stools from patients with bloody diarrhea be screened for the O157:H7 serotype. Antisera to the O157:H7 antigen can be used to screen isolates. Any isolates that screen positive should be sent to a reference laboratory for further characterization. Isolation of the bacteria is most likely during the first 6 days of diarrhea. Many times the O157:H7 serotype cannot be isolated from even bloody diarrheal stools that commonly have high concentrations of this pathogen.[20,21] Obtaining stool samples from multiple patients will increase isolation yield and assist with characterization of *E. coli* O157:H7 when present. Stool studies should include a search for other etiologic factors of the diarrheal disease, including those previously noted. Multiplex polymerase chain reaction (PCR) using multiple

TABLE 139-1 *E. coli* Causing Gastrointestinal Symptoms

TYPE OF *E. COLI*	SOURCE OR LOCATION	FEVER/ SYMPTOMS	TOXINS	INVASIVENESS	CLINICAL PICTURE	DIARRHEA
Enterotoxigenic Traveler's diarrhea (children and adult travelers)	Water sources	No, cholera-like	Cytotoxic heat stabile and/or heat labile	None, no cellular changes or bacteremia	Mild dehydration, self-limited	Watery, voluminous, originates in proximal small bowel
Enteroinvasive Dysentery syndrome (children and adults)	Asia	Yes, with tenesmus and abdominal cramps	*Shigella*-like	Epithelial cells of intestine	Dehydration	Blood-tinged with many polymorphonuclear lymphocytes
Enteroaggregative (children)	Less developed countries	No, stacked aggregates on cell surfaces	Some have a heat stabile	Aggregative adherence	Mild dehydration, self-limited	Watery, nonbloody, and persistent
Enteropathogenic (children and newly born)	Nurseries	No, localized adherence	None	Adherence, causing effacement	No fever, acute-onset diarrhea in neonates, dehydration	Nonbloody
Enterohemorrhagic (children and adults)	Foods, raw beef, and sewage	No	Shiga-like	Effacement of intestinal mucosa	Vomiting, no fever, nausea, chills, HUS, TTP	First nonbloody, then grossly bloody

HUS, Hemolytic uremic syndrome; *TTP*, thrombotic thrombocytopenic purpura.

primer studies, fingerprinting, and rapid identification[22,23] studies should be used to assist in determining the specific cause. If *E. coli* O157:H7 is identified, it is mandatory that it be reported to the CDC; this allows centralized monitoring of outbreaks.

PRE-INCIDENT ACTIONS

The greatest potential for limiting the effects of a terrorist attack involving the dissemination of *E. coli* O157:H7 is the readiness of the "front-line fighters" of the health care system: emergency medical personnel, outpatient clinics, and emergency departments. The presentation of an escalating number of patients with severe diarrheal disease along with similarities in medical, travel, or exposure history should alert medical and public health personnel to the possibility of a nonaccidental exposure.[24]

Continuous water and food production monitoring by the appropriate local, state, and federal agencies, as well as routine testing and retesting of in-place barriers to terrorism by Homeland Security task forces[25,26] will also contribute to the safety of citizens. Computer-aided programs, passive surveillance of foodstuffs, random testing of food processing areas, irradiation and filtration of airborne particles, and tighter control of treatment areas for national food and water supplies are all methods currently in place to decrease the effects of bioterrorism.[24,26] Hand washing and glove use at patient points of contact or before handling foodstuffs are ways spread can be minimized.

POST-INCIDENT ACTIONS

When an outbreak of *E. coli* O157:H7 infection is suspected, hospital laboratories should be alerted, and agent-specific cultures of stool samples should be obtained. Stool samples can also be tested for fecal leukocytes,[13,27] although results are not particularly sensitive or specific. Fecal lactoferrin assays have the potential to be beneficial, but their utility is also debated; use of fecal lactoferrin is considered more specific for bacterial

causes of diarrhea,[28] but it cannot help with determining the specific etiologic factor. If the source of the outbreak can be readily identified, it should be contained and eliminated immediately. Foodstuffs in the area should be incinerated to decrease perpetuation of the infection. Surface areas can be decontaminated with a 5% to 10% bleach solution.[29,30]

MEDICAL TREATMENT OF CASUALTIES

Oral rehydration solutions are helpful in patients with *E. coli* O157:H7 infection because most patients have minimal vomiting. The World Health Organization recommends solutions containing 2.6 g sodium chloride, 2.9 g trisodium citrate dihydrate, 1.5 g potassium chloride, and 13.5 g anhydrous glucose, all dissolved in 1 L of clean water for a total osmolarity of 245 mOsm/L solution. Recommendations have also been suggested to include zinc supplementation that varies by age because it has been shown in some studies to improve outcomes.[13,27,31–34] Appropriate infection control practices should be instituted for *E. coli* and include body substance isolation and hand washing. Masks are optional for *E. coli* because airborne spread is inconsequential (unless contaminated feces are aerosolized). Rehydration should include intravenous solutions if oral intake is poorly tolerated or if the patient fails to improve.

UNIQUE CONSIDERATIONS

E. coli O157:H7 infection is often not suspected early in outbreaks. Initial relatively benign symptoms of fevers, abdominal cramping, and diarrhea are commonly minimized, and thus fecal-oral spread continues before hemorrhagic diarrhea commences or *E. coli* O157:H7 infection is considered. Identification of *E. coli* O157:H7 requires specialized testing that may not be readily available at the local laboratory. Harbingers of a possible bioterrorism event with *E. coli* O157:H7 include a clustering of infectious diarrhea in a previously healthy population, all of whom have similar exposures (e.g., water or food). Travel to an area with a known outbreak of disease should also raise the clinician's level of suspicion.[24,35]

! PITFALLS

Several potential pitfalls may occur in response to an outbreak of *E. coli* O157:H7, which include the following:

- Failure to identify that a biological attack has occurred; dismissing a spike in gastrointestinal illnesses as a routine gastroenteritis outbreak
- Failure to have adequate supplies of the oral and intravenous rehydration solutions and supplies
- Failure to notify appropriate public health and law enforcement agencies when an outbreak is suspected or confirmed
- Failure to treat patients with oral rehydration solution instead of intravenous hydration, when possible (An excessive amount of intravenously treated patients will unnecessarily tie up resources needed by sicker patients in the event of a mass casualty event.)

REFERENCES

1. Eisenstein BI, Zaleznik DF. Enterobacteriaceae. In: Mandell GL, Bennett JE, Dolin R, eds. *Principals and Practice of Infectious Diseases*; vol 2. 5th ed. Philadelphia, PA: Churchill Livingstone; 2000:2294–2310.
2. U.S. Centers for Disease Control and Prevention. General Information: *Escherichia coli*. Available at: http://www.cdc.gov/ecoli/index.html. Accessed April 20, 2015.
3. Todar K. *Todar's Online Textbook of Bacteriology*. 2nd ed. Available at: http://www.textbookofbacteriology.net. Accessed 4/20/15.
4. Rhee MS, Lee SY, Dougherty RH, et al. Antimicrobial effects of mustard flour and acetic acid against *Escherichia coli* O157:H7, *Listeria monocytogenes*, and *Salmonella enterica* serovar Typhimurium. *Appl Environ Microbiol*. 2003;69:2959–2963.
5. Reinders RD, Biesterveld S, Bijker PGH. Survival of *Escherichia coli* O157:H7 ATCC 43895 in a model apple juice medium with different concentrations of proline and caffeic acid. *Appl Environ Microbiol*. 2001;67:2863–2866.
6. Cody SH, Glynn MK, Farrar JA, et al. An outbreak of *Escherichia coli* O157:H7 infection from unpasteurized commercial apple juice. *Ann Intern Med*. 1999;130:202–209.
7. U.S. Food and Drug Administration, Center for Food Safety & Applied Nutrition. *Foodborne Pathogenic Microorganisms and Natural Toxins Handbook. The Bad Bug Book*. Available at: http://www.fda.gov/food/foodborneillnesscontaminants/causesofillnessbadbugbook/default.htm. Accessed April 20, 2015.
8. Feng P. *Escherichia coli* serotype O157:H7: novel vehicles of infection and emergence of phenotypic variants. *Emerg Infect Dis*. 1995;1(2):47–52.
9. U.S. Centers for Disease Control and Prevention. Lake-associated outbreak of *Escherichia coli* O157:H7—Illinois, 1995. *Morb Mortal Wkly Rep*. 1996;45(21):437–439.
10. U.S. Centers for Disease Control and Prevention. Outbreaks of *Escherichia coli* O157:H7 infection and cryptosporidiosis associated with drinking unpasteurized apple cider—Connecticut and New York, October 1996. *Morb Mortal Wkly Rep*. 1997;45(21):4–8.
11. U.S. Centers for Disease Control and Prevention. Outbreak of *Escherichia coli* O157:H7 infections associated with drinking unpasteurized commercial apple juice-British Columbia, California, Colorado, and Washington, October 1996. *Morb Mortal Wkly Rep*. 1996;45(44):975.
12. Guerrant RL, Steiner TS. Principles and syndromes of enteric infections. In: Mandell GL, Bennett JE, Dolin R, eds. *Principals and Practice of Infectious Diseases*; vol 1. 5th ed. Philadelphia, PA: Churchill Livingstone; 2000:1080–1085.
13. Giannella RA. Infectious enteritis and proctocolitis and bacterial food poisoning. In: Feldman M, Friedman LS, Brandt LJ, eds. *Gastrointestinal and Liver Disease*; vol 2. 9th ed. Philadelphia, PA: Saunders; 2010:1843–1887.
14. Tauxe RV, Swerdlow DL, Hughes JM. Foodborne disease. In: Mandell GL, Bennett JE, Dolin R, eds. *Principals and Practice of Infectious Diseases*; vol 1. 5th ed. Philadelphia, PA: Churchill Livingstone; 2000:1150–1165.
15. U.S. Centers for Disease Control and Prevention. Preliminary report: foodborne outbreak of *Escherichia coli* O157:H7 infections from hamburgers—Western United States, 1993. *Morb Mortal Wkly Rep*. 1993;42 (4):85–86.
16. U.S. Centers for Disease Control and Prevention. Update: multi-state outbreak of *Escherichia coli* O157:H7 infections from hamburgers—Western United States, 1992-1993. *Morb Mortal Wkly Rep*. 1993;42 (14):258–263.
17. Weinstein RS, Alibek K. *Shigellosis*. In: *Biological and Chemical Terrorism—a Guide for Healthcare Providers and the First Responders*. New York, NY: Thieme Medical; 2003:96–97.
18. Weinstein RS, Alibek K. Biological weapon syndromic cross-references. In: *Biological and Chemical Terrorism—a Guide for Healthcare Providers and the First Responders*. New York, NY: Thieme Medical; 2003:13.
19. Richards A, Goodship JA, Goodship TH. The genetics and pathogenesis of haemolytic uraemic syndrome and thrombotic thrombocytopenic purpura. *Curr Opin Nephrol Hypertens*. 2002;11 (4):431–435.
20. Osterholm MT, Hedberg CW, Moore KA. Epidemiologic principles. In: Mandell GL, Bennett JE, Dolin R, eds. *Principals and Practice of Infectious Diseases*; vol 1. 5th ed. Philadelphia, PA: Churchill Livingstone; 2000:157–159.
21. Gill VJ, Fedorko DP, Witebsky FG. The clinician and the microbiology lab. In: Mandell GL, Bennett JE, Dolin R, eds. *Principals and Practice of Infectious Diseases*; vol 1. 5th ed. Philadelphia, PA: Churchill Livingstone; 2000:191–192.
22. Vidal R, Vidal M, Lagos R, et al. Multiplex PCR for diagnosis of enteric infections associated with diarrheagenic *Escherichia coli*. *J Clin Microbiol*. 2004;42(4):1787–1789.
23. Fratamico PM, Bagi LK, Pepe T. A multiplex polymerase chain reaction assay for rapid detection and identification of *Escherichia coli* O157:H7 in foods and bovine feces. *J Food Prot*. 2000;63(8):1032–1037.
24. Burkle FM. Mass casualty management of a large-scale bioterrorist event: an epidemiological approach that shapes triage decisions. *Emerg Med Clin North Am*. 2002;20(2):409–436.
25. Kahn AS, Swerdlow DL, Juranek DD. Precautions against biological and chemical terrorism directed at food and water supplies. *Public Health Rep*. 2001;116(1):3–14.
26. Filoromo C, Macrina D, Pryor E, et al. An innovative approach to training hospital-based clinicians for bioterrorist attacks. *Am J Infect Control*. 2003;31(8):511–514.
27. Lung E. Acute diarrheal diseases. In: Friedman SL, McQuaid KR, Grendell JH, eds. *Current Diagnosis and Treatment in Gastroenterology*. 2nd ed. New York, NY: Lange Medical Books/ McGraw-Hill; 2003:131–150.
28. Huicho L, Campos M, Rivera J, Guerrant RL. Fecal screening tests in the approach to acute infectious diarrhea: a scientific overview. *Pediatr Infect Dis J*. 1996;15(6):486–494.
29. Bosilevac JM, Arthur TM, Wheeler TL, et al. Prevalence of *Escherichia coli* O157 and levels of aerobic bacteria and Enterobacteriaceae are reduced when hides are washed and treated with cetylpyridinium chloride at a commercial beef processing plant. *J Food Prot*. 2004;67 (4):646–650.
30. Oldfield EC, 3rd. Emerging foodborne pathogens: keeping your patients and your families safe. *Rev Gastroenterol Disord*. 2001; 1(4):177–186.
31. World Health Organization. *The Selection and Use of Essential Medicines, Report of the WHO Expert Committee*; 2011 (including the 17th WHO Model List of Essential Medicines and the 3rd WHO Model List of Essential Medicines for Children). Available at: http://whqlibdoc.who.int/trs/WHO_TRS_965_eng.pdf. Accessed April 20, 2015.

32. World Health Organization. Enterohaemorrhagic *Escherichia coli* (EHEC) Fact Sheet. Available at: http://www.who.int/mediacentre/factsheets/fs125/en/index.html. Accessed April 20, 2015.

33. World Health Organization. Diarrhoea treatment guidelines including new recommendations for the use of ORS and zinc supplementation for clinic-based healthcare workers. Available at: http://www.who.int/maternal_child_adolescent/documents/a85500/en/index.html. Accessed April 20, 2015.

34. U.S. Centers for Disease Control and Prevention. Managing acute gastroenteritis among children. Oral rehydration, maintenance, and nutritional therapy. *Morb Mortal Wkly Rep.* 2003;52(RR16):1–16.

35. Weinstein RS, Alibek K. Basic bioterrorism. In: *Biological and Chemical Terrorism—a Guide for Healthcare Providers and the First Responders.* New York, NY: Thieme Medical; 2003:2–12.

140 | CHAPTER

Viral Encephalitis (Alphavirus) Attack

Khaldoon H. AlKhaldi

DESCRIPTION OF EVENT

Alphaviruses are one of the three families of the arthropod-borne viruses (arboviruses) that can cause encephalitis. There are currently three alphaviruses known to cause human disease in the United States: the Eastern equine encephalitis (EEE), Western equine encephalitis (WEE), and Venezuelan equine encephalitis (VEE) viruses. All three viruses are transmitted through mosquito bites, and all three cause similar initial presentations of illness, resembling a "flu-like" syndrome. However, many can include high fever, headache, photophobia, stiff neck, nausea, and vomiting. In cases of encephalitic invasion, symptoms can progress to confusion, obtundation, seizures, and focal neurologic deficits.

Eastern Equine Encephalitis

The EEE virus is maintained through a bird-mosquito-bird life cycle. The most important vector is the mosquito *Culiseta melanura*.[1] These mosquitoes are often found in coastal areas and near freshwater swamps. Thus most U.S. cases have been reported in Florida, Georgia, Massachusetts, and New Jersey. EEE has a high case fatality rate: 35%, reported by the Centers for Disease Control and Prevention (CDC). Of those who survive, an estimated 35% will have permanent mild to severe neurologic deficits. There have been approximately 200 human cases in the United States since 1964, with one fatality in 1990 and three in 2012 in Massachusetts.[2] The average is one to two deaths per year in that state.

In 2011, 80 of 4604 mosquito samples collected in Massachusetts were positive for EEE virus. One fatal case of EEE infection was identified in a Bristol County resident aged more than 60 years, with a clinical presentation of meningoencephalitis. A case was also identified in a Missouri resident aged more than 60 years with a clinical presentation of encephalitis. An epidemiological investigation determined that this individual was most likely exposed in Southeastern Massachusetts.[3] Just 1 year later, in 2012, 267 of 6828 mosquito samples collected in Massachusetts were positive for EEE virus. There were seven human cases of EEE reported in Massachusetts in 2012, one from Middlesex County (believed to have been acquired out of state), one from Worcester County, one from Franklin County, two from Plymouth County, and two from Essex County.[3]

Western Equine Encephalitis

WEE is closely related to EEE, but it has a lower case fatality rate: approximately 10%. As with EEE, it is a summertime disease, but WEE is found in states west of the Mississippi River and in some western Canadian provinces. It is also maintained by a bird-mosquito-bird life cycle, with its primary vector the mosquito *Culex tarsalis*. The worst outbreak recorded was 3336 human cases in 1941. Since 1955, a varied range of 0 to 200 cases per year have been reported, with no human cases reported since 1994.[1,2]

Venezuelan Equine Encephalitis

VEE is found in South and Central America. It is maintained by a rodent-mosquito life cycle and it claims at least 10 mosquito species as its vector. The fatality rates have been approximately 0.6% in reported outbreaks. Past epidemics include 32,000 human cases in Venezuela from 1962 to 1964, and, in 1971, more than 10,000 horses died from a VEE epidemic. Human cases have been sporadic since then.[1,2]

PRE-INCIDENT ACTIONS

Mitigation activities represent the principal pre-incident actions useful against the alphavirus encephalitides. Humans who live in high-risk areas or work or play outside frequently in these areas should be sure to wear mosquito repellant that contains DEET and wear long-sleeved shirts and pants. During outbreaks, outdoor activity should be limited. Widely available vaccines are being developed, and their validity is undergoing testing.

In preparation for potential biological terrorist attacks, the Institute of Medicine Committee on Research and Development to Improve Civilian Medical Response recommends that major hospitals conduct mass casualty planning and training, have isolation rooms available for infectious diseases, have decontamination capacity, and be fully supplied with drugs, ventilators, and personal protective equipment. The committee also encourages the CDC to help keep medical care providers up-to-date on the science related to current dangerous biological agents and materials.[4]

Providers should be made aware of the endemic viral infections in their region because the geographic range of the illnesses continues to spread. Providers should also consider alphavirus infections in their differential diagnoses for patients with suitable clinical presentations and test for the viruses in conjunction with infectious disease experts and public health authorities when appropriate.

POST-INCIDENT ACTIONS

Alphavirus infections should be reported to the appropriate local or state health authority, who in turn is responsible for reporting to the

CDC. Public health warnings may then be issued to limit the risks of further exposures. Public health authorities may also consider whether further measures, such as mosquito spraying or others, should be initiated. Eradicating potential arthropod vectors and vaccinating equine reservoirs may help to prevent the spread of encephalitis in the event of a biological attack.[5]

Because no person-to-person spread is possible, universal precautions are the only precautions that must be maintained with patients infected with one of these viruses.[5,6]

MEDICAL TREATMENT OF CASUALTIES

As in the case of most viral illnesses, treatment of the alphavirus encephalitides consists primarily of supportive care.[2,7–10] Patients suspected of having viral encephalitis should undergo an appropriate clinical workup for concomitant bacterial or fungal meningitis with lumbar puncture and possible computed tomography imaging of the head. Further serologic testing may also be necessary. As with all acute illness, the airway should be protected, especially if the patient's mentation is severely depressed. Nutrition, fluids, and electrolytes should be optimized, and pyrexia should be aggressively treated.[8,10] In the setting of increased known or suspected elevated intracranial pressure, patients should be managed in the intensive care setting with appropriate clinical measures, potentially including head elevation, administration of hypertonic saline or osmotic agents, and possibly steroids or intravenous immunoglobulin.[10] Prevention of seizures is important, and clinicians may wish to consider administration of anticonvulsant therapy.[2]

Consultation with neurology and infectious disease specialists is recommended for patients with viral encephalitis. Neurosurgical consultation may be necessary if the patient required active intracranial pressure monitoring or decompression, or if a brain biopsy is considered.[9] Although there is no specific medical treatment available for the alphaviruses, the use of ribavirin and recombinant interferon alpha is being assessed.[2,9]

Prognosis depends not only on the particular type of alphavirus responsible for the encephalitis, but also on the age and prior health of the individual infected. Children 1 year old or younger and adults 55 years old or older are at increased risk of life-threatening complications.

UNIQUE CONSIDERATIONS

Although the clinical effects of alphavirus encephalitis can be devastating, with persistent neurologic sequelae or death possible, the vast majority of patients exposed to these viruses will actually be asymptomatic or present for medical care with nonspecific "flu-like" symptoms.[5] An early alphaviral attack may be difficult to identify and distinguish from routine "viral syndrome" because of the similarity of illness presentation and lack of routine laboratory testing available for the viruses.

The viral encephalitides are CDC category B biological agents, which means that they are moderately easy to disseminate, but have lower mortality rates. In their natural state, these viruses require

arthropod vectors for transmission and have a variable seasonality that is dependent on the geography, local climate, and virus-specific life cycle. These qualities make the use of the alphaviruses as a terrorist agent more difficult to control and to disseminate to the public. That said, aerosol transmission of a weaponized (manufactured) form of the virus has been demonstrated, and it would represent the most likely route of mass infection if terrorists were able to produce large amounts of aerosolized virus.[4,9] Other characteristics of the alphaviruses lend themselves to weaponization: large amounts of stable alphaviruses could be produced inexpensively and native viruses could be genetically manipulated.[8]

One possible indicator that an alphavirus attack has occurred would be a large number of sick or dying equine animals in the vicinity.[10] As with seasonal alphavirus outbreaks, arthropod vector control and vaccinating equine reservoirs could help to prevent the spread of encephalitis during an outbreak.[5]

⚠ PITFALLS

- Failure to notify appropriate public health officials of a diagnosis of viral encephalitis
- Failure to prepare local emergency departments and clinics to respond appropriately in case of an outbreak
- Failure to disseminate mitigation information to local communities
- Failure to recognize that reports of sick or dying equine animals in the area may be related to a vector-borne disease

REFERENCES

1. Markhoff L. Alphaviruses. In: Mandell GL, Bennett JE, Dolin R, eds. *Principles and Practice of Infectious Diseases*. 5th ed. Philadelphia, PA: Churchill Livingstone; 2000.
2. US Centers for Disease Control and Prevention, Division of Vector-Borne Infectious Diseases. Arboviral Encephalitides. Available at: http://www.cdc.gov/ncidod/dvbid/arbor/index.htm.
3. Information about Eastern Equine Encephalitis (EEE). September 20, 2013. Available at: http://www.quincyma.gov/CityOfQuincy_Content/documents/EEE2013.pdf.
4. Katona P. Bioterrorism preparedness: a generic blueprint for health departments, hospitals, and physicians. *Infect Dis Clin Pract*. 2002;11(3):115–122.
5. Rajagopalan S. Deadly viruses. *Top Emerg Med*. 2002;24(3):44–55.
6. Cherry CL, Kainer MA, Ruff TA. Biological weapons preparedness: the role of physicians. *Intern Med J*. 2003;33:242–253.
7. Harwood-Nuss A. *The Clinical Practice of Emergency Medicine*. 3rd ed. Philadelphia, PA: Lippincott Williams & Wilkins; 2001.
8. Franz DR, Jahrling PB, Friedlander AM, et al. Clinical recognition and management of patients exposed to biological warfare agents. *JAMA*. 1997;278:399–411.
9. Kawamura N, Kizawa M, Ueda A, et al. Tatsuro Mutoh. *Future Virology*. 2012;7(9):901–909. Available at: http://reference.medscape.com/article/1166498-overview.
10. Sardesai AM, Brown NM, Menon DK. Deliberate release of biological agents. *Anesthesia*. 2002;57(11):1067–1082.

Tick-Borne Encephalitis Virus Attack

Heather Rybasack-Smith, Lawrence Proano, and Robert Partridge

DESCRIPTION OF EVENT

Tick-borne encephalitis (TBE) is a zoonotic illness caused by one of three identified subtypes of tick-borne encephalitis virus (TBEV): European (TBEV-Eu, formerly Central European encephalitis virus [CEEV]); Siberian (TBEV-Sib, formerly West Siberian virus); and Far Eastern (TBEV-FE, formerly Russian spring-summer encephalitis virus [RSSEV]). In Russia, where 5000 to 10,000 cases occur yearly, it is still commonly called spring-summer encephalitis. The viral genomes are relatively stable, without significant antigenic variation.[1] TBE is part of the mammalian group of flaviviruses, a family of about 70 viruses that includes yellow fever, dengue fever, and Japanese encephalitis. Although little known in North America, it is a reportable disease in 16 European countries,[2] and it is endemic from Japan and China through Russia and Europe.[3] The European Union deemed TBE a reportable disease in 2012. Approximately 10,000 to 12,000 cases of TBE are reported yearly, a number thought to be a gross underestimation of the actual incidence of disease.[1] Cases are largely limited to temperate, forested regions.

The incidence and distribution of TBE have increased dramatically over the last 30 years, with a 400% increased morbidity in Europe alone.[2] From 2004 to 2006, its incidence in Germany increased from 274 to 546/10,000 cases and in the Czech Republic from 507 to 1029/10,000 cases.[4] The causes of this increase are multifactorial, with climate change, changes in land use, and recreation patterns all likely contributing to an increase in vector to human interactions and an increase in human illness.[2]

TBE is transmitted primarily through several species of *Ixodes* tick, which act as both reservoirs and vectors for TBEV. There have been reports of transmission through unpasteurized goat milk,[5,6] but there are no reports of human-to-human transmission. Humans and other large-bodied mammals are dead-end hosts that do not participate in the cycle of viral transmission. Up to a third of patients who present with TBE do not recall having been exposed to ticks.[7]

TBEV-FE generally follows a monophasic course, whereas TBEV-Eu typically produces a biphasic pattern, beginning with several days of a nonspecific viral prodrome, including high fever, headache, myalgias, nausea, and vomiting.[3] After an incubation period of 2 to 10 days, neurologic symptoms begin and range from encephalitis to severe meningoencephalomyelitis.[3] One fourth to one third of patients will develop symptoms of central nervous system (CNS) dysfunction, including severe headache and meningismus, confusion, lethargy, delirium, convulsions, paralysis, coma, and death. The virus migrates from dermal cells through the reticuloendothelial system until it finally crosses the blood-brain barrier. In fatal cases, polioencephalomeylitis, primarily of the spinal cord, cerebellum, and brain, is characteristic.[1]

Once a person is infected, significant morbidity can occur. Long-term sequelae, including ataxia, occur in about one third of cases, with roughly 30% of patients reporting permanent CNS dysfunction.[8] The encephalitic form appears to carry the worst prognosis, but severity varies geographically, likely related to differing strains of the virus.[8] TBEV-FE has a reported case fatality rate of >20%[1]; however, this percentage likely reflects underreporting of less severe cases. Cases of a severe, hemorrhagic form of TBE have been reported in Russia,[9] highlighting the possibility that more virulent strains of TBE have yet to emerge.

Coinfection with other tick-borne diseases such as *Borrelia burgdorferi* occurs in about 15% of cases.[10] Once infected, the host develops IgG antibodies, which persist and appear to convey lifelong immunity.[1] Laboratory data are nonspecific and can include cerebrospinal fluid (CSF) studies consistent with aseptic meningitis, leukopenia, elevated inflammatory markers, and thrombocytopenia. CNS imaging is not likely to be useful except in ruling out other causes of meningismus or encephalitic syndromes.

PRE-INCIDENT ACTIONS

TBEV is classified by the National Institute of Allergy and Infectous Diseases (NIAID) as a category C bioterror agent and has the potential to be engineered for mass dissemination, with resulting high morbidity and mortality. Surveillance systems using government and hospital data may be used to detect clusters of encephalitis or meningitis. Given the nonspecific nature of TBE and its overlap with other tick-borne illness, identification of an attack will rely on epidemiological analyses.

Given the effectiveness of the available vaccinations, it is reasonable to recommend vaccination in persons living or traveling to endemic areas. TBE has been called a "neglected" travel disease[11] and is likely very underreported, given the nonspecific symptoms and frequently benign course.

Several countries with endemic TBEV have successfully reduced the incidence of cases with vaccination programs.[2] Available vaccines are 95% to 99% effective but are expensive and require repeat administrations to preserve immunity, which is likely not cost-effective in nonendemic areas.

In the event of an attack in a nonendemic area, it may be exceedingly difficult to identify TBE as a cause unless clinicians retain a high level of suspicion.

POST-INCIDENT ACTIONS

Confirmation of cases requires specialized laboratory testing due to the highly nonspecific clinical presentation. In the initial viremic phase, CSF and serum testing for viral RNA is possible but impractical. Most patients seek care only during the second phase of illness, when neurologic symptoms emerge; however, at this point there is no detectable viremia. Diagnosis is generally made via ELISA antibody detection. There is cross-reactivity with other flaviviruses, such as Japanese encephalitis, which may lead to underdiagnosis in endemic regions[12] or among vaccinated travelers. The geographic distribution of TBE overlaps with other tick-borne infections that cause similar disease profiles and may coinfect the same host. It is vital to exclude other causes of aseptic meningitis or encephalitis, such as herpes, which have effective treatments.

Prevention is the only means of stopping an attack once it is identified. If spread occurs via the natural tick-borne route, vector control, personal protection with permethrin or DEET-based repellants, and tick prevention education will be crucial measures in the event of an attack. Simple measures such as tight-fitting clothing, checking for ticks, and avoiding underbrush can be very effective in preventing exposure to ticks.

Person-to-person transmission has never been reported. Pasteurization of milk appears to inactivate the virus and should be encouraged in endemic areas. The case reports of hemorrhagic syndrome assiciated with TBE are concerning, and little is known about the variation in virus or transmission that may be associated with the hemorrhagic form.

MEDICAL TREATMENT OF CASUALTIES

There is no specific cure for TBE. Supportive therapy is the mainstay of therapy, with fever control and airway protection for severely affected individuals. Neuromuscular paralysis can develop in less than 1 hour.[13] Corticosteroids have been used by clinicians, but their benefit has not been formally investigated.[8] Passive postexposure prophylaxis with IgG has not been well studied and is no longer recommended, due to the significant theoretical risk of antibody-mediated enhancement of infection.[14]

UNIQUE CONSIDERATIONS

Flaviviruses and other vector-borne diseases can cause a wide range of nonspecific viral symptoms and a spectrum of severity. TBE is not as internationally recognized as other flaviviruses, such as yellow fever and dengue, and therefore might be an ideal agent for bioterrorism. Few places outside of endemic areas even have the laboratory capacity to screen for the TBE viruses. As civilization encroaches on wilderness and outdoor activities increase in popularity, the interface between humans and ticks will likely increase. The effects of climate change on vector distribution may result in significantly increased human exposure to tick vectors. The ability of TBE to infect humans through ingestion is also of concern, and raw milk consumption, another potential source, is on the rise.[15]

Although the United States and Canada have thus far been spared from the endemic outbreaks of TBEV found in Europe and Asia. North America has an endemic deer tick population. The rate of Lyme and other tick-borne illness has been on the rise in North America for decades, secondary to a multitude of factors, including reforestation, larger deer populations, and climate change. TBE viruses have been isolated from American deer ticks,[16] and there are case reports of fatal TBE transmitted by deer ticks in the United States.[17] Foci of other TBE-like viruses have been isolated and have the potential to spread along with the tick population.[18]

PITFALLS

- Failure to consider tick-borne viral encephalitis as a cause of an acute febrile illness with neurologic complications
- Failure to recognize two or more cases as representing a cluster of unusual infections that should be reported to health authorities
- If a case or cluster is recognized, failure to take proper respiratory, contact, and universal precautions when handling body fluid samples from patients
- Failure to send those samples to the appropriate state health agencies for further testing

REFERENCES

1. WHO. *Wkly Epidemiol Rec.* 2011;86(24):241–256.
2. Süss J. Tick-borne encephalitis in Europe and beyond—the epidemiological situation as of 2007. *Euro Surveill.* 2008;13(26).
3. Mansfield KL, Johnson N, Phipps LP, Stephenson JR, Fooks AR, Solomon T. Tick-borne encephalitis virus—a review of an emerging zoonosis. *J Gen Virol.* 2009;90:1781–1794.
4. Donoso Mantke O, Schädler R, Niedrig M. A survey on cases of tick-borne encephalitis in European countries. *Euro Surveill.* 2008;13(17).
5. Hudopisk N, Korva M, Janet E, et al. Tick-borne encephalitis associated with consumption of raw goat milk, Slovenia, 2012. *Emerg Infect Dis.* 2013;19 (5):806–808.
6. Holzmann H, Aberle SW, Stiasny K, et al. Tick-borne encephalitis from eating goat cheese in a mountain region of Austria. *Emerg Infect Dis.* 2009;15 (10):1671–1673.
7. Kaiser R, Holzmann H. Laboratory findings in tick-borne encephalitis. Correlation with clinical outcome. *Infection.* 2000;28:78–84.
8. Mickiene A, Laiškonis A, Gunther G, et al. Tickborne encephalitis in an area of high endemicity in Lithuania: disease severity and long-term prognosis. *Clin Infect Dis.* 2002;35:650–658.
9. Ternovoi VA, Kurzhukov GP, Sokolov YV, et al. Tick-borne encephalitis with hemorrhagic syndrome, Novosibirsk Region, Russia, 1999. *Emerg Infec Dis.* 2003;9(6):743–746.
10. Lotric-Furlan S, Petrovec M, Avsic-Zupanc T, et al. Prospective assessment of the etiology of acute febrile illness after a tick bite in Slovenia. *Clin Infect Dis.* 2001;33(4):503–510.
11. Haditsch M, Kunze U. Tick-borne encephalitis: a disease neglected by travel medicine. *Travel Med Infect Dis.* 2013;5:295–300.
12. Takashima I, Morita K, Chiba M, et al. A case of tick-borne encephalitis in Japan and isolation of the virus. *J Clin Microbiol.* 1997;35:1943–1947.
13. Dumpis U, Crook D, Oksi J. Tick-borne encephalitis. *Clin Infect Dis.* 1999;28:882–890.
14. Heyman P, Cochez C, Hofhuis A, et al. A clear and present danger: tick-borne diseases in Europe. *Expert Rev Anti Infect Ther.* 2010;8(1):33–50.
15. Oliver SP, Boor KJ, Murphy SC, Murinda SE. Food safety hazards associated with consumption of raw milk. *Foodborne Pathog Dis.* 2009;6(7):793–806.
16. Telford SR III, Armstrong PM, Katavolos P, Foppa I, Garcia ASO, Wilson ML. A new tick-borne encephalitis-like virus infecting New England deer ticks, Ixodes dammini. *Emerg Infect Dis.* 1997;3(2):165–170.
17. Tavakoli NP, Wang H, Dupuis M, et al. Fatal case of deer tick virus encephalitis. *N Engl J Med.* 2009;360(20):2099–2107.
18. Ebel GD, Foppa I, Spielman A, Telford SR III. A focus of deer tick virus transmission in the northcentral United States. *Emerg Infect Dis.* 1999;5 (4):570–574.

SUGGESTED READINGS

1. Kaiser R. Tick-borne encephalitis. *Infect Dis Clin North Am.* 2008;22 (3):561–575.

142 CHAPTER

Viral Hemorrhagic Fever Attack: Arenaviruses

Valarie Schwind

DESCRIPTION OF EVENT

To date, there have been no reports of the use of Arenaviruses as biological weapons. However, because certain viruses in this family can cause significant hemorrhagic viral syndromes, they could become attractive for use in terrorism. To recognize and respond effectively should a mass casualty incident involving one of these viruses occur, either weaponized or emerging as a natural outbreak, practical knowledge of Arenaviruses, including their presentation and treatment, is imperative.

Arenaviruses belong to a family of Arboviruses that are characterized by their similar viral structure, which includes enveloped, single-stranded RNA that are about typically 110 to 130 nm in diameter.[1] A few of these viruses cause hemorrhagic fevers. These include Lassa virus, Junín virus, Machupo virus, Guanarito virus, and Sabia virus, and these will be the center of our discussion in this chapter. In nature, Arenaviruses are found in rodent reservoirs. The type of rodent determines the geographic distribution of the virus. Because of this, many hemorrhagic fevers are named after the region or country in which they are found. In nature, the viruses are spread to humans through contact with infected rodent blood, urine, and feces, through inhalation of aerosolized fecal particles, direct contact, or contamination of food with the above-mentioned substances.[2] Person-to-person transmission has been reported but only through the direct spread of infected bodily fluids. There have been no proven cases of aerosol transmission from person to person.[3]

Arenaviruses are classified as either "Old World" or "New World" viruses, based on their geographic location and rodent reservoir. Of the viruses discussed in this chapter, Lassa virus is the only Old World Arenavirus. The other four viruses discussed in this chapter are referred to as New World Arenaviruses, and they may be grouped together for purposes of this discussion.[1,2] Collectively, all of these viruses are classified as category A biological agents by the Centers for Disease Control and Prevention (CDC).[4] This is because these viruses have a high mortality rate, are easily obtainable from natural hosts, are able to be developed for aerosol spread, and have the potential to cause wide-spread panic should an attack occur.[3]

Lassa Fever

Lassa fever is endemic to many countries in Northwest Africa including Sierra Leone, Nigeria, Liberia, and Guinea. Since the year 2000, cases have also been reported with growing frequency in the surrounding countries. Lassa fever received its name from the town in Nigeria where it was first discovered in 1969.[5] It is now responsible for nearly 500,000 infections annually, and of those cases, approximately 3000 to 5000 are fatal.[1] The virus is transmitted to humans by contact with the rodent *Mastomys natalensis* or its bodily fluids. Most cases of Lassa virus are relatively benign, with the disease course being either asymptomatic or with mild flu-like symptoms. Moderate or severe disease occurs in approximately 20% of those infected and is characterized by a somewhat flu-like illness including fever, headache, pharyngitis, lymphadenopathy, facial edema, myalgia, nausea, vomiting, diarrhea, and abdominal pain. Severe disease progresses into anasarca, bleeding diathesis, organ failure, encephalitis, and death.[1] Of those who survive the disease, approximately one third experience some level of hearing loss or deafness. The severity of the Lassa virus does not correlate with the level of hearing loss incurred by survivors, and even those with mild illness may have this complication. These effects may be permanent. Overall mortality from the disease is about 1%; however, among those who progress to severe disease, the mortality rate increases to nearly 20%.

Lassa virus has the potential to be a biological threat because it can be aerosolized and transmitted. This form of transmission from rodent excrement is well documented. Lassa could be manipulated for mass, aerosolized dissemination; however, its subsequent propagation after initial dissemination would be limited, as human-to-human spread occurs only through contact with infected bodily fluids and not via the air. Spread between humans can be prevented with proper use of personal protective equipment. Diagnosis of Lassa virus is usually clinical and based on an appropriate travel history or history of rodent exposure combined with the symptom constellation as stated above. Laboratory abnormalities may show hemoconcentration, thrombocytopenia, leukopenia, and elevated liver function tests. Coagulation abnormalities may also be present. It should be noted that Lassa fever has an incubation period of 1 to 3 weeks, and therefore initial symptoms may be quite delayed after exposure. Diagnosis can be made by polymerase chain reaction (PCR) testing. Enzyme-linked immunosorbent assay (ELISA) testing is also available, and it can detect IgG, IgM, and Lassa antigen. Testing for Lassa requires specialized laboratory facilities, and therefore laboratory results can be delayed. If Lassa is suspected, appropriate isolation and treatment should be initiated before the confirmatory results are received.[5]

Junín Virus

Junín virus was discovered in 1958 in remote agricultural regions of Argentina. Its clinical syndrome was appropriately named Argentine hemorrhagic fever. The virus is spread to humans through contact with bodily fluids and aerosolized excrement particles from the mammalian reservoir, *Calomys musculinus* (drylands vesper mouse).[6] Those most at risk are rural populations in endemic areas who come into contact with the mouse during agricultural work or in their homes.

The syndrome caused by the Argentine hemorrhagic fever virus is very similar to the other illnesses described in this chapter. The incubation period is approximately 7 to 14 days, after which patients develop fever, headache, myalgias, and anorexia. During days 3 to 5 of the disease, patients may develop petechial rashes on the soft palate and trunk. Disease may progress to generalized edema, with development of pleural effusions and bleeding from gums, nose, GI system, and uterus, as well as neurologic symptoms. Argentine hemorrhagic fever is also associated with autonomic instability, and patients often exhibit signs of postural hypotension, as well as intermittent flushing and diaphoresis. Argentine hemorrhagic fever is more likely to progress to a hemorrhagic phase than Lassa virus is,[7] and although there are fewer than 50 cases reported every year, approximately 15% to 30% of those cases are fatal.[8] Fortunately, a vaccine has been developed for endemic areas called Candid #1, which has been used successfully to treat thousands of people in rural Argentina at risk for the disease.[6,9]

Machupo Virus

The Machupo virus is an Arenavirus endemic to Bolivia that causes the disease commonly called Bolivian hemorrhagic fever. It was first discovered in 1959 in an outbreak in San Joaquin, Bolivia. This virus, like the other New World hemorrhagic viruses, is also spread by a murine vector, specifically, the *Calomys callosus*, also commonly known as the large vesper mouse.[10] Clinically, Bolivian hemorrhagic fever is very similar to Argentine hemorrhagic fever. It has a constellation of symptoms that can include signs of increasing capillary leak, proteinuria, mucosal hemorrhage, narrow pulse pressure, and resultant vasoconstriction causing shock.[11] With both the Junín and Machupo viruses, petechiae, facial edema, and hyperesthesia of the skin are more commonly observed than they are with the other New World hemorrhagic viruses.[12] Survivors often have no permanent sequelae, except for mild alopecia and orthostatic hypotension that can last for a few weeks.

Guanarito Virus

Gaunarito virus was discovered in 1989 in a small Venezuelan municipality, where it caused an outbreak of Venezuelan hemorrhagic fever among settlers moving into a previously unpopulated area. It is believed that contact with the cane mouse (*Zygodontomys brevicauda*) spread the disease to humans.[11] The virus occurs naturally and results in sporadic outbreaks.[1] It has been responsible for approximately 200 known cases of human illness since its discovery. It has many of the same clinical features as the other New World hemorrhagic viruses; however, in contrast to the Machupo and Junín viruses, pharyngitis, vomiting, and diarrhea are far more prominent in Venezuelan hemorrhagic fever.[12] Treatment is largely supportive for Venezuelan hemorrhagic fever. If untreated, case fatality can reach 30% to 40%.[8] For unknown reasons, the incidence of this disease has been decreasing over the past 20 years.[12]

Sabia Virus

Sabia virus was discovered in a rural area near São Paulo, Brazil, and, to date, there have only been three reported cases. Two of those cases involved laboratory workers. Only one case has been fatal. The disease reservoir is unknown, but it is thought to be a rodent, as with the other New World viruses.[8] It is difficult to draw conclusions on the potential of this little-known virus for use in bioterrorism.

Emerging Viruses

Many other viruses in the Arenaviridae family have not been found to cause human disease. Over the past 10 years, new hemorrhagic illnesses have begun to emerge, and newly discovered viruses are being added to the family. For example, in 1999-2000, three cases of Whitewater Arroyo virus were reported in California. The Arenavirus-caused illness appeared to have been carried by rodents in the United States, but not much information is available on its pathogenesis or epidemiology. In 2004, in a more mountainous area of Bolivia, the Chapare virus was isolated. Its symptoms were similar to that of the Machupo and Sabia viruses, but again, with only one reported case, not much information is known.[12] In South Africa in 2008, five cases of

hemorrhagic fever were reported, which lead to the discovery of the Lujo virus. The index case was a patient from Zambia, and the disease was spread nosocomially.[13] The disease has a very abrupt onset of symptoms that include rash, CNS symptoms, and bleeding diathesis. Among the small outbreak of cases, mortality was 80%.[14]

The ability of these Arenaviruses to be spread through the aerosol route means that they could potentially be weaponized for malicious intent. However, some people believe that the long incubation periods of many of these diseases may deter terrorists from using them because they would not get immediate results after distributing the virus.[15] This same feature, however, could make a terrorist use of the viruses very difficult to detect or investigate, because the clinical disease will not show up until weeks later when exposed and infected people have dispersed potentially all over the country, taking the disease with them to different hospitals and regions. Therefore, clinicians may not recognize a mass casualty event with only one or a few case presentations. The viruses are endemic to rural foreign countries and wild animals, so source control is difficult for the United States to achieve. The virus particles are found in nature, and they can be replicated easily in a laboratory. One characteristic that makes Arenaviruses less favorable for terrorist use is the that, after initial spread through the aerosol route, they are not spread from person to person in that same manner. Spread between humans occurs through contact with bodily fluids, and an outbreak can be contained using isolation and strict contact precautions.[15]

◀◀ PRE-INCIDENT ACTIONS

Bioterrorism is an ever-persistent threat. Hospitals must be vigilant for signs of an attack because they would be on the front lines of any mass casualty incident resulting from the use of a biological agent. Hospitals should provide targeted education to staff on how to suspect and detect strange disease patterns. If concerning patterns emerge or if the diagnosis of any viral hemorrhagic fever is made state government officials and the Centers for Disease Control and Prevention should be notified immediately. Hospital disaster plans must consider how the hospital would respond to an act of biological terrorism causing a large influx of patients. Hospitals should anticipate needs for increased staffing and supplies. For viral hemorrhagic fevers (VHF), resuscitative supplies such as IV fluids, antipyretics, antiemetics, blood products, and vasopressors will be in high demand. For Arenaviruses specifically, ribavirin will be the treatment of choice (until Lassa fever can be ruled out), and it may need to be stockpiled. A plan for appropriate isolation of numerous ill patients and both training and supplies to support strict contact precautions must be in place. In some disaster plans, it might be possible to select a certain hospital that could be designated to treat all cases, to concentrate expertise and prevent exposing other "well" patients to the disease.

▶▶ POST-INCIDENT ACTIONS

After a viral hemorrhagic fever outbreak has been identified, the CDC and other local, state, and national government officials should be immediately notified so that containment efforts can be coordinated. Because of the increased rate of travel, national-level help may be needed to perform appropriate risk mitigation and contact tracing. Patients with symptoms should be isolated initially, and strict contact precautions should be used, including impermeable gowns, eye protection, gloves, and shoe covers, which should be worn when health care workers have contact with them. Although the diseases are not spread by the airborne route, the use of negative pressure isolation rooms and respirators (N95 or PAPR) is generally recommended. Any contacts of patient within the past 3 weeks should be placed under public health surveillance, although the degree of the surveillance may be hotly debated, as seen in the 2014 Ebola outbreak. If any of the index patient's contacts develops signs of illness, they should be put in isolation and treated. If after 21 days a contact remains symptom free, he or she no longer requires surveillance. An outbreak can be considered controlled when no new cases are reported for two consecutive incubation periods; in the case of VHF, that translates to 42 days.[4]

Bodily fluid samples should only be sent to specialized and appropriately trained and equipped laboratories. Samples should be sealed in biohazard bags according to prespecified protocols. Coordination with Biosafety Level-4 labs may be required, because they are the only labs with appropriate safety mechanisms and machinery in place to confirm the presence VHF via PCR or ELISA testing. Two such laboratories are the CDC in Atlanta, Georgia, and the U.S. Army Medical Research Institute of Infectious Diseases in Frederick, Maryland.[4,15] After any contact with an infected patient or their bodily fluids, hospital rooms and equipment must be sanitized properly with bleach preparations. Disposable items should be incinerated. Linens should be either destroyed or washed in hot water and bleach. All laboratory testing and environmental remediation should be conducted under the guidance of appropriately skilled experts.

✚ MEDICAL TREATMENT OF CASUALTIES

The mainstay of treatment for VHF is mostly supportive. Ribavirin is currently the only drug proven to have any efficacy against viral hemorrhagic fevers in this class. Its use has only been proven effective against *Lassa* virus. Once a presumptive diagnosis of *Lassa* virus is made, ribavirin may be started, with the understanding that confirmatory testing can take up to 7 to 10 days. Case fatality can be significantly reduced if the drug is started early in the disease.[4,15] Ribavirin dosing is as follows:
1. Intravenous therapy:
   a. Loading dose: 30mg/kg (max 2g) followed by
   b. 15 mg/kg (max 1g) every 6 hours for 4 days followed by
   c. 7.5 mg/kg (max 500mg) every 8 hours for 6 days.
2. Oral therapy:
   a. 35mg/kg (max 2.5g) loading dose followed by
   b. 15mg/kg (max 1g) every 8 hours for 10 days

IV therapy is recommended; however, in a mass casualty situation, supplies may be limited, and oral therapy can be used if necessary.[4] Side effects of ribavirin therapy may include hemolytic anemia which occasionally requires transfusion and rigors if the medication is administered too quickly. Caution should be taken in all patients with known allergy, liver disease and kidney disease. The drug is technically contraindicated in pregnancy due to development of birth defects in lab studies but consideration may be given to the drug situations where the mothers life is in imminent danger.[14] In South America, the convalescent plasma of immune persons has also been used to treat Junín and Machupo viruses, but this may be difficult to obtain in a rapid manner should an outbreak occur outside of an endemic area. In 2014 we saw such therapy be administered with success during the Ebola outbreak.

Supportive therapy should be tailored to each individual patient. Careful attention must be paid to fluid and electrolyte balance because vasculature is very permeable and overhydration can lead to worsening edema. Intensive care units are usually the appropriate placement for these patients who can quickly develop respiratory failure, kidney failure, shock, and encephalopathy.

Vaccines against the Junín virus have been developed and dispersed in endemic areas with effective results.[6] Postexposure immunization and the effect that it might have on the control of an acute outbreak has not been studied. However, vaccines may be preventative in the case of ongoing exposure or a secondary attack.

💡 UNIQUE CONSIDERATIONS:

VHF have not been used as biological terrorism agents, but they may have the potential to be used as a weapon for terrorists seeking to cause mass disease, hysteria, and economic collapse. Even if an outbreak of viral hemorrhagic fever were discovered and easily contained, the effect on the population could be long lasting. Because VHF diseases are very rare in the United States, clinicians must always maintain an appropriate level of suspicion when dealing with unique disease patterns, such as unexplained bleeding.

⚠ PITFALLS

- Failure to recognize and correctly diagnose viral hemorrhagic illness early on
- Failure to contact local and national departmental agencies as soon as disease is discovered
- Failure to have unique bioterrorism disaster plans
- Failure to quarantine and use strict contact precautions
- Failure to start ribavirin treatment as soon as viral hemorrhagic fever is suspected

REFERENCES

1. Safronetz D, Feldmann H, Falzarano D. Arenaviruses and Filoviruses. In: Greenwood D, Barrer M, Slack R, Irving W, eds. *Medical Microbiology.* 18th ed. Philidelphia, PA: Elsevier; 2012:546–588.
2. Hensley L, Wahl-Jensen V, McCormick J, Rubins K. Viral hemorrhagic fevers. In: Cohen J, Opal S, Powderly W, eds. *Infectious Diseases.* 3rd ed. Philadelphia, PA: Elsevier; 2010:1247–1252.
3. Borio L, Inglesby T, Peters CJ, et al. Hemorrhagic fever viruses as biological weapons: medical and public health management. *JAMA.* 2002;287 (18):2391–2405.
4. Kman NE, Nelson RN. Infectious agents of bioterrorism: a review for emergency physicians. *Emerg Med Clin North Am.* 2008;26(2):517–547, x-xi.
5. U.S. Centers for Disease Control and Prevention: Lassa Fever. Available at: http://www.cdc.gov/vhf/lassa/index.html. Updated: 4 April 2014.
6. Grant A, Seregin A, Huang C, et al. Junín virus pathogenesis and replication. *Virus.* 2012;4(10):2317–2339.
7. Pfau CJ. Arenaviruses. In: Baron S, ed. *Medical Microbiology.* 4th ed. Galveston, TX: University of Texas Medical Branch at Galveston; 1996, Chapter 57. Available at: http://www.ncbi.nlm.nih.gov/books/NBK8193/
8. Bausch, Daniel G. Viral hemorrhagic fevers. In: Goldman L, ed. *Goldman's Cecil Medicine.* 24th ed. Philadelphia, PA: Elsevier; 2012: 2147–2156.
9. Abrosio A, Saavedra MC, Mariani MA, Gamboa G, Maiza A. Argentine hemorrhagic fever vaccines. *Hum Vaccin.* 2011;7(6):694–700.
10. Patterson M, Grant A, Paessler S. Epidemiology and pathogenesis of Bolivian hemorrhagic fever. *Curr Opin Virol.* 2014;5:82–90.
11. Seregin A, Yun N, Paessler S. Lymphocytic choriomeningitis, Lassa fever, and the South American hemorrhagic fevers (Arenaviruses). In: Bennett J, Dolin R, Blaser M, eds. *Mandell, Douglas, and Bennett's Principles and Practice of Infectious Diseases.* 8th ed. Philadelphia, PA: Elsevier; 2015: 2031–2037.
12. Charrel R, Lamballerie X. Arenaviral hemorrhagic fevers. In: Cherry JD et al eds. *Feigin and Cherry's Textbook of Pediatric Infectious Diseases.* Philadelphia, PA: Elsevier Saunders; 2014: 2466–2477.
13. Briese T, Paweska JT, McMullan LK, et al. Genetic detection and characterization of Lujo virus, a new hemorrhagic fever—associated Arenavirus from Southern Africa. *PLoS Pathog.* 2009;5(5):e1000455.
14. Bloomberg L, Enria D, Bausch D. Viral hemorrhagic fevers. In: Farrar J. ed. *Manson's Tropical Diseases.* 23rd ed. Philadelphia, PA: Elsevier; 2014: 171–194.
15. Peters CJ. Viral hemorrhagic fevers as agents of bioterrorism. In: Bennett J, Dolin R, Blaser M, eds. *Mandell, Douglas, and Bennett's Principles and Practice of Infectious Diseases.* 7th ed. Philadelphia, PA: Elsevier; 2010: 3995–3998.

CHAPTER 143

Viral Hemorrhagic Fever Attack: Bunyavirus

Andrea G. Tenner and Alexander P. Skog

DESCRIPTION OF EVENT

Four families of viruses classically cause hemorrhagic fever: Filoviridae, Arenaviridae, Bunyaviridae, and Flaviviridae. These viral agents all share similar characteristics: they are lipid-enveloped RNA viruses and they require an animal or insect host reservoir. Because of this, they are geographically restricted, and, therefore, human disease is sporadic, unanticipated, and generally occurring through accidental contact with the reservoir due to human encroachment on the environment.[1-3] Even though it is not common for naturally occurring viruses to be transmitted person to person, transmission through bodily fluids and small-particle aerosol has occurred with all of the hemorrhagic fever viruses (HFVs) (generally this has occurred in laboratory workers handling specimens or in persons exposed to the blood and tissues of infected animals).[2-4] Because most of these viruses tend to present with a nonspecific syndrome of fever, myalgia, headaches, and prostration,[1] a high index of suspicion should be maintained.

According to the Working Group on Civilian Biodefense, the key features of a dangerous biological weapon include: high morbidity and mortality, the potential for person-to-person transmission, low infective dose, the ability to be aerosolized (leading to the capacity to cause a large outbreak), no available vaccine (or ineffective or scarce vaccine), anxiety-provoking, readily available, able to be produced on a large scale, stable in the environment, and previously researched as a bioterrorist agent. Among the Bunyaviridae family, viruses with potential for large-scale epidemics and bioterrorism events are (in decreasing order of potential effect): Rift Valley fever (RVF), Crimean-Congo hemorrhagic fever (CCHF), and hantavirus.[2,5,6] However, a relatively new bunyavirus called severe fever with thrombocytopenia syndrome (SFTS) virus has emerged in China that also has the potential for significant effect.[7]

Several countries, including the former Soviet Union, Canada, North Korea, and the United States, have attempted to weaponize viruses causing hemorrhagic fever.[8] Bunyaviruses, in particular, are generally easily cultured in vitro, and they can be prepared in large quantities. Because of the high potential for these viruses to be weaponized, the case definition for a suspected deliberate release of HFV in Europe is =1 confirmed case that is not imported.[3]

The Bunyaviridae, specifically, tend to damage the vascular beds throughout the body and can produce capillary leak syndrome.[3] All viruses in this family may cause thrombocytopenia, leukopenia, decreased levels of coagulation factors, and disseminated intravascular coagulation (most notably in RVF).[2] The characteristics of these specific viruses will be reviewed below.

Rift Valley Fever

RVF is a zoonotic disease endemic to sub-Saharan Africa, with spread to the Arabian Peninsula that primarily affects domestic animals (sheep, goats, and cattle). It is spread by several genera of mosquito (*Aedes, Anopheles, Culex, Eretmapoites,* and *Mansonia*) as well as sand flies, but has also been shown to be infectious through aerosolization in workers handling the blood or body fluids of infected animals.[2-4] Additionally, it has the ability to utilize the predominant mosquito of any given location, making mosquitos in any country viable vectors.[4] Once domestic animals are infected with RVF, they can serve as a virus reservoir for transmission to mosquitos, and, while epidemic spread is limited to certain climatologic conditions (sufficient rain and/or water accumulation to allow vector proliferation), the virus is also capable of lying dormant in mosquito eggs, making eradication difficult. It is thought that a single infected human or animal (live or dead) entering a country could be sufficient to cause a major outbreak in a previously unexposed country, possibly before the RVF virus could even be detected.[4] Deliberate use of the agent could have devastating effects both through direct human infection, as well as through significant destruction to the livestock industry, severely limiting the food supply and disrupting the economy.[4,9]

The incubation period for RVF is 2 to 6 days. Patients initially present with abrupt onset of biphasic fever, with the first febrile period lasting about 4 days, followed by an afebrile period of 1 to 2 days, and a second bout of fever lasting 2 to 4 days. Epistaxis, hematemesis, melena, jaundice, retinitis, and meningoencephalitis may develop.[2,3] The virus leads to the destruction of infected cells and hemostatic derangements thought to occur through a combination of vasculitis and hepatic necrosis.[2]

Even though the mortality rate is generally reported to be less than 2%, recent outbreaks have had case fatality rates (CFRs) of 20% to 45% for unknown reasons.[4] A bioterrorist attack with the previous less-virulent strain would likely have a primary effect of causing public fear and creating economic loss from the death of livestock, given the 1% to 2% mortality rate; however, if the more-virulent strain is weaponized, RFV could pose a far-greater direct threat to humans.[9]

Crimean-Congo Hemorrhagic Fever

CCHF is endemic in Africa, Eastern Europe, the former Soviet Union, and Asia. It is transmitted through tick bites and contact with blood from infected livestock or infected patients (either direct inoculation or possibly aerosolized virus from the blood).[1,3,5] Even though CCHF does not achieve high viral numbers in cell culture and is difficult to produce in large quantities, its potential for person-to-person transmission, high CFR, and its ubiquitous presence in central Asia, sub-Saharan Africa, and the Middle East make it a real threat as a bioterrorism agent.[2]

The CCHF incubation period is 1 to 3 days.[3] Human disease is characterized by the sudden onset of fever with rigors and chills that wax and wane over the course of 7 to 9 days. Severe myalgia, nausea, vomiting, diarrhea, facial hyperemia, hepatomegaly, hemorrhage, and petechiae may be seen.[5] Other signs and symptoms include sore eyes and photophobia, mood swings, confusion, and aggression, followed by sleepiness and depression. Hepatitis is usually present, and multisystem organ failure (especially hepatorenal and pulmonary failure) may develop after the fifth day of illness.[3] CFRs range from 13% to 50%.[3,5]

Hantavirus

Hantaviruses are unique in that they are the only Bunyaviridae that do not have an arthropod vector; their vectors are rodents. The vector itself is unaffected but sheds virus in the urine, saliva, and feces; transmitting the virus via inhalation of aerosolized particles or rodent bite.[1,10] Despite that these viruses do not reproduce well in culture and are potentially harmful to those trying to produce them (Biosafety Level 3 or 4 laboratories are required for production),[11] there are some characteristics of Hantaviruses that make them potential biologic weapons. They exist worldwide; only a rudimentary understanding of virology is needed for laboratory reproduction; they are spread via aerosol; the general immunity in the population is low; and the number of viruses that can cause disease without cross-immunity is high.[11] Cleaning with detergents will kill Hantaviruses, but, in disaster conditions where hygiene is difficult to maintain, there is potential for rapid dissemination.[1]

Infection with hantavirus is generally classified as hemorrhagic fever with renal syndrome (HFRS) or hantaviral pulmonary syndrome (HPS), depending on the specific virus and the clinical syndrome it causes.[1,5] Both HFRS and HPS are characterized by increased vascular permeability and dysfunction. HPS presents with the rapid onset of a flu-like prodrome that is associated with gastrointestinal symptoms and lasts approximately 4 days, followed by pulmonary edema with an ARDS-like picture, cardiovascular collapse, and shock due to increased capillary permeability.[1] CFRs can be as high as 50% to 60% and the Andes virus, which can cause HPS, has shown person-to-person transmission.[10,12,13] The most severe forms of HFRS, however, are caused by Hantaan or Dobrova viruses and also start with fever, myalgia, and eye pain, which then progresses to renal failure with proteinuria, hypotension, and hemorrhage, with mortality rates of 5% to 10%. Laboratory investigations often show thrombocytopenia, but also an increased white blood cell count (in contrast to other Bunyaviruses) and blast cells.[1]

Severe Fever with Thrombocytopenia Syndrome

SFTS virus was identified in China in 2009.[7] Since that time, over 20 strains of viruses that can produce this syndrome have been isolated in six provinces in China, and two cases of a similar virus were reported in Missouri.[14] The SFTS viruses are thought to be transmitted by a tick vector, but there is evidence of potential reservoirs in domestic animals and person-to-person transmission via direct blood contact has occurred. The CFR is estimated to be 10% to 12%.[7,14] This coupled with the ease of culture of the virus and the lack of known effective antivirals or vaccines makes this virus another potential agent for bioterrorism.[7]

SFTS presents with the same nonspecific symptoms of high fever, thrombocytopenia, leukocytopenia, gastrointestinal symptoms, and lymphadenopathy. Three major stages of disease have been identified: the fever stage, the multiorgan dysfunction stage, and the convalescent

stage. Days 1 to 7 of illness comprise the febrile stage. During this stage, both fatal and nonfatal cases have high viral loads, fever, thrombocytopenia, and leukopenia, with evidence of hepatic dysfunction toward the later period of this stage. The second stage occurs between days 7 and 13 and, in nonfatal cases, is marked by a decreasing viral load and improvement in hepatic function followed by a convalescent recovery phase with resolution of disease as symptoms subside and laboratory markers return to normal. In fatal cases, the second stage is comprised of a persistently elevated viral load, increasing aminotransferase (AST), lactate dehydrogenase (LDH), creatine kinase (CK), and creatin kinase-MB (CK-MB) fraction, and declining platelet counts. In the third stage, fatal cases progress to multisystem organ dysfunction, disseminated intravascular coagulation (DIC), overt hemorrhage, and death.[7,14]

◀ PRE-INCIDENT ACTIONS

Hospitals should have disaster preparedness plans in place and run routine drills. As all of these viruses may be spread via aerosolization, personal protective equipment (PPE) should be available and disaster plans should include isolation of all affected patients. Drills should include identifying and rapidly isolating these patients, as well as coordinating local and states authorities and emergency medical services to protect the hospital environment, all responders, and as much of the general community as possible from contamination and exposure.

▶ POST-INCIDENT ACTIONS

Respiratory and contact isolation of symptomatic patients and their contacts in negative pressure rooms should be undertaken until the nature of the virus causing the outbreak is better understood. Access to the hospital should be limited to patients and trained health care providers with appropriate PPE. Additionally, state and local authorities and hospital infection control personnel and laboratory workers should be notified immediately.[2,7,15]

For all Bunyaviridae, identification of the specific virus often takes days, so the approach to these illnesses is the same. First, a high index of suspicion should be maintained. Patients who acquire these illnesses naturally will have some exposure to risk factors such as travel to Africa or Asia, handling of animal carcasses, contact with sick animals or people, mosquito/sand fly/tick bites within 21 days, or recent exposure to rodent urine/feces/saliva. However, in an intentional attack, the victims will have none of these risk factors.[2] Patients should be identified using the World Health Organization (WHO)'s recommended case definition: acute onset of fever (=101 °F or 38.3 °C) of less than 3 weeks duration in a severely ill patient and any two of the following: hemorrhagic or purpuritic rash, epistaxis, hematemesis, hemoptysis, blood in stools, other hemorrhagic symptoms, and no known predisposing host factors for hemorrhagic manifestations.[2,15] Strict isolation precautions should be initiated if HFVs are suspected. All health care workers should use double gloves, leg and shoe coverings, and N95 masks or powered air-purifying respirators (PAPRs). Environmental decontamination should be undertaken with Environmental Protection Agency-registered hospital disinfectant or a 1:100 dilution of household bleach. Linens should be washed in hot water with bleach, autoclaved, or incinerated. Bodies should be handled carefully because contact with cadavers has been known to cause transmission of HFVs. Trained personnel with the same PPE as those caring for live patients should handle the bodies. Autopsies should be performed only by trained personnel with respiratory protection in negative pressure rooms. Preferably, bodies should be promptly buried or cremated with as little handling as possible and no embalming performed.[2]

✚ MEDICAL TREATMENT OF CASUALTIES

Care for infections with Bunyaviruses is primarily supportive; however, it is important to be careful with the volume of intravenous fluids given because pulmonary edema can develop rapidly. In light of this, patients with hemodynamic instability should be started on vasopressor therapy early, with hemodynamic monitoring. Intramuscular injections, heparin, nonsteroidal antiinflammatory drugs, and other anticoagulant medications are contraindicated, and steroids are not effective.[2] However, ribavirin has been shown to inhibit many of the Bunyaviridae viruses in vitro and has some in vivo activity.[2,5] Even though human studies are lacking and this regimen is not Food and Drug Administration approved, current recommendations are to give (under an investigational new drug protocol) an intravenous loading dose of 30 mg/kg (max 2 g) initially, followed by 16 mg/kg (max 1 g per dose) every 6 hours for 4 days, followed by 8 mg/kg (max 500 mg per dose) every 8 hours for 6 days. In mass casualty situations, the recommendation is loading dose of 2 g orally once, followed by 600 mg twice a day (>75 kg) or 400 mg in the morning and 600 mg at night (=75 kg) for 10 days. In children, the recommended dose is a loading dose of 30 mg/kg orally, then 15 mg/kg per day in two divided doses for 10 days. Ribavirin is a pregnancy class X drug, but the benefit to the mother likely outweighs the risk in a viral hemorrhagic fever outbreak.

Interferon alpha has been shown to protect rhesus monkeys from viremia and hepatocellular damage, if given shortly before or after infection with RVF, but no human trials have been performed.[2]

❓ UNIQUE CONSIDERATIONS

Bunyaviridae, unlike Filoviridae or Flaviviridae, are sensitive to ribavirin. Therefore ribavirin should be given initially until the etiology of the HFV is elucidated.[2]

In general, the Bunyaviridae are easy to culture and mass produce (except for the Hantaviruses and CCHF) and many have livestock reservoirs and multiple vectors, which can allow for persistence even after the initial attack is over. Reemergence should be anticipated, and control measures implemented. There is a livestock vaccine available for RVF, as well as a human vaccine, but these are expensive, not readily available, and the human vaccine requires multiple doses and yearly boosters, making it impractical to be distributed for a large-scale attack or prevention.[4]

❗ PITFALLS

- Failure to consider the diagnosis, especially in an intentional attack, as patients will not have the usual risk factors
- Ignoring the livestock reservoir. These viruses "hide" in livestock and mosquito eggs and may return later once the acute epidemic is thought to be over.

- Not initiating ribavirin treatment—even though not Food and Drug Administration (FDA) approved, it is the only potential treatment for Bunyavirus infection
- Not containing the infection, isolating secretions, and placing on respiratory isolation—even though most naturally occurring Bunyaviridae are not spread via the respiratory tract, all can be spread via aerosol or contact with blood; weaponized viruses would likely be chosen for ease of transmission, so all patients should be isolated until the virus is characterized

REFERENCES

1. Bronze MS, Huycke MM, Machado LJ, et al. Viral agents as biological weapons and agents of bioterrorism. *Am J Med Sci.* 2002;323(6):316–325.
2. Borio L, Inglesby T, Peters CJ, et al. Hemorrhagic fever viruses as biological weapons: medical and public health management. *JAMA.* 2002;287 (18):2391–2405.
3. European Centre for Disease Prevention and Control (ECDC)-Health Comunication Unit-Eurosurveillance editorial team. Bichat guidelines for the clinical management of haemorrhagic fever viruses and bioterrorism-related haemorrhagic fever viruses [Internet]. 2004 [cited 2014 Apr 28]. Available from: http://www.eurosurveillance.org/ViewArticle.aspx? ArticleId=504.
4. Bouloy M, Flick R. Reverse genetics technology for Rift Valley fever virus: current and future applications for the development of therapeutics and vaccines. *Antiviral Res.* 2009;84(2):101–118.
5. Sidwell RW, Smee DF. Viruses of the Bunya- and Togaviridae families: potential as bioterrorism agents and means of control. *Antiviral Res.* 2003;57 (1–2):101–111.
6. Centers for Disease Control. CDC | Bioterrorism Agents/Diseases (by Category) | Emergency Preparedness & Response [Internet] [cited 2014 Apr 28]. Available from: http://emergency.cdc.gov/agent/ agentlist-category.asp.
7. Bao C, Guo X, Qi X, et al. A family cluster of infections by a newly recognized bunyavirus in eastern China, 2007: further evidence of person-to-person transmission. *Clin Infect Dis.* 2011;53(12):1208–1214.
8. James Martin Center for Nonproliferation Studies. CNS—Chemical and Biological Weapons: Possession and Programs Past and Present [Internet] [cited 2014 Apr 29]. Available from: http://cns.miis.edu/cbw/possess.htm.
9. Dar O, Hogarth S, McIntyre S. Tempering the risk: Rift Valley fever and bioterrorism. *Trop Med Int Health.* 2013;18(8):1036–1041.
10. Feldmann H, Czub M, Jones S, et al. Emerging and re-emerging infectious diseases. *Med Microbiol Immunol (Berl).* 2002;191(2):63–74.
11. Clement JP. Hantavirus. *Antiviral Res.* 2003;57(1–2):121–127.
12. Toro J, Vega JD, Khan AS, et al. An outbreak of hantavirus pulmonary syndrome, Chile, 1997. *Emerg Infect Dis.* 1998;4(4):687–694.
13. Figueiredo LTM, Souza WM de, Ferrés M, et al. Hantaviruses and cardiopulmonary syndrome in South America. *Virus Res.* 2014 Feb; [Internet] [cited 2014 Apr 29]. Available from: http://www-ncbi-nlm-nih-gov.proxy-hs.researchport.umd.edu/pmc/articles/PMC2640255/.
14. Li D. A highly pathogenic new bunyavirus emerged in China. *Emerg Microbes Infect.* 2013;2(1):e1.
15. WHO Recommended Surveillance Standards [Internet] [cited 2014 Apr 29]. Available from: http://www.who.int/csr/resources/publications/ surveillance/whocdscsrisr992syn.pdf.

Viral Hemorrhagic Fever Attack: Filo Viruses

William Porcaro

DESCRIPTION OF EVENT

The Ebola and Marburg viruses are members of the Filoviridae family of viral hemorrhagic fevers that have the ability to produce a high degree of morbidity and mortality, making them enticing candidates to be used as biological weapons. The Centers for Disease Control and Prevention (CDC) has classified filoviruses as category A biological agents because of their high degree of virulence, demonstrated aerosol infectivity, and ability to instill fear and anxiety in the population.[1] Concern exists about terrorist groups obtaining samples of filoviruses from existing laboratory stocks, rogue government agents, or natural outbreaks. Some research has confirmed that the Ebola virus may be capable of infecting via the aerosol route as the virus is likely able to traverse airway epithelial cells.[2] Some researchers have suggested that the Japanese cult group Aum Shinrikyo, which was responsible for the Sarin Subway Attack in Tokyo in 1995, sent members to Zaire in the 1990s to obtain samples of the Ebola virus.[3]

Viral hemorrhagic fevers are clinical syndromes characterized by acute onset of fever and generalized symptoms such as malaise, headache, myalgia, and diarrhea. In the majority of victims the syndrome progresses to a bleeding diathesis, septic shock, and multiple organ failure. Russia and the former Soviet Union produced and stockpiled large quantities of weaponized Marburg and possibly Ebola as recently as the 1990s.[4]

Marburg virus was first discovered in 1967 in Germany and Yugoslavia. African green monkeys originating from Uganda were determined to be the source animals that infected laboratory workers. Thirty-two cases were reported, with a 23% mortality rate. The Ebola virus, whose genome is remarkably homologous with the Marburg virus, was first identified in 1976 in Zaire and Sudan when simultaneous outbreaks occurred. In part because of poor infection control practices, the human impact was devastating, with rapid spread to patients, family members, and health care workers. The Ebola-Zaire outbreak involved 318 patients with an 88% mortality rate, and the Ebola-Sudan outbreak affected 284 people with a 53% mortality rate.[5] During the past quarter of a century, there have been numerous outbreaks of Ebola. Different strains of the virus have been identified, and several have been named according to the location of the outbreak.

The filoviruses are enveloped, negative-sense ribonucleic acid (RNA) viruses. They are generally grouped into "Marburg-like" or "Ebola-like" families. Several strains have been characterized in the Ebola family, including Ebola-Zaire, Ebola-Sudan, Ebola-Reston, and Ebola-Cote d'Ivoire. Microscopically, these viruses appear as thread-like filaments that have linear, circular, and U-shaped forms. Fig. 144-1 is an electron micrograph of the Ebola virus. Each of the viral genomes encodes nine protein products. Some demonstrate immuno-modulatory properties, and others cause vascular cell toxicity.[6] Various types of bats are considered to be the natural host of the Ebola and possibly Marburg viruses. Studies evaluating bats have shown that the virus may be harbored in reservoir animals in various parts of the world, including Africa and Asia.[7,8]

The Ebola and Marburg viruses produce similar clinical syndromes. Current epidemiologic evidence suggests that these viruses are spread through direct contact with blood, secretions, or infected tissues. The viruses may also be transmitted via mucosal contact; thus there is risk of human hand-to-mouth or conjunctiva spread. Although there is no conclusive documented evidence, several human and animal cases have raised some concern about airborne spread of the virus via droplet nuclei.[4,9] Ebola and Marburg viruses are relatively stable and may retain infectivity for some time at room temperature when exposed to the environment. Previous biological weapons programs have also succeeded in aerosolizing these viruses and proving aerosol transmission in animal models.[5] The incubation periods are 2 to 21 days for Ebola and 3 to 10 days for Marburg. Because of the possibly prolonged asymptomatic incubation period, the danger of delayed recognition and possible continued dissemination of disease exists. Initial clinical symptoms may include myalgia and arthralgia, fever, nausea and vomiting, abdominal pain, and a rash (petechiae, purpura, and ecchymosis) spreading distally from the trunk. As the hemorrhagic fever progresses, oliguria, hematemesis, melena, pericarditis, encephalitis, acute renal failure, and shock may occur. In severe cases the victim succumbs to disseminated intravascular coagulation.[4,5,10] The classic dermatologic manifestations are quite common as patients generally exhibit a maculopapular rash within 5 days of onset of illness. Although petechiae may be initially apparent, larger patchy lesions generally form and progress to confluent regions. Desquamation may occur and may be the first skin lesion noted in non-Caucasian individuals. Victims may also complain of burning and paresthesia over areas of their skin.

The other classic manifestation of viral hemorrhagic fever is bleeding. More than 70% of infected, symptomatic patients suffer from bleeding diatheses. Bleeding may be pronounced and present as melena, epistaxis, hematemesis, hemoptysis, bleeding gums, or puncture sites. The rate of bleeding complication does not appear to differ between survivors and nonsurvivors.[5] Individuals who survive acute viral hemorrhagic fever may be left with long-term sequelae, including arthralgia, uveitis, orchitis, and hearing loss. The virus has been isolated from the urine and seminal fluid of patients who were recovering from the disease up to 3 months after the onset of acute disease.[11]

Specific polymerase chain reaction (PCR) or antibody studies are required to identify infection. These tests are generally only available at specialized laboratories. Reverse transcription-PCR (RT-PCR) has been demonstrated to be effective in the rapid diagnosis of the Ebola virus. Studies have also shown a correlation between disease severity

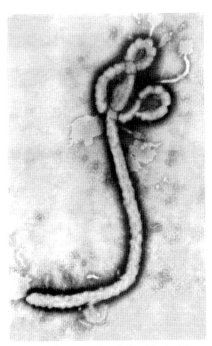

FIG 144-1 Electron Micrograph of the Ebola Virus. (Courtesy of Frederick A. Murphy, University of Texas Medical Branch, Galveston, Tex.)

and higher RNA copy levels.[12] The PCR technique has also been used with success in field settings during African Ebola outbreaks using TaqMan-RT-PCR on a portable SmartCycler.[13] The techniques of viral growth in tissue culture followed by electron microscopy and enzyme-linked immunosorbent assay (ELISA) testing have also been used to identify filovirus infection.[14] Immunohistochemical staining of skin biopsies may also prove to be an effective method for identifying infection.[15]

PRE-INCIDENT ACTIONS

As with any disaster or possible bioterrorism attack, hospitals and emergency departments should have preexisting disaster plans in place that are rehearsed before an event. In suspected cases of filovirus infection or terrorist attack, coordination of local, state, and federal agencies are required to diagnose and manage the incident. Notably, state departments of public health, the CDC, and the U.S. Army Medical Research Institute of Infectious Diseases (USAMRIID) need to be involved early in the process of identification and treatment. As always, universal precautions must be practiced. Health care workers must maintain a high level of vigilance when patients present in clusters with febrile illnesses. This vigilance must be even greater if a patient reports recent travel to an area endemic with viral hemorrhagic fever or if there is a report of a recent outbreak. In the event of suspected cases of filovirus infection, facilities must be prepared for proper isolation of the patient, bodily fluids, and specimens. Protective gowns, gloves, high-efficiency particulate air (HEPA) face masks, and eye protection should be used by clinical and laboratory personnel because of the theoretical risk of aerosol transmission.

POST-INCIDENT ACTIONS

Levels of suspicion for filovirus infection should be high when patients present with the aforementioned signs and symptoms, particularly when there are reports of recent cases or a terrorist attack with viral agents. When there is a high level of suspicion of a filovirus terrorist attack, state and federal authorities must be notified at once. If there are a limited number of patients, consideration should be given to transferring patients to dedicated Biosafety Level 4 facilities, namely the CDC in Atlanta or the USAMRIID in Fort Detrick, Maryland. In cases of suspected Ebola or Marburg infection, blood and bodily fluid samples must be handled with extreme caution. No material should be forwarded to the CDC or USAMRIID without prior consultation and arrangement. If a filovirus aerosol attack occurred, victims would begin presenting with illness about 1 week later; at this point, virtually no infectious virus should remain viable in the environment. Patients or staff contaminated with liquids or materials possibly containing a filovirus should be decontaminated via a vigorous hot shower with soap and water. Surfaces or items that may be contaminated should be sterilized with a dilute bleach solution or standard hospital quaternary ammonium or phenol disinfectants. Steam sterilization, where applicable, is the most effective method for inactivating filoviruses.[14]

If a significant event begins to evolve, consideration may be given to quarantine practices. In general, logistical, legal, and functional issues make frank quarantine likely to be an ineffective and impractical choice. Other less drastic measures, such as isolation, are likely to be used first and enjoy more success.[16]

MEDICAL TREATMENT OF CASUALTIES

Unfortunately, treatment for victims of filovirus hemorrhagic fever is largely supportive. As victims progress to disseminated intravascular coagulation and septic shock, usual treatment with blood, clotting products, and vasopressor medications should be instituted. Conventional antiviral agents such as ribavirin have not been shown to have any significant clinical benefit in either in vitro or in vivo studies. Interferon-alpha (INF-α) has shown some success in suppressing filovirus replication in cell culture and some promise in protecting Ebola-infected mice from the illness.[14] Attempts have been made to treat patients by passive immunization through the use of the convalescent blood and serum from recovered filovirus patients. After the transfer of immunoglobulin-G (IgG) Ebola antibodies to infected patients, a lower mortality rate was observed. However, there were a small number of patients in these studies, and questions have arisen about other confounders in their care.[17] Purified IgG from horses hyperimmunized with Ebola-Zaire was shown to protect baboons and guinea pigs from disease when given to them shortly after virus challenge.[18] Treatment with the anticoagulant rNAPc2 has shown some encouragement in the treatment of Ebola-infected monkeys.[2]

A concerted effort to develop an Ebola vaccine is under way. Ebola-related deoxyribonucleic acid, liposome-encapsulated irradiated Ebola virus, and Ebola protein segments are all being studied for possible use as vaccines. Ebola virus–like particles, when injected into mice, allowed the animals to develop Ebola-specific antibodies and conferred protection from the lethal virus.[19]

Protection of health care providers in both austere and tertiary settings is of utmost importance. A 2001 experience in Canada exemplifies a well-executed contingency plan for a patient found to be infected with a viral hemorrhagic fever. Through enhanced isolation precautions, contact tracing, laboratory work, and communication, an effective and feasible plan was carried out at a tertiary center.[20] The CDC has issued the *Interim Guidance for Managing Patients with Suspected Viral Hemorrhagic Fever in U.S. Hospitals* in which they address all aspects of care ranging from infection control to specimen handling to handling of remains.[21]

💡 UNIQUE CONSIDERATIONS

The filoviruses have the potential to be used as devastating biological weapons. Their high level of virulence and equally impressive mortality rate make them a tempting target for any terrorist organization wishing to obtain a weapon of mass destruction. Initial identification of a viral hemorrhagic fever attack will be difficult given the week-long incubation period and nonspecific signs and symptoms in the initial phase of disease. The high risk of transmission to health care providers is another factor that makes this threat even more ominous.

❗ PITFALLS

- Failure of health care personnel to recognize the nonspecific signs and symptoms of viral hemorrhagic fever, leading to delayed institution of containment procedures
- Delayed reporting of possible cases of viral hemorrhagic fever to state and federal officials, leading to delay in appropriate diagnostic procedures and isolation of materials and patients
- Failure to practice simple universal precautions, leading to uncontrolled spread of the viral agent
- General public fear and reaction over release of information regarding possible cases of viral hemorrhagic fever

REFERENCES

1. Rotz LD, Khan AS, Lillibridge SR, et al. Public health assessment of potential biological terrorism agents. *Emerg Infect Dis.* 2002;8(2):225–230.
2. Kagan E. Update on Ebola virus and its potential as a bioterrorism agent. *Clin Pulm Med.* 2005;12(2):76–83.
3. Kaplan D. Aum Shinrikyo. In: Tucker J, ed. *Toxic Terror: Assessing Terrorist Use of Chemical and Biological Weapons.* Cambridge, MA: MIT Press; 2000:207–226.
4. Borio L, Inglesby T, Peters CJ, et al. Hemorrhagic fever viruses as biological weapons: medical and public health management. *JAMA.* 2002;287(18):2391–2405.
5. Salvaggio MR, Baddley JW. Other viral bioweapons: Ebola and Marburg hemorrhagic fever. *Dermatol Clin.* 2004;22(3):291–302 (review).
6. Takada A, Kawaoka Y. The pathogenesis of Ebola hemorrhagic fever. *Trends Microbiol.* 2001;9(10):506–511.
7. Olival KJ, Islam A, Yu M, et al. Ebola virus antibodies in fruit bats, Bangladesh. *Emerg Infect Dis.* 2013;19(2):270–273.
8. Leroy EM, Kumulungui B, Pourrut X, et al. Fruit bats as reservoirs of Ebola virus. *Nature.* 2005;438:575–576.
9. Francesconi P, Yoti Z, Declich S, et al. Ebola hemorrhagic fever transmission and risk factors of contacts, Uganda. *Emerg Infect Dis.* 2003;9(11):1430–1437.
10. Easter A. Ebola. *Am J Nurs.* 2002;102(12):49–52.
11. Rowe AK, Bertolli J, Khan AS, et al. Clinical, virologic, and immunologic follow-up of convalescent Ebola hemorrhagic fever patients and their household contacts, Kikwit, Democratic Republic of Congo. *J Infect Dis.* 1999;179(Suppl 1):S28–S35.
12. Towner JS, Rollin PE, Bausch DG, et al. Rapid diagnosis of Ebola hemorrhagic fever by reverse transcription-PCR in an outbreak setting and assessment of patient viral load as a predictor of outcome. *J Virol.* 2004;78(8):4330–4341.
13. Weidmann M, Muhlberger E, Hufert FT. Rapid detection protocol for filoviruses. *J Clin Virol.* 2004;30:94–99.
14. Bray M. Defense against filoviruses used as biological weapons. *Antiviral Res.* 2003;57(1–2):53–60 (review).
15. Zaki SR, Shieh WJ, Greer PW, et al. A novel immunohistochemical assay for the detection of Ebola virus in skin: implications for diagnosis, spread, and surveillance of Ebola hemorrhagic fever. *J Infect Dis.* 1999;179(Suppl 1):S36–S47.
16. Barbera J, Macintyre A, Gostin L, et al. Large-scale quarantine following biological terrorism in the United States: scientific examination, logistic and legal limits, and possible consequences. *JAMA.* 2001;286:2711–2717.
17. Mupapa K, Massamba M, Kibadi K, et al. Treatment of Ebola hemorrhagic fever with blood transfusions from convalescent patients. *J Infect Dis.* 1999;179(Suppl 1):S18–S23.
18. Jahrling PB, Geisbert J, Swearengen JR, et al. Passive immunization of Ebola virus-infected cynomolgus monkeys with immunoglobulin from hyperimmune horses. *Arch Virol Suppl.* 1996;11:135–140.
19. Warfield KL, Bosio CM, Welcher BC, et al. Ebola virus-like particles protect from lethal Ebola virus infection. *Proc Natl Acad Sci U S A.* 2003;100(26):15889–15894.
20. Loeb M, MacPherson D, Barton M, et al. Implementation of the Canadian Contingency Plan for a case of suspected viral hemorrhagic fever. *Infect Control Hosp Epidemiol.* 2003;24(4):280–284.
21. CDC. Policy Statement, May 2005—Interim Guidance for Managing Patients with Suspected Viral Hemorrhagic Fever in U.S. Hospitals. US Centers for Disease Control and Prevention.

CHAPTER 145

Viral Hemorrhagic Fever Attack: Flaviviruses

Valarie Schwind

The viruses causing viral hemorrhagic fevers are classified into four separate families. One of the four families, flaviviruses, contains more than 60 species, 30 of which are known to cause human disease.[1] Flaviviruses are similar in structure, in that they are all enveloped, and have positive sense, single-stranded RNA that measures about 40 to 60 nm in diameter. Flaviviruses are easily transmitted in nature via arthropods, including ticks and mosquitos, from a natural mammalian reservoir.[2] This chapter will focus on five flaviviruses: yellow fever, Kyasanur Forest disease, Omsk hemorrhagic fever, Alkhurma hemorrhagic fever, and dengue fever. Each of these viruses is known to cause a syndrome of fever and concomitant bleeding diathesis. The Flavivirus family also contains many other viruses that can cause encephalitis, such as West Nile disease,[1] but these will not be discussed in this chapter.

Flaviviruses vary naturally in how they present, and case severity can range from mild to deadly. Clinically, most of the Flavivirus infections begin with fever and flu-like symptoms. Symptoms can progress, however, to a variety of bleeding diatheses, including petechiae, epistaxis, hemoptysis, hematemesis, melena, hematochezia, and hematuria. Vital signs may reveal hypotension with a relative bradycardia. Laboratory studies may show leukopenia, thrombocytopenia, elevated liver function tests, or abnormal coagulation studies. Death is usually the result of hypovolemic shock and organ failure.[3,4] Classically, Flavivirus-infected patients have a biphasic presentation, where the patient appears to recover from the flu-like stage of illness before the onset of the more severe symptoms. Illnesses that present similarly include influenza, hepatitis, gram-negative sepsis, meningococcemia, toxic shock syndrome, rickettsial infections, leptospirosis, typhoid fever, Q fever, malaria, collagen vascular diseases, acute leukemia, and platelet disorders.

Flaviviruses have a few important characteristics that make them a potential threat for use as a bioterrorism agent. First, the viruses can produce significant morbidity and mortality. Second, flaviviruses are also easily obtainable in nature and have already proven to be sustainable in a natural environment. Third, although no cases of person-to-person transmission have been reported, the viruses generally have low infective doses and could easily cause widespread illness if released into a population, if the virus was manipulated for aerosol dissemination. Lastly, there are currently no vaccines available for the flaviviruses.[3] Indeed, for these reasons, many of these viruses have been studied previously by multiple countries as potential bioterrorism agents. In fact, yellow fever was developed by the United States as a biological weapon until the program's cessation in the late 1960s.[5]

YELLOW FEVER

Endemic to sub-Saharan African countries and northern South America, yellow fever was first discovered in the 1600s.[1] Its usual mode of transmission occurs through the vector of Aedes and Haemagogus mosquitos, who bite infected monkeys and then transmit the virus to humans. The incubation period of yellow fever is usually 3 to 6 days, after which symptoms of fever, malaise, headache, photophobia, nausea, vomiting, and irritability may occur. Physical examination may reveal a febrile, toxic appearing patient who may be bradycardic relative to the high fever. The patient may also likely have hyperemic skin, injected conjunctiva, coated tongue, and epigastric/hepatic tenderness. After 3 to 5 days, the patient either recovers or enters the next stage of disease wherein the virus causes extensive hepatic injury and jaundice (thus the name *yellow fever*) after a typical 48-hour remission. At this point, hemorrhagic diathesis such as epistaxis, oozing at the gums, petechiae, ecchymosis, hematemesis, melena, hematuria, thrombocytopenia, and disseminated intravascular coagulation may occur. Myocarditis, encephalopathy, and shock may also ensue.[1,6,7] Yellow fever is the most deadly of Flaviviridae family, and, if untreated, the case fatality rate is 20%.[3,7]

In the tropics, diagnosis of yellow fever is usually clinical. Liver biopsy may provide further evidence of infection with characteristic pathological changes of Councilman bodies and midzonal necrosis; however, biopsy results are neither sensitive nor specific for the disease and should be used in conjunction with clinical findings. Given that these patients are also usually coagulopathic, liver biopsies may also lead to massive hemorrhage. In developed nations or larger hospitals, definitive diagnosis can be made by viral cultures, polymerase chain reaction (PCR) tests, or by enzyme-linked immunosorbent assay (ELISA) tests that identify immunoglobulin M (IgM) rise during acute infection or later immunoglobulin G (IgG) presence showing exposure to the disease.

KYASANUR FOREST DISEASE

This disease was first isolated in 1957 from a sick monkey in Karnataka, India. Since the discovery of the virus, there have been reportedly approximately 400 to 500 human cases per year. Similar to the other viruses discussed herein, patients exhibit an incubation period of 3 to 12 days before symptoms present. Initial symptoms include a severe febrile illness with headache, photophobia, myalgia, upper respiratory symptoms, vomiting, and diarrhea. Physical examination findings include fever with relative bradycardia (Faget sign), hypotension, facial erythema, conjunctivitis, palatal vesicles, lymphadenopathy, hepatosplenomegaly, as well as bleeding diatheses such as petechiae, epistaxis, hematemesis, hemoptysis, melena, and hematochezia. Patients might develop pulmonary edema, renal failure, or hepatic failure. Intermittent improvement might be seen, but between 20% and 50% of patients will progress to a second stage of illness, which can present with symptoms of encephalitis.[8]

Initial laboratory tests for Kyasanur Forest disease are nonspecific. Patients may appear hemoconcentrated while leukopenic and thrombocytopenic initially, and may have elevated renal and liver function tests in later stages. There are specific IgG and IgM tests available; however, this can sometimes be complicated with cross reactivity with other illnesses that can lead to false positives. The virus can be isolated from the blood in the first 12 days of illness.

OMSK HEMORRHAGIC FEVER VIRUS

Omsk hemorrhagic fever virus (OHFV) is a lesser-studied flavivirus found in central Russia. There are only about 100 to 200 cases annually in the endemic area. This virus is naturally harbored in small rodents and is spread to humans via *Dermacentor* spp. tick bites or from contact with rodent blood or excrement. There have been no reported cases of human-to-human transmission. OHFV presents similarly to Kyasanur Forest disease with an incubation period of 6 to 14 days, although it appears to be less virulent. Fewer patients progress toward the hemorrhagic complications of the disease, and thus the mortality is markedly lower than that of other flaviviruses, at around 0.5% to 3%. Detection of these viruses can be achieved by using ELISA and PCR methods similar to the other flaviviruses. Treatment is supportive. Vaccines for related tick-borne flaviviruses developed in Europe have shown some cross protection against OHFV.[9]

ALKHURMA HEMORRHAGIC FEVER VIRUS

Alkhurma hemorrhagic fever virus (AHFV) is a member of the Flavivirus family that emerged in Saudi Arabia in the 1990s. It is believed to be a genetic variant of the Kyasanur Forest disease virus. It is believed to be spread by soft tick bites, although the mammalian reservoir remains unknown. Endemically, risk factors include working with livestock or butchering livestock. Symptoms are very similar to that of the previously discussed hemorrhagic fevers, and treatment again is mostly supportive. Reportedly, case fatality rates are as high as 30%, but this may be an overestimation, because it is thought there is gross underreporting of less severe illness. This virus can be isolated and detected using PCR and ELISA methods.[10]

DENGUE FEVER

Dengue fever is probably the most widespread disease caused by the flaviviruses, with nearly 50 million cases reported yearly. Dengue is spread by the *Aedes aegypti* mosquito and is endemic in most tropical parts of the world. More than 50% of U.S. states reported cases in 2010; however, most of cases of dengue in the United States are actually in people who are returning from travel to endemic countries. A few native cases, however, have been reported in Texas, Hawaii, and Florida. Dengue fever has an incubation period that is typically 4 to 7 days. Patients then begin to develop high fevers, headache, classic retro-orbital pain, myalgias, and arthralgia. These last symptoms are usually so severe that the disease has been nicknamed break bone fever. A maculopapular rash that may coalesce develops, and it has been described as "islands of white on a sea of red." Patients may also have

mild respiratory or gastrointestinal (GI) symptoms. Occasionally a petechial or puerperal rash may develop, and patients may exhibit, conjunctivitis, epistaxis, or other mild mucosal bleeding.[11]

About 3% of patients progress to dengue shock syndrome (DSS). This usually happens after 4 to 7 days of illness. This syndrome is characterized by a rise in hematocrit of 20% and thrombocytopenia. Severe plasma leakage occurs, and patients may develop pleural or cardiac effusions, ascites, peripheral edema, and bleeding diatheses, resulting in circulatory collapse and end organ failure, which usually leads to death.[11]

Diagnosis is usually made clinically. The "tourniquet test" may be performed to pick up hemorrhagic manifestations. To perform this, inflate a blood pressure cuff on the person's upper arm to a pressure half-way between measured systolic and diastolic blood pressures. If after left inflated for 5 minutes, more than 20 individual petechial hemorrhages per square inch on the forearm are counted, then the patient is thought to have a propensity for hemorrhagic complications. ELISA testing for IgG and IgM may confirm the diagnosis. When treated, classic dengue fever is rarely fatal. However, if dengue has progressed to DSS and it is left untreated, the mortality approaches 20%. If resuscitative efforts are started early, the mortality can be reduced to less than 1%.[11]

◀◀ PRE-INCIDENT ACTIONS

Hemorrhagic viral illnesses are rarely seen in the United States, so if multiple cases are seen then bioterrorism must be considered as a possible cause. The viral hemorrhagic fevers can be difficult to diagnose because their initial presentation can be so similar to that of many diseases that are more common. Providers must maintain vigilance for abnormal patterns of illness that could be caused by the viral hemorrhagic fevers, such as increased incidence of severe febrile illness or multiple patients without bleeding diatheses especially in "non-flu" months. Hospitals should have disaster plans in place that are capable of managing increased patient volumes while providing for appropriate isolation, as well as an increased need for blood products and resuscitative supplies. In all cases of suspected viral hemorrhagic fever, the local and state health authorities, as well as the Centers for Disease Control and Prevention (CDC), should be notified early so that the specific disease can be diagnosed and an appropriate epidemiological investigation conducted. If available, it may be necessary to distribute a vaccine (yellow fever). It should be noted that in a bioterror situation, the severity and grotesque manifestations of these diseases have the potential to induce mass anxiety, cause psychological stress, and cripple economic infrastructure.

▶▶ POST-INCIDENT ACTIONS

Once an outbreak has been identified, it is important that government organizations be notified immediately. Viral hemorrhagic fevers may be difficult to detect, but if they are suspected, patients should be isolated. Proper isolation precautions include masks, gowns, gloves, and eye protection. Although the diseases are not spread by the airborne route, the use of a negative pressure room and respirators by caregivers is generally recommended. The patients' contacts since the exposure or for 2 weeks before disease presentation should be carefully monitored by public health authorities for signs of fever or bleeding diathesis for 21 days. If symptoms develop, those contacts must also be isolated. After 21 days of monitoring, if no symptoms develop, surveillance may be discontinued.

✚ MEDICAL TREATMENT OF CASUALTIES

Treatment for all diseases caused by the Flavivirus family is mostly supportive. Patients will need fever control, fluid resuscitation, electrolyte management, antiemetics, blood products, and likely vasopressor support. Drugs that suppress the immune system should be avoided, as should anticoagulants. Ribavirin may be started while diagnostic tests are pending, but because there has been little evidence that shows ribavirin is an effective treatment against flaviviruses and once diagnosis of any flavivirus is made, it should be discontinued.[3,12]

In the case of yellow fever, a vaccine is available that has been shown to offer immunity within a few days of administration. Stockpiles of the vaccine should be mobilized and given to patients showing signs of the disease, as well as to healthy exposed individuals. It is administered in 0.5 mL increments subcutaneously. Immunity lasts for 10 years. A vaccine exists for Kyasanur Forest disease, but it is not readily available in the United States. Omsk hemorrhagic fever does not have a vaccine, but cross immunity is thought to be obtained from vaccines formulated for other tick-borne illnesses in Eastern Europe.[9]

❓ UNIQUE CONSIDERATIONS

Flaviviruses are rarely spread from person to person. Vector and waste-product control and destruction are key in controlling an outbreak. Treatment is largely supportive, and vaccines are available for some of these diseases. Early detection can determine the severity and mortality of a biological terror attack, so frontline providers must always keep viral hemorrhagic fevers in their differential.

❗ PITFALLS

- Failure to keep viral hemorrhagic fever in the clinical differential for appropriate patients
- Failure to obtain a travel history for febrile patients
- Failure to make correct clinical diagnosis
- Failure to report suspected cases to public and governmental agencies for epidemiological and surveillance purposes

REFERENCES

1. Mandell G, Bennett J, Dolin R. Flaviviruses (yellow fever, dengue, dengue hemorrhagic fever, Japanese encephalitis, West Nile encephalitis, St. Louis encephalitis, tick-borne encephalitis). In: *Mandell, Douglas, and Bennett's Principles and Practice of Infectious Diseases 7th ed.* Philidelphia, PA: Churchill, Livingstone Elsevier; 2010: 2133-2156.
2. Bray M. Pathonegesis of viral hemorrhagic fever. *Curr Opin Immunol.* 2005;17:399–403.
3. Borio L, Inglesby T, Peters CJ, et al. Hemorrhagic fever viruses as biological weapons: medical and public health management. *JAMA.* 2002;287 (18):2391–2405.
4. Bausch D. Viral Hemorrhagic Fevers. In: *Cecil Medicine.* Philadelphia, PA: Elsevier Saunders; 2012:2147–2156.
5. Mandell G, Bennett J, Dolin R. Viral hemorrhagic fevers as agents of bioterrorism. In: *Mandell, Douglas, and Bennett's Principles and Practice of Infectious Diseases 7th ed.* Philidelphia, PA: Churchill Livingstone Elsevier; 2010: 3995–3998.
6. Paessler S, Walker DH. Pathogenesis of the viral hemorrhagic fevers. *Annu Rev Path Mech Dis.* 2013;8:411–440.
7. Ferri FF. Yellow fever. In: *Ferri's Clinical Advisor.* Philadelphia, PA: Elsevier Mosby; 2014:1185e2–1185e3.
8. Holbrook MR. Kyasanur Forest disease. *Antiviral Res.* 2012;96 (3):355–362.
9. Mandl C, Holbrook M. Tick borne encephalitis and omsk hemorrhagic fever. In: *Tropical Infectious Diseases: Principles, Pathogens and Practice.* Philadelphia, PA: Elsevier Saunders; 2011:505–518.
10. Memish ZA, Charrel RN, Zaki AM, Fagbo SF. Alkhurma haemorrhagic fever—a viral haemorrhagic disease unique to the Arabian peninsula. *Int J Antimicrob Agents.* 2010;36:553–557.
11. Ferri FF. Dengue fever. In: *Ferri's Clinical Advisor.* Philadelphia, PA: Elsevier Mosby; 2014:323e2–323e4.
12. Kman NE, Nelson RN. Infectious agents of bioterrorism: a review for emergency physicians. *Emerg Med Clin North Am.* 2008;26:517–547.

Chikungunya Virus Attack

Stephen P. Wood and Heather Long

DESCRIPTION OF EVENT

Chikungunya (CHIK) virus is an alphavirus-borne enzootic infection carried primarily by the *Aedes* mosquito.[1] The word *chikungunya* is from the Makone word *Kun qunwala*, meaning "that which bends up,"[1] and describes the contortions and contractions that can occur with this disease. The virus was first isolated in 1952 in a febrile patient during an outbreak of febrile illness on the Makinde plateau in Tanzania.[2]

The virus is endemic to many tropical and subtropical regions throughout the world, including sub-Saharan Africa, Southeast Asia, India, and the western Pacific. In the past several years, with a surge in 2014, chikungunya became endemic in the Caribbean, with many cases seen in Haiti, the Dominican Republic, and elsewhere in the region.[1] The most common route of transmission is vector-borne via mosquito to humans.[3] There has been no evidence of person-to-person transmission documented to date. CHIK virus, however, can be aerosolized, and there are case reports of laboratory workers having been infected while working with the virus.[4-7]

As an agent of biological terrorism, CHIK virus would most likely be dispersed as an aerosol or by the coordinated release of infected mosquitoes.[8] In the event of a CHIK virus attack, a large percentage of the exposed population could be expected to become ill after an incubation period of 2 to 10 days.[4] Illness associated with the CHIK virus is generally self-limited and short-lived; however, it may be temporarily debilitating, and a large number of affected patients would be expected to seek care for fever and severe arthralgias.[1-4]

Infection with the CHIK virus is characterized by a triad of fever, maculopapular rash, and arthralgia.[9] Nausea, headache, vomiting, and myalgia are also common. Sudden onset of fever is characteristically the first symptom to appear after the incubation period.[4] Arthralgia is the most prominent symptom. The severity of the illness ranges from mild weakness and stiffness to excruciating pain. The pain is typically symmetric and involves multiple joints. Previously injured joints, as well as fingers, wrists, elbows, toes, ankles, and knees, are most commonly affected.[8] Joints may appear swollen and are generally tender to palpation. The frequency and severity of symptoms are generally more mild in children. Complete resolution of all symptoms occurs in most patients after 2 to 5 days; however, about 12% of patients will have a persistent arthropathy that may last months to years.[7] Persistent arthropathy is generally associated with higher titers of CHIK virus antibodies.[7]

Although not classified as a hemorrhagic virus, hemorrhagic forms of the disease that mimic dengue fever and yellow fever have been reported.[10,11] In some outbreaks of CHIK virus infection, up to 10% of patients have been noted to have mild hemorrhage, including petechiae, epistaxis, and bleeding gums. Cases of myocarditis and cardiomyopathy after CHIK virus infection have also been reported.[12,13] Rare deaths among the elderly and children have been associated with CHIK virus outbreaks, and the CHIK virus was isolated from one Sri Lankan child who died.[14,15]

Diagnosis of the chikungunya virus is either by polymerase chain reaction (PCR) or by identification of virus-specific immunoglobulin G (IgG) and/or immunoglobulin M (IgM), which are apparent within 3 to 6 days of disease onset.[16]

PRE-INCIDENT ACTIONS

Prehospital services, hospitals, and local and state health departments should have implemented preparedness programs for bioterrorism and mass casualty events. Recognition of a CHIK virus event would require familiarity with the agent as well as a high degree of clinical suspicion. Maintaining a high level of alertness to abnormal patterns is critical to the recognition of any covert bioterrorist attack. Automated biosurveillance systems, which aggregate data from multiple medical care sites (such as emergency departments or community health centers) and/or laboratories, may also play a role in the early identification of unusual outbreaks of illness.

No current vaccine is available, but several trials have shown potential for the development of a useful vaccine. Low antigenic variation and lifelong protection after exposure to the native virus make the development of a vaccine promising.[17]

POST-INCIDENT ACTIONS

All suspected cases of CHIK virus infection should be reported to local and state health departments, who would then notify the CDC. Local infection control professionals and laboratory personnel should be notified immediately. Biosafety Level 3 practices should be maintained in handling specimens. If CHIK virus infection is suspected, 10 to 12 mL of serum from the affected patient(s) should be shipped cold or on dry ice in a plastic tube to the appropriate laboratory. Public health authorities, in conjunction with the CDC, should aid clinicians in preparing specimens for transport to a reference laboratory. (See "Packaging Protocols for Biological Agents/Diseases" at http://www.bt.cdc.gov/Agent/VHF/VHF.asp.) Laboratory personnel must be alerted to the possibility of small-particle aerosol generation to minimize their risk of infection. With prior notice, the CDC can offer a preliminary laboratory diagnosis after approximately 1 working day.[18]

MEDICAL TREATMENT OF CASUALTIES

The only available treatment for chikungunya virus infection is nonsteroidal antiinflammatory drugs (NSAIDs), in conjunction with usual supportive care.[1,19] No specific NSAID or dosing regimen has been identified as recommended, although there is some evidence that the combination of an NSAID with steroids is superior to NSAIDs alone.[19] Ribavarin and chloroquine have been suggested as possible therapeutic agents, although small trials have shown little to no benefit.[20-22] Because most cases are self-limited, supportive care along with analgesia is the only specific therapy that is required.

❓ UNIQUE CONSIDERATIONS

The CHIK virus is highly infectious; therefore a large percentage of people exposed to the agent would be expected to become ill. Illness with the CHIK virus is short-lived but temporarily debilitating and not considered lethal. Because there is no animal reservoir for the virus in Western countries and no person-to-person transmission, it is seen as a "clean" biological weapon that may be a desirable agent for use against a civilian site.[8]

❗ PITFALLS

- Failure to consider a CHIK virus infection or attack in patients presenting with the nonspecific symptoms of fever, rash, and arthralgia
- Failure to suspect CHIK virus in travelers returning from the Caribbean[23,24]
- Failure to alert laboratory personnel to the possibility of small-particle aerosolization in suspected cases
- Failure to notify local and/or state health departments of suspected cases

REFERENCES

1. Burt F, Rolph M, Rulli N, Mahalingham S, Heise M. Chikungunya: a re-emerging virus. *Lancet.* 2012;379:662–671.
2. Robinson MC. An epidemic of virus disease in Southern Province, Tanganyika territory, in 1952–1953. *Trans R Soc Trop Med Hyg.* 1955;49 (1):28–32.
3. Reller M, Akorada U, Nagahawatte A, et al. Chikungunya as a cause of acute febrile illness in southern Sri Lanka. *PLoS One.* 2013;8(12):e82259.
4. Tesh RB. Arthritides caused by mosquito-borne viruses. *Ann Rev Med.* 1982;33:31–40.
5. Shah KV, Baron S. Laboratory infection with chikungunya virus: a case report. *Indian J Med Res.* 1965;53:610–613.
6. Banerjee K, Gupta NP, Goverdhan MK. Viral infections in laboratory personnel. *Indian J Med Res.* 1979;69:363–373.
7. Ramachandra RJ, Singh KRP, Pavri KM. Laboratory transmission of an Indian strain of chikungunya virus. *Current Sci.* 1964;33:235–236.
8. CBWInfo. Factsheets on chemical and biological warfare. Chikungunya fever: essential data. Available at: http://www.cbwinfo.com/Biological/Pathogens/CHIK.html.
9. Brighton SW, Prozesky OW, de la Harpe AL. Chikungunya virus infection. A retrospective study of 107 cases. *S Afr Med J.* 1983;63:313–315.
10. Hammon WM, Rudnick A, Sather GE. Viruses associated with epidemic hemorrhagic fevers of the Philippines and Thailand. *Science.* 1960;131:1102–1103.
11. Sarkar JK, Chatterjee SN, Chakravarti SK, et al. Chikungunya virus infection with haemorrhagic manifestations. *Indian J Med Res.* 1965;53:921–925.
12. Maiti CR, Mukherjee AK, Bose B, et al. Myopericarditis following chikungunya virus infection. *J Indian Med Assoc.* 1978;70:256–258.
13. Obeyesekere I, Hermon Y. Myocarditis and cardiomyopathy after arbovirus infections (dengue and chikungunya fever). *Br Heart J.* 1972;34:821–827.
14. Rao AR. An epidemic of fever in Madras—1964: a clinical study of 4,223 cases at the Infectious Diseases Hospital. *Indian J Med Res.* 1965;53:745–753.
15. Hermon YE. Virological investigations of arbovirus infections in Ceylon, with special reference to the recent chikungunya fever epidemic. *Ceylon Med J.* 1967;12:81–92.
16. Litzbaa N, Schuffeneckerb I, Zeller H, et al. Evaluation of the first commercial chikungunya virus indirect immunofluorescence test. *J Virol Methods.* 2008;175–179.
17. Edelman R, Tacket CO, Wasserman SS, et al. Phase II safety and immunogenicity study of live chikungunya virus vaccine TSI- GSD-218. *Am J Trop Med Hyg.* 2000;62:681–685.
18. Borio L, Inglesby T, Peters CJ, et al. Hemorrhagic fever viruses as biological weapons: medical and public health management. *JAMA.* 2002;287:2391–2405.
19. Suhrbier A, Jaffar-Bandjee MC, Gasque P. Arthritogenic alphaviruses—an overview. *Nat Rev Rheumatol.* 2012;8(7):420–429.
20. Ravichandran R, Manian M. Ribavirin therapy for chikungunya arthritis. *J Infect Dev Ctries.* 2008;2:140–142.
21. de Lamballerie X, Boisson V, Reynier JC, et al. On chikungunya acute infection and chloroquine treatment. *Vector Borne Zoonotic Dis.* 2008;8:837–839.
22. Briolant S, Garin D, Scaramozzino N, et al. In vitro inhibition of Chikungunya and Semliki Forest viruses replication by antiviral compounds: synergistic effect of interferon-alpha and ribavirin combination. *Antiviral Res.* 2004;61:111–117.
23. Anderson KB, Pureza V, Walker PF. Chikungunya: acute fever, rash and debilitating arthralgias in a returning traveler from Haiti. *J Travel Med.* 2014;21(6):418–420.
24. Requena-Mendez A, Garcia C, Aldasoro E, et al. Cases of chikungunya virus infection in travellers returning to Spain from Haiti or Dominican Republic, April-June 2014. *Euro Surveill.* 2014;19(28):20853.

Variola Major Virus (Smallpox) Attack

Robert G. Darling

DESCRIPTION OF EVENT

Smallpox might be responsible for more human deaths throughout history than any other known disease, with estimates that it has killed more than 100 million people since the beginning of recorded history.[1] Smallpox was declared eradicated in 1980 by the World Health Organization, and there have been no cases of smallpox anywhere in the world since 1978. By treaty, there are only two official repositories of smallpox in the world today: one repository is at the Russian State Research Center of Virology and Biotechnology in Novosibirsk, Russia, and the other is at the Centers for Disease Control and Prevention (CDC) in Atlanta, Georgia. A single case of smallpox should be presumed to be intentional unless it can be shown to be the result of a laboratory accident.

Terrorist use of variola as a biological weapon could occur under one of several different scenarios. The simplest method might involve obtaining an illicit sample of the virus from a clandestine stock and then exposing a number of unsuspecting victims. These unfortunate individuals would then go about their daily business and serve as vectors for further spread of the disease once they become contagious. This might not be the most efficient manner to spread the infection because most victims become quite ill as symptoms develop and are unlikely to remain ambulatory. The most efficient manner to infect a large number of people would involve the deliberate spread of a weaponized aerosol of the virus.

The incubation period of smallpox averages 12 days, with a range of 7 to 17 days following exposure. Clinical manifestations begin acutely with malaise, fevers, rigors, vomiting, headache, and backache, and 15% of patients develop delirium. Approximately 10% of light-skinned patients exhibit an erythematous rash during this phase. Two to three days later, an exanthem appears concomitantly with a discrete rash about the face, hands, and forearms.

After eruptions on the lower extremities, the rash spreads centrally to the trunk over the next week. Lesions quickly progress from macules to papules and eventually to pustular vesicles. Lesions are more abundant on the extremities and face, and this centrifugal distribution is an important diagnostic feature. In distinct contrast to varicella, lesions on various segments of the body remain generally synchronous in their stages of development. From 8 to 14 days after onset, the pustules form scabs that leave depressed depigmented scars upon healing. Although variola concentrations in the throat, conjunctiva, and urine diminish with time, the virus can be readily recovered from scabs throughout convalescence. Therefore, patients should be isolated and considered infectious until all scabs separate.

For the past century, two distinct types of smallpox were recognized. *Variola minor* was distinguished by milder systemic toxicity and more diminutive pox lesions; it caused 1% mortality in unvaccinated victims. However, the prototypical disease, *variola major*, caused mortality of 3% and 30% in the vaccinated and unvaccinated populations, respectively.[2]

Smallpox must be distinguished from other vesicular exanthems, such as chickenpox, erythema multiforme with bullae, or allergic contact dermatitis. Particularly problematic to infection control measures would be the failure to recognize relatively mild cases of smallpox in persons with partial immunity. An additional threat to effective quarantine is that exposed persons may shed virus from the oropharynx without ever manifesting disease. Therefore, quarantine and initiation of medical countermeasures should be promptly followed by an accurate diagnosis to avert panic.

The usual method of diagnosis is demonstration of characteristic virions on electron microscopy of vesicular scrapings. Under light microscopy, aggregations of variola virus particles, called Guarnieri bodies, are found. Another rapid but relatively insensitive test for Guarnieri bodies in vesicular scrapings is Gispen's modified silver stain, in which cytoplasmic inclusions appear black.

None of the aforementioned laboratory tests is capable of discriminating variola from vaccinia, monkeypox, or cowpox. This differentiation has classically required isolation of the virus and characterization of its growth on chorioallantoic membrane. The development of polymerase chain reaction diagnostic techniques promises a more accurate and less cumbersome method of discriminating between variola and other orthopoxviruses.[3]

PRE-INCIDENT ACTIONS

Pre-Event preparations should focus on first responder and medical and public health personnel education. This is particularly important for health care providers because an astute clinician will be far more likely to diagnose a first case of smallpox before any surveillance system would lead public health authorities to suspect there is an epidemic in the community. Rapid identification and vaccination of contacts will be the keys to controlling an outbreak of smallpox.

Ideally, all first responders and medical and public health personnel will be vaccinated against smallpox before an outbreak and will have extensively drilled their local smallpox response plans. However, efforts by the CDC in 2003 to vaccinate up to 500,000 volunteers were unsuccessful, largely because of concerns about the side effects of the vaccine and a general belief among the public that the threat of terrorist use of smallpox was low. To date the U.S. military has vaccinated more than 600,000 of its personnel, with a relatively low rate of complications.[4]

A well-developed, integrated "all-hazards" hospital disaster-response plan should be in place and tested regularly. It should include provisions to care for a rapid influx of large numbers of contagious patients. The local plan should be linked to other regional, state, and federal disaster plans.

POST-INCIDENT ACTIONS

A single case of smallpox should be treated as an international public health emergency. Hospital infection control and laboratory personnel; law enforcement authorities, including the Federal Bureau of Investigation; and local, state, and federal public health authorities, including the CDC, must be notified immediately. An epidemiological investigation to identify all of those potentially exposed must be initiated so that a postexposure vaccination effort can commence. With a mortality rate of 30% and high morbidity, the vaccination risk-benefit ratio shifts markedly in favor of vaccination, even for patients with contraindications to receiving the vaccine. Patients who have been exposed to a smallpox patient should be vaccinated as soon as possible, even up to 5 to 7 days after exposure because the disease may either be prevented or ameliorated.[5]

The smallpox vaccine, using vaccinia virus, is most often administered by intradermal inoculation with a bifurcated needle. The current smallpox vaccine is the ACAM2000 (Smallpox [Vaccinia] Vaccine, Live), which is a licensed product plaque purification cloning from Dryvax (Wyeth Laboratories, Marietta, Pennsylvania, calf lymph vaccine, NY City Board of Health Strain).[6] Primary and repeat vaccinees receive 15 jabs from a bifurcated needle. A vesicle typically appears at the vaccination site 5 to 7 days after inoculation, with associated erythema and induration. The lesion forms a scab and gradually heals over the next 1 to 2 weeks; the evolution of the lesion may be more rapid, with less-severe symptoms in those with previous immunity.

Side effects include a low-grade fever and axillary lymphadenopathy. The attendant erythema and induration of the vaccination vesicle is commonly misdiagnosed as bacterial superinfection. More-severe vaccine reactions include inadvertent inoculation of the face, eyelid, or other parts of the body; generalized vaccinia; and transient, acute myopericarditis. Rare, but often fatal, adverse reactions include eczema vaccinatum (generalized cutaneous spread of vaccinia in patients with eczema), progressive vaccinia (systemic spread of vaccinia in immunocompromised individuals), and postvaccinia encephalitis.[6,7]

Vaccination is contraindicated in the following conditions: immunosuppression, HIV infection, history or evidence of eczema, other active severe skin disorders, during pregnancy, or current household, sexual, or other close physical contact with individuals possessing one of these conditions. In addition, vaccination should not be performed in breast-feeding mothers, in individuals with serious cardiovascular disease or three risk factors for cardiovascular disease, or individuals who are using topical steroid eye medications or have had recent eye surgery. Despite these caveats, most authorities state that with the exception of significant impairment of systemic immunity, there are no absolute contraindications to postexposure vaccination of a person with a confirmed exposure to variola. However, concomitant vaccine immune globulin (VIG) administration is recommended for pregnant and eczematous persons in such circumstances.[8]

VIG is indicated for treating some complications of the smallpox vaccine, including generalized vaccinia with systemic illness, ocular vaccinia without keratitis, eczema vaccinatum, and progressive vaccinia, and it should be available when administering vaccine. The dose for prophylaxis or treatment is 100 mg/kg for the intravenous formulation (first line), or 0.6 mL/kg for the intramuscular preparation (second line). Because of the large volume of the intramuscular formulation (42 mL in a 70-kg person), the dose would be given in multiple sites over 24 to 36 hours.

If VIG is not available, cidofovir may be of use for treating vaccinia adverse events. Limited data suggest that VIG may also be of value in postexposure prophylaxis of smallpox when given within the first week after exposure, and concurrently with vaccination. Vaccination alone is recommended for those without contraindications to the vaccine. If more than 1 week has elapsed after exposure, administration of both products, if available, is reasonable.[9]

In March 2013, the first shipment of a novel, proprietary antiviral drug, Arestvyr (tecovirimit), was delivered to the SNS (Strategic National Stockpile) via the Biomedical Advanced Research and Development Authority (BARDA), which was created under the post-9/11 legislative authority known as Project Bioshield. Arestvyr is an investigational new drug (IND), which is not approved by the Food and Drug Administration (FDA) except in emergencies, but it may be a useful treatment option for patients with active smallpox disease. This purchase of Arestvyr was a controversial decision because of the very high cost of the drug. The federal government purchased approximately 2 million doses at a cost of $463 million or over $200 per course of treatment.[10,11] Some argued the that cost-benefit ratio for Arestvyr is orders of magnitude higher than most other antiviral drugs on the market today and is therefore not cost effective.

In the event of a large-scale smallpox outbreak, the controversial issue of quarantine must be considered. (See Chapter 82 for a detailed discussion of this topic.) Historically, imposition of quarantine was a key element in the eventual control of a smallpox outbreak, but it has been more than 50 years since any such measure has been taken in the United States.

MEDICAL TREATMENT OF CASUALTIES

People who have been exposed to known cases of smallpox should be monitored for a minimum of 17 days from exposure. Regardless of their vaccination status, such individuals should be immediately isolated, using droplet and airborne precautions at the onset of fever. Strict quarantine of asymptomatic contacts may prove to be impractical and impossible to enforce. A reasonable alternative would be to require contacts to remain at home and to check their temperatures daily.[12] Any fever greater than 38 °C (101 °F) during the 17 days after exposure to a confirmed case would suggest the development of smallpox. The contact should then be isolated immediately, preferably at home, until smallpox is either confirmed or ruled out, and they should remain in isolation until all scabs separate. Immediate vaccination or revaccination should also be undertaken for all personnel exposed to a clinical case of smallpox. Caregivers should be vaccinated and should continue to wear appropriate personal protective equipment regardless of vaccination status. Vaccination with a verified clinical "take," defined as vesicle with scar formation, within the past 3 years is considered to render a person immune to smallpox.

Antivirals for use against smallpox are under investigation. Cidofovir has had significant in vitro and in vivo activity in animal studies.[13] Whether it would offer benefit superior to immediate postexposure vaccination in humans has not been determined. Even though cidofovir is a licensed drug, its use for treating smallpox is "off-label," and thus it should be administered as an IND. Topical antivirals such as trifluridine or idoxuridine may be useful for treating smallpox ocular disease.

Supportive care is imperative for successful management of smallpox victims; measures include maintenance of hydration and nutrition, pain control, and management of secondary infections.

UNIQUE CONSIDERATIONS

Smallpox (variola major) is categorized as a category A critical biological agent by the CDC because of its transmissibility, high morbidity and mortality, ability to cause panic in afflicted populations, and the extraordinary public health measures that would be required to contain an epidemic.[14] Of particular concern with smallpox is evidence that it can be transmitted person-to-person via airborne droplet nuclei. This has been seen among some smallpox patients who have prominent respiratory symptoms.[15]

Significant progress has been made in acquiring enough licensed smallpox vaccine for every American. As of 2015, the SNS reportedly has 300 million doses of ACAM2000, which is enough to vaccinate nearly every American. Moreover, Australian researchers have demonstrated an interleukin-2 modified poxvirus that was able to defeat the current smallpox vaccine in an animal model.[16] Research likewise continues on antiviral drugs that could be used to treat smallpox patients, and the drugs cidofovir and Arestvyr offer some promise.

⚠ PITFALLS

- Failure to recognize a case of smallpox on clinical grounds
- Failure to immediately institute airborne and droplet precautions among patients and hospital staff
- Failure to notify hospital laboratory personnel that clinical specimens might be from a smallpox patient
- Failure to notify law enforcement and public health authorities immediately of a suspected case of smallpox

REFERENCES

1. Fenner F, Henderson DA, Arita I, Jezek Z, Ladnyi ID. *Smallpox and Its Eradication.* Geneva: World Health Organization; 1988.
2. Dumbell DR, Huq F. The virology of variola minor: correlation of laboratory tests with the geographic distribution and human virulence of variola isolates. *Am J Epidemiol.* 1986;123:403–415.
3. Ibrahim M, Lofts R, Jahrling P, et al. Real-time microchip PCR for detecting single-base differences in viral and human DNA. *Anal Chem.* 1998;70:2013–2017.
4. Grabenstein J, Winkenwerder W. US military smallpox vaccination program experience. *JAMA.* 2003;289:3278–3282.
5. Wharton M, Strikas R, Harpaz R, et al. Recommendations for using smallpox vaccine in a pre-event vaccination program.

6. Supplemental recommendations of the Advisory Committee on Immunization Practices (ACIP) and the Healthcare Infection Control Practices Advisory Committee (HICPAC). *MMWR Recomm Rep.* 2003;52:1–16.
6. ACAM2000 Package insert. http://www.fda.gov/downloads/biologicsbloodvaccines/vaccines/approvedproducts/ucm142572.pdf. Accessed April 11, 2015.
7. Frey S, Couch R, Tacket C, et al. Clinical responses to undiluted and diluted smallpox vaccine. *N Engl J Med.* 2002;346:1265–1274.
8. Suarez V, Hankins G. Smallpox and pregnancy: from eradicated disease to bioterrorist threat. *Obstet Gynecol.* 2002;100:87–93.
9. Jahrling PB, Zaucha GM, Huggins JW. Countermeasures to the reemergence of smallpox virus as an agent of bioterrorism. In: Scheld WM, Craig WA, Hughes JM, eds. *Emerging Infections 4.* Washington, DC: ASM Press; 2000.
10. U.S. Stockpiling smallpox drug, first shipment of Arestvyr received. http://www.examiner.com/article/u-s-stockpiling-smallpox-drug-first-shipment-of-arestvyr-received. Accessed April 11, 2015.
11. Wary of Attack with Smallpox, U.S. Buys up a Costly Drug. http://www.nytimes.com/2013/03/13/health/us-stockpiles-smallpox-drug-in-case-of-bioterror-attack.html?pagewanted=all&_r=0. Accessed April 11, 2015.
12. Henderson D, Inglesby T, Bartlett J, et al. Smallpox as a biological weapon: medical and public health management. Working Group on Civilian Biodefense. *JAMA.* 1999;281:2127–2137.
13. De Clercq E. Cidofovir in the therapy and short-term prophylaxis of poxvirus infections. *Trends Pharmacol Sci.* 2002;23:456.
14. US Centers for Disease Control and Prevention. Bioterrorism Agents/Diseases. Available at: http://www.bt.cdc.gov/agent/agentlist.asp. Accessed April 11, 2015.
15. Wehrle PF, Posch J, Richter KH, Henderson DA. An airborne outbreak of smallpox in a German hospital and its significance with respect to other recent outbreaks in Europe. *Bull World Health Organ.* 1970;43:669–679.
16. Jackson R, Ramsay A, Christensen C, et al. Expression of mouse interleukin-4 by a recombinant ectromelia virus suppresses cytolytic lymphocyte responses and overcomes genetic resistance to mousepox. *J Virol.* 2001;75:1205–1210.

CHAPTER 148

Influenza Virus Attack

Majed Aljohani, Geoffrey D. Horning, and Anna I. Cheh

DESCRIPTION OF EVENT

Influenza is an acute infectious illness of viral etiology that primarily affects the respiratory tract, although it may have significant systemic effects as well. The influenza virus is a member of the *Orthomyxoviridae* family. There are three immunologic types of influenza: A, B, and C. Type A influenza is most commonly found among wild birds as its principal reservoir but can affect several other species and is the predominant form of influenza to cause illness in humans. Influenza A has two surface glycoproteins, hemagglutinin (HA) and neuraminidase (N), that determine both the host immunity and subtype designation (i.e., H1N1). Influenza types B and C are much less common. Type B influenza almost exclusively infects humans, although seals and ferrets may also become infected. Type B influenza circulates the globe widely with type A influenza, although it causes a much lower percentage of illnesses. Type C influenza can infect several species, but in humans it typically causes only mild illness.

The influenza genome contains eight segments of single-stranded, negative sense RNA. The virus is prone to frequent mutations, which leads to genetic "drift" of the virus and subtle changes in the immunogenicity of the virus nearly every year. Because of the high mutation rates, vaccination against influenza commonly provides protection for only a few years or less. The segmented structure of the virus also facilitates occasional genetic reassortment of the virus and alterations in the major HA and N surface glycoproteins, called genetic "shifts." These genetic shifts and antigenic variations lead to the genetic diversity of type A.[1] Major antigenic shifts underlie the development of worldwide pandemics, such as those of 1918, 1957, 1968, and 2009.

POTENTIAL AS A BIOTERRORISM WEAPON

Influenza is not classified as a bioterrorism agent by the U.S. Centers for Disease Control and Prevention (CDC) but is known to cause significant morbidity and mortality worldwide in its commonly circulating form every year.[2] Influenza is a highly contagious and highly mutable virus, and dissemination of certain novel types of influenza is well known to be able to cause worldwide social and economic disruption in addition to severe health effects, as has been evidenced in the pandemics of the past 100 or more years. Because of its ubiquity influenza virus is readily available to nefarious actors, unlike many other potential biothreat agents that are more difficult to obtain. Even more worrisome are advances that allow infectious agents to be directly produced in the laboratory without a natural template.[3]

Transmission of influenza occurs easily via respiratory droplets or fomites and surfaces,[4] with the virus able to survive on hard, nonporous surfaces for up to 48 hours and on porous surfaces, such as clothing and bed linens, for up to 12 hours. Aerosol transmission of influenza, a method likely to be used in a sophisticated attack, takes 27,000 times fewer virions than that required in direct respiratory contact to induce equivalent disease.[5] The incubation period of influenza is short, ranging from 18 to 72 hours, and a person typically becomes contagious within a day after infection and can remain so for a week after becoming symptomatic. Public health control measures are more difficult to institute for influenza because infected persons may be contagious and spread disease for up to 48 hours before they themselves begin to feel ill. This feature of influenza makes quarantine measures essentially ineffective at controlling the spread.

CLINICAL PRESENTATION

The classic presentation of influenza is the abrupt onset of fever, headache, myalgia, and extreme malaise. The virus targets and reproduces within the ciliated columnar epithelial cells of the respiratory tract.[1] Therefore signs of both upper and lower respiratory involvement can also be present. Constitutional symptoms are more pronounced during the acute phase, encompassing the first 3 to 5 days. The subsequent convalescent phase can last for weeks, with lingering respiratory symptoms and malaise, often termed postinfluenza asthenia.[6] Complicated influenza (requiring hospital admission) has a predilection for individuals who are immunocompromised, the elderly, and those with chronic underlying disease. High-risk groups include those with cardiovascular or pulmonary disease, diabetes mellitus, renal disease, or immunosuppression. Pneumonia is the complication most responsible for the excess fatalities associated with influenza outbreaks.

Although common, influenza can still be a formidable foe. Attack rates are commonly between 10% and 30% in the general population but can exceed 50% during pandemics. Institutionalized and close quartered populations are especially at increased risk, including those in dormitories or barracks. During nonpandemic years as many as 30,000 annual deaths and 100,000 hospitalizations have been attributed to influenza in the United States.[7]

The diagnosis of influenza is often based on diagnosis of the clinical syndrome, and this is especially appropriate within an epidemic. Rapid viral diagnostic tests, such as enzyme-linked immunosorbent assays (ELISAs), are now commonly available to assist with the diagnosis, although these tests commonly suffer from poor sensitivity of 70% or less. Polymerase chain reaction (PCR) is also increasingly available for diagnosis, and this method has a much higher sensitivity; however, neither the ELISA nor PCR is able to identify the responsible subtype strain. Tissue cultures can also be obtained within 48 to 72 hours of inoculation.[8]

PRE-INCIDENT ACTIONS

Influenza is possibly the most tracked virus in the world. The CDC and the World Health Organization (WHO) Global Influenza Network have an extensive worldwide surveillance system (WHO Flunet) in place to monitor disease activity and to identify the appropriate candidates for the development of the annual influenza vaccine. Effective surveillance and early detection of outbreaks is essential for agents, such as influenza, for which effective prophylaxis and immunization exist.[7] Establishing population immunity to influenza will also aid in distinguishing it from the more deadly biological agents that have a similar initial presentation.[9]

Vaccination against seasonal influenza is accomplished each year by predicting the most likely strains of influenza to be circulating in the coming year and contains either three antigens (in the trivalent vaccine) or four antigens (in the quadrivalent vaccine). The vaccines contain two type A influenza strains and either one or two influenza type B virus strains. Influenza vaccines may be administered as an injection or as a nasal spray. The trivalent and quadrivalent influenza vaccines make a person on average "60% less likely to have serious symptoms that require treatment by a health care provider."[10] The 2014 to 2015 CDC guidelines for influenza vaccination recommend the vaccine for all persons 6 months and older with special emphasis on persons at risk for medical complications attributable to severe influenza and on persons who live with or care for persons at high risk for influenza-related complications.[11] High rates of community vaccination against influenza are an important mitigation strategy against influenza, and efficient vaccine clinics and vaccine distribution systems are likely to speed delivery of medical countermeasures should a new strain of influenza emerge.

The use of nonpharmaceutical interventions (NPIs), such as social distancing, and population education on good hand and respiratory hygiene have also been shown to be important "in the mitigation of pandemic influenza."[11] Careful planning to consider the types of NPIs that may be employed in a novel influenza virus outbreak and how they would be implemented is an essential component of a community resiliency strategy.

⤸ POST-INCIDENT ACTIONS

Recognition of an emerging pandemic is aided by influenza's classic presentation and clustering epidemiology. The early deployment of countermeasures, such as antiviral medications, may be of some utility, but the national and international efforts to expedite vaccine development, production, and dissemination will be pivotal to the success of the response. Public awareness campaigns regarding public health measures to reduce transmission should be quickly instituted to blunt the mortality of an outbreak.[7,12] Good risk communication regarding when to seek medical care may help blunt the medical surge, although it is likely that medical facilities will need to implement their surge plans in response to any significant influenza outbreak.

✚ MEDICAL TREATMENT OF CASUALTIES

Treatment of influenza is largely supportive. Patients generally require antipyretics and good oral hydration. For more severe cases, intravenous hydration may be required and some persons may require aggressive ventilatory support. Patients with underlying pulmonary disease and/or other chronic medical conditions are at the greatest risk of hospitalization and of complications from influenza.

Specific antiviral agents, such as amantadine and rimantadine, have long been approved for both the treatment and prophylaxis for influenza type A but are generally no longer recommended due to resistance to these agents. Newer agents in the class of oral N inhibitors, such as oseltamivir and zanamivir, have proved effective for both types A and B, although some development of antiviral resistance has again been observed. Taking osltamivir early may prevent severe influenza infection and may reduce mortality.[13] Oseltamivir is typically administered to

adult patients with uncomplicated disease at a dose of 75 mg twice daily for 5 days. Patients with pneumonia or clinical worsening on the lower dose can optionally be given 150 mg twice daily for 10 days.[14] In 2014 the first intravenous N inhibitor was approved by the Food and Drug Administration (FDA). The optimum efficacy of these medications depends on starting the treatment regimen within 48 hours after symptom onset. Current data show significant underutilization of these medications for hospitalized persons with influenza. During possible acute outbreaks, these agents can potentially provide a delay in the spread of illness in the population until vaccine-induced immunity can be established, whether used in a treatment or a prophylactic strategy.[15] Because of the large amounts of medication that may be required in a prophylactic strategy, many experts recommend only a treatment strategy for most persons exposed to influenza.

"AVIAN" INFLUENZA

As mentioned above, type A influenza viruses are endemic to wild birds. Most type A influenza viruses that are found in birds, sometimes referred to as "avian" or "bird" flu, do not infect humans. However, some types, such as H5N1, H7N3, H7N7, H7N9, and H9N2, have been observed to cause serious infections in people.[16] In particular, influenza A/H5N1 has evolved into a virus strain that is highly lethal when infecting humans and has infected more species than any previously known strain. It was first recognized in Asia in 2003 and reached Europe in 2005 and Africa and the Middle East and North Africa (MENA) region the following year.[17] Although influenza A/H5N1 has thankfully not shown significant evidence of sustained human-to-human transmission, the emergence of H5N1 (and its human lethality) have raised significant questions globally about its potential as the source of a potential pandemic.

Health experts are especially concerned that a person or animal may become coinfected with one of the flu viruses that is easily transmissible from person to person and a novel avian flu virus (especially H5N1). This coinfection may provide an opportunity for genetic material to be exchanged between species-specific viruses, possibly creating a new virulent influenza strain that is easily transmissible between and also highly lethal to humans. Although millions of birds have become infected with the virus since its discovery, only 393 humans have died from the H5N1 in 12 countries, according to WHO data (as of October 2014) with 668 confirmed cases. The WHO has described the potential threat from H5N1 as a "public health crisis."[18]

Some limited data suggested a mortality benefit of oseltamivir in the treatment of H5N1 compared with no antiviral therapy. There are also two human H5N1 vaccines that have been approved by the U.S. FDA, with limited reports of their efficacy.

Vaccines for poultry have been formulated against several of the avian H5N1 influenza varieties. H5N1 has killed millions of birds in a growing number of countries. In affected East Asian nations 84% of affected bird populations are composed of chicken and farm birds, as opposed to wild birds.[19] Vaccination of poultry against the ongoing H5N1 epizootic outbreak is widespread in certain countries.

THE "SWINE" INFLUENZA PANDEMIC OF 2009

As mentioned above, some strains of influenza A virus are able to infect pigs. In 2009 a novel strain of H1N1 influenza, known commonly as "swine flu," emerged; it was a porcine variant of the influenza virus that made the jump from pigs to human through genetic mutation. The virus was a descendent of the 1918 H1N1 "Spanish Flu," which is thought to have been avian (as influenza naturally is) in nature. Viral H1N1 descendants of the 1918 pandemic strain had previously been known and detected in pigs but had never before mutated enough to allow them to infect a human host.[19,20] The novel H1N1 outbreak seen in 2009 caused approximately 60.8 million cases, more than 274,000 hospitalizations, and nearly 13,500 deaths.[21] The 2009 pandemic illustrates one of the most worrisome features about influenza—the ability to mutate in a host thereby producing novel strains that may then cross species and infect those for which immunity does not exist.

The ability of any individual influenza virus strain to cause such rapid spread and death on the scale of the 1918 "Spanish Flu," which caused an estimated 50 million deaths worldwide, is unknown. Although it is thought that viral spread may be facilitated more efficiently in modern society with global travel and urban concentrations of populations becoming ever more prominent, so are proper prevention measures, social distancing, and treatment.

UNIQUE CONSIDERATIONS

- Influenza pandemics have the potential to cause economic disasters even as medical advances help to avert direct fatalities.[22] Agricultural effects may be the most prominent because 3 million chickens were slaughtered to prevent further transmission of the Hong Kong avian influenza virus in 1997, but due to travel restrictions, lost productivity, higher health care costs, and other factors, the potential economic impact of an influenza pandemic is substantial.
- Because influenza is a virus that impacts certain segments of the population disproportionately, especially persons with advanced age and medical comorbidities, the demographic changes in society of an aging population and increasing numbers of patients with chronic medical concerns means that the health effects of a potential influenza pandemic may be even more pronounced.

⚠ PITFALLS

- Failure to consider terrorism during the early phase of a pandemic because of influenza's natural existence.
- Failure to diagnose accurately. The broad spectrum of influenza symptoms often overlaps with many other possible bioterrorism agents. Clinicians should be educated for greater utilization of confirmatory tests and reporting positive cases to a central tracking database.
- Failure to institute mechanisms to ensure adequate supply of antiviral medications, currently unlikely to be able to meet prolonged demand.
- Failure of existing vaccine infrastructure to respond quickly to a novel virulent strain. Currently, a vaccine is almost a year out of date by time of administration.
- Failure to update immunization strategy to better address the unique threats of terrorism.
- Failure to anticipate the social and economic impact of a pandemic outbreak.

REFERENCES

1. Schoch-Spana M. Implications of pandemic influenza for bioterrorism response. *Clin Infect Dis.* 2000;31:1409–1413.
2. Centers for Disease Control and Prevention. Bioterrorism Agents/Diseases. Available at: http://www.bt.cdc.gov/agent/agentlist-category.asp.
3. Cello J, Paul AV, Wimmer E. Chemical synthesis of poliovirus cDNA: generation of infectious virus in the absence of natural template. *Science.* 2002;297:1016–1018.
4. Rao BL. Epidemiology and control of influenza. *Nat Med J India.* 2003;16:143–148.
5. Madjid M, Lillibridge S, Mirhaji P, Casscells W. Influenza as a bioweapon. *J R Soc Med.* 2003;96:345–346.
6. Harrison's Internal Medicine On-Line (Chap 190). Available at: www.accessmedicine.com.
7. Lutz BD, Bronze MS, Greenfield RA. Influenza virus: natural disease and bioterrorism threat. *J Okla State Med Assoc.* 2003;96:27–28.
8. Covalciuc KA, Webb KH, Carlson CA. Comparison of four clinical specimen types for detection of influenza A and B viruses by optical immunoassay (FLU OIA Test) and cell culture methods. *J Clin Microbiol.* 1999;37:3971.
9. Irvin CB, Nouhan PP, Rice K. Syndromic analysis of computerized emergency department patients' chief complaints: an opportunity for bioterrorism and influenza surveillance. *Ann Emerg Med.* 2003;41:447–452.
10. Flu.gov, Vaccination & Vaccine Safety. Last modified 2014. http://www.flu.gov/prevention-vaccination/vaccination/.
11. Cowling BJ, Chan KH, Fang VJ, et al. Facemasks and hand hygiene to prevent influenza transmission in households a cluster randomized trial. *Ann Intern Med.* 2009;151(7):437–446.
12. Krug RM. The potential use of influenza virus as an agent for bioterrorism. *Antiviral Res.* 2003;57:147–150.
13. Writing Committee of the Second World Health Organization Consultation on Clinical Aspects of Human Infection with Avian Influenza A (H5N1) Virus, Abdel-Ghafar AN, Chotpitayasunondh T, Gao Z, et al. Update on avian influenza A (H5N1) virus infection in humans. *N Engl J Med.* 2008;358:261–273.
14. Uptodate.com. Last modified 2014. http://www.uptodate.com/contents/oseltamivir-drug-information?source=see_link.
15. Leong HK, Goh CS, Chew ST, et al. Prevention and control of avian influenza in Singapore. *Ann Acad Med Singapore.* 2008;37(6):504–509.
16. Monke J. *Avian Influenza: agricultural issues;* August 29, 2006, CRS Report for Congress. RS21747.
17. Stephenson I. Epidemiology, Transmission, and Pathogenesis of Avian Influenza. Uptodate.Com. last modified 2014. http://www.uptodate.com/contents/epidemiology-transmission-and-pathogenesis-of-avian-influenza.
18. First Human Avian Influenza A (H5N1) Virus Infection Reported in Americas. CDC. January 8, 2014.
19. Taubenberger JK, Morens DM. 1918 influenza: the mother of all pandemics. *Rev Biomed.* 2006;17:69–79.
20. Taubenberger JK. The origin and virulence of the 1918 "Spanish" influenza virus. *Proceedings of the American Philosophical Society.* 2006;150(1):86.
21. Shrestha S, Swerdlow D, Borse R, et al. Estimating the Burden of 2009 Pandemic Influenza A (H1N1) in the United States (April 2009-April 2010). *Clin Infect Dis [online].* 2010;52(Supplement 1):S75–S82. Available at: http://cid.oxfordjournals.org/content/52/suppl_1/S75.long.
22. Dennis Carroll. Avian Influenza: A Symposium Report: Political, Social and Economic Dimensions of the Continuing Threat from Emerging Infectious Diseases. In: Political, Social And Economic Dimensions Of TheContinuing Threat From Emerging Infectious Diseases. Washington D.C.: International Resources Group and The George Washington University Medical Center; 2005.

SUGGESTED READINGS

1. Simberkoff MS. Vaccines for adults in an age of terrorism. *J Assoc Acad Min Phys.* 2002;13:19–20.
2. Owens SR. Being prepared: preparations for a pandemic of influenza. *EMBO Rep.* 2001;21:1061–1063.
3. Webster RG, Shortridge KF, Kawaoka Y. Influenza: interspecies transmission and emergence of new pandemics. *FEMS Immun Med Microbiol.* 1997;18:275–279.
4. Longini IM, Halloran ME, Nizam A, Yang Y. Containing pandemic influenza with antiviral agents. *Am J Epidemiol.* 2002;159:623–633.
5. Ferguson NM, Fraser C, Donnelly CA, Ghani AC, Anderson RM. Public health risk from the Avial H5N1 influenza epidemic. *Science.* 2004;304:968–969.
6. O'Brien KK, Higdon ML, Halverson JJ. Recognition and management of bioterrorism infections. *Am Fam Phys.* 2003;67:1927–1934.

Monkeypox Attack

Nicole F. Mullendore, Benjamin J. Lawner, and John D. Malone

DESCRIPTION OF EVENT

Monkeypox is an orthopox virus that was recognized in 1958 in laboratory monkeys and found to cause human infection in 1970 by the World Health Organization (WHO). The natural host is unknown, but the virus can naturally infect squirrels, rodents, rabbits, and other nonhuman primates (NHP). Monkeypox is in the same genus as smallpox (*Variola major* and *minor*), *Molluscum contagiosum*, cowpox, and the vaccinia virus. Other nonhuman-associated animal orthopox infections include volepox, skunkpox, raccoonpox, camelpox, and buffalopox. Monkeypox was endemic in Ghana and Zaire, with a recent resurgence in the Democratic Republic of the Congo (DRC), and it is associated with the hunting, handling, and consumption of infected rodents and other NHP.[1,2]

In 2003, six infected African rodents, including the Gambian giant rat, were imported into the United States. They transferred the monkeypox virus to prairie dog rodents housed in adjacent cages. Within 2 months, human cases were reported in individuals with direct exposure to the infected prairie dogs. In the outbreak, there were 37 laboratory-confirmed cases and 10 probable cases. There was no laboratory-confirmed human-to-human transmission or deaths reported from these cases.[2]

Patients presented with fever greater than 38 °C and skin lesions. Skin manifestations ranged from nodular swellings in the wound margins to satellite and disseminated lesions. Papules progressed to vesicles and pustules. Significant symptoms included severe chills and sore throat. Lymphadenopathy and tonsillar hypertrophy were present. Along with the history of an intimate rodent animal exposure history 2 to 3 weeks before symptom onset, the presence of adenopathy helps clinicians to differentiate monkeypox from other viral illness that present with skin lesions and prodromal phases. The clinical course was self-limited for most of these cases; one patient required a corneal transplant from ocular sequelae, and another was intubated due to virus-associated oropharyngeal and mucosal edema.

With close cooperation from the Centers for Disease Control and Prevention (CDC) and multiple Midwestern state health authorities, the outbreak was controlled through an emergency embargo and quarantine orders against the "importation, sale, distribution, or display of prairie dogs or any mammals that had been in contact with prairie dogs after April 1, 2003."[3] Appropriate and aggressive animal control measures prevented the establishment of monkeypox in the North American rodent population.

The initial symptoms of monkeypox include a 2- to 3-day febrile illness, usually occurring from 10 to 14 days after initial exposure. The onset of skin lesions can occur at up to 16 days post exposure and are extremely similar to those for smallpox: monomorphic, hard and pea sized on an erythematous base. Lesions are often described as "dew drops on a rose petal." The rash begins as maculopapular lesions, progressing through vesicular, pustular, and crust phases over a 14-day period. The lesions can be located on all parts of the body including the palms, soles, and face. Beyond the initial days, the lesions spread to the trunk. The initial papules become umbilicated vesicles, with all of the lesions in the same stage at the same time. Skin vesicles result from viral invasion of terminal capillaries in the epithelium. The initial viremia is manifested by the sudden onset of fever, malaise, headache, and severe back pain. Gastrointestinal symptoms such as abdominal pain and vomiting occur less often. Multiple factors account for the disparity of disease course, including: prior smallpox vaccination, age, nutritional status, and relative immunocompetency.[2,4,5]

The clinician should formulate a broad-based differential diagnosis when confronted with a sick patient who presents with a generalized rash. Septic shock, bacterial meningitis, and disseminated intravascular coagulopathy are life-threatening conditions that present with alarming dermatologic sequelae such as purpura and petechiae. The differential diagnosis for a generalized pustular eruption is a bit narrower. For example, the "chickenpox" eruption associated with the varicella zoster virus (VZV) manifests with a similar distribution of pustules. The varicella exanthem starts centrally on the trunk, face, and proximal limbs. Varicella vesicles are also described as a "dew drop on a rose petal."[6] In contrast to monkeypox lesions, the varicella rash displays vesicles in various stages of maturation and appears up to three weeks after exposure to an infected contact.[6] Coxsackievirus infection is also included in the differential diagnosis of a generalized viral rash but involves an entirely different clinical course. Yellow-colored lesions appear on the surface of oral mucosa. Dorsal limb surfaces are more frequently affected, and the rash is usually self-limiting. In contrast to monkeypox, lesions are elliptical, vesicular, and not usually umbilicated or purulent.[7] Other similar rash illnesses may include secondary syphilis, erytherma multiforme, and drug eruptions, all of which produce less typical vesicular rashes on the palm and soles. Rocky Mountain spotted fever, a rickettsial illness, is associated with a spring/summer tick exposure in the Southeastern United States. Meningococcal infection is characterized by rapid progression to shock. Molluscum infection occurs in children and HIV-infected adults; the painless lesions do not cause fever. Table 149-1 compares the clinical features of the monkeypox exanthem to other viral eruptions.

Polymerase chain reaction (PCR) assay is the test of choice for definitive diagnosis of monkeypox. PCR assay reliably differentiates monkeypox from smallpox. This ensures an appropriate and scaled response from public health authorities. Electron microscopy of vesicular scrapings identifies the *Orthopoxvirus* species. The viruses appear as large brick-like boxes with rounded corners. Tissue from lymph nodes and blood specimens can also be evaluated. Specimen collection instructions are detailed by the CDC.[8,9]

TABLE 149-1 Clinical Features of Important Viral Eruptions

VIRUS	PRODROMAL PERIOD	PRODROMAL SYMPTOMS	RASH CHARACTERISTICS
Smallpox	2-4 days	High fever Headache Malaise Nausea Vomiting	Lesions start on the face then spread outward. The initial appearance of papules is followed by pustules over the entire body surface. All skin lesions appear at the same stage. Pustules are often umbilicated.
Monkeypox	1-10 days	Febrile illness Chills Sweats Headache Malaise Anorexia Shortness of breath Cough Lymphadenopathy a distinguishing feature	Skin lesions may appear in clusters and progress from macules to vesicles and then to pustules. In contrast to smallpox, lesions display less of a "centrifugal" distribution. The rash appears less dense on the face and extremities.
Chickenpox	Mild prodromal period of 1-2 days	Fever Malaise (Rash is often the first sign of disease in pediatric population)	"Dew drop on a rose petal" is the characteristic vesicle-erythematous halo that surrounds the vesicle. The trunk is most affected, and rash may spread to other areas and on the mucosal surface of the throat. Lesions present in active and healing stages.

Recent genomic studies show continuing evolution of the monkeypox virus and the emergence of four distinct lineages from endemic regions of Africa, including the DRC. These changes found within the genes may be due to the decrease in herd immunity with the eradication of smallpox since the 1980s. Nonetheless, the observed increase in human-to-human transmission in endemic areas demonstrates the progression of this potentially dangerous virus.[10]

It is not known whether the monkeypox virus has ever been weaponized. However, the process would probably be similar to the method used to weaponize the smallpox virus. If a stable, infectious monkeypox biological aerosol was produced and delivered as a fine particle aerosol under ideal atmospheric conditions over a targeted population, one would expect to see large numbers of casualties presenting at about the same time to local hospitals and doctor's offices with signs and symptoms as described here. Studies using aerosolized monkeypox virus suspensions have shown that it is a hardy virus that could potentially remain infectious for a long time, given the ideal environment.[11] One primate study discussed different exposure results; how a lethal aerosolized dose would lead to severe respiratory disease with or without skin reactions, but a lethal intravenous exposure would result in systemic reactions causing death.[12] Of course, these studies have evaluated nonhuman subjects and cannot predict the outcomes of monkeypox as a biological weapon used on humans.

PRE-INCIDENT ACTIONS

Emergency departments should have well-rehearsed standard operating procedures to evaluate potentially contagious infectious disease patients using airborne and contact transmission precautions (protective gowns, gloves, and N95 mask). A small contingent of smallpox-vaccinated health care workers should be available to initially evaluate and care for patients with any suspected orthopox infection. Along with concerns for patient transmissible bioterrorism agents, such as smallpox, pneumonic plague, and viral hemorrhagic fevers, clinical suspicion is necessary for the more common agents of SARS and rubeola virus in our highly mobile global society.

POST-INCIDENT ACTIONS

When presented with an initial case of monkeypox, great concerns about the possibility of smallpox are appropriate in this time of ongoing terrorist threats. In contrast to smallpox, monkeypox would be a poor agent for bioterrorism because of a very low mortality rate and respiratory transmission by large droplets that requires direct and prolonged face-to-face contact. Monkeypox is unlikely to be self-sustaining in human communities without small rodent populations. If monkeypox infection is suspected, the appropriate local and state health authorities must be notified early to assist with agent identification.

MEDICAL TREATMENT OF CASUALTIES

Supportive therapy with antipyretics and fluids are indicated. Monkeypox has a low lethality (1.5% in a 1996 DRC outbreak) and requires close family contact for transmission. Accumulating experience in the United States suggests a relatively low risk of person-to-person transmission. According to the CDC, all health care settings such as hospitals, emergency departments, and physician offices should have the capacity to care for monkeypox-infected patients and to protect health care workers and other patients from exposure.[1,13] A negative pressure room should be used if available. Quarantine of affected patients is advisable until a definitive diagnosis is made.

UNIQUE CONSIDERATIONS

Smallpox vaccination with the second generation vaccinia live virus (ACAM2000) is also protective against the monkeypox virus. During the 2003 monkeypox outbreak, CDC guidelines for vaccination included public health and animal control investigators, health care workers caring for monkeypox patients, or those who may be asked to care for infected patients or family members with close contact with someone who was symptomatic with monkeypox. In addition, veterinarians and their technicians who had direct physical exposure to an infected animal were also included. Vaccination up to 14 days after exposure will attenuate or prevent monkeypox illness.

In 2007 the Department of Defense started to utilize the product ACAM2000, a second generation smallpox vaccine. The ACAM2000 is derived from a clone of the previously used vaccine "Dryvax," and it is the first vaccine to have a medication guide through the U.S. Food and Drug Administration, with a screening protocol before injection. Precautions are similar to the previous "Dryvax" vaccine, as it can cause pericarditis and myocarditis and should not be administered to immunocompromised or pregnant patients. The risk of inadvertent smallpox transmission is low from vaccination sites covered by occlusive dressings.[14,15]

Fear and panic are major issues for monkeypox viral infection. Commonality in name with smallpox raises anxieties and misperceptions in the public, patients, and health care providers. Significant psychological and economic impacts result. Preliminary knowledge of monkeypox, personal protective equipment, and effective leadership of the health care team will ensure appropriate patient care and avoid crisis and closure of emergency departments.

⚠️ PITFALLS

- The skin lesions of monkeypox and smallpox are virtually identical, and the clinical course of the disease can help differentiate monkeypox from chickenpox.
- Lymphadenopathy, tonsillar hypertrophy, fever, and direct rodent exposure are more characteristic of monkeypox infection.
- Monkeypox has relatively low risk of person-to-person transmission; however, airborne and contact precautions (including N95 mask) are recommended.
- A high clinical suspicion and well-rehearsed standard operating procedures are needed to safely evaluate potentially contagious patients.
- Emergency departments should have a group of smallpox-vaccinated health care workers trained in initial response, decontamination, and treatment procedures.
- There are few labs that perform onsite analysis to differentiate between monkeypox and other systemic rash illnesses; collaboration with public health and governmental agencies (such as the CDC) is key to the mitigation of a monkeypox-related threat.

REFERENCES

1. Huntin Y, Williams R, Malfait P. Outbreak of human monkeypox, Democratic Republic of Congo. *Emerg Infect Dis.* 2001;7:434–438.
2. Damon IK. Status of human monkeypox: clinical disease, epidemiology and research. *Vaccine.* 2011;29(suppl 4):D54–D59. http://dx.doi.org/10.1016/j.vaccine.2011.04.014.
3. Centers for Disease Control and Prevension (CDC). Multistate outbreak of monkeypox-Illinois, Indiana, and Wisconsin, 2003. *MMWR Morb Mortal Wkly Rep.* 2003;52(23):537–540.
4. Reynolds MG, Emerson GL, Pukuta E, et al. Detection of human monkeypox in the Republic of the Congo following intensive community education. *Am J Trop Med Hyg.* 2013;88(5):982–985. http://dx.doi.org/10.4269/ajtmh.12-0758.
5. Graham M, Gunkel J. Monkeypox. *Emedicine.* 2014; Available at, http://emedicine.medscape.com/article/1134714-overview. Accessed 20.04.14.
6. Papadopoulos A, Janniger C. Chickenpox clinical presentation. *Emedicine.* 2013; Available at, http://emedicine.medscape.com/article/1131785-clinical.
7. Dyne P, Sawtelle S, Kesler DeVore H. Hand-Foot-and-Mouth disease in emergency medicine. *Emedicine.* 2014; Available at, http://emedicine.medscape.com/article/802260-overview.
8. Casebeer L, Nafsinger S, Katta S, et al. *Bioterrorism and Emerging Infections Education: Monkeypox;* 2004, Available at, http://www.bioterrorism.cme.uab.edu/aboutThisSite.html. Accessed 20.04.14.
9. Centers for Disease Control. *MONKEYPOX: Updated Interim CDC Guidance for Use of Smallpox Vaccine, Cidofovir, and Vaccinia Immune Globulin (VIG) for Prevention and Treatment in the Setting of an Outbreak of Monkeypox Infections;* 2003, 1–7.
10. Kugelman JR, Johnston SC, Mulembakani PM, et al. Genomic variability of monkeypox virus among humans, Democratic Republic of the Congo. *Emerg Infect Dis.* 2014;20(2):232–239. http://dx.doi.org/10.3201/eid2002.130118.
11. Verreault D, Killeen SZ, Redmann RK, Roy CJ. Susceptibility of monkeypox virus aerosol suspensions in a rotating chamber. *J Virol Methods.* 2013;187(2):333–337. http://dx.doi.org/10.1016/j.jviromet.2012.10.009.
12. Barnewall RE, Fisher DA, Robertson AB, Vales PA, Knostman KA, Bigger JE. Inhalational monkeypox virus infection in cynomolgus macaques. *Front Cell Infect Microbiol.* 2012;2(September):117. http://dx.doi.org/10.3389/fcimb.2012.00117.
13. Centers for Disease Control. *Updated Interim Infection Control and Exposure Management Guidance in the Health-Care and Community Setting for Patients with Possible Monkeypox Virus Infection;* 2003, 1–4. Available at, http://www.cdc.gov/ncidod/monkeypox/infectioncontrol.htm.
14. Department of Defense. Update to clinical policy for the department of defense smallpox vaccination program. 2008.
15. Centers for Disease Control. *ACAM2000 (Smallpox Vaccine) Questions and Answers;* 2000, Available at, http://www.fda.gov/BiologicsBloodVaccines/Vaccines/QuestionsaboutVaccines/ucm078041.htm.

CHAPTER 150

Hantavirus Pulmonary Syndrome Attack

Bryant Allen

DESCRIPTION OF EVENT

Hantavirus pulmonary syndrome (HPS) is characterized by the rapid onset of noncardiogenic pulmonary edema, which develops after infection with one of several subspecies of New World rodent-borne hantavirus. Early recognition of HPS is essential, given the potential of rapid progression from the initial flu-like symptoms (malaise, fever, myalgias) to shock and complete respiratory failure, sometimes within days.[1] Hantavirus has not been known to be weaponized or used for bioterrorism, but it is recognized by the Centers for Disease Control and Prevention (CDC) as a Category C Agent.[2] Its presumed ease of production and dissemination, as well as its high potential for severe morbidity and mortality, raise concern for the possibility that this emerging pathogen could be engineered for future mass exposures.[2]

Belonging to the family Bunyaviridae, hantavirus was first isolated in Korea in 1978 as the culpable agent in the Old World disease known as hemorrhagic fever with renal syndrome (HFRS), an acute prostrating febrile illness with associated renal failure and shock.[3,4] HFRS is thought to have affected more than 3000 soldiers during the Korean War and was also known at the time as Korean hemorrhagic fever.[5] More than 20 different serotypes or genotypes of hantavirus have been identified since the initial discovery, each maintained in nature by a single, unique rodent species host. Human infection occurs through inhalation of aerosolized virus shed in rodent saliva, urine, and feces, or by direct inoculation via rodent bites.[4] Hantavirus can be divided into two major groups: Old World and New World hantavirus. Old World hantaviruses can be found predominately in Asia and Europe and are thought to result in approximately 150,000 cases of HFRS each year, mainly seen in the country of China.[5] Importantly, however, although they have been linked to another minor disease, nephropathia epidemica (NE), Old World hantaviruses have not been linked to HPS.[5]

In 1993 a mysterious clinical entity causing fever, rapid respiratory failure, and cardiopulmonary dysfunction killed 29 people in the southwestern United States.[6] Linked by genetic sequencing to a previously unknown hantavirus species, the disease was named Four Corners disease and later HPS. The "Sin Nombre" virus, as it came to be known, became the first identified strain of New World hantaviruses, many of which were ultimately found to cause HPS, changing the recognized spectrum of hantavirus disease completely. The "Sin Nombre" virus, which is credited as the primary causative agent of the largest HPS outbreak in the United States, is carried by the deer mouse, *Peromyscus maniculatas*. Other hantaviruses known to cause HPS in the United States include the New York, Black Canal, and Bayou viruses hosted by the white-footed mouse (*Peromyscus leucopus*), the cotton rat (*Sigmodon hipidus*), and the rice rat (*Oryzomys palustris*), respectively. The rodent reservoir of the Seoul virus, the brown rat (*Rattus norvegicus*), thought to have been brought by cargo ship to the Western

hemisphere from Europe, has caused the only cases of HFRS documented in the United States.[7] Nearly all of the United States falls within range of one or more hantavirus-carrying rodent species, as does the majority of South and Central America.[5] As of 2011, more than 2000 total cases of HPS have been documented, with 587 cases being documented in the United States from 1993 to 2011.[5,8] The incubation period for human hantavirus infections has been documented to range from 4 to 42 days, with an average of 12 to 16 days from the suspected exposure.[9] Recent evaluation of the "Sin Nombre" virus found that virulence was eliminated when the virus was not first passed through a rodent host, but rather propagated through in vitro means.[10] However, certain outbreaks of HPS in South America have shown evidence of apparent human-to-human transmission, illustrating a great variation of potential for infectivity across strains.[11] Most notably, an outbreak of Andes virus, another New World hantavirus similar to the "Sin Nombre" virus, that occurred in 1996 showed apparent human-to-human transmission when a physician caring for a patient with HPS suffered from a delayed-onset case of HPS. This physician had no other identified exposures to the rodent host of the Andes virus.[11]

HPS progresses through four clinical phases: prodrome, pulmonary edema and shock, diuresis, and convalescence.[12] The initial prodrome lasts for 3 to 6 days and is characterized by malaise, myalgia, fever, tachypnea, and gastrointestinal symptoms such as nausea, vomiting, diarrhea, or abdominal pain. In 10% of cases the abdominal pain is reported to be severe enough to mimic appendicitis.[1] Presenting symptoms may overlap with more common viral infections, challenging early recognition by health care workers. One study that attempted to quantify a clinically distinct constellation of symptoms suggests excluding patients with rapid influenza A–proven infection from consideration.[13] Additionally, the presence of sore throat and nasal symptoms and the finding of an injected pharynx are less likely to be associated with HPS.[13]

The subsequent cardiopulmonary phase is heralded by the acute onset of noncardiogenic pulmonary edema.[14] Clinically, patients are noted to have progressive cough with shortness of breath. On the cellular level, significant capillary leak in pulmonary endothelial cells occurs.[9,14] The time interval from the development of dyspnea to the need for ventilator support is reported to be within 1 to 6 hours, underscoring the extremely rapid progression of respiratory collapse.[1,12] Other signs include hypoxia and copious amber-colored, nonpurulent secretions with secretion protein-to-serum protein ratio greater than 80%.[6,15] Specific laboratory and radiographic findings that are suggestive of HPS assist in diagnosis and should raise clinical suspicion. A peripheral blood smear triad of thrombocytopenia, leukocytosis with left shift, and circulating immunoblasts is unique to HPS in North America.[15] Elevated lactate levels and hemoconcentration up to 77% that corrects to anemic levels after fluid resuscitation are also observed.[16] Radiographically, HPS is distinguished by the central location of infiltrates rather than the peripheral pattern typically seen in acute respiratory distress syndrome (ARDS). HPS has typically also lacked the focal consolidation common in most community-acquired pneumonias.[13] The sepsis syndrome observed in HPS features a diminished cardiac index and normal or elevated systemic vascular resistance, the opposite of that typically seen in sepsis.[17] Hypotension, which may be seen initially, is often the result of diminished stroke volume, resulting from inadequate left ventricular preload and exacerbated by myocardial depression. Death rates range between 50% and 70% with cardiogenic shock and pulseless electrical activity as the proximate cause.[6] Survivors of the cardiopulmonary phase recover quickly, with a spontaneous diuresis occurring 2 to 5 days after the onset of pulmonary edema, usually facilitating extubation within 1 week of initiation of ventilator support. Convalescence ensues with minor residual respiratory impairment.[12] Identification of the virus is achieved through serologic testing in the acutely ill for immunoglobulin G (IgG) and immunoglobulin M (IgM) antibodies to viral nucleocapsid proteins.[1] ELISA assays are available at some state public health laboratories or by state health department referral at CDC.[7] These tests are effective for diagnosing either HFRS or HPS and take between 4 and 6 hours to yield results.[5] Because of the time delay associated with these forms of testing, a recombinant immunoblot assay in the form of a test strip is being evaluated.[1]

PRE-INCIDENT ACTIONS

Exposure of individuals or groups to hantavirus might occur naturally as a result of increased exposure caused by an environmental change such as increased rodent food production or decreased rodent predator population, or as the result of a planned bioterrorist attack. Similar to the epidemic that heralded the discovery of HPS in the southwestern United States in 1993, individuals or groups of people can be exposed through contact with contaminated material. The most recent outbreak of HPS in the United States occurred when visitors to Yosemite National Park in California came in contact with an increased deer mouse population while staying in close proximity to newly constructed insulated tents, ultimately found to be an ideal breeding location for the rodent host.[8] Increased rodent populations or high-risk activities such as cleaning enclosed rodent-infested areas can lead to infection. Disaster scenarios, either naturally occurring or as a result of terrorism, that displace populations, disrupt the sanitation infrastructure, or create living conditions where people are forced into closer proximity to rodent hosts significantly increase the risk of hantavirus exposure. The CDC has published a useful guide of risk reduction strategies in an effort to mitigate risk in the case of an outbreak. Actions to reduce exposure to rodents involve securing food and trash in rodent-proof containers; keeping items that attract rodents such as garbage cans, woodpiles, and bird feeders far from human dwellings; and using raised cement foundations in new construction of outbuildings or shelters.[18]

In addition, educating individuals on appropriate mask or ventilator usage while cleaning and using wet mopping instead of sweeping while cleaning in potential areas of rodent exposure have illustrated potential as a risk reduction method.[19] Hantavirus is recognized as an emerging pathogen for bioterrorism because of its relative ease of transmission and high mortality rate. Dissemination would most likely occur via aerosolization of infectious particles released over populated areas. Furthermore, given the documented cases illustrating possible human-to-human transmission of hantavirus in South America, the potential of epidemic is much greater than previously thought possible.[11] In the case of intentional dissemination, bioterrorists might use low-flying aircraft, munitions, or indoor contamination through air ducts to initiate exposure.

POST-INCIDENT ACTIONS

Suspicious and/or atypical patterns of disease presentation would be the first clue that an HPS outbreak has occurred at the hands of bioterrorists. An understanding of the demographic distribution of naturally occurring hantavirus infection will allow the health care professional to recognize unusual variations and to suspect bioterrorist activity. Infection caused by hantavirus and rodent hosts not recognized in the United States, an infectious disease consistent with HFRS in the New World, and disease in nonendemic areas or in patients with no travel history should all raise suspicion of an unnatural or deliberate infection. Virus isolation, genotyping, and comparison to known national and world prevalence data could unveil irregular geographic incidence patterns. Cases of natural hantavirus have generally occurred in young adults and previously healthy persons because of exposure occurred during activities like farming, cleaning, or camping.[6] An attack generated by terrorism with infectious particles in high concentration on the ground or in soil in densely populated areas might affect children, who are smaller and shorter, in greater proportion than observed naturally. Also, an increase in disease incidence without a rise in the endemic rodent population or in persons not exposed to rodents should raise suspicion.

Universal precautions and respiratory isolation of affected individuals is recommended. Although person-to-person transmission is generally not recognized, during a hantavirus outbreak in Argentina, five health care workers involved in treating HPS patients may have contracted the disease without known exposure to rodents.[3,11] This case helps to emphasize the importance of the use of proper personal protective equipment, including respirators when indicated, especially in the case of a suspected zoonotic or bioterrorist-related patient exposure.

MEDICAL TREATMENT OF CASUALTIES

Supportive care is the mainstay of treatment for HPS. Volume replacement must be cautious and conservative because of the potential for significant pulmonary capillary leak. Pulmonary artery occlusive pressures higher than 10 to 12 mm Hg are associated with significant pulmonary edema. Classic to HPS is a shock state characterized by decreased cardiac output and increased systemic vascular resistance, although frank hypotension is also documented. Use of inotropic agents such as dobutamine should usually be accompanied by judicious volume resuscitation. Despite the presence of severe pulmonary edema, adequate oxygenation can usually be achieved with mechanical ventilation and high levels of positive end-expiratory pressure.[1]

Further studies on the treatment of HPS are needed to assess the role of immunologic therapy and inflammatory mediators on vascular function. The use of antiviral agents such as ribavirin has illustrated some utility in HFRS, with an observed decrease in overall mortality after administration.[7] However, multiple studies on the use of ribavirin in the treatment of HPS have had inconclusive results.[5] It is also conceivable that some added benefit could be achieved by applying the principles of early goal-directed therapy, which has demonstrated effectiveness among patients with sepsis of other origins. However, at this time there are no Food and Drug Administration (FDA)-approved vaccines, medications, or immunotherapies for HPS or HFRS.[5]

UNIQUE CONSIDERATIONS

The importance of rapid recognition of HPS and the need for widespread dissemination of information between other health care institutions and health departments is the key to effective management. As nearly all infected patients become ventilator-dependent, the prospect of a mass casualty situation caused by HPS could prove catastrophic unless adequate intensive care unit capabilities were mobilized and appropriately staffed to augment local health care facilities.

! PITFALLS

- Failure to rapidly recognize the symptoms of HPS and include it in the differential diagnosis
- Failure to report a suspicion for HPS to the appropriate public health authority
- Failure to recognize the possibility for extremely rapid progression of respiratory failure and initiate appropriate ventilator support
- Failure to prepare for significant numbers of patients requiring ventilator support
- Failure to judiciously manage fluid balance and cardiovascular status

REFERENCES

1. Simpson SQ. Hantavirus pulmonary syndrome. *Heart Lung.* 1998;27:51–57.
2. Moran GJ. Threats in bioterrorism II: CDC category B and C agents. *Emerg Med Clin North Am.* 2002;20:311–330.
3. McCaughey C, Hart CA. Hantaviruses. *J Med Microbiol.* 2000;49:587–599.
4. Chapman LE, Khabbaz RF. Etiology and epidemiology of the Four Corners hantavirus outbreak. *Infect Agents Dis.* 1994;3:234–244.
5. Jonsson CB, Figueiredo LT, Vapalahti O. A global perspective on hantavirus ecology, epidemiology, and disease. *Clin Microbiol Rev.* 2010;23(2):412–441.
6. Levy H, Simpson SQ. Hantavirus pulmonary syndrome. *Am J Respir Crit Care Med.* 1994;149:1710–1713.
7. Doyle TJ, Bryan RT, Peters CJ. Viral hemorrhagic fevers and hantavirus infections in the Americas. *Infect Dis Clin North Am.* 1998;12:95–110.
8. Núñez JJ, Fritz CL, Knust B, et al. Yosemite Hantavirus Outbreak Investigation Team. Hantavirus infections among overnight visitors to Yosemite National Park, California, USA, 2012. *Emerg Infect Dis.* 2014;20 (3):386–393.
9. Butler JC, Peters CJ. Hantaviruses and hantavirus pulmonary syndrome. *Clin Infect Dis.* 1994;19:387–395.
10. Safronetz D, Prescott J, Feldmann F, et al. Pathophysiology of hantavirus pulmonary syndrome in rhesus macaques. *Proc Natl Acad Sci U S A.* 2014;111(19):7114–7119.
11. Wells RM, Sosa Estani S, Yadon ZE, et al. An unusual hantavirus outbreak in southern Argentina: person-to-person transmission? Hantavirus Pulmonary Syndrome Study Group for Patagonia. *Emerg Infect Dis.* 1997;3 (2):171–174.
12. Jenison S, Koster F. Hantavirus pulmonary syndrome: clinical, diagnostic, and virologic aspects. *Semin Respir Infect.* 1995;10:259–269.
13. Moolenaar RL, Dalton C, Lipman HB, et al. Clinical features that differentiate hantavirus pulmonary syndrome from three other respiratory illnesses. *Clin Infect Dis.* 1995;21:643–649.
14. Graziano KL. Hantavirus pulmonary syndrome: a zebra worth knowing. *Am Fam Physician.* 2002;66(6):1015–1020.
15. Duchin JS, Koster FT, Peters CJ, et al. Hantavirus pulmonary syndrome: a clinical description of 17 patients with a newly recognized disease. *N Engl J Med.* 1994;330:949–955.
16. Zakik SR, Greer PW, Coffield LM, et al. Hantavirus pulmonary syndrome, pathogenesis of an emerging infectious disease. *Am J Pathol.* 1995;146:552–579.
17. Hallin GW, Simpson SQ, Crowell RE, et al. Cardiopulmonary manifestations of hantavirus pulmonary syndrome. *Crit Care Med.* 1996;24:252–258.
18. Mills JN, Corneli A, Young JC, Garrison LE, Khan AS, Ksiazek TG. Hantavirus pulmonary syndrome—United States: updated recommendations for risk reduction. *MMWR Recomm Rep.* 2002;51 (RR-9):1–12.
19. McConnell MS. Hantavirus Public Health outreach effectiveness in three populations: an overview of northwestern New Mexico, Los Santos Panama, and Region IX Chile. *Viruses.* 2014;6(3):986–1003.

Henipavirus Attack: Hendra and Nipah Viruses

Stephen P. Wood

DESCRIPTION OF EVENT

In 1994 in the village of Hendra, a suburb of Brisbane in Queensland, Australia, 19 horses housed together in a stable became acutely ill with a rapidly developing respiratory illness.[1,2] The index case was a pregnant mare, who, 2 days after arrival in the stables, had developed an illness characterized by a fever, frothy nasal discharge, facial edema, and neurologic symptoms.[1,3] Eventually, thirteen of these horses died, and the remaining six were euthanized.[3] Two stable hands who cared for these horses also fell ill within 6 days of the index case; one of them died within a week after developing fever, pneumonitis, and eventually respiratory and renal failure.[1] A previously unidentified morbillivirus was identified as the likely causative agent. This was later characterized as a novel Paramyxoviridae virus, termed the *Hendra virus* after the village in which it was first manifested.[1–4]

In September 1998, in a suburb on the Malaysian Peninsula, a respiratory illness among pigs first thought to be classic swine fever then appeared in a cluster of pig farmers.[5–7] The swine developed a mostly respiratory illness, followed by symptoms suggesting encephalitis with a relatively low mortality. The human outbreak, however, was a rapidly progressing febrile encephalitis.[5–8] It was characterized by fever and headache, as well as clinical evidence of brainstem dysfunction.[5,6,9] This disease was initially believed to be Japanese encephalitis, but negative serum antibodies for this agent suggested another cause.[5] The agent was later identified as yet another novel Paramyxoviridae virus, later named the Nipah virus, again after the origin of the index cases.

The henipaviruses, including both Hendra and Nipah, are a genus of zoonotic, highly virulent, and highly pathogenic Paramyxoviridae viruses.[7,10,11] They are enveloped, negative-sense RNA viruses and are larger than most typical Paramyxoviridae viruses.[10] They are the only known zoonotic Paramyxoviridae, with bats considered as the natural reservoir.[4,5,7,12] These viruses are also known to infect humans, horses, swine, and rodents. The mechanism of action is a complex interaction of interferon and proinflammatory cytokine suppression via sequestration of signal transducer and activator of transcription 1 (STAT1).[7,13] Type 1 interferon is important to the innate immune cascade that involves the initial recognition of viral particles, and the subsequent release of interferons that can then activate Janus kinases (JAK).[14] JAK has many functions including increasing interferon transcription and activation of interferon responsive genes, as well as STAT1 phosphorylation.[7,14] Phosphorylation of STAT1 leads to downstream activation of a variety of antiviral cytokines and interferons. The henipaviruses suppress this cascade, leading to its significant virulence and pathogenicity.[7,13–16]

The clinical manifestations of Hendra virus are similar to an influenza-like illness, and they include fever, pneumonia, pneumonitis, and a delayed-onset encephalitis. The chest x-ray may reveal an infiltrate but is often nonspecific. The onset of this illness is typically days to weeks after exposure.[7] No other laboratory or imaging findings are specific or pathognomonic for this disease.

Nipah virus presents with a rapid onset of fever, chills, headache, confusion, and segmental myoclonus.[5] This can rapidly progress to lethargy, disorientation, and coma. Clinical signs of brainstem dysfunction are common, and they include an impaired doll's eyes reflex and pupil abnormalities. Hypertension and tachycardia are also common. Laboratory investigation may reveal leukopenia, thrombocytopenia, and a mild transaminitis.[5,6] Evaluation of the cerebral spinal fluid may reveal leukocytosis, as well as elevated protein.[5,6] The underlying pathology appears to be a necrotizing vasculitis.[5]

PRE-INCIDENT ACTIONS

Pre-incident preparedness for viral infection of zoonotic illnesses includes knowledge of potential agents and training in the use of personal protective equipment (PPV) and surveillance systems that utilize epidemiologic methods to identify potential epidemics early on. In zoonotic illnesses it is imperative that medical personnel and veterinarians work cooperatively to identify new and emerging diseases. At the hospital level, there needs to be well-identified protocols for managing viral outbreaks and regular exercises to practice these responses. Care providers need to be knowledgeable in the use of PPV. Hospitals and local and national governments need a means to provide the necessary medical hardware to take care of large volumes of critically ill patients. The Centers for Disease Control and Prevention (CDC) or other international agencies need to maintain laboratories capable of identifying the potential culprit agents, and the ability to develop diagnostics, vaccines, and treatments.

A vaccine is currently licensed for use in horses, as well as a monoclonal antibody for postexposure prophylaxis, which is still in animal trials at this time. There is no current vaccine available for human use.[17,22]

POST-INCIDENT ACTION

If an outbreak of *Henipavirus* is suspected, it is imperative that the nation-specific epidemiologic institution, such as the CDC in the United States, be notified promptly. These viruses require a Biosafety Level 4 lab for isolation and identification.[18] Standard and respiratory precautions should be undertaken when treating patients with suspected *Henipavirus* disease. Laboratory isolation of the virus or viruses can be performed on infected tissue utilizing a number of techniques, including immunohistochemistry, PCR, and ELISA.[19] The destruction of infected animals can help to decrease zoonotic transmission.[5] Thus far, no human-to-human transmission has been reported.[4]

✚ MEDICAL TREATMENT OF CASUALTIES

Supportive care that includes respiratory support, intravenous hydration, antipyretics, and sedation is important to the initial management of patients infected with *Henipavirus*. There is some evidence to support the use of the antiviral ribavirin. This drug did show some promise in limited use in the Malaysian Nipah virus outbreak, as well as some evidence of in vitro effectiveness against Hendra virus.[7,9,20] The side effect profile of this drug may limit its use, but, being one of the only specific therapies, the benefits may outweigh the risks of this pharmaceutical agent. If utilized, the adult dosing is 30 mg/kg IV (max 2 g) followed by 16 mg/kg IV (max 1 g) every 6 hours for 4 days, then 8 mg/kg (max 500 mg) every 8 hours for 6 days. The pediatric dose is the same except the oral agent is used. The oral agent may be substituted in adults as well using the following regimen: 2-g loading dose, followed by 600 mg twice a day for 10 days.[21]

💡 UNIQUE CONSIDERATIONS

Both of these illnesses share characteristics common to several other diseases, and thus high clinical suspicion is imperative to recognition, diagnosis, and management. In the case of Hendra virus, exposure to sick horses with suspicious symptoms is a key historical clue. Working with swine or swine products provides similar evidence for infection with Nipah virus. Even though bats are a known carrier, it is not yet fully understood how transmission occurs among this species and humans. As mentioned previously, there is no known human-to-human exposure risk.

❗ PITFALLS

- Failure to identify the potential for infection with either of these or other novel henipaviruses can lead to delayed recognition and treatment.
- Failure to alert the CDC or other nation-specific relevant government agencies early in the course of the outbreak so that the pathogen can be identified and the appropriate measures instituted.
- Failure to appropriately manage the infection with supportive care and antivirals if indicated.

REFERENCES

1. Selvey LA, Wells RM, McCormack JG, et al. Infection of humans and horses by a newly described morbillivirus. *Med J Aust.* 1995;162(12):642–645.
2. Murray K, Selleck P, Hooper P, et al. A morbillivirus that caused fatal disease in horses and humans. *Science.* 1995;268(5207):94–97.
3. Field H, Young P, Yob JM, Mills J, Hall L, Mackenzie J. The natural history of Hendra and Nipah viruses. *Microbes Infect.* 2001;4:307–314.
4. Eaton B, Broder C, Middleton D, Wang L. Hendra and Nipah viruses: different and dangerous. *Nat Rev.* 2006;4:23–35.
5. Chua KB. Nipah virus outbreak in Malaysia. *J Clin Virol.* 2003;26(3):265–275.
6. Goh KJ, Tan CT, Chew NK, et al. Clinical features of Nipah virus encephalitis among pig farmers in Malaysia. *N Engl J Med.* 2000;342:1229–1235.
7. Aljofan M. Hendra and Nipah infection: emerging paramyxoviruses. *Virus Res.* 2013;177:119–126.
8. Lee KE, Umpathi T, Tan CB, et al. The neurologic manifestations of Nipah virus encephalitis, a novel paramyxovirus. *Ann Neurol.* 1999;46:428–432.
9. Chong HT, Kunjapan SR, Thayaparan T, et al. Nipah encephalitis outbreak in Malaysia: clinical features in patients from Seremban. *Can J Neurol Sci.* 2002;29:83–87.
10. Wang L, Harcourt B, Yu M, et al. Molecular biology of Hendra and Nipah viruses. *Microbes Infect.* 2001;3:279–287.
11. Xu K, Rockx B, Xie Y, et al. Crystal structure of the Hendra virus attachment G glycoprotein bound to a potent cross-reactive neutralizing human monoclonal antibody. *PLoS Pathog.* 2005;9(10):e1003684.
12. Eaton B, Broder C, Middleton D, Wang L. Hendra and Nipah viruses: different and dangerous. *Nat Rev.* 2006;4:23–35.
13. Ciancanelli M, Volchkova V, Shaw M, et al. Nipah virus sequesters inactive STAT1 in the nucleus via a P gene-encoded mechanism. *J Virol Methods.* 2009;83(16):02610–02618.
14. Stark G, Kerr I, Williams B, et al. How cells respond to interferons. *Annu Rev Biochem.* 1998;67:227–264.
15. Rodriguez J, Cruz C, Horvath C. Identification of the nuclear export signal and STAT-binding domains of the Nipah virus reveals mechanisms underlying interferon invasion. *J Virol.* 2004;78:5358–5367.
16. Lo M, Peeples M, Bellini W, et al. Distinct and overlapping roles of Nipah virus P gene products in modulating the human endothelial cell antiviral response. *PLoS One.* 2012;7(10).
17. Broder C, Xu K, Nikolov D, et al. A treatment for and vaccine against the deadly Hendra and Nipah Viruses. *Antiviral Res.* 2013;100:8–13.
18. Corrigan K. Hendra and Nipah Virus Attack (Hendra virus disease and Nipah virus encephalitis). In: *Disaster Medicine,* Ciottone. Philadelphia: Mosby Elsevier; 2006:693–694.
19. Daniels P, Ksiazek T, Eaton B. Laboratory diagnosis of Nipah and Hendra virus infection. *Microbes Infect.* 2001;3:289–295.
20. Wright P, Crameri G, Eaton B. RNA synthesis during infection by Hendra virus: an examination by quantitative real-time PCR of RNA accumulation, the effect of ribavirin and the attenuation of transcription. *Arch Virol.* 2005;150(3):521–532.
21. Brown D, Lloyd G. Zoonotic viruses. In: Cohen JM, Powderly WC, eds. *Infectious Diseases.* Philadelphia: Elsevier; 2004:2095–2109.
22. Broder C, Xu K, Nikolov D, et al. A treatment for and vaccine against the deadly Hendra and Nipah viruses. *Antiviral Res.* 2013;100:8–13.

SARS-CoV Attack (Severe Acute Respiratory Syndrome)

David Freeman and Elizabeth Kenez

DESCRIPTION OF EVENT

As you are completing a patient's chart in the emergency department (ED), the emergency medical service(s) (EMS) telephone rings. You pick up the phone and introduce yourself. In a muffled tone, the paramedic begins to provide a thorough report. He states that he is wearing an N-95 mask due to concern that the patient onboard may have a communicable disease. Your sympathetic tone kicks in as you listen to the report. The paramedic provides you with the following information:

- Middle-aged woman complaining of high fever, neck stiffness, shortness of breath, and nonproductive cough, and who had visited the same ED 2 days prior, for similar symptoms, and was sent home with instructions for flu-like syndrome. Patient denies chest pain.
- History: Hypertension
- Allergies: No known allergies
- Medications: Metoprolol
- Vital signs: Blood pressure 148/90. Heart rate 120. Sinus tachycardia, respiratory rate 26 and diminished bilaterally. Blood oxygen saturation 93% on room air. Unable to obtain temperature in the ambulance.
- Physical assessment: Limited assessment in the ambulance reveals a patient that is diaphoretic, tachycardic, and tachypneic. Nuchal rigidity is noted. Patient is only alert and oriented to person and place (not to time) and appears fatigued. Pupils are equally round and reactive to light.

Based on this report, what is the possible ailment? Could this be meningitis? Pneumonia? Severe acute respiratory syndrome (SARS)? You advise the staff caring for the patient in the ED to wear N-95 masks. You assess the patient while labs are drawn. You quickly perform a lumbar puncture while antibiotics are started for meningitis. You are shocked, however, when the lumbar puncture results come back normal. Her chest x-ray shows a severe bilateral pneumonia. You recall that there was a SARS outbreak two weeks prior in a local suburb. What if this patient had SARS? How would you have provided medical care to this patient without exposing yourself and others? Have you received training and preparation in managing a patient infected with SARS?

Our recent history and current events (at the time of this publication) have shown that SARS is a formidable, evolving virus, able to withstand changing environmental and human-made conditions, with the potential of infecting hundreds or even thousands of people. The SARS pandemic, beginning in late 2002 through mid-2003, proved that the world was not ready for such a biological catastrophe. On November 16, 2002, a patient in Guangdong, China, presented with an atypical pneumonia. Over the next several weeks and into early 2003, this atypical pneumonia spread throughout the southern border of China to Hong Kong and Vietnam, and across the Atlantic Ocean into Canada. On March 17, 2003, the Centers for Disease Control and Prevention (CDC) conducted its first briefing showing that this new virus had landed in the United States. In June 2003, the outbreak was finally contained, and the CDC removed air travel alerts from Hong Kong. During the outbreak, more than 8000 individuals became infected with SARS. Approximately 774 died in 26 countries over 5 continents. This pandemic demonstrated that the world and the medical community had not been prepared for such an event. Nevertheless, the international medical community showed its resiliency and the ability to join together for one cause.

In May 2012, a new respiratory virus related to SARS, MERS-CoV (Middle East respiratory syndrome or MERS), evolved in the Middle East. Saudi Arabian officials detected this new virus causing flu-like symptoms that rapidly evolved into respiratory distress, similar to SARS. To date, 808 people have become infected with MERS, and 311 of those individuals have died. This virus has spread to 21 countries, including the United States, France, Germany, Italy, Tunisia, and Great Britain. Investigations are currently under way. A recently published study in *The Journal of American Medical Association* (JAMA) shows that transmission of MERS to humans originated from dromedary camels.[1] Even though MERS-CoV is considered to be distinct from SARS-CoV,[2] individuals who have contracted the virus in the Middle East have died from respiratory and/or kidney failure.[3]

Terrorist attacks using biological agents such as SARS can be described as a type of *asymmetric warfare*. In asymmetric warfare, a single individual or group can cause damage and destruction to massive numbers of objects and/or people, with a small amount of ammunition, such as a biological agent.[4] However, using biological agents in a terrorist attack is highly expensive and sophisticated, and it takes many years to develop. When a terrorist decides to develop a biological agent, the individual or group must first locate scientists who are willing and able to conduct the development of the agent without exposure to themselves, exposure to the terrorist organization, or others. Second, the terrorist(s) must acquire the equipment needed to facilitate the development of the agent in a safe manner. Third, the development of the agent in mass quantities requires many years. Finally, synthesized agents require certain environmental conditions that must be met for appropriate dissemination. Because of these conditions, the world has been fortunate to not have fallen victim to such a terrorist attack to date.

The origin, its transmission mechanisms, effective treatment modality, and the full extent of SARS have yet to be fully understood; however, much information about SARS has been discovered. SARS is caused by SARS-CoV, which belongs to the Coronaviridae family. Coronaviruses are a family of enveloped, single-stranded ribonucleic acid (RNA) viruses with the ability to affect humans and animals. SARS-CoV is a polyadenylated, single-stranded virus, containing 29,727 nucleotides, making their genome the largest of any RNA virus.[5] Within the SARS-CoV genome, there are four major open reading frames (ORFs) that encode the structural proteins such as the nucleocapsid protein (N), envelope (E), spike (S), and membrane glycoproteins (M) that all contribute to replication. At each proximal end of the virus, there is 5′ methylated cap on one end, and the 3′ polyadenylated tail that enables the virus to attach to ribosomes for translation. SARS-CoV genome also contains a replicase gene (rep gene) that enables the virus to be transcribed into new RNA copies. Once the virus enters its host, the virus has high affinity to and it uses angiotensin-converting enzyme 2 (ACE2) receptors to infect cells.[6] These receptors are predominantly found in the lungs, kidneys, and gastrointestinal (GI) tract.

SARS-CoV is a virus that is disseminated from person to person through respiratory droplets and is able to infect hosts through the mucous membranes of the mouth, nose, or eyes. Once the virus is inside the host, the virus will bind to the ACE2 receptors using the spike (S). Through endocytosis, the virus will enter the cell. Once in the cytoplasm, the virus is translated and then transcribed into immature virions. These immature particles will progress to become mature, icosahedral-shaped viruses. Within vesicles, the newly formed viruses are released via exocytosis, to begin the replication cycle again while infecting the host.

SARS can affect individuals of any age, gender, race, and socioeconomic status. Even though the clinical manifestation of the SARS-CoV virus is nonspecific, the manifestations present similar to influenza. Once infected, signs and symptoms may appear within 2 to 14 days. Patients begin to develop a high fever (>100.4 °F [>38 °C]), followed by body aches, headache, and a mild lower-respiratory infection. In the lungs, the virus causes atelectasis, gross edema, desquamation of epithelial cells on the respiratory tract, and the development of fibrous tissues within alveolar spaces.[7] Many patients may develop pneumonia and hypoxia, which may progress rapidly, within hours to several days, into respiratory failure secondary to acute respiratory distress syndrome (ARDS). These respiratory symptoms may appear rapidly, within hours or over several days. Within the central nervous system (CNS), neural edema and degeneration have been seen. In the kidneys, necrotic tubular epithelial cells may result in renal dysfunction or failure. There is evidence attained through immunohistochemistry that SARS increases IgG precipitation, causing an immune response and increasing temperature, resulting in orchitis and the destruction of germ cells within the testes.[8] The immune system may also suffer damage. There may be extensive splenic necrosis, atrophy of the lymph nodes, and lymphopenia. SARS also affects the cardiovascular system as patients may develop vasculitis, pericarditis, and coagulopathy. Coagulopathy may result in disseminated intravascular coagulopathy (DIC). Gastrointestinal symptoms involve a range from nausea and vomiting to diarrhea from inflammation caused by infected epithelial cells. Hepatic steatosis and centrilobular necrosis may also be seen.[9] Box 152-1 summarizes the signs and symptoms of SARS.

◀ PRE-INCIDENT ACTIONS

Preparation is of utmost importance, and it begins with information sharing. Throughout history, many of the failures and shortcomings in mitigating catastrophes involve the lack of information sharing among all parties. This lack of sharing originates from egos of an individual or a group of individuals wanting to be the "hero." To prevent this, all health care providers must first acknowledge that they are part of a national and international team united by medicine, having a duty not only to themselves, their peers, and colleagues, but also to all

---

BOX 152-1 Summary of Signs and Symptoms of SARS*

General	Immunological
High fever (>100.4 °F [>38 °C])	Lymphopenia
Body aches	Necrosis of the spleen
Headache	Lymph node atrophy

Cardiovasular	Gastrointestinal
Vasculitis	Nausea
Coagulopathy	Vomiting
Pericarditis	Diarrhea

Respiratory	Urinary
Mild lower-respiratory infection	Renal dysfunction or failure
Atelectasis	
Pulmonary edema	**Reproductive (Males)**
Dry cough	Hepatic steatosis
Hypoxia	Orchitis
	Centrilobular necrosis
	Destruction of germ cells

SARS, Severe acute respiratory syndrome.

---

patients, especially when a contagious and communicable virus is involved. Information sharing is best achieved through education. This education begins with prioritizing the development of a disaster plan addressing outbreaks or biological attacks. The disaster plan should be a "living" document, able to be edited on a yearly basis to include surveillance for communicable and contagious diseases; notification of and joint efforts with outside agencies; and personal protective equipment (PPE)/universal precautions guidelines for all health care providers. Terminology within the disaster plan should be a universal language that is shared among police departments, fire departments, EMS, and state, local, and federal government personnel. This universal language can be achieved through using documents such as the National Incident Management System (NIMS) and the National Response Framework (NRF) from the Federal Emergency Management Agency (FEMA). Using these documents will assist in creating a disaster plan with interoperable communications, as well as in defining leadership, chain of command, roles and responsibilities, and interdepartmental efforts. The disaster plan should be made available to all personnel, and frequent mock evolutions should be performed on a bi-yearly or yearly basis. Hospitals and outpatient facilities should perform frequent mock evolutions individually and with outside agencies. With each evolution, debriefing sessions should occur to learn the strengths and weakness, so that changes and enhancements to the plan can be made. Many fire, police, and EMS departments require personnel to complete online FEMA courses through its Independent Study Program (ISP), which covers these topics in more detail. These courses are free of charge; each course takes 3 to 8 hours to complete, and the health care provider will receive a certificate of completion. Hospital administration may also require their health care employees to complete these courses. When all parties involved in patient treatment and mitigation can work together systematically, more time and more patients will be saved. The FEMA ISP website address and the courses designed specifically for hospitals and health care providers are listed in Box 152-2.

In syndromic surveillance, hospitals and outpatient centers will need to allocate resources to monitor a possible influx of respiratory illnesses, especially those accompanied by a high fever. When a suspicion of a communicable disease is confirmed, the disaster plan should include policies and procedures in contacting outside agencies. The plan should also contain the contact information of agencies and individuals who will be involved in the investigation and mitigation process. Immediate notification is a priority upon confirmation.

Policies and procedures for PPE and universal precautions guidelines for all health care providers should exist and be strictly enforced. Hand washing is paramount and is a basic skill to lessen the possibility of exposure to SARS-CoV. All necessary equipment and supplies to mitigate a possible exposure should be accrued prior to patient arrival or an outbreak. The equipment to mitigate SARS-CoV exposures includes N-95 masks, gloves, gowns, eye protection, shoe covers, and disinfectant such as sodium hypochlorite. All health care providers should be properly fitted for N-95 masks prior to any exposure.[10] Hospitals also should have ventilation and filtration systems tested, repaired, or updated to be fully operational in the event of a SARS outbreak.

Health care providers who conduct patient assessments and provide treatment should incorporate additional questions while assessing the history of present illness, to develop an earlier working diagnosis. Questions should include inquiring about any recent international travel to countries prior to declaring a SARS outbreak, or any exposure to people who may have recently traveled to those countries. Asking patients about their employment history and personal relationships could also provide invaluable information. Patients who work in a facility containing SARS-CoV, or a patient who lives with a person who is employed in a SARS-CoV-containing laboratory could also provide the etiology for the outbreak. Since the first SARS outbreak involved animal-to-human transmission, it may also be beneficial to inquire about exposures to any infected animals. If a health care provider or hospital has evaluated an influx of patients suffering from atypical pneumonia, notification of the proper personnel should begin. A summary of these questions is given in Box 152-3.

▷▷ POST-INCIDENT ACTIONS

If there is a high index of suspicion that a SARS exposure is imminent or has already occurred, immediate notification of hospital infection-control personnel should occur to notify proper authorities and agencies, beginning the information sharing and mitigation process. The earlier the notification, the faster and more efficient the mitigation of the outbreak can occur. Infection-control personnel should notify agencies such as the CDC and local police, fire, and EMS agencies. The public should be notified immediately. Hospital personnel should be used to disseminate the correct message to the public. This will assure that the public receives the necessary information, and minimize

panic. All healthcare personnel should adhere to the strictest universal precautions, such as mucous membrane protection with N-95 mask and eye protection. Gowns and scrubs should be used and then discarded upon completion of a shift, and they should not be removed from the building because that could cause contamination to others. Shoes should be covered with shoe covers. Rooms, equipment, and supplies that may have had exposure to SARS-CoV should be disinfected prior to being placed back into service or properly disposed of based on disaster plans. If invasive procedures are required for patient survival, the most-experienced providers should perform these procedures, using strict, aseptic technique. Infected patients who are admitted should be placed into quarantine rooms. Health care employees who have become exposed and are showing signs and symptoms of a SARS-CoV infection should be placed off duty until resolution of the infection. Procedures should be created, ensuring that these employees receive treatment and monitoring as their symptoms persist. Hospital personnel should use ventilation and filtration systems to minimize or prevent additional exposures. Patients who have become infected with SARS should be quarantined and not allowed to have visitors until resolution of symptoms.

EMS providers should also practice strict universal precautions because their risk of exposure and contraction of SARS-CoV is high because they are the first providers to render medical treatment to infected individuals who use prehospital emergency services. In a prospective observational study of an Asian metropolitan EMS system that was involved in the transport of patients during the SARS outbreak, EMS providers who transported patients with SARS were at higher risk of contracting SARS in comparison with the general population.[11] Proper medical evaluation and treatment of EMS providers are also recommended when a fever of over 38 °C is present. Within days of Ontario's declaring a provincial emergency due to the 2003 SARS outbreak, Toronto fire and police departments created a medical unit that was designed to support, educate, and evaluate EMS providers regarding the SARS outbreak. In this collaboration with a hospital-based medical director, EMS providers received daily medical support and evaluation to determine the extent of their infection and whether further treatment was needed.[12]

✚ MEDICAL TREATMENT OF CASUALTIES

Unlike hurricanes, earthquakes, and other natural disasters, biological attacks and outbreaks bring about a unique dynamic to patient treatment. In such natural disasters, traumatic injuries are primarily seen. During an outbreak or biological attack, physicians may see a combination of traumatic injuries and medical and psychological complications.

Similar to first responders who must properly allocate limited resources to facilitate the initial, high volume of patient triage and treatment, hospitals may also be faced with the same dilemmas. One of the major goals is to treat as many patients as possible in the quickest amount of time without exposure to health care personnel. However, many lessons were learned from the SARS outbreak in 2003. For example, because many health care workers had to work under extreme conditions, staff suffered from infections secondary to physical and mental exhaustion.[13]

Hospital personnel must effectively and rapidly triage patients, provide treatment, and request assistance early when resources begin to become scarce. There are several reasons why there could be an influx of hospital visits during an outbreak. First, many patients who are ill will still come for medical treatment. Many patients who have flu-like symptoms during an outbreak will wonder if they have been infected by the SARS-CoV and seek out medical treatment. Second, many asymptomatic people may panic and seek out medical evaluations. The media will play a significant role in peoples' perceptions. Many people may not be aware of the outbreak, and the tone of the reporters can influence the actions of others. However, the opposite could occur in the ED. In the 2003 outbreak, Toronto-based community hospitals saw a decrease in ED visits during the SARS outbreak. Even though many people considered the ED as a place of safety, many viewed the ED as the etiology for the outbreak and therefore avoided the ED.[14] It was determined that human-to-human transmission in Toronto originated in hospitals and households of infected individuals.[15] In the current MERS-CoV outbreak in the Middle East, the human-to-human transmission has been originating primarily in hospital settings. Saudi Arabian hospital surveillance in 2013 demonstrated that the etiology for the majority of transmissions occurred in the ICU, dialysis centers, and hospital wards.[16]

Treatment of individual patients during a SARS-CoV outbreak also brings about unique obstacles. Therefore treatment of SARS-infected patients should be patient-centered. To date, there are no effective antivirals or anti-inflammatory medications for the treatment of SARS-CoV.[17,18] However, experiments have been performed in attempts to produce a vaccination. One experiment used a portion of the S glycoprotein from the virus, as the foundation of the vaccine, and it was injected into mice. Addressing the glycoprotein as foreign, the immune system of the mice created a cell-mediated response through the creation of T cells and antibodies. When the immunized mice received the virus, replication of the virus within the nostrils and lungs was reduced.[18]

As many SARS-infected patients will develop respiratory complications secondary to pneumonia, emphasis must focus on airway management, the treatment of hypoxemia, and the prevention of multiple organ failure. This encompasses the early recognition of disease and aggressive resuscitation of the patient. As emphasized earlier, because of the high-stress, low-resource atmosphere, it is imperative that the most-experienced health care providers perform invasive procedures such as endotracheal intubation.[19] Endotracheal intubation should be considered for patients with respiratory distress, using the recommended ventilatory support with low-tidal volume settings.[20] Postintubation management should include continued resuscitation, pain management, and consideration of the broad differential diagnosis of a patient with rapid-onset respiratory distress.

![] UNIQUE CONSIDERATIONS

Unfortunately, in the event of an outbreak or biological attack, most of the actions performed to mitigate the catastrophe will be reactive, even though preparedness may be emphasized. This reactive mitigation results from the incubation time of the virus and the time

required for investigational and epidemiological reports to declare such an event. Because of its complex and resilient structure, SARS-CoV has the ability to adapt to adverse environments. This resiliency enables SARS-CoV to spread across various types of environments with the capability to quickly infect hosts. As the presenting signs and symptoms are nonspecific, many health care providers may treat the virus as an isolated infection, such as pneumonia, and release the patient to recover at home or admit the patient to the hospital floor without isolation. Similar to the Tokyo Sarin subway attack in 1995, terrorists may use an aerosolized form of the SARS-CoV virus to disseminate into a highly populated area. To lessen the effects of an outbreak or biological attack, health care providers must continually "think outside the box," and remember to keep their differential diagnosis for a patient with rapidly progressing flu symptoms broad, considering viruses such as SARS-CoV and other potential agents of biological warfare.

[!] PITFALLS

- Failure to focus on preparation through the design of a comprehensive, "living" disaster plan that is modifiable based on up-to-date information
- Failure to practice disaster plans through training evolutions to evaluate interoperability, communications, and the integration of resources among agencies
- Failure to provide early notification and updates to public health agencies when there is a possible SARS outbreak
- Failure to notify the public of an outbreak or attack or failure to provide thorough and proper notification to guide the future actions of the mitigation process[21]
- Failure to assess resources prior to a SARS outbreak or biological attack
- Failure to quarantine patients who present with possible SARS-CoV infection: remember, one person with the infection can cause a major spread of the disease[22]
- Failure to educate health care providers on the clinical manifestations of SARS-CoV
- Failure to perform a comprehensive medical history including travel, living, and workplace arrangements
- Failure to adhere to strict universal precautions anytime while performing physical examinations and providing medical treatment
- Failure to sterilize or dispose of equipment used in the treatment of infected patients
- Ultimately, failure of health care providers to "think outside the box"

REFERENCES

1. Friedrich MJ. Dromedary camels and MERS. *JAMA*. 2014;311(51):1489.
2. *Genetic Sequence Information for Scientists about the Novel Coronavirus 2012*. London: Health Protection Agency; 2012. http://webarchive. nationalarchives.gov.uk/20140714084352/http://www.hpa.org.uk/webw/ HPAweb&HPAwebStandard/HPAweb_C/1317136246479.
3. Memish ZA, Zumla AI, Al-Hakeeem RF, et al. Family cluster of Middle East respiratory syndrome coronavirus infection. *N Engl J Med*. 2013;368 (26):2487–2494.
4. Cordesman A. *Terrorism, asymmetric warfare, and weapons of mass destruction: defending the U.S. homeland*. Center for Strategic and International Studies; 2002, 1–10.
5. Rota P, Oberste MS, Monroe SS, et al. Characterization of a novel coronavirus associated with severe acute respiratory syndrome. *Science*. 2003;300(5624):1394–1399.

6. Wenhui LI, Greenough T, Moore M, et al. Efficient replication of severe acute respiratory syndrome coronavirus in mouse cell is limited by murine angiotensin-converting enzyme 2. *J Virol.* 2004;78 (20):11429–11433.

7. Xu J, Lihua Q, Xiaochin C, et al. Orchitis: a complication of severe acute respiratory syndrome (SARS). *Biol Reprod.* 2005;74(2):410–416.

8. Shi X, Gong E, Zhang B, et al. Severe acute respiratory syndrome associated is detected in intestinal tissues of fatal cases. *Am J Gastroenterol.* 2005;100:169–176.

9. Seto WH, Tsang D, Yung RW, et al. Effectiveness of precautions against droplets and contact in prevention of nosocomial transmission of severe acute respiratory syndrome (SARS). *Lancet.* 2003;361 (9368):1519–1520.

10. Ko PC, Chen WJ, Ma M, et al. Emergency medical services utilization during an outbreak of severe acute respiratory syndrome (SARS) and the incidence of SARS-associated coronavirus infection among emergency medical technicians. *Acad Emerg Med.* 2004;11(9):903–910.

11. Silverman A, Simor A, Loutfy M. Toronto emergency medical services and SARS. *Emerg Infect Dis.* 2004;10(9):1688–1689.

12. Lai T, Yu W. The lessons of SARS in Hong Kong. *Clin Med.* 2010;10 (1):50–53.

13. Heiber M, Lou WY. Effect of the SARS outbreak on visits to a community hospital emergency department. *Can J Emerg Med.* 2006;8(5):323–328.

14. Svoboda T, Henry B, Shulman L. Public health measures to control the spread of the severe acute respiratory syndrome during the outbreak in Toronto. *N Engl J Med.* 2004;350(23):2352–2359.

15. Assiri A, McGeer A, Perl TM, et al. Hospital outbreak of Middle East respiratory syndrome coronavirus. *N Engl J Med.* 2013;369(5):407–416.

16. Peiris JSM, Yuen KY, Osterhaus ADME, et al. Current concepts: the severe acute respiratory syndrome. *N Engl J Med.* 2003;349(25):2431–2441.

17. Rubenfeld GD. Is SARS just ARDS. *JAMA.* 2003;290(3):397–399.

18. Johnston RE. A Candidate vaccine for severe acute respiratory syndrome. *N Engl J Med.* 2004;351(8):827–828.

19. Wong E, Ho KH. The effect of severe acute respiratory syndrome (SARS) on emergency airway management. *Resuscitation.* 2006;70(1):26–30.

20. Mazulli T, Farcas GA, Poutanen SM, et al. Severe acute respiratory syndrome-associated coronavirus in lung tissue. *Emerg Infect Dis.* 2004;10:20–30.

21. Anderson LJ, Baric RS. Emerging human coronavirus—disease potential and preparedness. *N Engl J Med.* 2012;367:1850–1852.

22. Weinstein RA. Planning for epidemics—the lessons of SARS. *N Engl J Med.* 2004;350(23):2332–2334.

Staphylococcal Enterotoxin B Attack

Robert G. Darling

DESCRIPTION OF EVENT

Staphylococcus aureus produces a number of exotoxins, including staphylococcal enterotoxin B (SEB). Such toxins are referred to as exotoxins because they are excreted from the organism that synthesizes them. Because they normally exert their pathological effects on the gastrointestinal tract, they are also called enterotoxins. SEB causes a markedly different clinical syndrome when inhaled than it characteristically produces when ingested. Significant morbidity is produced in persons who are exposed to this toxin by either portal of entry to the body.

SEB is one of the most common causes of food poisoning. It is a pyrogenic toxin, which commonly causes food poisoning in humans when improperly handled foodstuffs are contaminated with *S. aureus*, which in turn produces and releases SEB into the food that is subsequently ingested, causing illness. Often these outbreaks occur in a setting such as a picnic or other community event due to a common source exposure in which contaminated food is consumed. Although an aerosolized SEB toxin weapon would not likely produce significant mortality, it could render a significant percentage of an exposed population clinically ill for 1 to 2 weeks.[1] The demand on the medical and logistical systems could be overwhelming. For these reasons SEB was one of several biological agents stockpiled by the United States during its biological weapons program, which was terminated in 1969.[2]

Staphylococcal enterotoxins are proteins produced by coagulase-positive staphylococci. Up to 50% of clinical isolates of *S. aureus* produce exotoxins. They are produced in culture media and also in foods when there is overgrowth of the organism. SEB is one of at least seven antigenically distinct, moderately stable enterotoxins that have been identified. SEB causes symptoms in humans when inhaled at doses at least 100 times less than the lethal dose that would be sufficient to incapacitate 50% of those exposed.[1] This toxin could also be used to sabotage food or small-volume water supplies.

Staphylococcal enterotoxins belong to a class of potent immune stimulants known as bacterial superantigens.[3] Superantigens bind to monocytes at major histocompatibility complex type II receptors rather than the usual antigen-binding receptors. This leads to the direct stimulation of large populations of T-helper lymphocytes while bypassing the usual antigen processing and presentation pathway. This induces a brisk cascade of proinflammatory cytokines (such as tumor necrosis factor, interferon, interleukin-1, and interleukin-2), with recruitment of other immune effector cells and relatively deficient activation of counter-regulatory immune inhibitory mechanisms. This results in an intense inflammatory response that injures host tissues. These cytokines are thought to mediate many of the toxic effects of SEB.[4]

Symptoms of SEB intoxication begin after a latent period of 3 to 12 hours after inhalation or 4 to 10 hours after ingestion. It is important to note that SEB causes an intoxication, not an infection. The delay in onset of symptoms is the time for the SEB toxin to be absorbed and to cause clinical illness by its toxic effects. A similar delay in onset of illness (i.e., the incubation period) is seen with infectious agents (e.g., anthrax and tularemia) and is the time for the organism to multiply to a level that causes clinical illness. Symptoms include nonspecific flu-like symptoms (e.g., fever, chills, headache, and myalgias) and specific clinical features dependent on the route of exposure. Oral exposure results in predominantly gastrointestinal symptoms: nausea, vomiting, and diarrhea. Inhalation exposures produce predominantly respiratory symptoms: nonproductive cough, retrosternal chest pain, and dyspnea. Gastrointestinal symptoms may accompany respiratory exposure due to inadvertent swallowing of the toxin after normal mucociliary clearance of toxin-containing secretions from the respiratory tract. Exposure to aerosolized SEB may cause mucous membrane irritation (e.g., conjunctivitis).

Respiratory pathology is due to the activation of proinflammatory cytokine cascades in the lungs, leading to pulmonary capillary leakage and pulmonary edema. Severe cases may result in acute noncardiogenic pulmonary edema and respiratory failure.[5] Fever may last up to 5 days and range from 103 to 106 °F with variable degrees of chills and prostration. Patients may not fully recover for 2 weeks and the cough may persist up to 4 weeks.

Physical examination in patients with SEB intoxication is often unremarkable. Conjunctival injection may be present, and postural hypotension may develop due to fluid losses. Chest examination is unremarkable except in the unusual case in which pulmonary edema develops and rales may be heard on auscultation. Generally the chest x-ray is normal, but in severe cases increased interstitial markings, atelectasis, and possibly overt pulmonary edema or adult respiratory distress syndrome may be seen.

PRE-INCIDENT ACTIONS

It is essential that hospitals have a well-developed emergency response plan that is regularly exercised by hospital staff and is well integrated into community, state, and federal emergency response plans. There should be robust plans in place to expand patient care facilities to accommodate large numbers of sick patients who self-refer or who arrive by ambulance, possibly within a span of hours. At the present time there is no vaccine available for human use to protect against aerosol exposure to SEB. However, animals studies are promising and human trials may begin soon.[6,7]

POST-INCIDENT ACTIONS

Identifying aerosolized SEB as the cause of a mass casualty event will be difficult unless the health care provider considers exposure to this toxin early in the course of the event. One must maintain a high index of suspicion. The differential diagnosis for patients presenting with a febrile respiratory illness is quite large and involves most respiratory pathogens, including many bacteria and viruses. Diagnosis of SEB intoxication is based on clinical and epidemiologic features. The symptoms of SEB intoxication may be similar to several respiratory pathogens, such as influenza, adenovirus, and mycoplasma. Patients might present with fever, nonproductive cough, myalgias, and headache. The epidemiologic pattern of the illness outbreak is a critical clue for determining the causative agent of and the circumstances leading to the epidemic (i.e., naturally occurring vs. bioweapon attack). SEB attack would cause cases to present in large numbers over a very short period of time, probably within a single 24-hour period. Naturally occurring pneumonias or influenza would involve patients presenting over a more prolonged interval of time. Persons with naturally occurring staphylococcal food poisoning would not exhibit pulmonary symptoms. Because it is not an infection, SEB intoxication tends to plateau rapidly to a fairly stable clinical state, whereas inhalational anthrax, tularemia pneumonia, or pneumonic plague would all continue to progress if left untreated. Tularemia, plague, and Q fever would be associated with infiltrates on chest x-rays. Other diseases, including hantavirus pulmonary syndrome, chlamydia pneumonia infection, and chemical warfare agent (e.g., mustard and phosgene) inhalation, should also be considered.

Laboratory confirmation of SEB intoxication includes antigen detection enzyme-linked immunosorbent assay and electrochemiluminescence on environmental and clinical samples and gene amplification techniques (polymerase chain reaction to detect staphylococcal genes) on environmental samples.[8] SEB may not be detectable in serum by the time symptoms occur. However, a serum specimen should be drawn as early as possible after exposure. SEB accumulates in the urine and can be detected for several hours after exposure. Therefore urine samples should also be obtained and tested for SEB. Respiratory secretions and nasal swabs may demonstrate the toxin early (within 24 hours of exposure). Because most patients will develop a significant antibody response to the toxin, acute and convalescent sera should be drawn for retrospective diagnosis. Nonspecific findings include a neutrophilic leukocytosis, an elevated erythrocyte sedimentation rate, and chest x-ray abnormalities consistent with pulmonary edema.

Once a mass casualty situation is recognized as a possible bioterrorism event, the hospital's emergency plan should be activated. Simultaneously, public health and law enforcement officials should be notified. An epidemiologic investigation should begin immediately.

Standard precautions are sufficient because SEB intoxication is not contagious and secondary aerosol production is unlikely. Decontamination with soap and water is sufficient.

MEDICAL TREATMENT OF CASUALTIES

Supportive care is the current mainstay of treatment. Attention to oxygenation and hydration is essential. Most patients' conditions will quickly stabilize after the acute phase of the illness. Rarely, some patients may develop acute pulmonary edema requiring intubation and mechanical ventilation.

UNIQUE CONSIDERATIONS

SEB toxin is one of the most ubiquitous toxins in nature and in its natural state is one of the most common causes of human food poisoning. However, respiratory disease caused by exposure to an SEB aerosol is never a natural event and will almost certainly be due to either a laboratory accident or bioterrorism.

The U.S. government weaponized SEB in the 1960s and investigated its use on the battlefield as an incapacitating agent.[2] The toxin was especially attractive because of the extremely small doses required to cause incapacitating illness in soldiers. The incapacitating dose, or effective dose to produce 50% casualties (ED_{50}), was found to be 0.0004 µg/kg; the lethal dose (LD_{50}) was estimated to be 0.02 µg/kg. Both measurements were taken in terms of the inhalational route.[2]

Ingestion of SEB toxin causes classic food poisoning: nausea, vomiting, and diarrhea without fever. Aerosol exposure produces a far different clinical picture, consisting of fever, headache, severe respiratory distress, and sometimes nausea, vomiting, and diarrhea. The gastrointestinal symptoms seen after aerosol exposure are most likely due to the swallowing of toxin from respiratory tract secretions and are not likely to be as severe as those seen in primary gastrointestinal SEB exposure.

Prophylactic administration of an investigational vaccine protects laboratory animals against aerosol exposure and is nearing transition for study in humans.[6] However, it is not currently available for clinical use.

PITFALLS

Several potential pitfalls in response to an SEB attack exist, including the following:

- Failure to consider aerosolized SEB as the potential cause for large numbers of patients presenting with an acute febrile respiratory illness
- Failure to notify laboratory personnel of a suspected case of SEB intoxication and failure to collect appropriate clinical specimens to aid in the diagnosis, including nasal swabs and urine
- Failure to notify appropriate law enforcement and public health authorities in the event of a suspected biological attack

REFERENCES

1. Hursh S, McNally R, Fanzone Jr. J, Meshon M. *Staphylococcal Enterotoxin B Battlefield Challenge Modeling with Medical and Non-Medical Countermeasures. Technical Report MBDRP-95-2.* Joppa, MD: Science Applications International Corp; 1995.
2. Ulrich, Robert G., SHELDON SIDELL, and THOMAS J. TAYLOR. "Staphylococcal enterotoxin B and related pyrogenic toxins." Medical aspects of chemical and biological warfare (1997): 621–630.
3. Ulrich RG, Bavari S, Olson M. Bacterial superantigens in human diseases: structure, function and diversity. *Trends Microbiol.* 1995;3:463–468.

4. Stiles BG, Bavari S, Krakauer T, et al. Toxicity of staphylococcal enterotoxins potentiated by lipopolysaccharide: major histocompatibility complex class II molecule dependency and cytokine release. *Infect Immun.* 1993;61:5333–5338.

5. Mattix ME, Hunt RE, Wilhelmsen CL, et al. Aerosolized staphylococcal enterotoxin B–induced pulmonary lesions in rhesus monkeys (*Macaca mulatta*). *Toxicol Pathol.* 1995;23:262–268.

6. Coffman JD, Zhu J, Roach JM, et al. Production and purification of a recombinant staphylococcal enterotoxin B vaccine candidate expressed in Escherichia coli. *Protein Expr Purif.* 2002;24:302–312.

7. Lindsay CD, Griffiths GD. Addressing bioterrorism concerns: options for investigating the mechanism of action of *Staphylococcus aureus* enterotoxin B. *Hum Exp Toxicol.* 2013 Jun;32(6):606–619.

8. USAMRIID's Medical Management of Biological Casualties Handbook. 7th ed. August 2011. Fort Detrick, Md. Available at: http://www.usamriid .army.mil/education/bluebookpdf/USAMRIID%20BlueBook%207th% 20Edition%20-%20Sep%202011.pdf.

Clostridium botulinum Toxin (Botulism) Attack

Janna H. Villano and Gary M. Vilke

DESCRIPTION OF EVENT

Botulinum toxin has been used by terrorists as a bioweapon, although unsuccessfully, on several occasions. In these instances, Clostridium botulinum was obtained from soil and cultivated, and the toxin was then collected. The attacks likely failed because of faulty microbiologic techniques, deficient aerosol-generating equipment, or internal sabotage.[1] As with many biologic agents, it is not likely that a terrorist attack using botulinum toxin will be reported or even noticed at the time it occurs.

Adult botulism is usually contracted through consumption of contaminated food, though alternative routes are possible. There is a variable delay before the effects of poisoning become clinically apparent, depending on the route of exposure, with as little as 2 hours before onset of symptoms and up to a week or more after ingestion. The majority of patients will present between 12 and 72 hours, initially with symptoms of prominent bulbar palsies, including blurred vision, mydriasis, diplopia, ptosis, and photophobia. Dysarthria, dysphonia, and dysphagia also tend to present early in the clinical course and are commonly misdiagnosed. Patients will be afebrile with a clear sensorium and, as symptoms progress, will develop progressive, symmetric, descending skeletal muscle paralysis to the point of respiratory failure when muscles of respiration become involved. The degree of respiratory failure may not be readily apparent because of an inability to exhibit appropriate expressions of distress given paralysis of facial musculature.[2]

PRE-INCIDENT ACTIONS

Background knowledge of C. botulinum, the bacterium that produces botulinum toxin, is critical if diagnosis and treatment are to be rendered in a timely manner to prevent significant casualties from an exposure, either accidental or intentional. Botulinum toxins comprise a family of neurotoxic proteins produced and secreted by four different clostridium anaerobic bacteria, including C. botulinum.[3] There are seven serotypes, A through G, that are produced by different strains of the bacteria, all acting by similar mechanisms and with slight variations in their effects. Although technical factors would make such dissemination very difficult, a single gram of crystalline toxin, effectively weaponized and aerosolized, would kill more than 1 million people.[1] These toxins are the most poisonous substances known with an oral dose lethal to 50% of an exposed population (LD_{50}) estimated (based on primate studies) to be 1.3 to 2 ng/kg when given intravenously, 10 to 20 ng/kg inhaled, and 1 mcg/kg when given orally.[1] However, lower figures have been reported.[2,4] In outbreak situations, not all persons may be affected.[2,5]

Botulinum toxin acts within the presynaptic nerve terminal of the neuromuscular junction and at cholinergic autonomic synapses. Botulinum toxin is a simple dichain polypeptide that consists of a 100-kDa

"heavy" chain joined by a single disulfide bond to a 50-kDa "light" chain. The toxin's light chain is a zinc-containing endopeptidase that cleaves one or more fusion proteins, which blocks acetylcholine-containing vesicles from fusing with the terminal membrane of motor neurons, thereby preventing the presynaptic release of acetylcholine.[6] This cascade disrupts cholinergic neurotransmission, generating the clinical findings of descending flaccid paralysis. (These findings differentiate it from tetanus, which causes spastic paralysis.) Inhibition of acetylcholine release also causes dry mucous membranes, as is seen in anticholinergic poisoning. Although nerve agent poisoning also causes muscular paralysis, the cholinergic finding of copious secretions and rapidity of onset of symptoms typically differentiates this from botulism. Ganglionic adrenergic blockade also occurs, though without significant clinical effects.[2]

If an intentional threat is identified by intelligence with adequate lead time, botulinum toxin vaccines can be considered for use in the population at risk. The vaccine is developed by treating the toxin with formalin, destroying its toxicity but maintaining its antigenic properties. The pentavalent botulinum toxoid presently available is administered via an investigational protocol at 0, 2, and 12 weeks, followed by annual booster doses.[7] Eighty percent of patients receiving the vaccine will develop protective titers at 14 weeks, but almost all will not have any measurable titer just before receiving the first booster dose.[8] The 1-year booster dose will result in a robust response in almost all patients. Clinical experience with the investigational vaccine in many persons, mostly military personnel, reflects that it is safe and effective. A recombinant vaccine is also in developmental stages.[7]

It is also important to identify the closest source of any botulinum antitoxin via the local health department so that it can be located quickly if needed.

POST-INCIDENT ACTIONS

Post-incident actions include early diagnosis, initiation of treatment, and timely reporting. With the presentation of a single patient, the diagnosis can be challenging. The classic presentation is an acute, symmetric, descending flaccid paralysis with bulbar musculature involvement in an afebrile, alert patient. Vitals signs are usually unaffected, though mild hypotension may occur. Multiple cranial nerve palsies are always associated with symptomatic botulism exposures. The clinical presentation is often confused early with other neuromuscular disorders, such as myasthenia gravis, Guillain-Barré syndrome, or tick paralysis.[9] However, these medical conditions generally do not produce outbreaks, so multiple presentations with similar symptoms support the diagnosis.[2] In the evaluation of such a patient, the edrophonium (Tensilon) test for myasthenia gravis may have transiently positive results for botulism. Electromyelography testing characteristically shows normal nerve conduction velocity and sensory nerve function, small amplitude motor potentials, and an incremental response (facilitation) to repetitive stimulation. The cerebral spinal fluid analysis in patients with botulism is normal. Laboratory testing is of little utility in the clinical diagnosis of botulism.

Diagnosis is confirmed with a mouse bioassay neutralization test, which demonstrates botulinum toxin in bodily fluids or food, etc. This test is available at the Centers for Disease Control and Prevention (CDC) and a number of state and municipal public health laboratories. Samples used for this assay can include serum, stool, gastric aspirate, vomitus, and suspected contaminated foods. Serotyping of the botulinum toxin is by neutralization of the bioassay with the appropriate botulinum antisera (serotypes A through G). Because a terrorist attack is a criminal event, it is important to treat all laboratory samples collected as evidence, maintaining an appropriate chain of custody between collection and delivery to the testing agency. Serum samples must be obtained before therapy with antitoxin because it nullifies the diagnostic mouse bioassay. The mouse bioassay can detect as little as 0.03 ng of botulinum toxin and usually yields results in 1 to 2 days.[10] Fecal and gastric specimens can also be anaerobically cultured, with results typically available in 7 to 10 days. Toxin production by culture isolates is then confirmed by the mouse bioassay. Mass spectrometry can be used as well with limited availability.[11] Typically, the diagnosis of botulism will be made on clinical grounds, especially in the setting of an outbreak. Treatment should not be withheld while awaiting results of confirmatory testing.

If a respiratory route of exposure is suspected, then persons in the area where the patient was exposed should wear full-face respirators and follow universal precautions to protect themselves from residual aerosolized toxin. Environmental persistence of botulinum toxin is difficult to determine after an initial release. Conditions such as weaponization techniques, humidity, temperature, wind, and size of aerosol particles will determine the rate of atmospheric dissipation. The toxin does not penetrate intact skin, but toxin can be absorbed through mucosal surfaces, the eyes, and non-intact skin. While universal precautions should be exercised, special protective clothing is not necessary for caregivers. Botulism is not contagious, and no case of person-to-person transmission has been described.[2]

Local and state health authorities must be notified quickly for several reasons. They assist in obtaining botulinum antitoxin to treat current patients and to arrange for assay tests to confirm the toxin. Additionally, health authorities assess the route of exposure and initiate tracking of other potential victims in need of treatment. If a terrorist attack is suspected, local, state, and federal law enforcement and emergency management agencies must be notified as early as possible. This will facilitate criminal investigations and initiate activation of federal response assets, such as the Strategic National Stockpile (SNS), if needed.

The toxin is heat sensitive. Heating contaminated food or drink to an internal temperature of 85 °C for at least 5 minutes will detoxify contaminated products; contaminated food products should be removed from public access and submitted to health officials for testing. Decontamination of equipment can be accomplished by heating to 85 °C for 10 minutes or with 0.1% hypochlorite bleach solution, though contaminated surfaces should be avoided for hours to days to allow natural degradation to occur. Aerosolized toxin is degraded most quickly with extremes of temperature and humidity, though based on weather conditions, particles will dissipate.[1]

✚ MEDICAL TREATMENT OF CASUALTIES

The two main treatment modalities available for managing botulism patients are supportive therapy and antitoxin administration. Treatment of botulism is largely supportive, including ventilator support if respiratory failure develops. Some patients may be mildly affected, whereas others may become completely paralyzed, appear comatose, and require months of ventilatory support. The rapidity of onset is proportional to the amount of toxin absorbed into the circulation. Symptoms of foodborne botulism may begin as early as 2 hours or as long as 8 days after ingestion of toxin.[10] The time to onset of inhalational botulism in humans was approximately 72 hours after exposure in the three known cases reported of accidental inhalational exposure to reaerosolized toxin (botulinum toxin serotype A) in a laboratory setting.[12]

Supportive therapy involves mechanical ventilation when appropriate, and often long-term enteral feeding is necessary. However, enteral feeding is often difficult in paralyzed botulism patients because of smooth muscle paralysis in the gastrointestinal tract. Patients with protracted ileus may need prolonged parenteral nutritional support. In patients who do not require mechanical ventilation but have some degree of respiratory insufficiency, reverse Trendelenburg's position of 20 to 25 degrees with cervical stabilization on a rigid mattress is reported to potentially improve ventilation and respiratory excursion by reducing entry of oral secretions into the airway and by suspending more of the weight of the abdominal viscera from the diaphragm.[1] Up to 20% of patients involved in foodborne outbreaks require mechanical ventilation, and more than 60% of children suffering infant botulism require ventilation.[13,14] Frequently repeated bedside spirometry, including negative inspiratory force and vital capacity, is used to assess diaphragmatic function and respiratory status. Indication for intubation is a vital capacity less than 12 to 15 mL/kg or 30%.[15]

Antibiotics have no role in most cases of acute botulism; however, it is often recommended that patients suffering from wound botulism be treated with penicillin to eliminate the source of the toxin.[16] Patients with botulism are prone to secondary infections, particularly ventilator-associated pneumonia. If antibiotics are required for secondary infections, aminoglycosides and clindamycin are contraindicated because they can exacerbate neuromuscular blockade.[17,18] Use of activated charcoal has no reported benefit in the treatment of foodborne botulism.

Unlike nerve agent exposures that involve excess acetylcholine at the neuromuscular junction because of inhibition of acetylcholinesterase, botulism is caused by a lack of acetylcholine in the synapse. Therefore, pharmacologic treatments such as atropine are relatively contraindicated and could worsen the symptoms.

Beyond supportive therapy, the mainstay of treatment rests with the early use of botulinum antitoxin. Early administration of passive neutralizing antibody is critical, so that the agent might bind with circulating toxin before it becomes tissue-bound. Antitoxin will minimize subsequent nerve damage and severity of disease but will not reverse existent paralysis.[19] Antitoxin should be administered to patients with neurologic signs of botulism as soon as possible and must not be delayed for laboratory confirmatory testing. In the United States, botulinum antitoxin is available from the CDC via state and local health departments and the SNS. While there were previously multiple forms available, the CDC now offers only the heptavalent antitoxin (HBAT) to treat noninfant forms of foodborne botulism in the United States. This antitoxin was previously investigational and was recently approved by the FDA.[20] Equine-derived HBAT contains 1000 to 8500 IU of antibodies A-G, though 90% of the preparation is despeciated by cleaving the Fc fragments from the horse immunoglobulin molecules, eliminating or limiting the chance of allergic reaction. Because Fab fragments are cleared from circulation more quickly than intact immunoglobulines, repeat dosing may be indicated.[21] A human-derived immunoglobulin, BabyBIG, is available for treatment of infant botulism types A and B from the California Infant Botulism Treatment and Prevention Program.[22] However, BabyBIG is only FDA-approved for treatment of infantile botulism and is not available in large supply.

Use of the equine antitoxin requires skin testing for horse serum sensitivity prior to use. This is performed by injecting 0.1 mL of a 1:10 sterile dilution of antitoxin intradermally and observing for 20 minutes. The skin test result is considered positive if any of the following ensue: fever or chills; hypotension with a drop of 20 mm Hg in the systolic and diastolic blood pressures; hyperemic skin induration > 0.5 cm; nausea and vomiting; shortness of breath or wheezing; or skin rash or generalized itching. If any of these reactions occur, desensitization should be performed, and allergy specialist consultation is advised. Even if the skin test result is negative, anaphylaxis may still occur unpredictably. If no allergic reactions occur, then the dose of 10 mL of antitoxin is given as a single intravenous dose in saline over 20 to 30 minutes. Pretreatment with intravenous diphenhydramine 50 mg and possibly an H2 blocker is recommended as well as having epinephrine immediately available in case an anaphylactic reaction does occur.

Recovery results from new motor axon twigs that sprout to reinnervate paralyzed muscle fibers—a process that, in adults, may take weeks or months to complete.[23]

💡 UNIQUE CONSIDERATIONS

Multiple routes of exposure to botulism exist. Intestinal and wound botulism result from the production of botulinum toxin in devitalized tissue in a wound or the intestine. Neither is usually considered to be from an act of bioterrorism. Iatrogenic botulism by injection for cosmetic or therapeutic purposes has occurred but is considered to be an impractical terrorist vehicle because of low concentrations of toxin.[1] However, foodborne botulism can be either natural or intentional, and the aerosolized route is highly likely to be intentional. No cases of waterborne botulism have ever been reported.[24] A mathematical model of a cow-to-consumer supply chain release of bolutinum toxin for a single milk-processing facility indicates that a minimal amount of toxin is required to do damage. Researchers recommend increased investigation of heat pasteurization to decrease this threat.[25]

The rapidity with which patients present largely depends on the route of exposure and the dose absorbed. However during outbreaks, not all exposed persons may manifest symptoms.[2] Symptoms may not appear for several days if the toxin is inhaled in lower concentrations, but they may appear earlier if inhaled in higher concentrations or if absorbed by ingestion. With ingestion, the course from onset of symptoms to respiratory failure has progressed in less than 24 hours.

There is no indication that treatment of children, pregnant women, and immunocompromised persons with botulism should differ from standard therapy.[1] Children and pregnant women have received equine antitoxin without apparent short-term adverse effects; however, the risks to fetuses of exposure to equine antitoxin are unknown.[26–29] Human-derived neutralizing antibody, Botulism Immune Globulin, decreases the risk of allergic reactions that are associated with equine botulinum antitoxin, but use of this product is limited to suspected cases of infant botulism.[30]

⚠ PITFALLS

Several potential pitfalls in response to a botulism attack exist. These include the following:

- Failure to consider the diagnosis of botulism in a patient presenting with descending paralysis
- Failure to notify local and state health authorities as soon as possible to access botulism antitoxin in an expedited fashion
- Failure to make the clinical diagnosis of botulism if multiple patients present with bulbar and cranial nerve palsies and a descending paralysis
- Exacerbation and prolongation of neuromuscular blockade with use of aminoglycosides and clindamycin in patients with botulism

REFERENCES

1. Arnon SS, Schechter R, Inglesby TV, et al. Working Group on Civilian Biodefense. Botulinum toxin as a biological weapon: medical and public health management. *JAMA.* 2001;285:1059–1070.
2. Sobel J. Botulism. *Clin Infect Dis.* 2005;41:1167–1173.
3. Peck MW. Biology and genomic analysis of *Clostridium botulinum. Adv Microb Physiol.* 2009;55:183–265.
4. McNally RE, Morrison MB, Berndt JE, et al. *Effectiveness of Medical Defense Interventions Against Predicted Battlefield Levels of Botulinum Toxin A,* vol. 1 Joppa, MD: Science Applications International Corporation; 1994, 3.
5. Kalluri P, Crowe C, Reller M, et al. An outbreak of foodborne botulism associated with food sold at a salvage store in Texas. *Clin Infect Dis.* 2003;37(11):1490–1495.
6. Montecucco C, ed. Clostridial neurotoxins: the molecular pathogenesis of tetanus and botulism. In: *Curr Top Microbiol Immunol.* 1995;195:1–278.
7. Smith L. Botulism and vaccines for its prevention. *Vaccine.* 2009;27: D33–D39.
8. Middlebrook JL. Contributions of the U.S. Army to botulinum toxin research. In: Das Grupa B, ed. *Botulinum and Tetanus Neurotoxins and Biomedical Aspects.* New York: Plenum Press; 1993:515–519.
9. Schantz EJ, Johnson EA. Properties and use of botulinum toxin and other microbial neurotoxins in medicine. *Microbiol Rev.* 1992;56:80–99.
10. Terranova W, Breman JG, Locey RP, et al. Botulism type B: epidemiological aspects of an extensive outbreak. *Am J Epidemiol.* 1978;108:150–156.
11. Joseph B, Brown CV, Diven C, et al. Current concepts in the management of biologic and chemical warfare casualties. *J Trauma Acute Care Surg.* 2013;25(4):582–589.
12. Holzer VE. Botulism from inhalation. *Med Klinik.* 1962;57:1735–1738.
13. St Louis ME, Peck SH, Bowering D, et al. Botulism from chopped garlic: delayed recognition of a major outbreak. *Ann Intern Med.* 1988;108: 363–368.
14. Schreiner MS, Field E, Ruddy R. Infant botulism: a review of 12 years' experience at the Children's Hospital of Philadelphia. *Pediatrics.* 1991;87: 159–165.
15. Mehta S. Neuromuscular disease causing acute respiratory failure. *Resp Care.* 2006;51(9):1016–1021.
16. Bleck TP. *Clostridium botulinum* (botulism). In: Mandell GL, Bennett JE, Dolin R, eds. *Mandell, Douglas and Bennett's principles and practice of infectious diseases.* 6th ed. Philadelphia: Churchill Livingstone; 2005:2822–2828.
17. Santos JI, Swensen P, Glasgow LA. Potentiation of *Clostridium botulinum* toxin by aminoglycoside antibiotics: clinical and laboratory observations. *Pediatrics.* 1981;68:50–54.
18. Schulze J, Toepfer M, Schroff KC, et al. Clindamycin and nicotinic neuromuscular transmission. *Lancet.* 1999;354:1792–1793.
19. Tacket CO, Shandera WX, Mann JM, et al. Equine antitoxin use and other factors that predict outcome in type A foodborne botulism. *Am J Med.* 1984;76:794–798.
20. Centers for Disease Control and Prevention. Investigational heptavalent botulinum antitoxin (HBAT) to replace licensed botulinum antitoxin AB and investigational botulinum antitoxin E. *MMWR.* 2010;59(10):299.
21. Sevcik C, Salazar V, Diaz P, D'Suze G. Initial volume of a drug before it reaches the volume of distribution: pharmacokinetics of F(ab')2 antivenoms and other drugs. *Toxicon.* 2007;50:653–665.
22. Arnon SS, Schechter R, Maslanka SE, Jewell NP, Hatheway CL. Human botulism immune globulin for the treatment of infant botulism. *N Engl J Med.* 2006;354:462–471.
23. Duchen LW. Motor nerve growth induced by botulinum toxin as a regenerative phenomenon. *Proc R Soc Med.* 1972;65:196–197.

24. Centers for Disease Control and Prevention. *Botulism in the United States 1899–1996: Handbook for Epidemiologists, Clinicians, and Laboratory Workers.* Atlanta, Ga: Centers for Disease Control and Prevention; 1998.

25. Wein LM, Liu Y. Analyzing a bioterror attack on the food supply: the case of botulinum toxin in milk. *Proc Natl Acad Sci U S A.* 2005;102(28):9984–9989.

26. Weber JT, Goodpasture HC, Alexander H, et al. Wound botulism in a patient with a tooth abscess: case report and literature review. *Clin Infect Dis.* 1993;16:635–639.

27. Keller MA, Miller VH, Berkowitz CD, et al. Wound botulism in pediatrics. *Am J Dis Child.* 1982;136:320–322.

28. Robin L, Herman D, Redett R. Botulism in a pregnant woman. *N Engl J Med.* 1996;335:823–824.

29. St Clair EH, DiLiberti JH, O'Brien ML. Observations of an infant born to a mother with botulism. *J Pediatr.* 1975;87:658.

30. Krishna S, Puri V. Infant botulism: case reports and review. *J Ky Med Assoc.* 2001;99:143–146.

155 | CHAPTER

Clostridium perfringens Toxin (Epsilon Toxin) Attack

Mariann Nocera, Lynne Barkley Burnett, and Siraj Amanullah

DESCRIPTION OF EVENT

Biological warfare is the deliberate use of living organisms, or toxins derived from them, that cause disease in humans, animals, or plants, in conflict or terrorist attack.[1] Bioweapons, therefore, include living organisms and the toxins they produce. Toxins are biologically active compounds but do not grow or reproduce,[2] though once produced they can act alone without reliance on the organism.[3] In the case of a toxin bioweapon, it is the poison produced, rather than the microorganism, that is weaponized.[2]

Several bacteria in the genus *Clostridium* produce toxins and are considered potential bioterrorism agents.[4,5] Clostridia are gram-positive, nonencapsulated, spore-forming, fermentative, catalase-negative, rectangular-shaped bacilli.[6,7] Of approximately 90 species, fewer than 20 are known to be associated with clinical illness in humans,[5] including botulism, tetanus, gas gangrene, and food poisoning.[4,5] *Clostridium perfringens*, which may well be the most common bacterial pathogen,[5] is ubiquitous and found in soil, water, and the gastrointestinal tracts of mammals, including humans.[8,9] First described in 1892 the survival of these bacteria in nature (even in harsh environments) is due to its resilient endospores. These spores can germinate in an extremely short duration of less than 10 minutes into a vegetative organism.[10] There are five strains of *C. perfringens* (designated types A through E[4]) that produce more than 20 toxins,[11] the largest number by any bacteria.[12] The major lethal toxins identified with *C. perfringens* are alpha, beta, epsilon, iota, and enterotoxin.[6] Type A *C. perfringens*, which produces alpha toxin, is most commonly associated with uncomplicated gastroenteritis in humans and myositis and myonecrosis, also known as *gas gangrene*. Type C *C. perfringens* also causes disease in humans, specifically necrotizing enteritis and septicemia.[13] The only known reported use of *C. perfringens* as a bioweapon is during World War II by the Japanese biological weapons program, Unit 731, which used shrapnel contaminated with *C. perfringens* in an attempt to increase incidence and severity of wound infections in humans.

Epsilon toxin, the most potent clostridial toxin after botulinum and tetanus neurotoxins,[14] is a pore-forming toxin[9] made by *C. perfringens* types B and D.[4] These are commensal organisms whose primary host is sheep, although they are occasionally isolated from other herbivores, such as goats and cattle[15] and rarely humans.[16] Natural infection typically affects livestock, primarily sheep and goats,[9,15] in which it produces enterotoxemia[9] and pulpy kidney disease.[7,17] Though there are no reports of death in humans from epsilon toxin[15] and only few reports of disease in humans,[12] its toxicity and clinical pathogenesis extrapolated from animals make it a potential bioterrorism agent.[6] For this reason the U.S. Centers for Disease Control and Prevention (CDC) has designated epsilon toxin as a Category B biological agent along with staphylococcal enterotoxin B and ricin.[3,18,19]

Epsilon toxin is produced as a prototoxin, which is cleaved by trypsin, alpha-chymotrypsin, and lambda-chymotrypsin (the latter two of which are also produced by *C. perfringens*) into the active form.[8,9,12] This active form is approximately 1000 times more toxic than the prototoxin.[8,20] In a natural infection in herbivores a large dose of intraintestinal epsilon toxin results in increased intestinal permeability, facilitating entry of *C. perfringens* from the gut into the systemic circulation with hematogenous spread to all organs,[12,21] primarily the brain, lungs, and kidneys.[8,9] The toxin does not enter the cells and does not have any intracellular activity.[21] Rather, it binds to a receptor on the cell membrane[22] and oligomerizes to form a pore, creating a nonselective diffusion channel for hydrophilic solutes.[9,15,21,23] In this way it is similar to other pore-forming toxins, aerolysin in particular.[9,12] Ion shifts through this pore lead to a rapid decrease in intracellular potassium, increase in intracellular chloride and sodium, and a slower increase in intracellular calcium.[9,21] The efflux of intracellular potassium causes plasma membrane blebbing, cell swelling, lysis,[15] and cell death.[21] This disruption in the vascular endothelium leads to osmotic alterations, including extravasation of serum proteins and red blood cells and massive edema[18] involving the brain,[24,25] kidneys, lungs,[26] and liver,[27] clinically manifesting as cerebral edema,[24,25] pulmonary edema,[4,24,25] pericardial fluid collections,[15,25,28] kidney edema,[25] and gastrointestinal distress.[29]

In animal studies epsilon toxin administered intravenously accumulates preferentially in the brain. In addition to pore formation, epsilon toxin also disrupts the cellular cytoskeleton,[9] which allows it to effectively cross the blood-brain barrier.[9,30] Pathological changes are characterized by focal to diffuse[14] liquefactive necrosis and perivascular edema in the internal capsule, thalamus, cerebellar white matter,[12] and meninges.[7] At high doses the neurotoxicity of epsilon toxin is due to stimulation of presynaptic neurons, leading to excessive release of glutamate.[12,14,31] To a lesser degree, epsilon toxin also causes release of dopamine[14] and gamma-aminobutyric acid (GABA).[31] Though controversial, epsilon toxin has been reported to act directly on myelin in the peripheral and central nervous systems.[12,30] Other than the brain, epsilon toxin also accumulates in the kidneys,[26] where necrosis of the renal cortex (so called "pulpy kidney disease") may occur.[7,17]

The potential impact of an epsilon toxin bioweapon on humans must be extrapolated from animal studies. Studies in sheep, goats, and mice[4] suggest that inhalation by humans could lead to damage of pulmonary vascular endothelial cells, resulting in high-permeability pulmonary edema and hematogenous spread to the kidneys, heart, and central nervous system.[15] The central nervous system is the primary target of epsilon toxin.[14] Therefore the most clinically significant presentation in humans is neurological stimulation due to the release of the excitatory neurotransmitter glutamate.[30] This could manifest as ataxia, weakness, dizziness,[32] trembling,[27] and seizures.[30] Coma is a potential late presentation.[32] Pulmonary manifestations due to inhalational exposure may include respiratory irritation, cough, bronchospasm, dyspnea,[32] adult respiratory distress syndrome, and respiratory failure.[32] Cardiovascular abnormalities may include tachycardia, hypotension,[32] or hypertension,[12] leading to subsequent cardiovascular collapse.[24] Gastrointestinal distress may present as nausea, vomiting, diarrhea,[29,32] severe abdominal cramping and distention,[29] and decreased gut motility.[12] Epsilon-toxin toxicity may result in hyperglycemia and glycosuria[12] because of altered hepatic metabolism of glycogen.[27] Pancytopenia is a late complication resulting in bleeding, bruising, and immunosuppression.[32,33] Initial laboratory studies may reveal anemia caused by intravascular hemolysis, thrombocytopenia, elevation of serum aminotransferase levels, and hypoxia.[33] Renal cell toxicity has been demonstrated in in vitro studies using human kidney cell lines, suggesting that renal failure may be a clinical feature of human disease.[12,34,35]

Production of epsilon toxin as a bioweapon would most likely depend on chemical synthesis rather than fermentation from *C. perfringens* because of constraints of time and finances.[36] The anticipated primary routes for mass dissemination of epsilon toxin would be as an aerosol,[15,24,32,37] in foodstuffs, or in water.[32] As epsilon toxin is taken up from the gut in diseased animals, food contamination might be the most important and natural avenue for a bioterrorist attack. In an aerosol toxin attack the presumption is that the toxin retains its harmful potential for 8 hours once released.[38] To use epsilon toxin as an effective aerosolized biological weapon, terrorists would need to manufacture a respirable aerosol of the purified toxin,[39] with particles ranging from 0.5 to 5 μm in diameter—the "ideal" particle size for absorption into the circulatory system via the inhalational route. Particles within this size range remain airborne for a prolonged period of time and are optimal for being carried to the distal airways, where retention and absorption of a toxin are maximized. Furthermore, aerosolized agents need to be coated to overcome electrostatic forces and stabilized against environmental stressors, such as ultraviolet light, humidity shifts, and temperature. Similarly, aerosolized *infectious* biological agents (e.g., anthrax spores) achieve their highest rates of infection in the distal airways.[38] However, unlike the spores of *Bacillus anthracis*, there is no evidence that spores of clostridia can be aerosolized to produce disease. It is important to note that epsilon toxin has not been shown to have person-to-person transmission.[6]

The estimated lethal dose of epsilon toxin is 0.1 μg/kg intravenously[20] and 1 μg/kg[15] inhalationally, though the exact lethal dose of inhalational or oral routes depends in part on the interaction of the toxin with the respiratory or gastrointestinal mucosa[20] of humans. Onset of illness is anticipated to be within 1 to 12 hours of exposure.[29] Death can occur within 30 to 60 minutes of symptom onset in affected animals[20]; thus the abrupt onset of clinical illness could progress rapidly to death in humans.[15,20,32]

Recognition relies on clinical acumen and appreciation of the context of the presentation, especially when a cluster of patients presents with the same form of illness.[40] Immediate diagnosis of an epsilon-toxin attack would be clinical and epidemiological. Culture of *C. perfringens* is only useful if the organism itself, not the toxin alone, was used in the attack.[4] Epsilon toxin can be identified via polymerase chain reaction, enzyme-linked immunosorbent assay (ELISA),[9,39] mass spectroscopy,[3,9] or with the use of monoclonal antibodies.[39,41] Swabs of the nasal mucosa,[39] acute serum, and possibly tissue samples should be collected as soon as possible[42] in cooperation with the local or state health department or the CDC and sent to an appropriate reference facility[33,42] via the laboratory response network. They must be properly packaged to preserve their biological structure and/or activity. Because these samples are also evidence of a crime, they must be transported in a manner that maintains an appropriate chain of custody, as required for any such bioterrorism attack.

PRE-INCIDENT ACTIONS

Terrorist attacks are unpredictable, may vary due to number of infected or affected individuals, can occur in multiple sites simultaneously or be conducted sequentially, and will likely overtax resources at every level of response: local, state, and possibly national.[43] Thus although there are no pre-incident steps to be taken specifically for epsilon toxin, it is essential that emergency medical service(s) (EMS) agencies, hospitals, and health care professionals proactively plan, organize, train, and obtain the supplies necessary for responding to terrorist incidents involving any known or unknown biological agent. This is often referred to as the "all hazards" approach to preparedness.

POST-INCIDENT ACTIONS

It may be unclear whether the initial cases of an infectious disease outbreak are the result of a natural occurrence or an act of bioterrorism. Therefore it may be prudent to consider bioterrorism in any disease outbreaks, especially those that involve organisms not expected in a given geographic region or occur in a pattern not likely to be "natural." Steps of management include, but are not limited to, immediate reporting of suspicious or clustered disease syndromes to local, state, or federal public health officials for investigation, immediate implementation of respiratory protection and/or body fluid precautions for all responders, and recognition that biological samples and other materials (e.g., clothing) as well as laboratory results have potential forensic and clinical relevance.[40]

Decontamination of all involved is critical; for epsilon toxin the recommended approach is with soap and water.[29,38,39] There is no known *person-to-person* spread of epsilon toxin by air.[4] However, epsilon toxin is dermonecrotic[8] and can be transmitted via contaminated wound discharge[26]; thus body fluid precautions should be observed. Direct contamination of consumables, such as water, food,[32,38] or medications,[44] is a possible route of dissemination and would be difficult to detect prior to the onset of illness because it is unlikely that appearance, taste, or smell would be significantly affected.

MEDICAL TREATMENT OF CASUALTIES

Insofar as epsilon toxin is concerned, there are no vaccines, antitoxins,[4] or specific treatment[33] for humans. Supportive medical care, including airway management[45] and fluid replacement with particular attention paid to electrolyte status because of potassium loss, is the mainstay of therapy.[29] Critical care in an intensive care setting, including mechanical ventilation and vasopressors, may be needed for the treatment of multisystem organ failure and shock.[4]

No vaccine currently exists for humans, though a veterinary vaccine does exist.[8,20,25,46-48] This animal vaccine, however, is too crude for use in humans,[9,25] and therefore current research focuses on the creation of a recombinant vaccine for humans.[20,22,48]

If weaponized and aerosolized *C. perfringens* is the biological agent disseminated (as opposed to weaponized purified epsilon toxin), high-dose penicillin might be indicated, although a primary role for antibiotic therapy has not been established.[4] A study of guinea pigs with gas gangrene (caused by clostridial alpha toxin) showed that protein synthesis inhibitors were more effective inhibitors of cell wall active toxins than were antimicrobial agents with a different mechanism of action.[5] In the antimicrobial group, penicillin plus clindamycin is considerably more efficacious than penicillin alone.[49]

Adjunctive hyperbaric oxygen therapy for gas gangrene is based on blocking production of alpha toxin at a partial pressure of oxygen of more than 250 mm Hg.[47] However, use of hyperbaric oxygen and its effect on the production of epsilon toxin have not been reported.

❓ UNIQUE CONSIDERATIONS

The pediatric population is at a higher risk of any bioterrorism agent compared with adults. Children have a larger minute ventilation and therefore may inhale a larger relative dose of aerosolized bioweapons than adults. Furthermore, bioweapons that are heavier than air may have a larger concentration near the ground, allowing for children to inhale more particles than adults. Finally the skin of children is more permeable, and a proportionately larger body surface area in children may lead to a higher overall exposure to the toxin through the skin.[50]

❗ PITFALLS

Potential pitfalls in response to an epsilon toxin attack are generic to other agents that have the potential to be used in bioterrorism and include the following:

- Absence of familiarity with novel bioterroism agents on the part of medical personnel, public health officials, and disaster planners.[43] A high index of suspicion by health care providers is also essential for the preparedness and response to a terrorist incident.[40]
- Failure to recognize a bioterror incident early in its presentation may compromise the care of the affected individuals, proper removal or decontamination of the agent, and evidence collection for investigation.[40]

REFERENCES

1. Clarke S. Bacteria as potential tools in bioterrorism, with an emphasis on bacterial toxins. *Br J Biomed Sci.* 2005;62:40–46.
2. Biological Weapons. Chapter 4.3 Technical. The US Army Center for Health Promotion and Preventive Medicine USACHPPM Tech Guide. 244;2000:4-15.
3. Alam SI, Kumar B, Kamboj DV. Multiplex detection of protein toxins using MALDI-TOF-TOF tandem mass spectrometry: application in unambiguous toxin detection from bioaerosol. *Anal Chem.* 2012;84:10500–10507.
4. Lucey DR. A guide to the diagnosis and management of 17 CDC category B bioterrorism agents ("Beware of Germs"). Washington Hospital Center. Available at: http://bepast.org/docs/posters/beware_of_germs_full.pdf. Accessed April 10, 2003.
5. Lorber B. Gas gangrene and other *Clostridium*-associated diseases. In: Mandell GL, Bennett JE, Dolin R, eds. *Principles and Practice of Infectious Disease.* 5th ed. London: Churchill Livingstone; 2000:2549–2561.
6. Engelthaler DM, Lewis K. Zebra Manual. Chapter: Epsilon Toxin of Clostridium Perfringens. Phoenix, AZ: Arizona Department of Health Services, Division of Public Health Services; 2004:5.16–5.18.
7. Kitron UD. Anaerobic infections. Veterinary pathobiology 331 lectures. College of Veterinary Medicine, University of Illinois at Urbana-Champaign.
8. Bokori-Brown M, Savva CG, Fernandes da Costa SP, Naylor CE, Basak AK, Titball RW. Molecular basis of toxicity of *Clostridium perfringens* epsilon toxin. *FEBS J.* 2011;278:4589–4601.
9. Stiles BG, Barth G, Barth H, Popoff MR. *Clostridium perfringens* epsilon toxin: a malevolent molecule for animals and man? *Toxins.* 2013;5:2138–2160.
10. Lindstrom M, Heikinheimo A, Lahti P, Korkeala H. Novel insights into the epidemiology of *Clostridium perfringens* type A food poisoning. *Food Microbiol.* 2011;28:192–198.
11. Songer G. Clostridia causing enteric disease. Lecture notes: pathogenic bacteriology. Veterinary Science and Microbiology, The University of Arizona. Available at: http://microvet.arizona.edu:16080/courses/mic420/classnotes.html.
12. Popoff MR. Epsilon toxin: a fascinating pore-forming toxin. *FEBS J.* 2011;278:4602–4615.
13. Pons JL, Picard B, Niel P, et al. Esterase electrophoretic polymorphism of human and animal strains of *Clostridium perfringens. Appl Environ Microbiol.* 1993;59:496–501.
14. Miyamoto O, Minami J, Toyoshima T, et al. Neurotoxicity of *Clostridium perfringens* epsilon-toxin for the rat hippocampus via the glutamatergic system. *Infect Immun.* 1998;66:2501–2508.
15. Greenfield R, Brown BR, Hutchins JB, et al. Microbiological, biological, and chemical weapons of warfare and terrorism. *Am J Med Sci.* 2002;323:326–340.
16. Structural studies on epsilon toxin from *Clostridium perfringens.* Research in the School of Crystallography. Birkbeck College, The University of London. Available at: http://people.cryst.bbk.ac.uk/~toxin/cproj/eps.html.
17. Kit for the detection of *Clostridium perfringens* epsilon toxin in biological fluids or culture supernatants. Available at: http://www.biox.com/UDTData/13/UDTEnglishInsert/BIO%20K%20268%20-%20EPSILON%20Ag%20_Eng_.pdf.
18. Agrawal A, O'Grady NP. Biological agents and syndromes. In: Farmer JC, Jiminez EJ, Talmor DS, et al., eds. *Fundamentals of Diaster Management.* Des Plaines, IL: Society of Critical Care Medicine; 2003:72.
19. NIAID Category A, B, and C Priority Pathogens. 2013. Available at: http://www.niaid.nih.gov/topics/BiodefenseRelated/Biodefense/Pages/CatA.aspx.
20. Mantis NJ. Vaccines against the category B toxins: Staphylococal enterotoxin B, epsilon toxin and ricin. *Adv Drug Deliv Rev.* 2005;57:1424–1439.
21. Petit L, Maier E, Gibert M, et al. *Clostridium perfringens* epsilon toxin induces a rapid change of cell membrane permeability to ions and forms channels in artifical lipid bilayers. *J Biol Chem.* 2001;276:15736–15740.
22. Chassin C, Bens M, de Barry J, et al. Pore-forming epsilon toxin causes membrane permeabilization and rapid ATP depletion-mediated cell death in renal collecting duct cells. *Am J Physiol Renal Physiol.* 2007;293:F927–F937.
23. The channel-forming e-toxin family. Transport Classification Database. University of California San Diego. Available at: http://tcdb.ucsd.edu/tcdb/tcfamilybrowse.php?tcname=1.C.5.
24. Marks JD. Medical aspects of biologic toxins. *Anesthesiol Clin North America.* 2004;22:509–532.
25. McClain MS, Cover TL. Functional analysis of neutralizing antibodies against *Clostridium perfringens* epsilon-toxin. *Infect Immun.* 2007;75:1785–1793.
26. Structural studies on the epsilon toxin from *Clostridium perfringens.* Birkbeck College, The University of London. Available at: http://people.cryst.bbk.ac.uk/~toxin/cproj/eps.html.
27. Williamson L. *Clostridium perfringens* type D: young ruminant diarrhea. LAMS 5350 Large animal digestive system. Available at: http://goatconnection.com/articles/publish/article_38.shtml.
28. Garcia J, Adams V, Beingesser J, et al. Epsilon toxin is essential for the virulence of *Clostridium perfringens* type D infection in sheep, goats and mice. *Infect Immun.* 2013;81:2405–2414.
29. *Clostridium perfringens* epsilon toxins: essential data. CBWInfo.com. Available at: http://www.cbwinfo.com/Biological/Toxins/Cper.html. 1999;1-4.
30. Dorca-Arevalo J, Soler-Jover A, Gibert M, et al. Binding of epsilon-toxin from *Clostridium perfringens* in the nervous system. *Vet Microbiol.* 2008;131:14–25.
31. Lonchamp E, Dupont JL, Wioland L, et al. *Clostridium perfringens* epsilon toxin targets granule cells in the mouse cerebellum and stimulates glutamate release. *PLoS One.* 2010;5:e13046.
32. Hasbrook L. *Clostridium perfringens* Factsheet. In: Illinois Department of Public Health: Emergency Preparedness; 2014. http://www.idph.state.il.us/Bioterrorism/factsheets/clostridium.htm.
33. *Clostridium perfringens* toxins. NATO Handbook on the Medical Aspects of NBC Defense. Virtual Naval Hospital: FM8-9. Available at: http://www.vnh.org/MedAspNBCDef/2appb.htm.
34. Shortt S, Titball RW, Lindsay CD. An assessment of the in vitro toxicology of *Clostridium perfringens* type D epsilon-toxin in human and animal cells. *Hum Exp Toxicol.* 2000;19:108–116.

35. Fernandez Miyakawa ME, Zabal O, Silberstein C. *Clostridium perfringens* epsilon toxin is cytotoxic for human renal tubular epithelial cells. *Hum Exp Toxicol.* 2010;30:275–282.

36. Gorka S, Sullivan R. Biological toxins: a bioweapon threat in the 21st century. *Security Dialogue.* 2002;33:141–156.

37. Biological Weapons. Chapter 4.4 Biological Agent Operational Data Charts. The US Army Center for Health Promotion and Preventive Medicine USACHPPM Tech Guide. 244;2000:4-24.

38. Biological Weapons. Chapter 4.2 Operational issues. The US Army Center for Health Promotion and Preventive Medicine USACHPPM Tech Guide. 244;2000:4-8-13.

39. Franz DR. *Defense Against Toxin Weapons.* US Army Medical Research Institute of Infectious Diseases: Fort Detrick, MD; 1997.

40. Bogucki S, Weir S. Pulmonary manifestations of intentionally released chemical and biological agents. *Clin Chest Med.* 2002;23:777–794.

41. El-Enbaawy M, Abdalla YA, Hussein AZ, et al. Production and evaluation of monoclonal antibody to *Clostridium perfringens* type D epsilon toxin. *Egypt J Immunol.* 2003;10:77–81.

42. *Clostridium perfringens.* USAF pamphlet on the medical defense against biological weapons. Available at: http://www.gulflink.osd.mil/declassdocs/af/19970211/970207_aadcn_015.html.

43. Redlener I, Markenson D. Disaster and terrorism preparedness: what pediatricians need to know. *Dis Mon.* 2004;50:6–40.

44. Biological Weapons. Chapter 4.1 Intelligence. The US Army Center for Health Promotion and Preventive Medicine USACHPPM Tech Guide. 244;2000:4-6.

45. *Clostridium perfringens* toxins. Bioterrorism Treatment Guidelines. Illinois Department of Public Health. Available at: http://www.idph. state.il.us/Bioterrorism/pdf/bioterrorismcards.pdf.

46. Titball RW. *Clostridium perfringens* vaccines. *Vaccine.* 2009;27:D44–D47.

47. Van Unnik A. Inhibition of toxin production in *Clostridium perfringens* in vitro by hyperbaric oxygen. *Antonie Van Leeuwenhoek.* 1965;31:181–186.

48. Lobato FC, Lima CGRD, Assis RA, et al. Potency against enterotoxemia of a recombinant *Clostridium perfringens* type D epsilon toxoid in ruminants. *Vaccine.* 2010;28:6125–6127.

49. Franz DR. Defense against toxin weapons. In: Sidell FR, Takafuji ET, Franz DR, eds. *Medical Aspects of Chemical and Biological Warfare.* Washington, DC: Office of the Surgeon General at TMM Publications, Department of the Army, United States of America; 1997;608:616.

50. American Academy of Pediatrics, Committee on Environmental Health and Committee on Infectious Diseases. Chemical-biological terrorism and its impact on children: a subject review. *Pediatrics.* 2000;105:662–670.

156 CHAPTER

Marine Toxin Attack

Stephen P. Wood, Kate Longley-Wood, and Wende R. Reenstra

DESCRIPTION OF EVENT

Although there have been no recorded efforts to weaponize a marine toxin, these are agents that have potential for use as biological weapons. Marine toxins are produced by a wide array of organisms ranging from small microbes and invertebrates to fish. Naturally occurring marine toxins are typically a combination of several peptides that can produce a variety of effects, including dermatonecrosis, myonecrosis, hemolysis, neurotoxicity, and cardiotoxicity.[1] The toxins are typically introduced by some mechanism of envenomation, contact with a nematocyst, or ingestion.[1]

Common sources of marine toxins include *Cnidaria phylum* (jellyfish), *Mollusca* (octopus, squid, and snails), and *Echinodermata* (sea stars, urchins, sea snakes, and a number of fish). The effects on humans, as with any toxin, depend on the route and amount of exposure. The amount of toxin in some species, such as the puffer fish, can vary depending on the reproductive cycle stage, time of year, or even geography.[2,3] Many of the marine toxins are low-molecular weight, are stable, and can be introduced as an aerosol, which make them well suited for weaponization. To date, however, there is no way to synthesize these chemicals, and collection from natural sources would be both technically difficult and time consuming. This significantly limits their potential for use as weapons for mass chemical attack, but they could theoretically be used in smaller attacks or terrorist actions targeting an individual or small groups.[4,5] The most likely scenario would be the utilization of one or more of the several marine neurotoxins as a chemical agent in an attack, and that will be the focus of this chapter. These agents include saxitoxin, conotoxin, tetrodotoxin, and palytoxin.

PRE-INCIDENT ACTIONS

As in other toxin attacks a robust public health care system is of most benefit in the pre-incident phase. Hospitals should have disaster plans that would be adaptable to a toxin attack and the subsequent surge of patients demonstrating the characteristic symptoms of the exposure to marine toxins. Although there are no known antidotes to these marine toxins, adequate resuscitation equipment, including mechanical ventilators, should be part of the preparation for such an attack.

POST-INCIDENT ACTIONS

Epidemiology is one of the most important tools in the recognition of patients presenting en masse with specific toxidromes. This is made easier when the patients present acutely after exposure and to the same or neighboring institutions. This would be typical of an aerosolized marine toxin for which the onset is rapid. It is more difficult when there is a delay in presentation, such as what might be seen with contaminated food or water. It is imperative that there exists a means for hospitals to report and communicate unusual presentations or trends. In the setting of the use of weaponized marine toxins, emergency medical providers would see a rise in the number of patients exhibiting the characteristic parasthesias and progressive paralysis often seen in marine toxin exposure. Once a trend is recognized, notification should be made to local and regional public health departments, and the resources to handle large numbers of symptomatic patients should be gathered. It is also important to ensure that efforts are made to educate providers as to any issues, such as personal protective equipment, treatment, and recovery. Rising numbers of symptomatic patients should be an indicator of a potential terrorist attack using a marine toxin agent, especially in areas where such toxins are not commonly seen (e.g., inland regions). Once an attack is suspected, notification of law enforcement on the local and federal level should follow.

MEDICAL TREATMENTS OF CASUALTIES

Saxitoxin

Saxitoxin is a potent inhibitor of voltage-gated sodium channels, specifically Na_vs channels responsible for the intiation and propagation of action potentials in nerve and muscle cells.[6] Saxitoxin binds to voltage-gated sodium channels on nerve fibers and muscle cells. The binding of the toxin blocks conduction of the nerve impulse. General symptoms of saxitoxin poisoning are neurologic and respiratory paralysis.[7-9] The toxin is made by small, single-celled organisms called dinoflagellates, which contaminate filter-feeding shellfish (clams, scallops, oysters).[7-9] Rapid growth and dispersion of dinoflagellates can result in harmful algal blooms or "red tide" events. This may lead to widespread shellfish contamination, which can result in cases of paralytic shellfish poisoning via ingestion of contaminated shellfish.[1]

Clinical Features

General: There is an initial latent period varying from 30 minutes to several hours following ingestion, before the onset of neurologic symptoms.

Neurologic: Neurologic symptoms are typically the first to manifest and are the most pronounced symptoms from saxitoxin poisoning.[10] A tingling and burning sensation, initially occurring around the mouth and lips, is usually the first symptom. The numbness may be on the hands and spread over the chest and abdomen.[7,10-12] These symptoms may progress, with difficulty walking and arm and leg weakness.[7,10-12] Involuntary movements and tremors may occur.[7]

Cardiovascular: There are no specific cardiovascular effects, although in laboratory animals saxitoxin caused hypotension and conduction defects.[7-10]

Respiratory: Respiratory distress from muscular paralysis may occur up to 12 hours after intoxication. The respiratory paralysis from significant saxitoxin exposure may lead to death.[7,10]

Gastrointestinal: Gastrointestinal symptoms may appear hours to days after ingestion. These symptoms may include nausea, vomiting, abdominal pain, and diarrhea.[7,12]

There are no specific antidotes for saxitoxin poisoning.[7] Treatment is predominantly symptomatic. If oral ingestion is suspected, orogastric lavage may be helpful to remove unabsorbed toxin, but the efficacy of this is limited. Activated charcoal has also been recommended as an adsorbant.[12] Intubation and mechanical ventilation with monitoring to support respiration may be necessary.[7]

Identification: Clincial suspicion based on the type of exposure and the clinical presentation are likely to be the most helpful means for identifying exposure to this toxin. Routine laboratory studies are not helpful. Diagnosis can be confirmed by detection of the toxin in food, water, or environmental samples by means of enzyme-linked immunosorbent assay (ELISA) or high-performance liquid chromatography (HPLC), although lack of standardization makes this somewhat challenging.[13,14]

Conotoxin

The venom of the cone snail is composed of small substances termed conotoxins. There are more than 2000 peptides identified[15] that lead to a complex set of symptoms. The toxins are heat stable but are inactivated by the disinfectants glutaraldehyde and formaldehyde.[15]

The mechanism of action of conotoxins can be divided into presynaptic and postsynaptic pathways. The presynaptic conotoxin blocks the release of acetylcholine.[12,16] The postsynaptic conotoxin inhibits sodium, potassium, and calcium channels and blocks muscular contraction.[12] The toxicity of the venom is thought to result from additive effects and not the concentration of the toxin. Conotoxins are very small, stable toxins, which theoretically may be weaponized and disseminated as aerosols and by direct injection.

Clinical Features

General: The onset of symptoms is almost immediate upon injection. Common symptoms include localized pain, swelling, numbness, and ischemia at the injection site.[12,15,16] The numbness, swelling, and tingling may spread rapidly from the injection site to involve the entire body.[12,15,16] The clinical course is characterized by rapid onset and deterioration for the first 6 to 8 hours.[15] This is followed by improvement, and complete recovery may take 4 to 6 weeks.[15]

Cardiovascular: No specific cardiac effects are seen.

Respiratory: Respiratory depression is a significant feature of conotoxin exposure. Death results from respiratory paralysis.[12,15]

Gastrointestinal: Abdominal cramping and nausea are common effects.

Identification: Diagnosis is by clinical signs and symptoms, and there are no laboratory tests available. Treatment is to immobilize the limb or site of envenomation. Pressure dressings should be applied, and pain medication and tetanus prevention should be provided.[16] Intubation and mechanical ventilation may be necessary to support breathing.[12,16]

Tetrodotoxin

Tetrodotoxin is one of the best characterized marine toxins because of its historical involvement in fatal food poisoning. The toxin is named from the pufferfish family (*Tetraodontidae*), where it has been found to be concentrated in the liver and other organs.[17,18] The toxin can also be found in the blue-ringed octopus, parrotfish, crabs, newts, and algae.[8,12,18–20]

The toxin is made by a bacterium that forms a symbiotic relationship with the animals.[12,20] Tetrodotoxin is a neurotoxin that interferes with transmission of the nerve impulse at the nerve-muscle junction.[8,20] The toxin is heat stable and can be solubilized in acetic solutions.[12,20] This toxin specifically blocks sodium channels on nerve cells and inhibits transmission of the impulse.[8,12,20] The target molecular channels are thought to be very similar to saxitoxin.[18] Relatively little is known about tetrodotoxin as a possible toxin weapon. A company in Japan is known to produce the toxin.[20] It is not known to be made in large quantities that could be used in weapons, and little or nothing has been published about its inhalational toxicity.[20]

Clinical Features

General: The first symptom is increasing numbness and tingling in the face and around the mouth.[20] These may extend to the extremities or become generalized.[8,20]

Neurologic: The neurologic involvement may start as muscular twitching and proceed to complete skeletal muscle paralysis, interfering with speech and swallowing.[19,20] The pupils, after initially constricting, may become fixed and dilated. The victim may be completely paralyzed but conscious.

Cardiovascular: Chest pain, hypotension, and cardiac arrhythmias may occur.[8,20]

Respiratory: There is increasing respiratory distress. Exposed individuals typically exhibit difficulty breathing and cyanosis. Paralysis increases and convulsions, mental impairment, and cardiac arrhythmia may occur.[8,20]

Gastrointestinal: Nausea, vomiting, and/or diarrhea may develop.[8,20]

Other: Coagulopathy can occur and may lead to bleeding into the skin and mucosa, the formation of blood blisters, and desquamation of the skin.

When untreated, the death rate is 50% to 60% in some studies.[12,20] Death usually occurs within 4 to 6 hours, with a known range of approximately 20 minutes to 8 hours.[19,20] Management is supportive, and standard management of poison ingestion should be employed if intoxication is by the oral route. These include gastric lavage or emetics, particularly after control of the airway has been obtained. Intubation and mechanical ventilation may be required in severe intoxication.[12,20]

After weakness has become apparent, the treatment is symptomatic (e.g., maintenance of respirations, monitoring of vital signs and electrolytes).[12,19,20] Because of the likelihood of consciousness being maintained with complete paralysis, periodic administration of a sedative and analgesic is recommended along with continuous reassurance.[19,20]

Palytoxin

Palytoxin is one of most potent marine toxins known. It was isolated first from corals located in the South Pacific.[1,21,22] Originally it was thought that the toxin was made by the corals; now, however, it is known that the toxin is made by a dinoflagellate and that the corals concentrate the toxin.[8,21] It is estimated that the lethal dose for a human is less than 5 μg.[21,22] Palytoxins are stable in seawater and alcohols.

Extensive pharmacological research has determined that palytoxin is not a neurotoxin.[21,23] It instead acts on the sodium-potassium adenosine triphosphatase (ATPase) pump, effectively "locking" it in an open position. This allows for the diffusion of sodium and potassium across the cell membrane and effectively disrupts the normal intracellular ion gradient.[21,23,24] Without the gradients of these ions, cells are unable to function or maintain their shape.[22,23] Relatively little is known about palytoxin as a possible toxin weapon. It is not known to be made in large quantities that could be used in weapons, and little or nothing has been published about its inhalational toxicity.[21]

TABLE 156-1   Specific Effects of Marine Toxins

TOXIN	ORIGIN	EFFECT
Conotoxin	Marine snail	Blocks voltage-sensitive calcium channels; blocks voltage-sensitive sodium channels; blocks ACh receptors
Palytoxin	Soft coral	Activates sodium channels, disrupts Na-K-ATPase receptors
Saxitoxin	Dinoflagellate	Blocks voltage-sensitive sodium channels
Tetrodotoxin	Puffer fish	Blocks sodium channels

ACh, acetylcholine; *ATPase*, adenosine triphosphatase.

Clinical Features

General: Symptoms are rapid, with death occurring within minutes.[21]

Cardiovascular: An initial symptom may be chest pain from coronary vasoconstriction. This may lead to cardiac ischemia and myonecrosis of cardiac cells. An electrocardiogram may demonstrate peaked T waves or ST segment elevation.[21] Loss of consciousness can ensue as hypotension predominates, and there is reduced cerebral perfusion.[21]

Respiratory: Shortness of breath and wheezing can occur.

Gastrointestinal: There are no specific gastrointestinal effects.

Other: Hemolysis may occur as cell membranes become permeable to various ions, red blood cells swell, and membranes rupture. This results in decreased oxygen-carrying capacity. Death is thought to result from hypoxia and shock.[21]

There is no effective treatment for palytoxin poisoning. Supportive care, such as supporting respirations, providing intravenous fluids for hypotension, and antiarrythmics, may provide some benefit. There are animal studies that have used isosorbide to treat the intense vasoconstriction from this toxin, but these studies have demonstrated this treatment is likely to be ineffective.[25]

In summary these toxins act on a variety of sites. Table 156-1 summarizes their specific effects.

🔅 UNIQUE CONSIDERATION

Marine toxins should be considered when a number of patients present with the characteristic parasthesias and paralysis. It is highly unusual to have large numbers of such patients, particularly in noncoastal regions, and therefore a terrorist attack should be suspected when this is seen. Early intervention with supportive care, including mechanical ventilation if needed, can be lifesaving.

⚠ PITFALLS

Several potential pitfalls in response to a marine toxin attack exist. These include the following:

- Failure to prepare adequate systems to respond to possible terrorist attacks before an attack occurs
- Failure to consider marine toxins as the cause for paralysis in patients
- Failure to consider a marine toxin attack in the setting of a large number of otherwise healthy people presenting over several hours with acute paralysis

- Failure to rapidly support the respiratory system with urgent intubation and mechanical ventilation
- Failure to notify appropriate public health and law enforcement agencies when marine toxin exposure is suspected or confirmed among persons with no aquatic environment exposure or seafood ingestion

REFERENCES

1. Brush DE. Marine envenomations. In: *Goldfrank's Toxicologic Emergencies.* 9th ed. New York: McGraw-Hill; 2011.
2. Silva M, Azevedo J, Rodriguez P, et al. New gastropod vectors and tetrodotoxin potential expansion in temperate waters of the Atlantic Ocean. *Mar Drugs.* 2012;10(4):712–726.
3. Miyazawa K, Noguchi T. Distribution and origin of tetrodotoxin. *J Toxicol Toxin Rev.* 2001;20:11–33.
4. Franz D. Defense against toxin weapons. In: *Medical Aspects of Chemical and Biological Warfare.* Washington, DC: The Office of the Surgeon General at TMM Publications; 2007.
5. Williams P, Willens S, Anderson J, et al. Toxins—established and emergent threats. In: *Medical Aspects of Chemical and Biological Warfare.* Washington, DC: The Office of the Surgeon General at TMM Publications; 2007.
6. Thottumkara A, Parsons W, Dubois J. Saxitoxin. *Angew Chem Int.* 2014;53:5760–5784.
7. Saxitoxin: essential date. Available at: http://www.cbwinfo.com/Biological/Toxins/Saxitoxin.html.
8. Yasumoto T, Murata M. Marine toxins. *Chem Rev.* 1993;93:1897–1909.
9. Tu A, ed. *Handbook of Natural Toxins: Marine Toxins and Venoms.* Marcel Dekker; 1988.
10. Brett M. Food poisoning associated with biotoxins in fish and shellfish. *Curr Opin Infect Dis.* 2003;16:461.
11. Mines DM, Stahmer S, Shepherd S. Poisonings: food, fish, shellfish. *Emerg Med Clin North Am.* 1997;15:157–177.
12. Edmonds C. *Dangerous Marine Creatures: A Field Guide for Medical Treatment.* Best; 1995.
13. Tunik M. Food poisoning. In: *Goldfrank's Toxicologic Emergencies.* 9th ed. New York: McGraw-Hill; 2011.
14. Laycock MV, Thibault P, Ayer S, et al. Isolation and purification procedures for the preparation of paralytic shellfish poisoning toxin standards. *Nat Toxins.* 1994;152:2049.
15. Conotoxins: essential data. Available at: http://www.cbwinfo.com/Biological/Toxins/Conotox.html.
16. Halstead BW. *Poisonous and Venomous Marine Animals of the World.* 2nd rev ed. Darwin; 1988.
17. Kao C, Levinson SR, eds. *Tetrodotoxin, Saxitoxin and the Molecular Biology of the Sodium Channel.* New York, NY: The New York Academy of Sciences; 1986.
18. Hall S, Strichartz G, eds. *Marine Toxins, ACS Symposium series.* Washington, DC: American Chemical Society; 1990.
19. Underman AE, Leedom JM. Fish and shellfish poisoning. *Curr Clin Top Inf Dis.* 1993;13:203–225.
20. Tetrodoxin: essential data. Available at: http://www.cbwinfo.com/Biological/Toxins/TTX.html.
21. Palytoxin: essential data. Available at: http://www.cbwinfo.com/Biological/Toxins/Palytoxin.html.
22. Moore RE, Scheuer PJ. Palytoxin: a new marine toxin from a coelenterate. *Science.* 1971;172(982):495.
23. Haberman E. Palytoxin acts through Na+, K+-ATPase. *Toxicon.* 1989;27:1171–1187.
24. Wu CH. Palytoxin: membrane mechanisms of action. *Toxicon.* 2009;54(8):1183–1189.
25. Wiles JS, Vick JA, Christensen MK. Toxicological evaluation of palytoxin in several animal species. *Toxicon.* 1974;12(4):427–433.

CHAPTER 157

T-2 Toxin (Trichothecene Mycotoxins) Attack

Frederick Fung

DESCRIPTION OF EVENT

The 1972 Biological and Toxin Weapons Convention is a major international treaty to control biological and chemical warfare that prohibits state parties from developing, producing, and testing biological and toxic weapons.[1,2] However, Iraq admitted to the development of an aflatoxin bioweapon and may have used it during the *Al-Anfal* campaigns against the Kurds in the 1980s. With the expansion of terrorism, the possibility of using mycotoxins as a chemical weapon exists. In reality, there are three likely attack scenarios using T-2 mycotoxin as an agent of terrorism:

1. Product tampering: substantial human and economic damages caused by product tampering, such as the cyanide contamination of Tylenol in 1984, could happen. Use of T-2 mycotoxin to contaminate premade consumer products may be the most plausible attack scenario.

2. A second scenario is the use of T-2 mycotoxin as part of state-sponsored bioterrorism against a discrete population, group, or region.

3. The third scenario is related to food industry contamination: food, especially in the dairy industry (e.g., milk transported by tanker truck), is vulnerable to biological and chemical attack. An attack on the food industry could cause local outbreaks of disease within hours or days, as well as enormous economic damage.

Trichothecenes (Fig. 157-1) are a large group of sesquiterpenoid chemicals characterized by a tetracyclic 12,13-epoxy ring commonly known as the 12,13-epoxytrichothecene, which is responsible for the toxicological activity.[3] All trichothecenes are mycotoxins; however, some mycotoxins belong to other chemical groups and are not trichothecenes. They are classified into four groups. Group A includes T-2 toxin and diacetoxyscirpenol. Group B includes 4-deoxynivalenol and nivalenol. Many *Fusarium* species produce group A and B trichothecenes. *Baccharis megapotamica* produces the group C trichothecene baccharin. Group D mycotoxins include roridins produced by *Myrothecium roridum*, verrucarin produced by *M. verrucaria*, and satratoxins produced by *Stachybotrys atra* (also known as *S. chartarum* and *S. alternans*).[4]

It is important to point out that the more common and potent trichothecenes are produced by *Fusarium* species. There are over 190 toxins produced by fusaria and related fungi.[3] They infect wheat and other grains that are important as human food sources. They are highly resistant to heat. T-2 toxin has been the most extensively studied and is the most likely mycotoxin to be used as a weapon.[5]

T-2 is rapidly absorbed from the gastrointestinal (GI) tract. Although there are no human data on absorption through inhalational or dermal exposure, in vitro and animal studies have shown that trichothecenes are poorly absorbed through intact skin.[6] Trichothecenes undergo deepoxidation and glucuronidation, resulting in less toxic metabolites. The elimination half-life is estimated at 1.6 ± 0.5 hours after intravenous injection of the toxin in a canine model.[7] Another model using swine and cattle showed a half-life of 13 and 17 minutes, respectively.[8] T-2 does not require metabolic activation to exert its toxicity. The presence of the reactive electrophilic 12,13-epoxide moiety accounts for a rapid onset of toxicity. The mechanism of toxicity involves inhibition of protein and DNA synthesis.[9] It also produces general cytotoxicity by inhibiting the mitochondrial electron transport system.[10] The 12,13-epoxide of the trichothecenes is essential for the toxicologic activity. The deepoxidation of T-2 in mammalian systems results in loss of toxicity.[11]

The dose of trichothecene needed to cause symptoms in humans is unknown. There is great variability in the toxicity of these compounds in animal studies. The dose of trichothecenes that will be fatal to 50% of an exposed population (LD_{50}) ranges from 0.5 to 300 mg/kg, depending on the route of administration and animal model used.[12]

T-2 is a potent dermal blistering agent. Purified trichothecenes have been investigated because of their potential use in chemical warfare. T-2 toxin was implicated in the "yellow rain" attacks in Southeast Asia. However, further investigations have been inconclusive.[13]

Acute pulmonary hemorrhage in infants was purportedly associated with residential exposure to *S. chartarum* and other toxigenic fungi. A detailed analysis of this report was conducted by the Centers for Disease Control and Prevention, which found methodological shortcomings and concluded that the association was not confirmed.[14] A recent review on mycotoxin toxicology suggested an "incongruous" situation between the alleged seriousness of mycotoxin exposure from moldy homes in the United States and thousands of deaths in technologically less-developed countries, mostly from the consumption of highly mycotoxin-contaminated foods.[15]

An early report indicates that direct skin contact with trichothecenes produced irritant contact dermatitis.[16] Mild to moderate abdominal pain has been reported to develop within 15 minutes to 1 hour after ingestion of foods contaminated with significant levels of trichothecenes. Throat irritation and diarrhea have also been frequently described after ingestion. GI tract symptoms usually resolve within 12 hours.[17,18]

After a presumed T-2 attack, four clinical stages have been suggested.[19] The first stage includes irritation and inflammation of the GI mucosa, leading to abdominal pain, vomiting, and diarrhea, which may last 3 to 9 days. The second stage occurs on days 10 to 14 after exposure and is a latent period; symptoms are not prominent, but progressive anemia, thrombocytopenia, and leukopenia with relative lymphocytosis develop. The third stage occurs over the ensuing 3 to 4 weeks. Clinically, patients may show petechial hemorrhages on their skin and mucous membranes, and a hemorrhagic diathesis from mucous surfaces occurs. Varying degrees of necrotic lesions may

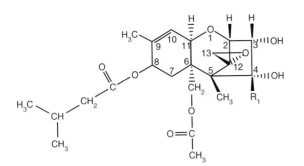

FIG 157-1 Structure of T-2 and HT-2. Trichothecenes: T-2 (R1 = OAc) and its metabolite HT-2 (R1 = OH).

develop in the GI tract or larynx, and generalized lymphadenopathy may appear. Blood abnormalities become more severe, and the erythrocyte sedimentation rate is elevated. Infections and sepsis during this stage are usually fatal. The fourth is the convalescence stage, when there is a rebound in the white blood count, the necrotic lesions of the mucous membranes resolve, and the patient recovers completely. The current weight of scientific evidence does not support a causal relationship between purported inhalation exposure to fungi capable of producing trichothecenes in the indoor environment and specific health effects.[20]

High-performance liquid chromatography, gas chromatography, and liquid chromatography mass spectrometry[21,22] have been used for trichothecene analysis in human blood and urine. However, these methods have not been validated by, or used in, sound epidemiologic studies. Serologic testing for antibodies specific to toxigenic fungi does not provide accurate information on exposure to trichothecenes or mycotoxins because the immunoglobulin is directed toward fungal antigens, not mycotoxins. Concerns on cross-reactivity in laboratory assays exist between *S. chartarum* antigens and fungi that are commonly found in outdoor environments.[23] Abnormalities in lymphocyte subset analysis have been reported in some studies, but consistent and specific findings have not been identified. The most appropriate diagnostic test to evaluate hematologic and immune status associated with trichothecene exposure is a complete blood count (CBC) with white blood cell differential.

PRE-INCIDENT ACTIONS

Hospital, emergency department, and ambulatory care facilities should have general disaster plans in place in the event of mycotoxin attack. The plan should be well thought out, should include an "all-hazards" approach, should be robust enough to respond to large numbers of victims, and should be tested by periodic and realistic exercises involving all essential personnel. The early detection of illness outbreaks requires surveillance systems that are capable of finding and validating the diagnosis and providing a means of communication between clinicians and health departments.[24] This would require coordination of local, state, and federal public health and safety resources. In the event of a large number of patients seeking medical care in a short timeframe, emergency medical services, hospital, and ambulatory care facilities need to be mobilized in a coordinated and expeditious fashion. Isolation and decontamination procedures should be in place and triage and decontamination personnel trained well before an attack occurs. As most physicians and health care providers, as well as first responders, may not be familiar with mycotoxin attack, close contact with the local

poison control center or local health department may be important to identify and treat the initial cases.

POST-INCIDENT ACTIONS

Medical providers should maintain a high level of suspicion for possible mycotoxin attack in the event of a sudden increase in the number of patients with similar symptoms and histories. Appropriate local, state, and federal public health and law enforcement authorities will need to be notified. Materials (e.g., clothing), bodily fluids, and surfaces possibly contaminated by mycotoxins should be decontaminated with 10% bleach (sodium hypochlorite) solution.[25] Proper environmental sampling may be necessary for mycotoxin identification and documentation. Further epidemiologic investigations in collaboration with state or local health authorities may be necessary. CBC and liver function tests are recommended. Analysis of blood or urine samples may provide information concerning the metabolites of the mycotoxin. All samples should be stored and shipped using strict chain of custody procedures to preserve their evidentiary value.

MEDICAL TREATMENT OF CASUALTIES

There are no specific antidotes for trichothecene or T-2 poisoning. Standard supportive care is indicated for symptomatic cases after removal from exposure and decontamination. These measures should include management of airways, breathing, and circulation. Supplemental oxygen can be given, if indicated. Contaminated clothing should be removed before skin decontamination occurs. The skin can be effectively decontaminated within minutes after T-2 exposure through washing with an aqueous soap solution. Polyethylene glycol 300 (PEG 300) is also effective at removing large doses of T-2 toxin from the skin.[26] An animal model has shown that dexamethasone may improve survival after low- and high-dose subcutaneous injection exposure to T-2 toxin.[27] T-2 toxin is tightly adsorbed onto activated charcoal; use of activated charcoal been associated with improved survival when administered with oral or parenteral doses of T-2 toxin in a mouse model.[28] These findings suggest that activated charcoal may decrease toxin absorption from the GI tract and may possibly enhance elimination of toxin via enterohepatic circulation. Although human data are lacking, a single dose of activated charcoal is probably warranted after acute trichothecene ingestion.

Laboratory testing should include serial CBC and differential evaluations for thrombocytopenia, anemia, and effects on the various white blood cell lines. The development of significant immune suppression, including pancytopenia, warrants neutropenic precautions and antibiotic coverage for fevers. After ingestion, careful examination of the oral mucous membranes and GI tract is warranted to evaluate for the presence of petechial, necrotic, or ulcerative lesions. In cases of airway compromise due to blistering effects of inhaled T-2 mycotoxin, patients should be monitored in a critical care setting with aggressive airway management readily available.

UNIQUE CONSIDERATIONS

Although skin blistering may be produced by dermal exposure to T-2 mycotoxin, it is most toxic when ingested. An attack using an aerosolized T-2 weapon is unlikely to produce sufficient inhalational dosages to cause significant morbidity or mortality.[29] The most probable sign that a T-2 toxin or related mycotoxin attack has occurred may be the presentation of a large number of previously healthy persons over a course of hours to days with nonspecific and systemic symptoms.

⚠ PITFALLS

Several potential pitfalls in response to a mycotoxin attack exist. These include the following:

- Failure to prepare adequate plans, to perform realistic training exercises, and to develop emergency response systems to respond to a possible terrorist attack before the incident occurs
- Failure to consider mycotoxin as the cause for nonspecific, as well as systemic, symptoms in previously healthy patients
- Failure to consider mycotoxin attack in the setting of a large number of otherwise healthy people presenting over hours to days with a similar range of general as well as specific complaints
- Failure to notify appropriate public health, safety, and law enforcement authorities when a possible biochemical agent attack is suspected, especially when animals are affected along with people
- Failure to provide basic supportive medical care when a patient is suspected to have undergone exposure to a biochemical warfare agent

REFERENCES

1. Zilinskas RA. Verifying compliance to the biological and toxin weapons convention. *Crit Rev Microbiol*. 1998;24: 195–218.
2. Zilinskas RA. Terrorism and biological weapons: inevitable alliance? *Perspect Biol Med*. 1990;34:44–72.
3. Li Y, Wang Z, Beier R, et al. T-2 toxin, a trichothecene mycotoxin: review of toxicity, metabolism and analytical method. *J Agric Food Chem*. 2011;59:3441–3453.
4. Fung F, Clark RF. Health effects of mycotoxins: a toxicological overview. *J Toxicol Clin Toxicol*. 2004;42:1–18.
5. Anderson PD. Bioterrorism: toxins as weapons. *J Pharm Prac*. 2012;25:121–129.
6. Kemppainen BW, Riley RT. Penetration of [H]T-2 toxin through excised human and guinea pig skin during exposure to [H]T-2 toxin adsorbed to corn dust. *Food Chem Toxicol*. 1984;22:893–896.
7. Barel S, Yagen B, Bialer M. Pharmacokinetics of the trichothecenes mycotoxin verrucarol in dogs. *J Pharm Sci*. 1990;79:548–551.
8. Beasley VR, Swanson SP, Corley RA, et al. Pharmacokinetics of the trichothecene mycotoxin, T-2 toxin, in swine and cattle. *Toxicon*. 1986;24:13–23.
9. Ueno Y. Mode of action of trichothecenes. *Ann Nutr Aliment*. 1977;31 (4–6):885–900.
10. Khachatourians GG. Metabolic effects of trichothecene T-2 toxin. *Can J Physiol Pharmacol*. 1989;68:1004–1008.
11. Yoshizawa T, Sakamoto T, Kuwamura K. Structure of deepoxytrichothecene metabolites from 3-hydroxy HT-1 toxin and T-2 tetraol in rats. *Appl Environ Microbiol*. 1985;50:67–69.
12. World Health Organization. *WHO Environmental Health Criteria 105. Selected Mycotoxins: Ochratoxins, Trichothecenes, Ergot*. Geneva: World Health Organization; 1990.
13. Marshall E. Yellow rain: filling in the gaps. *Science*. 1982;217:31–34.
14. CDC. Update: pulmonary hemorrhage/hemosiderosis among infants—Cleveland, Ohio, 1993–1996. *MMWR*. 2000;49:180–184.
15. Paterson RR, Lima N. Toxicology of mycotoxins. *Molecular Clin Environ Toxicol*. 2010;100:31–63.
16. Drobotko VG. Stachybotryotoxicosis: a new disease of horses and humans. *Am Rev Soviet Med*. 1945;2:238–242.
17. Wang ZG, Feng JN, Tong Z. Human toxicosis caused by moldy rice contaminated with Fusarium and T-2 toxin. *Biomed Environ Sci*. 1993;6:65–70.
18. Bhat RV, Beedu SR, Ramakrishna Y, et al. Outbreak of trichothecene mycotoxicosis associated with consumption of mould-damaged wheat production in Kashmir Valley, India. *Lancet*. 1989;1(8628):35–37.
19. Stahl CJ, Green CC, Farnum JB. The incident at Tuol Chrey: pathologic and toxicologic examinations of a casualty after chemical attack. *J Forensic Sci*. 1985;30:317–337.
20. Hardin BD, Kelman BJ, Saxon A. Adverse human health effects associated with molds in the indoor environment. ACOEM evidence-based statement. *J Occup Environ Med*. 2003;45:470–478.
21. Gilbert J. Recent advances in analytical methods for mycotoxins. *Food Addit Contam*. 1993;10(1):37–48.
22. Yagen B, Sintov A. New sensitive thin-layer chromatographic-high-performance liquid chromatographic method for detection of trichothecene mycotoxins. *J Chromatogr*. 1986;356:195–201.
23. Halsey J. Performance of a Stachybotrys chartarum serology panel. Abstract of presentation at the Western Society of Allergy, Asthma and Immunology Annual Meeting. *Allergy Asthma Proc*. 2000;21:174–175.
24. Buehler JW, Hopkins RS, Overhage JM, et al. Framework for evaluating public health surveillance systems for early detection of outbreaks. *MMWR*. 2004;53(RR05):1–11.
25. Stark AB. Threat assessment of mycotoxins as weapons. *J Food Protec*. 2005;68:1285–1293.
26. Fairhurst S, Maxwell SA, Scawin JW, et al. Skin effects of trichothecenes and their amelioration by decontamination. *Toxicology*. 1987;46:307–319.
27. Fricke RF, Jorge J. Beneficial effect of dexamethasone in decreasing the lethality of acute T-2 toxicosis. *Gen Pharmacol*. 1991;22:1087–1091.
28. Fricke RF, Jorge J. Assessment of efficacy of activated charcoal for treatment of acute T-2 toxin poisoning. *J Toxicol Clin Toxicol*. 1990;28:421–431.
29. Ciegler A. *Mycotoxins: A New Class of Chemical Weapons*. Department of Defense, Washington DC: NBC Defense and Technology International; 1986, 52-57.

158 CHAPTER

Ricin Toxin from *Ricinus communis* (Castor Bean) Attack

Brian J. Yun

📄 DESCRIPTION OF EVENT

The Centers for Disease Control and Prevention (CDC) classifies ricin as a category B biological warfare agent (i.e., moderately easy to disseminate with moderate morbidity rates and low mortality rates).[1] Ricin is a toxin derived from the castor oil plant, *Ricinus communis*, which most likely originated in Africa. Nowadays the plant grows wild in many tropical and subtropical regions.[2] It is cultivated commercially for its castor oil with major producers being India, China, and Brazil.[2] In the United States its use is primarily ornamental, and it can be found growing wild in the southwest.[3] Using some commonly available chemicals a knowledgeable person with access to laboratory equipment can purify ricin toxin from the castor bean.

Ricin toxin falls under the A-B family of toxins. Diphtheria, shiga, cholera, and anthrax toxins also belong in this family.[4,3] Ricin toxin works by inhibiting protein synthesis, which ultimately leads to cell apopotosis.[4] The active (A-chain) part is an enzyme, whereas the binding (B-chain) part navigates the toxin into the cell.[4] Because the ricin B-chain has a binding site for galactose, it can bind to many sites on the cell surface due to the abundance of cell surface proteins that contain galactose. The ricin B-chain binds to the surface of the cell and is endocytosed.[4] Once the ricin toxin reaches the endoplasmic reticulum the A-chain acts as a ribosome-inactivating protein by removing an adenine base of the 28S ribosomal RNA (rRNA).[4] Transfer RNA (tRNA) can no longer bind to the 28S rRNA, and as a result protein translation is stopped. Interestingly ricin does not have selectivity for specific cells.[4] Because all types of cells can be affected, clinical symptoms depend on the entry site of the toxin into the body (Table 158-1).

Ricin poisoning can occur through ingestion, inhalation, or injection. Depending on the dose in the context of the route of exposure, death may occur in 36 to 72 hours. Ricin toxin can be prepared in a liquid or crystalline form or as a dry powder, and it is water soluble, odorless, and tasteless. Although it is not contagious the ricin powder can spread through direct contact from an exposed person's clothing or skin to a person without protective clothing.

Ingestion

An intentional, mass, oral ricin poisoning would most likely occur by someone contaminating food, water, or commercial products. A scenario could involve contaminating a water supply, which would be extremely difficult to achieve covertly because of the amount of ricin toxin needed for a lethal dose as well as the neutralizing effects of water treatment with hypochlorite.[5] However, if a terrorist's goal was to only cause morbidity, a smaller amount of ricin toxin would suffice. Ingestion is thought to be the least toxic route due to poor gastrointestinal (GI) absorption and gastric acid deactivation of the toxin.[5] The median lethal dose (LD_{50}) for ingestion of ricin in mice is 30 mg/kg, which is 1000 times less toxic than poisoning through the parenteral or inhalation route.[6] The lethal oral dose in humans has been estimated to be 1 to 20 mg/kg (approximately 8 beans).[6] A review of castor bean seed intentional and unintentional ingestion by a statewide poison control system found 17 reported cases of ingestion of 10 or more castor bean seeds. Most developed GI symptoms, but all recovered.[7] It is important to realize that ricin doses estimated by number of beans ingested give an inaccurate estimate of dose due to variations in size, weight, and growth factors. In addition, chewing or crushing the beans facilitates more ricin release.

Autopsy findings of dead patients secondary to ricin poisoning include multifocal ulcerations and hemorrhages of gastric and small intestinal mucosa.[4,6] As a result most symptoms associated with ingestion relate to local injury in the GI tract. Onset of symptoms is usually 4 to 6 hours after ingestion. Symptoms of mild ricin poisoning include nausea, vomiting, and cramping abdominal pain. In moderate to severe toxicity, hypotension can occur secondary to fluid loss from third spacing from GI mucosal injury. Hematochezia and hematemesis may also occur.[7] In animal studies, ingested ricin toxin was found to accumulate in the liver and spleen. As a result, one may see elevated transaminases, hyperbilirubinemia, and anemia.[6] With modern supportive care the fatality rate for accidental ricin ingestion is fairly low at approximately 1.8%.[2] However, in a scenario in which a water supply were successfully contaminated with a sufficient quantity of ricin toxin, the fatality rate most likely would be higher because health care resources would be overwhelmed.

Inhalation

Of all the routes of exposure, inhalation of ricin has the most potential to hurt people. The LD_{50} in mice that have inhaled ricin particle sizes less than 5 μm is approximately 3 to 5 μg/kg. However, there are significant technical challenges in order to succeed in intentionally poisoning a large number of people. First, a sufficient quantity, estimated to be in excess of several metric tons, would need to be manufactured in order to cover a large enough area.[5] Second, the particles must be small enough to deposit into the alveoli of the respiratory tract. Large particles will be cleared by either the ciliary mechanism of the respiratory tract or by being swallowed. In order to meet these challenges, one would require advanced technical and logistical skill. The more likely scenarios, of which one hears and sees on the media, are targeted ricin poisonings through the postal service. The person who unseals the contaminated mail may agitate and then become subsequently exposed to aerosolized ricin powder.

Postmortem examination of monkeys exposed to inhaled ricin showed diffuse pulmonary edema with multifocal areas of necrosis and inflammation.[6] There are limited studies of human airborne exposure to ricin. In the 1940s eight people exposed to uncharacterized

TABLE 158-1 Summary of Human Clinical Presentations to Ricin Exposure

EXPOSURE ROUTE (ONSET)	SYMPTOMS
Mild ingestion (1-6 h)	Nausea, vomiting, diarrhea, abdominal pain, and cramping
Moderate to severe ingestion (1-6 h)	Vomiting and diarrhea (bloody or nonbloody), hypovolemic shock, hepatic and renal failure, hemolysis
Inhalational exposure (4-8 h)	Allergic symptoms (rhinitis and bronchospasm), flu-like symptoms, dyspnea, pulmonary edema
Intramuscular and subcutaneous (5 h)	Local necrosis, weakness, myalgias, fever, vomiting, shock, multiorgan failure

ricin-containing materials developed fever, nausea, cough, shortness of breath, chest pain, and arthralgias within 4 to 8 hours.[6] Unfortunately, these symptoms could easily be mistaken for influenza infection. Ricin toxin may also cause an allergic response leading to conjunctival irritation, rhinitis, and reactive airway inflammation.[6]

Parenteral

Injection is not considered a realistic route of delivery to a large population. However, parenteral delivery of ricin is associated with a greater mortality rate than ingestion.[5] The LD_{50} in mice is approximately 5 to 10 µg/kg. The clinical effects are nonspecific and include fever, headache, dizziness, nausea, anorexia, hypotension, and abdominal pain.[6] It may take up to 10 to 12 hours for symptoms to appear. There also may be focal tissue damage at the site of injection.

Dermal

Dermal exposure is also considered an unrealistic route of mass poisoning. Although an allergic reaction may occur, there is no evidence to show that toxicity can be achieved through the dermal route. This is most likely due to poor absorption of ricin through intact skin.

PRE-INCIDENT ACTIONS

At this time there is no approved vaccination or antidote for ricin. For a vaccine to be effective against ricin toxin it should be protective against damage from both GI and inhalational routes of exposure. There is ongoing research on potential vaccine candidates. For example, RiVAX, which consists of a genetically inactivated subunit, ricin A chain, completed a phase I clinical trial and is undergoing a second trial.[8]

POST-INCIDENT ACTIONS

Cases of suspected or known ricin poisoning should be reported to the regional poison control center (1-800-222-1222), local and state health department, Federal Bureau of Investigation (FBI), and the CDC. As a large-scale poisoning results from criminal activity, contaminated articles should be handled as evidence and in accordance with state and federal laws. Items should be double-bagged, labeled, and secured until they can be handed over to law enforcement. Chain of custody should be maintained. Per the recommendation of the CDC, 0.5% sodium hypochlorite solution prepared from household bleach with its pH lowered into the 6 to 8 range by adding distilled white vinegar can be used to decontaminate areas with heavy contamination, such as ambulances that transported patients who were not decontaminated on scene. Otherwise a 0.1% sodium hypochlorite solution may be used to wipe environmental surfaces and equipment in areas outside the prime area.[9]

There are currently no clinically validated tests for the detection of ricin that can be performed by the hospital clinical laboratory. As a result patient treatment would be initiated before confirmation. Testing would be conducted after the incident occurred. If a health care facility suspects a substance to be ricin toxin, the laboratory, after contacting the CDC or state health department, should ship the sample to the appropriate Laboratory Response Network (LRN) facility. The LRN will test the sample through time-resolved fluorescence immunoassay or polymerase chain reaction. Positive samples may then be sent to the CDC for additional testing. If a provider suspects that a patient has been exposed to ricin toxins, a urine specimen should be collected. The health care facility should send the urine specimen to the appropriate LRN facility where they will test for ricinine, an alkaloidal toxin also found on the castor bean plant that is used as a surrogate marker for the presence of ricin.[6]

MEDICAL TREATMENT OF CASUALTIES

At this time, there is no antidote for ricin poisoning. As a result medical management is primarily supportive and determined by the route of exposure. When taking care of decontaminated patients, health care providers should practice standard universal precautions, including gown, gloves, and respiratory and eye protection. For patients who arrive to the hospital without decontamination, the CDC recommends that staff who are responsible for decontaminating victims wear a full polyethylene suit with gloves, surgical mask, face shield, and goggles.[9] In order to decontaminate patients, use soap and copious amounts of water. Asymptomatic patients should be watched for at least 12 hours. Patients who remain completely asymptomatic for 12 hours after exposure are unlikely to develop toxicity and may be discharged home with appropriate return instructions.

Ingestion

A single dose of activated charcoal should be administered in a patient who presents within 1 hour of ingestion, has an intact airway, and a normal level of consciousness. Adults should receive 50 g and children should receive 1 g/kg of activate charcoal. Patients who exhibit cardiovascular instability should be treated with intravascular fluid resuscitation and vasopressors as needed. Patients who exhibit GI blood loss should be treated with blood transfusions as necessary. Electrolyte abnormalities should be corrected. Health care providers should watch for signs of hepatic and renal failure.

Inhalation

The patient should undergo decontamination along with removal of clothing and jewelry. For patients who develop pulmonary edema, a trial of continuous positive airway pressure can be performed. However, patients should be intubated as needed. Allergic reactions should be treated with steroids, antihistamines, and beta-2 adrenergic agonists. Electrolyte abnormalities should be corrected. Health care providers should watch for signs of hepatic and renal failure.

Parenteral

The patient should receive intravenous fluid resuscitation and vasopressors as needed. Electrolyte abnormalities should be corrected. In addition to watching for signs of hepatic and renal failure, health care providers should look out for rhabdomyolysis.

Dermal

The patient should undergo decontamination along with removal of clothing and jewelry. Patients with ocular exposure should have their eyes irrigated with copious amounts of water.

UNIQUE CONSIDERATIONS

Ricin is stable under room temperature conditions and can persist in soil or a dry environment for approximately 3 days.[9]

PITFALLS

Several potential pitfalls in response to a ricin attack exist. These include the following:

- Symptoms due to ingestion of ricin may mimic infectious agents, such as viral gastroenteritis, *Salmonella, Shigella,* or *Campylobacter*
- Symptoms due to inhalation of ricin may mimic infectious agents, such as influenza or pneumonia

REFERENCES

1. Balali-Mood M, Moshiri M, Etemad L. Medical aspects of bio-terrorism. *Toxicon*. 2013;69:131–142.
2. Worbs S, Köhler K, Pauly D, et al. Ricinus communis intoxications in human and veterinary medicine—a summary of real cases. *Toxins (Basel)*. 2011;3 (10):1332–1372.
3. Doan LG. Ricin: mechanism of toxicity, clinical manifestations, and vaccine development. A review. *Clin Toxicol*. 2004;42(2):201–208.
4. Bigalke H, Rummel A. Medical aspects of toxin weapons. *Toxicology*. 2005;214(3):210–220.
5. Schep LJ, Temple WA, Butt GA, Beasley MD. Ricin as a weapon of mass terror—separating fact from fiction. *Environ Int*. 2009;35(8):1267–1271.
6. Audi J, Belson M, Patel M, et al. Ricin poisoning: a comprehensive review. *JAMA*. 2005;294(18):2342–2351.
7. Thornton SL, Darracq M, Lo J, et al. Castor bean seed ingestions: a state-wide poison control system's experience. *Clin Toxicol (Phila)*. 2014;52(4):265–268.
8. Wolfe DN, Florence W, Bryant P. Current biodefense vaccine programs and challenges. *Hum Vaccin*. 2013;9(7):1591–1597.
9. Centers for Disease Control and Prevention. Response to a Ricin Incident: Guidelines for Federal, State, and Local Public Health and Medical Officials 2006. Available at: http://www.bt.cdc.gov/agent/ricin/pdf/ricin_protocol.pdf. Accessed May 1, 2014.

CHAPTER 159

Aflatoxin (*Aspergillus* Species) Attack

Frederick Fung

DESCRIPTION OF EVENT

Aflatoxins are metabolites produced by certain strains of the fungi *Aspergillus flavus* and *Aspergillus parasiticus*. They were discovered during a disease epidemic in Great Britain that killed more than 100,000 turkeys in 1960. The source of the illness was traced to aflatoxin-contaminated turkey feed made of moldy Brazilian peanuts. Eventually it was discovered that all crops and foodstuffs, including corn, rice, wheat, barley, and nuts, can contain naturally occurring mycotoxins.[1]

There are several aflatoxins and their metabolites (such as AFB1, AFG1, AFM1) that are capable of producing human disease.[2] Aflatoxins are named by their fluorescence under ultraviolet light as blue (AFB) or green (AFG) as well as other analytic characteristics. Aflatoxins M (AFM), in which M denotes milk or mammalian metabolites, are secreted in the milk of animals exposed to aflatoxins. There are two broad categories of aflatoxins according to their structures: aflatoxins B1 and M1 are within the difurocoumarocyclopentenone series (Fig. 159-1), and aflatoxin G1 is of the difurocoumarolactone series (Fig. 159-2).

Exposure to aflatoxins is typically via ingestion of contaminated foodstuff. Dermal exposure results in slow and insignificant absorption.[3] Inhalational exposure in humans has not been studied, but food supplies could be contaminated to cause economic damage and public panic.[4] Metabolism studies in vitro have shown the following metabolic reactions for AFB1: reduction produces aflatoxicol (AFL), hydroxylation produces AFM1, hydration produces AFB2a, and epoxidation produces AFB1-2,3-epoxide. The epoxide is the most reactive metabolite and is thought to be responsible for both the acute and chronic toxicity of AFB.[5] In an Indian report ingestion of an estimated 2 to 6 mg/kg/day of aflatoxin over 1 month produced hepatitis, with some fatalities.[6] However, a suicide attempt by acute ingestion of 1.5 mg/kg of pure aflatoxin resulted only in nausea, headache, and rash.[7]

The liver is the primary target of toxicity and may lead to hepatic failure.[8] Early symptoms of hepatic injury from acute poisoning include abdominal pain, anorexia, malaise, and low-grade fever.[9] Icterus and jaundice develop within several days, followed by abdominal distention, vomiting, ascites, and edema.[10] Mortality rates from acute aflatoxicosis range from 10% to 76%.[9] The chronic effects of aflatoxins are primarily carcinogenesis resulting in hepatocellular carcinoma. Laboratory tests of liver function confirm the extent of hepatic injury in acute aflatoxicosis. Elevated aspartate and alanine aminotransferase levels frequently exceed 5000 International System of Units/L. Bilirubin levels are also increased. Acute jaundice and death have been recently reported in an outbreak of aflatoxin poisoning in Kenya.[11] In cases of liver failure, elevation of the prothrombin time, metabolic acidosis, and hypoglycemia are the characteristic signs.[12] Pathologically there is

extensive centrilobular necrosis in the perivenular zone (zone 3) extending to periportal zones (zone 1) with giant cell infiltration and cholestasis.[13]

The 1972 Biological and Toxin Weapons Convention is a major international treaty seeking to control biological warfare. It prohibits state parties from developing, producing, stockpiling, and testing biological and toxic weapons.[14,15] However, with the expansion of terrorism, the use of mycotoxins as weapons is a real threat. Possible attack scenarios include the following:

1. *Product tampering:* Substantial human and economic damage could result from consumer product tampering, such as the cyanide poisoning of Tylenol in 1984.[15] Tampering by spiking premade consumer products with mycotoxins may be the most plausible attack scenario.
2. *Chemical weaponry:* A second scenario is large-scale terrorism using aflatoxins as chemical weapons against a population group or region, such as the Anfal Operations against the Kurds of Northern Iraq.
3. *Food tampering:* Another scenario is an attack on food industries. The dairy industry is especially vulnerable to biochemical agents probably because of the nature of the manufacturing process and reliance of animal feeds that could be contaminated with biochemical (mycotoxins) agents.[15] Such an attack would cause local outbreaks of disease within hours or days. In September 2004 the Hungarian government pulled paprika off the market due to excessive levels of aflatoxin detected in much of their product.[16,17]

PRE-INCIDENT ACTIONS

Hospitals, emergency departments, and ambulatory care facilities should have general disaster plans in place to respond to a biochemical (mycotoxin) attack. Early detection of a biological or chemical weapon attack requires a surveillance system that is capable of finding and confirming the diagnosis and serving as a means of communicating this information between clinicians and health departments in a timely fashion.[18] Current syndromic surveillance appears to be directed more toward respiratory and flu-like illness, although several monitor gastrointestinal illness.[19] Efforts should be made to include hepatitis syndromes in such monitoring efforts. This would require coordination of local, state, and federal public health and safety resources. In the event of an attack, emergency medical services, hospitals, and ambulatory care facilities need to be mobilized to care for potentially large numbers of patients seeking medical care in a short timeframe. Decontamination and triage procedures should be in place and personnel properly trained before an attack occurs. Because most physicians, health care providers, and first responders are not likely to be familiar

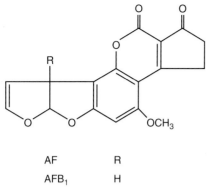

FIG 159-1 Structures of AFB_1 and AFM_1 (see text).

AF	R
AFB_1	H
AFM_1	OH

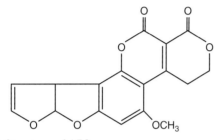

FIG 159-2 Structure of AFG_1.

with the characteristics of an aflatoxin terrorist attack, close contact with the local poison control center or local health department may be important in identifying the initial cases.

POST-INCIDENT ACTIONS

Medical providers should include aflatoxin toxicity in the differential of acute hepatitis. Appropriate local, state, and federal public health agencies and law enforcement authorities need to be notified. Aflatoxin-contaminated materials, body fluids, and surfaces should be decontaminated with a 10% bleach (sodium hypochlorite) solution.[8] Bleach should not be used to decontaminate patients. Proper sampling by a qualified industrial hygiene professional may be necessary for aflatoxin identification and evidence documentation. Further epidemiological investigations in collaboration with state or local health services may be necessary. Complete blood count and liver function tests are recommended. Analysis of blood or urine samples may provide information concerning the metabolites of the mycotoxin.

MEDICAL TREATMENT OF CASUALTIES

Treatment of acute aflatoxin exposure requires identification of and removal from the source of exposure. Activated charcoal is recommended in cases of recent ingestion. Aggressive supportive management, especially for acute liver failure, is indicated in all suspected cases. Hemodialysis and hemoperfusion are not expected to enhance elimination. Although there is no known antidote, *N*-acetylcysteine (NAC) may have a protective effect against aflatoxin carcinogenesis by increasing intracellular glutathione levels.[20] An animal model[21] found reduced hepatic injury when NAC was coadministered with high daily doses of AFB_1; however, efficacy in humans has not been demonstrated.

UNIQUE CONSIDERATIONS

Diseases caused by mycotoxins, such as aflatoxins, are most effective when they are ingested. Aflatoxin attack using an aerosolized mechanism is unlikely to produce sufficient levels to cause significant morbidity or mortality.[22]

! PITFALLS

Several potential pitfalls in response to an aflatoxin attack exist. These include the following:

- Failure to prepare adequate systems to respond to possible terrorist attacks before an incident occurs
- Failure to consider aflatoxin as the cause for nonspecific as well as systemic symptoms of acute hepatitis
- Failure to consider aflatoxin attack in the setting of a large number of otherwise healthy people presenting over hours and days with a wide range of general and specific complaints
- Failure to notify appropriate public health, safety, and law enforcement authorities when a biochemical agent attack is suspected, especially when animals fall sick along with people
- Failure to collect specimens for identification of aflatoxins
- Failure to provide basic supportive care when a patient is suspected to have been exposed to a biochemical warfare agent

REFERENCES

1. Pitt JI, Basilico JC, Abarca ML, et al. Mycotoxins and toxigenic fungi. *Med Mycol.* 2000;38(Suppl 1):41–46.
2. Fung F, Clark RF. Health effects of mycotoxins: a toxicological overview. *Clin Toxicol.* 2004;42:1–18.
3. Riley RT, Kemppainen BW, Norred WP. Penetration of aflatoxins through isolated epidermis. *J Toxicol Environ Health.* 1985;15:769–777.
4. Anderson PD. Bioterrorism: toxins as weapons. *J Pharm Prac.* 2012;25:121–129.
5. Hsieh DPH, Wong JJ. Metabolism and toxicity of aflatoxins. *Adv Exp Med Biol.* 1982;126(B):847–863.
6. Patten RC. Aflatoxins and disease. *Am J Trop Med Hyg.* 1981;30:422–425.
7. Willis RM, Mulvihill JJ, Hoofnagle JH. Attempted suicide with purified aflatoxin. *Lancet.* 1980;1(8179):1198–1199.
8. Stark AB. Threat assessment of mycotoxins as weapons. *J Food Prot.* 2005;68:1285–1293.
9. Ngindu A, Johnson BK, Kenya PR, et al. Outbreak of acute hepatitis caused by aflatoxin poisoning in Kenya. *Lancet.* 1982;1:1346–1348.
10. Krishnamachari KA, Bhat RV, Nagarajan V, et al. Hepatitis due to aflatoxicosis: an outbreak in Western India. *Lancet.* 1975;1:1061–1063.
11. Nyikal J, Misore A, Nzioka C, et al. Outbreak of aflatoxin poisoning: eastern and central provinces, Kenya, January-July, 2004. *MMWR Morb Mortal Wkly Rep.* 2004;53(34):790–793.
12. Olson LC, Bourgeois CH Jr, Cotton RB, et al. Encephalopathy and fatty degeneration of the viscera in northeastern Thailand: clinical syndrome and epidemiology. *Pediatrics.* 1971;47:707–716.
13. Chao TC, Maxwell SM, Wong SY. An outbreak of aflatoxicosis and boric acid poisoning in Malaysia: a clinicopathological study. *J Pathol.* 1991;164:225–233.
14. Zilinskas RA. Verifying compliance to the biological and toxin weapons convention. *Crit Rev Microbiol.* 1998;24(3):195–218.
15. Zilinskas RA. Terrorism and biological weapons: inevitable alliance? *Perspect Biol Med.* 1990;34:44–72.
16. Greenberg G. *Hungarian government temporarily prohibits sale of paprika.* November 3, 2004. Available at: (1) BBC: Hungarian Paprika Ban. Available at: http://www.bbc.co.uk/worldservice/learningenglish/newsenglish/witn/2004/10/041029_paprika.shtml. Accessed April 12, 2015. (2) Reuters: UT San Diego Hungary puts ban on sale of paprika http://www.utsandiego.com/uniontrib/20041028/news_1n28paprika.html.

Accessed April 12, 2015. http://www.utsandiego.com/uniontrib/20041028/news_1n28paprika.html. Accessed April 12, 2015.

17. Paterson RR, Lima N. Toxicology of mycotoxins. *EXS.* 2010;100:31–63.

18. Buehler JW, Hopkins RS, Overhage JM, et al. Framework for evaluating public health surveillance systems for early detection of outbreaks. *MMWR Morb Mortal Wkly Rep.* 2004;53(RR05):1–11.

19. Bravata DM, McDonald KM, Smith WM, et al. Systemic review: surveillance systems for early detection of bioterrorism-related diseases. *Ann Intern Med.* 2004;140:910–922.

20. De Flora S, Bennicelli C, Camoirano A, et al. In vivo effects of *N*-acetylcysteine on glutathione metabolism and on the biotransformation of carcinogenic and/or mutagenic compounds. *Carcinogenesis.* 1985;6:1735–1745.

21. Valdivia AG, Martinez A, Damian FJ, et al. Efficacy of *N*-acetylcysteine to reduce the effects of aflatoxin B1 intoxication in broiler chickens. *Poult Sci.* 2001;80:727–734.

22. Ciegler A. *Mycotoxins: A New Class of Chemical Weapons.* Washington, DC: NBC Defense and Technology International, Department of Defense; April 1986, 52-57.

160 | CHAPTER

Coccidioides immitis (Coccidioidomycosis) Attack

Robyn Wing and Siraj Amanullah

DESCRIPTION OF EVENT

Coccidioidomycosis, also known as "San Joaquin Valley Fever," "Valley Fever," or "desert rheumatism," is a fungal infection that results after inhalation of airborne spores of *Coccidioides immitis*. This soil-dwelling fungus is endemic primarily in six states in the United States: Arizona, California, New Mexico, Nevada, Texas, and Utah. The California Department of Public Health reported 25,217 coccidioidomycosis-associated hospitalizations for 15,747 patients from 2000 to 2011, making the San Joaquin Valley area the one with the highest incidence and prevalence of this illness.[1] Other endemic regions include Central and South America. The incidence in the endemic areas of United States has substantially increased from 5.3 per 100,000 in 1998 to 42.6 per 100,000 in 2011.[2] Of an estimated 150,000 annual reported cases, 50,000 are symptomatic.[3,4] Despite the majority of long-term residents in the endemic areas demonstrating evidence of prior *C. immitis* infection, there are still intermittent sharp seasonal increases in the number of cases, suggesting either infectivity of the disease or mutation by the organism.

C. immitis thrives in warm sandy soil in climates with hot summers, mild winters, and fewer than 20 inches of rainfall per year.[5] It exists as both a saprophyte and a parasite at different times during its life cycle. During the saprophytic stage, it grows in soil as a mold with septate hyphae. This mold ages to produce spores (arthroconidia) that can disperse in the air and are capable of resulting in epidemics of disease, especially after large-scale soil disturbances such as earthquakes, excavations, droughts, or dust storms.[6,7] Once inhaled, they start the parasitic phase of the life cycle in an animal or human as host. In the pulmonary alveoli, they grow into multinucleate spherules and large parasitic cells producing thousands of uninucleate endospores. Each endospore can in turn develop into a new spherule, further affecting the lungs.[8] Dissemination through the bloodstream has been shown to lead to deposition in perihilar, peritracheal, and cervical lymph nodes. Multisystem involvement can result in skin, soft tissue, joint, bone, or meningeal infection.

T cell immunity is pivotal for defense against coccidioidomycosis, although antibodies do not appear to confer protection against the organism.[9] Hence immunocompromised patients with T cell dysfunction such as human immunodeficiency virus (HIV) infection or patients on immunosuppressive agents are at high risk of severe primary infection, including disseminated illness or reactivation of latent disease.[10,11] Pregnant women, particularly those in the third trimester, are also at higher risk of disseminated disease possibly due to depressed cellular immunity and changes in hormone levels stimulating the growth of *C. immitus*.[12] There is also variation in susceptibility of disease among ethnic groups with African Americans and Filipinos having increased incidence of severe or disseminated disease.[13,14]

Approximately 60% of infected individuals are asymptomatic. In the remaining 40% of acutely exposed persons, the most common clinical manifestation is an acute respiratory infection that occurs 1 to 3 weeks after inhalation of spores.[15] Symptoms are similar to mild to moderate influenza-like illness or community-acquired pneumonia such as productive cough, fever, anorexia, weakness, myalgias, and arthalgias.[16] Severe headache, pleuritic chest pain, and profound fatigue with an acute respiratory illness are strongly suggestive of coccidioidal infection in endemic areas. Other pulmonary manifestations include pleural effusion, hilar lymphadenopathy, pulmonary nodules or cavities, and chronic progressive pneumonia.[15] The majority of infected individuals have spontaneous resolution of symptoms in 2 to 3 weeks, but median duration of illness has been found to be 120 days.[17–19] Less than 5% of immunocompetent patients develop disseminated extrapulmonary disease via lymphatics or blood. The most common extrapulmonary disease site is the skin, with superficial maculopapules, keratotic nodules, verrucous plaques, ulcers, and subcutaneous fluctuant abscesses being found.[18] Erythema multiforme has also been reported to be associated with *C. immitus* infection.[16] Erythema nodosum, characterized by painful subcutaneous red nodules on the lower extremities, may occur with a predilection for white and female patients.[16] Erythema nodosum may be the initial presentation of illness and reflects a vigorous cell-mediated immune response, which may confer a protective advantage against the organism.[20] Bone and joint infections may occur, in the company of dramatic effusions and synovial involvement, with dissemination. Coccidioidomycosis osteomyelitis may affect several bones, but common sites include the spine, tibia, skull, femur, and ribs.[18] Arthritis is unifocal in 90% of cases with the knee being the most commonly affected joint, followed by the ankle.[19]

The most feared and life-threatening form of disseminated disease is coccidioidal meningitis and is seen in one half of individuals with disseminated disease. Death within a few months was universal prior to the use of amphotericin B.[21] Presenting symptoms are fever, headache, vomiting, and altered mental status. Complications include hydrocephalus, cerebral vasculitis or infarction, and focal intracerebral coccidioidal abscesses.[21] Urgent neurosurgical consultation is important for shunting or incision and drainage. Rare presentations of disseminated coccidioidomycosis include fungemia, hepatitis, and intestinal infection.[22,23]

Diagnosis of coccidioidomycosis may be difficult and challenging, primarily due to a failure to consider the disease outside its endemic areas. A specific travel history is usually necessary in nonendemic areas to prompt suspicion of the diagnosis. Routine laboratory tests are not specific, although the erythrocyte sedimentation rate is usually elevated and the eosinophil counts are often increased.[24] Diagnosis of coccicioidal infection can be made in three ways: (1) identification of spherules in a cytology or biopsy specimen, (2) positive culture from any body fluid, or (3) serological testing. Direct microscopic examination of infected tissue samples will reveal the organism. Whereas culture and serologic testing are the most commonly available tests, direct microscopic examination of tissue samples is deemed safest. In histopathology specimens, a mature spherule with endospores is pathognomonic of infection and is easily recognizable on wet mounts using potassium hydroxide or Calcofluor white fluorescent stain. Spherules can also be seen with various staining techniques, for example, Grocott methenamine silver (GMS) and periodic acid-Schiff (PAS) stains.[24] The recovery of *Coccidioides* by culture is the most definitive diagnostic method but requires careful biosafety considerations. The organism can often be seen in, or grown from, pus, sputum, and body fluid aspirates (such as bronchoalveolar lavage). Not surprisingly, the respiratory tract yields the highest recovery rate.[24] The mycelial form of the fungus has minimal growth requirements, growing after 3 to 5 days on most mycologic or bacteriologic media under aerobic conditions and at most temperatures.[25] Mature colonies can have a myriad of appearances and can be confirmed using AccuProbe nucleic acid hybridization.[26] Serologic testing is useful for diagnosis and management of disease. Anticoccidioidal IgM and IgG are not protective but do indicate the organism's level of activity in the host and are highly specific but less sensitive. Serological response may be absent or compromised in immunosuppressed patients. Therefore, negative serological results cannot be used to rule out disease.[24,27] IgM antibodies are detected transiently in 50% of acutely infected persons in the first week and in 90% by the third week. Complement-fixing IgG becomes measurable 2 to 28 weeks after the acute infection and disappears in 6 to 9 months if symptoms resolve.[24] Persistently elevated IgG antibody is observed in disseminated disease when titer generally correlates with severity of disease.

In patients with *C. immitis* meningitis, cerebrospinal fluid (CSF) cultures are diagnostic, but are usually negative in 85% of early cases.[19] The CSF will show a marked mononuclear pleocytosis, low glucose level, and high protein level. A positive result of an IgG test of the CSF confirms the diagnosis, but a negative test cannot rule out the disease. There is currently no antigen detection method for *Coccidioides* infection.[21]

Imaging studies are nonspecific but can aid in the diagnosis. Chest radiographs may delineate pulmonary cavities, persistent nodules, and granulomas.[16] Magnetic resonance imaging may be useful to examine the brain for signs of meningitis, including typical basilar cistern enhancement or hydrocephalus, vasculitic infarction, or abscesses.[21] Skeletal lesions will have a lytic "punched out" appearance on plain radiographs, and radionuclide bone scanning may also be used to delineate bone lesions.[16]

C. immitis is the most virulent of the known primary fungal pathogens in humans and other animals. As such, it is the only fungus on the United States "Select Agent Rule" list due to its potential to cause widespread harm to human health.[28] It is classified as requiring Biosafety Level 3 (BLS3) practices for facilities handling this spore.[29] This fungus has many characteristics that would make it an ideal biological weapon. Spores are easily procured from their natural environment, and cultures are simple and inexpensive, resulting in a low cost of production. There is also a relative ease of dissemination (at least on a small scale) through aerosolization of spores. The fungus has a very high

virulence, with inhalation of only a few *C. immitis* spores required to produce primary coccidioidomycosis.[15] The high infectivity rate, especially with high levels of exposure, has been shown in some point-source outbreaks, with up to 100% of those exposed becoming infected.[30,31] Outbreaks have been demonstrated when coccidioidomycosis has been specifically grown in the laboratory setting, such as in the case of hospital laboratory personnel attempting to diagnose a patient. This occurrence demonstrates the increased virulence of the spore form of the organism when being grown in the laboratory. While *C. immitus* should be handled with great caution, perpetrators could protect themselves by taking prophylactic antifungal medications.[32]

Each year, 25,000 new cases are diagnosed with a crude mortality rate of 6% among adults and 7% among children.[33] These deaths almost always occur in those persons suffering from disseminated disease. The most common dissemination is to the skin, closely followed by the meninges. If meningitis occurs, the mortality rate is greater than 95% if not treated and 30% if treated.[21]

Coccidioidomycosis is potentially a lethal biological agent especially when it results in a disseminated illness. Health care workers in nonendemic areas may not initially recognize a coccidioidomycosis attack. With the majority of patients asymptomatic, and those who are symptomatic displaying a nonspecific upper respiratory infection, initial cases may be ignored or diagnosed as a self-limited viral disease. The long incubation period of 3 to 4 weeks may further hinder a clinician from making the connection from initial exposure to disease. For the sickest patients, an even longer incubation period of up to 1 year may be evident, further complicating the diagnosis and increasing the morbidity in the specific population of infected persons with the highest mortality. Although there has been no documented incidence of person-to-person spread through air droplets, the infectivity of these long-incubation patients is unknown. Use of *C. immitis* as a weapon could therefore cause a subtle increase in the workload of the health care system over time.

C. immitus could also be used an agent of agroterrorism as it is equally lethal in the animal population. Therefore an attack on farm animals could have economic consequences. In addition, an adversary may attempt environmental contamination through persistent contamination of soil, causing an indirect economic disruption.[32]

Despite the many concerning aspects of coccidioidomycosis, *C. immitus* has many properties that limit its desirability as a biological weapon. Most immunocompetent patients are asymptomatic, with only 40% of infected persons displaying any type of symptom. Among those who are symptomatic, the most common form is an upper or lower respiratory tract infection that usually resolves without specific therapy. Extrapulmonary manifestations have much higher morbidity and mortality but occur in only 0.5% of cases, may take up to a year to develop, and occur in specific subpopulations of at-risk persons. Lack of secondary transmission also limits the use of *C. immitis* as a biological weapon, as person-to-person spread does not occur. Problems with weaponization and delivery would have to be overcome in order for an attack to be successful. A large-scale attack would be complicated because airborne pathogens are difficult to control and disseminate over large areas, as wind, rain, and barometric pressures may affect dispersal of the agent.[28] Lastly, availability of effective treatment would limit the use of *C. immitis* as an effective bioweapon.

As with any potential bioterrorism agent, clinical suspicion due to the presence of a cluster of cases with similar illness is required. Such clusters then need to be worked up for a potential bioterrorism attack along with other possibilities to avoid undue morbidity and mortality of such an attack due to delayed diagnosis and management. The most likely scenario of a *C. immitis* attack would consist of a large urban population with a large number of persons presenting over a few weeks with a nonspecific upper respiratory infection. The most severely affected people would include minority populations, pregnant women, infants, immunocompromised patients (such as those with HIV or those having received an organ transplant), and patients taking steroids. An effective attack would require a large target population in one of these at-risk groups localized in a specific area that could be inoculated with airborne particles. Although evidence of prior infection may already be present in much of the population, a dramatic increase in clinical cases should alert health care workers, and once positive diagnoses are made, a biological attack should be considered. The population should be followed up for as long as 1 year after the incident for evidence of chronic severe infection; this requirement in itself will increase the load on the health care system and could increase public fear, as those exposed would constantly worry that they might develop delayed and serious illness. Indeed, the most profound effect of an attack using *C. immitus* is likely to be psychological.[32]

PRE-INCIDENT ACTIONS

In endemic areas, coccidioidomycosis can only be prevented by occupationally preventing susceptible persons from working in high-risk situations. In these specific areas, focused educational programs for construction and agricultural workers, students, military personnel, and health care workers should be in place. Documented cases of mass infection with *C. immitis* show occurrence in one of three ways: (1) recent visit to an endemic area, (2) reactivation of a prior infection, or (3) exposure to spores brought out of an endemic area.

The pre-incident actions include being prepared for any potential bioterrorism attack. Hospitals, emergency departments, and outpatient facilities should each have a disaster response plan in place. Coordination of local, state, and national public health and public safety resources are required in the event of a mass-casualty situation such as biological warfare. Both emergency medical services and hospital triage systems may need to be altered to account for the influx of patients with specific treatment requirements—in this case, respiratory ailments. Universal precautions should be in place, even though person-to-person transmission of coccidioidomycosis has never been documented. Diagnosis of the index case may be difficult, mainly due to a lack of suspicion for the agent in nonendemic areas. Special and specific care needs to be taken with the culturing of *C. immitis* with precautions including specialized training for laboratory technicians, universal precautions, Biosafety Level 3 procedures, and negative pressure rooms.[24,25] Physicians should be trained to highlight their suspicions for coccidioidomycosis when submitting culture specimens from suspect patients.

Although a real coccidioidomycosis attack or a major natural outbreak is unlikely, health care providers need to be aware of the disease and keep it on their list of differential diagnoses. The possibly long incubation period, nonspecific complaints, and multiple organ involvement may make initial diagnosis extremely difficult. Universal precautions need to be in place, as well as a surveillance system that can recognize a trend in patient syndromes. With documentation of trends over time, a specific index incident may be able to be identified.

An effective vaccine against coccidioidomycosis would be promising, as recovery from coccidioidomycosis results in apparent lifelong immunity to the disease.[34] Several vaccine preparations have been developed and proven useful in animal models, but a successful human vaccine has not yet been created.[34]

POST-INCIDENT ACTIONS

Health care providers with suspicion of, or a clear demonstrated case of, coccidioidomycosis need to contact specific public health officials because coccidioidomycosis became a nationally reportable disease in 1995.[35] Any medical providers or disaster responders that may have come into contact with the fungus need to be identified and possibly given fluconazole.[32] Such responders include any hospital or clinic worker, any physicians who treated patients from a specific location, emergency medical services personnel, police, fire personnel, cleanup crews, those working for the Red Cross and other relief organizations, and the military. While there are no data regarding use of antifungal prophylaxis in exposed individuals, fluconazole could be considered.[32] In cases of known soil contamination, workers should be encouraged to keep dust levels to a minimum and wear masks to prevent entry of spores into the airway.

Quarantine is of no value, as human-to-human and animal-to-human transmission does not occur. Disinfection of surfaces possibly contaminated with arthroconidia should be carried out with standard disinfectants or antiseptic agents.

MEDICAL TREATMENT OF CASUALTIES

Of the endemic fungal infections, coccidioidomycosis is the most resistant to therapy.[36] The treatment approach depends on three factors: (1) the severity of pulmonary infection, (2) the presence of dissemination, and (3) the individual patient's risk factors.[3,37] The treatment and care of primary uncomplicated respiratory infection is controversial, primarily due to the lack of controlled clinical trials. However, most authorities believe that antifungal therapy is not necessary in immunocompetent patients with mild pulmonary illness.[38] For these patients, care should include symptomatic treatment and careful reexamination to ensure the resolution of symptoms. Follow-up radiology for 1 to 2 years to monitor the resolution of pulmonary findings is also recommended.[37] Historically, initial pulmonary manifestations have a 95% spontaneous resolution rate. However, if risk factors for dissemination are present, rapid and high-dose antifungal medications should be given. Treatment is warranted for those with symptoms that persist longer than 2 months, weight loss greater than 10%, night sweats, extensive pulmonary infiltrates, certain ethnic backgrounds (Filipino, African American, or Mexican), pregnant female patients in their third trimester, or those with antibody titer greater than 1:16.[15] Treatments of choice are azole medications, such as fluconazole or itraconazole, for 3 to 6 months. Pregnant women, especially those in their third trimester, should be treated with amphotericin B as azoles are teratogenic.[16]

In cases of severe pulmonary or disseminated disease, antifungal therapy should always be initiated. No studies to date have directly compared amphotericin B with azole therapy. Although known for potent side effects, amphotericin B is preferred due to the more rapid onset when compared with the azoles.[39] Amphotericin B is usually administered for a total of 2 to 4 months, followed by maintenance azole therapy for 1 year or longer. Immunocompromised patients require indefinite azole therapy.[15] Future treatment may involve novel azole agents (e.g., posaconazole, voriconazole), caspofungin (an echinocandin that inhibits glucan synthetase), or sordarin derivatives (drugs that specifically inhibit fungal protein synthesis).[36] Surgical debridement of focal coccidioidomycosis infection is used sparingly, especially for infections with significant morbidity such as a paraspinal abscess. Surgery should be determined on a case-by-case basis and is an option in the case of extensive bone or skin involvement. The theory behind the use of debridement is that the spherule wall (1) is a strong stimulus for inflammation, (2) cannot be degraded by the body, and (3) cannot be cleared by macrophages. Thus, continued tissue damage can occur until the spherule is physically removed. Also, pulmonary cavities have been shown to react poorly to chemotherapy.[19]

The treatment of coccidioidal meningitis is challenging. Traditionally, a combination of intravenous and intrathecal amphotericin B has been used. However, several studies have reported comparable success with high-dose fluconazole.[21,40,41] Due to a high relapse rate, lifelong therapy is required. Alternative therapies for those who do not respond include voriconazole or intrathecal amphotericin B.[21] Hydrocephalus may require ventriculoperitoneal shunting, and brain abscesses may require drainage or excision.

❓ UNIQUE CONSIDERATIONS

Coccidioidomycosis is a fungal infection that usually causes self-limited upper respiratory or febrile illnesses. When disseminated, however, it can cause life-threatening extrapulmonary disease. Its manifestations are similar to many common nonspecific illnesses and thus may elude diagnosis. Although it is considered a possible biological weapon due to the high virulence of the arthroconidia and severe mortality of the disseminated disease, *C. immitis* would likely make a poor bioweapon due to its very long incubation period and the fact that it is not a virulent infection in normal hosts. Terrorists would need to either find a way to cause immune suppression in a normal population in advance of seeding the infection or target a compromised host population. The use of coccidioidomycosis as a biological weapon would be ineffective, and the identification of infected persons would be extremely difficult; a natural outbreak is far more likely but poses similar diagnostic pitfalls. The main points to remember are to keep this organism in the differential diagnosis and remember that appropriate therapy requires a multidisciplinary approach, using symptomatic therapy, antifungal chemotherapy, and surgery to produce the best outcome.

❗ PITFALLS

Several potential pitfalls in response to an attack exist. These include the following:

- Failure to have a disaster response plan
- Failure to consider coccidioidomycosis as a possible cause in patients with mild symptoms
- Failure to adequately diagnose persons suspected of having the disease process
- Failure to adequately treat patients with both surgical options as well as antifungal agents
- Failure to have adequately prepared and trained laboratory capabilities
- Failure to notify laboratory workers of a high suspicion for coccidioidomycosis in submitted specimens, so that they may take appropriate precautions to limit their own exposure
- Failure to notify and screen possibly infected persons who were involved with the index incident
- Failure to notify local, state, and federal agencies in the instance of a suspected case

REFERENCES

1. Sondermeyer G, Lee L, Gilliss D, Tabnak F, Vugia D. Coccidioidomycosis-associated hospitalizations, California, USA, 2000-2011. *Emerg Infect Dis.* 2013;19(10):1590–1597.
2. Centers for Disease Control. Increase in reported coccidioidomycosis—United States, 1998-2011. *MMWR.* 2013;62(12):217–221.
3. Galgiani JN, Ampel NM, Blair JE, et al. Coccidioidomycosis. *Clin Infect Dis.* 2005;41(9):1217–1223.
4. Hector RF, Rutherford GW, Tsang CA, et al. The public health impact of coccidioidomycosis in Arizona and California. *Int J Environ Res Public Health.* 2011;8(4):1150–1173.
5. Fisher FS, Bultman MW, Johnson SM, Pappagianis D, Zaborsky E. Coccidioides niches and habitat parameters in the southwestern United States: a matter of scale. *Ann N Y Acad Sci.* 2007;1111:47–72.
6. Laniado-Laborin R. Expanding understanding of epidemiology of coccidioidomycosis in the Western hemisphere. *Ann N Y Acad Sci.* 2007;1111:19–34.
7. Schneider E, Hajjeh RA, Spiegel RA, et al. A coccidioidomycosis outbreak following the Northridge, Calif, earthquake. *JAMA.* 1997;277(11):904–908.
8. Hung CY, Xue J, Cole GT. Virulence mechanisms of coccidioides. *Ann N Y Acad Sci.* 2007;1111:225–235.
9. Borchers AT, Gershwin ME. The immune response in coccidioidomycosis. *Autoimmun Rev.* 2010;10(2):94–102.
10. Bergstrom L, Yocum DE, Ampel NM, et al. Increased risk of coccidioidomycosis in patients treated with tumor necrosis factor alpha antagonists. *Arthritis Rheum.* 2004;50(6):1959–1966.
11. Blair JE, Smilack JD, Caples SM. Coccidioidomycosis in patients with hematologic malignancies. *Arch Intern Med.* 2005;165(1):113–117.
12. Crum NF, Ballon-Landa G. Coccidioidomycosis in pregnancy: case report and review of the literature. *Am J Med.* 2006;119(11):993, e11-7.
13. Ruddy BE, Mayer AP, Ko MG, et al. Coccidioidomycosis in African Americans. *Mayo Clin Proc.* 2011;86(1):63–69.
14. Crum NF, Lederman ER, Stafford CM, Parrish JS, Wallace MR. Coccidioidomycosis: a descriptive survey of a reemerging disease. Clinical characteristics and current controversies. *Medicine (Baltimore).* 2004;83(3):149–175.
15. Parish JM, Blair JE. Coccidioidomycosis. *Mayo Clin Proc.* 2008;83(3):343–348, quiz 348–349.
16. DiCaudo DJ. Coccidioidomycosis: a review and update. *J Am Acad Dermatol.* 2006;55(6):929–942, quiz 943–945.
17. Tsang CA, Anderson SM, Imholte SB, et al. Enhanced surveillance of coccidioidomycosis, Arizona, USA, 2007-2008. *Emerg Infect Dis.* 2010;16(11):1738–1744.
18. Welsh O, Vera-Cabrera L, Rendon A, Gonzalez G, Bonifaz A. Coccidioidomycosis. *Clin Dermatol.* 2012;30(6):573–591.
19. Stevens DA. Coccidioidomycosis. *N Engl J Med.* 1995;332(16):1077–1082.
20. Braverman IM. Protective effects of erythema nodosum in coccidioidomycosis. *Lancet.* 1999;353(9148):168.
21. Johnson RH, Einstein HE. Coccidioidal meningitis. *Clin Infect Dis.* 2006;42(1):103–107.
22. Keckich DW, Blair JE, Vikram HR. Coccidioides fungemia in six patients, with a review of the literature. *Mycopathologia.* 2010;170(2):107–115.
23. Smith G, Hoover S, Sobonya R, Klotz SA. Abdominal and pelvic coccidioidomycosis. *Am J Med Sci.* 2011;341(4):308–311.
24. Saubolle MA. Laboratory aspects in the diagnosis of coccidioidomycosis. *Ann N Y Acad Sci.* 2007;1111:301–314.
25. Sutton DA. Diagnosis of coccidioidomycosis by culture: safety considerations, traditional methods, and susceptibility testing. *Ann N Y Acad Sci.* 2007;1111:315–325.
26. Padhye AA, Smith G, Standard PG, McLaughlin D, Kaufman L. Comparative evaluation of chemiluminescent DNA probe assays and exoantigen tests for rapid identification of *Blastomyces dermatitidis* and *Coccidioides immitis*. *J Clin Microbiol.* 1994;32(4):867–870.
27. Pappagianis D. Serologic studies in coccidioidomycosis. *Semin Respir Infect.* 2001;16(4):242–250.
28. Warnock DW. Coccidioides species as potential agents of bioterrorism. *Future Microbiol.* 2007;2(3):277–283.
29. Services UDoHaH. *Biosafety in microbiological and biomedical laboratories.* 4th Ed Washington, DC: US Government Printing Service; 1999.
30. Cairns L, Blythe D, Kao A, et al. Outbreak of coccidioidomycosis in Washington state residents returning from Mexico. *Clin Infect Dis.* 2000;30(1):61–64.
31. Petersen LR, Marshall SL, Barton-Dickson C, et al. Coccidioidomycosis among workers at an archeological site, northeastern Utah. *Emerg Infect Dis.* 2004;10(4):637–642.
32. Deresinski S. *Coccidioides immitis* as a potential bioweapon. *Semin Respir Infect.* 2003;18(3):216–219.

33. Chu JH, Feudtner C, Heydon K, Walsh TJ, Zaoutis TE. Hospitalizations for endemic mycoses: a population-based national study. *Clin Infect Dis.* 2006;42(6):822–825.

34. Yoon HJ, Clemons KV. Vaccines against Coccidioides. *Korean J Intern Med.* 2013;28(4):403–407.

35. Centers for Disease Control and Prevention. Increase in coccidioidomycosis—Arizona, 1998-2001. *JAMA.* 2003;289(12):1500–1502.

36. Deresinski SC. Coccidioidomycosis: efficacy of new agents and future prospects. *Curr Opin Infect Dis.* 2001;14(6):693–696.

37. Galgiani JN, Ampel NM, Catanzaro A, Johnson RH, Stevens DA, Williams PL. Practice guideline for the treatment of coccidioidomycosis. Infectious Diseases Society of America. *Clin Infect Dis.* 2000;30(4):658–661.

38. Chiller TM, Galgiani JN, Stevens DA. Coccidioidomycosis. *Infect Dis Clin North Am.* 2003;17(1):41–57, viii.

39. Johnson RH, Einstein HE. Amphotericin B and coccidioidomycosis. *Ann N Y Acad Sci.* 2007;1111:434–441.

40. Galgiani JN, Catanzaro A, Cloud GA, et al. Fluconazole therapy for coccidioidal meningitis. The NIAID-Mycoses Study Group. *Ann Intern Med.* 1993;119(1):28–35.

41. Segal BH, Herbrecht R, Stevens DA, et al. Defining responses to therapy and study outcomes in clinical trials of invasive fungal diseases: Mycoses Study Group and European Organization for Research and Treatment of Cancer consensus criteria. *Clin Infect Dis.* 2008;47(5):674–683.

CHAPTER 161

Histoplasma capsulatum (Histoplasmosis) Attack

Wendy Hin-Wing Wong, Robert Partridge, and Lawrence Proano

DESCRIPTION OF EVENT

Histoplasmosis is caused by a small dimorphic fungus, *Histoplasma capsulatum*, a systemic mycosis with a worldwide distribution. It is endemic to the Americas, Africa, Asia, Australia, and some areas of Central Europe.[1,2] Histoplasmosis is the most common primary systemic mycosis in America and the most common fungal lung infection in the world.[3-6] In endemic areas, it is so common that up to 80% of adults have already been unknowingly infected.[3,7] Spores thrive in soil enriched with bird or bat excrement and are found in caves, trees, chicken coops, mines, water tanks, farms, abandoned buildings, basements, and attics. Outbreaks of histoplasmosis occur after travel to endemic areas and after activities that disturb contaminated soil. Histoplasmosis is an opportunistic infection in the immunosuppressed, with a reported frequency of over 10% in HIV/AIDS patients in endemic areas.[6]

The majority of infections occur through inhalation of *H. capsulatum* spores. Once inhaled, spores will germinate and progress to yeast-like forms, multiplying within alveolar macrophages in the lower respiratory tract and disseminating systemically. Within 2 to 3 weeks the infection is controlled by cell-mediated immunity, which encases infected tissue in a fibrous capsule or granuloma. Small numbers of viable yeast can be contained within a granuloma for decades, forming a reservoir for relapsing disease or possible foci of reactivation in latent disease.[1,8]

Disease presentation and clinical severity are highly varied because they depend on the host's immune status and the amount of organisms inhaled. Asymptomatic infections or self-limited pulmonary disease comprise 95% of all histoplasmosis infections.[1] When present, symptoms tend to appear within 3 to 17 days after exposure. Histoplasmosis has no unique clinical findings.[9] Most acute pulmonary histoplasmosis infections are mistaken for the flu as symptoms are nonspecific and include low-grade fever, myalgias, cough, headache, and fatigue. Pallor is a common sign.[5] Severe disease can cause dyspnea, weight loss, pneumonitis, or adult respiratory distress syndrome (ARDS).

Cell-mediated immunity is the key defense against *H. capsulatum*.[10,11] Increased disease severity and likelihood of dissemination tend to occur in people with defective or immature cellular immunity, such as infants and those with HIV or chronic immunosuppression. The most severe form of histoplasmosis is progressive disseminated histoplasmosis (PDH), which can occur in primary or reactivated infection but rarely occurs in otherwise well individuals. PDH is fatal if left untreated. However, with prompt recognition and therapy, mortality decreases from 100% to less than 20%.[1,12] PDH is defined as persistent clinical illness for at least 3 weeks with evidence of infection in extrapulmonary tissues.[12] Prolonged symptoms for months can commonly present as fever of unknown origin.[3] Patients may present with an overwhelming infection with pancytopenia, elevated serum ferritin, hepatosplenomegaly, gastrointestinal involvement with progressive transaminitis, increased lactate dehydrogenase, or mucosal ulcers and skin lesions.[12]

CNS histoplasmosis occurs in 5% to 10% of PDH cases, manifesting as meningitis, brain or spinal cord lesions, encephalitis, or stroke syndromes.[13] Meningitis is common in infants with PDH.[12] Complications of histoplasmosis can cause an inflammatory response resulting in pericarditis, pericardial effusion, cardiac tamponade, or rheumatologic syndromes (arthritis, arthralgias, and erythema nodosum).[1,5] Mediastinal lymphadenitis can cause compression of adjacent structures. Children are more prone to present with airway obstruction, and up to 60% of mediastinal masses in children from endemic areas are due to histoplasmosis.[1] In patients with comorbid lung disease such as emphysema, a chronic form of pulmonary histoplasmosis exists but is not of concern in the acute setting. In the central United States, histoplasmosis is the most common cause of mediastinal fibrosis.[14] Other complications include mediastinal granulomas, histoplasmomas, broncholithiasis, or chorioretinitis.

Although there are no reports of *H. capsulatum* being weaponized, a 1994 congressional report revealed that the United States government approved the sale of potentially lethal biological agents including *H. capsulatum* to Iraq from 1985 through 1989, which could have contributed to their biological warfare program.[15,16] A disaster from an intentional release of infective spores would not be difficult as spores can be aerosolized and carried for miles in air currents.[12] Forced-air ventilation systems that recirculate spores for days after the initial contamination have been implicated in the three largest histoplasmosis outbreaks.[8] Heating of histoplasma spores in conjunction with fire-related air currents (such as through burning of contaminated bamboo) may increase the infectivity rate.[17]

Despite the ability of *H. capsulatum* to be an undetectable, airborne infectious agent with the potential to cause life-threatening illness, it is not an ideal biologic weapon. People from endemic areas may be resistant to infection because of immunity from previous contact or subclinical infection.[4] Even though exposure to a large inoculum of inhaled spores can cause severe disease in otherwise healthy individuals, the toxic exposure limit is unknown.[11] Mortality and morbidity from histoplasmosis are generally low once it is properly treated. During one of the largest outbreaks in the United States, there were only 15 fatalities out of 120,000 infected patients.[8]

Because clinical manifestations of histoplasmosis is nonspecific, it has been called the "fungal syphilis," and diagnosis requires a high clinical suspicion as symptoms often go unnoticed.[6] The differential diagnosis is broad and includes influenza; upper respiratory disease such as pneumonia, tuberculosis, or other systemic mycosis; meningitis; lung cancer; or other viral/parasitic infections such as toxoplasmosis or malaria. Histoplasmosis can present as a solitary pulmonary nodule that often mimics lung cancer.

The most common radiographic finding is bilateral hilar or mediastinal lymphadenopathy with lobar or patchy infiltrates; hilar lymphadenopathy is helpful in differentiating histoplasmosis from bacterial pneumonia.[11] However, the chest x-ray may be normal in 40% to 50% of patients with disseminated disease.[3] Chest CT scan may show small single or multiple nodules, granulomas, mediastinal fibrosis, or cavitations.[5]

Diagnostic testing includes antigen detection, serology for antibody detection, cultures, polymerase chain reaction (PCR), and histopathology. In the acute setting, antigen detection in blood or urine is the most pertinent diagnostic test. Results are available within 24 to 48 hours and are more sensitive than antibody testing. Urine antigen is positive in 92% of disseminated disease and over 75% of acute histoplasmosis cases.[5] However, antigen testing is not available in all countries, and both antigen and serology tests may be positive in patients with other systemic mycoses due to cross-reactivity.[2,5]

In immunocompetent patients who are symptomatic, seropositivity will correlate with disease severity; antibodies are detected in only 18% of asymptomatic patients, 75% to 86% of symptomatic patients, and up to 100% of patients with severe symptoms.[1,5] Two antibody assays that are available are the immunodiffusion (ID) test and complement fixation test (CFT); the former is more specific in acute disease.[8] Even in endemic areas, serologic testing has been reliable.[9] However, antibody detection has important limitations during an attack because: (1) seroconversion takes time—antibody levels are not detectable until 2 to 6 weeks after exposure, and (2) immunosuppressed patients have a weak cell-mediated response and may not develop detectable antibodies.[5]

Culture of bodily fluids and tissue is the most definitive way of diagnosing histoplasmosis but is impractical in the disaster setting as growth of the organism is slow, with a delay of 2 to 4 weeks. It is most useful in disseminated disease, because 80% to 90% become positive, but has poor sensitivity in acute disease.[1,8] PCR is rapid and well suited for detection of low concentrations of yeast, but accuracy or significance in patient management has not been validated and remains inconsistent.[9,13] Histopathology is impractical as it requires specialized stains, and sensitivity is highly dependent upon the pathologist. Although skin testing was useful for epidemiologic studies, manufacture of the histoplasmin skin test was discontinued in January 2000 because it falsely elevated antibody titers, was not useful in patient management, and indicated prior infection without evidence of immunity.[3,5]

◀◀ PRE-INCIDENT ACTIONS

A histoplasmosis outbreak tends to present gradually with a diverse range of symptoms and disease manifestations because of the variability in disease severity, exposure level, and host immune response. Once spores are inhaled, the majority of the population will be asymptomatic with only a small fraction of symptomatic individuals seeking medical attention or requiring treatment. Patients will present 1 to 2 weeks after exposure to clinics, urgent care centers, and emergency departments.

Health care providers, especially in endemic areas, should maintain a high level of clinical suspicion for histoplasmosis and utilize electronic resources to rapidly communicate the possibility of an outbreak. In one multinational outbreak from a bat-infested tree in Uganda, the case patient discovered that other close contacts were presenting with similar respiratory complaints in other countries. Through the response of physicians to an alert in ProMED-mail, other exposed patients from the same trip across the world were questioned, the inciting event was identified, and efficient treatment of histoplasmosis patients across multiple nations was coordinated.[18]

Pre-incident actions can focus on prevention of H. capsulatum contamination of soil from bird or bat activity. This may involve clearing groves to reduce roosting and restricting access to certain caves or nesting areas. However, removal of bats, birds, and guano (a habitat for many arthropod species) can affect the ecosystem and is often not feasible.

In a disaster situation in which sites of soil enriched in H. capsulatum spores were disturbed (such as a large explosion with aerosolization of infected dust), there would be a high risk of histoplasmosis as a secondary threat. Many air handling systems in modern buildings fail to remove histoplasma spores.[1]

▷▷ POST-INCIDENT ACTIONS

Histoplasmosis is not contagious. No isolation precautions are needed because person to person or animal to person transmission does not occur.[3] Critical post-incident actions include: (1) identifying H. capsulatum as the causative organism, (2) protecting health care workers and patients from secondary exposure, and (3) containing or decontaminating infective spores in the environment.

Diagnostic testing in an acute attack should focus on antigen detection, then serology and culture. Personal protective equipment including disposable clothing, shoe covers, and a powered air-purifying respirator with a full facepiece should be worn by anyone entering an enclosed area in which the amount of contamination is unknown.[8] In highly contaminated areas, the large amount of airborne organisms has resulted in infection even in experienced researchers who used appropriate equipment.[4] Every effort must be made to avoid transporting spores away from a contaminated area because spores can recirculate and travel. Aerosolization of spores should be prevented by adding a surfactant or wetting agent, such as a water spray, prior to collection and removal of soil. Professional cleaning of mechanical air and heating systems will avoid inoculating additional patients.

Eradication of H. capsulatum may not be feasible as it is a resilient fungus, able to survive in extreme conditions.[4] Once contaminated, the soil can yield spores for many years.[3] The only disinfectant proven to be effective in eliminating spores from soil is fumigation with 3.8% formaldehyde. Multiple formaldehyde formulations exist; however, none is Environmental Protection Agency (EPA)-registered as a soil disinfectant and are not generally recommended. There are high environmental risks, and exposure to formaldehyde alone will cause additional health risks.[8] Restricting human access to highly contaminated areas may be the most effective containment strategy.

✚ MEDICAL TREATMENT OF CASUALTIES

Most pulmonary histoplasmosis is self-limiting and resolves spontaneously without treatment within a month. In an intentional histoplasmosis attack, antifungal agents should be reserved for those with severe or persistent pulmonary histoplasmosis, PDH, CNS histoplasmosis, and pregnant women. Nonsteroidal antiinflammatory agents (NSAIDs) are used to manage pericarditis and rheumatologic symptoms. Pericarditis with hemodynamic compromise or without improvement after NSAIDs may benefit from 6 to 12 weeks of oral itraconazole and 1 to 2 weeks of prednisone (0.5 to 1 mg/kg daily, max 80 mg daily). Mediastinal complications of histoplasmosis do not require treatment unless there is a mass effect on adjacent structures.[12]

In patients with persistent pulmonary histoplasmosis (continued symptoms for >1 month), oral itraconazole is recommended for 6 to 12 weeks (children: 5 to 10 mg/kg/day divided into 2 doses, max 400 mg daily; adults: 200 mg TID daily × 3 days then 200 mg daily or BID). In severe pulmonary histoplasmosis with respiratory distress, intravenous (IV) amphotericin B (AmpB) should be used for the initial 1 to 2 weeks (lipid complex AmpB 3 to 5 mg/kg daily in adults, deoxycholate AmpB 1 mg/kg daily in children) followed by oral itraconazole for a total of 12 weeks antifungal therapy. Adjunctive corticosteroids tapered over 1 to 2 weeks can be added to provide additional symptom relief (IV methylprednisolone 0.5 to 1 mg/kg IV daily).[12] However, steroids should be avoided if there is a possibility of concomitant malignancy and only used with antifungal therapy to avoid dissemination of acute pulmonary histoplasmosis into PDH.[1]

In adults with PDH, 1 year of antifungal therapy is required. Oral itraconazole is used in mild to moderate PDH and IV AmpB followed by oral itraconazole is recommended for severe PDH (e.g., requiring hospitalization). In children with PDH, either 4 to 6 weeks of IV AmpB or 2 to 4 weeks of IV AmpB followed by oral itraconazole for a total of 3 months of therapy is acceptable.[12]

In both adults and children, CNS histoplasmosis is treated with high-dose liposomal AmpB 5 mg/kg daily for a total of 175 mg/kg over 4 to 6 weeks followed by oral itraconazole (adults: 200 mg BID or TID, children: 10 mg/kg daily, max 400 mg) for a total of 1 year of antifungal therapy.[12]

Pregnant women should be treated for 4 to 6 weeks with lipid complex AmpB only, because azoles are teratogenic. Although there is inadequate evidence, transplacental transmission may be prevented if antifungal therapy is initiated prior to delivery.[12]

In AIDS patients, there is a paradoxical worsening of symptoms from therapy because of immune reconstitution syndrome, and it is important to continue antifungal treatment.[13] Although lifelong prophylaxis with itraconazole was formerly recommended for AIDS patients with PDH, current guidelines suggest itraconazole can be safely discontinued after 1 year of antifungal treatment in some patients with a good response to antiretrovirals and antifungals.[13,19] To monitor for relapse in immunosuppressed patients, antigen levels should be measured during therapy and for 12 months after treatment completion.[19]

Treatment monitoring: Because AmpB is notoriously nephrotoxic, electrolyte levels, blood counts, and renal function need to be measured several times a week. Azoles may be hepatotoxic, and liver function should be tested at baseline and during treatment. After at least 2 weeks of itraconazole therapy, random serum levels should be between 1.0 and 10 mcg/mL. Levels should be monitored for the first month of treatment to ensure correct therapeutic range or dosage changes, as well as drug compliance.[12,13]

💡 UNIQUE CONSIDERATIONS

The challenge in a histoplasmosis attack is not the treatment but in the recognition of the disease by first responders and initial health care providers because histoplasmosis can resemble many other pulmonary, malignant, inflammatory, and infectious processes. With a high variability in disease presentation and severity, individuals most at risk for severe or disseminated disease are the immunosuppressed, those with chronic lung disease, or those at the extremes of age. Symptoms, when present, are often nonspecific and cause an indolent illness which can then lead to significant morbidity and mortality in untreated patients. Because histoplasmosis has an overall low mortality once it is treated, a thorough history of travel, recreational, and occupational activities and any symptomatic close contacts is essential for identifying and mitigating a histoplasmosis attack.

⚠ PITFALLS

Several potential pitfalls in response to a histoplasmosis attack exist. These include:

- Failure to include histoplasmosis in the differential of nonspecific complaints based on history and risk factors

- Failure to diagnose histoplasmosis with appropriate and rapid diagnostic testing
- Failure to identify the inciting event, question other exposed contacts, and notify other providers through available electronic resources
- Failure to monitor treatment and drug levels, side effects, and interactions
- Failure to recognize histoplasmosis as a secondary cause of morbidity and mortality in disaster situations that involve aerosolization of contaminated soil, especially in endemic areas
- Failure to wear appropriate personal protective equipment when exposure to *H. capsulatum* spores is a possibility
- Failure to reduce the likelihood of transporting spores away from a contaminated area
- Failure to decontaminate or restrict access to a contaminated environment

REFERENCES

1. Adderson E. Histoplasmosis. *Pediatr Infect Dis J.* 2006;25(1):73–74.
2. McLeod DS, Mortimer RH, Perry-Keene DA, et al. Histoplasmosis in Australia: report of 16 cases and literature review. *Medicine (Baltimore).* 2011;90(1):61–68.
3. Fischer GB, Mocelin H, Severo CB, et al. Histoplasmosis in children. *Paediatr Respir Rev.* 2009;10(4):172–177.
4. Rocha-Silva F, Figueiredo SM, Silveira TT, et al. Histoplasmosis outbreak in Tamboril cave—Minas Gerais state, Brazil. *Med Mycol Case Rep.* 2014;4:1–4.
5. Aide MA. Chapter 4—histoplasmosis. *J Bras Pneumol.* 2009;35(11): 1145–1151.
6. Chang P, Rodas C. Skin lesions in histoplasmosis. *Clin Dermatol.* 2012;30(6): 592–598.
7. Edwards JA, Rappleye CA. Histoplasma mechanisms of pathogenesis—one portfolio doesn't fit all. *FEMS Microbiol Lett.* 2011;324(1):1–9.
8. Lenhart SW, Schafer MP, Singal M, et al. Histoplamosis—protecting workers at risk. http://www.cdc.gov/niosh/docs/2005-109/pdfs/2005-109.pdf. Accessed 25.05.14.
9. Hage CA, Knox KS, Wheat LJ. Endemic mycoses: overlooked causes of community acquired pneumonia. *Respir Med.* 2012;106(6):769–776.
10. Sahaza JH, Perez-Torres A, Zenteno E, et al. Usefulness of the murine model to study the immune response against *Histoplasma capsulatum* infection. *Comp Immunol Microbiol Infect Dis.* 2014;37(3):143–152.
11. Smith JA, Kauffman CA. Pulmonary fungal infections. *Respirology.* 2012;17(6):913–926.
12. Wheat LJ, Freifeld AG, Kleiman MB, et al. Clinical practice guidelines for the management of patients with histoplasmosis: 2007 update by the Infectious Diseases Society of America. *Clin Infect Dis.* 2007;45(7): 807–825.
13. Wheat LJ, Musial CE, Jenny-Avital E. Diagnosis and management of central nervous system histoplasmosis. *Clin Infect Dis.* 2005;40(6): 844–852.
14. Akman C, Kantarci F, Cetinkaya S. Imaging in mediastinitis: a systematic review based on aetiology. *Clin Radiol.* 2004;59(7):573–585.
15. Riegle DW. Arming Iraq: the export of biological materials and the health of our gulf war veterans. http://www.gpo.gov/fdsys/pkg/CREC-1994-02-09/ html/CREC-1994-02-09-pt1-PgS6.htm. Accessed 17.06.14.
16. Blum W. US companies sold Iraq billions of NBC weapons materials. http:// www.rense.com/general21/bil.htm. Accessed 17.06.14.
17. Haselow DT, Safi H, Holcomb D, et al. Histoplasmosis associated with a bamboo bonfire—Arkansas, October 2011. *MMWR Morb Mortal Wkly Rep.* 2014;63(8):165–168.
18. Cottle LE, Gkrania-Klotsas E, Williams HJ, et al. A multinational outbreak of histoplasmosis following a biology field trip in the Ugandan rainforest. *J Travel Med.* 2013;20(2):83–87.
19. Knox KS, Hage CA. Histoplasmosis. *Proc Am Thorac Soc.* 2010;7(3): 169–172.

Cryptosporidium parvum (Cryptosporidiosis) Attack

Benjamin Graboyes, Miriam John, and Carol Sulis

DESCRIPTION OF EVENT

Human cryptosporidiosis is a disease caused by the ubiquitous protozoan *Cryptosporidium*, an obligate intracellular parasite. The human pathogens *Cryptosporidium hominis* and *C. parvum* (previously referred to as *C. parvum* genotype 1 and 2, respectively) are the most important agents in human disease, but other species have been identified in immunocompromised hosts.[1] Reservoirs for cryptosporidia include humans, domesticated animals (e.g., cows, goats, and sheep), and wild animals (e.g., deer and elk). Tyzzer and Clarke discovered cryptosporidia in the stomach of a mouse in 1907. The first human case was reported by Nime in 1976 in a child with diarrhea.[2] Since 1982 and the beginning of the acquired immune deficiency syndrome (AIDS) epidemic cryptosporidia have been increasingly recognized as a cause of diarrheal illness in both immunocompromised and immunocompetent human hosts. Cryptosporidiosis has frequently been recognized as the leading cause of diarrhea due to protozoal infections worldwide.[3]

Cryptosporidium is classified by the Centers for Disease Control and Prevention (CDC) as a category B bioterrorism threat agent and more specifically as a water safety threat. Cryptosporidia are highly infectious enteric pathogens, which are resistant to chlorine and difficult to filter. Cryptosporidia are present in the feces of many animals, making them a persistent threat to any water supply.[4] It is a hardy organism that can survive for 18 months at 4 °C in surface water and for 2 to 6 months in groundwater.[5] Oocysts have been found in 87% of untreated water samples tested in the United States and Canada, and in a CDC surveillance study cases were reported in all 50 states.[5,6] Cryptosporidia are resistant to common water disinfection techniques, such as chlorination, treatment with sodium hypochlorite, and filtration (if the filter pore size is greater than 1 μm).[1]

Cryptosporidium infection occurs after ingestion of fecally contaminated food or water. Transmission can also occur directly from animal to person or person to person. The infectious form of *Criptosporidium* is the thick-walled (4 to 6 μm) oocyst and the median infective dose is 132 oocysts.[1,7] Ingested oocysts undergo excystation in the upper small intestine after being exposed to reducing conditions, proteolytic enzymes, and bile salts. Sporozoites invade the intestinal brush border epithelial cells and mature into merozoites, leading to inflammation, villous blunting, malabsorption, and diarrhea. Merozoites undergo sexual reproduction to produce thin-walled oocysts (which continue autoinfection in the host) or thick-walled oocysts (which are excreted and can then infect other hosts).[4,5] *Cryptosporidium* infection can be found at rates of 2.2% to 6.1% in immunocompetent persons with diarrhea in industrialized and developing countries, respectively. Human immunodeficiency virus (HIV)-positive persons with diarrhea show *Cryptosporidium* infection in 14% to 24% of cases in industrialized and developing areas, respectively.[4,8]

There have been numerous well-documented outbreaks of cryptosporidiosis in the United States. Most are water-borne outbreaks due to contamination of drinking water or recreational water, such as swimming or wading pools. There were approximately 1 dozen documented outbreaks of cryptosporidiosis in the United States between 1993 and 1998. The largest water-borne outbreak in U.S. history occurred in March and April 1993 in Milwaukee, Wisconsin, affecting an estimated 403,000 persons. This constituted a 52% cryptosporidiosis attack rate among those served by the South Milwaukee water works plant. The second largest outbreak occurred in Östersund, Sweden, in November 2010 infecting 27,000 residents (45% attack rate) by *C. hominis*.[9] Person-to-person spread has also been documented in institutions, such as daycare centers and hospitals, and may be especially difficult to control because infectious oocysts may be excreted for up to 5 weeks after the diarrheal illness ends.[4,8]

The clinical manifestations of *Cryptosporidium* infection are largely host dependent. In an immunocompetent host, cryptosporidiosis is primarily an intestinal disorder with a 1- to 2-week incubation period followed by symptoms of watery diarrhea, abdominal cramps, anorexia, nausea, vomiting, and possibly a low-grade fever. The disease is self-limited with an average duration of 9 to 12 days, and the main health risk is predictably dehydration. In the immunocompromised host cryptosporidiosis can be an acute dehydrating diarrheal syndrome or a chronic diarrheal and wasting syndrome. Patients with CD4 counts greater than 180 cells/mm^3 tend to have the self-limited syndrome. *Cryptosporidium* infection of biliary and pancreatic ducts leading to cholangitis or acalculous cholecystitis has been documented in patients with CD4 counts less than 50 cells/mm^4.[1,5] There are also infrequent reports of pulmonary and tracheal cryptosporidiosis in immunocompromised hosts, which manifests as cough with low-grade fever, usually accompanying severe intestinal illness.[3]

Diagnosis of cryptosporidiosis is made using modified acid-fast staining on unconcentrated fecal smears. It is likely underdiagnosed in industrialized countries because relatively few laboratories routinely process stool ova and parasite specimens for *Cryptosporidium* or other acid-fast enteric pathogens. Direct fluorescent antibody (DFA), enzyme-linked immunosorbent assay (ELISA), and polymerase chain reaction (PCR) testing are more sensitive and less user-dependent than routine acid-fast testing. However, these tests are newer and less commonly available.[1,5]

PRE-INCIDENT ACTIONS

Because cryptosporidia are ubiquitous and persistent in the environment, as well as highly transmissible, these organisms are well suited to be used in a covert biological attack. Mortality in a bioattack would be low, except among immunocompromised patients. However, morbidity could be extremely high, especially because there can be person-to-person transmission of cryptosporidiosis. Physicians, particularly those working in emergency departments, must remain vigilant to distinguish cryptosporidiosis from routine viral gastroenteritis. Large numbers of persons can be affected in an outbreak and may seek medical attention because of the frequency of stools (average of 12 to 15 per day), prolonged course of diarrheal illness (average of 9 to 12 days), or severity of illness if the person is immunocompromised.[5] Patients with suspected cryptosporidiosis should undergo laboratory analysis of stool samples, including modified acid-fast staining or DFA to confirm the diagnosis. Examples of pre-event public health surveillance might include monitoring the volume of antidiarrheal medication sold, monitoring health maintenance organization (HMO) and hospital logs of patient chief complaints, and monitoring the incidence of diarrhea in places such as nursing homes, daycare centers, and infectious disease clinics.[10]

To protect against widespread outbreaks the public water supply should be monitored closely. Water filtration and flocculation techniques that can eradicate oocysts are not routinely performed at many plants. Water-borne outbreaks have occurred even when the water supply met required turbidity levels. Methods such as reverse osmosis, membrane filtration, ozone treatment, or irradiation can eradicate infectious oocysts from the water supply but are not cost-effective. Ozone treatment is likely the most effective chemical means of inactivating *Cryptosporidium* oocysts.[4]

POST-INCIDENT ACTIONS

Public health authorities should be notified when cryptosporidia are confirmed by laboratory analysis of a stool sample. In the 2010 outbreak in Östersund, Sweden, multiple factors facilitated detection and control of the outbreak. Initially pathology staff suspected oocysts in smears of unstained fecal specimens and performed further staining (not originally requested) to identify *C. hominis*. Second, data from a local health advice line were linked with address data and identified those affected as residing within city limits. A water-boil advisory was immediately initiated, and epidemiology was followed closely via an electronic survey. Survey results showed a peak in incidence three days after the water-boil advisory with rapid decrease in reported cases.[10]

Similar strategies to those used in Sweden should be employed in future suspected outbreaks. An epidemiologic investigation involving appropriate public health authorities should be initiated promptly to identify the source of an outbreak and to rapidly institute corrective measures. In addition to standard precautions in hospitals, contact precautions should be instituted for diapered children and incontinent adults. Rigorous hand washing by hospital staff is necessary to prevent nosocomial spread. Information and education about *Cryptosporidium* species should be provided to the general public and should include instructions specific to immunocompromised groups. Boiling water is the most certain method of eradicating *Cryptosporidium* oocysts. Use of sterile water and microstraining water filters capable of removing particles less than or equal to 1 micron can also reduce the risk of cryptosporidiosis.[10-12]

MEDICAL TREATMENT OF CASUALTIES

Cryptosporidiosis is self-limited in immunocompetent hosts requiring only supportive care and monitoring hydration and volume status.

The disease is often severe in immunocompromised hosts warranting specific medical treatment. Nitazoxanide, a nitrothiazole benzamide compound, has been shown to reduce both diarrhea and oocyst shedding and was approved for use in cryptosporidiosis in 2005 by the U.S. Food and Drug Administration (FDA).[13] Immune reconstitution in HIV disease using highly active antiretroviral therapy (HAART) results in decreased stool frequency, weight gain, and fecal oocyst clearance. However, there is rapid relapse after discontinuation of HAART, suggesting that cryptosporidial infection had been suppressed rather than cured.[1]

UNIQUE CONSIDERATIONS

Cryptosporidium is a small, highly infectious and transmissible protozoan. These features make it a possible bioweapon and water safety threat. Although there is low mortality, there is substantial morbidity associated with cryptosporidiosis. A *Cryptosporidium* attack will be extremely difficult to identify and distinguish from routine viral gastroenteritis due to the similarity of illness presentation and lack of routine laboratory stool testing for *Cryptosporidium*. Health care providers must be vigilant in identifying a potential outbreak when treating larger numbers of patients with diarrheal illness, particularly identifying those who are immunocompromised. Without appropriate supportive care and institution of nitazoxanide treatment, cryptosporidiosis can lead to high mortality levels in this particular patient population.

PITFALLS

Several potential pitfalls in response to a cryptosporidiosis attack exist. These include the following:

- Failure to consider cryptosporidiosis as the cause of diarrheal illness
- Failure to request specific laboratory analysis of stool samples for *C. parvum* or *C. hominis*
- Failure to aggressively treat immunocompromised patients with diarrheal illness
- Failure to notify public health authorities about suspected or confirmed cases of cryptosporidiosis
- Failure to notify public health authorities about a suspected or confirmed cluster of patients with diarrheal illness

REFERENCES

1. Davies AP, Chalmers RM. Cryptosporidiosis. *BMJ.* 2009;339:b4168.
2. Nime FA, Burek JD, Page DL, Holscher MA, Yardley JH. Acute enterocolitis in a human being infected with the protozoan *Cryptosporidium*. *Gastroenterology.* 1976;70:592–598.
3. Butt A, Aldridge K, Sanders C. Infections related to the ingestion of seafood. Part II: parasitic infections and food safety. *Lancet Infect Dis.* 2004;4:294–300.
4. Guerrant RL. Cryptosporidiosis: an emerging, highly infectious threat. *Emerg Infect Dis.* 1997;3:51–57.
5. Katz D, Taylor D. Parasitic infections of the gastrointestinal tract. *Gastroenterol Clin North Am.* 2001;30:797–815.
6. Yoder J. Cryptosporidiosis surveillance—United States, 2009–2010. *Surveillance Summaries.* 2012;61(SS05):1–12.
7. DuPont HL, Chappell CL, Sterling CR, Okhuysen PC, Rose JB, Jakubowski W. The infectivity of *Cryptosporidium parvum* in healthy volunteers. *N Engl J Med.* 1995;332:855–859.
8. Chen X, Keithly JS, Paya CV, et al. Cryptosporidiosis. *N Engl J Med.* 2002;346:1723–1731.

9. Widerström M, Schönning C, Lilja M, et al. Large outbreak of *Cryptosporidium hominis* infection transmitted through the public water supply, Sweden. *Emerg Infect Dis [Internet].* 2014 Apr;[date cited].

10. Addiss D, Arrowood M, Bartlett M, et al. Assessing the public health threat associated with waterborne cryptosporidiosis: report of a workshop. *MMWR.* 1995;44:1–19.

11. Bongard J, Savage R, Dern R, et al. Cryptosporidium infections associated with swimming pools—Dane County, Wisconsin. *MMWR.* 1994; 43:561–563.

12. Weber DJ, Rutala WA. Cryptosporidiosis. *N Engl J Med.* 2002;347:1287.

13. Fox LM, Saravolatz LD. Nitazoxanide: a new thiazolide antiparasitic agent. *Clin Infect Dis.* 2005;40(8):1173–1180.

Explosions: Conventional

Robert Partridge

DESCRIPTION OF EVENT

Conventional explosions are common occurrences and result in numerous injuries every year worldwide. Explosions occur when solid or liquid material is rapidly transformed into a gas with sudden energy release. Conventional explosions and blasts occur as a result of unintentional civilian incidents (e.g., explosive detonation during ship or truck transport), intentional and unintentional detonation of military ordnance, and terrorist attacks. Powerful explosions have the potential to inflict many different types of traumatic injuries; such injuries can vary depending on the type and amount of explosive agent, the location of the victims (inside or outside), and whether the blast occurs in the air or in water.

High-order explosives, such as trinitrotoluene (TNT) and other nitrate compounds, detonate very quickly. The rapid expansion of explosive gases under extremely high pressure produces a supersonic overpressurization shock wave capable of causing catastrophic blast injuries as well as severe structural damage. Low-order explosives are composed of propellants, such as pyrotechnics, that deflagrate rather than detonate, resulting in a slower energy release. Low-order explosives produce subsonic explosions that do not cause overpressurization blast waves and only rarely cause the primary blast injuries associated with high-order explosives.

Conventional explosions from high-order explosives cause physical trauma through four mechanisms. *Primary* blast injury (PBI) results from the damage to human tissue from the sudden change in atmospheric pressure that propagates from the explosion (i.e., blast wave). *Secondary* blast injury occurs as debris accelerated by the blast strikes the victim, causing blunt or penetrating trauma. *Tertiary* blast injury occurs as the body of the victim is thrown onto the ground or into fixed objects as a result of the blast. In addition, *quaternary* injury can occur from carbon monoxide poisoning, fire, structural collapse, or inhalation of smoke or hot gases.

The damage caused by PBI is a type of barotrauma that primarily affects gas-containing organs—the lungs, ears, and gastrointestinal tract. The degree of tissue injury is directly related to the magnitude and duration of the maximum overpressure of the blast wave. Most victims of primary blast lung injury are killed immediately, often as a result of massive coronary or cerebral air embolism. Other immediate deaths are attributed to severe multisystem injury due to secondary and tertiary blast injury.

The majority of survivors will experience trauma caused by secondary, tertiary, or quaternary blast injury. In the last decade, PBI has also been shown to cause mild traumatic brain injury (TBI) that can eventually result in multiple adverse outcomes, including neuropsychiatric disorders such as posttraumatic stress disorder (PTSD) and long-term cognitive disability.[1]

PBI must be considered in all victims exposed to an explosion, even if there are no external signs of injury. Severe pulmonary manifestations include hemorrhage, barotrauma, and arterial air embolism. Gastrointestinal manifestations include hemorrhage and hollow viscous perforation. Of the small number of survivors of the initial explosion with lung PBI, deaths may occur by progressive pulmonary insufficiency, something comonly referred to as "Blast Lung." These lesions appear similar to pulmonary contusion, both radiographically and pathologically.[2,3]

Indoor detonations or explosions within a vehicle appear to cause more severe PBIs than open-air bombings because the blast wave is magnified rather than dissipated as it is reflected off the floor, walls, and ceiling.[4,5] The type of explosion and victim location at the time of the blast must be considered when managing blast injury.

PRE-INCIDENT ACTIONS

Conventional explosions can occur anywhere, at any time, with variable numbers of casualties. For these reasons, individuals can do little to prepare for a conventional explosion. However, communities can be prepared for such an event. Other than safety and law enforcement measures designed to prevent an explosion, the most effective pre-incident actions involve establishing an effective security, rescue, and medical infrastructure.

One of the major determinants of mortality from conventional bombings is the availability of medical resources at the disaster scene. Explosions occurring in or near major cities with established prehospital systems, emergency departments, and advanced trauma care would be expected to have lower mortality rates than remote areas or areas with less advanced medical systems and longer rescue and transport times. Medical management of blast victims is also enhanced if help is available beyond the community affected and if there is an ability to transfer victims to other medical facilities.

In addition, the panic, chaos, and emotional trauma of large conventional explosions can worsen morbidity and mortality. A plan for prompt leadership; coordination of security, rescue, and medical agencies involved in the disaster; and a preexisting plan for rapid rescue, disposition, and treatment of casualties can reduce this risk.[4,6–9] These concepts were clearly demonstrated after the Boston Marathon bombings in 2013. Training for mass casualty incidents, availability of prehospital and other medical professionals at the scene of the bombing, and an extensive network of trauma-receiving facilities unquestionably minimized the mortality rate from this tragic event.[10]

▶▶ POST-INCIDENT ACTIONS

Previous disasters involving conventional explosions have demonstrated that safety and protection of first responders and medical personnel is the most important initial action. In both terrorist bombings and other nonmilitary explosions, scene safety is the first priority for all responders, because of the risk of being struck by falling or unstable debris or becoming victims of an intentionally delayed secondary explosion.[8] Keeping medical personnel away from the scene of an explosion reduces their risk of injury from such events. Because first responders are trained to rescue and help victims, any secondary explosion and incapacitation of these persons would greatly impair subsequent rescue efforts.[11] These recommendations are evolving, however, due to positive results from the rapid response of bystanders and prehospital personnel at the Boston Marathon bombings and other mass casualty incidents. In the future, medical personnel may be sent into "warm zones" before bombs have been disarmed and the area is secured, given that fast and aggressive treatment, especially in controlling hemorrhage, may be critical in saving lives.[12,13]

Immediately after a blast, rescue, police, and emergency medical services (EMS) personnel will be the first to care for casualties. They may also be joined by trained and experienced bystanders, though other responders should not enter the blast scene until the incident commander has declared the area safe. Most victims will have traumatic injuries resulting from secondary and tertiary blast injury. EMS personnel should observe standard trauma protocols for management of these injuries.

EMS personnel should assess casualties for PBI. A careful assessment of the scene can give clues to the potential for PBI. A crater or a building collapse indicates high blast strength. An assessment of crater size and structural damage as well as the location and time of the explosion may be useful in estimating the number of casualties and the likelihood of PBI. Blast peak overpressures in unobstructed open-air explosions are directly related to the explosive force of the blast and inversely proportional to the distance from the explosion.[14] The farther away a person is from a blast, the less likely he or she is to develop severe PBI. The location and position that victims were in at the time of the blast should be noted. Reflected blast waves are even more likely to cause PBI. Solid surfaces that can reflect blast waves create a zone of very highly pressurized air as the blast wave is reflected back on itself.[15,16] Rigid shields between a person and an explosion may reduce the risk of secondary blast injury but may not prevent significant PBI.[17,18] Victims in close proximity to an explosion may have PBI only and may initially appear uninjured. Because physical activity after PBI can result in a poorer outcome, EMS personnel must ensure that these persons are not physically active until evaluation and observation for PBI is complete.

Injuries sustained from underwater PBI are different from those in open-air blasts. Because blast waves are reflected back underwater from the water-air surface boundary and interact with direct blast waves, greater blast loads are transmitted to the more deeply submerged parts of the victim. If a victim is submerged in a vertical position, particular concern should be raised for the possibility of PBI in the lower segments of the lungs or gastrointestinal tract. PBI to the bowel, including acute or delayed presentations of bowel perforation in addition to lower gastrointestinal bleeding, may occur in partially submerged victims of underwater blasts.[2,19]

✚ MEDICAL TREATMENT OF CASUALTIES

Management of casualties after a blast event initially involves gathering as much information as possible to assess the potential for PBI, including the force of the blast, victim location (proximity to the blast, inside or outside, in air or underwater), and whether there was any post-event strenuous activity. A thorough trauma evaluation is mandatory for all victims of explosive blasts. Standard trauma management for secondary and tertiary injury will be familiar to prehospital personnel, emergency physicians, and traumatologists, so this section will focus on management of PBI and other injuries commonly occurring in blast victims.

The most critically injured patients after an exposure to a conventional blast succumb to their injuries at the scene. For those patients killed immediately after an explosion, death results from head injuries, PBI of the lung, abdominal injuries, or chest injuries.[20,21] Among survivors, non–life-threatening injuries, including fractures, soft tissue injuries, and blast injuries to ears and eyes, are common.[1,6,8,20,22] Of those who survive a conventional explosion, only a few will have severe chest and abdominal injuries, including blast lung. These injuries should be recognized as prognostic markers of severity, and it is important to identify and treat them early because patients with such injuries have a significantly increased mortality rate.

Evaluation of prior blast injuries indicates certain patterns of morbidity and mortality from which conclusions about future events may be drawn. Immediate deaths appear to be related to the strength of the explosion, an associated building collapse, or a blast location that is indoors. The Beirut bombing in 1983 illustrates some important principles of medical management of casualties after an explosion. Most survivors had noncritical injuries, and for those critically injured, death occurred days to weeks later. Most of these deaths (86%) occurred in victims who were rescued and treated more than 6 hours after the blast event. A short interval between blast event and treatment and early aggressive resuscitation are good prognostic factors for survival.[20,23]

Pulmonary PBI may have an acute or delayed presentation. Patients with acute pulmonary PBI will present with chest pain, dyspnea, and tachypnea with rapid and shallow respirations, dry cough, wheezing, and hemoptysis. Breath sounds will be diminished on the affected side, making the diagnosis of PBI difficult unless pneumothorax, hemothorax, and pulmonary contusion have been excluded. Inspiratory rales, dullness to percussion, and poor chest wall expansion may also be present.[1] A chest radiograph is mandatory for all patients with respiratory difficulty or suspected PBI or chest trauma. Computed tomography (CT) scans of the chest may be useful to detect small pneumothoraces or pulmonary contusions, either of which may not be well visualized on a plain radiograph of the chest.

Massive hemoptysis resulting from PBI can be managed by preferentially intubating the unaffected lung with a cuffed endotracheal tube, thus protecting the function of that side. Patients with PBI of the lung may have concurrent pneumothorax, tension pneumothorax, or hemothorax. Emergent decompression with a tube or needle thoracostomy is indicated.[24] Patients with pulmonary PBI who are not having ventilatory problems are at risk for hypoxemia and should be managed with high-flow oxygen through a non-rebreather mask or continuous positive airway pressure. Patients able to ventilate spontaneously reduce their risk for arterial gas embolism. It has been suggested that patients requiring mechanical ventilation should be managed with low ventilatory pressures and permissive hypercapnia to reduce the risk of air embolism.[25,26]

Air embolism resulting from PBI may cause coronary vessel occlusion with subsequent myocardial infarction or cerebral infarction with altered mental status or stroke symptoms. Other organ systems may also be affected. Coronary artery air embolism after PBI can be difficult to diagnose but should be suspected in any blast victim who has electrocardiographic evidence of a myocardial infarction or is in shock with all other likely reasons for shock excluded. A head CT scan is mandatory in any patient with altered mental status, seizures, or focal neurologic deficits. Air embolism should be managed with hyperbaric oxygen therapy. Transferring patients to hyperbaric chambers may be problematic, given the risks of worsening the condition during aeromedical transportation and patient deterioration due to worsening pulmonary PBI.

The abdominal evaluation for PBI should focus on the search for perforation and signs of lower gastrointestinal hemorrhage and shock. The presentation and diagnosis of these conditions may be delayed. Diagnostic peritoneal lavage (DPL) is indicated in hemodynamically unstable patients with abdominal findings. Ultrasonography of the abdomen may be considered in patients with suspected intraabdominal trauma or hypotension and may be especially valuable in managing mass-casualty incidents. Abdominal CT scanning in stable patients to detect abdominal injury due to PBI may be useful in detecting small gastrointestinal perforations or hemorrhage. An abdominal CT scan performed after a DPL may have false-positive results because air and fluid will have been introduced into the peritoneum during the DPL procedure.[1]

Animal studies have demonstrated that the blast level necessary to cause a mild to moderate brain injury may be similar to that needed for pulmonary injury, so the clinician should have a high index of suspicion for TBI in the setting of possible lung PBI.[27] TBI resulting from PBI can range from mild to severe. Blast-related mild PBI and neuropsychologic sequelae, including postconcussive syndrome, PTSD, and chronic pain, have been increasingly recognized in military service members returning from modern war zones.[28]

Tympanic membrane (TM) rupture is a relatively common injury as a result of blast waves, as the ear is the organ most susceptible to PBI. Although a ruptured TM indicates exposure to a blast wave, its absence does not preclude PBI in other organs, especially in the military setting where victims may have been wearing hearing protection. Recent studies have suggested that a ruptured TM is a poor biomarker for other PBI. In addition, the absence of TM perforation should not be used to exclude the possibility of PBI in other organs.[29,30] Patients with TM rupture may have acute pulmonary PBI but are unlikely to have delayed-onset pulmonary PBI.[31]

Patients who appear stable but may be at risk for delayed PBI—including those in close proximity to the blast, who were knocked unconscious, or who felt the blast wave hit them—should be admitted for observation. Patients who have abdominal pain or tenderness, even if initial studies have normal results, may develop life-threatening bowel complications and should also be admitted.[24]

Patients can be discharged home if they have no chest complaints, normal chest radiographs, and no evidence of hypoxia, provided they have been observed for at least 6 hours. The risk of pulmonary PBI is low in these patients, and onset of any PBI-related complications in such patients should present slowly. These patients can safely return to the hospital for a secondary evaluation. Additionally, patients with isolated TM rupture only, with no other signs or symptoms after a period of observation and normal chest radiography, may be discharged home because they do not appear to be at risk of delayed-onset pulmonary PBI.[32] These patients should be given standard instructions on care of ear perforations and provided with otolaryngologic follow-up.

🔦 UNIQUE CONSIDERATIONS

Conventional blasts are unique because blast waves can cause PBI in persons physically separated from the epicenter of the explosion. Blast waves travel around walls and can be magnified by traveling down corridors. Persons in enclosed spaces frequently have the highest incidence of PBI regardless of whether the explosion occurred within that space or outside it.[18,25,33] The risk of PBI also increases as the volume of the enclosed space decreases. Persons located next to walls or in corners at the moment of the blast are also more likely to sustain PBI.[12]

Persons wearing body protection, such as Kevlar, at the time of the blast may be protected against secondary blast injury from flying objects but are still at risk for PBI. These garments transmit and may even amplify blast waves, so it should not be assumed that a blast victim wearing body protection has no PBI, even if he or she has no secondary blast injury.[34] Similarly, persons protected from secondary blast injury by a physical structure or water may have sustained PBI. Because their injuries are not as immediately apparent as those with external injuries from secondary blast injury, they may still be active and helping with the relief effort in the aftermath of the blast. As noted, strenuous activity after PBI may result in poorer outcome. EMS and other medical personnel on the scene must ensure that apparently uninjured persons in close proximity to an explosion do not engage in physical activity.

Survivors of conventional blasts perpetrated by suicide bombers are at risk for human projectile implantation injuries. Biological foreign bodies such as bone fragments or blood may have originated from the bodies of the suicide bombers or other nearby victims. In these cases, hepatitis B virus prophylaxis, antiretroviral prophylaxis against HIV, and baseline serological testing for future action against hepatitis C should be strongly considered, in addition to appropriate tetanus prophylaxis.[35]

⚠️ PITFALLS

The most significant pitfall in the evaluation of blast victims is failing to consider PBI in a person exposed to an explosion, whether near or far from the blast, indoors or outdoors, or in air or water.

REFERENCES

1. Koeissy F, Mondello S, Tumer N, Toklu HZ, et al. Assessing neuro-systemic & behavioral components in the pathophysiology of blast-related brain injury. *Front Neurol.* 2013;21(4):186.
2. Argyros GJ. Management of primary blast injury. *Toxicology.* 1997;121:105–115.
3. Huller J, Bazini Y. Blast injuries of the chest and abdomen. *Arch Surg.* 1970;100:24–30.
4. Cooper GJ, Maynard RL, Cross NL, et al. Casualties from terrorist bombings. *J Trauma.* 1983;23:955–967.
5. Leibovici D, Gofrit ON, Stein M, et al. Blast injuries: bus vs. open-air-bombings—a comparative study of injuries in survivors of open-air versus confined space explosions. *J Trauma.* 1996;41:1030–1035.
6. Brismar B, Bergenwald L. The terrorist bomb explosion in Bologna, Italy, 1980: an analysis of the effects an injuries sustained. *J Trauma.* 1982;22:216–220.
7. Rignault DP, Deligny MC. The 1986 terrorist bombing experience in Paris. *Ann Surg.* 1989;209:368–373.
8. Mallonee S, Shariat S, Stennies G, et al. Physical injuries and fatalities resulting from the Oklahoma City bombing. *JAMA.* 1996;276:382–387.
9. Ammons MA, Moore ME, Pons PT, et al. The role of a regional trauma system in the management of a mass disaster: an analysis of the Keystone, Colorado chairlift accident. *J Trauma.* 1988;28:1468–1471.
10. Walls RM, Zimmer MJ. The Boston Marathon response. Why did it work so well? *JAMA.* 2013;309(23):2441–2442.
11. Stein M, Hirshberg A. Medical consequences of terrorism: the conventional weapon threat. *Surg Clin North Am.* 1999;79:1537–1552.
12. Schmidt M. In mass attacks, new advice lets medics rush in. *New York Times.* December 8 2013;CLXIII.
13. Jacobs LM, McSwain NE Jr, Rotondo MF, et al. Improving survival from active shooter events: the Hartford Consensus. *J Trauma Acute Care Surg.* 2013;74(6):1399–1400.

14. Stuhmiller JH, Phillips YY, Richmond DR. The physics and mechanisms of primary blast injury. In: Bellamy RF, Zajtchuk R, eds. *Conventional Warfare: Ballistic, Blast and Burn Injuries*. Washington, DC: Office of the Surgeon General of the US Army; 1991:241–270.

15. Iremonger MJ. Physics of detonations and blast-waves. In: Cooper GJ, Dudley HAF, Gann DS, et al., eds. *Scientific Foundations of Trauma*. Oxford, UK: Butterworth-Heinemann; 1997:189–199.

16. Yelverton JT. Blast biology. In: Cooper GJ, Dudley HAF, Gann DS, et al., eds. *Scientific Foundations of Trauma*. Oxford, UK: Butterworth-Heinemann; 1997:200–213.

17. Wiener SL, Barrett J. Explosions and explosive device-related injuries. In: Wiener SL, Barrett J, eds. *Trauma Management for Civilian and Military Physicians*. Philadelphia: Saunders; 1986:13–26.

18. Mellor SG. The pathogenesis of blast injury and its management. *Br J Hosp Med*. 1988;39:536–539.

19. Paran H, Neufeld D, Shwartz I, et al. Perforation of the terminal ileum induced by blast injury: delayed diagnosis or delayed perforation? *J Trauma*. 1996;40:472–475.

20. Frykberg ER, Teppas JJ, Alexander RH. The 1983 Beirut Airport terrorist bombing: injury patterns and implications for disaster management. *Am Surg*. 1989;55:134–141.

21. Pyper PC, Graham WJH. Analysis of terrorist injuries treated at Craigavon Area Hospital, Northern Ireland, 1972-1980. *Injury*. 1982;14:332–338.

22. Frykberg ER, Tepas JJ. Terrorist bombings: lessons learned from Belfast to Beirut. *Ann Surg*. 1988;208:569–576.

23. Rignault DP. Recent progress in surgery for the victims of disaster, terrorism and war. *World J Surg*. 1992;16:885–887.

24. Wightman JM, Gladish SL. Explosions and blast injuries. *Ann Emerg Med*. 2001;37:664–678.

25. Pizov R, Oppenheim-Eden A, Matot I, et al. Blast lung injury from an explosion on a civilian bus. *Chest*. 1999;115:165–172.

26. Sorkine P, Szold O, Kluger Y, et al. Permissive hypercapnia ventilation in patients with severe pulmonary blast injury. *J Trauma*. 1988;45:35–38.

27. Rafaels KA, Bass CR, Panzer MB, et al. Brain injury from primary blast. *J Trauma Acute Care Surg*. 2012;73(4):895–901.

28. Rosenfeld JV, McFarlane AC, Bragge P, Armonda RA, Grimes JB, Ling GS. Blast-related traumatic brain injury. *Lancet Neurol*. 2013;12:882–893.

29. Harrison CD, Bebarta VS, Grant GA. Tympanic membrane perforation after combat blast exposure in Iraq: a poor biomarker of primary blast injury. *J Trauma*. 2009;67(1):2010–2011.

30. Peters P. Primary blast injury: an intact tympanic membrane does not indicate the lack of a primary blast injury. *Mil Med*. 2011;176(1):110–114.

31. Mellor SG. The relationship of blast loading to death and injury from explosion. *World J Surg*. 1992;16:893–898.

32. Leibovici D, Gofrit ON, Shapira SC. Eardrum perforation in explosion survivors: is it a marker of pulmonary blast injury? *Ann Emerg Med*. 1999;34:168–172.

33. Katz E, Ofek B, Adler J, et al. Primary blast injury after a bomb explosion on a civilian bus. *Ann Surg*. 1989;209:484–488.

34. Cooper GJ, Townend DJ, Cater SR, et al. The role of stress waves in thoracic visceral injury from blast loading: modification of stress transmission by foams and high density materials. *J Biomech*. 1991;24:273–285.

35. Patel HD, Dryden S, Gupta A, Stewart N. Human body projectiles in victims of suicide bombings and implications for health and emergency care providers: the 7/7 experience. *Ann R Coll Surg Engl*. 2012;94(5):313–317.

CHAPTER 164

Explosions: Fireworks

David V. Le and Craig Sisson

DESCRIPTION OF EVENT

This chapter will address the preparation for and response to explosions involving fireworks. According to the U.S. Consumer Products Safety Commission in 2012, most fireworks injuries in the U.S. were caused by fireworks sold to the general public. Only about 2% of all fireworks injuries were related to public fireworks displays.[1] In contrast, injuries associated with the production, storage, or distribution of fireworks are rare, but they warrant special consideration from a disaster medicine perspective. There have been multiple reports of large-scale explosions of fireworks facilities around the world, manifesting unique patterns of injury. This will be the focus of the chapter.

The inherent risk of manufacturing and storing fireworks are large-scale explosions and fire disasters. On May 13, 2000, in Enschede, Netherlands, several explosions at a fireworks storage depot destroyed the building along with the surrounding residential area. The explosions and ensuing fire killed 22 people, injured almost 1000, and caused over 1200 people to lose their homes.[2] Chen and colleagues[3,4] analyzed retrospective data from 339 patients involved in fireworks factory explosions from January 1987 to December 1999. They report a 13% mortality rate among victims, a significant percentage when compared with other causes of burns during the same period. The types of injuries caused by fireworks in this setting will be addressed later in the chapter.

Black powder, the basic component of fireworks, remains mostly unchanged since its invention by the Chinese approximately 1000 years ago. Historically, it is composed of a milled mixture of potassium nitrate, sulfur, and charcoal.[5] Black powder is considered a "low explosive"; it burns by a process known as deflagration.[6] Compared to high explosives (e.g., TNT), the chemical reaction of black powder is relatively slow, releasing energy over a longer period. If the chemical reaction is enclosed within a contained space, pressure can build rapidly, leading to an explosion. This property makes black powder very useful as a propellant, which has eventually led to its use as "gunpowder." Numerous uses of black powder now exist, including ammunition for various weapons and fireworks.

The current classification system for explosive materials was developed by the U.S. Department of Transportation. Fireworks are included in this classification system under divisions 1.3 and 1.4, which include large display fireworks and "common" publicly available fireworks, respectively.

PRE-INCIDENT ACTIONS

The U.S. Department of Health and Human Services summarizes a list of desired outcomes to support the prevention and mitigation of environmental threats to our health.[7] Using this model, there are four elements that a community can apply to prepare for a disaster such as one involving a large-scale fireworks explosion. These elements are: risk analysis and research, detection and reporting, prevention and mitigation, and response and recovery.

The first element describes the use of risk analysis and research to improve the understanding and anticipation of threats. What factors were associated with accidental explosions in the past? How likely is it that a facility will have an accident? In case of an accident, what are potential complications that need to be acknowledged? What training should be implemented to address a potential disaster? What resources are available? The goal is to anticipate threats through research and risk analysis to utilize resources effectively. Site selection, which includes consideration regarding proximity to residential areas, emergency responders, and medical facilities, should be thoroughly analyzed before approval for fireworks manufacturing operations begin.

The second element describes the process of detecting and reporting threats early and characterizing them fully. A surveillance program should be developed to ensure compliance to safety standards. What hazards are encountered during operations? What type of monitoring system will be used to detect these hazards? What materials are stored at the facility? Are material safety data sheets (MSDS) available for all materials in the facility? First responders in the area should have a thorough understanding of materials and hazards involved in case of disaster. The process of early detection and reporting of threats ensures that hazards are appropriately addressed before accidents happen.

The third element describes the development of mechanisms to prevent and mitigate threats. After detection of potential threats, systems should be implemented to mitigate hazards. Personal protective equipment should be used. Safety and rescue equipment should be available. Strict adherence to safety guidelines should be priority.

The last element describes the phase of response and recovery to an incident. In case of disaster, emergency response and evacuation procedures should be aimed at maximizing efficiency and reducing the number of casualties. Accountability of personnel, maintaining effective communication, and ensuring a safe and timely response from emergency responders are vital to the success of the post-incident phase.

POST-INCIDENT ACTIONS

In the immediate aftermath of a fireworks emergency, first responder personnel should be dispatched through predetermined communication pathways. This ensures that information and resources are disseminated in the most organized and effective manner. Medical facilities must be made aware of potential trauma and burn victims so that space may be allocated and the appropriate supplies and personnel are made available. During the Enschede, Netherlands, fireworks disaster, medical transport of casualties was uncoordinated and unrecorded during the first hour after the explosion. At the request of the first ambulance driver on scene, all 20 regional ambulances were dispatched for casualty transport to surrounding hospitals. Casualties were also transported to hospitals in private cars, police vehicles, and buses. Initially, there was no field triage system and no system for accountability of victims.[8]

First responders initially on scene at a fireworks storage facility explosion should be extremely cautious. One should immediately assess the scene for any potential hazards to the victims and rescuers.[9] The American Pyrotechnics Association instructs that emergency responders should never attempt to fight a fire that involves a building used in the manufacture of fireworks.[10] Efforts to evacuate all persons from the facility must be a priority including all employees, victims, and emergency responders. Firefighters are to focus their efforts on the prevention of secondary fires away from the initial site. The surrounding residential community should be evacuated and casualty-clearing stations should be deployed at a safe distance from the disaster site. All victims should be evaluated at casualty-clearing stations for triage, treatment, and transport in order to ensure optimal utilization of potentially limited resources and assets.[11]

✚ MEDICAL TREATMENT OF CASUALTIES

The National Fire Protection Association reports that in 2011, there were 9600 fireworks-related injuries treated in U.S. emergency departments. Of these cases, 89% of the injuries were caused by fireworks authorized for consumer use by federal regulations.[12] Reports pertaining to public fireworks disasters and the management of the specific injuries they cause are rare, but the literature suggests a higher mortality rate associated with fireworks facility explosions. A study by Navarro-Monzonis and others reports a mortality of 47% in casualties of industrial gunpowder explosions.[11] A 13-year retrospective study of fireworks factory injuries by Chen and colleagues[4] revealed a 13% overall mortality rate, with greater than 50% mortality in those with inhalation injury.[5]

The high morbidity and mortality rates associated with fireworks factory explosions are a result of multisystem injuries. Victims often succumb to hypovolemic shock, septicemia, acute respiratory distress syndrome, acute renal failure, and multiorgan system failure.[4] The pattern of injuries seen in survivors was a combination of burns, blast injuries, trauma, and inhalation injury.[5] In comparison with other blast injury disasters, fireworks disasters have a higher incidence of thermal injury. The burns characteristically involve a large total body surface area, and the majority of the burns are deep dermal or full thickness.[4,5,11] Wounds suffered by casualties near the primary blast may be severely contaminated with gunpowder residue.[5] The explosion of gunpowder in combination with the smoke generated by secondary fires makes inhalation injury a common finding.[4,5]

For the initial treatment of burn victims, remove all of the patients' clothing to prevent further thermal or chemical injury. Jewelry and watches should be removed to prevent a tourniquet effect from tissue swelling. First responders must evaluate the ABCs (i.e., airway, breathing, and circulation) of each victim, taking time only to perform interventions that are immediately required on salvageable patients.[13,14] Airway management is vitally important given the high incidence of inhalation injury and risk of blast lung injury. Indications for immediate definitive airway management include voice hoarseness, brassy cough, and stridor.[15] If a patient was in an enclosed space, has facial burns, or has carbonaceous sputum, early definitive airway management should be considered. Early tracheostomy is the preferred option for long-term management of ventilated patients.[4]

Intravenous access and aggressive fluid resuscitation with crystalloids such as normal saline or Ringer's lactate solution should be a priority in medical management. These patients will require extensive fluid resuscitation, given the frequency of deep dermal and full-thickness burns, large burn surface area, inhalation injury, and potential delays in treatment.[15-19] The Parkland formula may underestimate the fluid requirement and should only be used as a starting point for resuscitation. Urine output of 0.5-1.0 mL/kg/h, a heart rate of less than 120, and a clear sensorium are goals for resuscitation in adults.[16] For children, a goal urine output of 1.0 mL/kg/h and age-appropriate heart rate should be maintained.[15]

To decrease the temperature of the burned skin, cool tap water or a water-soaked towel should be used.[14] Ice should be avoided because it can cause decreased circulation to already damaged tissue. Nguyen and colleagues[20,21] report that cooling the burn wounds helps prevent progression to deep partial-thickness or full-thickness burns, and it reduces expanding injury. Medical providers must use sterile dressings to cover the wounds. Efforts should be made to ensure that the patient stays warm.

Primary blast injury is more severe when the victim is exposed to the blast wave over-pressurization while inside an enclosed space.[22-26] Leibovici and others[25] make a specific comparison between open-air and enclosed-space explosions, showing an increased incidence of primary blast injury, more severe injuries, and higher mortality rate in enclosed-space explosions. Intuitively, victims who are located in the collapsed portions of buildings are far more likely to die.[27,28] Most fireworks today are manufactured by hand inside of enclosed buildings. One can expect a high incidence of immediate death among victims in close proximity to the initial blast.[25,26]

A rapid and complete secondary survey of all patients will reduce missing associated injuries. Chen and colleagues[4] report 10% of burn victims to have an associated injury. The most common in decreasing frequency were limb fracture, blast lung injury, fractured rib with hemopneumothorax, and tympanic membrane rupture. The incidence of associated injuries among those who survived versus those who died was 5% and 48%, respectively. Leibovici and colleagues[25] report psychological stress, tinnitus, mild hearing loss, minor penetrating trauma, and simple fractures as associated injuries for patients not requiring hospital admission in open-air bombings.

Patients should be provided with adequate analgesia after initial stabilization, either in the prehospital setting or in the emergency department. Once a patient has reached the hospital, aggressive early debridement of devitalized tissue and topical antimicrobial treatment should begin as soon as possible.[16,17] Foreign bodies, such as paper fireworks covers and shrapnel from the blast, can increase the risk of infection and should be removed.[11] Chen and others show that 68% of victims required surgery with an average of 2.7 surgeries per patient.[5] There is a high risk of barotrauma in blast lung injury patients requiring mechanical ventilation.[24,26] They also show decreased mortality in patients undergoing early tracheostomy and subsequent mechanical ventilation.[4] Sepsis, multiple organ failure, hypovolemic shock from inadequate resuscitation, and pulmonary infection were common causes of death in hospitalized patients.[4] Long-term management of these patients requires an experienced intensive care specialist, preferably within a burn unit setting.

？ UNIQUE CONSIDERATIONS

Fireworks contain various chemical compounds and elements for the purpose of producing colored spectacles. One of these chemicals is elemental phosphorus. Elemental phosphorus is used in the military in various weapons due to its unique chemical properties. There are three allotropic forms of phosphorus: white, red, and black.[29] White phosphorus is sometimes included in the manufacture of fireworks. It burns spontaneously at 34° C, producing a bright greenish light, copious amounts of white fumes, and a garlic-like odor. A wound that is smoking white and exuding a garlic-like odor is characteristic of this substance. When placed in contact with oxygen, white phosphorus is oxidized to phosphorus pentoxide, which then combines with water to form phosphoric acid. This chemical sequence releases heat into the environment, causing burns. The phosphoric acid formed lowers the pH of tissues, causing chemical burns.[30] This chemical reaction sequence will continue until all of the phosphorus has reacted or until the phosphorus is deprived of its oxygen fuel.

When an explosion occurs with a device containing white phosphorus, immediate steps must be taken to stop the chemical reaction. Treatment should focus on wound irrigation, phosphorus neutralization, and wound debridement.[31] The victim's clothing should be removed immediately, to prevent any retained phosphorus particles from burning through to the skin or igniting the clothing. Once the clothing has been removed, the wounds should be irrigated with copious amounts of water. This will cut off the oxygen supply and cool the wound to below the ignition temperature, effectively stopping the reaction.[29,31-33] Before transport, the wounds should be covered with saline-soaked gauze to prevent them from drying and spontaneously igniting again. Oily dressings should not be used because white phosphorus is lipid-soluble and may penetrate into tissues.[30,31]

Once at the hospital, prompt debridement of all wounds is necessary to remove retained phosphorus particles. A Wood's lamp causes retained phosphorus to fluoresce, aiding in removal.[33] A second option is to wash the wound with a 1% copper sulfate solution, which reacts with elemental phosphorus and covers the particles with dark-colored copper phosphate. This easily identifies sites the need for further debridement and theoretically may slow the oxidation process. One concern is that copper itself is toxic and has never been shown to improve wound healing over normal saline washes alone.[30-32] As a result of phosphorus absorption, rapid changes in serum calcium and phosphorus levels can occur. Animal models have linked this to cardiac electrical abnormalities with increased risk of sudden death.[34] Therefore, continuous telemetry should be initiated for the patient, and his or her serum calcium and phosphorus levels should be monitored. Phosphorus absorption may also damage the kidneys and liver and cause other systemic effects.[29,35]

Magnesium and aluminum powders and pellets are also used in the production of fireworks. The chemical reactions are similar, producing a brilliant white light, intense heat, and loud noise effects if ignited in the presence of oxygen. Magnesium has an ignition temperature of 623° C, and it burns at roughly 3600° C. Once the oxygen source is removed, the reaction will stop.[36] Magnesium can react with oxygen, nitrogen, carbon dioxide, and water. The reaction with carbon dioxide produces magnesium oxide and carbon, and the reaction with water produces magnesium oxide and hydrogen gas. These reactions are important information for first responders. Applying water to a fire containing magnesium will increase the severity of the fire.[37] Hydrogen gas will be liberated and ignite, with the potential for a secondary explosion. Metal-extinguishing powders, such as graphite powder, powdered talc, and powdered sodium chloride present in class D fire extinguishers must be used to fight these fires.

All explosions can spread flaming debris, but fireworks are unique. Many class 1.4 fireworks are designed as self-propelled projectiles. Class 1.4 fireworks, although not at risk of initiating an explosive event, can spread fire throughout the storage facility and surrounding environment. They can also cause projectile injuries during the initial stages of a fire similar to secondary blast injuries but preceding an explosion.

This may inhibit a person's ability to evacuate the site and put that person at risk for more severe injury.

! PITFALLS

Several potential pitfalls in response to a fireworks disaster exist. These include the following:

- First responders not addressing scene safety; priority should be to evacuate all persons on premise
- Failure to decontaminate to stop the chemical burning process
- Not performing an ABCs evaluation with early definitive airway management
- Failure to complete the secondary survey; missed injuries increase morbidity and mortality
- Failure to administer appropriate resuscitative fluids
- Inadequate pain management
- Failure to deploy field triage sites at a safe distance from the primary event site

REFERENCES

1. Tu Y. Fireworks-related deaths, emergency department-treated injuries, and enforcement activities during 2012. *Fireworks Annual Report.* 2012;1–41.
2. Roorda J, Van Stiphout WAHJ, Huijsmans-Rubingh RRR. Post-disaster health effects: strategies for investigation and data collection. Experiences from the Enschede firework disaster. *J Epidemiol Community Health.* 2004;58:982–987.
3. Chen X, Wang Y, Wang C, et al. Gunpowder explosion burns in fireworks factory: causes of death and management. *Burns.* 2002;28:655–658.
4. Chen X, Wang Y, Wang C, et al. Burns due to gunpowder explosions in fireworks factory: a 13-year retrospective study. *Burns.* 2002;28:245–249.
5. Russell M. *The Chemistry of Fireworks.* 2nd ed. Cambridge, UK: Royal Society of Chemistry; 2009.
6. Bailey A, Murray SC. The explosion process: detonation shock effects. In: *Explosives, Propellants, and Pyrotechnics.* London: Brassey; 1989:21–47.
7. *The National Health Security Strategy of the United States of America.* Washington, DC: Department of Health and Human Services; 2012. www.phe.gov.
8. De Boer J, Debacker M. A more rational approach to medical disaster management applied retrospectively to the Enschede fireworks disaster, 13 May 2000. *Eur J Emerg Med.* 2003;10:117–123.
9. Delaney J, Drummond R. Mass casualties and triage at a sporting event. *Br J Sports Med.* 2002;36:85–88.
10. American Pyrotechnics Association. *Emergency Response Guidelines.* 2013. http://www.americanpyro.com/emergency-response.
11. Navarro-Monzonis A, Benito-Ruiz J, Baena-Montilla P, et al. Gunpowder-related burns. *Burns.* 1992;18:159–161.
12. Hall J. *NFPA's "Fireworks."* June 2013. www.nfpa.org.
13. Bar-Joseph G, Michaelson M, Halberthal M. Managing mass casualties. *Curr Opin Anaesthesiol.* 2003;16:193–199.
14. Allison K, Porter K. Consensus on the prehospital approach to burns patient management. *J Emerg Med.* 2004;21:112–114.
15. Monafo W. Initial management of burns. *N Engl J Med.* 1996;335:1581–1586.
16. Tang H, Xia Z, Lui S, et al. The experience in the treatment of patients with extensive full-thickness burns. *Burns.* 1999;25:757–759.
17. Rose J, Herndon D. Advances in the treatment of burn patients. *Burns.* 1997;23:S19–S26.
18. Navar P, Saffle J, Warden G. Effect of inhalation injury on fluid resuscitation requirements after thermal injury. *Am J Surg.* 1985;150:716–720.
19. Cancio L, Chavez S, Alvarado-Ortega M, et al. Predicting increased fluid requirements during the resuscitation of thermally injured patients. *J Trauma.* 2004;56:404–414.
20. Nguyen N, Gun R, Sparnon A, et al. The importance of immediate cooling—a case series of childhood burns in Vietnam. *Burns.* 2002;28:173–176.

21. Nguyen N, Gun R, Sparnon A, et al. The importance of initial management: a case series of childhood burns in Vietnam. *Burns.* 2002;28:167–172.

22. Wrightman J, Gladish S. Explosions and blast injuries. *Ann Emerg Med.* 2001;37:664–678.

23. Frykberg E. Medical management of disasters and mass casualties from terrorist bombings: how can we cope? *J Trauma.* 2002;53:201–212.

24. Gans L, Kennedy T. Management of unique clinical entities in disaster medicine. *Disaster Med.* 1996;14:301–326.

25. Leibovici D, Gofrit O, Stein M, et al. Blast injuries: bus versus open-air bombings—a comparative study of injuries in survivors of open-air versus confined-space explosions. *J Trauma.* 1996;41:1130–1135.

26. Pizov R, Oppenheim-Eden A, Matot I, et al. Blast lung injury from an explosion on a civilian bus. *Chest.* 1999;115:165–172.

27. Mallonee S, Shariat S, Stennies G, et al. Physical injuries and fatalities resulting from the Oklahoma City bombing. *JAMA.* 1996;276:382–387.

28. Biancolini C, Del Bosco C, Jorge M. Argentine Jewish community institution bomb explosion. *J Trauma.* 1999;47:728.

29. Chau T, Lee T, Chen S, et al. The management of white phosphorous burns. *Burns.* 2001;27:492–497.

30. Summerlin W, Walder A, Moncrief J. White phosphorous burns and massive hemolysis. *J Trauma.* 1967;7:476–484.

31. Konjoyan T. White phosphorus burns: case report and literature review. *Mil Med.* 1983;148:881–884.

32. Eldad A, Simon G. The phosphorous burn: a preliminary comparative experimental study of various forms of treatment. *Burns.* 1991;17:198–200.

33. Davis K. Acute management of white phosphorous burn. *Mil Med.* 2002;167:83–84.

34. Bowen T, Whelan T, Nelson T. Sudden death after phosphorus burns: experimental observations of hypocalcemia, hyperphosphatemia and electrocardiographic abnormalities following production of a standard white phosphorus burn. *Ann Surg.* 1971;174:779–784.

35. Ben-Hur N, Giladi A, Neuman Z, et al. Phosphorus burns: a pathophysiological study. *Br J Plast Surg.* 1972;25:238–244.

36. Mendelson J. Some principles of protection against burns from flame and incendiary munitions. *J Trauma.* 1971;11:286–294.

37. Madrzykowski D, Stroup W. *Magnesium Chip Fire Tests Utilizing Biodegradable, Environmentally Safe, Nontoxic, Liquid Fire Suppression Agents.* Gaithersburg, Md: Underwriters Laboratories Inc; 1995.

SUGGESTED READINGS

1. Reed JL, Pomerantz WJ. Emergency management of pediatric burns. *Pediatr Emerg Care.* 2005;21(2):118–129.

CHAPTER 165

Rocketpropelled Grenade Attack

Mark Greve and Joseph Lauro

Rocketpropelled grenades (RPGs) are shoulder launched weapon systems utilizing a rocket motor to deliver an explosive charge. The weapons system was originally designed to attack armored vehicles and thus the majority of explosive charges it delivers are high explosive anti-tank (HEAT) warheads. Additional types of warheads include fragmentation, illumination, smoke, tear gas, white phosphorus, and enhanced blast weapons (EBWs).

A significant amount of the risks associated with this weapon system are its propagation and relative ease of use. The RPG is most commonly associated with the Russian (Ruchnoy Protivotankovy Granatomyot) RPG-7 and has been used in virtually every conflict since the mid-1960s and has been a weapon of choice for a variety of terrorist organizations. The RPG-7 and its variants are a rugged, cheap, and simple weapon system produced by a variety of countries including Russia, Bulgaria, Pakistan, China, and Iran.[1] Virtually every army in the world has some form of RPGs in its arsenal. They have been used to attack personnel, military vehicles, civilian vehicles, helicopters, fixed wing aircraft, buildings, and ships. In October 1996 the Bandito's Motorcycle Club attacked a Hells Angels clubhouse in Sweden killing one of its members and decimating the residence with a Swedish anti-tank RPG.[2]

The Russian RPG-7 has a range around 500 m against static targets and 300 m against moving targets. The maximal range of the antitank HEAT round is 920 m and antipersonnel rounds have a maximal range of 1100 m and a blast radius of 4 m.[11] The weapon is widely used, aimed through traditional static sights and takes a minimal amount of training. During the Soviet-Afghan conflict the Mujahideen refined and expanded the tactics and targets of the RPG. These refinements continued during ensuing conflicts in Iraq, Afghanistan, and other conflicts particularly in the Middle East. During Operation Iraqi Freedom, 14.5% of battlefield injuries were due to RPGs.[3]

DESCRIPTION OF EVENTS

The RPG is a weapon system capable of delivering a variety of warheads. The injuries these impart can be due to thermal, blast, or ballistic trauma. All explosions and any of the warheads can have any of these effects. The types of injuries imparted are dependent on the nature of the warhead and circumstances of their use either via primary, secondary, or tertiary mechanisms. Understanding how these weapons work will help us understand the types of injuries that may be encountered and how to treat victims of such weapons.

White phosphorous and illuminating rounds have significant potential for thermal burns. White phosphorous (commonly known as Willie Pete) creates painful chemical burns which continue to burn through tissue to bone until it is expired.

Heat rounds are historically the most common type of RPG warhead. They use a shaped charge to focus blast energy resulting in a high velocity stream of molten metal which penetrates armor. This effect can impart massive thermal burns to personnel. The warhead carries more explosive but has a smaller metal casing and imparts less fragmentation effect. It can create a greater blast but in a more focused direction relative to a fragmenting warhead.

EBWs are powerful weapons whose primary mechanism is via blast effect. EBWs, or thermobaric weapons, are akin to a fuel air bomb which disperses explosive vapors or particles and uses oxygen from the surrounding atmosphere to generate an intense, high-temperature explosion. The fuel can permeate buildings, bunkers, and other facilities before exploding. The destructive power of a shoulder launched EBW is akin to a 152 mm artillery shell.[4] There is increasing concern over their propagation and the emerging global threat they pose.[5]

Fragmenting or ballistic RPG warheads feature a metal casing around an explosive charge. The explosive charge can be ignited by a delayed fuse or by impact. The resultant blast disperses fragments designed to kill and maim personnel. Explosions create fragments and the secondary effect of creating missiles from structures the RPG warhead impacts such as walls, vehicles, and other objects. These are the most common form of injury encountered in RPG attacks. For survivors blood loss is the greatest risk if the fragments do not critically damage vital organs.

The pressure wave from a blast injury renders the greatest destructive force to tissues with variable density such as the lung, intestines, heart, liver, and kidneys. The typical damage from the primary blast injury comes in the form of barotrauma effecting air containing organs. This overpressure wave, traveling in excess of 3000 m/sec, may cause a subsequent vacuum rupturing the lungs. Damage such as this can lead to rapid blood loss contributing to morbidity and mortality. Air embolism can also occur in coronary and cerebral vasculature.

Secondary blast injuries result from limited fragmentation of the warhead as well as the debris displaced by the blast. Such injuries can affect victims not in the immediate blast radius. Open areas reduce the effect but victims in enclosed areas such as buildings and bunkers have increased likelihood of secondary blast injuries. Typical secondary blast injuries are perforations of the body, fractures, injuries to the eyes (from dirt or dust), and lacerations. A characteristic skin finding in the secondary phase of a blast injury is spalling which occurs as high velocity debris interacts with the skin.

Tertiary blast injury results from the blast throwing the victim against solid objects with injuries resulting from deceleration and structural collapse. Typical injuries include blunt trauma, fractures, and amputated limbs. Rapid blood loss is of utmost concern.

PRE-INCIDENT ACTIONS

Once the force and destructive power of RPGs are understood preparation seems difficult. A well-developed and rehearsed disaster response plan will aid response, there are no specific preplanning actions to be taken. Body armor helps cut down on secondary injuries from fragmentation but may enhance primary blast injuries in enclosed spaces.[6,7]

▶▶ POST-INCIDENT ACTIONS

Prehospital trauma life support (PHTLS) and mass casualty incident response are the mainstays of response to an RPG incident. The simple triage and rapid assessment (START) algorithm is an ideal method of triaging, caring for and appropriately dispositioning MCI patients including victims of RPG injuries.

Prehospital personnel should document injuries that occurred within an enclosed space to highlight the possibility of secondary and tertiary injuries when the casualty reaches the emergency department. Post-incident actions include notification of the trauma team in anticipation of requiring increasing hospital-based resources such as operating room personnel and blood. Plans should be in place for casualties who may have unexploded ordnance embedded in their bodies, may still be alive, and require care. These weapons can be handled relatively safely during removal from patients, but they will need ultimate disposal by appropriately trained personnel. Police bomb disposal personnel should be involved if there are any unexploded RPGs or EBWs retained in the patient's body. Other considerations consist of mobilization of un-crossmatched blood and massive transfusion protocols. The police department and hospital security personnel should be used for crowd and media control.

➕ MEDICAL TREATMENT OF CASUALTIES

Blast injuries may be difficult to diagnose in the prehospital setting and can take time to manifest, especially in the case of chest and abdominal blast injuries. Initially injuries to the torso and abdomen may be indistinguishable from benign causes of respiratory distress such as hyperventilation, breathlessness, or agitation due to stress reaction. It is difficult to recognize clinically subtle colorectal lesions, particularly when these injuries are overshadowed by other obvious external wounds.[8]

Other subtle signs of primary blast injury include deafness secondary to middle ear barotrauma, bleeding from the ears, chest or abdominal pain, confusion, and difficulty breathing. Suspected blast casualties should be transported by stretcher if feasible because exercise has been shown to worsen pulmonary injuries.[9] Inappropriate use of intravenous fluids in patients with primary blast injury can cause rapid development of pulmonary problems due to pulmonary contusion (i.e., blast lung). Fluids should not be withheld for resuscitation but should be used based on clinical parameters such as level of consciousness, urine output, and peripheral pulses. Patients who show obvious signs of severe or ongoing blood loss should be transfused immediately with type O blood; women of childbearing age are transfused with O negative blood. Potentially unstable patients may be treated with isotonic crystalloid in lieu of blood, although unnecessary infusion of crystalloid should be avoided.[10] The type of crystalloid infusion is an area of ongoing debate.[11] Normal saline may be an appropriate initial consideration secondary to Ringer's lactate incompatibility with blood in the IV tubing.

❓ UNIQUE CONSIDERATIONS

Victims of an RPG attack may have sustained multiple mechanisms of injury (e.g. crush, lacerations, penetrating trauma, and blast injury). These are high energy military weapons. When compared with civilian modes of wounding, damage imparted and energy transferred by RPGs are likely to be far greater than injury sustained from civilian weaponry.

The RPO-A EBW uses isopropyl nitrate as an energetic material in the warhead. Isopropyl nitrate can be absorbed into the skin, ultimately causing formation of methemoglobin.[12] Isopropyl nitrate is also a carcinogen. Ordinarily, isopropyl nitrate is a clear fluid, but it may have been dyed pink for ease of identification during maintenance. If a pink fluid is present when the RPO-A malfunctions, avoid contact with this fluid.

⚠ PITFALLS

Blast injuries from RPG attacks may result in a wide variety of injuries ranging from tympanic membrane rupture to pneumothorax and even gastrointestinal bleeding from hollow viscous injury. Maximal destruction from the pressure wave itself tends to damage air-filled organs with greater propensity than solid organs and should always be considered during assessment. The damage to patients in enclosed spaces tends to be greater. A higher index of suspicion must be maintained including a greater risk of pulmonary injury in such cases.

The anxious patient with no outward evidence of trauma may have sustained barotrauma to the lungs which should be ruled out before discharging the patient.

Secondary injuries may be incurred by victims not in the direct vicinity of the blast.

Tertiary injuries and structural instability pose a risk to rescue workers, the blast scene should thus be entered with caution and appropriate resources.

The START algorithm is an appropriate responder approach to enhance patient care and disposition.

It is better to transfuse blood early to those patients with evident hemorrhage and hemodynamic instability in lieu of large volume crystalloid infusion.

REFERENCES

1. Gander T, Hogg IV. *Jane's Infantry Weapons.* Alexandria, VA: Jane's Information Group; 1995, 303–305.
2. Biker Sentenced to Life for Grenade Attack. Highbeam.com. Retrieved 2011-10-05.
3. Dunemn KN, Oakley CJ, Gamboa SR, et al. *Profile of Casualties Treated in US Army Medical Treatment Facilities During Operation Iraqi Freedom: 10 March-30 November 2003.* Washington, DC: Center for AMEDD Strategic Studies; 2004, 1–98.
4. New RPO. Shmel-M Infantry Rocket Flamethrower Man-Packable Thermobaric Weapon. defensereview.com. 2006-07-19. Retrieved 2012-08-27.
5. Dearden P. New blast weapons. *J Roy Army Med Corps.* 2001;147(1):80–86.
6. Grau LW, Smith T. A "crushing" victory: fuel-air explosives and Grozny 2000. Quantico, VA: Marine Corps Gazette; 2000, 84(8):30.
7. Directorate of army doctrine: the threat from blast weapons. Grodzinski J, ed. *The Bulletin, for Soldiers by Soldiers.* 2001;7(3):1–10.
8. Bortolin M, Baldari L, Sabbadini MG, Roy N. Primary repair or fecal diversion for colorectal: injuries after blast: a medical review. *Prehosp Disaster Med.* 2014;29(3):1–3.
9. Hamit HF, Bulluck MH, Frumson G, Moncrief JA. Air blast injuries: report of a case. *J Trauma.* 1965;5:117–124.
10. Ley EJ, Clond MA, Srour MK, et al. Emergency department crystalloid resuscitation of 1.5 L or more is associated with increased mortality in elderly and nonelderly trauma patients. *J Trauma.* 2011;70(2):398.
11. Cotton BA, Jerome R, Collier BR, et al. Eastern Association for the Surgery of Trauma Practice Parameter Workgroup for prehospital fluid resuscitation. *J Trauma.* 2009;67(2):389.
12. Safety (MSDS) data for isopropyl nitrate. October 27, 2003. Available at: http://ptcl.chem.ox.ac.uk/MSDS/IS/isopropyl_nitrate.html.

CHAPTER 166

Conventional Explosion at a Hospital

Stephen Grosse

DESCRIPTION OF EVENT

The experience gained from damage to health care facilities by earthquakes and other incidents provides some insight into the response phase to this type of emergency.[1-3] This chapter will discuss the types of explosions that may affect a hospital and the associated injuries to be anticipated. Potential pitfalls and successes from similar events will also be discussed. In 2004, the United States Department of Homeland Security implemented the National Incident Management System (NIMS), the first attempt at a national standardized approach to incident management and response.[4,5] Incident command is a very strong pillar of NIMS and hospitals must have well-developed Incident Command Systems (ICS) if they are to be resilient in responding to explosions on campus. The UK, Europe, Australasia, and NATO forces use and train to a different system, The Major Incident Medical Management and Support (MIMMS) system for out-of-hospital mass casualty incidents, and Hospital Major Incident Medical Management and Support (HMIMMS), a specific course for hospital staff.[6-8] Many of the concepts are the same, although the emphasis and training are quite different with more focus on practical experience in the MIMMS approach. Whichever system is in use, training has been highlighted repeatedly as being key to optimal response and performance during an incident.[7,9]

There have been many descriptions of the hospital impact of external mass casualty bombing incidents such as the Boston Marathon Bombing in Boston Massachusetts, in 2013.[10-13] Little has been written about explosions on site of health care facilities. Although an explosion at a hospital is an unlikely event, the impact of such an event on the infrastructure, patients, staff, and community must be considered. The hospital setting is rich in flammable and toxic materials, making it a potentially hazardous environment. The common use of hazardous materials, nuclear agents, and toxic substances makes most medical centers vulnerable to explosions.[14] There are a small number of published reports regarding explosions occurring on a hospital site, some relate to equipment failure[15] with a resultant explosion while others relate to bombings of hospital facilities themselves.[16,17] Hodgetts describes the impact of the 1991 IRA Bombing of the military wing of Musgrave Park Hospital, Belfast, where nine staff were killed or injured.[16]

Conventional explosions in hospitals are exceedingly rare. When a hazard vulnerability analysis is performed, the probability of such an event would be given a low score; however, the impact of the event on the institution warrants a high score, making the overall score low to intermediate. Explosions can result from either a terrorist event or an internal mishap, such as a ruptured gas line. Regardless of the source, the result is essentially the same.

A terrorist incident may involve the detonation of an improvised explosive device (IED). These devices come in a variety of shapes and sizes, ranging from small pipe bombs composed of metal pipe and rapidly burning gunpowder to large truck bombs such as the one used to destroy the Alfred P. Murrah Federal Building in Oklahoma City, Oklahoma, in 1995.[18] Secondary devices, which are devices timed to detonate after the primary explosion to injure first responders, also should be considered until the source of the explosion has been determined.

The storage of compressed gases, including oxygen and air, also can be the source of an explosion at a health care facility. Unlike terrorist bombings, explosions caused by flammable gases or liquids may continue to burn, resulting in secondary explosions and projectiles causing further damage to personnel and the structure. Large cylinders of medical gases can cause significant damage to structures either by exploding secondarily or from a "missile effect."[19]

Regardless of the source of the initial explosion, damage to the building may compromise structural components or infrastructural components (e.g., ventilation, water supply, and sprinkler systems). Secondary fires ignited from the initial explosion may continue to cause additional injuries, even among those who avoided direct injury from the initial event. Damage to anything other than a small confined area requires consideration of partial or facility-wide evacuation.

PRE-INCIDENT ACTIONS

As described earlier, ICS is the foundation of emergency operation planning for U.S. hospitals. The ICS itself is a predominantly U.S.-based system, while internationally other systems, such as HMIMMS, are in use. Ideally, all hospital personnel should have some training with respect to familiarization of how the facility will function during a mass casualty incident. For staff with the potential to occupy a critical command role, such training is essential.[20] Regularly scheduled drills using the localized ICS are vital to familiarize hospital staff with the procedures for organizing personnel, facilities, equipment, and communications during an emergency response.[7,9,21-23] A full discussion of the ICS can be found in previous chapters. Box 166-1 briefly outlines the immediate tasks of the sector chiefs for the ICS system.

POST-INCIDENT ACTIONS

The Incident Commander (IC) will determine when the incident is over or determined to be under control. The post-incident goal is to restore continuity of operations and for the hospital to return to its pre-incident state. Partial restoration of services may begin as soon as the building is

---

BOX 166-1   Immediate Tasks of Sector Chiefs in Emergency Response

Title Tasks to Consider

Incident Commander
1. Activate Emergency Operations Center
2. Set agenda for status report by sector chiefs (i.e., operations, logistics, planning, and finance)
3. Assign liaisons to coordinate with responding agencies
4. Assign a public information officer
5. Prepare staff for extended operations
6. Determine whether patient evacuation will be required

Logistics Sector Chief
1. Determine the structural integrity of the affected building and advise the Incident Commander
2. Secure the utilities, including medical gases
3. Ensure adequate supplies to treatment area
4. Activate emergency communications plan

Planning Sector Chief
1. Consider alternative care sites
2. Secure transportation for patients to alternative care sites
3. Ensure accurate patient tracking
4. Develop a plan for convergent volunteerism

Operations Sector Chief
1. Organize triage and treatment of all casualties
2. Ensure continued care of all unaffected patients

Finance Sector Chief
1. Immediately track all costs associated with response, recovery, and mitigation of event

---

deemed structurally sound. The determination of whether severely damaged structures can be repaired or will have to be razed must be addressed. After the 1994 Northridge, California, earthquake, four of the eight hospitals that evacuated patients because of that disaster required demolition.[24]

Immediate real-time cost tracking may become important for reimbursement. The finance officer should work closely with outside agencies, including the institution's insurance carrier, to provide accurate costs. This must include personnel costs as well as replacement costs for material. Determining what types of disaster relief or grant money will be available and how best to access these funds will assist the institution in returning to its pre-incident condition.

In the event the source of the explosion is unknown and possibly the result of a terrorist attack, the facility is now a crime scene. Evidence preservation and limited access to the scene are critical. Jurisdictional issues, particularly with law enforcement agencies, may become complicated. All agencies should understand that safety issues take priority, but responders should try to minimize their impact on the scene. Working with these agencies during drills and appreciating one another's roles and capabilities will greatly enhance the working relationship and allow both missions to be accomplished in overlapping timeframes.

Because hospitals have large amounts of hazardous and radioactive material, patient decontamination may be required. Contaminated patients cannot enter the general population without first being decontaminated. Depending on the location of the explosion and the damage sustained, the hospital's own decontamination facility may be unavailable. Even if the facility is undamaged, the personnel who usually provide decontamination may be unavailable. Contamination with radioactive material has some special considerations. Working closely with the hospital physicist or the radiation safety officer will greatly enhance decontamination efforts. In addition, educating staff about radioactive decontamination will reduce the anxiety of treating these patients.

Although explosions at hospitals are rare, they must be considered during the hazard vulnerability analysis. The best way to prepare for these and all types of events is to implement an Incident Command-based hospital emergency management plan. This plan should be exercised frequently and should involve as many community agencies as possible. Tabletop exercise drills have proved to be a very low cost and efficient way of drilling personnel regularly, ensuring that key concepts remain to the fore. This experience will be invaluable no matter what type of emergency disrupts the function of a hospital.

✚ MEDICAL TREATMENT OF CASUALTIES

Victims of a conventional explosion at a hospital will display the types of injuries seen in blasts and structural collapse. The care of these victims will follows guidelines described thoroughly in other chapters. In a hospital setting, however, some casualties may have underlying medical conditions for which they are being hospitalized. The management of such patients should also take into account these underlying conditions.

？ UNIQUE CONSIDERATIONS

There are unique considerations with hospital explosions. Ruptured medical gas lines can create an oxygen-rich environment with a significant increase in fire potential. It should be an absolute priority of the operations sector chief to have the oxygen lines shut down as soon as possible. This may mean shutting down the entire facility until the affected area of the building can be isolated and contingency planning for oxygen and medical gas supply should account for such eventuality.

Radioactive agents may be dispersed during an explosion, leading to contamination that will add a level of complexity to incident management. Decontamination will have to be executed in consultation with the facility's radiation safety officer. If the explosion is the result of a terrorist event, the involvement of law enforcement personnel adds yet another level of complexity. To ensure that potential radiation contamination is considered, the radiation safety officer should be notified whenever the emergency operations plan is implemented. He or she is a staff officer or liaison to the IC and needs to be incorporated into the operations plan. The IC can quickly dismiss him or her if the officer's services are not required, or the officer can be reassigned to the operations sector as needed.

The risk of evacuating patients from a structure that is potentially unstable must be considered. These risks include moving unstable patients through an environment that is of immediate danger to life and health. If the building sustains damage similar to facilities in Oklahoma City, technical rescue experts will be required and the evacuation will be lengthy. Sheltering in place is an option that also has its own risks, including a potentially stable structure becoming unstable as a result of any secondary explosions necessitating an emergency evacuation. The important point to determine is whether a patient is going to be exposed to greater risk during evacuation than he or she would face if sheltered in place.

! PITFALLS

Several potential pitfalls exist in responding to an explosion at a hospital. These include the following:
- Lack of an ICS-based emergency operations plan
- Failure to drill regularly pre-incident
- Failure of communication systems
- Failure to include local response agencies in pre-incident drills and planning
- Operating outside the ICS, allowing "freelancing" to occur
- Not incorporating ICS into all facets of drills, tabletop scenarios, and events
- Not getting to know all of the responders' capabilities and limitations before an event occurs

REFERENCES

1. Schreeb von J, Riddez L, Samnegård H, Rosling H. Foreign field hospitals in the recent sudden-onset disasters in Iran, Haiti, Indonesia, and Pakistan. *Prehospital Disaster Med.* 2008;23:144–151, discussion 152–153.
2. Djalali A, Corte Della F, Foletti M, et al. Art of disaster preparedness in European Union: a survey on the health systems. *PLoS Curr.* 2014;6.
3. Ardalan A, Kandi M, Talebian MT, et al. Hospitals safety from disasters in I.R.iran: the results from assessment of 224 hospitals. *PLoS Curr.* 2014;6.
4. National Incident Management System. Jones & Bartlett Learning; 2005:1.
5. Walsh DD, Walsh DW, Christen T, Lord GC. *National Incident Management System: Principles and Practice.* Sudbury, MA: Jones & Bartlett Learning; 2011.
6. Sammut J, Cato D, Homer T. Major Incident Medical Management and Support (MIMMS): a practical, multiple casualty, disaster-site training course for all Australian health care personnel. *Emerg Med.* 2001;13:174–180.
7. Hodgetts TJ. *Major Incident Medical Training: A Systematic International Approach.* UK: Informa UK; 2009;1:13–20.
8. Group ALS. *Major Incident Medical Management and Support.* Wiley; 2013, 1.
9. Graham CA, Hearns ST. Major incidents: training for on site medical personnel. *J Accid Emerg Med.* 1999;16:336–338.
10. Brunner J, Singh AK, Rocha T, Havens J, Goralnick E, Sodickson A. *Terrorist bombings: foreign bodies from the Boston Marathon Bombing. Semin Ultrasound CT MR.* Elsevier; 2015, 36:68–72.
11. Brunner J, Rocha TC, Chudgar AA, et al. The Boston Marathon bombing: after-action review of the Brigham and Women's Hospital emergency radiology response. *Radiology.* 2014;273:78–87.
12. Mirza FH, Parhyar HA, Tirmizi SZA. Rising threat of terrorist bomb blasts in Karachi—a 5-year study. *J Forensic Leg Med.* 2013;20:747–751.
13. Mekel M, Bumenfeld A, Feigenberg Z, et al. Terrorist suicide bombings: lessons learned in Metropolitan Haifa from September 2000 to January 2006. *Am J Disaster Med.* 2009;4:233–248.
14. Aghababian R, Lewis CP, Gans L, Curley FJ. Disasters within hospitals. *Ann Emerg Med.* 1994;23:771–777.
15. Hayt E. Hospital liable for anesthetic explosion due to defective equipment. *Hosp Manage.* 1957;83:78–79.
16. Hodgetts TJ. Lessons from the Musgrave Park Hospital bombing. *Injury.* 1993;24:219–221.
17. Piletić M. The bombing of the hospital for infectious diseases in Jasikovac in February 1943. *Vojnosanit Pregl.* 1966;23:866–868.
18. Mallonee S, Shariat S, Stennies G, Waxweiler R, Hogan D, Jordan F. Physical injuries and fatalities resulting from the Oklahoma City bombing. *JAMA.* 1996;276:382–387.
19. Gupta S, Jani CB. Oxygen cylinders: "life" or "death"? *Afr Health Sci.* 2009;9:57–60.
20. Reilly M, Markenson DS. Education and training of hospital workers: who are essential personnel during a disaster? *Prehosp Disaster Med.* 2009;24:239–245.
21. Williams MJ, Lockey AS, Culshaw MC. Improved trauma management with advanced trauma life support (ATLS) training. *J Accid Emerg Med.* 1997;14:81–83.
22. Carley S, Mackway-Jones K. Are British hospitals ready for the next major incident? Analysis of hospital major incident plans. *BMJ.* 1996;313:1242–1243.
23. Mackway-Jones K, Carley SD, Robson J. Planning for major incidents involving children by implementing a Delphi study. *Arch Dis Child.* 1999;80:410–413.
24. Schultz CH, Koenig KL, Lewis RJ. Implications of hospital evacuation after the Northridge, California, earthquake. *N Engl J Med.* 2003;348:1349–1355.

167 CHAPTER

Conventional Explosion in a High-Rise Building

James J. Rifino

DESCRIPTION OF EVENT

Historically, high-rise building construction dates back more than 2000 years to ancient Rome and possibly earlier. Similar structures have been built in Egypt, Italy, and the Yemeni city of Shibam as well. These were poorly built, by modern standards, and typically used to house people on the upper floors and to rent out the lower levels for commerce purposes with an added benefit of protection from attackers.[1] With the invention of the elevator, true high-rise buildings became possible. Large buildings were designed using steel, concrete, and other more durable materials. With the end of World War II, there was a need for more affordable and cheaper housing making the "high-rise building" very attractive as an answer. London experienced significant destruction and the opportunity for developing larger buildings that could support the large population needing housing as well as reconstruct the city was popular. Legislation in the United States allowed for affordable housing funding and the need for more consolidated living. Modern twentieth century high-rise buildings are typically residential sculptures designed to enhance the skylines of cities throughout the world. Developers and architects compete to design bigger, taller, more structurally sound structures capable of withstanding the environment associated with such great heights. To date, the tallest building in the world is the Burj Khalifa in Dubai standing 828 m tall with 163 floors.[2,3] While beautiful to look at, these structures are challenging with respect to emergency response, fire suppression, and protection from terrorist organizations who increasingly target such famous landmarks. The majority of the worst building collapses in history (Royal Plaza Hotel in Thailand, 1993; Hotel New World in Singapore, 1986; three high-rise buildings in Rio de Janeiro, Brazil, 2012; Sampoong Department Store in Seoul, South Korea, 1995; Katowice Trade Show in Silesia, Poland, 2006) were a result of poor construction, illegal construction, and/or bad engineering. Other causes of building collapse include flooding or other environmental issues, fire, or human mistakes. A gas explosion on May 16, 1968, resulted in the collapse of Ronan Point, a high-rise building in East London. Just 5 days after the completion of this building, a woman on the eighteenth floor lit a match to heat up a cup of tea on her stove. An explosion from this single match resulted in the complete collapse of the southeast corner of the building. All 22 floors came down in a "domino effect." It was found that unlicensed gas fitters had improperly secured the gas lines and poor construction did not allow for any support.[4] A turning point in building safety and security came in 1993 when high-rise structures became targets of terrorism. Health care workers and emergency managers worldwide have since learned the need for mass casualty training, disaster expertise, and emergency management familiarity and protocols specifically for high-rise buildings.

The first of three notorious large-scale attacks on high-rise buildings occurred on February 26, 1993. The bombing of the World Trade Center in New York City, New York, by an Islamist terrorist group using a truck bomb resulted in six deaths and 1042 injuries.[5] Less than 1 month later, on March 12, 50 people were killed in Bombay, India, after a car bomb exploded in the Bombay Stock Exchange Building followed by a series of suitcase bombs detonated in a number of other hotels, killing hundreds of additional people. The second attack in the United States was in Oklahoma City, Oklahoma, in 1995, when a truck bomb exploded adjacent to the Alfred P. Murrah Federal Building, killing 167 people and injuring more than 750 more.[6] The worst single act of terrorism in the history of the United States was the attack on the World Trade Center towers in New York City on September 11, 2001. There were 1527 bodies identified, and it is predicted that the actual death toll is between 2726 and 2742 people.[7,8] Thousands of others suffered injuries from the attack, and 1103 people were treated in hospitals for their injuries.[9] This single act of terrorism ignited the desire to prevent another such attack worldwide. Communication of relevant information between local and international governments was enhanced, and the concepts of emergency management and disaster preparedness grew quickly out of its infancy.

Many different types of explosives can be used to collapse high-rise buildings. In the correct amounts, ammonium nitrate, trinitrotoluene (TNT), Semtex, dynamite, nitroglycerin, and composite C-4 all are powerful enough to cause a building to collapse. These are all known as "high-order explosives" (HEs). Advancements in structural design have helped mitigate complete collapse; the World Trade Center Towers were a classic example. The original 1993 truck bomb did not take down the tower, though it created a large crater and significant damage, because of redundancy in the structural design. The 2001 attack involved large commercial airplanes, which themselves did not take out the tower because of improved engineering. The towers remained erect after the explosions, until the resulting fires from the planes aviation fuel weakened the structure, causing the steel to lose half of its strength and buckle, resulting in a domino collapse of the above floors.[10] The lessons learned from 9/11 have spawned heightened interest in new engineering and building design to withstand such issues. There are a number of international grants dedicated to designing buildings of the future that can withstand climate challenges as well as withstand explosive situations. The University of California, Berkeley College of Engineering program identified the need for "Bomb-Resistant Buildings." Their students have been tasked with this challenge.[11] In 2009, the New York City Police Department authored a 130-page document, "Engineering Security: Protective Design for High Risk Buildings." The document was published as a resource for New York City developers and security personnel. It provides guidelines pertaining to perimeter security, the risk-tiering system for buildings in New York, emergency preparedness, and building design issues.[12]

Blast Injuries

Blast injuries can be differentiated into four categories (primary, secondary, tertiary, and quaternary). Primary blast injuries are due to the direct effect of the pressure (blast) wave on the victim.[13] The most sensitive organ affected by the primary blast is the ear.[14] Other systems that are affected include the respiratory, circulatory, and digestive systems, as well as the eye and orbit. This is due to the fact that pressure affects air and can result in air embolization and hollow viscous injury.

Secondary blast injuries result from objects propelled by the blast (bomb fragments, glass, nails, shrapnel). These projectiles can be very significant in a high-rise building explosion and may extend far beyond the distance of the initial blast effect. The objects and debris become projectiles that can penetrate the body, cause significant blunt trauma, and also can result in fragment injuries to the extremities. Current building design uses a significant amount of glass, and chards of glass can travel great distances, resulting in eye injuries.

Tertiary blast injuries occur when a person is propelled by the blast against another structure. These are typically blunt injuries, including soft tissue injuries, lacerations, head injuries, fractures, and amputations. Less commonly seen are flash burns and thermal injuries.

Quaternary blast injuries include all other injuries as a result of the blast (crush injuries, burns, closed and open brain injury, asphyxia, toxic exposures, chronic illness exacerbations).[15] Crush injuries are common if a building explosion results in structural collapse, and these frequently cause immediate death. In the Oklahoma City Bombing, 97% of fatalities were immediate, and most were killed in the building collapse.[6] This was also true in the World Trade Center attack.[7] The risk of building collapse and resultant high fatality rates distinguish explosions in high-rise buildings from other types of explosions. Medical personnel are unlikely to care for crush victims who occupied the structure during a high-rise collapse because survival is rare.

PRE-INCIDENT ACTIONS

Prevention is the most effective method of reducing morbidity and mortality arising from an explosion in a high-rise building. Constructing high-rise buildings to withstand an explosion without structural failure should also reduce mortality. There is literature and research with respect to military injury mitigation as products are developed for personal protection as well as vehicle reinforcement (from IEDs, roadside bombs, pipe bombs, etc.), but there is still need for development of products that will not shatter and become sharp, penetrating objects when propelled.

Currently, significant focus is being placed on design guidance, including site location, layout, building envelope and interior, and on the mechanical and electrical systems used in high-rise construction. When designing a new building, design guidance is provided for limiting or mitigating the effects of terrorist attacks. It is beyond the scope of this chapter to discuss each of these methods. The U.S. Federal Emergency Management Agency's website (http://www.fema.gov) extensively outlines an infrastructure protection series to mitigate potential terrorist attacks against buildings in its second edition reference manual, October 2011.

Another critical element to have in place in the aftermath of a building explosion is a disaster plan that involves all medical and rescue personnel of a given area. Any city or large community must have a well-rehearsed disaster plan in place in case of a mass-casualty event.

In addition, it should have an emergency medical services (EMS) system that is able to surge appropriately for the event and respond in an expedient manner. All agencies (prehospital and within the hospital) need to have regular drills that test the system as well as engage all rescuers and emergency management personnel. The bombings at the Boston Marathon are a prime example of this. Although it was beneficial that medical, fire, and police personnel were very local to the incidents, the fact that this scenario had been drilled multiple times by the participants was key to the decreased morbidity and mortality associated with the event. There were unfortunate deaths as a result of this cowardly act, but lives were saved as a result of an instant shift to "emergency mode" with restaging equipment, communication changes, command designation, and immediate medical management of the situation…all a result of significant training or drilling.

Finally, pre-incident actions should include gathering information for the buildings themselves. In the United States, the National Fire Protection Association published a 38-page document, "Guidelines to Developing Emergency Action Plans for All-Hazard Emergencies in High-Rise Office Buildings." This encourages building management to collect data that local emergency service personnel can access if called to rescue large numbers of people as a result of a catastrophic issue involving the building. It encourages tabletop exercises, building information cards, occupant-tracking tables according to floors, and a record of those with disabilities who are in the building.[16]

POST-INCIDENT ACTIONS

Immediately after a conventional explosion in a high-rise building, there need to be individual and coordinated efforts between prehospital personnel, emergency department personnel, and personnel within the hospital who will be receiving these patients. While EMS personnel respond to the scene and prepare for the worst, hospital wards and emergency departments must prepare for an influx of patients. This includes the need to expedite patient movement out of the emergency department (ED) to clear the area for incoming patients. Such movements require significant preplanning and drilling by all hospital personnel at least annually. In addition, all personnel must be prepared for the possibility of secondary attack if the explosion is deemed to be of a possible terrorist etiology. Hospitals must go on "lock down," ambulances should be inspected quickly before being allowed near the building, and security forces must be on heightened alert. This takes extreme coordination and familiarity with procedures and protocols.

Prehospital management starts with the notification of all local agencies that an event (mass casualty incident [MCI]) has occurred. A standardized message system will ensure efficient transfer of such alerts. The METHANE message as used in the UK Major Incident Medical Management and Support (MIMMS) system is an example of an easily taught and repeatable message structure:

M—Major incident/mass casualty incident declared
E—Exact location (grid reference if known or GPS)
T—Type of incident (fire, crash, explosion, etc.)
H—Potential hazards involved (smoke, oil, chemicals, fire, etc.)
A—Access roads to the scene from various directions
N—estimated number of casualties
E—Emergency services present and required

In addition, the CSCATTT tool used in MIMMS for prioritizing actions is a useful reminder for early on-scene first responders and this system is used widely by NATO services, ensuring that civilian and military responders are using the same terminology:

C—Command and control
S—Safety/security

C—Communications
A—Assessment
T—Triage
T—Treatment
T—Transport

If the event is anticipated to outstrip local resources, activation of other agencies must occur. This may include other outside local agencies as well as regional and state agencies. Some countries may have federal resources to respond in the event of a declared disaster. Knowing one's local resources and protocols with regard to emergency management is of the utmost importance in advance of an event. "Scene Safety" is of the utmost importance, there exists significant potential for toxic chemicals, unstable structures, and hazardous materials. In addition, secondary explosive devices designed to explode on a delay, and directed at the personnel trying to rescue the victims, are unfortunately very common in terrorist attacks.[17] At the scene, the safety of the remaining structure must always be assessed. Building collapse is a significant risk after any explosion, and it is not uncommon for rescuers to become victims when attempting to do their job. Once the building is secured, the rescuers must quickly triage victims according to standard protocols determining who has salvageable life-threatening injuries. Scene command must be determined, patient-staging areas must be designated, and appropriate transfer of patients to designated facilities must be coordinated so as to not overwhelm one facility.

Prehospital and ED staff must be prepared to triage patients appropriately. Every hospital and region should have a disaster plan in place ahead of time. Typically, the first round of patients are the less severe and can "self-extricate" and transport themselves to the hospital. The more severely injured patients are typically the second round of patients. If there is a collapse of the structure, the hospital should expect increased severity and delayed arrival of casualties. Centers for Disease Control (CDC) advice in the United States outlines that an ED should double the first hour's casualties for a rough prediction of the total "first wave" of casualties.[15]

Prehospital personnel should expect to see familiar injuries, including blunt, penetrating, and thermal injuries. After an explosion, all medical personnel need to maintain a high index of suspicion for primary blast injury. Presence of a crater, injuries to closer victims, and building collapse are important observations regarding blast strength. Likewise, assessment of damaged objects near a casualty situation might yield a gross estimate of the pressures that existed in the vicinity. For example, shockwaves able to rupture a tympanic membrane are about the same as that needed to shatter automobile glass.[18]

It is also important to get a quick history. Phillips and Zajtchuk[19] recommend the following questions when evaluating a bombing casualty:

1. What type of ordnance was used? How large was the explosion?
2. Where was the casualty located with respect to the blast?
3. Did the blast occur inside an enclosed space, such as a room or vehicle?
4. What was the casualty's activity after exposure?
5. Were fires or fumes that might lead to an inhalation injury present?
6. What was the orientation of the casualty's head and body in relation to the blast?

Prehospital medical personnel should be ready to perform lifesaving interventions including intubations, field amputations, and chest decompressions. The most common procedures performed include spinal immobilization, field dressings, and intravenous fluid administration.[20] Prehospital personnel also should be trained and equipped for extrication of victims after complete or partial building collapse. Extricating these victims as quickly as possible greatly improves their chance of survival by reducing the occurrence of acute kidney injury

from crush syndrome. The concept of "scene safety" with respect to rescuers cannot be overemphasized.

ED personnel should be involved in helping to direct prehospital personnel with respect to patient transfer to the appropriate facility. In some U.S. regions, this concept is known as "medical direction." Designated trauma centers should be predesignated, and this concept should be used by all systems daily. EMS and hospitals should be considered a "continuum" of patient care, and thus ED personnel should consider themselves partners in EMS. Trauma centers should receive the most severely injured patients, even if they are not the closest hospital. It actually may be beneficial to take the more seriously injured to the further hospitals (if appropriate) because those less severely injured usually transport themselves to the more local hospitals. Upon arrival to the ED, staff must assess for the many types of injuries occurring as a result of a blast. Emergency staff must be prepared for victims, most of whom will have only minor injuries, to arrive by all modes of transportation. In the Oklahoma City Bombing, Hogan and colleagues report that 55% of victims came by private vehicle, whereas only 33% came by EMS transport. In addition, 80% were discharged that day.[20]

ED staff must activate the hospital disaster plan and mobilize the equipment necessary to treat mass casualty victims immediately upon notification of any MCI, including: wound care trays, tetanus immunizations, antibiotics, fracture care, endotracheal tubes, thoracostomy tubes, cricothyroidotomy trays, and all medications required for conscious sedation, rapid sequence induction, and advanced cardiac life support. Trauma teams must be notified, transport of admitted patients out of the ED must be expedited, and personnel from inside the hospital must be activated to the ED in anticipation of receiving injured patients requiring rapid assessment. This expedited "throughput" will create much needed ED space for incoming patients. The need for drills in preparation for this type of disaster by all hospital staff cannot be stressed enough. Communication between EMS and the ED is essential and can have positive or negative consequences with respect to morbidity and mortality associated with the disaster event.

✚ MEDICAL TREATMENT OF CASUALTIES

The treatment of casualties after an explosion in a high-rise building can be very challenging. Some injuries will be very apparent, whereas others will have to be "found" depending on the astute clinician evaluating the patient. There may be delayed presentation of an injury. Health care professionals need to be prepared to evaluate all four types of blast injuries as discussed previously.

Timely and repeated triage is essential for patients who arrive from a blast event. As discussed previously, the first wave of patients usually consists of those able to self-extricate and self-transport with minor injuries (such as abrasions and lacerations). Health care providers must assess and examine each patient, fully utilizing standard trauma protocols, while being mindful of delayed symptoms. Blast injuries (particularly primary blast injuries) differ from many other types of injuries because serious injury may not manifest immediately, therefore necessitating a period of observation. Primary blast injury may result after any explosion and can be amplified if it occurs in an enclosed building or next to a sturdy wall structure that will deflect the energy off the wall and toward the victims. The full management of blast injuries is discussed in more depth in other chapters.

Secondary blast injuries are caused from projectiles due to the blast. These types of injuries make high-rise building explosions different from other conventional blasts. Many of the modern high-rise buildings are constructed with significant amounts of glass and steel. These projectiles travel at high speed and are very dangerous. Shrapnel from a high-rise building can reach victims well outside the reach of the primary blast zone, as seen during the Oklahoma City Bombing. Glass laceration injuries occurred as far as 10 blocks from the site of the explosion. After more serious injuries have been ruled out, lacerations should be treated as time and resources allow. Delayed closure can be used if resources are not available to treat both the critically ill and those with minor injuries. Injury to the eye often results from secondary blast injuries and should not be overlooked. Of the surviving victims of the Oklahoma City Bombing, 8% sustained eye injuries including lid lacerations, open globe injuries, orbital fractures, corneal abrasions, retinal detachment, and intraocular foreign bodies.[21] Data from the Centers for Disease Control indicate up to 10% of all blast survivors have significant eye injuries. Due to the fact that they can cause minimal discomfort, it is recommended that patients be referred liberally for ophthalmologic screening.[15]

The most worrisome type of secondary blast injury is the penetrating injury. Every part of the building and its contents has the ability to become shrapnel moving at high velocity. Victims with penetrating injuries should be treated promptly and with the involvement of the surgical trauma team. As with all penetrating injuries, the practitioner should be ready to treat hemorrhagic shock. In a stable patient, deep penetrating shrapnel should only be removed in a safe, controlled environment such as an operating room.

While penetrating injuries are obvious, blunt trauma must not be overlooked. Blunt trauma can occur from secondary or tertiary blast injury after a high-rise explosion. Blast lung injury (BLI) is the most common fatal primary blast injury among initial survivors and is characterized by a clinical triad of apnea, bradycardia, and hypotension in its more severe state. Anyone with dyspnea, cough, hemoptysis, or chest pain should be considered for an earlier stage of BLI.[15] Severe entrapment or crush injuries are rare in survivors, but may be seen in the emergency department. Patients with crush injuries are at risk for amputation, compartment syndrome, rhabdomyolysis, and acute kidney injury. Air emboli can occur as a result of blast injuries presenting as a stroke, acute myocardial infarction, spinal cord injury, blindness, acute abdomen, pneumothorax, and pulmonary embolism. These patients should be treated according to standard trauma protocols. Flash burns and thermal injuries are usually superficial injuries and should be treated with standard burn care.

UNIQUE CONSIDERATIONS

Blast injuries were once thought to be associated only with the battlefield. As technology develops, buildings increase in height, and terror acts occur across our globe, penetrating and blunt trauma pathology are seen more commonly. Preparing for a conventional bombing in a high-rise building is a difficult task because of the wide variety of injuries seen and the potential for large numbers of victims. The harsh reality is that complete collapse of a building usually results in significant occupant mortality and minimal live presenting patients. As discussed, it is usually the second wave of patients that are more critical. High-rise explosions may result in exposure to toxic substances (carbon monoxide, cyanide, methemoglobin, etc.) for both survivors and rescuers, necessitating decontamination of victims and rescuers at the scene or outside the ED. A final consideration is emergency department patient flow. A triage system needs to be in place that will properly direct the large flow of injured victims. For emergency personnel responding to the scene, high-rise buildings have unique challenges, including longer access and egress times, specific need for evacuation strategies, fire control issues, confined vertical egress, fire control (access to water, specifically), and ventilation issues associated with smoke control. Materials

burning may expose rescuers and evacuees to different toxic chemicals. Fire suppression systems may be different from those used by emergency fire services. Finally, communication, as well as command and control, during a large event can be difficult depending on the building's height, concrete structure, and steel infrastructure.

⚠ PITFALLS

Several potential pitfalls in response to an explosion in a high-rise building exist. These include the following:

1. Failure to make sure the building is secure and safe for rescue personnel
2. Failure of a hospital and EMS to have a rehearsed disaster plan in place for a mass-casualty incident involving an explosion in a high-rise building
3. Failure of the building management to have a rehearsed pre-incident plan
4. Underestimation of the severity of injuries sustained by victims as a result of a conventional explosion in a high-rise building
5. Failure to test fire suppression systems in all buildings resulting in a nonworking system
6. Failure to engage with building managers with regard to building maintenance, logs of disabled people, and risk stratification with respect to the structure
7. Failure to recognize the possibility of a secondary attack by terrorists specifically targeting rescue personnel
8. Failure to disperse patients to appropriate hospitals to not overwhelm one hospital completely

REFERENCES

1. Aldrete GS. *Daily Life in the Roman City: Rome, Pompeii and Ostia.* Westport, CT: Greenwood Press; 2004, 79.
2. New York Times, Dubai Opens a Tower to Beat All; January 4, 2010.
3. Emporis Standards Committee. Available at: www.emporis.com/statistics/worlds-tallest-buildings; 2014.
4. Pearson C, Delatte N. Ronan Point Apartment Tower collapse and its effect on building codes. *J Perform Constr Facil.* 2005;19:172–177.
5. Federal Bureau of Investigation Bomb Data Center. *General Information Bulletin 96-1: 1996 Bombing Incidents.* Washington, DC: US Department of Justice; 1996.
6. Mallonee S, Shariat S, Stennies G, et al. Physical injuries and fatalities resulting from the Oklahoma City bombing. *JAMA.* 1996;276:382–387.
7. Schwartz SP, Li W, Berenson L, Williams RD. Deaths in World Trade Centers terrorist attacks: September 11th, 2001. *MMWR.* 2002;51:16–18.
8. Hirschkorn P. *New York reduces 9/11 death toll by 40.* October 29, 2003. Available at: www.cnn.com/2003/US/Northeast/10/29/wtc.deaths/.
9. Centers for Disease Control and Prevention. Rapid assessment of injuries among survivors of the terrorist attack on the World Trade Center—New York City, September 2001. *MMWR.* 2002;51:1–5.
10. Eagar TW, Musso C. Why did the World Trade Center collapse? Science, engineering and speculation. *JOM.* 2001;53(12):8–11.
11. *"Lab Notes," Research from the College of Engineering.* Volume 3, Issue 2, Berkeley: University of California; March 2003. Available at: www.coe.berkeley.edu/labnotes/0303/index.html.
12. New York City Police Department. *Engineering Security: Protective Design for High Risk Buildings;* 2009. Available at: www.nyc.gov/html/nypd/downloads/pdf/counterterrorism/nypd_engineeringsecurity_full_res.pdf.
13. Phillips YY. Primary blast injuries. *Ann Emerg Med.* 1986;15:1446–1450.
14. Adler OB, Rosenberger A. Blast injuries. *Acta Radiol.* 1988;29:1–5.
15. CDC Injury Prevention. *Explosions and Blast Injuries: A Primer for Clinicians.* Available at: www.cdc.gov/masstrauma/preparedness/primer.pdf.

16. NFPA National Fire Protection Association, High Rise Building Safety Advisory Committee. *Guidelines to Developing Emergency Action Plans for All-Hazard Emergencies in High-Rise Office Buildings.* January 2014. Available at: www.nfpa.org/highrise; 2013.

17. Boffard KD, Macfarlane C. Urban bomb blast injuries: patterns of injury and treatment. *Surg Annu.* 1993;25:29–47.

18. Wightman JM, Gladish SL. Explosions and blast injuries. *Ann Emerg Med.* 2001;37:6.

19. Phillips YY, Zajtchuk JT. The management of primary blast injury. In: Bellamy RF, Zajtchuk R, eds. *Conventional Warfare: Ballistic, Blast, and Burn Injuries.* Washington, DC: Office of the Surgeon General of the US Army; 1991:295–335.

20. Hogan DE, Waeckerle JF, Dire DJ, et al. Emergency department impact of the Oklahoma City terrorist bombing. *Ann Emerg Med.* 1999;34:160–167.

21. Mines M, Thach A, Mallonee S, et al. Ocular injuries sustained by survivors of the Oklahoma City Bombing. *Ophthalmology.* 2000;107:837–843.

Conventional Explosion at a Nuclear Power Plant

Stephen Grosse

DESCRIPTION OF EVENT

On March 11, 2011, a magnitude 9.0 earthquake struck off the eastern coast of Japan, producing a massive tsunami with waves greater than 10 m striking the coastline. The seawall barriers protecting the Fukushima Daiichi Nuclear Power Plant were overwhelmed by the tsunami causing damage to the power plant. The cooling system was severely damaged, leading to a meltdown of fuel rods and several hydrogen explosions that scattered radioactive nucleotides into the air, land, and sea surrounding the power plant. Emergency response was complicated by the earthquake and subsequent tsunami, including damage to hospitals that had been designated as radiation emergency facilities. Undamaged hospitals that had not been designated as radiation emergency facilities sometimes refused to accept possibly contaminated patients due to concerns about radiation exposure further complicating evacuation and treatment of those injured during the incident.[1]

In addition to damage resulting from natural disasters, there has been increased concern over the safety of nuclear power plants after the attacks on the World Trade Center in New York City on September 11, 2001, and the frequency of terrorist attacks worldwide. In the United States, there are over 100 such plants.[2] Security has been heightened around nuclear power plants, barricades are in place, and armed guards are present.[3] All commercial nuclear power plants in the United States house the reactor core in a thick stainless steel vessel within a concrete building.[4] Nonetheless, studies have shown that if a jet aircraft crashed into a nuclear reactor and only 1% of its fuel ignited after impact, the resulting explosion could compromise the integrity of the reactor core containment building. Thus these reactor core containment buildings, although designed to withstand impacts, are certainly destructible and vulnerable to large-scale explosions. Nuclear power plants harbor additional radioactive materials in the form of spent fuel pools. The spent fuel pools are housed in corrugated steel buildings, which are much more vulnerable to attack than the reactor core containment structure.[5]

Another example of a conventional explosion at a nuclear power plant took place at the Chernobyl Nuclear Power Plant in the former USSR in 1986. An accidental steam explosion during a safety test destroyed the reactor core. A plume of radioactive substances was released into the atmosphere during the explosion and fire.[6] Approximately 600 persons were hospitalized within a week due to injuries and illness linked to the explosion, with several immediate deaths and dozens more over the following months.[6]

At the time of the explosion, approximately 100,000 persons lived within a 30-km radius around the Chernobyl Nuclear Power Plant. When the explosion occurred, radioactive substances were released into the atmosphere and continued to do so for 10 days, until the fire was finally contained. Winds and rainfall distributed the radioactive substances throughout the northern hemisphere, with the highest concentration around the power plant. Contamination of the area around the power plant was patchy, in that distribution of the fallout depended largely on where it happened to rain. The volatile radioisotopes of iodine and cesium were the most important in terms of health risk.[7] Radioactive iodine has a half-life of just 8.05 days, but radioactive cesium has a half-life of approximately 30 years.[6,8] A total of 350,400 persons were resettled due to concerns over contamination caused by the Chernobyl explosion.[6]

Long-term effects of exposure to radiation, mainly carcinogenesis, are being seen in the population affected by the Chernobyl explosion. Increased rates of thyroid cancer, leukemia, and solid cancers (i.e., breath, lung, and urological) have been seen among inhabitants of contaminated areas and cleanup workers.[6,9] The long-term health effects of the explosion at Fukushima Daiichi have yet to be determined.

PRE-INCIDENT ACTIONS

Each nuclear power plant is required to have an emergency response plan, as are the local and state government agencies in which the power plant is housed. Some federal agencies have emergency response plans in the event of a power plant explosion.[2] Control and command procedures must be clarified before an incident occurs, as must organizational responsibilities. Assessment of the type and quantity of materials and equipment needed, along with decontamination plans and health care worker protection, should be addressed. The location of Geiger meters and other radiation survey instruments should be posted, along with reference material on what the various readings mean in terms of patient care. An adequate supply of potassium iodide to combat exposure to radioactive iodine should be available for the entire affected population.[4]

Each community surrounding a nuclear power plant should have a designated official who makes decisions about evacuation and other issues concerning the population at risk for possible radiation exposure. Communication during the incident is of vital concern, and emergency communication systems must be tested in advance.[4] There are two emergency planning zones: the first is within a 10-mile radius of the event, where the threat of direct radiation is highest, and the second is within a 50-mile radius, where the radioactive plume may threaten residents. A warning system, such as sirens or flashing lights, is required to be provided by the nuclear power plant to alert all inhabitants within a 10-mile radius of an event. Each year, the nuclear power plant is required to distribute emergency information materials to all people who live within this zone so that in the event of an explosion the public in the vicinity of the plant is prepared.[2]

Every hospital, regardless of its proximity to a nuclear power plant, should have a radiation control officer. This officer is responsible for monitoring all patients and medical personnel with radiation counters, supervising cleanup of the potentially radioactive waste, and devising a plan to minimize contamination. Training for physicians to prepare for a disaster involving radiation exposure is offered by the Radiation Emergency Assistance Center/Training Site in Oakridge, Tennessee.

The World Health Organization suggests that the general population, particularly those in the vicinity of nuclear power plants, should be prepared for a nuclear incident. One recommendation is to become aware of possible solid shelter areas in the local area. A second is to have disaster supplies on hand; these include food and water for 3 to 5 days, a first-aid kit, respiration protection, flashlights and batteries, a battery-operated radio with extra batteries, and stable iodine.[10]

►► POST-INCIDENT ACTIONS

Immediately after a conventional explosion at a nuclear power plant, the local emergency response will be activated. The disaster area safe for entry by emergency personnel must be designated. Geiger counters and other devices to detect radiation should be used. If the level is 0.1 Gy/hour or above, emergency personnel should not enter the area and should return to the control point until further notice. Specialized protective equipment will be needed to enter the area safely.

As with any mass casualty event, on-scene triage should be performed. Those with life-threatening injuries are to be taken directly to the hospital.[4] For these patients, emergency personnel should use gloves and gowns, remove the patients' clothes, cover their hair with surgical caps if available, and wrap the patients in sheets for transport. Simply removing the clothes reduces the patient's contamination by approximately 80%.[11] Those who are uninjured or suffering from minor injuries should be relocated upwind, and decontamination should be performed. Decontamination in these situations consists of removing the victim's clothes and placing them in hazardous material bags and washing the person's skin and hair with soap and warm water.[12] All those with nausea, vomiting, diarrhea, or rash should be referred to the emergency department for evaluation of possible acute radiation syndrome.[4]

In mass casualty situations, approximately 80% of victims are decontaminated at hospitals; thus, the hospital facility must be prepared to decontaminate patients both inside and outside the emergency department.[11] For those whose conditions are stable, decontamination should be done immediately and, if possible, outside of the hospital. Those who must be brought into the emergency department immediately should be treated in an area roped off from the rest of the department. Hospital personnel should wear disposable clothing, gowns, gloves, and shoe covers when treating these patients.[13]

The radiation control officer is responsible for monitoring the exposure of hospital staff. Personnel involved with care of contaminated patients should wear dosimeters to monitor radiation exposure.[11] The dose limit for persons providing emergency services other than lifesaving actions is 5 rem per event, whereas for lifesaving activities the recommended maximum dose is 25 rem per event. In the event of a disaster, the recommended limit increases to 150 rem per event.[4]

The U.S. Federal Bureau of Investigation (FBI) is the lead federal agency during crisis management, that is, during the period when the focus is on ensuring that there is no further threat and establishing the site of attack as a crime scene. The Federal Emergency Management Agency (FEMA) takes the lead during consequence management, where the focus is on limitation of damage, protection of the public, decontamination, and disposal of the radioactive material. These two agencies will be lead coordinating organizations and should be contacted with questions. Also, the Radiation Emergency Assistance/Training Site should be contacted with any concerns.[4]

✚ MEDICAL TREATMENT OF CASUALTIES

A conventional explosion at a nuclear power plant will lead to a variety of injuries. Blast, thermal burns, and smoke inhalation will be responsible for most immediate deaths. Radiation injuries will include whole-body or localized exposure (i.e., irradiation) and internal deposition of radioactive substances (i.e., contamination).[13]

Whole-body irradiation by gamma rays can lead to acute radiation syndrome. The most susceptible cells to radiation damage are rapidly dividing cells such as those in the intestinal mucosa and bone marrow.[3] However, with massive irradiation, even the central nervous system, with its relatively low cellular turnover rate, will show the effects.[13] The degree of whole-body radiation exposure is estimated using clinical signs and symptoms, the minimal lymphocyte count within the first 48 hours, the severity of thrombocytopenia and reticulocytopenia, and cytogenic studies of chromosomal abnormalities in bone marrow and red blood cells.[4,13] Lymphocytes are the most radiosensitive cells in the blood, and a substantial dip is apparent within the first 8 to 12 hours.[14] The faster the fall and the lower the nadir of lymphocytes, the greater the whole-body radiation dose.[4] Furthermore, the sooner the onset of signs and symptoms for each phase of radiation illness, the greater the whole-body irradiation.[2] Nausea, vomiting, diarrhea, and rash are the first presentation after gamma irradiation. Later, the clinical manifestations of acute radiation syndrome are related to the level of leukocytes and platelets (Table 168-1). Fever, infections, and hemorrhaging occur. Also, with sloughing of the intestinal mucosal surface, mucositis and enteritis occur.[4]

TABLE 168-1	Clinical Manifestations and Treatment of Gamma Radiation Exposure		
DOSE (GY)	SYMPTOMS	LYMPHOCYTE NADIR	TREATMENT
>30	Hypotension, high fever, mental status change, syncope, seizures	<100	Palliative
>10	Immediate nausea, vomiting, diarrhea	<100	Palliative
4-10	Delayed (by hours) nausea, vomiting, diarrhea	100-499	Protective isolation, TPN, gut sterilization, hematopoietic growth factors, antimicrobials
2-4	Delayed (by days) nausea and vomiting, or no symptoms	500–999	Antiemetics, pain control, fluids, close monitoring
<1	Less than 10% with delayed (by days) nausea and vomiting	>1000	Symptomatic care

TPN, Total parenteral nutrition.

In addition to the whole-body gamma ray irradiation, the skin is susceptible to local radiation injury. The distribution tends not to be uniform, and the skin radiation dosage absorbed is estimated to be 10 to 20 times greater than the bone marrow doses. The signs of a radiation burn are very similar to those of a thermal burn, with the difference being that signs of radiation burns appear after a period of days in contrast to thermal burns, where the results appear immediately.[4] In the Chernobyl explosion, a period of primary erythema was seen in the first few days, followed by a 3- to 4-day period of latency. In severe cases, secondary erythema and the full extent of the burn manifested as early as 5 to 6 days, and as late as 3 weeks in milder cases. The most frequent locations early on were the wrists, face, neck, and feet. As time went on, burns were also seen on the chest and back, and later on the knees, hips, and buttocks.[13] Vascular insufficiency can develop at any time after the radiation exposure, even years later, with necrosis occurring. Treatment includes control of pain, vasodilator therapy, and prophylaxis against infection.[3] Surgery and plastic surgery consultants should be involved because extensive debridement, skin grafting, and amputation are often required.[14] Burns to the eyelids and eyes are often seen and require an ophthalmology consultation.

Internal contamination occurs through inhalation, ingestion, and absorption through open skin. Inhalation can lead to radiation pneumonitis. Early bronchopulmonary lavage may be helpful in removing some of the radioactive contaminants. Chronic low-level inhalation of radioactive substances is more common and was seen among those involved in the cleanup efforts from the Chernobyl explosion. Radiation fibrosis was seen, and treatment with interferon was of some benefit.[13]

Ingestion of radioactive substances is either treated with specific antidotes and/or general measures to decrease absorption, both of which should be instituted as soon as possible after exposure. Specific antidotes include blocking agents that saturate a tissue with a nonradioactive element, thus reducing the uptake of the radioisotope. Another example is chelating agents, which bind metals into complexes, preventing tissue uptake and allowing urinary excretion.[13] As in all poisonings, the local or regional poison control center should be contacted.[4]

Contaminated wounds should be rinsed with saline until the Geiger meter reads no evidence of radioactive material. If the patient has received a dose of whole-body radiation that leads to decreased lymphocyte count (above 1 or 2 Gy to the bone marrow), the wound should be closed as soon as possible to decrease the chance of the wound serving as a portal of entry for infection.[4] Surgical debridement is necessary for the usual indications of dirt and nonviable tissue, as well as for continued high readings of radioactive contamination despite saline rinses.[13]

UNIQUE CONSIDERATIONS

A conventional explosion at a nuclear power plant differs from all other explosions because of the risk of radiation exposure, illness, and death to large populations. Decontamination is imperative and must be undertaken on a massive scale. Psychosocial issues are very important after the release of radioactive material, as fear and stress responses resulting from the incident can lead to symptoms in the general population that mimic radiation exposure, such as nausea, vomiting, and rash. The psychosocial effects can be quelled by communication with the general public in an honest and open manner about the event and the short-term and long-term health risks.[4]

! PITFALLS

Several potential pitfalls in response to an explosion at a nuclear power plant exist:

- Many of the victims most severely affected by radiation exposure are emergency personnel and those who were involved in cleanup activities.
- In the event of a conventional explosion at a nuclear power plant, radiation-safe and contaminated areas must be identified. Those with the proper personal protective equipment will be able to enter the designated contaminated area and bring patients to emergency personnel located in the designated radiation-safe areas. Once the patients are removed from the area of high radiation and are decontaminated, they no longer pose a significant risk to health care workers using universal precautions.[4]

REFERENCES

1. Tominaga T, Hachiya M, Tatsuzaki H, Akashi M. The accident at Fukushima Daiichi Nuclear Power Plant in 2011. *Health Phys.* 2014;106 (6):630–637.
2. *Are You Ready? A Guide to Citizens Preparedness.* Washington, DC: Federal Emergency Management Agency; 2002.
3. *Chernobyl: Ten Years After, Causes Consequences, Solutions.* Greenpeace International; 1996. Available at: http://skeptictank.org/treasure/GP1/CHTENAF.TXT.
4. Mettler F, Volez G. Current concepts: major radiation exposure: what to expect and how to respond. *N Engl J Med.* 2002;346:1554–1561.
5. Helfand I, Forrow L, Tiwari J. Nuclear terrorism. *BMJ.* 2002;324:356–359.
6. UNDP/UNICEF. *The Human Consequences of the Chernobyl Nuclear Accident: A Strategy for Recovery.* New York: United Nations; 2002.
7. United Nations Scientific Committee on the Effects of Atomic Radiation. *Exposures from the Chernobyl Accident: UNSCEAR Report to the General Assembly, with Specific Annexes.* New York, NY: United Nations; 1988.
8. United Nations Scientific Committee on the Effects of Atomic Radiation. *Acute Radiation Effects in Victims of the Chernobyl Accident: UNSCEAR Report to the General Assembly, with Specific Annexes.* New York, NY: United Nations; 1988.
9. *Fifteen Years After the Chernobyl Accident. Lessons Learned: Executive Summary of an International Conference, Kyiv, April 18–20, 2001.* Minsk, Belarus: Committee on the Problems of the Consequence of the Catastrophe at the Chernobyl Nuclear Power Plant; 2001.
10. *Health Protection Guidance in the Event of a Nuclear Weapons Explosion.* Geneva: World Health Organization; 2003.
11. Blackwell T. Weapons of mass destruction. In: Marx J, Hockberger R, Walls R, eds. *Rosen's Emergency Medicine: Concepts and Clinical Practice.* 5th ed. St Louis, MO: Mosby; 2002:2616–2649.
12. *What You Should Know if There Is an Attack Involving Radioactive Materials. Fact Sheet #16.* Olympia, WA: Washington State Department of Health; 2002.
13. Markovchick V. Radiation injuries. In: Marx J, Hockberger R, Walls R, eds. *Rosen's Emergency Medicine: Concepts and Clinical Practice.* 5th ed. St Louis, MO: Mosby; 2002:2056–2063.
14. Goans R, Holloway E, Berger M, et al. Early dose assessment in criticality accidents. *Health Phys.* 2001;81:446–449.

SUGGESTED READINGS

1. Aslan G, Terzioglu A, Tuncali D, et al. Consequences of radiation accidents. *Ann Plast Surg.* 2004;52:325–328.

Tunnel Explosion

Hazem H. Alhazmi and Michael Sean Molloy

DESCRIPTION OF EVENT

Tunnel importance in modern society cannot be overestimated. Transportation directly through mountainous terrain, under waterways, and through urban areas make tunnels an invaluable component of modern travel. These aspects also make tunnels themselves a hazard arising from the challenges of providing medical assistance to victims of a tunnel disaster. There have been many documented incidents of tunnel disasters illustrating the devastating consequences. In April 1982, a drunk driver collided with a wall in the Caldecott Tunnel in California, setting in motion a chain of events which resulted in a multivehicle collision involving a gasoline tanker and bus with seven fatalities. The Salang tunnel in Afghanistan was the scene of one of the worst tunnel explosions in history, where two Soviet military convoys allegedly collided, with reports of an explosive chain reaction involving a fuel tanker and munitions truck with 64 reported military deaths and 112 civilian deaths.

In 2014 there were multiple major tunnel explosions in the Syrian cities of Aleppo and Homs with rebels targeting government bases with large amounts of explosives set in tunnels under military facilities. China's Shanxi province was also the site of a major tunnel explosion on March 1, 2014, as a result of collision between two methanol tankers with 31 lives lost. An explosion at Calumet City, Illinois, arose after heavy rain overwhelmed the deep sewer tunnel system. In the year 2000, a deadly tunnel fire in Kitzsteinhorn, Austria, resulted in the death of 155 passengers on a shuttle train. Another tragic tunnel disaster occurred in Mont Blanc, France, in 1999 with 39 deaths in a 10-car accident. Although these examples demonstrate terrible outcomes of tunnel tragedies, they do not come close to the size of disaster associated with a large-scale tunnel explosion.[1]

In the changing world in which we live, an obvious source of tunnel explosions is domestic or international terrorism. Traditionally, explosive weapons used by terrorists have been of limited size, usually a few kilograms, resulting in a low mortality rate. However, due to advanced technology and more elaborate planning, the potential exists for much greater damage. Three primary factors increase the risk of morbidity and mortality from explosions: larger explosive devices, confined space, and structural collapse. All three of these possibilities exist in a tunnel explosion incident.[2] Although terrorist activity is a realistic possibility, other potential causes of tunnel explosions must be considered also, including construction, demolition, mining, and multivehicle collisions resulting in explosions. A gas explosion in 1995 in an underground railway in Daegu, South Korea, claimed the lives of 101 people and injured another 143. In 1919 there were two devastating tunnel explosions in the United States on the same day: a dynamite explosion in the Baltimore Tunnel (Maryland) that claimed the lives of 92 people, and a mining tunnel explosion in Wilkes Barre, Pennsylvania, that killed 83

people. Other possible causes of explosive events occurring in tunnels include tanker truck explosions and multivehicle accidents.

Tunnel explosions represent a significant challenge to emergency personnel due to many unique characteristics, and risks should be assessed in a hazard vulnerability assessment.[3] The purpose of this chapter is to understand the broad scope of preparedness that is essential to a successful emergency response.

PRE-INCIDENT ACTIONS

In addition to normal disaster preparation, there are some key areas that deserve specific attention in preparing for the possibility of tunnel explosion. A multi-agency, well-drilled incident command system will ensure effective management at the event site and strategic command levels. The U.S.-based National Response Plan was introduced to standardize a national approach to responding to natural or human-made threats.[4] Establishing command and control is vital in the early stages of a disaster to ensure a coordinated approach to management. First responders on scene will, by definition, be the command until a more appropriately trained person arrives, at which point command may be turned over to another individual who should be clearly identified by his tabard. Command does not need to be in the hands of the most senior person but it commonly is; the most appropriate commander is the person who has been trained for the role.

Command and control is the first of the seven priority pillars in Major Incident Medical Management and Support (MIMMS). MIMMS is the system used in United Kingdom, Europe, Australasia, and NATO for mass casualty incident management. The pillars are:

C—Command and control
S—Safety
C—Communication
A—Assessment
T—Triage
T—Treatment
T—Transport

In some jurisdictions, first responders activate the disaster plan, Incident Command System (ICS), and emergency procedures. In others, this requires a management function. Responsibilities of a first responder are to establish on-scene command, size up the event, and broadcast a report to appropriate personnel within and outside the agency. Having a standard method of delivery of such a report will greatly assist personnel and minimize the chance of message failure by "speaking a different language." The METHANE message (Major Incident Medical Management and Support system), as used in the United Kingdom, is an example of an easily taught and repeatable message structure:

M—Major incident declared

E—Exact location (grid reference, if known, or GPS)

T—Type of incident (fire, crash, explosion, etc.)

H—Potential hazards involved (smoke, oil, chemicals, fire, etc.)

A—Access roads to the scene from various directions

N—estimated number of casualties

E—Emergency services present and required

Due to the variety of tunnel locations, it is common for multiple hospitals and rescue teams to serve the impacted area of a tunnel explosion. Having regular interagency and interfacility drills will improve capabilities. Scene safety is vital in tunnels, with particular emphasis on the structural integrity of the tunnel and effective ventilation. A well-drilled, all-hazards integrated response plan that maximizes the effectiveness of triage, treatment, disposition, and evacuation will reduce mortality, morbidity, and incident stress. Such a response plan must be fluid with the ability to adjust based on actual event development. In previous mass casualty incidents such as the bombing of Centennial Park at the Atlanta Olympics in 1996, and the bombing of the World Trade Center in 1993, adhering to a coordinated response plan presented challenges. With many hospitals involved in the recovery process, effective coordination and communication are essential before, during, and after incidents to use all available resources effectively and avoid overburdening one particular agency. Additional communication challenges arise with tunnel explosions due to the complexities of tunnel design. With multiple entry and exit sites, several control points will be required. Walkie-talkies, cell phones, and landlines should all serve a role in establishing effective communication; however, some or all of these modalities may not function as planned deeper into a tunnel system, and written message transmission by individuals may be required. In addition, site flags should be used to explain the purpose of each organizational area in the most common languages of the area. This itself can be challenging in multicultural cities with pockets of residents who may not have any ability to converse in the city's native tongue. Translators should be available, both on-site and by phone, to assist with such circumstances.

Tunnel explosions are associated with an increased risk of smoke and toxin exposure. Tunnel explosions may involve nuclear, biological, or chemical toxins in transport for peaceful purposes or criminal acts. Equipment readiness should address the need for respiratory equipment, not only to aid victims suffering from inhalation injuries, but for response teams as well. It is also important for assistance teams to wear proper protective equipment (PPE) to limit additional injuries. Therapeutic agents, including atropine, pralidoxime chloride, oral prophylactic antibiotics, and potassium iodide, should be available to treat victims as well as health care providers who may be exposed. Readiness for a possible tunnel explosion includes preparation of site maps to determine the best locations for command posts and triage sites. As was previously stated, multiple entry and exit points increase the need for multiple control points. As a result, it is vital to have accurate maps available in advance of the incident, modern technology such as GPS mapping and Google Maps may prove invaluable on-site for rescue personnel. Finally, response transportation plans must include alternative methods of travel due to the likelihood that a tunnel explosion will result in vital city route closures and rerouting.

▶▶ POST-INCIDENT ACTIONS

The effective use of law enforcement is vital. Site security, as mentioned earlier, is an essential and often overlooked aspect of disaster response planning. A cordon should be established as quickly as possible to keep victims from leaving the disaster scene without assessment and to prevent injuries to outsiders entering the disaster area. It is also important

to set up a staging point for equipment and personnel with logistics staff to log staff in and out of the disaster scene. This will help with control of resources and rescuer safety. Distribution of site layout information should occur as rapidly as possible among the response team members. Security should be considered not only at the site of the explosion, but also at the receiving hospitals because they are a prime target for secondary explosions if the initial disasters are intentional.

A major post-event challenge with tunnel explosions relates to multiple access or egress points. Multiple primary and secondary triage points may be required. A subway explosion could occur where there are multiple underground-to-surface exit stairways allowing minimally injured passengers to exit at several locations. If triage personnel are not located at or near each of these sites, there is potential for significant delay in disposition of victims, as well as the increased likelihood that victims will leave the scene without evaluation. This can result in uneven distribution of injured persons to local hospitals and can also increase the risk of morbidity and mortality in those with delayed symptoms. At each of these triage sites, there should also be treatment stations for immediate administration of medical assistance if required.

A large percentage of patients treated in hospital facilities will self-present to the emergency department by nonemergency transportation. Establishing triage outside ED at the receiving facilities is important to prevent the ED from being overwhelmed by minor injuries which should be treated elsewhere. In addition, triage outside of the ED will involve initially triaging those who have not been assessed on-scene and performing secondary triage of those who have been assessed but whose condition has now changed, resulting in either up- or down-triage. Quickly identifying serious injuries in this group is essential because time is of the essence for those who may suffer from previously unrecognized life-threatening injuries. In addition, these external triage sites should quickly direct victims in need of decontamination to isolated decontamination sites to avoid further exposure to others and contamination of medical facilities.

✚ MEDICAL TREATMENT OF CASUALTIES

The majority of victims after tunnel explosions will present with blast injuries. The incidence of primary blast injury correlates directly to blast size and proximity to the blast, while correlating indirectly to the amount of open space surrounding the blast. In tunnels, it is important to consider the effects of an explosion in the confined longitudinal space of the tunnel with respect to the frequency and severity of injuries expected. Primary blast injuries are most likely to occur with victims located closest to the explosion due to the dissipation of shock waves with progression away from the blast source. The confined tunnel space increases reflection of blast forces and, therefore, increases the frequency of primary blast injury. The reflection of shock waves can increase the destructive potential by 2 to 20 times that of the incident wave, thereby increasing the severity of primary blast injuries.[5]

Secondary injury is the result of hurled objects causing blunt or penetrating trauma. This involves soft tissue, orthopedic, and head injuries, with traumatic head or limb amputations occurring in those closest to the blast source.[6] Tertiary injury is the result of two broad causative factors: the physical displacement of victims (those hurled from the blast source) and the structural collapse of buildings or tunnel walls (crush injuries) as a result of the force of the blast. Quaternary injury is a collection of other injuries resulting from the blast. This includes thermal injury (hot gases and secondary fires), inhalation injury (dust, smoke, carbon monoxide, and chemicals), and water injury (underwater tunnels).[6] The occurrence rate of quaternary injuries is likely to be increased in tunnel explosions because the length of the confined space may make it difficult to escape, prolonging exposure. People far from the explosion may still be exposed to smoke and gases that vent from the tunnel.

Primary blast injury to the lung or gastrointestinal (GI) blast injury may occur as a result of a tunnel explosion. GI blast injury is more common when victims are submerged or partially submerged in water. A secondary explosion in a tunnel flooded from the primary blast raises the possibility of underwater blast waves striking victims while submerged, resulting in GI blast injury. Blast injury to the GI system can result in hemorrhage, shock, and/or perforation. The colon, as the major site of intestinal gas accumulation, is the most common site for GI blast injury.[6] Physical evidence of GI blast injury includes absent bowel sounds, bright red blood from the rectum, guarding, rebound tenderness, abdominal pain, nausea, vomiting, diarrhea, and tenesmus.[7] This nonspecific presentation makes it necessary to maintain a high index of suspicion for GI blast injury. The risk of extensive bleeding makes fluid and blood transfusions vital to maintenance of cardiovascular stability before definitive surgical care. Due to the limitations of computed tomography scans in the recognition of hollow viscous injury, judicious use of more invasive diagnostic procedures, including diagnostic peritoneal lavage and laparotomy, should be used to maximize treatment success.[7]

Secondary and tertiary blast injuries may have a wide differential of typical and atypical traumatic injuries. Due to the large amount of fragmented materials projected from the blast site in tunnels, a large number of soft tissue injuries, penetrating injuries, head injuries, and traumatic amputations are to be expected. Secondary, tertiary, and quaternary injuries resulting from tunnel explosions should be managed according to standard treatment protocols.

UNIQUE CONSIDERATIONS

Tunnel explosions increase the risk of primary blast injury because the explosion occurs within a confined space, which magnifies the intensity of the blast wave. Tunnel explosions also increase the risk of quaternary injury. Thermal injuries and toxic inhalations are common, with increased incidence in direct proportion to proximity to the blast source. The extent and severity of these injuries depend greatly on the explosives, chemicals, and materials present at the site of the blast, as well as each victim's proximity to the blast and duration of exposure.[6] Multiple triage and tracking sites must be established because there are often many routes out of a tunnel, including stairs to the surface, ventilation shafts, connections to separate tunnels for traffic moving in the other direction, and obvious entrance and exit points. Body armor increases the severity of primary blast injuries. A high index of suspicion for severe primary blast injury should be maintained when caring for injured tunnel or subway security personnel.[7]

⚠ PITFALLS

Several potential pitfalls in response to a tunnel explosion exist. These include the following:

- Failure to recognize primary blast injury in victims who are asymptomatic or have only mild symptoms. Victims of primary blast injury who sustain minimal secondary and tertiary injuries may be inappropriately triaged based on initial evaluation.
- Failure to recognize associated physical examination findings that may signify otherwise occult injury. These findings include tympanic membrane rupture, hypopharyngeal petechiae, or ecchymosis, retinal artery air emboli, and subcutaneous emphysema.[7]
- The risk of blast lung is greater in tunnel explosions than in open-air explosions. In addition, the risk of gastrointestinal injury is greater in underwater tunnels due to the risk of secondary explosions occurring after the influx of significant volumes of water.

REFERENCES

1. Forsén R. Tunnel explosion characteristics. *SP RAPPORT*. 2008;2008:11.
2. Maevski IY. Design Fires in Road Tunnels. *Transportation Research Board*. 2011;1.
3. Doro-on AM. *Risk Assessment and Security for Pipelines, Tunnels, and Underground Rail and Transit Operations*. Boca Raton, FL: CRC Press; 2015, 1.
4. Couig MP, Martinelli A, Lavin RP. The National Response Plan: Health and Human Services the lead for Emergency Support Function #8. *Disaster Manag Response*. 2005;3:34–40.
5. Frykberg ER. Medical management of disasters and mass casualties from terrorist bombings: how can we cope? *J Trauma*. 2002;53:201–212.
6. Wightman JM, Gladish SL. Explosions and blast injuries. *Ann Emerg Med*. 2001;37:664–678.
7. Argyros GJ. Management of primary blast injury. *Toxicology*. 1997;121:105–115.

CHAPTER 170

Liquefied Natural Gas Explosion

Anas A. Khan and Michael I. Greenberg

DESCRIPTION OF EVENT

The chemical composition of natural gas is methane (with small quantities of other hydrocarbons), water, and compounds containing carbon dioxide, nitrogen, oxygen, and sulfur.[1-5] Upon cooling natural gas to less than −259 °F (−161 °C), any present substances will be eliminated, and the natural gas will turn into a clear liquid. The colorless and odorless reaction outcome material is known as liquefied natural gas (LNG). LNG is a cryogenic substance, which is noncorrosive and relatively harmless. LNG is lighter than water, which causes it to float on the surface if spilled in water.[2-5]

LNG is not an explosive material in itself and when properly stored will not spontaneously combust. However, if converted to a vapor, LNG can become suddenly explosive, especially if it is released in an enclosed space. For LNG to explode, its concentration in an air mixture "flammable range" should be 5% to 15%. LNG may combust if its vapor within the flammable range contacts air that is relatively warm in temperature. If large quantities of LNG spill into water rapidly, it will create "rapid phase transition." The heat will rapidly transfer from the water to the much colder LNG, causing rapid LNG transforming from a liquid to gaseous state. This transformation will release large amounts of energy in a boiling liquid expanding vapor explosion (BLEVE) type event. Such explosions carry a serious threat to life and nearby property.[1-5]

LNG is considered a potentially hazardous material that requires strict safety measures around its handling and transport. It can cause cold-related skin injury, creation of oxygen-poor environments, and risks of explosion and burns.[1-5] There is a cryogenic hazard from direct contact arising from the excessively cold temperatures at which LNG is stored. In addition, LNG vapor may displace oxygen from the air mixture causing risk of asphyxia. This hazard might manifest if LNG is released into an enclosed space. Lastly LNG vapor can ignite within parts of the cloud where the flammability range is achieved. Nonetheless, an ignition source is a must for conflagration. The large-scale potential hazard as a spill of LNG in water can impose a disaster. Effective containment will mostly be impossible. LNG rapidly vaporizing will form a cloud that potentially can explode. Terrorist attack against an LNG tanker at or near a port or harbor is another constant threat.[6]

PRE-INCIDENT ACTIONS

In dealing with LNG transport the most important pre-incident action is protection of LNG tankers and storage facilities from terrorist attack.[6]

LNG is usually transported by double-hulled tanker ships, which are specifically designed to accommodate the very low storage temperatures necessary to maintain LNG in its liquid state. Furthermore, all LNG tankers must be compliant with rigorous federal and international regulations from agencies, such as the U.S. Coast Guard, U.S. Department of Transportation, and International Maritime Organization.[6-9]

Currently there are 33 LNG export (liquefaction) terminals, more than 100 import (regasification) terminals, and 360 LNG ships. These numbers are expected to grow to meet the expanding demand for the energy, especially because it is economical "clean energy" and has achieved an excellent overall record in safety.[10]

Catastrophic accidents involving LNG plants have been modeled calculating the weights of different factors on the size of the catastrophe.[4,11,12] The model predicted a downwind spread of intense heat after the catastrophic loss of a four-tank LNG storage vessel.[4] Validated consequence models were also used to determine the vapor cloud dispersion exclusion zones in LNG releases, mainly using computational fluid dynamics (CFD) methods. This method takes into consideration the atmospheric conditions, LNG evaporation rate and pool area, source turbulence, and ground surface temperature and roughness height.[11] Other approaches to anticipate LNG events were validated, such as risk analysis of a regasification system of LNG on board a regasification unit, where the risk analysis must be performed under considerable uncertainty based on hybrid Bayesian networks.[12]

First responders working in areas that may store, receive, or transport LNG should be aware of the potential hazards and should train for hazardous materials incidents that may involve LNG.

POST-INCIDENT ACTIONS

Actions following an explosion and conflagration from an accident or terrorist attack depend to some extent on the incident location. If an incident involved an LNG tanker on the high seas, damage and loss of life would be limited to the ship itself and its staff. However, if an incident occurred in or near a port or at a fixed storage facility, the degree of property destruction, human injury, and death could be significant. A fire resulting from the explosion and ignition of LNG could be extremely difficult to control, especially in cases involving the phenomenon known as *burn back*, in which the entire transported load of LNG combusts. In this situation, the resultant fire may burn uncontrolled until the supply of LNG that was fueling the fire was fully consumed by the burning process.[9,13,14]

Vapor hazard, a flammable vapor cloud at the ground level, due to rapid vaporization and dense gas formation, is another significant hazard. This immediate hazard reveals the existence of a blocking effect (blocking convection and radiation to the pool) to reduce the vaporization rate. The water drainage rate of high expansion foam is essential to determine the effectiveness of the blanketing effect because water provides a boil-off effect.[15]

✚ MEDICAL TREATMENT OF CASUALTIES

As with most hazardous materials incidents, immediately removing exposed survivors from the scene is paramount. If the patients' skin came in contact with LNG, it requires immediate removal of LNG and initiating standard therapies for cold injuries, including immediate rewarming of cold-injured skin by immersion in warm water. Exposure to oxygen-poor environments caused by displacing LNG vapor cloud may require cardiopulmonary resuscitation after removal from the environment. First responders must not enter such environments without the use of appropriate respiratory protection with external supplied air. Persons who may be injured or burned in an explosion involving LNG should be evaluated and treated using standard trauma and burn protocols.

❓ UNIQUE CONSIDERATIONS

The excellent safety record for LNG is somewhat unique among potentially hazardous materials. International transport of LNG via tanker ship started in 1959, and since then there are no reports of serious explosions at sea or ports.[5] However, for fixed facilities the first documented case was the Cleveland Explosion in 1944, in which 128 people died. Experts claimed that its circumstances are not reproducible today. Historically, there have been many small incidents involving LNG in the United States.[16] The news displayed varieties of individual burns or explosions requiring evacuation of nearby areas, and some produced fatalities. They were attributed to technical or human failure. Internationally many significant incidents at on-shore LNG terminals have been documented. One accident occurred in Algeria in 1977 and resulted in at least one fatality.[5] In 2004 a fire at the LNG processing facility in Skikda, Algeria, resulted in the death of approximately 27 workers with injuries sustained by an additional 74 persons.[17] Another incident with a gas pipeline explosion took place in Saudi Arabia in 2007 with the fatality toll announced to be 28 people.[18] Such incidents illustrate that LNG is a potentially hazardous material that can cause major disasters and that its overall excellent safety record for the LNG industry should be monitored.

⚠ PITFALLS

It is common to confuse LNG with liquefied petroleum gas (LPG) or compressed natural gas (CNG). LPG is a mixture of propane and butane in a liquid state at room temperature and moderate pressure. LPG is highly flammable and requires storage far from sources of ignition and in a well-ventilated area, so that any leak can disperse safely away from populated areas. An additive, mercaptan, is mixed in to give LPG a distinctive and unpleasant smell, making leaks readily detectable. The concentration of the added mercaptan is such that an LPG leak can be detected when the concentration is below the lower limit of flammability.[5]

LNG also differs from the material known as CNG. CNG is a form of pressurized natural gas and is usually the same composition as pipeline-quality natural gas. CNG is often misrepresented as the only form of natural gas that can be used as vehicle fuel. However, LPG and LNG may also be used as transport fuels.[5]

REFERENCES

1. Fialka J, Gold R. Fears of terrorism crush plans for liquefied gas terminals. *Wall Street J.* 2004;A1.
2. Fay JA. Model of spills and fires from LNG and oil tankers. *J Hazard Mater.* 2003;B96:171–188.
3. Gerasimov VE, Kuz'menko IF, Peredel'skii VA, Darbinyan RV. Introduction of technologies and equipment for production, storage, transportation, and use of LNG. *Chem Petrol Eng.* 2004;40:31–35.
4. Havens J. Maintaining security in an era of heightened awareness. In: *GTI New Frontiers in LNG Shipping Conference*; 2002, London.
5. Institute for Energy, Law & Enterprise. *Introduction to LNG: An Overview on Liquefied Natural Gas, Its Properties, the LNG Industry, Safety Considerations.* Houston: University of Houston; 2003.
6. Wassel JJ. Public health preparedness for maritime terrorist attacks on ports and coastal waters. *Am J Disaster Med.* 2008;3(6):377–384.
7. Lehr W, Simecek-Beatty D. Comparison of hypothetical LNG and fuel oil fires on water. *J Haz Mater.* 2004;107:3–9.
8. Natural Transportation Safety Board Report. *Columbia LNG Corporation Explosion and Fire.* Cove Point, MD, October 6, 1979, NTSB-PAR-80-2, April 16,1980.
9. Parfomak P. Liquefied natural gas (LNG) import terminals: siting, safety and regulation. *CRS Report for Congress.* January 2004.
10. Foss M. An overview on liquefied natural gas (LNG), its properties, the LNG industry, and safety considerations. *Energy Economics Research.* January 2012.
11. Qi R, Ng D, Cormier BR, Mannan MS. Numerical simulations of LNG vapor dispersion in Brayton Fire Training Field tests with ANSYS CFX. *J Hazard Mater.* 2010;183(1–3):51–61.
12. Martins MR, Schleder AM, Droguett EL. A methodology for risk analysis based on hybrid Bayesian networks: application to the regasification system of liquefied natural gas onboard a floating storage and regasification unit. *Risk Anal.* 2014;34(12):2098–2120. http://dx.doi.org/10.1111/risa.12245.
13. Shook B. Despite recent explosion, BP and shell expanding LNG efforts. *Natural Gas Week.* February 13, 2004.
14. U.S. Bureau of Mines. *Report on the Investigation of the Fire at the Liquefaction.* Cleveland, OH: Storage, and Regasification Plant of the East Coast Gas Co; October 20, 1944, February 1946.
15. Zhang B, Liu Y, Olewski T, Vechot L, Mannan MS. Blanketing effect of expansion foam on liquefied natural gas (LNG) spillage pool. *J Hazard Mater.* 2014;280:380–388.
16. List of Pipeline accidents in the United States in the 21st Century. Available at: http://en.wikipedia.org/wiki/List_of_pipeline_accidents_in_the_United_States_in_the_21st_century.
17. Kemezis P. Algeria blast has officials rethinking LNG safety. *Engineering News Record.* 2004;252:17.
18. Abbot S. Saudi gas pipeline explosion kills 28. *Washington Post.* November 18, 2007.

SUGGESTED READING

Fisher D, Helman C. If you think that oil spill is bad. *Forbes.* June 10, 2010.

CHAPTER 171

Liquefied Natural Gas Tanker Truck Explosion

Nawfal Aljerian and Rakan S. Al-Rasheed

DESCRIPTION OF EVENT

The explosion of a liquid natural gas tanker is a boiling liquid expanding vapor explosion (BLEVE). A BLEVE occurs when a pressurized liquid evaporates rapidly, leading to explosion of the tank containing the liquid. Either mechanical damage to the tank shell or intense heat from a fire outside the tank causes the liquid to evaporate. In the case of fire the extreme heat weakens the walls of the tank, the tank is unable to withstand the rising pressure within, and the tank fails.[1] In either case the resulting explosion leads to a blast wave, fireball, and flying tank fragments. BLEVEs typically occur within 8 to 30 minutes of the start of a fire, with an average of 15 minutes.[2] This duration can be significantly shorter inside a tunnel.[3] Damage to the tank (as with impact in a traffic crash) usually results in an immediate BLEVE. Relief valves that are located on the top of the tanker truck are designed to vent vapor, reducing pressure in the vapor space of the tank but may not function properly if the tanker is on its side, as in a traffic crash. In this situation the valves will vent liquefied natural gas (LNG) and will not reduce the pressure inside the tank.

The risk related to this kind of transportation has increased with increasing traffic and the quantities transported.[4] It is estimated worldwide that between 1940 and 2005 there has been approximately 1000 fatalities, 10,000 victims injured, and billions of dollars in property damage.[5] Since 1993 in the United States and Canada only three significant BLEVE incidents have occurred (Table 171-1).[6]

A survey carried out using the database MHIDAS (Major Hazard Incident Data Service) of all incidents involving hazardous substances revealed a significant number of accidents occurred during transportation.[7] This information along with the occurrence of several severe accidents has encouraged efforts to advance safety in transport, especially in developed countries.

PRE-INCIDENT ACTIONS

Safety standards and codes related to LNG and propane have been established by the American National Standards Institute, the National Fire Protection Association (NFPA), and the American Society of Mechanical Engineers. These standards address safety issues related to tank design and manufacturing, relief valves, transportation, and fire and hazardous materials response. In addition, federal agencies, such as the U.S. Department of Labor and U.S. Department of Transportation, have established rules and regulations pertaining to the transportation of LNG and other flammable gases. In 2012 the U.S. Department of Transportation published "A guidebook for First Responders During the Initial Phase of a Dangerous Goods/Hazardous Materials Transportation Incident." This guidebook contains a detailed approach to hazardous material coding, public and first responders' safety, emergency response and decontamination.[8] Educational programs sponsored by the National Propane Gas Association and NFPA have also raised the awareness of emergency responders about appropriate decisions in managing LNG incidents. These efforts are all intended to enhance the safe transport of LNG and to ensure the enactment of the appropriate emergency response to an incident involving an LNG tanker.

At the incident scene, truck placards and color schemes can be used to identify tanker contents, such as the HAZCHEM Code system that is used by the United Kingdom, Australia, New Zealand, and Malaysia for use on vehicles transporting dangerous substances to provide instant action advice when arriving at an incident.[9,10]

The types of flammable gas as well as the size of the tank are important considerations for the Incident Commander. The size of a BLEVE depends on the weight of the container pieces and how much liquid vaporizes when the container fails.[2] The condition of the tank must also be evaluated; structural damage and the presence of fire are essential considerations. In addition to the type of fuel present, a consideration during scene assessment is the incident location. A BLEVE inside a tunnel or other closed space results in more devastating effects than one occurring in an open area.[2] If fire is present at the incident scene the decision to evacuate the scene may be more prudent than committing firefighting personnel to extinguish the fire. This decision must be based on the length of time the fire has been burning and knowledge of the usual time course for BLEVE occurrence.[2] The potential for a BLEVE should be considered any time there is direct flame impingement on an LNG tank, when venting through relief valves is not adequate to relieve the rising pressure.[2]

POST-INCIDENT ACTIONS

Once a BLEVE occurs, the resulting explosion typically burns up the fuel source, causing a large fireball. At this point the fire usually burns itself out as the fuel source is consumed, but extinguishing the fire may be necessary. The containment and clean up of leaked, unburned fuel may also be required, although LNG typically evaporates quickly. Casualties with burns and/or explosion injuries will necessitate field triage and treatment as well as transport to the hospital.

The incident area should be divided into three zones with access control points and establishing a contamination reduction corridor as recommended by the National Institute for Occupational Safety and Health (NIOSH), Occupational Safety and Health Administration (OSHA), U.S. Coast Guard (USCG), and Environmental Protection Agency (EPA).[11] The first zone is the exclusion zone or "hot zone" and includes all the hazardous material contamination. The second zone is the contamination reduction zone or "warm zone" and contains all the decontamination stations. The last zone is the support zone or "cold zone," which should be free from all hazardous material contamination and contains the command post.[11]

TABLE 171-1   Significant North American BLEVE Incidents, 1993-2004

DATE	LOCATION	DESCRIPTION	CASUALTIES
June 27, 1993	Ste. Elisabeth de Warwick, Quebec, Canada	1055-gallon propane tank	4 fatalities, 7 injured
October 2, 1997	Burnside, Illinois	1000-gallon propane tank	2 fatalities, 2 injured
April 9, 1998	Albert City, Iowa	18,000-gallon propane tank	2 fatalities, 7 injured

✚ MEDICAL TREATMENT OF CASUALTIES

Injuries occurring in conjunction with a BLEVE fall into two categories: (1) burns and thermal injuries and (2) trauma from fragments thrown from the explosion and blast injuries.[12] The fundamentals of management remain airway control, assuring effective breathing, and hemorrhage control through use of direct pressure in mild to moderate hemorrhage because it is the standard of care. Tourniquets can be used in the setting of major hemorrhage when standards of care have failed, given that the provider has the skill and knowledge needed.[12]

Once the secondary survey is completed, care can be undertaken with minimal wound debridement, copious irrigation, prevention of hypothermia, and early administration of antibiotics for prolonged transport times, especially in rural emergency medical service(s) (EMS) settings.[12]

Fragments causing penetrating injuries and burns are often associated with severe pain; the literature has shown that failure to recognize and appropriately treat such acute pain may result in an increased incidence of chronic pain and posttraumatic stress disorder.[13,14] Pain medications for delayed or prolonged extrication time and distances may decrease such unwanted outcomes.[12]

The potential for exposure to a leaking fuel source before the BLEVE also exists. In this case patients will require decontamination and evaluation for potential toxic effects. Toxic affects mainly affect the respiratory and nervous systems and include dizziness, drowsiness, and asphyxia. LNG in its liquid form may cause frostbite.[15]

❓ UNIQUE CONSIDERATIONS

Projectiles from a BLEVE are a major hazard. A Queens University study showed that projectiles are dispersed more than 300 feet away from an exploding tank.[2] Failure to take this into consideration can greatly increase the number of casualties and fatalities at the incident scene.

❗ PITFALLS

Past practice was based on the belief that debris fragments only come from the ends of the tank. BLEVE research and experience have shown that this is not accurate: any part of the tank can break and become a projectile. The U.S. Department of Transportation now recommends that emergency responders stay away from tanks engulfed in fire.[8]

REFERENCES

1. Herrig Brothers Propane Tank Explosion. *CSB Investigation Digest.* Washington, DC: U.S. Chemical Safety and Hazard Investigation Board; June 23, 1999.
2. Albert City. Iowa. *NFPA: Alert Bulletin.* 1998;98(1), Quincy, MA: National Fire Protection Association.
3. Ciambelli P. The risk of transportation of dangerous goods: BLEVE in a tunnel. *Ann Burns Fire Disasters.* 1997;10:241–247.
4. Van der Torn P, Pasman HJ. How to plan for emergency and disaster response operations in view of structural risk reduction. In: Pasman HJ, Kirillov IA, eds. *Resilience of Cities to Terrorist and Other Threats.* 1st ed. Dordrecht: Springer; 2008:343–379.
5. Abbasi T, Abbasi SA. The boiling liquid expanding vapour explosion (BLEVE): mechanism, consequence assessment, management. *J Hazard Mater.* 2007;141(3):489–519.
6. Noll GG, Hildebrand MS, Schnepp R, Rudner G. Implementing response objectives. In: Noll GG, Hildebrand MS, eds. *Hazardous Materials: Managing the Incident.* 4th ed. Burlington, MA: Jones & Bartlett Learning; 2012:366.
7. Planas-Cuchi E, Gasulla N, Ventosa A, Casal J. Explosion of a road tanker containing liquified natural gas. *J Loss Prev Proc.* 2004;17(4):315–321.
8. U.S. Dept. of Transportation, Pipeline and Hazardous Materials Safety Administration, 2012 emergency response guidebook: a guidebook for first responders during the initial phase of a dangerous goods/hazardous materials transportation incident. Available at: http://www.phmsa.dot.gov/hazmat/library/erg.
9. Safework.sa.gov.au. SafeWork SA. 2014. Available at: http://www.safework.sa.gov.au.
10. Hartac.com.au. Home—Hartac Signs & Safety Solutions. 2014. Available at: http://www.hartac.com.au.
11. Managing Hazardous Material Incidents (MHMI). *Volumes 1, 2 and 3. Agency for Toxic Substances and Disease Registry (ATSDR).* Atlanta, GA: U.S. Department of Health and Human Services, Public Health Service; 2001. http://www.atsdr.cdc.gov/MHMI/index.asp.
12. McManus J, Schwartz RB. Explosive and burn injuries. In: *Emergency Medical Services Clinical Practice and Systems Oversight.* Dubuque, IA: Kendall Hunt; 2009:191–202.
13. Otis JD, Keane TM, Kerns RD. An examination of the relationship between chronic pain and post-traumatic stress disorder. *J Rehab Res Dev.* 2003;40(5):397–405.
14. Asmundson GJ, Coons MJ, Taylor S, Katz J. PTSD and the experience of pain: research and clinical implications of shared vulnerability and mutual maintenance models. *Can J Psych.* 2002;47(10):930–937.
15. Cdc.gov. CDC—NIOSH Pocket Guide to Chemical Hazards—L.P.G. 2014. Available at: http://www.cdc.gov/niosh/npg/npgd0679.html.

CHAPTER 172

Petroleum Distillation and Processing Facility Explosion

Rakan S. Al-Rasheed and Sami A. Yousif

DESCRIPTION OF EVENT

The petroleum industry concentrates on obtaining and refining crude oil into usable compounds (i.e., gasoline or petrol, other fuel oil, plastics, and polymers). Crude oil or crude petroleum is a liquid or semisolid mixture of hydrocarbons that often contain sulfur, nitrogen, and oxygen, as well as metals such as iron, vanadium, nickel, and chromium. As crude oil is refined into fuels and gasoline, other useful products that are not fuels can also be manufactured (e.g., lubricants and asphalt for road paving). There are more than 4000 different petrochemical products, but those that are considered as basic products include ethylene, propylene, butadiene, benzene, ammonia, and methanol. The main groups of petrochemical end products are plastics, synthetic fibers, synthetic rubbers, detergents, and chemical fertilizers.

The chemical constitution of crude oil varies widely and can vary in consistency from a light volatile fluid to a semisolid substance. Crude oil can be classified into three broad chemical groups: aliphatic and paraffin compounds with saturated hydrocarbon chemical structures, naphthalene-type compounds with saturated cyclic chemical structure, and aromatic compounds. Crude oil may also be categorized as asphalt base, paraffin base, or mixed base. Sweet crude oils have less than 5 ppm of hydrogen sulfide, and sour crude oils have significantly more hydrogen sulfide; drilling site wellhead concentrations of hydrogen sulfide may range from 50,000 to 180,000 ppm.[1,2]

Refining crude oil can be grouped by several stages, each with certain characteristics, and disasters have occurred in all stages:

1. Obtaining and extracting crude oil, often by heavy machinery drilling and pumping, usually in an isolated area
2. Transporting crude oil, often involving large volumes
3. Refining, usually requiring heat and multiple other potentially toxic chemicals
4. Transporting products of refinement, usually through population centers

In the extraction phase, subterranean crude oil must be obtained by means of wells. Typically, an exploratory well, known as the wildcat, is dug. Once oil is located, full-scale drilling commences. Oil drilling is a complex and risky process involving exposure to high temperatures and pressurized systems. Initially the petroleum from a new well will come to the surface under its own pressure. Later, the crude oil must be pumped out or forced to the surface by injecting water, gas, or air into the deposits. Exposure to toxic gases released from the initial contact with oil field deposits frequently occurs.[3,4]

In the second stage of transportation, crude oil must be brought from the extraction site to refineries. Many of these wells are located in isolated areas of extreme environmental conditions that challenge the most advanced transportation systems. The main methods of transporting crude oil and natural gas from the oil fields to refineries are usually by ocean tanker or pipelines.

The petroleum-refining phase consists of three basic steps: distillation, conversion, and treatment. Fractional distillation involves using the difference in boiling point to separate the hydrocarbons in crude oil, and the process typically occurs in a vacuum distillation column. A large amount of heat is expended during this stage. As the distillate exits the column, it often requires further processing to make other fractions and to convert crude into basic petrol and other useful chemicals.

Conversion involves three main processes: cracking, unification, and alteration. Cracking is the most widely used conversion method. It is the process for breaking down larger molecules into smaller ones. Unification is the process of combining smaller molecules to make larger ones. Then, alteration is the process of rearranging various molecules to make the desired hydrocarbon product. These processes typically involve the use of significant amounts of heat, as well as an additional hydrogen source and a catalytic unit.

Finally, the distillate undergoes finishing treatments to make it into products that meet specific requirements. Such processes can include solvent extraction, dewaxing, and hydrogenation. Distillated and chemically processed fractions are further treated to remove impurities, such as organic compounds containing sulfur, nitrogen, oxygen, water, dissolved metals, and inorganic salts. Treating is usually done by passing the fractions through the following methods:

1. A column of sulfuric acid removes unsaturated hydrocarbons (those with carbon-carbon double bonds), nitrogen compounds, oxygen compounds, and residual solids (e.g., tars and asphalt).
2. An absorption column filled with drying agents removes water.
3. Sulfur treatment and hydrogen-sulfide scrubbers remove sulfur and sulfur compounds.

Ultimately, the refined products are transported to the consumer. Because of this, many refineries are located near large-population centers. Large customers, such as airports, are supplied directly from the refinery by pipelines. A disaster at a refinery may involve a nearby high-volume consumer, such as a petrochemical plant or a power station. Smaller consumers, such as gasoline stations, are supplied by a road tanker originating from terminals, which act as storage depots and distribution centers. The terminals are supplied by rail or pipeline if they are inland or by coastal tanker if they are on the coast or a river estuary.

The main process of the petroleum industry is to obtain and convert a relatively flammable product to a highly flammable one. Thus the majority of deaths reported in the petroleum industry disasters are caused by explosive blast injuries and burns (Tables 172-1 and 172-2). The petroleum industry makes use of various chemicals in the process of refining crude oil, including chlorine, chromium-containing corrosion inhibitors,

TABLE 172-1   Refinery Incidents in the United States (1999-2007)

INCIDENT TYPES	1999	2000	2001	2002	2003	2004	2005	2006	2007
Fires	18	25	20	19	14	26	26	18	23
Explosions	5	6	2	4	3	3	3	4	3
Spills	41	58	58	55	31	9	4	23	38
Injury, illness, or fatality	2	12	12	4	9	6	6	7	3
Total	66	101	92	82	57	44	39	52	67

Data from 2007 Process Safety Performance Measurement Report, American Petroleum Institute Statistics Department, June 2008.

TABLE 172-2   Refinery Major Accident Losses, 1979-2012

DATE	LOCATION	TYPE OF ACCIDENT
July 21, 1979	Texas City, Texas	Vapor-cloud explosion
September 1, 1979	Deer Park, Texas	Explosion
January 20, 1980	Borger, Texas	Vapor-cloud explosion
August 20, 1981	Shuaiba, Kuwait	Fire
April 7, 1983	Avon, California	Fire
July 23, 1984	Romeville, Illinois	Explosion
August 15, 1984	Las Piedras, Venezuela	Fire
March 22, 1987	Grangemouth, United Kingdom	Explosion
May 5, 1988	Norco, Louisiana	Vapor-cloud explosion
April 10, 1989	Richmond, California	Fire
September 5, 1989	Martinez, California	Fire
December 24, 1989	Baton Rouge, Louisiana	Vapor-cloud explosion
April 1, 1990	Warren, Pennsylvania	Explosion and fire
November 3, 1990	Chalmette, Louisiana	Vapor-cloud explosion
November 30, 1990	Ras Tanura, Saudi Arabia	Fire
January 12, 1991	Port Arthur, Texas	Fire
November 3, 1991	Beaumont, Texas	Fire
March 3, 1991	Lake Charles, Louisiana	Explosion and fire
April 13, 1991	Sweeney, Texas	Explosion
December 10, 1991	Westphalia, Germany	Explosion and fire
October 8, 1992	Wilmington, California	Explosion and fire
October 16, 1992	Sodegaura, Japan	Explosion and fire
November 9, 1992	La Mede, France	Vapor-cloud explosion
August 2, 1993	Baton Rouge, Louisiana	Fire
February 25, 1994	Kawasaki, Japan	Fire
July 24, 1994	Pembroke, United Kingdom	Fire
October 16, 1995	Rouseville, Pennsylvania	Fire
October 24, 1995	Cilacap, Indonesia	Explosion and fire
January 27, 1997	Martinez, California	Explosion and fire
September 14, 1997	Visakhapatam, India	Explosion and fire
June 9, 1998	St. John, New Brunswick	Explosion and fire
October 6, 1998	Berre l'Etang, France	Fire
February 19, 1999	Thessaloniki, Greece	Explosion and fire
March 25, 1999	Richmond, California	Explosion
December 2, 1999	Sri Racha, Thailand	Explosion
June 25, 2000	Mina Al-Ahmadi, Kuwait	Explosion and fire
April 9, 2001	Aruba, Caribbean	Fire
April 16, 2001	Killingholme, United Kingdom	Explosion and fire
April 23, 2001	Carson City, California	Fire
April 28, 2001	Lemont, Illinois	Fire
September 21, 2001	Lake Charles, Louisiana	Fire
November 22, 2002	Mohammedia, Morocco	Explosion and fire
January 6, 2003	Fort McMurray, Alberta	Explosion and fire
January 4, 2005	Fort McKay, Alberta	Explosion and fire
March 23, 2005	Texas City, Texas	Explosion and fire
October 12, 2006	Mazeikiu, Lithuania	Explosion and fire
August 16, 2007	Pascagoula, Mississippi	Explosion and fire
February 18, 2008	Big Spring, Texas	Explosion and fire
January 6, 2011	Fort McKay, Alberta	Explosion and fire
August 25, 2012	Falcon state, Venezuela	Explosion

Continued

and biological additives. Byproducts of the refining process, including carcinogenic polyaromatic hydrocarbons such as benzene, can also cause significant toxicity. Hydrogen sulfide is another byproduct produced in the drilling and refining processes that can cause significant injury. Hydrogen-sulfide gas has been reported to be a significant problem for oil fields in Alberta, Canada, because of its high concentration of sulfur.[5]

Highly hazardous chemical (HHC)- related incidents have resulted in many catastrophes in the petroleum refining industry around the world. In 1992 the U.S. Occupational Safety and Health Administration (OSHA) implemented the process safety management (PSM) standard in an attempt to reduce the frequency and severity of such incidents.[6] Nevertheless, HHC-related incidents continue to occur, with more than 36 fatal incidents reported between 1992 and 2007 in the United States alone. The Texas City British Petroleum refinery explosion in 2005 is considered one of the worst petroleum refining industry incidents, killing 15 workers and injuring 180 others, in addition to financial losses exceeding $1.5 billion.[7]

◀◀ PRE-INCIDENT ACTIONS

Explosions in petroleum distillation and processing facilities can happen without warning and with significant effects on life, property, and the surrounding environment. Therefore emergency planners should make every effort to prepare in advance for such devastating incidents.

This is best done through implementing a robust safety management system to identify and assess potential hazards that can lead to explosions, followed by establishing control measures and implementing emergency response plans to mitigate and reduce their effects. The emergency response plan should be distributed widely, practiced, easy to use, and in compliance with local laws and regulations. At minimum, these plans should address protective actions for life safety, warning, notification, communication, incident command, and roles and responsibilities, facility plans, and information. Conducting regular drills for on-site fire brigade service, emergency response teams, and volunteer personnel is essential to ensure effective implementation. Full-scale exercises should be completed at least every 3 years, to test the breadth of the plan and tabletop exercises, as well as the individual elements. They should occur much more frequently and be incorporated into the routine workflow. More importantly, emergency response plans should be fully integrated with public emergency services and key organizations that will be involved in responding to explosion incidents. Memoranda of understanding and mutual aid agreements must be executed beforehand, and joint exercises and training activities must focus on unified command and control, communication, and environmental protection procedures.

POST-INCIDENT ACTIONS

The first order of action is to confirm the site of the disaster and the access and egress routes for the emergency medical services (EMS) providers, who will also want to know about current and potential hazards present at the particular site. Use of a standardized message structure should be considered, such as the METHANE message taught on the Major Incident Medical Management and Support (MIMMS) course (Box 172-1). Although the majority of disasters reported are from explosions and fires, various parts of the petrochemical refining process are susceptible to specific scenarios. Disasters occurring in the process of obtaining crude oil often occur when an oil well ignites. Oil wells are often distant from major population centers. In contrast, refineries are often close to major population centers. In the former scenario, health care workers may have to get to a remote location such as an offshore oil rig.[4] In the latter situation, health care workers must address the demands of the local community.

The materials involved in an explosion must also be identified. Many refineries use and store toxic compounds. Hydrofluoric acid is a compound used during the refining process. It is a lethal substance and is toxic on contact to the lungs, skin, and eyes, producing profound hypocalcemia. It may be present in liquid form but turns into gas quickly. In significant releases of hydrofluoric acid, prehospital care providers will require personal protective equipment. Treatment of injuries caused by hydrofluoric acid exposure requires unique antidotes, such as calcium-containing dermal, inhalational, and intravenous treatments.[8,9]

BOX 172-1	Components of METHANE Message
M	Major incident declared or standby
E	Exact location (grid reference or GPS)
T	Type of incident (fire, explosion, bomb)
H	Hazards (fire, gas, debris, unsound structures)
A	Access (road access with options for approach)
N	Number of casualties, estimated
E	Emergency services required and present

An important early factor for victims and rescuers is identification of blast-resistant portable buildings. These buildings are structures developed to provide temporary safe haven to personnel from the potential hazards associated with the petroleum industry. They are designed to resist the explosive forces that can cause sliding and overturning of buildings during a blast. They are also designed to be easily sealed and airtight to provide a shelter during a toxic gas release. They are often the size and shape of shipping containers and are positioned to be easily accessed by personnel. During disasters, health care personnel should identify and seek out these structures to locate potential victims, and also to provide shelter if secondary incidents occur.[10]

A unified command and control structure and a joint operation center should be activated to ensure smooth operations and effective response. After making sure that the scene is safe and taking appropriate precautions as dictated by the safety officer, EMS personnel will be responsible for triaging victims, providing first aid, and transferring patients to nearby medical facilities, as soon as possible. The police will secure the perimeter and aid in evacuation of residential areas that could be affected by the incident. Local fire departments will commence fire suppression activities and establish a decontamination unit as needed. Depending on the magnitude and complexity of the incident, other governmental agencies, nongovernmental organizations, and mutual aid assistance will be necessary to conduct the response operations.

After the explosion at a petroleum distillation or processing facility, possible contaminants must be identified. A disaster at an Eastern European oil storage depot was reported to cause significant environmental contamination with heavy metals (e.g., lead, arsenic, cadmium, nickel, chromium, and copper), polyaromatic hydrocarbons, and polychlorinated biphenyls.[11–13]

It is important to identify and address psychological issues of victims, health care workers, and the community. Many of the reported disasters in the oil industry have involved a significant number of patients with burns, and there are multiple documented reports of significant effects on the mental health of health care workers.[9,14–22]

MEDICAL TREATMENT OF CASUALTIES

Disasters at petroleum facilities typically involve exposure to blast injuries and high-temperature burn. Blast injuries are either penetrating or blunt traumatic injuries, of which blast lung is the most common fatal injury. Abdominal blast injuries may initially be silent before developing signs of an acute condition of the abdomen. Higher morbidity and mortality are seen when explosions occur in an enclosed area, and care should be given to the possibility of structural collapse.[23]

The management of the trauma patient may be complicated by burn injuries, but the initial resuscitation and stabilization does not change; it is focused on stabilizing the airway with C-spine control, breathing, and circulation. The presence of a burn injury should not interfere with the resuscitation of the multitrauma patient, and its management should not take precedence over penetrating or blunt traumatic injuries.[24–26]

All burned clothing, debris, and wearable accessories should be removed as soon as possible, to prevent further injury and for a more accurate assessment of the burn injury. Cooling burned areas using cool water can reduce the area of injury and should be done as soon as possible. The cooling duration ranges from 15 minutes to 3 hours.[27–29] After cleaning and cooling the burn wound, a topical antibiotic is applied to all nonsuperficial burns, which are then covered with a nonadherent mesh gauze.[26]

Chemical exposures in a petroleum refinery are common. Hydrofluoric acid is a relatively common toxic chemical that requires specific treatments and antidotes. Patients should be immediately removed from the area and evaluated for signs of respiratory failure resulting from pulmonary edema, pneumonitis, pulmonary hemorrhage, or systemic toxicity. Administering 2.5% or 3% calcium gluconate inhalational solution by nebulizer as a therapy has been suggested for respiratory exposures.[30,31] Treatment of hydrofluoric acid dermal injury consists of immediate irrigation with copious amounts of water for at least 15 to 30 minutes, removal of all blisters because they may harbor fluoride ions, and application of calcium gluconate (2.5%) gel to the debrided skin surface.[31] Systemic toxicity from hydrofluoric acid exposure can cause dysrhythmias and hypocalcemia, thus warranting cardiac and electrolyte monitoring. A 10% calcium gluconate solution should be administered intravenously or intraarterially in patients exhibiting significant hydrofluoric acid systemic toxicity.

Ammonia is another compound found throughout the refining process. Ammonia is widely used as a cleaning agent and as a coolant. The release of ammonia causes injury to the patient in two ways: (1) because of its low freezing point ($-33\ °C$), frostbite injury occurs to any skin in direct contact; and (2) ammonia vapors readily dissolve in the moisture of the skin, eyes, and mucosa, causing chemical burns through liquefactive necrosis. Exposure requires prompt irrigation of the eyes and skin with water, as well as management of inhalation injury. Symptoms of ammonia inhalation include stridor, wheezing, rales, and hemoptysis. With high concentrations of inhaled ammonia, respiratory distress resulting from pulmonary edema can occur rapidly, leading to acute lung injury (ALI) or acute respiratory distress syndrome (ARDS). In some cases, laryngospasm and respiratory arrest may occur suddenly.[32]

Management of ammonia inhalation is supportive with the administration of 100% humidified oxygen and performing an endotracheal intubation to assist ventilation when necessary. Inhaled bronchodilators and corticosteroids may have a role in treating pulmonary edema induced by ammonia, but no strong evidence is available.[32]

❓ UNIQUE CONSIDERATIONS

A common scenario in a petroleum industry disaster is the explosion of oil and gasoline drums. Bak and colleagues[33] reported a series of incidents where these containers were inappropriately handled. The typical scenario was that in which a worker attempted to divide or cut through a presumably empty 55-gallon drum with a grinder or a blowtorch. These drums often contain residual quantities of flammable material in liquid or vapor form. Once the container is penetrated, the metal drum explodes, and proximate workers risk significant trauma from projectiles, blast force, or burns.

❗ PITFALLS

Pitfalls in responding to petroleum distillation and processing facility explosions include the following:

- Failure to train facility personnel on personal protective actions and emergency response plans
- Delay in the recognition of hazardous condition and community notification
- Delay in containing toxic chemical leaks and collecting air-monitoring data
- Premature fire suppression before identifying potential hazard and appropriate protective gear
- Delay in transitioning from a single to a unified command and control and in establishing a joint operations center
- Failure to use interoperable communication systems between responding agencies

REFERENCES

1. Snodgrass WR. Petroleum industry. In: Greenberg MI, Phillips SD, eds. *Occupational, Industrial, and Environmental Toxicology.* 2nd ed. St Louis, MO: Mosby; 2003.
2. U.S. Environmental Protection Agency. Types of petroleum oil. 2004. Available at: http://www.epa.gov/oilspill/oiltypes.htm.
3. Yapa PD, Zheng L, Chen F. A model for deepwater oil/gas blowouts. *Mar Pollut Bull.* 2001;43:234–241.
4. Leese WL. Some medical aspects of North Sea oil industry. *Scott Med J.* 1977;22:258–266.
5. Gabbay DS, De Roos F, Perrone J. Twenty-foot fall averts fatality from massive hydrogen sulfide exposure. *J Emerg Med.* 2001;20:141–144.
6. ABS Consulting, Inc., 2006. BP America Refinery Explosion Texas City, TX, March 23, 2005, Explosion Incident Investigation, Final Report, ABSC Project No. 1428551, October 31, 2006.
7. United States Department of Labor Occupational Safety and Health Administration. Process Safety Management. Available at: https://www.osha.gov/SLTC/processsafetymanagement/.
8. Trevino MA, Herrmann GH, Sprout WL. Treatment of severe hydrofluoric acid exposures. *J Occup Med.* 1983;25:861–863.
9. Dayal HH, Brodwick M, Morris R, et al. A community-based epidemiologic study of health sequelae of exposure to hydrofluoric acid. *Ann Epidemiol.* 1992;2:213–230.
10. Harrison BF. Blast resistant modular buildings for the petroleum and chemical processing industries. *J Hazard Mater.* 2003;104:31–38.
11. Skrbic B, Miljevic N. An evaluation of residues at an oil refinery site following fires. *J Environ Sci Health A Tox Hazard Subst Environ Eng.* 2002;37:1029–1039.
12. Skrbic B, Novakovic J, Miljevic N. Mobility of heavy metals originating from bombing of industrial sites. *J Environ Sci Health A Tox Hazard Subst Environ Eng.* 2002;37:7–16.
13. Attias L, Bucchi AR, Maranghi F, Holt S, Marcello I, Zapponi GA. Crude oil spill in seawater: an assessment of the risk for bathers correlated to benzopyrene exposure. *Cent Eur J Public Health.* 1995;3:142–145.
14. Hull AM, Alexander DA, Klein S. Survivors of the Piper Alpha oil platform disaster: long-term follow-up study. *Br J Psychiatry.* 2002;181:433–438.
15. Alexander DA. Burn victims after a major disaster: reactions of patients and their care-givers. *Burns.* 1993;19:105–109.
16. Campbell D, Cox D, Crum J, Foster K, Christie P, Brewster D. Initial effects of the grounding of the tanker Braer on health in Shetland. The Shetland Health Study Group. *BMJ.* 1993;307:1251–1255.
17. Crum JE. Peak expiratory flow rate in schoolchildren living close to Braer oil spill. *BMJ.* 1993;307:23–24.
18. Dayal HH, Baranowski T, Li YH, Morris R. Hazardous chemicals: psychological dimensions of the health sequelae of a community exposure in Texas. *J Epidemiol Community Health.* 1994;48:560–568.
19. Palinkas LA, Petterson JS, Russell J, Downs MA. Community patterns of psychiatric disorders after the Exxon Valdez oil spill. *Am J Psychiatry.* 1993;150:1517–1523.
20. Qiao B. Oil spill model development and application for emergency response system. *J Environ Sci (China).* 2001;13:252–256.
21. Qiao B, Chu JC, Zhao P, Yu Y, Li Y. Marine oil spill contingency planning. *J Environ Sci (China).* 2002;14:102–107.
22. Li J. A GIS planning model for urban oil spill management. *Water Sci Technol.* 2001;43:239–244.
23. Centers for Disease Control and Prevention. *Explosions and blast injuries: a primer for clinicians;* 2003. Available at: www.cdc.gov.
24. Shamir MY, Rivkind A, Weissman C, Sprung CL, Weiss YG. Conventional terrorist bomb incidents and the intensive care unit. *Curr Opin Crit Care.* 2005;11:580–584.
25. Wolf SE. Overview and management strategies for the combined burn trauma patient. In: Post TW, ed. *UpToDate.* Waltham, MA: UpToDate.
26. Phillip LR Jr, Dennis PO. Emergency care of moderate and severe thermal burns in adults. In: Post TW, ed. *UpToDate.* Waltham, MA: UpToDate.
27. Pushkar NS, Sandorminsky BP. Cold treatment of burns. *Burns Incl Therm Inj.* 1982;9:101–110.

28. Hartford CE. Care of outpatient burns. In: Herndon D, ed. *Total Burn Care*. Philadelphia, PA: Saunders; 1996:71.

29. Allwood JS. The primary care management of burns. *Nurse Pract*. 1995;20:74, 77.

30. Lee DC, Wiley JF 2nd., Synder JW 2nd. Treatment of inhalational exposure to hydrofluoric acid with nebulized calcium gluconate. *J Occup Med*. 1993;35(5):470.

31. Su M. Hydrofluoric acid and fluorides. In: Nelson LS, Lewin NA, Howland MA, Hoffman RS, Goldfrank LR, Flomenbaum NE, eds.

Goldfrank's Toxicologic Emergencies. 9th ed. New York, NY: McGraw-Hill; 2011:1374–1380.

32. Chemical Hazards Emergency Medical Management: CHEMM. U.S. Department of Health & Human Services, Office of the Assistant Secretary for Preparedness and Response, National Library of Medicine. Available at http://chemm.nlm.nih.gov/ammonia_hospital_mmg.htm. Accessed December 1, 2014.

33. Bak B, Juhl M, Lauridsen F, Pilegaard J, Roeck ND. Oil and petrol drum explosions: injuries and casualties by exploding oil and petrol drums containing various inflammable liquids. *Injury*. 1988;19:81–85.

173 CHAPTER

Introduction to Fires and Burns

Diana Clapp and Benjamin J. Lawner

Burn injuries can result from multiple mechanisms but are commonly found following an emergency response to incidents such as fires, explosions, motor vehicle collisions, industrial accidents, and transit incidents, among others. During 2003-2007, the National Fire Protection Association found that vehicle fires alone accounted for more than 400 civilian deaths and 1300 injuries.[1] Similarly, structure fires cause death and injury daily. The Centers for Disease Control and Prevention estimated that in 2010, a fire-related injury occurred every 30 minutes, and a death occurred every 169 minutes.[2] Emergency responders must therefore maintain a high level of awareness about the various mechanisms and types of burn injuries. This chapter reviews the core principles of incident response and patient management as they relate to burn-victim care.

PREPARATION

Emergency clinicians and prehospital personnel can expect to encounter victims from a fire- or burn-related event relatively frequently in their clinical practice. Preplanning is essential to effective incident management and the use of available specialty resources at both the individual and community level.[3] Because burn- and fire-related incidents may produce multiple casualties, availability of unique resources such as regional burn and trauma centers should inform the development of any mass casualty plan. The New York City Department of Health and Mental Hygiene conducted a study to examine the effect of a large-scale burn event (>400 patients) upon existing emergency medical resources. The study affirmed the need for a scalable plan that describes, catalogs, and incentivizes regional resource use.[4] Emergency responders should also plan to use a formalized system of triage when planning for patient prioritization and distribution. The "Simple Triage and Rapid Treatment (START/JumpSTART) and Sort, Assess, Lifesaving Interventions, Treatment, and Transport (SALT)" methods are commonplace in emergency medical service(s) (EMS) systems. The use of a common triage language minimizes confusion during a large-scale incident response.[3] The importance of a coordinated, system-wide approach to mass burn and mass casualty care cannot be overestimated.

PREHOSPITAL MANAGEMENT

Initial Actions and Primary Survey

The initial priority in burn patient management is to stop the burning process.[5] This strategy may require the extinguishing of flames, removal of the patient from the electrical source once safe, and/or removal of dry chemical through dusting or liquid chemical through thorough irrigation and dilution.[5] It is essential to gather any known information about chemicals involved, duration and type of electricity exposure, length of duration within confined a space, and/or the history and mechanisms of additional trauma. Once the risk of immediate and ongoing burn injury is addressed, providers should undertake a systematic approach to patient assessment. The curricula contained within courses such as Advanced Burn Life Support and Prehospital Trauma Life Support, Advanced Trauma Life Support, and other nationally endorsed courses specifically address the common essential prehospital actions such as airway support, assurance of adequate breathing and circulation, maintenance of adequate core body temperature, and fluid resuscitation.[6] As with all cases in emergency medical care, the patient assessment begins with a primary survey that is focused on airway patency, breathing, and circulation (ABC). Following the assessment and support of the ABCs, a thorough secondary assessment must be performed to examine the patient in a head-to-toe manner to identify all burns and other traumatic injuries.

Prehospital Treatment

Patient treatment begins with the administration of high-flow oxygen. Oxygen may mitigate the effects of airway edema, and it addresses potential lethal gas exposures such as carbon monoxide and hydrogen cyanide.[5] Placing the patient in a semi-Fowler's position optimizes respiratory mechanics.[7] Patients who have evidence of airway burn injury, such as a hoarse or raspy voice, stridor, indications of inhalation injury such as soot in the nares or mouth, altered mentation, or signs of respiratory distress, should receive early and swift airway management.[5-7] Patients requiring intubation should be evaluated and supported by the most experienced airway clinician, as rapid decompensation is possible. Ideally, the largest caliber endotracheal tube possible should be placed, given the potential for progressive airway edema and sloughing of the airway mucosa, as well as the need for possible bronchoscopy in patient management.[6] Intravenous or interosseous access should be obtained, ideally in a nonburned area if possible. Large bore peripheral catheters represent the ideal prehospital method for crystalloid administration. Although patients may present with initial hemodynamic stability, burn patients warrant continuous reassessment of airway, breathing, and circulation because of the potential volatility of their illness.

Prehospital providers should begin fluid resuscitation for all patients with a significant percentage (>10%) of their body surface area

---

BOX 173-1   American Burn Association Criteria for Referral to a Burn Center

1. Partial thickness burns greater than 10%
2. Burns involving critical areas such as the hands, feet, genitals, or perineum
3. Burns overlying major joints
4. Electrical burns and lightning injury
5. Chemical burns
6. Inhalation injury

7. Burn injury in association with a complex medical condition that could affect mortality or prolong recovery
8. Buns with concomitant trauma (traumatic injuries in which the burn injury poses the greatest risk for mortality and morbidity)
9. Pediatric burn patients
10. Burn injuries in patients who require specialized social, emotional, or rehabilitative care

---

(BSA) involved in the burn. Even though total BSA (TBSA) can be calculated by the rule of nines, it is not as accurate as the rule of palms or the Lund and Browder chart is.[8] Multiple studies cite the lack of accuracy of BSA calculations performed at the accident scene.[9,10] Prehospital responders should therefore focus their efforts on evidence-based interventions such as airway control, temperature management, wound care, and transport. A recent review article affirmed the correlation between airway compromise, hypothermia, and mortality.[11] Initial wound management involves covering affected areas with dry and sterile dressings, if available. Criteria developed by the American Burn Association assists providers with decisions about referral to burn specialty centers (Box 173-1). Prehospital protocols should authorize and encourage clinicians to assess accurately and treat adequately burn-related pain.[12]

EMERGENCY DEPARTMENT MANAGEMENT

The initial patient assessment and management in the emergency department (ED) should follow the same systematic approach as that discussed in the prehospital section.[5,7,13] Within the ED, the care of a burn patient should be focused on maintaining a secure airway, ensuring adequate oxygenation and ventilation, identifying and treating shock and related injuries, evaluating the burn severity, and considering the need for referral to a burn specialty center.[13] Table 173-1 describes the clinical features specific to partial and full thickness burns. In the event that thoracic burns are circumferential, escharotomy should be considered in an attempt to increase thoracic compliance and allow for ventilation.[13] If needed, additional central or peripheral access should be established. Laboratory tests to assess for the possibility of toxic inhalations, especially carbon monoxide inhalation, should be included with the standard chemistry and hematology panels commonly drawn in the ED.[5,13] It is important to remove all patient clothing, jewelry, and watches because edema will develop as the resuscitation progresses and may cause these items to become

constrictive, thus acting as tourniquets and thereby restricting blood flow and causing additional complications during care. While removing clothing, it is key to protect the patient from hypothermia. The injured tissue of a burn patient loses its ability to protect thermoregulation, and it leaves the patient at high risk of hypothermia and its associated complications.[5–7,13] Finally, the provision of adequate analgesia is also key to comprehensive and humane burn care.[12]

UNIQUE CONSIDERATIONS

Direct Inhalation Injury

Care should be taken to evaluate the patient for the possibility of inhalation injuries, which can be described in three phases, the first of which is direct thermal injury. Thermal insult to the upper airways may produce edema, bronchospasm, airway occlusion, decreased chest wall compliance, and intrapulmonary shunting.[7,13,14] Patients with inhalational injuries may present with singed nasal hairs, carbonaceous sputum or debris, a cough, hoarseness, stridor, retractions, or the presence of soot or facial burns.[7] Care for these patients can be monitored through bronchoscopy or chest radiographs.[7]

Cyanide and Carbon Monoxide

Systemic toxicity may occur following the inhalation of toxic gases, such as hydrogen cyanide and carbon monoxide, which are produced in the combustion of certain fuels and plastics.[13,14] Burn patients with a history of being enclosed in a confined space should undergo testing for carboxyhemoglobin and lactic acidosis.[13] Carbon monoxide (CO), a gas formed as a result of incomplete oxidization of carbon, binds with an affinity 240 times that of oxygen, to the hemoglobin molecules and leads to profound cellular and tissue hypoxemia.[13,15] Symptoms of exposure include altered mental status, decreased responsiveness, headache, nausea, and vomiting. With carbon monoxide toxicity, the patient may exhibit continued symptoms of hypoxia despite a potentially normal SpO_2. High-flow oxygen should be administered to all patients with suspected or confirmed CO exposure, because the half-life of CO is reduced to 40 minutes from 60 minutes in the presence of high-flow oxygen.[9] The use of hyperbaric oxygen in CO poisoning remains contested, and data to support its use are sparse and inconsistent.[14–17] Potential indications for hyperbaric referral include:
(1) significantly elevated carboxyhemoglobin level (>30%),
(2) evidence of cardiac instability such as new dysrhythmia or cardiac enzyme elevation, and
(3) altered mental status.

Hydrogen cyanide, a product of the combustion of plastics, is rapidly absorbed through inhalation. Hydrogen cyanide causes cellular changes and disruption ultimately leading to changes in consciousness, neurotoxicity, and seizures. Multiple treatment methods exist for the management of cyanide poisoning and are aimed at binding the cyanide to remove it from the circulatory system.[18] The key decision in the management of cyanide poisoning is the timely

TABLE 173-1   Characteristics of Burn Depth and Severity

DEGREE	DEPTH DESCRIPTION	WOUND DESCRIPTION
First degree	Partial thickness	Superficial, red, wet appearance, painful Not generally used in the calculation of burned surface area
Second degree	Partial thickness	Red, blisters, swollen, painful
Third degree	Full thickness	Whitish, charred, translucent, lacking sensation, cherry red, nonblanching
Fourth degree	Full thickness	Muscle, bone, and tendon involvement, insensate areas

administration of the selected antidote. Hydroxocobalamin is often preferred as current therapy, as the bound cyanide is renally excreted in the form of cyanocobalamin, which is nontoxic.[18] This is now largely preferred over the use of sodium thiosulfate, which is associated with the formation of methemoglobin, which can potentiate decreased oxygenation.[18] Given the rapid onset of symptoms, the antidote may be best administered to at-risk patients in the prehospital setting. In either the prehospital or ED setting, the decision to administer therapy for presumptive hydrogen cyanide toxicity will be a clinical one because serum laboratory values will not be available in time to guide therapeutic decisions.

Fluid Resuscitation in the Burned Patient

Ideally, intravenous access should be initiated in nonburned areas of the patient. Aggressive fluid resuscitation is generally indicated to maintain end organ perfusion in the patient with major burns. The initial volume resuscitation is achieved with crystalloid solutions, primarily Ringer's lactate, because of membrane permeability, which is thought to resolve in the first 12 hours.[8] Burn patients may experience massive interstitial fluid shifts and are at risk for intravascular hypovolemia, which in turn, reduces cardiac output and causes an increase in systemic vascular resistance. These unchecked compensatory mechanisms can result in a worsening of the shock state and will always require the clinician to pay careful attention to physiological parameters. Several formulas exist to guide the administration of intravenous fluids within the first 24 hours of a massive burn injury, the best known of which is the Parkland Formula. The initial volume of fluid as predicted by the Parkland Formula (4 cc × wt. in kg × % TBSA burned) may not accurately predict the patient's actual fluid requirements, and therefore the resuscitation should be goal directed.[5,13] Parameters such as mean arterial pressure and urine output may inform lifesaving efforts and prevent complications such as pulmonary edema, compartment syndrome, and hypothermia.[6,7,13,19]

⚠ PITFALLS

Estimating Burn Depth and Size

Clinicians are notoriously poor at estimating burn depth accurately at the initial time of injury. Burn depth assessment has been found to have more than 60% variation among experts in the field.[8] Unfortunately, clinicians are also often poor at estimating the actual size of the burn area on the patient, as well. A 2013 survey that included physician specialists, nurses, and medical students demonstrated significant inconsistencies, including "high deviations of TBSA of up to 62%."[20] Recent studies have suggested that there might be a potential role for computer modeling and three-dimensional (3D) visual simulation tools to try to solve this problem.[20]

Incident Management

Major burn events have historically been plagued by problems of poor incident management and poor resource utilization. Mackie has suggested that medical personnel should not be dispatched to the disaster scene[21] because doing so may put health care workers at risk of personal injury and delay patient transport and definitive treatment. Similar opinions were documented by reviewers of the 2001 World Trade Center disaster.[22] To this end, the American Burn Association (ABA) has made major strides following the New York City World Trade Center attack, in developing a national response to fire and burn disasters. The ABA has identified burn

centers and burn beds across the country. Via e-mail, this system can be activated as necessary to respond to major burn disasters. It is estimated that 350 to 500 beds could be filled during a disaster. This system would require judicial movement of patients to verified regional burn centers from the burn center nearest the disaster rather than the movement of trained personnel. Consensus of the ABA board after an evaluation of the September 11, 2001, disaster response is that local burn nursing corps would yield greater efficiency when remaining stationary, as opposed to transferring personnel to already overloaded burn centers.[23]

Proactive incident planning for burn events should be undertaken regionally to maximize the available resources and support the best achievable clinical outcomes. Dunbar reported on the Rhode Island nightclub fire that resulted in 200 injuries and 100 deaths. The author, an ED nurse, was present at a receiving ED in a hospital with a burn center. Activation of the Hospital Incident Command System (HICS) allowed an orchestrated response that enabled the staff to meet their goals of providing life-sustaining procedures and comfort measures. In a matter of hours, the hospital received 67 victims, admitted 43 patients, and intubated 22. The HICS activation, while key to incident mitigation, resulted in the convergence of a large amount of hospital personnel in areas in and around the ED.[24]

REFERENCES

1. National Fire Protection Association. Vehicle fire trends and patterns. Available at: http://www.nfpa.org/research/reports-and-statistics/vehicle-fires/vehicle-fire-trends-and-patterns.
2. Centers for Disease Control. Fire deaths and injuries: fact sheet. 2011. Available at: http://www.cdc.gov/homeandrecreationalsafety/fire-prevention/fires-factsheet.html.
3. Nelson S. Information management during mass casualty events. *Respir Care*. 2008;53(2):232–238.
4. Yurt RW, Lazar EJ, Leahy NE, et al. Burn disaster response planning: an urban region's approach. *J Burn Care Res*. 2008;29(1):158–165.
5. Price L, Milner S. The totality of burn care. *Trauma*. 2013;15(1):16–28.
6. White CE, Renz EM. Advances in surgical care: management of severe burn injury. *Crit Care Med*. 2008;36(7 Suppl):S318–S324.
7. Sheridan R. *Burns: A Practical Approach to Immediate Treatment and Long Term Care*. London: Manson; 2012.
8. Jeschke M, Kamolz L, Shahrokhi S, eds. *Burn Care and Treatment: A Practice Guide*. London: Springer; 2013.
9. Berkebile B, Goldfarb W, Slater H. Comparison of burn size estimates between pre-hospital reports and burn center evaluation. *J Burn Care Rehabil*. 1986;7:411–412.
10. Laing J, Morgan B, Sanders R. Assessment of burn injury in the accident and emergency department: a review of 100 referrals to a regional burn unit. *Ann R Coll Surg Engl*. 1991;73:329–331.
11. Muehlberger T, Ottomann C, Toman N, Daigeler A, Lehnhardt M. Emergency pre-hospital care of burn patients. *Surgeon*. 2010;8(2):101–104.
12. Gausche-Hill M, Brown K, Oliver ZJ, et al. An evidence based guideline for prehospital analgesia in trauma. *Prehosp Emerg Care*. 2014;18(Suppl 1):25–34.
13. Rowley-Conwy G. Management of major burns in the emergency department. *Nurs Stand*. 2013;27(33):66–68.
14. Dries D, Endorf F. Inhalation injury: epidemiology, pathology, treatment strategies. *Scand J Trauma, Resusc Emerg Care*. 2013;21(31):21–31.
15. Shochat G, Lucchesi M. *Carbon Monoxide Toxicity. Emedicine*; 2012. Available at: http://emedicine.medscape.com/article/819987-overview#a0104.
16. Buckley N, Juurlink D, Isbister G, Bennett M, Lavonas E. Hyperbaric oxygen for carbon monoxide poisoning. *Cochrane Database Syst Rev*. 2011;13(4), CD002041.
17. Smollin C, Olson K. Carbon monoxide poisoning (acute). *Clin Evid*. 2010;10:1–11.

18. Hamel J. A review of acute cyanide poisoning with a treatment update. *Crit Care Nurse.* 2011;31(1):72–82.

19. Mosier M, DeChristopher P. Use of therapeutic plasma exchange in the burn unit: a review of the literature. *J Burn Care Res.* 2013;34(3):289–298.

20. Giretzlehner M, Dirnberger J, Owen R, Haller HL, Lumenta DB, Kamolz LP. The determination of total burn surface area: how much difference? *Burns.* 2013;39:1107–1113.

21. Mackie D. Mass burn casaulties: a rational approach to planning. *Burns.* 2002;28:403–404.

22. Kirschenbaum L, Keene A, O'Neill P, Westfal R, Astiz ME. The experience at St. Vincent's Hospital, Manhattan on September 11, 2001: preparedness, response, and lessons learned. *Crit Care Med.* 2005;33: S48–S52.

23. Jordan M. 9/11 This is not a drill! *J Burn Care Rehabil.* 2004;25:15–24.

24. Dunbar J. The Rhode Island nightclub fire: the story from the perspective of an on-duty ED nurse. *J Emerg Nurs.* 2004;30:464–466.

Structure Fires

James P. Phillips

📄 DESCRIPTION OF EVENT

A structure is defined by the National Fire Protection Association (NFPA) as "that which is built or constructed, an edifice or building of any kind, or any piece of work artificially built up or composed of parts joined together in some definite manner."[1] Structures include any habitable space, such as residential, business, high-rise, multifamily and single family homes, and temporary buildings of varying complexity. Referring to a fire as a "structure fire" typically implies that the components of the building itself are involved, not just the contents of the structure. The NFPA also categorizes buildings into five major construction types by their different building materials and construction techniques and their corresponding susceptibility to fire damage and risk of structural collapse (Box 174-1).

Structure fires account for the majority of fire-related deaths in the United States each year. The incidence of human injuries and financial value of property damage is also dramatically higher when compared with other types of fires (Table 174-1). In 2013 there were more than 1.3 million fires reported in the United States, 487,500 of which were classified as structure fires by the NFPA. In that year 88% of fire-related civilian deaths were the direct result of structure fires.[2] Structure fires are deadly, are destructive, can create an overwhelming number of victims in a short period of time, and can require more firefighting resources than are locally available. Therefore they can represent the epitome of a disaster.

Structure fires are complex, and many variables contribute to the lethality of any particular event, including but not limited to: type of structure, cause of fire, materials burned, options for escape, presence of structural collapse, and various patient characteristics. To illustrate this point, it is interesting to note that three of the deadliest structure fires in the history of the United States were all quite different in regards to these variables. The Great Chicago Fire of 1871, with a death toll estimated at 300, started one evening in a single barn and quickly spread overnight to engulf more than 17,500 buildings. The fire easily spread through the city comprised mostly of wooden buildings with tar and shingle roofs that experienced high winds and had previously had prior months of drought conditions. Over one third of the city's population was left homeless by the fire, which started after ten o'clock in the evening. The Great Chicago Fire led to wide-ranging changes in fire codes and requirements for fire-resistant building materials.

Another of America's deadliest structure fires happened in Boston in 1942 when the Cocoanut Grove caught fire, killing 492 in the city's most popular nightclub.[4] The fire began in a basement bar and spread rapidly via combustible hanging decorations and quickly cut off the stairs for escape. The published reports highlighted a deficiency in escape routes from the one-story restaurant and bar, which undoubtedly increased the number of casualties. The main doorway contained a revolving door, which quickly jammed under pressure and was where approximately 200 dead bodies were located trying to escape. The flames then spread to the Broadway Cocktail Lounge where 100 more victims were trapped behind a door swinging the wrong way, which blocked access to the outside doorway, and other egresses were both hidden by decorations and locked.[4,5] This disaster required the mobilization of the Civilian Defense preparations that were already in place at Massachusetts General Hospital due to fear of wartime airplane attacks and which saved many lives. It demonstrated that disaster preparedness can help to reduce morbidity and mortality and that a flexible "all-hazards" approach to mass casualty incidents can be effective. At trial it was revealed that after building permits had been issued for the club and its renovations, the designer's plans had been modified and that the required automatic fire doors had simply not been built.[6]

When discussing structure fires, there is another key concept that must be remembered as a leading cause of death and injury: structural collapse. The two airliners that struck the World Trade Center towers in September 2001 caused the death of more than 2600 people located in and around the buildings. The heat-related weakening of the structural elements of the skyscraper itself led to loss of integrity and collapse. Once a single-floor collapse began, the dynamic weight load exceeded the static weight load capacity of the structural steel, leading to total loss of both buildings. Although the aircraft impacts and the resulting fires led to the immediate deaths of many, most are presumed to have died from blunt force trauma during the building collapse caused by the structure fire.

⏪ PRE-INCIDENT CONSIDERATIONS

Mitigation

One of the key concepts in disaster preparedness is mitigation—having in place important systems, responses, preparations, and infrastructure designed to lessen the impact of a deleterious event. Perhaps in no other area of disaster science has such an effect been made on human mortality and property protection than in the area of structure fire mitigation and prevention. Statistics published by the NFPA clearly show significant reductions in the total number of house fire deaths from 1977 through 2013.[7] The statistics presented in this article tout the reduction in deaths to the dramatically increased use of home smoke alarm devices. Although smoke alarms have certainly increased the chance of surviving a structure fire at home, further analysis of these data shows the true risk reduction is probably less than claimed, though still significant.[8] In addition to smoke alarms, deaths have been reduced by a combination of better building codes (marked, lighted exits, fire doors, and automatic alarms), fire-resistant materials for building as well as upholstery and mattress materials, a reduction in the percentage of Americans who smoke cigarettes, sprinkler systems, improved safety

BOX 174-1 NFPA Construction Types, from Least to Most Combustible

Type I	Fire resistive	All walls, roofs, floors, and supporting elements must be made of or coated with noncombustible or limited combustible materials. Concrete and cement are examples. Structural collapse is unlikely.
Type II	Noncombustible	Same as Type I, but with a lower hourly fire-resistance rating designation. Unprotected structural steel may be present and is susceptible to heat effects and can lead to collapse.
Type III	Ordinary construction	Exterior walls must be noncombustible, most commonly masonry or stone. Interior walls and structural elements are typically wood framed, which may have a fire-resistance rating of up to 1 hour.
Type IV	Heavy timber	Exterior walls are masonry or stone and use large-dimension lumber for structural members. Commonly seen in industrial plans before 1960, many have now been renovated for new use.
Type V	Wood-framed	Walls and roofs are made of combustible materials, most commonly wood, and is the type used in most single- and multiple-family homes. This lightweight construction can fail within minutes of direct fire exposure.

Data from National Fire Protection Association, *Standard on Types of Building Construction*

TABLE 174-1 NFPA Statistics on Structure Fires for 2013

2013 STATISTICS	NUMBER OF FIRES	DEATHS	FIRE INJURIES	PROPERTY DAMAGE
Structure	487,500 (39%)	2855 (88%)	14,075 (88%)	$9.5 billion (83%)
Vehicle	188,000 (15%)	320 (10%)	1050 (7%)	$1.3 billion (12%)
Outside or other	564,500 (46%)	65 (2%)	800 (5%)	$607 million (5%)
Total fires	1,240,000	3240	15,925	$11.5 billion

Data from NFPA Fire Loss in the U.S. During 2013.[3]

of household appliances, better firefighting equipment and tactics, and certainly better emergency medical service(s) (EMS) and emergency department care for injured patients.

➕ MEDICAL TREATMENT OF CASUALTIES

Medical treatment of victims of a fire begins immediately upon arrival of first responders. As in all responses, scene safety for the first responders is the first and most important consideration. When permitted by the incident commander to enter the scene, EMS professionals and other first responders may begin triage and treatment. Of the ambulatory victims outside the structure the majority of patients are likely to have respiratory complaints secondary to inhalation of fumes, plus or minus burns. Smoke inhalation is the leading cause of fire-related deaths, according to death certificate analysis in 1999; the

BOX 174-2 American Burn Association Burn Center Referral Criteria[12]

- Partial thickness burns greater than 10% total body surface area
- Burns that involve the face, hands, feet, genitalia, perineum, or major joints
- Third-degree burns in any age group
- Electrical burns, including lightning injury
- Chemical burns
- Inhalation injury
- Patients with preexisting medical disorders that could complicate management, prolong recovery, or affect mortality
- Patients with burns and concomitant trauma (such as fractures) in which the burn injury poses the greatest risk of morbidity or mortality
- Children in hospitals without qualified personnel or equipment for the care of children
- Patients who will require special social, emotional, or rehabilitative intervention

smoke inhalation to burns ratio was 2 to 1.[9] Smoke itself is composed of particulate matter, heated gases, irritants (such as hydrochloric acid, sulfur dioxide, and ammonia), asphyxiates (such as carbon dioxide), and toxins (such as hydrogen sulfide, carbon monoxide, and hydrogen cyanide).[10] Victims of structure fires should be assessed for signs of potential inhalational injury on scene (respiratory distress, facial burns, and soot in nasopharynx), provided oxygen, and rapidly transported to an emergency department. Victims with severe dyspnea and impending respiratory failure should be intubated before transport.

On scene the burn care should consist of wound coverage with sterile gauze, hypothermia countermeasures, and rapid transport. Intravenous fluid replacement should begin en route, if possible, using Ringer's lactate, but normal saline is adequate if this is not available. EMS providers should record the amount of fluid administered to allow the receiving physicians to calculate fluid needs, typically using the Parkland formula.[11] Pain should be treated with intravenous opiate analgesia, as needed.

EMS must decide where to transport victims who have burn injuries. Ideally each patient with significant burn injury would be sent directly to a burn center, although this is unrealistic given the paucity of such facilities and potentially significant transport times in many areas of the country. Factors for EMS to consider when choosing an appropriate destination should include patient stability (unstable patients should go to the nearest emergency department before transfer to a specialized burn center), patient age, size and depth of the burn, presence of traumatic injuries, and other clinical factors. In the event of a mass casualty incident, patient distribution to nonburn centers may be required. Emergency department care for burns, inhalation injuries, and crush injuries are beyond the scope of this chapter but can be found in all major emergency medicine textbooks. Receiving hospitals should consider transferring patients who meet American Burn Association referral criteria (Box 174-2) to burn centers after stabilizing treatment and transfer to facilities with hyperbaric treatment capabilities in the case of severe carbon monoxide poisoning. If blunt trauma or crush injury from structural collapse is present, a decision may need to be made as to whether burn injuries or the trauma are more severe, and patients should be transported accordingly.

▷▷ POST-INCIDENT ACTIONS

Large numbers of casualties will require immediate distribution among surrounding emergency departments, trauma centers, and burn

BOX 174-3 Primary Distribution Methods

Controlled primary	This method, controlled by the medical command and control center (MCCC), is the best method for primary distribution of casualties. The MCCC should use an information system that provides ongoing updates of hospital capacities and capabilities and helps EMS determine the optimal destination for each casualty.
Semicontrolled primary	In the absence of a functioning MCCC, this method can promote equitable distribution of casualties. Rather than trying to match the specialized needs of each victim to the appropriate hospital, the event commander distributes equal numbers of casualties to each regional hospital on a rotating basis.
Spontaneous primary	Although the least desirable, this distribution method is the most common. Ambulances and other vehicles transport victims to the closest hospital, with no connectivity, control, or coordination.

Data from Ashkenazi I, Hunt RC, Sasser SM, et al. *Preparedness and Response to a Mass Casualty Event Resulting from Terrorist Use of Explosives.* 2010.[14]

centers, as available. Some will subsequently require transfer to higher or lower care facilities. It has been shown in academic review that distributing burn victims to a nonburn center for stabilizing treatment in lieu of direct transport to a burn center does not significantly alter the mortality of the victim.[13] Following a mass casualty incident, such as a large structure fire with multiple victims, there are two levels of patient distribution called primary and secondary.

Primary distribution refers to moving patients from the scene to the hospital. There are three methods currently in use for primary distribution, and they are not equal in their desirability (Box 174-3). Secondary distribution refers to moving patients from the first receiving hospital to a second medical facility, as needed. Through secondary distribution, casualties can be redistributed from overloaded hospitals and care sites to less affected ones and/or more specialized facilities. All hospitals must develop formal and practical relationships with designated trauma and specialty centers to ensure that, when necessary, casualties will have access to appropriate levels of care.[14]

From the perspective of the fire department, the post-incident phase of a structure fire begins when the fire is extinguished and the patients have been transported to medical facilities. The fire department will be the lead agency for fire investigation, with law enforcement involvement as needed for criminal prosecution. Particular care must be taken by fire, police, and EMS personnel to prevent spoliation of critical evidence that may lead to discovery of the cause of the fire. Spoliation is the loss, destruction, or material alteration of an object or document that is potential evidence in a legal proceeding by one who has the responsibility for its preservation. Spoliation of evidence may occur when the movement, change, or destruction of evidence or the alteration of the scene significantly impairs the opportunity of other interested parties to obtain the same evidentiary value from the evidence, as did any prior investigator.[15]

❓ UNIQUE CONSIDERATIONS

Terrorism

An analysis by the Heritage Foundation evaluating 40 years of terrorism against the United States shows that of all domestic terrorism incidents between 2001 and 2009, arson was the cause of 46.2% of incidents, whereas the second and third most prevalent tactics were "other" tactics (20.9%) and bombings (18.7%). The majority of domestic arson attacks were conducted by the activist organizations Earth Liberation Front and Animal Liberation Front.[16] An all-hazards approach to facility preparedness, especially those who consider terrorism to be a significant threat by hazard vulnerability analysis, should include mitigation against arson.

It is notable that on September 11, 2012, the first murder of an American ambassador since 1988 took place in Benghazi, Libya. Although guns, homemade explosives, and military ordnance were used, it was not bullets or explosives that killed the U.S. ambassador, but rather smoke from an arson fire. During the attack on the U.S. mission in Benghazi, which killed four Americans, terrorists used fuel from jerry cans to start a fire in the main villa where Ambassador Christopher Stevens was sheltering with his diplomatic security detail.[17]

Extremes of Age

Very young children and older adults face the highest risk of fire death.[18] Only 7% of the U.S. population is under 5 years of age, but from 2003 to 2007 10% of the home fire fatalities were under 5 years. These children were almost 1.5 times as likely to die in fire as the general population and were at greatest risk of dying in home structure fires caused by playing with heat source, cooking equipment, and heating equipment. Adults more than 65 years of age have the highest risk of fire death, and this risk increases with age. During the same time period 28% of the people fatally injured in home fire were 65 or older, but only 12% of the population was that old. They were at highest risk of dying in home structure fires caused by smoking materials, electrical distribution and lighting equipment, and heating equipment.[9,18]

⚠ PITFALLS

A mass casualty incident involving multiple burn patients is likely to overwhelm local resources quickly, even in the event that there is a burn center in close proximity. As shown in a University of Michigan study in 2013 hospital utilization is constrained within the first 120 minutes due to the limited number of beds. The first bottleneck is attributable to exhausting critical care beds, followed by floor beds.[19] In fact in the case of a large national disaster causing very large numbers of burn patients, it could be expected that even with national distribution of patients to verified and unverified burn centers, the surge would overwhelm available burn care beds very quickly. As of 2014 there are 128 burn care facilities in the United States. Of them, 64 are verified by the American Burn Association and the American College of Surgeons.[20] Even fewer are verified as pediatric burn centers.

REFERENCES

1. National Fire Protection Association. *NFPA Glossary of Terms*; 2003.
2. NFPA. Fires-in-the-US. Available at: http://www.nfpa.org/research/reports-and-statistics/fires-in-the-us.
3. Karter MJ. National Fire Protection Association. Fire Analysis and Research Div. *Fire Loss in the United States During 2013*; 2014. Available at: http://www.nfpa.org/~/media/Files/Research/NFPA%20reports/Overall%20Fire%20Statistics/osfireloss.pdf.
4. Faxon NW. The problems of the hospital administration. *Ann Surg.* 1943;117(6):803–808.
5. Faxon NW, Churchill ED. The Cocoanut Grove disaster in Boston. *JAMA.* 1942;120(17):1385–1388.
6. Blackington AH. Trial proves criminal negligence at Cocoanut Grove fire. *Fire Eng.* 1943;96(5):242–246.
7. Ahrens M. National Fire Protection Association. Fire Analysis and Research Division. *Smoke Alarms in U.S. Home Fires*; 2014. http://dx.doi.org/10.1007/s10694-008-0045-9.

8. Dubner SJ. How many lives do smoke alarms really save? Freakonomics .com. Available at: http://freakonomics.com/2012/02/06/how-many-lives-do-smoke-alarms-really-save/.

9. Flynn JD. National Fire Protection Association. Fire Analysis and Research Division. *Characteristics of Home Fire Victims [2003-2007]*; 2010.

10. Riddle K. Smoke Inhalation and Hydrogen Cyanide Poisoning: The Danger Posed to Firefighters and Victims in Structure Fires. San Diego, CA: Jems Communications; 2004.

11. Scheulen JJ, Munster AM. The Parkland formula in patients with burns and inhalation injury. *J Trauma*. 1982;22(10):869–871.

12. American Burn Association: Burn Center Referral Criteria. 2010:1–1. Available at: http://ameriburn.org/BurnCenterReferralCriteria.pdf.

13. Bell N, Simons R, Hameed SM, Schuurman N, Wheeler S. Does direct transport to provincial burn centres improve outcomes? A spatial epidemiology of severe burn injury in British Columbia, 2001-2006. *Can J Surg*. 2012;55(2):110–116.

14. Ashkenazi I, Hunt RC, Sasser SM, et al. Preparedness and Response to a Mass Casualty Event Resulting from Terrorist Use of Explosives; 2010.

15. National Fire Protection Association. *NFPA 921 Guide for Fire & Explosion Investigations 2014*; 2014.

16. Muhlhausen DB, McNeill JB. The Heritage Foundation. *Terror Trends: 40 Years' Data on International and Domestic Terrorism*; 2011. 1–16. Available at: http://report.heritage.org/sr0093.

17. Pfeifer JW. Combating terrorism center at Westpoint. Fire as a weapon in terrorist attacks. *CTC Sentinel*. 2013;6(7):5–8.

18. National Fire Protection Association. Fire Analysis and Research Division. Demographic and Other Characteristics Related to Fire Deaths or Injuries. 2010.

19. Abir M, Davis MM, Sankar P, Wong AC, Wang SC. Design of a model to predict surge capacity bottlenecks for burn mass casualties at a large academic medical center. *Prehosp Disaster Med*. 2013;28(1):23–32.

20. Lentz CW, Bessey PQ, Phillips BD, et al. 2014 National Burn Repository Report of Data From 2004-2013. 2014. Chicago, IL, Available at: http://www.ameriburn.org/2014NBRAnnualReport.pdf.

SUGGESTED READINGS

1. Bales RF. The Great Chicago Fire and the Myth of Mrs. O'Leary's Cow. Jefferson, NC: McFarland; 2002.

2. National Fire Protection Association. *NFPA J*. 2008;220.

Wilderness and Forest Fire

John Moloney

DESCRIPTION OF EVENT

Fire is a natural phenomenon that has been a part of our ecosystem for millions of years.[1] Fire in an uninhabited area may have environmental and ecological consequences, but most remote fires per se do not have health or medical consequences. Although an unplanned fire of any size is a potentially challenging and frightening thing, it only becomes a hazard to human life when it interacts with people. When fire threatens numerous lives, homes, communities, and livelihoods, it has the potential to become a disaster. Recognizing this, fire authorities can prospectively advise communities on how to protect themselves and mitigate the effects of fire.[2]

Before the ability of humans to light fires, most forest fires occurred because of lightning strikes. Lightning strikes the Earth an average of 100 times per second or more than 3 billion times per year.[3] Lightning tends to strike at the tops of ridges, where there is often higher humidity, lower temperatures, and less fuel. These fires therefore may often be less severe than human-caused fires. Some other parts of the globe are too wet or too sparsely vegetated[4] for significant naturally occurring fires.

Due to the importance of fire for agriculture as well as for heat and cooking, humans have historically largely lived in fire-prone areas. Burning kills local flora and soil microfauna, leaving a cleared space in which to plant crops. Indeed a study identified a substance in smoke that stimulates the germination of many plant species.[5] Farmers often allow a field to lie fallow for a season, after which it is burnt to regenerate the area.[4]

Ninety percent of fires in the United States are caused by humans and their activities.[6] Accidental causes include the use of faulty machinery releasing sparks (e.g., chain saws), discarded cigarettes, burning of garden debris, and children playing with matches. Loss of control of an intentionally lit fire, including campfires and fuel reduction burns, have historically been another contributor. Between 2000 and 2008 in the Forestry Commission Wales district *Coed y Cymoedd*, there were more than 55,527 forest fires or grassfires. The South Wales Fire and Rescue Service (SWFRS) suggests that 95% are the result of deliberate actions.[6] In May 2000 the U.S. Park Service deliberately lit a fire to clear brush at the Bandelier National Monument. After getting out of control the fire burned for 2 weeks, destroying 200 homes and 47,000 acres of forest.[7]

There have been a number of large fires involving the interface between forest and urban areas that have had large costs in terms of lives lost and economic costs. U.S. government federal agencies spent $3 billion suppressing 170,000 fires during the 2-year period from 2002 to 2003. In 2014 the cost to suppress fires in the United States was $1.8 billion.[8]

PRE-INCIDENT ACTIONS

Management of forest resources can reduce the likelihood and impact of fire. Local communities in areas at risk for forest fires need to take preventive action to minimize the risk of fire involving their properties. Fuel loads can be assessed and reduced if appropriate. Controlled burning can reduce fuel levels and can be used to create buffer strips or firebreaks. These controlled burns should be carried out in lower hazard periods, such as the cooler months of the year. Long-term issues include setting up firebreaks around housing and other buildings and preventing vegetation from growing up to the edge of structures. Potential fuel for fires (e.g., fuel for farm machinery, piles of dry firewood) should not be stored next to housing. Buildings should be kept in a good state of repair, with the guttering clear of leaves and other flammable debris.

Local governments should also develop local plans to facilitate people moving away from fire danger at times of high risk and/or designating areas to be used as fire refuges (e.g., sporting grounds). They should identify facilities where vulnerable people are likely to be situated (e.g., aged care facilities, hospitals, schools, and child care centers).[9]

After the 2009 Black Saturday Fires in Victoria, Australia, a Royal Commission recommended an enhanced role of warning systems, including providing for timely and informative advice about the predicted passage of a fire and the actions to be taken by people in areas potentially in its path. The warnings should emphasize that all fires are different in ways that require an active awareness of fire conditions, local circumstances, and personal capacity. Community leaders are recommended to warn that the heightened risk on the worst days demands a different response. It is therefore vital to ensure that local solutions are tailored and known to communities through local bushfire planning arrangements.

With forest fires, visibility on the roads can be significantly impaired by smoke. Roads also may be blocked by fire or falling trees, and there may be high numbers of emergency vehicles on the road, further complicating evacuation and population movement. The lack of effective traffic management during the Berkeley Hills Tunnel Fire in California in 1991 is said to have directly contributed to loss of life.[10] The Royal Commission noted that "the greatest proportion of civilian deaths in bushfires occurred during attempts at late evacuation."[2] By way of contrast, it should be noted that 26,000 people were successfully evacuated in 2 hours from the Laguna Beach area in 1993, following detailed local planning that included planning for separate fire service access and civilian egress.

Individuals in areas of high fire risk should be encouraged to develop personal fire plans. These plans should include a considered opinion about whether in high-risk conditions to stay and defend the house or to leave the area early. The decision to evacuate when the fire is very close can be a deadly decision. Plans should include notification of relatives and a plan for children and pets. A fire plan should also include checks on neighbors who, because of age or illness, are less able to care for themselves. At times of high risk, such as hot dry summer days with dangerous winds, fire action plans should be invoked.

An example of a personal fire plan can be accessed at http://www.cfa.vic.gov.au/residents/living/index.htm.

If fire does invade an area, other personal actions can be taken to further minimize the risks to life and property. Appropriate clothing reduces the risk from radiant heat. As a fire approaches, people should move to the inner parts of the house away from windows and the radiant heat. Garden hoses, which may be used to put out small fires after the main fire front has passed, may be damaged by the main fire front and so should be protected.

Michael Rhode[11] undertook a review of incident command of fires at the interface between wild land and the urban environment and noted that command decisions and actions could and should be pre-planned both for firefighter safety and efficiency. He reviewed the response to six fires in California between 1990 and 1996. The initial command post locations were inadequate. Command posts burned in three of the six fires. In all fires, public volunteerism proved unmanageable. Communications centers and fire radio systems were overwhelmed. Before an incident, local emergency managers must develop and publicly communicate their strategies and tactics for managing the incident. Planning of evacuation routes and fire refuges should be communicated to the local population as well as emergency managers.

▶▶ POST-INCIDENT ACTIONS

With wilderness fires, effective control of the fire may not be possible for days or weeks. Nonetheless, during this time effective and efficient incident management must continuously occur. As is often seen in emergencies, maintenance of command can be difficult. This is especially so if the incident is spread geographically and there are impaired communications. In the 1993 fires around Malibu, 20 separate entrapments of firefighters occurred. These resulted from actions independent of command.[10] It should be noted that the birth of the Incident Command System itself stems from lessons learned in response to wildfires in California in the 1970s and the problems of command and control with such incidents.

Forest fires may cause displacement of people from their homes or from their local areas, often with inadequate preparation for the evacuation. Areas may become isolated because of road closure, affecting the ability to provide routine medical care and pharmaceuticals, regardless of any increase in requirements related to the fire. Local plans should include methods for provision of this routine care to isolated communities or displaced people.

Managers of health care facilities and prehospital medical services may not be able to access extra staff because these staff may either be protecting their homes[11] or may be unable to safely travel to their place of work. Most wilderness fires will continue for hours, days, or weeks. The provision of adequate staffing levels with adequate rest breaks will stretch the personnel resources of many institutions.

Management of the media in the post-incident phase is crucial. Media, particularly the radio and television, can provide up-to-date information to communities over a large area. In the case of radio, this can also include members of the community who are not at home because they are moving or after they have reached a refuge. Increasingly, social media is being used as an effective and efficient method of communication. Emergency managers could examine potential roles before the incident.

✚ MEDICAL TREATMENT OF CASUALTIES

Common medical complaints in patients who have been involved in forest fires include burns, heat-related injuries, smoke inhalation,

TABLE 175-1 Presenting Complaints of Emergency Department Patients Following the Canberra, Australia, Fire of 2003

CONDITION	PRESENTATIONS	ADMISSIONS
Breathing problems and smoke inhalation	65	10
Eye problems (irritation, ulcer, and foreign bodies)	43	0
Trauma (falls and motor vehicles)	45	6
Burns	24	10
Medication issues*	21	0
Accommodation and chronic diseases	5	5†
Other	30	5
Total	233	36

*Supply of usual medications required by people unable to return home. These included insulin, antipsychotics, antihypertensives, and home oxygen.
†Persons with chronic disease requiring emergency accommodation.
Adapted from Richardson DB, Kumar S. Emergency response to the Canberra Bushfires. *Med J Aust.* 2004;181:40–42. © Copyright 2004. The Medical Journal of Australia - reproduced with permission. The *Medical Journal of Australia* does not accept responsibility for any errors in translation.

and bronchospasm. After the fires around Canberra, Australia, in 2003 there were 233 presentations to the emergency department of the Canberra Hospital (Table 175-1). An analysis of the Black Saturday Fires found that most victims either died or survived with minor injuries. There were comparatively few survivors with major injuries.[11] Poor air quality was a major contributing factor for the increase in patients presenting for health care after the San Diego Fires in 2003.[12]

Important in the initial management of burn victims are the decisions about where patients should be managed. Patients with burns may be managed in an ambulatory setting, general hospital, or specialized burns unit, depending on the size and thickness of the burn, location of burns (e.g., face, perineum), comorbidities, and extremes of age.

💡 UNIQUE CONSIDERATIONS

Wilderness fires are unique among disasters. It is possible to predict in most cases when the conditions are suitable for a fire to develop. Preventive actions, such as fuel reduction and early evacuation can significantly reduce the impact of a fire on the population. Most disasters that cause "trauma," with the exception of war-like activities, have a beginning and an end to "new" injuries with a well-localized geography. Wilderness fires, however, are often ongoing events with the potential to continue for weeks or months and to spread to adjacent areas or to commence elsewhere. Another unique consideration of wilderness fires is their ability to destroy or threaten health care facilities at a time when these facilities are needed to manage casualties. Communication can also be disrupted because of loss of cell phone towers and landline infrastructure.

! PITFALLS

Several potential pitfalls in response to a wilderness fire exist. These include the following:

- Failure to prepare adequate systems to respond to large numbers of low-acuity patients (e.g., those with smoke inhalation or ocular foreign bodies)
- Failure to consider unavailability of staff to respond due to personal involvement in an incident or restricted ability to travel
- Failure to prepare adequate systems to deliver commonly used pharmaceuticals to members of the population displaced from their homes or communities
- Failure to consider that health care facilities may be directly threatened by the fire or smoke
- Failure to appreciate that wilderness fires are an ongoing incident that may last for days to weeks and that may change rapidly
- Failure to appreciate the extent of a burn injury; this may result in inadequate fluid resuscitation or triage to an inappropriate facility

REFERENCES

1. Wildland Fires: A Historical Perspective. In: *U.S. Fire Administration*; October 2000: Topical Fire Research Series; vol. 1 issue 3, Available at: http://nfa.usfa.dhs.gov/downloads/pdf/statistics/v1i3-508.pdf.

2. Victoria's Bushfire Safety Policy. Available at: http://www.royalcommission.vic.gov.au/finaldocuments/volume-2/PF/VBRC_Vol2_Chapter01_PF.pdf.

3. Ainsworth J, Doss TA. *Natural History of Fire and Flood Cycles.* Santa Barbara, CA: University of California; 1955.

4. Pyne S. *The long burn. Whole Earth Mag*; Winter 1999. Available at: http://www.wholeearth.com/issue/2099/article/173/the.long.burn.

5. Flematti GR, Ghisalberti EL, Dixon KW, Trengove RD. A compound from smoke that promotes seed germination. *Science.* 2004;305(5686):977.

6. Jollands M, Morris J, Moffat AJ. *Wildfires in Wales.* Report to Forestry Commission Wales. Forest Research, Farnham, 2011. http://www.forestry.gov.uk/fr/wildfiresinwales#finalreport.

7. Fire in the Forest - Fairbanks Museum and Planetarium. Available at: http://www.fairbanksmuseum.com/uploads/1212783347.pdf.

8. United States Department of Agriculture. Washington, DC. News Release No. 0075.14. Available at: http://www.usda.gov/wps/portal/usda/usdamediafb?contentid=2014/05/0075.xml&printable=true&contentidonly=true.

9. Recommendation 3. FINAL REPORT 2009 Victorian Bushfires Royal Commission. Available at: http://www.royalcommission.vic.gov.au/Assets/VBRC-Final-Report-Recommendations.pdf.

10. Rhode MS. Fires in the wildland—urban interface: best command practices. *Fire Manag Today.* 2004;64:27–31.

11. Cameron PA, Mitra B, Fitzgerald M, et al. Black Saturday: the immediate impact of the February 2009 bushfires in Victoria, Australia. *Med J Aust.* 2009;191:11–16.

12. Hoyt KS, Gerhart AE. The San Diego County wildfires: perspectives of healthcare providers. *Disaster Manag Response.* 2004;2:46–52.

CHAPTER 176

Tunnel Fire

Sami A. Yousif and Nawfal Aljerian

DESCRIPTION OF EVENT

People have been constructing tunnels for thousands of years, under rivers, through mountains, and beneath cities. Sometimes hailed as an engineering marvel, construction of tunnels requires the displacement of huge amounts of earth while still supporting enormous weight above them. Communities often depend on tunnels as a vital component of the transportation system, allowing movement of vehicular traffic, subways, and rail cars. Many large metropolitan areas depend on tunnels for large portions of their subway systems. Some cities depend on tunnels for major portions of their routine commuter traffic as well. For example, more than 42 million people traveled through the Fort McHenry tunnel in Baltimore, Maryland, in 2003.[1] Persistently high volumes of traffic, vehicle congestion, and mechanical failures, combined with sometimes flammable cargo, make tunnel fires almost inevitable. In addition, although less visible to the public, rail systems actively use many tunnels in both urban and rural settings; because freight train tunnels lack the hazardous materials restrictions and, in many cases, the adequate ventilation or fire-suppression systems required of passenger traffic tunnels,[2] freight train fires may have significant destructive potential.[3] Because of limited physical access and the potential for significant disruption to infrastructure, an intentional tunnel fire or explosion as a means of terrorism is a concerning possibility.

Tunnel fire safety requirements have changed dramatically in recent years, with some of the most important work coming from Europe. In 2001 the European Thematic Network FIT (Fire in Tunnels) was established by the European Union in response to major tunnel fire incidents between 1996 and 2001.[4] The main goal of the network was to harmonize the various European requirements regarding tunnel safety and develop consensus on fire safety for road, rail, and metro infrastructure in tunnels. The project was concluded in 2004 with recommendations on fire scenarios and guidelines for fire safe design and fire response management, along with a common paper titled *General Approach to Tunnel Fire Safety*. The FIT network has sparked major tunnel safety legislative changes in Europe and worldwide.

One of the greatest challenges in attempting to prevent and mitigate tunnel fires is the fact that the designs, materials, and features of tunnel construction are substantially different. Technology and materials have changed markedly, so emergency responders that respond to tunnel emergencies may be faced with a wide range of possible variables, depending on the specific design elements of the tunnel in question. Most older tunnels were excavated using drills, dynamite, and substantial manual labor. Many were constructed using horseshoe geometry and lined with brick and mortar. Modern tunnels, in contrast, are generally round, lined with steel and concrete, and are carved from the earth using enormous hydraulic tunnel-boring machines, which create

clean cylindrical tubes in which reinforced liners have been placed. These variances in construction materials and geometry call for different types of systems for evacuation, ventilation, and fire suppression.

Many older tunnels consist of a single-tube construction, whereas most modern roadway tunnels are built in connected pairs. Lengthy single-tube tunnels constructed for passenger traffic often have escape-route stairways that provide access to the surface, whereas paired tunnels usually contain cross-tunnel adits,[5] that is, airtight passageways connecting the two tubes. The adits are usually recognizable as doorways lining one side of a tunnel, spaced at regular intervals. While sometimes labeled (but sometimes not), these doorways provide essential refuge to tunnel victims from rapidly expanding smoke and heat. The doorways to these adits must be closed, however, to permit the paired tunnel to serve as a parallel escape route with a separate air supply and shielding from heat. If an adit door is left open, the adit will permit contamination of the unaffected tunnel and possible spread of smoke and fire.

Subway tunnels vary with regard to single-tunnel and cross-tunnel ventilation. Some circulate air mostly through the movement of the rail cars. Others have more modern fans and ventilation systems. Subway tunnels may also contain an additional hazard for escaping passengers—the electrified third rail. These rails generally operate on direct current of approximately 750 V. During an emergency, electrified rails must be shut off for the safety of evacuating passengers and emergency responders. Rescuers should be provided with "hotsticks" (voltage detectors) and trained in their use to ensure the track is de-energized before working in close proximity to it. The track should be rechecked repeatedly and always treated as if energized to minimize the chance of electrocution. If staffing permits, dedicated personnel should be assigned to continuously monitor tracks for electricity. This provides a greater level of safety for crews and evacuating passengers.

Once fires ignite, large plumes of smoke and superheated gas can rapidly fill a tunnel's confined spaces.[6] Within minutes, victims can be overcome with smoke at temperatures of more than 1000 °F. To provide a safe environment for escaping motorists and passengers, tunnel engineers have therefore designed and instituted various types of ventilation systems. The simplest system is a longitudinal one. Longitudinal ventilation systems are used in many older tunnels, as well as subway, rail, and smaller vehicular tunnels. In a longitudinal system, air is injected into a tunnel at one end, where it travels within the same compartment as passenger traffic, then exits at the other end. Depending on the specific system, airflow is driven by supply fans or pulled by exhaust fans. In most systems, a combination of both types operates in a push-pull fashion. When a fire is identified, manual or automated systems activate the fans to direct plumes of smoke and heat away from the majority of people. If these systems can generate adequate air velocities in the tunnel, they provide a temporary safe environment on the supply side of the fire. However, the exhaust side becomes significantly more dangerous because of a "burner effect"[6] generated by winds blowing past fires with superheated exhaust fumes. People trapped on the exhaust side of a fire in a longitudinal ventilated tunnel may succumb rapidly from the intense heat and smoke exposure.

In longitudinal systems, the fans can generally be reversed to direct exhaust in either direction; however, this feature may not always be effective. Tunnels have a natural air flow that is perpetuated by the flow of traffic. As vehicles travel through the tunnel, air is pushed along with them. This creates a "piston effect" that can take several minutes to diminish, even after traffic stops. Depending on the capacity and location of supply and exhaust fans, the natural air flow may be too strong to overcome for some time. In fact, attempts to do so would result in an increase in turbulent flow within the tunnel and dispersion of superheated gases and smoke.

Another method of tunnel ventilation is the transverse-ventilation system, which is used in many large metropolitan vehicular tunnels. In these systems, the (modern) circular tunnel tube is divided into three horizontal sections. The portion of the tube used by commuters occupies the center section. Two adjacent, large semicircular sections remain hidden from sight, but contain equipment and ventilation support systems that serve several important purposes. The adjacent semicircular sections often contain communications antennae, a water-drainage system, and the supply and exhaust ventilation system. Large buildings stationed near both entrances to the tunnel house enormous fans that funnel air through the tunnels via large cement conduits. New York's Holland tunnel is one such tunnel and is ventilated with 84 of these fans. The four tubes of Baltimore's Fort McHenry tunnel are ventilated with 24 even larger fans. Exhaust fumes are suctioned through vents in the steel-plate ceiling and blown out of stacks located in the ventilation buildings.

Transverse ventilation systems generally have much greater air flow capacity and have been shown to function quite effectively in real fire situations. Unlike longitudinal flow systems, transverse-flow ventilation has not been shown to exacerbate fires or create dangerous conditions for escaping motorists. Modern systems are now also incorporating adjustable dampers that focus exhaust air flow over or surrounding a fire to further speed evacuation of smoke and superheated gases.

Once ventilation is addressed and evacuation is ensured, fire suppression activities are the next priority. The decision by fire and rescue services over whether to enter a tunnel to attack a fire is neither a simple one nor one that should be made hastily. In general, there is no way to know with certainty what hazards exist at the source of a tunnel fire. Video cameras may permit eyes on the scene, but the presence of hazardous gases, oxygen levels, and other features must usually be assessed manually. As noted above, hazardous materials restrictions exist for most vehicular tunnels, but the same restrictions do not apply to most rail tunnels. In addition, despite laws regarding transport of hazardous materials, it is possible that trucks may knowingly or unknowingly transport hazardous materials through restricted tunnels.

The threat of terrorism brings with it unpredictability and the additional potential for intentional secondary explosive devices. While tunnels are designed to withstand fires of great intensity, most are not designed to withstand large explosions. Great care must be exercised when entering a tunnel with the intent of fire suppression. If available, material safety data sheets carried by all carriers should be inspected. All freight train conductors carry a "consist," which contains a detailed accounting of all rail car locations on the train, their contents, hazard potential, and specific instructions on suppression. The rail industry also has many hazardous materials specialists on-staff. Their expertise and that of local and regional experts should be requested for evaluating

hazards before blindly attacking a fire. At a minimum, all responders should have access to and familiarity with the Department of Transportation's *Emergency Response Guidebook*, which lists most industrial hazards, their placard identification numbers, and suppression information.

Although tunnels themselves are confined spaces, tunnel areas and operations generally affect a much broader expanse. As a tunnel fire burns, smoke, accompanied by possibly toxic gases, will be released out of the tunnel ends or ventilation buildings. This smoke should be monitored continuously for possible community hazards. If the potential for toxic releases is recognized, early consideration and planning for resident evacuation should be undertaken. Closure of major vehicular or subway routes can cause major traffic delays and delays in travel for emergency vehicles. In addition, tunnels are often lined with communications and Internet data cables. Fires often destroy these lines and can cause significant disruption of telecommunications traffic on a regional or national scale.[7]

◀ PRE-INCIDENT ACTIONS

Ideally, emergency response planning for tunnel fires should start from the design phase and continue throughout the lifetime of the tunnel.[8] In established tunnels, all emergency operation plans should be updated and amended to address specific hazards associated with fires and explosions. Plans should specifically address evacuation, ventilation, and fire suppression for all of the tunnels located in a given jurisdiction. Because each tunnel's construction is different, it is imperative that emergency operations personnel become familiar with each tunnel's infrastructure. Site visits, tabletop drills, and exercises should be coordinated with tunnel officials. These training sessions serve many purposes, including conducting hazard analysis, validating operating procedures, identifying and correcting flaws, testing communications equipment, practicing unified incident command, and improving relationships between agencies. Ventilation systems and water-delivery systems should be tested on a regular basis. Because of the hazardous materials potential, a network of specialists who can respond to any significant event should be formed, if one does not already exist. Personnel and agencies that should be included in the preparation for tunnel fires are fire service personal, hazardous materials responders and structural rescue specialists, emergency medical service(s) (EMS), governmental officials responsible for environmental protection, railroad and transportation officials, industrial hygienists, toxicologists, structural tunnel engineers, utility companies, and public works officials. This list is not inclusive and will likely vary by jurisdiction and local risk potential.

▶ POST-INCIDENT ACTIONS

Second only to ensuring responder safety, the next most important priority during a tunnel fire is to evacuate all of the people trapped inside. In large roadway tunnels and subway systems, there may be hundreds or thousands of people who need evacuation.[9] In contrast, if used strictly for freight, trains commonly travel with only a two- or three-person crew. Early establishment of incident command and a coordinated response among tunnel authorities and the responding emergency services is essential. Tunnel control center officials can help locate the fire and direct appropriate application of ventilation to provide a safe environment for evacuating people. Rapid identification of possible hazardous materials should be sought before the initiation of conventional fire-suppression activities. Most tunnel fires involve single vehicles and do not represent a significant threat to other motorists or the tunnel; however, larger trucks and fires involving flammable liquids can present a much greater hazard. A rapid but informed and methodical approach is warranted when dealing with unknown hazards in a confined space such as a tunnel.

✚ MEDICAL TREATMENT OF CASUALTIES

Most injuries occurring as a result of a tunnel fire will be related to smoke inhalation. If people are able to escape the fire by crossing over to an adjacent tube, they may avoid potentially fatal exposure to smoke and superheated gases. Any people trapped on the exhaust side of a substantial fire, once longitudinal ventilation has been initiated, may not survive. Rescuers should concentrate on rapid evacuation of motorists and passengers to a safe location outside the tunnel. Rescue operations should focus on checking abandoned vehicles and subway cars for people unable to ambulate to safety. EMS personnel should follow standard protocols for triage and transportation of the injured. Burn centers and centers with hyperbaric capabilities may be warranted in some circumstances.

? UNIQUE CONSIDERATIONS

Tunnel fires present numerous unique challenges that make emergency response dangerous and, at times, frustrating. Access to the fire is often hampered by several factors. Because of the confined space and dense smoke, visibility will likely be nonexistent. Many tunnels are quite long, and depending on the tunnel, a reliable water supply may not be available close to the fire. Once a fire breaks out, people will abandon their vehicles, obstructing the tunnel and making access by any means other than walking impossible. Firefighters may have great distances to cover by foot, reducing their available air from self-contained breathing apparatuses once they reach the fire.

Other conditions make suppression activities very dangerous. Ambient oxygen levels may be significantly diminished. The confined space may make rapid evacuation impossible, and usually there are no areas of refuge should the fire flash over or explode. If flammable liquids are extinguished, their vapors remain volatile and could saturate the tunnel, creating a dangerous explosive condition. In Swiss tunnel fire simulations using an abandoned rail tunnel, a gasoline fire spontaneously exploded 19 minutes after it was initially extinguished by sprinklers.[2] Another factor complicating suppression activities can be the development of dangerous steam clouds within the tunnel. Without effective means of escape, application of water to intensely burning fires can create a hazard to firefighters and evacuating victims far greater than the fire itself.

The possibility of terrorist acts should be taken into consideration when responding to a tunnel fire incident.[10,11] For instance, tunnel ventilation may need to be stopped in the unlikely event of a biological attack involving airborne agents. Also, it may be possible that the tunnel's fire suppression systems could be used for gross decontamination in special circumstances. These incidents should be dealt with individually and in consultation with subject matter experts.

⚠ PITFALLS

Several potential pitfalls in response to a tunnel fire exist. These include the following:

- Failure to proactively familiarize operations personnel with specific tunnel features, systems, and hazards
- Inappropriate management of the ventilation system, which can endanger evacuating people and complicate suppression activities
- Failure to test the capacity of ventilation and standpipe systems before a fire
- Failure to coordinate a network of hazardous materials specialists who can respond and aid in hazard analysis, mitigation, and clean-up
- Premature initiation of fire suppression activities before all potential hazards are identified
- Failure to verify that abandoned vehicles are empty and do not contain living, nonambulatory patients

REFERENCES

1. The Fort McHenry Tunnel, a Toll Facility of the Maryland Transportation Authority. *The Maryland Transportation Authority, Office of Media and Customer Relations*; 2004. Baltimore, MD.
2. Bajwa C. *An Analysis of a Spent Fuel Transportation Cask Under Severe Fire Accident Conditions. ML022340066.* Washington, DC: Spent Fuel Project Office, U.S. Nuclear Regulatory Commission; 2002.
3. Styron HC. CSX Tunnel Fire, Baltimore, MD. USFA-TR-140. Technical Report Series, U.S. Fire Administration, Federal Emergency Management Agency. July 2001.
4. Thematic Network Fire in Tunnels. *Fire in Tunnels: General Report.* Available at: http://www.wtcb.be/homepage/index.cfm?cat=services&sub=standards_regulations&pag=fire&art=library&niv01=fit.
5. Hay RE. Publication no. FHWA-RD-83-032 U.S. Department of Transportation, Federal Highway Administration—Office of Bridge Technology *Prevention and Control of Highway Tunnel Fires.* Springfield, VA: National Technical Information Service; May 2000, 22161.
6. CFD (Computational Fluid Dynamics) analysis of fire growth and smoke spread in tunnels. ARUP Fire Safety Engineering for Tunnels. Available at: http://www.arup.com/fire/skill.cfm?pageid=4383.
7. Media Advisory—Keynote. *The Internet Performance Authority.* San Mateo, CA: Keynote Systems; 2001.
8. English G. *Incident Management and Tunnel System;* March 2010, Fourth International Symposium on Tunnel Safety and Security, Frankfurt, Germany.
9. *Facts at a Glance.* Chicago: Chicago Transit Authority, 2004. Available at: http://www.transitchicago.com/welcome/overview.html#a.
10. Woodall J. Tokyo subway gas attack. *Lancet.* 1997;350(9073):296.
11. Carresi AL. The 2004 Madrid Train Bombings: an analysis of prehospital management. *Disasters.* 2008;32(1):41–65.

177 CHAPTER

Gunshot Attack: Mass Casualties

Leon D. Sanchez and Matthew R. Babineau

DESCRIPTION OF EVENT

In 2010 there were 31,672 deaths due to firearm injuries in the United States, 11,085 of which were due to homicide.[1] Gunshot injuries include violence-related, accidental, and self-inflicted injuries.[2] The majority of these injuries are caused by handguns. Although most gunshot attacks involve only one victim, there have been several well-publicized cases in which multiple persons were killed and injured in a single event. On December 14, 2012, it took less than 10 minutes to complete the deadliest school shooting in United States history, resulting in 27 dead including the shooter, at Sandy Hook Elementary School in Newtown, Connecticut.

Firearms include two basic types: rifled firearms and shotguns (Fig. 177-1). A rifled firearm (i.e., pistol or rifle) has spiral grooves in its barrel. When the cartridge is fired, the burning of the powder generates gas in a contained space, and the pressure generated by the gas propels the bullet forward. The bullet accelerates while inside the barrel, reaches its maximum speed upon exit (muzzle velocity), and heads toward its target. As the bullet enters tissue, it will begin to tumble and deform. Depending on the makeup of the bullet and the properties of the tissue through which it travels, it may expand, fragment, or remain in one piece.[3-6]

Shotguns differ from rifles and pistols in that they have a smooth barrel that discharges hot gases, wad, and either multiple projectiles or a single projectile (rifled slug). Shot charges containing multiple projectiles spread out from the muzzle in a cone-like pattern. The distance from the muzzle of the shotgun to the point of impact of the projectiles is a key determinant of the magnitude of injury. At short range (less than 6 m), the shot charge containing multiple projectiles results predominantly in a single-hole wound (diameter of less than or equal to 6 cm) that communicates with a deep underlying wound with massive tissue destruction. At this short range, soft-tissue impact deforms the individual pellets, increasing their original cross section with a concomitant increase in tissue crush or hole size. The multiple pellets result in severe disruption between the multiple wound channels. A gradual decrease in the amount of pellet deformation and tissue destruction occurs as the distance of the impact range increases. When the impact range exceeds 7 m, the multiple projectiles result in numerous discrete wounds that are not associated with underlying massive tissue destruction.[3]

Shotguns also can discharge rifled slugs that are designed for killing larger animals. The muzzle velocity of rifled slugs (487 m/s) is approximately half that of nonexpanding, fully jacketed rifle projectiles. The rifled slug does not hold the point orientation that it has as it is propelled from the muzzle of the gun, but drifts toward a sideways orientation as it moves toward the target. The rifled slugs experience a 25% decrease in velocity as the impact range increases from 5 to 45 m. At short range (less than or equal to 45 m), the slug deforms on striking the tissue, thereby enhancing the size of the permanent and temporary cavities.

PRE-INCIDENT ACTIONS

Hospital, emergency department, and outpatient facilities should all have general disaster plans in place in the event of an attack. Mass-casualty events require coordination of local, state, and federal public safety resources. Both emergency medical service (EMS)- and hospital-based triage systems may need to be altered in the event of a large number of patients seeking medical care within a brief period of time. Health care providers should practice universal precautions. In the event of multiple casualties, triaging of the victims at the scene and on arrival to the hospital will be necessary. Protocols for triaging of victims are part of a properly prepared disaster plan. Disaster plans should be in place, and personnel should be familiar with the plans so that when an event does occur, a minimum of confusion will ensue.

POST-INCIDENT ACTIONS

First responders and EMS personnel should confirm the scene is safe before evaluating casualties at the site of the event. Increasing numbers of state and local EMS departments have Tactical EMS-trained personnel who are able to provide initial first aid procedures to victims and first responders before the scene has been secured.[7,8] A joint commission between the American College of Surgery and the Federal Bureau of Investigation created the "Hartford Consensus," which describes methods to minimize loss of life in these instances. Their core recommendations are contained in the acronym THREAT (Threat Suppression, Hemorrhage control, Rapid Evacuation to safety, Assessment by medical providers, Transport to definitive care).[7,9]

If a large number of casualties are identified and a disaster needs to be declared, the proper channels must be notified and triage protocols instituted. Receiving hospitals should be given as much advance notice as possible to ensure that hospital personnel will be ready to handle the influx of patients. A "reverse triage" scenario may develop in which individuals with minor injuries rapidly self-extricate and self-present to first responders or local hospitals, straining resources before the

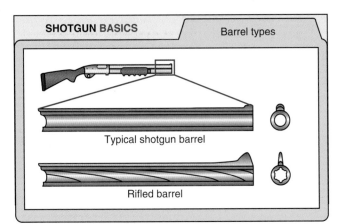

FIG 177-1 Rifles and handguns have grooves in the barrel (called rifling), which make bullets spin when fired. Shotgun barrels typically have no grooves and are called smooth bore. (Redrawn from Information for Firearms. Revolver Publishing, LLC, Berlin, Germany.)

more severely injured patients arrive.[7,9] Early psychological assessment and intervention for victims, bystanders, and personnel responding to the scene may help mitigate long-term mental health consequences from the incident.[10]

CLINICAL PRESENTATION

Tissue is injured by a bullet via two mechanisms: tissue crush and tissue stretch. These two mechanisms correspond to the permanent and temporary cavities created by passage of the projectile.[4,11] As the bullet travels through tissue, it will crush tissue that is directly in its path. This is the primary method of injury from gunshot wounds. The most important determinant of injury is the tissue the bullet crushes. The tissue that is crushed corresponds to the permanent cavity formed by the bullet. Injury created by the temporary cavity becomes more important with higher-energy bullets (see Chapter 178).

✚ MEDICAL TREATMENT OF CASUALTIES

Initial evaluation of persons with gunshot wounds is similar to that of any multiple-trauma victim, with initial evaluation of the ABCs (i.e., airway, breathing, circulation), followed by the secondary survey and ongoing monitoring, including vital signs, electrocardiographic monitoring, and pulse oximetry. The focus of the examination is the detection of penetrating or perforating injuries. A careful examination of the patient including the back, under the hair, the axillae, and the gluteal fold will help identify injuries. Radiographs of the areas the bullet is thought to have traversed are indicated to identify the position of the projectiles. Laboratory studies should be ordered as clinically indicated.

Evaluation, resuscitation, and ongoing management should proceed as for any other multi-trauma victim in both the prehospital setting and the emergency department. The management of gunshot wounds is best conducted in consultation with a trauma surgeon. If adequate resources are unavailable, the decision to transfer the patient should be made early in the course of treatment.

Wounds that may have crossed the mediastinum require a thorough evaluation even in the stable patient. In this setting, injury to the aorta, heart, pericardium, and esophagus must be ruled out. Patients who present with unstable vital signs or become unstable during evaluation should receive bilateral chest tubes. The presence of pericardial tamponade should also be considered; using bedside ultrasound is a fast way to identify cardiac tamponade. Surgical exploration is often indicated in these patients.[5]

Patients with penetrating gunshot wounds to the abdomen require exploratory laparotomy even in the presence of stable vital signs. Stable patients with back or flank wounds can be evaluated by computed tomography and observation, but these patients may also benefit from surgical exploration. This decision must be made in conjunction with the trauma surgeon.

Injuries to the extremities require evaluation of the distal neurovascular status. A bullet does not need to transect a vessel to cause injury. The development of compartment syndrome resulting from swelling of the injured area should be considered. Angiography is indicated if arterial injury is suspected. Fractures from a gunshot wound should be treated as open fractures with early administration of antibiotics. Debridement of devitalized soft tissue is often necessary.[5]

Penetrating gunshot wounds to the head are often not survivable. For patients with this type of injury who arrive at the hospital alive, consultation with a neurosurgeon is indicated. Injuries to the spine can occur even when the bullet does not actually pass through the vertebral canal. Use of steroids is not indicated for penetrating cord injuries. Additionally, the presence of a central nervous system injury should not delay assessment for the presence of thoracoabdominal injuries that can be rapidly fatal.

❓ UNIQUE CONSIDERATIONS

Gunshot wounds must be reported to the appropriate authorities. In most cases, shootings become the subject of a criminal investigation by law enforcement authorities. Therefore the medical record and patient property should be preserved as evidence. If patient clothing is cut, care should be used to avoid cutting through portions a bullet might have gone through. Any material that needs to be saved for law enforcement authorities should be placed in paper bags because plastic bags will trap moisture, which can degrade evidence. The location of all wounds identified should be recorded in the medical record, including comments on the presence of any powder residue observed surrounding the wound. It is often difficult to differentiate entrance from exit wounds. Although it is often thought that the smaller wound must be the entrance wound, this is not always true. If a bullet is recovered, avoid making any markings on the sides of the bullet because this will interfere with forensic evaluation of rifling patterns.[3] Any marking of recovered bullets that may be necessary for the preservation of chain of custody should be at the nose or base.

⚠ PITFALLS

Several potential pitfalls in response to a gunshot attack exist. These include the following:

- Allowing EMS personnel to enter the scene before it is secured
- Failure to have a disaster plan in place prior to the event
- Failure to involve a trauma surgeon early in the management of the patient
- Failure to consider transfer of the patient to another facility
- Delays in the evaluation of stable patients with thoracoabdominal injuries

REFERENCES

1. Murphy SL, Xu J, Kochanek KD. Deaths: Final Data for 2010. *National Vital Statistics Reports*, vol. 61. Atlanta: U.S. Department of Health and Human Services, Public Health Service. Centers for Disease Control and Prevention; May 8, 2013, No. 4.
2. Weapon Related Injury Surveillance System. *Weapon Related Injury Update Oct 1999*. Boston: Massachusetts Department of Public Health, Bureau of Health Statistics, Research and Evaluation; 1999.

3. Di Maio V. *Gunshot Wounds.* Boca Raton, Fla: CRC Press LLC; 1999.

4. Fackler ML. Ballistic injury. *Ann Emerg Med.* 1986;15:1451–1455.

5. Swan KG. Missile injuries: wound ballistics and principles of management. *Mil Med.* 1987;152:29–34.

6. Zajychuck R, ed. *Textbook of Military Medicine. Part I, Volume 5. Conventional Warfare: Ballistics, Blast and Burn Injuries.* Washington, D.C: TMM Publications; 1989.

7. U.S. Fire Administration. *Fire/Emergency Medical Services Department Operational Considerations Guide for Active Shooter and Mass Casualty Incidents;* September 2013. https://www.usfa.fema.gov/fireservice/ops_tactics/disasters/.

8. Callaway DW, Smith ER, Cain J, et al. Tactical emergency casualty care (TECC): guidelines for the provision of prehospital trauma care in high threat environments. *J Spec Oper Med.* 2001 Summer;11(3):104–122.

9. Jacobs LM, Wade DS, McSwain NE, et al. The Hartford consensus: THREAT, a medical disaster preparedness concept. *J Am Coll Surg.* 2013;217(5):947–953.

10. Stevens G, Byrne S, Raphael B, Ollerton R. Disaster medical assistance teams: what psychosocial support is needed? *Prehosp Disaster Med.* 2008;23(2):202–207.

11. Fackler ML. Wound ballistics: a review of common misconceptions. *JAMA.* 1980;259:2730.

CHAPTER 178

Sniper Attack

Shawn E. Johnson and Leon D. Sanchez

DESCRIPTION OF EVENT

News reports will often (inaccurately) use the term sniper to describe anyone shooting with a rifle at another person. A sniper is a concealed, usually skilled shooter who fires at exposed persons. These attacks typically occur using powerful high-energy, military-style assault rifles.[1] A true sniper is a highly trained marksman with acquired field craft used to disguise their movements and location. Snipers generally deliver lethal wounds while creating chaos and fear in a demoralizing fashion. To avoid being discovered, snipers generally engage their targets from a distance (i.e., 100 to 2000 yards), depending on their skill level and the type of rifle used. In general, a sniper will take as few shots as possible to inflict damage without the risk of being discovered. The more shots fired by a sniper, the greater the chances he can be located from his firing position. With all this being said, the only true sniper attacks in recent history which fulfilled the criteria above were the Beltway sniper attacks that covered a span of 3 weeks in October 2002. Whether a case of a "true sniper" or a layman with a rifle, innocent victims can be targeted and inflicted with devastating physical and psychological injuries.

PRE-INCIDENT ACTIONS

As with the sniper attacks in the Washington, DC, area in October 2002, confusion and panic may ensue if a sniper attack were to occur. The most effective way emergency departments can prepare for these types of incidents is to have a universal all-hazards disaster casualty management plan. Personnel at every echelon of care should be familiar with the plans in order to minimize confusion. This may require coordination of local, state, and federal public safety resources.

Health care providers should always practice universal precautions. In the event of mass casualties, protocols for triaging victims must be used. It is important for hospitals to periodically conduct practical exercises to test assumptions and current protocols. The exercise should not just focus on emergency department actions, but to also include other services (e.g., surgery, psychiatric and chaplain services) to enhance organizational and community preparedness.[2]

POST-INCIDENT ACTIONS

Situational awareness (SA) refers to the capability to maintain constant vigilance of current environmental surroundings and being able to anticipate making critical decisions of potential outcomes. If a sniper attack is suspected and the shooter has not been identified, prehospital personnel and first responders should approach with an escort of appropriate security force (i.e., police) or after the scene has been rendered safe by law enforcement. It is critical to approach the scene with keen SA and avoid tunnel vision while rendering aid to casualties.

Victims of sniper attack should be transported and treated behind cover if any threat is suspected.[3] Medical personnel at the scene should continually assess the environment to detect and protect against any perceived threats. If patients are conscious, they should be asked how many shots they heard and any other information they have relating to the event, such as their position and that of the assailant.

There should be close communication with emergency medical services personnel and the receiving hospitals to give as much lead time as possible for health care facilities to prepare for casualties. It is also important to be prepared to offer psychological help for victims and their families.

CLINICAL PRESENTATION

Injuries from a gunshot are the product of two mechanisms: tissue crush and tissue stretch. As the bullet travels through tissue, it will crush tissue that is directly in its path, which results in a permanent cavity. This is the primary method of injury from most gunshot wounds. Passage of the projectile at a high rate of speed also displaces tissue surrounding the direct path away from the path of the projectile. As this tissue stretches away from the path, a temporary tissue cavity is formed. This a more significant mechanism of injury with higher-velocity bullets, such as those encountered in a sniper attack.[4,5]

The degree of tissue stretch and the size of the temporary cavity that is formed vary depending on the elastic properties of the injured tissue. Elastic tissues such as muscle, skin, and lung are good energy absorbers. Their elastic properties allow them to maintain a lot of their structure and function, even after temporary cavitation. Inelastic tissue, including liver, heart, and brain, will be fractured and rendered nonviable to a much greater degree by a temporary cavity.[6]

Because the brain is encased in a solid container (the skull), brain tissue is even more susceptible to injury from temporary cavitation than other inelastic tissue. The solid container prevents tissue displacement during tissue cavitation, resulting in increased pressure inside the skull as a bullet penetrates. This pressure can only be relieved either through the entrance or exit wounds. The brain is also very sensitive to structural disruption. This combination makes high-velocity gunshots to the head very destructive.

MEDICAL TREATMENT OF CASUALTIES

Initial evaluation of persons with gunshot wounds in the prehospital setting and the emergency department is similar to that for any trauma victim. Initial assessment of the ABCs (i.e., airway, breathing, circulation) should be followed by the secondary survey and ongoing monitoring of vital signs. The focus of the examination is the detection of penetrating or perforating injuries. All clothing should be removed, and careful examination for entrance and exit wounds must include the back, under the hair, the axillae, the perineum, and the gluteal fold. Radiographs can be useful to identify the position of bullets. Radiographs and laboratory studies should be ordered when clinically indicated. Evaluation and treatment of gunshot wounds are best conducted in consultation with a trauma surgeon. Patients should be stabilized and transferred as quickly as possible if appropriate resources are unavailable where they are being treated.

Injury to the aorta, heart, pericardium, and esophagus must be suspected when wounds cross the mediastinum. These wounds require a thorough evaluation, even in stable patients. Surgical exploration is often indicated in these patients. Those who present with unstable vital signs or who become unstable during evaluation should receive bilateral chest tubes, and the presence of pericardial tamponade should be considered. Ultrasound is a fast way of identifying cardiac tamponade.[7]

Patients with gunshot wounds to the flank or back can be evaluated by computed tomography and observed if their conditions are stable. The decision to observe a patient must be made in conjunction with a trauma surgeon because these patients may benefit from surgical exploration. Patients with gunshot wounds to the abdomen require exploratory laparotomy.

Gunshot wounds to the extremities may cause neurovascular damage and fractures. Neurovascular function should be assessed carefully. There should be close monitoring for the development of compartment syndrome from swelling of the injured area. Angiography is indicated whenever arterial damage is suspected. High-velocity wounds should be debrided and closed secondarily. Fractures from a gunshot wound are considered open fractures, and early antibiotics should be instituted.[7]

Evaluation of gunshot wounds to the head should be done in consultation with a neurosurgeon. These injuries are often not survivable. Spinal cord injuries can result from direct penetrating injuries, but the spine can be injured by temporary cavitation even in the absence of direct passage of the bullet through the vertebral canal. Steroids are not indicated in direct penetrating injury to the spinal cord. Although injuries to the central nervous system can be distracting to the physician, it is important not to delay the assessment and treatment of thoracoabdominal injuries.

❓ UNIQUE CONSIDERATIONS

Gunshot wounds must be reported to the appropriate authorities. Special care must be taken because the medical record and patient property often become evidence. Paper bags should be used to collect material to be saved for law enforcement because plastic bags can trap moisture, resulting in damage to the evidence. If a bullet is recovered and it must be marked, this should be done at the nose or base rather than on the side. Marking the side will interfere with the evaluation of

rifling patterns. Care should be taken during clothing removal to avoid cutting through portions of clothing that a bullet might have gone through. The location of all wounds identified should be recorded in the medical record, with comment on the presence of any powder residue observed surrounding the wound. Attempts to differentiate between entrance and exit wounds are often educated guesses. The smaller wound is often thought to be the entrance wound, but this is not always the case.[8]

❗ PITFALLS

Several potential pitfalls in response to a sniper attack exist. These include the following:

- Failure to ensure that a scene is secure prior to approaching victims
- Failure to fully examine the patient and identify multiple injuries
- Failure to apply an effective tourniquet[9]
- Failure to recognized and treat a tension pneumothorax[10]
- Failure to consult a surgeon early in the management of the patient
- Failure to consider transfer to another facility
- Failure to fully evaluate stable patients with thoracoabdominal injuries

REFERENCES

1. Barach E, Tomlanovich M, Nowack R. Ballistics: a pathophysiologic examination of the wounding mechanisms of firearms, Part I. *J Trauma.* 1986;26:225–235; Part II. *J Trauma.* 1986;26:374–383.
2. Swienton R, Subbarao I, Markenson D, et al. *Basic Disaster Life Support Version 3.0 Course Manual.* 1st ed. American Medical Association; 2012, Chp 1, 14-28.
3. McSwain N, Salomone J. Prehospital Trauma Life Support. In: McSwain N, Salomone J, Butler FK, eds. military edition Revised 5th ed. St. Louis, Missour: Mosby Inc; 2005, Chp 16.
4. Fackler ML. Ballistic injury. *Ann Emerg Med.* 1986;15:1451–1455.
5. Fackler ML. Wound ballistics: a review of common misconceptions. *JAMA.* 1980;259:2730.
6. Zajychuck R, ed. Conventional warfare: ballistics, blast and burn injuries. In: Bellamy F, ed. *Textbook of Military Medicine. Part I,* vol. 5. Falls Church, VA: TMM Publications; 1989.
7. Swan KG. Missile injuries: wound ballistics and principles of management. *Mil Med.* 1987;152:29–34.
8. Di Maio V. *Gunshot Wounds: Practical Aspects of Firearms, Ballistics, and Forensic Techniques.* Boca Raton, Fla: CRC Press LLC; 1999.
9. Kragh JF. Emergency tourniquet effectiveness in four positions on the proximal thigh. *J Spec Op Med.* Spring 2014;14(1):26–29.
10. Butler FK, McSwain N, Adkisson G, et al. Management of open pneumothorax in tactical combat casualty care. *J Spec Op Med.* 2013, TCCC Guidelines change 13-02.

CHAPTER 179

Grenade and Pipe Bomb Injuries

Charles Stewart

DESCRIPTION OF EVENT

Recent terrorism has included an increasing use of explosives. The weapon of choice of these terrorists is often the grenade, pipe bomb, or explosive vest. Other groups may use a rocket-propelled grenade originally designed for military applications to defeat armor.

Pipe Bombs

Design of a pipe bomb is quite simple: a piece of pipe is filled with explosives, and end caps on the pipe are used to contain the explosives and the force of the explosion.[1] The fragments of the exploding pipe are propelled by the explosion and can cause lethal injury at a considerable distance. As pipe comes in many sizes and materials, the shape and size of a pipe bomb are quite variable. The explosives used for pipe bombs are also quite variable and may range from improvised explosives such as match heads or powder scavenged from fireworks to black powder or commercial gunpowder. These devices often either contain scrap metal or are wrapped in scrap metal to increase the number of fragments and resultant injuries.

Pipe bombs can be carried in a satchel, briefcase, or backpack. The Centennial Park terrorist explosive device in the 1996 Olympics was a backpack containing pipe bombs.

Pressure Cooker Bombs

A pressure cooker bomb is a variant of the pipe bomb made by placing explosive material into a pressure cooker and attaching an initiating device. This type of bomb is a popular terrorist weapon.[2,3] The bomb can be ignited using a simple command electronic device, such as a cell phone or pager, a timing device (e.g., a kitchen timer or alarm clock), or a thermal fuse. The power of the explosion, as always, depends on the explosives used (both type and amount) and on the size of the pressure cooker. The fragmentation of the pressure cooker provides potentially lethal fragments, but the bomber can add additional material such as nails, nuts, and bolts to increase lethality. Other than the increased size of the container and hence increase in potential size of the explosion, little difference exists between a pipe bomb and a pressure cooker bomb.

Pressure cooker bombs can be carried in a satchel or backpack. The 2006 Mumbai train bombing explosive devices were seven pressure cooker bombs that killed 209 people.[4] In 2010, the Times Square car bombing attempt was a pressure cooker bomb that failed to explode. The 2013 Boston Marathon bombers used two backpacks containing pressure cooker bombs built with nails and ball bearings and using black powder as the explosive.[5]

Grenades

In World War II (WWII), the grenade was a cast-iron segmented oval device designed to fit the thrower's hand. This is often called the *pineapple* grenade because of its shape. After the Vietnam War, the American army deployed an egg-shaped grenade that was constructed by wrapping scored steel wire around a high-explosive core. This wire would fragment much more reliably and in smaller pieces than the older cast-iron bodies. This design has been copied and improved and is widely available throughout the world. The United States M-26 grenade weighs 425 g and has a fuse delay of 5 seconds. The average throwing distance is about 40 m. Its blast radius is 10 m, with a killing distance of 5 m and a wounding distance of up to 25 m.

Two special forms of grenade have evolved that are now widely dispersed. These are the rifle grenades designed to project the grenade beyond the soldier's ability to throw and the antitank grenade, which has evolved into the rocket-propelled grenade discussed below.

Other types of grenades are also produced, but most of these have lesser wounding potential. These include concussion grenades (flashbang grenades), illuminating grenades, smoke grenades, incendiary grenades, and chemical or gas grenades.

Rifle Grenades

The grenade launcher has evolved into a weapon that projects a grenade with good accuracy for about 200 m. First employed during the Vietnam War, the M-79 grenade launcher resembles a short, fat (40-mm), breech-loading, break-open single-shot shotgun. The military also designed a grenade launcher that clamps onto the infantryman's M-16 rifle (the M-203 grenade launcher) that uses the same ammunition as the M-79 weapon. Numerous similar designs now exist for these weapons and are used both by NATO and former Warsaw Pact nations. Comparable devices are often used by police forces to project riot-control agents, "nonlethal" beanbag rounds, and smoke. Multiple different rounds exist for both military and civilian grenade-launching weapons, and the emergency physician may well see the use of these devices. Grenade rounds contain about as much explosive and cause as much damage as the more common baseball grenade.

Rocket-Propelled Grenades

The need for an antitank weapon that could reliably defeat enemy armor has been present since the tank was first used in World War I. One solution to this problem was to upsize the grenade and mount it atop a rocket—the rocket-propelled grenade or RPG for short. Warsaw Pact countries manufactured these devices in the millions and sold the inexpensive RPG to hundreds of countries, rebels, and terrorist groups. The former Soviet RPG-7 launcher is reloadable (Fig. 179-1). There are four basic loads for the RPG-7: the high explosive anti-tank (HEAT), two-stage HEAT for defeating reactive armor, antipersonnel fragmentation, and a thermobaric explosive round. The United States distributes a similar light antitank weapon (the M-72 LAW or the M-136 AT4) that is not reloadable.

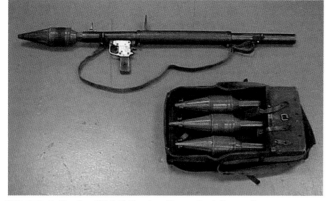

FIG 179-1 Soviet RPG-7 Rocket-Propelled Grenade.

Although illegal for civilians to possess in the United States and most other countries, the RPG device is portable and can cross borders easily. The RPG is designed to defeat the armor on a tank and carries substantially more explosive than most other devices discussed in this chapter. Although designed to defeat tank armor, any RPG and variant rounds are effective against personnel in the open.

CLINICAL PRESENTATION

Trauma caused by explosions traditionally has been divided into injuries caused by the direct effect of the blast wave (primary injuries), the effects caused by other objects that are accelerated by the explosive wave (secondary injuries), the effects caused by movement of the victim (tertiary injuries), and miscellaneous effects caused by the explosion or explosives or the byproducts of the explosion.

The victims of primary blast injury almost always have other types of injuries, such as penetrating wounds from flying debris or blunt trauma from impact on immovable objects.[6] The number of victims of primary blast injury due to a grenade, pipe bomb, pressure cooker bomb, or suicide vest will likely not be large, as the quantities of explosives contained are much smaller than most explosive devices. This phenomenon is covered in other sections or chapters in this book; the reader should refer to the section on blast injury.

With both grenades and pipe bombs, secondary blast injuries are both the most common and the intended injury mechanism. Terrorist devices often add additional objects such as nails, nuts, and bolts to the explosive mixture in order to increase the effects of secondary blast injury.[7] Military devices such as grenades are designed to increase the number of fragments flung by the explosion. The penetrating injuries occur most often in exposed areas such as the head, neck, and extremities.

Tertiary blast injuries are caused when the victim's body is propelled into another object by the blast winds.[8,9] This is unlikely to occur from the relatively small amounts of explosives found in a grenade. It may be possible to note these effects from the larger amount of explosive in an RPG, pipe bomb, or suicide vest.

◀◀ PRE-INCIDENT ACTIONS

It is difficult to plan for the consequences of an explosive device that can be carried in a backpack briefcase, or even a pocket. The use of these devices in the United States is not common, but several events have occurred as discussed previously. The emergency physician is increasingly likely to see the effects of these devices and must be prepared to treat the victims of these explosive hazards.

▶▶ POST-INCIDENT ACTIONS

The predominant injury found after an explosion of a grenade or pipe bomb will be penetrating trauma from fragment wounds. Those who are quite close to the blast may sustain either primary blast injury or traumatic amputations.

Guidelines for field medical care include the following:

- Initial care is similar to regular trauma care.
- Rapid evacuation increases the chance of survival.
- Do not do definitive care in triage.
- Arterial bleeding from traumatic amputations should be controlled with tourniquets until the area is entirely safe and the casualty can have definitive care.
- Do not do extensive resuscitation in the field.
- CPR at the scene of a mass casualty is not indicated.

An explosion that occurs in a confined space (including vehicles, mines, buildings, and subways) is associated with greater morbidity and mortality.

✚ MEDICAL TREATMENT OF CASUALTIES

Most of the injuries seen after the explosive in a grenade or pipe bomb detonates are blunt, penetrating, and thermal trauma that is well known to prehospital providers, emergency physicians, and trauma surgeons.[10] Much of this trauma is soft-tissue, orthopedic, or head injuries.[11–13] The initial approach to the casualty with blast-related injury from grenades or pipe bombs is the same as any other trauma victim.

The first and most important step of management is assessing life support needs and ensuring that the patient has an adequate airway, appropriate ventilation, and adequate circulation. As noted above, use of tourniquets can buy time to evacuate the victim to a safe area where appropriate care can be rendered.

A thorough physical examination should be performed. Most of the wounds will be fragments from the device or metal surrounding the device.

There are few screening studies that are of any benefit in the casualty with primary blast injury. Indeed, for these smaller devices, studies should be directed toward the effects of multiple penetrating fragments. A seemingly small abrasion or wound may mask the entrance wound for a substantial fragment. The physician should also remember that blast fragments may be traveling up to 5 times as fast as a military bullet.

A chest x-ray (CXR) should be obtained in all patients who have been near a significant explosion. If the casualty is not wearing body armor, presume that there are fragments in the chest until CXR is negative for both pneumothorax and intrathoracic fragments. A CXR may also show fragments or free air under the diaphragm, signifying hollow viscous rupture in the abdomen. Long-bone films are indicated in traumatic amputation or if wounds are found in the patient's extremities.

A computed tomography (CT) study of the head, chest, or abdomen should be obtained if the history or physical examination suggests pathology in these areas. If the patient is unconscious, these CT studies are not optional. All debris that is flung by the explosion is not radiopaque, and the wise provider should carefully explore injuries and consider CT or ultrasound of wounds to evaluate for radiolucent foreign bodies.

The only laboratory studies that are immediately useful are serial hemoglobin or hematocrit determinations and urinalysis. The urinalysis may be useful in detecting casualties who have severe ureteral, bladder, or kidney injuries. The hemoglobin or hematocrit data may be used as a guide for blood transfusion requirements. Multichannel electrolytes, clotting studies, and serum enzyme determinations may be useful as baseline studies, but will not change any immediate management.

Hypotension in blast injury victims can be due to several mechanisms:

- Blood loss due to wounds otherwise not related to the cardiovascular system. This is particularly common with traumatic amputations and the multiple fragments sustained at close range from a modern fragmentation grenade.
- Blood loss due to gastrointestinal hemorrhage.
- Blood loss due to intraabdominal solid organ rupture.
- Hypotension from compression of vessels and heart by pneumothorax.
- Hypotension due to the cardiovascular effects of an air embolism.
- Hypotension due to vagal reflexes.

The disposition of these patients depends on the injury sustained by each victim. Those who were close to the center of the explosion should be considered for observation for at least 24 hours, even if they have no obvious injuries.

🔍 UNIQUE CONSIDERATIONS

Expect that the most severely injured patients will arrive after the less injured.[14] The less injured often skip emergency medical services (EMS) and proceed directly to the closest hospitals. For a rough prediction of the "first wave" of casualties, double the first hour's casualty count.

Ensure that physical activity of the victims is minimized after the blast explosion. Exertion after the blast explosion can increase the severity of primary blast injury. This was seen in WWII where some blast casualties appeared well, but died after vigorous exercise.[15]

⚠ PITFALLS

Interior versus Exterior Blast

Explosions in a closed area are significantly more dangerous than explosions that occur outdoors. Fragments can travel significantly farther in open air. In closed spaces, fragments can be absorbed or may ricochet from walls and ceilings. In the open air, the blast energy dissipates rapidly as the inverse cube of the distance from the source. Conversely, indoor blast waves can reflect from walls, floors, and ceilings with significant exacerbation of blast effects on the trapped victims.

Secondary and Multiple Devices

Recent bombings have often included simultaneous or near-simultaneous use of multiple devices. Suicide bombers frequently have either a partner or a monitor who can initiate a secondary device to increase casualties involving fire, police, and EMS responders. Remember to check all victims for weapons, booby traps, and explosives. It is quite common for a bomber to become a victim of his own device. It is also common for a secondary device to be concealed under a casualty.

Eye Injuries

Up to 10% of all blast survivors have significant eye injuries. These injuries involve perforations from high-velocity projectiles and may have minimal initial discomfort. Indeed, the patient may present for care days, weeks, or months after the event.[14] Findings can include decreased visual acuity, hyphema, globe perforation, subconjunctival hemorrhage, foreign body, or lid lacerations. Patients with eye complaints after a blast injury or with potential eye injuries should have a thorough eye exam.

Blast Lung

If the clinician does not consider the possibility of primary blast injury, it may further complicate the patient's care. Almogy et al. described a

retrospective analysis of 15 suicide bomb attacks treated over a 3-year period in Israeli hospitals.[16] The authors found that patients with >10% burn surface area, skull fracture, or penetrating injuries to head or torso were more likely to also suffer a blast lung injury. This entity is more thoroughly covered elsewhere in this section.

If a patient with a blast lung injury abruptly decompensates, the clinician should presume that the patient has a tension pneumothorax and evaluate or treat accordingly.[17] This is particularly true when the patient has thoracic fragment wounds from a grenade or pipe bomb.

Wound Care

There is about an 80% rate of infection when fragment wounds are sutured.[18] Delayed primary closure with cleansing, irrigation of the wound, and closure of the wound after 72 hours of observation is associated with significantly fewer infections.

Air Transportation

The potential from pneumothorax that results from grenade or pipe bomb explosion can be exacerbated by air evacuation. This creates a controversy. Some authors feel that regardless of the altitude and distance of the flight, casualties with evidence of pneumothorax must have a chest tube placed. Others have noted that when the change in altitude is minimal, there is little risk of worsening of the pneumothorax. Evacuation aircraft should fly at the lowest possible altitude consistent with safety.

REFERENCES

1. Bors D, Cummins J, Goodpaster J. The anatomy of a pipe bomb explosion: measuring the mass and velocity distributions of container fragments. *J Forensic Sci.* Oct 22 2013.
2. The AQ Chef. Make a bomb in the kitchen of your mom. *Inspire.* 2010;1 (1):33–40.
3. Spencer R. Boston Marathon bombs: al-Qaeda's Inspire magazine taught pressure cooker bomb-making techniques. *The Telegraph.* April 16, 2013.
4. CBC News. *A History of Pressure Cooker Bombs.* April 6, 2013, http://www .cbc.ca/news/world/a-history-of-pressure-cooker-bombs-1.1301728.
5. CNN. *Boston Marathon Terror Attack Fast Facts.* 2013, http://www.cnn .com/2013/06/03/us/boston-marathon-terror-attack-fast-facts/. Accessed 22.12.13.
6. Cernak I, Savic J, Ignjatovic D, Jevtic M. Blast injury from explosive munitions. *J Trauma.* 1999;47(1):96–103, discussion 103–104.
7. Caldwell J. *Understanding the Basics of Improvised Explosive Devices (IED).* Civil-Military Fusion Center; 2011.
8. de Candole C. Blast injury. *Can Med Assoc J.* 1967;96:207–214.
9. Stuhmiller J, Phillips Y, Richmond D. The physics and mechanisms of primary blast injury. In: Bellamy R, Zajtchuk R, eds. *Conventional Warfare: Ballistic, Blast, and Burn Injuries.* Washington, DC: Office of the Surgeon General of the US Army; 1991:241–270.
10. Weiner S, Barrett J. Explosions and explosive device-related injuries. In: Weiner SL, Barrett J, eds. *Trauma Management for Civilian and Military Physicians.* Philadelphia, PA: Saunders; 1986:13–26.
11. Hadden W, Rutherford W, Merrett J. The injuries of terrorist bombing: a study of 1532 consecutive patients. *Br J Surg.* 1978;65:525–531.
12. Mallonee S, Shariat S, Stennies G, Waxweiler R, Hogan D, Jordan F. Physical injuries and fatalities resulting from the Oklahoma City bombing. *JAMA.* 1996;276(5):382–387.
13. Frykberg E, Tepas J, Alexander R. The 1983 Beirut airport terrorist bombing: injury patterns and implications for disaster management. *Am Surg.* 1989;55:134–141.
14. *Explosions and Blast Injuries: A Primer for Clinicians.* Atlanta, GA: CDC; 2006.

15. Hutton JJ. Blast lung: history, concepts, and treatment. *Curr Conc Trauma Care.* 1986;9:8–14.

16. Almogy G, Luria T, Richter E, et al. Can external signs of trauma guide management? Lessons learned from suicide bombing attacks in Israel. *Arch Surg.* 2005;140(4):390–393.

17. Biocina B, Sutlic Z, Husedzinovic I, et al. Penetrating cardiothoracic war wounds. *Eur J Cardiothorac Surg.* 1997;11(3):399–405.

18. Almogy G, Rivkind AI. Surgical lessons learned from suicide bombing attacks. *J Am Coll Surg.* 2006;202(2):313–319.

Introduction to Structural Collapse (Crush Injury and Crush Syndrome)

Pier Luigi Ingrassia, Marco Mangini, Luca Ragazzoni, Ahmadreza Djalali, and Francesco Della Corte

DESCRIPTION OF EVENT

Earthquakes cause the majority of deaths related to natural disasters. The building collapse and damages that occur during such events are responsible for the majority of fatalities.[1] Poverty, ignorance, avoidance of building codes by contractors, and higher-risk land-use practice are among the determinants of structural collapse, especially in poor countries.[1,2] Anbarci and co-workers found an inversely proportional ratio between pro capita country income and earthquake deaths.[3] The 1988 Armenian Earthquake released half of the energy of the Loma Prieta (California, USA) Earthquake, but caused 250 times more deaths.[1]

Earthquakes, hurricanes, tornados, bombings, and landslides are a common cause of collapsed structures and subsequent crush injuries.[4-6] Major earthquakes such as Christchurch and L'Aquila are followed by a substantial number of crush syndrome injuries, the victims of which may develop rhabdomyolysis and heme pigment-induced acute renal failure (ARF).[7,8] Approximately 50% of patients suffering crush syndrome (with an estimated incidence of 2% to 5%) may develop ARF, and some 50% of those with ARF require renal replacement therapy.[9]

Dialysis capability in the aftermath of a catastrophe may be deficient for several reasons, including damage to the dialysis facilities themselves[10]; damage to urban systems, such as electricity and water, causing loss of dialysis machine efficiency[11]; and a considerable drop in dialysis personnel.[10]

Crush syndrome is the systemic manifestation of muscular tissue lysis (rhabdomyolysis) resulting from a continuous and prolonged pressure.[12,13] It is a reperfusion injury phenomenon secondary to traumatic rhabdomyolysis.

Bywaters and Beal were the first to describe crush syndrome.[14] They reported on the injuries of London's entrapped bombing victims of World War II. The Armenian Earthquake in 1988 was one of the first documented catastrophes to produce numerous casualties requiring dialysis as a consequence of crush injuries.[15] The typical clinical presentation of crush syndrome is caused by a traumatic rhabdomyolysis and the subsequent release of muscle cell contents. The mechanism behind crush syndrome is leakiness of the sarcolemmal membrane triggered by pressure or stretching. Because of the sarcolemmal membrane widening, calcium, sodium, and water leak into the sarcoplasm, and the extracellular fluid flows into the muscle cells. Moreover, potassium and other toxic substances such as myoglobin, phosphate, and urate are released into the circulation by damaged cells.[9,16,17] Injury to other cells may release lactic acid, histamine, leukotrienes, peroxides, free radicals of oxygen, superoxides, lysozyme, and enzymes (such as creatine phosphokinase).

These events may result in hypovolemic and distributive shock, hyperkalemia, metabolic acidosis, compartment syndrome, and ARF. Kidney injury develops early, often before extrication, because of a decrease in blood volume and to third spacing of fluids. The heme protein released by myoglobin has several nephrotoxic effects. Prerenal ARF is exacerbated by the nitric oxide–scavenging effect of myoglobin, which increases vasoconstriction. Iron contained in the heme group, promotes formation of free radicals, leading to intrarenal failure. Finally, myoglobin, together with Tamm-Horsfall protein, precipitates in renal tubules, forming a cast, decreasing glomerular filtration. Compartment syndrome occurs when injured skeletal muscle contained within fascia-bound compartments develops swelling because of increased fluid uptake by injured muscle cells. Once the compartment pressure exceeds capillary perfusion pressure (at around 30 mm Hg), tissue inside the compartment becomes ischemic and compartment syndrome develops.

PRE-INCIDENT ACTION

Emergency physicians, general practitioners, surgeons, and pediatricians should be familiar with the diagnosis and management of crush injuries and crush syndrome. As part of disaster preparedness to treat these patients, a simple portable medical kit for on-scene treatment of patients with crush injury should be organized. These kits would contain materials and means to treat at least five critically ill patients and also maps and telephone numbers of all medical aid centers in the region to which patients should be moved as soon as possible, theoretically within the first hour.[18]

The medical aid centers would be established at no further than an hour's walk from any location, to ensure accessibility even if the road transportation system were to fail.

Because crush syndrome is a common cause of death in large-scale events, hemodialysis facilities and their capacity should be identified in advance, locally, and a register of the same should be maintained.[19]

The front-line intensive care unit for a prompt on-spot monitoring and treatment should be prepared and assembled to be deployable quickly, close to the epicenter of the earthquake. Previous experience has demonstrated the benefits of this in decreasing both mortality rate and complications in patients with severe crush injury.[20]

After a disaster, challenges in communication should be anticipated. Consequently, one of the first priorities must be to establish an independently powered short-wave communication network. The hospitals, especially emergency departments and intensive care units, must be prepared to receive multiple critically ill patients, including crush injuries.

Triage practices are of vital importance during mass casualty disaster.[20]

▶▶ POST-INCIDENT ACTION

It is imperative that medical and rescue personnel harmonize their efforts in caring for victims of crush injury. Serious morbidity and mortality may occur with delay in treatment of a crush victim. Prevention of renal and cardiac crush injury complications can be obtained with an aggressive medical treatment. Those measures must be started as early as possible, even during the extrication of the patient from the debris.

Crush syndrome is among the most important reasons for increasing morbidity and mortality, and triage guidelines must incorporate this into patient assessments, to facilitate the strategic use of hemodialysis resources. Triage should also consider all patients with preexisting end-stage renal disease.[21]

In the field, disaster medical personnel can obtain relevant physiological parameters from crush victims, without using any specific equipment. An initial field triage model for determining which patients might require early intervention for crush syndrome could consist of the following three factors:

- Pulse rate
- Time-to-rescue or extrication (>3 hours)
- Macroscopic urine findings

Experts have recommended the use of urine dipsticks to check myoglobin and subclinical rhabdomyolysis.[12,22]

A more detailed triage model, applicable in health care facilities, was developed to predict the risk of renal replacement therapy and in-hospital mortality. It is easily calculated with readily available clinical, demographic, and laboratory values.[23]

Hemodialysis machines and filters, together with nephrologists, nurses, and technicians, should arrive within 36 hours, as national and international resources are mobilized. Emergency dialysis units should be set up in easily accessible areas to avoid problems of transport for those patients who might have other serious injuries requiring major surgery. On-scene doctors treating disaster victims could consult with remote renal experts using telemedicine or Internet linkages, for advice on treating particularly complex cases. In making decisions about which type of dialysis modalities to use, the health care provider should consider the hypercatabolic state of the victims, the degree of electrolyte disturbances, the presence of polytrauma and bleeding tendency, specific geographic and local conditions, transport problems, and other logistical difficulties. Conventional hemodialysis allows efficient solute removal, treatment of multiple patients, and application without anticoagulants.

In patients with abdominal trauma, peritoneal dialysis is not easy to perform and often inefficient for removal of potassium and other catabolic metabolites. It might offer temporary help, however, especially

during disaster scenarios where conventional hemodialysis equipment is not ready available.[24] In the case of extreme needs, measures such as isolated ultrafiltration and sorbent technology could be used as a bridge to more efficient therapies.[21]

✚ MEDICAL TREATMENT OF CASUALTIES

The treatment of crushed victims should begin as soon as they are discovered. Concomitant injuries, such as fractures, solid organ damage, or spinal injury, should be suspected and assessed. Intravenous large-bore catheters should be placed, and the patient should receive fluid as soon as possible.[25–27] Multiple intravenous lines are necessary because these patients require large fluid volumes, and individual intravenous lines may dislodge during extrication. Normal saline is an appropriate initial choice for intravenous fluid resuscitation. A saline infusion of 1000 mL/h should be initiated during extrication and afterward tailored to clinical and environmental factors (e.g., bleeding, time spent under the rubble, and dimensions of the disaster).[28] Because electrolyte abnormalities, such as hyperkalemia, are common in crush injured patients, the use of intravenous solutions that contain potassium should be avoided.[22] Hyponatremia is common in patients with crush syndrome, and associated with poor prognosis.[29] When urine flow has been established, a compulsory mannitol-alkaline diuresis equal to 8 L/day should be maintained (urine pH > 6.5). Once the patient reaches the hospital, 5% dextrose ought to be alternated with normal saline to reduce the potential sodium load. Because a large volume of intravenous fluids may not be available in the first 2 days after a major incident, it has been reported that hypertonic saline is also safe and effective in a variety of trauma patients.[30] Placement of a Foley catheter is also recommended to measure urine output accurately.

Alkalization increases the urine solubility of acid hematin and aids in its excretion. This therapy should be continued until myoglobin is no longer detectable in the urine, because it may prevent the onset of renal failure. Mannitol is effective as osmotic diuretic and scavenger of oxygen free radicals, and it could help reduce the reperfusion-related component of this injury by this mechanism.[16,17] However, its real efficacy is questioned.[31] It is contraindicated in anuric and hypovolemic patients, and treatment with mannitol must be monitored closely.

At hospital admission, electrolytes, arterial blood gases, and muscle enzymes should be measured. Electrocardiograms should be frequently performed to detect hyperkalemia-associated changes early.[22] Empirical treatment with potassium-binding resins should be considered for those victims who have to wait to receive dialysis.[32]

Clinicians should monitor for early signs and symptoms of compartment syndrome (disproportionate pain, paresthesia, and a swollen and tense limb) and intervene as appropriate.[33]

A recent review shows that the fasciotomy in victims with crush injuries is controversial. Active decompression to improve circulation and reverse muscle necrosis is the favorable result of performing this procedure.[34] On the contrary, the risk of infection is the motivation to avoid it.[25] Other experts recommend fasciotomy only under specific circumstances, such as imminent distal gangrene or difficult clearing of necrotic tissue.[35]

Performing a simple dipstick test on the urine for hemopositivity in the mildly injured patients can diagnose subclinical rhabdomyolysis and be useful in identifying this critical condition. If these patients are discharged because of limited facilities, they should be advised to check the color and the volume of their urine daily and note other symptoms of ARF, such as weight gain and edema.[12]

The type of trauma, concomitant events, and complications observed during the clinical course can influence the outcomes of earthquake casualties with renal injury. For example, age, distance to reference hospitals, and time delay between disaster and admission to reference hospitals can affect the outcome.[36] The earlier that intravenous therapy is initiated, the better the chance of preventing ARF.[37] When fluid treatment is delayed for 6 hours following extrication, ARF is almost inevitable[38] If the anticipated urinary output cannot be achieved, the use of diuretics, preferably furosemide should be considered. Attention should be paid to those crush injury victims who do not receive intravenous therapy early enough and who do not respond to enforced alkaline diuresis, because of the high risk of developing renal failure and the requirement for hemodialysis.[39] In case the nephrology services become overwhelmed by a great number of patients who require dialysis, highest priority should be given to individuals with oliguric renal failure. Those with hyperkalemia could be medically managed and should be delayed.[40] Rather than haul mobile dialysis units in the stricken area, transporting the patients to a secure area with functionally active infrastructure is a possibility to be considered.[28]

The use of hyperbaric oxygen has been shown to improve the outcome of crush injury victims.[41,42] The use of this modality is obviously limited in disaster situations because of lack of access to hyperbaric chambers.

UNIQUE CONSIDERATIONS

There is no doubt that the majority of disaster-related deaths occur immediately after structural collapse or catastrophic event such as earthquakes.[43] Among survivors, short-term mortality dramatically increases in line with the duration of their being buried under the rubble. During the first few hours, a number of trapped earthquake victims are still alive. After 24 to 48 hours buried, the survival curve dramatically falls, and, after 5 days, it is very likely that all who are dug out are dead.[44] Disaster medical plans should comprise a medical care chain in which casualties receive life-supporting measures at the accident scene, with subsequent transport to a hospital for more definitive care within a few hours of their rescue. The development of crush syndrome after a crush injury is preventable and treatable. Crush injury patients may present with few signs or symptoms; thus medical personnel must maintain a high index of suspicion in treating crush victims.

PITFALLS

Several potential pitfalls in response to structural collapse exist. These include the following:

- Destruction of medical centers in the disaster-affected area, which diminishes the possibility of providing rapid hospital treatment of crush syndrome patients
- Damage to health facilities and urban facilities with electricity and water supply issues causing loss of efficiency of dialysis machines
- Considerable drop in available professional staff, such as dialysis personnel
- Failure to plan evacuation routes before an event
- Failure to know who is in command of disaster operations within your local area
- Delayed treatment after victim extrication
- Delay in starting intravenous fluids
- Low index of suspicion for crush injuries
- Failure to continue monitoring patients with high risk for ARF

REFERENCES

1. Kenny C. Disaster risk reduction in developing countries: costs, benefits and institutions. *Disasters*. 2012;36(4):559–588.
2. Bilham R, Gaur V. Buildings as weapons of mass destruction. *Science*. 2013;341:618–619.
3. Anbarci N, Escaleras M, Register C. Earthquake fatalities: interaction of nature and political economy. *J Publ Econ*. 2005;89(9–10):1907–1933.
4. Kopp JB, Ball LK, Cohen A, et al. Kidney patient care in disasters: lessons from the hurricanes and earthquake of 2005. *Clin J Am Soc Nephrol*. 2007;2:814–824.
5. Scapellato S, Maria S, Castorina G, Sciuto G. Crush syndrome. *Minerva Chir*. 2007;62(4):285–292.
6. Anderson AH, Cohen AJ, Kutner NG, Kopp JB, Kimmel PL, Muntner P. Missed dialysis sessions and hospitalization in hemodialysis patients after Hurricane Katrina. *Kidney Int*. 2009;75:1202–1208.
7. Irvine J, Buttimore A, Eastwood D, Kendrick-Jones J. The Christchurch earthquake: dialysis experience and emergency planning. *Nephrology (Carlton)*. 2014;19(5):296–303.
8. Bonomini M, Stuard S, Dal Canton A. Dialysis practice and patient outcome in the aftermath of the earthquake at L'Aquila, Italy, April 2009. *Nephrol Dial Transplant*. 2011;26(8):2595–2603.
9. Erek E, Sever MS, Serdengeçti K, et al. An overview of morbidity and mortality in patients with acute renal failure due to crush syndrome: the Marmara earthquake experience. *Nephrol Dial Transplant*. 2002;17:33–40.
10. Sever MS, Erek E, Vanholder R, et al. Features of chronic hemodialysis practice after the Marmara earthquake. *J Am Soc Nephrol*. 2004;15:1071–1076.
11. Naito H. The basic hospital and renal replacement therapy in the Great Hanshin Earthquake. *Ren Fail*. 1997;19:701–710.
12. Sever MS, Erek E, Vanholder R, et al. Clinical findings in the renal victims of a catastrophic disaster: in the Marmara Earthquake. *Nephrol Dial Transplant*. 2002;17:1942–1949.
13. Visweswaran P, Guntupalli J. Rhabdomyolysis. *Crit Care Clin*. 1999;15:415–428.
14. Bywaters EGL, Beall D. Crush injuries with impairment of renal function. *BMJ*. 1941;1:427–432.
15. Sever MS, Vanholder M, Lameire N. Management of crush-related injury after disaster. *N Engl J Med*. 2006;354:1052–1063.
16. Better OS. Rescue and salvage of casualties suffering from the crush syndrome after mass disasters. *Mil Med*. 1999;164:366–369.
17. Smith J, Greaves I. Crush injury and crush syndrome: a review. *J Trauma*. 2003;54:S226–S230.
18. Schultz CH, Di Lorenzo RA, Koenig KL, et al. Disaster medical direction: a medical earthquake response curriculum. *Ann Emerg Med*. 1991;20:470–471 [Abstract].
19. Vanholder R, Stuard S, Bonomini M, Sever SM. Renal disaster relief in Europe: the experience at L'Aquila, Italy, in April 2009. *Nephrol Dial Transplant*. 2009;24:3251–3255.
20. Li W, Qian J, Liu X, et al. Management of severe crush injury in a front-line tent ICU after 2008 Wenchuan earthquake in China: an experience with 32 cases. *Crit Care*. 2009;13:R178.
21. Perkins M, Yuan CM. Renal replacement therapy in austere environments. *Int J Nephrol*. 2011;2011:748053.
22. Yoshimura N, Nakayama S, Nakagiri K, Azami T, Ataka K, Ishii N. Profile of chest injuries arising from the 1995 southern Hyogo Prefecture earthquake. *Chest*. 1996;110:759–761.
23. McMahon GM, Zeng X, Waikar SS. A risk prediction score for kidney failure or mortality in rhabdomyolysis. *JAMA Intern Med*. 2013;173 (19):1821–1828.
24. Vanholder R, Sever MS, Erek E, Lameire N. Rhabdomyolysis. *J Am Soc Nephrol*. 2000;11:1553–1561.
25. Better OS, Stein JH. Early management of shock and prophylaxis of acute renal failure in traumatic rhabdomyolysis. *N Engl J Med*. 1990;322:825–829.
26. Better OS, Rubinstein I. Management of shock and acute renal failure in casualties suffering from crush syndrome. *Ren Fail*. 1997;19(5):647–653.
27. Noji EK. Prophylaxis of acute renal failure in traumatic rhabdomyolysis. *N Engl J Med*. 1990;323(8):550–551.
28. Sever MS, Vanholder R. Management of crush victim in mass disaster: highlights from recently published recommendation. *Clin J Am Soc Nephrol*. 2013;8:328–335.
29. Zhang L, Fu P, Wang L, et al. Hyponatraemia in patients with crush syndrome during the Wenchuan earthquake. *Emerg Med J*. 2013;30(9):745–748.
30. Vassar MJ, Fisher RP, O'Brien PE, et al. A multicenter trial for resuscitation of injured patients with 7.5% sodium chloride: the effect of added dextran

70: the Multicenter Group for the Study of Hypertonic Saline in Trauma Patients. *Arch Surg.* 1993;128:1011–1013.

31. Brown CV, Rhee P, Chan L, Evans K, Demetriades D, Velmahos GC. Preventing renal failure in patients with rhabdomyolysis: do bicarbonate and mannitol make a difference? *J Trauma.* 2004;56(6):1191–1196.

32. Jagodzinski N, Weerasinghe C, Porter K. Crush injuries and crush syndrome—a review. Part 1: the systemic injury. *J Trauma.* 2010;12:69–88.

33. Genton A, Wilcox SR. Crush syndrome: a case report and a review of literature. *J Emerg Med.* 2014;46(2):313–319.

34. Duman H, Kulahci Y, Sengezer M. Fasciotomy in crush injury resulting from prolonged pressure in an earthquake in Turkey. *Emerg Med J.* 2003;20:251–252.

35. Michealson M. Crush injury and crush syndrome. *World J Surg.* 1992;16:899–903.

36. Sever MS, Erek E, Vanholder R, et al. Lessons learned from the catastrophic Marmara earthquake: factors influencing the final outcome of renal victims. *Clin Nephrol.* 2004;61:413–421.

37. Leung LP. A potentially life-threatening complication of university orientation activities. *World J Emerg Medn.* 2012;3(1):71–73.

38. Gunal AI, Celiker H, Dogukan A, et al. Early and vigorous fluid resuscitation prevents acute renal failure in the crush victims of catastrophic earthquakes. *J Am Soc Nephrol.* 2004;15:1862–1867.

39. Castañer Moreno J. Insuficiencia renal aguda postraumática. *Rev Cubana Med Milit.* 1999;28(1):41–48.

40. Amundson D, Dadekian G, Etienne M, et al. Practicing internal medicine onboard the USNS COMFORT in the aftermath of the Haitian earthquake. *Ann Intern Med.* 2010;152:733–737.

41. Siriwanij T, Vattanagomgs V, Sitprija V. Hyperbaric oxygen therapy in crush injury. *Nephron.* 1997;75(4):484–485.

42. James PB. Hyperbaric oxygen treatment for crush injury. *BMJ.* 1994;309 (6967):1513.

43. Pointer JE, Michaelis J, Saunders C, et al. The 1989 Loma Prieta earthquake: impact on hospital patient care. *Ann Emerg Med.* 1992;21:1228–1233.

44. Macintyre AG, Barbera JA, Smith ER. Surviving collapsed structure entrapment after earthquakes: a "time-to-rescue" analysis. *Prehospital Disaster Med.* 2006;21(1):4–19.

CHAPTER 181

Train Derailment

Srihari Cattamanchi and J. Scott Goudie

DESCRIPTION OF EVENTS

Railways have a long history of providing vital passenger travel. They provide important means of transportation for both passengers and goods. Industrialization and technological innovations increased the influence of railways in the last two centuries by enabling faster movement of goods and passengers over long distances more cheaply than other means of transport.[1] In 1804 the first locomotive-hauled train was powered by a steam engine, whereas the first passenger rail line opened in England in 1825.[2] Steam engines were the standard propulsion method until the 1950s.[1,3] The first electrified railway began service in 1902 in Italy.[4] In the 1950s high labor costs associated with the steam engine led to diesel engines becoming more popular.[3,5] By the 1970s, in part because of the 1973 oil crisis, many countries began electrifying their railways.[1] Maglev, which uses magnetic levitation, was developed as a propulsion technology between the late 1940s and early 1970s. The first commercial Maglev train was introduced in Birmingham, Britain, in 1984 and is available to a limited extent in China, Japan, and Germany.[1,6]

When railway passenger traffic began in the mid-nineteenth century, there were only a few major train accidents due to limited traffic and lower speeds.[7] In the second half of the twentieth century, railways gained significant advances in safety and technology, which led to a continuous increase in train speed. The first steam engine reached an approximate speed of 31 mph (50 km/h).[2] More than half of the trains now operate at a top speed of 100 mph (160 km/h) or more.[8] The high-speed electrified Train à Grande Vitesse (TGV) had an average speed of 132 mph (213 km/h) when introduced in France in 1979.[1,9] As of 2014, the TGV operates at speeds of 173 to 200 mph (279 to 320 km/h), with the highest recorded speed of 357 mph (575 km/h) in 2007.[9] Several Maglev trains operate at speeds of 186 mph (300 km/h), but in Shanghai, the Maglev transrapid train runs at speeds of 267 mph (450 km/h) in regular traffic.[10] In 2003 Maglev trains had the highest recorded speed of 361 mph (581 km/h).[11] Severe morbidity and mortality are to be expected in any modern high-speed train accident.

Emergency Events Database (EM-DAT) maintains a worldwide database on disasters. Between 1900 and 2014, 585 train accidents were reported, killing 26,919 people, and injuring another 54,083, according to data retrieved from the EM-DAT.[12] About 88% of all train accidents recorded in the database occurred in the four and half decades between 1970 and 2014 (Figure 181-1). A majority of events since the 1970s occurred in Africa, Asia, and Central and South America, combined, whereas only 33% occurred in Oceania, America, and Europe (Table 181-1).[12] Although there has been a decrease in the annual number of train accidents in Europe since the 1980s, there has been a marked increase in train accidents in Asia and Africa. The number of victims killed per disaster (1970 to 2014 data) was highest in Africa and lowest in North America. The number of people injured per train accident on average was 2 to 3 times the number of fatalities (Table 181-1). Since the 1970s, more people were injured than killed in train crash events. Among the 585 train accidents, India reported the highest number of train accidents (117, 20%) followed by the United States (33, 6%), and Pakistan (26, 4%). India also had the highest number of people killed due to rail disasters (4830, 18%) (Table 181-2).[12] In addition, India reported the highest rail passenger kilometers traveled in 2013, that is, 1098.10 billion passenger kilometers,[13] in part explaining the high number of train accident deaths and injuries.

Only 26% of the train accidents in the database were reported in the first seven decades of the EM-DATA database (Figure 181-1).[12] Train accidents may have occurred less frequently due to fewer passenger kilometers traveled and also due to lower speeds. However, these data are probably not as complete as it should be for the early half of the twentieth century.[7] In the early 1900s, train carriages were made of wood to protect the passengers from cold, the passengers involved in a train crash more often suffered fatal injuries as a result. During a train accident, due to the dissipated kinetic energy, the wooden carriages disintegrated in a manner called "telescoping" (Figure 181-2).[7] Telescoping was an important cause of death and injury in a train crash at that time. In a French train accident of 1933, a locomotive collided with a slow-moving passenger train from behind, ripping through almost the entire length of the train, and killing about 230 people.[14] Additionally, train crashes were commonly complicated by fire, and the rescue techniques and resources were very much limited in comparison to modern rescue and Emergency Medical Services (EMS) protocols.[7]

By the 1950s, wooden carriages began being replaced by metal carriages. As the kinetic energy in a collision is absorbed better by metal carriages, such carriages may emerge relatively intact from a crash.[7] The metal carriage minimized the telescoping problem, but created another dangerous phenomenon called "overriding" (Figure 181-2), where one carriage overrides another and crashes down on the passenger below.[7] In the Clapham, England, three-train collision in the 1980s, one train overrode another, crashing down on the passengers below and killing 33 people.[15] Later, "anti-climb" devices (corrugated plates) and crash zones were introduced to minimize the overriding risk in metal carriages.[7] The corrugated plates fitted to the ends of each rail carriage hook the carriages together in an accident. When train carriages derail on impact, it develops a phenomenon called "jack-knifing" or lateral-buckling (Figure 181-2).[7] The carriages collide against each other's side, making the sidewalls collapse inward and injure the passengers inside in the carriage. An example is the 1989 Purely train accident, where two trains bound for London collided, and the rear

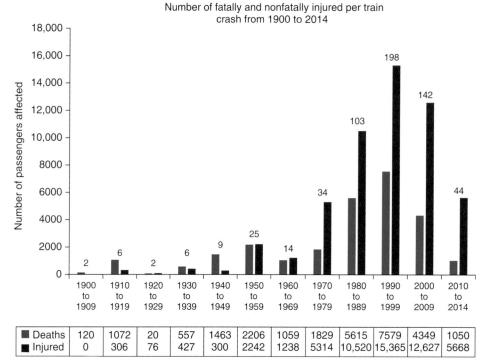

Number of fatally and nonfatally injured per train crash from 1900 to 2014

	1900 to 1909	1910 to 1919	1920 to 1929	1930 to 1939	1940 to 1949	1950 to 1959	1960 to 1969	1970 to 1979	1980 to 1989	1990 to 1999	2000 to 2009	2010 to 2014
■ Deaths	120	1072	20	557	1463	2206	1059	1829	5615	7579	4349	1050
■ Injured	0	306	76	427	300	2242	1238	5314	10,520	15,365	12,627	5668

FIG 181–1 The number of fatally and nonfatally injured per train crash from 1900 to 2014. (Reproduced from D. Guha-Sapir, R. Below, Ph. Hoyois—EM-DAT: International Disaster Database - www.emdat.be - Université Catholique de Louvain - Brussels - Belgium).

carriages of the train rolled down the railway embankment and jack-knifed against a tree.[16] The passengers were thrown about the carriage against the roof, floor, and sides, either seriously injuring or killing them. Currently, overriding and jack-knifing are the most common phenomenon of train accidents worldwide.[7]

In the four decades between 1970 and 2014, despite new safety measures, the number of train accidents has increased, as has the number of fatalities and injuries.[7] These increases may be due to more passenger kilometers traveled, more passengers inside each train carriage, and higher train speeds. Events inside a train carriage during a crash are as critical as events happening outside.[17] The interior of the carriage and loose objects inside have a significant impact on passengers as during a crash, unsecured seat cushions, luggage and unrestrained passengers are all thrown around inside the carriage.[16] Structural elements such as folding tables, tables located between chairs, and luggage racks, also have a significant impact on the injury profile.[18] Safer interior design and more secure baggage stowage will reduce injuries and facilitate rescue and evacuation. Use of seat belts and head restraint prevents or mitigates fatal injuries in a train accident, but the debate on seat belts still continues and they have not been installed as a standard feature on trains.[17] In some regions including South Asia, window bars and locked doors are used. In a fire incident, the locked doors and window bars make access and egress difficult and inhibit passenger rescue.[7]

Trains carrying hazardous materials crashing into a passenger train or a derailment pose a significant hazard with the potential to kill more people than a train accident alone. This also places large populations at risk where such trains are routed through major population centers.[17] The downtown Baltimore 2001 freight derailment, with subsequent hazardous material spill and fire is such an example.[19]

Ensuring safer trains remains a concern in an era of ever-increasing speed, as the energy involved in collisions is a factor of velocity squared ($KE = \frac{1}{2}MV^2$). Consider the 267-mph Shanghai Maglev train in commercial operation in China.[10] Engineers are focused on developing lighter, smoother, and faster trains, and this increases the risk of a

major train disaster.[20] In Eschede, in 1981 a carriage wheel failure left the most technologically advanced German ICE Train in ruins. The train derailed and crashed straight into a concrete bridge at speeds of 125 mph (200 km/h), disintegrating on impact and killing 101 passengers and injuring 103.[20]

Increased safety standards, new design, and advanced technologies could not prevent a train from being swept off the tracks by the South Asian Tsunami in Sri Lanka on December 2004.[21] All 1700 passengers on the train were killed in the world's worst train disaster to date.[21] Hostile acts such as the 2004 Madrid subway bombings, the 2005 London subway bombings, and 2006 and 2008 Mumbai Metro bombings indicate rising new threats to mass transit safety.[22–26] Explosions in confined spaces such as within railway carriages have a higher incidence of blast injuries with greater severity and mortality than those in open areas.[17]

Train travel is relatively safe, but the rail industry is growing rapidly with a significant increase in rail traffic and train speeds, so we are seeing increasing numbers of train accidents.[17] The challenge is to find ways to control the conditions inside the train carriages during crashes to better absorb the shock and to protect passengers by taking into consideration the effects of kinetic energy generated during crashes. With the existing state of technology and safety practices, there are substantial challenges that remain in the issue of train safety, so further improvements and higher vigilance are needed both in designing trains and in maintaining them.[17]

PRE-INCIDENT ACTIONS

In the event of a railway emergency, routine day-to-day operations are affected, giving way to a dedicated, trained, and resilient crisis management approach which requires specialized skills of the emergency first responders, people from outside agencies, and multiple transit disciplines.[27] Effectively establishing the skills to direct an all-hazards railway disaster response and recovery requires adequate preplanning,

TABLE 181-1 Number of Fatal and Nonfatally Injured Classified by Decade and Continent from 1970 to 2014[12]

	1970-1979	1980-1989	1990-1999	2000-2009	2010-2014
Africa					
Dead	115	980	1783	1483	214
Injured	390	1473	2714	2586	2016
No of Events	3	14	31	33	9
America					
Dead	580	616	519	95	124
Injured	2505	1441	2053	1476	1444
No of Events	7	13	27	13	7
Asia					
Dead	333	3026	4678	2268	526
Injured	1122	5076	8779	7070	1393
No of Events	7	47	110	72	18
Europe					
Dead	718	993	587	492	186
Injured	1206	2530	1768	1352	815
No of Events	16	29	29	22	10
Oceania					
Dead	83	0	12	11	0
Injured	91	0	51	143	0
No of Events	1	0	1	2	0

Data from D. Guha-Sapir, R. Below, Ph. Hoyois—EM-DAT: International Disaster Database. www.emdat.be. Université Catholique de Louvain, Brussels, Belgium.

TABLE 181-2 Number of Railway Disasters Among Top 15 Countries from 1900 to 2014[12]

COUNTRY	OCCURRENCE	DEATHS	INJURED
India	117	4830	6857
United States	33	798	3653
Pakistan	26	1583	2335
United Kingdom	24	943	3936
China—Peoples Republic	23	1601	3669
Indonesia	22	603	1189
South Africa	20	331	3133
Mexico	19	1148	2417
Russia	18	612	971
Germany	17	724	800
Bangladesh	15	492	2732
Egypt	14	827	1058
France	11	1083	982
Belgium	11	153	891
Italy	10	696	767

Data from D. Guha-Sapir, R. Below, Ph. Hoyois—EM-DAT: International Disaster Database. www.emdat.be. Université Catholique de Louvain, Brussels, Belgium.

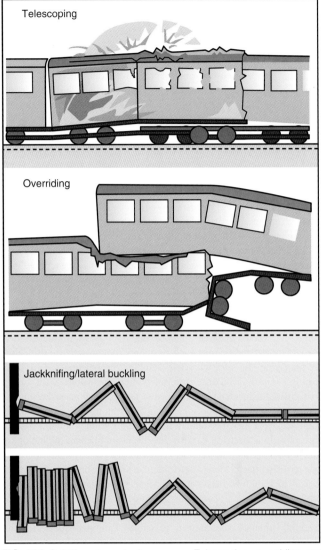

FIG 181–2 Different crash-phenomena: Telescoping, overriding and jackknifing or lateral buckling. Reproduced with permission from Forsberg R, Björnstig U. One hundred years of railway disasters and recent trends. Prehosp Disaster Med. 2011;26(05):367-373. Cambridge University Press.

internal coordination, resourcing and prestaging of critical assets, and coordination with external agencies.[28]

A hazard vulnerability assessment (HVA) should be completed to identify risk factors for train disasters in the community. An HVA is completed considering the frequency of trains, characteristics of train services (high-speed commuter, subway, hazardous waste, industrial freight), population density adjacent to the tracks, route vulnerabilities (tunnels, bridges, falling rocks, landslides, avalanche risk, etc.), and vulnerable facilities (schools, hospitals, apartments, nursing homes, military bases) adjacent to the tracks.

Even though the relative risk of a train disaster in the community is low, emergency response organizations should plan and prepare for them. A high-speed train accident dissipates enormous kinetic energy with the potential for severely injured mass casualties.[17] The complex nature of responding to such accidents makes pre-incident action planning essential.[17] To respond adequately to these incidents, hospitals, emergency departments, emergency medical services, fire departments, law enforcement agencies, and the department of transportation should develop All Hazard multiagency disaster response plans for mass casualty and hazardous material incidents. Specific elements to be considered include terrorist attacks, sabotage, and chemical, biological, radiological, nuclear, or explosive (CBRNE) attacks directed toward railway infrastructure. Such preparedness plans should be drilled, tested, and updated annually and should be supported with proper equipment and training.

Responding to a train crash site may expose rescue personnel to hazards requiring mandatory use of personal protective equipment (PPE), HazMat suits with self-contained breathing apparatus (SCBA), insulated gloves, aprons, mats, and blankets to provide protection from electrical shock.[17,29] First responders should be provided with communications that function in subways and tunnels.[17] Responders must be supplied with the appropriate rescue tools effective against the rugged steel in today's high-speed trains. Even if the railway company disconnects the high-voltage electric power lines, rescue personnel need such skills and equipment to perform protective grounding. Gangways may be required to access the carriage and evacuate passengers. Heavy lift cranes may be required to lift and move carriages to search for entrapments under the carriages themselves. Lack of heavy rescue equipment could hamper rapid extrication of victims and be detrimental to the survival rate of casualties.[17] Rescue personnel should have access to essential tools including emergency evacuation carts, emergency headlights and floodlights, emergency ladders and planks, airbag rescue and lifting system, hydraulic jacks, and "jumpers" or "stingers" for third rail power.[29]

`Each train disaster presents its own unique problem sets, whether it is the high volume of injured persons, the varied nature of the cargo, hazardous material spill, or the remoteness of the accident scene. Unprepared or untrained personnel may experience difficulties in managing the disaster scene resulting in potentially "avoidable deaths."[7] Crash avoidance and safety measures alone were unable to decrease the incidence of railway disasters, placing increasing emphasis on pre-incident response planning and training.[7] In responding to train accidents, first responders need training to identify and manage threats such as electrical hazards, fire, exposure to chemical, biological, and nuclear agents, and secondary explosions, especially in the aftermath of a terrorist attack.[17] Rapid extrication techniques should be taught and drilled to minimize delays in providing appropriate medical care to injured victims.[17,30,31] Confined-space medicine techniques also require consideration by those training first responders and rescue personnel to medically manage the trapped passenger. Confined-space medicine training provides the skills required to perform a medical evaluation and to provide necessary treatment to a victim entrapped in a confined space, thus preventing crush syndrome.[17,27,31]

Periodic unannounced exercises will enhance the capabilities of first responders and rescue personnel while allowing for continuous capability assessments.[27] Training should be provided in emergency procedures (first aid, evacuation, emergency access or egress), emergency protocols, communications and logistics, train carriage safety, and PPE use. Such training may be conducted through orientation and education sessions, games, tabletop exercises, walkthrough drills, functional drills, confined-space drills, evacuation drills, or full-scale exercises.[27] Regular tabletop exercises have proven to be an effective, low-cost method for organizations to improve their capabilities.

Emergency responders should familiarize themselves during drills with the primary train systems vehicles, facilities, and equipment.[32] First responders should be familiar with automatic vehicle location (GPS), evacuation plans and staging areas, train station street-level ventilation grates, tunnels and their emergency exits, subway emergency ventilation fans and controls, and emergency control panels.[32] Familiarity with overhead power sources, third rail, rail traction power shut-off systems, fire detection and suppression systems, and hazardous gas and chemical detection systems will be necessary to effectively manage a live scene. Emergency personnel must know how to access or egress a passenger train car, shut it down, isolate the power, and switch on the emergency lighting in the car.[32]

▶▶ POST-INCIDENT ACTION

In the event of a train disaster, a variety of agencies and personnel are called upon to provide individual actions to manage the disaster.[27] First responders from a number of disciplines may initiate this process. These responders include transit police, transit operations and safety personnel, law enforcement agencies, fire department, emergency medical services, medical examiner or coroner, staff from utility companies, nonprofit and volunteer organizations, other local government officials, and insurance companies.

In some jurisdictions, first responders activate the disaster plan, Incident Command System (ICS), and emergency procedures, whereas in others this requires a management function. Responsibilities of a first responder are to establish on-scene command, size up the situation on the ground, and broadcast a report to appropriate personnel within and outside the agency. Having a standard method of delivery of such a report will greatly assist personnel and minimize the chance of message failure through "speaking a different language." The METHANE message as used in the UK Major Incident Medical Management and Support system is an example of an easily taught and repeatable message structure:

M—Major incident declared
E—Exact location (grid reference, if known, or GPS)
T—Type of incident (fire, crash, explosion, etc.)
H—potential Hazards involved (smoke, oil, chemicals, fire, etc.)
A—Access roads to the scene from various directions
N—estimated Number of casualties
E—Emergency services present and required

In addition, the CSCATTT tool used in Major Incident Medical Management and Support (MIMMS) for prioritizing actions is a useful reminder for early on-scene first responders. This is a system used widely by NATO services, ensuring that civilian and military are using the same terminology:

C—Command and control
S—Safety and security
C—Communications
A—Assessment
T—Triage
T—Treatment
T—Transport

Establishing command and control is vital in the early stages of a disaster to ensure a coordinated approach to management. First responders on-scene will, by definition, be the command until a more appropriately trained person arrives, at which point command may be turned over to another individual who should be clearly identified by tabard. Command does not need to be in the hands of the most senior person but it commonly is; the most appropriate commander is the person who has been trained for the role.[27]

"Size Up" or a METHANE message situation assessment is the most important part of early disaster response. Critical information that should be conveyed with respect to train-related mass casualty incidents is the type of emergency (fire, accident, derailment, hazardous material spill, or a bomb threat), location of emergency (milepost, track designation, or the street address), type of vehicle involved, train serial number and length, station and exact location of the station, size of the area involved, number and type of casualties or injuries; and assistance required from other emergency services including ambulances, fire, public utility, and other.[27] Making an initial assessment of the number and severity of injuries at the disaster site is difficult if the incident is in a tunnel or a subway.[17] Sometimes no passenger list exists, making it difficult to estimate the number of passengers onboard, the number of fatalities or injured, the number of passengers trapped in debris, and when to call off rescue operations.[17] Remote location of a crash site makes it difficult to reach and mobilize resources to the scene, making it necessary to use helicopter emergency medical services in addition to other emergency responders.[7]

An important role of a first responder is to set up a command post.[27] The command post is the location where the primary incident command functions and should be located in a safe place near the crash site, but not too close or within the area of the incident (Figure 181-3).[27] When local police, fire, or EMS personnel arrive first on the scene, they usually take control of managing the event; activating and establishing the unified command system (UCS).[27] Usually, the fire department heads the unified command structure, but this may differ depending on the country or the disaster situation itself where other military or federal authorities may have command.

In a rail disaster, command and control at the scene can be particularly problematic if the victims injured or killed are scattered throughout the incident area.[17] An example is the Eschede train disaster where the victims were scattered over approximately 3 miles of track length, and with communication lines down, the medical team had to act independent of command.[33,34] Simultaneous coordinated terror attacks in various locations can create difficulties in command and control and cause responders to lose the global perspective in regards to the disaster

as was seen in the 2004 Madrid subway terrorist attack.[22] Absence of an overarching emergency response plan can create problems in command and control of the rescue operations as was noted in the 2005 Amagasaki train crash in Japan.[31] A well-established system of communication and coordination between the command and local emergency services is vital as is maintaining points of contact with the regional, state, and federal disaster response agencies.[17]

Rescue operations near a rail track endanger rescue personnel and may expose them to kinetic, thermal, electrical, and chemical hazards at the incident site.[17,35] It is hazardous to approach tracks unless cleared by railway supervisors, as it takes more than 2 km for a full speed train to come to a stop. Bridges, tunnels, narrow cuttings, concrete cable ducts, high voltage electric lines, and moving blades of switch tracks further contribute to unsafe environments and may threaten the emergency first responder.[35] Obtaining access to a carriage from the ground level is always difficult due to its height, especially in an overriding crash, necessitating the use of ladders, gangways, and the need to walk on a sloped surface, which also contributes to the hazards. Moving blades of switch tracks that are controlled remotely can trap a foot without warning and create another hazard.[35] Emergency personnel may sustain burn injuries during rescue operations as some parts of the train

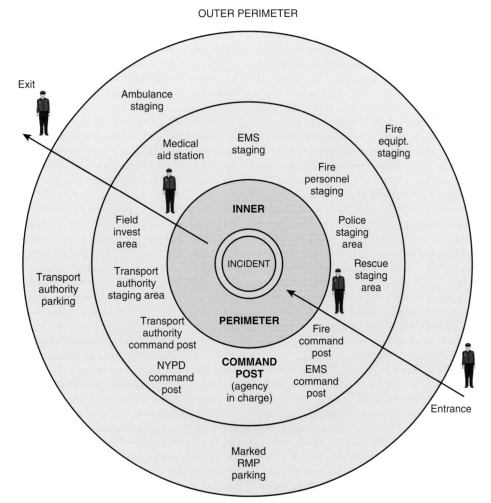

FIG 181–3 Illustration showing an overview of the staging area for a train disaster. Incident area is the Hot Zone. Inner Perimeter is the Warm Zone. The middle circle with various command posts and staging areas is the Cold Zone. The outer perimeter is the incident management area where the ambulances and other rescue vehicles are parked. (Reproduced from Boyd AM, Maier PM, Caton JE. Critical incident management guidelines U.S. Department of Transportation, Research and Special Programs Administration–Volpe National Transportation Systems Center. 1998;FTA-MA-26-7009-98-1.)

are extremely hot during operations and may not have had time to cool after derailment. Transportation of chemicals in a train further complicates the safety of emergency personnel.[35] High voltage power lines carry up to 25,000 V of electricity and require a person to maintain 3 m of safe distance from a live cable waiting until the power is disconnected and cables grounded to approach the tracks.[35] Overriding or jack-knifing carriages tend to slide and make it difficult to lift the carriage without causing further damage.[17,33] Metal cutters and similar rescue equipment cannot be used in the presence of a gasoline leak or chemical spill in crash situations where there are high risks of ignition.[17,31,35] The safety officer should search for these hazards. Measures should be taken by the safety officer to keep all emergency rescue personnel, passengers, and any crowd safe and secure from these dangers.

All rescue personnel working at the site of the crash should mandatorily use PPE including hard hats, insulated gloves, aprons, mats, blankets, and boots to provide protection from electrical shock. HazMat suits with self-contained breathing apparatus (SCBA) should be used in case of risk of exposure to toxic or chemical agents. Appropriate PPE use should be verified on entry to the site by the safety officer or deputy.

Early identification and confirmation of hazardous material spillage in a train disaster are required to determine the applicable decontamination measure and medical treatment.[27] Sensors such as colorimetric tubes, detection papers (M8/M9), electronic detectors, pesticide tickets, and military detection kits may be employed to detect hazardous agents by appropriately trained personnel. HAZCHEM or Kemmler plates, train shipment papers, labels or markings on the containers, and shape of the containers may also be used to identify hazardous materials and their risks.[27] With hazardous material, spills-trained HazMat personnel must secure the area to ensure safety of victims and rescuers.[27]

Rescue personnel should quickly recognize and perform a rapid assessment of the hazard, determine quickly if victims are alive and accessible, and what level of PPE is required to make an early entry and to extricate victims to a safe zone.[36] No emergency rescue personnel are allowed in the "hot zone" without appropriate PPE.[27] Once survivors are extricated to a safe area, triage can be done only after emergency decontamination of survivors.[27] If a contaminated passenger comes in contact with crew or equipment, all of them, including any equipment, should be decontaminated.[27] If triage and treatments need to be initiated urgently before emergency decontamination, the emergency personnel should triage and treat survivors only after donning the appropriate PPE.[36] In addition, once patients are decontaminated, secondary triage needs to be performed and, if the person was not triaged earlier, primary triage.[36] In mass casualty incidents, victims can occasionally only be grossly decontaminated to reduce the time to definitive medical care, and details regarding the number of passengers and victims and decontamination status should be conveyed to the receiving hospital, the transport officer, and EMS personnel.[27]

Responding to terrorist train disasters is complex and involves police and fire departments, EMS, and the local HazMat teams, along with agencies such as the FBI, FEMA, DoD, and EPA in the United States.[27] Responsibilities of first responders and rescue personnel are to secure the scene of train disaster and to rescue or extricate the victims. Victims should be checked for any potential secondary devices, decontaminated, and then triaged, treated, and transported to an appropriate medical facility. Crowds should be moved to a safe area. Emergency rescue personnel should be protected and avoid secondary contamination. The crime scene and evidence should be secured, and steps taken to protect against secondary attack.[27]

A staging area should be established in the "cold zone," safe from the incident area for responding personnel and equipment (Figure 181-3).[27] The incident command center and its command posts—police, fire, EMS, and transit agency, along with staff from various emergency

response agencies, a medical field hospital, and equipment for rescue operations—are located in the staging area. Ambulances, fire engines, police cruisers, and transit agency vehicles are parked outside the staging area with a clear circuit for transport access and egress. Vehicles should be parked with keys in ignition to facilitate vehicle movement as required and should never block access to the circuit (Figure 181-3). It is important to establish the staging area at safe distance from the disaster zone and hot zone, to avoid exposure risk to hazardous chemicals, toxic agents, fires, electrocution, or secondary bomb explosions.[17,27]

Emergency evacuation of passengers from the train car poses another major safety issue.[17] The sliding doors between the vestibules and the compartment may become jammed or crushed in a crash, preventing passengers from escaping.[17,37] Doors used in carriages are heavy and are harder to open if the carriage is overturned, trapping the passengers inside.[17] In some countries, carriages have window bars, and doors are usually locked, making it difficult to evacuate the train.[7] Stairways in a double-decker carriage may be damaged or destroyed in a crash, entrapping the passengers on the upper deck.[17] Suitcases, seat cushions, and clothes obstruct exit routes, and usually power is lost in the accident, making evacuation more difficult.[7,17]

Normally, passengers enter and exit a train at a station from a platform through the side doors. The preferred method of evacuating passengers to safety in a train crash is either by moving all or undamaged cars of the train to the nearest station, or moving the passengers to a rescue train through the front, rear, or side door when the disabled train cannot be moved.[27] The side doors or the back door of the rescue train and the disabled trained are aligned, and the passengers are moved directly to the rescue train. In an emergency, the doors may be opened without electric power from the outside.[27] Locking of doors should be discouraged and sealing of windows with grills should be avoided to facilitate emergency access and egress. A train station should have an adequate number of entrances and exits and should be located strategically to provide entry for fire and rescue personnel and for evacuating passengers safely in an emergency.[27] Except for a third rail hazard, the additional hazards present in an elevated track or a confined tunnel are absent while evacuating passengers from ground level train disasters.[27]

Provision of fresh air and smoke and fire management are crucial aspects of emergency preparedness in the rail industry.[27] Ventilation purges heat and smoke providing fresh air and visibility to passengers and rescue and fire personnel in a fire. For this reason, ventilation is an essential component of emergency preparedness and should be installed in every train, subway, and train station.[27] Ventilation and air conditioning systems dissipate heat and remove noxious odors while providing fresh air to passengers. A portable or uninterruptable backup power source should be supplied to maintain ventilation operations even when power is lost during a train disaster.[27]

Lessons learned from major disasters in the two decades between 1990 and 2014 highlight the lack of communication and coordination between different agencies and stress the importance and need for well-established communication and coordination between all emergency services.[7,17,27,36] During a disaster, cell phone networks may become overloaded with additional rescuer communication complexities if the accident site is in a deep tunnel or subway, potentially impacting rescue operations and endangering lives of rescue personnel and passengers.[17]

Efficient triaging of victims is crucial to maximizing use of scarce on-scene resources and health care infrastructure in a large multi casualty incident such as a train disaster.[36] Triaging passengers inside a deformed and unstable train carriage at the site of train disaster is controversial and puts emergency personnel at risk. It is reasonable to triage passengers once they are evacuated or extricated from the train carriage at the triage collection zone. On-scene triage of victims according to an established system, such as the Simple Triage and Rapid Treatment system or the Sieve and Sort system as used in Europe, allows for prioritizing medical evacuation of victims back to the medical center according to the severity of injury.[38] Even though the difference between minor and severe injuries are evident in a train disaster, all passengers should be triaged and tagged appropriately, even if a large number of passengers are walking unwounded and appear not to have been injured at all.[17,22,31] The responding emergency personnel must have an adequate supply of triage tags as the number of passengers involved may be significant, as observed in 2004 Madrid subway terrorist attack where 1500 people were injured and responders ran out of triage tags.[22] Immediately after the train disaster and before effective incident management is established with adequate resources, there will be a substantial degree of victim self-triage and self-transport, observed both in developing countries with low-resourced EMS systems and also in industrialized societies with highly resourced EMS systems.[36] Usually, the self-triaged and self-transported victims present to the nearest health care facility or those hospitals with which they are familiar, as observed in the 9/11 World Trade Center terrorist attack in New York City, the 1999 Oklahoma terrorist bombing, and the 2006 coordinated terrorist bombings of Mumbai trains.[24,39,40]

Remoteness of the accident site poses difficulties in transporting victims to appropriate health care facilities quickly and may require aeromedical support for effective EMS transport.[7,17] In an intercity train crash, there is a possibility of passengers being trapped in isolated, inaccessible areas.[15,17] Emergency responders may be required to climb over carriages using ladders, extricate victims, and potentially transport victims over rough terrain for some distance or up train embankments to the nearest road.[15,17] Train tracks do not always run parallel to road networks, and there may be a considerable distance from the nearest road to the track, particularly where tracks skirt along riverbanks in valleys or mountainous terrain. Bystander volunteers may help improve outcomes in countries where an EMS system is absent or underdeveloped. Bystanders may help transport victims to nearby hospitals using taxis, personal vehicles, and public transport as observed in the 2006 coordinated terrorist blasts on Mumbai commuter trains.[17,24] If ambulances are not available in sufficient numbers immediately or if the magnitude of the disaster exceeds local resources, a treatment center should be set up in the staging area.[36] As per triage priority, victims are transported to the treatment center with secondary transport in ambulances, buses, or vans to definitive medical facilities as and when resources become available.[36]

In a developed EMS system, there should be an ambulance-loading officer to manage logistics of patient loading and transportation to assigned hospitals or specialty center destination assignments as they are exiting the incident from the medical communications coordinator.[36] Even though most developed EMS systems have a robust patient distribution mechanism in place, a disproportionate number of casualties may be transported to the closest general or specialty trauma or burns center.[24,39,40] Even if on-scene managers use a robust patient distribution system, victims and walking wounded who self-transport usually present to the closest hospitals, overwhelming a few health care facilities, while others receive only a few victims.[17,36]

Recovery should integrate early, beginning once the incident shifts from initial response phase to rescue operations phase.[27] Recovery operations focus on repairing the damage and restarting train services as early as possible after EMS evacuation of all passengers, medical examiner or coroner clearing the scene, and investigating agencies completion of enquiries and clearing the scene.[27]

MEDICAL TREATMENT OF CASUALTIES

Victims may present with a broad spectrum of traumatic injuries, ranging from simple lacerations and fractures to severe head and deceleration injuries (e.g., aortic or mesenteric avulsions).[41] Patterns of injury may vary considerably depending on the victims' location (e.g., seated versus standing, forward- versus rear-facing seats) at the time of the injury. Standing patients have a higher incidence of neck and craniofacial injuries.[42] Seated patients have a higher incidence of thoracoabdominal injuries, those in forward-facing seats having a greater potential for facial injuries and deceleration injuries.[18] In prolonged extrication, victims may be prone to crush syndrome and hypothermia or hyperthermia from exposure.[17,31] Burn or blast injuries also may manifest, depending on the presence of combustible materials or if the incident relates to terrorist explosion.

Emergency medical responders should consider confined-space therapeutic techniques to treat trapped survivors with an emphasis on securing intravenous access and administering fluids to prevent crush syndrome, endotracheal intubation where indicated, and needle decompression of tension pneumothoraces.[17,27,31]

Traumatic injuries to passengers and railway workers is the primary medical challenge, however, in cases of hazardous material exposures, the potential exists for the exposure of residents living near the disaster. The most frequent injuries sustained by railroad employees second to trauma are respiratory irritation, nausea, vomiting, and headache—all suggestive of hazardous material exposure.[43] Residents near the derailment and first responders are most likely to present with respiratory, dermatologic, or ophthalmic complaints due to exposure.[4] Correct use of PPE for rescue workers, decontamination of both victims and rescuers upon leaving the scene, and evacuation of any nearby residents can mitigate the consequences of a hazardous material spill.

Psychological first aid is an oft-forgotten element in dealing with the consequences of train derailment. Psychological casualties may present both immediately and delayed.[44] Victims may present with psychological complaints, somatic symptoms, or both. Posttraumatic stress disorders have been identified in both train passengers and nearby residents after a major train derailment.[45] Establishment of a critical incident stress debriefing support center to provide stress management, chaplain services, and psychological counseling for victims and their families, as well as the community, is helpful in minimizing the short- and long-term psychological sequelae after a railway disaster. Emergency responders responding to widespread devastation also suffer from emotional trauma.[27] Emergency responders should be afforded the opportunity to participate in a critical incident stress debriefing program, both individually and as a team, provided by a mental health professional, however, not all will avail of same.[27]

❓ UNIQUE CONSIDERATIONS

Derailment may occur in an urban environment with the subsequent risk of injury to the many people living and working nearby, or it may manifest in an isolated, rural location with challenges in response to the accident as well as other logistical difficulties. The number of casualties can vary from only a handful of railway workers to hundreds of passengers on board a commuter rail service. The possibility of hazardous material exposure exists in every train derailment, which may delay extrication of victims, as well as present serious problems for rescue workers and those nearby. An effective train disaster response plan must take into account all of these diverse possibilities.

❗ PITFALLS

Several potential pitfalls in response to a train derailment exist. These include the following:

- Failure to develop and practice a disaster response plan
- Failure to coordinate response with other agencies

- Failure to recognize hazardous material release
- Failure to maintain the integrity of a crime scene for investigators
- Failure to communicate with the public regarding risk and need for evacuation
- Failure to improve the interior design of trains to reduce injuries to passengers
- Failure to address the safety issues in the rail sector similar to the aviation industry
- Failure to implement passenger screening system similar to the aviation sector to reduce vulnerability of the rail industry to terrorist incidents
- Failure to implement seat belt and head restraint in trains for passenger safety
- Failure to develop early and rapid passenger extrication techniques and equipment
- Failure to address identification of both victims and deceased

REFERENCES

1. Forsberg R. *Train crashes: consequences for passengers;* 2012. Available at: http://www.surgsci.umu.se/digitalAssets/119/119614_rebecca-forsberg.pdf.
2. Kirby MW. *The Origins of Railway Enterprise: The Stockton and Darlington Railway 1821-1863.* Cambridge: Cambridge University Press; 2002.
3. Train History. History of steam locomotives. Train History website. Available at: http://www.trainhistory.net/railway-history/history-of-steam-locomotive/.
4. Óbuda University. Kálmán kandó. Óbuda University—Pro Scientia et Futuro website. Available at: http://uni-obuda.hu/en/munkatarsak/2297/kalman-kando.
5. Train History. Railway timeline—important moments in railway history. Train History website. Available at: http://www.trainhistory.net/railway-history/railroad-timeline/.
6. Ross Edgar. AirRail link: Birmingham International airport. The Gondola Project website. Available at: http://gondolaproject.com/2013/02/13/airrail-link-birmingham-international-airport/. Updated 2013.
7. Forsberg R, Björnstig U. One hundred years of railway disasters and recent trends. *Prehosp Disaster Med.* 2011;26:367–373.
8. Amtrak. Amtrak National Fact Sheet—2013. Amtrak website. Available at: http://www.amtrak.com/servlet/ContentServer?c=Page&pagename=am%2FLayout&cid=1246041980246. Updated 2013.
9. Railway Technology. TGV, France. Railway-Technology.Com website. Available at: http://www.railway-technology.com/projects/frenchtgv/.
10. Gebicki M. What's the world's fastest passenger train? Available at: http://www.stuff.co.nz/travel/news/63558825/whats-the-worlds-fastest-passenger-train Updated 2014.
11. Taylor CJ. Speed survey. *Railway Gazette International*; 2007. Available at: http://www.railwaygazette.com/fileadmin/user_upload/railwaygazette.com/PDF/RailwayGazetteWorldSpeedSurvey2007.pdf.
12. EM-DAT—the international disaster database. Center for Research on Epidemiology of Disasters—CRED website. Available at: http://emdat.be/advanced_search/index.html. Updated 2014.
13. Indian Railways. *Statistical summary—Indian railways;* 2013. Available at: http://www.indianrailways.gov.in/railwayboard/uploads/directorate/stat_econ/IRSB_2012–13/PDF/Statistical_Summary/Summary%20Sheet_Eng.pdf.
14. Lagny-pomponne—1933. Danger Ahead! Historic Rail Disasters website. Available at: http://danger-ahead.railfan.net/accidents/lagny/home.html. Updated 1999.
15. Stevens KLH, Partridge R. The Clapham rail disaster. *Injury.* 1990;21:37–40.
16. Fothergill NJ, Ebbs SR, Reese A, et al. The Purley train crash mechanism: injuries and prevention. *Arch Emerg Med.* 1992;9:125–129.
17. Björnstig U, Forsberg R. Transportation disasters. In: Koenig KL, Schultz CH, eds. *Koenig and Schultz's Disaster Medicine: Comprehensive Principles and Practices.* 1st ed. New York, NY: Cambridge University Press; 2009:253–274. Available at: http://www.cambridge.org/us/academic/

18. Ilkjær LB, Lind T. Passengers' injuries reflected carriage interior at the railway accident in Mundelstrup, Denmark. *Accid Anal Prev.* 2001;33:285–288.
19. Hsu EB, Grabowski JG, Chotani RA, Winslow JA, Alves DW, VanRooyen MJ. Effects on local emergency departments of large-scale urban chemical fire with hazardous materials spill. *Prehosp Disaster Med.* 2002;17:196–201.
20. Oestern H, Huels B, Quirini W, Pohlemann T. Facts about the disaster at Eschede. *J Orthop Trauma.* 2000;14:287–290.
21. Steele J. One train, more than 1,700 dead. *The Guardian*: 2004. World News—Indian Ocean Tsunami 2004. Available at: http://www.theguardian.com/world/2004/dec/29/tsunami2004.srilanka.
22. Carresi AL. The 2004 Madrid train bombings: an analysis of pre-hospital management. *Disasters.* 2008;32:41–65.
23. Mohammed AB, Mann HA, Nawabi DH, Goodier DW, Ang SC. Impact of London's terrorist attacks on a major trauma center in London. *Prehosp Disaster Med.* 2006;21:340–344.
24. Rai S, Sengupta S. Series of bombs explode on 7 trains in India, killing scores. *New York Times*: 2006. Asia Pacific. Available at: http://www.nytimes.com/2006/07/12/world/asia/12india.html?pagewanted=all&_r=0.
25. Rabasa A, Blackwill RD, Chalk P, et al. *The Lessons of Mumbai.* Santa Monica, CA: RAND; 2009, 249.
26. Roy N, Kapil V, Subbarao I, Ashkenazi I. Mass casualty response in the 2008 Mumbai terrorist attacks. *Disaster Med Public Health Prep.* 2011;5:273–279.
27. Boyd AM, Maier PM, Caton JE. *Critical incident management guidelines U.S. department of transportation, Research and special programs administration—volpe national transportation systems center;* 1998. FTA-MA-26-7009-98-1. Available at: http://transit-safety.volpe.dot.gov/publications/emergency/criticalincidents/html/cimg.htm.
28. Frazier ER, Ekern DS, Smith MC, Western JL, Bye PG, Krentz MA. *Managing catastrophic transportation emergencies: A guide for transportation executives;* 2014. NCHRP Project 20-59(36). Available at: http://onlinepubs.trb.org/onlinepubs/nchrp/nchrp_w206.pdf.
29. Hathaway WT, Markos SH, Pawlak RJ. *Recommended emergency preparedness guidelines for rail transit systems;* 1999. UMTA-MA-06-0152-85-1. Available at: http://transit-safety.volpe.dot.gov/publications/Emergency/Rec_EmerPrep/repg_rts.htm.
30. Hambeck MW, Pueschel MK. Death by railway accident: incidence of traumatic asphyxia. *J Trauma.* 1981;21:28–31.
31. Nagata T, Rosborough SN, VanRooyen MJ, Kozawa S, Ukai T, Nakayama S. Express railway disaster in Amagasaki: A review of urban disaster response capacity in Japan. *Prehosp Disaster Med.* 2006;21:345–352.
32. Security Emergency Management Group. *Recommended practice for first responder familiarization of transit systems;* 2008. APTA-SS-SEM-RP-002-08. Available at: http://www.apta.com/resources/standards/Documents/APTA-SS-SEM-RP-002-08.pdf.
33. Esslinger V, Kieselbach R, Koller R, Weisse B. The railway accident of Eschede—technical background. *Eng Failure Anal.* 2004;11:515–535.
34. Iselius L, Nilsson P, Riddez L. KAMEDO report no. 79 train accident in Germany, 1998. *Prehosp Disaster Med.* 2006;21:119–120.
35. Calland V. A brief overview of personal safety at incident sites. *Emerg Med J.* 2006;23:878–882.
36. Miller KT. Emergency medical services—scene management. In: Koenig KL, Schultz CH, eds. *Koenig and Schultz's Disaster Medicine: Comprehensive Principles and Practices.* 1st ed. New York, NY: Cambridge University Press; 2010:275–284.
37. Braden GE. Aircraft-type crash injury investigation of a commuter train collision. *Aviat Space Environ Med.* 1975;46:1157–1160.
38. Super G, Groth S, Hook R. *START: simple triage and rapid treatment plan.* Newport Beach, CA: Hoag Memorial Presbyterian Hospital; 1994, 199.
39. Centers for Disease Control and Prevention (CDC). Rapid assessment of injuries among survivors of the terrorist attack on the world trade center—New York City, September 2001. *MMWR Morb Mortal Wkly Rep.* 2002;51:1–5.
40. Hogan DE, Waeckerle JF, Dire DJ, Lillibridge SR. Emergency department impact of the Oklahoma City terrorist bombing. *Ann Emerg Med.* 1999;34:160–167.

41. Prabhakar T, Sharma Y. Ghaisal train accident. *Indian J Anaesth.* 2002;46:409–413.

42. Cugnoni H, Fincham C, Skinner D. Cannon Street rail disaster—lessons to be learned. *Injury.* 1994;25:11–13.

43. Orr MF, Kaye WE, Zeitz P, Powers ME, Rosenthal L. Public health risks of railroad hazardous substance emergency events. *J Occupat Environ Med.* 2001;43:94–100.

44. Hagström R. The acute psychological impact on survivors following a train accident. *J Trauma Stress.* 1995;8:391–402.

45. Chung MC, Easthope Y, Farmer S, Werrett J, Chung C. Psychological sequelae: post-traumatic stress reactions and personality factors among community residents as secondary victims. *Scand J Caring Sci.* 2003;17:265–270.

Subway Derailment

Asaad Alsufyani and Michael Sean Molloy

DESCRIPTION OF EVENT

In 1863 the first underground railway opened in London. The Metropolitan Railway—now known as the London Underground—featured gas-lit carriages hauled by steam locomotives. New York City celebrated a century of its subway in 2004.[1,2] The first deep lines in London (not cut-and-cover construction)[3] opened with electrified trains in 1890. Since then, worldwide, subways have become an ordinary means of mass transit transporting hundreds or even thousands of people per train, often at frequent intervals per station of 5 minutes or less. In some cities, subways transport more than 6 million passengers per day. Thus, the potential for mass casualty incidents is significant. Subways run on tracks underground, although in the late nineteenth century, there was some experimentation with pneumatic tubes in New York. Derailment is a serious risk that must be mitigated and planned for. Recent developments in railroad car safety should help in preventing derailments in the future.[4] Derailment can present as a thump barely noticed by passengers or as catastrophic failure resulting in mass casualty injuries and death. A subway train may derail because of mechanical failure of the train,[5] mechanical failure of the rail,[5] external objects on the tracks, sabotage,[6] natural disaster,[7] maintenance failure,[2] driver error, or terrorist attack on the train system or the city above. Kyriakidis reviewed precursors for metro accidents and found the 27 precursors analyzed, for the period 2002-2009, fall into six categories: human performance, technical failures, passengers, fires, malicious action, and management action.[8] One of the worst accidents in subway history occurred in New York City on November 1, 1918. An inexperienced dispatcher (filling in for striking motormen) who was tasked with driving a train after only 2 hours of instruction entered a tunnel too fast, causing the wooden train to derail. The train struck a wall, killing 97 people and injuring 200. This incident led to the Brooklyn Rapid Transit Company going out of business a month later.[9] Subways have become considerably safer in the intervening period, with considerable emphasis on education and safety, but accidents including derailments still occur. Gershon reviewed medical records of 668 subway fatalities in New York City between 1990 and 2003, finding that 343 related to suicide; 10 to homicide; and 315 to accidents.[10] Operator error remains the most common cause of derailment.[11] Intentional sabotage of tracks or cars can also lead to derailment.[6] On March 29, 2010, 40 people were killed, and more than 100 injured when two bombs exploded in separate Moscow Metro stations, with a roughly 40-minute interval between explosions.[12]

The location of derailment events or underground rail emergencies can present unique challenges for emergency responders.[13,14] Consider the course of a subway ride in a large city; the journey may encompass travel aboveground and underground, on elevated platforms, on city streets, and on bridges over bodies of water, gorges, or ravines. An underground subway derailment necessitates evacuation of the train in a dark tunnel with possibly a long walking distance to access points. During an aboveground derailment, train cars may tip over, override, or telescope.[15] Underground telescoping has been reduced by the introduction of metal carriages with anticlimb devices and crush zones.[15] Train derailment on an elevated railway may result in carriages falling from the bridge. Passengers and emergency responders face similar risks during the response phase to such an event. Elevated railways passing over water present additional hazards, including drowning and exposure to cold for victims falling into the water. A common hazard to all electrified train incidents is the risk of electrocution from contact with the third rail providing several hundred volts of direct current power to the train, Contact with the third rail can be fatal. Hazardous materials being transported also pose significant risks to responders, passengers, and residents in the environs.[16]

PRE-INCIDENT ACTIONS

Emergency managers completing a hazard vulnerability analysis (HVA) for their hospital should include a survey of subway or train stations located in the catchment area. Historic rail accidents within the hospital catchment area should be reviewed carefully to determine whether there are "danger zones" requiring mitigation efforts or where future accidents may be more likely to occur.[17] Where rail accidents feature highly on the HVA, preparation for rail accidents should be made in the form of multiagency tabletop drills, communication exercises and real-time-real-size drills with casualties to test individual elements of the response system.[18,19] This will also preempt response issues such as failure of interagency communication underground because of equipment designed to be used over ground.

The kinetic energy of a traveling train is proportional to the number of cars (mass) and the velocity of the train squared. An increase in speed from 50 to 70 km/h doubles the kinetic energy involved in collisions. An increase from 50 to 100 km/h increases the energy involved in a collision fortyfold. The higher the kinetic energy, the greater the risk of injury to passengers in the event of a derailment event.[20] An estimate of the potential number of victims that could result from a subway derailment can be obtained by multiplying the number of cars per train traveling through local stations and rail routes by the passenger capacity of each car. If the potential number of patients that could result from such a rail accident exceeds the capacity of local prehospital and hospital resources, multiagency disaster plans should be developed and drilled for such a scenario. In a rail disaster, command and control at the scene can be particularly problematic if the victims injured or killed are scattered throughout the incident area, multiple forward commanders may be required. An example was the Eschede train disaster, where the victims were scattered over approximately 3 miles of track length.

POST-INCIDENT ACTIONS

The earliest priority is to recognize the event as a mass casualty incident and declare that the incident has occurred. Once notification occurs then the incident command structure should be instituted. In the United States, the National Incident Management System (NIMS)[21,22] will be used, whereas in other jurisdictions, the Major Incident Medical Management and Support (MIMMS)[23] system will be used. Early appropriate transmission of the initial message can influence development of the response phase, having a message structure template will assist this process.

The METHANE (Hodgetts 2013)[24] message as used in the UK's MIMMS system is an example of an easily taught and repeatable message structure for responders to declare a mass casualty incident. The transmitter begins his transmission by asking the receiver to prepare to receive a METHANE message:

M—Major incident declared
E—Exact location (grid reference if known or GPS)
T—Type of incident (fire, crash, explosion, etc.)
H—Potential hazards involved (smoke, oil, chemicals, fire, etc.)
A—Access roads to the scene from various directions
N—Estimated number of casualties
E—Emergency services present and required

The advantage of such a message structure is that both receiver and transmitter are aware of the sequence reducing the chance that a vital portion of the message will be missed on either side.

The CSCATTT tool as both outlined below and used in MIMMS for prioritizing actions on scene is useful for first responders.[25]

C—Command and control
S—Safety/security
C—Communications
A—Assessment
T—Triage
T—Treatment
T—Transport

Responders need to set up a command post, the location where the incident command functions, early, and this should be located in a safe place near the crash site, but not too close to prevent becoming involved in the incident or being at risk from the potential hazards.[26] HazMat teams should be involved as early as possible to rule out toxic exposures. Usually, the fire department heads the unified command structure when there are entrapped victims and active hazards, but this may differ depending on the country or the disaster situation itself where other military or federal authorities may have command.

Considering the variety of possible disaster scenes and hazards after a subway event, the responder must pay particular attention to scene safety issues and the use of personal protective equipment (PPE). Adequate resources should be mobilized to address the specific scenarios faced, and predetermined evacuation plans for survivors should be implemented. When victim rescue operations are completed, assessment of the rail bed must be made to determine structural integrity before the reestablishment of service along that route. Train cars must likewise be inspected to determine future usability.

Debriefing or "hotwash" with emergency responders should be undertaken soon after the event and rescue operation, with senior members of involved agencies and specialized organizations, to understand any difficulties that may have been encountered during the rescue and recovery operations.

MEDICAL TREATMENT OF CASUALTIES

In low-speed derailments, musculoskeletal injuries such as ankle and wrist injuries, and injuries caused by falls are predominantly seen. In high-speed derailments, in which deceleration forces may be significant, the spectrum of traumatic injuries presenting is similar to that seen in other groups suffering high-speed blunt trauma. High-speed derailments in tunnels may result in collision with tunnel support stanchions, which may remain intact but cause passenger cars to collapse, presenting risks from falling debris or unstable structures.[27] Fire, smoke, and release of toxic gases may complicate injuries resulting from blunt trauma.[12]

Rail accident scenes are prone to multiple hazards, of which emergency responders must be aware and must take precautions to avoid. Live electrical wires or the train's electrified third rail present risk of electrocution leading to burns and respiratory and cardiac arrest. Fire in a subway tunnel can result in hypoxia and the possibility of exposure to toxic fumes. If fire is present, active suppression must take place before rescue attempts can be made.

When scene safety is assured, victims should be evacuated from the accident zone as quickly as possible to minimize further risk from on-scene hazards and to allow for appropriate triage,[28] on-scene treatment, and transportation to hospital if required.[29] High-angle rope rescue or confined-space medical rescue techniques may be required in specific instances. Spinal immobilization and extrication of hundreds of patients on long boards presents enormous technical and logistical challenges for emergency responders. In this situation, deployment of appropriately trained prehospital physicians to the field to evaluate and triage patients without evidence of cervical spine injuries can significantly expedite the safe extrication of patients at risk for cervical spine injuries, avoiding overtriage and excess use of spinal immobilization if it can be avoided.

The triage area should be established upwind and outside of the accident zone, away from potential hazards, ideally in an area that is accessible to transporting ambulances. Responders should consider using intact tunnels as an evacuation route. Patients should be triaged using standard algorithms for a mass casualty incident.

Basic trauma stabilization of injured patients can be initiated on scene, in preparation for transport to hospital. Patients with smoke inhalation or exposure to other toxic fumes should receive supplemental oxygen.

UNIQUE CONSIDERATIONS

Subway derailments, when they occur underground or on elevated platforms, may be associated with difficult access issues for rescuers. Underground accidents may be associated with fire, smoke, and toxic gas hazards that present risks to victims and rescuers alike. Rescuers may have to walk long distances through tunnels to reach the accident scene, carrying extrication and other rescue equipment, and then transport patients out on foot along the same route. The extrication of passengers from severely damaged or crushed train cars may require the use of heavy equipment outside the scope of standard emergency medical service(s) (EMS) or fire department capabilities. Planning for such scenarios should occur in advance and involve representation from all relevant response agencies, including the Transit Authority.

⚠ PITFALLS

Several potential pitfalls in response to a subway derailment exist. These include but are not limited to the following:

- Failure to complete multiagency drills covering underground derailment for all response services
- Failure to develop and practice a disaster response plan for underground derailment
- Failure to implement passenger screening to reduce vulnerability to terrorism
- Failure to address identification of victims and the deceased
- Failure to logically track victims when transported off site
- Failure to consider underground derailment in hazard vulnerability plans for emergency first response services
- Failure of hospitals to consider their role in responding to underground derailments, including training staff in prehospital elevated- and confined-space rescue techniques
- Inadequate implementation of an emergency plan with sufficient elements, including fire, police, EMS, and government agencies (e.g., the National Transportation Safety Board [NTSB])
- Slow or incomplete discontinuation of track electricity supply and commuter service on the line
- Failure to recognize hazardous material release
- Failure of ventilation systems with accumulation of toxic gases underground
- Underground communication failures
- Technically difficult rescues and extrication, either because of entrapment in machinery, conditions other than on level ground, or remote locations underground

REFERENCES

1. Transit A. New York City's Subway Century. *TR News*. 2006.
2. Cudahy B. *A Century of Subways*. 1st ed. Fordham University Press; 2003.
3. Edwards JT. *Civil Engineering for Underground Rail Transport*. Butterworth-Heinemann; 1990.
4. Shanley TE. *E ST. Railroad Car Derailment Safety Device*; 1993. Available at: http://patft.uspto.gov/netacgi/nph-Parser?Sect2=PTO1&Sect2=HITOFF&p=1&u=/netahtml/PTO/search-bool.html&r=1&f=G&l=50&d=PALL&RefSrch=yes&Query=PN/5188038.
5. Evans AW. Rail safety and rail privatisation in Britain. *Accid Anal Prev*. 2007;39(3):510–523.
6. Murphy GK. Death in the desert: the sabotage-derailment of "The City of San Francisco." *Am J Forensic Med Pathol*. 1983;4(2):145–148.
7. Xiao X, Ling L, Jin X. A study of the derailment mechanism of a high-speed train due to an earthquake. *Vehicle Syst Dynam*. 2012;50(3):449–470.
8. Kyriakidis M, Hirsch R, Majumdar A. Metro railway safety: an analysis of accident precursors. *Saf Sci*. 2012;50(7):1535–1548.
9. Scores Killed or Maimed in Brighton Tunnel Wreck. *NY Times*. 1918.
10. Gershon RRM, Pearson JM, Nandi V, et al. Epidemiology of subway-related fatalities in New York City, 1990-2003. *J Safety Res*. 2008;39(6):583–588.
11. NTSB. *Railroad Accident Report RAR-97/02 [Internet]*. NTSB: Washington; 1997. Available at: http://www.ntsb.gov/investigations/AccidentReports/Reports/RAR9702.pdf.
12. Moscow Metro Hit by Deadly Suicide Bombings [Internet]. news.bbc.co.uk. 2010. Available at: http://news.bbc.co.uk/2/hi/europe/8592190.stm.
13. Bessant GT. King's Cross underground station, London: an overview. *Proc ICE—Transport*. 2004;157(4):211–220.
14. Haack A, Schreyer J. Emergency scenarios for tunnels and underground stations in public transport. *Tunnelling and Underground Space Technology*. 2006.
15. Forsberg R, Bjornstig U. One hundred years of railway disasters and recent trends. *Prehosp Disaster Med*. 2011;26(5):367–373.
16. Gibson C, Fowler R, Foltas W. 11 November 1979—a day to remember: the Mississauga disaster. *Can J Hosp Pharm*. 1980;32(6):178–180.
17. Lennquist S. *Medical Response to Major Incidents and Disasters*. Berlin, Heidelberg: Springer; 2012.
18. Klima DA, Seiler SH, Peterson JB, et al. Full-scale regional exercises: closing the gaps in disaster preparedness. *J Trauma Acute Care Surg*. 2012;73(3):592–597, discussion 597–598.
19. Hodgetts TJ. Major Incident Medical Training: A Systematic International Approach. *Intl J Disaster Med*. 2009;1(1):13–20. Available at: http://dx.doi.org/10.1080/15031430310013429.
20. Jussila J, Kjellström BT, Leppäniemi A. Ballistic variables and tissue devitalisation in penetrating injury—establishing relationship through meta-analysis of a number of pig tests. *Injury*. 2005;36(2):282–292.
21. Stopford BM. The National Disaster Medical System: America's medical readiness force. *Disaster Manag Response*. 2005;3(2):53–56.
22. Dr. Donald W. Walsh, Dr. Hank T. Christen Jr., Graydon C. Lord, Geoffrey T. Miller. *National Incident Management System*. 2nd ed Jones & Bartlett Learning, 2010.
23. Kevin Mackway-Jones, ed. Advanced Life Support Group. *Major Incident Medical Management and Support*, 3 ed. BMJ Books; 2012.
24. Hodgetts TJ, Porter C, eds. *Major Incident Management System (MIMS)*. 1st BMJ Books; 2013.
25. Wachira BW, Abdalla RO, Wallis LA. Westgate Shootings: an emergency department approach to a mass-casualty incident. *Prehosp Disaster Med*. 2014;29(5):538–541.
26. Brinker K, Lumia M, Markiewicz KV, et al. Assessment of emergency responders after a vinyl chloride release from a train derailment: New Jersey, 2012. *MMWR Morb Mortal Wkly Rep*. 2015;63(53):1233–1237.
27. www.nycsubway.org. Available at: http://www.nycsubway.org/wiki/Subway_FAQ:_Accidents.
28. Jenkins JL, McCarthy ML, Sauer LM, et al. Mass-casualty triage: time for an evidence-based approach. *Prehosp Disaster Med*. 2008;23(01):3–8.
29. Oswald M, Kirchberger H, Lebeda C. Evacuation of a high floor Metro train in a tunnel situation: experimental findings. In: *Pedestrian and Evacuation Dynamics 2008*. Berlin, Heidelberg: Springer; 2010:67–81.

CHAPTER 183

Bus Accident

Eike Blohm and Kavita Babu

DESCRIPTION OF EVENT

Americans travel by bus approximately six billion times a year.[1] An estimated 480,000 school buses transport 26 million schoolchildren to and from school each weekday[2] for an annual total of 5.8 billion miles.[2] Despite these extraordinary numbers, serious bus crashes are still uncommon events. There were 118 school bus–related fatalities in 2009, and all but three of the victims were outside the bus (e.g., a struck pedestrian). Of the 2508 deaths associated with American school bus crashes between 1977 and 1992, 10.8% affected school bus occupants.[3] A study of Iowa (United States) school buses estimated approximately 320 school bus crashes for every 100 million bus miles traveled,[4] resulting in approximately 0.2 deaths.[5] Limited data exist for commercial buses; 55 deaths were reported to the U.S. Bureau of Transportation Statistics in 2012, but the number of miles driven is unknown.[6] Overall, the risk of fatal injury for a bus passenger is significantly lower than that of an automobile occupant in the United States.[6]

The maximum occupancy of buses varies depending on size. In regard to school buses in the United States, up to three small children may sit on each bench.[5] A single type D school bus filled to its stated capacity may therefore hold more than 70 passengers.[7] In some developing countries, the maximum occupancy of buses is frequently exceeded.[8] Given the capacity of a typical bus, a crash may cause an instant mass casualty event, as was the case with the 2011 World Wide Tours bus crash in New York City. After the driver lost control, the bus toppled onto its right side and slid into a sign pole, tearing the bus open along the window line. Fifteen people died, and 17 were injured.[9]

The U.S. Department of Transportation recorded 54 deaths of bus occupants in 2011.[6] While transit and charter bus data are available, the most complete data on bus crashes are derived from analyses of school bus crashes. The characteristics of the crashes that produced fatalities included front-end and side-impact crashes, overturned buses, and collisions with trains.[10] According to the U.S. National Highway Traffic Safety Administration (NHTSA), death and significant injury were often attributed to being seated at the point of impact.[10]

In general, there are two approaches to reducing harm to bus occupants: active safety and passive safety. Active safety aims to prevent motor vehicle crashes from happening by means of traffic laws, driver training, designated bus lanes, vehicle maintenance, etc. Passive safety focuses on minimizing damage to passengers during and after a collision. This approach is embodied in passenger restraints, cabin stability, and medical response.

Analyses of individual crashes have guided the bus industry safety standards. The primary passenger safety feature of school buses is called "compartmentalization." Given the size of buses and the crash forces imparted to passengers, legislation was passed in 1977 to make compartmentalization standard in new production of school buses in the United States.[10] Padded seats create a compartment for the passenger between high-seat backs and the seat in front, protecting the rider in sudden deceleration events, as is the case in a head-on collision. The seats themselves are constructed of steel designed to absorb energy by bending. However, this method of protection is particularly limited in rollovers, when passengers may be thrown from their seats.[11] A study analyzing a 14-year period of commercial bus crashes in Uppsala, Sweden, found that 35% to 40% of crashes involved a side impact to the bus.[12]

As of 2013, the NHTSA in the United States mandates that all new commercial buses be outfitted with seat belts. Currently, there is no mandate for passengers to wear them.[13] Continued controversy exists over the use of seat belts in school and city transit buses.[7] Proponents for seat belts cite that only about 65% of school bus crashes are frontal or rear-end collisions in which children are protected by "compartementalization."[3] New York, New Jersey, Florida, California, Louisiana, and Texas require seat belts on school buses or are in the process of passing such legislation.[14] Federal transportation authorities argue that the cost of the seat belt implementation may be better allocated for other safety measures, such as driver training and increasing safety during loading and unloading.[15] This idea was echoed by an observational study (a video camera in a bus), which found that only just above 60% of students would wear the provided seat belts. The study took place in the state of Alabama, which does not require seat belts to be worn in school buses.[7]

It is the primary goal of emergency preparedness to prevent or minimize harm to occupants of buses, especially schoolchildren. The American College of Emergency Physicians released a statement[16] that encourages further investigation of the utility of passenger restraints but also advocates for safer loading and unloading zones and increased school bus visibility. Yet the reality is that a balance must be struck between money invested and the number of lives saved. For example, seat belts would decrease the capacity of each school bus by 5% to 18%, as three small children could no longer occupy the same bench. Subsequently, an increase in the bus fleet and personnel to operate them might result. The total cost (seat belt installation, buses, and wages) over the 10-year life span of the bus fleet divided by the number of fatalities over the same time period would result in an estimated $32 to $38 million per life saved.[7] Yet among all fatalities from bus crashes in the United States, only 13% occurred within the bus compartment. Most fatalities are pedestrians or occupants of other vehicles.[17] Turner associates concluded that costs far exceed benefits, and school bus seat belts appear to be less cost-effective than other types of safety treatments, such as increasing safety during loading and unloading of students, a time period when 69% of pedestrian student fatalities occur.[3,7] From a utilitarian perspective, the same amount of money is likely to do greater good elsewhere, such as teaching children how to swim.[18] Moreover, seat belts in buses may be less efficacious compared to those in cars. The primary purpose of a seat belt is to prevent ejection, an uncommon event in bus crashes.[19] Proponents state that seat belts are an essential intervention for preventing injury to passengers during a rollover and lateral impact collisions.[19] Rollovers account for approximately 0.5% of bus crashes and lateral impacts for approximately 10%.[4] Currently, only six states in the United States require seat belts on school buses.[20] The European Union mandates three-point restraints for all new buses since 2002.[21] No commercial or school buses in the United States feature airbags for passengers.

PRE-INCIDENT ACTIONS

Given the nearly ubiquitous presence of buses, every public safety system, emergency department, and hospital must have a comprehensive plan in place for managing a bus crash with multiple casualties. A serious bus crash may rapidly overwhelm the resources of a single hospital.[22] Activation of local, state, and even federal resources may be required. Prehospital triage is critical to avoiding saturation of the nearest hospital. On-scene personnel should transport unstable patients to the nearest hospital, while patients with minor injuries can be diverted to outlying facilities.

One unique difficulty faced by prehospital personnel at the scene of a bus crash is the difficulty of extricating victims. This was highlighted in 2012 by a bus crash in Sierre, Switzerland, where extrication of some passengers took up to 8 hours.[23] The standard extrication tools and techniques used at car crashes may not be effective in evacuating victims from a bus. Particular difficulties with extrication were also noted in an Omaha, Nebraska, crash in 2003. As a consequence of this accident, the National Transportation Safety Board (NTSB) issued a recommendation that all fire and rescue personnel undergo specialized training in bus extrication techniques.[24]

Rapid extrication of bus crash victims is particularly vital in cases where the bus ends up submerged in a body of water. Recent crashes in China and India resulted in massive death tolls after buses left the road and entered nearby rivers.[25] High numbers of bus crash fatalities in developing countries may also be attributed to older equipment, bus overcrowding, lack of standardized driver training, and hazardous road conditions.

POST-INCIDENT ACTIONS

In recent years, the United States NHTSA has identified the collection and assimilation of transit and charter bus crash data as a priority in creating applicable safety interventions. The efforts of clinicians, local rescue personnel, and law enforcement to report all bus crashes are critical for surveillance. One established surveillance system in the United States is the National Trauma Data Bank (NTDB).[26]

If the bus crash involves a large number of fatalities, part of the disaster response must involve quick activation of local, state, and national mortuary teams to identify remains in a rapid and accurate manner.[27]

MEDICAL TREATMENT OF CASUALTIES

There are five main mechanisms that are responsible for the vast majority of killed or severely injured (KSI) bus passengers: internal collision (in which the passenger collides with a piece of the bus or another passenger), complete ejection, partial ejection, intrusion of an outside object into the passenger cabin, or smoke inhalation.[21] Of those, partial ejection caused the vast majority (71%) of fatalities.[28] A review of bus-related injuries in Europe revealed that extremity injuries occurred in two thirds of patients, head injuries in one third, and torso injuries in less than 10%.[21] An Australian study reviewing school bus–related

fatalities in children identified head injury and blood loss as the most common causes of death.[29]

In a mass casualty event, triage protocols such as SALT, Jump-START, Smart triage, or Sieve and Sort help identify patients that require emergent treatment. As with other reasons for blunt trauma, immediate attention must be directed to controlling massive hemorrhages, airways with cervical spine control, breathing, and circulation. Rapid airway management may be required in patients with a depressed Glasgow Coma Score, traditionally advocated as being below 8. Significant burns or chest wall trauma may lead to a rapid decline of respiratory function. Spinal immobilization must be maintained until injury can either be ruled out clinically or radiologically. The secondary survey for injuries should be performed rapidly. Patients with life- or limb-threatening injuries must be addressed emergently, while other patients may be suitable for instant transfer or triage to a less urgent level of care. Some patients may not require any medical care and can be discharged by authorized personnel (depending on local emergency medical service(s) [EMS] protocols or physician availability). In most bus crashes, there are far more "walking wounded" than patients with incapacitating injuries.[30] In the case of multiple serious casualties, the physician, or his or her staff, must be able to mobilize both hospital and prehospital resources without failing to provide care to all patients.

UNIQUE CONSIDERATIONS

In many ways, the traumatic injuries sustained by any individual during a bus crash are not markedly different from those found in a simple motor vehicle collision. However, bus crashes have the potential to generate far more patients than individual car crashes, depending on the capacity of the bus in question and the severity of the crash. Local resources may become quickly overwhelmed. The nature of patient injuries may be specialized, with school bus crashes representing a potential pediatric mass casualty, while a charter bus may represent a geriatric mass casualty or a group of tourists unable to give histories due to language barriers.[31] Moreover, multiple documented bus crashes recorded large numbers of burn victims, creating the need for aggressive airway management and resuscitation.[32]

PITFALLS

- Failure to develop adequate mass casualty protocols at the emergency services, hospital, community, and state levels
- Failure to train community EMS in specialized techniques for bus extrication
- Failure to educate schoolchildren and public transportation passengers regarding emergency exit operation and utilization
- Failure to anticipate a large number of trauma victims
- Failure to anticipate a large number of pediatric victims
- Failure to anticipate a large number of burn victims requiring definitive airway management
- Failure to inform national registries (NTSB or NHTSA in the United States) regarding bus crashes (of all severity) to provide better data and improve overall safety

REFERENCES

1. American Public Transportation Association. *America Rides the Bus*; 2009. Available at: http://www.apta.com/resources/reportsandpublications/Documents/bus_w_cov_a.pdf. Accessed 12.05.14.
2. American School Bus Council. Environmental benefits. Fact: you can go green by riding yellow. Available at: http://www.americanschoolbuscouncil.org/issues/environmental-benefits. Accessed May 12, 2014.

3. Hall WL. Seat belts on school buses: a review of issues and research. In: *North Carolina School Bus Safety Conference*: 1996. Raleigh, NC.

4. Yang J, Peek-Asa C, Cheng G, Heiden E, Falb S, Ramirez M. Incidence and characteristics of school bus crashes and injuries. *Accid Anal Prev.* 2009;41(2):336–341.

5. U.S. Department of Transportation. *NHTSA Sends School Bus Report to Congress* [press release]; 2002. Available at: http://www.nhtsa.gov/About +NHTSA/Press+Releases/2002/NHTSA+Sends+School+Bus+Report+to +Congress. Accessed 04.12.15.

6. U.S. Department of Transportation, Bureau of Transportation Statistics, Office of the Assistant Secretary for Research and Technology. *Table 2-1; Transportation Fatalities by Mode;* 2013. Available at: http://www.rita.dot .gov/bts/sites/rita.dot.gov.bts/files/publications/national_transportation_ statistics/html/table_02_01.html_mfd. Accesed 12.05.14.

7. Turner D. *Summary Report: Alabama School Bus Seat Belt Pilot Project.* Birmingham, AL: University of Alabama; 2010.

8. Gomes Rocha N. *Case Report of Overcrowded Buses and a Possible Solution. Urban Transport XIV: Urban Transport and the Environment in the 21st Century;* 2008. http://trid.trb.org/view.aspx?id=873597.

9. McFadden R. Carnage on I-95 After Crash Rips Bus Apart. *New York Times;* 2011.

10. Hinch J, Elias J, Hott C, Willke D, Sullivan L, Prasad A, McCray L. *Report to congress: School Bus Safety: Crashworthiness Research.* 2002.

11. Sibbald B. MDs call for new safety features after death in school bus crash. *Can Med Assoc J.* 2003;169(9):951.

12. af Wåhlberg AE. Characteristics of low speed accidents with buses in public transport. *Accid Anal Prev.* 2002;34(5):637–647.

13. National Highway Traffic Safety Administration. *NHTSA Announces Final Rule Requiring Seat Belts on Motorcoaches.* 2013.

14. Wiegand DM, Bowman D, Hanowski RJ, Daecher C, Bergoffen G. *Special Safety Concerns of the School Bus Industry: A Synthesis of Safety Practice. Commercial Truck and Bus Safety. Synthesis 17.* Transportation Research Board of the National Academies; 2010, Vol. 17.

15. *National Highway Traffic Safety Administration, U.S. Department of Transportation. Federal Motor Vehicle Safety Standards; Denial of Petition for Rulemaking; School Buses. Federal Register* 76(165):2011.

16. American College of Emergency Physicians. School bus safety. Policy statement. *Ann Emerg Med.* 2013;62(4):445.

17. Cafiso S, Di Graziano A, Pappalardo G. Road safety issues for bus transport management. *Accid Anal Prev.* 2013;60:324–333.

18. Rahman F, Bose S, Linnan M, et al. Cost-effectiveness of an injury and drowning prevention program in Bangladesh. *Pediatrics.* 2012;130(6): e1621–e1628.

19. Lapner PC, Nguyen D, Letts M. Analysis of a school bus collision: mechanism of injury in the unrestrained child. *Can J Surg.* 2003;46 (4):269–272.

20. Frisman P. 2010. *State laws requiring seat belts in school buses; Connecticut General Assembly Office of Legislative Research Report 2010-R-0055.* Available at: http://www.cga.ct.gov/2010/rpt/2010-R-0055.htm. Accessed 04.12.15.

21. Albertsson P, Falkmer T. Is there a pattern in European bus and coach incidents? A literature analysis with special focus on injury causation and injury mechanisms. *Accid Anal Prev.* 2005;37(2): 225–233.

22. Wright P. Dissecting a disaster. *Blue Mountain Eagle;* 2013, Grant County, OR. Available at http://www.bluemountaineagle.com/news/ state_national/20130628/dissecting-a-disaster. Accessed 04.12.15.

23. Pietsch U. The Swiss bus accident on 13 March 2012: lessons for pre-hospital care. *Crit Care.* 2013;17(1):416.

24. National Transportation Safety Board. 2004. School Bus Run-off-Bridge Accident, Omaha, Nebraska, October 13, 2001. Highway Accident Report NTSB/HAR-04/01. Washington, DC.

25. Pratab A. *India Bus Accident Kills 28 Children;* CNN, 11/18/1997.

26. Nance M. *National Trauma Data Bank Annual Report 2012.* 2013, American College of Surgeons. Available at https://www.facs.org/~/media/ files/quality%20programs/trauma/ntdb/ntdb%20annual%20report% 202012.ashx. Accessed 04.12.15.

27. Valenzuela A, Martin-de las Heras S, Marques T, Exposito N, Bohoyo JM. The application of dental methods of identification to human burn victims in a mass disaster. *Int J Legal Med.* 2000;113(4):236–239.

28. Albertsson P. *Occupant Casualties in Bus and Coach Traffic: Injury and Crash Mechanisms;* UMEÅ UNIVERSITY MEDICAL DISSERTATIONS. 2005. Available at: http://www.diva-portal.org/smash/get/diva2:143554/ FULLTEXT01.pdf. Accessed 04.12.15.

29. Cass DT, Ross F, Lam L. School bus–related deaths and injuries in New South Wales. *Med J Aust.* 1996;165(3):134–137.

30. National Highway Traffic Safety Administration. *Occupant Fatalities in School Buses;* 2002.

31. Duchateau FX, Verner L. K-plan for patient repatriation after mass casualty events abroad. *Air Med J.* 2012;31(2):92–94.

32. Martin-de las Heras S, Valenzuela A, Villanueva E, Marques T, Exposito N, Bohoyo JM. Methods for identification of 28 burn victims following a 1996 bus accident in Spain. *J Forensic Sci.* 1999; 44(2):428–431.

184 CHAPTER

Aircraft Crash Preparedness and Response

Peter B. Pruitt and Paul D. Biddinger

DESCRIPTION OF EVENT

More than 30,000 commercial flights carry more than 2 million passengers in the United States daily.[1] With only 72 fatal accidents between 2004 and 2014, commercial jet air travel is one of the safest means of mass transportation per mile traveled.[2] The previous flight statistics do not account for private aircraft. A crash involving either a fixed-wing aircraft (i.e., airplane) or rotor-wing aircraft (i.e., helicopter) is a highly visible event that garners intense public and media scrutiny. The event response taxes local first responders, emergency managers, and local leaders. With more than 3355 significant public-use airports in the United States, the potential for response in any given community is more than just theoretical.[3] A registry review revealed more than 700 aviation-related deaths per year, although only 7% of those are related to commercial airliners.[4] In communities without an airport, there remains potential for an aircraft flying overhead to either crash or make an emergency landing with little warning and the potential for significant injuries to passengers and the local populace.

PRE-INCIDENT CONSIDERATIONS

The most important factor related to planning an initial response phase to an aircraft crash is to note the vast majority of aircraft accidents (80%) occur during takeoff and landing at an airport or in close proximitiy.[5] Such statistics highlight the importance of both airport emergency operations planning as well as off-airport planning. Water-based response plans must be robust for those airports adjacent to large bodies of water. Response to aviation emergencies on the airport site begins with the airport rescue firefighting (ARFF) resources but will often quickly escalate to a mutual aid response event. In the event of an off-airport crash the affected jurisdiction will have initial responsibility for providing fire and rescue response. Fire departments in close proximity to airports must plan responses to crashes with attention to how such events are different from the usual fires to which they respond. Even jurisdictions not located close to airports must be prepared to handle these major events because a small but significant number of aircraft crashes occur remote from airports.

Planners should consider size, capabilities, and ability of medical facilities closest to airports in their region to receive mass patient transports. Airports located close to a major trauma center may require fewer transportation resources to manage the incident with shorter transfer times and single transport required to definitive care. If there is no major trauma center close to the airport, a larger number of ambulances may be required both for primary transfers from the incident scene to the nearby trauma center and subsequent secondary transfers from those initial hospitals to trauma and burn centers for definitive care.

Active patient tracking is essential in aircraft incidents to enable timely repatriation and reconciliation with families. The Federal Aviation Authority (FAA) has developed special requirements for airlines to facilitate patient and passenger identification and communication with families and to establish family support centers. These systems depend ideally on an efficient flow of information between emergency medical service(s) (EMS), hospitals, and airline, airport, and public health authorities to locate and identify patients and passengers. Concerns surrounding the privacy of health information may adversely affect such dynamic information flow. EMS providers and hospitals should work with the relevant aviation authority and emergency managers to test emergency plans and patient tracking systems on a regular basis. Public health authorities and other agencies, such as the American Red Cross, should also be included in such reviews.

Under U.S. Federal Aviation Regulations (FAR Part 139.325) each airport operator must conduct a full-scale airport emergency plan exercise once every 3 years.[6] Exercises enable responding agencies to fulfill their responsibilities under the plan and are intended to improve proficiency in execution. Because air crashes are often large-scale events requiring assistance from neighboring jurisdictions, exercises should include local and regional hospital providers, emergency managers, EMS, fire departments, police departments, and public health services. Drills provide an excellent opportunity for community mass casualty planning; local medical and disaster leaders should be invited to participate in such training exercises.

The anticipated type of aircraft involved is important in planning emergency response to aircraft crashes. This may be predicted based on the size of the airport and the capabilities of its runways, although this is not always the case because aircraft sometimes are forced to divert to airports with smaller runways or may accidentally land at the wrong airport.[7] Planners in the area of a large, regional, or international airport must be prepared for any type of aircraft, ranging from large commercial jet airliners to small private planes. Although large aircraft carry more passengers than smaller aircrafts, their speed of travel and fuel loads often mean that there are fewer survivors following a crash. Smaller aircraft crashes will involve fewer passengers, although with a smaller amount of fuel onboard may be more likely to have survivors. Although almost any area may experience a rotor-wing aircraft crash, such crashes tend to occur more frequently around helipads and roadways. Passengers involved in small aircraft crashes are more likely to have orthopedic injuries and less likely burns due to the relatively smaller amount of fuel on these aircraft.[8]

Analysis of National Transportation Safety Board (NTSB) data with regard to aircraft size and the severity of injuries in "hull loss" events demonstrate a declining trend in aviation accident rates over time.[9] This can be ascribed to the augmented use of wide-bodied, larger commercial aircraft. This allows for improved structural integrity, enhanced occupant protection mechanisms, improved fuel cutoff and fire extinguishing capabilities, and the suppression of toxic fumes from burning cabin materials.[10] An analysis of 473 civilian airplane crashes with survivors between 1977 and 1986 demonstrated only eight crashes with more than 50 injured victims. Moreover, there were only three crashes in which more than 50 severely injured casualties occurred.[11] Another study of eight commercial aviation aircraft crashes between 1983 and 2000 revealed initial fatality rates of approximately 56%.[12] The number of injured passengers surviving a plane crash incident has averaged more than 60 passengers per event.[13] However, the potential for significantly greater numbers of casualties rises as passenger capacity increases. Two loaded Boeing 747 jets collided on the runway in Tenerife, Canary Islands, on March 27, 1977, bursting into flames; 500 people were killed on the tarmac and a further 60 critically injured, many of whom later died. This remains the deadliest aviation accident in history. However, with the introduction of the Airbus A380, aircraft capacity is further increasing, creating the possibility of even higher numbers of casualties.

A critical aspect in the survivability of an airplane crash has to do with the aircraft conditions during and immediately after the crash event. An airframe that endures an impact alone will likely yield many more survivors than an airframe that sustains an impact followed by fire and explosion. Avianca Flight 52 ran out of fuel and crashed on the north shore of Long Island, New York, in January 1990. There were 158 passengers on board, of whom 85 survived.[14,15] The majority of deaths were due to trauma, not as a result of fire or smoke inhalation. The remarkably high survival rate in this accident illustrates that the risk to passenger safety increases with the presence of fire or explosion on impact. Even in what may be an otherwise survivable event, fire contributes to significant morbidity and mortality of passengers, primarily from the rapid incapacitation of passengers by heat, smoke, and toxic fumes. Review of the British Airtours Boeing 737 accident on August 22, 1985, at the Manchester International Airport demonstrates that passengers died within 4.5 minutes of declaring an emergency and probably within 2 minutes of smoke and flames entering the fuselage.[16] This exemplifies the aggressive nature of fire and smoke within the confined space of the cabin especially in the setting of a large reservoir of jet fuel.

In today's environment of increased terrorist threats, deployment of a rocket-propelled grenade (RPG) at an aircraft has become a growing concern. On November 29, 2002, there was a near miss involving an RPG and an Arkia Airlines Boeing 757 departing from Mombassa, Kenya.[17] The 2014 missile attack on Malaysian Airlines Flight 17 highlights how aircraft even at significant altitude are at risk of being taken down by ground-based weapon systems. In the setting of current security risks, any aviation disaster is likely to be considered the result of terrorist action until proven otherwise. Responses to off-airport incidents are likely to include the airport, aviation authorities, local community, state, and federal emergency responders, and a large contingent of law enforcement officials.[18] Disaster planning for an airport located near or adjacent to bodies of water must incorporate an offshore or inshore response strategy for an aircraft downed in the water. This response is likely to include airport-based water rescue resources along with municipal, Coast Guard, and other Defense Department rotor wing and water-based rescue assets.[19] This type of response was prominently on display during the 2009 crash of U.S. Airways Flight 1549 into the Hudson River.[20] Although not routinely handled by civil authorities, personnel responding to military air crashes must be aware of the potential presence of weapons, including unexploded ordnance.

▶▶ POST-INCIDENT CONSIDERATIONS

Regardless of the location of an air crash event, disaster operations are likely to follow four distinct operational phases (Box 184-1). The initial phase, *emergency response*, is primarily focused on life-saving, firefighting, and safety-related operations. It is during this phase that control and perimeter security are established, fire suppression is engaged, emergency medical care/search and rescue services are initiated, and traffic redirected. The first arriving emergency personnel will establish a unified command post and staging areas to provide on-scene management of the incident. If there are multiple crash sites or if there is a significant wreckage scattered over a wide geographic area, multiple area commands may be established to provide effective command and control of the disaster scene. This phase of aircraft disaster operations will be considered complete when the last surviving passengers are transported from the scene and all life safety hazards at the crash site have been stabilized or eradicated. During this phase it is essential to ensure that living patients are identified and a method of patient tracking is established. As patients arrive at hospitals, continuity of tracking should support reuniting them with their families. Patient identification information should be shared with governmental crash investigators and public health authorities. It is crucial for disaster medical planners to be familiar with the unique tracking and information sharing systems used in responses to commercial airline crashes.

The second phase of operations, the *transition and stabilization* phase, will often occur simultaneously with the emergency response phase. It is intended to serve as a bridge between the initial response to the air crash event and the investigative and recovery aspects of the incident. It is during this phase that the disaster site is assessed, and long-term strategic and recovery plans are developed. This includes the anticipation of necessary staffing and resource requirements over time. In coordination with the local or state health departments, law enforcement officials, and other forensic experts, morgue operations are established, and provisions are made for the chief medical examiner's office. The process of establishing a forensic support area in which remains may be collected and tested to support victim identification can be a complicated one. A family assistance center will likely be established if there are multiple fatalities arising from the crash. The family assistance center is a site where support and counseling is provided to families affected by the crash but also where information and occasionally DNA and other materials are collected to facilitate identification. Family assistance centers can require a large amount of space for both counseling and forensic operations. Airline representatives and local, state, and federal public health, law enforcement, and transportation officials all need to collaborate to provide the breadth of forensic services, victim identification, translation services, family counseling, and communication with foreign governments required following a major aviation disaster.[21]

In the United States it is also likely that personnel from the NTSB will begin arriving on the scene during this phase of operations. Operational control of the scene is passed from the fire department to law enforcement authorities at the end of the stabilization phase.

BOX 184-1 **Post-incident Operational Phases**
• Phase 1: Emergency response
• Phase 2: Transition and stabilization
• Phase 3: Investigation
• Phase 4: Recovery

The *investigation* phase, which begins at the conclusion of the stabilization of the crash site, may last for several days, weeks, or months and includes all aspects of the investigation to determine the cause and origin of the crash. The NTSB retains primary responsibility for coordinating all aspects of the investigation, with significant assistance provided by the FAA, local, state, and federal law enforcement agencies, and representatives of the involved airline(s). The NTSB may assume direction and control of the "wreckage site" to conduct an investigation into the cause of the crash. This is accomplished in close coordination with law enforcement organizations to manage the incident scene. The NTSB also works with the airline carrier(s) involved in the crash, other appropriate airline organizations, and local and state governments to coordinate federal resources required to meet needs of aviation disaster victims and their families. The NTSB leads the investigation of aviation accidents. If the crash is determined to have been caused by a criminal act, the Federal Bureau of Investigation takes the lead role in coordinating crisis management response. The U.S. Department of Homeland Security may elect to send a representative to help coordinate the overall federal response to the incident.[22]

The final phase of the incident, the *recovery* phase, starts at the conclusion of the investigative phase and similarly may last for several days, weeks, or months. It begins with the transition toward normal flight operations. This also includes completion of the clean-up operations at the crash site, demobilization of staff, equipment, and other resources, and the finalization of all reports, incident records, and other documentation. It is completed by the preparation of an after-action report detailing all four phases of the operational response to the air crash event.

✚ MEDICAL TREATMENT OF CASUALTIES

The mechanisms of injury in aircraft accidents are primarily related to a combination of blunt, penetrating, and thermal injuries. Multiple mechanisms of injury can occur simultaneously, resulting in multisystem traumatic injuries. Explosive decompression, crush, and entrapment, passenger restraint systems, burn and thermal exposure, and events associated with evacuation are some of the major causes of injury.

Rapid and explosive decompression may be one of the initial events occurring in a loss of aircraft integrity leading to ground impact. Decompression particularly affects air-filled structures that are predisposed to injury from barotrauma, such as the lungs, sinuses, and gastrointestinal tract. Lung injuries are the most serious and are caused by rapidly increasing positive pressure leading to tearing of lung tissue and subsequent pneumothorax. Traumatic sinus rupture and tympanic membrane rupture can result from increased pressure in the sinuses. Gas expansion within the gastrointestinal tract can lead to bowel perforation with subsequent ventilatory compromise due to elevation of the diaphragm. Hypoxia and loss of consciousness are also common when an aircraft depressurizes rapidly at altitudes greater than 10,000 feet.

Crush and entrapment within the airframe wreckage is likely to result in post-incident casualties. When a plane impacts a surface, there is compression of cabin space, leading to entrapment and crush injuries. Long bone fractures and head and spinal trauma are commonly seen in the acute setting. Prolonged extrication time combined in the setting of crush injuries commonly leads to rhabdomyolysis. The evacuation process is also a frequent cause of injuries because friction burns, fractures, and sprains may occur when using the evacuation slide.[23]

Passenger restraint systems may cause patterns of injury similar to those seen in motor vehicle crashes; however, the velocity of the impact is greatly increased. This leads to a high incidence of blunt force injuries to the head, thorax, pelvis, and abdomen. The lack of shoulder restraints with lap belts allows for greater bodily movement and therefore increases the risk of injury to lower abdominal structures similar to those seen in nonshoulder-belted, motor vehicle collision passengers. Untethered objects within the cabin may become projectiles, resulting in blunt or penetrating injuries.

Thermal and burn injuries can cause severe injury even after survivable impact. This is due to the confined space of the aircraft and the inability to egress in rapid fashion. Toxic fumes, especially carbon monoxide, pose a major risk. In a study of military aircraft fatalities occurring between 1986 and 1990, 535 cases were analyzed for carboxyhemoglobin. There were 23 cases (4%) having elevated levels of carboxyhemoglobin (above 10% saturation). In each case the victim survived the crash and died in the post-crash fire.[24]

Many injuries arise during the evacuation process from the aircraft. The crash environment will be chaotic, with high auditory stimulus and diminished visual perception, resulting in risk of collision with other passengers or exposed wreckage. Fractures, sprains, and soft tissue injuries predominate. Flash and chemical burns from either jet fuel or hydraulic fluid can cause significant injury after exiting the airplane.

Specific patterns of injuries in survivors can be divided into three major categories. Fractures are the most common injury grouping, representing greater than a quarter of all injuries.[4] Fractures range from isolated closed fractures requiring minimal medical attention to complex vertebral, pelvic, and open long bone fractures associated with hemodynamic instability and risk of fat embolism. Head trauma is also a major cause of morbidity, making up the second largest injury grouping.[4] Thermal and burn injuries are another major cause of morbidity in surviving passengers, including the risk of inhalation injury. Blunt and penetrating trauma to intrathoracic and intraabdominal organs can result in major bleeding and shock. These are usually related to direct impact or the movement of large objects within the cabin post-disaster. In catastrophic accidents, such as crashes from high altitude, severe, devastating head, thorax, and abdomen injuries with no chance of survival are to be expected.[25]

❓ UNIQUE CONSIDERATIONS

The response to all air crash events will necessarily invoke a significant law enforcement component, particularly in the initial investigative phase of the event, to rule out a terrorist attack. The TWA Flight 800 crash off the southern coast of Long Island, New York, in the summer of 1996 and the crash of American Airlines Flight 587 immediately upon takeoff from New York Kennedy International Airport in October 2001 typified such law enforcement involvement. Of course 9/11 also had a tremendous amount of law enforcement involvement. The implication of such a response is that patients brought to the hospitals may eventually need to undergo law enforcement questioning and evaluation. All clothing and other personal items transported with the patient from the disaster scene will be considered as evidence and therefore must be collected and stored according to agreed-upon procedures in conjunction with local law enforcement officials. Firearms found on survivors or in the wreckage would have traditionally been associated with possible hijackers. However, with the reintroduction of armed federal air marshals on board an increasing number of flights, particularly those departing or arriving from key high-threat urban areas, such weapons may in fact be attributable to law enforcement personnel.

Aircraft crashes or accidents are always subject to media scrutiny. A small crash may only generate interest in the local community, whereas the crash of a commercial airliner is a major national and international event. Uncoordinated release of unverified, unvetted information can be devastating for families. Alternatively uninformed speculation will result if there is no coordinated release of information by a designated public information officer. This is especially true in the age of social media, when it is difficult to determine which reports are valuable and which are speculative. It should be noted that social media is often the first place where the public (and sometimes even hospitals) may begin to receive information about a disaster.[26]

⚠ PITFALLS

Most disaster scene triage decisions are predicated upon the application of an appropriate triage decision-making algorithm. Although this triage approach works for the majority of mass casualty situations, it needs to be adapted for use in air crash disasters, particularly those in which there has been a fire or explosion. For example, patients who may present with only mild throat irritation without any other injuries would likely be placed in the lowest transport priority group by someone inexperienced in trauma. However, such symptoms may be the harbinger of a more serious developing inhalation injury, either due to an explosion and fire through the passenger cabin, exposure to toxic fumes, or aspiration of water or toxic fluids in the event of a water ditching. Such patients must be frequently reassessed because triage is a dynamic process, and the triage status must be upgraded as signs of airway compromise become evident. If transport resources are plentiful consideration should be given to early transport of this group. These patients can sometimes benefit from early aggressive airway management if the index of suspicion of an inhalation injury remains high based on the assessment of the initial out-of-hospital care providers.

The most effective way to identify possible issues requiring correction in one's own regional response plan is to examine after action reports to prior air crashes. Key issues identified by after-action review of Sioux City, Iowa, crash response include the following[27]:

- No identified entry and exit way was available for emergency vehicles. This caused some traffic jams and indecision regarding how to exit the area.
- There were inadequate emergency equipment and resource management. Ambulances had extra equipment, including portable oxygen, intravenous supplies, and pressure dressings, that would have been tremendously valuable to the on-scene response. However, these were not left at the scene; the equipment remained on the individual transport units.
- Uncoordinated release of public information led to inconsistent reporting by media and news organizations.
- Failure of the water pump in the fire engine resulted in inadequate water supply for 10 minutes.
- First responders and disaster planners could not get an accurate count of the passengers. Children who sat on a guardian's lap were not counted on the passenger manifest.
- Many different languages were spoken without available interpreters, leading to miscommunication during the rescue efforts.

REFERENCES

1. Mouawad J, Drew C. Airline industry at its safest since the dawn of the jet age. *New York Times*; 2013. 11 Feb:Sect.A(1).
2. *Statistical Summary of Commercial Jet Airplane Accidents Worldwide Operations (1959–2013).* Seattle, WA: Boeing; August 2014. Available at: http://www.boeing.com/news/techissues/pdf/statsum.pdf. Accessed 05.05.15.
3. *National Plan of Integrated Airport Systems (NPIAS) 2013–2017.* Washington, DC: US Department of Transportation; October 5, 2012.
4. Baker SP, Brady JE, Shanahan DF, Li G. Aviation-related injury morbidity and mortality: data from U.S. health information systems. *Aviat Space Environ Med.* 2009;80(12):1001–1005.
5. Distefano N, Leonardi S. Risk assessment procedure for civil airport. *IJTTE.* 2014;4(1).
6. Airport Emergency Plan (§139.325), 139.325. US Code of Federal Regulations. Available at: http://www.gpo.gov/fdsys/browse/collectionCfr.action?collectionCode=CFR. Accessed 05.05.15.
7. *Cargo Jet Takes Off from Wichita on Short Runway.* [Internet] Atlanta: CNN; 2013. November 21, 2014. Available at: http://www.cnn.com/2013/11/21/travel/kansas-cargo-plane-wrong-airport/. Accessed 10.12.14.
8. Friedman A, Floman Y, Sabatto S, Safran O, Mosheiff R. Light aircraft crash—a case analysis of injuries. *Isr Med Assoc J.* 2002;4(5):337–339.
9. *Review of U.S. Civil Aviation Accidents: Review of Aircraft Accident Data.* Washington, DC: National Transportation Safety Board; 2011 January. Report No.: NTSB/ARA-11/01. Available at: http://www.ntsb.gov/doclib/reports/2011/ara1101.pdf. Accessed 10.12.14.
10. Abelson LC, Star LD, Stefanki JX. Passenger survival in wide-bodied jet aircraft accidents vs. other aircraft: a comparison. *Aviat Space Environ Med.* 1980;51(11):1266–1269.
11. Rutherford WH. An analysis of civil aircrash statistics 1977–1986 for the purposes of planning disaster exercises. *Injury.* 1988;19(6):384–388.
12. *Survivability of Accidents Involving Part 121 U.S. Air Carrier Operations, 1983 Through 2000.* Washington, DC: National Transportation Safety Board; 2001 March. Report No.: NTSB/SR-01/01. Available at: http://www.ntsb.gov/doclib/safetystudies/SR0101.pdf. Accessed 09.12.14.
13. Anderson PB. A comparative analysis of the emergency medical services and rescue responses to eight airliner crashes in the United States, 1987–1991. *Prehosp Disaster Med.* 1995;10(03):142–153.
14. van Amerongen RH, Fine JS, Tunik MG, Young GM, Foltin GL. The Avianca plane crash: an emergency medical system's response to pediatric survivors of the disaster. *Pediatrics.* 1993;92(1):105–110.
15. Dulchavsky SA, Geller ER, Iorio DA. Analysis of injuries following the crash of Avianca flight 52. *J Trauma.* 1993;34(2):282–284.
16. Hill IR. An analysis of factors impeding passenger escape from aircraft fires. *Aviat Space Environ Med.* 1990;61(3):261–265.
17. *MANPADS: Combating the Threat to Global Aviation from Man-Portable Air Defense Systems.* [Internet]. 2011. US Department of State; 2011. Updated July 27. Available at: http://www.state.gov/t/pm/rls/fs/169139.htm, Accessed 09.12.14.
18. *Fairfax County Emergency Operations Plan—Aircraft Crash Appendix for Off Airport Incidents*; October 24, 2003. Available at: http://www.fairfaxcounty.gov/oem/offairport_crash.pdf. Accessed 05.05.15.
19. Bush R, Rutley JG. *Multi-Agency Ocean Rescue Disaster Plan and Drill.* Washington, DC: Federal Emergency Management Agency; December 1994. Available at: http://www.usfa.fema.gov/downloads/pdf/publications/tr-079.pdf, Accessed 05.05.15.
20. *Aircraft Accident Report: Loss of Thrust in Both Engines after Encountering a Flock of Birds and Subsequent Ditching on the Hudson River: US Airways Flight 1549.* Washington, DC: National Transportation Safety Board; May 4, 2010. Report No. NTSB/AAR-10/03. Available at: http://www.ntsb.gov/doclib/reports/2010/aar1003.pdf. Accessed 09.12.14.
21. *Federal Family Assistance Plan for Aviation Disaster.* National Transportation Safety Board; December 2008. Available at: http://www.ntsb.gov/tda/TDADocuments/Federal-Family-Plan-Aviation-Disasters-rev-12-2008.pdf. Accessed 05.05.15.
22. Michell A. The crash of flight 587: first test for a disaster response plan. *New York Times.* November 13, 2001;13.
23. Motevalli V, Monajemi L, Rassi M. *Evaluation and Mitigation of Aircraft Slide Injuries.* Washington, DC: Transportation Research Board; 2008. Report No. 2. Available at: http://onlinepubs.trb.org/onlinepubs/acrp/acrp_rpt_002.pdf, Accessed 05.05.15.
24. Klette K, Levine B, Springate C, Smith ML. Toxicological findings in military aircraft fatalities from 1986–1990. *Forensic Sci Int.* 1992;53(2):143–148.
25. Vosswinkel JA, McCormack JE, Brathwaite CE, Geller ER. Critical analysis of injuries sustained in the TWA flight 800 midair disaster. *J Trauma.* 1999;47(4):617.
26. Beaumont C. New York plane crash: Twitter breaks the news, again. *Telegraph.* January 16, 2009;16.
27. *Aircraft Accident Report: United Airlines Flight 232.* (PBSO-910406 NTSB/AAR-SO/06). Washington, DC: National Transportation Safety Board; November 1, 1990. Available at: http://www.airdisaster.com/reports/ntsb/AAR90-06.pdf. Accessed 05.05.15.

Air Show Disaster

Joshua J. Solano and Peter D. Panagos

DESCRIPTION OF EVENT

Air shows are mass gathering events where aviators display their aircraft and skills. Air shows are typically held between spring and fall in colder climates and often year round in warmer areas, during daytime hours. The gatherings are sponsored by military, civilian, or commercial entities and may be used to raise funds, gather local support, for entertainment, or for patriotic reasons. Air shows are typically held at military or civilian airfields, not at commercial ones. These often tend to be in less populated areas and may be at the outskirts of urban or suburban centers. They may also be held in waterfront areas like beaches, lakes, or riverfronts. Acts performed at these events may include crowd flyovers, aerial acrobatics, pyrotechnics, and demonstration of military aircraft special capabilities, like vertical takeoff. There may also be static displays of historical, experimental, or other aircraft for spectators to visit. Spectators can range from hundreds to hundreds of thousands at the largest gatherings.

In the United States the International Council for Air Shows (ICAS) sets guidelines on safety and standards for air shows for civilian or commercial purposes, while in Europe the European Airshow Council sets standards. Decades of experience with accidents has led to increased preparedness and attention to safety during these events. Local and national authorities also produce standards for safety practice. The National Transportation and Safety Administration and Federal Aviation Authority both have multiple mandates in place for air show organizers.

A disaster at an air show is often a multiple casualty event involving morbidity and mortality to those on the ground and in the aircraft, without effect to the local community infrastructure. Over the last 40 years there have been many crashes at air shows involving only the aircrew, but as shown in Table 185-1, there has also been a significant amount of accidents involving multiple casualties. As with any mass gathering event planning, incident response and post-event action must be taken in order to deal with ground accidents, aircraft crashes, or terrorism.

PRE-INCIDENT ACTIONS

As with other mass gatherings, when planning an air show, organizers should coordinate with local emergency medical services (EMS) authorities in the event of a crash, explosion, or fire. The ICAS has multiple protocols dedicated to these events, including evacuation. A disaster plan devised from a hazard vulnerability analysis should include a risk analysis of the local area for nearby population centers, environment, responding personnel available, and other local resources (Box 185-1).[1-7] Specialized fire units and aviation safety personnel

are typically on hand as part of the air show in the event of a crash or fire.[8] These units should have training in the hazardous materials that are carried on the aircraft and the ordinance that may be on military aircraft. EMS on the ground should have training on usual local protocols in the event of a mass casualty. Local EMS along with the Medical Reserve Corps (MRC), Disaster Medical Assistance Teams (DMAT), specialized fire units, and aviation safety personnel should be prestaged at the air show as part of the pre-incident plan if possible.

The disaster plan should include the above elements, and there should be discussions beforehand regarding likely scenarios with the parties who will be responsible for the safety of the event along with local authorities. This can take the form of a tabletop drill prior to the event. Communication during an accident is especially important so synchronization of radio and cellular communication should be established pre-event. Implementation of an incident command system should also be in place prior to the opening of the air show. Tabletop and real-time drills should be conducted before the event or as part of local training, and should be a part of community disaster planning in areas where regular mass gatherings like air shows occur.

POST-INCIDENT ACTIONS

After an incident has occurred local resources should be mobilized, through a unified command structure with efficient communication between the first responders, EMS, police, fire department, and other resources. The alert mechanism must be expeditious because the survival of severely traumatized patients, as typically seen in air show disasters, is time sensitive. In an air show disaster involving ground casualties on the airfield, knowledge of the disaster will often be immediate. Notification of a crash may come over primary or secondary communication networks, and a crash message is disseminated to include aircraft type, nature of the emergency, location of crash or landing runway, number of persons onboard, hazardous cargo, ground casualties, and other pertinent information.[9] If there are survivors at the scene, the urge by first-responders to rush in and render care should be prevented. Trained rescue teams knowledgeable in airfield scene safety will bring casualties to a neutral area or allow the medical team into the area when it is deemed safe.

When multiple casualties are involved, a system of triage is required (a more detailed discussion of Disaster Triage can be found in Chapter 54).[3] Specific areas for casualty management should be predesignated with standard nomenclature. It is the medical leader's responsibility to keep the Incident Commander abreast of numbers and types of casualties, the need for additional support, and any other facts required to make decisions.[9,10]

TABLE 185-1   Fatal Crashes at Air Shows over the Last 40 Years

DATE	LOCATION	DESCRIPTION	INJURED/ KILLED
October 2013	Secunda, Mpumalanga	Extra EA-300 crashed	0/1
June 2013	Finowfurt, Germany	Zlin Z-526AFS Akrobat crashed	0/1
June 2013	Vandalia, Ohio	Boeing-Stearman IB75A crashed doing aerobatics	0/2
May 2013	Adana, Turkey	Light biplane crashed doing aerobatics	0/1
May 2013	Madrid, Spain	Hispano HA-200 Saeta crashed during flyby	3/1
April 2013	Santo Domingo, Dominican Republic	ENAER T-35 Pillan crashed into water	0/2
September 2012	Bandung City, Indonesia	AS/SA 202 Bravo crashed doing aerobatics	0/2
September 2012	Quad City, Iowa	Aero L-39 Albatros crashed	0/1
July 2012	Bedfordshire, Great Britain	de Havilland DH 53 Hummingbird crashed	0/1
June 2012	Klerksdrop, South Africa	Aero L-39 Albatros crashed doing aerobatic	0/1
April 2012	Erfurt, Germany	Zlin T Trener 6 crashed in formation maneuver	0/1
October 2011	Wei Nan City, China	Xian JH-7A crashed on flyby	1/1
September 2011	Martinsburg, West Virginia	T-28C Trojan crashed doing maneuver	0/1
September 2011	Reno, Nevada	P-51D Mustang crashed after mechanical failure	69/11
August 2011	Dorset, United Kingdom	BAE Hawk T1 crashed performing aerobatics	0/1
August 2011	Kansas City, Kansas	Pitts 12 crashed	0/1
September 2010	Nuremberg, Germany	de Havilland Tiger Moth crashed into a crowd	38/1
April 2010	Santa Cataina, Brazil	Embraer EMB 312 Tucano crashed during aerobatics	0/1
March 2010	Hyderabad, India	HAL Kiran crashed performing aerobatics	0/2
November 2009	Bredasdorp, South Africa	English Electric Lightning crashed from mechanics issue	0/1
September 2009	Montichiari, Italy	CAP-10B crashed during aerobatics	1/1
August 2009	Radom, Poland	Sukhoi Su-27 crashed after bird strike	0/2
July 2009	Tehachapi, California	L-29 Deflin crashed in flyby	0/2
August 2008	Upper Rhinebeck, New York	Neiuport 24 biplane crashed after simulated dogfight	0/1
June 2008	Rome, Italy	NH 90 helicopter crashed performing aerobatics	1/1
June 2008	Kindel, Germany	Zlin Z-37 Cmelak crashed on takeoff into a crowd	10/1
September 2007	West Sussex England	Hawker Hurricane failed to pull up during a dogfight	0/1
September 2007	Radom, Poland	Two Zlin Z-525 s had a midair collision	0/2
July 2007	Dayton, Ohio	S2S Bulldog crashed performing aerobatics	0/1
July 2007	Oshkosh, Wisconsin	P-51D Mustang crashed while landing	0/1
April 2007	Beaufort, South Carolina	F/A 18 Hornet crashed on maneuvering	0/1
March 2007	Titusville, Florida	Aero L-39 Albatros crashed performing a loop	0/1
October 2006	Tucumcari, New Mexico	Extra 300 L crashed while performing a loop	0/1
September 2006	Marsamxett Harbour, Malta	Yak-55 collided with an Extra 200	1/1
July 2006	Oshkosh, Wisconsin	RV-6 was struck by a TBM-3 Avenger	0/1
July 2006	Hillsboro, Oregon	HS Hunter Mk 58 crashed into a home	0/1
May 2006	Suwon, South Korea	A-37B Dragonfly crashed during stunt	0/1
July 2005	Moose Jaw, Canada	Waco UPF-7 and Wolf-Samson collided midair	0/2
October 2004	Miramar, California	Cabo Wabo Skyrocker crashed during a dive	0/1
July 2003	Duxford, England	Fairey Firefly crashed on nosedive	0/1
May 2003	Coventry, England	Replica of Spirit of St. Louis broke apart midair	0/1
July 2002	Western Ukraine	Russian Sukhoi Su-27 performing maneuvers crashed into crowd	84/115
June 1999	Bratislava, Slovakia	British Royal Air Force Hawk 200 crashed	1/1
September 1997	Baltimore, MD	F-117A crashed during flyby	5/0
July 1997	Ostend, Belgium	Light aircraft mounting an aerobatics display crashed into crowd around a Red Cross tent	9/57
August 1988	Ramstein Air Force Base, West Germany	Three Italian Air Force jets collided midair and crashed into crowd	70/100 s
June 1988	Mulhouse-Habsheim, French-Swiss border	New Airbus A320 crashed during low-level demonstration flight	3/133
September 1982	Mannheim, West Germany	U.S. Army Chinook helicopter carrying multination sky divers crashed	46 killed
June 1973	Paris, France	Prototype Russian Tupolev Tu-144 exploded midair	15 (6 crew, 9 ground)

(Source: Patricia L. Meinhardt, MD, MPH, MA, Adjunct Associate Professor, Department of Environmental and Occupational Health, Drexel University School of Public Health, Drexel University, Philadelphia, Pennsylvania.)

If an aircraft crashes in a remote setting, all responding personnel from the airfield will proceed to a prearranged assembly point for the convoy to the area.[11] In any disaster, medical personnel should enter the area only when it is declared safe. The high temperatures found in aviation disasters can not only lead to thermal injuries but also to the firing off of ordinance originally deemed to be safe.[12]

The recovery phase begins once all casualties are cared for, the deceased removed, and the scene returned to its original condition.

BOX 185-1 Pre–Air Show Risk Analysis

Security Requirements
- Isolation of air show and base operations
- Terrorism/vandalism/theft concerns

Parking Plan and Traffic Control
- General public
- Handicapped
- VIP
- Crowd arrival and departure plan

FAA Coordination
- Schedule practice for dynamic shows
- Airspace coordination

Emergency Planning and Drills
- Published and practiced
- Community resources informed

Communications and PA System
- Many methods and backup communication systems available
- Phonebook of key personnel and services

Crowd Control Barriers
- No-smoking signs in hazardous areas
- Parking away from sensitive areas

Pedestrian Concerns
- Trip hazards
- Sound and sun mitigation options
- Comfort stations
- Lost-parent stations
- Published safety guidelines
- Medical response plan

Medical Response Plan
- First-aid stations clearly identified
- Medical personnel placed in crowd
- Airfield and local EMS transportation
- LZ identified for rotary ring evacuation

Restroom Facilities
- Sufficient numbers for crowd
- Contract for routine cleaning

Vendor Setup
- Area and infrastructure available to support

EMS, Emergency medical services; *FAA,* Federal Aviation Administration; *LZ,* landing zone; *PA,* public address.

A debriefing of the event, with all participating agencies involved (referred to as a "hotwash"), should be undertaken within 1 to 2 days of conclusion of response activities. A further discussion of measures of effectiveness in disaster response can be found in Chapter 62. Psychological care for both victims and responders should be addressed as soon as possible following the event. If possible and when feasible, psychosocial first aid and other modalities should be implemented concurrently with medical care. This care should also be extended to family and close friends of those who died or were severely wounded.[13,14]

✚ MEDICAL TREATMENT OF CASUALTIES

Injury patterns seen in air show disasters are predominantly traumatic in nature, with a mix of blunt trauma, ballistic impact, and thermal injury. Scene safety issues in air show disasters are of particular importance due to the proximity of extremely flammable and explosive materials, in particular jet fuel and military ordinance. Refueling trucks should be immediately displaced to an area distant from the accident. After the scene is secured, triage of the victims is based on the locally agreed-upon method, such as the Simple Triage and Rapid Treatment (START) protocol.[1] Care should be taken to move the victims to safer areas if there are continued issues of scene safety. Multisystem life-threatening injuries with blunt and penetrating trauma, burns, and amputations are common in aircraft crashes involving ground personnel. The sudden deceleration of the aircraft and ignition and disbursement of aircraft ordnance and fuel cause the majority of injuries. The field management consists of triage, stabilization, and transportation of victims to definitive care providers.[12]

Typically if aircrew are unable to eject, they will be killed by the initial impact despite advances in aircraft safety. The pattern of injuries relates to four specific types: thermal, blunt, penetrating, and deceleration-trauma. Thermal injury, particularly to flight crews, can be devastating despite the flame-retardant clothing they may be wearing. These injuries manifest as dermal-soft tissue burns, inhalational burns, and carbon monoxide inhalation. The blunt trauma can cause internal injuries as well as traumatic amputations, necessitating the rapid application of tourniquets. Intrusive injuries from the loss of occupiable space due to the intrusion of main rotor blades, propellers, trees, or wires are also common types of severe injury. Finally, impact and deceleration forces cause injuries based on the position during deceleration and the distribution of force over the body parts (Table 185-2). For example, a pilot who ejects before impact may survive but may sustain extremity fractures resulting from the violent extremity movements involved in a high-speed ejection.

Spectators on the ground experience thermal injuries, blunt and penetrating trauma, amputations, ocular injuries, and exposure to toxic

TABLE 185-2 Decelerative Injuries and Approximate G Forces Involved

BODY PART/INJURY	DECELERATIVE FORCE (G)
Pulmonary contusion	25
Nose fracture	30
Vertebral body compression	20-30 (less in thoracic region or if poor body position)
Fracture dislocation of	20-40 C-1 or C-2
Mandible fracture	40
Maxilla fracture	50
Aorta intimal tear	50
Aorta transection	80-100 (at ligamentum arteriosum)
Pelvic fracture	100-200
Vertebral body transection	200-300 (through body, not intervertebral disc)
Total body fragmentation	350
Concussion	60 G over 0.02 s
	100 G over 0.005 s
	180 G over 0.002 s

Adapted from *The U.S. Naval Flight Surgeon's Pocket Reference to Aircraft Mishap Investigation.* 4th ed. Pensacola: The Naval Safety Center, Aeromedical Division in conjunction with The Society of United States Naval Flight Surgeons; 1995.

materials. Air show disasters have a number of amputations, and recent experience has shown that the use of tourniquets will minimize blood loss and mortality in mass casualty events.[15] Also in air show disasters, there will be a disproportionate need for burn units due to the number of burn injuries.[16]

Aircraft wreckage sites can have multiple hazards. Personnel involved in the recovery, examination, and documentation of the wreckage may be exposed to physical hazards posed by such things as hazardous cargo, flammable and toxic fluids, sharp or heavy objects, and disease. Hazardous materials, such as cartridge-actuated devices, tires, and oxygen bottles are major concerns. Explosive ordnance disposal personnel should target items such as pressurized bottles, hydraulic reservoirs, and canopy detonation cord to secure the scene and prevent further injury.[17–21]

Finally, once all injured or trapped victims have been cleared from the crash site, the area should be considered a crime scene. Wreckage and cargo should not be disturbed or moved except to the extent necessary for personnel safety. Arrangements should be made for security at the accident scene to protect the wreckage from additional damage and to protect rescue personnel and the public from injury.

🛈 UNIQUE CONSIDERATIONS

Most advanced military aircraft contain composite structures consisting of light, strong, stiff fibers embedded in a matrix material. Although these materials offer a significant structural advantage, they present a danger to rescue and medical personnel. Studies have shown that composite fibers can cause mild short-term skin, eye, and respiratory problems, but the long-term carcinogenic potential is unknown. Therefore, prudence is required in using personal protective equipment (PPE).

The reinforcing fibers most commonly used in aircrafts are graphite, bismaleimide, and boron fibers such as Kevlar. For example, in the F-18A/B, there are 1000 lb (9.8% total aircraft structural weight) of composite material.[22] When these fibers are released from an epoxy matrix they become fine splinters that can easily be driven into the skin and will cause irritation. Graphite fibers are very small and light and pose a respiratory threat similar to asbestos. While the aircraft is still burning or smoking, only firefighters should be in the immediate vicinity. Once the fire is completely extinguished and cooled, the composite material is normally sprayed with a fixant, such as polyacrylic acid or aircraft firefighting foam, to contain the release of composite fiber material. Finally, it is recommended that all personnel around the released fibers wear a National Institute for Occupational Safety and Health (NIOSH)-approved disposable air-filtering mask, Tyvek disposable overalls, and puncture-resistant gloves and goggles while on scene and shower before leaving the airfield.[22–29]

Additionally, the risk of being exposed to blood and body fluids is possible in any mishap involving human injury. Human immunodeficiency virus, hepatitis B, Lyme disease, and tetanus pose a threat to rescue personnel. Hepatitis B virus can survive in a dried state for several weeks. Therefore, it is recommended that all crash scene rescue and medical personnel become familiar with potential onscene hazards, adhere to Occupational Safety and Health Administration work practice controls,[30] and make use of PPE.[31]

⚠ PITFALLS

Several potential pitfalls in response to an air show disaster attack exist. These include the following:
- Failure to identify, prepare for, and properly train for a mass-casualty event by not developing contingency plans and periodically reviewing and correcting errors in the plans as local experience and resources change

- Failure to plan for the medical needs of a mass gathering including both geriatric and pediatric persons, many with significant preexisting diseases, exposed to a wide range of environmental elements, hazards, and stresses unique to an airfield
- Failure to recognize the unique injuries sustained by ground personnel from explosive and thermal forces in close proximity to an aircraft crash
- Failure to appreciate that emergency responders may become casualties themselves if they do not recognize the hazardous dangers of a modern aircraft crash scene containing composite materials, biologic hazards, and unexploded ordnance (Use of PPE is paramount to avoid responder injury.)
- Failure to recognize the unique injury patterns of aircraft crash survivors who have experienced sudden deceleration forces (high G) and exposure to hazardous materials

REFERENCES

1. Wolfson AB, Hendey GW, Ling LJ, et al. *Harwoood-Nuss' Clinical Practice of Emergency Medicine.* 5th ed. Philadelphia: Lippincott Williams and Wilkins; 2010.
2. Schultz CH, Koenig KL, Noji EK. A medical disaster response to reduce immediate mortality after an earthquake. *N Engl J Med.* 1996;334:438–444.
3. Schultz CH, Koenig KL, Noji EK. Disaster preparedness and response. In: Rosen P, Barkin RM, eds. *Emergency Medicine: Concepts and Clinical Practice.* 8th ed. St Louis: Mosby; 2010.
4. Hogan DE, Burstein JL, eds. *Disaster Medicine.* 2nd ed. Philadelphia: Lippincott Williams and Wilkins; 2007.
5. Waeckerle JF. Disaster planning and response. *N Engl J Med.* 1991;324:815.
6. Levitin HW, Siegelson HF. Hazardous materials: disaster medical planning and response. *Emerg Med Clin North Am.* 1996;14:327.
7. Edwards M. Airshow disaster plans. *Aviat Space Environ Med.* 1991;62:1192–1195.
8. de Boer J. Tools for evaluating disasters: preliminary results of some hundred of disasters. *Eur J Emerg Med.* 1997;4:107–110.
9. Christen H, Maniscalco P. *The EMS Incident Management System.* Upper Saddle River, NJ: Prentice-Hall Inc; 1998, 1–15.
10. Irwin RL. The incident command system (ICS). In: Auf der Heide E, ed. *Disaster Response: Principles of Preparation and Coordination.* St Louis: Mosby; 1989.
11. Postma IL, Weel H, Heetveld MJ, et al. Mass casualty triage after an airplane crash near Amsterdam. *Injury.* 2013;44:1061–1067.
12. Mozingo DW, Barillo DJ, Hoolcomb JB. The Pope Air Force Base aircraft crash and burn disaster. *J Burn Care Rehabil.* 2005;26(2):132–140.
13. Burkle FM Jr. Acute-phase mental health consequences of disasters: implications for triage and emergency services. *Ann Emerg Med.* 1996;28:119–128.
14. Linton JC, Kommor MJ, Webb CH. Helping the helpers: the development of a critical incident stress management team through university/community cooperation. *Ann Emerg Med.* 1993;22:663.
15. Caterson EJ, Carty MJ, Weaver MJ, et al. Boston bombings: a surgical view of lessons learned from combat casualty care and the applicability to Boston's terrorist attack. *J Craniofac Surg.* 2013 Jul;24(4):1061–1067.
16. Weissman O, Israeli H, Rosengard H, et al. Examining disaster planning models for large scale burn incidents-theoretical plane crash into a high rise building. *Burns.* 2013;39:1571–1576.
17. Pepe PE, Kvetan V. Field management and critical care in mass disasters. *Crit Care Clin.* 1991;7:321–327.
18. Dunne MJ Jr., McMeekin RR. Medical investigation of fatalities from aircraft accident burns. *Aviat Space Environ Med.* 1977;48:964–968.
19. Mason JK. *Aviation Accident Pathology.* London: Butterworths; 1962.
20. McMeekin RR. Patterns of injury in fatal aircraft accidents. In: Mason JK, Reals WJ, eds. *Aerospace Pathology.* Chicago: College of American Pathologists Foundation; 1973.
21. Shanahan DF, Mastroianni GR. Spinal injury in a U.S. Army light observation helicopter. *Aviat Space Environ Med.* 1984;55:32–40.

22. Boyarsky I, Shneiderman A. Natural and hybrid disasters—causes, effects, and management. *Top Emerg Med.* 2002;24:1–25.

23. SUSAFS. *Aircraft Mishap Investigation Handbook.* Brooks Air Force Base, TX: The Society of USAF Flight Surgeons; 2002.

24. SUSNFS. *The US Naval Flight Surgeon's Pocket Reference to Aircraft Mishap Investigation.* 6th ed. Pensacola: Society of United States Naval Flight Surgeons; 2006.

25. DON. *US Naval Flight Surgeon Manual.* 3rd ed. Washington, DC: The Bureau of Medicine and Surgery, Department of the Navy; 1991.

26. McMeekin RR. Aircraft accident investigation. In: DeHart RL, ed. *Fundamentals of Aerospace Medicine.* Philadelphia: Lea & Febiger; 1985.

27. Ernsting J, Nicholson AN, Rainford DJ, eds. *Aviation Medicine.* 3rd ed. London: Arnold; 2003.

28. Department of the Air Force Human Systems Center. *Response to Aircraft Mishaps Involving Composite Materials (Interim Guidance).* Consultative Letter, AL-OE-BR-CL-1988-0108 Brooks Air Force Base, Tex: AFMC; 1998.

29. Olson JM. *Mishap Risk Control Guidelines for Advanced Aerospace Materials: Environmental, Safety, and Health Concerns for Advanced Composites.* McClellan Air Force Base, CA; October 1993.

30. OSHA. *Bloodborne Pathogens 29 CFR Part 1910.1030.* Washington, DC: Occupational Safety & Health Administration; 2001.

31. National Institute of Justice. *Guide for the Selection of Personal Protective Equipment for Emergency First Responders, NIJ Guide 102–00*; Vols. I, IIa, IIb, and IIc. November 2002. Available at: http://www.osha.gov.

CHAPTER 186

Asteroid, Meteoroid, and Spacecraft Reentry Accidents

Jay Lemery, Faith Vilas, and Benjamin Easter

Who knows whether, when a comet shall approach this globe to destroy it, as it often has been and will be destroyed, men will not tear rocks from their foundations by means of steam, and hurl mountains, as the giants are said to have done, against the flaming mass? – and then we shall have traditions of Titans again, and of wars with Heaven.

—*Lord Byron*

DESCRIPTION OF EVENT

From our planet's origins 4.6 billion years ago, its natural history was replete with evidence of extraterrestrial impacts. Asteroids, meteoroids, and comets are believed to be the source of the organic molecules necessary for the development of terrestrial life.[1] Subsequently, they have continued to mold the planet. The Chicxulub crater off the Yucatan Peninsula appears to be the impact site of a 10 km asteroid that led to the extinction of the dinosaurs 65 million years ago.[2] Although impacts of such magnitude are exceedingly rare, as recently as February 2013, an 18 m asteroid exploded over Chelyabinsk, Russia, with an energy equivalent to 20 to 30 times the strength of the atomic bomb dropped on Hiroshima.[3] The airburst caused the atmosphere to sustain a substantial portion of the impact energy; nevertheless, approximately 1200 people were injured (mostly by glass broken by the shockwave) and 50 were hospitalized; 4500 buildings were damaged, including 34 hospitals and clinics.[4] Estimates of damage exceeded $30 million.[5] While this is the only impactor known to have caused human injury, approximately 100 tons of cosmic material fall to Earth daily, mostly in the form of tiny dust particles.[6] As our understanding and interaction with the cosmos has broadened over the last few decades, we have realized that there are quantifiable risks to humanity from impactors, ranging from locally traumatic to globally cataclysmic. These risks fall into three categories:

1. Local-effect near-Earth object (NEO) impacts
2. Global-effect NEO impacts
3. Reentry of artificial orbital debris

The risk posed by an impactor is directly proportional to its size[1] (Table 186-1). Those less than 50 m in diameter will most likely incinerate. Impactors 1 to 2 km in diameter will devastate the area surrounding the impact site. Impactors larger than 2 km in diameter have the potential to cause obliterative local damage, as well as displace large amounts of dust into the stratosphere. The consequent effects would resemble a "nuclear winter" that would affect the entire globe and disrupt entire ecosystems, with a resultant drop in global temperature, loss of agricultural productivity, and possible societal breakdown.[1] Because more than 70% of the Earth is covered with water, an ocean impact could cause tsunamis with inland flooding extending tens of kilometers into the coastal plains.

Orbital debris, the artificial residual of the last 60 years of human endeavors in space, is another source of potential terrestrial impactors. According to the Orbital Debris Program of the National Aeronautics and Space Administration (NASA), there are more than 21,000 objects wider than 10 cm orbiting Earth and approximately 500,000 objects between 1 and 10 cm.[7] Although the vast majority of orbital debris pieces incinerate upon reentry, some components could survive, whether due to heat-resistant material (e.g., shuttle tiles) or a design that sheds heat fast enough to keep object temperatures below the component's melting point. In fact, 2012 saw more than 400 uncontrolled entries of spacecraft and debris.[8] As the *Columbia* space shuttle tragedy demonstrated, even controlled reentry can fail, in which case suborbital debris would be expected to survive reentry in greater quantity, with a commensurate impact potential on life and property.

PRE-INCIDENT ACTIONS

A near-Earth object (NEO) is an asteroid, comet, or piece of debris whose orbit is close to the sun and therefore Earth (technically, it is an object whose closest approach to the sun is less than 1.3 times the average distance between the sun and Earth).[9] More than 90% of NEOs larger than 1 km have already been discovered, and work is under way to identify 90% of objects greater than 140 m by 2020.

As of January 2014, 10,598 NEOs have been discovered: 864 of these are asteroids with diameters larger than 1 km, and 1446 are classified as "potentially hazardous," which involves more stringent criteria.[9] The Torino Scale, an impact hazard scale, has only one current NEO whose score is not the lowest possible category, which indicates "zero . . . or effectively zero risk." In the long run, the actuarial risk of an NEO impact is estimated at 91 deaths per year, larger than the U.S. average of 20 deaths per year from earthquakes.[10] However, this is a mathematical calculation of long-run risk from events that are quite infrequent but highly destructive. In addition, there is significant uncertainty around this estimate; perhaps the highest residual risk results from the inability to model the environmental and human psychosocial and behavioral consequences of an impact.

Near-Earth Objects 50 to 1000 m in Diameter

An impactor with a diameter larger than 50 m will reach Earth's surface on average once every 100 years. The composition of the impactor could determine the extent of local damage. If the object has less physical coherence, such as a loosely bound, low-density comet body containing ice, it might not remain whole before impact and could explode in the atmosphere over earth's surface. Scientists believe this happened in the Tunguska explosion over Siberia on June 30, 1908.

TABLE 186-1   Impactor Category and Diameter

ENVIRONMENTAL EFFECTS	REGIONAL DISASTER 300 m	CIVILIZATION ENDER 2 km	K/T EXTINCTOR (CRETACEOUS-TERTIARY EXTINCTION) 10-15 km
Fires Ignited by fireball and/or reentering ejecta	Localized fire at ground zero	Fires ignited only within hundreds of km of ground zero	Fires ignited globally; global firestorm assured
Stratospheric dust Obscures sunlight	Below catastrophic levels	Sunlight drops to "very cloudy day" (nearly globally): global agriculture threatened by summertime freezes	Global night; vision is impossible. Severe, multiyear "impact winter"
Other atmospheric effects Sulfate aerosols, water injected into stratosphere, ozone destruction, nitric acid, smoke, etc.	None (except locally)	Sulfates and smoke augment effects of dust; ozone layer may be destroyed	Synergy of all factors yields decade-long winter. Approaches level that would acidify oceans (more likely by sulfuric acid than nitric acid)
Earthquakes	Local ground shaking	Significant damage within hundreds of km of ground zero	Modest to moderate damage globally
Tsunamis	Flooding of historic proportions along shores of proximate ocean	Shorelines of proximate ocean flooded inland tens of km	Primary and secondary tsunamis flood most shorelines ~100 km inland, inundating low-lying areas worldwide
Total destruction in crater zone	Crater zone ~5-10 km across	Crater zone ~50 km across	Crater zone several hundred km across

From Chapman CR, Durda DD, Gold R. The comet/asteroid impact hazard: a systems approach. Office of Space Studies, Southwest Research Institute. Available at: http://www.internationalspace.com/pdf/NEOwp_Chapman-Durda-Gold.pdf.

The diametrical sizes at which incoming objects will break apart when they enter Earth's atmosphere are 540 m for icy objects, 330 m for rocks, and 200 m for solid iron. These objects will change shape, flattening out to 5 to 10 times their original diameters because of the immense heat and pressure generated as they pass through the atmosphere. A surface impact will excavate material dependent on the incoming velocity and angle of impact, resulting in a crater 10 to 25 times the size of the impactor. One model estimates that the Puchezh-Katunky crater in Russia (40 km in diameter) was created by a rocky asteroid 2 km in diameter moving at a velocity of 20 km/second with a 45-degree angle of impact.[11–13] This impact destroyed near-surface layers of land to a depth of 100 m up to 40 km from the center of the impact.

Impactors less than 1 km in size are expected to have locally devastating effects, including total destruction within the resulting crater, thermal radiation surface fires, air blast compression, tidal wave flooding of low-lying areas, and compression wave injuries well beyond the crater zone. The Tunguska explosion occurred with minimal impact on humanity; however, if it had been delayed by only a few hours, the most populous regions of Europe (and millions of lives) would have been in jeopardy.

Near-Earth Objects 1 to 2 km in Diameter

Impacts from NEOs larger than 1 km in diameter are thought to occur, on average, every few hundred thousand years. NEOs of this size can have globally devastating effects; the resulting crater could reach 50 km in diameter. Debris would be launched into the stratosphere, blocking sunlight and threatening agricultural production globally. Superheated impact debris would rain back down on Earth's surface. An ocean impact would produce flooding tens of kilometers inland. Although rare, we have witnessed such impacts recently within our solar system. The impactors of comet Shoemaker-Levy 9 on Jupiter in 1994 were a series of 20 discernible fragments ranging up to 2 km in diameter. Had this comet hit Earth, it would have killed billions of people and risked most species on our planet.[14]

Near-Earth Objects 10 to 15 km in Diameter

NEOs 10 to 15 km in diameter will strike Earth even less frequently, on the order of once every 500,000 years. Global "earthquakes" from the impact, tsunamis, and total destruction over hundreds of kilometers would culminate in a nuclear winter that would ensue for decades. The effect of such an impact would result in major global climate change, such as that which triggered the demise of the dinosaurs.

Orbital Debris

Orbital debris is the artificial byproduct of the last 60 years of human endeavors in space. According to U.S. Strategic Command, orbital debris can be categorized as 7% operational satellites, 15% rocket bodies, and about 78% fragmentation and inactive satellites.[15] The further degradation of these objects is facilitated by solar heating and solar radiation, component explosions, and debris collisions. Recently, the population of orbital debris has seen a substantial increase from two events. On January 11, 2007, China tested an antisatellite missile on its own Fengyun-1C weather satellite. The successful strike and the resulting explosion resulted in the addition to orbital debris of approximately 2600 objects larger than 10 cm and 150,000 objects larger than 1 cm.[16] Approximately 2 years later, an accidental collision between a Russian Cosmos satellite and an American Iridium satellite further contributed to the problem. Together, these events doubled the amount of cataloged fragmentation debris.[17]

Although the intense pressure and heat of reentry will incinerate much of the mass of orbital debris, some satellite components can withstand this process. Components that have a sufficiently high melting temperature or a shape that allows rapid heat dispersal will have a higher probability of persisting. When debris pieces enter the lower regions of the atmosphere, they will lose velocity, begin to cool, and fall virtually straight down from the sky at relatively low speeds (terminal velocity); these are clearly a potential hazard to life and property.

Although NASA attempts to track orbital debris and predict where debris from a randomly reentering satellite will hit Earth, it is an uncertain science: the atmospheric density varies greatly at high altitudes, thus confounding the calculation of reentrant drag. Other confounding factors include variations in the gravitational field, solar radiation pressure, and atmospheric drag. The predicted time to reentry is accurate to within 10% of the actual time, although this translates to a margin of error of several miles on the ground. Over the last 40 years, more than 1400 metric tons of materials are believed to have survived reentry without report of injury.[16]

In the event that Earth becomes at risk of being hit by a moderate-to-large impactor, we would likely know well in advance, perhaps several years to decades. There would be an immediate, intense psychological reaction among the public, with likely intense media coverage and speculation. An incredible challenge would be posed to scientists, public health officials, and political leaders to relay the known risks and possible solutions to the public accurately. A discordance between calculated risks and publicly perceived risks can be expected, contributing to widespread fear and even mass hysteria.[18] Familiar doomsday scenario patterns of behavior are likely to emerge on the fringes of society. Mental health providers could expect an increase in anxiety, depression, or both in a large portion of the population.

POST-INCIDENT ACTIONS

As previously discussed, the risk of damage of an impactor is related to its size. Casualties and property damage should be treated as they would be in other mass casualty incidents.

Meteorites are classified as "irons" (nickel-iron metal) or "stones." Stones can be divided into two subgroups: chondrites and achondrites. Chondrites (about 86% of stones) are aggregates of early solar system materials that have not been significantly altered since formation of the solar system. Achondrites (about 8% of stones) are the products of melting and recrystallization of mostly magnesian silicates. One percent of meteorites are a conglomerate of those two types (called "stony irons").

When a meteorite strikes, it does so at terminal velocity and has therefore cooled from the intense temperatures of atmospheric entry. The outer layer, or fusion crust, is usually 1 to 2 mm thick, the rest having burned off during entry and posing no risk of burn from contact (silicate materials are traditionally poor conductors of heat). There are reports of eyewitnesses picking up an object that has fallen, cracking it in two, and discovering ice particles. Meteorites are composed of materials that are abundantly found on Earth and pose no toxic or radiation risk.

Historically, the controlled reentry of large components of artificial orbital material (Skylab, Mir) has been directed to remote, uninhabited parts of the planet (oceans). As seen with *Columbia*, however, spacecraft components can return to Earth relatively intact. Beyond the risk of impact, they can pose a toxicologic risk. Rocket propellants such as hydrazine and nitrogen tetroxide pose a chemical burn and inhalation risk. Structural materials such as beryllium have been known to cause pulmonary damage. Other potential hazards include ammonia, radiation sources (e.g., radioactive altimeters), live ordnance (e.g., pyrotechnics for emergency hatch opening), and other exotic compounds (e.g., scientific payloads, solar arrays, environmental control items such as lithium perchlorate and permanganate). On January 24, 1978, the malfunctioning Russian Kosmos 954 satellite reentered Earth's atmosphere with its nuclear reactor still intact. Radioactive debris spread across an approximately 800 km region of northwest Canada, requiring a months-long cleanup.[19] There are, however, currently no known nuclear-powered devices (e.g., powered by uranium) in orbit.

Once an orbital debris piece is committed to a reentrant trajectory, it will fracture and scatter over a predictable pattern based on mass. The "footprint" of debris will consist of heavier objects at the "heel" of the footprint and lighter objects at the "toe."

In certain cases of reentry events, forensic and possibly national security concerns will necessitate the mobilization of law enforcement personnel across several jurisdictions. As seen with *Columbia* in 2003, a concerted effort between law enforcement agencies in several states and NASA, coupled with direct appeals to the public, were initiated to preserve the integrity of the debris sites and to preclude souvenir hunters from disturbing debris fields. In such cases, mobilization of the military (national security concerns or naval salvage) may be deemed necessary, as may international coordination if debris fields cross international borders.

MEDICAL TREATMENT OF CASUALTIES

There is nothing unique to the medical treatment of casualties from the events discussed in this chapter. Blunt trauma is the likely mechanism of smaller impactors, expanding to burn and blast injuries for larger impactors. Blast injuries are of particular concern given the significant amount of energy involved in impacts. Areas of gas-tissue interface, such as the tympanic membrane, lungs, and gastrointestinal tract, are at particular risk. However, the duration of the overpressure wave in impact events is relatively short, approximately 0.001 to 0.1 seconds, in comparison to approximately 1 second for a nuclear explosion.[20] Consequently, despite the significantly higher energy that may be involved in a large impact event in comparison to a nuclear explosion, there is a relative paucity of blast injuries.

The Chelyabinsk meteorite also saw significant numbers of patients reporting flash blindness and lacerations from broken glass. An ambient temperature of −15 °C also placed victims at significant risk for hypothermia from broken windows and structural damage. For large-scale impactors approaching 1 km in diameter, humanitarian and refugee crises will be a major concern.

Psychological treatment will be another important consideration in any impactor scenario. Often even the smallest meteorite impacts are covered widely in the news media and may trigger anxiety and concern in otherwise unaffected portions of society. Mental health will be a major concern in the event of an orbital debris impact involving the loss of life. The scope of such a tragedy on the national psyche can affect all segments of the population, and there is a risk of depression and posttraumatic stress disorder.

Special concern should be made for those suffering personal loss. Despite efforts to shield them from further anguish, astronauts and other NASA staff (not unlike New York City firefighters after the World Trade Center bombings on September 11, 2001) played a major role in the search for the remains of *Columbia*, prompting concerns of exacerbating already severe mental trauma.

UNIQUE CONSIDERATIONS

Perhaps unique to this chapter is the potential scope of the disaster. If a NEO larger than 1 to 2 km in diameter were identified as a probable Earth impactor, humanity would face an existential crisis. Few disasters have the potential for such widespread and devastating consequences. The need for international coordination would be unprecedented.

The logistical scope of such an endeavor would be daunting. Whereas protocols are in place among astronomers to verify impactors and their risks before a public announcement, the ramifications of living in the age of the Internet could easily unglue efforts to sequester such proceedings. Initial efforts would likely focus on understanding the shape, configuration, mineral composition, and spin state of an impactor. These characteristics would further clarify the risk and, potentially, a strategy for deflection using existing technology of conventional rockets and explosives.[10] Future strategies could include attaching solar sails or engines to the NEO to deflect its path.

A final consideration should be mentioned. As space-related technology proliferates and becomes more accessible over the next decades, satellites and space vehicles may become susceptible targets for terrorists, particularly as an impactor over urban areas, power or chemical complexes, or military targets.

! PITFALLS

One pitfall that should be anticipated with any impactor event is relying on uninterrupted global communication. The effects of an impactor entering the ionosphere may disrupt satellite communication and possible security networks. It is reported that those who have observed meteor "fireballs" before impact experience a metallic taste sensation, possibly due to electromagnetic disturbance.[21]

REFERENCES

1. Chyba CF, Owen TC, Ip W-H. Impact delivery of volatiles and organic molecules to earth. In: Gehrels T, ed. *Hazards Due to Comets & Asteroids.* Tucson, AZ: University of Arizona Press; 1994:9–58.
2. Morrison D, Chapman CR, Slovic P. The impact hazard. In: Gehrels T, ed. *Hazards Due to Comets & Asteroids.* Tucson, AZ: University of Arizona Press; 1994:59–92.
3. Yeomans D, Chodas P. *Additional details on the large fireball event over Russia on Feb. 15, 2013. NASA/JPL Near-Earth Object Program Office.* Available at: http://neo.jpl.nasa.gov/news/fireball_130301.html. Accessed November 30, 2014.
4. RT News. Meteorite hits Russian Urals: fireball explosion wreaks havoc, up to 1,200 injured. Available at: http://rt.com/news/meteorite-crash-urals-chelyabinsk-283/. Accessed November 30, 2014.
5. Zhang M. *Russia Meteor 2013: Damage to Top $33 Million; Recuse, Cleanup Team Heads to Meteorite-Hit Urals.* Available at: http://www.ibtimes.com/russia-meteor-2013-damage-top-33-million-rescue-cleanup-team-heads-meteorite-hit-urals-1090104. Accessed November 30, 2014.
6. Kyte FT, Wasson JT. Accretion rate of extraterrestrial matter: iridium deposited 33 to 67 million years ago. *Science.* 1986;232:1225–1229.
7. NASA Orbital Debris Program Office. Orbital Debris Frequently Asked Questions. Available at: http://orbitaldebris.jsc.nasa.gov/faqs.html. Accessed November 30, 2014.
8. NASA Orbital Debris Program Office. US Launch Vehicle Components Land in Africa. *Orbital Debris Quarterly News.* 2013;17(4):1.
9. NASA Near Earth Object Program. NEO Groups. Available at: http://neo.jpl.nasa.gov/neo/groups.html. Accessed November 30, 2014.
10. Committee to Review Near-Earth-Object Surveys and Hazard Mitigation Strategies Space Studies Board. *Defending Planet Earth: Near-Earth-Object Surveys and Hazard Mitigation Strategies.* Washington, DC: National Academies Press; 2010.
11. Ivanov BA. *Geomechanical models of impact cratering. Presented at the International Conference on Large Meteorite Impacts and Planetary Evolution.* Sudbury, Canada, 1992, 40 [Abstract].
12. Pevzner LA, Kirijakov A, Vorontsov A, et al. Vorotilovskay drill hole: first deep drilling in the central uplift of large terrestrial impact crater. *Lunar Planet Sci.* 1992;XXIII:1063–1064 [Abstract].
13. Shoemaker EM. Interpretation of lunar craters. In: Kapal Z, ed. *Physics and Astronomy of the Moon.* New York: Academic Press (Elsevier); 1962:283–359.
14. A'Hearn M. The impacts of D/Shoemaker-Levy 9 and bioastronomy. Bologna, Italy: Editrice Compositori; 1997:165. Astronomical and Biochemical Origins and the Search for Life in the Universe, Proceedings of the 5th International Conference on Bioastronomy, Capri, Italy, July 1-5, 1996, IAU Colloquium 161.
15. McCall, GH. Space Surveillance. U.S. Air Force Space Command. Available at: http://fas.org/spp/military/program/track/mccall.pdf. Accessed November 30, 2014.
16. NASA Orbital Debris Program Office. Fengyun-1C Debris: One Year Later. *Orbital Debris Quarterly News.* 2008;12(1):3.
17. Committee for the Assessment of NASA's Orbital Debris Programs. *Limiting Future Collision Risk to Spacecraft: An Assessment of NASA's Meteoroid and Orbital Debris Programs.* Washington, DC: National Academies Press; 2001.
18. Benjamin GC. Managing terror: public health officials learn lessons from bioterrorism attacks. *Physician Exec.* 2002;28:80–83.
19. Portree DSF, Loftus JP. Orbital debris: a chronology. National Aeronautics and Space Administration. Available at: http://ston.jsc.nasa.gov/collections/trs/_techrep/TP-1999-208856.pdf. Accessed November 30, 2014.
20. Kring DA. Air blast produced by the Meteor Crater impact event and a reconstruction of the affected environment. *Meteorit Planet Sci.* 1997;32:517–530.
21. Associated Press. Scientist: Check your rooftops for meteor fragments. Available at: http://www.katu.com/news/local/16431791.html. Accessed November 30, 2014.

CHAPTER 187

Building Collapse

Mai Alshammari, Catherine Y. Ordun, and Timothy E. Davis

DESCRIPTION OF EVENT

The attacks on September 11, 2001, shocked the American public with the destruction of the World Trade Center towers. It also brought to the forefront the danger of building collapse, or progressive collapse, a significant, if not leading, cause of injury and death in building failures.[1] In the engineering world, progressive collapse has been studied for 40 years since the 1968 Ronan Point disaster.[2] Progressive collapse is a "chain reaction of structural failures that follow from damage to a comparatively small portion of a structure"[3] or "the spread of an initial local failure from element to element that eventually results in the collapse of an entire structure or a disproportionately large part of it."[4] Simply stated, progressive collapse is a "domino effect," causing the sequential collapse of one floor on top of lower floors.[3] In this chapter, the terms building collapse, structural collapse, and progressive collapse are used interchangeably.

There are six causes of building collapse: bad design, faulty construction, foundation failure, unusual loads, unexpected failure, and a combination of these causes. Some causes of bad design are errors in engineering computation, failure to consider all stresses and weights, reliance on inaccurate data, and poor choice of materials.[5] Faulty construction is the most common reason for building collapse around the world. It results from the use of inferior material, bad riveting, infirm fastening or securing, and bad welds.[5] In the case of foundation failure, the earth beneath a building may be unsuitable to support the weight of the building. During an earthquake, such buildings are shaken off their mountings if built on top of unstable soil or not properly secured to their foundations.[6] Loads exceeding calculated stress tolerances may occur during natural disasters such as earthquakes, tornados, and tsunamis. Human-made events such as a motor vehicle striking an essential support pillar, a gas explosion, or a bombing also can exceed tolerated stresses.[4] Blast and overpressure waves resulting from explosions damage buildings.[3] Depending on the force of explosion, distance from building, and sturdiness of building construction, an explosion can induce progressive collapse in milliseconds.[3] The blast will first target the weakest point of the building closest to the detonation and push onto the exterior walls of the lower floors, leading to wall failure and window breakage.[3] While the shock wave expands, it enters the structure and pushes upward and downward, onto all floors of the building, inducing collapse.[3] The reflection of the oncoming, or "incident," blast wave against hindering structures including hard surfaces of a building's exterior, can lead to additional pressures up to 13 times greater than the peak incident pressure.[3,7] Laboratory tests have shown that surfaces exposed perpendicularly to the incident blast wave may experience pressures up to 5000 psi. Typical window glass breaks at an incident overpressure of 0.15 to 0.22 psi.[3]

PRE-INCIDENT ACTIONS

Although engineers note that the progressive collapse cannot be entirely prevented from occurring, they agree that tools can be designed to improve building performance to resist or better withstand against collapse.[1,8] National institutes encourage designing multihazard resistance and mitigation suitable to withstand progressive collapse from all threats, including natural and technological disasters.[1] Specific mitigation against terrorist bombings focuses more on window and glass hazards, stand-off distancing, and "hardening" of the building's exterior. Site design and modification for perimeter defense uses soil, bollards, planters, and retaining walls as mitigation strategies. Increasing stand-off distance between the facility and possible threats (such as a truck bomb) can deter and delay terrorist attacks capable of initiating building collapse.[3] Strategies to limit parking, vehicular entry, and limitation of access adjacent to the structure are additional mitigation strategies.[3] If the latter measures fail, structural "hardening" to fortify the building's exterior will mitigate the effects of an explosion once it has occurred. The objective of exterior wall design is to ensure that structures (walls, doors, and windows) fail in a flexible mode. Failure in flexible mode avoids the shear stresses which result in multiple fragments of cement, glass, and other materials capable of serious injury with a brittle mode failure.[3] In the 1998 bombings of the U.S. Embassies in Kenya and Tanzania, the U.S. Department of State found, "Although there was little structural damage to the five-story reinforced concrete building, the explosion reduced much of the interior to rubble destroying windows, window frames, internal office partitions and other fixtures on the rear side of the building. The secondary fragmentation from flying glass, internal concrete block walls, furniture, and fixtures caused most of the embassy casualties."[1,8,9] Nonstructural components such as ceiling fixtures, lights, windows, office equipment, and objects stored on shelves and hung on walls can also become an injury hazard.[3,6] In an earthquake, these nonstructural elements are likely to be unhooked, dislodged, and flung, causing injury and damage.[3] The U.S. Federal Emergency Management Agency (FEMA) recommends that building design be optimized to facilitate emergency rescue and response through effective placement, structural design, and redundancy of emergency exits and electrical and mechanical systems.[3]

POST-INCIDENT ACTIONS

After a building collapse, trapped survivors requiring quick rescue "where minutes count" are rare. An expeditious poorly planned ingress into the "hot zone" can risk valuable human assets with limited potential benefit. The rules for traumatic arrest still apply—attempts to resuscitate persons with blunt traumatic arrest are typically futile.

The bulk of surviving casualties will arrive over a 60-minute period at the closest hospital(s), either self-transported or transported by emergency medical service(s) (EMS). The majority of early presenters will self-transport. Disaster managers should expect high resource utilization from hospitalized survivors, far exceeding the benchmark comparisons for similar injury severity score (ISS) casualties. Critically injured progressive collapse survivors can be compared with casualties of explosive injury, and they require an extraordinary amount of hospital resources. Hospitalized explosion survivors have longer than usual hospital and intensive care unit length of stay, more surgeries, and more ventilator time. They are more often discharged to a rehabilitation facility compared with ISS-equivalent casualties of motor vehicle or gunshot wounds.[10,11]

Some general emergency management options apply:

1. Follow your hospital and regional disaster system plan.
2. Expect increased severity and delayed arrival of casualties.
3. Expect an "upside-down" triage—the most critically wounded arrive after the less injured, as they bypass EMS triage and go straight to the nearest hospitals.[12]
4. Double the first hour's number of casualties to estimate the total number of patients during the "first wave."[12]
5. Obtain and record details about the nature of the event, potential toxic exposures, environmental hazards, and casualty location. The details are collected using all reliable informants including local police and fire departments, EMS, incident command system, regional emergency management agency, local health department, and eyewitness casualties. The need for epidemiological injury data are an imperative national agenda.[13]

✚ MEDICAL TREATMENT OF CASUALTIES

Progressive structural collapse produces casualty and injury patterns similar to earthquakes and can be more severe than blast injuries alone.[14] The final casualty toll and injury pattern depend most on pre-existing circumstances such as time of day, occupancy, warning, evacuation proficiency, individual health status, and building design and materials. The most common injury seen among survivors is penetrating and blunt trauma. The most severely injured sustain burns, traumatic amputations, and head, chest, and abdominal injuries.[14-16] Frykberg notes a substantial immediate mortality rate and a constant critical mortality rate among victims of a terrorist bombing building collapse, despite differences in TNT-equivalents of the blast force.[16]

Those that are in the direct path of building collapse die immediately or in the ER. Those found within the rubble alive are trapped in partially collapsed spaces. Most injuries affecting survivors relate to head, torso, and long bones. Transport of these patients to trauma centers should follow local protocols. Crush syndrome is a risk for patients entrapped for more than 1 hour with the potential to develop rhabdomyolysis and subsequent acute kidney injury.

❓ UNIQUE CONSIDERATIONS

Traumatic amputation of any limb may be a marker for multisystem injuries since such injuries usually result from proximity to the blast.[17,18] Since wounds may be grossly contaminated, consider delayed primary closure. Close follow-up of wounds is essential to prevent the formation of sepsis.[19] Primary blast lung and abdominal injuries after explosions are associated with high mortality rates.[20,21] The symptoms of mild traumatic brain injury (e.g., concussion) and posttraumatic stress disorder may be difficult to distinguish in the early stages.[22] Auditory complaints and injuries can easily be missed. It is prudent to provide patients with specific written instructions with respect to follow-up regarding deafness (temporary or permanent) or tinnitus.[23] Consider the possibility of exposure to inhaled toxins and poisonings (e.g., carbon monoxide, cyanide, methemoglobin) in both industrial and criminal explosions.[9,11,24]

In New York City, March 2014, two apartment buildings collapsed when a gas leak caused an explosion; eight were killed and 70 were injured. The buildings, although built over a period of 100 years previously, were inspected routinely the month before the explosion, revealing no problems. The buildings were leveled within 20 minutes of the explosion.[25]

⚠ PITFALLS

- Do not discourage buddy rescue and self-transport of casualties. Survivors and bystanders conduct the majority of rescue. Self-evacuation clears the scene and moves the bulk of the exposed population out of harm's way.
- Strict interpretation of The U.S. Federal Emergency Medical Treatment and Active Labor Act may limit the expeditious movement of excess outpatient casualties to hospitals that may have the capacity to care for them.[26]
- Another pitfall is activating an entire hospital's disaster plan for a distant regional event and not releasing recalled staff in a timely manner. Only the closest one to three hospitals receive the majority of the casualties, and half of all casualties arrive over a 60-minute period.[9]
- It should not be assumed that all ambulatory casualties are "worried well." All have been exposed to a degree of physical trauma and environmental hazards. Israeli pediatric traumatologists have proposed eliminating "Green" or "Minimal" from the triage protocol.[27]
- Adult casualties in cardiopulmonary arrest are either dead or unsalvageable. No attempt should be made to resuscitate beyond confirming the absence of vital signs.

REFERENCES

1. National Research Council. *Blast Mitigation for Structures: 1999 Status Report on the DTRA/TSWG Program.* Washington, DC: National Academy Press; 1999.
2. Failed Architecture. *The Downfall of British Modernist Architecture.* Available at: http://failedarchitecture.com/the-downfall-of-british-modernist-architecture/; 2011.
3. U.S. Federal Emergency Management Agency. *Risk Management Series: Reference Manual to Mitigate Potential Terrorist Attacks Against Buildings.* Washington, DC: FEMA; 2003.
4. International Risk Management Institute, Inc. (IRMI). *Quantifying the Risk for Progressive Collapse in New and Existing Buildings;* 2003. Available at: http://www.irmi.com/expert/articles/2003/gould03.aspx.
5. Calvert JB. *The Collapse of Buildings.* Available at: http://mysite.du.edu/~jcalvert/tech/failure.htm; 2001.
6. Federal Emergency Management Agency. *Earthquake Fast Facts.* Available at: https://www.fema.gov/earthquake/earthquake-fast-facts; 2014.
7. Boffard KD, MacFarlane C. Urban bomb blast injuries: patterns of injury and treatment. *Surg Annu.* 1993;25:29–47.
8. Multi hazard Mitigation Council. *Prevention of Progressive Collapse: Report on the July 2002 National Workshop and Recommendations for Future Efforts.* Washington, DC: Multi hazard Mitigation Council of the National Institute of Building Sciences; 2003.
9. U.S. Department of State Archive. *Report of the Accountability Review Boards on the Embassy Bombings in Nairobi and Dar es Salaam on August 7, 1998;* 1999. Available at: http://1997-2001.state.gov/www/regions/africa/accountability_report.html.

10. Peleg K, Aharonson-Daniel L, Stein M. the Israeli Trauma Group (ITG). Gunshot and explosion injuries: characteristics, outcomes, and implications for care of terror-related injuries in Israel. *Ann Surg.* 2004;239:311–318.

11. Peleg K, Aharonson-Daniel L, Michael M, Shapira SC, the Israel Trauma Group. Patterns of injury in hospitalised terrorist victims. *Am J Emerg Med.* 2003;21:258–262.

12. Centers for Disease Control and Prevention. *Explosions and Blast Injuries: A Primer for Clinicians;* 2003. Available at: http://emergency.cdc.gov/masscasualties/explosions.asp.

13. National Research Council. *Protecting People and Buildings from Terrorism Technology Transfer for Blast-Effects Mitigation.* Washington, DC: National Academy Press; 2001.

14. Butcher TP. Explosive emergencies treating blast injuries in the field. *JEMS.* 1991;50–54.

15. Frykberg ER, Tepas JJ 3rd. Terrorist bombings: lessons learned from Belfast to Beirut. *Ann Surg.* 1988;208:569–576.

16. Frykberg ER. Medical management of disasters and mass casualties from terrorist bombings: how can we cope? *J Trauma.* 2002;53:201–212.

17. Hull JB. Traumatic amputation by explosive blast: pattern of injury in survivors. *Br J Surg.* 1992;79:1303–1306.

18. Hull JB, Bowyer GW, Cooper GJ, Crane J. Patterns of injuries in those dying from traumatic amputation caused by bomb blast. *Br J Surg.* 1994;81:1132–1135.

19. Wightman JM, Gladish SL. Explosions and blast injuries. *Ann Emerg Med.* 2001;37:664–678.

20. Leibovici D, Gofrit ON, Stein M, et al. Blast injuries: bus versus open-air bombings—a comparative study of injuries in survivors of open-air versus confined-space explosions. *J Trauma.* 1996;41:1030–1035.

21. Stuhmiller LH, Phillips YY, Richmond DR. The physics and mechanisms of primary blast injury, a brief history. In: Bellamy RF, Zajtcjuk JT, eds. *Conventional Warfare: Ballistics, Blast, and Burn Injuries. Textbook of Military Medicine series.* Washington, DC: Office of the Surgeon General at TMM Publications; 1991:241–270.

22. Barrow DW, Rhoades HT. Blast concussion injury. *JAMA.* 1944;125:900–902.

23. Hirsch FG. Effects of overpressure on the ear: a review. *Ann NY Acad Sci.* 1968;152:147–162.

24. Quenemoen LE, Davis YM, Malilay J, et al. The World Trade Centre bombing: injury prevention strategies for high-rise building fires. *Disasters.* 1996;20:125–132.

25. The New York Times. *At Least 3 Killed as Gas Explosion Hits East Harlem.* Available at: http://www.nytimes.com/2014/03/13/nyregion/east-harlem-building-collapse.html?hpw&rref=nyregion&_r=2; 2014.

26. ACEP.org. 2014. EMTALA. Available at: http://www.acep.org/News-Media-top-banner/EMTALA/.

27. Waisman Y, Aharonson-Daniel L, Mor M, et al. The impact of terrorism on children: a two-year experience. *Prehospital Disaster Med.* 2003;18:242–248.

Bridge Collapse

Mai Alshammari, Laura Diane Melville, and Najma Rahman-Khan

DESCRIPTION OF EVENTS

On the morning of May 9, 1980, the *Summit Venture* had just entered a difficult portion of the shipping channel leading directly into Tampa Bay that passed under the Sunshine Skyway Bridge. The boat was a tanker the size of two football fields. A sudden squall blew up and created almost zero visibility, and the ship's radar ceased to function. Based on a number of factors, the captain made the choice to go ahead and try to pass under the bridge. The ship rammed the south pier 700 feet from the center of the channel, causing the center span of the Skyway to collapse into the channel below. Several cars and a Greyhound bus disappeared into the bay. Thirty-five people died in the disaster.[1]

There is such a dearth of medical or disaster planning literature specifically addressing bridge collapse that information must be gathered from news media and websites. The most common reason for bridge collapse is structural failure, other causes include weather (including floods, tornados, earthquakes), explosions (both accidental or nonaccidental), acts of war or terrorism, and objects crashing into the bridge (such as a barge). Since the events of September 11, 2001, in New York City, we should consider symbolic bridges (such as the Brooklyn Bridge or the Golden Gate Bridge) with significant passenger loads (including pedestrian, motor, and rail) as potential terrorist targets. During war, bridges as vital infrastructure become targets for similar reasons. The T shaped Aioi Bridge was the target for "Little Boy," the atomic bomb dropped on Hiroshima. Bridge collapse over water will require skilled water rescue personnel as well as standard EMS rescuers.

Not all bridges cross water, highway overpasses are essentially bridges, and the collapse of such structures also occurs. This kind of collapse requires interventions more like those required for structural collapses, such as urban search and rescue teams and personnel experienced in confined-space medical interventions.

A brief description of the different types of bridges may be useful in understanding the types of risks to which they are subject. There are several different types of bridges, including arch, cable-stayed, suspension, draw span, truss, and beam, with the first three being the most common. Arch bridges are relatively small, usually 130 to 500 feet in length. This type of bridge allows no movement in horizontal bearing, so these bridges are usually located on stable ground and cross over valleys and rivers.

Cable-stayed bridges range from 300 to 1600 feet long with a continuous bridge that has one or two towers erected in the middle with support cables attaching the bridge to the towers. The towers bear the brunt of the load. This design provides strong support against earthquakes and strong winds but remains vulnerable to shifting or uneven sinking ground. The Sunshine Skyway Bridge is an example of a single-tower cable-stayed bridge.

Suspension bridges, such as the Golden Gate Bridge, have a span ranging from 2000 to 7000 feet. These bridges have cables that are attached to either end to transmit the load to either anchorage. These anchorages at either side provide strong support, but the construction makes the bridge vulnerable to strong winds. The collapse of the Galloping Gertie, otherwise known as the Tacoma Narrows Bridge is a famed example of the failure of a suspension bridge.[2–4]

The Tacoma Narrows Bridge is a case of a suspension bridge gone wrong. It collapsed in 1940 because of strong winds and harmonic resonance. The bridge's undulations were an attraction to locals and tourists for years before the actual collapse. Due to its suspension wire construction, there were both vertical and horizontal undulations in the bridge that contributed to its failure. During some winds, there was as much as a 28-foot disparity between the left and right sides of the bridge. Before that event, there was pressure to construct bridges to maximize "lightness, grace, and flexibility"; however, this collapse forced a reevaluation of this in favor of safety and stability.[2] The impressive amateur video taken just before the collapse can be viewed on the Internet.[3]

A serious event that took place in 2007 was the collapse of the I-35 W Mississippi River Bridge. The bridge collapsed August 1 during rush hour, killing 13 people and injuring 145. The failure happened after the bridge experienced a catastrophic failure in the main span of the deck truss. 111 vehicles fell into the 15-foot river after a portion of the bridge collapsed.[5]

Pedestrian bridges also collapse. Once such occurrence was in Istanbul on September 3, 2014, where a pedestrian was killed after a dump truck mechanism was mistakenly activated, destroying a bridge support pillar. Reports say that a vehicle may have smashed into the side of the bridge during rush hour.[6,7] Another example of a pedestrian bridge collapse occurred over water in China on the September 26, 2013. There were no fatalities and only minor injuries recorded as life preservers were dispersed immediately by onlookers. Both major and minor traumas are to be expected with pedestrian bridge collapses, particularly if the bridge is elevated. Drowning and near drowning may also be seen if the bridge traverses water.[8]

PRE-INCIDENT ACTIONS

Each U.S. government agency (state, county, city, township) that manages a public bridge is required by the Federal Highway Administration to have a crisis management plan.[2] These involve such agencies as the police, sheriff, fire, rescue, emergency medical service(s), Coast Guard, Army Corp of Engineers, Federal Aviation Administration, and railroads.

Hospitals should be aware of the plans for bridges in their area and should have an understanding of how loss of the specific transportation route and potential influx of patients will affect their facilities. This should be one of the many scenarios envisioned in the all-hazards hospital disaster plan. A critical factor in this planning should be an expectation that staff members may not be able to get to work. This could mean anyone from cleaning staff to the hospital's only two trauma surgeons. Hospital representatives should be involved in the creation of the federal state and local plans because emergency departments can expect to be the center point of any medical consequences. Important issues will be traffic rerouting, designation of receiving hospitals, etc.

Software programs such as the Geographical Resource Intranet Portal, created by the Oklahoma Department of Transportation (ODOT), can overlay all area roads with information about their ability to handle trucks and high traffic volume, locations of hospitals, and other information facilitating a timely return of traffic flow. This program allowed the ODOT to effectively reroute traffic within 2 hours after the 2002 collapse of the I-40 bridge.[9] Hospitals with hyperbaric chambers should be identified in case they are required for victims or rescuers.

Communication issues, both within the hospital and with outside agencies, are paramount and must be addressed before the event itself. This is often one of the most challenging parts of developing and implementing a disaster plan, and it should be emphasized in planning and drilling. Search and rescue teams, with divers, will be required for recovery of victims trapped under structures and underwater. There must be planned routes for emergency vehicles and rescue personnel to get to and from the event site. Knowledge of the body of water (e.g., currents and pollutants) also could be critical to effective rescue efforts. If the collapse occurs due to weather, earthquake, or terrorism, there may be damage to other critical structures and resources including the hospital itself.[10] Those performing triage must be clear about the rules of a mass casualty triage, taking into consideration the available resources and the number of victims.

If the bridge collapse is part of a large event, the Federal Emergency Management Agency and disaster medical assistance teams (DMATs) may become part of the response after the first 48 to 72 hours. Those teams are rapid-response teams used to augment local resources until federal responses are mobilized or the situation is resolved.[11]

POST-INCIDENT ACTIONS

Rescue attempts may pose a risk to the rescuer(s) and such risk must be weighed on each occasion. It is vital to secure the area as much as possible and to ensure the maximum possible safety for everyone on-scene. This is the second of the seven priority pillars in Major Incident Medical Management and Support (MIMMS) system. MIMMS is the system used in the United Kingdom, Europe, Australia, and NATO for mass casualty incident management. The pillars are:

C—Command and control
S—Safety and security
C—Communication
A—Assessment
T—Triage
T—Treatment
T—Transport

A collapsed bridge can be particularly dangerous because the elevated structure may continue to be a hazard with risk of further collapse of the remaining unstable structure. Large amounts of debris underwater can endanger divers, as can weather and current conditions. Under certain circumstances, this may include evaluation for any coincidental biological, chemical, or radiation terrorism.

Plans that are in place must be implemented in an orderly fashion. It is paramount that communication between agencies occurs as smoothly as possible with vertical and horizontal channels of communication. As in all of the situations addressed in this book, coordination of federal, state, and local resources will lead to the most effective and efficient handling of the situation. The conventional wisdom is that a response team must be able to stand alone for 12 to 24 hours.[10,12] This isolation may be prolonged if a bridge has collapsed due to severe weather conditions or a geologic event such as an earthquake.

Urban search and rescue teams will require activation, and preliminary medical care may have to be delivered at the scene for victims who are trapped alive. If there are large numbers of victims, it will be important to bring stable patients to hospitals farthest from the scene. The walking wounded and the worried well often self-transport to the closest hospital, and the severely injured also will be transported to the closest hospital unless there is a well-rehearsed priority dispatch system in operation.[10]

Other emergency management issues that warrant inclusion in hospital disaster plans for bridge collapse include how to manage medical and nonmedical volunteers, hospital capabilities regarding trauma and pediatrics, how and where to transfer patients who require care that cannot be provided either on scene or locally, and how to get staff to the facility if the usual traffic routes are not available.

MEDICAL TREATMENT OF CASUALTIES

The detailed medical treatment of bridge collapse victims is not going to be covered in this chapter. Near drowning is an important injury mechanism to be considered. Drowning can sometimes be a reason for the demise after a major trauma, For example, an open femur fracture after a car crash can prevent the victim from swimming to safety.

Other issues to be considered include blast injuries if the bridge collapse occurred due to an explosion. Primary, secondary, and tertiary injuries can all be seen in these situations, along with near drowning, singly or combined.

The saying "not dead till warm and dead" may not be easily applicable once disaster triage is implemented. Those without any pulse or respiratory effort are considered unsalvageable without any consideration to their body temperature. Such patients will pose an ethical challenge to those making the decision not to actively intervene. With limited rescuers greatly outnumbered by the numbers of critically injured victims, the "expectant" triage category may however be used in some European jurisdictions this requires authorization by local government.

Crush injuries, exposure to known or unknown chemicals, and psychological stress all complicate the treatment of those affected.

UNIQUE CONSIDERATIONS

Bridges are most likely to collapse due to a combination of severe environmental circumstance, structural flaws, or wear and tear. However, sudden collapse caused by structural failure, impact, or attack can occur. Staff may not be able to get to work or return home if the bridge is critical for access to that area or if traffic becomes congested.

Although drowning victims rarely have concurrent traumatic injuries other than cervical spine injuries, passengers in vehicles or pedestrians falling from bridges and submerging may be multiply injured. Most are unlikely to survive severe traumatic injury followed by submersion, but these types of injuries should be anticipated in this circumstance. Collapse of bridges that do not cross water may lead to trapped and crushed victims requiring confined-space medicine intervention more like those for other structural collapses. In addition, exposure to polluted water could lead to chemical toxicity and overwhelming sepsis.

PITFALLS

- Failure to plan for the collapse of any local or important bridge
- Failure to be aware of and incorporate plans already in place by state and local authorities

- Failure to have hospital disaster plans in place before the incident
- Failure to include the possibility of the bridge collapse in plans for larger events such as earthquakes, flooding, or a terrorist attack
- Failure to consider larger events (e.g., earthquake or flood) when planning for a possible bridge collapse
- Failure to consider that such larger events (e.g., earthquake or flood) may compromise the functioning of the hospital itself
- Lack of knowledge regarding water conditions, including level of pollution and chemical content of polluted water
- Failure to plan alternate ways for staff to get to the hospital

REFERENCES

1. A blinding squall, then death. *St. Petersburg Times.* Available at: http://www.sptimes.com/StormWatch/SW.2.html.
2. Washington State Department of Transportation, Tacoma Narrows Bridge. Available at: http://www.wsdot.wa.gov/tnbhistory/connections/connections3.htm.
3. Mark Ketchum's Bridge Collapse Page. Available at: http://www.ketchum.org/bridgecollapse.html.
4. NOVA Online. Super Bridge: Resources. Available at: http://www.pbs.org/wgbh/nova/bridge/resources.html.
5. Hick JL. Hospital response to a major freeway bridge collapse. *Disaster Med Public Health Preparedness.* 2008;(Suppl 1):6–11.
6. BBC news. Istanbul Bridge Collapse Kills One. September 3, 2014. Available at: http://www.bbc.com/news/world-europe-29051597.
7. canoe.ca. Fatal Bridge Collapse in Istanbul. September 3, 2014. Available at: http://cnews.canoe.ca/CNEWS/Microgalleries/2014/09/03/21915826.html#1.
8. MailOnline. A Bridge Too Far: Dozens of Tourists Plummet into Lake After Ignoring "Maximum Capacity of 40" Warning Sign. October 14, 2013. Available at: http://www.dailymail.co.uk/news/article-2458589/Stampeding-tourists-dumped-sea-footbridge-collapses-China.html.
9. Adams J. *ODOT gets a GRIP on transportation.* May 1, 2003. Available at: http://connection.ebscohost.com/c/articles/9705294/odot-gets-grip-transportation.
10. Hogan DE, Burnstein JL, eds. *Disaster Medicine.* Philadelphia, PA: Lippincott, Williams & Wilkins; 2002.
11. U.S. Department of Health & Human Services. National Disaster Medical System. Available at: http://www.phe.gov/Preparedness/responders/ndms/Pages/default.aspx.
12. Lovejoy JC. Initial approach to patient management after large-scale disasters. *Clin Pediatr Emerg Med.* 2002;3:217–223.

CHAPTER 189

Human Stampede

Bader S. Alotaibi, Michael Sean Molloy, C. Crawford Mechem, and Angela M. Mills

DESCRIPTION OF EVENT

The word *stampede* is derived from the Spanish word *estampida*, meaning *crash*, and it is a vivid term to describe a sudden rush of animals (e.g., buffaloes or cattle).[1] *Human stampede* may be defined as a sudden collective movement of a crowd of people induced by panic, which often leads to injuries and death from suffocation and trampling. What has not been defined though is the velocity or acceleration involved in determining whether or not an incident could be classified as a stampede. The Hillsborough tragedy at Sheffield in April 1989 is an example of a low-velocity high-volume crowd surge. Gates were opened late to alleviate crowding outside the stadium and a large number of supporters entered a terrace, causing those at the front of the terrace to be crushed against the safety barriers.[2] Eighty-one people died at the scene. The game was abandoned after a few minutes, when people realized how serious the crushing was. Wardrope has published images taken just before kick off, showing overcrowding in two pens, with free space in adjacent pens.[3] In July 2000 at a World Cup qualifying soccer match in Harare, Zimbabwe, a bottle was thrown from the crowd, striking a goal scorer on the head. Police responded by using tear gas on the crowd, which resulted in the crowd rushing the exits to get away. Thirteen people died on scene, with hundreds more injured.[4] The absence of a clear definition for *human stampede* has resulted in such events being classified and reported in a number of ways, such as riot, crowd crush, or stampede. Some of the reported stampede events involve very large crowds, exceeding a million or more, traveling through narrow (relative to the crowd size and density) corridors at low speed, so that when individuals fall, the weight of the following crowd ensures that the fallen cannot get back to their feet. A crush ensues, usually with multiple fatalities.[5–7]

On November 28, 1942, a fire started at a famous Boston nightclub, the Cocoanut Grove, that caused widespread panic and a stampeding crowd. Inward-opening doors and locked doors prevented escape. As a result, 491 people died, and more than 400 were injured.[8] On August 31, 2005, more than 950 people were killed, and hundreds more were injured, in the Al-Aaimmah Bridge Stampede in Baghdad as approximately 1 million Shias marched to a shrine during a religious festival.[9] There had been an earlier mortar attack locally, and a rumor had started that there was a suicide bomber in proximity. When the gate to the bridge opened, pilgrims rushed through; some fell, and the ensuing crush caused massive suffocation.

Human stampedes have resulted in more than 7000 deaths and 14,000 casualties during the past 30 years.[10] In a review of the human stampede literature, Hsieh noted that the origins of human stampedes are multifactorial and that stampedes occurred at various types of mass gathering events: religious,[11–13] sports,[4,14–18] musical,[19,20] political, and other gatherings.[21] Among these different types of events, individual variables affect the magnitude of the stampede, such as crowd size, economic development of the country, time of day, indoor versus outdoor activity, and the mechanism of the crowd flow, either unidirectional or turbulent.[21]

Religious events are associated with the highest median number of fatalities occurring within human stampedes. This is most likely due to characteristically large crowd sizes and events held in outdoor locations.[11] A human stampede with one of the highest recorded fatality rates occurred in 1990 during the annual Muslim Hajj in Mecca, which was attended by millions of pilgrims.[22] More than 1400 people died, and hundreds were injured in the Al-Mua'asem tunnel. Over the past four decades, human stampede incidents were reported as the most frequent type of disaster event during the Hajj.

A model for crowd disasters can be used to understand the causes, prevention, and alleviation of an ongoing incident. The four elements of this model form the acronym *FIST* and include the following: force (F) of the crowd or crowd pressure; information (I), whether real or perceived, on which the crowd acts; physical space (S) involved in the disaster; and time (T) or duration of the event.[23] Forces are produced by persons pushing and leaning against each other. There is often a lack of communication from front to back in a crowd, with the result that persons in the rear push forward and injure those in front. As individuals are injured or fall, they become obstacles to the movement of others. Access to the fallen becomes impossible.[19,23] Large numbers of persons involved in a disaster tend to exhibit mass behavior and do what others do. As people crowd against one another and jamming occurs, alternative exits are frequently overlooked or not used adequately, resulting in additional injuries.[24]

Escape panic has been studied extensively, and it exhibits the following characteristics. Panicking persons attempt to move faster than usual and begin pushing and having physical contact with others. This movement, especially around bottlenecks, becomes uncoordinated. Exits become clogged. The pressures generated by a crowd may exceed 4500 N (1000 lb), allowing steel railings to bend and brick walls to fall.[23–25]

The widening of the corridor has been demonstrated in some circumstances to slow down movement of panicked persons rather than facilitating faster movement. In a study performed with mice, the most efficient escape was a door large enough for only one mouse to fit through at a time. As door widths were increased, the mice ceased lining up and began competing with one another, prolonging the escape rate.[26] This behavior also pertains to rushing pedestrians who will block an exit that they could safely pass through at walking speed. Jamming and clogging may be minimized in the construction of venues by avoiding bottlenecks and placing columns asymmetrically in front of exits to improve outflow.

A human stampede may result in casualties with multiple injuries and possibly even fatalities. Traumatic asphyxia is the most common cause of death and serious injury. The majority of deaths are due to compressive asphyxia as persons are stacked vertically on top of one another or horizontally with associated pushing and leaning forces. A severe crush injury force causes pressure to the chest and/or upper abdomen, resulting in asphyxia if the pressure is not relieved.[27] The mechanism is believed to be acute, severe venous hypertension.[16,27] The various presentations include asystolic cardiac arrest, status epilepticus, prolonged confusion, and cortical blindness.[2] Clinical manifestations include facial edema and petechiae, cranial cyanosis, subconjunctival hemorrhage, exophthalmos, and ecchymotic hemorrhages of the face and upper chest.

Life-threatening pulmonary, cardiac,[28] renal,[29] and gastrointestinal injuries may occur, along with traumatic asphyxia. Injuries in survivors can include pulmonary contusion, pneumothorax, myocardial contusion, flail chest, liver and splenic lacerations, and gastrointestinal hemorrhage. Superior vena cava syndrome may mimic the features of traumatic asphyxia, and should be ruled out. Basilar skull fractures may also present similar symptoms that should be considered. Skull fractures are rare in traumatic asphyxia because the compressive force is usually to the chest or upper abdomen. Morbidity and mortality are associated with the severity and duration of compression and the high incidence of associated injuries. These injuries may be identified by a computed tomography scan, duplex ultrasound, or echocardiogram as dictated by the physical examination. Long-term neurologic sequelae are rare, and full recovery may be achieved with early reestablishment of ventilation and correction of hypoxia.[16,27]

Other injuries that may occur as a result of crush or stampede include musculoskeletal trauma, soft tissue crush injuries, acute right heart strain, and brachial plexus injuries.[2,28] Crush injuries include crush syndrome, compartment syndrome, and acute traumatic ischemia leading to hemorrhage, edema, and hypoperfusion with resulting tissue hypoxia and ischemia. Although any tissue may be affected, nerve and muscle located in myofascial compartments are at increased risk. Cellular death leads to the release of potassium, phosphate, and myoglobin as part of crush syndrome with rhabdomyolysis.[30] Most cases of crush syndrome occur because of compression lasting for 4 or more hours. Complications include hypovolemia, hypotension, and disseminated intravascular coagulation. Renal failure is the most severe complication. The magnitude of elevation of the creatine kinase level has been shown to correlate with the occurrence of renal failure and mortality.[30-32]

◀◀ PRE-INCIDENT ACTIONS

Human stampedes can occur at venues with or without organized medical care. Mass gathering events require extensive coordination of various agencies (e.g., emergency medical services, fire and police departments, local emergency departments and hospitals, and local government agencies including public health departments) as discussed in the National Association of EMS Physicians (NAEMSP) position paper on mass gathering medical care and Medical Directors Checklist.[33-35] Factors to be considered when planning for large events include the type and duration of the event, climate, predicted weather patterns, physical plant and location characteristics, routes of ingress and egress, age and baseline health of attendees, availability of beds in local hospitals, trauma destination protocols, and levels of care to be provided on site. These latter considerations are required for the efficient running of any event, but of themselves, they do not encompass what is required in the event of a mass casualty event such as a stampede. A sophisticated command system must be in operation that will aid in managing the early stage of the disaster effectively. All staff and particularly those expected to operate as command staff at the site of the

mass gathering should be well trained for the roles they could occupy. Unfortunately, this is not always the case.[36-38] In the United States, the National Incident Management System was introduced in the 1990s and updated in 2008 to introduce a national system of preparedness and response to disasters in the United States.[39] In the rest of the world, other systems are in use, the most widely used being the Major Incident Medical Management and Support (MIMMS) system.[40-43]

The MIMMS has seven pillars or priorities. It is the system used in the United Kingdom, Europe, Australasia, and NATO for mass casualty incident management. This system is now mandatory for stadium medical staff who provides medical services to crowds at English Premiership soccer games because of the history of stadium disasters in the United Kingdom.[14,44] The pillars of this system are progressive, building on the previous pillar, but some may be achieved simultaneously. These include the following:

C—Command and control
S—Safety
C—Communication
A—Assessment
T—Triage
T—Treatment
T—Transport

Individuals who provide services at mass gatherings where there is a predictable stampede risk should also avail themselves of MIMMS training in their region to maximize their effectiveness if a disaster occurs.

Stampede mitigation methods may include providing reserved seating rather than general admission to large events, avoiding the use of fixed barricades, ensuring availability of multiple exits, minimizing bottlenecks, limiting access to alcohol and illicit drugs, and having the crowd form into queues.[23,45,46] However, having reserved seating does not completely prevent crowd crush or stampede. In Victoria Hall in Sunderland, UK, 183 children died in 1983 when at the end of the show an announcement was made that gifts would be distributed to children on exit. An estimated 1000 children stampeded toward the staircase, worried about missing the opportunity. Inward-opening doors that were bolted shut resulted in crush and subsequent fatalities. This event led to the introduction of push bars for exit doors. Similarly, forming queues does not prevent disasters, as was shown in the PhilSports Arena, Manila, Philippines, in 2006, where a barrier collapsed as patrons were queuing to enter a televised game show, resulting in 74 fatalities and more than 600 injuries.

▶▶ POST-INCIDENT ACTIONS

The Incident Command System, or MIMMS, both standard emergency management systems, should be activated as early as possible, to coordinate the response to a human stampede. Establishment of effective communication is vital, beginning with the initial message from scene to EMS or other relevant command structure agency. The MIMMS system has a standardized message process, which ensures that both transmitter and responder are aware of what the information and sequence to be transmitted will be, thus aiding the communication process.

The METHANE message is an example of an easily taught and repeatable message structure.

M—Major incident declared
E—Exact location (grid reference if known or GPS)
T—Type of incident (fire, crash, explosion, stampede, etc.)
H—Potential hazards involved (smoke, oil, chemicals, fire, gas, unstable structures, etc.)
A—Access roads to the scene from various directions
N—Estimated number of casualties
E—Emergency services present and required

Prehospital providers must commence triage and rapid treatment, and determine the most sensible distribution or transport of patients to area hospitals. Hospitals, and in particular emergency departments, should have disaster protocols available to handle mass casualty events efficiently, and should be able to anticipate injury patterns associated with human stampede.[20,47–50]

MEDICAL TREATMENT OF CASUALTIES

Standard trauma protocols should be followed when caring for victims of human stampede. Treatment of traumatic asphyxia is mainly supportive and aimed at the associated injuries, which include pulmonary and myocardial contusion, pneumothoraxes, intraabdominal injuries, and neurologic injuries. Prompt delivery of oxygen and efficient ventilation compose the mainstay of treatment, as well as elevation of the head. Prognosis is excellent for those who survive the initial crush injury. The recovery rate is approximately 90% for patients surviving the initial hour.[27]

If massive compression occurs in a stampede, patients should be evaluated for crush injuries and compartment syndromes. The goal of therapy is to prevent renal failure by avoiding hypotension and maintaining adequate urine output. The administration of appropriate intravenous fluid therapy with crystalloid solution should be initiated as early as possible, even before extrication, to maximize intravascular volume and renal perfusion. Staged release protocols as developed by Van der Velde may assist in preventing development of crush syndrome.[51,52] Urine output should be maintained at approximately 200 mL/h in adults. Alkalization of the urine has been shown to increase the solubility and excretion of myoglobin and prevent renal failure. If employed, the urine pH level should be maintained between 6 and 7. The use of mannitol is controversial, but it may aid in diuresis. If compartment syndrome is suspected, compartment pressures should be measured directly, and if elevated, fasciotomy may be required.[30–32] Hyperbaric oxygen therapy has also been shown to be effective in treating severe extremity crush injuries.[53]

UNIQUE CONSIDERATIONS

In the event of a human stampede, access to patients, as well as patient extrication, during early stages may be difficult if not impossible. The safety of emergency responders must be considered. Traumatic asphyxia and crush syndrome are anticipated clinical entities that may be associated with high morbidity and mortality. Early and aggressive therapy, often initiated in the prehospital setting and even before extrication, may be required to ensure the best possible outcome. Adequate planning, public education, and interagency cooperation play key roles in minimizing the risk of human stampede and its associated injuries and deaths.

PITFALLS

Several potential pitfalls for response to a human stampede exist. These include the following:

- Failure to plan appropriately for the mass gathering event with an all-hazards approach
- Failure to train staff in the incident command system
- Failure to conduct tabletop drills of stampede management in advance
- Failure to identify and mitigate stampede threats
- Failure to plan adequately and coordinate the necessary agencies needed to respond to mass gathering events

- Failure to initiate the major incident or mass casualty plan early enough
- Failure to alert appropriate persons, hospitals, and emergency departments to a human stampede event
- Failure to rapidly restore oxygenation and ventilation to victims of a human stampede
- Failure to identify and aggressively treat associated injuries of traumatic asphyxia and massive compression
- Failure to review a stampede incident to identify improvement opportunities

REFERENCES

1. Pearsall J. *The Concise Oxford English Dictionary.* Oxford University Press; 2002, 1.
2. Wardrope J, Hockey MS, Crosby AC. The hospital response to the Hillsborough tragedy. *Injury.* 1990;21(1):53–54, discussion 55–57.
3. Wardrope J, Ryan F, Clark G, Venables G, Crosby A, Redgrave P. The Hillsborough tragedy. *BMJ.* 1991;303(6814):1381–1385.
4. Madzimbamuto FD. A hospital response to a soccer stadium stampede in Zimbabwe. *Emerg Med J.* 2003;20(6):556–559.
5. Ahmed QA, Arabi YM, Memish ZA. Health risks at the Hajj. *Lancet.* 2006;367(9515):1008–1015.
6. Alshinkity I. Hajj: the oldest and largest mass gathering. *Prehosp Disaster Med.* 2005;20(S1):40.
7. Soomaroo L, Murray V. Disasters at mass gatherings: lessons from history. *PLoS Curr.* 2012;4, RRN1301.
8. Saffle JR. The 1942 fire at Boston's Cocoanut Grove nightclub. *Am J Surg.* 1993;166(6):581–591.
9. 2005 Al-Aaimmah bridge stampede [Internet]. Wikipedia [cited Mar 2, 2015]. Available at: http://en.wikipedia.org/wiki/2005_Al-Aaimmah_bridge_stampede.
10. Hsieh Y-H, Ngai KM, Burkle FM, Hsu EB. Epidemiological characteristics of human stampedes. *Disaster Med Public Health Prep.* 2009;3(4):217–223.
11. Burkle FM, Hsu EB. Ram Janki Temple: understanding human stampedes. *Lancet.* 2011;377(9760):106–107.
12. Greenough PG. The Kumbh Mela stampede: disaster preparedness must bridge jurisdictions. *BMJ.* 2013;346:f3254.
13. Hsu EB, Burkle FM. Cambodian Bon Om Touk stampede highlights preventable tragedy. *Prehosp Disaster Med.* 2012;27(5):481–482.
14. Shiels RS. 1971 Ibrox disaster [Internet]. *The Sports Historian.* 2009;148–155. Wikipedia Available at: http://en.wikipedia.org/wiki/1971%20Ibrox%20disaster.
15. Inquiry GASSDCO. *Accra Sports Stadium Disaster Commission of Inquiry final report.* 2001, 1.
16. DeAngeles D, Schurr M, Birnbaum M, Harms B. Traumatic asphyxia following stadium crowd surge: stadium factors affecting outcome. *WMJ.* 1998;97(9):42–45.
17. Madzimbamuto F, Madamombe T. Traumatic asphyxia during stadium stampede. *Cent Afr J Med.* 2004;50(7–8):69–72.
18. Delaney JS, Drummond R. Mass casualties and triage at a sporting event. *Br J Sports Med.* 2002;36(2):85–88, discussion 88.
19. Johnson NR. Panic at "The Who Concert Stampede": an empirical assessment. *Soc Problems.* 1987;34(4):362–373.
20. Stardust fire [Internet]. Wikipedia.org. Wikipedia; 2005 [cited Feb 14, 2015]. Available from: http://en.wikipedia.org/wiki/Stardust_fire.
21. Hsieh Y-H, Ngai KM, Burkle FM, Hsu EB. Epidemiological characteristics of human stampedes. *Disaster Med Public Health Prep.* 2009;3(4):217–223.
22. Ahmed QA, Arabi YM, Memish ZA. Health risks at the Hajj. *Lancet.* 2006;367(9515):1008–1015.
23. Fruin J. The causes and prevention of crowd disasters. In: Smith RA, Dickie JF, eds. *Engineering for Crowd Safety.* Amsterdam: Elsevier; 1993:99–108.
24. Helbing D, Farkas I, Vicsek T. Simulating dynamical features of escape panic. *Nature.* 2000;407(6803):487–490.

25. Low DJ. Statistical physics. Following the crowd. *Nature*. 2000;407 (6803):465–466.

26. Saloma C, Perez GJ, Tapang G, Lim M, Palmes-Saloma C. Self-organized queuing and scale-free behavior in real escape panic. *Proc Natl Acad Sci U S A*. 2003;100(21):11947–11952.

27. Dunne JR, Shaked G, Golocovsky M. Traumatic asphyxia: an indicator of potentially severe injury in trauma. *Injury*. 1996;27(10):746–749.

28. Grech ED, Bellamy CM, Epstein EJ, Ramsdale DR. Traumatic mitral valve rupture during the Hillsborough football disaster: case report. *J Trauma*. 1993;35(3):475–476.

29. Sheikh IA, Shaheen FA, El-Aqeil NA, Al-Khader A, Karsuwa S. Acute renal failure due to rhabdomyolysis following human stampede. *Saudi J Kidney Dis Transpl*. 1994;5(1):17–22.

30. Smith J, Greaves I. Crush injury and crush syndrome: a review. *J Trauma*. 2003;54(5 Suppl):S226–S230.

31. Malinoski DJ, Slater MS, Mullins RJ. Crush injury and rhabdomyolysis. *Crit Care Clin*. 2004;20(1):171–192.

32. Delaney JS, Drummond R. Mass casualties and triage at a sporting event. *Br J Sports Med*. 2002;36(2):85–88, discussion 88.

33. Jaslow D, Yancy A, Milsten A. Mass gathering medical care. National Association of EMS Physicians Standards and Clinical Practice Committee. *Prehosp Emerg Care*. 2000;359–360.

34. Jaslow D, Yancy A, Milsten A. *Mass Gathering Medical Care: The Medical Director's Checklist;* 2000.

35. Advanced Life Support Group. Major Incident Medical Management and Support. *Wiley*. 2013;1.

36. Graham CA, Hearns ST. Major incidents: training for on site medical personnel. *J Accid Emerg Med*. 1999;16(5):336–338.

37. Lennquist S. Medical Response to Major Incidents and Disasters. In: Lennquist S, ed. Berlin, Heidelberg: Springer; 2012, 1.

38. Djalali A, Carenzo L, Ragazzoni L, et al. Does hospital disaster preparedness predict response performance during a full-scale exercise? A pilot study. *Prehosp Disaster Med*. 2014;29(5):441–447.

39. Walsh DW, Christen T, Lord GC, et al. National Incident Management System. *Principles and Practice;* Jones & Bartlett Publishers, 2011.

40. Sammut J, Cato D, Homer T. Major Incident Medical Management and Support (MIMMS): a practical, multiple casualty, disaster-site training course for all Australian health care personnel. *Emerg Med*. 2001;13 (2):174–180.

41. Jenkins JL, McCarthy ML, Sauer LM, et al. Mass-casualty triage: time for an evidence-based approach. *Prehosp Disaster Med*. 2008;23(01):3–8.

42. Hodgetts TJ. Major incident medical training: a systematic international approach. *Int J Disast Med*. 2009;1(1):13–20. Available at: http://dx.doi.org/10.1080/15031430310013429.

43. Group ALS. Major Incident Medical Management and Support. *Wiley*. 2011;1.

44. Walker E. Not all those who died after Hillsborough did so by 3:15 pm. *BMJ*. 1997;314(7089):1283.

45. Grange JT. Planning for large events. *Curr Sports Med Rep*. 2002;1(3):156–161.

46. Milsten AM, Maguire BJ, Bissell RA, Seaman KG. Mass-gathering medical care: a review of the literature. *Prehosp Disaster Med*. 2002;17(03):151–162.

47. Amiri M, Chaman R, Raei M, Nasrollahpour Shirvani SD, Afkar A. Preparedness of hospitals in north of Iran to deal with disasters. *Iran Red Crescent Med J Kowsar*. 2013;15(6):519–521.

48. Valesky W, Silverberg M, Gillett B, et al. Assessment of hospital disaster preparedness for the 2010 FIFA World Cup using an Internet-based, long-distance tabletop drill. *Prehosp Disaster Med*. 2011;26 (3):192–195.

49. Carley S, Mackway-Jones K. Are British hospitals ready for the next major incident? Analysis of hospital major incident plans. *BMJ*. 1996;313 (7067):1242–1243.

50. Williams DJ. Major disasters. Disaster planning in hospitals. *Br J Hospital Med*. 1979;22(4), 308-313-4, 316-7 passim.

51. Nutbeam T, Boylan M. ABC of Prehospital Emergency Medicine. *Wiley*. 2013;1.

52. Van der Velde J, Serfontein L, Iohom G. Reducing the potential for tourniquet-associated reperfusion injury. *Eur J Emerg Med*. 2013;20 (6):391–396.

53. Bouachour G, Cronier P, Gouello JP, Toulemonde JL, Talha A, Alquier P. Hyperbaric oxygen therapy in the management of crush injuries: a randomized double-blind placebo-controlled clinical trial. *J Trauma*. 1996;41(2):333–339.

CHAPTER 190

Mining Accident

Dale M. Molé

DESCRIPTION OF EVENT

The Industrial Revolution significantly increased the demand for fossil fuels. In America, outcrop deposits of coal along the James River in Virginia supplied fuel for blacksmith forges as early as 1702, and when surface supplies diminished, miners followed the coal seams underground. Deeper mines combined with poor ventilation increased the formation of explosive mixtures of methane. The inevitable occurred in 1810 with the first coal mine explosion.[1]

Mine disasters in the first half of the twentieth century involved hundreds of deaths in each accident. Advances in mine technology and safety have greatly reduced the hazard of underground occupations since the early days, but they have not completely eliminated danger. As recently as 2010, 29 miners were killed in a coal dust explosion at the Upper Big Branch Mine in West Virginia.[2] This was the worst mining disaster in the United States in 40 years. China currently leads the world in mining deaths; 2631 miners died in mining accidents in 2009, which was an improvement over the 6995 who lost their lives in 2002.

In the immediate aftermath of a mine accident, surviving until rescue is the first priority of trapped miners. Obstacles to survival include poor communication, extreme darkness, confined space, hypothermia, toxic atmosphere, and injuries. The development of inflatable safety chambers that provide breathable air, water, food, and sanitary facilities for trapped miners may save many lives in the future.

One of the most challenging aspects of any rescue operation is establishing the existence, location, and condition of any survivors. Mine communication systems are often damaged or unreachable in a disaster. Low-frequency radio waves can penetrate rock and offer promise for minewide alarm and communication devices. Seismic locators can detect the vibrations produced by trapped miners in some circumstances. If a survival borehole is drilled, tapping on the drill using prearranged tap codes provides useful information.

Shutting off electricity to reduce ignition sources for fires or explosions is often the first action after a mine accident. Plunged into absolute darkness, the miners must rely on limited-duration, battery-powered helmet lights, making survival efforts more arduous.

Cool ambient mine temperatures combined with water from mine operations, aquifers, rain, or flooding create a major problem for miners who get wet. Immersion in water increases conductive heat loss by as much as fivefold, hastening the onset of hypothermia. Adaptive survival mechanisms (e.g., shivering thermogenesis) increase metabolic heat production by two to five times, but they also significantly increase oxygen consumption and carbon dioxide production—a major problem in small, airtight spaces.[3] Hypothermia depresses the central nervous system, impairs judgment, and prevents the accomplishment of appropriate survival actions.

The atmosphere within a mine is composed of many gases. Early miners used canaries as biologic atmosphere monitors because the birds are overcome by relatively small amounts of noxious gases or damps. The word *damp*, originally derived from the German word *dampf* meaning "fog" or "vapor," is the mining vernacular to describe any mixture of gases in an underground mine, usually noxious or oxygen deficient.[4]

Firedamp primarily refers to methane resulting from the decomposition of coal or other carbonaceous material in an anoxic environment and is explosive when present in air in concentrations of 5% to 15%. The Davy safety lamp, one of the earliest detection devices, detects concentrations as low as 1%. Flame color and height indicate the amount of methane present. Low oxygen levels extinguish the flame entirely. Special colorimetric detectors are now used.

Blackdamp, referring to an anoxic mixture of nitrogen and carbon dioxide, extinguishes flame and causes death by suffocation. Carbon dioxide is produced by the complete combustion of carbonaceous material, metabolism of miners and animals, decay of organic matter, oxidation of coal, or the chemical action of acid water on carbonates.

Chokedamp is any anoxic mixture of mine gases. *Whitedamp* contains large amounts of carbon monoxide; is found in the exhaust of diesel engines, detonated explosives, and wood or coal fires; and is the result of the incomplete combustion of carbonaceous materials. This colorless, tasteless, odorless gas competes with oxygen for hemoglobin binding sites and binds with an affinity 218 times greater. The oxyhemoglobin dissociation curve is transformed from the normal sigmoid to an asymptotic shape, impairing or preventing oxygen transport to the tissues. Tissues with high oxygen demands (e.g., brain and heart) are among the first affected. Symptoms include fatigue, dizziness, headache, seizures, unconsciousness, and hypotension.

Afterdamp is the gas produced by an explosion. It almost always contains dangerous amounts of carbon monoxide and oxides of nitrogen, reported in terms of nitrogen dioxide that can form nitric acid in the lungs. *Stinkdamp*, or hydrogen sulfide gas, has a characteristic pungent smell of rotten eggs. The byproduct of organic decomposition, the action of mine acid on sulfur minerals, or the burning of explosives containing sulfur such as black powder or dynamite, it is soluble in water and may be liberated whenever a mine pool is agitated. It is extremely poisonous and has a mechanism of action similar to cyanide. High concentrations produce loss of consciousness, seizures, and death with just a few breaths.

Other gases include highly explosive hydrogen gas from battery-charging stations; sulfur dioxide, which creates sulfuric acid in the lungs; and acetylene resulting from methane heated in a low-oxygen atmosphere or the interaction of calcium carbide with water.

Oxygen is essential for survival. It is the partial pressure of oxygen, not the absolute percentage, that determines whether the ambient atmosphere can sustain life. Fire or metabolic activity can rapidly consume the available oxygen in a confined, airtight space. Flooding can compress air pockets, raising the total pressure and therefore the partial pressure of oxygen to dangerous levels. Since air is 21% oxygen and normal atmospheric pressure (1 atmosphere absolute [ata]) is equivalent to 760 torr, the partial pressure of oxygen is 760 times 0.21, or 160 torr. Expressed in atmospheres absolute, this would be 1 ata times 0.21, or 0.21 ata. If the atmospheric pressure were doubled to a total pressure of 1520 torr, or 2 ata, the partial pressure of oxygen could be expressed as (1520 torr × 0.21) = 320 torr, or (2 ata × 0.21) = 0.42 ata. Pulmonary oxygen toxicity results from prolonged exposure to high-oxygen partial pressures in excess of 0.5 ata. Breathing 0.6 ata oxygen produces respiratory symptoms in the majority of humans in less than 24 hours.[5] Conversely, as survivors in a closed space consume the available oxygen, the partial pressure of oxygen falls, producing signs and symptoms of hypoxia such as dyspnea (i.e., air hunger), cyanosis, impaired cognition, poor muscle coordination, and unconsciousness.

Nitrogen comprises 79% of our atmosphere and is generally considered an inert (metabolically inactive) gas. When breathed at increased pressure, however, it produces a narcotic effect in a dose-dependent fashion; that is, the higher the partial pressure of nitrogen, the greater the narcosis. Nitrogen narcosis causes both cognitive and psychomotor disturbances. Breathing room air at 4 to 7 ata results in exposure to elevated partial pressures of nitrogen high enough to cause delayed response to auditory and visual stimuli, impaired neuromuscular coordination, a loss of clear thinking, and a tendency toward idea fixation. The effect is similar to ethanol intoxication, and it can significantly impair the ability of miners to take the necessary steps to ensure survival.

Carbon dioxide comprises only 0.001 ata, or one tenth of 1% of the atmosphere. It is a byproduct of cellular metabolism, and for each standard cubic foot of oxygen consumed an almost equal amount of carbon dioxide is produced. If the carbon dioxide level climbs past 0.10 ata, unconsciousness is soon followed by death. In an airtight space, it is the carbon dioxide level that limits survival, not the amount of oxygen.[6]

In prolonged survival situations, food and water also become important considerations. Inadequate caloric intake can produce starvation diarrhea, making survival less likely.[7]

PRE-INCIDENT ACTIONS

One of the most significant advances in mine rescue operations occurred in 1856 with the introduction of self-contained breathing apparatus, allowing rescuers to conduct operations with increased safety. Part 49 of Title 30 of the Code of Federal Regulations requires every mine in the country to have mine rescue teams. It stipulates how many members each team should have and outlines physical and training standards and required equipment, maintenance, and storage. Modern mine rescue, with enhanced team training and improved equipment, has transformed chaotic, uncoordinated rescue attempts into efficient, well-coordinated group efforts. The full integration of medical elements into the team is essential for a successful outcome to rescue operations.

Today's teams use modern gas detection and communication equipment, seismic locators, geophones, and other devices to locate miners. Rescue vans are outfitted with breathing apparatus, recharging facilities, hand tools, medical supplies, and gas analysis equipment. A qualitative and quantitative knowledge of constituent gases within the mine provides important clues to past events, as well as current atmosphere conditions such as elevated carbon monoxide levels suggestive of a fire.

Mine emergency operations teams can drill boreholes down from the surface to reach miners. Once a small-diameter "survival hole" is drilled, rescuers can lower microphones, lights, and cameras into the mine to help locate the miners, determine their situation, and lend support and assistance while a rescue hole is drilled. Trapped miners can be safely hauled to the surface in specially designed "rescue capsules," as was successfully demonstrated in the 2002 Quecreek Mine disaster with the rescue of all nine miners.[8]

POST-INCIDENT ACTIONS

The first few hours after the emergency are the most critical. Coordination of mine rescue teams, mine personnel, and local, state, and federal officials is essential. A command center forms the hub of mine rescue operations and contains communications equipment, underground diagrams, and local area maps. As mine rescue teams arrive, a rotation schedule is prepared, designating which teams are to be the exploration team, backup team, and standby team. A bench area with running water allows breathing apparatus to be cleaned, tested, and prepared.

Establishing perimeter security is essential to keep roads open for emergency personnel and to ensure that curious bystanders do not hinder rescue efforts or become injured while on mine property. Company personnel or police officers should guard all routes to the mine.

A press center should be established away from the disaster site and should be the only area where news media receive information. A public affairs officer will authorize, issue, and ensure the accuracy of the information being released to the public. The family waiting area should be away from any rescue activity and the media center.

Provision should be made to feed and house rescue personnel during an emergency. Food can be catered or brought in from a nearby restaurant. The American Red Cross is skilled at providing disaster relief services. Nearby motels can often provide sleeping quarters, or if none is available, tents and cots can be set up at the rescue site. Ensuring adequate field hygiene is critical to preventing infectious disease outbreaks among rescue personnel.

Mine exploration is the process of assessing conditions underground and locating miners during a rescue or recovery operation. The safest route into the mine is determined before anyone goes underground. In a shaft mine, the cage (i.e., elevator) is thoroughly tested for proper operation, and the shaft is tested for the presence of gases, smoke, or water.

In some disaster situations, conditions may make it possible to begin the initial exploration without self-contained breathing apparatus. This "barefaced" exploration is conducted only when the ventilation system is operating properly and gas tests demonstrate a safe atmosphere. Backup crews with apparatus are stationed nearby, ready to perform a rescue if necessary. Barefaced exploration stops where disruptions in ventilation are discovered, when gas analysis indicates the presence of noxious or explosive gases or an oxygen deficiency, or when smoke or damage is encountered. A "fresh air base" is usually established at the point where conditions no longer permit barefaced exploration. Teams equipped with breathing apparatus continue exploration from the fresh air base. Typical mine rescue equipment includes gas detectors, oxygen indicators, communication equipment, thermal imaging cameras or heat-sensing devices, link-line, map board and marker, scaling bar, walking stick, stretcher, first aid kit, fire extinguisher, tools, blankets, and extra breathing apparatus. Before going underground, each team is briefed about what has happened in the mine and what conditions currently exist.

Because every underground coal mine contains harmful gases, dust fumes, and smoke, a ventilation system draws air from the surface via the main intake shaft. Ventilation controls force air to move in certain directions and at certain velocities to safely ventilate all sections of the mine. The main fan creates a pressure differential and must be monitored or guarded to ensure the rescue team's safety while underground after the fresh air base is established and exploration is under way. Changes in ventilation are only made by the command center. As the team advances through the mine, all ventilation controls are examined. Team members must be able to recognize damaged ventilation controls, determine the direction and velocity of ventilation air by using an anemometer or smoke tube, measure the cross-sectional area of a mine entry, and calculate the volume of air by using the area and velocity. The quantity of air (measured in cubic feet) is equal to the area (in square feet) multiplied by the velocity (in feet per minute).

Fires in underground mines are especially hazardous because they pose explosion hazards, consume oxygen, and produce smoke, toxic gases, and heat. Ventilation is always maintained during a fire to carry off explosive gases and distillates away from the fire area and to direct the smoke, heat, and flames away from the team. The most frequent cause of explosions in coal mines is the ignition of methane gas, coal dust, or a combination of the two. Explosions can blow out roof supports, damage ventilation controls, twist or scatter machinery, and ignite numerous fires. Roof and ribs can be weakened, and fires can be spread. Further explosions may occur because of damage to the ventilation system during the initial explosion.

✚ MEDICAL TREATMENT OF CASUALTIES

In a disaster in which several miners are trapped underground, or in which injuries are sustained after an explosion, roof fall, or fire, a temporary medical treatment facility should be established. After initial stabilization, a carefully considered means of patient transport may include ambulances or evacuation aircraft, with medical crew on standby. If large numbers of corpses are being recovered from the mine, a temporary morgue is necessary.

❓ UNIQUE CONSIDERATIONS

Delayed care for contaminated wounds and crush injuries, as well as the synergistic effects of toxic gases, hypothermia, and inadequate nutrition make medical management of the victims of a mining accident especially challenging. Provision for decontamination is essential after prolonged underground dwelling. Carbon monoxide poisoning may require treatment with hyperbaric oxygen.

⚠ PITFALLS

Potential pitfalls in response to a mining accident include:
- Inadequate training and equipment familiarization
- Inadequate integration of medical personnel into mine rescue team training
- Failure to optimize ventilation following a mine explosion or fire
- Failure to maintain proper communication channels to family members and the media
- Failure to consider the effects of elevated pressure in mine flooding situations

REFERENCES

1. Kravitz J. *An Examination of Major Mine Disasters in the United States and a Historical Summary of MSHA's Mine Emergency Operations Program.* Available at: http://www.msha.gov/S&HINFOTECHRPT/MED/MAJORMIN.pdf.
2. NRC. *April 2010 Upper Big Branch Mine Explosion—29 Lives Lost. Safety Culture Communicator of the Nuclear Regulator Commission;* March 2012. Available at: http://pbadupws.nrc.gov/docs/ML1206/ML12069A003.pdf.
3. Danzl D. Accidental hypothermia. In: Auerbach P, ed. *Wilderness Medicine.* 6th ed; 2012:116–142.
4. MSHA. *Advanced Mine Rescue Training—Coal Mines.* Washington: Mine Safety and Health Administration; 2013.
5. Dougherty J, Styer D, Eckenhoff R. *The Effects of Hyperbaric and Hyperoxic Conditions on Pulmonary Function During Prolonged Hyperbaric Chamber Air Saturation Dives.* Bethesda, Md: Undersea Biomedical Research; 1981.
6. Molé D. *Submarine Escape and Rescue: An Overview.* San Diego, Calif: Submarine Development Group One; 1990.
7. House C, House J, Oakley H. Findings from a simulated disabled submarine survival trial. *Undersea Hyperb Med.* 2000;27(4):175–183, Winter.
8. Molé D. Steaming to assist at the Quecreek Mine disaster. *Navy Med.* 2002;93:18–29.

Submarine or Surface Vessel Accident

Dale M. Molé

Ours is a water planet. Water covers 70% of the earth's surface. Humans first crossed bodies of water by swimming or clinging to floating objects.[1] Technology eventually advanced from log rafts and dugout canoes to modern ships and submarines. Before the nineteenth century, culture, conflict, commerce, and contagion rapidly spread by sea and ocean.[2] Great sea powers, such as the Dutch, Spanish, British, and United States, successively led the world in trade and influence. Humans still depend upon the oceans to connect us. Ninety percent of the world's commerce moves by sea. The oceans are used for pleasure, profit, and power projection in support of national foreign policy. Maritime exploration and discovery still continue today. Even the Arctic Ocean, shrouded in a permanent mantle of ice impenetrable to surface ships, reveals its secrets to submarines.[3] Deep submergence vehicles plumb the abyss of the deep ocean trenches,[4] and tourist submarines display the wonders of the "silent world" to the general public. Fishing vessels are a life-sustaining source of food and income for many around the world. The oceans influence our daily life in myriad ways, from terrestrial weather patterns to the cost and availability of the merchandise we use.

As with aviation the sea is unforgiving of poor design or human error. Maritime disasters too frequently capture world news headlines. Ferry disasters, such as the April 2014 capsizing of the Korean MV Sewol[5] with the loss of hundreds of young lives, or the events of January 2012, when the Italian cruise ship Costa Concordia with more than 4000 passengers aboard struck a rock and sank in shallow water resulting in 32 deaths,[6] are stark reminders that misfortune can beset even the most modern vessels.

Many mishaps are the result of poor communications between crew members. The patient safety acronym "SBAR" (situation, background, assessment, and recommendation) familiar to many medical professionals had its origin in the nuclear submarine community as a means to flatten the organizational hierarchy and improve communication of critical information.[7]

Ships are high-risk industrial environments with little margin for error. Large vessels have power plants generating enough energy to light several neighborhoods, machinery capable of handling tons of material a day, and engineering spaces filled with loud, high-pressure, high-voltage, rotating machinery. Because volume and weight are at a premium aboard ship, all this equipment is located in small, often cramped spaces that are difficult to access. Marine engineering design dictates high-pressure air, inert gas, and hydraulic systems run the length of the ship, often through living, eating, and recreational spaces, posing an immediate hazard if rupture occurs. Add ladders or steep stairs, heavy steel doors and hatches, wet and slippery decks, rolling, rocking, heaving, and pitching wave action, high winds, and sea spray; it is easy to see why injuries or mass casualties occur aboard ships despite safety regulations, procedures, and equipment.[8]

Fire, collision, and grounding remain the top causes for loss of a vessel at sea.[9] Given the various sources of combustion and combustible materials aboard, fires of all types represent an omnipresent and often fatal danger. Fire requires a source of ignition (electrical arcing, overloaded wiring, open flames, smoking materials, and hot surfaces) and fuel (gasoline, diesel, hydraulic fluid, engine oil, wood, plastics, canvas, and furniture). Although fires can occur anywhere, the engine room and hydraulic systems represent the primary locations.[10] Fire rapidly consumes oxygen in enclosed spaces while producing toxic fumes, thick smoke, and a significant potential for burn injuries. Hazardous cargo that is combustible, toxic, corrosive, or radioactive adds additional complexity to an already challenging situation. This is especially true in the case of container ships in which container content is not always properly declared and cargo located above deck have no fixed fire suppression systems; they must be extinguished manually by firefighting teams often with little experience fighting container fires.[11] Given the unique operating environment, conventional fire fighting techniques are sometimes difficult to implement aboard ship. The priority of the crew in the event of a fire is to first extinguish the fire, after which any casualties are treated. This may result in significant treatment delays, especially if the fire occurs at sea rather than pier side.

Collisions and groundings can compromise the watertight integrity of the hull and result in uncontrolled flooding. The rate of flooding and the reserve buoyancy of the vessel ultimately determine how long the ship remains afloat or if the submarine is able to return to the surface rather than sink to below crush depth. Collisions between surface ships or a surface ship and a submarine occur more commonly than one would suspect. While practicing an emergency ascent ("emergency blow") in 2001 the submarine U.S.S. Greenville collided with Japanese surface vessel Ehime Maru, causing the ship to sink resulting in death for nine of the 35 crew.[12,13] Two years later the submarine U.S.S. San Francisco collided with an underwater seamount while on a high-speed run in the Pacific, injuring scores of crew members and killing one.[14]

In most maritime settings, pipes for engine cooling and sanitation penetrate the hull. A pipe rupture or stopcock failure can result in forceful, massive flooding and physical trauma to those in the vicinity, including direct blunt trauma, falls on slippery decks, and drowning.

Submarine disasters provide their own unique challenges. Submarines sink because of uncontrolled flooding. Only marginally buoyant by design, relatively small amounts of flooding can prevent a submarine from surfacing, especially if propulsion is lost.[15] If this happens in the deep ocean, there are no medical issues because the submarine implodes once crush depth is exceeded. However, because most collisions are more likely to occur over the continental shelf in heavily traveled and congested sea lanes, having survivors trapped in a sunken submarine is a real possibility. The Peruvian submarine Pacocha was returning to port on the evening of August 26, 1988 when it was struck by a

Japanese fishing vessel. With the hull breached, the submarine sank in 140 feet of water 6 nautical miles from shore. Twenty-two crew members were trapped in the forward compartment of the submarine.[16]

The decision to await rescue or to begin escape depends on the external as well as the internal environment of the submarine. In water deeper than 180 m (600 feet), escape is not currently an option, despite a hostile internal submarine environment (i.e., high pressure, low oxygen, toxic gases). Rapid geometric compression (a doubling of pressure every 2 seconds) in the escape trunk of the submarine is required for the submariner to "outrun" the lethal physiological effects of breathing normal atmospheric constituents (oxygen and nitrogen) at significantly elevated partial pressures. Once outside the submarine, the submariner is exposed to the ambient high-pressure, cold, and dark deep ocean environment. Any delay in escape trunk compression or delay in ascent would prove fatal. Weather over the disaster site may prevent the timely rescue of survivors. The ability for a submarine crew to survive at least 5 to 7 days is the ideal goal because time is required to mobilize rescue assets and deploy them to a remote disaster site. The nature of the disaster, such as loss of electrical power or carbon dioxide scrubbing capability, may result in significantly shorter survival times.

Barriers to survival are many. The ingress of water reduces the internal submarine volume, compressing the air and subjecting the crew to an elevated atmospheric pressure. As total pressure increases, the partial pressure of constituent gases increases as well. Oxygen and nitrogen, the primary constituents of air, are lethal at high partial pressures. Central nervous system oxygen toxicity can cause death in a matter of minutes. High partial pressures of nitrogen produce narcosis in a dose-dependent fashion as well as loading tissue with excess nitrogen. Survivors with nitrogen-saturated tissues must be decompressed or slowly returned to normal atmospheric pressure to avoid potentially fatal decompression sickness. Carbon dioxide produced by human metabolism is the limiting factor for submariners trapped in an airtight compartment because carbon dioxide climbs to lethal levels before oxygen becomes insufficient to sustain life. Because the average ocean temperature is 4 °C, clothing wet from flooding can quickly lead to hypothermia. Shivering helps to maintain core temperature, but markedly increases the consumption of oxygen and the production of carbon dioxide. Toxic gases from fire or chlorine produced by flooded batteries may force the crew to use emergency breathing apparatus or escape under unfavorable conditions.[17]

Submarine escape is potentially hazardous even under the most ideal conditions. Pulmonary barotraumas resulting in arterial gas embolism, as well as fulminate decompression sickness, are conditions that may occur and require immediate hyperbaric oxygen treatment.[18] Submarine rescue via rescue chamber or deep submergence rescue vehicle is the preferred method of saving trapped submariners because it avoids exposing them to ambient underwater conditions and allows medical treatment during transit to the surface.

◀◀ PRE-INCIDENT ACTIONS

Providing medical care at sea is challenging even in the best of circumstances. The open ocean is a remote, austere environment with limited personnel, few treatment options, and long or impossible evacuation opportunities. Dedicated medical personnel exist only on larger ships. More often the "ship's doctor" is a layperson with limited first aid training and a small medical kit. Even for trained clinicians the lack of medical imaging, laboratory, or the other ancillary services traditionally found in most clinical settings makes caring for seriously sick or injured crew members or passengers extremely difficult.

Federal, state, and port authorities responsible for maritime safety and rescue should have a well-established, well-practiced integrated emergency response plan that includes any Coast Guard and naval bases in the area. Essential elements of the plan are a robust and reliable communication network, a realistic casualty (sea, air, and land) transportation system, geographically assigned areas of responsibility for primary receiving medical facilities, and identified secondary facilities based upon requirements for specialty care or overwhelming numbers of casualties at the primary facility. Casualty decontamination from exposure to hazardous substances must also be considered.

▶▶ POST-INCIDENT ACTIONS

Shipboard crew must take immediate action to address the incident, which hopefully was previously drilled. If the incident cannot be contained, the decision as to when to abandon ship can be critical depending on ambient environmental conditions. Provisions should be made for passengers with reduced mobility to enter lifeboats early. All those leaving the ship should be wearing personal floatation devices. If habitable the ship or vessel is the best lifeboat. Some pleasure craft are virtually unsinkable. Catamarans have buoyant foam cores sandwiched between layers of fiberglass, as well as watertight compartments, in addition to having two separate hulls. Although completely flooded and perhaps capsized, one is much better off remaining on or near a capsized catamaran because it presents a much bigger target for search efforts than a small rubber raft.[19] Larger vessels should be abandoned before sinking to avoid becoming entangled or trapped. Eddy currents or air bubbles from a rapidly sinking large ship may affect buoyancy, making it difficult for nearby survivors in the water to remain on the surface. Lifeboats must be lowered before the vessel achieves a list (tilt) of 20° or a pitch of 10°, otherwise they may not be able to be properly deployed.

Very high frequency (VHF) radios and an Emergency Position Indicating Radio Beacon (EPIRB) are required by many maritime nations on certain vessels.[20] The EPRIB operates on the exclusive international beacon distress frequency (406 MHz), monitored by the National Oceanographic and Atmospheric Agency's (NOAA) Search and Rescue Satellite Aided Tracking (SARSAT) system. Class I EPIRBs have a special bracket with hydrostatic release which automatically activates and releases the device to float to the surface from depths of 3 to 10 feet of seawater. Class II EPIRBS can only be manually activated. Once a distress signal is received, the NOAA notifies the appropriate authority, such as the Coast Guard, Navy, or Air Force Pararescue Service.

✚ MEDICAL TREATMENT OF CASUALTIES

A wide variety of mechanisms of injury may both be a cause and a result of a maritime disaster. The mechanism of injury may include blunt and penetrating trauma, burns, inhalation injuries, and near-drowning. Treatment should follow current medical practice. Major complicating factors include hypothermia, hazardous material exposure, and preexisting medical conditions.

Except in the most tropical of waters, hypothermia is a significant problem. Accidental hypothermia is defined as the unintentional decrease in normal core temperature of at least 2 °C (3.6 °F).[21] Cold water immersion survival time is difficult to accurately predict and depends upon many factors, such as the amount and type of clothing, percent body fat, activity, heat loss attenuating positions, age, and gender. Even after leaving the water, wet clothing reduces survival odds. During the 1982 Falklands war, sailors from the torpedoed Argentine cruiser *General Belgrano* died from hypothermia after climbing into life rafts.[22] The clinician needs to prevent further heat loss and vigilantly monitor body temperature in recently rescued patients.

Contamination with hazardous material (petroleum distillates, chemicals, radioactive materials) can complicate the treatment of patients. The provision for and practicing of decontamination procedures is an essential part of disaster medical treatment planning. The ability to perform emergent "life and limb" saving procedures on heavily contaminated patients while maintaining medical staff safety is possible and should be incorporated into medical response plans.

Preexisting medical conditions are common in older civilian mariners and are sometimes not disclosed because they directly influence employment opportunities. The age distribution among passengers on cruise ships is skewed toward the older and therefore sicker population.[23] With less physiological reserve, less physical strength, and more problems with mobility, even those without significant underlying medical conditions are at a disadvantage in a maritime disaster as compared with a younger, healthier population.

UNIQUE CONSIDERATIONS

Transporting nonambulatory patients from the point of injury to an area of medical treatment or evacuation is particularly difficult in the confined spaces, narrow passageways, and steep stairs aboard ship. Location, initial assessment, extraction, and patient movement require more time and more "muscle" than a similar land-based scenario. Getting the patient off a ship at sea is fraught with difficulty and danger, making the risk of patient evacuation a variable in the decision equation.

PITFALLS

Several potential pitfalls in response to a ship or submarine accident exist. These include the following:

- Failure to fully exercise the sea disaster mass casualty plan
- Failure to consider radiological or toxic contamination in the process of providing medical treatment
- Allowing low-level radioactive contamination to delay life and limb saving medical treatment
- Poor communications hampering efforts to properly coordinate patient transport
- Failure to anticipate and properly treat hypothermia in casualties exposed to the environment
- Failure to adequately communicate instruction for basic medical care to on-scene personnel lacking medical expertise
- Lack of knowledge regarding the location of hyperbaric facilities for treating submarine disaster victims

REFERENCES

1. Lavery B. *Ship: The Epic Story of Maritime Adventure.* New York, NY: DK; 2008.
2. Paine L. *The Sea & Civilization: A Maritime History of the World.* New York, NY: Alfred A. Knopf; 2013.
3. Leary W. *Under Ice: Waldo Lyon and the Development of the Arctic Submarine.* College Station, TX: Texas A&M University Press; 1999.
4. Forman W. *The History of American Deep Submersible Operations.* Flagstaff, AZ: Best; 1999.
5. Sinking of MV Sewol. Available at http://en.wikipedia.org/wiki/Sinking_of_the_MV_Sewol. Accessed 30.11.14.
6. Costa Concordia Disaster. Available at http://en.wikipedia.org/wiki/Costa_Concordia. Accessed 30.11.14.
7. Heinrichs W, Bauman E. SBAR "flattens the hierarchy" among caregivers *Stud Health Technol Inform.* 2012;173:175–182.
8. Thomas T, Parker A, Horn W, et al. Accidents and injuries among U.S. Navy crewmembers during extended submarine patrols, 1997 to 1999. *Mil Med.* 2001;166(6):534–540.
9. *Allianz Global Corporate Specialty Safety & Shipping Review 2014.* Available at: https://www.allianz.com/v.../AGCS_Shipping_Review_2014_5mb.pdf. Accessed 30.11.14.
10. Tyrell D. Accidental fire causes. In: *Guide for Conducting Marine Fire Investigations;* Marine Accident Investigators' International Forum 2000:25–37.
11. Tosseviken A, Bregmann J. Cargo fires on container carriers. *Det Norske Veritas Technical Paper.* No.2003-P013.
12. Lewis J, Shiroma C, Von Guenther K, et al. Recovery and identification of the victims of the Ehime Maru/USS Greeneville collision at sea. *J Forensic Sci.* 2004;49(3):539–542.
13. Roberts K, Tadmor C. Lessons learned from non-medical industries: the tragedy of the USS Greeneville. *Qual Saf Health Care.* 2002;11(4):355–357.
14. Jankosky C. Mass casualty in an isolated environment: medical response to a submarine collision. *Mil Med.* 2008;173(8):734–737.
15. Friedman N. *Submarine Design and Development.* Annapolis, MD: U.S. Naval Institute Press; 1984.
16. Harvey C, Carson J. *The B.A.P. Pacocha (SS-48) Collision: The Escape and Medical Treatment of Survivors.* San Diego, CA: Submarine Development Group One; 1988.
17. Molé D. Submarine medicine. In: Edmonds C, Lowry C, Pennefather J, eds. *Diving and Subaquatic Medicine.* 3rd ed; 1992: 499–512.
18. Harvey C, Stetson D, Burns M, et al. *Pressurized Submarine Rescue: A Manual for Undersea Medical Officers.* Naval Submarine Medical Research Laboratory; June 22, 1992, NSMRL Report. 1178.
19. Tarjan G. *Catamarans: The Complete Guide for Cruising Sailors.* New York, NY: McGraw-Hill; 2006.
20. Title 46 U.S. Code of Federal Regulations Subpart 25.26—Emergency Position Indicating Radio Beacons (EPIRB).
21. Danzl D. Accidental hypothermia. In: Auerbach P, ed. *Wilderness Medicine.* 6th ed; 2012:116–142.
22. Gerding E. Accidental immersion hypothermia in the South Atlantic. *Int Rev Armed Forces Med Service.* 1996;LXIX 4/5/6:126–139.
23. ACEP. *Heath Care Guidelines for Cruise Ship Medical Facilities, Rev;* Jul 2014, Available at: http://www.acep.org/Physician-Resources/Clinical/Health-Care-Guidelines-for-Cruise-Ship-Medical-Facilities/. Accessed 30.11.14.

Aircraft Hijacking

Leon D. Sanchez, Laura Ebbeling, and Kurt R. Horst

DESCRIPTION OF EVENT

Aircraft hijacking is defined as the armed takeover of an aircraft.[1] Prior to the events involving the World Trade Center in New York City on September 11, 2001, most hijackings involved using the aircraft as transportation and the passengers as hostages. The hijackers would then typically present specific demands, which would be negotiated.[1]

The first recorded aircraft hijacking occurred in 1931 in Peru when a group of armed revolutionaries approached a Ford tri-motor aircraft and attempted to force the pilot to fly them to their destination.[1,2] The pilot refused, and after a 10-day standoff during which the revolution succeeded, the pilot was released.[1,2] Unfortunately, many aircraft hijackings do not end so peacefully. A few noteworthy incidents are presented in Box 192-1.

Before the events of September 11, 2001, antihijacking training followed what was termed the "Common Strategy." This philosophy was based on prior experiences with hijackers. It instructed aircrews to avoid attempts to overpower these persons and encouraged actions to resolve hijackings peacefully, even by accommodating the hijackers when necessary. But the goal of the September 11 hijackings was to use the aircraft to perform a suicide attack, rendering the Common Strategy obsolete.[5]

Since this attack, training has been altered and now follows what is referred to as the "Crew Training Common Strategy." It instructs pilots to not open the cockpit door, and new Federal Aviation Administration regulations require reinforcement of those doors. However, if the door is breached, the flight crew will attempt to protect the aircraft from being taken over.[6] New legislation, including the Arming Pilots Against Terrorism Act of 2002, has opened the way for the training and deputization of pilots.[6,7] Federal flight deck officers are sworn, deputized federal law enforcement officers commissioned by the Department of Homeland Security/Transportation Security Administration (TSA) Law Enforcement Division, meaning pilots are allowed to carry firearms, providing added safeguards to the security of the flight deck.[6,7]

In November 2001, the Aviation and Transportation Security Act was passed, and the TSA was created to oversee travel security.[8,9] Initially placed under the U.S. Department of Transportation, the TSA now falls under the Department of Homeland Security[9] and is responsible for overseeing the screening of passengers, baggage, and cargo to detect possible threats, including explosives.[8,9]

As in historical aircraft hijackings, many hostage situations are resolved with force. The emergence of the field of tactical emergency medical support over the past decade provides a key role in such operations. Emergency medical providers, preferably trained at the paramedic level, serve as members of special weapons and tactics (SWAT) teams, which often have a role in resolving hostage situations involving aircraft. The ability to provide immediate, high-level medical attention to hostage victims after entry is made can increase survival of those injured in the incident.[10,11]

PRE-INCIDENT ACTIONS

Much of the focus on aircraft hijackings has centered on modalities to detect and prevent them. The TSA was developed to spearhead many of the changes that have occurred since the September 11, 2001, hijackings in the United States.[8,9]

Medical personnel should be aware of the various injury patterns that can be seen in victims involved in an aircraft hijacking with hostages. Knowledge of and participation in tactical emergency medical support operations will improve survivability.[10,11] Acute exacerbations of pre-event medical conditions among victims may occur during the hostage situation. This may be precipitated either by the stress of the event or the lack of availability of the patient's routine medications. For example, a diabetic might develop hyperglycemia because his insulin was in his checked luggage. Therefore, emergency responders should be prepared to treat a myriad of primary medical conditions.

Continued training of airline personnel using the Crew Training Common Strategy will be imperative in preventing future suicide hijackings.[6,7] The arming of pilots is a controversial issue. Proper training in firearms safety and use is required.[7] The presence of air marshals, law enforcement officers who fly aboard commercial flights, can also provide added protection because they have specialized training in the prevention of hijackings.[12] As seen on September 11, 2001, the actions of private citizens can prevent a hijacked airliner from reaching its target.[5] Aircraft passengers may find themselves in a position where they must act. This will certainly be a hard decision, and providing specific advice is difficult.

POST-INCIDENT ACTIONS

Once on the ground, negotiations can occur between the hijackers and law enforcement. Alternatively, specialty teams can enter the aircraft, using an array of techniques to gain entry and incapacitate the

---

BOX 192-1 Selected Aircraft Hijackings

1968 Three members of the Popular Front for the Liberation of Palestine (PFLP) hijack an El Al plane. After 40 days, the hostages and hijackers are released.[1,2]

1969 Eight U.S. airliners are hijacked to Cuba in 1 month. This leads to development of a Federal Aviation Administration task force that creates a hijacker "profile" used in conjunction with weapons-screening devices.[2]

1970 Four airliners, including one operated by a U.S. carrier, are hijacked by the PFLP. Three are successful and force landings in the Jordanian desert, where they are exploded after the passengers deplane. All hostages are subsequently freed after seven PFLP members are released from prison.[1–3]

1970 A copilot is fatally wounded by a hijacker on an Eastern Airlines flight. Another copilot shoots and severely wounds the hijacker. The pilot, who was also injured, safely lands the aircraft.[2]

1976 Palestinians hijack an Air France aircraft. After the plane lands in Uganda, Israeli commandos free 105 passengers after they storm a building where the hijackers had relocated the hostages. Three passengers, all the hijackers, and one commando are killed.[1]

1982 Fifty-nine people die when Egyptian commandos infiltrate an Egypt Air plane after it is hijacked by Palestinians and flown to Malta.[2]

1984 Four Arab hijackers aboard a Kuwait Airways jetliner force the aircraft to land in Iran. Once there, they kill two American citizens and commit other brutalities against the passengers. Iranian forces storm the aircraft, freeing the remaining hostages.[3]

1985 Lebanese Shiite Moslems hijack a TWA airliner in Athens and kill a U.S. serviceman onboard the flight. The rest of the passengers are released in stages over the course of 2 weeks. The International Security and Development Cooperation Act of 1985 is signed 2 months later and provides monies for development of new airport security devices and hiring of additional security inspectors to serve as air marshals.[3,4]

1986 After a 16-hour standoff, 22 people are killed when Pakistani forces storm a hijacked Pan Am flight in Karachi.[1,2]

1988 The explosion of a Pan American jetliner over Lockerbie, Scotland, by an explosive device in a cassette player prompts the institution of a number of security measures, including installation of devices to detect explosives and stricter penalties for trying to take a gun through airport screening sites.[3,4]

1996 One hundred twenty-five passengers are killed when an Ethiopian Airlines flight crashes into the Indian Ocean after hijackers refuse to allow the pilot to land and refuel. Fifty passengers survive.[2]

2001 On September 11, three American aircraft are hijacked and deliberately used to cause destruction at the World Trade Center towers in New York City and the Pentagon in Washington, DC. A fourth hijacked aircraft crashes in Pennsylvania after passengers attempt to retake the plane.[1,2,4]

---

hijackers. Medical personnel must be readily available to treat injuries to hijackers and hostages alike.

✚ MEDICAL TREATMENT OF CASUALTIES

A variety of injury patterns are likely among victims of aircraft hijackings. With more stringent passenger and luggage screening, there is a lesser chance of seeing gunshot wounds compared with previous hijackings. However, because some pilots now carry weapons and armed rescue attempts by military special forces and SWAT teams are possible once the aircraft is on the ground, this type of injury remains plausible. Emergency personnel attached to these teams and in emergency departments must be prepared to provide appropriate immediate care. Additionally, penetration trauma by an array of instruments such as knives, screwdrivers, and other sharp objects is possible.

Evaluation in the field and the hospital should begin with an assessment of the airway, breathing, and circulation, then progress to a secondary survey. Intubation should be performed as needed, and intravenous resuscitation should begin with crystalloid solutions.

Penetrating trauma to the chest can result in cardiac injury leading to pericardial tamponade, which must be immediately recognized and treated with fluid boluses and needle aspiration in the field, followed by subsequent surgical intervention in the hospital.[13,14] Beck's triad, while not always present, is indicative of pericardial tamponade and consists of hypotension, distended neck veins, and muffled heart sounds. Ultrasonography is used to confirm the diagnosis but may not be available in the field. Thoracotomy can also play a role in treatment once the patient arrives in an emergency department.[14] If a tension pneumothorax is suspected (evidenced by hypotension, distended neck veins, unilateral decreased breath sounds, and tracheal deviation), immediate needle decompression must be performed before obtaining a chest radiograph, regardless of setting.[13,15] A tube thoracotomy may then be performed.[15] Simple pneumothorax, hemothorax, and a variety of injuries to the great vessels and lung

parenchyma can also occur and must be identified early because surgical therapy may be indicated.[13,14]

Penetrating abdominal trauma can be recognized by identification of a penetrating wound, evisceration, and the presence of tenderness and peritoneal signs on physical examination. Any aberration in vital signs can also point to the presence of internal hemorrhage.[16] In the field, management is predominately stabilization and resuscitation while transferring for definitive care. Diagnostic peritoneal lavage, focused abdominal sonography for trauma (FAST), and computed tomography (CT) play roles in the management of a stable patient once in the emergency department; however, emergent exploratory laparotomy may be required, especially if the patient becomes unstable.[16,17]

Penetrating trauma to the neck can result in damage to a number of structures including the vasculature, esophagus, or trachea. Specialty services are necessary to further evaluate these injuries because surgical intervention might be required.[18] Penetrating head wounds produce brain injury and hemorrhage and require CT scans and neurosurgical evaluations. Complications include infection, seizure disorders, and various neurologic dysfunctions.[19]

The potential for blunt trauma also exists. Blows to the head can result in an array of injuries, including epidural and subdural hematomas and intraparenchymal hemorrhages, which are diagnosed by CT and should prompt neurosurgical consultation.[19] Blows to the chest can result in rib fractures, or possibly pneumothorax or hemothorax, which are treated using needle decompression and tube thoracotomy when necessary.[15] Blunt trauma to the abdomen can cause solid organ injury and internal hemorrhaging. Physical examination can reveal abdominal tenderness, peritoneal signs, and abdominal abrasions or areas of ecchymosis. Evaluation using FAST, CT, or diagnostic peritoneal lavage is indicated, and positive findings may warrant monitoring or surgical intervention.[20] The management of extremity trauma includes control of hemorrhage and stabilization of possible fractures until the patient reaches definitive care.

Exposure to chemical incapacitants such as 1-chloroacetophenone (Mace) and oleoresin capsicum (i.e., pepper spray) can also occur. These agents are irritants that affect the eyes, respiratory tract, and skin.

Rescuers and health care providers should wear appropriate protective equipment to avoid exposure to the irritant, which may be more persistent in enclosed spaces. The victim should be removed immediately from the area of release, and his or her skin should be washed with soap and water. Respiratory symptoms can require treatment with inhaled beta2-agonists such as albuterol.[21] Eye symptoms should be treated with irrigation once contact lenses, if present, are removed. After improvement of symptoms, the eyes should be examined using a slit lamp to detect corneal abrasions, and a topical antibiotic should be prescribed if abrasions are present.[22]

Another consideration during hijackings is altitude illness. The standard flight level for commercial airliners is about 12 km with air pressure of roughly 200 hPa.[23] Flight level is higher on longer flights.[24] In a hijacking, terrorists can damage the aircraft, leading to loss of structural integrity and depressurization. This can lead to hypoxia with loss of consciousness or minimal side effects, depending on whether loss of pressurization was gradual or sudden. The effects will also vary depending on the patient's age and underlying cardiopulmonary status.[25–27] While hypoxia is the most common effect of sudden depressurization, other decompression barotraumas include musculoskeletal involvement, chokes, skin manifestations, paresthesias, and frank neurologic features.[28,29] In extreme cases, a hyperbaric oxygen chamber can be used for treatment, as in dive injuries.[29]

A number of victims will likely have underlying medical conditions that may require treatment. A major area of concern among all victims is that of psychological trauma. This may take the form of acute stress reactions, and some may develop posttraumatic stress disorder. One possible method of intervening to prevent this disorder or decrease its symptoms is a debriefing of the event soon after its occurrence. After the December 1994 hijacking of an Air France plane, passengers underwent a debriefing of the incident by a team of psychiatrists. During the hijacking, two passengers were killed by hijackers in front of passengers in the first 5 hours, and a third was executed the next day. Thirty-five passengers were released before the aircraft departed for Marseilles. The other 188 were released after a total of 54 hours following a military assault of the aircraft. It was found that the group of passengers who were initially released suffered from more psychological reactions, perhaps as a result of concern over being executed immediately after being freed.[30] Unfortunately, this study did not follow up with patients to determine whether this single debriefing prevented worsening or occurrence of psychological symptoms. Although many support the use of an immediate debriefing technique (e.g., critical incident stress debriefing), some reviews have not found this form of single-session therapy to be beneficial.[31] A better technique may be to use the debriefing as a bridge to further outpatient therapy if it is determined that the patient would benefit from ongoing care.

UNIQUE CONSIDERATIONS

Elements of an aircraft hijacking that are unique include the following:

- The possibility of suicide hijackings even though historical examples involve hostage-taking and negotiating demands.
- An airplane represents a relatively small, closed space, and when in flight, hostages are prevented from attempting to escape.
- The flight deck must remain locked down at all times, irrespective of events occurring in the passenger compartment.
- Pilots on the flight deck may be carrying guns to prevent hijackers from taking over the aircraft.
- Air marshals may be present to assist in overcoming a would-be hijacker.

- Because of the confined space, an increased number of injuries may be expected if special teams gain entry to eliminate the threat posed by the hijackers.
- Exposure to chemical incapacitants in this closed space may result in a large number of occupants becoming symptomatic after exposure.
- Many passengers will experience some form of psychological reaction after the event.
- Passengers may experience acute exacerbations of underlying medical conditions.

⚠ PITFALLS

Several potential pitfalls exist in response to an aircraft hijacking. These include the following:

- Not having appropriate and rigid screening practices in place to detect potential weapons that may be placed on the aircraft
- Assuming that hijackers only wish to divert the flight and land at another locale
- Allowing hijackers to overtake the flight deck by opening the flight deck door
- Improper training of the flight crew regarding the Crew Training Common Strategy on how to deal with an attempted hijacking
- Not incorporating medical assets into special response teams that may gain entry into the aircraft in an attempt to rescue hostages
- Medical personnel not wearing appropriate protective equipment, especially when exposure to chemical incapacitants is likely

REFERENCES

1. Wikipedia. Aircraft hijacking. Available at: http://en.wikipedia.org/wiki/Aircraft_hijacking.
2. Worldhistory.com. Aircraft hijacking. Available at: http://www.worldhistory.com/wiki/a/aircraft-hijacking.htm.
3. Federal Aviation Administration. *FAA historical chronology: civil aviation and the federal government, 1926-1996.* 1998, Available at: http://www.faa.gov/docs/b-chron.doc.
4. Rumerman J. Aviation security. U.S. Centennial of Flight Commission. Available at: http://www.centennialofflight.gov/essay/Government_Role/security/POL18.htm.
5. National Commission of Terrorist Attacks upon the United States. Staff statement no. 4: the four flights. Initially presented January 26-27, 2004, in Washington, DC, at the Seventh Public Hearing of the Commission. Available at: http://news.findlaw.com/hdocs/doc/terrorism/911comm–SS4.pdf.
6. Loy J. *Statement of Admiral James M. Loy Administrator, Transportation Security Administration before the Committee on Commerce, Science, and Transportation. United States Senate;* September 9, 2003. Available at: http://www.tsa.dot.gov/public/display?theme=47&content=0900051980069a68.
7. Homeland Security Act of 2002. Title XIV—Arming Pilots against Terrorism. Available at: http://thomas.loc.gov/cgi-bin/query/z?c107:h.r.5005.enr.
8. Aviation and Transportation Security Act. *Public Law 107-71;* November 19, 2001. Available at: http://frwebgate.access.gpo.gov/cgi-bin/getdoc.cgi?dbname=107_cong_public_laws&docid=f:publ071.107.pdf.
9. Transportation Security Administration. *Report to Congress on transportation security;* March 31, 2003. Available at: http://www.tsa.gov/interweb/assetlibrary/Report_to_Congress_on_Transportation_Security_Final_March_31_2003.pdf.
10. Heck J, Pierluisi G. Law enforcement special operations medical support. *Prehosp Emerg Care.* 2002;5:403–406.
11. Heiskell L, Carmona R. Tactical emergency medical services: an emerging subspecialty of emergency medicine. *Ann Emerg Med.* 1994;23:778–785.

12. Federal Aviation Administration. FAA federal air marshal program. September 2001. Available at: http://www.faa.gov/Newsroom/factsheets/2001/factsheets_0109.htm.

13. Shahani R, Galla JD. *Penetrating chest trauma.* Updated, June 11, 2004. Available at: http://www.emedicine.com/med/topic2916.htm.

14. Schouchoff B. Penetrating chest trauma. *Top Emerg Med.* 2001;23:12–19.

15. Schouchoff B, Rodriguez A. Blunt chest trauma. *Top Emerg Med.* 2001;23:1–11.

16. Kaplan L, Alson R, Talavera F, et al. *Abdominal trauma, penetrating.* Updated, May 16, 2003. Available at: http://www.emedicine.com/emerg/topic2.htm.

17. Kirkpatrick A, Sirois M, Ball C, et al. The hand-held ultrasound examination for penetrating abdominal trauma. *Am J Surg.* 2004;187:660–665.

18. Thompson E, Porter J, Fernandez L. Penetrating neck trauma: an overview of management. *J Oral Maxillofac Surg.* 2002;60:918–923.

19. Shepard S, Dulebohn SC, Talavera F, et al. *Head trauma.* Updated, July 26, 2004. Available at: http://www.emedicine.com/med/topic2820.htm.

20. Salomone JA, Salomone JP. *Abdominal trauma, blunt.* Updated, May 16, 2003. Available at: http://www.emedicine.com/emerg/topic1.htm.

21. Smith J, Greaves I. The use of chemical incapacitant sprays: a review. *J Trauma.* 2002;52:595–600.

22. Rega PP, Mowatt-Larssen E, Sole DP. *CBRNE-irritants: Cs, Cn, Cnc, Ca, Cr, Cnb PS.* Updated, June 29, 2004. Available at: http://www.emedicine.com/emerg/topic914.htm.

23. Muehlemann T, et al. The effect of sudden depressurization on pilots at cruising altitude. *Adv Exp Med Biol.* 2013;765:177–183.

24. Hampson NB, et al. Altitude exposures during commercial flight: a reappraisal. *Aviat Space Environ Med.* 2013;84(1):27–31.

25. Aerospace Medical Association; Aviation Safety Committee; Civil Aviation Subcommittee. Cabin cruising altitudes for regular transport aircraft. *Aviat Space Environ Med.* 2008;79(4):433–439.

26. Cottrell JJ. Altitude exposures during aircraft flight. Flying higher. *Chest.* 1988;93(1):81–84.

27. Roubinian N, et al. Effects of commercial air travel on patients with pulmonary hypertension air travel and pulmonary hypertension. *Chest.* 2012;142(4):885–892.

28. Johnston MJ. Loss of cabin pressure in a military transport: a mass casualty with decompression illnesses. *Aviat Space Environ Med.* 2008;79(4):429–432.

29. Ryles MT, Pilmanis AA. The initial signs and symptoms of altitude decompression sickness. *Aviat Space Environ Med.* 1996;67(10):983–989.

30. Cremniter D, Crocq L, Louville P, et al. Posttraumatic reactions of hostages after an aircraft hijacking. *J Nerv Ment Dis.* 1997;185:344–346.

31. Rose S, Bisson J, Wessely S. Psychological debriefing for preventing post traumatic stress disorder (PTSD) [systematic review]. Cochrane Depression, Anxiety and Neurosis Group. *Cochrane Database Syst Rev.* 2004; Volume 3. Available at: http://www.cochrane.org/cochrane/revabstr/AB000560.htm.

CHAPTER 193

Aircraft Crash into a High-Rise Building

Ilaria Morelli and Michelangelo Bortolin

DESCRIPTION OF EVENT

According to the National Fire Protection Association (NFPA), a high-rise is a "building where the floor of an occupied story is greater than 75 feet (23 m) above the lowest level of fire department vehicle access."[1] Alternatively, according to Emporis, a global provider of building information, a high-rise building is a "multi-story structure between 35 and 100 meters tall, or a building of unknown height with a minimum of 12 floors," whereas a skyscraper is a "multi-story building whose architectural height is at least 100 meters."[2]

In the last decades the development of metropolises and megacities has contributed to designing increasingly taller high-rise building areas with many skyscrapers that are increasingly close to air traffic and airports. For example, Hong Kong with its 1251 skyscrapers has the most high-rise buildings as well as some of the busiest air traffic of any city worldwide.

From a historical perspective the World Trade Center (WTC) towers are not the first skyscrapers in New York City involved in an aircraft crash: in 1945 and 1946, respectively, the Empire State Building and 40 Wall Street (now the Trump Building) were damaged during accidental crashes, resulting in a small number of victims.[3,4] Several tower blocks have been involved in aircraft crashes during the twentieth and twenty-first centuries (Table 193-1). Some of these were accidental crashes due to human error, fuel exhaustion, or breakdowns, as in the 2002 Pirelli Tower plane crash in Milan.[5]

On the other hand, after the September 11 attacks, hijacked planes were used as destructive weapons.[6] The reports on patterns of injury following these attacks provide basic information on how to plan a response to this kind of human-made disaster. These mass casualty incidents (MCI) are typically characterized by the sequence of crash, explosion, fire, and possible collapse.[7] This succession leads to specific types of traumatic injuries that responders have to treat in the early phase: deep wounds and lacerations, closed head injuries, contusions, sprains, strains, fractures, ocular irritations, and injuries caused by the blast, burns, inhalation, and crushing.[8]

However, death and injury tolls are variable both in accidental crashes and suicide attacks. In some cases, such as the 2002 Tampa tower suicide attack or the 2006 Belaire building accident[9] in New York City, crashes resulted in very few victims. In other cases, such as the 1992 Bijlmermeer accident,[10] even an unintentional crash resulted in an MCI. The number of victims and injured people depends on four variables:

1. Aircraft
2. Location (building and surrounding area)
3. Rescuers
4. Time

In the case involving aircraft, it is evident that the larger the plane is, the heavier the losses resulting from the incident will be

- A larger plane has a greater number of passengers and crew: people on board are unlikely to escape death (as shown in Table 193-1).
- It causes a more serious impact on the building, involving more floors and thus more people.
- It is usually designed to cover greater distances, so it has more powerful engines, which may result in high-speed impacts, and more capacious fuel tanks, resulting in wider explosions and fires.

With respect to location, the building type affects the disaster severity

- The larger the building is, the greater the number of injured people will be.
- The higher a tower is, the more likely it is to collapse (increasing death toll), particularly if the plane crashes into its lower floors. In fact, depending on building design and materials, the lower the crash point is, the greater the weight borne by the underlying floors is if the floors above collapse.[7]
- The sooner the high-rise collapses, the less time rescuers will have to complete the evacuation.[7]

The WTC towers were characterized by a redundant structure: each floor was able to hold up 1,300 t beyond its own weight, so they were able to support the plane crash at first, even if some of the external steel columns were destroyed by the impact. Crashes were followed by fuel-rich diffuse flame fire, unable "to burn at a temperature high enough to melt the steel. However, its quick ignition and intense heat caused the steel to lose at least half of its strength and to deform, causing buckling or crippling. This weakening and deformation caused a few floors to fall, while the weight of the stories above caused the crushing of the floors below, initiating a domino collapse."[7]

- Another important factor to be considered is the efficiency of the evacuation plan, which depends on the relationship of building stairways and emergency exits to the number of people to be evacuated. This directly impacts the time rescuers have, which may affect the number of victims.
- The building density of the surrounding area may also contribute to morbidity and mortality. If the area is highly populated, there could be victims outside the building from falling debris. Explosions and collapses also result in the emission of airborne particulate matter, such as dust, debris, fumes, and smoke, causing ocular and respiratory tract irritations. The diffusion of asbestos and other carcinogenic or otherwise dangerous matter into the air may

TABLE 193-1   Examples of Aircraft Crashes into High-Rise Buildings in the Past Decades.

DATE	LOCAL TIME	PLACE AND BUILDING	TOTAL FLOORS	CRASH FLOORS	COLLAPSE	AIRCRAFT TYPE	PEOPLE ON BOARD	FATALITIES TOTAL	FATALITIES ON BOARD	INJURED PEOPLE	ACCIDENT/ATTACK	CAUSE
Sun., Oct. 4, 1992	6:36 pm	Bijlmermeer, Groeneveen and Klein-Kruitberg flat complexes	11	Apex	Partial	Boeing 747-258 F	4	43	4	26	UFIT	Engine detachment
Thu., Sept. 11, 2001	8:46 am	NYC, WTC North Tower	110	93-99th	Yes	Boeing 767-223ER	92	2819	92	>6000	Suicide hijacking	Al Qaeda terrorist attacks
Thu., Sept. 11, 2001	9:03 am	NYC, WTC South Tower	110	77-85th	Yes	Boeing 767-222	65	(10 hijackers)	65		Suicide hijacking	Al Qaeda terrorist attacks
Sat., Jan. 5, 2002	5:15 pm	Tampa, Bank of America Tower	42	23-24th	No	Cessna 172	1	1	1	0	Suicide attack	Possible Al Qaeda attacks emulation
Thu., Apr. 18, 2002	5:48 pm	Milan, Pirelli Tower	30	26th	No	Rockwell Commander A112	1	3	1	60	CFIT	Pilot inability to manage technical problems
Wed., Oct. 11, 2006	2:42 pm	NYC, The Belaire apartments	42	40th	No	Cirrus SR20	2	2	2	3	CFIT	Pilot inability to perform a 180° turn inside a limited space

CFIT, Controlled flight into terrain; NYC, New York City; UFIT, uncontrolled flight into terrain; WTC, World Trade Center.

increase the number of injured people and victims, even years after the disaster.[11] Pursuant to the WTC attacks, eye and respiratory tract irritations were the most frequent admission complaints to NYC emergency departments.[8] Respiratory symptoms and ocular irritations were reported by lower Manhattan residents and workers even months after the attacks.[12,13] The Environmental Protection Agency reported the presence of asbestos, particulate matter, and volatile organic compounds at the WTC site.[13]

- The quality and organization of the emergency response also influence the resilience capacity to this type of disaster. In a metropolitan area, there will be more hospitals and perhaps more organized rescue programs, which lead to a more efficient surge capacity.

- If emergency medical service (EMS) workers are not well trained to protect themselves first[14] or if personal protective equipment (PPE) is not available early on,[15] a great number of rescuers risk turning into victims either during the immediate response or some time after the event.

After the 9/11 attacks, 343 Fire Department of New York City (FDNY) rescue workers died and 240 (158 firefighters and 82 EMS workers) requested emergency medical treatment during the first 24 hours.[16] Most of them did not have such severe injuries to require hospital admission (ocular and respiratory tract irritation, dehydration, exhaustion). Twenty-eight rescue workers required hospitalization for traumatic injuries (a cervical spine fracture requiring surgical stabilization, other fractures, meniscus tears, back traumas, facial burns) or life-threatening inhalation injuries.[16] Reports highlight that many rescuers did not wear adequate PPE.[15]

Furthermore, many articles describe the development of chronic illness following a disaster. For example, acute and prolonged exposures were associated with asthma development and persistence of chronic cough years after the 9/11 attack.

- It is important to stress a phenomenon well characterized by the 9/11-related medical literature called *convergent volunteerism*. This expression defines "the arrival of unexpected or uninvited personnel wishing to render aid at the scene of a large-scale emergency incident."[17] Among these volunteers are physicians, called *freelancers* because they operate "at an incident without knowledge or direction from the on-scene command authority." Even if well intentioned, these people are often untrained and unequipped to provide medical care under austere conditions, and they may interfere with scene operations and jeopardize their own lives, exposing themselves to physical hazards in disaster areas, such as fires and unstable structures. Volunteers are not part of the local accountability system, and therefore incident commanders are unable to track, communicate with, and help them when in danger.[17]

Time of day and building occupancy levels may also influence disaster severity:

- Offices are more populated during the daytime working hours. A night attack on the WTC would not have resulted in such a high number of victims.

- Residential towers follow the opposite rule: a night crash could cause heavier losses, because most of the occupants are at home in the evening.

- Time influences the number of out-of-building victims too: at night, there would probably be fewer people walking or working in the surrounding area, so fewer people would be exposed to the hazards.

PRE-INCIDENT ACTIONS

The analysis of past events is useful to prevent future incidents and limit the damages in case of terrorism. Routine maintenance of planes has to be performed in order to avoid in-flight breakdowns. Pilots' licenses should be reviewed often and revoked if necessary, especially if pilots are shown to be too careless,[5] insufficiently experienced to fly,[9] or alcohol or drug impaired. Pilots must also undergo ongoing physical evaluation. Considering that an aircraft may turn into a weapon in the wrong hands, candidates should undergo a compulsory psychiatric assessment before getting a license and when it is renewed.[18] Pilot-recognition systems are needed on private planes to prevent theft for terrorist activities (as with the Cessna theft before the 2002 Tampa tower attack).[18]

In case of suspected hijacking, the Air Force should escort the plane and consider shooting it down, especially if it is flying toward a built-up area.[19] The WTC lesson teaches us that building structural redundancy is not the only factor to consider. Future skyscrapers should be designed in consideration of mitigating against the possibility of collapse due to a fuel-rich diffuse fire caused by a plane crash, in order to allow for a complete evacuation.[7] Engineers should focus on designing better evacuation systems,[7] which should take the maximum number of people occupying the building into consideration. The estimation should include not only "the population of employees in offices, shops, and restaurants," but also "rush-hour figures and the additional burden of holidays," and "if a train or bus station is present in the building, the number of passengers and workers in the vicinity during normal and peak hours."[20]

MCI protocols have to be ready for use and effectively applied when an event happens. For different disaster types, each tower block should have an individualized protocol outlining patient distribution to the nearest hospitals and involving more medical centers located further away as the injury toll increases.[21] Medical freelancing should be prevented, instead enlisting volunteer physicians in disaster response programs, such as the Medical Reserve Corps. There they should be trained to provide medical care during an MCI in coordination with the overall response and following the incident commander's instructions.[17] Thus if more physicians are needed at a possible disaster scene, officers could call trained volunteers from this registry.[17] As a consequence the depletion of either first-wave or second-wave emergency department capabilities could be prevented,[17] which is a top priority, considering the possibility of a prolonged disaster response.

Explosions, fires, and falling structures boost the number of critical and burned patients needing admission to intensive care units (ICUs) and burn units.[20] Unfortunately, both such wards usually have few (and often already occupied) hospitalization beds. Thus an assessment of surge capacity, health care worker qualifications, the number of functional beds routinely available, and their normal occupancy, should be carried out in advance.[20] This information should be made available to national emergency authorities promptly upon need. Personnel needs and allocation in hospitals should be planned in advance as well. The possible institution of an emergency burn care corps, including plastic surgeons, anesthesiologists, and nurses from the private sector and perhaps other countries, should be taken into consideration.[20] Disaster response leaders should be nominated in advance, and each one should have an established role.

POST-INCIDENT ACTIONS

The development of an organized disaster response is fundamental. The incident command post should be placed near the scene, but buildings at risk for collateral damage or further terrorist attacks (as with the other WTC buildings after the 9/11 attacks) should be avoided. Chiefs and officers have to coordinate medical field teams, police officers, security teams, and firefighter brigades.[20] An area should be secured and cordoned off around the incident site by police officers to prevent walking casualties from going away and to prevent access by unauthorized people and convergent volunteers.[17] In the event of terrorist attacks, even unharmed bystanders should be detained until a radiological or chemical attack is excluded in order to avoid spreading hazards.

Ingress-egress routes for ambulances have to be located promptly. Airspace restrictions should be established, and military air assets should monitor air traffic. The safety of the scene has to be ensured before rescuer access. Unified Command must consult with engineers first and prevent firefighters and rescuers from entering the building if a collapse is possible. Firefighters should carry out building evacuation rapidly when possible, provided that rescuer safety comes first.[14] For this reason, PPE should be developed to offer protection from debris and biological and respiratory hazards.[15] Rescuers should be provided with appropriate PPE and trained to use it correctly before assignments.[15] The establishment of several supply staging areas near the incident site might be very useful to store a large amount of different levels of PPE and send them immediately to incident sites when needed. An Advanced Medical Post (AMP) should be set in the nearest safe location. Triage should be performed rapidly and accurately as patients are carried to the medical post.[22] A rapid assessment of dead victims, as well as the number, type, and severity of injuries of casualties should be carried out and communicated to the Unified Command as soon as possible in order to alert the nearest hospitals and organize the transfer of injured people.[20,8]

In the event of an MCI, triage should be performed in an effective and well-organized way. Critical (red) individuals must be transported first and allocated to the nearest hospitals[21] using authorized helicopters. Urgent but not critical (yellow) patients may be transferred via ambulance to hospitals farther away, but EMS vehicles should be equipped to address possible changes in patients' conditions. The walking wounded (green) should be registered and monitored in case their status worsens. Green patients should be transferred to hospitals as well. After initial care and stabilization, victims might undergo a secondary transfer to referral hospitals, depending on their injury type.[21]

The Unified Command has to divide rescuers into layered response waves to prevent rescuer depletion if prolonged disaster operations are required. Considering the hazards mentioned, hospitals should stockpile adequate supplies of drugs and instruments needed from manufacturers and other sources, including tetanus vaccine.[11] A surveillance committee should be established as soon as possible in order to assess the degree of air and water pollution consequent to explosion, fires, and collapse.[11] In case of a terrorist attack this presence of toxic substances, such as radioactive isotopes, should be considered.[23]

➕ MEDICAL TREATMENT OF CASUALTIES

Appropriate resuscitation measures, including airway maintenance, spinal immobilization, and peripheral venous access, should be provided as soon as possible to all patients with possible life-threatening injuries once the scene is safe to do so. Further care is provided during transport and at the receiving hospital as needed.

Blunt Trauma

Most injuries encountered will be from blunt trauma and worked-up as any other trauma patient. Unconscious patients with stable vital signs and signs of head, chest, or abdomen trauma should undergo the appropriate radiological examination (FAST scans, as well as head, chest, and abdomen CT scans as required) in order to exclude life-threatening injuries.[24] Priority should be given to patients with active bleeding symptoms or with altered or worsening neurologic signs. Therefore traumatic head injuries, intracranial bleeding requiring emergent evacuation, open or depressed skull fractures with more than 1 cm of inward displacement, and cervical spine fractures with spinal cord injuries must be immediately attended to with neurosurgery consultation.[25,26] Less urgent neurosurgical referral may be needed for delayed decompressive craniectomy in the event of refractory intracranial pressure elevation.[25] Patients with suspected cervical spine fractures should always be transported from the scene on a backboard wearing a semi-rigid cervical collar until the time of their surgical fixation, if needed.[26]

Tension pneumothorax should be clinically diagnosed and immediately treated with needle thoracostomy at the AMP.[27] Blunt chest traumas have to be managed conservatively with analgesics, oxygen therapy, and possibly tube thoracostomy.[27] Pulmonary contusion toilet and flail chest plate fixation as well as ventilation supports may be necessary in case of respiratory distress.[27] However, immediate surgery is recommended in the event of massive hemothorax, massive air leak following chest tube insertion, and major bronchial, tracheal, esophageal, pericardial, cardiac, or thoracic vessel injuries.[27] Short-acting beta-blockers are useful for temporizing medical treatment of aortic injuries.[27]

For blunt or penetrating abdominal trauma, surgery is recommended for peritoneal signs, uncontrolled hemorrhage or shock, hemoperitoneum, or clinical deterioration: patients' general condition should guide in choosing "damage control" surgery rather than an "observation" strategy.[28,29] For unstable pelvic fractures, external compression with a sheet at the incident scene and external fixation are recommended.[30] Urethral injuries have to be ruled out before inserting a catheter.[30] If bleeding continues after fracture fixation, intraaortic/intrailiac balloon occlusion, transcatheter embolization, and/or pelvic packing is required for massive bleeding control.[30] Antibiotics should be administered if bowel, vagina, or urinary tract injuries are associated.[30]

Fractured limbs should be splinted and followed by orthopedic referral.

Asthma Exacerbation

Asthma exacerbation should be treated in a typical fashion with oxygen or helium-oxygen therapy, inhaled short-acting beta-agonists (and muscarinic antagonists, such as ipratropium, when the acute episode is severe), and systemic corticosteroids, such as prednisone. Endotracheal intubation and ICU hospitalization may be needed.[31]

Inhalation Injuries

A 24- to 48-hour observation of patients exposed to toxic smoke, even if asymptomatic, is mandatory because of a possible delayed clinical presentation. Oxygen supply in case of hypoxia, cardiac monitoring, and specific antidotes depending on the type of toxic smoke should be provided.[32] Hyperbaric oxygen therapy may be necessary in case of carbon monoxide (CO) poisoning.[33] Pentoxifylline and heparin systemically or via aerosol are sometimes useful in case of pulmonary irritation,[34] as well as brief use of corticosteroids for severe lower airway obstruction provoked by some toxic smokes (oxides of nitrogen, zinc oxide, red phosphorus, sulfur trioxide, titanium tetrachloride, and polytetrafluoroethylene). Patients have to be monitored for development of bacterial pneumonia. Bronchodilators are indicated for inhalation-caused bronchospasm and respiratory arrest (especially in patients already suffering from asthma or chronic obstructive pulmonary disease [COPD]).[32]

Thermal Burns

Intravenous fluids and humidified oxygen via a nonrebreathing reservoir mask are a useful starting point, but early intubation is mandatory if signs of upper airway injury are present. Burn treatment includes moistening with cool sterile saline, open blister debridement, wrapping of single fingers and toes, cleaning of other parts with mild soap and gentle scrubbing, and partial thickness wound covering with antibiotic ointment.[35] Escharotomy is needed in case of full-thickness neck burns, chest burns limiting respiratory excursion, and circumferential full-thickness burns involving extremities and the chest.[36]

Ocular Injuries

Ocular irritations are treated only with topical nonsteroidal antiinflammatory drugs (NSAIDs) and irrigation with sterile saline solution.[37] Ocular burn therapy includes irrigation, analgesics, topical antibiotics, cycloplegic mydriatics, tetanus immunization, surgical debridement of necrotic tissue, amniotic membrane patching, and conjunctival reconstruction for patients with ocular burns.[38] Antibiotics, topical steroids, and surgical removal are needed to treat intraocular foreign bodies. In the case of corneal laceration, eye covering, antiemetics, analgesics (to reduce intraocular pressure), and antibiotics are useful.[39] Surgical repair is necessary for globe ruptures.[40]

❓ UNIQUE CONSIDERATIONS

Long-lasting physical and psychological issues are frequent among civilians and rescuers who witness a disaster scenario. Psychological problems include posttraumatic stress disorder (PTSD),[12,41] temporarily increased alcohol consumption,[13,42] depression and panic disorder,[43] psychosomatic symptoms, and unspecific psychological distress.[41] Psychiatric assessment and psychological counseling should be provided to these patients not only in the first weeks after but years after the MCI.[44] People exposed to the 9/11 attacks report an increased risk of chronic respiratory conditions,[45] chronic heart disease,[45] and hospitalization for heart and cerebrovascular diseases, especially in patients suffering from PTSD.[46] Other commonly seen conditions include gastroesophageal reflux disease, obstructive sleep apnea, and musculoskeletal complaints.[43]

The September 11, 2001, attacks taught us that many terrorist attacks may come in succession, leading to a chaotic response. This was also seen in the Boston Marathon Bombing. Disaster responders to terrorist events should be ready to manage a rapid increase of victims with varying injuries.

⚠ PITFALLS

Different disasters have several pitfalls in common. Nevertheless, the characteristic issues with an aircraft crash into a high rise include the following:

- Incident command (IC) or AMP location associated with unsafe structures, such as adjacent buildings that may undergo collateral damage or that are possible terrorist targets
- Rescuer access to the building before the possibility of a collapse has been excluded with certainty
- Delay in building evacuation, when possible
- Inadequate supply of PPE or inadequate training in how to use them
- Lack of correct, redundant, and frequent communication between field rescuers (physicians, firefighters, police officers) and the Unified Command, as well as among the Unified Command, national authorities, and hospitals[44,47]

- Over- and under-triage: increased critical mortality rate has been directly related to over- and under-triage in several disasters.[48] Furthermore, under-triage may delay the recognition and care of red and yellow codes with good survival chances if treated[22]
- Failure to prevent people from reaching the scene until all hazards have been removed[13]

REFERENCES

1. U.S. National Fire Protection Association. *Guidelines to Developing Emergency Action Plans for All-Hazard Emergencies in High-Rise Office Buildings;* 2013. Retrieved from: http://www.nfpa.org/~/media/files/safety-information/for-consumers/occupancies/highrise/emergencyactionplanhighrise.pdf?la=en. Accessed April 13, 2015.
2. Emporis. *High-Rise Building (ESN 18727);* 2014. Retrieved from: http://www.emporis.com/building/standard/3/high-rise-building. Accessed April 13, 2015.
3. The Minerals, Metals & Materials Society. Empire state building withstood airplane impact. *JOM.* 2001;53(12):4–7.
4. 40 Wall Street—The Trump Building. Wired New York. Retrieved from: http://wirednewyork.com/skyscrapers/40wall/. Accessed April 13, 2015.
5. Agenzia Nazionale per la Sicurezza del Volo. *Relazione D'inchiesta (deliberata dal Collegio nella riunione del 12 dicembre 2002) Incidente occorso all'aeromobile Rockwell Commander 112TC, MARCHE HB-NCXLocalità Milano—Palazzo della Regione ("Grattacielo Pirelli") 18 aprile 2002;* 2002. Retrieved from: http://www.ansv.it/cgi-bin/ita/Rel.%20A_18_02HB-NCX.pdf. Accessed April 13, 2015.
6. Centers for Disease Control and Prevention. Deaths in World Trade Center terrorist attacks—New York City, 2001. *MMWR Morb Mortal Wkly Rep.* 2002;(51 SpecNo):16–18.
7. Eagar TW, Musso C. Why did the World Trade Center collapse? Science, engineering, and speculation. *JOM.* 2001;53(12):8–11.
8. Centers for Disease Control and Prevention. Rapid Assessment of Injuries Among Survivors of the Terrorist Attack on the World Trade Center—New York City, September 2001. *MMWR Morb Mortal Wkly Rep.* 2002;51 (1):1–5.
9. National Transportation Safety Board. *Aircraft Accident Brief;* 2007. Retrieved from: http://libraryonline.erau.edu/online-full-text/ntsb/aircraft-accident-briefs/AAB07-02.pdf. Accessed April 13, 2015.
10. Nederlands Aviation Safety Board. *Aircraft Accident Report 92-1 1 El Al Flight 1862 Boeing 747-258f 4x-Axg Bijlmermeer, Amsterdam, October 4, 1992.* Retrieved from: http://web.archive.org/web/20090205093738/http://verkeerenwaterstaat.nl/kennisplein/uploaded/MIN/2005-07/39448/ElAl_flight_1862.pdf. Accessed April 13, 2015.
11. Centers for Disease Control and Prevention. New York City Department of Health response to terrorist attack, September 11, 2001. *MMWR Morb Mortal Wkly Rep.* 2001;50:821–822.
12. Centers for Disease Control and Prevention. Impact of September 11 attacks on workers in the vicinity of the World Trade Center—New York City. *MMWR Morb Mortal Wkly Rep.* 2002;(51 Spec No):8–10.
13. Centers for Disease Control and Prevention. Community needs assessment of lower Manhattan residents following the World Trade Center attacks—Manhattan, New York City, 2001. *MMWR Morb Mortal Wkly Rep.* 2002;(51 Spec No):10–13.
14. Garrison HG. Keeping rescuers safe. *Ann Emerg Med.* 2002;40:633–635.
15. Centers for Disease Control and Prevention. Use of respiratory protection among responders at the World Trade Center site—New York City, September 2001. *MMWR Morb Mortal Wkly Rep.* 2002;(51 Spec No):6–8.
16. Centers for Disease Control and Prevention. Injuries and illnesses among New York City Fire Department rescue workers after responding to the World Trade Center attacks. *MMWR Morb Mortal Wkly Rep.* 2002;(51 Spec No):1–5.
17. Cone DC, Weir SD, Bogucki S. Convergent volunteerism. *Ann Emerg Med.* 2003;41:457–462.
18. Benny DJ. Flight school security. *FA Aviat News.* 2002;41:13–14.
19. The 9/11 commission report. Retrieved from: http://www.9-11commission.gov/report/911Report.pdf. Accessed April 13, 2015.

20. Weissman O, Israeli H, Rosengard H, et al. Examining disaster planning models for large scale burn incidents—a theoretical plane crash into a high rise building. *Burns*. 2013;39:1571–1576.

21. Postma IL, Weel H, Heetveld MJ, et al. Patient distribution in a mass casualty event of an airplane crash. *Injury*. 2013;44:1574–1578.

22. Frykberg ER. Principles of mass casualty management following terrorist disasters. *Ann Surg*. 2004;239:319–321.

23. Centers for Disease Control and Prevention. Syndromic surveillance for bioterrorism following the attacks on the World Trade Center—New York City, 2001. *MMWR Morb Mortal Wkly Rep*. 2002;51:13–15.

24. Jang T. *Focused Assessment with Sonography in Trauma (FAST)*; 2011. Retrieved from: http://emedicine.medscape.com/article/104363-overview. Accessed April 13, 2015.

25. Crippen DW. *Head Trauma. Treatment and Management*; 2012. Retrieved from: http://emedicine.medscape.com/article/433855-treatment. Accessed December 29, 2014.

26. Davenport M. *Cervical Spine Fracture. Treatment and Management*; 2013. http://emedicine.medscape.com/article/824380-treatment. Accessed April 13, 2015.

27. Mancini MC. *Blunt Chest Trauma*; 2014. http://emedicine.medscape.com/article/428723-overview#a11. Accessed April 13, 2015.

28. Legome EL. *Blunt Abdominal Trauma. Treatment and Management*; 2014. Retrieved from: http://emedicine.medscape.com/article/1980980-treatment. Accessed April 13, 2015.

29. Stanton-Maxey KJ. *Surgical Therapy for Penetrating Abdominal Trauma*; 2014. Retrieved from: http://emedicine.medscape.com/article/2035661-overview. Accessed April 13, 2015.

30. Crawford Mechem C. *Pelvic Fracture in Emergency Medicine. Treatment and Management. Prehospital Care*; 2013. http://emedicine.medscape.com/article/825869-treatment. Accessed April 13, 2015.

31. Morris MJ. *Asthma. Treatment and Management. Acute Exacerbation*; 2014. Retrieved from: http://emedicine.medscape.com/article/296301-treatment#aw2aab6b6b7. Accessed April 13, 2015.

32. Lafferty KA. *Smoke Inhalation Injury. Treatment and Management. Carbon Monoxide Poisoning*; 2013. Retrieved from: http://emedicine.medscape.com/article/771194-treatment#aw2aab6b6b1aa. Accessed April 13, 2015.

33. Lafferty KA. *Smoke Inhalation Injury. Treatment and Management. Approach Considerations*; 2013. Retrieved from: http://emedicine.medscape.com/article/771194-treatment#aw2aab6b6b5. Accessed April 13, 2015.

34. Lafferty KA. *Smoke Inhalation Injury. Treatment and Management. Pulmonary Irritants*; 2013. Retrieved from: http://emedicine.medscape.com/article/771194-treatment#aw2aab6b6b8. Accessed April 13, 2015.

35. Jenkins JA. *Emergent Management of Thermal Burns. Practice Essentials*; 2014. Retrieved from: http://emedicine.medscape.com/article/769193-overview#aw2aab6b2. Accessed April 13, 2015.

36. Jenkins JA. *Emergent Management of Thermal Burns. Treatment of Special Burn Types*; 2014. http://emedicine.medscape.com/article/769193-overview#aw2aab6b7. Accessed April 13, 2015.

37. Denniston PL, Kennedy CW. *Eye*. Retrieved from: http://www.guideline.gov/content.aspx?id=47578&search=acute+eye+irritation. Accessed April 13, 2015.

38. Solano J. *Ocular Burns. Treatment and Management. Approach Considerations*; 2013. Retrieved from: http://emedicine.medscape.com/article/798696-treatment. Accessed December 29, 2014.

39. Aronson AA. *Corneal Lacerations. Treatment and Management. Emergency Department Care*; 2013. Retrieved from: http://emedicine.medscape.com/article/798005-treatment#a1126. Accessed December 29, 2014.

40. Acerra JR. *Globe Rupture. Treatment and Management. Emergency Department Care*; 2014. Retrieved from: http://emedicine.medscape.com/article/798223-treatment#a1126. Accessed April 13, 2015.

41. Witteveen AB, Bramsen I, Twisk JW, et al. Psychological distress of rescue workers eight and one-half years after professional involvement in the Amsterdam air disaster. *J Nerv Ment Dis*. 2007;195:31–40.

42. North CS, Adinoff B, Pollio DE, et al. Alcohol use disorders and drinking among survivors of the 9/11 attacks on the World Trade Center in New York City. *Compr Psychiatry*. 2013;54(7):962–969.

43. Lucchini RG, Crane MA, Crowley L, et al. The World Trade Center health surveillance program: results of the first 10 years and implications for prevention. *G Ital Med Lav Ergon*. 2012;34:529–533.

44. Dasgupta S, French S, Williams-Johnson J, et al. EMS response to an airliner crash. *Prehosp Disaster Med*. 2012;27:299–302.

45. Brackbill RM, Cone JE, Farfel MR. Chronic physical health consequences of being injured during the terrorist attacks on World Trade Center on September 11, 2001. *Am J Epidemiol*. 2014;179(9):1076–1085.

46. Jordan HT, Stellman SD, Morabia A, et al. Cardiovascular disease hospitalizations in relation to exposure to the September 11, 2001 World Trade Center disaster and posttraumatic stress disorder. *J Am Heart Assoc*. 2013;2(5):e000431.

47. Simon R, Teperman S. The World Trade Center attack. Lessons for disaster management. *Crit Care*. 2001;5:318–320.

48. Postma IL, Weel H, Heetveld MJ, et al. Mass casualty triage after an airplane crash near Amsterdam. *Injury*. 2013;44:1061–1067.

CHAPTER 194

Airliner Crash into a Nuclear Power Plant

Patrick M. Jackson

DESCRIPTION OF EVENT

The terrorist attacks of September 11, 2001, have forever changed the perception of the people of the United States as far as feeling secure. In particular, there has been an increased awareness among the public, governmental agencies, and the health care community that nuclear power plant facilities are a vulnerable target for terrorist organizations using hijacked commercial passenger jets as weapons.[1] Although nuclear power plants have not been designed to protect against airliner crashes, they do have general protective mechanisms designed to prevent nuclear catastrophes. All nuclear power plants in the United States are required to have containment buildings to protect their reactor cores. The power plants are also designed with "fail-safe" systems to stop the nuclear fission reaction and cool down in the event of an incident. However, it is theoretically possible for a commercial airliner crash to penetrate the containment building and damage the reactor core and cooling systems. This cascade of events would result in the release of an atmospheric plume of radioactive substances leading to immediate health effects on the nearby population.[2] The planning required for an emergency response to an airliner crash into a nuclear power plant requires an all-hazards approach, not simply a radiological response.[3]

After the 1979 nuclear accident at Three Mile Island near Harrisburg, Pennsylvania, the U.S. Congress enacted legislation mandating that all nuclear power plants be covered by emergency contingency plans. New attention was given to these contingency plans following the recent increase in terrorist attacks. These contingency plans now account for the possible use of airliners destroying the protective mechanisms of nuclear reactors.[4] The U.S. Nuclear Regulatory Commission (NRC), the federal agency responsible for security at the 100-plus nuclear power plants in the United States, has issued several regulatory orders to meet the increased security threat.[4] Disaster planning and response beyond the nuclear power plant boundaries are the responsibility of the Federal Emergency Management Agency (FEMA).[5]

Nuclear power plants are designed to withstand extreme natural disasters, such as earthquakes, tornadoes, and hurricanes.[6] Deliberate impacts by large, high-speed passenger jets filled with jet fuel were not considered when designing nuclear power plants and their containment buildings. The NRC requires that all new nuclear power plants incorporate design features to ensure that impacts by large commercial aircraft will not result in radioactive releases. However, the NRC does not require that existing reactors should be redesigned or retrofitted with systems able to withstand impacts from airplane crashes.[7] A core meltdown and subsequent contamination leading to mass exposure to escaping radiation by a large number of people can only occur if the structural integrity of the containment building is compromised.[8] Sizable explosions are required to inflict even minor damage to the reinforced concrete walls at nuclear power plants, which is why aerial attacks are viewed as a greater risk than ground attacks.[9] Large-scale damage to the containment walls could occur either as a direct consequence of the impact itself or through a delayed loss of strength of the structural membranes from a sustained and intense conflagration, similar to the reaction that melted the steel beams of the World Trade Center buildings. In addition to damage to the containment walls, the reactor vessel, its control equipment, or the cooling mechanism must be damaged or disrupted in order for a meltdown to occur.[8,10]

The NRC conducted a detailed engineering analysis from 2002 to 2006 of the possible effects of various airliner crash scenarios. Because of the sensitive nature of the information contained in these analyses, the NRC did not release specific details of the security updates that were put into place in the nuclear power plants reviewed. The NRC reports that the majority of plane crashes into containment buildings following the completion of these security updates would not result in significant releases of radiation.[7] However, as was demonstrated by the 2011 events at the Fukushima reactor in Japan, release of radioactive materials will still occur under severe circumstances.[11] In addition, the NRC reports that there would be sufficient time to implement the emergency response strategies in the unlikely event of radiological release due to a terrorist attack.[6]

PRE-INCIDENT ACTIONS

Emergency plans mandated by Congress after the Three Mile Island accident require that each nuclear power plant have an emergency planning zone with a radius of approximately 10 miles. The NRC requires each plant operator to maintain warning systems and evacuation plans to cover these zones. At least every 2 years, the NRC and FEMA evaluate evacuation and emergency shutdown exercises performed by the plants to prepare for a plant malfunction, accident, or terrorist attack. The NRC also requires that each plant operator have plans in place to prevent ingestion of radioactive material after an incident by persons within a 50-mile radius, typically by banning possibly contaminated food and water.[6]

Maintaining public awareness of the potential for a nuclear power plant accident and how people should prepare and react is a critical part of emergency planning. Large numbers of persons who have little to no significant radiation exposure, but remain concerned about the impact to their health, have the potential to inundate emergency departments and hospitals if they are not properly informed of the action plan prior to the incident.[2] In addition, hospitals need to plan to have areas away from the emergency department for the assessment of those who do not require acute medical care, while still assessing for minor injuries and need for potential decontamination and counseling.[10] Persons living in close proximity to power plants must also be able to recognize the sound of a warning siren, know its relevance, and be ready to begin evacuation in a timely and orderly fashion. Residents around nuclear power plants are encouraged to keep emergency supplies available for possible loss of power and to consider stocking iodine pills in their households.

The security of nuclear power plants and their vulnerability to deliberate attacks by airliners remains an important concern over a decade after the 9/11 attacks, and the NRC has spearheaded planning to ensure the safety of the power plants. The NRC has addressed several aspects of updating the emergency plans and incorporating a new comprehensive security plan, including increased patrols, augmented security forces, installation of additional physical barriers, enhanced coordination with law enforcement agencies, and more restrictive access for all personnel. The NRC regularly communicates with the Department of Homeland Security, the Federal Aviation Administration, and the Department of Defense to protect and restrict airspace above nuclear power plants.[6] The NRC is also attempting to maintain a state of constant readiness and response through increased inspections and random force-on-force exercises at the plants.

POST-INCIDENT ACTIONS

Once an incident has occurred, it is crucial that emergency plans are activated immediately. Using appropriate personal protective equipment for radiation exposure, rescue personnel should evacuate victims who are not able to leave the scene of the incident by themselves in an orderly fashion. Victims presenting with blast, burn, or crush injuries should be treated with typical emergency trauma care. The care of mass casualties from blast, burn, and crush injuries has been discussed previously in this book. All victims should be evacuated to a location upwind from the site and evaluated for degree of exposure. If the patient's condition permits, decontamination should be performed at the scene, as many community hospitals are not equipped for decontamination. Contaminated clothing should be removed from victims and placed in sealed plastic bags, and exposed skin and hair should be cleansed with soap and water. Removal of clothing can reduce contamination on the patient by 90%.[10,12] Receiving hospitals should be notified early during post-incident actions to facilitate preparations. Victims of radiation poisoning should be separated from other patients in the treatment area. If decontamination occurs inside the emergency

department, isolated water and ventilation systems should be used in designated containment and decontamination areas. Security personnel should be used to control access and minimize the spread of contamination.[12,13]

All rescue and medical personnel should use universal precautions with gowns, gloves, masks, and shoe covers. Respirators are not required at the hospital, but should be used by first responders or anyone entering a highly contaminated area. The risk to medical personnel from radioactive contamination is minimal with universal precautions, so lifesaving treatments should be prioritized. Radiation survey monitors (Geiger-Mueller meters) should be used to detect and prevent contamination beyond known areas. All hospitals designated as decontamination zones should have Geiger-Mueller survey meters available.[12,13]

A radioactive form of iodine would be a significant component of a release event from a nuclear power plant. Radioactive iodine is absorbed and remains concentrated in the thyroid glands of humans, thus posing a long-term increased risk of cancer of the gland.[11,14] All exposed persons, especially within the emergency planning zone, should take potassium iodide pills within 1 hour of exposure to prevent absorption of the radioactive iodine.[12,14]

MEDICAL TREATMENT OF CASUALTIES

If a terrorist attack is successful in releasing large-scale nuclear contamination, radiation exposure would first affect the rapidly dividing radiosensitive cells in the gastrointestinal tract and integument. The central nervous system can also be affected indirectly, secondary to edema. If the immediate effects of radiation poisoning are survived, delayed hematopoietic effects are the major cause of mortality.[12] The typical presentation of acute radiation syndrome occurs in four phases and follows a predictable course, with onset ranging from hours to weeks depending on the dose of radiation received by the body (Table 194-1). The prodromal phase consists of gastrointestinal symptoms followed by the latent phase. The time to onset of the manifest illness stage is days to weeks. The final phase is recovery or death. Survival, even with appropriate medical treatment, is highly unlikely for doses above 1000 roentgen equivalent man (rem).[10]

Gastrointestinal Manifestations

Gastrointestinal manifestations can occur within 30 minutes of a severe exposure or after 6 hours with a lesser exposure. Higher doses of

---

TABLE 194-1   Findings of Acute Radiation Syndrome by Approximate Dose of Acute Whole Body Exposure

	MILD (1-2 GY)	MODERATE (2-4 GY)	SEVERE (4-6 GY)	VERY SEVERE (6-8 GY)	LETHAL (>8 GY)
Onset of prodromal phase and signs	2 h or later. Slight headache, no diarrhea.	1-2 h after exposure. Mild headache, no diarrhea, fever.	<1 h. Mild diarrhea, moderate headache, fever.	<30 min. Profuse diarrhea, severe headache, possible altered consciousness, high fever.	<10 min. Profuse diarrhea, severe headache, high fever, unconsciousness.
Onset of manifest illness phase and signs	>30 days. Fatigue, weakness.	18-28 days. Fever, infections, bleeding, weakness, epilation.	8-18 days. High fevers, infections, bleeding, epilation.	<7 days. High fever, diarrhea, vomiting, dizziness, disorientation, hypotension.	<3 days. High fever, diarrhea, unconsciousness.
Mortality	0%	0-50%	20-70%	50-100%	100%
Medical response	Prophylactic and outpatient observation.	Observation in hospital. Prophylactic treatment days 14-20.	Treatment in specialized hospital. Prophylactic treatment days 7-10.	Specialized hospital. Prophylactic treatment from day 1.	General hospital. Palliative and symptomatic treatment only.

Data from Koenig K, Goans R, Hatchett R, et al. Medical treatment of radiological casualties: current concepts. *Ann Emerg Med.* 2005;45:643–652.
Gy, Gray unit (absorption of 1 J of radiation energy by 1 kg of matter).

radiation (>10 gray [Gy]) typically result in an earlier onset of symptoms and a more protracted course. Initial symptoms include nausea, anorexia, and diarrhea. Significant dehydration often results from transudation of plasma into the gastrointestinal tract. Pancytopenia combined with the denuded intestinal tract is a major source of septicemia and death.[12]

Integument

Increasing exposure leads to epilation, erythema, and desquamation of the skin. Erythema and blistering with necrosis can develop within hours of a severe exposure, or within 1 to 2 days after a lesser exposure.[12] Patients presenting with burns immediately after a terrorist event are more likely to have suffered thermal burns rather than radiation burns.[10]

Central Nervous System

Massive radiation exposure can lead to edema of the brain. Presenting complaints include headache and vertigo. Ominous signs are altered mental status and possible development of seizures.[12]

Unlike contamination by biological and chemical hazardous materials, decontamination of radioactive material should not take precedent over resuscitation, stabilization, and transportation. Decontamination is the secondary objective; all patients should be cared for per standard trauma protocol with decontamination only occurring once the patient is stabilized. Treatment should be tailored to the degree of exposure to radiation and the manifestation of symptoms. However, there are core measures common to all victims of radiation exposure. All wounds should be irrigated with saline followed by 3% hydrogen peroxide or soapy solution. Gastrointestinal decontamination with whole-bowel irrigation with activated charcoal is indicated within 2 hours of exposure for those with moderate or greater levels of exposure. Supportive treatment with intravenous antiemetic agents, intravenous fluids to replace gastrointestinal losses, and the dressing of open wounds and burns is indicated. Evaluate time of onset and degree of nausea, vomiting, diarrhea, and fatigue to gauge dose of radiation received. Obtain a complete blood count (CBC) with absolute lymphocyte count every 6 hours for those manifesting symptoms. The main focus of treatment of acute radiation syndrome is prevention of infection, see Table 194-1 for details. Antibiotics and antivirals should be given as needed for neutropenia. If advised, hematopoietic growth factors should be given within the first 24 hours and then daily. Finally, early transport to an advanced medical facility should be arranged for all victims exposed to high doses of radiation.[10,13]

UNIQUE CONSIDERATIONS

Gross structural failure of the containment building is essential for a large-scale contamination event occurring from a reactor material release. Although the containment building may not be compromised by the direct impact of an airliner, the effect of a subsequent jet fuel fire or explosion could cause further mechanical and thermal damage to the containment facility, resulting in a structural collapse of the building.

Nuclear power plants house many more times the amount of radioactive substances than is present in stored nuclear weapons. If a deliberate act of sabotage is successful in releasing even only a small portion of material, there can still be severe consequences.

Radiation cannot be detected by sight, smell, or any other sense. This should be a consideration of responders and other personnel. Another element to be kept in mind is that the prompt ingestion of a nonradioactive iodine pill will prevent the absorption and concentration of radioactive iodine during a nuclear power plant meltdown.

Although there have been no incidents of an airliner crash into a nuclear power plant, the possibility of this type of terrorist attack cannot be excluded. Increased vigilance and preparedness of local, regional, state, and federal agencies, as well as of the medical staff in areas with operational nuclear power plants, is indicated.

PITFALLS

Severe potential pitfalls in response to an aircraft crashing into a nuclear power plant exist. These include the following:
- Failure of rescue personnel to use appropriate personal protective equipment
- Failure to quickly isolate affected persons
- Failure to notify receiving hospitals in a timely manner
- Failure to identify and treat emergent traumatic injuries prior to decontamination
- Failure to create an emergency plan prior to an incident

REFERENCES

1. Behrens CE. Nuclear power plants: vulnerability to terrorist attack. *Congressional Research Service Report for Congress.* 2003.
2. Mettler F, Voelz G. Major radiation exposure: what to expect and how to respond. *N Engl J Med.* 2002;346:1554–1561.
3. Mettler F. Medical resources and requirements for responding to radiological terrorism. *Health Phys.* 2005;89:488–493.
4. United States Nuclear Regulatory Commission. Nuclear reactors. Available at: http://www.nrc.gov/reactors.html.
5. U.S. Federal Emergency Management Agency. Radiological emergency preparedness program. Available at: http://www.fema.gov/radiological-emergency-preparedness-program.
6. Nuclear Regulatory Commission. Frequently asked questions about security assessments at nuclear power plants. Available at: http://www.nrc.gov/security/faq-security-assess-nuc-pwr-plants.html.
7. Holt M, Andrews A. *Nuclear Power Plant Security and Vulnerabilities.* Congressional Research Services; January 3, 2014. Available at: http://www.fas.org/sgp/crs/homesec/RL34331.pdf.
8. Lyman ES. *The Vulnerability of Nuclear Power Plant Containment Buildings to Penetration by Aircraft.* Nuclear Control Institute; September 21, 2001. Available at: http://www.nci.org/01nci/09/aircrashab.html.
9. Cepin M, Cizelj L, Leskovar, et al. Vulnerability analysis of a nuclear power plant considering detonations of explosive devices. *J Nucl Sci Technol.* 2006;43:1258–1269.
10. Bushber J, Kroger L, Hartman M, et al. Nuclear/radiological terrorism: emergency department management of radiation casualties. *J Emerg Med.* 2007;32:71–85.
11. Parfitt T. Chernobyl's legacy. 20 years after the power station exploded, new cases of thyroid cancer are still rising, say experts. *Lancet.* 2004;363:1534.
12. Marx J, Hokberger R, Walls R. *Rosen Emergency Medicine: Concepts and Clinical Practice.* 8th ed. Philadelphia: Elsevier Inc; 2010, 1945–1953.
13. Koenig K, Goans R, Hatchett R, et al. Medical treatment of radiological casualties: current concepts. *Ann Emerg Med.* 2005;45:643–652.
14. Kahn LH, Von Hippel F. Nuclear power plant emergencies and thyroid cancer risk: what New Jersey physicians need to know. *N Engl J Med.* 2004;101:22–27.

Explosion at a Nuclear Waste Storage Facility

Jonathan E. Slutzman

DESCRIPTION OF EVENT

An explosion at a nuclear waste storage facility raises unique challenges for the first responder and medical provider. From safety concerns of explosions, including fire, debris, and structural instability, at the scene to the medical concerns of primary through tertiary blast injuries, these events add the factor of the presence of radioactive materials. Nuclear wastes pose a threat to both the victims of an event and to subsequent personnel tending to those victims.

Nuclear or radioactive waste is the byproduct of various processes that use radionuclides. These wastes can be generated in industry (electricity generation, manufacturing), medicine (diagnostic and therapeutic settings), research (small reactors), and defense (weapons manufacturing and dismantling). There are, broadly speaking, three categories of radioactive waste: high-level, low-level, and mill tailings. High-level wastes are irradiated or used nuclear reactor fuel or weapons components. Low-level wastes are materials that have been contaminated by radioisotopes and are, as a result, radioactive. Mill tailings are residues from processing ore to extract naturally occurring radioactive minerals. Most of this final category of waste is stored at mine sites.[1]

There is no single long-term repository of nuclear waste in the United States. All users of radioisotopes also store their wastes, at least for short periods of time, until disposed. In addition, many facilities store large quantities of wastes for longer times. Most high-level waste is produced in nuclear power generators, with the waste stored in either water pools (majority) or dry casks. There are currently high-level wastes stored in 33 states.[2] Low-level wastes are stored at sites where they are generated and then either disposed as nonradioactive wastes (if they contain short-lived radioisotopes and have decayed to background levels of radiation) or sent to low-level waste disposal facilities.[1] There are currently four such facilities in the United States, located in Barnwell, South Carolina; Richland, Washington; Clive, Utah; and Andrews, Texas.[3] Although the U.S. government once planned to store high-level wastes indefinitely in a single large site in Nevada (the Yucca Mountain Nuclear Waste Repository), the construction project was terminated in 2011 with no existing replacement scheme.

A nuclear waste facility explosion can be accidental or purposeful. Accidental explosions can be a result of the underlying physical risks inherent in storing spent nuclear fuel. Fuel rods generate heat and, if not sufficiently cooled, can ignite. In addition, wet storage facilities present a risk of hydrogen production and subsequent explosion in certain circumstances. There is also a small risk of spent fuel spontaneously maintaining a nuclear reaction, potentially leading to criticality and explosion. The probability of a spontaneous explosion occurring is certainly not zero.[4] Either a spontaneous or a purposeful explosion would be analogous to a dirty bomb (see Chapter 76), as the explosion could disperse radioactive materials.

All wastes are stored in containment structures, usually concrete or metal. An explosive event may remain within a containment structure, which would potentially concentrate any exposures within the structure and limit the number of victims. If containment structures are breached, however, radioactive materials would be released into the environment, affecting more people, although those farther away would likely receive lower doses.

The radiological at risks related to such an event are due to decay of the radioisotopes involved. In general, radioactive material decays by emission of particles: alpha (helium nuclei), beta (electrons released after a neutron splits), and gamma (generated from electromagnetic waves). Often a mix of all particles is released.[5] Each radioisotope has a different penetration distance and decays at its own rate. Through combination of the rate and type of emission, each isotope presents different risks to human health and the environment. If an event were to occur, authorities would need to identify which radioisotopes were involved and share that information with responders in order to tailor the response and therapy needed.[6]

PRE-INCIDENT ACTIONS

Storing nuclear wastes entails certain responsibilities, including taking steps to prevent ill effects and mitigate the impacts of any hazardous events. Engineered and administrative controls should be implemented to protect radionuclides. These controls would likely include ensuring adequate containment structures, proper ventilation, and cooling mechanisms to prevent spontaneous explosions, as well as site security and access controls. Conventional materials that could contribute to an explosion should be stored safely away from radionuclides. Response plans should be developed and shared with local first responders. For nuclear power plants, these may be coordinated with the Federal Emergency Management Agency's Radiological Emergency Preparedness (FEMA REP) Program (www.fema.gov/radiological-emergency-preparedness-program). Facilities should make available all necessary personal protective equipment (PPE) for potential response to incidents. Finally, practice is the cornerstone of good disaster planning. Frequent drills should be held to ensure that all personnel know how to respond.

Local and regional first responders and emergency teams also need to develop response plans. First, they should identify any nuclear waste storage facilities in their jurisdictions. This task may be facilitated by identifying any potential users of radioisotopes, including electric generators, industrial manufacturers, medical facilities, research institutes, and universities. Various government agencies, including the U.S. Environmental Protection Agency (EPA), Department of Energy (DOE), Nuclear Regulatory Commission (NRC), and their state counterparts, may have information from permitting and other activities that will help identify potential sources of radioisotopes. Once facilities have been identified, responders should coordinate efforts with them, review mitigation and response plans, tour locations, and participate in drills (including with FEMA REP, as appropriate). Response teams should also attempt to identify which radioisotopes are be likely to be involved at each facility, as this will help in determining which PPE and medical care may be most appropriate. Finally, responders should obtain and regularly use radiation detection equipment to help determine when an incident involves radioisotopes.

All personnel, including first responders and hospitals, should be familiar with their local emergency planning committee (LEPC). These committees are a regulatory requirement under the Emergency Planning and Community Right to Know Act and are administered by the EPA. While they are designed for chemical emergency management, there is overlap with jurisdiction with this kind of an incident, and their expertise would be valuable. LEPCs can be found by contacting the appropriate State Emergency Response Commission. Response and mitigation plans should be coordinated with LEPCs.

In addition to LEPCs, responders should become familiar with the resources offered by the Radiation Emergency Assistance Center/Training Site (REAC/TS) at Oak Ridge National Laboratory. As specialists in nuclear incidents, they can provide guidance on how to manage specific nuclear incidents. Plans should include contacting REAC/TS at the first sign of a nuclear incident.

Hospitals and other medical facilities represent the third line of defense in the treatment of casualties from a nuclear waste facility explosion. Much as local and regional emergency teams need to coordinate planning and training with waste repositories and generators, medical facilities should coordinate their efforts with local first responders. Hospitals must have disaster plans that address management of casualties from radiological incidents.[5] They should acquire and test decontamination facilities and procedures. Hospitals need to provide adequate PPE to personnel in order to ensure their safety. As generators of nuclear waste, they should perform the actions noted above, including implementing engineering and administrative controls to protect their own wastes. Medical personnel should also familiarize themselves with assessment and treatment protocols for blast and radiological casualties. One useful resource is the U.S. Department of Health and Human Services' Radiation Emergency Medical Management (REMM) System, which can be found at www.remm.nlm.gov.

⏩ POST-INCIDENT ACTIONS

In the event of an incident, the first step will be to recognize that a potential radiological event has occurred. Notification may be formal, from higher authorities down to emergency responders and hospitals, or may more likely be informal, in the form of contaminated and injured patients arriving at health care facilities. Once responders and hospitals are aware of an event, the next step will be to activate disaster plans and mobilize resources. In addition to local resources, REAC/TS should be contacted at (865) 576-1005 as soon as possible, so they can mobilize personnel and equipment to assist.

First responders and emergency teams need to ensure scene safety for themselves and bystanders. This will include restricting access to the event location; establishing hot, warm, and cool zones of activity; and assessing structural integrity of the site before permitting rescue activities. Any radioactive isotopes involved will need to be identified, either through an inventory of site contents or through direct sampling. This information will be helpful in directing optimal PPE use and casualty treatment and prophylaxis. In the absence of reliable risk information, comprehensive PPE against inhalation, ingestion, and dermal

transmission should be used. This will likely require masks or, in the event of an explosion, supplied air breathing apparatus and physical barrier protections like turnout gear. Individual dosimeters and radiation meters will be useful to direct operational rotations and ensure that responders are not exposed to radiation greater than established guidelines.[7] Scene responders will also commence decontamination procedures, enabling people to move from the hot to the cool zones for further assessment and treatment. Decontamination will require, at a minimum, removal of clothing and washing with high-volume, low-pressure water from head to toe.[6]

Hospitals, upon activating disaster plans, will need to clear adequate patient space in the emergency department to treat expected casualties. This will require expedited disposition decisions for patients currently in the department and coordination with inpatient providers to facilitate discharges and admissions. Even if the number of expected casualties is low, hospital planners should expect a large number of worried well patients to arrive at hospitals in the event of a radiological incident. Facility access controls will need to be implemented to direct patients and visitors to the appropriate areas within the hospital. In particular, any potentially contaminated individuals will need to be processed through decontamination prior to entry to the hospital, clinical condition permitting. Any life-threatening injuries should be addressed prior to decontamination. Hospital personnel will need to receive and don PPE. At a minimum, this will include a cap, surgical mask, eye protection, gown, and gloves. X-ray shielding (lead aprons) may also be worn to protect against x-rays and gamma rays. Providers should also have radiation dosimeters to monitor how much exposure they face. Health care providers should also review REMM algorithms to remind themselves of proper assessment and treatment of exposed and contaminated patients.

✚ MEDICAL TREATMENT OF CASUALTIES

People exposed to explosions at nuclear waste facilities can suffer a wide range of injuries and will require multidisciplinary treatment. Casualties will have blast injuries, burns, and radiation exposure and contamination.

The priority is immediate treatment of life-threatening conditions. Decontamination should be performed as soon as possible and will likely be performed first for most patients. However, given the expectation that contaminated patients pose a low risk to medical providers, priority is given to initial resuscitative measures.[6] These measures include the "X-ABCs" of trauma care, representing control of exsanguinating injuries, airway, breathing, and circulation, in that order.

Following primary control of immediate threats to life, patients can then move to decontamination. Even if decontamination is performed at the scene of an incident, it should be confirmed and will likely need to be more comprehensively completed at the medical facility. Radiation detectors should be used to identify and measure any continued contamination of patients prior to entering the emergency department.[5]

Once decontaminated, patients should be fully assessed again in a primary and secondary survey to identify potential injuries. If the number of patients is low, full and complete assessments should be done, identifying all injuries prior to disposition. However, in the event of a mass casualty event, evaluations in the emergency department may need to be truncated in order to care for as many people as possible. Re-triage procedures should be in place to ensure that clinically significant injuries are not missed.

Blast injuries can be classified as primary, secondary, tertiary, and quaternary, and providers should be alert to typical injury patterns.

Primary injuries result from the over-pressurization wave from explosives and typically include blast lung, hollow viscous injuries, intracranial injuries, and ear injuries. Secondary injuries result from impact with flying debris and typically include penetrating trauma to all parts of the body. Tertiary injuries result from patients being thrown into other objects by a blast wind and include blunt trauma to all parts of the body. Quaternary injuries are all other explosion-related injuries and, in this case, include burns and radiation exposure.[8]

Burns should be managed as usual, with slight changes. Skin should be irrigated for decontamination prior to any dressings. Otherwise, patients should receive fluid resuscitation as needed, generally per the Parkland formula (4 mL/kg/% total body surface area [TBSA] burned, divided between the first 8 hours and the next 16 hours) for partial and full-thickness burns of more than 20% TBSA. Patients who have not had a booster within the previous 5 years should have tetanus immunizations administered.[9]

There are a number of considerations surrounding radiation exposure and contamination. Exposure is absorption of penetrating ionizing radiation from a source external to the body. Contamination is the ingestion, inhalation, or deposition of radioisotopes on or in the body. The former only causes effects to the patient related to direct cellular damage from the ionizing radiation. The latter does the same, but continues to release radiation as long as the patient remains contaminated.[5]

For patients who are exposed to radiation, the key concern is acute radiation syndrome (ARS). The body systems typically involved are hematologic, gastrointestinal, cutaneous, and neurological.[6] Effects are directly related to received radiation dose; calculators are available on the REMM site to help estimate dose from signs, symptoms, lab tests, and time (www.remm.nlm.gov). The site also provides guidance on specific therapies, such as blood transfusions, bone marrow stimulators, and symptomatic medications.

Decontamination is the key treatment for patients who are contaminated with radioisotopes. A contamination survey should be performed to identify any particular areas of the body that require greater attention. Skin should be decontaminated as described above, with low-pressure, tepid water and mild soap wash.[5] In the future, additional products such as decontamination lotions may be available.[10] Wounds should be copiously irrigated, taking care to avoid spreading effluent to other parts of the body. Any remaining radioactive shrapnel that cannot be removed with bedside irrigation and extraction should be referred for surgical debridement. Eyes should be decontaminated with irrigation as well. The nose can be cleaned with moistened cotton swabs. The mouth should be decontaminated via tooth brushing and rinsing with dilute hydrogen peroxide solution. Ears with intact tympanic membranes should be irrigated.[6]

Table 195-1 shows specific antidotes for many radioisotopes that may be involved in an event. Some of these are Food and Drug Administration-approved for these uses, but many are not. Health care providers should consult toxicology and medical physics experts regarding their use.

UNIQUE CONSIDERATIONS

As with many environmental and toxicological effects, children will likely be impacted more than adults. Their rapidly dividing cells are more susceptible to DNA damage from ionizing radiation. A higher surface area-to-body mass ratio makes temperature regulation in the setting of burns more difficult for them. Smaller size can also result in a larger radiation received dose in children.

Similar concerns exist for pregnant women. The effects of radiation on a developing fetus are not entirely known, presenting challenging

risk management. Following an event, a pregnant woman should be encouraged to discuss the risks to the fetus with her obstetrician, a maternal-fetal medicine specialist, pediatric toxicologist, or geneticist in order to make the best decisions and plans she can.

Nuclear disasters can result in severe mental health needs among the population. At least in one prior incident, people who had very low risk of radiation exposure suffered no increase in cancer incidence, but did have a higher rate of suicide.[6] Counselors and other mental health professionals are necessary for adequate long-term response and recovery.[5] Critical incident stress debriefing for responders is one tool among many to assist with the mental health needs of those directly involved in incident response. In addition, public health authorities will need to be involved to mobilize mental health resources for the general public.

One method to help reduce general panic and concern in the public is ensuring the unity of messages from all providers about real risks and mitigation strategies. It is important that people hear the same message from all providers: governments, health care providers, first responders, and public health authorities. In general, public health personnel will likely take the lead on public risk information, and public communications should be conveyed through appropriate channels, including the public information officer within an incident command system.

Regarding other, longer-term impacts and needs, radioactive fallout can persist in the environment, raising risks associated with food and water supplies. Health care providers will need to be in touch with authorities to ensure the best recommendations are disseminated among patients and the general population. Furthermore, although an event may occur in one small location, with time radioactive contaminants can spread, so downwind and downstream jurisdictions will need to be notified.

It is also likely that a nuclear waste facility explosion will be heavily investigated, whether accidental or a purposeful attack. Preserving evidence and clearly and accurately documenting findings will be helpful to investigating authorities.

! PITFALLS

Perhaps the greatest potential pitfall in responding to an explosion at a nuclear waste storage facility is not recognizing early that the incident involves nuclear waste. While many facilities obviously present the risk of radioisotopes (such as nuclear power generators), there are many unlikely sources of nuclear material. First responders must be vigilant and suspicious in responding to explosions, using their monitoring and testing equipment to assess the risk of radiation as early in response activities as possible.

There is also a risk of health care providers and other staff, particularly at sites away from the incident, being concerned about their own safety. If staff do not feel protected, they may be reluctant to provide needed care to casualties. Adequate training, drills, and PPE are key to ensuring that all staff feel comfortable in their roles.

Many of the procedures outlined here are rarely needed, which raises the risk of not being able to complete tasks effectively. Caring for these casualties is a high-risk, low-frequency event that requires regular training, exercises, and checklists to maintain proficiency.

As the control of life-threatening conditions trumps decontamination, it is possible for treatment areas to become contaminated themselves, reducing their availability to treat additional casualties. Providers must be careful to prevent contamination of these areas as much as possible, and decontamination procedures must be available to ensure rapid turnaround of care spaces.

TABLE 195-1	**Radiation Countermeasures for Treatment of Internal Contamination**				
MEDICAL COUNTERMEASURE	**ADMINISTERED FOR**	**MECHANISM OF ACTION**	**ROUTE OF ADMINISTRATION**	**DOSAGE**	**DURATION OF TREATMENT**
Aluminum carbonate	Phosphorus (P-32)	Phosphate binder	PO	600 mg tablet TID or 400 mg/5 mL TID	
Aluminum hydroxide	Radium (Ra-226) Strontium (Sr-90)	Blocks intestinal absorption	PO	*Adults:* 60-100 mL (1200 mg) *Children:* 50 mg/kg, not to exceed the adult dose	Give one dose within 24 h of radionuclide intake
	Phosphorus (P-32)	Phosphate binder	PO	600 mg tablet TID or 320 mg/5 mL TID	
Barium sulfate	Radium (Ra-226) Strontium (Sr-90)	Blocks intestinal absorption	PO	100-300 g (as a single dose in 250 mL water)	Give one dose within 24 h of radionuclide intake
Calcium carbonate	Radium (Ra-226) Strontium (Sr-90)	Competes for bone binding sites	PO	Use as directed on label	Begin therapy within 12 h of radionuclide intake if possible
Calcium gluconate	Radium (Ra-226) Strontium (Sr-90)	Competes for bone binding sites; phosphate binder	IV	5 ampoules (500 mg Ca/ amp) in 500 mL 5% D5W; infuse over 4-6 hours	6 days; begin therapy within 12 h of radionuclide intake if possible
Calcium phosphate	Radium (Ra-226) Strontium (Sr-90)	Increases excretion	PO	1200 mg	Give one dose within 24 h of radionuclide intake
Deferoxamine (DFOA)	Plutonium (Pu-239)	Chelating agent	IM (preferred route)	2 ampoules (500 mg DFOA/ amp)	• Give a single dose, then obtain bioassay to assess residual body burden of Pu-239
			IV (slow infusion)	2 ampoules (500 mg DFOA/amp) at 15 mg/kg/h	• Repeat as indicated: 500 mg IM (preferred) or IV q 4 h × 2 doses, then 500 mg IV q 12 h for 3 days
DTPA (calcium and zinc)	Americium (Am-241) Californium (Cf-252) Cobalt (Co-60) Curium (Cm-244) Plutonium (Pu-238 and Pu-239) Yttrium (Y-90)	Chelating agent	IV (give once daily as a bolus or as a single infusion, i.e., do not fractionate the dose)	*Adults:* 1 g in 5 mL 5% D5W or 0.9% NS slow IV push over 3-4 minutes or 1 g in 100-250 mL D5W or NS as an infusion over 30 minutes *Children < 12 years:* 14 mg/ kg/day slow IV push over 3-4 minutes (not to exceed 1 g/day)	• Begin treatment with Ca-DTPA, then change to Zn-DTPA for maintenance, as indicated • Duration of therapy depends on total body burden and response to treatment
			Nebulized inhalation (for use in adults only)	1 g in 1:1 dilution with sterile water or NS over 15-20 minutes	
			Wound irrigation fluid	1 g Ca- or Zn-DTPA and 10 mL 2% lidocaine in 100 mL 5% D5W or 0.9% NS	• Irrigation can be amLompanied by IV or inhaled DTPA • Amount of DTPA absorbed by wound tissues cannot be measured • Avoid overdosing with DTPA and/or 2% lidocaine
Dimercaprol (BAL)	Polonium (Po-210)	Chelating agent	IM (300 mg/vial for deep IM injection only)	2.5 mg/kg QID × 2 days (days 1 and 2), then BID × 1 day (day 3), then QD (days 4-10)	10 days
EDTA	Cobalt (Co-60)	Chelating agent	IV	1000 mg/m²/day in 500 mL 5% D5W or 0.9% NS; infuse over 8-12 h	Given as a single dose

Continued

TABLE 195-1	Radiation Countermeasures for Treatment of Internal Contamination—cont'd				
MEDICAL COUNTERMEASURE	**ADMINISTERED FOR**	**MECHANISM OF ACTION**	**ROUTE OF ADMINISTRATION**	**DOSAGE**	**DURATION OF TREATMENT**
			IM	Divide IV dose equally into two doses and administer 8-12 h apart	Given as a divided dose
D-penicillamine	Polonium (Po-210)	Chelating agent	PO	*Adults:* 0.75-1.5 g (250 mg/capsule) QD *Children:* 30 mg/kg/day (250 mg/capsule) divided into 4 doses	• Obtain bioassay to assess • Continue only if clinically indicated • D-penicillamine has a narrow therapeutic index; use is associated with high risk of toxicity
Potassium iodide (KI)	Iodine (I-131)	Blocking agent	PO	*Adults >40 years:* 130 mg/day (for projected thyroid dose ≥500 cGy) *Adults 18-40 years:* 130 mg/day (projected thyroid dose ≥10 cGy) *Pregnant or lactating women of any age:* 130 mg/day (for projected thyroid dose ≥5 cGy) *Adolescents ≥ 70 kg:* 130 mg/day (for projected thyroid dose ≥5 cGy) *Children & adolescents 3-18 years:* 65 mg/day (projected thyroid dose ≥5 cGy) *Infants & toddlers 1 month-3 years:* 32.5 mg/day (projected thyroid dose ≥5 cGy) *Neonates from birth to 1 month:* 16 mg/day (projected thyroid dose ≥5 cGy)	• Some incidents will require only a single dose of KI. • Incident managers may recommend additional daily doses if ongoing radioactive iodine ingestion or inhalation represents a continuing threat.
Potassium phosphate	Phosphorus (P-32)	Phosphate binder	PO	600-1200 mg, given in divided doses	
Potassium phosphate, dibasic	Phosphorus (P-32)	Phosphate binder	PO (take with full glass of water with meals and at bedtime)	*Adults:* 1-2 tablets (250 mg/tab) QID *Children > 4 years:* 1 tablet (250 mg/tab) QID	
Propylthiouracil	Iodine (I-131)	Blocking agent	PO	*Adults:* 2 tablets (50 mg/tab) TID	8 days
Prussian blue, insoluble	Cesium (Cs-137)	Ion exchange; inhibits enterohepatic recirculation in GI tract	PO	*Adults, children > 12 years:* • 1-3 g (2-6 capsules; 0.5 g insoluble Prussian blue per cap) TID; up to 10-12 g/day (based on Goiânia incident data) • 3 g (6 capsules; 0.5 g insoluble Prussian blue per cap) TID (see FDA package insert) *Children 2-12 years:* • 1 g (2 capsules; 0.5 g	• Minimum 30 day course per FDA • Obtain bioassay and whole body count to assess treatment of efficacy • Duration of therapy depends on total body burden and response to treatment

TABLE 195-1	Radiation Countermeasures for Treatment of Internal Contamination—cont'd				
MEDICAL COUNTERMEASURE	**ADMINISTERED FOR**	**MECHANISM OF ACTION**	**ROUTE OF ADMINISTRATION**	**DOSAGE**	**DURATION OF TREATMENT**
				insoluble Prussian blue per cap) TID • Capsules may be opened and contents mixed with food • See FDA package insert for pediatric prescribing information *Children < 2 years:* Prussian blue is not FDA-approved for use (IND or EUA may be required)	
Sevelamer	Phosphorus (P-32)	Phosphate binder	PO	• 2-4 tablets (400 mg-800 mg/tab) TID • Not to exceed 1600 mg TID	5 days if possible; first dose is the most important
Sodium alginate	Radium (Ra-226) Strontium (Sr-90)	Blocks intestinal absorption	PO (take with a full glass of water)	5 g BID × 1 day, then 1 g QID	
Sodium bicarbonate	Uranium (U-235)	Facilitates increased renal excretion	IV PO	• 2 amps (44.3 mEq bicarbonate/amp) in 1000 mL 5% D5W or 0.9% NS • 250 mL (1-2 mEq/kg) slow infusion 2 tablets/q 4 h	Administer therapy until urine pH is 8-9; continue for 3 days
Sodium glycerophosphate	Phosphorus (P-32)		PO	600-1200 mg, given in divided doses	
Sodium phosphate	Phosphorus (P-32)		PO	600-1200 mg, given in divided doses	
SumLimer (DMSA)	Polonium (Po-210)	Chelating agent	PO	• 100 mg capsules • Administer 10 mg/kg or 350 mg/m² every 8 h for 5 days, then reduce; safety and efficacy in children < 12 years has not been established	Reduce frequency of administration to 10 mg/kg or 350 mg/m² every 12 h for an additional 2 weeks of therapy; typical treatment course 19 days
Water	Tritium (H-3)	Facilitates excretion	PO	>3-4 L/day	3 weeks

References for use:
a. Management of Persons Contaminated with Radionuclides: Handbook (NCRP Report No. 161, Vol. I), National Council on Radiation Protection and Measurements, Bethesda, MD, 2008.
b. Population Monitoring and Radionuclide Decorporation Following a Radiological or Nuclear Incident (NCRP Report No. 166), National Council on Radiation Protection and Measurements, Bethesda, MD, 2011.
c. FDA drug information related to radiation emergencies.
BID, Twice a day; *D5W,* 5% dextrose in water; *EUA,* Emergency Use Authorization; *FDA,* Food and Drug Administration; *IND,* investigational new drug; *IV,* intravenous; *IM,* intramuscular; *NS,* normal saline; *PO,* by mouth; *q,* daily; *QD,* one per day; *TID,* three times a day.
From Radiation Emergency Medical Management: REMM [US Department of Health and Human Services] at www.remm.nlm.gov/int_contamination.htm#blockingagents.

REFERENCES

1. U.S. Nuclear Regulatory Commission. *Radioactive Waste: Production, Storage, Disposal. NUREG/BR-0216, Rev 2;* May 2002.

2. U.S. Government Accountability Office. *Spent Nuclear Fuel: Accumulating Quantities at Commercial Reactors Present Storage and Other Challenges. GAO-12-797;* August 2012.

3. U.S. Nuclear Regulatory Commission. Locations of Low-Level Waste Disposal Facilities. http://www.nrc.gov/waste/llw-disposal/licensing/locations.html. Accessed June 10, 2014.

4. Butler D. Call for better oversight of nuclear-waste storage. *Nature.* 2014;509 (7500):267–268.

5. Wolbarst AB, Wiley AL Jr, Nemhauser JB, Christensen DM, Hendee WR. Medical response to a major radiologic emergency: a primer for medical and public health practitioners. *Radiology.* 2010;254(3):660–677.

6. Yamamoto LG. Risks and management of radiation exposure. *Pediatr Emerg Care.* 2013;29:1016–1029.

7. FEMA. *Radiological Emergency Preparedness Program Manual;* June 2013, Available at, www.fema.gov/reference-library.

8. Plurad DS. Blast injury. *Mil Med.* 2011 Mar;176(3):276–282.

9. Enoch S, Roshan A, Shah M. Emergency and early management of burns and scalds. *BMJ.* 2009 Apr 8;338:b1037.

10. Rana S, Dutta M, Sharma N, et al. Scintigraphic evaluation of decontamination lotion for removal of radioactive contamination from skin. *Disaster Med Public Health Prep.* 2014 Mar;31:1–6.

CHAPTER 196

Maritime Disasters

Michael Sean Molloy, John Mulhern, and Lucille Gans

DESCRIPTION OF EVENT

Maritime disasters or major incidents involving loss of vessel at sea are rare, they no longer occur with the frequency of centuries past when shipping was the main form of mass transport and significant loss of life was common. However, such disasters remain a major source of tragedy and loss for the transportation industry.[1] Seafarers must be aware that the next major disaster or serious incident may be aboard their vessel. Oldenburg found that 28.6% of the seagoing crew they interviewed, who were participating in a medical refresher course at the Institute of Occupational and Maritime Medicine in Hamburg, reported that they had been confronted with at least one serious medical emergency at sea.[2] Large oceangoing passenger vessels exhibit the potential for mass casualty incidents involving thousands with significant challenges as the traditional first response from emergency services will not be available and far more emphasis must be placed on crew resilience in responding to the disaster. Maritime disasters include incidents involving cruise ships, yachts, ferries, barges, container and cargo vessels, fishing boats, submarines, offshore oil platforms, and other watercraft. The initiating event of the disaster may relate to weather, terrorism, war, infectious disease outbreak, vessel structural integrity and seaworthiness, collision, grounding, submersion, or fire. The effect of maritime disasters extends further than the initial loss of life and injury; it can leave a legacy that many of those involved spend the rest of their lives coming to terms with as described by Maeda, who states, "investigations into maritime disasters have outlined that approximately two thirds of survivors from two major car ferry accidents had symptoms of serious traumatic responses."[3] Líndal and Stefánsson,[4] in another study of maritime disasters, found that crew involved in incidents with fatal outcomes had more long-lasting negative effects than those where there were no fatalities.

Every incident at sea is a learning experience, whatever the size of vessel or number of people carried. The majority of nations have signed on to the recommendations of the Convention for Safety of Lives at Sea (SOLAS) since its introduction in 1974 and subsequent amendments in 1981.[5,6] The loss of seaworthiness of a ship can result from several causes, often occurring in combination. Disasters are most often caused by storms, fires, and explosions, although loss of life generally results from human error. Contributing factors may include excessive reliance on technology, which can result in the loss of basic and advanced sailing techniques, plus underestimation of potential vessel vulnerabilities and risks posed by weather and sea conditions. Technological advances have meant increases in the size and carrying capacity of ships, with concomitant increased potential for loss of life and property. Human factors also include: failure to establish or follow procedures to enhance the safety of ships, passengers, and crew; inexperience; and "cutting corners" to save time and money. If commercial concerns such as

competitiveness, maintaining schedules, and cargo take precedence over passenger and crew safety, disasters can and do result. Survival is enhanced by diligent compliance with appropriate procedures and standards combined with knowledge, experience, and resourcefulness.[7]

Drowning is the most common cause of death due to maritime disasters, followed by hypothermia,[7] although traumatic injuries may also occur because of the event that produced the disaster. These injuries include but are not limited to burns, blast injuries from explosions, and both blunt and penetrating trauma.[8] In addition, victims who survive the initial sinking of the ship but who are not rescued in a timely manner may ultimately die from dehydration, starvation, or exposure while occupying life rafts or floating in the sea.

Maritime disasters also include events when no human lives are lost but loss of the ship's cargo results in pollution and damage to the ocean waters, marine life, and shoreline. Such situations have most often involved oil tankers, as in the cases of the *Exxon Valdez* in Alaska and the *Sea Empress* in Australia. Other cargo ships carrying hazardous materials that have been damaged while near shore and habitation include the *Multitank Ascania*, carrying highly explosive vinyl acetate, and the *Bilboa*, carrying ferrosilicon (which can release toxic and explosive gases when exposed to moisture), to list only a few of the hundreds of incidents that have occurred in recent decades.[9] There are huge costs associated with rescue, salvage, and recovery in such situations. For example, the cost for cleanup after the *Exxon Valdez* spill is estimated at $2.2 billion (U.S.).

Those who have earned their living at sea know well the importance of emergency preparedness. In 2006, a maritime disaster occurred aboard the MV *Star Princess*, an oceangoing passenger vessel carrying 2690 passengers and 1123 crew. A fire started on a balcony and quickly spread. The crew at every level from the Master to the waiters used their emergency preparedness training to save the 4000 people onboard. The incident, cause, and subsequent recommendations are fully explained in the report (28/2006) published by the Marine Accident Investigation Branch of the Department of Transport, UK.

At 03:09 AM on March 23, 2006, the crew of MV Star Princess were awakened by the announcement "Assessment party, assessment party proceed to ..." the standard bridge response to a potential fire or a fire alarm activation, calling the few designated responders within the ship's crew to check the alarm. Within a few minutes, all crew were signaled by a continuous ringing of the ship's crew alarm to muster with life jacket in hand at designated emergency muster stations preparing to carry out their emergency duties. Among the mustered crew were the ship's medical team, consisting of two doctors and four nurses practiced and certified in advanced cardiac life support (ACLS) and prehospital emergency care. The medical team with several crew trained in "stretcher party" duties was prepared and capable of handling the many sick and injured that presented to them. Soon after the crew alarm, the

General Emergency Stations (GES) alarms were sounded, seven short followed by one long blast of the ship alarms and whistle. This GES signal was the call to all passengers to muster at designated gathering points for role call, as was practiced before voyage commencement and as part of the normal safety drill for newly boarded passengers.

Fire spread quickly, engulfing several decks and passenger staterooms with many casualties, some of whom required immediate resuscitations and lifesaving interventions. Many of the casualties suffered from noxious smoke inhalation requiring oxygen and monitoring. The final report commended the crew firefighting teams for bringing the fire under control within about 1 hour (Marine Accident Investigation Branch [MAIB], 2006).[7a] It is the fact that they drilled frequently, understood their responsibilities, and were well trained in the disaster premise of "prevention, preparedness, response, and recovery" that there were so few fatalities. Temperature of the fire exceeded over 500 °C on the balconies inside the metal boxes which joined together to make up the framework of a modern passenger vessel.

The medical center was full with one deceased casualty in the medical mortuary refrigerator. Oxygen supply was at a premium with air concentrators for the least sick and high flow oxygen for the critical. When medical center stores of oxygen ran low, the "stretcher party" had to go out on deck, risking injury, to collect further large oxygen bottles from storage. The "Secondary Medical Center," a further area occupying what was usually a restaurant was now unapproachable due to the levels of smoke. In hindsight, a tertiary medical center designated in advance would have been beneficial, particularly if casualty numbers had increased any further. The medical team's own sleeping quarters adjacent to the medical center were commandeered to house some of the lesser-injured casualties. Triage was essential with many minor nonserious injured sent to their muster station with other passengers for safety and, if necessary, treatment later. Soon the fire was extinguished, the ship had reached port, and the seriously injured ferried to hospital by ambulance and, in some cases, flown by helicopter to trauma centers.

◀◀ PRE-INCIDENT ACTIONS

Before leaving port, both cargo and passenger vessels are subject to various laws and maritime agreements. These requirements include the national laws of the country under which the ship is registered. Many oceangoing vessels are registered under "flags of convenience" to take advantage of national marine laws that may be less stringent than those of the country from which the passenger or cargo company most often sails.[8] Regulations exist for SOLAS ships with respect to radio installation, capabilities, antenna installation, energy sources, and alternates as well as navigation and global positioning services.[10]

In addition, there are further security requirements imposed by the individual ports that the ship enters. The International Maritime Organization (IMO) is the specialized agency of the United Nations that has the responsibility for the safety of shipping and the prevention of marine pollution by ships.[11] Following the September 11, 2001, terrorist attacks on the World Trade Center in New York City, the IMO developed and adopted port security measures as outlined in the International Ship and Port Facility Security Code which came into effect in 2004.[12]

Managing any disaster situation effectively requires an Incident Command System, which has been drilled and is familiar to all the relevant players. Establishing command and control is vital in the early stages of a disaster to ensure a coordinated approach to management. First responders on scene will, by definition, be the command until a more appropriately trained person arrives, at which point command may be turned over to another individual who should be clearly identified by tabard. Command does not need to be in the hands of the most

senior person but it commonly is; the most appropriate commander is the person who has been trained for the role.

In the United States, the National Incident Management System was introduced in the 1990s and updated in 2008 to introduce a national system of preparedness and response within the United States.[13] In the rest of the world, other systems are in use, the most widely used being the Major Incident Medical Management and Support system.[14–17]

Command and control is the first of the seven priority pillars in the Major Incident Medical Management and Support (MIMMS) system. MIMMS is the system used in United Kingdom, Europe, Australasia, and NATO for mass casualty incident management. The pillars are:

C—Command and control
S—Safety and security
C—Communication
A—Assessment
T—Triage
T—Treatment
T—Transport

This approach should be regularly drilled on vessels using tabletops and live drills to ensure that response to an incident is fluid among the crew.

All ships should be required to sail with adequate life jackets and lifeboats or rafts aboard for all passengers and crew. National standards for life jackets or personal flotation devices (PFDs) vary among countries. In addition, PFDs designed to allow greater freedom of movement for participation in water sports, such as windsurfing, may provide lesser degrees of buoyancy. PFDs should be adjustable to fit various body shapes and statures and volumes of clothing, including specialized protective gear. Ideally, the PFD should be self-righting, should maintain the wearer at the water surface, and should keep the airway clear of water, which requires a minimum of 34 lb (150 N) of buoyancy. PFDs should be fitted with a crotch strap to prevent the device from riding up over the shoulders. Even with a properly fitted PFD, however, the dependent legs of the wearer act as a sea anchor, turning the face toward the waves. A person with impaired consciousness, a condition that may develop with hypothermia after immersion in cold water, may be unable to coordinate breathing with the irregular pattern of wave splash over face, and death by drowning may occur.[7]

Lifeboat drills and other safety instruction should be provided once the vessel leaves port. However, there is no guarantee that such information will be provided in multiple languages or that passengers will understand, remember, or comply with directions at the time of an emergency.

Lifeboats, life rafts, and their launch equipment must be maintained to ensure that they are functional and seaworthy. At the bare minimum, each lifeboat should be supplied with a container of survival supplies including water, food rations, raft repair equipment, a sea anchor, and signaling equipment such as flares, lights, and mirrors. The IMO stipulates the equipment that the survival craft must carry, based on the number of persons to be carried. Anyone aboard a vessel should consider assembling a grab bag containing additional supplies, clothing, and medications should it become necessary to abandon ship, using as a guide the requirements listed by maritime regulators or sailing race authorities.[7,18]

Because factors external to the ship, such as weather and sea conditions, can affect the safe passage of the vessel, technological advances, such as Doppler weather radar and global positioning systems, combined with enhanced global communication systems, have contributed greatly to improved ocean safety records in recent years.[18]

▶▶ POST-INCIDENT ACTIONS

Once the integrity of a ship is breached, or as soon as some other threat to passenger or crew safety is recognized, it is essential that rescue procedures are initiated. Alarms both onboard and via radio transmission to appropriate sea- and land-based rescue facilities should be raised. The extent of the potential danger to the ship and those onboard should be assessed, with consideration for potential worsening of conditions.

If the problem can be adequately managed with onboard resources, appropriate personnel should be advised and intervention measures initiated. Procedures for fire suppression must be well understood and initiated immediately once a fire is detected. If the incident is thought to be manageable with the resources available onboard, a "Pan Pan" message should be sent via radio transmission. If the vessel is in immediate danger, a "Mayday" message should be transmitted. In both cases, the radio message should include the vessel name, nature of the incident, number of persons onboard, and geographic location with latitude and longitude. Maritime history includes many cases in which rescue was delayed by either incomplete information or failure of notification from the stricken vessel, often resulting in loss of life.[7]

Generally, those onboard will be better off remaining on the ship unless the captain determines that the ship is in danger of sinking. Before leaving the ship, each person should put on a lifejacket or PFD. If available, survival suits also should be worn. Lifeboats and rafts are smaller and less comfortable than a full-size ship, especially in rough cold ocean waters, with no mechanism for steering or sailing most rafts.

The crew should instruct passengers on how to get into lifeboat or rafts and the procedures for launching them. Once afloat, occupants should attempt to rescue survivors in the water, which may be hampered greatly by hypothermia of both parties. Therefore bailing and drying procedures must be adopted early on in the survival craft.[7] Rationing of food and water should be initiated, even if rescue is anticipated in a short time.[18] No one should drink seawater, in any quantity, as this markedly reduces the chance of survival.[7] Measures should be taken to reduce seasickness, including taking anti-nausea medications, if available, because seasickness will worsen most medical conditions and has further negative effects on hygiene and morale for all persons in a survival craft.[18]

➕ MEDICAL TREATMENT OF CASUALTIES

Rescuers may include those specially equipped and trained for water rescues, for example, the U.S. Coast Guard Search and Rescue (SAR) program or other international resources such as the German SAR services.[19,20] Often, however, rescue comes from those closest who may not have the knowledge or gear to mount the most effective rescue or resuscitation.

The most common conditions suffered by those rescued from the water are near drowning and hypothermia. Rescuers should remove wet clothing and dry the skin and hair of victims before providing warm and dry clothing. If survival suits are available, it may be adequate to dress the victims in these for passive rewarming. However, particularly in the setting of multiple victims rescued from cold ocean waters, the rescuing vessel may not have enough gear for all persons rescued. It may be necessary to put two persons into each suit, and in this case, a warmer victim should be paired with a colder one.[7]

Although hypothermia causes deterioration more commonly and more rapidly, victims rescued from lifeboats and rafts may suffer heat illnesses, including sunburn, heat exhaustion, and heat stroke, the last of which requires urgent medical intervention.[7] Survivors who are rescued after a prolonged time adrift at sea may be suffering from dehydration or starvation plus exposure and may require intensive or prolonged resuscitation and medical care.

❓ UNIQUE CONSIDERATIONS

Maritime rescues are frequently complicated by the very factors that caused the incident. Poor visibility, strong winds, and rough seas may prevent rescuers from reaching or finding damaged ships or floating victims. Once located, high waves and cold temperatures further endanger both rescuers and victims and may damage rescue and medical equipment. Salt water can reduce the effectiveness of equipment immediately or over time. Noise, impaired visibility, and hypothermia can interfere with communications between rescuer and victim, and language barriers may exist. Victims are often hypothermic, dehydrated, and exhausted, any of which reduce their ability to assist with their own rescue.

Victims who are rescued from immersion in cold water may experience temperature afterdrop as a complication of hypothermia, with this postimmersion collapse often resulting in death. This condition occurs when chilled blood from peripheral tissues circulates to the body core with rewarming, causing a drop in the core temperature and a drastically worsened clinical practice.[21,22] The clinical status of survivors rescued after near-drowning may worsen gradually or abruptly due to the development of respiratory distress syndrome with hypoxia and subsequent respiratory failure. Pulmonary edema, cardiovascular complications, and multisystem organ failure may develop, even with intensive medical care.[23] Supportive care and prompt transport to a tertiary care center are essential.

Victims may be covered with fuel oil or may have swallowed or aspirated oil while immersed. They may develop vomiting, aspiration pneumonia or pneumonitis, or conjunctivitis.[7] Oil contamination also complicates the healing of skin wounds, such as abrasions or punctures, as does seawater containing bacteria or other contaminants. Prolonged exposure to damp conditions or clothing in a lifeboat may allow saltwater boils, pustules, or even ulcers to develop. Immersion foot can occur in survivors aboard lifeboats and rafts when feet remain cool, damp, dependent, and inactive, with the development of blood stagnation and tissue swelling.[7]

Survivors rescued from the sea may have swallowed significant quantities of saltwater and may develop osmotic diarrhea and hypernatremia, which will require volume replacement and careful monitoring of electrolyte levels.[7]

After rescue from the sea, there may be delays in reaching definitive medical care. Although the rescue vessel may have adequate personnel and equipment to provide first aid or even major resuscitation for victims, weather and sea conditions may delay transport to a site where surgery or intensive care could be provided, such as a mainland tertiary care center. In addition, distances to the nearest appropriate health care facility may be significant, particularly in the case of mid-ocean rescues.

The same conditions that complicate rescue also make investigation of ship and submarine accidents difficult and hazardous. Evidence may be scattered over the ocean floor, resting several kilometers below the surface in cold, dark water, subject to strong ocean currents.[24] There may be no survivors to describe the events leading up to a tragedy or any actions taken in response, whether or not they were effective, heroic, or foolhardy. There may be no conclusive determination of the cause of a tragic event at sea—rather, only conflicting theories and conjecture—but experts must nevertheless attempt to identify what went wrong so that they may recommend methods to prevent future disasters.[25]

❗ PITFALLS

Several potential pitfalls exist in response to a maritime disaster. These include:

- Failure to appreciate dangerous weather and sea conditions, especially when combined with ship weaknesses or damage
- Failure to adapt course or sailing techniques to changing conditions
- Failure to follow rules of sailing, navigation, and sea transport

- Excessive reliance on technology and failure to identify deficiencies or weakness in ship structure and function
- Failure to request assistance or rescue in a timely manner
- Failure to follow safety procedures and lack of familiarity with evacuation and emergency exits and equipment
- Failure to abandon ship or deploy emergency escape equipment, such as lifejackets or PFDs, survival suits, and lifeboats
- Failure to activate the emergency position indicator rescue beacon before abandoning ship
- Failure to ration water and food supplies after abandoning ship
- Failure to drill evacuation procedures regularly
- Failure to plan for loss of primary and secondary medical centers on large vessels

REFERENCES

1. Bonsall TE. *Great Shipwrecks of the Twentieth Century.* New York, NY: Gallery Books; 1988, 1.
2. Oldenburg M, Rieger J, Sevenich C, Harth V. Nautical officers at sea: emergency experience and need for medical training. *J Occup Med Toxicol.* 2014;9(1):19.
3. Maeda M, Kato H, Maruoka T. Adolescent vulnerability to PTSD and effects of community-based intervention: Longitudinal study among adolescent survivors of the Ehime Maru sea accident. *Psychiatry Clin Neurosci.* 2009;63 (6):747–753.
4. Líndal E, Stefánsson JG. The long-term psychological effect of fatal accidents at sea on survivors: a cross-sectional study of North-Atlantic seamen. *Soc Psychiatry Psychiatr Epidemiol.* 2011;46(3):239–246.
5. International Convention for the Safety of Life at Sea. *Texts of Amendments Relating to Passenger Ro-Ro Ferries Adopted on 21 April and 28 October 1988;* 1989, 1.
6. IMO. *Amendments to the International Convention for the Safety of Life at Sea, 1974;* 1982, 1.
7. Golden F, Tipton M. *Essentials of Sea Survival.* Champaign, IL: Human Kinetics; 2002, 1.
7a. Safety Digest, Lessons from Marine Accident Reports, Department of Transport, Marine Accident Invesitigation Branch, United Kingdom, 2006.

Available at: https://www.gov.uk/government/uploads/system/uploads/attachment_data/file/373790/SafetyDigest__01_06.pdf.
8. Roberts SE. Work-related mortality among British seafarers employed in flags of convenience shipping, 1976-95. *Int Marit Health.* 2003;54(1–4):7–25.
9. Australian Maritime Safety Authority. Available from: http://www.amsa.gov.au.
10. Johnson B. *Global Maritime Distress and Safety System.* 1994, Wikipedia Available at: http://en.wikipedia.org/wiki/Global%20Maritime%20Distress%20and%20Safety%20System.
11. International Maritime Organization. Available at: http://www.imo.org.
12. IMO adopts comprehensive maritime security measures. Available at: http://www.imo.org/blast/mainframe.asp?topic_id=583&doc_id=2689.
13. National Incident Management System. *Principles and Practice;* 2011.
14. Sammut J, Cato D, Homer T. Major Incident Medical Management and Support (MIMMS): a practical, multiple casualty, disaster-site training course for all Australian health care personnel. *Emerg Med.* 2001;13 (2):174–180.
15. Jenkins JL, McCarthy ML, Sauer LM, et al. Mass-casualty triage: time for an evidence-based approach. *Prehosp Disaster Med.* 2008;23(01):3–8.
16. Hodgetts TJ. Major Incident Medical Training: A Systematic International Approach. *Int J Disast Med.* 2009;1(1):13–20. Available at: http://dxdoiorg/101080/15031430310013429.
17. Group ALS. *Major Incident Medical Management and Support.* Chichester: Wiley; 2011, 1.
18. Howorth F, Howorth M. *The Grab Bag Book.* London: A&C Black; 2013, 1.
19. Buschmann C, Niebuhr N, Schulz T, Fox UH. "SAR-First-Responder Sea"— backgrounds to a medical education concept in German SAR service. *Int Marit Health.* 2009;60(1–2):43–47.
20. United States of America Coast Guard Website. Available at: http://www.uscg.mil.
21. Giesbrecht GG, Bristow GK. A second postcooling afterdrop: more evidence for a convective mechanism. *J Appl Physiol.* 1992;73(4):1253–1258.
22. Giesbrecht GG. Prehospital treatment of hypothermia. *Wilderness Environ Med.* 2001;12(1):24–31.
23. Volturo GA. Submersion injuries. In: Harwood-Nuss A, Wolfson AB, Linden CH, eds. *The Clinical Practice of Emergency Medicine.* 3rd ed. Philadelphia, PA: Lippincott Williams & Wilkins; 2001:194–196.
24. Bird L. *The Wreck Diving Manual.* Marlborough: Crowood Press; 1997, 1.
25. Krieger M. *All the Men in the Sea.* 1st ed. New York, NY: Simon & Schuster; 2003, 1.

CHAPTER 197

Cruise Ship Infectious Disease Outbreak

Nadine A. Youssef and Scott G. Weiner

DESCRIPTION OF EVENT

For centuries, infectious diseases that travel by boat have affected the course of history. For instance, the plague (also known as the Black Death), which was caused by *Yersinia pestis*, was carried by boats traveling from Asia to Europe. The plague caused the death of approximately one third of the European population during the 1300s. This epidemic led to the practice of refusing the landing of ships with suspected plague cases for 40 days; this practice was the first practice of "quarantine," which is derived from the Italian word "*quaranta*" for "*forty*."[1] Ship-borne smallpox also played a role in history, as this disease saved England from a French invasion in 1779 after an outbreak spread among the French sailors.[2] The closed environment of the ships and the prolonged duration of the voyages led to a high infection rate.

In modern times, airplanes have replaced ships for long-range passenger transportation; however, a steadily increasing number of people choose to go on cruises as a form of vacation. Every year, the cruise industry attracts more travelers from around the world. Over 16 million passengers traveled on the major cruise lines in 2011.[3] The length of these cruises ranges from a few hours to several months, and the average cruise ship carries 2200 passengers. "Mega" cruise ships with more than 5000 passengers are also becoming more common. On cruise ships, passengers with different ages and comorbidities and crew members from around the world are brought together in close proximity for extended periods of time, facilitating the spread of communicable diseases.[4]

On cruise ships, gastrointestinal and upper respiratory infections are the most commonly encountered infectious disease problems. Other frequently reported medical illnesses include sunburns, intoxication, seasickness, orthopedic injuries, and the exacerbation of chronic medical illnesses.[4] Infections can spread easily on a cruise ship, where passengers encounter crowded conditions with common facilities and food and water supplies. Infections can also have serious operational and financial consequences for the ships and the cruise ship companies involved. Cruise ships usually stop at a number of ports, transferring diseases across international lines, either through infected individuals or through disease vectors, such as insects and rodents.[4] The infectious diseases that affect cruise ships can be divided into three broad categories: gastrointestinal, respiratory, and other miscellaneous infections.

Gastrointestinal Illness

Gastrointestinal illness is by far the most common result of cruise ship outbreaks. Because of this frequency, the Centers for Disease Control and Prevention maintains the Vessel Sanitation Program (VSP). The VSP assists the cruise ship industry to prevent and control the introduction, transmission, and spread of gastrointestinal illnesses on cruise ships. Cruise ships that carry 13 or more passengers and have a foreign itinerary with U.S. ports are required to participate.[4] An *outbreak* is defined as events in which 3% or more of the passengers or crew report symptoms of diarrheal disease to the ship's medical staff during the voyage. Between 2009 and 2013, 68 outbreaks were reported; of these outbreaks, 51 (75%) were caused by norovirus.[5] The predominance of norovirus outbreaks represents a shift in epidemiology from infections before the turn of the twentieth century, when a larger proportion of outbreaks were due to bacterial sources.[6]

Norovirus is highly infectious and can spread rapidly on a cruise ship because of its survivability, low infective dose, easy transmissibility, prolonged viral shedding, and the absence of long-term host immunity. Norovirus can spread from person to person or through contaminated food or water.[7] Other causes of gastrointestinal outbreaks on cruise ships include *Salmonella*, enterotoxigenic *Escherichia coli*, *Shigella*, *Vibrio*, *Staphylococcus aureus*, *Clostridium perfringens*, *Cyclospora*, hepatitis E virus, and *Trichinella*.[4] Outbreaks of gastrointestinal illnesses can be caused by contaminated water supplies, inadequate water disinfection, or improper food handling. Proper ship design and construction, especially of potable water storage tanks, is paramount for water safety. The encouragement of hand washing or hand gel disinfectant use by passengers and crew as well as isolation of passengers with gastroenteritis symptoms are methods employed by cruise ships to control the spread of these highly infectious, transmittable illnesses.[7]

Respiratory Illness

Even though the most common illness that afflicts passengers and crew aboard cruise ships is gastroenteritis, respiratory infections comprise about one third of sick bay visits.[8] Respiratory infections, including viral upper respiratory infections and influenza, are common among cruise ship passengers. These viruses can occur year-round on cruise ships because passengers and crew members come from different regions of the world, where climate differences make these viruses prevalent during different seasons. Outbreaks of pandemic (H1N1) and other strains of influenza have been reported on cruise ships.[9,10]

Legionella species can invade a ship's water, including showers and whirlpool spas.[11] This infection has the potential to cause significant outbreaks of pneumonia (i.e., Legionnaire's disease), especially for travelers who are older or have underlying medical problems. *Legionella* is spread through aerosolized water, not person to person, and symptoms can take 2 to 10 days to present, making diagnosis and prompt antibiotic treatment difficult.[4] Over 200 cases and 50 incidents of *Legionella* cases on cruise ships have been reported over the last 30 years. Cruise ships may do urine antigen testing for *Legionella*, and sputum cultures can also be performed to confirm the diagnosis.

Other Diseases

Vaccine-preventable and vector-borne illnesses comprise the final category. Diseases that are encountered infrequently in most developed countries may occur on cruise ships, as crew members may come from countries with low immunization rates. Approximately 11% to 13% of cruise ship crew members who have been tested for rubella or varicella have been shown to have susceptibility.[4] A 1997 outbreak of rubella among crew members mostly from countries that did not have routine immunization programs serves as a reminder that unanticipated outbreaks can arise in close quarters.[12]

Vector-spread diseases, such as malaria, dengue, and yellow fever, can be endemic at ports where cruise ships dock and patients disembark.[2] This risk can be minimized by encouraging passengers to use insect repellant, to wear appropriate protective clothing, and to take chemoprophylactic medications when traveling to endemic areas. Fortunately, it is unlikely that these pathogens will cause an outbreak.

◀◀ PRE-INCIDENT ACTIONS

Prevention is the single most important action that can be taken to avoid an infectious disease outbreak. The VSP inspects cruise ships with both periodic and unannounced sanitation inspections, monitors gastrointestinal illnesses, investigates/responds to outbreaks, trains cruise ship employees on public health practices, and provides general health education.[4] Under the VSP, each cruise ship medical staff member is required to maintain a log of reported cases of gastrointestinal illness. These reports must be submitted 24 to 36 hours prior to arriving in the United States or closer to the arrival time if an outbreak is identified; these reports must be made even when no cases of diarrheal illness occur. Cruise lines are also responsible for developing an outbreak prevention and response plan that includes a trigger that determines when the plan is to be activated and provides detailed infection control procedures for the ship.[13]

It is essential that cruise lines use adequate infection control measures, including proper disinfection, filtering, and storage of water and regular maintenance of spas and ventilation systems to prevent the spread of airborne infections. The World Health Organization (WHO) maintains a *Guide to Ship Sanitation*, which was last updated in 2011 and includes detailed preventative measures.[7]

The provision of onboard health care facilities that are capable of treating patients during outbreaks is another important pre-incident step. The American College of Emergency Physicians has a section dedicated to cruise ship medicine.[14] This organization has published guidelines for cruise ship medical facilities, which were last updated in 2013, that delineate recommended practices.[15] Although the guidelines do not identify specifics regarding outbreaks, they do recommend that ships have properly trained physicians and nurses, adequate medical equipment, an isolation room, gastrointestinal and respiratory system medications (including appropriate antibiotics and the ability to provide oral or intravenous hydration), and an emergency preparedness plan. The guidelines also recommend an infection control program, including screening crew for tuberculosis and providing immunizations for hepatitis B and seasonal influenza.

▶▶ POST-INCIDENT ACTIONS

Once an outbreak is identified, it is crucial that a predetermined decontamination plan is initiated immediately.[6] Rapid implementation of control measures at the first sign of a suspected outbreak is fundamental for three important reasons: (1) many people share the same water, food, and environment and are at risk for infection; (2) the ship's medical resources can quickly become overwhelmed in an outbreak; and (3)

without intervention, the infection can spread to subsequent cruises.[16] The VSP and WHO operation manuals both delineate detailed steps in the case of an outbreak.[16,7]

After an outbreak, international quarantine regulations dictate that the master of the ship traveling to a U.S. port report to the closest quarantine station. The VSP's investigation is composed of three phases: (1) an epidemiologic investigation, in which interviews and questionnaires are performed; (2) a laboratory investigation to determine the causative agent; and (3) an environmental health investigation, in which the source of transmission, which is usually water, food, or air, is analyzed. After the investigation is complete, the information, including recommendations for control and prevention, is sent to the cruise line.

Once an outbreak occurs, prompt disinfection of the ship and, if possible, isolation of ill crew members and passengers for 72 hours after clinical recovery are ideal. Suitable disinfectants, such as chlorine, phenol-based compounds, or accelerated hydrogen peroxide products, should be used to disinfect the ship.[6] Further, the staff should remind passengers and crew members to perform frequent, rigorous hand washing with soap and water. Healthy disembarking passengers should be informed of the incident and provided with advice and information about the outbreak should they become sick.[17]

✚ MEDICAL TREATMENT OF CASUALTIES

The first problem facing the medical staff and crew of the ship is the logistics of treating hundreds of casualties onboard and finding an appropriate docking port. The ship's medical staff members will be forced to ration care as they balance resources with the number of afflicted patients. The most seriously affected victims should receive care first. For instance, those who are very young, very old, or significantly dehydrated should receive intravenous fluid before others. The crew should locate a suitable port where hundreds of casualties can most easily obtain care. If there is a choice, the ship should not dock at a small port if a larger port near a large city is available. Calling ahead and warning the receiving port is also crucial.

The treatment of the casualties should be tailored to the individual disease process. For patients with viral gastroenteritis, only supportive care is necessary. Norovirus illness lasts 12 to 60 hours and is typically accompanied by the sudden onset of nausea, vomiting, and watery diarrhea. The incubation period of this illness is 12 to 48 hours. No specific treatment or vaccine exists.[6] Even though the disease is generally self-limited, viral gastroenteritis may cause more severe illness in children, elderly persons, and persons with serious underlying medical conditions. Treatment should include oral rehydration for mild cases and intravenous fluid for patients with more significant dehydration. If the cause is determined to be bacterial, appropriate antibiotics (e.g., ciprofloxacin) should be administered to the affected passengers.

Other treatments will depend on the infectious agent. Legionnaires disease may present with symptoms that range from a mild febrile illness to a severe pneumonia with malaise, cough, and gastrointestinal symptoms.[18] Standard pneumonia antibiotic therapies, such as azithromycin or levofloxacin, are curative, and these medications should be stocked on the ship. Regardless of the etiology, air evacuation is indicated for very ill patients.[19]

❓ UNIQUE CONSIDERATIONS

Cruise ships are closed spaces, and the combination of thousands of people contained for several days in this space represents an opportunity for infection to spread rapidly. Only limited resources are available onboard, so a ship's medical bay may quickly become overwhelmed during an outbreak. Ships often visit ports in countries where infectious disease is more prevalent than it is in the United States, so the potential for bringing an agent onboard is elevated. In addition, the background of the crew is often diverse, and some crew members may have increased susceptibility to diseases, depending on immunization status.

Although there have been no reported incidents of bioterrorism on cruise ships, this possibility cannot be excluded. A cruise ship might become a means for an infectious disease agent to be purposefully transmitted into a country. Increased vigilance among the ship's crew and medical staff is indicated.

An infectious disease outbreak may represent a huge financial loss to a cruise line because cruises may need to be cancelled and future passengers may be less likely to travel on an affected line. Again, preventative measures are essential.

! PITFALLS

Several potential pitfalls exist in response to an outbreak of infectious disease aboard a cruise ship. These include the following:
- Failure to properly staff and supply the ship's medical clinic
- Failure to recognize or report an infectious disease outbreak
- Failure to quickly isolate and treat affected passengers and crew
- Failure to properly sanitize the ship after an outbreak
- Failure to create a plan for mass treatment in the event of an outbreak, including provisions for airlifting patients out or supplies in

REFERENCES

1. Quarantine. Available at: http://en.wikipedia.org/wiki/Quarantine.
2. Minooee A, Rickman LS. Infectious diseases on cruise ships. *Clin Infect Dis.* 1999 Oct;29(4):737–743.
3. Cruise Lines International Association, Inc. Available at: http://www.cruising.org/regulatory/industry-welcome.
4. Slaten DD, Mitruka K. Cruise ship travel. Available at: http://wwwnc.cdc.gov/travel/yellowbook/2014/chapter-6-conveyance-and-transportation-issues/cruise-ship-travel.
5. Centers for Disease Control and Prevention. Outbreak updates for international cruise ships. Available at: http://www.cdc.gov/nceh/vsp/surv/gilist.htm.
6. Centers for Disease Control and Prevention. Outbreaks of gastroenteritis associated with noroviruses on cruise ships—United States, 2002. *MMWR Morb Mortal Wkly Rep.* 2002;51:1112–1115.
7. World Health Organization. Guide to ship sanitation (third edition). Available at: http://www.who.int/water_sanitation_health/publications/2011/ship_sanitation_guide/en.
8. Peake DE, Gray CL, Ludwig MR, et al. Descriptive epidemiology of injury and illness among cruise ship passengers. *Ann Emerg Med.* 1999;33:67–72.
9. Ward KA, Armstrong P, McAnulty JM, et al. Outbreaks of pandemic (H1N1) 2009 and seasonal influenza A (H3N2) on cruise ship. *Emerg Infect Dis.* 2010 Nov;16(11):1731–1737.
10. Brotherton JM, Delpech VC, Gilbert GL, et al. A large outbreak of influenza A and B on a cruise ship causing widespread morbidity. *Epidemiol Infect.* 2003;130:263–271.
11. Centers for Disease Control and Prevention. Cruise-ship—associated Legionnaires disease, November 2003-May 2004. *MMWR Morb Mortal Wkly Rep.* 2005 Nov 18;54(45):1153–1155.
12. Centers for Disease Control and Prevention. Rubella among crew members of commercial cruise ships—Florida, 1997. *MMWR Morb Mortal Wkly Rep.* 1998 Jan 9;46(52-53):1247–1250.
13. Centers for Disease Control and Prevention. Gastrointestinal illness surveillance and outbreak investigations. Available at: http://www.cdc.gov/nceh/vsp/desc/about_investigations.htm.
14. American College of Emergency Physicians. Cruise Ship Medicine Section. Available at: https://www.acep.org/content.aspx?id=24928.
15. American College of Emergency Physicians. Health care guidelines for cruise ship medical facilities. Available at: http://www.acep.org/Content.aspx?id=29980.
16. Centers for Disease Control and Prevention. About the Vessel Sanitation Program. Available at: http://www.cdc.gov/nceh/vsp/desc/aboutvsp.htm.
17. Sedgwick J, Joseph C, Chandrakumar M, et al. Outbreak of respiratory infection on a cruise ship. *Euro Surveill.* 2007 Aug 9;12(8), E070809.1.
18. de Jong B, Payne Hallström L, Robesyn E, et al. Travel-associated Legionnaires' disease in Europe, 2010. *Euro Surveill.* 2013 Jun;6:18(23).
19. Prina LD, Orzai UN, Weber RE. Evaluation of emergency air evacuation of critically ill patients from cruise ships. *J Travel Med.* 2001;8:285–292.

Massive Power System Failures

M. Kathleen Stewart and Charles Stewart

📄 DESCRIPTION OF EVENT

A massive power outage is a widespread interruption or loss of electrical service caused by accident, sabotage, natural hazards, or equipment failure. A *significant power failure* is defined as any incident of a long duration that would require the involvement of the local and/or state emergency management organizations to coordinate provision of food, water, heating, shelter, etc. This is not an uncommon event (a Wikipedia entry on major power outages lists 77 such power outages, causing greater than 1,000,000 people-hours of electrical disruption in the past 10 years).[1] Causes of electric power outages can be natural, such as lightning, high winds, ice storms, hurricanes, floods, and human error, as well as either accidents or deliberate sabotage or attack of the power system.[2-7] In some cases, these power failures have been massive and prolonged, creating their own addition to an ongoing disaster such as a flood. In other cases, they have been the sole contributor to the disaster. Clinical operations within the health care facility are dependent on electronic equipment, electrically operated devices, and electrically controlled and powered environmental conditioning. Injuries due to the direct effect of a power failure, hypothermia and hyperthermia, and indirect effects and injuries as citizens attempt to cope with generalized loss of electrical power will occur.

This chapter will discuss the potential causes of these massive power failures, how it may affect disaster operations, and some selected actions that a physician involved in the disaster might encounter. It should be stressed that this chapter is not exhaustive but rather is intended only to illustrate how the technology base of the world, and emergency medical services (EMS) in particular, is vulnerable.

A modern electric power system consists of six main components[8]:
1. The power station (may be hydroelectric, fossil fuel, nuclear, solar, wind-driven, or some other central power generation technique)
2. A set of large transformers to raise the generated power to the high voltages used on the transmission lines—may include substations to direct power along alternative pathways (the grid)
3. The transmission lines
4. The substations at which the transmitted power is stepped down to the voltage on the distribution lines and distributed to the local area
5. The distribution lines (overhead or underground neighborhood power-distribution wiring)
6. The transformers that lower the distribution voltage to the level used by the consumers' equipment

Electricity generation stations throughout the United States are interconnected via power grids. This allows electricity generated in one state to be sent to users in another state. It also allows distant power generation stations to provide electricity for cities and towns whose power generators may have failed or been destroyed by some accident or sabotage. This distribution, of course, requires surplus power generation capacity in one or more areas.

In the United States, the electric system is divided into three grid systems: the northeastern grid, the western grid, and the Texas grid. Two major power subgrids, the Ontario-New York-New England pool and the Pennsylvania-New Jersey-Maryland pool (the PJM interconnection), together make up the northeast power grid. Power from these stations is moved around the country on almost a half million miles of bulk transmission lines that carry high-voltage electricity.

In a typical system, the generators at the power station deliver a voltage of 1000 to 26,000 V of alternating current power. (Alternating current is used because it is technically much easier to step up and step down for economy of transmission.) From the high-voltage transmission lines of the power grid, electric power is transmitted to regional substations. Transformers step this voltage up to values ranging from 120,000 to 750,000 V for the long-distance primary transmission line because higher voltages can be transmitted more efficiently over long distances. At the regional substation, the voltage can be transformed down to levels of 69,000 to 138,000 V. Another set of transformers at neighborhood substations step the voltage down again to a distribution level such as 2400 or 4160 V or 15, 27, or 33 kV. Finally, the voltage is transformed once again at the distribution transformer near the point of use to a voltage that can be used in homes, hospitals, and offices (220 to 1200 V).

Power transmission may be lost or destroyed at any point during the transmission process. Natural hazards such as earthquakes; tsunami and other floods; windstorms such as hurricanes and tornados; and ice storms can destroy the transmission of power and affect wide swaths of the populace. Solar flares can cause widespread destruction of power generation and transmission.

Natural Hazards

The Japanese earthquake and subsequent tsunami caused widespread damage at all levels of the power-distribution grid. Local distribution lines, substations, long-distance transmission lines, and even power sources, such as the Fukushima reactors, were destroyed by the combination of quake damage and subsequent flooding.[9,10] (A visual graphic from NASA shows this widespread power loss and is available at: http://earthobservatory.nasa.gov/NaturalHazards/view.php?id=49773.) Similar destruction of generating capability, long-distance transmission lines, step down substations, and local distribution lines occurs because of the widespread windstorms and subsequent flooding seen with hurricanes and cyclones.[11-15] Destruction that may involve all parts of the power transmission system occurs in the pathway of a tornado.[16]

Ice storms, however, destroy local distribution lines and long-distance lines preferentially. A half inch of ice on a tree branch or on power lines can add hundreds of pounds of weight, resulting in breakage of either the tree branch or the power line. More ice can topple transmission line towers. As the ice-laden bough breaks, it can damage power lines, power poles, and even substation transformers.

In addition, these ice-laden boughs are conductive and may result in transformer overload and subsequent failure or even destruction. Freezing rain in Oklahoma led to over 1 million customers without power in 2007.[17] Repair of lines and damaged poles/towers kept some customers without power for up to 47 days during the middle of winter.

An electromagnetic pulse (EMP) induced by a solar flare or coronal mass ejection was described in 1849 by Richard Carrington.[18] Ground currents induced during severe geomagnetic storms can actually melt the copper windings of transformers at the heart of many power-distribution systems. Sprawling power lines act like antennas, picking up the currents and spreading the problem over a wide area.[19] Similar, smaller, events have caused massive power failure in multiple areas, with damage to all parts of the power generation and distribution chain. The most recent severe solar flare event occurred in 1989, causing widespread damage to the power grid in Quebec. In March of 1989, a solar flare struck North America, 90 seconds after the flare struck, the entire province of Quebec was without power.[18] It is estimated that a coronal mass ejection event of Carrington size occurs somewhere between every 200 and 500 years.

Terrorism and Military Actions

The towers that carry high-voltage lines present the easiest pathway for a terrorist to destroy the power system.[20] Only modest amounts of conventional explosives detonated at two to three transmission towers are sufficient to interrupt a high-voltage transmission line. Recent vandalism (or possible localized terrorism) has shown that this can be accomplished with only a tractor.[21] Repair and replacement of the towers and connecting high-voltage lines may take days to weeks.

Simple explosives can easily be used to sabotage any above-ground high-voltage power-distribution system. A below-ground system is somewhat more difficult to access and has some additional security afforded by this limited access. Although this tactic will destroy the distribution system, it will not destroy the equipment that it powers. In this regard, the consequences will be similar to those of a naturally occurring event.

Rifle fire appears to be a greater threat than cyberterrorism.[22] Other possible terrorist incidents have also shown that long-distance rifle fire can destroy transformers simply by causing them to leak cooling oil through bullet holes.[22] When the transformer overheats, it may simply shut down, or it may be destroyed. For larger transformers, replacements may not be readily available; they have long lead times for construction and may be technically difficult to replace. The leakage of complex cooling oils lends another dimension to the act of sabotage: cleanup of the environment may be expensive and prolonged.

Another device, graphite bombs, works by exploding a cloud of thousands of electrically conducting carbon-fiber wires over electric installations and power-distribution systems. This short-circuits the electric systems. A graphite bomb (sometimes called a G-bomb) was used in the 1991 Gulf War to successfully disable 85% of Iraq's power supply. The North Atlantic Treaty Organization (NATO) used a later version in May 1999, to successfully disable 70% of Serbia's power supply.[23] These bombs will destroy the distribution system, but not the equipment that it powers.

ELECTROMAGNETIC PULSE

Finally, EMP devices can be used to cause massive power failures similar to those caused by a "Carrington Event."[19] When "detonated," an EMP weapon (also known as an E-bomb) generates a powerful pulse of energy capable of short-circuiting a wide range of electronic equipment, including computers (even those contained in ignition circuits in cars and trucks and those that operate traffic lights), radios, and public utility power supplies. These weapons can disable practically any non-shielded modern electronic device within the effective range of the weapon. (Some military-grade electronics are designed to resist EMPs, but most civilian equipment is not adequately shielded from this type of attack.) The damage from burnout or overload of the electronic circuits would extend far beyond the area directly affected by the blast and radiation of the EMP.

Commercial computer equipment is particularly sensitive to EMPs, as are UHF and VHF radio receivers, televisions, and cell phones.[24] The consequences of disabling such equipment are mind boggling for the now technology-dependent health care community.[25] However, although devastating to electronic equipment, EMPs, at least in theory, do not hurt humans.[25]

Three basic types of EMP weapons exist: nuclear weapons, flux compression generators, and high-power microwave generators.[24,26-31] Although an in-depth discussion of each is beyond the scope of this chapter, each weapon would create differing levels of havoc, ranging from continent-wide to relatively local effects. Those who have only basic engineering and technical skills can harness EMP technology. EMP weapons can be built with materials available to governments and terrorists alike. Fully developed, ready-to-deploy weapons may be available to clandestine markets at any time. Because the United States has actually deployed such a weapon (in Desert Storm, an EMP designed to mimic the flash of electricity from a nuclear bomb was used), it is quite possible that the design is available to terrorist nations today.[24,26-30] EMP devices are highly portable and can even be operated from a distance. Detonating the EMP in the air or near the top floors of a skyscraper maximizes the effects of the weapon, and the effects may occur at quite some distance from the detonation.

◀ PRE-INCIDENT ACTIONS

Even before the terrorist attacks of September 2001, disaster planning in U.S. hospitals was designed primarily for external disasters involving large-scale trauma or mass casualties; for example, airline crashes, radiation accidents, or outbreaks of infectious diseases. Although it is certainly necessary to plan for such events, catastrophic power failures are actually more likely to involve in-hospital scenarios. By the 1960s, engineers and architects began sealing off buildings from the outdoors, constructing mechanical environments solely controlled by electric power. When this power supply fails, the modern hospital may become totally uninhabitable. When windows cannot be opened, and the only heat or cooling is electrical, power failure may rapidly degrade available medical care.

Preparation for an Unscheduled Power Outage

In the United States, each health care facility must have an emergency power testing program that includes generator load testing and emergency power supply system (EPSS) maintenance. The Joint Commission revised its standards in 2007 to require hospitals to test their emergency generators at least once every 36 months for a minimum of four continuous hours.[32] This testing is over and beyond the prior requirement to test emergency generators for 30 continuous minutes, 12 times each year. The National Fire Protection Association (NFPA) establishes codes and standards on the minimum design, installation, and testing of these systems in the National Electric Code (NFPA 70 contains wiring requirements for standby power supplies), the Standard on Health Care Facilities (NFPA 99), and the Standard for Emergency and Standby Power Systems (NFPA 110).[33-35] EPSSs meeting the NFPA codes and standards are designed for immediate life safety: in other words, to complete surgical or other procedures where lives are in balance or to evacuate the building in case of fire. These systems should be designed to "hold out" until normal power is restored.

The disaster planner must not only consider the usual devices such as lights and power to critical areas but also take steps to ensure against unintended actions when power is restored.[36] Fiscal restraints often prevent hospitals from spending adequately on emergency power protection. Hospital accountants do not consider absolutely fail-safe 24-hour power for hospitals to be cost-effective. Ironically, when hospitals do provide power protection, it is often used to protect their data systems, not their critical care systems.

Devices expected to operate when the power fails need to be inspected, maintained, and tested as part of an equipment preventive maintenance program. Plans and checklists to maintain critical services need to be prepared, implemented, and tested. This includes rapid deployment of battery-powered equipment such as suction units and lights to appropriate hospital locations and ensuring that critical equipment is actually plugged into the protected power outlet and that critical refrigerators have both appropriate power supply and appropriate monitoring of ongoing temperatures to make sure that power is actually being delivered to these areas.

Many hospitals test their EPSSs at night or early in the morning before the bulk of the hospital's daily activities begin. This test time is often chosen because it is one of low clinical activity and will, therefore, cause less disruption, but normal or peak clinical loads will not be reflected in this EPSS test loading. Many hospitals do not test their EPSSs when their operating rooms are in use. In addition, the mechanical, building, radiology, and other clinical processes all vary during a typical hospital day.

Protective Measures Against an Electromagnetic Pulse Device or Carrington Event

It is difficult to protect against an EMP weapon without purchasing military-grade communications equipment.[37,38] Vehicles require computers to satisfy U.S. Environmental Protection Agency requirements, and these computers are vulnerable. Some anti-EMP measures that EMS providers can take include the following:

1. Build a Faraday cage. A Faraday cage can be made from fine metal mesh that is connected to a ground wire and completely encloses the items to be protected. If any power cables, data cables, or antennas go into the cage, it may be rendered worthless. Keep all equipment in the cage disconnected from batteries and other power supplies and not in contact with the Faraday cage.
2. Maintain a supply of spare radio, monitor, and engine ignition spare parts, including spare automotive computer boards of the type used in the most common ambulance and/or fire vehicle. Keep the spare parts in the Faraday cage.
3. Use one system at a time during a threat period. Disconnect other systems from power and antennas and keep them in the Faraday cage.
4. If your vehicle ignition fails, disconnect the negative battery terminal, wait 2 minutes, and attempt to restart the vehicle. Some computerized ignition systems on late-model cars might be reset in this way.

Continuity of Critical Services

Backup power generators and uninterruptible power supplies should be selected and installed by qualified electric service contractors and then coordinated with the electric utility company. It is particularly important to avoid improper switching from one power supply to another. This can lead to power feedback into the regular power system, resulting in damage to equipment and the generator itself. These requirements are covered in the NFPA codes cited above.

As plentiful and redundant as backup power sounds, diesel generators alone cannot provide fail-safe backup power to protect hospital

patients. The lag between utility shutdown and generator power startup may destroy computerized diagnostic and life-support equipment. Even a 3-second disruption can be perilous to this sensitive electronic equipment. For this same reason, electric engineers and contractors like to specify uninterruptible power supplies to protect vital equipment from even brief disruptions.

Finally, preparation for long-term power outage must include provision of fuel for the emergency generator(s) and maintenance of the generators. As hospitals in Oklahoma rapidly found out, emergency fuel suppliers may be compromised when the roads are blocked with fallen branches, and fuel may not be readily available due to failure of pumps to load trucks, of pumps for diesel fuel for the truck, or of foresight of the emergency manager to arrange for refueling beyond 72 hours after initiation of the emergency. After 72 hours of continuous operation, emergency generators start to require service and maintenance (such as oil changes). This leads to periods of generator down time.

Assess the need for additional redundancy through portable, truck-mounted generators, and develop procedures to isolate generators from problem areas and to tie in supplemental equipment not normally fed by emergency power. In addition, consider designing in emergency connection panels. These might, for example, be used to hook up a truck-mounted unit during maintenance or repair of the main emergency generator.

▶▶ POST-INCIDENT ACTIONS

When the power is restored, the following equipment and checklists will be useful:

- List manually operated switches that may need to be placed in the *off* position.
- List valves that need to be checked for proper position.
- List utilities such as steam, radio, telephone, computers, and pager communications that need to be verified for operability after the power is restored.
- List automatic starting equipment that should be shut down for safety and to minimize load demand when the power is restored.
- To prevent carbon monoxide poisoning, use generators, pressure washers, grills, and similar items outdoors only.
- If the power is out longer than 2 hours, throw away food that has a temperature higher than 40 °F.
- Check with local authorities to be sure that your water is safe.
- In hot weather, stay cool and drink plenty of fluids to prevent heat-related illness.
- In cold weather, wear layers of clothing, which help to keep in body heat.
- Avoid power lines and use electric tools and appliances safely to prevent electrical shock.

✚ MEDICAL TREATMENT OF CASUALTIES

Power outages may cause differing types of injuries. In more rural areas, victims may be trapped for prolonged periods of time without adequate food, water, and medications. In colder climates, this may also result in casualties due to exposure. The risk and type of injury to the general population will be determined by the area in which the power outage strikes. Long-term power outage in hot weather may lead to a spike in heat-associated illnesses, while long-term power outage in cold weather may lead to spikes in burns and carbon monoxide poisoning, as well as cold-related injuries and hypothermia. Those with respiratory diseases are at particular risk as nebulizers, and oxygen concentrators fail. Likewise, the elderly are often significantly affected by hypothermia caused by power outage.

Risks to Worker Safety and Health

Workers operate machines and power tools and are engaged in chemical processes. These workers could be at risk of injury, exposure to dangerous chemicals, or death from a sudden loss of power without immediate restoration of power for vital systems.

People may sustain injuries when trapped in elevators, subways, and mass transit systems. Many of these injuries are sustained during attempts to get out of the local environment to a "safer" area.

During recovery from the 2007 ice storm, a marked increase in chainsaw-related injuries occurred as residents and day-labor workers who were untrained in chainsaw use attempted to remove fallen limbs. Likewise, an increase in fall-related injuries occurred not just due to the ice on the ground, sidewalks, and streets but also from workers who were attempting to remove fallen tree limbs from overhead structures under icy and cold conditions. Similar injuries were seen following Hurricane Katrina during cleanup operations.

Risks to Hospital Patients

Ventilator-dependent patients will need supplemental breathing equipment, such as a bag-valve-mask operated by qualified personnel. Some ventilators have built-in, short-term uninterruptible power supplies and may supply oxygen to patients for a few moments after the power fails. Operating room equipment may fail, and patients within the operating room may be subjected to increased danger as surgeons attempt to complete operations with failing light. Some equipment, such as a heart-lung bypass machine, is mission critical and should be protected by an uninterruptible power supply. Other equipment, such as lights, can be operated by battery power after a short interval of power outage without damage. Infants and critical patients such as burn patients may be subject to hypothermia or hyperthermia as incubator and heating/air conditioning fails. Dialysis may become problematic. Laboratory equipment, particularly computerized equipment, may not adequately survive a power loss of only a few seconds. This equipment must be protected by uninterruptible power supply to ensure that data being tested are not lost or degraded.

? UNIQUE CONSIDERATIONS

During extended power outage in cold weather, residents may turn to alternative methods of heating and food preparation. These alternative methods will cause a marked increase in patients with carbon monoxide poisoning and household/apartment fires with subsequent burns. Carbon monoxide may also be produced by running small generators indoors or in attached garages. During the 2007 ice storm, a larger number of Latino patients were seen with carbon monoxide poisoning. Subsequent interventions included directing warnings in Spanish over radio and TV stations that normally serviced the Spanish-speaking population.[39]

Alternative heating methods also increase the number of household/apartment fires as residents attempt to heat local areas with kerosene or other heaters. Food preparation with grills brought indoors can lead to either fire or carbon monoxide poisoning.

Qualified electrician services will be at a premium after an ice storm, tornado, or hurricane destroys local electrical service connections. Amateur efforts to reconnect services can cause electrocutions, fires, and injuries due to falls.

Catastrophic power failure caused by EMP devices or to a lesser degree by flooding may require replacement of all computerized circuitry within the equipment. This means that ambulances may not be operable until the computer ignition control circuitry has been replaced. It may also mean that every computerized piece of equipment from cardiac monitors to laboratory devices within the hospital may need to be replaced.

During the Oklahoma ice storm of 2007, hospital emergency departments were havens with a warm building, warm water, warm food in the hospital cafeteria, and working TVs. Many people congregated in the ED simply for these services.

! PITFALLS

Several potential pitfalls exist in the response to a massive power system failure. These include the following:

- Ensure that the hospital standby generator is neither located in the basement in a flood-prone area nor on the upper floor where fuel cannot be pumped up with available devices. Ensure that the generator and fuel supplies have adequate security to prevent vandalism, sabotage, and pilferage.
- Check to ensure that automated drug supply cabinets will actually function during adverse power supply conditions or that keys to open them are readily available.
- Ensure that critical refrigerators are actually connected to backup power supplies and have appropriate monitoring devices to maintain safety for blood bank supplies and pharmacy supplies that require continuous refrigeration.
- Check that backup generators will run for prolonged periods at anticipated full load. This should be checked at least twice a year for at least 12 hours. As noted above, several hospital generators during the 2007 ice storm were required to operate for prolonged periods exceeding 72 hours and this has been addressed in Joint Commission requirements.
- Existing generators will fail under harsh conditions and extended use. Backup generator failure may be due to battery failure, insufficient fuel supplies, overheating, mechanical failure, or fuel pump failure. Many generators are *standby rated*, meaning that they can reliably perform for only 2 out of 24 hours. Ensure that plans for supplemental generators (truck- or trailer-mounted units) exist and that adequate preparations for connection of these units have been made.
- Ensure that contracts with fuel vendors place hospitals as high-priority customers during extended power outage.
- Ensure that crisis communication messages are prepared in advance for the dangers of carbon monoxide poisoning and fires due to inappropriate alternative heating/cooling techniques. Make sure that these messages are appropriately targeted in the intended recipients' language and communication venues.

REFERENCES

1. Major Power Outages. 2014. http://en.wikipedia.org/wiki/List_of_major_power_outages. Accessed 10.01.14.
2. Nates JL. Combined external and internal hospital disaster: impact and response in a Houston trauma center intensive care unit. *Crit Care Med*. Mar 2004;32(3):686–690.
3. Franklin C. What we learned when Allison turned out the big light. *Crit Care Med*. Mar 2004;32(3):884–885.
4. Lewis CP, Aghababian RV. Disaster planning, Part I. Overview of hospital and emergency department planning for internal and external disasters. *Emerg Med Clin North Am*. May 1996;14(2):439–452.
5. Dealing with power failure: how Spokane hospitals survived the ice storm. *Hosp Secur Saf Manage*. Mar 1997;17(11):3–4.
6. Milsten A. Hospital responses to acute-onset disasters: a review. *Prehosp Disaster Med*. Jan-Mar 2000;15(1):32–45.
7. Fawcett WJ, Blowers H, Wilson G. Complete power failure 2. *Anaesthesia*. Mar 2001;56(3):274.

8. Generator grid connection guide: an introduction to power systems and the connection process. In: Bones D, ed. *Perth*. Australia: Western Power; 2011. https://http://www.google.com/url?q=http://www.westernpower.com.au/documents/reportspublications/generator_grid_connection_guide.pdf&sa=U&ei=ykrYUpbEA9KxoQT-qoGIAQ&ved=0CAUQFjAA&client=internal-uds-cse&usg=AFQjCNGhAj0065rXeetOj_R6-_gHdKQE0Q, Accessed 10.01.14.

9. NASA. Japan earthquake and tsunami March 2011. *Earth Observatory*. http://earthobservatory.nasa.gov/NaturalHazards/view.php?id=49773. Accessed 15.01.14.

10. Defense Meteorological Satellite Program. Japan earthquake and tsunami March 2011. *National Geophysical Data Center*. Accessed 19.03.11.

11. Powers R, Evidence-based ED. Disaster Planning. *J Emerg Nurs*. Jun 2009;35(3):218–223, quiz 272–213.

12. Comstock RD, Mallonee S. Comparing reactions to two severe tornadoes in one Oklahoma community. *Disasters*. Sep 2005;29(3):277–287.

13. Han SR, Guikema SD, Quiring SM. Improving the predictive accuracy of hurricane power outage forecasts using generalized additive models. *Risk Anal*. Oct 2009;29(10):1443–1453.

14. Norcross ED, Elliott BM, Adams DB, Crawford FA. Impact of a major hurricane on surgical services in a university hospital. *Am Surg*. Jan 1993;59(1):28–33.

15. Congress US. *Office of Technology Assessment. Physical Vulnerability of Electric System to Natural Disasters and Sabotage OTA-E-453*. Washington, DC: U.S. Government Printing Office; 1990.

16. Brown SP, Kruger E, Bos J. *Investigation of the deaths and injuries resulting from the May 3rd, 1999 tornadoes. Injury Update*. Oklahoma City, OK: Injury Prevention Service, Oklahoma State Department of Health; 2000.

17. Almon SC. *December 2007 Ice Storm Summary*. Tulsa: 211 Heartline; 2008.

18. Solar Carrington Event Repeat Today Would Collapse Civilization. 2009. http://www.futurepundit.com/archives/006079.html. Accessed 26.06.11.

19. *High-Impact, Low-Frequency Event Risk to the North American Bulk Power System. A Jointly-Commissioned Summary Report of the North American Electric Reliability Corporation and the U.S. Department of Energy's November 2009 Workshop*. 2010.

20. Rose A, Oladosu G, Liao S-Y. *Regional Economic Impacts of Terrorist Attacks on the Electric Power System of Los Angeles 2005*. create.usc.edu/assets/pdf/51840.pdf. Accessed 10.01.14.

21. Anderson N. Hackers in the electric grid? Meh! Fear the dude with the stolen tractor. *ArsTechnica*. 2013. http://arstechnica.com/tech-policy/2013/10/hackers-in-the-electric-grid-meh-fear-the-dude-with-the-stolen-tractor/. Accessed 10.01.14.

22. CBS San Francisco. Vandalism At San Jose PG&E Substation Called. http://sanfrancisco.cbslocal.com/2013/04/16/gunshots-cause-oil-spill-at-san-jose-pge-substation/.

23. Rogers K. Are electromagnetic pulses terrorists' next weapon of choice? *Las Vegas Review-Journal*. 30, September, 2001.

24. McNeill JB, Weitz R. Electromagnetic pulse (EMP) attack: a preventable homeland security catastrophe. *Backgrounder*. 2008;2199:1–7.

25. Ross LH Jr, Mihelic FM. Healthcare vulnerabilities to electromagnetic pulse. *Am J Disaster Med*. Nov-Dec 2008;3(6):321–325.

26. McNeill JB. *Understanding the EMP threat could save your life. Family Security Measures.*; 2010, http://www.familysecuritymatters.org/publications/id.5801,css.print/pub_detail.asp.

27. Stewart S, Hughes N. *Gauging the Threat of an Electro-Magnetic Pulse Attack in the US*. 2010. http://www.businessinsider.com/gauging-the-threat-of-an-electro-magnetic-pulse-attack-in-the-us-2010-9. Accessed 16.07.11.

28. Thompson M. EMP: the next weapon of mass destruction? *Time*. 2010. http://www.time.com/time/printout/0,8816,1976224,00.html. Accessed 16.07.10.

29. Vandre RH, Klebers J, Tesche FM, Blanchard JP. Electromagnetic pulse (EMP), Part II: field-expedient ways to minimize its effects on field medical treatment facilities. *Mil Med*. 1993;158(5):285–289.

30. Vandre RH, Klebers J, Tesche FM, Blanchard JP. Electromagnetic pulse (EMP), Part I: effects on field medical equipment. *Mil Med*. 1993;158(4):233–236.

31. Glasstone S, Dolan PJ. Declassified data on effects of nuclear weapons and effective countermeasures against them: EMP radiation from nuclear space bursts in 1962. http://glasstone.blogspot.com/2006/03/emp-radiation-from-nuclear-space.html. Accessed 16.07.11.

32. Joint Commission. Preventing adverse events caused by emergency electrical power system failures. *Sentinel Event Alert*. 2006;(37). http://www.jointcommission.org/sentinel_event_alert_issue_37_preventing_adverse_events_caused_by_emergency_electrical_power_system_failures/. Accessed 10.01.14.

33. NFPA 70. *National Electric Code*. 2014 ed. Quincy, MA: NFPA; 2014.

34. NFPA 99. *Health Care Facilities Code*. 2012 ed. Quincy, MA: NFPA; 2012.

35. NFPA 110. *Standard for Emergency and Standby Power Systems*. 2013 ed. Quincy, MA: NFPA; 2013.

36. CBS News. Blackout by the numbers. 2003. http://www.cbc.ca/news/background/poweroutage/numbers.html.

37. Manto CL. Introduction to EMP all-hazards public safety planning and emerging requirements for 9-1-1 emergency communications centers. In: *2006 Congress for Technology Leadership*. Chicago, Ill; 2006.

38. Chapter 5: electromagnetic pulse protection. Department of Defense: United States Army, 2002 ed. *Vol TM 5-690: Grounding and Bonding in Command, Control, Communications, Computer, Intelligence, Surveillance, and Reconnaissance (C4ISR) Facilities*. Washington, DC: Government Printing House; 2002.

39. Ahlborn L, Franc JM. Tornado hazard communication disparities among Spanish-speaking individuals in an English-speaking community. *Prehosp Disaster Med*. Feb 2012;27(1):98–102.

SUGGESTED READINGS

1. Anderson GB, Bell ML. Lights out: impact of the August 2003 power outage on mortality in New York, NY. *Epidemiology*. Mar 2012;23(2):189–193.

CHAPTER 199

Hospital Power Outages

Marc C. Restuccia

DESCRIPTION OF EVENT

Loss of electrical power is likely to be a catastrophic event for a hospital. Electricity is necessary for the safe operation of all hospitals, for lighting; for equipment to diagnose conditions and treat patients, document medical records, and enter and acknowledge treatment orders; and for cooling and heating the environment. Hospitals are more dependent than ever on their information technology (IT) systems, which are sometimes housed several miles away and supplied by a different portion of the power grid. Without power, IT does not operate, resulting in a serious disruption in the operational capabilities of the hospital.

PRE-INCIDENT ACTIONS

Hospitals are required to have easily accessible disaster plans in place. Plans must be understood by all staff members, who ideally should participate in drills routinely. Such drills should not only occur during daylight hours on weekdays but also during all shifts, on all days. Among the scenarios envisioned, electrical power loss must be included in disaster plans. Ideally, a robust backup electricity-generating system should be available to the hospital at all times; however, events have shown that such systems are not always as reliable as assumed.[1] The disaster plan should include information on whether any power loss will be isolated, meaning that the hospital is surrounded by an infrastructure and facilities that retain their own power supplies, or if an outage will be a more widespread event, with adjacent facilities and populations losing power. Planning must include local and regional governments, emergency medical service(s) (EMS) agencies, and contiguous medical facilities. Loss of power may necessitate movement of patients, some of them potentially critically ill or injured, to other medical facilities, as well as triaging of incoming patients away from the affected institutions. Advanced planning with local, regional, state, and potentially even national agencies will ensure that implementation of the disaster plan is as smooth as possible during a significant power outage.

Loss of Electrical Power

A loss of electrical power can be extraordinarily disruptive to patient care and operations. In health care facilities, the number of critical patient-care and ancillary devices that are electrically powered is enormous. Interruption of reliable electrical power, even for a very short time, can be catastrophic. Computers, monitoring systems, laboratory instruments, and many more computer-driven devices do *not* function well with even a short loss of power. This vital dependence on electrical power creates a source of potential trouble in the event of a natural disaster, such as a hurricane, and it makes a hospital an inviting target for terrorist activities.

Multiple redundancies in the delivery of uninterrupted electrical power must be *immediately* available in the event of a power loss. As seen in the twenty-first-century "superstorm" hurricanes in Louisiana (Katrina, 2005) and New York (Sandy, 2012), placement of hospital backup generators on a ground floor or basement left them susceptible to flooding.[2] Systems and equipment that cannot function for even a short time without power must be identified in advance, and a contingency plan must be tried and tested for them. Uninterruptible power supplies should be in place for all patient-critical and "power-critical" pieces of equipment. Potential disasters (e.g., an extraordinary heat wave, a tornado, a hurricane, or a human-made event) must be identified and prepared for in advance, along with coping protocols. In the best-case scenario, a plan for mitigating risk is ready before a disaster occurs. Concerning loss of electrical power, advance planning is infinitely preferable to improvising after a disaster.

Pre-incident plans for the loss of electrical power should

- Be robust, well thought out, and well practiced
- Identify the primary source of electrical power and potential scenarios for its loss
- Identify alternative sources of electrical power, including uninterruptible power supplies for equipment unable to tolerate the time elapsed until emergency generators begin working, which is usually at least 3 seconds[1]
- Identify the locations of emergency generators, usually diesel motors, and determine that they are available in adequate numbers and/or capacity
- Provide for continued interfacing with electrical utilities and suppliers of electricity-generating equipment to ensure prompt response to a loss of power
- Provide for testing of the primary electric source and all emergency systems on an ongoing basis
- Mandate ongoing training of hospital personnel in the use of all of emergency backup electrical systems
- Ensure that adequate fuel is on hand or immediately accessible for any emergency electricity-generating systems
- Identify alternative methods of delivering care to patients and allowing staff members to function in the event of the failure of all electricity-generation capability
- Identify the command structure that would ultimately order the evacuation of the hospital patients to another facility, and drill all hospital personnel on using the designated incident command system (ICS)
- Identify and equipping a hospital emergency operations center (EOC), making allowances for the loss of all electrical power
- Identify alternative facilities for care of currently hospitalized patients and for the public who may seek routine or emergency care in the event of the loss of all electrical power

- Identify personnel to run alternative-care facilities, if needed
- Develop memoranda of understanding with other facilities covering such contingencies, including transfer of patients to those institutions
- Involve local EMS personnel in planning for the transfer of large numbers of patients
- Determine what group of patients, if any, can continue to be cared for at the affected facility
- Identify the means of informing the public about the nature of the emergency, its effect on the hospital, what services will and will not be available, and the expected duration of the emergency
- Identify which medications and vaccines are temperature dependent (most are) and make alternative plans for those thought to be most critical for the immediate care of inpatients
- Identify alternative means of feeding patients and staff

Loss of Heating and Cooling Capacity

Whether emergency loss of heating or cooling capacity is due to a natural event or a human-made event, the complexity of the disaster increases if multiple contiguous health care facilities are involved, thus greatly increasing the number of patients affected. In addition, the number of people in the local population requiring routine, ongoing, and especially emergency medical care would also increase substantially. Regional, state, and most likely federal responses would be required to mitigate the disaster.

Hospitals in colder climates must have emergency plans in place to protect staff members and patients should it become impossible to heat the buildings. In colder climates during the winter months, such a loss would affect quickly and adversely the ability of staff members to care for patients. In remote hospitals with no contiguous medical facilities, the difficulties in transferring patients would be magnified when there is no heating.

In the case of hospitals in warm, humid climates, loss of the ability to air condition effectively all buildings would lead to similar considerations. Staff members would find it harder to care for their patients, and patients themselves could easily become hyperthermic. In such climates, environmental conditions could quickly become problematic, with moisture accumulating on surfaces and mildew rapidly making conditions intolerable.[3]

Pre-incident actions necessary to prepare for a loss of heating or cooling consist of the following:
- Forming a well-planned and drilled disaster strategy
- Regularly testing the hospital's heating and cooling systems and identifying alternative mechanisms for regulating the facility's environment
- Identifying supplemental means to heat patient-care areas in the event of failure of all primary heating capabilities and identifying similar cooling mechanisms in the event of failure of the air-conditioning system
- Adopting the hospital ICS and drilling personnel in it; this must include identifying who should report to the EOC and developing a chain of command with clear functions, reporting lines, and expectations for each individual, including those in the EOC and those throughout the facility
- Identifying and equipping an EOC, being aware that communication is the weak link in most plans
- Identifying potential alternative sites or facilities for the care of currently hospitalized patients and for members of the public seeking health care during the emergency
- Identifying personnel to staff these alternative facilities (if needed)
- Developing memoranda of understanding with other institutions covering such contingencies, including local, regional, statewide,

and other facilities; contingency plans should include means of transferring patients to unaffected facilities
- Involving local EMS personnel in planning for the transfer of large numbers of patients
- Determining for which groups of patients, if any, care might be continued at the affected facility
- Determining how to best notify the public about the nature of the emergency, how it will affect them, what the capabilities are of the affected facility, and when a return to normal operations can be expected

✚ MEDICAL TREATMENT OF CASUALTIES

Electricity Loss

In the event of a loss of electrical power to a hospital, the first priorities are patients dependent on electrically driven life-support systems, such as breathing ventilators, intraaortic balloon pumps, intravenous infusion pumps for critically important medications (e.g., vasopressors), and operating-room equipment. In many cases, if all electrical power is lost, battery backup will be available for most of these devices. For patients using ventilators, lifesaving alternative means of ventilating include hand-powered bag-valve-mask ventilation and the Oxylator (Lifesaving Systems, Inc., Roswell, Georgia), an oxygen-powered nonelectrical ventilation device. Contingency plans for alternative, often portable, sources of electrical power for other devices should be in place. Preplanning, strong leadership, good communication, contingency plans, and commitment from all members of the hospital staff are essential.[4]

Cooling and Heating Loss

The loss of cooling power for a medical institution would not usually be expected to lead to an influx of new patients. The exception would be if the loss of cooling were due to an accident, human-made or natural, affecting a local or regional area, such as explosions, fires, earthquakes, hurricanes, and tornadoes. In such cases, local resources would be overwhelmed, and outside resources would be needed. It would take time to get these resources into place, so contingency plans should already exist to cover this gap so that the hospital can care for inpatients and new patients from the community and prepare for transferring patients to other unaffected facilities.

A loss of heating power engenders most of the same difficulties and issues occurring with a loss of cooling. A key difference is that in most cases, loss of the ability to heat the hospital in a colder climate will lead to the need to evacuate all inpatients and divert incoming patients.

❓ UNIQUE CONSIDERATIONS

Medical facilities are uniquely dependent on the continued availability of heating, cooling, and, most especially, electrical power. Loss of any of these is most certainly a cause for the implementation of the institution's disaster plan. Prior planning, contingency identification, practice, and commitment of all facility leaders and staff members are crucial to a positive outcome after an emergency.

❗ PITFALLS

Several potential pitfalls exist in the response to a hospital power outage, including the following:
- Failure of the disaster plan to address adequately the loss of heat, cooling, or electricity

- Failure to address alternative sources of cooling, heating, and, most especially, electrical power
- Lack of memoranda of understanding with other health care facilities regarding provision of support for the stricken institution
- Failure to inform and train medical and support staff members adequately in their expected roles during an electrical power loss
- Lack of training of staff members before a disaster occurs
- Failure to include the prehospital (EMS) system in predisaster planning
- Failure to continually test the system's response to a failure of heating, cooling, or electrical power; this would include failure to test backup systems
- Failure to evacuate the hospital soon after attempts to remedy the problem have failed

REFERENCES

1. Ornstein C. Why do hospital generators keep failing? *ProPublica*; 2012. Nov 1; Available at: http://www.propublica.org/article/why-do-hospitals-generators-keep-failing.
2. Rettner R. Why power is so tricky for hospitals during hurricanes. *LiveSciencecom*; 2012. Nov 1; Available at: http://www.livescience.com/24489-hospital-power-outages-hurricane-sandy.html.
3. CDC.gov [Internet]. *Indoor environmental quality: dampness and mold in buildings*. Atlanta, GA: Centers for Disease Control and Prevention; 2013. [updated October 13, 2013; cited December 16, 2014]. Available at: http://www.cdc.gov/niosh/topics/indoorenv/mold.html.
4. Beatty ME, Phelps S, Rohner MC, Weisfuse MI. Blackout of 2003: public health effects and emergency response. *Public Health Rep.* 2006;121:36–44.

Intentional Contamination of Water Supplies

Anas A. Khan and Patricia L. Meinhardt

DESCRIPTION OF EVENT

The terrorist events of September 11, 2001, followed by the multiple thwarted attempts of further attacks on Western society, have forced the public health and medical community, federal security and regulatory agencies, and state and local water utilities to consider the possibility of intentional contamination of U.S. water supplies as part of an organized effort to disrupt and damage important elements of the nation's infrastructure.[1-4] Water supplies and water distribution systems represent potential targets for terrorist activity in the United States because of the critical need for water in every sector of industrialized society.[2] Even short-term disruption of water services can significantly affect a community, and intentional contamination of a municipal water system as part of a terrorist attack could lead to serious medical, public health, and economic consequences. The magnitude of water service disruption for a community has been vividly demonstrated by the destruction of water supply systems in the Gulf of Mexico region as a result of Hurricane Katrina in 2005. As this massive hurricane illustrated, contamination of water with biological, chemical, or radiological agents has generally resulted from natural disasters, industrial pollution, or unintentional human-made accidents in the United States. However, the deliberate contamination of the wells, reservoirs, and other water sources for civilian populations has been used as a method of attack by opposing military forces throughout the history of war. Many armies have resorted to using this method of warfare, including the Romans, who contaminated the drinking water of their enemies with diseased cadavers and animal carcasses.[4] With enhanced technology and modern scientific advances, the mechanisms of dispersal of biological, chemical, and radiological warfare agents have expanded considerably and currently include water as a delivery mechanism. Whether advanced scientific techniques or ancient warfare methods are used by terrorists, overt and covert contamination of water supplies remains a potential public health threat for the U.S. population.

The plausibility of intentional contamination of water supplies as part of a terrorist attack has been reinforced by a congressional testimony, a consensus statement by a governmental review panel, and a joint Centers for Disease Control and Prevention (CDC) and Environmental Protection Agency (EPA) water advisory health alert.[5,6] As part of its 2002 congressional report, the National Research Council of the National Academy of Sciences concluded that water supply system contamination and disruption should be considered a possible terrorist threat in the United States.[5] On February 7, 2003, the national terrorism threat level was increased to "high risk" because of information received and analyzed by the federal intelligence community. Subsequent to this heightened alert, the CDC and EPA issued *Water Advisory in Response to the High Threat Level*, which describes the need for enhanced vigilance by the public health, medical, and water utility communities regarding the risk of a terrorist attack on the nation's water infrastructure.[6] Apprehension regarding a terrorist assault on drinking water systems has also been reinforced by arrests of suspects in 2002 and 2003 who were charged with threatening to contaminate municipal water supplies in the United States.[3,4]

Spectrum of Disease Resulting from Intentional Water Contamination

The biological, chemical, and radiological agents that have been designated as potential terrorist weapons may be dispersed through multiple exposure pathways, including water.[2,4,7-9] Recognizing and managing a waterborne disease outbreak and the health effects of exposure to water contaminants are diagnostic challenges under normal circumstances, but the challenge will be even more significant during an act of water terrorism.[10] Intentional contamination of water supplies with biological, chemical, or radiological agents may produce a broad spectrum of disease and involve virtually every organ system including, but not limited to, the gastrointestinal, respiratory, dermatologic, hematopoietic, immunologic, and nervous systems. In addition, waterborne agents may enter the body through various portals, including the following: (1) ingestion and aspiration of contaminated water, (2) dermal absorption of contaminated water during bathing activities, (3) inoculation of skin lesions from direct contact with contaminated water, (4) consumption of food directly contaminated by water during food preparation, and (5) consumption of contaminated food indirectly contaminated by water through uptake in the food chain or through agricultural practices.[4]

A key factor in the accurate diagnosis and appropriate management of disease resulting from intentional contamination of water supplies is inclusion of water by the health care provider as one possible exposure pathway for the dissemination of biological, chemical, and radiological agents at the time of initial case presentation. The categories of compounds that may cause a diverse spectrum of water-related disease during an act of water terrorism include many of the agents traditionally associated with other modes of delivery. Biological, chemical, and radiological agents that have been designated as possible terrorist agents of public health concern and include the potential for waterborne route of exposure and weaponized agent delivery are presented in Box 200-1.

PRE-INCIDENT ACTIONS

Although medical practitioners may not be able to prevent the first cases of illness or injury resulting from an act of intentional water contamination, they are positioned to play a critical role in minimizing the impact of such an event by practicing medicine with an increased index of suspicion that such an attack may occur in their community. To

BOX 200-1 Selected Biological, Chemical, and Radiological Agents That Include Water as a Potential Mode of Dispersal for Terrorism

Biological Agents
Bacterial Pathogens
Anthrax (*Bacillus anthracis*)
Brucellosis (*Brucella melitensis, Brucella suis, Brucella abortus, Brucella canis*—undulant or Malta fever)
Cholera (*Vibrio cholerae*)
Clostridium perfringens
Glanders (*Burkholderia mallei*—formerly *Pseudomonas mallei*)
Melioidosis (*Burkholderia pseudomallei*—formerly *Pseudomonas pseudomallei*)
Plague (*Yersinia pestis*)
Salmonella (*Salmonella typhimurium* and *Salmonella typhi*—acute gastroenteritis and typhoid fever)
Shigellosis (Shigella *dysenteriae* and other *Shigella* spp.)
Tularemia (*Francisella tularensis*)

Viral Pathogens
Hepatitis A virus (HAV)
Smallpox (*Variola major*)
Viral encephalitides (e.g., Venezuelan equine encephalomyelitis [VEE])
Viral hemorrhagic fevers (e.g., Ebola, Marburg, Lassa fever, Rift Valley fever, yellow fever, Hantavirus, and dengue fever)

Parasitic Pathogens
Cryptosporidiosis (*Cryptosporidium parvum* and other *Cryptosporidium* spp.)

Rickettsial and Rickettsial-Like Pathogens
Psittacosis (*Chlamydia psittaci*)
Q fever (*Coxiella burnetti*)
Typhus (*Rickettsia prowazekii*)

Biological Toxins
Bacterial Biotoxins
Clostridium botulinum toxins (collectively BTX)
Clostridium perfringens toxins
Staphylococcus enterotoxin B (SEB) (e.g., protein toxin from *Staphylococcus aureus*)

Fungal-Derived Biotoxins (Mycotoxins)
Aflatoxin (metabolite of *Aspergillus flavus*)
T-2 mycotoxin (extract from *Fusarium* spp.)
Anatoxin A (product of cyanobacteria, *Anabaena flos-aquae*)
Microcystins (products of cyanobacteria, *Microcystis* spp.)

Plant- and Algae-Derived Biotoxins
Ricin (extract from castor bean)

Marine Biotoxins
Saxitoxin (paralytic shellfish poisoning [PSP] or product of dinoflagellate, *Gonyaulax*)
Tetrodotoxin (neurotoxin from pufferfish spp.)

Chemical Agents
Nerve Agents ("Gases")
G agents (volatile)
GA (Tabun), GB (Sarin), GD (Soman)
V agents (nonvolatile)
VX

Vesicant and Skin-Blistering Agents
Lewisite L, L-1, L-2, L-3
Nitrogen mustards HN-1, HN-2, HN-3

Industrial and Agricultural Agents
Pesticides, persistent and nonpersistent
Dioxins, furans, polychlorinated biphenyls (PCBs)

Blood Agents (Asphyxiant or Systemic Agents)
Cyanide compounds
Hydrogen cyanide (AC)
Cyanogen chloride (CK)
Arsine compounds (arsenicals)
Ethyldichloroarsine (ED)
Phenyldichloroarsine (PD)

Incapacitating Agents (Psychotropic or Behavior-Altering Compounds)
CNS depressants (e.g., BZ [3-quinoclinidinyl benzilate] and similar compounds)
CNS stimulants (e.g., LSD [D-lysergic acid and diethylamide])
Dioxins, furans, polychlorinated biphenyls (PCBs)
Explosive nitro compounds and oxidizers (e.g., ammonium nitrate combined with fuel oil)
Flammable industrial gases and liquids (e.g., gasoline and propane)
Poisonous industrial gases, liquids, and solids (e.g., cyanides and nitriles)
Corrosive industrial acids and bases (e.g., nitric acid and sulfuric acid)

Radiological Agents
Radiation Terrorism Threat Scenarios
Nuclear blast
Detonation of suitcase-sized nuclear bomb
Nuclear reaction
Sabotage of nuclear power plant or "meltdown"
Radiation dispersal device (RDD or "dirty bomb" release)

Potential Exposure Pathways and Agent Source
External exposure
External radiation exposure from nuclides in the plume after detonation
External radiation and contamination from surface-deposited contamination and activation products
Personal contamination of skin and clothing
Internal contamination
    Internal contamination from plume inhalation due to nuclides in plume after detonation
    Internal contamination due to inhalation of resuspended contamination
    Internal contamination due to inhalation or ingestion from personal contamination
    Internal exposure due to ingestion of contaminated food and water
    Internal contamination through skin or wound absorption or deposition from contact with contaminated material, including water

Modified and reprinted with permission from *Physician Preparedness for Acts of Water Terrorism: An On-line Readiness Guide.* Available at: http://www.waterhealthconnection.org/bt.

prevent a missed diagnosis of a case of terrorism-related waterborne disease, it is vital that medical practitioners understand how water could act as a potential exposure pathway or mode of dispersal for biological, chemical, and radiological agents *before* an incident occurs.[4] Pre-incident preparedness by the medical community will be critical to reduce the following: (1) the public health impact of a water terrorism incident, (2) the secondary disruption to potable water availability and distribution, and (3) the psychological impact of the public's lack of confidence in water safety and quality after an incident of intentional contamination of water.[2,4] If pre-incident actions include terrorism preparedness and disaster readiness, educated medical and public health professionals may make the difference between a controlled response to a water terrorism event versus a public health crisis.[4,11]

It is important to note that a major effort has been undertaken to improve and enhance the ability to detect and characterize deliberate contamination of water systems in the United States as part of a collaborative effort by local water utilities and several federal public health agencies.[3,4,12] As a result, U.S. water systems are more physically secure than ever before, with multiple layers of enhanced protection. However, there are several potential points of contamination that could be targeted for acts of water terrorism. Therefore it is critically important for the medical community to have a basic understanding of these water system vulnerabilities in order to be able to complete an accurate exposure history when evaluating a suspected case of water-related disease. Various scientific consensus groups, public health agencies, and water utility specialists have outlined a series of potential points of contamination of the U.S. water supply and distribution system.[4,5] This information is summarized in Box 200-2 and acts as a valuable resource for health care providers and public health professionals when evaluating an unusual symptoms complex or an atypical illness pattern that may represent a case of waterborne terrorism.

▶▶ POST-INCIDENT ACTIONS

Although environmental monitoring of water supplies is improving rapidly, the most likely *initial indication* that a water terrorism incident has occurred may be an increased number of patients presenting to their health care providers or emergency department with unusual or unexplained illness or injury, a change in local disease trends and illness patterns, or a community-wide waterborne disease outbreak. Therefore health care providers and public health practitioners may be the first to discover that a waterborne release of biological, chemical, or radiological agents has occurred in a targeted population and must understand their critical role as "front-line responders" in detecting water-related disease resulting from terrorist activity.[4]

Certain clinical manifestations and disease syndromes may be characteristic of a terrorist attack in which biological, chemical, or radiological agents are used via a waterborne route. A heightened level of alertness and awareness by the medical community of these patterns of illness and clusters of disease may enhance the initial discovery of a waterborne terrorist attack and are critical to any post-incident action plan. Early and accurate clinical detection of a suspicious case of terrorism-related disease will be especially important for timely follow-up epidemiological investigations to be initiated and appropriate remediation and prevention efforts to be instituted by the public health and water utility communities.[4] During the post-incident period, health care practitioners will need to "think like an epidemiologist" when evaluating any suspect case or unusual pattern of disease in their clinical practice.[13] A medical practitioner's diagnostic acumen for recognizing waterborne disease resulting from intentional contamination of water can be augmented significantly by embracing this epidemiological approach. Several epidemiological patterns and sentinel clues

---

BOX 200-2 Possible Points of Intentional Contamination of U.S. Water

Health care providers should keep these sources of potential water contamination and unusual modes of delivery of biological, chemical, and radiological agents in mind when evaluating a suspected case of terrorism-related disease:

- *Upstream of a community water supply system or collection point:* Water supply systems are composed of small streams and bodies of water, rivers, service reservoirs, aquifers, wells, and dams that may act as points of deliberate contamination of water.
- *Community water supply intake access point or water treatment plant:* Many water supply systems are designed to receive water from source water reserves at a central intake point, with this source water being subsequently filtered and sanitized at the community water treatment facility for eventual distribution as potable water. Both a water intake point and a community water treatment plant may be targeted for terrorist activity and deliberate water contamination.
- *Selected points in the posttreatment water distribution system:* Treated water is distributed to water consumers or end users through transmission pipelines to homes and businesses. Selected portions of a water distribution system or water main are another potential point of water contamination that may be targeted by terrorists and could affect a subdivision, specific neighborhood, school, medical center, or nursing home.
- *Private home or office building water supply connection, individual building water supply, water tanks, cisterns, or storage tanks:* Treated water that is stored very close to the water consumer or end user as well as individual house or building connections may serve as points of contamination of water by terrorists.
- *Water used in food processing, bottled water production, or commercial water:* Water used for food processing or preparation as well as bottled water production also represent points of potential water contamination by terrorists.
- *Deliberate contamination of recreational waters and receiving waters:* Both treated and untreated recreational waters may serve as a point of potential contamination of water, including swimming pools, water parks, and natural bodies of water (small lakes and ponds). Receiving waters, such as rivers, estuaries, and lakes, may be secondarily contaminated with wastewater from sanitary and storm sewer systems that may have been environmentally contaminated by a biological, chemical, or radiological agent used in a terrorist assault.

Modified and reprinted with permission from *Physician Preparedness for Acts of Water Terrorism: An On-line Readiness Guide*. Available at: http://www.waterhealthconnection.org/bt.

---

have been published and provide a valuable resource for the medical and public health community facing the challenges of diagnosing terrorism-related disease that may result from multiple exposure pathways, including water, and have universal application in a clinical and public health setting (Box 200-3).

Post-incident actions also require that health care providers become familiar with the appropriate mechanisms for communicating with law enforcement agencies, public utilities, the media, and the concerned public. If a health care provider suspects that an act of water terrorism is responsible for a patient's symptom complex or an unusual illness pattern in his or her practice, *immediate action* to contact the appropriate public health authority is essential, even before laboratory confirmation or final diagnosis. This contact is the critical first step necessary for the public health authority to (1) initiate a prompt investigation; (2) provide guidance to health care providers and the affected community; (3) establish communication and cooperation with other local, state, and federal agencies as warranted; and (4) contact local

BOX 200-3   Epidemiological Indicators and Sentinel Clues Indicating Possible Terrorism-Related Exposure and Disease

Several epidemiological patterns have been identified as possible sentinel clues of a terrorist attack. However, none of these indicators alone is pathognomonic for terrorism-related disease. These indicators and sentinel clues are presented here as an educational tool for use by health care providers and public health practitioners as possible disease trends that may warrant further investigation:

- Point source illness and injury patterns with record numbers of severely ill or dying patients presenting within a short period of time
- Very high attack rates, with 60% to 90% of potentially exposed patients displaying symptoms or disease from possible biological, chemical, or radiological agent exposure
- Severe and frequent disease manifestations in previously healthy patients
- Increased and early presentation of immunocompromised patients and vulnerable-population patients with debilitating disease since the dose of inoculum or toxic exposure required to cause disease less than would be expected for the general healthy population
- "Impossible epidemiology" with naturally occurring diseases diagnosed in geographic regions where the disease has not been encountered previously
- Higher-than-normal number of patients presenting with gastrointestinal, respiratory, neurologic, or fever diagnoses
- Record number of fatal cases with few recognizable signs and symptoms, indicating lethal doses of biological, chemical, or radiological agents near a point of dissemination or dispersal source
- Localized areas of disease epidemics that may occur in a specific neighborhood or sector, possibly indicating contamination of a selected point in a posttreatment water distribution system
- Multiple infections at a single location (school, hospital, nursing home) with an unusual or rare biological pathogen
- Lack of response or clinical improvement of presenting patients to traditional treatment modalities
- Near-simultaneous outbreaks of similar or different epidemics at the same or different locations, indicating an organized pattern of intentional biological or chemical agent release
- Endemic disease presenting in a community during an unusual time of year or found in a community where the normal vector of transmission is absent
- Unusual temporal or geographic clustering of cases with patients attending a common public event, gathering, or recreational venue
- Increased patient presentation with acute neurologic illness or cranial nerve impairment with progressive generalized weakness
- Unusual or uncommon route of exposure of a disease such as illness resulting from a waterborne agent not normally found in the water environment

Modified and reprinted with permission from *Physician Preparedness for Acts of Water Terrorism: An On-line Readiness Guide*. Available at: http://www.waterhealthconnection.org/bt.

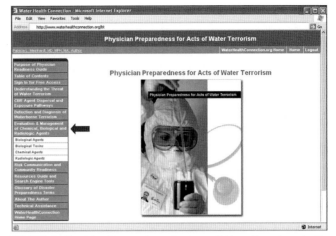

FIG 200-1 *Physician Preparedness for Acts of Water Terrorism: An On-line Readiness Guide* is a free online medical resource accessible at: http://www.waterhealthconnection.org/bt.

Individual host susceptibility and differences in biological, chemical, and radiological agent virulence and toxicity may result in a wide variation in the severity of disease resulting from a waterborne terrorist event.[16] Water-related disease resulting from intentional contamination may present as benign symptoms or self-limited illness in a healthy patient population, whereas the same waterborne exposure in a vulnerable patient population may result in serious morbidity and mortality. In addition, as is apparent from the 50 agents that may be dispersed in water (Box 200-1), the medical management and treatment protocols for water terrorism–related disease vary significantly depending on the agent used.[4]

An online clinical management guide has been developed for health care practitioners and public health specialists faced with addressing the evaluation and management of water-related disease resulting from terrorist activity.[4,10] This free resource, *Physician Preparedness for Acts of Water Terrorism: An On-line Readiness Guide*, which is accessible at www.waterhealthconnection.org/bt, is highlighted in Figure 200-1 and provides "24/7" access to medical management guidelines addressing water-related disease resulting from intentional contamination of water supplies from biological, chemical, and radiological agents.

UNIQUE CONSIDERATIONS

1. Even though environmental monitoring of water supplies continues to improve, the most likely initial indication that an intentional water contamination event has occurred in a population may be a change in disease trends and illness patterns. Therefore health care providers may be the first to recognize that an act of water terrorism has occurred in their community.
2. Use of water as a mode of dispersion for terrorist agents may confound diagnosis, delay treatment, and impede protective public health measures if clinical evaluations and epidemiological investigations do not include the possibility of a waterborne route of exposure or mode of dispersal.
3. Prompt identification of waterborne disease resulting from water terrorism may be difficult as the signs and symptoms of waterborne disease and the health effects of water contamination are often nonspecific and mimic more common medical conditions and disorders unrelated to water contamination.
4. Coinfections with waterborne pathogens, coupled with multiple chemical agent exposure during an act of water terrorism, may result in exposed patients presenting with both acute and delayed

water utilities for prompt remediation and protective measures. Attention to this post-incident procedure by health care providers is mandatory to initiate the appropriate response to a potentially high-risk public health event that may indicate intentional contamination of drinking water supplies.

MEDICAL TREATMENT OF CASUALTIES

The nature of the medical sequelae resulting from exposure to intentional contamination of water supplies depends on a multitude of factors including the following: (1) agent characteristics, including toxicity and virulence; (2) individual host susceptibility and level of immunity; and (3) movement and dilution of the agent in the environment.[14,15]

symptoms from mixed agent exposure, complicating accurate and timely diagnosis.

5. Waterborne exposure to biological, chemical, or radiological agents may result from both direct and indirect environmental contamination, including contamination through wastewater from sanitary and storm sewer systems receiving run-off from an aerosolized terrorist attack or through decontamination wastewater generated during patient decontamination procedures.

❗ PITFALLS

- Failure to include water as a possible exposure pathway or mode of transmission during initial case presentation of a suspected terrorist incident
- Failure to identify site where contamination occured[17]
- Failure to recognize that more than 50 potential terrorist agents of public health concern may be distributed through water as a mode of dispersal
- Failure to notify appropriate public health authorities immediately of a suspected case of waterborne disease, preventing timely remediation efforts and protective public health measures
- Failure to consider the special needs of susceptible populations most at risk for morbidity and mortality from intentional water contamination
- Failure to identify alternative sources of drinking water as part of disaster preparedness plans in order to ensure that affected communities have adequate drinking water for days to weeks after a water contamination event
- Failure to provide effective risk communication regarding water safety to concerned patients and the public

REFERENCES

1. Clark RM, Deininger RA. Protecting the nation's critical infrastructure: the vulnerability of US water supply systems. *J Contingencies Crisis Manag.* 2000;8:73–80.
2. Krieger G. Water and food contamination. In: Chase KH, Upfal MJ, Krieger GR, et al. *Terrorism: Biological, Chemical and Nuclear from Clinics in Occupational and Environmental Medicine.* Philadelphia, PA: Saunders; 2003:253–262.
3. States S, Scheuring M, Kuchta J, Newberry J, Casson L. Utility-based analytical methods to ensure public water supply security. *Am Water Works Assoc J.* 2003;95:103–115.
4. Meinhardt PL. *Physician Preparedness for Acts of Water Terrorism: An On-line Readiness Guide.* Environmental Protection Agency, Arnot Ogden Medical Center. Available at: http://www.waterhealthconnection.org/bt/index.asp.
5. National Research Council. *Making the Nation Safer: The Role of Science and Technology in Countering Terrorism.* Washington, DC: Committee on Science and Technology for Countering Terrorism, National Academies Press; 2002.
6. Centers for Disease Control and Prevention. CDC and EPA Water Advisory in Response to High Threat Level. Available at: http://stacks.cdc.gov/view/cdc/25035.
7. Franz DR, Jahrling PB, Friedlander AM, et al. Clinical recognition and management of patients exposed to biological warfare agents. *Clin Lab Med.* 2001;21:435–473.
8. Inglesby TV, O'Toole T. *Medical Aspects of Biological Terrorism.* American College of Physicians. Available at: http://www.acponline.org/bioterro/medicalaspects.htm.
9. Headquarters, Departments of the Army, Navy and the Air Force, and Commandant, Marine Corps. *Field Manual: Treatment of Biological Warfare Agent Casualties.* Available at: http://www.med.navy.mil/directives/Pub/5042.pdf.
10. Meinhardt PL. *Recognizing Waterborne Disease and the Health Effects of Water Pollution: Physician On-line Reference Guide.* Environmental Protection Agency, American Water Works Association, Arnot Ogden Medical Center. Available at: http://www.waterhealthconnection.org.
11. Henderson DA. Bioterrorism as a public health threat. *Emerg Infect Dis.* 1998;4(3).
12. Environmental Protection Agency. Safe Drinking Water Act (SDWA). Available at: http://water.epa.gov/lawsregs/rulesregs/sdwa/index.cfm.
13. Burkle FM. Mass casualty management of a large-scale bioterrorist event: an epidemiological approach that shapes triage decision. *Emerg Med Clin North Am.* 2002;20:409–436.
14. World Health Organization. *Public Health Response to Biological and Chemical Weapons: WHO Guidance.* Available at: http://www.who.int/csr/delibepidemics/biochemguide/en/.
15. Kaufmann AF, Meltzer MI, Schmid GP. The economic impact of a bioterrorist attack: are prevention and postattack intervention programs justifiable? *Emerg Infect Dis.* 1997 Apr-Jun;3(2):83–94.
16. Burrows WD, Renner SE. Biological warfare agents as threats to potable water. *Environ Health Perspect.* 1999;107:975–984.
17. McKay C, Scharman EJ. Intentional and inadvertant chemical contamination of food, water, and medication. *Emerg Med Clin North Am.* 2015;33(1):153–177.

CHAPTER 201

Food-Supply Contamination

Marc C. Restuccia

📄 DESCRIPTION OF EVENT

Despite the many improvements made in overseeing the U.S. food supply, foodborne illness remains a serious cause of morbidity and mortality throughout the world, including the United States.[1] Many factors contribute to an ideal chain for amplification of foodborne pathogens, including mass-production farming, the scale of modern water supplies, importation of food from other countries that may lack the strict food-handling and food-shipping guidelines present in the United States, use of immense industrial food-processing plants, and the distances (sometimes quite lengthy) over which food is transported to consumers. The scale of the problem has not been described in detail. It is estimated that millions of people are affected worldwide. The majority experience only temporary discomfort. However, for the young, the very old, patients with concomitant systemic illness, and increasingly for the immunocompromised (patients with cancer, AIDS, and organ transplants), foodborne illness can be fatal. Each year in the United States approximately 48 million people contract foodborne illnesses, and approximately 56,000 hospitalizations and 3000 deaths are attributable to foodborne illness.[2]

Foodborne illnesses are virtually always the result of human actions or omissions that occur routinely in daily life or as intentional attacks on the food chain of a given population. In 2013 a couple in India poisoned a free school lunch program with the pesticide monocrotophos, resulting in the death of 23 children (ages 4 to 12 years). There was also the well-publicized London poisoning of the author Alexander Litvinenko in 2006 by placing radioactive polonium in his tea, resulting in his death.

Typical Food Poisoning

Improper handling, leading to fecal contamination of food, is the usual cause of most foodborne illnesses. Agents typically causing such illness include bacteria, viruses, parasites, and toxins.

Natural events such as earthquakes, tornados, hurricanes, and floods disrupt the food-supply chain by causing food contamination during production, processing, transportation, or preparation, which can have severe consequences on the affected population. Fortunately in such an event, unaffected areas of the state, region, country, or world can supply untainted food to the stricken area.

The diagnosis of foodborne illness in a typical scenario is difficult.[3] An individual health care provider may have difficulty identifying a foodborne epidemic, unless multiple persons present with symptoms and a clearly identifiable source can be determined. The incubation period can range from a few hours (bacterial toxins) to days (many bacterial, viral, parasitic, and protozoan agents) to years (prion-induced illness). Multiple other causes of gastrointestinal dysfunction may mimic foodborne illness, making diagnosis exceedingly difficult.

If multiple persons are affected by a typical foodborne illness and have a common point in their recent activities, such as attending a particular event, eating at a specific restaurant, or buying a specific food item at a single food market, the diagnosis may quickly become evident. However, if patients present at multiple emergency departments, physician offices, and urgent care facilities, the appropriate questions may not be asked or accurately answered, and the diagnosis may not be made in a timely manner. The typical signs and symptoms of foodborne illness—nausea, vomiting, diarrhea, abdominal pain, fever, and dehydration—may be seen with many nonfoodborne illnesses and require an astute clinician to make the connection.

Intentional Attack on the Food Supply

In the current climate of worldwide terrorist activities, the potential for an individual or group to deliberately contaminate a population's food supply cannot be discounted.[4] Because of this concern, the U.S. Congress enacted the Public Health Security and Bioterrorism Preparedness and Response Act of 2002. The U.S. Food and Drug Administration is charged with developing guidelines to ensure the safety of food produced in the United States and food imported from outside U.S. borders. In addition, when the U.S. Department of Homeland Security was created, it was recognized that U.S. agriculture and food industries had to be included in the list of critical parts of infrastructure needing protection. The expanding aggregation of food growers, suppliers, and long lines of transportation, often stretching across international boundaries, made this chain of supply susceptible to intentional contamination.

A terrorist seeking to sabotage a nation's food supply, especially in a highly industrialized nation like the United States, has many potential vectors to target: crops, livestock, fertilizer, cattle feed, the food-processing and food-distribution chain, storage facilities, transport modes, and food and agricultural research laboratories. As the U.S. Government Accountability Office (GAO) noted in a 2003 report, individuals or groups seeking to cause economic disruption may well target livestock and crops.[3] Conversely, if such groups seek to cause human illness, they might contaminate finished food products at the processing stage, at the distribution or transportation stage, or at the site of consumption. An example of the latter was a cult in the 1980s that, seeking to sway the outcome of a local election, contaminated a local restaurant's salad bar with *Salmonella*.[4] The cult envisioned this act sickening the local populace and rendering enough persons unable to vote that the cult could gain the majority of votes.

The GAO report noted that significant gaps in federal controls for protecting agriculture and the food supply, including inadequate education of border inspectors about hand-foot-and-mouth disease, numbers of inspectors to handle the large number of international passengers, and scanning technology or inconsistency in its use at cargo and bulk mail facilities.[5]

The potential costs of a bioterrorist attack on the food supply, especially if it involved livestock, would be much greater than simply the cost of the livestock and disposal of the animals. As was seen in Great Britain with the outbreak of hand-foot-and-mouth disease (a nonterrorist incident), the loss of confidence in British food suppliers and tourism income significantly multiplied losses to the U.K. economy. If there had been a terrorist-sponsored food-contamination attack, the economic disruption and losses could have been magnified many times. The mere threat or suggestion of a biological attack on the food supply would be sufficient to seriously disrupt the economy and the lives of the targeted population. Lack of confidence in the safety of the food available would have unimaginable consequences for the area targeted.

The speed at which contamination of the food supply would be recognized varies according to the agent(s) used. For long-incubating agents, such as bovine spongiform encephalopathy (mad cow disease), the first indication would be positive test results for the disease in sample livestock. It would not, however, appear in the at-risk human population for years. With other agents targeted at the human population and introduced at later stages of the food-production chain, such as the *Salmonella* attack previously described, it would take only hours to a few days for the population to show signs and symptoms of food poisoning, which would mirror those of a typical foodborne illness, potentially magnified many times. It is entirely conceivable that health care facilities and providers would be overwhelmed with the numbers of patients and severity of their illness, and it is extremely likely that health care providers also would become ill. A calculated terrorist act might very well target the health care infrastructure *first* to maximize the disruption, loss of life, and productivity of the affected populace.

PRE-INCIDENT ACTIONS

Planning for the possible contamination of any part of the food-supply chain, whether due to deliberate acts of terrorism or simply to human carelessness, must be performed in advance. Plans must include strategies for the following aspects: rapid identification of the altered food supply, limitation of its health and economic impact, treatment of affected persons, and identification of alternative sources of noncontaminated food. Adequate numbers of unaffected public safety and health care workers must be available to identify the outbreak, limit its expansion, maintain public safety, and treat patients. Local, state, and federal officials must identify beforehand those links in the food-supply chain that are particularly vulnerable to contamination and must implement plans for prevention.

Educating the entire population about foodborne illnesses would be beneficial. Farmers, distributors, retailers, and consumers must be informed about the potential for foodborne illnesses, how to recognize signs and symptoms, how to identify when the food-supply chain is compromised, and how to act decisively if such a situation arises. Legislators at local, state, and federal levels need to understand the vulnerability of the food supply and be proactive in initiating and funding legislation to protect the food supply, treat patients, and limit the economic devastation caused by any disruption in the food-supply chain.

Syndromic surveillance is a method of rapidly tracking and identifying disease trends. It allows cities, regions, states, and even wider communities to share via computer the background health of a population. An example would be a surveillance system that receives data on a daily basis on symptoms and diagnoses of patients admitted to area emergency departments. This system in theory would quickly identify unusual disease clusters and alert boards of health, triggering a preplanned response. This powerful tool has implications beyond that of food-supply contamination and could well be invaluable in any disease outbreak or bioterrorist attack.[6]

Every hospital, locality, state, and nation should have predeveloped disaster plans to cover the eventuality of a food-supply disruption. These plans should address (1) access and distribution of needed medications; (2) methods for communicating with local boards of health, public safety agencies, the medical community, and especially the general public; and (3) identification of alternative food supplies. Although state and federal assistance can be expected, such responses will take some time, and each entity should have a detailed plan for dealing with the first few hours of the disaster or possibly even as long as the first 3 days.

Greater state and federal oversight of the food supply is critical to prevent and limit the impact of a widespread foodborne illness. Improved inspection of all food products during both production and shipping (including over international borders) is desirable. Rapid containment of such an outbreak will limit its progression, minimize its economic impact, and restore the public's confidence in the food supply.

POST-INCIDENT ACTIONS

After an outbreak of foodborne poisoning a high degree of suspicion is necessary, especially on the part of medical professionals, to determine whether a cluster of illnesses is something out of the ordinary. Open lines of communication and the use of tools like syndromic surveillance will be essential for early identification of the problem, limitation of a burgeoning outbreak, and prompt and appropriate treatment of patients. The impact of foodborne poisoning on critical social-protection elements, such as police, firefighters, and health care providers, must be considered along with restoration of more normal function of the affected area(s). Early notification and clear lines of communication will be vital in controlling the situation.

MEDICAL TREATMENT OF CASUALTIES

For the majority of people with foodborne illness the treatment is primarily supportive. With some diseases the addition of appropriate antibiotics can be lifesaving or at least shorten the duration of the illness.

UNIQUE CONSIDERATIONS

The main difficulty in determining whether food-supply contamination has occurred is the way in which patients present. Early on, medical practitioners generally will see a few cases each of what appears to be viral gastroenteritis. Only if the health care community, food-supply industry, and government agencies are communicating and ready to act will it be possible to identify and address contamination before serious health and economic consequences occur.

PITFALLS

There are several potential pitfalls in the response to food-supply contamination, including the following:

- Failure to have a disaster plan in place that specifically details the steps to be taken
- Failure to communicate to the health care community and boards of health regarding new trends in disease appearance
- Failure to protect the health care community and public safety agencies from being ravaged by a contamination outbreak
- Failure to identify alternative means of feeding the population if the primary food supply is contaminated or unavailable
- Failure of legislators at all levels to be proactive in preventing and limiting the effects of a contamination outbreak

REFERENCES

1. Wallace RB, Oria M. *Institute of Medicine and National Research Council. Enhancing Food Safety: The Role of the Food and Drug Administration.* Washington, DC: National Academies Press; 2010.
2. Braden CR, Tauxe RV. Emerging trends in foodborne diseases. *Infect Dis Clin North Am.* 2013;27:517–533.
3. Arendt S, Rajagopal L, Strohbehn C, et al. Reporting of foodborne illness by U.S. consumers and healthcare professionals. *Int J Environ Res Public Health.* 2013;10:3684–3714.
4. Moran GJ, Talan DA, Abrahamian FM. Biological terrorism. *Infect Dis Clin North Am.* 2008;22:145–187.
5. *Bioterrorism: a threat to agriculture and the food supply.* Washington, DC: U.S. General Accountability Office, GAO-04-259T; November 19, 2013. Available at: http://www.gao.gov/assets/90/82077.pdf.
6. Smith S, Elliot AJ, Mallaghan C, et al. Value of syndromic surveillance in monitoring a focal waterborne outbreak due to an unusual *Cryptosporidium* genotype in Northamptonshire, United Kingdom, June-July 2008. *Euro Surveill.* 2010;15:19643.

Mass Gatherings

Majed Aljohani and Katharyn E. Kennedy

DESCRIPTION OF EVENT

Thousands of mass gathering events take place worldwide each year. In the United States, as many as 65 million attend National Basketball Association (NBA), National Football League (NFL), and/or National Collegiate Athletic Association (NCAA) events. The inauguration of President Obama on January 20, 2009, attracted a crowd of 1.8 million to the National Mall in Washington, D.C.; a state of emergency was declared to allow the release of federal money and resources. Protests during the Arab Spring in 2011 drew millions of largely peaceful protesters to central locations of Tunis, Tunisia, and Cairo, Egypt. More than 5 million were present when the departure of Egypt's President Hosni Mubarak was announced in February, 2011.[1] Millions of people celebrated the 2014 World Cup in Brazil without significant problems; it seems that lessons have been learned from previous soccer disasters (Table 202-1).

There is no consensus on a definition of a "mass gathering." The World Health Organization (WHO) defines it as "an organized or unplanned event where the number of people attending is sufficient to strain the planning and response resources of the community, state, or nation hosting the event."[2] The National Association of Emergency Medical Services Physicians (NAEMSP) defines it as "organized emergency health services provided for spectators and participants at events in which at least 1000 persons are gathered at a specific location for a defined period of time."[3]

There are two types of mass gatherings: the *traditional*, such as religious festivals, sporting events, music concerts, fairs, and parades; and the *nontraditional*, which have not been researched very well, including metropolitan subway systems, large shopping complexes, airports, cruise ships, public demonstrations, and refugee camps.[4] Medical care of some sort has been provided at such gatherings for the last 30 years in both the United States and Europe. Event organizers everywhere need to take responsibility for the safety and well-being of the participants at an event.

Considerable variation exists in the type of medical care provided to both participants and spectators at these gatherings. General standards have been proposed for the provision of primary care, emergency and disaster care, and means of evacuation. Both the American College of Emergency Physicians (ACEP)[5] and NAEMSP[6] have addressed the previous lack of guidelines and standardized care. A survey in 1998[7] showed that only six U.S. states provided regulatory guidance for the provision of care at mass gatherings, although many are now starting to address this omission.

Terrorist threats have become an unfortunate reality, as shown by the bombing at Centennial Park during the 1996 Olympics in Atlanta, Georgia, and the targeting of nontraditional mass gatherings, such as the Madrid train bombings in 2004, the Kenyan shopping mall mass shootings in 2013, and the Boston Marathon Bombing that same year. Such events pose unique issues regarding the care and evacuation of patients, particularly in unsafe or unsecure scenes.

PRE-INCIDENT ACTIONS

Mass Gatherings Overall

At organized mass gatherings, predictable medical problems and an unpredictable wide variation in medical care exist worldwide. Preplanning and prediction of resource requirements, based on careful needs assessment of anticipated medical care usage and public health risks, may lead to a standardized optimal provision of medical care (Box 202-1).[8]

Provision of medical care is the responsibility of the event planners. Public health officials need to be involved early in the planning process, especially for large events, such as the Olympics, world fairs, and pilgrimages. The local health department should be involved in overseeing the preparation, storage, and serving of food and sanitation requirements. Once identified, those providing medical care at mass gatherings need to liaise with local emergency medical services (EMS), fire, and law enforcement officials. Ground and building plans, close estimates of possible attendance, and identification of any specific hazards should be shared among these providers. Multiple variables interact to make planning for a mass gathering event challenging. An understanding of these may allow for a more efficient and effective planning process. Some of these variables will be discussed below.

Security and Crowd Control

Estimates of attendance may be gleaned from advanced ticket sales or from attendance at previous similar events. However, previous history is notoriously unreliable, as demonstrated by the papal mass in Denver (1993) where 250,000 people were predicted but 500,000 turned up. An adequate ticketing system is essential, as well as public address measures to inform crowds of no further access to an event once capacity is reached.[9]

Mass gathering venues should have multiple access points for entering and exiting the site. During the 1990 Hajj, 1426 people lost their lives due to a stampede as all the pilgrims were trying to leave the city of Mecca at the same time through a tunnel.[10] Planners should promote a unidirectional flow of the crowd, which would significantly reduce the risk of crowd convergence. Training of security staff in crowd control should be implemented before an event to improve crowd safety and avoid panic should overcrowding occur. During a football match in Ellis Park, South Africa, tear gas was thrown into a crowd by event security in an effort to disperse intense overcrowding. This, unfortunately, served to incite panic and caused a stampede (Table 202-1).[9] Keeping the crowd comfortable and relaxed is also essential, therefore awnings,

TABLE 202-1	**Major Soccer Disasters**	
YEAR	**MONTH, DAY**	**DISASTER**
1985	May 11	*Bradford, England:* 56 burned to death, 200 injured due to a fire at Bradford soccer stadium.
1985	May 26	*Mexico City:* 10 trampled to death and 29 injured forcing their way into a match.
1985	May 29	*Brussels, Belgium:* British soccer fans attack rival Italian supporters at Heysel Stadium. A concrete retaining wall collapses, resulting in 39 deaths and more than 400 injured.
1988	March 12	*Kathmandu, Nepal:* 80 fans seeking shelter during a violent hailstorm are trampled to death.
1989	April 15	*Sheffield, England:* 96 died at Hillsborough Stadium. Many were crushed to death when a barrier collapsed on an overcrowded area.
1992	May 5	*Bastia, Corsica:* 17 killed when a grandstand collapsed.
1996	October 16	*Guatemala City:* 84 killed and 147 injured by stampeding fans at Mateo Flores National Stadium.
2001	April 11	*Johannesburg, South Africa:* 43 dead, 250 injured at Ellis Park Stadium due to crushing as crowds pushed into an already overcrowded stadium.
2001	May 9	*Accra, Ghana:* More than 120 killed in a stampede at a soccer match.
2004	March 12	*Qamishli, Syria:* A riot erupted at a soccer match, killing more than 25.
2007	Nov 25	*Salvador, Brazil:* 7 died and about 40 were injured when a stand collapsed.
2012	Feb 1	*Port Said Stadium, Egypt:* 79 killed and more than 1000 injured as a result of riots.

BOX 202-1 Requirements for Medical Care at Mass Gatherings

- Medical oversight by a physician
- Medical reconnaissance
- Medical equipment
- Negotiations for event medical services
- Human resources
- Level of care
- Treatment facilities
- Transportation resources
- Communication
- Public health elements
- Access to care
- Emergency medical operations
- Command and control
- Documentation
- Continuous quality improvement (CQI)

Adapted from data from NAEMSP.

TABLE 202-2	**Anticipating Medical Needs at Mass Gatherings Based on Type of Event**
TYPE OF EVENT	**INJURIES TO BE EXPECTED**
Political events	Minor and major trauma
Religious events	Minor injuries, heat-related problems, cardiac problems
Musical events	Drug or alcohol use, minor trauma
Sporting events	Minor trauma, heat-related problems, and cardiac issues
Auto racing	Severe trauma, heat- and alcohol-related problems

cooling fans (in hot weather), and entertainment are sometimes helpful and should be part of the preplanning.

On-Site Medical Care

It is crucial to establish goals for medical services. These include the following:

- Establishing rapid access to injured or ill patients and providing triage
- Stabilizing and transporting seriously injured or acutely ill patients in a timely manner
- Providing on-site care for injured or ill patients[4]

The type of medical care to be provided at the event needs to be considered beforehand (Table 202-2).[11-15] Primary medical care, such as first aid, emergency care, and preparation for a possible disaster, should be addressed. Staffing levels and type of staffing also need to be anticipated. Recommended ratios include one to two physicians per 50,000 attendees, two paramedics or one paramedic and one emergency medical technician per 10,000 attendees, and one basic first aid provider per 1000 participants at the event.[16] On-site physicians have been shown to reduce ambulance transfers to local hospitals by as much as 89%.[17]

significantly lessening the impact of an event on local EMS services and hospitals. The majority of nondisaster injuries and medical complaints at a mass gathering can be effectively treated at the scene, which reduces the number of hospital referrals and patient presentation rates to the hospital. Physician presence should be strongly encouraged at events where significant trauma may occur or where there is a long distance to definitive care. Cardiac arrest cases are rare in mass gatherings, with reports of 0.5 to 1 per 500,000, though on-site resuscitation and early defibrillation are important and can improve patient survival rates.[18]

A prediction tool for expected medical needs considering five different variables (attendance, heat index, crowd age, crowd mood, and availability of alcohol) was developed and tested in 55 mass gathering events (Tables 202-3 and 202-4).[19] After the anticipated usage rates and staffing levels have been addressed, the positioning, number, and type of aid stations should be considered. Fixed events at stadiums may have areas specially designed and designated for medical care. For other events, aid station locations should be no more than a 5-minute walk for attendees. Stations should be clearly visible, and the locations should be known to participants and other event personnel. These areas need to be adequately and appropriately staffed before the anticipated start of the event, and remain so until the event is completed. Consideration needs to be given to providing medical care in the crowd for occurrences such as cardiac arrest or lower extremity fractures, including how to transport these patients to aid stations. Thought needs to be given regarding provision of ambulances for hospital transport and access and egress for these vehicles. The organizers of medical care need to know the capabilities of local hospitals and should liaise with hospital personnel before the event. All patient encounters should be

TABLE 202-3	Prediction of Patient Presentation Rates at Mass Gathering Events				
ATTENDANCE	WEATHER (HEAT INDEX)	CROWD AGE	CROWD MOOD	AVAILABILITY OF ALCOHOL	POINT VALUE
>15,000	>90 °F (>32.2 °C)	Older	Animated	Significant	2
1000-15,000	<90 °F (<32.2 °C)	Mixed	Intermediate	Limited	1
	Climate not controlled				
<1000	Climate controlled	Supervised younger	Calm	None	0

TABLE 202-4	Recommendations for Medical Need
EVENT CLASSIFICATION	RECOMMENDATIONS
Major (total score >5 or scores of 2 in two different categories)	Multiple ALS personnel, specialized equipment, physicians
Intermediate (total score >3 but <5 or score of 2 in any one category)	Two transport units with 1-3 ALS and 1-6 BLS providers
Minor (total score <3)	Single transport vehicle with 1 ALS and 1 BLS provider

ALS, advanced life support; *BLS*, basic life support.
Modified from reference 19.

documented. Use of noncarbon record (NCR) paper will facilitate a copy accompanying a patient who needs transport to a medical facility. Records are needed for medical and legal reasons and may also be useful for research purposes.

Environmental Factors

There is a positive correlation between temperature and humidity and patient presentation rates.[20] Heat indexes, which take into account the temperature and the humidity, are probably a better indicator of medical need, as it has been shown that with every 10° rise in the heat index, the number of patients per 10,000 spectators (PPTT) tripled.[21] Thirty-one percent of physician encounters at the 1996 California AIDS ride were for heat-related problems.[22] The Denver papal visit resulted in an unanticipated 21,000 patient encounters at a mainly youthful gathering, due in part to the 14-mile walk and high temperatures.[23] Preplanning for the Atlanta Olympics in 1996, in the form of education about preventing heat-related illnesses given to those who purchased advance tickets, might have led to a decrease in the number of patient encounters, despite the high heat and humidity.[24] Cold weather events generally lead to lower medical usage rates by participants and spectators.[25] Use of weather surveillance, early warning systems, and evacuation to shelter protocols is important in cases of storms and lightning.

Alcohol and Illicit Drug Usage

An increase in the number of patient medical encounters may be related to alcohol and illicit drug usage. Historically the consumption rate of alcohol and drugs may be higher at music festivals, rock concerts, and raves. Open-air music events in the United Kingdom have resulted in a primary diagnosis of alcohol intoxication in 4% of patient encounters.[26] Banning the consumption of alcohol at Wembley Stadium led to a 50% reduction in alcohol-related problems.

Crowd Density and Demographics

An increase in crowd size does not necessarily mean an increase in medical usage. One study has shown that the overall medical usage rate decreases with overall crowd size. Patient encounters at events with

more than 1 million participants average 10 per 10,000 participants. Events with fewer participants average 41 per 10,000 spectators. One interpretation of this is that it is easier to seek medical care at a less crowded venue. The medical usage rate can vary even within an event itself. At the Los Angeles Olympics, soccer events had usage rates of 68 per 1000, and rowing and canoeing, 6.8 per 1000 spectators.

Anticipated crowd demographics may be useful in the preplanning stage. Older groups may be expected at papal visits, classical music concerts, and large sporting events.[27] Younger groups frequently attend rock concerts and auto-racing events.[28] The needs of children also must be considered. Most children present with minor injuries, but medical teams need to be prepared to deal with serious medical emergencies and trauma. Overall medical usage at a children's fair was 19.2 per 10,000 participants, and half of those who presented were younger than 14 years old. Protocols need to be in place for the provision of care to minors who present without an accompanying adult.[14]

Event Type

Event type is an unpredictable variable. Certain types of music, known team rivalries, and religious furor may lead to disruptive behavior and an increase in medical usage rates. Crowded events may lead to a "too-close-for-comfort" feel among attendees. Environmental conditions, such as inclement weather, squalid conditions, poor sanitation, and lack of access to drinking water, may lead to ugly crowd dynamics.

Despite the many variables to be considered, it has been shown that event type and temperatures are the ones that best predict medical usage rates.[12] Examples of event types will be discussed later in this chapter. Other variables to consider include event duration and time of occurrence.

Command Structure and Communication

Attention to the location, staffing, and communication needs of a medical command center should be addressed. Communication needs should be considered for event medical providers, other event planners, and local EMS, police, and fire personnel. Backup communication in the form of handheld devices or cell phones should be decided on, and medical personnel must be able to connect with local dispatch centers.

An incident command structure for medical personnel may be used. The event medical officer oversees all aspects of medical care provided at the site. The event triage officer conducts and directs medical assessment of casualties at designated treatment areas or while roving through the crowds and transporting patients to a central area. The event treatment officer oversees treatment to the sick and injured. The event transport officer directs transport to other facilities, and the logistics officer provides the necessary support for EMS at the event. Consideration may be given to the need for hazardous material teams, decontamination, wilderness medicine, or use of amateur radio groups.

The NAEMSP addressed 15 components on which event planners must focus (Box 202-1). For a detailed review of these elements, the NAEMSP produced a comprehensive document entitled "Mass Gathering—Medical Care; The Medical Director's Checklist."[8]

Concerts and Sports Gatherings

The medical usage rate may vary by type of music, with rhythm and blues having rates of 1.3 per 10,000 and gospel or Christian 12.6 per 10,000 attendees. The overall median usage for concerts is 2.1 per 10,000 attendees.[27] Rock concerts typically have rates 2.5 times that of other concerts. The anticipated audience participation in "moshing," crowd surfing, and stage diving may lead to a dramatic increase in medical incidents.[29] Other problems encountered include minor trauma and alcohol or illicit drug intoxication.[30]

Surgical problems may be caused by falls, assaults, being crushed against barriers, and assorted "missiles" causing head injuries. Severe trauma may occur in up to 1.4% of attendees at rock concerts. Medical issues include headache, syncope, asthma, and hypoglycemia. Cardiac arrest is uncommon, with a rate of 0.01 to 0.04 per 10,000 attendees. Asthma may be very common at rodeos.[31]

The ultimate sporting event is probably the Olympics. Planning for the medical care of both spectators and participants begins as soon as the host city has been announced. Around 10 million spectators attended the 2012 London Olympics. Apart from routine medical care, there exists a potential for transmission of infectious diseases, risk of injury from crowd crushing, and now the very real risk of terrorist activity or political protests. Extensive planning at local, state, and federal levels is vital to ensure the health and safety of all concerned.[32-34]

At the 1996 Atlanta games, specialized incident assessment teams were set up to analyze terrorist risks and to address issues such as stockpiling of antibiotics and antidotes. Medical providers of all levels received training in awareness of chemical, biological, and radiological weapons.[35] Local hospitals were updated to include mass decontamination units. Local EMS providers were given uniform operational plans and procedures, enhanced communications were agreed on, protocols were developed for the management of heat-related illnesses, and guidelines for response to mass casualties were issued. Public health initiatives to address heat-related illnesses included a media campaign; packets sent to ticket purchasers; shelters; and provision of water, wide-brimmed hats, sunscreen, and water misters at the most crowded sites. These, plus the cooler-than-normal temperatures, may have led to a decrease in the expected number of hyperthermia victims. Organizers of the 2010 World Cup in South Africa developed an infectious disease surveillance system for the event, which reported to a national health operations center. Despite taking place over a month during the peak of the influenza season in South Africa (in anticipation of which WHO donated 3.5 million doses of pandemic H1N1 vaccine), only 30 communicable disease events were reported.[36]

Marathons

More than 300 marathons are staged each year, along with countless half marathons, triathlons, and 5K and 10K events. Pre-Event considerations include course layout, number of runners, climate, and medical team experience. Earlier start times and the addition of half marathons have led to a decreased risk of injury.[37,38] Encouraging runners to seek help early has also reduced serious medical problems.[39] Educating runners before the event on issues such as dehydration, hypoglycemia, exhaustion, blisters, the importance of good preparation and training, and the use of energy drinks may lessen the need for medical intervention. Runners with a history of asthma are encouraged to carry their inhalers and not to run if they feel ill. Accessible, visible first aid stations along the route, use of mobile paramedic teams, and a medical control center should provide adequate medical coverage. Radio communication is essential between medical providers, and a treatment tent at the finish line should include paramedic and triage teams, massage therapists, and podiatrists. The use of computer tracking chips may be used to identify how many runners use medical treatment and help in the planning of the provision of care and supplies in the future.

On April 15, 2013, while thousands of spectators were celebrating the Boston Marathon, two pressure cooker bombs exploded, killing three people and injuring an estimated 264 others. The bombs exploded about 13 seconds and 190 m (210 yards) apart, near the finish line. Many of the victims suffered serious injuries, and at least 16 people lost limbs as a result of the blast and its debris. Many lives were saved that day because of good planning. The perfectly located medical treatment areas were well staffed and were immediately converted into a mass casualty triage unit, serving as a direct egress point for the ambulances. Only lifesaving procedures were done, without delaying the transfer of the seriously injured patients to hospitals. Victims were distributed equally to six Level 1 trauma centers surrounding the area, which avoided overwhelming a single center. Pre-Event coordination and planning among all agencies and hospitals, along with regular joined training and drills, were huge factors in the success of patient care.

Pilgrimages

Millions of people perform pilgrimages every year. The Muslim pilgrimage, the Hajj, to the Holy Land of Makkah (Mecca) in Saudi Arabia, may have up to 2.5 million participants from 160 countries for a period of 5 to 7 days. The pilgrimage involves a 24-mile round trip from Makkah through the plains of Arafat. Many of the pilgrims are elderly, come from poor countries, live in tents in extreme conditions, and perform physically exhausting religious rituals. The Hajj season varies every year because it follows the lunar Islamic calendar. Therefore likely diseases also vary, depending on the temperature, which is a huge challenge for those involved in planning. In India, millions of pilgrims visit Lord Ayyappa at Sabarimala each year. This occurs over a 41-day period and involves a 90-minute trek uphill to the temple.

Kumbh Mela is a mass Hindu pilgrimage of faith in which people gather to bathe in sacred rivers. It is considered the largest peaceful gathering in the world; more than 100 million people visited during the Maha Kumbh Mela in 2013, a 55-day event. Thirty-six people died in a stampede at the Allahabad Railway Station the same year. A massive rush of passengers, returning from a dip in the waters of the Ganga and Yamuna rivers at the Maha Kumbh, contributed to the tragic event. Many other pilgrimages on a smaller scale take place throughout the world.

Several of the problems encountered may be anticipated. Many of the participants are not in good health and may have chronic medical problems. Heat exhaustion is common during the hot cycle of the Hajj. Cases of heat stroke doubled from 1980 to 1981. This could be overcome by educating pilgrims before and during the event. Infectious disease outbreaks are also common. These include meningococcal meningitis; gastroenteritis; hepatitis A, B, and C; and various zoonotic diseases. The implementation of vaccination policies, infection control policies, and public health initiatives have proven successful in addressing these problems.[40] Pilgrims need proof of appropriate vaccinations to obtain a visa for travel to Saudi Arabia. Face mask use is encouraged to reduce the spread of respiratory infections. Some of the mitigation actions taken at the Hajj are discussed in Table 202-5. The 2014 Hajj faced particular infectious threats with both Middle East Respiratory Syndrome (MERS) and Ebola virus outbreaks in nearby regions.

Free medical care is provided at the holy site in Makkah. In 1997 and 1998 a "treat and release" program commenced, leading to a 73% reduction in ambulance transports.[41] In India at Sabarimala, a medical center is provided at the site. Typically 8000 pilgrims receive medical care over the 41-day period.

TABLE 202-5	Hajj Mitigation Actions		
TYPE	**INCIDENT**	**EXAMPLES OF MITIGATION ACTIONS**	**RESULTS**
Communicable diseases	Meningitis outbreak (1987)	• Bivalent A and C meningococcal vaccines required for attending the Hajj	No further outbreaks to serogroup A
	Hepatitis B and C outbreaks due to head shaving by unlicensed barbers (shaving is part of Hajj completion rituals)	• Full hepatitis B vaccine encouraged for all pilgrims • Only licensed barbers with strict hygiene measures are allowed to shave pilgrims	No published results
	Cholera outbreak (1989), 109 pilgrims affected	• Improvement in water supply and sewage treatment • Strict regulation of food importation by pilgrims	No further outbreaks reported
	H1N1 pandemic (2009)	• Discouraged pilgrims with high risk from participating in Hajj • Thermography screening for febrile pilgrims at the airport • Encouraged H1N1 vaccines • Public health campaign (masks and hand hygiene)	Limited documentation of H1N1 cases in 2009 Hajj season
Non-communicable hazards	Stampede: 1990 (1426 deaths) 1994 (270 deaths) 2006 (350 deaths)	• Construction of Jamarat Bridge reduced crowding from 10 people per m^2 to fewer than 4 • Unidirectional flow of pilgrims • Antipanic systems and automated human stream networking	No major events after 2006
	Fire in Mina: 1995 (150 deaths) 1997 (350 deaths)	• Fiberglass tents • Use of electrical stoves instead of cooking gas	Only limited cases

POST-INCIDENT ACTIONS

In the wake of various disasters at mass gatherings, it is vital to learn from previous mistakes. The European Convention on Spectator Violence and Misbehavior met in 1985 to address issues rising largely from the Heysel Stadium Disaster. It identified the need for police and sports authorities to cooperate in ensuring segregation of rival supporters, controlling access to stadiums, and banning the consumption of alcohol. After the 1989 Hillsborough disaster in England, the Gibson Report recommended medical care at stadiums for the first time. All-seat stadiums were to be phased in, leading to safer stadiums with greater attendance. The Boston Marathon has instituted a post-event clinic that is open for 3 days after the event to meet the delayed medical needs of runners.

MEDICAL TREATMENT OF CASUALTIES

The need for a mass gathering triage system is clear, because these events, by their very nature, have the potential to turn into mass casualty incidents (MCIs). Also, the current prehospital disaster triage systems are biased toward traumatic victims without considering medical complaints, drugs and alcohol, and environmental exposures, making these systems imperfect instruments for use in mass gatherings. Having a unified triage system that is agreed upon among all local agencies and hospitals is essential. Frequent training on triage is important for the success of any response plan.

In general, most participants require minor medical interventions that may be addressed by trained first responders or paramedics.[11] Paramedics may use triage protocols to identify casualties who should

be transported to a hospital after initial stabilization rather than waiting for treatment by an on-site physician.[42]

At rock concerts, 1.4% of attendees may experience severe trauma. Major and minor trauma results from falls, assaults, being crushed against barriers, and head injuries from assorted "missiles." Anticipated medical problems include headaches, syncope, hyperventilation, asthma, epilepsy, and hypoglycemia. At the Atlanta Olympics, most of the injuries were sprains or strains (13%) and contusion abrasions (7%); bronchitis was common (9%), and heat cramps and dehydration accounted for 7% of those seeking medical care.[33] In addition, three cardiac arrests were reported; the provision of defibrillators at mass gatherings is an important consideration.[43]

Hyponatremia is increasingly prevalent among marathon runners. It is defined as a serum sodium level of less than 136 mmol/L and is commonly caused by overhydration. Mild cases may be treated by fluid restriction and consumption of salty foods until urination resumes. In moderate cases the patient's sodium level may need to be checked hourly and, in critical cases, intravenous access will be required and diuretics and hypertonic saline may be administered. Complications such as seizures, pulmonary edema, and coma should be treated appropriately. Runners should be encouraged to replace only 16 ounces of fluid along with salt for every pound of weight lost. Exercise-associated collapse may occur at the finish due to venous pooling. This may be treated by laying the patient supine with the legs elevated and rehydrating with oral electrolyte or carbohydrate solution. Dehydration should be assessed clinically and treated with oral fluids. Heat-related illnesses are addressed in the usual fashion. Hypoglycemia is treated with oral or intravenous glucose replacement.

Many pilgrims are in poor health before the event and may need more than minor first aid. Many suffer from heat-related illnesses or infectious diseases. Provision of free medical care and on-site medical facilities with capabilities of providing even an intensive care unit level of care may meet these needs.

Disasters do occur at mass gatherings, and appropriate medical care needs to be available. Frequently, the cause of death is traumatic asphyxia,[44] for which rapid interventions may make a difference.

UNIQUE CONSIDERATIONS

Every mass gathering should be considered as a unique event. Careful and exhaustive preplanning may reap many benefits. It is important for those providing medical care at the event not to do so in a vacuum. Local EMS providers may well be needed and certainly will be required if a mass casualty event occurs. Mass gatherings occurring in urban settings will have different characteristics and requirements from those in more rural or remote settings. Even though it may be difficult to predict all the medical needs of the crowd, prior studies have started to use a more scientific approach to addressing these needs. Event type, duration, expected attendance, and weather conditions need to be taken into careful consideration in the planning process.

PITFALLS

- Lack of legislation regulating minimum standards for provision of medical care at mass gatherings
- Lack of a coordinated, integrated preplanning process
- Lack of funding to provide needed public health initiatives and medical resources
- Failure to identify a medical director for the event
- Failure to learn from previous experiences
- Underestimating expected attendance
- Failure to consider all variables, such as crowd size, demographics, event duration, and environmental factors
- Failure to consider and prepare for a terrorist event or MCI
- Inability to allow capacity crowd ingress to a stadium in a 1-hour period
- Failure to consider ambulance access and egress at an event
- Lack of training of security personnel, leading to failure to recognize and control potentially dangerous situations

REFERENCES

1. Memish ZA, Stephens GM, Steffen R, Ahmed QA. *Lancet Infect Dis.* 2012;12:56–65.
2. De Lorenzo RA. Mass gathering medicine: a review. *Prehosp Disaster Med.* 1997;12:68–72.
3. World Health Organisation. *Communicable Disease Alert and Response for Mass Gatherings: Key Considerations,* June 2008, Available at: http://www.who.int/csr/Mass_gatherings2.pdf.
4. Arbon P. Mass gathering medicine: a review of the evidence and future directions for research. *Prehosp Disast Med.* 2007;22(2):131–135.
5. Leonard RB, Petrilli R, Noji EK, et al. *Provision for Emergency Medical Care for Crowds.* Dallas: ACEP Publications; 1990, 1–25.
6. Jaslow D, Yancy A, Milsten A. Mass gathering medical care. *Prehosp Emerg Care.* 2000;4(4):359–360.
7. Jaslow D, Drake M, Lewis J. Characteristics of state legislation governing medical care at mass gatherings. *Prehosp Emerg Care.* 1999;3(4):316–320.
8. Jaslow D, Yancy A, Milsten A. *Mass Gathering Medical Care: The Medical Director's Checklist for the NAEMSP Standards and Clinical Practice Committee.* Lenexa, Kan: National Association of Emergency Medical Services Physicians; 2000.
9. Soomaroo L, Murray V. Disasters at mass gatherings: lessons from history. *PLoS Curr.* 2012 Feb 2;4:RRN1301[revised 2012 Mar 12].
10. Ahmed QA, Arabi YM, Memish ZA. Health risks at the Hajj. *Lancet.* 2006;367:1008–1015.
11. Varon J, Fromm RE, Chanin K, et al. Critical illness at mass gatherings is uncommon. *J Emerg Med.* 2003;25(4):409–413.
12. Arbon P, Bridgewater F, Smith C. Mass gathering medicine: a predictive model for patient presentation and transport rates. *Prehosp Disast Med.* 2001;16(3):109–116.
13. Zeitz KM, Schneider DP, Jarrett D, et al. Mass gathering events: retrospective analysis of patient presentations over seven years at an agricultural and horticultural show. *Prehospital Disaster Med.* 2002;17(3):147–150.
14. Thierbach AR, Wolcke BB, Piepho T, et al. Medical support for children's mass gatherings. *Prehospital Disaster Med.* 2003;18(1):14–19.
15. Milsten AM, Maguire BJ, Bissell RA. Emergence of medicine for mass gatherings: lessons from the Hajj. 2002;17(3):151–162.
16. Football Licensing Authority. *Guide to Safety at Sports Grounds.* 4th ed. London: The Stationery Office; 1997.
17. Grange JT, Baumann GW, Vaezazizi R. On-site physicians reduce ambulance transports at mass gatherings. *Prehosp Emerg Care.* 2003;7(3):322–326.
18. Dutch MJ, Senini LM, Taylor DJ. Mass gathering medicine: the Melbourne 2006 Commonwealth Games experience. *Emerg Med Australas.* 2008;20:228–233.
19. Hartman N, Williamson A, Sojka B, et al. Predicting resource utilisation at mass gatherings using a simplified stratification scoring model. *Am J Emerg Med.* 2009;27(3):337–343.
20. Baird MB MDa, O'Connor RE MDa, Williamson AL RNb, Sojka BBA, EMT-Pc, Alibertis KBA, EMT-Pd, Brady WJ MDa. The impact of warm weather on mass event medical need: a review of the literature. *Am J Emerg Med.* 2010;28:224–229.
21. Perron AD, Brady WJ, Custalow CB, et al. Association of heat index and patient volume at a mass gathering event. *Prehosp Emerg Care.* 2005;9:49–52.
22. Friedman LJ, Rodi SW, Krueguer MA, et al. Medical care at the California AIDS Ride 3: experiences in event medicine. *Ann Emerg Med.* 1998;31(2):219–223.
23. De Lorenzo RA. Mass gathering medicine: a review. *Prehospital Disaster Med.* 1997;12(1):68–72.
24. Centers for Disease Control and Prevention. MMWE: prevention and management of heat-related illness in many spectators and staff during the Olympic Games—Atlanta, July 6–23, 1996. *JAMA.* 1996;45(29):631–633.
25. Eadie JL. Health and safety at the 1980 Winter Olympics, Lake Placid, New York. *J Environ Health.* 1981;43(4):178–187.
26. Hewitt S, Jarrett L, Winter B. Emergency medicine at a large rock festival. *J Accid Emerg Med.* 1996;13(1):26–27.
27. Grange JT, Green SM, Downs W. Concert medicine: spectrum of problems encountered at 405 major concerts. *Acad Emerg Med.* 1999;6(3):202–207.
28. Nardi C, Bettini M, Brazoli C, et al. Emergency medical services in mass gatherings: the experience of the Formula 1 Grand Prix 'San Marino' in Imola. *Eur J Emerg Med.* 1997;4(4):217–223.
29. Janchar T, Samaddar C, Milzman D. The mosh pit experience: emergency medical care for concert injuries. *Am J Emerg Med.* 2000;18(1):62–63.
30. Erickson TB, Koenigsberg M, Bunney E, et al. Prehospital severity scoring at major rock concert events. *Prehospital Disaster Med.* 1997;12(3):195–199.
31. Fromm RE, Varon J. Frequency of asthma exacerbations at mass gatherings. *Chest.* 1999;116(4):251S.
32. Meehan P, Toomey KE, Drinnon J. Public health response for the 1996 Olympic Games. *JAMA.* 1998;279(18):1469–1473.
33. Wetterhall SF, Coulombier DM, Herndon JM, et al. Medical care delivery at the 1996 Olympic games. *JAMA.* 1998;279(18):1463–1468.
34. Flynn M. More than a sprint to the finish: planning health support for the Sydney 2000 Olympic and Paralympic Games. *ADF Health.* 2000;1:129–132.
35. Sharp TW, Brennan RJ, Keim M, et al. Medical preparedness for a terrorist incident involving chemical or biological agents during the 1996 Atlanta Olympic Games. *Ann Emerg Med.* 1998;32(2):214–223.
36. Report on WHO support to the 2010 FIFA World Cup South Africa™ Pretoria, South Africa, 27 January 2011.

37. Crouse B, Beattie K. Marathon medical services: strategies to reduce runner morbidity. *Med Sci Sports Exerc.* 1996;28(9):1093–1096.

38. Roberts WO. A 12-year profile of medical injury and illness for the Twin Cities Marathon. *Med Sci Sports Exerc.* 2000;32(9):1549–1555.

39. Ridley SA, Rogers PN, Wright IH. Glasgow marathons 1982–1987. A review of medical problems. *Scott Med J.* 1990;35(1):9–11.

40. Memish ZA. Infection control in Saudi Arabia: meeting the challenge. *Am J Infect Control.* 2002;30(1):57–65.

41. Al-Bayouk M, Seraj M, Al-Yamani I, et al. Treat and release: a new approach to the emergency medical needs of the oldest mass gatherings—the pilgrimage. Presented at: 11th World Congress on Emergency and Disaster Medicine. Free Paper Session Topics and Abstracts, May 10–13, 1999, Osaka, Japan; 2002.

42. Salhanick SD, Sheahan W, Bazarian JJ. Use and analysis of field triage criteria for mass gatherings. *Prehospital Disaster Med.* 2003;18(4):347–352.

43. Crocco TJ, Sayre MR, Liu T, et al. Mathematical determination of external defibrillators needed at mass gatherings. *Prehosp Emerg Care.* 2004;8(3):292–297.

44. Orue M, Pretell R. Mass Casualty in a Pop Music Concert Instead of Being a Programmed Event: Home Fair 1997, Lima, Peru. Available at: http://pdm.medicine.wisc.edu/moncerrat.htm.

CHAPTER 203

Ecological Terrorism*

George A. Alexander

DESCRIPTION OF EVENT

Ecological terrorism or *ecoterrorism* may be defined as the use of force directed at the environment or ecosystem to terrorize, frighten, coerce, or intimidate governments or societies.[1] The scenario of a terrorist or rogue nation group using nuclear, radiological, biological, or chemical agents or weapons as a means of ecoterrorism is plausible. Radiological agents can be obtained readily through legal and illegal means. Chemical and biological agents are easy and cheap to develop and use. In addition to the devastating human effects of such agents, they can have destructive environmental consequences. For these reasons, global terrorists are more likely to resort to ecological terrorism.

As for nuclear targets, ecological terrorism may occur as a result of sabotage or attack on commercial nuclear power reactors, spent fuel storage depots, or nuclear fuel reprocessing facilities. There are 107 nuclear power plants in the United States and more than 429 nuclear reactors worldwide.[2]

The 1986 Chernobyl nuclear power plant accident in the former Soviet Union serves as a harsh reminder of potential scenarios in which terrorists could engage in ecological terrorism by trying to release radioactive nuclear materials into the environment. As a result of the Chernobyl accident, 28 people died from acute radiation exposure, 134 patients suffered from acute radiation syndrome, hundreds of thousands of people were evacuated, and almost as many people were involved in cleanup efforts.[3] The extensive atmospheric fallout caused considerable concern far from the accident site. Within 10 days after the accident, elevated levels of radioactivity were reported in Israel, Kuwait, Turkey, Japan, China, the United States, and Canada.[4] In addition, radioactive fallout contaminated large forested areas in Europe.[5]

A large radiological dispersal device (RDD) also has the potential to contaminate the environment or ecosystems. The environmental hazards from dispersal of highly radioactive fuel in a large RDD would be similar to that which occurred at Chernobyl, but on a smaller scale.[6] Radioactive gases, liquids, and particulates would cause considerable environmental contamination. The areas of risk from radioactive contamination can extend many miles away from the explosion site.

Biological pathogens may be used to perpetrate ecological terrorism. For example, *Bacillus anthracis*, the organism that causes anthrax, is very stable because of its ability to sporulate. This characteristic makes anthrax spores attractive for terrorists to use to contaminate the environment. Dormant spores are known to have survived in some archaeological sites for perhaps hundreds of years.[7] An aerosol release of anthrax spores in parks, playgrounds, or sports fields using a portable cropduster sprayer would contaminate these areas and may infect unsuspecting people who come in contact with the spores. A public acknowledgment of such a release by a terrorist group would cause widespread distress, panic, and fear. Bioterrorism has become a great public health and infection control threat.[8]

During the Gulf War of 1990, the Iraqis deliberately released oil from the Kuwaiti oil fields with the intention of polluting and contaminating Saudi Arabian waters and coastlines. These acts were tantamount to ecological terrorism.[1] Approximately 400 miles of Persian Gulf shoreline were contaminated with oil.[9] The environmental consequences of these oil spills will adversely affect these shorelines and coastal waters for many years to come. Similar acts of oil dispersal on land resulted in much larger oil-polluted areas in Kuwait.

The burning of Kuwaiti oil fields by the Iraqis was another form of ecological terrorism. More than 700 oil wells in Kuwait burned for about 10 months.[10] These fires consumed up to 6 million barrels of oil per day and engulfed the entire region with massive clouds of smoke.[11] These acts of ecological terrorism resulted in a level of environmental pollution that exceeded that of any other previous human-made disaster.[12] The long-term environmental impact of this ecological catastrophe is unknown.[13]

The estimated deaths of more than 10,000 people and morbidity of approximately 200,000 persons from the accidental release of methyl isocyanate in Bhopal, India, in 1984[14] serve as a bleak reminder of potential scenarios in which terrorists could engage in ecological terrorism by attempting to release toxic industrial chemicals into the environment.[1] Unlimited possibilities of threats exist from chemical ecoterrorism. An estimated 70,000 chemicals are used commonly worldwide, and an additional 200 to 1000 new synthetic chemicals are introduced and marketed by the chemical industry each year.[10]

PRE-INCIDENT ACTIONS

Public health emergencies are profound and dynamic situations that may overwhelm existing health care and public health infrastructure, resulting in adverse community health effects.[15] Ecoterrorism clearly involves a public health emergency. The first challenge for medical and public health providers in preparing for ecological terrorism is to make an assessment of potential environmental targets and ecological threats from nuclear, radiological, biological, and chemical agents. Medical response plans for a variety of likely targets should be developed. These should contain descriptions of the types of possible ecological terrorism, including the identification of anticipated hazards and the response actions that can be taken to minimize them. The medical resources needed for each threat situation and a plan for augmenting those resources should be specified. Consultation should be sought

---

*The views expressed in this chapter are those of the author and do not necessarily represent the official policy or position of the National Cancer Institute, the National Institutes of Health, or the Department of Health and Human Services.

with specialists who have experience in the management of terrorist threats. Management response plans should have scenarios based on each particular type or category of agent. Planning should be coordinated with local and state hazardous-material response teams as well as medical and environmental laboratories. Effective preparedness, response, and recovery from disastrous terrorist attacks require a well-planned effort involving experienced professionals who can apply detailed knowledge and specialized skills in precarious situations.[16]

POST-INCIDENT ACTIONS

Awareness of ecological terrorism is the second challenge and should focus on recognizing that an act of terrorism has occurred. Early detection of an ecological hazard should be the goal to prevent or reduce adverse human and environmental health risks. Any assessment of potential hazards or risks from chemical or radiological exposures should consider not only the innate toxicity of the substance, but also the nature of the exposure.

Once aware of the threat, executing a credible medical response to any attack is the third challenge. An ecological risk assessment should be performed to estimate the probability that untenable ecological health effects may occur in populations as a result of exposure to a specified hazard. The basic elements of an ecological risk assessment include defining the problem, obtaining the necessary information and data, assessing the hazard potential, assessing the exposure potential, integrating the hazard and exposure assessment (risk characterization), and summarizing and presenting the results.[17]

MEDICAL TREATMENT OF CASUALTIES

The management of specific human injuries associated with various forms of ecological terrorism is beyond the scope of this chapter and is readily available elsewhere in this book. An intentional release of nuclear, radiological, biological, or chemical agents or weapons into the environment has the potential to cause a major public health disaster. Such incidents pose special features that require specific considerations by emergency responders. A latent period may occur between release of the agent and the development of symptoms associated with illness. Symptoms of acute disease may be seen within minutes or hours, whereas chronic exposure can be insidious and continue undetected until large numbers of people develop catastrophic illness. Universal precautions including gowns and gloves[18] as well as facial masks are considered adequate protection for medical personnel coming into contact with contaminated persons. Several months may pass without people knowing that they have been exposed and are at risk. The long-term effects of these exposures may be the most important consideration, particularly if there are no acute effects.[19]

Clinical and pathological effects of the terrorist weapons previously mentioned are well known. Certain syndromes with specific symptomatology may arise as the focus of a known or suspected incident. Acute radiation syndrome is clearly associated with nuclear or radiological incidents. Specific biological syndromes are associated with a variety of infectious disease agents. Chemical syndromes also exist for numerous toxic chemical agents.

UNIQUE CONSIDERATIONS

As already indicated, the medical, public health, and environmental consequences of ecological terrorism require specialized considerations. Emergency responders and health care providers should apply similar medical and public health management principles regardless of the ecological threat. Exposure to pollutants from ecological terrorism

may or may not result in acute illness requiring the treatment of large numbers of people. In fact, after exposure to any terrorist ecological hazard, people may present with nonspecific symptoms such as headache, fatigue, skin rashes, fever, eye and respiratory irritation, gastrointestinal problems, tiredness, and poor concentration.

Depending on the agent involved, evacuation from the scene of a terrorist toxic release contaminating the environment may need to be made immediately after the release. Unfortunately, the information needed to fully evaluate the risk and on which to base an evacuation decision may not be readily available. In this situation, a health risk assessment should be considered to help decide whether evacuation is necessary immediately after the terrorist release or to predict long-term health consequences. The health risk assessment includes hazard identification, dose-response assessment, exposure assessment, and risk characterization.[1]

Although decontamination plans describe methods for providing decontamination, the plans must be multidisciplinary and integrated; they require planning, retraining, and teamwork to be effective.[20] First responders, first receivers, and institutions must be adequately protected, and decontamination must be performed quickly and safely.

! PITFALLS

Obstacles to the provision of optimal medical and public health management include the following:

- Lack of adequate preparedness, emergency response, and recovery planning for possible ecological terrorist attacks before they occur
- Lack of coordination with local and state medical, public health, and environmental response agencies
- Lack of consultation with health professionals who have the expertise to manage specific types of ecological terrorism
- Lack of recognition that reporting of nonspecific symptoms among an affected population may be associated with various forms of ecological terrorism
- Lack of involvement by behavioral and social health professionals to address the psychosocial consequences of ecological terrorism

REFERENCES

1. Alexander GA. Ecoterrorism and nontraditional military threats. *Mil Med.* 2000;165:1–5.
2. King G. *Dirty Bomb: Weapon of Mass Disruption.* New York, NY: Penguin Group; 2004.
3. Soloviev V, Ilyin LA, Baranov AE, et al. Radiation accidents in the former U.S.S.R. In: Gusev I, Guskova AK, Mettler Jr. FA, eds. *Medical Management of Radiation Accidents.* 2nd ed. Boca Raton, FL: CRC Press; 2001:157–194.
4. Guskova AK, Gusev IA. Medical aspects of the accident at Chernobyl. In: Gusev I, Guskova AK, Mettler Jr FA, eds. *Medical Management of Radiation Accidents.* 2nd ed. Boca Raton, FL: CRC Press; 2001:195–210.
5. Linkov I, Morel B, Schell WR. Remedial policies in radiologically-contaminated forests: environmental consequences and risk assessment. *Risk Anal.* 1997;17:67–75.
6. National Council on Radiation Protection and Measurement. *Management of Terrorist Events Involving Radioactive Material.* Report No. 138, Bethesda, MD: National Council on Radiation Protection and Measurement; 2001.
7. Knobler SL, Mahmoud AAF, Pray LA, eds. *Biologic Threats and Terrorism: Assessing the Science and Response Capabilities.* Washington, DC: National Academy Press; 2002.
8. Lippi D, Conti AA. Plague, policy, saints and terrorists: a historical survey. *J Infect.* 2002;44:226–228.
9. Overton EB, Sharp WD, Roberto P. Toxicity of petroleum. In: Cockerham LG, Shane BS, eds. *Basic Environmental Toxicology.* Boca Raton, FL: CRC Press; 1994:133–156.

10. Moeller DW. *Environmental Health.* Cambridge, MA: Harvard University Press; 1997.

11. Warner F. The environmental consequences of the Gulf War. *Environ.* 1991;33:5–7.

12. Johnson DW, Kilsby CG, McKenna DS, et al. Airborne observations of the physical and chemical characteristics of the Kuwait oil smoke plume. *Nature.* 1991;353:617–621.

13. Small RD. Environmental impact of fires in Kuwait. *Nature.* 1991;350:11–12.

14. Murthy RS. Bhopal gas leak disaster: impact on mental health. In: Havenaar JM, Cwikel JG, Bromet EJ, eds. *Toxic Turmoil: Psychological and Societal Consequences of Ecological Disasters.* New York, NY: Kluwer Academic/Plenum; 2002:129–148.

15. Clements BW. *Disasters and Public Health: Planning and Response.* Amsterdam: Elsevier; 2009, 1–25.

16. Walsh L, Subbarao I, Gebbie K, et al. Core competencies for disaster medicine and public health. *Disaster Med Public Health Prep.* 2012;6:42–52.

17. Rodier DJ, Zeeman MG. Ecological risk assessment. In: Cockerham LG, Shane BS, eds. *Basic Environmental Toxicology.* Boca Raton, FL: CRC Press; 1994:581–604.

18. Reynolds SL, Crulcich MM, Sullivan G, Stewart MT. Developing a practical algorithm for a pediatric emergency department's response to radiological dispersal device events. *Pediatr Emerg Care.* 2013;29:814–821.

19. Hyams KC, Murphy FM, Wessely S. Responding to chemical, biological, or nuclear terrorism: the indirect and long-term health effects may present the greatest challenge. *J Health Polit Policy Law.* 2002;27:273–291.

20. Levitin HW, Kahn CA. Decontamination. In: Koenig KL, Schultz CH, eds. *Koenig and Schultz's Disaster Medicine: Comprehensive Principles and Practices.* Cambridge: Cambridge University Press; 2010:195–202.

Computer and Electronic Terrorism and Emergency Medical Services

M. Kathleen Stewart and Charles Stewart

DESCRIPTION OF EVENT

Every machine connected to the Internet is potentially a printing press, a broadcasting station, and a place of assembly. With the advent of the Internet, anyone can disseminate information that is undiluted by the media and untouched by government censors.[1] It should come as no surprise, then, that terrorists have used the Internet to spread instructions, propaganda, and plans for both devices, such as improvised explosives, and for attacks.[2] The use of computers for terrorism is a real, true threat to societies.[3]

Unfortunately, actual terrorist use of computers, networks, information architectures, and the Internet has been largely ignored by the media. The reality of our weaknesses and vulnerabilities is both more chilling and far less reassuring. A *cyber attack* is deliberate exploitation of computer systems, technology-dependent enterprises, and networks. In cyber attacks, malicious code is used to alter computer code, logic, or data, resulting in disruptive consequences that can compromise data and lead to cybercrimes, such as information and identity theft. Cyber attacks may include the following consequences:

- Identity theft, fraud, and extortion
- Malware, pharming, phishing, spamming, spoofing, spyware, Trojans, and viruses
- Stolen hardware, such as laptops or mobile devices that may contain sensitive information in readily retrievable forms
- Denial-of-service and distributed denial-of-service attacks
- Breach of access
- Social-engineering attacks to retrieve/access data for nefarious purposes
- Private and public Web-browser exploits
- Instant messaging abuse
- Intellectual property (IP) theft or unauthorized access

Four major venues of attack that would affect emergency medical services (EMS) are a "viral" attack, a denial-of-service attack, theft of laptops or other devices with sensitive information, and a "social-engineering" attack to retrieve secure or restricted data for nefarious purposes. Another target that indirectly effects EMS is the Supervisory Control and Data Acquisition (SCADA) controller units connected to the Internet. *SCADA* is a term for the industrial control system that monitors and controls industrial processes that exist in the physical world through the Internet, wired, or wireless connections. SCADA systems that tie together decentralized facilities such as power, oil, and gas pipelines and water distribution and wastewater collection systems were designed to be open, robust, and easily operated and repaired, but not necessarily secure. SCADA controllers can include multiple sites with large distances between the controller and the process machine. The number of connections between SCADA systems, office networks, and the Internet has made them vulnerable to types of network attacks, such as Stuxnet, which is discussed later.

Viruses/Worms

Malignant computer programs are often called *viruses* because they share some of the traits of biological viruses. The computer virus requires a functioning "host machine" to replicate, works only with the proper "host," and passes from computer to computer like a biological virus passes from person to person.

There are other similarities. A biological virus is a fragment of deoxyribonucleic acid (DNA) inside a protective jacket. A computer virus must piggyback on top of another program, document, or E-mail to get into the computer, and it often must disguise itself from antiviral software with a surrounding innocuous package, like its biological counterpart.

People create computer viruses. A person has to write the code for the virus and test it to make sure that it functions as intended and spreads as designed.

A computer that has an active copy of a virus is considered *infected*. The way that the virus is activated depends on the design (coding) of the virus. Some viruses become active if the user simply opens an infected document. Others require specific actions on the part of the user.

Traditional computer viruses were first noted in the 1980s. During that decade, computers were found in not only large centralized areas but also small businesses and homes because of the availability of small computers—the advent of the personal computer (PC). The first viruses were "Trojan horse" viruses. A *Trojan horse* is a malignant computer program that claims to do one thing (often a game or a utility) but actually does something else instead, such as erase your disk. A Trojan horse program has no way to replicate automatically.

Another early virus was the *boot sector virus*. The boot sector is a small program that initializes the computer and the process of loading the operating system, thus "booting" it into the memory. By putting code in the boot sector, the virus guarantees that it will be loaded into memory immediately and will be able to run whenever the computer is on.

Modern viruses are much more insidious in their invasions. Attachments that come as word files (.doc), spreadsheets (.xls), and images (.gif and .jpg) can contain viral attachments. Even opening a contaminated website may download a viral program. A file with an extension such as .exe, .com, or .vbs is executable and can do any damage the designer wants. Many viruses disguise themselves by doubling the suffix of the program name, such as stuff.gif.vbs.

Once the virus is active on the computer, it can copy itself to files, disks, and programs as they are used by the computer, whether automatically or by the computer user. The big difference between a computer virus and other programs is that the computer virus is specifically designed to make a copy of itself. When the viral programs are executed, the virus examines the hard drives to see whether there is a susceptible program on the disk. If found, the virus adds the viral code to the program or replaces the program or file with its own code. The virus has now reproduced itself so that two or more programs are infected. Every time the user runs any infected program, the virus has the chance to reproduce by attaching to other programs, and the cycle continues. This replication often occurs without the knowledge of the computer user (sometimes the programs infected are system programs that the user does not control).

A virus often contains a "*payload*," or an additional program that the virus will carry out in addition to replicating itself. Payloads vary from trivially annoying to destructive. The payload is often termed *malware*, short for *malicious software*. Some nondestructive and non-trivial payloads include logging programs that record every keystroke typed in, programs that automatically send E-mail to every address in the computer, and programs that open portals for strangers to examine and use your computer. If the payload is well designed, the user may not even be aware that the computer is infected. Public machines, nonsecure business or office machines, and some secure systems can be used as remote intelligence gathering devices. Locating the offending program is often difficult because many of the keylogging programs are titled or disguised as necessary system files or folders.

A *worm* is simply a virus that has the ability to copy itself from machine to machine. A copy of the worm looks around and infects other machines with the same security defect through any available computer network. Using the networks and the Internet, worms can infect other machines incredibly quickly.

Modern computer viruses can be found in programs available on USB drives, floppy disks, CDs, and DVDs; hidden in multiple kinds of E-mail attachments; and found in material that is downloaded from the Internet.[4,5]

Examples of Recent Destructive Viruses/Worms

Code Red (now with multiple variants) first appeared in July 2001 and ultimately infected more than 300,000 computers in the United States.[6] The worm exploited a security opening in Microsoft's IIS Web servers. No one knows where this worm originated or by whom it was written. The worm was time sensitive, based on dates. From days 1 to 19 of the month, the worm would propagate. From days 20 to 27, it would launch a denial-of-service attack against a particular site. From day 27 through the end of the month, the worm would "sleep" in the computer.[7] Some variants have opened covert access ports (back doors) in operating systems that allow other intrusions.

The concept of the covert access port (back door) is important. These covert ports of entry allow a malicious programmer remote access and even control of programs running on the affected computer. The access may be gained by contaminating programs with a virus, as part of the "remote help" services in some operating systems or by being built into a program by the designer or a programmer (either disgruntled or operating under instructions).

Even though Microsoft provided a patch for Code Red, many system administrators did not obtain or apply the patch to their systems. These unprotected computers remain vulnerable to this virus.

The newer intrusions using similar exploits may have a more malignant purpose:

For example, the *Nimda* worm appeared 1 week after the September 11, 2001, terrorist attacks on the United States, and it targeted the financial sector.[8] A more "intelligent" worm, Nimda could replicate itself in several ways: by infecting E-mail programs, by copying itself onto the computer servers, or by affecting users who downloaded infected pages from the infected Web servers. The Nimda affected millions of computers and brought the Internet to a crawl. The Nimda worm replicated itself much faster than the Code Red worm did, and it caused billions of dollars in damage.[9]

The *Slammer* worm, or *Sapphire* worm as it is also known, surfaced January 25, 2003, on Super Bowl weekend.[10] The Slammer exploited a vulnerability in the servers delivering Web pages to users. It was the fastest cyber attack in history. The number of Slammer infections doubled every 8.5 seconds, and the Slammer did more than 90% of its damage in the first 10 minutes of its release. Slammer incapacitated parts of the Internet in Korea and Japan; disrupted phone service in Finland; and markedly slowed airline reservation systems, credit card networks, and ATM machines in the United States.[9]

Slammer could have been much more destructive had it been properly programmed. When the next "new, improved Slammer" is released, it could do much more damage. It could even affect phone and other trunking communication systems (including some radio links) for a city or larger region of the country. Although control systems are unlikely to be directly damaged by an Internet virus like Slammer, the denial-of-service to control points for water distribution systems, railroad switch points, power grids, chemical plants, and telephone systems may cause widespread nondestructive failures. Since the "mapping" (remote identification) of the covert access points previously described, terrorists may well have targeted specific weak spots for harassment.

Stuxnet is a 500-kilobyte computer worm that infected the software of at least 14 industrial sites in Iran, including a uranium-enrichment plant.[11] This worm was an unprecedentedly masterful and malicious piece of code that attacked in three phases. First, it targeted Microsoft Windows machines and networks, repeatedly replicating itself. Then it sought out Siemens Step7 SCADA software, which is also Windows-based, and used to program industrial control systems that operate equipment, such as centrifuges. Finally, it compromised the programmable logic controllers of the control systems embedded in the equipment. The worm's authors could thus spy on the industrial systems using these controllers and even cause the fast-spinning centrifuges to tear themselves apart, unbeknownst to the human operators at the plant. Apparently the initial target was uranium-enrichment centrifuges in Iran's nuclear program. It is unknown if these centrifuges were damaged by the worm.

Any of the modern viruses/worms could be redesigned to destroy, or at least severely cripple, the 911 emergency response system in the United States. If a similar worm were to be used to alter SCADA systems at a refinery, chemical plant, or a power generation or distribution station, the results clearly could be devastating.[12] A Stuxnet-like worm could also cripple or destroy transportation and telecommunications systems, as well as disrupt water supplies and perhaps our defense systems.[13,14] Although these attacks do not directly target EMS, the resultant carnage would clearly affect EMS functions.

Social-Engineering Attacks

"Social engineering" is the exploitation of the "weakest link" in the security chain of an organization: the human.[15] The aim is to trick people into revealing passwords or other information that compromises a target system's security. The infamous Kevin Mitnick, for example, conducted most of his corporate intrusions by using the telephone, relying on the gullibility and friendly helpfulness of real people to gain access to corporate networks.[16] Hackers may call an organization and pretend to be users who have lost their password or show up at a site and simply wait for someone to hold a door open for them.[17,18]

Techniques to mitigate a social-engineering attack include the following:

- Activate caller ID at work. Match the name given by the caller with the number and extension.
- Set your organization's outbound caller ID to display only the front desk's phone number, not individual phone extensions.
- Implement an organizational call-back policy. If someone calls asking for information about the organization, say you will call them back, then look up and dial the number or go through their company's switchboard operator.
- Be mindful of information posted in out-of-the-office messages.
- Never allow another person to piggyback his or her physical access into a secured room or facility on your security ID card, even if the person apparently has his or her own card.
- Confront strangers. Ask whether you can take them to someone's office or help escort them outside. If they balk, contact security.
- Get to know your information technology (IT) support staff.
- Never write down your network password on a sticky note or tape it to the bottom of your keyboard. "Crackers" (experts at finding and cracking passwords) know where to look.
- Beware of E-mail that asks for verification of your password. This is often a practice called "phishing," which solicits passwords for illicit use.
- Periodically perform a Google search on your organization and scrutinize whether sensitive information is available outside your organization's firewall.
- Institute a security alert system. Have anyone who receives a suspicious phone call report it to a simple E-mail address, something like securityalert@company.com. If someone calls saying he or she is from IT and asks for your network password, say "no," hang up, and contact IT and security.

Denial-of-Service Attack

A denial-of-service (DoS) attack is not a virus but a method hackers use to prevent or deny legitimate users access to a computer or servers. The loss of service may be as simple as the inability of a particular network service to use E-mail or the loss of all network connectivity and services for every computer attached to the Internet in any way.

The most common DoS attack is simply to send more traffic to a network address than the programmers who planned its data buffers anticipated someone might send. The attacker may be aware that the target system has a weakness that can be exploited, or the attacker may simply try the attack in case it might work. For example, a terrorist creates a computer program that automatically calls 911. The 911 operator answers the telephone but discovers it is a prank call. If the program repeats this task continuously, it prevents legitimate customers from using 911 because the telephone line is busy. This is a DoS.

Many DoS attack tools are also capable of executing a distributed DoS (DDoS) attack. For example, imagine the terrorist now plants his or her program onto many computers on the Internet and has them all call 911 at once. This would have a bigger impact because there would be more computers calling the 911 operators. It would also be more difficult to locate the attacker, since the program is not running from the attacker's computer; the attacker is only controlling the computer that secretly had the program installed. This is a DDoS attack. A DoS attack can also destroy programming and files in a computer system.

In the worst case, an Internet-connected site can be forced to cease operation. If this is a critical control system, the organization will lose the use of the control functions that are connected to the Internet.

How Can Antivirus Software Help Against a Denial-of-Service Attack?

Using a virus, the DoS attack tools can be secretly installed onto a large number of innocent computer systems. Systems that unknowingly have DoS attack tools installed are called *Zombie* agents, or *Drones*. These "Zombie" systems can be centrally managed by a hacker to initiate DoS attacks at targeted computers. Zombies are not the victims of the DoS attack, but they are used to perform the actual attack.

Antivirus software detects viruses that can inject the DoS agents, but it does not detect the DoS attacks. By extracting a pattern or a signature from known Zombie agents, antivirus products can detect malevolent software on the compromised system. Antivirus software may also detect when a hacker is secretly installing Zombie agents.[19]

It is difficult to trace the origin of the request packets in a DoS attack, especially if it is a DDoS attack. It is impossible to prevent all DoS attacks, but there are precautions server administrators can take to decrease the risk of being compromised by a DoS attack. These precautions are beyond the scope of this chapter. By keeping the antivirus software up-to-date and using good computing practices, previously listed, the IT service can keep the system from becoming a Zombie and aiding a DoS attack.

◤ PRE-INCIDENT ACTIONS

A significant protective action is to install a commercial virus protection program on all computers and to update this virus protection frequently, almost "religiously." Set up a schedule to perform operating system updates and run a virus scan. If a virus is found, eliminate it.

Each virus is tailored for a specific operating system and/or program. If the computer is using a variation of Windows (e.g., Windows 98, 2000, or XP), then a virus tailored for UNIX will *not* affect this computer. Likewise, if the computer uses Linux, a Windows virus will *not* affect the computer. Some viruses are built to exploit known weaknesses in popular programs. If Microsoft Outlook, for example, is the target of such a virus, then computer users who do *not* use Outlook as their E-mail program will not be troubled by the virus.

- Have the virus protection set to scan each document before it is opened. Do not open any file or attachment unless you were expecting that file from someone you know and trust. The file will execute as soon as it is open, and if it contains a harmful or destructive virus/worm, you have just infected your system and anyone else you may send E-mail to.[19]
- Do not use macros in application programs unless they come from a known source. Macros are common ways to introduce viruses into systems.
- Ensure that the system administrator has a solid backup plan that can rapidly restore the operating system and essential programs in an emergency. Make sure that he or she keeps these backup copies readily available and updated to reflect new operating system and program updates.[20]
- Essential operating systems, such as dispatch centers, should have an expert evaluate their computers for the presence of covert back doors that allow other intrusions.
- Ensure that all available updates for the operating system have been applied to ensure that known weaknesses are limited in scope, and that security services within the operating system have been properly activated.[20]

POST-INCIDENT ACTIONS

- Essential operating systems should require that known uninfected working copies of all necessary software be immediately available should a disruption occur. Trained personnel able to "revive" the computer system should be on-duty, in-house, 24 hours a day, every day, for just this type of problem.
- Perhaps the most important action is to report any suspicious E-mail or unusual computer activity to the person in charge, the system administrator, or other designated person. Establish an on-call point-of-contact with your Internet service providers and appropriate law enforcement officials should you discover a launching of a cyber attack by either someone in your organization or an external operator.

MEDICAL TREATMENT OF CASUALTIES

Direct medical casualties from a "cyber" attack would not be expected. The only direct casualties that would result would be those deprived of services due to an inability to dispatch emergency vehicles or to communicate with those vehicles. Medical care would consist of treatment of the underlying illness that originally prompted the call for help. In addition, some institutions use an Internet-based patient care and tracking system. In the event of an attack, these systems may be rendered inoperable or, worse, made to give inaccurate data. All medical facilities that rely on computer and Internet-based systems should have adequate backups in place.

UNIQUE CONSIDERATIONS

Our Internet-enabled (net-centric) society is easy prey for two reasons. First, the growing technological sophistication of terrorists includes not only weapons of mass destruction and casualties but also a growing use of computers. Second, our own economic and technological systems have an increasing vulnerability to carefully timed attacks as we increase our dependence on computers to include those that are critical to safety.[21]

The entire critical infrastructure of the United States, including electrical power, telecommunications, health care, transportation, water, and the Internet, is vulnerable to a cyber attack. Many control systems, communication systems, and dispatch systems are now connected to the Internet and, thus, are potentially open to intrusion. This does not include the possible effects that a cyber attack could cause to the financial sector or to national defense.

PITFALLS

- Do not use weak passwords, such as "admin," "administrator," or "password."[16]
- Do not leave passwords on sticky notes or taped to computers or desks.
- Do not ever give out passwords in E-mail or on the phone.
- Ensure that virus protection is updated frequently (set virus protection software to automatic updates for the most rapid protection).
- Do not use wireless networking for secure communications.[19]

REFERENCES

1. Conway M. Reality bytes:cyberterrorism and terrorist "use" of the Internet. *First Monday.* 2002;7(11). http://firstmonday.org/ojs/index.php/fm/article/view/1001/922. Accessed 11.03.14.
2. Minei E, Matusitz J. Cyberspace as a new arena for terrorist propaganda: an updated examination. *Poiesis & Praxis: International Journal of Ethics of Science and Technology Assessment.* Nov 2012;9(1–2):163–176.
3. Technical Analysis Group. Examining the Cyber Capabilities of Islamic Terrorist Groups. Hanover, NH: Institute for Security Technology Studies at Dartmouth College, Technical Analysis Group; 2004. Available at: http://www.ists.dartmouth.edu/library/164.pdf. Accessed 11.03.14.
4. Meinal C. How hackers break in. *Sci Am.* 1998;279:98–105.
5. Scandariato R, Knight JC. The Design and Evaluation of a Defense for Internet Worms. In *23rd IEEE International Symposium on Reliable Distributed Systems,* 2004;164–173.
6. CERT Advisory CA-2001-19 "Code Red" worm exploiting buffer overflow in IIS indexing service DLL. Carnegie Mellon Software Engineering Institute.
7. Cyberwar! The warnings? http://www.pbs.org/wgbh/pages/ frontline/shows/cyberwar/warnings/.
8. CERT Advisory CA-2001-26 Nimda worm. 2001. http://www.cert.org/historical/advisories/ca-2001-26.cfm? Accessed 11.03.14.
9. Cyberwar! Introduction. http://www.pbs.org/wgbh/pages/frontline /shows/cyberwar/etc/synopsis.html.
10. Moore D, Paxson V, Savage S, Shannon C, Staniford S, Weaver N. Inside the Slammer Worm. *IEEE Security and Privacy.* 2003;1(4):33–39.
11. Cyberwarfare challenge. *Nature.* 2011;474(7350):127.
12. Weinberger S. Computer security: is this the start of cyberwarfare? *Nature.* 2011;474(7350):142–145.
13. Moya JM, Araujo A, Bankovic Z, et al. Improving security for SCADA sensor networks with reputation systems and self-organizing maps. *Sensors.* 2009;9(11):9380–9397.
14. Nicoul DM. Hacking the lights out. Computer viruses have taken out hardened industrial control systems. The electrical power grid may be next. *Sci Am.* Jul 2011;305(1):70–75.
15. Arthurs W. A proactive defence to social engineering. http://www.sans.org/rr/papers/51/511.pd.
16. Gragg D. A multi-level defense against social engineering. *Inside the Slammer Worm. IEEE Security and Privacy.* 2003;1(4):33–39. 2003. http://www.sans.org/reading-room/whitepapers/engineering/multi-level-defense-social-engineering-920. Accessed 11.03.14.
17. Allen M. The use of "social engineering" as a means of violating computer systems. http://www.sans.org/rr/papers/51/529.pdf.
18. Gulati R. The threat of social engineering and your defense against it. http://www.sans.org/rr/papers/51/1232.pdf.
19. Orvis WJ, Krystosek P, Smith J. Connecting to the Internet securely; protecting home networks. http://www.vialardi.org/VdSF/pdf/Websecurity.pdf.
20. Streufert J. Business continuity strategies for cyber defence: battling time and information overload. *J Bus Contin Emer Plan.* Nov 2010;4(4):303–316.
21. Greenwell WS. Learning lessons from accidents and incidents involving safety-critical software systems [master's thesis presentation]. http://www.cs.virginia.edu/colloquia/event310.html.

VIP Care

Saleh Fares and Lynne Barkley Burnett

📄 DESCRIPTION OF EVENT

It might be necessary to manage a "very important person" (VIP) during a disaster. This can happen in planned or unplanned events. Although medical care should not be different from one person to another, the presence of a VIP can affect the flow of operations and require adequate planning and response. The literature presents many experiences in dealing with this elite group of patients and the challenges surrounding their care. Several lessons have been learned during those events that can be used when preparing a response plan.

Within the medical context, a *VIP* has been variously defined as any patient who can exert unusual influence on the treating staff[1] and, more broadly, as "anyone whose presence in the hospital, by virtue of fame, position, or claim on the public interest, may substantially disrupt the normal course of patient care."[2] Included would be those with public, financial, or political influence, as well as individuals with unusual professional influence,[1,3] such as the president of the United States or another major political figure, visiting dignitaries, a famous actor, a well-known sports figure, or a chair of the hospital board.[2] Although it is true that any of the aforementioned persons could potentially disrupt the normal course of patient care in the everyday activities of a hospital, the degree to which they would have such an effect in a disaster would, in large part, be a function of their prominence within society.

◀◀ PRE-INCIDENT ACTIONS

The Joint Commission requires health care organizations to have a disaster plan for incidents of a magnitude that can be expected to overwhelm the standard operating procedures of the emergency department and hospital.[4] Such a document should include a written plan for treatment of VIP patients and should address, at a minimum, the following questions[2]:

- Is the event planned or unplanned?
- What medical care will be needed or expected?
- Which hospital personnel are to be notified of a VIP's impending arrival, and in what sequence?
- What is the plan for security during the hospitalization of the VIP?
- Who decides whether a command center needs to be established? What will be the makeup of its staff? What is the function of the center?
- Who will lead the care?
- In what clinical setting will care be administered?
- How will the press receive necessary information?
- How will the patient information be protected?
- How will other related services such as police and government agencies be involved?

- What type of care will other patients receive?
- Is there a contingency plan?

If the VIP is a high-ranking politician protected by the U.S. Secret Service, and time so permits, an advance team will assess hospital capabilities, choosing one or more to receive the VIP in the event of injury or illness, while also selecting travel routes that are safest and most secure.[5] Advanced planning also entails working with local emergency medical services (EMS) systems, hospitals, and trauma centers on various "what if" scenarios to ensure preparation for the visit[6]; for example, if the president or vice president is to be more than 20 minutes from a trauma unit, capability for helicopter evacuation is a priority.

Different aspects of the security plan can be established by following proper steps such as risk assessment planning, walk-through survey, development of the security services needs assessment, and finally framing of a contingency plan.[7] This ensures that adequate decisions are made, including what doors, corridors, and elevators can and should be sealed, and which areas can and should be evacuated, if such becomes necessary. If possible, one elevator is selected for movement of the VIP and, following an electronic sweep, continuously guarded. Clinical conditions permitting, it is best to have the VIP patient stay in a room (or suite of rooms) in the safest area of the hospital, where equipment may be brought in.[3,7] The hospital should also be prepared to provide the VIP's security detail, a complete personnel roster with the Social Security number and date of birth of all employees.[3,7]

▶▶ POST-INCIDENT ACTIONS

Several components need to be implemented immediately once an incident has occurred. Consistent with the planned response, the emergency department (ED) and hospital must be quickly secured, appropriate to the anticipated level of need or threat, as well as the demands imposed by the disaster itself. The usual procedure of activating the VIP plan needs to be followed. This can be institution dependent. Commonly, the Hospital Incident Command System (HICS) is activated if necessary. In an assassination attempt, the VIP's security detail has no way of knowing the extent of the plot and who may be involved.[2] In such a circumstance, it may be necessary to grant them control over the hospital environment. In the unlikely event that the hospital must be closed for security reasons, notification of EMS dispatch is essential.

Presentation of a VIP often engenders crowd control problems, from not only the media or well-wishers but also chiefs of service, other medical staff members, administrators, nurses, and hospital personnel who want to see the VIP or observe what is going on.[2] The problem of too many hands, rather than not enough, makes control of access essential and problematic.[2] Hospital security officers must often play a role in keeping unnecessary hospital personnel out of the VIP's area, as well as ensuring the VIP's safety. Restricting access may best be accomplished by placing a senior emergency medicine physician in a strategic location, in case security is unable to identify who should be allowed access to the ED or is hesitant to bar senior physicians or administrators. This is preferred to be coordinated with the VIP's security team. If the VIP patient is hospitalized, a list of those allowed access to the VIP should be generated and updated daily, with enforcement of access limited only to those so authorized (e.g., frequently changed coded pins).[8]

Care of a VIP entails a need to coordinate and organize, lest chaotic care and diffusion of responsibility result.[9] Clinical and administrative responsibilities should be separated.[2] In the ED, the patient's condition will be the determinative factor as to whether a senior emergency medicine physician assumes clinical control, delegating administrative control to a more junior physician or charge nurse, or vice versa.

Another consideration the hospital must address is the immense media interest generated by a disaster, which is then magnified by involvement of a VIP. The media policy should ensure that the release of information is well controlled and that the VIP patient's privacy is appropriately protected.[2,3,10] The goal should be the orderly flow of accurate, timely information and the provision of a forum in which reporters' questions may be asked and answered. Consideration should be given to establishment of a press area at a site separate from the hospital. A single physician, who is knowledgeable, should be designated to serve as spokesperson. This spokesperson is expected to receive some form of specialized training on dealing with the media, especially in disasters. All other hospital staff should be instructed not to talk with the media and should be cautioned about hallway or elevator conversations.[3,10]

✚ MEDICAL TREATMENT OF CASUALTIES

One of the first considerations in disaster medical care is triage, with establishment of priority for care. When a VIP is among many patients, determination of who will be treated first has medical, practical, and moral facets. Triage was developed to meet the needs of the military in time of war; thus, priority for care sometimes went to soldiers with more minor conditions over those more gravely injured. Such an approach has been extended from soldiers to, for example, medical personnel with minor injuries, so that they could care for other patients in earthquakes.[3,11]

It is considered ethically justifiable for a person to receive priority for treatment based on social utility only if his or her contribution is indispensable to attaining a major social goal.[3,11] Thus, someone who achieved VIP status because of fame as an actor would be triaged as would anyone else, based on the disaster triage[12] factors of medical condition and the availability of personnel and equipment to meet the actor's specific needs, within the context of caring for the needs of everyone else. In contradistinction would be the VIP who is a government official and whose leadership is needed to respond to the crisis or whose death would significantly affect the resolve of the community, state, or nation. Such a VIP fulfills the criterion of a "mission-essential" role and, thus, would be triaged, per the military approach, as highest priority irrespective of the severity of the physiologic insult.

A VIP syndrome has been described in which treating staff alter their usual operating procedures because a patient's power and influence cause them to lose their objectivity and thereby the ability to make the cool, rational, detached decisions necessary for good medical care. VIP syndrome may prompt decisions to do fewer tests, diagnostic procedures, or therapeutic maneuvers to save the patient from pain[13] or embarrassment. Spouses of physicians, for example, are less likely to have a pelvic examination than are other patients.[14] The result may be a missed diagnosis.[13] On the contrary, if too aggressive an approach is used, the patient may unnecessarily undergo painful and potentially

dangerous procedures. Treat the VIP first as a patient and secondarily as a VIP,[2] evaluating him or her in a standard manner, including any embarrassing invasive procedures. "There is nothing biologically different between a pope or president, and there is no need to alter one's thinking in caring for them."[13]

To facilitate an orderly and uneventful transfer of care, it is essential that there be coordination between emergency physicians and specialists who will care for the patient in the hospital,[11] bringing up yet another "syndrome" that has been identified in the care of a VIP patient. The "chief syndrome" occurs when senior physicians who do not routinely work in the ED respond because the patient is a VIP, and they intervene in an uncoordinated manner, upsetting the way in which the emergency team normally works together.[2] It is essential that health care providers function in familiar roles. The attending physician must take command and explain that the care given will be identical to that given to all other patients with a similar condition because, "Usual medical care is correct care."[13] Consults should be obtained as appropriate, but, at all times, it should be clear which physician is responsible for the patient's clinical care,[2] whether it be an emergency medicine attending physician, trauma surgeon, or other specialist. Guzman and colleagues presented "nine principles" to follow when caring for a VIP. Many of the presented principles are applicable to disaster situations. The authors highlighted the importance of maintaining the same level of clinical wisdom and practices, despite the pressure to "bend" the rules in these situations, because bending the rules may lead to worse outcome and misdiagnoses. Another important principle is to work as a team, given the complexity of the situation, and not to work alone. Communication was also presented as a key principle when dealing with a VIP situation. This includes the patients, relatives, accompanying physicians, or any other involved individuals. As highlighted earlier, they also recommend careful management of communication with the media, which can be a "friend or a foe." In some VIP situations, there might be a request to involve the "chairperson" as the primary physician. The authors recommend resisting this unless the chairperson is the clinician with most expertise in the patient's clinical case. Another situation that might occur is pressure to transfer the VIP to a special setting. This might actually compromise the care provided when critical monitoring is needed, for example. Other principles talk about the need to protect patient's security, about dealing with gifts, and, finally, about working with the patient's personal physician.[10]

❓ UNIQUE CONSIDERATIONS

As stated earlier, the VIP may be traveling with a physician.[2,10] If the VIP is a primary protectee of the U.S. Secret Service, it is the responsibility of the Secret Service to protect and, if necessary, rescue the principal. Several countries provide special medical coverage for their officials. In the United States, the White House Medical Unit (WHMU), in conjunction with first responders who may be on scene, has the responsibility to evaluate, resuscitate, and evacuate the patient to a suitable site for definitive care.[15] The WHMU, all of whose members are military personnel, is a team consisting of a physician and emergency or critical care nurse who accompany primary protectees at all times, for provision of initial medical care.[5] Physicians who have completed Advanced Cardiac Life Support (ACLS) and Advanced Trauma Life Support (ATLS)[8] represent the specialties of family medicine, internal medicine, or emergency medicine. All WHMU personnel, whether officer or enlisted status, have completed chemical, biological, radiological, nuclear, and explosive (CBRNE) training, and some of the physicians have completed tactical medicine courses to support SWAT teams.

In a life-threatening situation, the attending physician in the hospital bears the responsibility for patient care decisions,[2] but diplomacy, collegiality, and good judgment are always required concerning participation by the VIP's physician in patient care. For example, the physician in the ED may be an internist who is called on to provide initial care to an injured VIP who is accompanied by a board-certified emergency physician. Conversely, the ED physician who may be board-certified in emergency medicine may be responsible for providing emergent obstetric (OB) care to a VIP in the company of a family physician with considerable OB experience.

If the VIP is the president of the United States, among the myriad of factors needing to be addressed may be the issue of whether the president is capable of making the decisions necessary to fulfill the responsibilities of office. Carried in the "Football," the briefcase in the custody of a military aide who is always near the president, are the codes necessary to launch a nuclear war. Also contained therein is an "emergency action plan" for devolution of presidential powers to the vice president, including the requisite paperwork for its emergency execution.[15]

The 25th Amendment to the U.S. Constitution sets forth the mechanism whereby the vice president may assume presidential powers and duties as acting president. In such a situation, the White House physician plays a critical role in the constitutional process of deciding whether the president is, on the basis of medical judgment, fit to govern.[8] Even though the White House physician has an obligation to preserve the confidentiality of the president's condition, that may, and in fact must, be broken "if the health of the president interferes with his or her ability to do the job."[15] "Impairment is a medical judgment, disability is a political decision"[15]; thus the findings and opinion of the White House physician are reported to a classified group of White House and Cabinet officials[8] who make the final decision, if the president is unable to do so or if there is a question about the president's decision.

⚠ PITFALLS

- Failure to have a written plan for VIP situations
- Not involving outside organizations, such as the police, security apparatus, professional media associations, and governmental bodies in the planning
- Not providing medical treatment to the VIP like any other patient (too much or too little care)
- Bending rules for the VIP, which will likely result in worse outcomes
- Failure to appoint a lead physician to manage the care
- Overlooking the importance of drills of VIP plans

REFERENCES

1. Strange RE. The VIP, with illness. *Mil Med*. 1980;45(7):473–475.
2. Smith MS, Shesser RF. The emergency care of the VIP patient. *N Engl J Med*. 1988;319(21):1421–1423.
3. Mariano EC, McLeod JA. Emergency care for the VIP patient. *Intensive Care Medicine*. New York: Springer; 2007, 969-975.
4. The Joint Commission Environment of Care Standard EC.02.01.01 in 2014. Available at: http://www.jointcommission.org/standards_information/standards.aspx.
5. NurseZone.com. Nurses a heartbeat away from the president. Available at: http://www.nursezone.com/Stories/SpotlightOnNurses.asp?articleID=5067.
6. Clark AA. All the president's medics. *J Emerg Med*. 1992;17(8):57–58, 62.
7. Luizzo A, Scaglione BJ, Walsh M. Aspects of hospital security: protecting the VIP. *J Healthc Protect Manag*. 2011;27(1):43.
8. Nelsen V. VIP protection and executive protection in hospitals. *J Healthc Prot Manage*. 1989;6(1):56–68.
9. O'Leary DS, O'Leary MR. Care of the VIP patient. *N Engl J Med*. 1989;320 (15):1016.
10. Guzman JA, Sasidhar M, Stoller JK. Caring for VIPs: nine principles. *Cleve Clin J Med*. 2011;78(2):90–94.
11. Beauchamp TL, Childress JF. Justice. In: *Principles of Biomedical Ethics*. 5th ed. New York: Oxford University Press Inc; 2001:225–282.
12. Hogan DE, Lairet J. Triage. In: Hogan DE, Burstein JL, eds. *Disaster Medicine*. Philadelphia: Lippincott Williams & Wilkins; 2002:10–15.
13. Block AJ. Beware of the VIP syndrome. (When status of a person affects medical care decisions) [editorial]. *Chest*. 1993;104(4):989.
14. Diekema DS. It's wrong to treat VIPs better than other patients. *ED Manag*. 2000;12(8):92–93.
15. Julie Bulson MPA, Bulson T. A systematic approach to very important person preparedness for a trauma center. *J Trauma Nurs*. 2012;19(1):11–14.

Note: Page numbers followed by *b* indicate boxes, *f* indicate figures, and *t* indicate tables.